PRINCIPLES AND PRACTICE OF

Palliative Care and Supportive Oncology

FOURTH EDITION

PRINCIPLES AND PRACTICE OF

Palliative Care and Supportive Oncology

FOURTH EDITION

EDITORS

Ann M. Berger, MSN, MD
Pain and Palliative Care
Bethesda, Maryland

John L. Shuster, Jr., MD
Chief Medical Officer, Alive Hospice
Nashville, Tennessee
Clinical Professor of Psychiatry and Medicine
Vanderbilt University Medical Center
Nashville, Tennessee

Jamie H. Von Roenn, MD
Professor of Medicine,
Division of Hematology/Oncology
Department of Medicine
The Feinberg School of Medicine
Robert H. Lurie Comprehensive Cancer Center of
Northwestern University
Chicago, Illinois

Wolters Kluwer | Lippincott Williams & Wilkins
Health
Philadelphia · Baltimore · New York · London
Buenos Aires · Hong Kong · Sydney · Tokyo

Senior Executive Editor: Jonathan W. Pine, Jr.
Senior Product Manager: Emilie Moyer
Senior Manufacturing Manager: Benjamin Rivera
Director of Marketing: Caroline Foote
Creative Director: Doug Smock
Production Service: Integra Software Services Pvt., Ltd.

© 2013 by LIPPINCOTT WILLIAMS & WILKINS, a WOLTERS KLUWER business
Two Commerce Square
2001 Market Street
Philadelphia, PA 19103 USA
LWW.com

3rd edition © Lippincott Williams & Wilkins, 2007;. 2nd edition © 2002 by Lippincott Williams & Wilkins; 1st edition © 1998 by Lippincott-Raven Publishers.

All rights reserved. This book is protected by copyright. No part of this book may be reproduced in any form by any means, including photocopying, or utilized by any information storage and retrieval system without written permission from the copyright owner, except for brief quotations embodied in critical articles and reviews. Materials appearing in this book prepared by individuals as part of their official duties as U.S. government employees are not covered by the above-mentioned copyright.

Printed in China

Library of Congress Cataloging-in-Publication Data

Berger, Ann (Ann M.)
  Principles and practice of palliative care and supportive oncology/editors, Ann M. Berger, John L. Shuster, Jr., Jamie Von Roenn. —4th ed.
    p. ; cm.
  Includes bibliographical references and index.
  ISBN 978-1-4511-2127-8 (alk. paper)
  I. Shuster, John L. II. Von Roenn, Jamie H. III. Title.
  [DNLM: 1. Neoplasms—therapy. 2. Neoplasms—complications. 3. Pain Management—methods. 4. Palliative Care—methods. QZ 266]
  616.99'406—dc23

                                                                          2012028570

Care has been taken to confirm the accuracy of the information presented and to describe generally accepted practices. However, the authors, editors, and publisher are not responsible for errors or omissions or for any consequences from application of the information in this book and make no warranty, expressed or implied, with respect to the currency, completeness, or accuracy of the contents of the publication. Application of the information in a particular situation remains the professional responsibility of the practitioner.

The authors, editors, and publisher have exerted every effort to ensure that drug selection and dosage set forth in this text are in accordance with current recommendations and practice at the time of publication. However, in view of ongoing research, changes in government regulations, and the constant flow of information relating to drug therapy and drug reactions, the reader is urged to check the package insert for each drug for any change in indications and dosage and for added warnings and precautions. This is particularly important when the recommended agent is a new or infrequently employed drug.

Some drugs and medical devices presented in the publication have Food and Drug Administration (FDA) clearance for limited use in restricted research settings. It is the responsibility of the health care provider to ascertain the FDA status of each drug or device planned for use in their clinical practice.

To purchase additional copies of this book, call our customer service department at (800) 638-3030 or fax orders to (301) 223-2320. International customers should call (301) 223-2300.

Visit Lippincott Williams & Wilkins on the Internet: at LWW.com. Lippincott Williams & Wilkins customer service representatives are available from 8:30 am to 6 pm, EST.

10 9 8 7 6 5 4 3 2 1

RRS1210

*To our spouses and children, whose love and support
make our work possible*

CARL, STEPHEN, REBECCA

SUSAN, MARY GRACE, BEN, MOLLY, JOSEPH,

KELVIN (IN MEMORY), ERIKA, ALEXANDER, KARL

Contributing Authors

Amy P. Abernethy
Associate Professor
Division of Medical Oncology
Department of Medicine
Duke Cancer Care Research Program,
  Duke Cancer Institute
Duke University Medical Center
Durham, North Carolina

Sunil Kumar Aggarwal, MD, PhD
Housestaff Physician, PGY-3
Department of Physical Medicine and
  Rehabilitation
New York University Langone Medical
  Center
New York, New York

Timothy Ahles, PhD
Director of the Neurocognitive Research
  Laboratory
Memorial Sloan Kettering Cancer Center
New York, New York

Faisal Ahmed, MD
Resident
Department of Urology
George Washington University Hospital
Washington, D.C.

Jörg Albert, PD Dr. med
Department of Internal Medicine I
Johann Wolfgang Goethe-University
  Hospital
Frankfurt am Main, Germany

Robert M. Arnold, MD
Professor of Medicine
Chief, Section of Palliative Care and
  Medical Ethics
Assistant Director
Institute to Enhance Palliative Care
Director, Institute for Doctor-Patient
  Communication
Leo H Criep Chair in Patient Care
UPMC Montefiore Hospital
Pittsburgh, Pennsylvania

Noreen M. Aziz, MD, PhD, MPH
Senior Program Director
Bethesda, Maryland

Justin N. Baker, MD, FAAP, FAAHPM
Chief
Division of Quality of Life and Palliative Care

Director, Hematology/Oncology
  Fellowship Program
Memphis, Tennessee

Yevgeniy Balagula, MD
Dermatology Service
Department of Medicine
Memorial Sloan-Kettering
  Cancer Center
New York, New York

Justin Banerdt
Center for Psychosocial Epidemiology
  and Outcomes Research
Dana-Farber Cancer Institute
Boston, Massachusetts

Emma Bateman, MD
Laboratory Manager
Mucositis Research Group
School of Medicine
University of Adelaide
Australia

Compton J. Benjamin, MD, PhD
Department of Urology
George Washington University Medical
  Center
Washington, D.C.

James R. Berenson, MD
Chief of Cancer Research
Associate Director of Research
West Los Angeles VA Medical Center
West Hollywood, California

Ann M. Berger, MSN, MD
Pain and Palliative Care
Bethesda, Maryland

**Andrea Bezjak, BMedSc, MDCM,
MSc, FRCPC**
The Addie MacNaughton Chair in
  Thoracic Radiation Oncology
Associate Professor
Department of Radiation Oncology
Princess Margaret Hospital
University of Toronto
Toronto, Ontario
Canada

Elizabeth Blanchard, MD
Southcoast Centers for Cancer Care
Fairhaven, Massachusetts

Susan K. Bodtke, MD, FAAFP
Medical Director
San Diego Hospice and Institute for
  Palliative Medicine
San Diego, California

Joanne M. Bowen, PhD, NHMRC
Lecturer/Laboratory Head
School of Medicine
The University of Adelaide
Adelaide, South Australia
Australia

Nina L. Bray, MD
Attending Physician
Hospice and Palliative Medicine
Washington, D.C.

Eduardo Bruera, MD
Professor and Chair
Department of Palliative Care and
  Rehabilitation Medicine Unit 8
UT, M.D. Anderson Cancer Center
Houston, Texas

Gary T. Buckholz, MD
Fellowship Director
Hospice and Palliative Medicine
San Diego Hospice and the Institute for
  Palliative Medicine
San Diego, California

Gayle L. Byker, MD, MBA
Hospice Medical Director
Capital Caring
Falls Church, Virginia

John A. Carucci, MD, PhD
Chief
Mohs Micrographic and Dermatologic
  Surgery
NYU Langone Medical Center
New York, New York

David Casarett, MD, MA
Associate Professor of Medicine
University of Pennsylvania Chief Medical
  Officer
Penn-Wissahickon Hospice
Philadelphia, Pennsylvania

M. Jennifer Cheng, MD
Post-Doctorate Fellow
Department of Palliative Medicine

Johns Hopkins School of Medicine
Baltimore, Maryland

Caroline Chung, MD, FRCPC, CIP

Department of Radiation Oncology
Princess Margaret Hospital
Toronto, Ontario

James F. Cleary, MB, BS, FRACP, FAChPM

Associate Professor of Medicine
Department of Medicine
University of Wisconsin School of
  Medicine and Public Health
Madison, Wisconsin

Melissa DeLario, MD

Assistant Professor of Pediatrics
Division of Hematology Oncology
Scott and White Children's Hospital and
  Clinics
Texas A&M Health Science Center College
  of Medicine
Temple, Texas

Paul Duberstein, PhD

Professor of Psychiatry
Department of Psychiatry
University of Rochester Medical Center
Rochester, New York

Deborah Dudgeon, MD, FRCPC

W. Ford Connell Professor of Palliative
  Care Medicine
Queen's University
Director of Palliative Care Medicine
Kingston General Hospital
Kingston, Ontario
Canada

Alexandra M. Easson, MD, MSc

Department of Surgery
Princess Margaret Hospital
Toronto, Ontario
Canada

Michael K. Eichler, MD

Institute for Diagnostic and Interventional
  Radiology
Johann Wolfgang Goethe-University Frankfurt
Frankfurt am Main, Germany

**Paula Erwin-Toth, MSN, RN,
  CWOCN, CNS**

Director
WOC Nursing Education
Cleveland Clinic
Cleveland, Ohio

Egidio del Fabbro, MD

Program Director, Palliative Care
Division of Hematology/Oncology and
  Palliative Care
Massey Cancer Center
Richmond, Virginia

**Jane M. Fall-Dickson, RN,
  PhD, AOCN**

Associate Professor
Assistant Chair, Research
Georgetown University School of Nursing
  and Health Studies
Washington, D.C.

Leonard A. Farber, MD

Founder/Director
The Faber Center for Radiation Oncology
New York, New York

Parviz Farshid, MD

Institute for Diagnostic and Interventional
  Radiology
Johann Wolfgang Goethe-University
  Frankfurt
Frankfurt am Main, Germany

Betty Ferrell, PhD, MA, FAAN, FPCN

Professor and Research Scientist
Department of Nursing Research and
  Education
City of Hope National Medical Center
Duarte, California

Frank D. Ferris, MD, FAAHPM, FAACE

Director, International Program
San Diego Hospice and the Institute for
  Palliative Medicine
San Diego, California

Debra L. Friedman, MD

Associate Professor of Pediatrics
E. Bronson Ingram Chair of Pediatric
  Oncology
Director
Pediatric Hematology-Oncology
Medical Director
REACH for Survivorship Program Leader
Vanderbilt-Ingram Cancer Division of
  Hematology-Oncology
Nashville, Tennessee

Kenneth D. Friedman, MD

Medical Director-Hemostasis Reference
  Laboratory
The Blood Center of Wisconsin
Milwaukee, Wisconsin

Juan Carlo Gea-Banacloche, MD

Chief
Infectious Diseases Consultation Service
NIH Clinical Research Center
Experimental Transplantation &
  Immunology
Bethesda, Maryland

Hans Gerdes, MD

Attending Physician
Director of GI Endoscopy
Memorial Sloan-Kettering Cancer Center
Professor of Clinical Medicine

Weill Medical College of Cornell
  University
New York, New York

Rachel Jane Gibson, Ph.D

Senior Lecturer
School of Medical Sciences
University of Adelaide
Adelaide, South Australia
Australia

Paul A. Glare, MD

Chief, Pain and Palliative Care Service
Department of Medicine
Memorial Sloan-Kettering Cancer Center
New York, New York

Shari Goldfarb, MD

Department of Medicine and Department
  of Epidemiology and Biostatistics
Memorial Sloan-Kettering Cancer
  Center and Weill Cornell Medical
  College
New York, New York

Christine Grady, MSN, PhD

Chief
Department of Bioethics, Clinical Center,
  National Institute of Health
Bethesda, Maryland

Donna B. Greenberg, MD

Program Director
Psychiatric Oncology
Department of Psychiatry
Massachusetts General Hospital Cancer
  Center
Boston, Massachusetts

Hunter Groninger, MD

Bethesda, Maryland

James L. Hallenbeck, MD

Associate Professor
Stanford University School of Medicine
Associate Chief of Staff, Extended Care
VA Palo Alto HCS
Palo Alto, California

Julie R. Hamrick, PsyD

Postdoctoral Research Fellow
Department of Psychosomatic Medicine
Vanderbilt University Medical Center
Nashville, Tennessee

Daniel L. Handel, MD

Hospice and Palliative Medicine
Gaithersburg, Maryland

Jo Hanson, RN, MSN, CNS, OCN

Senior Research Specialist
Nursing Research & Education
City of Hope
Duarte, California

Jeremy M. Hirst, MD

Director, Psychiatry Clinical Program
San Diego Hospice and the Institute for
   Palliative Medicine
San Diego, California

Mary K. Hughes, BS, MS, RN, CNS, CT

Department of Psychiatry
MD Anderson Cancer Center
Houston, Texas

Scott A. Irwin, MD, PhD

Chief of Psychiatry & Psychosocial Services
San Diego Hospital and the Institute for
   Palliative Medicine
San Diego, California

Jessica Israel, MD

Division Chief, Palliative Care
Monmouth Medical Center
Drexel University College of Medicine
Long Branch, New Jersey

Albert L. Jochen, MD

Associate Professor of Medicine
Endocrinology, Metabolism and Clinical
   Nutrition Medicine
Medical College of Wisconsin
Milwaukee, Wisconsin

Liza-Marie Johnson, MD, MPH, MBE

Fellow, Department of Pediatric Oncology
Division of Palliative and End-of-Life Care
St Jude Children's Research Hospital
Memphis, Tennessee

Kunal C. Kadakia, MD

Department of Internal Medicine
The Mayo Clinic
Rochester, Minnesota

Javier R. Kane, MD

Professor of Pediatrics
Section Chief, Pediatric Hematology
   Oncology
Director, Hospice and Palliative Care
Scott and White Children's Hospital and
   Clinics
Texas A&M Health Science Center College
   of Medicine
Temple, Texas

Mohana B. Karlekar, MD

Director Vanderbilt University Palliative
   Care
Vanderbilt University Medical Center
Nashville, Tennessee

**Dorothy M. K. Keefe, MBBS, MD,
   FRACP, FRCP**

Service Director
Department of SA Cancer Service
SA Health

Royal Adelaide Hospital, RAH Cancer
   Centre
North Terrace, Adelaide
Australia

Vaughan I. Keeley, PhD

Consultant in Palliative Medicine/
   Lymphoedema
Department of Palliative Medicine
Royal Derby Hospital
Derby, United Kingdom

Sally A. Kelley, MD

Assistant Medical Director
Midwest Palliative & Hospice Care Center
Glenview, Illinois

Philip S. Kim, MD

Medical Director
Center for Interventional Pain and Spine,
   LLC
Newark, Delaware

Kenneth L. Kirsh, PhD

Director
Behavioral Medicine and Ancillary
   Services
The Pain Treatment Center of the
   Bluegrass
Lexington, Kentucky

Elizabeth Kvale, MD

Assistant Professor of Medicine
University of Alabama at Birmingham
Birmingham, Alabama

Mario E. Lacouture, MD

Associate Attending Physician
Dermatology Service
Department of Medicine
Memorial Hospital for Cancer and Allied
   Disease
New York, New York

**Normand Laperriere, MD, FRCPC,
   FRANZCR (Hon)**

Department of Radiation Oncology
   Princess Margaret Hospital/University
   Health Network
Toronto, Ontario
Canada

Tanya J. Lehky, MD

Director, Clinical EMG Lab
EMG Section, OCD
National Institutes of Neurological
   Diseases and Stroke
Bethesda, Maryland

Dona Leskuski, DO

Palliative Care Consultant
Capital Caring
Falls Church, Virginia

Jerilyn A. Logemann, PhD

Ralph and Jean Sundin Professor,
   Northwestern University
Department of Communication Sciences
   and Disorders
Evanston, Illinois

Russell R. Lonser, MD

Chief, Surgical Neurology Branch
National Institute of Neurological
   Disorders and Stroke
National Institutes of Health
Bethesda, Maryland

Charles L. Loprinzi, MD

Regis Professor of Breast Cancer
   Research
Department of Oncology
The Mayo Clinic
Rochester, Minnesota

Matthew J. Loscalzo, MSW

Executive Director
Sheri & Les Biller Patient and Family
   Resource Center
Supportive Care Medicine
City of Hope National Medical Center
Duarte, California

Fade Mahmoud, MD

Fellow, Hematology and Oncology
UAMS Winthrop P. Rockefeller Cancer
   Institute
Little Rock, Arkansas

Andrew Mannes, MD

Chief
Department of Perioperative Medicine
National Institutes of Health
Bethesda, Maryland

Patrick W. Mantyh, PhD, JD

Professor
Research Service
VA Medical Center, Minneapolis,
   Minnesota
Department of Pharmacology, College of
   Medicine, University of Arizona
Tucson, Arizona

Sara F. Martin, MD

Assistant Professor
Department of Internal Medicine
Vanderbilt University Medical Center
Nashville, Tennessee

Laura McGevna, MD

Department of Dermatology
The University of Vermont
Burlington, Vermont

Sebastiano Mercadante, MD

Professor of Palliative Medicine
University of Palermo

Director of Anesthesia & Intensive Care
and Pain Relief & Palliative Care
La Maddalena Cancer Center
Palermo, Italy

Adam R. Metwalli, MD

Urologic Oncology Branch
National Cancer Institute, NIH
Bethesda, Maryland

Benjamin J. Miriovsky, MD, MS

Divisions of Medical Oncology,
Hematology, & Hematologic
Hematologic Malignancies, Department of
Medicine
Duke University Medical Center
Durham, North Carolina

Sumi K. Misra, MD, MPH, CMD

Chief of Palliative Care Program
Vanderbilt University Medical Center
Nashville, Tennessee

R. Sean Morrison, MD

Hermann Merkin Professor of Palliative Care
Professor of Geriatrics and Medicine
Vice-Chair for Research
Brookdale Department of Geriatrics and
Adult Development
Mount Sinai School of Medicine
New York, New York

Mary F. Mulcahy, MD

Division of Hematology/Oncology
Department of Medicine
Robert H. Lurie Comprehensive Cancer
Center
Northwestern University
Feinberg School of Medicine
Chicago, Illinois

Ryan R. Nash, MD, MA

Assistant Professor
Director, Palliative Care Leadership Center
UAB Center for Palliative and Supportive
Care
Birmingham, Alabama

Lori L. Olson, MD

Assistant Professor
Department of Internal Medicine
University of Kansas Medical Center
Kansas City, Kansas

Irene M. O'Shaughnessy, MD, FACP

Department of Endocrinology, Diabetes
and Metabolism
Medical College of Wisconsin
Milwaukee, Wisconsin

Judith A. Paice, PhD, RN, FAAN

Research Professor of Medicine
Department of Hematology-Oncology

Northwestern University; Feinberg School
of Medicine
Chicago, Illinois

Steven D. Passik, PhD

Professor of Psychiatry and
Anesthesiology
Vanderbilt University Medical Center
Department of Psychosomatic Medicine
Nashville, Tennessee

Jenny H. Petkova, MD

Assistant Professor
Hematology-Oncology
MUSC
Charleston, South Carolina

Peter A. Pinto, MD

Urologic Oncology Branch
Principal Investigator
National Cancer Institute
Bethesda, Maryland

Rosene D. Pirrello, BPharm, RPh

Executive Director of Pharmacy
San Diego Hospice and the Institute for
Palliative Medicine
San Diego, California

Holly G. Prigerson, PhD

Director
Center for Psychosocial Epidemiology &
Outcomes Research
Dana-Farber Cancer Institute
Medical Oncology, Division of Population
Sciences
Boston, Massachusetts

Christina M. Puchalski, MD, FACP

Director
The George Washington Institute of
Spirituality and Health;
Associate Professor of Medicine
School of Medicine and Health Sciences
The George Washington University
Washington, D.C.

Thomas J. Raife, MD

Clinical Professor
Medical Director-Transfusion Medicine
Department of Pathology
University of Iowa Hospitals and Clinics
Iowa City, Iowa

Alvin L. Reaves, III, MD

Emory Palliative Care Center
Department of Medicine
Emory University
Atlanta, Georgia

Carla Ida Ripamonti, MD

Head
Supportive Care in Cancer Unit

Fondazione IRCCS, Istituto Nazionale dei
Tumori
Via Venezian, 1
Milano, Italy

Christine S. Ritchie, MD, MSPH

Director, Center for Palliative Care
University of Alabama at Birmingham
Birmingham, Alabama

James C. Root, PhD

Assistant Attending Neuropsychologist
Neurocognitive Research Laboratory
Memorial Sloan Kettering Cancer
Institute
New York, New York

Jennifer M. Cuellar-Rodrìguez, MD

Staff Clinician
Laboratory of Clinical Infectious Diseases
National Institute of Allergy and Infectious
Diseases, NIH
Bethesda, Maryland

Alyx Rosen, MD, BSE

Clinical Research Fellow
Dermatology Service, Department of
Medicine
Memorial Sloan-Kettering Cancer Center
New York, New York

Paul Rousseau, MD

Associate Professor of General Internal
Medicine and Geriatrics
Medical Director
Palliative and Supportive Care Program
Medical University of South Carolina
Charleston, South Carolina

Elizabeth Ryan, PhD

Assistant Attending Neuropsychologist
Department of Psychiatry and Behavioral
Sciences
Memorial Sloan-Kettering Cancer Center
New York, New York

Vaibhav Sahai, MD, MSc

Hematology/Oncology Fellow
Department of Medicine
Northwestern Memorial Hospital
Chicago, Illinois

Nabeel Sarhill, MD

Division of Hematology/Oncology
Department of Medicine
The UT Health Sciences Center at San
Antonio
Harlingen, Texas

Lee Steven Schwartzberg, MD, FACP

Medical Director
The West Clinic
Memphis, Tennessee

Lauren Shaiova, MD

Chief of Palliative Care and Pain Medicine
Metropolitan Hospital Center Medicine
New York, New York

John L. Shuster , Jr., MD

Chief Medical Officer, Alive Hospice
Nashville, Tennessee
Clinical Professor of Psychiatry and Medicine
Vanderbilt University Medical Center
Nashville, Tennessee

Eric A. Singer, MD, MA

Assistant Professor
Section of Urologic Oncology
The Cancer Institute of New Jersey
New Brunswick, New Jersey

David A. Slosky, MD

Assistant Professor of Medicine
Vanderbilt Heart and Vascular Institute
Nashville, Tennessee

Eliezer Soto, MD, DABPM

Beth Israel Medical Center
Department of Pain Medicine and
    Palliative Care
New York, New York

**Linda J. Stricker, MSN/ED, RN,
    CWOCN**

Director WOC Nursing Education
The Cleveland Clinic
Cleveland, Ohio

Thomas Strouse, MD

Maddie Katz Professor of Palliative Care
    Research and Education
UCLA David Geffen School of Medicine
Medical Director, Vice Chair for Clinical
    Affairs
Department of Psychiatry and
    Biobehavioral Sciences
UCLA Resnick Neuropsychiatric Hospital
Los Angeles, California

Joan M. Teno, MD, MS

Professor of Health Services, Policy and Practise
Brown University

Center for Gerontology and Health Care
    Research
Providence, Rhode Island

James A. Tulsky, MD

Professor of Medicine and Nursing
Chief, Center for Palliative Care
Duke University and VA Medical Centers
Durham, North Carolina

Martha L. Twaddle, MD, FACP, FAAHM

Chief Medical Officer
Midwest Palliative and Hospice Care
    Center
Glenview, Illinois

Leigh Vaughan, MD

Assistant Professor
College of Medicine
Medical University of South Caroline
    Hospitalist Program
Charleston, South Carolina

Jaya Vijayan, MD

Palliative Medicine Physician
Department of Medicine
Holy Cross Hospital
Silver Spring, Maryland

Thomas J. Vogl, MD

Chief of Radiology
Department of Radiology
Universitätsklinik Frankfurt

Charles F. von Gunten, MD, PhD, FACP

Clinical Professor of Medicine
Division of Hematology/Oncology,
    Department of Medicine
Moores Cancer Center, University of
    California, San Diego
La Jolla, California

Jamie H. Von Roenn, MD

Professor of Medicine
Division of Hematology/Oncology
Department of Medicine
The Feinberg School of Medicine
Robert H. Lurie Comprehensive Cancer
    Center of Northwestern University
Chicago, Illinois

Xiao-Min Wang, MD, PhD

NINR/NIH
Bethesda, Maryland

Xin Shelley Wang, MD, PhD

Department of Symptom Research
Division of Internal Medicine
M.D. Anderson Cancer Center
Houston, Texas

Sharon M. Weinstein, MD, FAAHPM

Professor of Anesthesiology
Adjunct Associate Professor of Neurology
    and Oncology
Program Leader, Support Oncology-Pain
    Medicine and Palliative Care
Huntsman Cancer Institute, University of
    Utah
Salt Lake City, Utah

Howard Su-Hau Yeh, MD

Hematologist and Medical Oncologist
Berenson Oncology
West Hollywood, California

Christopher B. Yelverton, MD, MBA

Assistant Professor
Department Med-Dermatology
Division of Dermatology
Burlington, Vermont

James R. Zabora, ScD

Dean, Associate Professor
The Catholic University of America
National Catholic School of Social
    Services
Washington, D.C.

Stefan G. Zangos, MD

Institute for Diagnostic and Interventional
    Radiology
Johann Wolfgang Goethe-University
    Frankfurt
Frankfurt am Main, Germany

Shali Zhang, MS

Department of Dermatology
NYU Langone Medical Center
New York, New York

I had the pleasure of being present at the birth of the current textbook as I worked with one of the editors and had the opportunity to discuss the structure of the first edition with her. From the beginning, this text stretched the definitions and concept of palliative care beyond care for the terminally ill and led the way in visualizing palliation as supporting patients with cancer, and their families, from diagnosis to return to a normal life, or to a more comfortable ending to their life. I have to admit I was one of those physicians concerned with focusing on a separate specialty of palliative care. I was worried that some patients would be lost in the crevice between those who focus on treatment and those who are interested in palliation, as new opportunities arose both in treatment and in supportive care. The more comprehensive view of palliative and supportive care in this text was a strong defense against that happening. The first three editions served as the launching pad for the concept of integrating palliative care into the training and thinking of all cancer specialties. This book is a text for all health-care providers in the cancer field.

We find ourselves in an extraordinary time in the history of oncology. As the famous comic strip character, Pogo, said, "We are faced with insurmountable opportunities." New targeted treatments of a wholly different type are being developed against previously unresponsive tumors; national mortality rates have been falling since 1990 coincident with the application of this new information; and, in 2005, for the first time, overall deaths from cancer decreased in the United States, despite the increased size and age of the US population. Yet the diagnosis of cancer is still a devastating event in the life of a patient and their families and it is likely to remain that way for some time to come.

When editors plan a book they must take care to provide complete coverage by selecting the appropriate subject matter and also editing the content for completeness, selecting authors who work at the cutting edge of the field and are able to provide a complete and fresh look at the information offered to the reader. In this edition the editors have selected an impressive array of new authors to insure freshness. Good textbooks are supplemented by current literature but not replaced by it because only a small fraction of current literature in any field alters the way medicine is practiced. The editors of this compendium have once again done all of that. I like textbooks. I believe, if they are done well, the role they play in advancing a field and translating advances into clinical practice is underestimated. Cancer doctors, more than ever, need to be complete physicians and the information provided in this text will go a long way to assure that happens.

Vincent T. DeVita, Jr., MD

Preface to the Fourth Edition

The fourth edition of *Principles and Practice of Palliative Care and Supportive Oncology* is the product of months of work by a large number of contributors, all aimed at helping those who care for patients with cancer. As with previous editions, the editors and authors have endeavored to create authoritative and up-to-date reviews of research and clinical care best practices in palliative care and supportive oncology, presented with a focus on practical, clinical application. We continue to emphasize integrated interdisciplinary care, collaborating with the patient and family to shape care that respects and prioritizes the patient's goals, values, and preferences. It is our hope that this effort will be a source of both help and inspiration to all who practice palliative care and supportive oncology.

The fourth edition contains updated and revised chapters throughout. The section on pain has been extensively revised, with new chapters on interventional approaches to pain, pathobiology of bone metastases, and pathobiology of chemotherapy-induced neuropathy. There are a total of 19 new chapter topics, including chapters on the dermatologic toxicity of cancer treatment, the impact of hepatic and renal dysfunction on the pharmacology of palliative care drugs, infectious complications common in palliative oncology and their management, care for patients with brain and meningeal metastases, the cognitive impact of cancer treatments, running family meetings for setting goals of care, and the toxicity and supportive care of patients undergoing bone marrow and stem cell transplantation.

This is an exciting time to practice palliative care and supportive oncology. Since the preparation and publication of the third edition, our field has continued to grow and mature. In 2006, the American Board of Medical Specialties announced that 10 of its member boards—anesthesiology, emergency medicine, family medicine, internal medicine, obstetrics and gynecology, pediatrics, physical medicine and rehabilitation, psychiatry and neurology, radiology, and surgery—would offer subspecialty certification in hospice and palliative medicine. Advances in cancer therapies are making supportive care of cancer patients ever more important and integral to good care and favorable outcomes. The knowledge base continues its steady advance. For those who practice, teach, or perform research in palliative care and supportive oncology, the unique opportunities to blend scientific knowledge with the primary role of the therapeutic relationship, to witness and be inspired by occasions of genuine healing and growth, and to participate in "doctoring" at its most authentic are special rewards of the work. It is our hope that we have captured the essence of this with the text you hold in your hand.

As always, we wish to thank our contributors, without whose efforts this book would not have been possible. We are grateful that they have so generously shared their gifts in these pages. Thanks also go to the publisher and production staff for their diligent efforts in producing this volume. We are also grateful for the patient forbearance of our families, allowing us the time and offering us the support needed to get the work done. Finally, special thanks are due to Zia Raven, Editorial Assistant, whose tireless effort, professionalism, and gentle clarity of focus simultaneously organized and inspired us.

Ann M. Berger, MSN, MD
John L. Shuster, Jr., MD
Jamie H. Von Roenn, MD

The term supportive oncology refers to those aspects of medical care concerned with the physical, psychosocial, and spiritual issues faced by persons with cancer, their families, their communities, and their health-care providers. In this context, supportive oncology describes both those interventions used to support patients who experience adverse effects caused by antineoplastic therapies and those interventions now considered under the broad rubric of palliative care. The term palliative is derived from the Latin pallium: to cloak or cover. At its core, palliative care is concerned with providing the maximum quality of life to the patient-family unit.

In 1990, the World Health Organization (WHO) published a landmark document, Cancer Pain Relief and Palliative Care, which clearly defined the international barriers and needs for improved pain and symptom control in the cancer patient. The WHO definition of palliative care is

> The active total care of patients whose disease is not responsive to curative treatment. Control of pain, of other symptoms, and of psychological, social, and spiritual problems is paramount. The goal of palliative care is achievement of the best quality of life for patients and their families. Many aspects of palliative care are also applicable earlier in the course of the illness in conjunction with anti-cancer treatment.

In 1995, the Canadian Palliative Care Association chose a somewhat broader definition that emphasizes a more expanded role of palliative care:

> Palliative care, as a philosophy of care, is the combination of active and compassionate therapies intended to comfort and support individuals and families who are living with a life-threatening illness. During periods of illness and bereavement, palliative care strives to meet physical, psychological, social, and spiritual expectations and needs, while remaining sensitive to personal, cultural, and religious values, beliefs, and practices. Palliative care may be combined with therapies aimed at reducing or curing the illness, or it may be the total focus of care.

In developing this textbook, the editors have brought together those elements of palliative care that are most applicable to the health-care professional caring for cancer patients and have combined this perspective with a detailed description of related therapies used to support patients in active treatment. The editors view these interventions as a necessary and vital aspect of medical care for all cancer patients, from the time of diagnosis until death. Indeed, most patients will have a significant physical symptom requiring treatment at the time of their cancer diagnosis. Even when cancer can be effectively treated and a cure or life prolongation is achieved, there are always physical, psychosocial, or spiritual concerns that must be addressed to maintain function and optimize the quality of life. For patients whose cancer cannot be effectively treated, palliative care must be the dominant mode, and one must focus intensively on the control of distressing symptoms. Planning for the end of life and ensuring that death occurs with a minimum of suffering and in a manner consistent with the values and desires of the patient and family are fundamental elements of this care. Palliative care, as a desired approach to comprehensive cancer care, is appropriate for all health-care settings, including the clinic, acute care hospital, long-term care facility, or home hospice.

Palliative care and the broader concept of supportive care involve the collaborative efforts of an interdisciplinary team. This team must include the cancer patient and his or her family, care givers, and involved health-care providers. Integral to effective palliative care is the opportunity and support necessary for both care givers and health-care providers to work through their own emotions related to the care they are providing.

In organizing this textbook, the editors have recognized the important contributions of medical research and clinical care that have emerged from the disciplines of hospice and palliative medicine; medical, radiation, and surgical oncology; nursing; neurology and neuro-oncology; anesthesiology; psychiatry and psychology; pharmacology; and many others. The text includes chapters focusing on the common physical symptoms experienced by the cancer patient; a review of specific supportive treatment modalities, such as blood products, nutritional support, hydration, palliative chemotherapy, radiotherapy, and surgery; and finally, a review of more specialized topics, including survivorship issues, medical ethics, spiritual care, quality of life, and supportive care in the elderly, pediatric, and AIDS patients.

There are many promising new cancer treatments on the horizon. No matter what these new treatments will offer in terms of curing the disease or prolonging life, cancer will remain a devastating illness, not only for the affected patients but also for their families, community, and health-care providers. Providing excellent, supportive care will continue to be a goal for all health-care providers.

The authors would like to thank the many contributors for their efforts. We are also grateful to our publisher and secretaries, whose oversight and gentle prodding were essential to our success. Finally, we want to express our gratitude to our families and colleagues, who accommodated our needs in bringing the volume to fruition and provided the support we needed throughout the process.

Ann M. Berger, MSN, MD
Russell K. Portenoy, MD
David E. Weissman, MD

Acknowledgments

We would like to thank all of the contributors for their tireless effort. We are also very grateful to Zia Raven, whose oversight, gentle prodding, and years of experience were essential to the success of the book. We would like to thank Jonathan W. Pine at Lippincott Williams & Wilkins for his efforts in helping us get the book completed. We want to express our gratitude to our families and colleagues for their unstinting support for all of our efforts. Finally, we would like to express appreciation to the patients who continuously teach us, and who are the true heroes.

Contents

SECTION VI:

Research Issues in Supportive Care and Palliative Care

Symptoms and Syndromes

CHAPTER 1

Difficult Pain Syndromes: Neuropathic Pain, Bone Pain, and Visceral Pain

Lauren Shaiova ■ Leonard A. Farber ■ Sunil Kumar Aggarwal

Nociception is what occurs physiologically in our bodies during the activation and sensitization of tissue nociceptors, also known as A-delta and C-nerve fibers. Pain corresponds to our awareness of nociception and has been defined by the International Study for Pain as "an unpleasant sensory and emotional experience associated with tissue damage or described in terms of such damage" (1).

In the clinical setting, pain may occur as a response to a noxious event in the tissue, for example, tissue inflammation due to a burn injury, or as a response to an abnormal pathologic process occurring within the nervous system pain pathways. In the first case, the pain signal presumably originates from "healthy" tissue nociceptors activated or sensitized by the local release of algogenic substances (e.g., protons, prostaglandins, bradykinin, adenosine, and cytokines). This type of pain is called *nociceptive* and is characterized by gnawing and visceral aching pain. In the second case, the pain signal is generated ectopically by abnormal peripheral nerve fibers involved in pain transmission and/ or by abnormal pain circuits in the central nervous system (CNS); this type of pain has been called *neuropathic*, it is characterized by sharp electrical-like, burning or lancinating pain. However, the separation between nociceptive and neuropathic pain states is often blurred. Indeed, as discussed in the subsequent text, neuropathic pain may arise from inflammation (i.e., inflammatory neuropathic pain) (2). Inflammatory and neuropathic mechanisms may be present at the same time or at different times in patients who have been diagnosed with cancer pain syndromes of bone or visceral origin. In fact, cancer pain, whether arising from viscera, bone, or any other somatic structure, is more often than commonly thought the result of a mixture of pain mechanisms. When cancer pain becomes a clinical challenge to treatment, it has been labeled as a difficult pain syndrome or refractory pain.

DIFFICULT PAIN SYNDROMES: PERIPHERAL AND CENTRAL MECHANISMS

The pain signal is transmitted from the peripheral nociceptors, through the dorsal horn of the spinal cord and the thalamus, up to the cortex. In the periphery, nociceptors can be activated by chemical products of tissue damage and inflammation, which include prostanoids, serotonin, bradykinin, cytokines, adenosine, adenosine-5'-triphosphate, histamine, protons, free radicals, and growth factors. These agents can activate afferent fibers or sensitize them to a range of mechanical, thermal, and chemical stimuli. Notably, a proportion of the afferent fibers that are normally unresponsive to noxious stimuli ("silent" or "sleeping" nociceptors) can be "awakened" by inflammatory chemicals and be stimulated to contribute to pain and hyperalgesia. The products of tissue damage and inflammation interact with receptors located on the A-delta fibers and C-nerve fibers to initiate membrane excitability and intracellular transcriptional changes.

Most neuropathic pain conditions develop after partial injuries to the peripheral nervous system (PNS). For example, as observed in animal models of partial nerve injury, both injured and uninjured primary sensory neurons acquire the ability to express genes de novo and, therefore, change their phenotype (phenotypic shift). Nerve endings develop sensitivity to a number of factors, such as prostanoids and cytokines (e.g., tumor necrosis factor-α [TNF-α]) (3–6). One example is the upregulation or induction of catecholamine receptors in undamaged nociceptors; in this condition, nociceptors are activated by noradrenaline and the resulting neuropathic pain has been called *sympathetically maintained pain* (*SMP*) (7,8). Reversal of the phenotypic shift is associated with the reduction of neuropathic pain (9).

Recent findings suggest that during cancer (and other pathologic inflammatory conditions), a number of diffusible factors might be involved in causing a "neuropathic spin" in the cancer-related pain state. Tissue-related growth factors (e.g., nerve growth factor [NGF]) in combination with specific proinflammatory cytokines (e.g., TNF-α, interleukin [IL]-1β (10)) might sensitize nociceptors and generate ectopic and spontaneous activity in tissue nociceptors. In these instances, pain caused by cancer could be classified more properly as inflammatory neuropathic pain. There is considerable hope that the identification of the diffusible factors causing altered gene expression in the dorsal root ganglia sensory neurons will direct research to discover more effective treatments. Early and aggressive pain interventions and the use of specific therapies that disengage gene expression might be sufficient to uncouple the phenotypic shift and reverse a difficult pain syndrome into an easy-to-treat condition.

Peripheral and Central Mechanisms of Pathological Pain

In the PNS, several elements of the cellular "machinery" that are thought to be relevant to the development of pathologic pain have been identified as potential targets for analgesic drugs.

In the CNS, in particular within the spinal cord, a variety of neurobiologic events can occur during the course of an ongoing peripheral tissue damage and inflammation (15).

NEUROPATHIC PAIN

Clinical Findings and Diagnosis

The clinical interview of a patient with cancer pain should focus on questions about onset, duration, progression, character, and nature of complaints suggestive of neurologic deficits (e.g., persistent numbness in a body area, limb weakness, such as tripping episodes, and the progressive inability to open jaws), as well as complaints suggestive of sensory dysfunction (e.g., touch-evoked pain, intermittent abnormal sensations, spontaneous burning, and shooting pains). Notably, patients may report only sensory symptoms and have no neurologic deficits. The interview should also focus on relieving factor if any that the patient has realized during the pain process.

Patients with neuropathic pain may present with some or all of the following abnormal sensory symptoms and signs:

■ *Paresthesias*: spontaneous, intermittent, painless, and abnormal sensations
■ *Dysesthesias*: spontaneous or evoked unpleasant sensations, such as annoying sensations elicited by cold stimuli or pinprick testing
■ *Allodynia*: pain elicited by nonnoxious stimuli (i.e., clothing, air movement, and tactile stimuli) when applied to the symptomatic cutaneous area; allodynia may be mechanical (static, e.g., induced by application of a light pressure, or dynamic, e.g., induced by moving a soft brush) or thermal (e.g., induced by a nonpainful cold or warm stimulus)
■ *Hyperalgesia*: an exaggerated pain response to a mildly noxious (mechanical or thermal) stimulus applied to the symptomatic area
■ *Hyperpathia*: a delayed and explosive pain response to a stimulus applied to the symptomatic area

Allodynia, hyperalgesia, and hyperpathia represent positive abnormal findings, as opposed to the negative findings of the neurologic sensory examination, that is, hypesthesia and anesthesia. Heat hyperalgesia and deep mechanical allodynia (i.e., tenderness on soft tissue palpation) are findings that are commonly present in the cutaneous epicenter of an inflammatory pain generator, also known as the *zone of primary hyperalgesia*. These findings are indicative of PNS sensitization and are related to a local inflammatory state. On the other hand, the skin surrounding the site of inflammation, also known as the *zone of secondary hyperalgesia*, may present the finding of mechanical allodynia, which can be elicited, for example, by stroking the area with a soft brush. Secondary hyperalgesia is indicative of CNS sensitization. Patients affected by SMP typically complain of cold allodynia/hyperalgesia. This is assessed by providing a cold stimulus, such as placing a cold metallic tuning fork, to the painful region for a few seconds.

Clinical and research tools to assess and measure the intensity and quality of neuropathic pain include the Brief Pain Inventory (BPI) and the Neuropathic Pain Scale (NPS) (18). The BPI is a well-validated instrument that consists of 15 items asking the patient about average pain, worst pain in the past week, whether the patient has received relief from pain treatment, and whether the pain has interfered with daily activities (19). The NPS is a self-report scale for measuring neuropathic pain. It consists of 12 distinct questions, which ask about intensity and quality of the patient's pain. In validation studies, it has been found to have a good predictive power in discriminating between major subgroups of patients with neuropathic pain (19).

Table 1.1 (20) lists the most common neuropathic pain syndromes that have been reported in association with cancer. Neuropathy may result from one or more cancer-related mechanisms (21), for example, compression, mechanical traction, inflammation, or infiltration of nerve trunks or plexi caused by the progression of the primary cancer or by metastatic disease affecting bone or soft tissues. Head and neck cancer and skull-based tumors can cause painful cranial neuropathies by direct nerve compression. Salivary gland cancers may cause painful facial neuropathies. Breast or lung cancer can infiltrate the brachial plexus and cause painful plexitis. Pelvic or retroperitoneal cancer may invade the lumbosacral plexus. If the meninges are affected (meningeal carcinomatosis), the involvement of adjacent roots, spinal nerves, and plexi can occur. Metastatic disease or lymphoma can cause meningeal carcinomatosis and affect multiple spinal roots. Peripheral neuropathies with pain and dysesthesia may also be observed in the presence of lymphomas. Acute inflammatory demyelinating polyneuropathy of the Guillain-Barré syndrome type may occur with lymphomas, particularly Hodgkin's disease.

Antineoplastic therapeutic agents such as platinum-based agents, taxoids, and vincristine may cause painful neuropathies; these are usually distal symmetrical polyneuropathies, but can manifest as a mononeuropathy. Postradiation plexopathies may arise when >60 Gy (6,000 rad) of irradiation is given to the patient as a radiation dose. Surgical resection of cancers may result in traumatic injuries to peripheral nerves, with the development of painful neuromas. For example, postthoracotomy pain can be caused by injury to the intercostal nerves and postmastectomy pain may arise through injury to the intercostobrachial nerve.

Compression or entrapment neuropathies occur in the presence of cachexia; for example, patients with cancer who have lost substantial fat and muscle body weight are prone to develop peroneal neuropathies.

Paraneoplastic autoimmune syndromes due to antineuronal antibodies may present as painful neuropathies.

TABLE 1.1	Neuropathic pain syndromes related to cancer

Neuropathic Pain Syndromes	Clinical Examples
Cranial nerve neuralgias	Base of skull or leptomeningeal metastases and head and neck cancers
Mononeuropathy and other neuralgias	Rib metastases with intercostal nerve injury
Radiculopathy	Epidural mass and leptomeningeal metastases
Cervical plexopathy	Head and neck cancer with local extension and cervical lymph node metastases
Brachial plexopathy	Lymph node metastases from breast cancer or lymphoma and direct extension of Pancoast tumor
Lumbosacral plexopathy	Extension of colorectal cancer, cervical cancer, sarcoma, or lymphoma and breast cancer metastases
Paraneoplastic peripheral neuropathy	Small cell lung cancer and antineuronal nuclear antibodies type 1
Central pain	Spinal cord compression
Cachexia	Compression or entrapment neuropathies

Adapted from Martin LA, Hagen NA. Neuropathic pain in cancer patients: mechanisms, syndromes, and clinical controversies. *J Pain Symptom Manage.* 1997;14:99-117.

Patients who complain of burning dysesthesias in their feet, hands, and face (in the setting of diagnosed or undiagnosed carcinoma) may have antineuronal nuclear antibodies type 1 (ANNA-1), also known as *anti-Hu*. Most patients who present with sensory neuronopathy and small cell carcinoma of the lung have significantly elevated titers of anti-Hu. All patients with burning dysesthesias of face, hands, and legs and positive titers for anti-Hu should undergo a computed tomography (CT) or magnetic resonance imaging (MRI) of the chest. In fact, small cell carcinoma of the lung may remain undetected by plain chest x-ray. In any case, anti-Hu positivity should prompt a careful search for malignancy, especially for a small cell carcinoma of the lung. Painful dysesthesias develop first in one limb and then progress to involve other limbs, face, scalp, and trunk over weeks or months. In these patients, deep tendon reflexes are reduced or absent and muscle strength is preserved. Patients may be disabled in their ambulation because of the sensory ataxia that is often associated with the painful symptoms.

Therapeutic Interventions for Neuropathic Pain

Management of severe neuropathic pain can be a challenge, and a combination of therapies employing agents from a variety of pharmacologic classes and pain procedures represent the contemporary standard approach. Treatment includes a wide range of modalities, ranging from opioid and nonopioid analgesics, neuropathic adjuvant medication to implantable devices and surgery. Table 1.2 tabulates the pharmacotherapy used in neuropathic pain.

Antiepileptic Drugs

Antiepileptic drugs (AEDs) are the most effective agents for the management of neuropathic pain. The gabapentinoid anticonvulsants gabapentin and pregabalin have both established efficacy in treating neuropathic pain. In May 2002, gabapentin gained U.S. Food and Drug Administration (FDA) approval for the treatment of postherpetic neuralgia (PHN), a state characterized by allodynia and burning pain. However, gabapentin is also known to be effective in treating neuropathic pain from diabetic neuropathy, a state predominantly characterized by spontaneous burning pain (22–24). In December 2004, the gabapentin analog pregabalin gained FDA approval for the treatment of PHN and painful diabetic neuropathy. Gabapentinoids act on neither γ-aminobutyric acid (GABA) receptors nor sodium channels. Recent evidence suggests that gabapentin and pregabalin may modulate the cellular calcium influx into nociceptive neurons by binding to voltage-gated calcium channels, in particular to the α-2-Δ subunit of the channel (25). Trigeminal neuralgia (a neuropathic condition characterized by a brief excruciating, lancinating pain) responds extremely well to carbamazepine or oxcarbazepine, while another AED, lamotrigine, has shown some efficacy in treating carbamazepine-resistant trigeminal neuralgia (26). Topiramate has been anecdotally used in the treatment of complex regional pain syndrome (CRPS) type 1 (27). Several new AEDs (e.g., levetiracetam, zonisamide, oxcarbazepine, and tiagabine) have become available for medical use, and some of these, along with topiramate, may have analgesic effect in primary headache and perhaps in neuropathic pain (28, 29). Interestingly, in a recent randomized, double-blind, active placebo-controlled, crossover trial, patients with neuropathic pain received lorazepam (active placebo), controlled-release morphine, gabapentin, and a combination of gabapentin and morphine, each treatment given orally for 5 weeks. The study indicated that the best analgesia was obtained from the gabapentin–morphine combination, with each medication given at a

TABLE 1.2	Pharmacotherapy of neuropathic pain	
Agent/Class	**Initial Dose**	**Dose Increment**
Gabapentin	100–300 mg/d	100–300 mg every 3–5 d
Pregabalin	50–150 mg/d	25–50 mg every 3 d
Topiramate	25–50 mg/d wk	50 mg/d increase every wk
Carbamazepine	100–200 mg bid	100–200 mg every 2 d
Tricyclic antidepressants	10–25 mg/d	10–25 mg every wk
Duloxetine	20–60 mg/d	20–30 mg every 1–3 d
Venlafaxine	37.5 mg/d	37.5 mg every 1–3 d
Tramadol	25–50 mg/d or bid	50–100 mg every 1–3 d
Opioid analgesics	Morphine sulfate 5–15 mg or equivalent short-acting opiate every 4 h p.r.n	Convert to long-acting agent after 1–2 wk
Capsaicin	0.075% qid	
Topical lidocaine 5%	Maximum 3 patches daily for 12 h	
Mexiletine	150 mg/d	150 mg/d

Blank spaces indicate no dose increment.

Freeman R. The Treatment of Neuropathic Pain. *CNS Spectr.* 2005;10(9):698-706.

lower dose when given as a combination than when given as a single agent (30).

Opioids

Opioids are currently the most potent and effective analgesics used to treat acute and chronic pain, and, as such, they have been prescribed to patients suffering from intractable pain. Morphine, a μ-agonist, represents the mainstay for the treatment of moderate to severe nociceptive cancer pain (31). Long considered to be ineffective for neuropathic pain, opioids have demonstrated efficacy in several recent clinical trials (32–37). A double-blind, placebo-controlled, crossover trial (34) in which 76 patients with PHN received opioids (e.g., controlled-release morphine or methadone), tricyclic antidepressants (TCAs) (e.g., amitriptyline or nortriptyline), and placebo found that both opioids and TCAs provided significantly better pain relief than placebo. Among patients completing the study, most preferred opioids (50%) to TCAs (30%; $p = 0.02$). The results indicate that opioids are as effective as TCAs in the treatment of PHN. This is important because among medical professionals, there is a myth that opioids are not effective for neuropathic pain.

The analgesic action of the pure opioid agonists (e.g., morphine, methadone, fentanyl, oxycodone, hydromorphone, and oxymorphone) is well known and utilized clinically. Among all the analgesic medications currently available, the most powerful and effective drugs are still the agents acting on the μ-, κ-, and Δ-opioid receptors. Opioid receptors are located not only in the CNS (primarily in the dorsal horn) but also peripherally on the nociceptors. Opioids may have a relevant peripheral analgesic effect during painful inflammatory states (38).

The pure opioid agonists are the mainstay for the treatment of severe disabling pain. Mixed agonists or partial agonist–antagonist are not recommended for use in cancer pain. The treatment of chronic pain may rely on the use of long-acting agents (i.e., methadone and levorphanol) or controlled-release preparations of morphine, fentanyl, oxycodone, oxymorphone, and hydromorphone. Many pure opioid agonists are also available in short-acting forms for breakthrough cancer pain and rapid onset opioids that are available in a transmucosal preparation and in an intranasal preparation for rapid "rescue" of breakthrough cancer pain.

Among the pure opioid agonists, methadone has peculiar properties. The methadone used clinically is a racemic mixture of the d and l isomers. In research the isomers are separated: the d isomer has more N-methyl-d-aspartate (NMDA) properties and the l isomer has more opioid properties. The methadone has an intrinsic NMDA receptor antagonistic effect, which may add adjuvant analgesic effect in case of neuropathic pain (see subsequent text). Interestingly, recent animal studies suggest that the addition of an extremely low dose of an opioid receptor antagonist (e.g., naltrexone) to morphine in a ratio of 1:1,000 may enhance the analgesic efficacy of the opioid agonists (39). Tramadol is an analgesic agent with a weak μ-opioid agonistic effect. Its potency is comparable to that of a codeine–acetaminophen preparation.

Notably, in controlled trials, tramadol has shown efficacy in the treatment of neuropathic pain (39–41).

Clinicians should be careful during opioid titration because the requirement for neuropathic pain may be high. The opioid dose should be increased until analgesia is achieved or till side effects become intolerable. Common side effects are constipation, sedation, pruritus, and nausea/vomiting. Although rare, confusion may develop and it is very important to rule out a medical cause if a patient has been stable on an opioid and develops sudden change in mental status. Except for constipation, tolerance occurs for most of the opioid-related side effects (e.g., nausea, vomiting, respiratory depression, and drowsiness). The most feared complication of respiratory depression is rare, especially in patients who are somewhat tolerant to opioids, which is anywhere from 3 to 5 days. Unlike anti-inflammatory drugs, opioid agonists have no true "ceiling dose" for analgesia and do not cause direct organ damage. Opioids that are in combination with acetaminophen or a nonsteroidal drug exhibit ceiling effect, wherein the nonopioids confer the ceiling effect. Side effects can often be managed with additional pharmacotherapy, and the clinician may choose to treat the side effects and continue the opioid dose or "rotate" to another opioid. When converting to another opioid, it is wise to refer to an opioid conversion table such as in Table 1.3 or a similar reference and reduce the dose by 50% to avoid incomplete cross-tolerance. Opioid titration and opioid rotation are essential concepts in the management of neuropathic pain. To determine adequate opioid responsiveness, a careful titration of the opioid dose is necessary. However, the development of tolerance to opioid side effects, degree of analgesia, and the development of analgesic tolerance are extremely variable among patients with pain receiving these medications. If severe pain persists or side effects become intolerable during the initial drug trial, trials of different opioids (i.e., opioid rotation) are recommended. Studies indicate that patients on a stable opioid regimen do not report significant impairment in their driving ability, attention, mood, and general cognitive functioning (42).

Antidepressants

Antidepressants also play an important role in the treatment of chronic pain. TCAs, such as amitriptyline, nortriptyline, and desipramine (43), have established efficacy in the treatment of neuropathic pain. They have been used successfully for the treatment of painful diabetic neuropathy and PHN and provided pain relief in nondepressed patients affected by neuropathic pain. Notably, TCAs such as amitriptyline, doxepin, and imipramine have been found to have potent local anesthetic properties. Amitriptyline appears to be more potent than bupivacaine as a sodium channel blocker (44). TCAs frequently have poorly tolerated adverse effects, including cardiotoxicity, confusion, urinary retention, orthostatic hypotension, nightmares, weight gain, drowsiness, dry mouth, and constipation. These medications are difficult to titrate and at times patients may need to stop the medication because of side effects that are untoward.

Duloxetine and venlafaxine are both antidepressants that lack the anticholinergic and antihistamine effects of the TCAs (45–47). Duloxetine has recently been approved

TABLE 1.3	Equianalgesic potency conversion for cancer pain	
Drug	**Equianalgesic Dose (mg)**	
	Intramuscular[a,b]	**Oral**
Morphine	10	60[c]
Codeine	130	200
Heroin	5	60
Hydromorphone	1.5	7.5
Levorphanol	2	4
Meperidine	75	300
Methadone	10	20
Oxycodone	15	30
Oxymorphone	1	10 (rectal)

[a]Based on single-dose studies in which an intramuscular dose of each drug listed was compared with morphine to establish relative potency. Oral doses are those recommended when changing from a parenteral to an oral route.

[b]Although no controlled studies are available, in clinical practice it is customary to consider the doses of opioid given intramuscularly, intravenously, or subcutaneously to be equivalent.

[c]The conversion ratio of 10 mg of parenteral morphine to 60 mg of oral morphine is based on a potency study in patients with acute pain.

Note: All intramuscular and oral doses listed are considered to be equivalent in analgesic effect to 10 mg of intramuscular morphine.

by the FDA for the treatment of pain secondary to diabetic neuropathy (47,48). Duloxetine and venlafaxine appear to possess an analgesic mechanism of action, with similar TCA-like beneficial properties but fewer side effects. Also, a slow-release preparation of bupropion, an atypical antidepressant, at the dose of 150 mg twice a day, was found to be effective for the treatment of neuropathic pain (49). Selective serotonin reuptake inhibitors (SSRIs), such as paroxetine and fluoxetine, are effective antidepressants, but these are quite ineffective analgesics. While being used for the management of comorbidities such as anxiety, depression, and insomnia, which frequently affect patients with chronic neuropathic pain, SSRIs have not shown the same efficacy as TCAs in the treatment of neuropathic pain (43).

Local Anesthetics

The FDA has approved transdermal lidocaine for the treatment of postherpetic pain (50). In a controlled clinical trial, the transdermal form of 5% lidocaine relieved pain associated with PHN without significant adverse effects (51). There is also early evidence to suggest that the patch provides benefit for other neuropathic pain states (52), including diabetic neuropathy (53), CRPS, postmastectomy pain, and HIV-related neuropathy (54).

Intravenous lidocaine and oral mexiletine have also been utilized in patients with neuropathic pain (55). Mexiletine, an antiarrhythmic local anesthetic, is a sodium channel blocker with analgesic properties for the treatment of neuropathic pain, similar to the properties of some AEDs (e.g., lamotrigine and carbamazepine). Mexiletine is contraindicated in the presence of second-degree and third-degree atrial–ventricular conduction blocks. Also, the incidence of gastrointestinal side effects (e.g., diarrhea and nausea) is quite high in patients taking mexiletine.

Sodium channel–blocking properties are found not only in the traditional local anesthetics, such as bupivacaine and lidocaine, and in the oral antiarrhythmic agent mexiletine but also in several AEDs, such as carbamazepine, oxcarbazepine, and lamotrigine, and in the TCAs, such as amitriptyline, doxepin, and imipramine (13,56,57).

Adjuvants and Nonopioid Analgesics for Neuropathic Pain

In addition to the agents discussed in the preceding text, many drugs from a variety of pharmacologic classes can be classified as adjuvant analgesics and used "off label" in the management of patients with chronic intractable pain. In many cases, the mechanisms supporting this analgesic enhancement are still unknown. At present, the evidence that adjuvants and emerging analgesics may possess analgesic properties for the treatment of neuropathic pain has mostly been derived from preliminary clinical investigations and observations.

α_2-Adrenergic Agonists

Drugs acting on the α_2-adrenergic spinal receptors (e.g., clonidine and tizanidine) have been clinically recognized as analgesics (9,58). α_2-Adrenergic agonists are known to have a spinal antinociceptive effect. Controlled trials have shown the effectiveness of intraspinal clonidine for controlling pain (58,59). Clonidine has been found to potentiate intrathecal opioid analgesia. Moreover, transdermal clonidine has a local antiallodynic effect in patients with SMP (60). Topical clonidine, an α_2-adrenergic agonist, has an analgesic effect in SMP. Clonidine causes local inhibition of noradrenaline release by acting on the adrenergic α_2-autoreceptors of the sympathetic endings (60). Tizanidine is a relatively short-acting, oral α_2-adrenergic agonist with a much lower hypotensive effect than clonidine. Tizanidine has been used for the management of spasticity. However, animal studies and clinical experience indicate the usefulness of tizanidine for a variety of painful states, including neuropathic pain disorders (61–63). The most common side effects of the α_2-adrenergic agonists are somnolence and dizziness (to which tolerance usually develops).

Capsaicin

Capsaicin is the natural substance present in hot chili peppers. Capsaicin activates the recently cloned vanilloid neuronal membrane receptor (64). A single administration of a large dose of capsaicin, after an initial depolarization, appears to produce a prolonged deactivation of capsaicin-sensitive nociceptors. The analgesic effect is dose dependent and may last for several weeks. Capsaicin must be compounded topically at high concentrations (>1%) and administered under local or regional anesthesia (65). Over-the-counter creams must be applied several times a day for many weeks. Controlled studies at low capsaicin concentrations (0.075% or less) have shown mixed results, possibly because of noncompliance.

NMDA Antagonists

Evidence gleaned from animal experiments shows that NMDA receptors play an important role in the central mechanisms of hyperalgesia and chronic pain (16,17). Dextromethorphan, memantine, and ketamine are NMDA antagonists that may be considered as adjuvants in the management of hyperalgesic neuropathic states poorly responsive to opioid analgesics (47,66–70). Ketamine and dextromethorphan may be used in conjunction with opioids in the prevention and treatment of analgesic tolerance and the management of allodynia and hyperalgesia. Recent studies indicate that ketamine may have a particular role in the management of cancer pain in those patients who are poorly responsive to opioids. Ketamine as an adjuvant to opioids increases pain relief by 20% to 30% and allows opioid dose reduction by 25% to 50% and can be used in both adult and pediatric patients (67,68). Ketamine is able to alter the nociceptive input at the spinal level. Because of the potential neurotoxicity of intrathecal racemic ketamine, the administration of the active compound $S(+)$-ketamine may be a valuable alternative (70). Topical ketamine can provide effective palliation of mucositis pain induced by radiation therapy (69). However, ketamine has a very narrow therapeutic window. Parenteral ketamine can cause intolerable side effects, such as hallucinations and memory impairment.

Methadone

The opioid methadone is a racemic mixture of the isomers d-methadone and l-methadone. d-methadone, although reportedly lacking the opioid agonistic effect, has been shown to possess NMDA receptor antagonist activity (71). Methadone's role in the treatment of neuropathic pain (71) may be limited by its long and unpredictable half-life, interindividual variations in pharmacokinetics, and lack of knowledge about appropriate use. Of interest is the possibility that NMDA antagonists may prevent or counteract opioid analgesic tolerance (72,73).

There has been some concern recently about intravenous methadone and prolongation of the QTc. Current recommendations are to perform an ECG before starting intravenous methadone and carry out serial ECGs when the dose is escalated or when another class of drug that has the potential to prolong the QTc is added, such as antifungals, quinolone antibiotics, phenothiazines, and antidepressants. (75) Oral methadone lacks the preservative chlorobutanol and is thus not as much a concern for the risk of QTc prolongation. Although at the basis of any treatment, goals of care must be discussed with patients and families.

Cannabinoids

Evidence from preclinical and clinical studies indicates that cannabinoids have analgesic properties (71,73,74) that are chiefly mediated via the endocannabinoid signaling system (73). Cannabinoids are a class of drugs that take their name from the cannabinoid botanical *Cannabis sativa* from which they were first isolated and include herbal preparations of cannabis as well as synthetic, semisynthetic, and extracted cannabinoid preparations (73,74). Historically, in oncology, the main approved therapeutic use of cannabinoids has been in the prevention of nausea and vomiting caused by chemotherapy. In patients with cancer or acquired immunodeficiency syndrome, Δ-9-*trans*-tetrahydrocannabinol (Δ-9-THC) can be used to increase the appetite and treat weight loss. Several studies have now been carried out to assess the therapeutic effectiveness of cannabinoids as analgesics. Cannabis and the major active constituent of cannabis, Δ-9-THC, have been shown to have antinociceptive effects. Cannabinoids appear to have a predominant antiallodynic/antihyperalgesic effect (71,73–75). Interestingly, the addition of inactive doses of cannabinoids to low doses of μ-opioid agonists appears to potentiate opioid antinociception (76,77).

Δ-9-THC is the most widely studied cannabinoid, but a number of clinical trials of inhaled herbal cannabis and cannabis extracts in the treatment of pain have been recently conducted. Analgesic sites of action have been identified in brain areas, the spinal cord, and the PNS, which correspond with cannabinoid receptor tissue distributions. Cannabinoids appear to have a peripheral anti-inflammatory action and induce antinociception at lower doses than those needed for psychoactivity. Cannabinoids have been shown to suppress neuropathic nociception in at least nine different animal models of surgically induced traumatic nerve or nervous system injury, including partial ligations of sciatic and saphenous nerves, spinal cord injury, spinal nerve ligation, and others (78). In humans, the results of a series of randomized, placebo-controlled clinical trials performed by regional branches of the University of California have demonstrated that inhaled cannabis holds therapeutic value in the treatment of neuropathic pain. Two studies examined neuropathic pain resulting from painful HIV sensory neuropathy (79,80). One examined neuropathic pain of varying causes, including HIV neuropathy, diabetic neuropathy, brachial plexus avulsion, and CRPS (81), while the other used an experimental model of neuropathic pain with heat and capsaicin tested in healthy volunteers (82). The largest study, by Abrams et al. (79), involved 55 patients with HIV-associated neuropathic pain who were randomized in a double-blind fashion to inhaled cannabis of up to three cannabis (3.56% THC) cigarettes daily for 5 days or placebo. Results showed that smoked cannabis relieved chronic neuropathic pain (34% reduction, $p = 0.03$), and more than 50% of patients experienced at least a 30% reduction in pain intensity ($p = 0.04$). Anxiety, sedation, disorientation, confusion, and dizziness occurred more often in cannabis recipients, but these effects were rated as between "none" and mild.

Overall, the three separate University of California clinical trials of inhaled cannabis for chronic neuropathic pain involved a total of 127 patients. The results from these studies have been convergent, with all demonstrating a significant decrease in pain after cannabis administration. The magnitude of effect in these studies, expressed as the number of patients needed to treat to produce one positive outcome, was comparable to current therapies. A recent outpatient randomized controlled trial of patients with chronic posttraumatic or post-surgical refractory neuropathic pain using inhaled cannabis conducted by researchers at McGill showed favorable results in concordance with the University of California studies (83).

Synthetic cannabinoids have also been studied in clinical trials. For example, in chronic neuropathic pain, 1′,1′-dimethylheptyl-Δ8-tetrahydrocannabinol-11-oic acid (CT-3), a THC-11-oic acid analog, at a dose of 40 mg/d, was shown to be more effective than placebo and without major unfavorable side effects. Twenty-one patients with chronic neuropathic pain were randomized to a double-blind, placebo-controlled, crossover trial. Three hours after the administration, the visual analog scale values of CT-3 differed significantly from those of the placebo ($p < 0.02$), whereas, after 8 hours, the differences between the two groups were less marked. Dry mouth and fatigue were the most common CT-3-related side effects ($p < 0.02$) (73).

Recently, a trial of a transmucosal *C. sativa* extract known as nabiximols was under investigation on advanced cancer patients in several countries. The study was specifically for breakthrough cancer pain syndromes on subjects who were started on a long-acting opioid for chronic cancer pain.

Preliminary results demonstrate that nabiximols in the dose range encompassed by the low and medium dose groups of this study has analgesic efficacy and is well tolerated. This suggests the optimum dose range for the next trial, the results of which should provide stronger evidence of analgesic efficacy, effect on opioid dose, adverse events, and potential impact on other outcomes that may improve the quality of life in advanced cancer (84). Confirmation of analgesic efficacy of cannabinoid medicines as adjunctive therapy for pain related to advanced cancer may provide an opportunity to address a significant clinical challenge in the future of cancer care.

In summary, neuropathic pain is an indication for which cannabinoids appear to have a stronger evidence base. However, most studies are of short trial duration and enrolled small sample sizes. High-quality trials of cannabinergic pain medicines, with large sample sizes, long-term exposure, including head-to-head trials with other analgesics, and focused on pain relief and functional outcomes, are needed to further characterize safety issues and efficacy with this class of medications.

Anti-inflammatory and Immunomodulatory Agents

Steroid therapy may be considered for severe inflammatory pain due to cancer-infiltrating structures such as the brachial or lumbosacral plexus, roots, or nerve trunks. Nonsteroidal anti-inflammatory drugs (NSAIDs), for example, cyclooxygenase (COX) type-1 and type-2 inhibitors, and acetaminophen have been of little benefit in the treatment of severe neuropathic pain. Several lines of evidence indicate that TNF-α, as well as other proinflammatory interleukins, may play a key role in the mechanism of pathologic intractable pain. Neutralizing antibodies to TNF-α and IL-1 receptor may become an important therapeutic approach for severe inflammatory pain resistant to NSAIDs, as well as for other forms of neuropathic inflammatory pain. Thalidomide has been shown to prevent hyperalgesia caused by nerve constriction injury in rats (80,85) and is known to inhibit TNF-α production. TNF-α antagonists or newly developed thalidomide analogs with a better safety profile may play a relevant role in the prevention and treatment of otherwise intractable painful disorders (86). Finally, inhibitors of microglia activation and nuclear factor-κB are being explored, and these lines of research may open new exciting treatment avenues.

Bisphosphonates (e.g., pamidronate and clodronate) have been reported to be efficacious in the treatment of not only bone cancer pain but also CRPS, a neuropathic inflammatory pain syndrome (87,88). The analgesic effect of bisphosphonate is poorly understood. It may be related to the inhibition and apoptosis of activated cells such as osteoclasts and macrophages. This leads to a decreased release of proinflammatory cytokines in the area of inflammation. In animal models of neuropathic pain (sciatic nerve ligature), bisphosphonates reduced the number of activated macrophages infiltrating the injured nerve, reduced Wallerian nerve fiber degeneration, and decreased experimental hyperalgesia (89).

GABA Agonists

Baclofen is an analog of the inhibitory neurotransmitter GABA and has a specific action on the GABA-B receptors. It has been used for many years as an effective spasmolytic agent. Baclofen also has shown effectiveness in the treatment of trigeminal neuralgia (38). Clinical experience supports the use of low-dose baclofen to potentiate the antineuralgic effect of carbamazepine in trigeminal neuralgia. Baclofen has also been used intrathecally to relieve intractable spasticity and may have a role as an adjuvant when added to spinal opioids for the treatment of intractable neuropathic pain and spasticity. The most common side effects of baclofen are drowsiness, weakness, hypotension, and confusion. It is important to note that discontinuation of baclofen always requires a slow tapering to avoid the occurrence of seizures and other severe neurologic manifestations.

Benzodiazepines (e.g., alprazolam, lorazepam, and diazepam) are GABA-A agonists. Their clinical use in patients with chronic pain is controversial. In a controlled trial, patients with PHN did worse when treated with lorazepam than with placebo or amitriptyline (90). Benzodiazepine-related side effects include depression and disruption of physiologic sleep. In combination with opioids, benzodiazepines cause significant cognitive impairment (42).

Invasive Interventions

Implantable devices, such as intrathecal pumps (IPs), have recently become available for the treatment of neuropathic pain that responds poorly to standard pharmacologic and conservative therapeutic modalities. Among the most commonly utilized implantable devices are spinal cord stimulators (SCSs) and IPs. SCSs have been used successfully in patients with severe limb pain that does not respond to conventional methods. IPs are used to deliver a variety of agents, such as opioids, clonidine, local anesthetics, ziconotide, and baclofen, into the cerebrospinal fluid. Clinical experience and several reports indicate that clonidine and/or local anesthetics administered intrathecally can potentiate opioid analgesia for neuropathic pain (12). Intrathecal morphine is currently the most commonly used analgesic administered by pump. However, before implantation of an intrathecal morphine pump, treatment trials must show that the patient's pain is somewhat responsive to opioids. Combination of intrathecal opioids and bupivacaine enhances the effectiveness of the analgesic regimen and reduces the need for ablative or neurolytic techniques for cancer pain, particularly for visceral and pelvic pain. Pumps can be implanted permanently once trials are successful.

Intraspinally implanted tunneled catheters are also being used for the administration of opioids and/or local anesthetics. Neuraxial analgesia through implanted tunneled catheters can be considered in patients with advanced oncologic disease and pain intractable to standard intervention. Intraspinally implanted tunneled catheters can provide a safe, reliable means of long-term administration of drugs into the epidural space. Utilization of bupivacaine in combination with opioids allows for enhanced pain relief in those patients with pain that is poorly responsive to opioid analgesics. Successful pain management through an intraspinal tunneled catheter system requires a careful education of the patient and caregiver, repeated follow-ups with pain assessment and monitoring of side effects, and close interaction between the patient, caregiver, pharmacist, home care nurse, and physician (91).

Motor cortex stimulation may relieve neuropathic pain. Many publications have corroborated this finding. The mechanism by which stimulation in this area relieves pain is unclear, but long-term results are encouraging. For some specific intractable neuropathic pain disorders, neuroablative procedures might be considered. For example, the dorsal root entry zone (DREZ) lesion has been recommended for the treatment of intractable pain from painful brachial plexopathy. DREZ can also be useful for relieving pain from head and neck cancer. The decision to perform neuroablative surgery should be made only after a thorough comprehensive assessment has been carried out by a multidisciplinary team of pain medicine specialists and after conservative management has failed to produce any improvement in the patient's quality of life. Cordotomy can be an effective treatment for unilateral pelvic and leg pain due to cancer. By sectioning the anterolateral quadrant of the spinal cord, interruption occurs in the spinothalamic tract with subsequent loss of contralateral pain and temperature sensation. The procedure can be done as a percutaneous radiofrequency ablation at C1-2 or through laminectomy. Cordotomy appears to be more effective in addressing intermittent shooting pain than steady burning pain. Unfortunately, the benefit tends to subside with time, and, therefore, its use in treating chronic pain receives little attention. Dorsal root rhizotomies may be beneficial for patients with chest wall pain. It has been hypothesized that malignancies may induce pain through somatic and visceral mechanisms. Midline myelotomy has been advocated as a way of treating visceral pain associated with cancer. Discrete midline myelotomies have also been performed in patients with abdominal/pelvic pain due to cancer and encouraging results have been reported (92).

BONE PAIN

Metastasis to bone is the most common cause of pain in patients with cancer (93). Bone pain is usually associated with direct tumor invasion of the bone and is often severe and debilitating. Tumors that metastasize to bone most commonly originate in the breast, lung, prostate, thyroid, and kidney; these may be blastic or lytic. Multiple myeloma causes painful bone lesions that are lytic. More than two-thirds of patients with radiographically detectable lesions will experience bone pain, although many patients experience pain even before skeletal metastases become radiographically apparent.

Immunohistochemical studies have revealed an extensive network of nerve fibers in the vicinity of and within the skeleton, not only in the periosteum but also in the cortical and trabecular bone, as well as in the bone marrow (11). Thinly myelinated and unmyelinated peptidergic sensory fibers, as well as sympathetic fibers, occur throughout the bone marrow, mineralized bone, and periosteum. Although the periosteum is the most densely innervated tissue, when the total volume of each tissue is considered, the bone marrow receives the greatest total number of sensory nerve fibers (94). These sensory fibers express multiple signaling molecules, including neuropeptides and neurotrophins. The presence of receptors for some neuropeptides (e.g., calcitonin gene–related peptide and substance P) on osteoclasts and osteoblasts and the capacity of these receptors to regulate osteoclast formation and bone formation and resorption have recently been described. Because NGF has been shown to modulate inflammatory neuropathic pain states, in most recent animal models of cancer bone pain, NGF antibody antagonist therapy has also been shown to produce significant reduction in both ongoing and movement-related pain behavior. This treatment was more effective than morphine (14).

It is believed that skeletal lesions result, at least in part, from a disruption of the normal balance between bone formation and bone resorption. In the process, bone nociceptors respond to changes in the bone marrow, as well as cortical, trabecular, and periosteum microenvironments. Inflammatory, immunologic, and neuropathic mechanisms develop in the bone in response to the cancer insult and the patient experiences pain. As osteolysis continues, the bone integrity declines and patients become vulnerable to other complications, including pathologic fractures, nerve compression syndromes, spinal instability, and hypercalcemia.

Although the mechanisms by which these neurochemical pathways cause bone pain are still not completely understood, the prospective for a better understanding of bone pain is thought to be provoking and exciting (95). Moreover, the progress in this field will promote the development of newer and more targeted therapies for pathologic pain.

Clinical Findings and Diagnosis

Pain is commonly the presenting symptom of bone metastases, and the presence of focal pain in a patient with cancer should trigger an investigation. Patients may experience a deep powerful throbbing pain punctuated by sharper intense pain, often triggered by movement (incident or breakthrough pain). On examination, there may also be focal tenderness and swelling at the affected sites. Range of motion is usually severely limited, especially if the joint space is involved. In many patients, normal activities such as deep breathing, coughing, or moving an affected limb can cause intense, often unbearable, pain. Pain may be localized or referred to various sites. Bone pain due to metastases must be differentiated from other bone pain syndromes that are caused by non-neoplastic conditions such as osteoarthritis, osteoporotic fractures, and osteomalacia.

Accurate history and physical examination are the first step in diagnosing bone metastases. Clinicians must remember that pain is generally underassessed. The assessment of pain intensity should rely on the patient's own report of pain.

Many different pain scales have been developed, including numeric (0 to 10) and pictorial scales, among others. The specific pain scale used is less important than using the same scale consistently.

Bone pain may be focal, multifocal, or generalized. Multifocal pain is commonly experienced by patients with multiple sites of bony metastases. Approximately 25% of patients with bone metastases do not complain of pain. Additionally, a patient with multiple sites of osseous metastases may only have a few painful sites (96,97). There is a well-described generalized bone pain syndrome that occurs when there is replacement of bone marrow by tumor. This is observed with myeloproliferative malignancies and less commonly with solid tumors (98).

The vertebral bodies are the most common sites of osseous metastases; more than two-thirds of vertebral metastases are found in the thoracic spine, because there is a valveless plexus of epidural veins called the *Batson's plexus* in which blood flows rostrally or caudally. This may serve as a route for the metastatic spread of some cancers. The lumbosacral and cervical spine account for approximately 20% and 10% of bone metastases, respectively. Additionally, 85% of patients have multiple-level involvement. Early recognition of pain syndromes of the vertebral bodies is essential because the pain serves as an indicator that compression of adjacent neural structures could be imminent and that neurologic compromise, that is, spinal cord compression, could ensue (99,100). MRI is the best diagnostic tool that can be used, given its best accuracy of extent of disease; clinically, CT can also be diagnostic. Plain films reveal a "moth-eaten" appearance of a bone that has lytic bone metastases. However, plain films and bone scans (scintigraphy) should only be regarded as adjuncts to the former tests.

Occipital pain can indicate the destruction of the atlas or fracture of the odontoid process and the pain can radiate over the posterior aspect of the skull. This can result in a pathologic fracture and subsequent spinal cord compression at the cervicomedullary junction (99).

Bone metastases at the level of C7-T1 vertebral bodies can cause a pain referral pattern at the infrascapular area, with upper back pain and muscle spasm (100). When T12 or L1 is affected by bone metastases, the referral pattern can often be at the iliac crest or sacroiliac joint; imaging could miss the metastases if it is directed at the pelvis. Sacral syndrome can develop from bone metastases, and referred and/or radiating pain can arise in the buttock, posterior thigh, or perineum (101,102). In addition to this skeletal component, involvement of adjacent structures, such as nerves or muscles, may produce other types of pain. Involvement of adjacent nerve tissue of the peripheral system, such as the lumbar plexus, or central system, such as the spinal cord, can produce not only worrying neurologic deficits but also neuropathic pain syndromes. Many times, epidural disease is the first sign of malignancy in a community setting. Severe back pain is the initial symptom in almost all patients who present with epidural compression. Back pain precedes epidural compression for a prolonged period. Clinically, there is a rapid and crescendo type of pain with epidural disease, and there may or may not be a lancinating quality to the pain or a band-like tightness that wraps around the chest or abdomen. If epidural disease is not diagnosed and treated in a timely manner, paraplegia or quadriplegia may occur. Large lytic metastases present with localized severe pain in the affected bone. The risk of fracture is high; Fidler reported a fracture incidence of 3.7% when 25% to 50% of the cortex was involved, 61% when the degree of cortical involvement ranged between 50% and 75%, and 79% when >75% of the cortex was involved (102,103). Although any tumor can metastasize to the bone and result in a pathologic fracture, mammary carcinoma is responsible for 50% of such fractures. Multiple myeloma is the second most common cancer to cause pathologic fractures.

In any patient with cancer, the development of an unexplained focal pain should trigger an investigation into the cause, should the goals of care allow it. Clinicians should keep in mind that pain may be referred in numerous patterns, for example, involvement of the hip may refer the pain to the knee or the groin. Plain radiography, CT, MRI, and bone scintigraphy are all measures to image metastatic lesions. In many cases, plain radiography will be adequate in identifying skeletal lesions. MRI is more sensitive at detecting very early skeletal metastases. CT scanning is also more sensitive than plain films and is often used for patients who cannot tolerate or are not candidates for MRI. Bone scintigraphy is more useful when identifying the extent of bone lesions throughout the body.

Therapeutic Interventions for Bone Pain

There are numerous options for the treatment of pain related to bone metastases, including opioid therapy, specific pharmacotherapy, radiotherapy, systemic radionuclide therapy, and surgery (Table 1.4). With the skillful and compassionate use of these measures, even patients with severe pain can expect to achieve adequate relief.

Anti-inflammatory Drugs

Corticosteroids. Steroid therapy may be considered for severe inflammatory pain, especially when bone cancer infiltrates or compresses adjacent nerve tissue structures, such as the brachial or lumbosacral plexi, roots or nerve trunks, or spinal cord. High-dose steroids are used in epidural disease for pain control and for decompression while definitive treatment is planned (104,105). High-dose steroids are also necessary for patients with increased intracranial pressure secondary to a mass effect of intracranial tumors that are primary or metastatic.

Nonsteroidal Anti-inflammatory Drugs. NSAIDs, for example, COX type-1 and type-2 inhibitors, and acetaminophen are commonly used in the treatment of mild to moderate pain evolving from inflammation. NSAIDs share a common mechanism of action, which is the inhibition of COX and, therefore, prostaglandin (PG) production. PGs play

TABLE 1.4	Therapeutic interventions for bone pain		
	Denosumab	**Zoledronic Acid**	**Pamidronate**
Agent class	- Fully human monoclonal antibody to RANKL	- Nitrogen-containing bisphosphonate	- Nitrogen-containing bisphosphonate
Indications	- Prevention of SREs from bone metastases due to solid tumors	- Bone metastases from solid tumors, MM, and HCM - For prostate cancer with progression after ≥1 previous hormonal therapy	- Bone metastases in solid tumors, MM, and HCM
Dosing and administration	- 120 mg s.c. every 4 wk	- 4 mg i.v. every 3–4 wk. - HCM 4 mg, potential for retreatment if inadequate response (allow minimum of 7 d between treatments)	- Bone metastases, 90 mg i.v. over 4 h every 4 wk - HCM, 60–90 mg i.v. as single dose over 2–24 h
Adverse events	- Fatigue/asthenia, hypophosphatemia, nausea, dyspnea, hypocalcemia, and ONJ	- Fatigue, nausea, bone pain and myalgias, fever, hypocalcemia, subtrochanteric fracture, ONJ, and renal toxicity	- Monitor serum calcium, phosphate, magnesium, and potassium levels in patients with HCM; transient fever; renal toxicity; ONJ; and musculoskeletal symptoms
Safety information	- Can cause severe hypocalcemia; calcium levels lower if CrCl < 30 mL/min - Calcium and vitamin D supplementation recommended - ONJ rate 2.2% in clinical trials; oral exam recommended before starting therapy; avoid invasive dental procedures during therapy	- Due to potential renal toxicity, must obtain baseline CrCl; ZA dose based on CrCl and serum creatinine - Measure serum creatinine level before each dose; withhold treatment for renal deterioration - Calcium and vitamin D supplementation recommended - ONJ rate 1.3% in clinical trials; oral exam recommended before starting therapy; avoid invasive dental procedures during therapy	- Due to potential renal toxicity, assess baseline and subsequent serum creatinine levels before treatment - Oral exam recommended before starting therapy; avoid invasive dental procedures during therapy - Calcium and vitamin D supplementation recommended - Closely monitor patients with preexisting anemia, leukopenia, or thrombocytopenia for first 2 wk after treatment
FDA approval date	-2010: bone metastases -Not approved for HCM or MM	-2001: HCM -2002: broad bone metastases including MM	-1991: HCM -1995: MM and breast cancer

MM, multiple myeloma; ONJ, osteo necrosis of the jaw; HCM, hypercalcemia of malignancy; SRE, skeletal related events; RANKL, Rank Ligand.

important roles in a variety of tissues. For example, PGs, specifically PGE_2 and PGI_2, are responsible for maintaining renal perfusion in patients with compromised kidney function. PGs also act to protect the gastric mucosa and initiate platelet aggregation. Furthermore, PGs function to generate pain by stimulating peripheral sensory neurons during inflammation. The mechanism of action of NSAIDs has been further elucidated by the discovery of two distinct isoforms of COX (COX-1 and COX-2). COX-1 is the constitutive isoform present in, for example, the stomach, kidney, and platelets, and its inhibition is responsible for producing the common side effects of NSAIDs. Conversely, the inducible isoform, COX-2, usually becomes expressed in cells after being activated by proinflammatory cytokines. COX-1 and COX-2 inhibition results in both the adverse and beneficial effects of the NSAIDs. The anti-inflammatory and analgesic effects of the NSAIDs are generally considered equal when comparing agents within the class. However, the frequency with which they produce side effects varies greatly. Caution must be exercised when using NSAIDs in patients with hypertension, impaired renal function, or heart failure. A well-known benefit of the COX-2 inhibitors and acetaminophen is their gastrointestinal safety. However, highly specific COX-2 inhibitors are not void of adverse effects, in particular, the vascular prothrombotic effect. Acetaminophen has a dose-dependent hepatotoxic effect (not to be used at a dose higher than 4 g/d). With the large number of COX inhibitors being available, one must consider the patient's history of response and the efficacy, safety, and cost effectiveness of the agent to be prescribed.

Bone Metabolism Modulators

Bisphosphonates. Some of the most important drugs that have emerged in the battle against bone pain are the bisphosphonates, the synthetic analogs of pyrophosphate that bind hydroxyapatite crystals of the bone with a high affinity. They reduce resorption of bone by inhibiting osteoclastic activity and osteolysis. Bisphosphonate therapy has proved to be highly valuable in the management of numerous bone-related conditions, including hypercalcemia, osteoporosis, multiple myeloma, and Paget's disease. Earlier bisphosphonates, such as etidronate, have been largely replaced by second-generation bisphosphonates, including pamidronate, as well as third-generation bisphosphonates, including zoledronic acid and ibandronate. Multiple studies have demonstrated the efficacy of second- and third-generation bisphosphonates in reducing pain in bone metastases (106–108). Zoledronic acid significantly reduces the overall risk of developing a skeletal-related pathologic event in patients with bone metastasis by an additional 20% in comparison with pamidronate and significantly improves pain and quality of life (109). Ibandronate has been shown to provide significant and sustained relief from metastatic bone pain, improving patient functioning and quality of life. The oral and intravenous formulations of ibandronate appear to have comparable efficacy (110). With a favorable long-term safety profile and the added convenience and flexibility offered by its efficacious oral formulation, ibandronate represents a new therapeutic option for metastatic bone disease management. Recently, a conjugated bisphosphonate, rhenium 186–labeled MAG3-bisphosphonate (^{186}Re-MAG3-HBP), has been developed as a bifunctional radiopharmaceutical (see subsequent text) for the palliation of metastatic bone pain (111). This conjugated form is stable and is expected to be a valuable tool for the palliation of bone pain in the future. However, further research on this drug is necessary.

Rank Ligand Inhibition. Rank ligand is a protein that stimulates osteoclasts, the cells that resorb bone, in patients with metastatic bone disease. Increased Rank ligand helps drive a vicious cycle of bone destruction, which can lead to devastating skeletal-related events. (112) Rank ligand inhibitor denosumab is used for solid tumor bone metastases, with the exclusion of multiple myeloma. This medication is recently available for the treatment of bone metastases. If skeletal-related events are decreased, it is then thought that there may be less pain from pathologic fracture or impending fracture. One large study in *Lancet*, November 2011, enrolled 1,432 subjects who had hormone-resistant prostate cancer. The patients received either placebo or denosumab. During the 2-year study, it was evident that treatment with denosumab had delayed symptoms of metastases, extended the time to the first bone metastases, and increased bone metastasis-free survival by an average of more than 4 months (113,114). However, there was no survival difference between the two groups.

The most common adverse reaction was dyspnea, and the most common reason for stopping this medication was osteoradionecrosis and hypocalcemia. (112).

Calcitonin. Calcitonin may have several pain-related indications in patients who have bone pain, including osseous metastases. The most frequent routes of absorption are intranasal and subcutaneous injection. Calcitonin reduces resorption of bone by inhibiting osteoclastic activity and osteolysis (112).

Radiotherapy

Radiation therapy is a valuable tool in managing pain from bone metastases. Based on the evaluation of pain by the physician, partial pain relief with radiotherapy is seen in 80% to 90% of patients and complete pain relief in 50% of patients. Using patient evaluation, between 60% and 80% of patients with bone metastases will experience a substantial pain reduction after irradiation of the affected area with complete pain relief seen in 15% to 40% of patients. Response to radiation treatment, as well as duration of response, is dependent on a variety of factors, including the primary tumor, histology, type of lesion, location of metastases, number of sites treated, the pain level prior to radiation therapy, and the radiation fractionation scheme utilized.

The radiation treatment process itself is relatively quick and the treatment painless. Setup time in general is several minutes in duration and the actual beam on time likewise only a few minutes long per anatomical site being treated. The additive use of bisphosphonates to radiotherapy may also improve the palliative effects of radiation as well as bone healing outcome. Pain scores have been shown to be diminished and decreased use of opioid pain medication has been seen with the combined use of bisphosphonates and external beam radiotherapy. Bone density in the metastatic treatment area has been shown to increase and in select patients complete radiographic responses have been seen.

For a few discrete areas of painful bony metastases, local-field external beam radiation therapy is typically used. Radiation therapy can be delivered with a variety of fractionation schemes. The first large randomized study evaluating the different dose and fractionation schemes was the Radiation Therapy Oncology Group (RTOG) 74-02 trial

(113). Patients with multiple painful bony metastases were treated in 1 of 4 schedules: 30 Gy in 10 fractions, 15 Gy in 5 fractions, 20 Gy in 5 fractions, or 25 Gy in 5 fractions. Patients with solitary bone metastases were randomized to 40.5 Gy in 15 fractions versus 20 Gy in 5 fractions. After initial analysis and with adjustment in response definition, analysis revealed a significant difference in response in favor of the longer treatment fractionation regimens: 30 Gy in 10 fractions for multiple metastases and 40.5 Gy in 15 fractions for the solitary metastases. There have been multiple, randomized prospective trials evaluating various radiation doses and fractionation schemes (136–139,142,143). The earlier studies focused on different multifraction treatment schemes (113–116). In these studies, no significant difference was seen between the course durations.

Several randomized studies have also evaluated single radiation therapy doses for palliation of bone metastases, with randomization of 4 versus 8 Gy (117) and 4 versus 6 versus 8 Gy (118). In both of these trials, the higher dose arm (8 Gy) was superior to 4 Gy. In the more recent subsequent trials that have used a multiple fraction treatment regimen as the control arm, single doses of 8 or 10 Gy are used as the study arm (137,139,142,143).

There have been two large recent studies examining the comparison between a single-dose treatment and longer multifractionated radiation treatment. In the Dutch trial (119), 1,171 patients with bone metastases from solid tumors (primarily breast [39%], prostate [23%], and lung [25%]) were randomized to 8 Gy in single fractions versus 24 Gy in 6 fractions; 53% of patients received systemic therapy and approximately half of the patients received narcotic pain management prior to randomization. There was no difference in median survival after treatment (30 weeks) between the two groups. No difference in overall response rate or complete response rates was seen between the single-dose arm and the longer course treatment arms, with 71% of patients achieving a response to therapy and 35% achieving a complete response at follow-up. The majority of responses were seen within the first 4 to 6 weeks following therapy, with higher complete response rates for patients with breast and prostate cancers (44% and 41%, respectively) compared with lung and other primary sites (21% and 16%, respectively). There were significant differences noted between the two treatment groups. The rate of retreatment was significantly higher in the single treatment group. Patients who received 24 Gy in 6 fractions had a retreatment rate of 7%, while the 8-Gy single fraction group received a second course of treatment 25% of the time, with evidence suggestive of a willingness to re-irradiate after a single dose or increased reluctance to re-irradiate after a higher initial dose of radiation treatment. A significant difference was also observed in the rate of pathologic fracture between the two treatment arms, although the rates were low. The rate of pathologic fracture in the initially treated area was higher for the single fraction group: 4% for the 8-Gy single treatment arm versus 2% for the 24 Gy in 6 fractions arm. The median time to fracture was similar between the two groups, at 21 and 17 weeks.

The second large study comparing single dose versus longer course treatment was RTOG 9714 (120). This study included patients with painful bony metastases from breast or prostate primary sites and with up to three painful sites permissible. At study entry, more than 70% of patients had severe pain (pain scores of 7 to 10) based on the BPI 11-point scale system. Randomization was to a single fraction of 8 Gy versus 30 Gy in 10 treatments. At 3-month follow-up, there were no significant differences in complete response rates (17%) and partial response rates (49%) between the two treatment arms. Similar to the Dutch trial, retreatment rates were higher in the single fraction (8 Gy) treatment arm compared with 9% in the 30 Gy in 10 fractions group. There were no significant differences noted in stability rates (26% vs. 24%), progressive pain scores (9% vs. 10%), and rates of narcotic usage. Overall toxicity rates were low. Unlike the Dutch trial, there was no significant difference in the rate of pathologic fractures between the treatment groups; 5% for the single-arm group and 4% for the multifraction group. Further subgroup analysis suggested that social support factors may significantly impact on the retreatment for painful bone metastases, especially with declining health status (121). In this analysis, married men and single and married women were more likely to receive retreatment after single fraction treatment versus 30 Gy in 10 fractions, and no difference was noted in retreatment rates in single men. The authors concluded that such subgroups of patients may benefit from the longer multifractionated radiation treatment course.

These comparisons have demonstrated that single-dose treatments of 8 Gy provide similar pain relief to those of longer treatment regimens of 30 Gy in 10 fractions, 20 Gy in 5 fractions, or 24 Gy in 8 fractions (122). Also impacting on a patient's level of palliation is sustainability of pain relief. After a short course of radiotherapy, retreatment rates are higher, sometimes by a factor of 2 or 3. When pretreatment pain scores are initially reported as mild or minor (i.e., lower than moderate or severe), response rates with radiotherapy are typically better than seen with higher pain scores. Furthermore, these studies have concluded that there is no consistent dose–response relationship seen. What this suggests is that the mechanism of acute pain relief from radiotherapy is more likely to be related to a change in the regional environment causing osteoclastic bone resorption activation rather than to a reduction in overall tumor burden. Pain relief by this mechanism may therefore account for the higher retreatment rates seen after the delivery of a single dose of 8 Gy compared with 30 Gy in 10 fractions because of an expected lower cell kill with the former approach. For patients with a good performance status and longer life expectancy, there exists a greater proclivity for tumor regrowth, leading to osteoclast activation. On the other hand, for patients with a poor performance status, shorter life expectancy, extensive nonosseous metastases, and limited access to radiation facilities, a single 8-Gy fraction may be the most appropriate treatment option. It is important to note that a single high-dose fraction of radiation treatment may cause a paradoxical flare-type reaction with a temporary increase in pain at the treatment site, which may be diminished by the use of nonsteroidal anti-inflammatory medications or corticosteroids.

The role of radiation therapy is most appropriate in patients with single or few osseous metastases. For patients with widespread metastatic disease, hemibody radiation therapy and intravenous radiopharmaceuticals have been used with effective palliative response.

Radiopharmaceuticals

Pain palliation with bone-seeking radiopharmaceuticals has proved to be an effective treatment modality in patients with metastatic bone pain. Bone-seeking radiopharmaceuticals are extremely powerful in treating scattered painful bone metastases, for which external beam radiotherapy is impossible because of the large field of irradiation (123,124). Generally, the effectiveness of radioisotopes is satisfactory, but it can be greater when they are combined with chemotherapeutic agents such as cisplatin. The most common and major safety concern related to the adverse effects from radiopharmaceuticals is bone marrow toxicity. These medications are not used as readily as they were in the past for reasons of toxicity, they are worth a mention; however, other modalities mentioned in this chapter are standard of care.

Strontium 89, Samarium 153 (^{89}Sr, ^{153}Sm). The radioisotopes ^{89}Sr and ^{153}Sm have been used for the palliation of pain from metastatic bone cancer. Repeated doses are effective in providing pain relief in many patients, with response rates between 40% and 95%. Pain relief usually starts 1 to 4 weeks after the initiation of treatment, continues for up to 18 months, and is associated with a reduction in analgesic use in many patients. Thrombocytopenia and neutropenia are the most common toxic effects, but they are generally mild and reversible. Some studies with ^{89}Sr and ^{153}Sm indicate a reduction of hot spots on bone scans in up to 70% of patients and suggest a possible tumoricidal action (123).

Samarium-153 Ethylene Diamine Tetramethylene Phosphonate. ^{153}Sm-ethylene diamine tetramethylene phosphonate (^{153}Sm-EDTMP) is a widely available and extensively tested radiopharmaceutical for systemic therapy in patients with multiple skeletal metastases. Its use is approved for any secondary bone lesion that has been shown to accumulate the traditional marker in bone scans, that is, technetium Tc 99 m-methylene diphosphonate (Tc 99 m-MDP). The short half-life, the relatively low-energy β-emissions, and the γ-emissions make the ^{153}Sm an attractive radionuclide, allowing therapeutic delivery of short-range electrons at relatively high dose (125).

Rhenium-186 Hydroxyethylidene Diphosphonate. Rhenium-186 hydroxyethylidene diphosphonate (^{186}Re-HEDP) is a potentially useful radiopharmaceutical agent for the palliation of bone pain, having numerous advantageous characteristics. Bone marrow toxicity is limited and reversible, which makes repetitive treatment safer. Studies using ^{186}Re-HEDP have shown encouraging clinical results of palliative therapy, with an overall response rate of about 70% in painful bone metastases (120). It is effective for fast palliation of painful bone metastases from various tumors, and the effect tends to last longer if patients are treated early in the course of their disease. It is preferred to radiopharmaceuticals with a long half-life in patients who have been pretreated with bone marrow–suppressive chemotherapy.

Surgery

In general, patients with only skeletal metastases have a longer survival than those with visceral metastases. When weighing the risks and benefits of surgery, it is critical to assess the patient's ability to tolerate the procedure. In patients for whom the prognosis is less than a month, surgery is rarely indicated. Patients with cardiopulmonary disease (even unrelated to the cancer) should have a thorough operative assessment. Orthopedic stabilization of the affected skeletal segment can be helpful for patients with large lytic lesions who are at risk for fracture and can improve the overall quality of life for many patients. However, it should not be used as a substitute for dedicated and effective pain management. Vertebroplasty and kyphoplasty are relatively new techniques that may be efficacious in treating painful vertebral metastasis. These techniques are currently used to treat vertebral compression fractures due to osteoporosis or painful hemangiomas. Vertebroplasty is the injection of bone cement, generally poly (methyl methacrylate), into a vertebral body. Kyphoplasty is the placement of a balloon into the vertebral body, followed by an inflation/deflation sequence to create a cavity before the cement injection. These procedures are most often performed in a percutaneous manner on an outpatient or short-stay basis. The risks associated with the procedures are low, but serious complications, such as spinal cord compression, nerve root compression, venous embolism, and pulmonary embolism, including cardiovascular collapse, may occur (126).

VISCERAL PAIN

Visceral pain is common in patients with cancer and becomes evident during cancer infiltration, compression, distention, or stretching of thoracic and/or abdominal viscera. It may be an early or late manifestation of cancer. Visceral nociceptors are activated by noxious stimuli, including inflammation of the mucosa and omentum and stretching of hollow viscera, as well as organ capsule. Visceral pain is generally diffuse and caused by obstructive syndromes due to tumor involvement of the organ or the organ capsule. Pain can be caused by a primary tumor or metastatic disease to an organ.

Clinical Findings and Diagnosis

Visceral pain may be described as dull, squeezing, colicky, sharp, and deep aching, intermittent or continuous, and can often be perceived as generalized lassitude. Visceral pain is poorly localized and can be accompanied by other symptoms such as nausea, fatigue, and diaphoresis. It may frequently be referred to cutaneous areas overlying or adjacent to the affected structure; referral patterns may vary and actually be distant from the underlying malignancy. The clinician must be knowledgeable about the pain referral patterns to treat the syndrome with precision. An example might be an aching and gnawing right shoulder pain; this may indicate the presence of hepatic metastases or diaphragmatic irritation (127,128). Pancreatic and endometrial cancers may manifest as back pain. Pain from prostate cancer may appear in the abdomen or lower extremities. Hepatic capsular pain may occur with a primary hepatocellular carcinoma or, more commonly, with liver metastases. The inflammation caused by the disease may result in capsular stretching and produce pain, which is dull and aching in the right subcostal region. Movement may exacerbate the pain; deep breaths cause right diaphragmatic irritation. The treatment for this syndrome is analgesic doses of corticosteroids given in divided dose and opioid analgesics (129,130). Retroperitoneal pain syndrome is most common in pancreatic cancer and retroperitoneal lymphadenopathy. The pain is exacerbated on recumbency and alleviated with forward flexion. The pain is dull, diffuse, and poorly localized. This type of pain should be differentiated from epidural metastasis, and a careful examination and appropriate imaging can confirm the diagnosis. Intestinal obstruction can be the result of gastrointestinal tumor, adhesions, and intra-abdominal or pelvic space-occupying lesions. The pain is characterized as colicky. It is usually associated with nausea and/or vomiting, anorexia, and bloating. Another cause of this syndrome can be an atonic bowel due to ischemia, autonomic denervation, or primary cancer therapies including radiotherapy. Visceral carcinomatosis can cause pain because of multiple mechanisms: peritoneal inflammation, malignant adhesions, and ascites. Tense ascites produce discomfort from abdominal wall stretching and can also manifest as low back pain. Pelvic and perineal pain can occur in malignancies that arise in the pelvis, including colorectal and genitourinary tumors. The tumor invades the pelvic floor and is frequently both nociceptive and neuropathic pain. Occasionally, patients experience painful spasms in the rectum, bladder, or urethra. The visceral component of this pain syndrome can be marked by tenesmus.

Therapeutic Interventions for Visceral Pain

Treatment includes a wide range of modalities, including opioid analgesics (which should be considered for visceral organ pain), steroids, anticholinergics, octreotide (which relieves bowel obstructive symptoms by decreasing gastric secretions) (131,132), and adjuvant analgesics given for the neuropathic component.

The pharmacologic treatments for painful spasms are many; the standard treatment may be the anticholinergic medications. Donnatal, which is a combination of atropine, phenobarbital, scopolamine, and hyoscyamine given by mouth three to four times daily, is an old preparation that is still used for spasms or colicky pain. The anticholinergic medication hyoscyamine has been used as a single agent to treat gastrointestinal spasms at the usual dose of 0.125 mg, 1 to 2 tablets every 4 hours as needed. The old antispasmodic combination of chlordiazepoxide (a benzodiazepine) and clidinium (an anticholinergic), Librax, has also been used to relieve intestinal spasms or cramps.

There are other anticholinergic medications such as propantheline and glycopyrrolate used for much of the same purpose; however, as with all the drugs in this class, the side effects may limit their use excessively. The anticholinergic drugs can be used for bladder spasm due to overactive bladder pathology. Side effects can include mucous membrane dryness, dizziness, gastrointestinal sluggishness, constipation, and, rarely, obstructive symptom.

Steroids are one of the most common medications used for visceral pain syndromes; a dose of 16 mg of dexamethasone followed by 4 mg every 6 hours is standard for relieving capsular pain syndromes.

Opioids through IPs or tunneled intraspinal catheter systems, neurolytic blockades, neuroablative procedures, and palliative surgery, i.e., bowel resection, percutaneous endoscopic gastrostomy tube inserted for the purpose of nutrition, paracentesis, and palliative ostomies, might be an option to relieve the pain associated with the physical obstruction. There are studies underway evaluating the use of peripheral opioid antagonists in the treatment of severe constipation; however, exclusion criteria would include frank obstruction.

Neurolytic Blockade for Visceral Pain

Neurolytic blockade can be efficacious for visceral-related pain in cancer; however, it is usually reserved for patients with a limited prognosis and well-localized pain syndromes. Nerve blocks that are specifically for visceral pain lack durability and have an analgesic benefit of 6 months or less in some cases. Neurolytic blocks are primarily viewed as adjuvant therapy and not as replacing systemic pharmacotherapy for cancer pain. Alcohol and phenol are the most widely used agents (133,134).

Intrapleural phenol block has been reported to be helpful in managing visceral pain associated with esophageal cancer (135). Certain types of thoracic pain from invasion of the chest wall secondary to a pleural tumor may respond to intercostal neurolytic blocks or paravertebral blockade.

Neurolytic block of the celiac plexus is well described in the literature and has proven efficacy in patients with pancreatic cancer and epigastric and/or back pain. Celiac plexus block has also been used successfully in treating visceral pain from upper abdominal malignancies. In one prospective randomized trial of patients with pancreatic cancer, the pain relief provided by a neurolytic celiac plexus block was equal to that provided by systemic opioids with fewer side effects. (137,137). Data also support the use of intraoperative neurolytic blockade of the celiac plexus for unresectable pancreatic tumor (138,139). *Neurolysis of the superior hypogastric plexus* has been used for the treatment of visceral pain from cancer of the lower abdomen and pelvis, including gynecologic, colorectal, and genitourinary malignancies. However, some of these cancers may have a significant retroperitoneal

TABLE 1.5	Adjuvant medications for visceral cancer pain	
Drug	**Usual Dose**	**Indications**
Octreotide	Octreotide 100–600 mg/d via s.c. bolus or infusion	Useful for secretory diarrhea and malignant bowel obstruction
Calcium channel blockers	Diltiazem	
Scopolamine	0.8–2 mg/d s.c. 1.5–3 mg/g 3 d transdermally	

pain component, which may lead to poor results with this type of neurolysis. Reportedly, the procedure seems to carry minimal risks in terms of complications (140). *Neurolysis of the ganglion impar* is used for intractable rectal and perineal pain in patients who often suffer from urgency. The ganglion is located at the sacrococcygeal junction. There are limited published data on this procedure. *Intrathecal neurolytic blockade* might be indicated for patients with advanced or terminal malignancy, with intractable, unilateral pain affecting only a few dermatomes (preferably of the thoracic region). The most common complications of intrathecal neurolysis are persistent pain, limb weakness, and urinary and rectal dysfunction.

Epidural neurolytic blockade can be performed by the insertion of a catheter, so that multiple repeated injections can be administered. Epidural neurolysis has been used successfully for unilateral or bilateral pain of thoracic and abdominal visceral origin. It has been described as a procedure safer than intrathecal neurolysis. The duration of analgesia may vary from 1 to 3 months (141).

ANALGESIC ALGORITHMS

The management of severe neuropathic, bone, and visceral cancer pain often represents a difficult treatment challenge. Combination of therapies employing medications from a variety of pharmacologic classes and, at times, procedures corresponds to the contemporary standard approach. Specific agents can be used as treatment trials and courses can be escalated according to the proposed analgesic algorithms for neuropathic, bone, and visceral cancer pain described in Tables 1.2, 1.4, and 1.5, respectively. The number and variety of options can be confusing and intimidating, even for physicians specializing in the treatment of pain. Dose titration is an important principle to be familiar with when using analgesics, in particular, opioids, AEDs, and antidepressants. Physicians must know how to titrate the dose appropriately while assessing the pain and recognizing and managing drug-related side effects. Patients suffering from difficult cancer pain syndromes need to have treatment plans tailored to their individual problems. As patients become less

functional, a more aggressive intervention based on titration and combination therapy will be necessary. The treating physician needs to balance efficacy, safety, and tolerability of several drugs, often used on an "off-label" basis. Moreover, the physician who wishes to utilize the analgesic algorithms should

1. know how to assess the quality and features of the pain,
2. determine the predominant mechanism(s) underlying the difficult cancer pain syndrome,
3. understand the pharmacology of the analgesics and the indications for the procedures, and
4. recognize and manage side effects of medications and procedure-related adverse events.

CONCLUSION

Difficult and refractory cancer pain syndromes are challenging pain states to treat. Advances are being made in the comprehension of the various mechanisms underlying neuropathic, bone, and visceral pain. If a patient presents with a difficult cancer pain syndrome, a more comprehensive pain assessment and a much more aggressive intervention are going to be needed. Therapeutic interventions can be employed in an escalating regimen to counteract the intensity and the disabling nature of the patient's difficult cancer pain syndrome. Patients suffering from these disorders need to have treatment plans tailored to their individual problems. The employment of agents from a variety of pharmacologic classes represents a contemporary standard approach to pain management. At present, the management of the difficult cancer pain syndrome calls for a balanced combination of therapies that will include analgesic medications, adjuvants, and procedures. What has proven to be very useful is the expanding field of pain medicine and palliative care that has identified cancer pain syndromes as well as other symptoms that are bothersome to cancer patients either receiving active anticancer treatment or are hospice appropriate. Along the trajectory of cancer care there are best practices employed to overall better the quality of life of this patient population.

ACKNOWLEDGMENT

We wish to acknowledge Jason Georgekutty, DO, our Research Fellow in the Department of Pain and Palliative Medicine, who helped with table organization and proofreading.

REFERENCES

1. Merskey H, Bogduk N, eds. *Classification of Chronic Pain*. 2nd ed. *IASP Task Force on Taxonomy*. Seattle, WA: IASP Press; 1994:209-214.

2. Pappagallo M. Peripheral neuropathic pain. In: Pappagallo M, ed. *The Neurological Basis of Pain*. New York , NY: McGraw-Hill; 2005:321-341.

3. Allan SM, Tyrrell PJ, Rothwell NJ. Interleukin-1 and neuronal injury. *Nat Rev Immunol*. 2005;5:629-640.

4. Empl M, Renaud S, Erne B, et al. TNF-alpha expression in painful and nonpainful neuropathies. *Neurology* 2001;56:1371-1377.

5. Lindenlaub T, Sommer C. Cytokines in sural nerve biopsies from inflammatory and non-inflammatory neuropathies. *Acta Neuropathol (Berl)*. 2003;105:593-602.

6. Schafers M, Lee DH, Brors D, et al. Increased sensitivity of injured and adjacent uninjured rat primary sensory neurons to exogenous tumor necrosis factor-alpha after spinal nerve ligation. *J Neurosci*. 2003;23:3028-3038.

7. Raja SN, Turnquist JL, Meleka S, et al. Monitoring adequacy of alpha-adrenoceptor blockade following systemic phentolamine administration. *Pain*. 1996;64(1):197-204.

8. Ali Z, Raja SN, Wesselmann U, et al. Intradermal injection of norepinephrine evokes pain in patients with sympathetically maintained pain. *Pain*. 2000;88:161-168.

9. Scholz J, Woolf CJ. Mechanisms of neuropathic pain. In: Pappagallo M, ed. *The Neurological Basis of Pain*. New York, NY: McGraw-Hill; 2005:71-94.

10. Schafers M, Brinkhoff J, Neukirchen S, et al. Combined epineurial therapy with neutralizing antibodies to tumor necrosis factor-alpha and interleukin-1 receptor has an additive effect in reducing neuropathic pain in mice. *Neurosci Lett*. 2001;310:113-116.

11. Lerner UH. Neuropeptidergic regulation of bone resorption and bone formation. *J Musculoskelet Neuronal Interact*. 2002;2:440-447.

12. Katz N. Neuropathic pain in cancer and AIDS. *Clin J Pain*. 2000;16:S41-S48.

13. Lai J, Hunter JC, Porreca F. The role of voltage-gated sodium channels in neuropathic pain. *Curr Opin Neurobiol*. 2003;13:291-297.

14. Sevcik MA, Ghilardi JR, Peters CM, et al. Anti-NGF therapy profoundly reduces bone cancer pain and the accompanying increase in markers of peripheral and central sensitization. *Pain*. 2005;115:128-141.

15. Watkins LR, Milligan ED, Maier SF. Glial activation: a driving force for pathological pain. *Trends Neurosci*. 2001;24(8):450-455.

16. Bennett G, Deer T, Du PS, et al. Future directions in the management of pain by intraspinal drug delivery. *J Pain Symptom Manage*. 2000;20:S44-S50.

17. Bennett GJ. Update on the neurophysiology of pain transmission and modulation: focus on the NMDA-receptor. *J Pain Symptom Manage*. 2000;9:S2-S6.

18. Galer BS, Jensen MP. Development and preliminary validation of a pain measure specific to neuropathic pain: the Neuropathic Pain Scale. *Neurology*. 1997;48:332-338.

19. Cleeland CS, Ryan KM. Pain assessment: global use of the Brief Pain Inventory. *Ann Acad Med Singapore*. 1994;23:129-138.

20. Martin LA, Hagen NA. Neuropathic pain in cancer patients: mechanisms, syndromes, and clinical controversies. *J Pain Symptom Manage*. 1997;14:99-117.

21. Amato AA, Collins MP. Neuropathies associated with malignancy. *Semin Neurol*. 1998;18:125-144.

22. Backonja M, Beydoun A, Edwards KR, et al. Gabapentin for the symptomatic treatment of painful neuropathy in patients with diabetes mellitus: a randomized controlled trial. *JAMA*. 1998;280:1831-1836.

23. Rice AS, Maton S. Gabapentin in postherpetic neuralgia: a randomised, double blind, placebo-controlled study. *Pain*. 2001;94:215-224.

24. Rowbotham M, Harden N, Stacey B, et al. Gabapentin for the treatment of postherpetic neuralgia: a randomized controlled trial. *JAMA*. 1998;280:1837-1842.

25. Matthews EA, Dickenson AH. Effects of spinally delivered N- and P-type voltage-dependent calcium channel antagonists on dorsal horn neuronal responses in a rat model of neuropathy. *Pain*. 2001;92:235-246.

26. Zakrzewska JM, Chaudhry Z, Nurmikko TJ, et al. Lamotrigine (lamictal) in refractory trigeminal neuralgia: results from a double-blind, placebo controlled, crossover trial. *Pain*. 1997;73:223-230.

27. Pappagallo M. Preliminary experience with topiramate in the treatment of chronic pain syndromes. Poster presented at: The 17th annual meeting, American Pain Society, 1998, San Diego, CA.

28. Shi W, Liu H, Zhang Y, et al. Design, synthesis, and preliminary evaluation of gabapentin–pregabalin mutual prodrugs in relieving neuropathic pain. *Arch Pharm (Weinheim)*. 2005;338:358-364.

29. Pappagallo M. Newer antiepileptic drugs: possible uses in the treatment of neuropathic pain and migraine. *Clin Ther*. 2003;25:2506-2538.

30. Gilron I, Bailey JM, Tu D, et al. Morphine, gabapentin, or their combination for neuropathic pain. *N Engl J Med*. 2005;352:1324-1334.

31. Portenoy RK. Opioid therapy for chronic nonmalignant pain: a review of the critical issues. *J Pain Symptom Manage*. 1996;11:203-217.

32. Dellemijn PL, Vanneste JA. Randomised double-blind active-placebo-controlled crossover trial of intravenous fentanyl in neuropathic pain. *Lancet*. 1997;349:753-758.

33. Gimbel JS, Richards P, Portenoy RK. Controlled-release oxycodone for pain in diabetic neuropathy: a randomized controlled trial. *Neurology*. 2003;60:927-934.

34. Raja SN, Haythornthwaite JA, Pappagallo M, et al. Opioids versus antidepressants in postherpetic neuralgia: a randomized, placebo-controlled trial. *Neurology*. 2002;59:1015-1021.

35. Rowbotham MC, Twilling L, Davies PS, et al. Oral opioid therapy for chronic peripheral and central neuropathic pain. *N Engl J Med*. 2003;348:1223-1232.

36. Suzuki R, Chapman V, Dickenson AH. The effectiveness of spinal and systemic morphine on rat dorsal horn neuronal responses in the spinal nerve ligation model of neuropathic pain. *Pain*. 1999;80:215-228.

37. Watson CP, Babul N. Efficacy of oxycodone in neuropathic pain: a randomized trial in postherpetic neuralgia. *Neurology.* 1998;50:1837-1841.

38. Pappagallo M. Aggressive pharmacologic treatment of pain. In: Pisetsky DS, Bradley L, eds. *Pain Management in the Rheumatic Diseases. Rheumatic Disease Clinics of North America.* Philadelphia, PA: WB Saunders; 1999:193.

39. Crain SM, Shen KF. Antagonists of excitatory opioid receptor functions enhance morphine's analgesic potency and attenuate opioid tolerance/dependence liability. *Pain.* 2000;84:121-131.

40. Harati Y, Gooch C, Swenson M, et al. Double-blind randomized trial of tramadol for the treatment of the pain of diabetic neuropathy. *Neurology.* 1998;50:1842-1846.

41. Sindrup SH, Madsen C, Brosen K, et al. The effect of tramadol in painful polyneuropathy in relation to serum drug and metabolite levels. *Clin Pharmacol Ther.* 1999;66:636-641.

42. Haythornthwaite JA, Menefee LA, Quatrano-Piacentini AL, et al. Outcome of chronic opioid therapy for non-cancer pain. *J Pain Symptom Manage.* 1998;15:185-194.

43. Max MB, Lynch SA, Muir J, et al. Effects of desipramine, amitriptyline, and fluoxetine on pain in diabetic neuropathy. *N Engl J Med.* 1992;326:1250-1256.

44. Sudoh Y, Cahoon EE, Gerner P, et al. Tricyclic antidepressants as long-acting local anesthetics. *Pain.* 2003;103:49-55.

45. Grothe DR, Scheckner B, Albano D. Treatment of pain syndromes with venlafaxine. *Pharmacotherapy.* 2004;24:621-629.

46. Marchand F, Alloui A, Pelissier T, et al. Evidence for an antihyperalgesic effect of venlafaxine in vincristine–induced neuropathy in rat. *Brain Res.* 2003;980:117-120.

47. Rowbotham MC, Goli V, Kunz NR, et al. Venlafaxine extended release in the treatment of painful diabetic neuropathy: a double-blind, placebo-controlled study. *Pain.* 2004;110:697-706.

48. Goldstein DJ, Lu Y, Detke MJ, et al. Duloxetine vs. placebo in patients with painful diabetic neuropathy. *Pain.* 2005;116:109-118.

49. Semenchuk MR, Sherman S, Davis B. Double-blind, randomized trial of bupropion SR for the treatment of neuropathic pain. *Neurology.* 2001;57:1583-1588.

50. Galer BS, Rowbotham MC, Perander J, et al. Topical lidocaine patch relieves postherpetic neuralgia more effectively than a vehicle topical patch: results of an enriched enrollment study. *Pain.* 1999;80:533-538.

51. Rowbotham MC, Davies PS, Verkempinck C, et al. Lidocaine patch: double-blind controlled study of a new treatment method for post-herpetic neuralgia. *Pain.* 1996;65:39-44.

52. Devers A, Galer BS. Topical lidocaine patch relieves a variety of neuropathic pain conditions: an open-label study. *Clin J Pain.* 2000;16:205-208.

53. Hart-Gouleau S, Gammaitoni A, Galer B, et al. Open label study of the effectiveness and safety of lidocaine patch 5% (Lidoderm) in patients with painful diabetic neuropathy [abstract]. Program and abstracts of the IASP 10th World Congress of Pain. Seattle, WA: IASP; 2002.

54. Berman SM, Justis JV, HO M, et al. Lidocaine patch 5% (Lidoderm) significantly improves quality of life (QOL) in HIV-associated painful peripheral neuropathy [abstract]. Program and abstracts of the IASP 10th World Congress of Pain. Seattle, WA: IASP; 2002.

55. Wallace MS. Calcium and sodium channel antagonists for the treatment of pain. *Clin J Pain.* 2000;16:S80-S85.

56. Hains BC, Klein JP, Saab CY, et al. Upregulation of sodium channel Na(v)1.3 and functional involvement in neuronal hyperexcitability associated with central neuropathic pain after spinal cord injury. *J Neurosci.* 2003;23:8881-8892.

57. Roza C, Laird JM, Souslova V, et al. The tetrodotoxin-resistant Na+ channel Na(v)1.8 is essential for the expression of spontaneous activity in damaged sensory axons of mice. *J Physiol.* 2003;550:921-926.

58. Khan ZP, Ferguson CN, Jones RM. Alpha-2 and imidazoline receptor agonists. Their pharmacology and therapeutic role. *Anaesthesia.* 1999;54:146-165.

59. Eisenach JC, Rauck RL, Buzzanell C, et al. Epidural clonidine analgesia for intractable cancer pain: phase I. *Anesthesiology.* 1989;71:647-652.

60. Davis KD, Treede RD, Raja SN, et al. Topical application of clonidine relieves hyperalgesia in patients with sympathetically maintained pain. *Pain.* 1991;47:309-317.

61. Fogelholm R, Murros K. Tizanidine in chronic tension-type headache: a placebo controlled double-blind cross-over study. *Headache.* 1992;32:509-513.

62. Fromm GH, Aumentado D, Terrence CF. A clinical and experimental investigation of the effects of tizanidine in trigeminal neuralgia. *Pain.* 1993;53:265-271.

63. McCarthy RJ, Kroin JS, Lubenow TR, et al. Effect of intrathecal tizanidine on antinociception and blood pressure in the rat. *Pain.* 1990;40:333-338.

64. Caterina MJ, Schumacher MA, Tominaga M, et al. The capsaicin receptor: a heat-activated ion channel in the pain pathway. *Nature.* 1997;389:816-824.

65. Robbins WR, Staats PS, Levine J, et al. Treatment of intractable pain with topical large-dose capsaicin: preliminary report. *Anesth Analg.* 1998;86:579-583.

66. Bell RF, Eccleston C, Kalso E. Ketamine as adjuvant to opioids for cancer pain. A qualitative systematic review. *J Pain Symptom Manage.* 2003;26:867-875.

67. Fitzgibbon EJ, Viola R. Parenteral ketamine as an analgesic adjuvant for severe pain: development and retrospective audit of a protocol for a palliative care unit. *J Palliat Med.* 2005;8:49-57.

68. Lossignol DA, Obiols-Portis M, Body JJ. Successful use of ketamine for intractable cancer pain. *Support Care Cancer.* 2005;13:188-193.

69. Slatkin NE, Rhiner M. Topical ketamine in the treatment of mucositis pain. *Pain Med.* 2003;4:298-303.

70. Vranken JH, van der Vegt MH, Kal JE, et al. Treatment of neuropathic cancer pain with continuous intrathecal administration of S+-ketamine. *Acta Anaesthesiol Scand.* 2004;48:249-252.

71. Davis AM, Inturrisi CE. d-Methadone blocks morphine tolerance and *N*-methyl-d-aspartate-induced hyperalgesia. *J Pharmacol Exp Ther.* 1999;289:1048-1053.

72. Price DD, Mayer DJ, Mao J, et al. NMDA-receptor antagonists and opioid receptor interactions as related to analgesia and tolerance. *J Pain Symptom Manage.* 2000;19:S7.

73. Russo EB. The role of cannabis and cannabinoids in pain management. In: Weiner RS, ed. *Pain Management: A Practical Guide for Clinicians*, 6th ed. Boca Raton, FL: CRC Press; 2002:357-337.

74. Aggarwal SK, Carter GT, Sullivan MD, ZumBrunnen C, Morrill R, Mayer JD. Medicinal use of cannabis in the United States: historical perspectives, current trends, and future directions. *J Opioid Manag.* 2009; 5:153-168.

75. Shaiova L, Berger A, Pappagallo M, Bruera E, Perlov E. Consensus guidelines on parenteral use in pain and methadone palliative care. *J Palliat Support Care.* November 2008;34(6):1897s-1902s.

76. Cichewicz DL. Synergistic interactions between cannabinoid and opioid analgesics. *Life Sci.* 2004 Jan 30; 74(11):1317-1324.

77. Narang S, Gibson D, Wasan AD, et al. Efficacy of dronabinol as an adjuvant treatment for chronic pain patients on opioid therapy. *J Pain.* March 2008;9(3):254-264.

78. Rahn EJ and Hohmann AG. Cannabinoids as pharmacotherapies for neuropathic pain: from the bench to the bedside. *Neurotherapeutics.* 2009;7(4):713-737.

79. Abrams DI, Jay CA, Shade SB, et al. Cannabis in painful HIV-associated sensory neuropathy: a randomized placebo-controlled trial. *Neurology.* 2007;68:515-521.

80. Ellis R, Toperoff W, Vaida F, et al. Smoked medicinal cannabis for neuropathic pain in HIV: a randomized, crossover clinical trial. *Neuropsychopharmacology.* 2008;34(3):672-680.

81. Wilsey B, Marcotte T, Tsodikov A, et al. A randomized, placebo-controlled, crossover trial of cannabis cigarettes in neuropathic pain. *J Pain.* April 2008;9(6):506-521.

82. Wallace M, Schulteis G, Atkinson JH, et al. Dose-dependent effects of smoked cannabis on capsaicin-induced pain and hyperalgesia in healthy volunteers. *Anesthesiology.* November 2007;107(5):785-796.

83. Ware MA, Wang T, Shapiro S, et al. Smoked cannabis for chronic neuropathic pain. *Can Med Asso J.* October 2010;182(14):E694-E701.

84. Portenoy R, Ganae-Motan E, Allende S, et al. Nabiximols (Sativex`) for opioid-treated cancer patients with poorly-controlled chronic pain: a randomized, placebo-controlled, graded-dose trial. *J. Pain.* 2012;13(5):438-449.

85. Sommer C, Marziniak M, Myers RR. The effect of thalidomide treatment on vascular pathology and hyperalgesia caused by chronic constriction injury of rat nerve. *Pain.* 1998;74:83-91.

86. Ribeiro RA, Vale ML, Ferreira SH, et al. Analgesic effect of thalidomide on inflammatory pain. *Eur J Pharmacol.* 2000;391:97-103.

87. George A, Marziniak M, Schafers M, et al. Thalidomide treatment in chronic constrictive neuropathy decreases endoneurial tumor necrosis factor-alpha, increases interleukin-10 and has long-term effects on spinal cord dorsal horn met-enkephalin. *Pain.* 2000;88:267-275.

88. Cortet B, Flipo RM, Coquerelle P, et al. Treatment of severe, recalcitrant reflex sympathetic dystrophy: assessment of efficacy and safety of the second generation bisphosphonate pamidronate. *Clin Rheumatol.* 1997;16:51-56.

89. Varenna M, Zucchi F, Ghiringhelli D, et al. Intravenous clodronate in the treatment of reflex sympathetic dystrophy syndrome. A randomized, double blind, placebo controlled study. *J Rheumatol.* 2000;27(6):1477-1483.

90. Liu T, van Rooijen N, Tracey DJ. Depletion of macrophages reduces axonal degeneration and hyperalgesia following nerve injury. *Pain.* 2000;86:25-32.

91. Max MB, Schafer SC, Culnane M, et al. Amitriptyline, but not lorazepam, relieves postherpetic neuralgia. *Neurology.* 1988;38:1427-1432.

92. Mercadante S. Problems of long-term spinal opioid treatment in advanced cancer patients. *Pain.* 1999;79(1):1-13.

93. Campbell JN, Sciubba DM. Neurosurgical approaches to the treatment of pain. In: Pappagallo M, ed. *The Neurological Basis of Pain.* New York, NY: McGraw-Hill; 2005:631-639.

94. Banning A, Sjogren P, Henriksen H. Pain causes in 200 patients referred to a multidisciplinary cancer pain clinic. *Pain.* 1991;45:45-48.

95. Mach DB, Rogers SD, Sabino MC, et al. Origins of skeletal pain: sensory and sympathetic innervation of the mouse femur. *Neuroscience.* 2002;113:155-166.

96. Jonsson OG, Sartain P, Ducore JM, et al. Bone pain as an initial symptom of childhood acute lymphoblastic leukemia: association with nearly normal hematologic indexes. *J Pediatr.* 1990;117:233-237.

97. Constans JP, De Divitiis E, Donzelli R, et al. Spinal metastases with neurological manifestations. Review of 600 cases. *J Neurosurg.* 1983; 59:111-118.

98. Sorensen S, Borgesen SE, Rohde K, et al. Metastatic epidural spinal cord compression. Results of treatment and survival. *Cancer.* 1990;65:1502-1508.

99. Sundaresan N, Galicich JH, Lane JM, et al. Treatment of odontoid fractures in cancer patients. *J Neurosurg.* 1981;54:187-192.

100. Stark RJ, Henson RA, Evans SJ. Spinal metastases. A retrospective survey from a general hospital. *Brain.* 1982;105:189-213.

101. Portenoy RK, Galer BS, Salamon O, et al. Identification of epidural neoplasm. Radiography and bone scintigraphy in the symptomatic and asymptomatic spine. *Cancer.* 1989;64:2207-2213.

102. Ruff RL, Lanska DJ. Epidural metastases in prospectively evaluated veterans with cancer and back pain. *Cancer.* 1989;63:2234-2241.

103. Fidler M. Incidence of fracture through metastases in long bones. *Acta Orthop Scand.* 1981;52:623-627.

104. Ettinger AB, Portenoy RK. The use of corticosteroids in the treatment of symptoms associated with cancer. *J Pain Symptom Manage.* 1988;3:99-103.

105. Vecht CJ, Haaxma-Reiche H, van Putten WL, et al. Initial bolus of conventional versus high-dose dexamethasone in metastatic spinal cord compression. *Neurology.* 1989;39:1255-1257.

106. Watanabe S, Bruera E. Corticosteroids as adjuvant analgesics. *J Pain Symptom Manage.* 1994;9:442-445.

107. Mystakidou K, Katsouda E, Stathopoulou E, et al. Approaches to managing bone metastases from breast cancer: the role of bisphosphonates. *Cancer Treat Rev.* 2005;31:303-311.

108. Smith MR. Osteoclast-targeted therapy for prostate cancer. *Curr Treat Options Oncol.* 2004;5:367-375.

109. Wardley A, Davidson N, Barrett-Lee P, et al. Zoledronic acid significantly improves pain scores and quality of life in breast cancer patients with bone metastases: a randomised, crossover study of community vs hospital bisphosphonate administration. *Br J Cancer.* 2005;92:1869-1876.

110. Gordon DH. Efficacy and safety of intravenous bisphosphonates for patients with breast cancer metastatic to bone: a review of randomized, double-blind, phase III trials. *Clin Breast Cancer.* 2005;6:125-131.

111. Pecherstorfer M. Efficacy and safety of ibandronate in the treatment of neoplastic bone disease. *Expert Opin Pharmacother.* 2004;5:2341-2350.

112. Ogawa K, Mukai T, Arano Y, et al. Development of a rhenium-186-labeled MAG3-conjugated bisphosphonate for the palliation of metastatic bone pain based on the concept of bifunctional radiopharmaceuticals. *Bioconjug Chem.* 2005;16:751-757.

113. Tong D, Gillick L, Hendrickson FR. The palliation of symptomatic osseous metastases: final results of the study by the Radiation Therapy Oncology Group. *Cancer.* 982;50:893-899.

114. Hirokawa Y, Wadasaki K, KashiwadoK, et al. A multiinstitutional prospective randomized study of radiation therapy of bone metastases [in Japanese]. *Nippon Igaku Hoshasen Gakkai Zasshi.* 1988;1099;58:793-796.

115. Rasmusson B, Vejborg I, Jensen AB, et al. Irradiation of bone metastases in breast cancer patients: a randomized study with 1 year follow-up. *Radiother Oncol.* 1995;34:179-184.

116. Niewald M, Tkocz HJ, Abel U, et al. Rapid course radiation therapy vs. more standard treatment: a randomized trial for bone metastases. *Int J Radiat Oncol Biol Phys.* 1996;36:1085-1089.

117. Hoskin PJ, Price P, Easton D, et al. A prospective randomized trial of 4 Gy or 8 Gy single doses in the treatment of metastatic bone pain. *Radiother Oncol.* 1992;23:74-78.

118. Jeremic B, Shibamoto Y, Acimovic L, et al. A randomized trial of three single-dose radiation therapy regimens in the treatment of metastatic bone pain. *Int J Radiat Oncol Biol Phys.*1998;42:161-167.

119. Steenland E, Leer JW, van Houwelingen H, et al. The effect of a single fraction compared to multiple fractions on painful bone metastases: a global analysis of the Dutch Bone Metastases Study. *Radiother Oncol.* 1999;52:101-109.

120. Hartsell WF, Scott CB, Bruner DW, et al. Randomized trial of short- versus long-course radiotherapy for palliation of painful bone metastases. *J Natl Cancer Inst.* 2005;97:798-804.

121. KonskiA, DeSilvio M, Harsell W, et al. Continuing evidence for poorer treatment outcomes for single male patients: retreatment data from RTOG 97 14. *Int J Radiat Oncol Biol Phys.* 2006;66:229-2333.

122. Roodman GD. Mechanisms of bone metastasis. *N Engl J Med.* 2004;350:1655-1664.

123. Mundy GR. Metastasis to bone: causes, consequences and therapeutic opportunities. *Nat Rev Cancer.* 2002;2:584-593.

124. Kantoff PW, Higano CS, Shore ND, et al. Sipuleucel-T immunotherapy for castration-resistant prostate cancer. *N Engl J Med.* 2010;363:411-422.

125. Szanto J, Ady N, Jozsef S. Pain killing with calcitonin nasal spray in patients with malignant tumors. *Oncology.* 1992;49:180-182.

126. Finlay IG, Mason MD, Shelley M. Radioisotopes for the palliation of metastatic bone cancer: a systematic review. *Lancet Oncol.* 2005;6:392-400.

127. Nilsson S, Larsen RH, Fossa SD, et al. First clinical experience with alpha-emitting radium-223 in the treatment of skeletal metastases. *Clin Cancer Res.* 2005;11:4451-4459.

128. Maini CL, Bergomi S, Romano L, et al. 153Sm-EDTMP for bone pain palliation in skeletal metastases. *Eur J Nucl Med Mol Imaging.* 2004;31(suppl 1):S171-S178.

129. Lam MG, de Klerk JM, van Rijk PP. 186Re-HEDP for metastatic bone pain in breast cancer patients. *Eur J Nucl Med Mol Imaging* 2004;31(suppl 1):S162-S170.

130. Smith MR, Saad F, Coleman R, Shore N, et al. Denosumab and bone metastasis-free survival in men with castration-resistant prostate cancer: results of a phase 3, randomised, placebo controlled trial. *Lancet.* 2012;379(9810):39-46.

131. Burton AW, Rhines LD, Mendel E. Vertebroplasty and kyphoplasty: a comprehensive review. *Neurosurg Focus.* 2005;18(3):e1.

132. Milne RJ, Foreman RD, Giesler GJ Jr, et al. Convergence of cutaneous and pelvic visceral nociceptive inputs onto primate spinothalamic neurons. *Pain.* 1981;11:163-183.

133. Cherny NI. Cancer pain: principles of assessment and syndromes. In: Berger A, Portenoy RK, Weissman D, eds. *Principles and Practice of Supportive Oncology,* 1st ed. Philadelphia, PA: Lippincott Williams & Wilkins; 1998:3-42.

134. Farr WC. The use of corticosteroids for symptom management in terminally ill patients. *Am J Hosp Care.* 1990;7:41-46.

135. Ripamonti C, Mercadante S, Groff L, et al. Role of octreotide, scopolamine butylbromide, and hydration in symptom control of patients with inoperable bowel obstruction and nasogastric tubes: a prospective randomized trial. *J Pain Symptom Manage.* 2000;19:23-34.

136. Cousins MJ. Techniques for neurolytic neural blockade. In: Cousins MJ, Bridenbaugh PO, eds. *Neural Blockade in Clinical Anesthesia and Management of Pain,* 3rd ed. Philadelphia, PA: Lippincott Williams & Wilkins; 1998:1007-1061.

137. Lema MJ, Myers DP, Leon-Casasola O, et al. Pleural phenol therapy for the treatment of chronic esophageal cancer pain. *Reg Anesth.* 1992;17:166-170.

138. Mercadante S, Nicosia F. Celiac plexus block: a reappraisal. *Reg Anesth Pain Med.* 1998;23:37-48.

139. Mercadante S. Celiac plexus block versus analgesics in pancreatic cancer pain. *Pain.* 1993;52:187-192.

140. Plancarte R, Leon-Casasola OA, El Helaly M, et al. Neurolytic superior hypogastric plexus block for chronic pelvic pain associated with cancer. *Reg Anesth.* 1997;22:562-568.

141. Korevaar WC. Transcatheter thoracic epidural neurolysis using ethyl alcohol. *Anesthesiology.* 1988;69:989-993.

2 Opioid Pharmacotherapy

Judith A. Paice

Opioids and their derivatives have been used to relieve pain for centuries, and their contribution to relief of suffering is well established. Many of the earliest recorded reports of opioid use are attributed to the Egyptians and extend back many centuries. In the 1600s, Thomas Sydenham promoted the use of laudanum, a mixture of opium, saffron, cinnamon, and cloves in wine (1). Two centuries later, the pharmacist Wilhelm Sertürner extracted morphine from poppy juice, calling this substance morphium after Morpheus, the Greek god of sleep (1). Since that time, many new opioids have been developed, and information about the pharmacodynamics, pharmacokinetics, and pharmacogenomics of these compounds has increased greatly. This understanding has led to improvements in their clinical application, for relief not only of pain but also of dyspnea, cough, and intractable diarrhea. Yet, more than any other agent, opioids generate fear, misunderstanding, and controversy. To address these misconceptions and provide optimal relief, those caring for patients with pain and other symptoms associated with cancer or other life-threatening illnesses must have a strong knowledge base regarding the pharmacology and clinical application of opioids.

PHARMACOLOGY OF OPIOIDS

To fully appreciate the optimal clinical use of opioids, the clinician must understand the pharmacodynamics (the mechanism of opioid analgesia) and the pharmacokinetics (the process by which opioids are absorbed, distributed, metabolized, and excreted) of this class of drugs. The pharmacogenomics of opioids helps explain the variability in response seen in the clinical setting.

Pharmacodynamics

Opioids act through three major types of opioid receptors, including μ (MOR for μ-opioid receptor), δ (DOR for δ-opioid receptor), and κ (KOR for κ-opioid receptor). These receptors are distributed widely throughout the nervous system, including the peripheral nerves, spinal cord, and brain (2). The highest density of opioid receptors appears in laminae I and II of the dorsal horn of the spinal cord (3). Opioid receptors are also found in the brainstem, including the periaqueductal gray, nucleus raphe magnus, and locus coeruleus, areas known to be involved in the mediation of opioid analgesia (4). Opioid receptors have also been found on immune cells.

Opioid receptors are G protein–coupled, activating a complex cascade of events. These include increased conduction through potassium channels, which hyperpolarizes the sensory neuron. Opioid receptor binding results in diminished conduction through calcium channels, resulting in decreased release of neurotransmitters involved in nociception. Finally, opioid receptor binding leads to inhibition of adenylate cyclase. Together, these actions contribute to the analgesia that results when an opioid agonist binds to the above receptors.

Pharmacokinetics

As with all other compounds, the absorption, distribution, metabolism, and elimination of an opioid influence the efficacy of the drug. Alterations are of particular concern when caring for patients with advanced malignancy or other life-threatening illnesses because any of these phases of the opioid may be altered by extensive disease.

Absorption

Absorption is influenced by the lipophilicity of an agent. Morphine and hydromorphone have a partition coefficient (octanol/water) of 1 compared with 115 for methadone and 820 for fentanyl (5). Therefore, fentanyl can cross biologic membranes more avidly when compared with morphine, making it the more appropriate agent for transdermal delivery. The lipophilicity affects the time to maximal serum concentration (C_{MAX}). The C_{MAX} for a hydrophilic drug, such as morphine, is approximately 60 minutes after oral administration, 30 minutes after subcutaneous (s.c.) delivery, and 6 minutes or more after intravenous (i.v.) delivery. The half-life of oral morphine is approximately 4 hours. Because steady state is reached in approximately 4 to 5 half-lives, it will be reached within approximately 16 to 20 hours of regular immediate-release oral morphine administration. Little is known about the alterations in absorption of opioids that occur when patients have extensive disease. For example, factors such as shortened transit time may delay the absorption of oral opioids, particularly long-acting or sustained-release compounds.

Distribution

Plasma proteins and lipid solubility of a particular opioid affect the distribution of the drug throughout the vasculature (5). Other mediating factors include body fat stores and total body water. All of these factors listed above can be significantly altered in older adults or in persons with cachexia and dehydration, the common sequelae of advanced disease.

Metabolism

Most opioids are metabolized through glucuronidation, dealkylation, or other processes and are then excreted by the kidneys. Although some metabolites produce analgesia (e.g., morphine-3-glucuronide [M3G]), they may also contribute to neurotoxicity (6). Myoclonus has been associated with both M3G and hydromorphone-3-glucuronide (H3G), metabolites that appear to pose a risk for accumulating in patients receiving high doses of opioid for extended periods or in those with renal disease (7). Metabolism is known to be affected by advanced age, liver disease, genetics, and other factors that are prominent in palliative care.

Elimination

Most opioids are excreted renally, with only methadone being eliminated fecally. Experience suggests that patients with renal failure or those receiving dialysis might benefit from the use of agents that are more readily dialyzable, such as fentanyl, as opposed to morphine or codeine (8). However, even in patients who have undergone a successful renal transplantation, the large variability in the kinetics of fentanyl after surgery supports the axiom that all opioid therapy must be individualized (9). Much more research is needed on the interaction between advanced disease and the pharmacokinetics of opioids.

Pharmacogenomics

The field of pharmacogenomics is rapidly growing and much evidence for the variability in response to opioids seen in the clinical setting is related to inborn properties caused by genetic variability (10). The MOR was cloned in 1993 and was called *MOR-1*. Additional work has identified splice variants of the MOR-1 receptor, with different localization of the splice variants within the nervous system (11). The efficacy of morphine varies among the variants, and this may explain, in part, the variability in response to opioids seen in the clinical setting, including efficacy and adverse effects. The translation of this information to the clinical experience includes the practice of opioid rotation when a particular opioid agonist is either ineffective or produces unmanageable adverse effects.

Another clear clinical example of the contribution of pharmacogenomics to the variability in analgesia from opioids is related to codeine. People who are poor metabolizers of the enzyme CYP2D6 derive little analgesic effect from codeine, a prodrug that must be metabolized to morphine to produce analgesia. Approximately 5% to 10% of Whites, 1% of Asians, and 0% to 20% of African Americans are poor metabolizers (12). Conversely, case reports have described overdose in a patient taking a small dose of codeine. Analysis also revealed the patient to be an ultrarapid metabolizer of CYP2D6, which theoretically resulted in a rapid, extensive

conversion of the drug to morphine (13). Another report described toxicity in a breastfed neonate when the mother was prescribed codeine; the mother was found to be an ultra-rapid metabolizer of codeine (14).

One example of the role of pharmacogenomics in cancer pain control is related to the catechol-*O*-methyltransferase (*COMT*) gene, which inactivates dopamine, epinephrine, and norepinephrine in the nervous system. A study of 207 white patients with cancer found that polymorphism of the *COMT* gene contributes to variability in response to morphine in pain control (15). A common functional polymorphism (Val158Met) leads to a significant variation in the COMT enzyme activity, with the Met form displaying lower enzymatic activity. Patients with the Val/Val genotype needed more morphine when compared with the Val/Met and the Met/Met genotype groups. The investigators could not explain these differences by other factors such as duration of opioid treatment, performance status, time since diagnosis, perceived pain intensity, adverse symptoms, or time until death. Much more research is needed to fully understand the pharmacogenetics of opioids and their implications for those with cancer or other life-threatening illnesses.

CLINICAL APPLICATION

Opioids are a critical component of the armamentarium used to control pain in palliative care. They are indicated in moderate to severe pain, as well as in the management of cough, dyspnea, and severe diarrhea. Because opioids alter pain signal transmission and perception throughout the nervous system, they have an analgesic effect despite the underlying pathophysiology of pain. In fact, despite earlier beliefs, opioids have been shown to be effective in providing relief of neuropathic pain.

Specific Opioids

Opioids are generally categorized as agonists, partial agonists, and mixed agonist–antagonists. Additionally, antagonists to opioids may be used to counteract adverse effects of opioids.

Agonists

Numerous opioid agonists are available for clinical use. These agents can be subcategorized as alkaloids and synthetic opioids (Table 2.1). Attributes associated with the more commonly used opioids are described in the following text and in Table 2.2.

Codeine. Codeine is a relatively weak opioid that is more frequently administered in combination with acetaminophen. Codeine is metabolized by glucuronidation primarily to codeine-6-glucuronide and to a much lesser degree to norcodeine, morphine, M3G, morphine-6-glucuronide, and normorphine (16). As described earlier in the section Pharmacogenomics, codeine is converted to morphine by

TABLE 2.1	Opioids by classification
Agonists	
Alkaloids	
Morphine	
Codeine	
Semisynthetic opioids—hydrocodone, hydromorphone, oxycodone, and oxymorphone	
Synthetic opioids	
Phenylpiperidine derivatives—fentanyl, sufentanil, alfentanil, remifentanil, and meperidine	
Diphenylheptane derivatives—methadone	
Morphinan derivatives—levorphanol	
Novel formulations—tramadol and tapentadol	
Partial Agonists	
Semisynthetic—buprenorphine	
Mixed Agonist–Antagonists	
Semisynthetic alkaloid—nalbuphine	
Synthetic benzomorphan derivative—pentazocine	
Synthetic morphinan derivative—butorphanol	
Antagonists	
Naloxone	
Naltrexone	
Methylnaltrexone	

CYP2D6. The polymorphism seen in this enzyme between various ethnic groups, and between individuals, leads to a significant percentage obtaining reduced analgesia.

Fentanyl. Fentanyl is a highly lipid-soluble opioid (partition coefficient 820) that has been administered parenterally, spinally, transdermally (including an iontophoretically administered patient-controlled device), transmucosally, intranasally, and by a nebulizer for the management of dyspnea (17,18). Dosing units are usually in micrograms because of the potency of this opioid. Questions arise about the efficacy of fentanyl and related compounds, alfentanil, remifentanil, and sufentanil, in the face of extremes in body weight. A study of i.v. fentanyl for acute postoperative pain in lean and obese patients found no relationship between plasma levels required for analgesia and total body weight. Therefore, using i.v. dosing on the basis of weight (or milligram per kilogram dosing) in patients with cachexia could lead to underdosing, whereas the same practice in the obese patient could lead to overdosing (19). A more recent small study of cancer patients receiving fentanyl patches revealed that cachectic patients had lower plasma concentrations when compared with normal weight patients (20). This does not preclude the use of fentanyl patches in cachectic patients, but it reinforces the need for individualized dosing and reassessment.

Hydrocodone. Hydrocodone is more potent than codeine, and it is found not only in combination products, primarily acetaminophen, but also with ibuprofen. Liquid cough formulations of hydrocodone also contain homatropine. These additives limit the use of hydrocodone in palliative care when higher doses of opioid are required. Hydrocodone is metabolized through demethylation to hydromorphone. Laboratory evidence suggests that CYP2D6 polymorphism may alter the analgesic response to hydrocodone (21).

Hydromorphone. Hydromorphone is a derivative of morphine, with similar properties, and is available as oral tablets, liquids, suppositories, and parenteral formulations (22). Because it is highly soluble and approximately 5 to 10 times more potent than morphine, hydromorphone is used frequently in palliative care when small volumes are needed for s.c. infusions. A long-acting formulation is now available in the United States. Hydromorphone undergoes glucuronidation and the primary metabolite is H3G (16). Recent experience suggests that this metabolite may lead to opioid neurotoxicity, similar to that seen with morphine metabolites, including myoclonus, hyperalgesia, and seizures (7,23,24). This appears to be of particular risk with high doses, prolonged use, or in persons with renal dysfunction (25).

TABLE 2.2	Properties of commonly used opioids					
Agent	Routes	Formulations	i.v./s.c.* (mg)	Oral Dose (mg)	Starting Dose for Adults[a]	Other
Codeine*	Oral Parenteral (uncommon)	Codeine sulfate 15,30, or 60 mg tablets Tylenol No. 2 (15 mg codeine/300 mg acetaminophen) Tylenol No. 3 (30 mg codeine/300 mg acetaminophen) Tylenol No. 4 (60 mg codeine/300 mg acetaminophen) Codeine/guaifenesin liquid (5 mL = 10 mg codeine/100 mg guaifenesin)	130	200	Oral: 30-60 mg	Converted to morphine by CYP2D6; poor metabolizers obtain little pain relief
Fentanyl	Intraspinal i.v. Transdermal Transmucosal	Fentanyl solution for i.v. Fentanyl patch (Duragesic, generics) 12, 25, 50, 75, or 100 µg/h Fentanyl oral transmucosal (Actiq) 200,400, 600, 1,200, or 1,600 µg units Fentanyl transmucosal (Fentora) 100, 200, 400, 600, 800 mcg buccal tablets Fentanyl transmucosal (Abstral) 100, 200, 300, 400, 600, 800 mcg sublingual tablets Fentanyl transmucosal (Onsolis) 200, 400, 600, 800, 1200 mcg buccal strips Fentanyl nasal (Lazanda) 100, 400 mcg/ spray	0.1	NA	NA	Transdermal fentanyl 25 µg/h approximately equal to 50 mg oral morphine
Hydrocodone*	Oral	Norco (5,7.5, or 10 mg hydrocodone/ 325 mg acetaminophen) Vicodin Hycodan (5 mL = 5 mg hydrocodone/ 1.5 mg homatropine)	NA	15-30	Oral: 5-10 mg	Role of CYP2D6 unclear

(Continued)

TABLE 2.2	Properties of commonly used opioids (Continued)				
Agent	Routes	Formulations	i.v./ s.c.* (mg)	Oral Dose (mg)	Starting Dose for Adults[a]	Other
Hydromorphone	Oral Parenteral	Hydromorphone 2,4, or 8 mg (Dilaudid, generics) Hydromorphone 3 mg suppository Exalgo 8,12,16 mg once/day	1.5	7.5	Oral: 4-8 mg	Toxicity may be due in part to hydromorphone-3-glucuronide
Levorphanol	Oral Parenteral (uncommon)	Levo-Dromoran 2 mg	2	4	Oral: 2-4 mg	Long half-life; repeated dosing may lead to accumulation Increased incidence of psychotomimet-ic effects
Meperidine	Oral Parenteral	Demerol	75-100	300	Not recommended	Not recommended because of toxic metabolite, normeperidine
Methadone	Oral Parenteral	Dolphine and generics (5,10,40 mg tablets; 1 mg/mL solution; 10 mg/mL solution)	See text	See text	See text	See text and Tables 3.3 and 3.4
Morphine	Intraspinal Oral Parenteral	Morphine immediate release (15,30 mg) Morphine sustained release q12h (15, 30,50,60, 100, 200 mg) (MS Contin, Kadian, Oramorph, generics) Moraphine sustained release q24h (Avinza) (30, 60,90, 120 mg) Morphine liquid 1 mg/mL, 20 mg/mL Morphine suppository 5, 10,20, 30 mg	10	30	Oral: 15-30 mg	Avinza and Kadian may be used as sprinkles Toxicity may be due in part to morphine-3-glucuronide

Oxycodone*	Oral	Oxycodone immediate release (5,15,30 mg) (OxyIR, generics) Oxycodone 5 mg/325 mg acetaminophen (Percocet) Oxycodone sustained release (10, 15, 20,30, 40,60 80 mg) (OxyContin) Oxycodone liquid 20 mg/mL	NA	20-30	Oral: 5-20 mg
Oxymorphone	Oral	Oxymorphone immediate release (5,10 mg) Oxymorphone controlled release (5,10, 20, 30, 40 mg) (Opana) Oxymorphone injection (5,10 mg s.c., i.v.) (Opana)	1	10	Oral:10-20 mg
Tapentadol	Oral	Tapentadol immediate release (50,75,100 mg) (Nucynta) Tapentadol extended release (50, 100, 150, 200, 250 mg) (Nucynta ER)	NA	100 mg	Oral: 50-100 mg
Tramadol	Oral	Tramadol immediate release (50 mg) (Ultram) Tramadol extended release (100, 200, 300 mg) (Ultram ER)	NA	50-100	Oral: 25 mg

aStarting doses are approximations for opioid-naive adult patients.

*Recent FDA mandate will result in lower acetaminophen doses- doses > 325 mg will no longer be available in US after 2012.

Methadone. Methadone has been gaining renewed popularity in the management of severe, persistent pain, yet it has several characteristics that complicate its use. Methadone is a μ- and δ-agonist and is an antagonist to the *N*-methyl-d-aspartate (NMDA) receptor, with affinity similar to that of ketamine (26). This antagonism is believed to be of particular benefit in neuropathic pain and in the management of hyperalgesia. A double-blind study in palliative care patients revealed its efficacy in the management of neuropathic pain, although a Cochrane review of existing studies found no obvious clinical effects (27,28). Methadone also blocks the reuptake of serotonin and norepinephrine, another potentially favorable attribute to its use in treating neuropathic pain. The prolonged plasma half-life of methadone (ranging from 15 to 60+ hours) allows for a relatively convenient dosing schedule of every 8 hours. Furthermore, methadone is much less expensive than comparable doses of commercially available continuous-release formulations.

Another advantage of the use of methadone in palliative care is the variety of available routes that can be used, including oral, rectal, s.c., i.v., and epidural (29). Nasal and sublingual administration have been reported to be effective, but preparations are not currently available commercially. The ratio of oral to parenteral methadone is 2:1 and of oral to rectal is 1:1. Subcutaneous methadone infusions may produce local irritation, although using a more dilute solution or changing the needle more frequently can mediate this.

Despite the many advantages, much is unknown about the efficacy of methadone when compared with other agents, the appropriate dosing ratio between methadone and morphine, or the safest and most effective time course for conversion from another opioid to methadone. Despite much anecdotal support for the use of methadone, Bruera et al. conducted a randomized controlled trial in patients with cancer and found no significant difference when compared with morphine (30). Early reports suggested that the analgesic ratio of morphine to methadone might be 1:1, yet this appears to be true only for individuals without recent prior exposure to opioids (31). For individuals currently taking another opioid, the dose ratio increases as the dose of oral opioid equivalents increases (32,33). The oral morphine to oral methadone ratio may be 2:1 for patients on <30 mg of oral morphine equivalent daily doses (MEDD) but may be 10:1 or 20:1 for patients on >300 mg oral MEDD (Tables 2.3 and 2.4). An additional complicating factor in the use of methadone is the limited experience in reverse rotation from methadone to another opioid (31,32).

The kinetics of methadone varies greatly between individuals, and causes for the variability include protein binding, CYP3A4 activity, urinary pH, and other factors. Methadone binds avidly to α_1-glycoprotein, the level of which is increased in advanced cancer, leading to decreasing amounts of unbound methadone and initially delaying the onset of effect. As a result, the interindividual variability of the pharmacokinetics of methadone is more pronounced in patients with cancer (26).

| TABLE 2.3 | **Methadone dose ratios** |

Oral Morphine Equivalent (mg/d)	Dose Ratio (Morphine:Methadone)
<30	2:1
30–99	4:1
100–299	8:1
300–499	12:1
500–999	15:1
>1,000	20:1 or greater

Note: These ratios are generally accepted in clinical practice, although these serve only as a guide to converting an opioid to methadone. Many factors can increase or decrease serum methadone levels and caution is advised. Frequent assessment of pain and sedation are warranted when converting to methadone or when increasing the dose.

Methadone is metabolized primarily by CYP3A4, but also by CYP2D6 and CYP1A2 (26,34,35). Drugs that induce CYP3A4 enzymes accelerate the metabolism of methadone, resulting in reduced serum levels of the drug. Patients report shortened analgesic periods or reduced overall pain relief (36). Drugs that inhibit CYP3A4 enzymes slow down methadone metabolism, potentially leading to sedation and respiratory depression. Table 2.5 lists many agents commonly used in palliative care that are CYP3A4 inducers and inhibitors.

Urinary pH can account for a significant amount of the variability seen in methadone plasma levels. Clearance of methadone is greater when the pH is more acidic (<6). As a result, urinary alkalizers, such as sodium bicarbonate, will decrease methadone excretion. Other factors that alter methadone kinetics include drug interactions. In addition to the CYP3A4 interactions listed previously, others have been described. For example, the proton pump inhibitor omeprazole increases gastric pH, thereby increasing the rate of absorption.

Although the extended half-life of methadone allows longer dosing intervals, it also increases the potential of drug accumulation, leading to delayed sedation and respiratory depression. This may occur 2 to 5 days after initiating the drug or increasing the dose. Another consequence of prolonged or high-dose opioid administration, myoclonus, has been reported with methadone use (37). Finally, controversy exists about the role of methadone in QT-wave interval prolongation (Torsade de pointes). Some question whether this is due to preservatives in the parenteral formulation, although the syndrome has been reported with oral administration of methadone (38). A study of 100 patients taking methadone found that one-third had prolonged QT-wave intervals on electrocardiogram, occurring more frequently in men, yet there did not appear to be a risk of serious prolongation

TABLE 2.4	Protocols for the conversion from other opioids to methadone

Protocol 1—Three- to Five-Day Method

- Calculate an equianalgesic dose of methadone
- Reduce the existing opioid dose by approximately one-third and administer one-third of the predicted methadone dose (give in three doses or every 8 h); continue to use the existing short-acting opioid for rescue
- On day 2, reduce the existing morphine by another third and increase the methadone dose by one-third
- On day 3, discontinue the existing opioid and increase the methadone dose by the remaining third; use a short-acting opioid or methadone for rescue

Protocol 2—Conservative Approach

- Start a fixed dose of methadone, 5 or 10 mg, orally q8h for 4–7 d
- Increase the dose by 50% in case of inadequate pain control and continue for another 4–7 d
- Continue increasing the methadone dose by 50% every 4–7 d until pain is relieved
- For rescue, use a short-acting oral opioid every 1 h as needed

Protocol 3—For Patients on Higher Doses of Opioids (>600 mg oral morphine equivalents/d)

- Stop the original opioid
- Start methadone at a dose of 5–10 mg orally every 4 h, with rescue doses of 5–10 mg every hour allowed as needed
- After 2–3 d, increase the methadone dose by approximately 30% every 4 h
- After 3 d following the switch to methadone, the dose is changed from every 4 h to every 8 h; the rescue doses are administered every 3 h, as needed, at the same single dose as established on days 2 and 3
- The dose can then be increased by up to 30% if further upward titration is required

Protocol 4—For Opioid-Naive Patients or Those on Lower Doses

- Start methadone at 3–5 mg every 8 h if the patient is opioid naive or at a dose equivalent to 50% of the daily morphine dose
- Continue for 3 d
- When the patient has pain relief for 6–8 h, change the dose to once daily and allow rescue doses as needed

Note: These are just a few of the many methods for conversion to methadone that have been recommended. Clinicians are advised to carefully assess patients for any signs of sedation; if these appear, reduce or stop the dose of methadone. If at all possible, avoid adding or discontinuing any other medications during conversion or dose escalation, particularly those metabolized by CYP3A4 because these may alter plasma methadone levels.

(39,40). This was confirmed in a prospective study of cancer patients receiving methadone that revealed elevated QTc to be common at baseline and that elevations beyond 500 milliseconds after initiating therapy were rare (41).

Patients currently on methadone as part of a maintenance program for addictive disease will have developed cross-tolerance to the opioids and, as a result, will require higher doses than naive patients when the drug is used for pain control (42). Prescribing methadone for addictive disease requires a special license in the United States. As a result, prescriptions provided for methadone to manage pain in palliative care should include the statement "for pain."

Morphine. In the past, morphine was considered the "gold standard." We now recognize that because of the wide variability in response, the most appropriate opioid is the agent that works for a particular patient. Morphine is a useful compound for many patients, in that there are a wide range of formulations and routes available for its use (43,44). Initial adverse effects are similar to all other opioids, including sedation and nausea that should be anticipated and treated appropriately. These generally resolve within a few days (45). Long-term effects, such as constipation, should be prevented. An active metabolite of morphine, M3G, may contribute to myoclonus, seizures, and hyperalgesia (increasing pain), particularly when clearance is impaired because of renal impairment (6,16,46). In differentiating adverse effects and metabolic effects, the time course of onset should be determined. Adverse effects generally occur soon after the drug has been absorbed, whereas metabolite-induced effects are generally delayed by several days. When adverse effects do not respond to appropriate management, conversion to an equianalgesic dose of a different opioid is recommended.

TABLE 2.5 Agents used in palliative care that may interact with methadone	
Inhibitors of CYP3A4 (May Increase Serum Methadone Levels)	Inducers of CYP3A4 (May Lower Serum Methadone Levels)
Amiodarone	Carbamazepine
Aprepitant	Dexamethasone
Clarithromycin	Efavirenz
Cimetidine	Ethanol (acute use)
Ciprofloxacin	Isoniazid
Delavirdine	Lopinavir
Diazepam	Nevirapine
Dihydroergotamine	Oxcarbazepine
Diltiazem	Pentobarbital
Disulfiram	Phenobarbital
Erythromycin	Phenytoin
Ethanol (chronic use)	Rifampin
Fluconazole	Risperidone
Fluoxetine	Spironolactone
Haloperidol	St. John's wort
Ketoconazole	Topiramate
Nicardipine	
Norfloxacin	
Omeprazole	
Paroxetine	
Thioridazine	
Venlafaxine	
Verapamil	

Oxycodone. Oxycodone is a synthetic opioid available in a long-acting formulation, as well as immediate-release tablets (alone or with acetaminophen) and liquid. A recent systematic review found the equianalgesic ratio between morphine and oxycodone to be 1.5:1 (47). Metabolites of oxycodone include noroxycodone and oxymorphone. In addition to binding to the MOR, oxycodone binds to the KOR. Side effects appear to be similar to those experienced with morphine. One study comparing these two long-acting formulations in persons with advanced cancer found that oxycodone produced less nausea and vomiting; however, a recent systematic review found no difference between these agents (48,49).

Oxymorphone. Oxymorphone is a semisynthetic derivative of morphine that is available in the United States as both long-acting and immediate-release oral formulations, as well as a parenteral solution and a rectal suppository (50). Oxymorphone is thought to be twice as potent as morphine,

and it does not appear to induce or inhibit the CYP2D6 or CYP3A4 enzyme pathways (51,52). The prevalence of adverse effects appears to be similar to other opioids (53).

Tapentadol. Tapentadol is a new opioid that binds to the MOR and inhibits norepinephrine reuptake. In clinical trials, there appear to be fewer gastrointestinal adverse effects when compared with oxycodone (54,55).

Tramadol. Tramadol is a synthetic analog of codeine that binds to the MOR and blocks the reuptake of serotonin and norepinephrine. As a result of the monoamine action, naloxone will not completely reverse respiratory depression. Furthermore, because of the inhibited reuptake of monoamines, the use of tramadol should be avoided in patients on serotonin selective reuptake inhibitors or tricyclic antidepressants. Tramadol is thought to be approximately one-tenth as potent as morphine in patients with cancer (56). Analgesia may be reduced in poor metabolizers of CYP2D6 (56). Individuals on higher doses of tramadol or who have a history of seizures may be at increased risk for seizures. The ceiling dose of tramadol is 400 mg/d. Both long-acting and immediate-release products are available. In a double-blind study of tramadol in cancer patients, adverse effects, including vomiting, dizziness, and weakness, were more likely when compared with hydrocodone and codeine (57).

Other Opioids. Meperidine is not recommended in palliative care or cancer pain management because of the neurotoxic effects of its metabolite, normeperidine. Levorphanol is an analog of morphine that binds to MOR, KOR, and DOR; is an antagonist at NMDA receptors; and is a monoamine reuptake inhibitor. It is not widely used, in part because of limited availability.

Partial Agonists

Case reports and open-label trials suggest that transdermal buprenorphine, a partial agonist, is useful in cancer pain (58). Additionally, a randomized placebo-controlled study in patients with cancer pain revealed an analysis effect of this therapy (59). However, breakthrough medication consisted of sublingual buprenorphine, a product not commercially available in the United States. A recent consensus panel endorsed its use for cancer pain (60), and a small open-label study's suggestion of using i.v. morphine for breakthrough pain did not alter the analgesic effects of the transdermal buprenorphine (61). The interaction of pure and partial opioid agonists may lead to reduced analgesia. Furthermore, studies of buprenorphine suggest that there is a ceiling effect for analgesia, limiting the efficacy of this agent in palliative care (62).

Mixed Agonist–Antagonists

Mixed agonist–antagonist opioid analgesics, including butorphanol, nalbuphine, and pentazocine, exhibit a ceiling effect for analgesia, are more likely to cause psychotomimetic effects, and can precipitate the abstinence syndrome if given to a patient physically dependent on a pure opioid agonist (63). As a result, these agents are not recommended in cancer pain management.

Antagonists

Opioid antagonists, such as parenteral naloxone, have been used to reverse acute adverse effects, primarily respiratory depression, caused by opioids. Oral naloxone has been described as being effective in relieving opioid-induced constipation, although one must use bad-tasting solutions intended for parenteral administration (64). Furthermore, higher doses, up to 8 to 12 mg, can reverse analgesia. Agents such as methylnaltrexone act peripherally to block opioid receptor binding within the gastrointestinal tract and will be discussed in *Constipation* (65).

Definitions

Misconceptions about terms such as tolerance, physical dependence, and addiction contribute to inadequate management of pain (Table 2.6). Education of professionals,

TABLE 2.6	Definitions associated with opioids (66,67)
Addiction	
Addiction is a primary, chronic, neurobiologic disease, with genetic, psychosocial, and environmental factors influencing its development and manifestations. It is characterized by behaviors that include one or more of the following: impaired control over drug use, compulsive use, continued use despite harm, and craving	
Physical Dependence	
Physical dependence is a state of adaptation that is manifested by a drug class–specific withdrawal syndrome that can be produced by abrupt cessation, rapid dose reduction, decreased blood level of the drug, and/or administration of an antagonist	
Tolerance	
Tolerance is a state of adaptation in which exposure to a drug induces changes that result in a diminution of one or more of the drug's effects over time	
Pseudoaddiction	
Pseudoaddiction is the mistaken assumption of addiction in a patient who is seeking relief from pain	
Pseudotolerance	
Pseudotolerance is the misconception that the need for increasing doses of drug is due to tolerance rather than disease progression or other factors	

patients, family members, and the public is needed to overcome the many misconceptions and biases that limit the effective use of this class of analgesics (68). See Chapter 44 for specific information on substance abuse issues in palliative care.

Routes of Opioid Administration

Numerous routes of opioid administration that are of particular benefit in palliative care are available. In a study of patients with cancer at 4 weeks, 1 week, and 24 hours before death, the oral route of opioid administration was continued in 62%, 43%, and 20% of patients, respectively (69). When oral delivery is no longer useful, many alternative routes exist. Sublingual, buccal, rectal, transdermal (including iontophoretic), s.c., intramuscular (i.m.), i.v., pulmonary, nasal, spinal, and peripheral (topical) routes of administration have all been described. However, the fact that a drug can be administered by a particular route does not imply that it is effective. Lipid solubility and the size of the molecule influence the transport of the opioid across biological membranes, affecting the pharmacokinetics of the agent. The unique clinical challenge of caring for a person unable to swallow because of anatomic abnormalities or loss of consciousness at the end of life leads to the desire to find alternative routes. Yet, the attributes of the compound must first be considered.

Oral, Sublingual, and Buccal

Numerous options are available when patients are able to swallow tablets or pills, including immediate-release or long-acting tablets, as well as liquids. Morphine's bitter taste may be prohibitive, especially if immediate-release tablets are left in the mouth to dissolve if the patient cannot normally swallow. For patients with dysphagia, several options are available. The 24-hour, long-acting morphine capsule can be broken open and the "sprinkles" placed in applesauce or other soft foods. Oral morphine solution can be swallowed or small volumes (0.5 to 1 mL) of a concentrated solution (e.g., 20 mg/mL) can be placed sublingually or buccally in patients whose voluntary swallowing capabilities are more significantly limited (70). However, buccal or sublingual uptake of morphine is slow and not very predictable because of its hydrophilic chemical nature (71). In fact, most of the analgesic effect of morphine administered in this manner is due to the drug trickling down the throat and the resultant absorption through the gastrointestinal tract. Topical morphine mouthwash has been studied to treat chemotherapy-induced oral mucositis (72).

Enteral and Rectal

If already in place, enteral feeding tubes can be used to access the gut when patients can no longer swallow opioids. The size of the tube should be considered when placing long-acting morphine "sprinkles" to avoid obstruction of the tube. The rectal, stomal, or vaginal route can be used to administer medication when oral delivery is unreasonable. Commercially prepared suppositories, compounded suppositories, or microenemas can be used to deliver the drug into the rectum or stoma. Sustained-release morphine tablets have been used rectally, with resultant delayed time to peak plasma level and approximately 90% of the bioavailability being achieved by oral administration (73). Rectal methadone has a bioavailability approximately equal to that of oral methadone (29). Thrombocytopenia or painful lesions preclude the use of these routes. Additionally, delivering medications through these routes can be difficult for family members, especially when the patient is obtunded or unable to assist in turning.

Oral Transmucosal

Oral transmucosal fentanyl citrate (OTFC) is composed of fentanyl on an applicator that patients rub against the oral mucosa for rapid absorption of the drug (74). Clinicians must be aware that, unlike other breakthrough pain drugs, the around-the-clock dose of opioid does not predict the effective dose of OTFC. Patients should use OTFC for over a period of 15 minutes, because too rapid use will result in more of the agent being swallowed rather than being absorbed transmucosally. Fentanyl buccal soluble film and buccal tablets are also available (75–77). Pain relief can usually be expected to be more rapid when compared with immediate-release morphine.

Nasal

Nasal fentanyl, hydromorphone, and morphine have been investigated (23,78,79). A fentanyl nasal spray for breakthrough cancer pain was recently approved in the United States (80).

Parenteral

Parenteral administration includes both s.c. and i.v. delivery, routes that are frequently used in palliative care when other methods are ineffective (43). Intramuscular opioid delivery is inappropriate in the palliative care setting because of the pain associated with this route and the variability in systemic uptake of the drug (63). The i.v. route provides rapid drug delivery, but it requires vascular access. Subcutaneous boluses have a slower onset and a lower peak effect when compared with i.v. boluses (81), although continuous infusions are equianalgesic (68,82). Subcutaneous infusions may include rates of up to 10 mL/h (83) (although most patients absorb 2 to 3 mL/h with least difficulty). Volumes of s.c. drug delivery greater than these are poorly absorbed.

Spinal (Epidural/Intrathecal)

Intraspinal routes, including epidural and intrathecal delivery, may allow administration of drugs, such as opioids, local anesthetics, and/or α-adrenergic agonists, in palliative care settings (84). A randomized, controlled trial demonstrated benefit for patients with cancer who experience pain (85). One must consider the complexity of the equipment used to deliver these medications and the potential caregiver burden. Additionally, not all centers have healthcare professionals on staff with the specialized knowledge to provide these therapies. Finally, cost is a significant concern related to high-tech procedures.

Intraspinal delivery should be considered when patients experience intolerable adverse effects to opioids and other analgesics, despite aggressive management. Additionally, patients who do not obtain adequate relief from aggressive titration of systemic opioids and other analgesics should be considered for intraspinal drug administration (86). When systemic opioids are relatively ineffective, this suggests the need for the addition of a local anesthetic, such as bupivacaine, to the infusion. Additionally, pain that is bilateral or midline and is not responsive to systemic analgesics might best be treated with intraspinal drug administration because nerve blocks or other ablative procedures are generally not indicated in these circumstances.

Spinal Delivery Systems. Percutaneous catheters attached to an external infusion device can be used to deliver medications through the epidural or intrathecal space. Patients with a longer life span would likely benefit from a more permanent catheter that is tunneled to reduce the risk of infection. Dislodgement and infection are the most common complications. Subcutaneous ports, similar to those used to access the venous system, can be implanted and are approved for epidural delivery. Although technically an implanted system, the port must be constantly accessed with a deflected tip needle to allow continuous infusions by an external pump. Implanted pumps are battery driven and programmable, allowing more precise delivery of the drug. There is a potential for reduced risk of infection because the pump is entirely implanted. However, they are more expensive and require specially trained staff to refill the device as well as equipment to make programming changes that allow changes in the rate of drug delivery.

Agents Administered Spinally. Opioids given intraspinally typically include morphine, hydromorphone, fentanyl, remifentanil, and sufentanil. The more lipophilic compounds, such as fentanyl, remifentanil, and sufentanil, are likely to be administered epidurally, whereas more hydrophilic agents, including morphine and hydromorphone, are delivered intrathecally. Adverse effects include those seen with systemic administration of an opioid, with a greater prevalence of pruritus and urinary retention. Local anesthetics are beneficial when treating neuropathic pain, particularly in the pelvis and lower extremities. Clonidine, an α_2-adrenergic agonist, has been shown to be of benefit in providing relief of postoperative, cancer, and labor pain. Hypotension is a potentially dose-limiting adverse effect. The N-specific calcium channel blocker, ziconotide, has been shown to produce analgesia when delivered intrathecally, although the therapeutic window is narrow and adverse effects can be significant.

Topical

Because of the hydrophilic nature of morphine, creams and patches that contain morphine are unlikely to provide analgesia when applied to intact skin. An analysis of the bioavailability of topical morphine gel applied to the intact skin of the wrist, identical to the formulation used in some hospices, revealed no measurable serum levels (87). Controversy exists about whether topical morphine or other opioids might be useful in providing pain relief when applied to open areas, such as burns, pressure ulcers, or skin lesions due to venous stasis or sickle cell disease. Several case reports and open-label trials indicate that this might be an effective route (88–90). However, a randomized controlled trial of topical morphine used to treat painful skin ulcers found no benefit when compared with placebo (91). An analysis of the bioavailability of morphine when delivered to open ulcers found little systemic uptake, a possible explanation for the lack of efficacy (92).

Transdermal

Transdermal fentanyl has been used extensively, and a wide range of dosing options (12.5, 25, 50, 75, and 100 µg-per-hour patches) makes this route particularly useful in palliative care (93). Fever, diaphoresis, cachexia, morbid obesity, and ascites may have a significant impact on the absorption, predictability of blood levels, and clinical effects of transdermal fentanyl, although studies are lacking. There is some suggestion that transdermal fentanyl may produce less constipation when compared with long-acting morphine; yet, the studies demonstrating this effect are small and not sufficiently powered to evaluate this effect (93). A small subset of patients will develop skin irritation because of the adhesive in any patch. Most topical antihistamines have an oil base and would preclude adherence by the patch. Spraying an aqueous steroid inhaler (intended to treat asthma) on the skin and allowing it to dry before applying the patch will often prevent rashes.

A small proportion of patients will experience decreased analgesic effects after only 48 hours of applying a new patch; this should be accommodated by determining whether a higher dose is tolerated with increased duration of the effect or a more frequent (q48h) patch change should be scheduled. As with all long-acting preparations, breakthrough pain medications should be made available to patients using immediate-release opioids.

Adverse Effects

The adverse effects associated with opioids are generally well known, although the underlying mechanism for each of these effects might not be fully articulated. More common adverse effects include constipation, cognitive impairment, nausea and vomiting, and sedation. Less common effects include myoclonus, pruritus, and respiratory depression.

Constipation

Patients in palliative care frequently experience constipation, in part because of opioid therapy. Little data exist on the prevalence of opioid-induced constipation or the symptoms that accompany this phenomenon (e.g., bloating, cramping, early satiety and reflux). There is also no evidence-based consensus on the appropriate management of opioid-induced constipation. A prophylactic bowel regimen should be started when commencing opioid analgesic therapy (94). Bulking or high-fiber agents (e.g., psyllium) are rarely effective and may contribute to worsening constipation, particularly in patients who cannot take in sufficient amounts of fluid. Oil-based products, such as mineral oil, are not indicated, because they prevent the absorption of fat-soluble vitamins and cause incontinence. A daily combination of stimulant laxative and softener (e.g., senna and docusate) titrated upward is generally warranted. Methylnaltrexone, an opioid antagonist that acts at the opioid receptors within the gastrointestinal tract without affecting analgesia, administered subcutaneously is highly effective when constipation is due to opioids (95). See Table 2.7 for a list of agents used to prevent and treat opioid-induced constipation. See Chapter 14 for a complete discussion on the management of constipation.

TABLE 2.7   Opioid-induced constipation

Prevention

Stimulant Laxatives	Stool Softeners
Senna	*Docusate Sodium*
Recommended dose: 0.5–2 g	Recommended dose: 100–300 mg/d
Onset of laxative effect: 6–24 h	Onset to softening: 1–3 d
Bisacodyl	
Recommended dose: 10–30 mg/d oral or 1–2 suppositories	
Combination products include (as well as many generics):	
Peri-Colace—Docusate sodium 100 mg and senna 8.6 mg	
Senokot-S—Docusate sodium 100 mg and senna 8.6 mg	

Management of Preexisting or Intermittent Constipation

Category	Agent and Dose
Methylnaltrexone	.15 mg/kg s.c. every other day
Sugars	Lactulose 15–30 mL orally/d
Saline laxative	Magnesium citrate 1–2 bottles/d
	Milk of magnesia 15–60 mL/d
Osmotic laxative	Polyethylene glycol 17–34 g (1–2 heaping teaspoons in 240–480 mL of water)

- If patients are unable to swallow or too weak to assist in evacuation of the stool, laxative suppositories (such as bisacodyl) are indicated; s.c. methylnaltrexone may be useful when opioids are implicated

- Glycerin suppositories coat the rectal mucosa, providing some pain relief when stools are painful and preventing tissue damage

- For patients with neuromuscular dysfunction affecting the bowel (e.g., spinal cord compression), bowel training may be helpful; this includes preventive agents, along with the use of bisacodyl at the same time each day

- Saline-type enemas (e.g., Fleet) may be indicated if suppositories are ineffective

TABLE 2.8	Management of opioid-induced nausea and vomiting

- Rule out other causes of nausea and vomiting and treat accordingly
  - A. Other medications (antibiotics and anticonvulsants)
  - B. Tumor (increased intracranial pressure)
  - C. Treatment (radiation to thorax or upper abdomen; chemotherapy)
  - D. Bowel obstruction or constipation
- Treat with centrally acting antiemetics
  - A. Butyrophenones
    - i. Haloperidol 0.5–5 mg every 4–6 h orally or 0.5–2 mg every 3–4 h i.v.; fewer adverse effects at lower doses; as effective as phenothiazines
  - B. Phenothiazines
    - i. Trimethobenzamide 300 mg orally every 6–8 h or 200 mg per rectum every 6–8 h
    - ii. Prochlorperazine 5–25 mg orally every 3–4 h or 25 mg per rectum every 6–8 h; side effects may limit routine use
  - C. Prokinetic agents
    - i. Metoclopramide 5–10 mg orally or i.v. every 6 h
- Consider dexamethasone 4–8 mg every day (although optimal dose is unknown)
- If vestibular component to the nausea is present, add cyclizine 25–50 mg every 8 h orally or 25–50 mg per rectum
- Administer antiemetics on a schedule for the first 2–3 d of opioid therapy, then slowly withdraw to determine whether the patient has developed tolerance to this effect
- If these interventions are inadequate, consider opioid rotation

Cognitive Impairment

Anecdotally, patients taking opioids for pain control often report "fuzzy" thinking and an inability to concentrate or perform simple cognitive tasks (such as balancing a checkbook). Few studies have been conducted to explore this phenomenon. A double-blind, crossover, controlled trial of patients on sustained-release opioids for pain control examined cognitive performance and memory after administration of oral immediate-release morphine or placebo. There were significant differences in pain reduction, but little effect on sedation. Interestingly, both transient anterograde and retrograde memory impairment and reduced performance on a complex tracking task were observed in those receiving morphine (96). More studies are needed to fully understand the effects of opioids on cognitive functioning.

Nausea and Vomiting

Nausea and vomiting as a result of initial opioid administration are relatively common because of the activation of the chemoreceptor trigger zone in the medulla, vestibular sensitivity, and delayed gastric emptying. Habituation occurs in most cases within several days. Around-the-clock antiemetic therapy can be effective during this period. If persistent, assess for other causes. Table 2.8 provides recommendations for the management of opioid-induced nausea and vomiting. See Chapter 13 for a thorough discussion on the assessment and treatment of persistent nausea and vomiting.

Sedation

Excessive sedation may occur with the initial doses of opioids. If sedation persists, the use of psychostimulants may be beneficial. Starting doses include dextroamphetamine 2.5 to 5 mg p.o. every morning and midday or methylphenidate 5 to 10 mg p.o. every morning and 2.5 to 5 mg midday (97). Adjust both the dose and the timing to prevent nocturnal insomnia and monitor for undesirable psychotomimetic effects (such as agitation, hallucinations, and irritability). A recent study conducted in patients with cancer allowed "as-needed" dosing of methylphenidate to manage opioid-induced sedation. Doses up to 20 mg/d did not result in sleep disturbances or agitation, although most subjects took doses in the afternoon and evening (98).

Modafinil, an agent approved to manage narcolepsy, has been reported to relieve opioid-induced sedation with once daily dosing (99).

Myoclonus

Myoclonic jerking occurs more commonly with high-dose opioid therapy. Opioid rotation may be useful because metabolite accumulation may be implicated, particularly in case of renal dysfunction (6,37,46). A lower relative dose of the substituted drug may be possible because of incomplete cross-tolerance. Benzodiazepines, such as clonazepam 0.5 to 1 mg p.o. q6-8h, to be increased as needed and tolerated, may be useful in patients who are able to take oral preparations. Lorazepam can be given sublingually if the patient is unable to swallow. Parenteral administration of lorazepam or midazolam may be indicated if symptoms progress. Grand mal seizures associated with high-dose parenteral opioid infusions have been reported, requiring aggressive interventions that include benzodiazepines, barbiturates, and propofol (24).

Pruritus

Pruritus is less common with chronic opioid therapy. When pruritus occurs in the palliative care patient, other etiologies should also be explored. Opioid rotation may be indicated because there appears to be variability in the prevalence of pruritus associated with various opioids (68). Antihistamines (such as diphenhydramine) are the most common first-line approach to this opioid-induced symptom when treatment is indicated, although these agents produce sedation and are rarely totally effective. Ondansetron has been reported to be effective in relieving opioid-induced pruritus, but no randomized controlled studies exist. Chapter 23 provides a thorough review of pruritus.

Respiratory Depression

Respiratory depression is greatly feared, although in palliative care, this occurs rarely because most patients are opioid tolerant. Clinicians and family members often fear "giving the last dose" of an opioid. Existing data suggest a lack of correlation between opioid dose, timing of opioid administration, and patient death (100,101).

When respiratory depression (rate < 8/min and/or hypoxemia [O_2 saturation < 90%]) occurs and the cause is clearly associated with opioid use, cautious and slow titration of naloxone should be instituted. Standard doses of naloxone may cause abrupt opioid reversal with pain and autonomic crisis. Dilute one ampule of naloxone (0.4 mg/mL) in 10 mL of injectable saline (final concentration 40 µg/mL) and inject 1 mL every 2 to 3 minutes while closely monitoring the level of consciousness and respiratory rate. Because the duration of effect of naloxone is approximately 30 minutes, the depressant effects of the opioid will recur at 30 minutes and persist until the plasma levels decline (often 4 or more hours) or until the next dose of naloxone is administered (68). If the patient has been on methadone, an infusion of naloxone may be warranted because of the long half-life of this opioid.

Principles of Opioid Use

Effective pain control requires interdisciplinary care that incorporates a thorough assessment, which informs the development of a multimodal treatment plan. Optimally, the plan includes pharmacologic and nonpharmacologic therapies. Because opioids are the mainstay of this treatment plan, clinicians caring for patients must understand the basic principles of opioid use that build on the information previously presented in this chapter (Table 2.9).

Prevent and Treat Pain

As much as possible, pain should always be prevented and managed aggressively once it occurs. Prevention includes adequate premedication before invasive procedures and also incorporates patient education to take an immediate-release opioid before a painful activity (e.g., bathing and riding in car).

When in the hospital setting, opioids should be ordered around the clock rather than p.r.n. As-needed dosing of an opioid requires the patient to determine when the pain is sufficiently intense to call the nurse. Furthermore, there is great reluctance to "bother" the nurse coupled with a fear of appearing to be "addicted" to the medication. In a study conducted on an inpatient medicine unit, around-the-clock dosing provided significantly lower pain intensity with no increased risk of adverse effects (102).

Use of Long-Acting and Breakthrough Opioids

Long-acting or sustained-release oral opioid preparations allow convenience and are believed to enhance adherence to the treatment. There are a number of formulations currently available in the United States, including once daily morphine, twice daily morphine, twice daily oxycodone, twice daily oxymorphone, and transdermal fentanyl and buprenorphine. Methadone is often included in this list because it can be given every 8 hours. Selection is based on the patient's ability to obtain relief with a particular opioid; the need for an oral, enteral, or transdermal delivery method; support in the home to adhere to a particular regimen; and preference. When using these sustained-release oral formulations, as well as transdermal agents, several principles should be considered:

1. First, titrate with a short-acting product, such as immediate-release morphine, oxycodone, or hydromorphone; then determine the dose that provides relief during a 24-hour period and convert this dose to an equivalent sustained-release opioid.
2. Immediate-release opioids should be available for breakthrough pain, with each dose calculated as approximately

TABLE 2.9	Principles of opioid administration in palliative care

- Screen for pain frequently; conduct a thorough assessment when the patient reports experiencing pain
- Consider symptoms that frequently occur with pain, including fatigue, depression, and others
- Use opioids as part of a multimodal treatment plan that incorporates nonopioids, adjuvant analgesics, cancer therapies when appropriate, nerve blocks, and other ablative procedures as warranted, as well as nonpharmacologic strategies
- Because pain includes physical, emotional, social, spiritual, and other factors, multidisciplinary care is required
- Prevent pain whenever possible
- Prevent and manage opioid-related adverse effects
- Use sustained-release opioids combined with short-acting opioids for rescue doses
  - A. Rescue doses are generally 10–20% of the 24-h sustained-release dose
  - B. Rescue doses for parenteral administration are 50–100% of the hourly i.v. or s.c. rate
- Rotate opioids when unmanageable adverse events occur or when relief is inadequate despite aggressive titration
  - A. Calculate the appropriate dose using an equianalgesic chart
  - B. Reduce the dose by approximately 25–50% to account for cross-tolerance
- Consider patient-related factors when selecting the route of administration
  - A. If the patient has dysphagia, choose transdermal or parenteral delivery
  - B. Determine whether equipment and cost of parenteral or spinal administration will place a hardship on family caregivers
- Educate patients and families about the most effective strategies for using pharmacologic and nonpharmacologic management
  - A. Diaries, flow sheets, and pill boxes will help promote adherence
  - B. Knowing how and when to use p.r.n. medications is particularly difficult for many patients and family members; reinforce this information repeatedly
  - C. Differentiate p.r.n. medications for pain, nausea and vomiting, and anxiety through color-coding or copying pictures of the pills onto a small poster that explains their use
  - D. Consider the patient and family's literacy level when providing any instructional material
- When financial barriers to obtaining opioids exist, explore patient assistance programs
  - A. www.needymeds.com
  - B. www.togetherrxaccess.com
  - C. www.pparx.com
  - D. www.cancer.org/Treatment/index
- Never abruptly discontinue an opioid
  - A. Gradually reduce the dose by approximately 25–50% to prevent distressing symptoms associated with the abstinence syndrome: agitation, sleeplessness, abdominal cramping, diarrhea, lacrimation, yawning, and piloerection

5% to 20% of the 24-hour total sustained-release opioid and administered as frequently as every hour.

3. If the patient consistently requires more than two or three doses of breakthrough medication in a 24-hour period, the total breakthrough dose needed during that time should be added to the sustained-release dose (63).

There is great variability in opioid requirements, so the dose of the opioid necessary to relieve pain is the correct dose for that individual.

Opioid Rotation

When the treatment of opioid-induced adverse effects is not successful, changing to an alternative opioid, also called *opioid rotation* or *switching*, can be useful. Convert the daily dose of the current opioid, such as morphine, to the equivalent dose of an alternate opioid, such as hydromorphone, using equianalgesic tables as a guide. The 24-hour equianalgesic dose is usually reduced by approximately 20% to 25% because of incomplete cross-tolerance and is titrated as needed (63). Ongoing evaluation of the efficacy of any analgesic regimen is essential and doses of drug must be titrated on the basis of the patient's self-report of pain.

Multimodal Therapy

For the complicated pain syndromes often seen in advanced disease, opioids alone are rarely sufficient. Adjuvant analgesics, nonsteroidal anti-inflammatory drugs, and interventional approaches, along with cognitive–behavioral and physical approaches, are warranted (63). See Chapters 2 to 4 for information on other pharmacologic therapies, nonpharmacologic approaches, and interventional procedures for pain control.

CONCLUSION

For most patients with pain associated with cancer or advanced disease, relief is possible through the use of opioids and other therapies. An understanding of opioid pharmacotherapy is a critical component of pain management in those with cancer or other life-threatening illnesses. The evolving field of pharmacogenomics reinforces and informs the clinical observation that all regimens must be individualized to the patient's needs and responses. One envisions a time when screening to determine the optimal response to a particular opioid will be widely available, preventing the trial and error approach currently required.

Although the science of pain mechanisms and opioid pharmacotherapy is advancing rapidly, myths and misperceptions about addiction persist. In fact, there appears to be an even greater fear of addiction as media attention to celebrity addictive disease increases. To address these misunderstandings, patients, family members, and, often, other clinicians need extensive education. Pain in people with life-threatening illness is a serious problem in healthcare that can be addressed only through the combined efforts of scientists, clinicians, regulators, and the public to ensure the availability of opioids to provide relief.

REFERENCES

1. Zimmerman M. The history of pain concepts and treatment before IASP. In: Mersky H, Loeser J, Dubner R, eds. *The Paths of Pain 1975-2005.* Seattle: International Association for the Study of Pain; 2005:1-21.
2. Snyder SH, Pasternak GW. Historical review: opioid receptors. *Trends Pharmacol Sci.* 2003;24(4):198-205.
3. Yaksh TL, Rudy TA. Analgesia mediated by a direct spinal action of narcotics. *Science.* 1976;192(4246):1357-1358.
4. Jensen TS, Yaksh TL. Comparison of antinociceptive action of morphine in the periaqueductal gray, medial and paramedial medulla in rat. *Brain Res.* 1986;363(1):99-113.
5. Jackson KC II. Opioid pharmacokinetics. In: Davis M, Glare P, Hardy J, eds. *Opioids in Cancer Pain.* New York, NY: Oxford University Press; 2005:43-52.
6. Smith MT. Neuroexcitatory effects of morphine and hydromorphone: evidence implicating the 3-glucuronide metabolites. *Clin Exp Pharmacol Physiol.* 2000;27(7):524-528.
7. Thwaites D, McCann S, Broderick P. Hydromorphone neuroexcitation. *J Palliat Med.* 2004;7(4):545-550.
8. Dean M. Opioids in renal failure and dialysis patients. *J Pain Symptom Manage.* 2004;28(5):497-504.
9. Koehntop DE, Rodman JH. Fentanyl pharmacokinetics in patients undergoing renal transplantation. *Pharmacotherapy.* 1997;17(4):746-752.
10. Klepstad P, Dale O, Skorpen F, et al. Genetic variability and clinical efficacy of morphine. *Acta Anaesthesiol Scand.* 2005;49(7):902-908.
11. Pasternak GW. Molecular biology of opioid analgesia. *J Pain Symptom Manage.* 2005;29(suppl 5):S2-S9.
12. Rogers JF, Nafziger AN, Bertino JS Jr. Pharmacogenetics affects dosing, efficacy, and toxicity of cytochrome P450-metabolized drugs. *Am J Med.* 2002;113(9):746-750.
13. Gasche Y, Daali Y, Fathi M, et al. Codeine intoxication associated with ultrarapid CYP2D6 metabolism. [see comment] [erratum appears in *N Engl J Med.* 2005;352(6):638]. *N Engl J Med.* 2004;351(27):2827-2831.
14. Koren G, Cairns J, Chitayat D, Gaedigk A, Feeder SJ. Pharmacokinetics of morphine poisoning in a breastfed neonate of a codeine-prescribed mother. *Lancet.* 2006;38:704.
15. Rakvag TT, Klepstad P, Baar C, et al. The Val158Met polymorphism of the human catechol-*O*-methyltransferase (*COMT*) gene may influence morphine requirements in cancer pain patients. *Pain.* 2005;116(1-2):73-78.
16. Lotsch J. Opioid metabolites. *J Pain Symptom Manage.* 2005;29(suppl 5):S10-S24.
17. Sathyan G, Jaskowiak J, Evashenk M, et al. Characterisation of the pharmacokinetics of the fentanyl HCl patient-controlled transdermal system (PCTS): effect of current magnitude and multiple-day dosing and comparison with IV fentanyl administration. *Clin Pharmacokinet.* 2005;44(suppl 1):7-15.
18. Mystakidou K, Katsouda E, Tsilika E, et al. Transdermal therapeutic fentanyl-system (TTS-F). *In Vivo.* 2004;18(5):633-642.
19. Shibutani K, Inchiosa MA Jr, Sawada K, et al. Pharmacokinetic mass of fentanyl for postoperative analgesia in lean and obese patients. *Br J Anaesth.* 2005;95(3):377-383.
20. Heiskanen T, Matzke S, Haakana S, Gergov M, Vuori E, Kalso E. Transdermal fentanyl in cachectic cancer patients. *Pain.* 2009;144:218-222.
21. Hutchinson MR, Menelaou A, Foster DJR, et al. CYP2D6 and CYP3A4 involvement in the primary oxidative metabolism of hydrocodone by human liver microsomes. *Br J Clin Pharmacol.* 2004;57(3):287-297.
22. Murray A, Hagen NA. Hydromorphone. *J Pain Symptom Manage.* 2005;29(suppl 5):S57-S66.

23. Finn J, Wright J, Fong J, et al. A randomised crossover trial of patient controlled intranasal fentanyl and oral morphine for procedural wound care in adult patients with burns. *Burns.* 2004;30(3):262-268.

24. Golf M, Paice JA, Feulner E, et al. Refractory status epilepticus. *J Palliat Med.* 2004;7(1):85-88.

25. Lee M, Leng M, Cooper R. Measurements of plasma oxycodone, noroxycodone and oxymorphone levels in a patient with bilateral nephrectomy who is undergoing haemodialysis. *Palliat Med.* 2005;19(3):259-260.

26. Benmebarek M, Devaud C, Gex-Fabry M, et al. Effects of grapefruit juice on the pharmacokinetics of the enantiomers of methadone. *Clin Pharmacol Ther.* 2004;76(1):55-63.

27. Nicholson AB. Methadone for cancer pain. *Cochrane Database Syst Rev.* 2004;(2):CD003971, http://gateway.ut.ovid.com/gw2/ovidweb.cgi.

28. Morley JS, Bridson J, Nash TP, et al. Low-dose methadone has an analgesic effect in neuropathic pain: a double-blind randomized controlled crossover trial. *Palliat Med.* 2003;17(7):576-587.

29. Dale O, Sheffels P, Kharasch ED. Bioavailabilities of rectal and oral methadone in healthy subjects. *Br J Clin Pharmacol.* 2004;58(2):156-162.

30. Bruera E, Palmer JL, Bosnjak S, et al. Methadone versus morphine as a first-line strong opioid for cancer pain: a randomized, double-blind study. *J Clin Oncol.* 2004;22(1):185-192.

31. Manfredi PL, Houde RW. Prescribing methadone, a unique analgesic. *J Support Oncol.* 2003;1(3):216-220.

32. Moryl N, Santiago-Palma J, Kornick C, et al. Pitfalls of opioid rotation: substituting another opioid for methadone in patients with cancer pain. *Pain.* 2002;96(3):325-328.

33. Santiago-Palma J, Khojainova N, Kornick C, et al. Intravenous methadone in the management of chronic cancer pain: safe and effective starting doses when substituting methadone for fentanyl. *Cancer.* 2001;92(7):1919-1925.

34. Kharasch ED, Hoffer C, Whittington D, et al. Role of hepatic and intestinal cytochrome P450 3A and 2B6 in the metabolism, disposition, and miotic effects of methadone. *Clin Pharmacol Ther.* 2004;76(3):250-269.

35. Wang J-S, DeVane CL. Involvement of CYP3A4, CYP2C8, and CYP2D6 in the metabolism of (*R*)- and (*S*)-methadone in vitro. *Drug Metab Dispos.* 2003;31(6):742-747.

36. Ferrari A, Coccia CPR, Bertolini A, et al. Methadone—metabolism, pharmacokinetics and interactions. *Pharmacol Res.* 2004;50(6):551-559.

37. Sarhill N, Davis MP, Walsh D, et al. Methadone-induced myoclonus in advanced cancer. *Am J Hosp Palliat Care.* 2001;18(1):51-53.

38. Krantz MJ, Kutinsky IB, Robertson AD, et al. Dose-related effects of methadone on QT prolongation in a series of patients with torsade de pointes. *Pharmacotherapy.* 2003;23(6):802-805.

39. Cruciani RA, Sekine R, Homel P, et al. Measurement of QTc in patients receiving chronic methadone therapy. *J Pain Symptom Manage.* 2005;29(4):385-391.

40. Reddy S, Fisch M, Bruera E. Oral methadone for cancer pain: no indication of Q-T interval prolongation or torsades de pointes. *J Pain Symptom Manage.* 2004;28(4):301-303.

41. Reddy S, Hui D, El Osta B, et al. The effect of oral methadone on the QTc interval in advanced cancer patients: a prospective pilot study. *J Palliat Med.* 2010;13:33-38.

42. Peles E, Schreiber S, Gordon J, et al. Significantly higher methadone dose for methadone maintenance treatment (MMT) patients with chronic pain. *Pain.* 2005;113(3):340-346.

43. Mercadante S. Intravenous morphine for management of cancer pain. *Lancet Oncol.* 2010;11:484-489.

44. Swarm R, Abernethy AP, Anghelescu KL, et al. Adult cancer pain. *J Natl Compr Canc Netw.* 2010;8:1046-1086.

45. Hanks GW, Conno F, Cherny N, et al. Morphine and alternative opioids in cancer pain: the EAPC recommendations. *Br J Cancer,* 2001;84(5):587-593.

46. Andersen G, Jensen NH, Christrup L, et al. Pain, sedation and morphine metabolism in cancer patients during long-term treatment with sustained-release morphine. *Palliat Med.* 2002;16(2):107-114.

47. Mercadante S, Caraceni A. Conversion ratios for opioid switching in the treatment of cancer pain: a systematic review. *Palliat Med.* 2011;5:504-515.

48. Lauretti GR, Oliveira GM, Pereira NL. Comparison of sustained-release morphine with sustained-release oxycodone in advanced cancer patients. [see comment]. *Br J Cancer.* 2003;89(11):2027-2030.

49. King SJ, Reid C, Forbes K, Hanks G. A systematic review of oxycodone in the management of cancer pain. *Palliat Med.* 2011;5:454-470.

50. Gabrail NY, Dvergsten C, Ahdieh H. Establishing the dosage equivalency of oxymorphone extended release and oxycodone controlled release in patients with cancer pain: a randomized controlled study. *Curr Med Res Opin.* 2004;20(6):911-918.

51. Sloan P. Review of oral oxymorphone in the management of pain. *Ther Clin Risk Manag.* 2008;4:777-787.

52. Adams M, Pieniaszek HJ Jr, Gammaitoni AR, Ahdieh H. Oxymorphone extended release does not affect CYP2C9 or CYP3A4 metabolic pathways. *J Clin Pharmacol.* 2005;45:337-345.

53. Prommer E. Oxymorphone: a review. *Support Care Cancer.* 2006;14:109-115.

54. Prommer EE. Tapentadol: an initial analysis. *J Opioid Manag.* 2010;6:223-226.

55. Wade WE, Spruill WJ, Tapentadol hydrochloride: a centrally acting oral analgesic. *Clin Ther.* 2009;31:2804-2818.

56. Grond S, Sablotzki A. Clinical pharmacology of tramadol. *Clin Pharmacokinet.* 2004;43(13):879-923.

57. Rodriguez RF, Bravo LE, Castro F, et al. Incidence of weak opioids adverse events in the management of cancer pain: a double blind comparative trial. *J Palliat Med.* 2007;10:56-60.

58. Muriel C, Failde I, Mico JA, et al. Effectiveness and tolerability of the buprenorphine transdermal system in patients with moderate to severe chronic pain: a multicenter, open-label, uncontrolled, prospective, observational clinical study. *Clin Ther.* 2005;27(4):451-462.

59. Sittl R, Griessinger N, Likar R. Analgesic efficacy and tolerability of transdermal buprenorphine in patients with inadequately controlled chronic pain related to cancer and other disorders: a multicenter, randomized, double-blind, placebo-controlled trial. *Clin Ther.* 2003;25(1):150-168.

60. Pergolizzi JV Jr, Mercadante S, Echaburu AV, et al. The role of transdermal buprenorphine in the treatment of cancer pain: an expert panel consensus. *Curr Med Res Opin.* 2009;25:1517-1528.

61. Mercadante S, Villari P, Ferrera P, et al. Safety and effectiveness of intravenous morphine for episodic breakthrough pain in patients receiving transdermal buprenorphine. *J Pain Symptom Manage.* 2006;32:175-179.

62. Johnson RE, Fudala PJ, Payne R. Buprenorphine: considerations for pain management. *J Pain Symptom Manage.* 2005;29(3):297-326.

63. Miaskowski C, Cleary J, Burney R, et al. *Guideline for the Management of Cancer Pain in Adults and Children.* APS Clinical Practice Guidelines Series No. 3. Glenview, IL: American Pain Society; 2005.

64. Meissner W, Schmidt U, Hartmann M, et al. Oral naloxone reverses opioid-associated constipation. *Pain.* 2000;84(1):105-109.

65. Yuan C-S. Clinical status of methylnaltrexone, a new agent to prevent and manage opioid-induced side effects. *J Support Oncol.* 2004;2(2):111-117; discussion 119-22.

66. American Pain Society Glossary of Pain Terminology. http://www.ampainsoc.org/resources/pain_glossary.htm, accessed July 6, 2012.

67. Weissman DE, Haddox JD. Opioid pseudoaddiction—an iatrogenic syndrome. *Pain.* 1989;36(3):363-366.

68. Miaskowski C, Blair M, Chou R, et al. *Principles of Analgesic Use in the Treatment of Acute Pain and Cancer Pain.* 6th ed. Glenwood, IL: American Pain Society; 2008

69. Coyle N, Adelhardt J, Foley KM, et al. Character of terminal illness in the advanced cancer patient: pain and other symptoms during the last four weeks of life. [comment]. *J Pain Symptom Manage.* 1990;5(2):83-93.

70. Zeppetella G. Sublingual fentanyl citrate for cancer-related breakthrough pain: a pilot study. *Palliat Med.* 2001;15(4):323-328.

71. Weinberg DS, Inturrisi CE, Reidenberg B, et al. Sublingual absorption of selected opioid analgesics. *Clin Pharmacol Ther.* 1988;44(3):335-342.

72. Cerchietti LCA, Navigante AH, Korte MW, et al. Potential utility of the peripheral analgesic properties of morphine in stomatitis-related pain: a pilot study. *Pain.* 2003;105(1-2):265-273.

73. Gourlay GK. Sustained relief of chronic pain. Pharmacokinetics of sustained release morphine. *Clin Pharmacokinet.* 1998;35(3):173-190.

74. Hanks GW, Nugent M, Higgs CMB, et al. Oral transmucosal fentanyl citrate in the management of breakthrough pain in cancer: an open, multicentre, dose-titration and long-term use study. *Palliat Med.* 2004;18(8):698-704.

75. Rauck R, North J, Gever LN, et al. Fentanyl buccal soluble film (FBSF) for breakthrough pain in patients with cancer: a randomized, double-blind, placebo-controlled study. *Ann Oncol.* 2010;21:1308-1314.

76. Taylor DR. Fentanyl buccal tablet: rapid relief from breakthrough pain. *Expert Opin Pharmacother.* 2007;8:3043-3051.

77. Vasisht N, Gever LN, Tagarro I, Finn AI. Single-dose pharmacokinetics of fentanyl buccal soluble film. *Pain Med.* 2010;11:1017-1023.

78. Rudy AC, Coda BA, Archer SM, et al. A multiple-dose phase I study of intranasal hydromorphone hydrochloride in healthy volunteers. *Anesth Analg.* 2004;99(5):1379-1386 (table of contents).

79. Fitzgibbon D, Morgan D, Dockter D, et al. Initial pharmacokinetic, safety and efficacy evaluation of nasal morphine gluconate for breakthrough pain in cancer patients. *Pain.* 2003;106(3):309-315.

80. Mercadante S, Radbruch L, Davies A, et al. A comparison of intranasal fentanyl spray with oral transmucosal fentanyl citrate for the treatment of breakthrough cancer pain: an open-label, randomized, crossover trial. *Curr Med Res Opin.* 2009;25:2805-2815.

81. Parsons HA, Shukkoor A, Quan H, et al. Intermittent subcutaneous opioids for the management of cancer pain. *J Palliat Med.* 2008;11:1319-1324.

82. Nelson KA, Glare PA, Walsh D, et al. A prospective, within-patient, crossover study of continuous intravenous and subcutaneous morphine for chronic cancer pain. *J Pain Symptom Manage.* 1997;13(5):262-267.

83. Anderson SL, Shreve ST. Continuous subcutaneous infusion of opiates at end-of-life. *Ann Pharmacother.* 2004;38:1015-1023.

84. Baker L, Lee M, Regnard C, et al. Evolving spinal analgesia practice in palliative care. *Palliat Med.* 2004;18(6):507-515.

85. Coyne PJ, Viswanathan R, Smith TJ. Nebulized fentanyl citrate improves patients' perception of breathing, respiratory rate, and oxygen saturation in dyspnea. *J Pain Symptom Manage.* 2002;23(2):157-160.

86. Myers J, Chan V, Jarvis V, et al. Intraspinal techniques for pain management in cancer patients: a systematic review. *Support Care Cancer.* 2010;18:137-149.

87. Paice JA, Von Roenn JH, Hudgins JC, et al. Morphine bioavailability from a topical gel formulation in volunteers. *J Pain Symptom Manage.* 2008:35:314-320.

88. Zeppetella G, Paul J, Ribeiro MDC. Analgesic efficacy of morphine applied topically to painful ulcers. *J Pain Symptom Manage.* 2003;25(6):555-558.

89. Ballas SK. Treatment of painful sickle cell leg ulcers with topical opioids. *Blood.* 2002;99(3):1096.

90. Long TD, Cathers TA, Twillman R, et al. Morphine-infused silver sulfadiazine (MISS) cream for burn analgesia: a pilot study. *J Burn Care Rehabil.* 2001;22(2):118-123.

91. Vernassiere C, Cornet C, Trechot P, et al. Study to determine the efficacy of topical morphine on painful chronic skin ulcers. *J Wound Care.* 2005;14(6):289-293.

92. Ribeiro MDC, Joel SP, Zeppetella G. The bioavailability of morphine applied topically to cutaneous ulcers. *J Pain Symptom Manage.* 2004;27(5):434-439.

93. Muijsers RB, Wagstaff AJ. Transdermal fentanyl: an updated review of its pharmacological properties and therapeutic efficacy in chronic cancer pain control. *Drugs.* 2001;61(15):2289-2307.

94. Ishihrara M, Iihara H, Okayasu S, et al. Pharmaceutical interventions facilitate premedication and prevent opioid-induced constipation and emesis in cancer patients. *Support Care Cancer.* 2010;12:1531-1538.

95. Thomas J, Karver S, Cooney GA, et al. Methylnaltrexone for opioid-induced constipation in advanced illness. *N Eng J Med.* 2008;358:2332-2343.

96. Kamboj SK, Tookman A, Jones L, et al. The effects of immediate-release morphine on cognitive functioning in patients receiving chronic opioid therapy in palliative care. *Pain.* 2005;117(3):388-395.

97. Rozans M, Dreisbach A, Lertora JJL, et al. Palliative uses of methylphenidate in patients with cancer: a review. *J Clin Oncol.* 2002;20(1):335-339.

98. Bruera E, Driver L, Barnes EA, et al. Patient-controlled methylphenidate for the management of fatigue in patients with advanced cancer: a preliminary report. *J Clin Oncol.* 2003;21(23):4439-4443.

99. Webster L, Andrews M, Stoddard G. Modafinil treatment of opioid-induced sedation. *Pain Med.* 2003;4(2):135-140.

100. Sykes N, Thorns A. The use of opioids and sedatives at the end of life. *Lancet Oncol.* 2003;4(5):312-318.

101. Thorns A, Sykes N. Opioid use in last week of life and implications for end-of-life decision-making. *Lancet.* 2000;356(9227):398-399.

102. Paice JA, Noskin GA, Vanagunas A, et al. Efficacy and safety of scheduled dosing of opioid analgesics: a quality improvement study. *J Pain.* 2005;6(10):639-643.

CHAPTER 3

Nonpharmacologic Management of Pain

Gayle L. Byker ■ Dona Leskuski

A recent meta-analysis revealed that 64% of patients with cancer experience pain (1). Medications are currently the mainstay of treatment for cancer pain. Despite internationally accepted guidelines for the medical treatment of cancer pain, the fact remains that patients' symptoms are often inadequately treated (2). In 1986, the World Health Organization developed an analgesic ladder that makes recommendations for the appropriate and effective treatment of cancer pain with the use of nonopioid and opioid analgesic medications in addition to adjuvant medications based on pain intensity and the escalating severity of pain. While this ladder has been the subject of some debate, the concept of a guideline-based approach that emphasizes pharmacologic management of cancer pain has not.

Another approach has been growing in popularity in recent years, namely, nonpharmacologic management of pain as an adjunct or a complement to traditional medication-based treatment. Nonpharmacologic therapies are widely used among cancer patients (3–5). In 2001, the American Cancer Society and the National Comprehensive Cancer Network published cancer pain control guidelines for patients and families that recommend nonpharmacologic modalities for cancer pain as an adjunct to medications (6). The American Pain Society has also developed guidelines for cancer pain management that emphasize the combination of pharmacologic and nonpharmacologic modalities (7).

Numerous nonpharmacologic modalities are employed for the treatment of cancer pain, more than could be adequately described in the context of this chapter. Further, many of these modalities lack a rigorous evidence base for their efficacy (8). Most of the studies that have been performed to date are small and biased. Like conventional medications, nonpharmacologic treatments carry with them the risk of side effects and adverse reactions and should be subject to the same standard of clinical scrutiny.

This chapter focuses on the most widely used and accepted nonpharmacologic interventions for cancer pain. Particular attention will be paid to those modalities for which there is an empirical evidence of efficacy in treating cancer-related pain. Broadly, these modalities fall under the categories of psychosocial and physiatric interventions. Psychosocial interventions can be further conceptualized as self-regulatory approaches, psychoeducation, and cognitive-behavioral therapies (CBTs). More commonly used physiatric approaches fall under the categories of nociceptive modulation and restoration of normal biomechanics. Finally, the chapter highlights promising new directions in the field of nonpharmacologic cancer pain management.

RATIONALE FOR NONPHARMACOLOGIC INTERVENTIONS

In his *Treatise of Man* published in 1664, French philosopher René Descartes described the "pain pathway" as a simple matter of a single neural thread relaying information about a stimulus in the body to the brain (9). Cancer pain specialists now believe the experience of pain to be far more complex. Melzack's neuromatrix theory broadens the concept of a single neural thread to include a neural network that integrates input from somatosensory, limbic, and thalamocortical systems (10,11). The complex experience of pain is therefore understood to reflect the activity of numerous brain inputs. It is thought to be the result of information relayed to the brain not only from peripheral nociception but also from other aspects of sensorimotor, cognitive, and emotional processing (12) (Figure 3.1).

There is a broad and expanding volume of literature on the psychosocial factors that influence the experience of pain. First, psychological distress is known to directly impact the experience of pain (13). Specifically, studies have shown that depression, anxiety, anger, and mood disturbances are correlated with higher levels of perceived cancer-related pain (13,14). Conversely, patients with higher levels of social support report lower levels of cancer pain intensity (15,16).

Additionally, there are numerous coping styles that have been shown to influence the experience of pain. Self-efficacy is the belief that one has the capability to achieve a desired outcome, such as coping with pain. One study revealed that

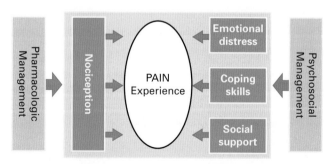

Figure 3.1. The complex experience of pain. (Adapted from Breitbart W, Gibson C. Psychiatric aspects of cancer pain management. *Primary Psychiatry* 2007;14:81-91.)

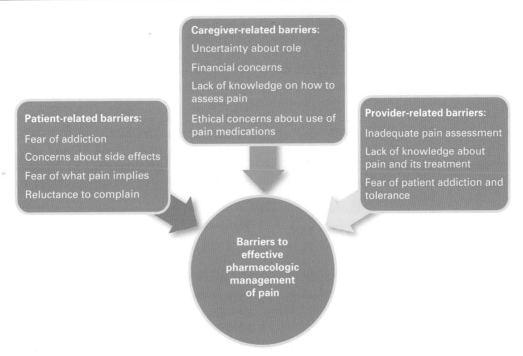

Figure 3.2. Barriers to effective pharmacologic pain management.

self-efficacy is a significant predictor of the development of pain during bone marrow transplantation (17). Passive coping is another psychosocial factor that influences the perceptions of pain. This coping mechanism is characterized by helplessness and uses strategies that relinquish control of pain to others or allow other areas of life to be adversely affected by pain (18). The use of this maladaptive method of coping has been shown to increase the experience of cancer-related pain (19).

Of the various forms of coping that have been studied, pain catastrophizing has proven to be one of the most consistent predictors of pain and disability (20). This method of coping refers to a negative response style characterized by a tendency to ruminate on aspects of the pain experience, to exaggerate the threat value of pain, and to adopt a helpless orientation toward pain (21). A study of 70 patients with gastrointestinal cancer showed that caregivers of patients who catastrophized rated the patient as having significantly more pain and engaging in more pain behaviors than patients who did not engage in catastrophizing (22).

Other important psychosocial factors contributing to the pain experience are the beliefs and attitudes of patients, caregivers, and healthcare providers that function as barriers to effective pharmacologic pain management. Patient-related barriers include fear of addiction, concern about side effects, fear of what pain implies, and reluctance to complain or distract their physicians (23,24). Barriers experienced by caregivers include uncertainty about their role in pain management, financial concerns, lack of knowledge of how to assess pain, and ethical concerns about the use of pain medications (25,26). Healthcare provider–related barriers include inadequate pain assessment, inadequate knowledge about pain and its treatment, and fear of patient addiction and tolerance (27) (Figure 3.2).

Clearly, the experience of pain is affected not only by direct injury to tissue but also by cognitive, emotional, and psychosocial contributions. It stands to reason, therefore, that a pain management approach that includes therapies to address these various dimensions of suffering will more effectively treat the whole patient with cancer who is experiencing pain.

PSYCHOSOCIAL INTERVENTIONS FOR CANCER PAIN

Psychosocial interventions have been shown to lead to improved pain control in patients with cancer-related pain (28). There are several psychosocial approaches that have strong or promising empirical evidence to support their efficacy in treating such patients. These approaches can be grouped into three broad categories: self-regulatory approaches, psychoeducation, and CBTs. All of these modalities can be used safely and effectively in combination with pharmacologic approaches to cancer-related pain treatment.

Self-regulatory Approaches

Relaxation

Relaxation is the central theme running through many self-regulatory techniques employed for pain management in patients with cancer. Relaxation therapies, techniques, and training will be referenced frequently in subsequent sections of this chapter as important components of most self-regulatory approaches, including biofeedback, hypnosis, and CBT. Relaxation focuses on the identification of sources of tension within the mind and body, followed by the practice of systematic methods such as deep or diaphragmatic breathing, progressive muscle relaxation, and visualization or imagery to reduce tension and alter the perception of physical pain (29). It may improve pain symptoms by reducing the physical tension and emotional stressors and by facilitating the ability to become comfortable, rest, and fall asleep (30). Relaxation has been shown to be effective for chronic pain management of a variety of noncancer illnesses, including migraine (31), musculoskeletal pain (32), and low back pain (33).

Studies have repeatedly found relaxation to be one of the most frequently used complementary therapies by cancer survivors (34). A controlled study in hospitalized oncology patients performed in the 1990s examined the efficacy of relaxation techniques involving deep breathing, muscle relaxation, and imagery compared with no relaxation (35). Results showed a significant reduction in subjective pain ratings and in nonopiate, as-needed analgesic intake. Previous studies also support the use of relaxation in the context of hypnosis and imagery as effective adjunctive pain interventions in terminally ill cancer patients (36).

Although the implications for relaxation in treating cancer-related pain are promising, the data remain inconsistent. A recent review found that pain was the primary focus of four efficacy trials of relaxation in cancer patients, with beneficial effects demonstrated in three (30). Samples included inpatients and outpatients with cancer-related pain as well as women with early-stage breast cancer. One study randomized 58 women with breast cancer to practice progressive muscle relaxation or receive massage therapy for 30-minute sessions 3 times a week for 5 weeks (37). The control group received standard treatment. Pain assessments were completed after the first and last sessions. Both the progressive muscle relaxation group and the massage group had significantly lower pain scores after the first and last sessions compared with the standard treatment group.

A second study randomized 57 patients taking opiates for chronic cancer-related pain to relaxation, distraction, positive mood interventions, or wait-list control (38). Patients in the three intervention groups were given audiotapes describing the cognitive-behavioral techniques and written instructions on practicing regularly at home. Patients who practiced relaxation and distraction reported significantly lower pain intensity immediately after listening to the cognitive-behavioral tapes as compared with the control group. The pain reduction was not long-lasting, however, with no significant difference in pain intensity or pain interference found between groups 2 weeks after the intervention.

A third smaller study examined pain in patients with advanced cancer (39). Twenty-four patients were randomized to receive either six electromyography biofeedback-assisted relaxation sessions over a 4-week period or conventional care. They found that relaxation training supplemented with electromyography biofeedback was effective

in reducing cancer-related pain in patients with advanced cancer. They postulated that this pain reduction is achieved through attenuation of physiologic arousal.

The earliest of the four studies, however, found no significant differences in pain between daily relaxation and distraction alone in patients undergoing surgical skin cancer resection (40). Forty-nine patients with skin cancer were randomly assigned to practice relaxation techniques 20 minutes per day prior to surgical excision versus reading a book for 20 minutes a day. There was no significant difference in pain scores between the two groups either before or after skin cancer removal surgery.

Biofeedback

Biofeedback is a process for monitoring physiologic functions such as breathing, heart rate, and blood pressure and then altering that function, most commonly through relaxation therapy. Instrumentation is used to measure and relay information to the patient regarding their vital signs, electroencephalography or brain waves, electromyography or muscle tension, and peripheral skin temperature. Over time and with the guidance of a trained practitioner, the patient learns to control these physiologic functions without the need for instrumentation in order to improve symptoms including pain (41).

A National Institutes of Health Technology Assessment Panel recognized the benefits of biofeedback for the treatment of chronic pain in 1996 (42). Since then a number of studies have shown biofeedback to be effective in the treatment of specific pain syndromes. Biofeedback has been shown to help reduce chronic low back pain, joint pain, headache, and procedural pain (43). A recent large meta-analysis of 94 trials studying biofeedback for migraine and tension headaches found medium to large effect size for all types of biofeedback that remained stable for an average of 15 months (44,45).

A review of the use of mind–body interventions for chronic pain in older adults found that these modalities are feasible and likely safe in older patients (46). Another examination of the use of biofeedback for chronic pain in older adults found ample evidence that older adults respond well to behavioral interventions such as biofeedback (47). Comparisons of older versus younger patients reveal that older patients are as capable as younger patients of readily acquiring the physiologic self-regulation skills taught in biofeedback-assisted relaxation training. In fact, one study comparing 58 older and 59 younger patients found that older participants achieved increases in skin temperature and decreases in respiration rate that were similar to those of younger participants, using the same training protocol and an equal number of training sessions (47). Older patients also reported a significantly greater decrease in current and maximum pain scores compared with their younger counterparts.

The body of evidence supporting biofeedback specifically for the treatment of cancer-related pain is still small. A randomized controlled trial referenced earlier in this chapter studied the effect of electromyography biofeedback-assisted relaxation in cancer-related pain in patients with advanced cancer (39). Results showed that patients in the treatment arm had significantly lower pain intensity scores than those receiving conventional care. Patients receiving biofeedback had a pain score reduction of 2.29 points from baseline on the 0 to 10 Brief Pain Inventory scale, which was statistically significant when compared with the control group. Sixty-seven percent of patients in the study groups reported a reduction of at least 30% in pain intensity from baseline and 50% obtained a reduction of at least 50% in pain intensity from baseline. In contrast, patients in the control arm reported an average increase of 14% in pain intensity from baseline.

An earlier analysis of the biofeedback literature suggested that the improvement in pain with biofeedback is confounded by the use of relation techniques in order to achieve the desired alterations of physiologic functions (48). In fact, relaxation techniques are usually an integral component of biofeedback training, and whether biofeedback can independently improve pain without relaxation may be difficult to examine.

Hypnosis and Imagery

Hypnosis is the induction of a deeply relaxed state, with increased suggestibility and suspension of critical faculties (49). Once in this state of heightened and focused concentration, known as a hypnotic trance, patients can be given therapeutic suggestions to change their perception of pain (14). One study demonstrated that the hypnotic effects on postsurgical pain are mediated in part by response expectancies and emotional distress (50). The efficacy of hypnosis has been well established for procedural pain (51,52), anticipatory nausea and vomiting (53), and various types of chronic pain (54–56).

Hypnosis for cancer-related pain has also become the subject of considerable research. A study published in 1983 by Spiegel and Bloom randomized 58 patients with metastatic breast cancer to group therapy with or without imagery-guided hypnosis and found that women receiving hypnosis experienced significantly less pain sensation and suffering than the control group (57). There was no difference in pain frequency or duration. In two studies in the early 1990s, Syrjala et al. found that hypnosis with guided imagery improved mucositis pain associated with bone marrow transplantation (36,58). Additionally, the National Institutes of Health Technology Assessment Panel found a strong evidence for hypnosis in alleviating cancer-related pain (42).

Hypnosis and imagery have an established role in the management of acute procedural pain in patients with cancer, particularly in pediatric patients. Liossi et al. examined venipuncture-induced pain in children with cancer in the age group of 6 to 16 (59). Forty-five pediatric patients were randomized to receive local anesthetic, local anesthetic plus hypnosis, or local anesthetic plus attention. Patients receiving local anesthetic plus hypnosis reported significantly less procedure-related pain and demonstrated less behavioral distress during the procedure than patients in the other two groups. The same group of researchers performed two trials examining hypnosis in pediatric cancer patients undergoing

lumbar puncture for hematologic malignancies and obtained similar results (60,61).

In a study of adult patients with cancer, Montgomery et al. randomized 200 women undergoing excisional breast biopsy or lumpectomy to a 15-minute presurgical hypnosis session with a psychologist versus nondirective empathic listening prior to surgery (62). On a scale of 0 to 100, women in the hypnosis group reported significantly less pain intensity (mean of 22.43 versus 47.83), less pain unpleasantness (mean of 21.19 versus 39.05), and less discomfort (mean of 23.01 versus 43.20) compared with control. Hypnosis patients also required significantly less propofol and lidocaine than patients who did not receive hypnosis.

Elkins et al. conducted a prospective randomized study of 39 patients with advanced stage cancer and malignant bone disease (63). Patients were randomized to receive either supportive attention or weekly hypnosis sessions followed by instructions and audiotapes for self-hypnosis. All participants received four individual sessions and rated their pain pre- and post-session. Patients who received the hypnosis intervention demonstrated a significant decrease in pain compared with those receiving supportive attention. There was a significant reduction in post-session pain by the second session which remained significant across all remaining sessions.

Overall, hypnosis is effective in alleviating pain in patients with cancer, particularly those undergoing brief procedures and bone marrow transplantation. When practiced by experienced hypnotherapists, hypnosis can serve an important role in the nonpharmacologic management of cancer pain.

Psychoeducation

Education programs are among the most common methods of addressing barriers to cancer pain management (64). This intervention, which is intended to improve knowledge and attitudes about cancer pain and analgesia, has been extensively researched (65). Pain education is provided to patients, their caregivers, or both and consists of a variety of methods, including didactic or coaching sessions, role modeling, and audio, video, and written material. In a series of papers, de Wit et al. reported on the effectiveness of a tailored pain education program, which included education about basic principles of pain and pain treatment, instruction in the use of a pain diary, instruction in simple nonpharmacologic pain management techniques, as well as encouragement to contact healthcare providers to talk about the pain experience (66–69).

Patient Education

There is a substantial body of literature in the area of patient education for cancer-related pain. A recent meta-analysis quantified the benefit of patient-based educational interventions in the management of cancer pain (70). Twenty-one controlled trials (19 randomized) totaling 3,501 patients were examined, with 15 included in the meta-analysis. Compared with usual care or control, educational interventions reduced average pain intensity by more than 1 point on a 0 to 10 scale and reduced worst pain intensity by just under 1 point. There was no significant benefit of education on reducing interference with daily activities.

A recent randomized controlled study included in the meta-analysis examined 93 patients with cancer-related pain and a life expectancy of less than 6 months (71). Patients were randomized to control or to watching an educational video followed by a 20-minute manual, standardized training session with an oncology nurse. Assessments of Brief Pain Inventory, opioid use, barriers to pain relief, and physician and nurse ratings of patient pain were made prior to the training session and 1, 3, and 6 months post-training. Compared with the control group, trained patients reported significantly reduced barriers to pain relief, lower usual pain, and interestingly, greater opioid use. Also notable was the fact that physician and nurse ratings were significantly closer to patient ratings of pain for trained versus control groups.

Another study included 64 outpatients with cancer treated by radiation therapy (72). Patients were randomly assigned either to a clinical intervention arm that included an information session, the use of a pain diary, and the possibility to contact a physician to adjust pain medications or to a control arm involving the usual treatment of pain by the staff radiation oncologist. Patients reported their average and worst pain levels prior to the information session and 2 and 3 weeks after intervention. After 3 weeks, the clinical intervention group reported significantly less average pain than the control group (2.9/10 versus 4.4/10) and less worst pain than the control group (4.2/10 versus 5.5/10).

Caregiver Education

Caregivers of patients with cancer experience significant psychological distress (73), particularly those who care for patients with cancer-related pain (74). There are few studies examining the efficacy of caregiver pain education. One study of 50 caregivers of patients with cancer-related pain found that pain education programs improved caregiver knowledge and attitudes regarding pain management (26). More recently, Keefe et al. published a study testing the effects of a caregiver-guided pain management intervention in patients with cancer at end of life (75). Seventy-eight patients with cancer-related pain were randomized to usual care or to caregiver-assisted intervention which integrated educational information about cancer pain with training in three pain-coping skills (relaxation, imagery, and activity pacing). Education was provided by a nurse in the patient's home. Caregivers in the experiment group did show significant improvements in sense of self-efficacy in helping the patient control their pain and they tended to report improvements in their level of caregiver strain. While results indicated a trend toward reported improvement in cancer-related pain for patients in the caregiver-assisted intervention group, this finding was not statistically significant.

Cognitive-Behavioral Therapy

CBT is an empirically supported psychotherapeutic treatment whose purpose is to help individuals improve or resolve their maladaptive emotions, thoughts, and behaviors through a goal-oriented, systematic procedure (29). The theory behind CBT is that what an individual thinks and believes about his or her symptoms, including thoughts about a symptom's meaning, controllability, and consequences, influence how that symptom is experienced (30). Through systematic counseling, patients learn cognitive strategies and coping skills to change their thoughts and behaviors. Treatment sessions are meant to be interactive and use a combination of instruction, review of home practice, positive reinforcement, guided practice, behavioral rehearsal, and problem solving (64) (Table 3.1).

TABLE 3.1	Cognitive-behavioral pain management protocol	
Session	**Topics**	**Pain Management Goals**
1	Rationale for CBT	
2	Progressive relaxation training	Diverting attention away from pain
3	Guided imagery	
4	Using focal points	Altering activity patterns
5	Activity pacing	
6	Pleasant activity scheduling	Reducing negative pain-related emotions
7	Identifying negative thoughts	
8	Challenging negative thoughts	
9	Goal setting	Applying and maintaining skills in everyday situations
10	Skills maintenance	

CBT, cognitive-behavioral therapy.

Adapted from Keefe FJ, Abernethy AP, Campbell LC. Psychosocial approaches to understanding and treating disease-related pain. *Annu Rev Psychol* 2005;56:601–630.

Numerous studies support the efficacy of CBT for chronic pain. A recent *Cochrane Review* examined the effect of CBT on all types of chronic pain (76). Twenty-three studies of 1,199 patients reported that the effect of CBT on chronic pain reduction was significantly greater than the treatment as usual. And 12 studies with 935 participants found that CBT was effective for chronic pain when compared with active control.

Controlled studies of the effect of CBT on cancer-related pain have only relatively recently been performed. Syrjala et al. conducted some of the first randomized controlled trials comparing CBT with treatment as usual for mucositis pain in patients receiving bone marrow transplantation for hematologic cancers (36,58). Only in the second study did CBT result in lower reported pain than those who did not receive CBT (36). In this study, 94 patients with oral mucositis were randomized to 5 weeks of training in a "package" of cognitive-behavioral copings skills, which included relaxation and imagery, training solely in relaxation and imagery, therapist support, or treatment as usual. Patients who received either relaxation and imagery or the package of cognitive-behavioral coping skills reported significantly less pain than patients who received therapist support or treatment as usual. However, there was no significant additive benefit of the package of cognitive-behavioral skills beyond that of relaxation and imagery alone.

More recent randomized studies of the effect of CBT on cancer-related pain have also shown mixed results. One study of 131 patients with cancer-related pain evaluated the efficacy of a profile-tailored CBT program compared with either standard CBT or usual care (77). CBT patients received five 50-minute treatment sessions. Compared with standard CBT and usual care patients, profile-tailored CBT patients reported significant improvements in worst pain, least pain, and interference of pain with sleep immediately after intervention. However, 6 months after intervention, standard CBT patients had significantly less average pain and current pain than profile-tailored CBT, although both interventions were significantly better than usual care.

A recently published feasibility study investigated a cognitive-behavioral pain management program for cancer patients with chronic treatment-related pain (78). Thirteen patients completed the study which consisted of a combination of interventions, including education, relaxation, exercise training, and goal setting. They found a significant trend toward improvement in many variables, including coping with pain. Vilela et al., however, found no significant difference in pain perception in patients with head and neck cancer using a variant of CBT known as coping skills training (CST) compared with control (79). One hundred and thirty-eight patients were matched either to no intervention or to a short-term psychoeducational coping strategies program. After 3 to 4 months, the intervention group had improved physical and social functioning, quality of life, fatigue, sleep disturbance, and depressive symptoms compared with the control group. Reported pain intensity, however, did not differ between the two groups.

PHYSIATRIC AND BODY-BASED INTERVENTIONS FOR CANCER PAIN

As this chapter highlights, the experience and treatment of cancer-related pain are complex in nature. An integrated approach, which may include pharmacologic, psychosocial, as well as physiatric and body-based intervention, is often required for effective pain management. Physiatry, or physical medicine and rehabilitation, is a field of medicine that traditionally treats patients with anatomic injuries or deformities with the goal of returning the patient to function. However, the physiatric model can also be employed effectively as a nonpharmacologic means of enhancing pain control in patients with cancer-related pain. Many of the physiatric approaches to pain management have yet to be extensively studied in the specific context of cancer-related pain. However, several of these modalities have been shown to be effective in noncancer-related pain and are becoming more prevalent in the cancer patient population. One category of physiatric intervention that this chapter addresses is nociceptive modulation, which includes the practice of massage, myofascial release, transcutaneous electrical nerve stimulation (TENS), acupuncture, and touch therapy. Other physical or body-based modalities that may be helpful in treating cancer-related pain include restoration or preservation of normal biomechanics, such as with therapeutic exercise as well as the use of adaptive orthotics to allow pain-free mobility and self-care. Special issues of safety and comfort for patients with cancer will also be discussed.

Nociceptive Modulation

Massage Therapy

The National Comprehensive Cancer Network recommends the use of massage in its treatment guidelines for refractory cancer pain (80). Major cancer centers such as Memorial Sloan-Kettering have been using and studying the use of massage for cancer-related pain since the 1990s (81). It is among the most popular complementary therapies used by cancer survivors (31). Massage encompasses a multitude of therapies, each with the goal of calming the patient and promoting the generalized well-being, with different forms having slightly different styles (82). The most commonly used techniques include traditional Swedish massage, Thai massage, shiatsu, myofascial release, reflexology, and manual lymphatic drainage. Experts recommend consulting with a licensed professional massage therapist to determine the best method to utilize for individual patients (82).

Massage is believed to affect pain by reducing muscle tension, improving circulation, promoting general relaxation, and through the nurturing effect of touch (83). A recent review of the literature found four randomized controlled trials that used pain as an outcome for massage in patients with cancer (84). Two studies showed a non-significant trend toward pain improvement in the massage group (85,86). A 10-minute back massage was shown to be an effective short-term nursing intervention for cancer patients, but only for males (87). A second relatively large study of 87 hospitalized cancer patients found that a 10-minute foot massage significantly reduced pain compared with control (88).

A crossover study of 23 inpatients with breast or lung cancer compared foot massage reflexology with usual care (89). Patients with breast cancer reported a significant decrease in pain compared with control. In the largest study to date, Cassileth and Vickers retrospectively examined massage and symptom control in 1,290 inpatients and outpatients with cancer (81). Patients were self- or provider-referred for massage therapy and there was no control. Pre-treatment and post-treatment pain and symptom surveys were completed for a combination of Swedish massage, foot massage, and light touch. Results showed an impressively large reduction in pain for patients who received massage, with a 40.2% mean post-treatment reduction in pain for all patients and 47.8% mean decrease for those with moderate to severe pre-treatment pain.

Although widely considered to be safe, certain considerations and precautions must be taken for the cancer patient. Deep tissue massage should be avoided in cancer patients with coagulopathy (i.e., thrombocytopenia, warfarin, or heparin therapy) due to the risk of bleeding or bruising (90). Therapists should perform only light massage in the area of bony metastasis to avoid fracture. An open wound, rashes, and radiation dermatitis should not be massaged due to the risk of increased pain and infection (82).

Myofascial Release

Myofascial release is a commonly used subtype of massage therapy. The technique is used to restore normal length–tension relationships of muscles and fascia. The capacity of hypertonic muscles to function as pain generators is well established (91). The potential contribution of contracted fascia to musculoskeletal pain is less understood.

Fascia occurs ubiquitously throughout the body's supporting muscles, joints, and viscera. It is densely innervated with nociceptors and can therefore serve as an independent pain generator. Ideally, fascia moves freely in synchrony with the motion of muscles and joints. Many conditions that are associated with cancer can produce fascial contractures. Examples include radiation fibrosis, immobility, postsurgical scarring, and pain-engendered muscle spasms. Contracted fascia may become painful at rest or with the minimal tension required by routine daily activities. Fascial release techniques are used to release the contracted fascia. Practitioners use vigorous "hands-on" compression and stretching to alter the mobility of affected tissues. Multiple sessions with a skilled practitioner are generally required. Often fascial contractures must be addressed before patients can tolerate therapeutic exercise or aerobic conditioning. Trigger point release is a type of myofascial release that involves the strategic

application of pressure to discrete foci of increased muscle tone called *trigger points*. Sustained pressure is applied to a circumscribed, symptomatic area in conjunction with passive range of motion.

Transcutaneous Electrical Nerve Stimulation

TENS is the application of electrical stimulation to the skin for purposes of pain control (92). A recent *Cochrane Review* determined that while experts suggest that TENS plays an important role in the treatment of cancer-related pain, there is currently insufficient evidence for or against the use of TENS in the oncology and palliative care setting (93). However, TENS is generally well tolerated without serious side effects and a trial can be considered when pharmacologic and/or procedural approaches fail to control pain.

Acupuncture

The practice of acupuncture has its roots in ancient Chinese traditional medicine. It involves the insertion of very fine sterile needles into the skin at precise locations (acupuncture points) to treat various diseases and symptoms (94). Although the mechanism is not fully understood, acupuncture has been shown to increase the release of calcitonin gene-related peptide, neuropeptide Y, and vasoactive intestinal peptide in saliva during and after treatment (95). MRI studies have shown that acupuncture can induce brain activation in the hypothalamus and nucleus accumbens while also inducing deactivation of the amygdalae and hippocampus (96). There is substantial evidence supporting the use of acupuncture for low back pain (97), dental pain (98), headache (99), and chemotherapy-induced nausea and vomiting (100). Acupuncture should be avoided in patients with severe thrombocytopenia, coagulopathy, or neutropenia due to the risk of bleeding or infection.

Several systematic reviews have recently been conducted to evaluate the efficacy of acupuncture, specifically for cancer-related pain (94,101,102). There are four oft-cited randomized controlled studies examining the effects of acupuncture on pain in patients with cancer (103–106). Most recently, Chen et al. randomized 66 patients with late-stage cancer to receive acupuncture at three to five of their most severe tender points or to receive medication according to the World Health Organization three-step analgesic ladder (103). Acupuncture and medication patients were divided and matched into groups of mild, moderate, and severe pain. Patients in the medication group with mild pain took aspirin, moderate pain took codeine, and severe pain took morphine. While each group achieved significant pain relief, those receiving acupuncture had significantly greater pain relief than those receiving medication (94% versus 87.5%).

Alimi et al. randomized 90 patients with cancer who had neuropathic pain to receive true auricular acupuncture, auricular acupuncture at placebo sites, or auricular seeds implanted at placebo sites (104). After 2 months of treatment, patients receiving true auricular acupuncture reported a decrease in pain intensity of 36% from baseline compared with 2% in the placebo groups. While the two acupuncture groups were blinded to the intervention, neither the acupuncturist nor the auricular seed groups could be randomized.

Touch Therapies

Touch therapies consist of healing touch, therapeutic touch, and Reiki, which are closely related touch-mediated therapies that have considerable overlap in theory and application (107). All of these therapies are based on the principle that the body is a complex energy system that can be affected by another to promote well-being, healing, and symptomatic relief (108). These therapies involve use of a practitioner's hands on or above a patient's body with the intention of promoting physical healing and emotional, mental, and spiritual balance (109). A recent Cochrane systematic review found that all three types of touch therapies have a modest effect in pain relief (110). While the lack of sufficient data made the results inconclusive, the authors assert that the existing evidence supports the use of touch therapies in pain relief.

Post-White et al. assessed healing touch as an intervention for pain in patients receiving chemotherapy (109). Two hundred and thirty patients were randomized to healing touch, massage therapy, or caring presence. Results showed that after 4 weekly sessions, patients receiving either healing touch or massage therapy had significantly lower pain ratings than those receiving caring presence alone. Cook et al. studied 78 women receiving radiation therapy for gynecologic and breast cancer (111). Patients were randomized to either healing touch by a certified provider or mock treatment by someone who had never been trained in or received healing touch. Patients received 6 weekly sessions occurring immediately after radiation treatment. Patients were blinded by a curtain between their head and body. Results revealed a near-significant reduction in pain for women receiving healing touch versus mock touch.

A small study by Olson et al. randomized 24 patients with cancer pain to either standard opioid management plus rest or opioids plus Reiki (112). Participants either rested for 1.5 hours or received two Reiki treatments on days 1 and 4, 1 hour after their first afternoon analgesic dose. Participants receiving Reiki experienced significantly improved pain control on days 1 and 4 following treatment compared with standard opioid management alone. There was no overall reduction in opioid use in either group. Another small study by Tsang et al. compared 16 patients in a crossover study who received multiple Reiki sessions versus rest sessions (113). Comparing pain reports pre-session 1 to post-session 5, patients receiving Reiki indicated significantly lower pain than those who rested.

The results for touch therapies in reducing cancer pain are mixed, however. Frank et al. randomized 82 patients undergoing stereotactic core biopsy of suspicious breast lesions to either therapeutic touch or sham touch during their procedure (114). They found no significant difference in pain outcomes between the two groups.

Restoration and Preservation of Normal Biomechanics

Therapeutic Exercise

While exercise therapy has not been studied specifically for the treatment of cancer-related pain, it is widely used in the treatment of various pain syndromes. Therapeutic exercise has been extensively studied in adults with low back pain and has been found to be slightly effective in treating pain and improving function in this population (115). This modality encompasses a range of interventions, including general physical fitness, aerobic exercise, muscle strengthening, and flexibility and stretching exercises. Unfortunately, patients with advanced cancer are often excluded from exercise therapy due to their degree of infirmity. However, such patients may benefit significantly from conservative, incremental strengthening and conditioning programs despite their precarious health.

Orthotics

Orthotics are braces designed to alter articular mechanics when their integrity is compromised. They may be used therapeutically to provide support, restore normal alignment, protect vulnerable structures, address soft tissue contractures, substitute for weak muscles, or maintain joints in positions of least pain. This latter application can be very helpful as an adjunct in cancer pain, particularly in the case of bone metastases. The use of orthotics for patients with cancer-related pain must always be considered within the framework of patient comfort. For example, a molded body jacket may provide maximal stability for a patient with vertebral metastases; however, the cumbersome nature of these particular devices and the discomfort they sometimes cause may make them inappropriate for patients with advanced cancer. Similarly, orthotics designed to elongate soft tissue contractures related to radiation therapy may cause more short-term physical discomfort than long-term functional benefit.

It is important to refer patients to orthotists or physical medicine and rehabilitative specialists to ensure that they are provided with appropriate orthoses. Since many rehabilitative specialists are not experienced in dealing with patients with cancer-related pain, it is important to communicate the patients' symptom burdens, prognoses, goals of care, and financial constraints. This will help patients to receive the orthoses that best meet their unique needs and pain symptoms (Table 3.2).

FUTURE DIRECTIONS

There appear to be many patients with cancer who might benefit from nonpharmacologic interventions for their pain but are not currently receiving them (64). One barrier to access for these interventions is that patients with cancer who require treatment for their pain may be too sick or immobile to travel to their provider's clinic. In addition, many patients live in rural areas with limited providers or lack the financial

TABLE 3.2	Common orthoses for spinal stabilization in patients with cancer	
Orthotic	**Description**	**Indication for Patients with Cancer**
Cervical Orthoses		
Collars Soft collar	• Constructed of soft foam affording little constriction of neck movement • Functions as reminder to avoid neck movement	• Used in the *absence of instability* for pain and muscle spasm
Rigid collar Philadelphia Newport Miami J California Stiff-neck Malibu	• Constructed of firm Plastazote or polyethylene • Incorporates head through occiput and chin supports • Offers some control of extension, but little limitation of rotation or lateral bending	• For use during soft tissue healing after cement and pin stabilization
Post appliances Two-poster orthosis Three-poster orthosis Sternal occipital mandibular immobilizer	• Constructed of anterior sternal and posterior interscapular plates, and chin and occipital supports connected by rigid anterior–posterior metal struts • Flexion–extension and rotation well controlled • Lateral bending restricted by only 34%	• During radiation if pain and minor instability are present • After bone grafting with fixation
Halo Vest	• Four posts fixed to a vest, rostrally attached to a graphite ring held in place by pins inserted into the skull	• For significant instability of cervical spine after stabilization or grafting • Rarely indicated in malignancy
Minerva	• Total contact device that may offer more rotatory and lateral bending motions • Extends from head to thorax	• For stabilization during radiation or after surgery when greater control of lateral and rotatory cervical movement is required
Thoracolumbosacral Orthoses		
Corsets Lumbosacral Thoracolumbosacral	• Constructed of canvas with posterior rigid or semirigid struts • Laced or Velcro closure • Off-the-shelf availability very convenient • Abdominal constriction may not be tolerated by patients with malignancy	• Provides pain control during radiation in the *absence of instability*
Thoracolumbosacral Braces Jewett	• Prevents flexion • No abdominal apron • Three-point pressure system over sternum, hypogastrum, and lumbar spine • May place excessive hyperextension forces on lumbar vertebrae	• Pain reduction and support for patients with anterior compression fractures, often when conservative measures indicated
Knight Taylor	• Reduces flexion at thoracolumbar junction • Poor restriction of extension and lateral bending • Axillary straps must be very tight for brace to function	• Pain relief for a stable or mildly unstable spine

(Continued)

TABLE 3.2	Common orthoses for spinal stabilization in patients with cancer (*Continued*)	
Body Jacket	• Usually constructed out of polypropylene • Total contact design distributes pressure over wide area • Challenging to take off and on	• Postoperatively after stabilization or for an unstable spine
Lumbosacral Braces		
Chairback Brace	• Controls flexion–extension and lateral motion • Consists of two paraspinal uprights and two uprights in midaxillary line	• May provide relief for mild instability during or after radiation therapy

resources necessary to commute to a provider's clinic. Since the emergence of the Internet, researchers have been investigating approaches to deliver pain management interventions using this virtual avenue. While a number of well-designed studies have been performed examining Internet-delivered treatment for various types of pain, very few have examined this modality specifically for cancer-related pain, making it an exciting direction for future research.

Lorig et al. have conducted a number of studies examining the effects of alternative settings on chronic disease management (116–118). In a randomized controlled trial of 580 patients with chronic back pain, they studied the effects of a closed, moderated email discussion group on pain outcomes (118). Participants also received a book and a videotape about back pain. Patients in the control group received a subscription to a non–health-related magazine of their choice. After 1 year of intervention, patients in the email group reported significant improvements in pain and disability compared with the control group.

Another study examined the feasibility and efficacy of providing online mind–body self-care techniques to 78 older adult patients with chronic pain (119). Patients were randomized to wait-list control versus access to online self-care modules that included exercises in each of the following: abdominal breathing, relaxation, writing about positive experiences, writing about difficult experiences, creative visual expression, and positive thinking. Intervention participants also received supplemental online audio, video, and written materials as well as worksheets to encourage reflection and develop a plan of action. At a 6-week follow-up the online intervention group reported significant improvements in awareness of responses to pain, pain intensity, and pain interference compared with wait-list control. Researchers also found reductions in mean pain scores reported by the intervention group at log on and log off, which suggested an immediate impact of the online modules on pain reduction.

In one of the few studies of cancer-related pain, Kroenke et al. investigated whether centralized telephone-based care coupled with automated symptom monitoring via voice recording or Internet could improve depression and pain in patients with cancer (120). Two hundred and seventy-four participants were randomized to usual care versus intervention, which included regularly scheduled telephonic care management by a nurse care manager as well as automated symptom monitoring using either interactive voice-recorded telephone calls or Internet-based surveys depending on patient preference. Compared with usual care, patients in the intervention group reported significantly lower pain severity and interference at 1, 3, 6, and 12 months.

CONCLUSION

Patients with cancer-related pain are increasingly turning to nonpharmacologic methods as adjuncts to traditional medication-based treatments. Recent theory and research suggest that psychosocial factors play an important role in the experience of pain. As this chapter highlights, randomized clinical trials suggest that interventions designed to address psychosocial factors may benefit many patients with cancer-related pain. Additionally, physiatric and body-based approaches have been shown to be an effective means of nonpharmacologic management for many patients with cancer who suffer from pain. As always, larger studies are needed to further explore the full potential of this field of cancer pain management. Nevertheless, the fact that an evidence base has been established for nonpharmacologic cancer pain management is important and should enhance clinicians' confidence in recommending these interventions to their patients.

REFERENCES

1. van den Beuken-van Everdingen MH, de Rijke JM, Kessels AG, Schouten HC, van Kleef M, Patijn J. Prevalence of pain in patients with cancer: a systematic review of the past 40 years. *Ann Oncol.* 2007;18:1437-1449.
2. Fairchild A. Under-treatment of cancer pain. *Curr Opin Support Palliat Care.* 2010;4:11-15.
3. Ernst E, Cassileth BR. The prevalence of complementary/alternative medicine in cancer: a systematic review. *Cancer.* 1998;83:777-782.
4. Eisenberg DM, Davis RB, Ettner SL, et al. Trends in alternative medicine use in the United States, 1990–1997: results of a follow-up national survey. *JAMA.* 1998;280:1569-1575.

5. Richardson MA, Sanders T, Palmer JL, Greisinger A, Singletary SE. Complementary/alternative medicine use in a comprehensive cancer center and the implications for oncology. *J Clin Oncol.* 2000;18:2505-2514.

6. http://www.cancer.org/Treatment/TreatmentsandSide Effects/PhysicalSideEffects/Pain/PainDiary/pain-control-non-medical-pain-treatments. Accessed September 12, 2011.

7. Gordon DB, Dahl JL, Miaskowski C, et al. American Pain Society recommendations for improving the quality of acute and cancer pain management: American Pain Society Quality of Care Task Force. *Arch Intern Med.* 2005;165: 1574-1580.

8. Bardia A, Barton DL, Prokop LJ, Bauer BA, Moynihan TJ. Efficacy of complementary and alternative medicine therapies in relieving cancer pain: a systematic review. *J Clin Oncol.* 2006;24:5457-5464.

9. Descartes R. *L'homme et un traitté de la formation du foetus du mesme autheur.* Paris: C. Angot; 1664.

10. Melzack R. From the gate to the neuromatrix. *Pain.* 1999; 82(suppl 1):S121-S126.

11. Melzack R, Wall PD. Pain mechanisms: a new theory. *Science.* 1965;150:971-979.

12. Cassileth BR, Keefe FJ. Integrative and behavioral approaches to the treatment of cancer-related neuropathic pain. *Oncologist.* 2010;15(suppl 2):19-23.

13. Zaza C, Baine N. Cancer pain and psychosocial factors: a critical review of the literature. *J Pain Symptom Manage.* 2002;24:526-542.

14. Breitbart W, Gibson C. Psychiatric aspects of cancer pain management. *Primary Psychiatry.* 2007;14:81-91.

15. Ferrell BR, Grant MM, Funk BM, Otis-Green SA, Garcia NJ. Quality of life in breast cancer survivors: implications for developing support services. *Oncol Nurs Forum.* 1998;25:887-895.

16. Koopman C, Hermanson K, Diamond S, Angell K, Spiegel D. Social support, life stress, pain and emotional adjustment to advanced breast cancer. *Psychooncology.* 1998;7:101-111.

17. Syrjala KL, Chapko ME. Evidence for a biopsychosocial model of cancer treatment-related pain. *Pain.* 1995;61:69-79.

18. Snow-Turek AL, Norris MP, Tan G. Active and passive coping strategies in chronic pain patients. *Pain.* 1996;64(3):455-462.

19. Utne I, Miaskowski C, Bjordal K, Paul SM, Jakobsen G, Rustoen T. Differences in the use of pain coping strategies between oncology inpatients with mild vs. moderate to severe pain. *J Pain Symptom Manage.* 2009;38:717-726.

20. Sullivan MJ, Thorn B, Haythornthwaite JA, et al. Theoretical perspectives on the relation between catastrophizing and pain. *Clin J Pain.* 2001;17:52-64.

21. Sullivan MJL, Bishop SR, Pivik J. The pain catastrophizing scale: development and validation. *Psychol Assessment.* 1995; 7:524.

22. Keefe FJ, Lipkus I, Lefebvre JC, et al. The social context of gastrointestinal cancer pain: a preliminary study examining the relation of patient pain catastrophizing to patient perceptions of social support and caregiver stress and negative responses. *Pain.* 2003;103:151-156.

23. Sun V, Borneman T, Koczywas M, et al. Quality of life and barriers to symptom management in colon cancer. *Eur J Oncol Nurs.* 2011;16(3):276-280.

24. Ward SE, Goldberg N, Miller-McCauley V, et al. Patient-related barriers to management of cancer pain. *Pain.* 1993;52:319-324.

25. Berry PE, Ward SE. Barriers to pain management in hospice: a study of family caregivers. *Hosp J.* 1995;10:19-33.

26. Ferrell BR, Grant M, Chan J, Ahn C, Ferrell BA. The impact of cancer pain education on family caregivers of elderly patients. *Oncol Nurs Forum.* 1995;22:1211-1218.

27. Jacobsen R, Sjogren P, Moldrup C, Christrup L. Physician-related barriers to cancer pain management with opioid analgesics: a systematic review. *J Opioid Manag.* 2007;3: 207-214.

28. Abernethy A, Keefe F, McCrory D, Scipio C, Matchar D. *Technology Assessment on the Use of Behavioral Therapies for Treatment of Medical Disorders: Part 2. Impact on Management of Patients with Cancer Pain.* Durham, NC: Duke Center for Clinical Health Policy Research; 2005:1-103.

29. Kerns RD, Sellinger J, Goodin BR. Psychological treatment of chronic pain. *Annu Rev Clin Psychol.* 2011;7:411-434.

30. Kwekkeboom KL, Cherwin CH, Lee JW, Wanta B. Mind–body treatments for the pain–fatigue–sleep disturbance symptom cluster in persons with cancer. *J Pain Symptom Manage.* 2010;39:126-138.

31. Kaushik R, Kaushik RM, Mahajan SK, Rajesh V. Biofeedback assisted diaphragmatic breathing and systematic relaxation versus propranolol in long term prophylaxis of migraine. *Complement Ther Med.* 2005;13:165-174.

32. Middaugh SJ, Woods SE, Kee WG, Harden RN, Peters JR. Biofeedback-assisted relaxation training for the aging chronic pain patient. *Biofeedback Self Regul.* 1991;16:361-377.

33. McCauley JD, Thelen MH, Frank RG, Willard RR, Callen KE. Hypnosis compared to relaxation in the outpatient management of chronic low back pain. *Arch Phys Med Rehabil.* 1983;64:548-552.

34. Bell RM. A review of complementary and alternative medicine practices among cancer survivors. *Clin J Oncol Nurs.* 2010;14:365-370.

35. Sloman R, Brown P, Aldana E, Chee E. The use of relaxation for the promotion of comfort and pain relief in persons with advanced cancer. *Contemp Nurse.* 1994;3:6-12.

36. Syrjala KL, Donaldson GW, Davis MW, Kippes ME, Carr JE. Relaxation and imagery and cognitive-behavioral training reduce pain during cancer treatment: a controlled clinical trial. *Pain.* 1995;63:189-198.

37. Hernandez-Reif M, Field T, Ironson G, et al. Natural killer cells and lymphocytes increase in women with breast cancer following massage therapy. *Int J Neurosci.* 2005;115:495-510.

38. Anderson KO, Cohen MZ, Mendoza TR, Guo H, Harle MT, Cleeland CS. Brief cognitive-behavioral audiotape interventions for cancer-related pain: immediate but not long-term effectiveness. *Cancer.* 2006;107:207-214.

39. Tsai PS, Chen PL, Lai YL, Lee MB, Lin CC. Effects of electromyography biofeedback-assisted relaxation on pain in patients with advanced cancer in a palliative care unit. *Cancer Nurs.* 2007;30:347-353.

40. Domar AD, Noe JM, Benson H. The preoperative use of the relaxation response with ambulatory surgery patients. *Hosp Top.* 1987;65:30-35.

41. http://www.nlm.nih.gov/medlineplus/ency/article/002241. htm. Accessed September 13, 2011.

42. Integration of behavioral and relaxation approaches into the treatment of chronic pain and insomnia. NIH Technology Assessment Panel on Integration of Behavioral and Relaxation Approaches into the Treatment of Chronic Pain and Insomnia. *JAMA.* 1996;276:313-318.

43. Astin JA. Mind–body therapies for the management of pain. *Clin J Pain.* 2004;20:27-32.

44. Nestoriuc Y, Martin A. Efficacy of biofeedback for migraine: a meta-analysis. *Pain.* 2007;128:111-127.

45. Nestoriuc Y, Martin A, Rief W, Andrasik F. Biofeedback treatment for headache disorders: a comprehensive efficacy review. *Appl Psychophysiol Biofeedback.* 2008;33:125-140.

46. Morone NE, Greco CM. Mind–body interventions for chronic pain in older adults: a structured review. *Pain Med.* 2007;8:359-375.

47. Middaugh SJ, Pawlick K. Biofeedback and behavioral treatment of persistent pain in the older adult: a review and a study. *Appl Psychophysiol Biofeedback.* 2002;27:185-202.

48. Burish TG, Jenkins RA. Effectiveness of biofeedback and relaxation training in reducing the side effects of cancer chemotherapy. *Health Psychol.* 1992;11:17-23.

49. Vickers A, Zollman C, Payne DK. Hypnosis and relaxation therapies. *West J Med.* 2001;175:269-272.

50. Montgomery GH, Hallquist MN, Schnur JB, David D, Silverstein JH, Bovbjerg DH. Mediators of a brief hypnosis intervention to control side effects in breast surgery patients: response expectancies and emotional distress. *J Consult Clin Psychol.* 2010;78:80-88.

51. Lang EV, Berbaum KS, Faintuch S, et al. Adjunctive self-hypnotic relaxation for outpatient medical procedures: a prospective randomized trial with women undergoing large core breast biopsy. *Pain.* 2006;126:155-164.

52. Lang EV, Berbaum KS, Pauker SG, et al. Beneficial effects of hypnosis and adverse effects of empathic attention during percutaneous tumor treatment: when being nice does not suffice. *J Vasc Interv Radiol.* 2008;19:897-905.

53. Richardson J, Smith JE, McCall G, Richardson A, Pilkington K, Kirsch I. Hypnosis for nausea and vomiting in cancer chemotherapy: a systematic review of the research evidence. *Eur J Cancer Care (Engl).* 2007;16:402-412.

54. Elkins G, Jensen MP, Patterson DR. Hypnotherapy for the management of chronic pain. *Int J Clin Exp Hypn.* 2007;55:275-287.

55. Jensen M, Patterson DR. Hypnotic treatment of chronic pain. *J Behav Med.* 2006;29:95-124.

56. Patterson DR, Jensen MP. Hypnosis and clinical pain. *Psychol Bull.* 2003;129:495-521.

57. Spiegel D, Bloom JR. Group therapy and hypnosis reduce metastatic breast carcinoma pain. *Psychosom Med.* 1983;45:333-339.

58. Syrjala KL, Cummings C, Donaldson GW. Hypnosis or cognitive behavioral training for the reduction of pain and nausea during cancer treatment: a controlled clinical trial. *Pain.* 1992;48:137-146.

59. Liossi C, White P, Hatira P. A randomized clinical trial of a brief hypnosis intervention to control venepuncture-related pain of paediatric cancer patients. *Pain.* 2009;142:255-263.

60. Liossi C, Hatira P. Clinical hypnosis in the alleviation of procedure-related pain in pediatric oncology patients. *Int J Clin Exp Hypn.* 2003;51:4-28.

61. Liossi C, White P, Hatira P. Randomized clinical trial of local anesthetic versus a combination of local anesthetic with self-hypnosis in the management of pediatric procedure-related pain. *Health Psychol.* 2006;25:307-315.

62. Montgomery GH, Bovbjerg DH, Schnur JB, et al. A randomized clinical trial of a brief hypnosis intervention to control side effects in breast surgery patients. *J Natl Cancer Inst.* 2007;99:1304-1312.

63. Elkins G, Cheung A, Marcus J, Palamara L, Rajab H. Hypnosis to reduce pain in cancer survivors with advanced disease: a prospective study. *J Cancer Integrat Med.* 2004;2:167-172.

64. Keefe FJ, Abernethy AP, Campbell LC. Psychological approaches to understanding and treating disease-related pain. *Annu Rev Psychol.* 2005;56:601-630.

65. Raphael J, Hester J, Ahmedzai S, et al. Cancer pain: part 2: physical, interventional and complimentary therapies; management in the community; acute, treatment-related and complex cancer pain: a perspective from the British Pain Society endorsed by the UK Association of Palliative Medicine and the Royal College of General Practitioners. *Pain Med.* 2010;11:872-896.

66. de Wit R, van Dam F. From hospital to home care: a randomized controlled trial of a Pain Education Programme for cancer patients with chronic pain. *J Adv Nurs.* 2001;36:742-754.

67. de Wit R, van Dam F, Loonstra S, et al. Improving the quality of pain treatment by a tailored pain education programme for cancer patients in chronic pain. *Eur J Pain.* 2001;5:241-256.

68. de Wit R, van Dam F, Loonstra S, et al. The Amsterdam Pain Management Index compared to eight frequently used outcome measures to evaluate the adequacy of pain treatment in cancer patients with chronic pain. *Pain.* 2001;91:339-349.

69. de Wit R, van Dam F, Zandbelt L, et al. A pain education program for chronic cancer pain patients: follow-up results from a randomized controlled trial. *Pain.* 1997;73:55-69.

70. Bennett MI, Bagnall AM, Jose Closs S. How effective are patient-based educational interventions in the management of cancer pain? Systematic review and meta-analysis. *Pain.* 2009;143:192-199.

71. Syrjala KL, Abrams JR, Polissar NL, et al. Patient training in cancer pain management using integrated print and video materials: a multisite randomized controlled trial. *Pain.* 2008;135:175-186.

72. Vallieres I, Aubin M, Blondeau L, Simard S, Giguere A. Effectiveness of a clinical intervention in improving pain control in outpatients with cancer treated by radiation therapy. *Int J Radiat Oncol Biol Phys.* 2006;66:234-237.

73. Northouse LL, Mood D, Templin T, Mellon S, George T. Couples' patterns of adjustment to colon cancer. *Soc Sci Med.* 2000;50:271-284.

74. Miaskowski C, Kragness L, Dibble S, Wallhagen M. Differences in mood states, health status, and caregiver strain between family caregivers of oncology outpatients with and without cancer-related pain. *J Pain Symptom Manage.* 1997;13:138-147.

75. Keefe FJ, Ahles TA, Sutton L, et al. Partner-guided cancer pain management at the end of life: a preliminary study. *J Pain Symptom Manage.* 2005;29:263-272.

76. Eccleston C, Williams AC, Morley S. Psychological therapies for the management of chronic pain (excluding headache) in adults. *Cochrane Database Syst Rev.* 2009;(2):CD007407.

77. Dalton JA, Keefe FJ, Carlson J, Youngblood R. Tailoring cognitive-behavioral treatment for cancer pain. *Pain Manag Nurs.* 2004;5:3-18.

78. Robb KA, Williams JE, Duvivier V, Newham DJ. A pain management program for chronic cancer-treatment-related pain: a preliminary study. *J Pain.* 2006;7:82-90.

79. Vilela LD, Nicolau B, Mahmud S, et al. Comparison of psychosocial outcomes in head and neck cancer patients receiving a coping strategies intervention and control subjects receiving no intervention. *J Otolaryngol.* 2006;35:88-96.

80. www.nccn.org/professionals/physician_gls/f_guidelines.asp. Accessed September 12, 2011.

81. Cassileth BR, Vickers AJ. Massage therapy for symptom control: outcome study at a major cancer center. *J Pain Symptom Manage.* 2004;28:244-249.

82. Corbin L. Safety and efficacy of massage therapy for patients with cancer. *Cancer Control.* 2005;12:158-164.

83. Ahles TA, Tope DM, Pinkson B, et al. Massage therapy for patients undergoing autologous bone marrow transplantation. *J Pain Symptom Manage.* 1999;18:157-163.

84. Wilkinson S, Barnes K, Storey L. Massage for symptom relief in patients with cancer: systematic review. *J Adv Nurs.* 2008;63:430-439.

85. Wilkie DJ, Kampbell J, Cutshall S, et al. Effects of massage on pain intensity, analgesics and quality of life in patients with cancer pain: a pilot study of a randomized clinical trial conducted within hospice care delivery. *Hosp J.* 2000;15:31-53.

86. Sims S. Slow stroke back massage for cancer patients. *Nurs Times.* 1986;82:47-50.

87. Weinrich SP, Weinrich MC. The effect of massage on pain in cancer patients. *Appl Nurs Res.* 1990;3:140-145.

88. Grealish L, Lomasney A, Whiteman B. Foot massage. A nursing intervention to modify the distressing symptoms of pain and nausea in patients hospitalized with cancer. *Cancer Nurs.* 2000;23:237-243.

89. Stephenson NL, Weinrich SP, Tavakoli AS. The effects of foot reflexology on anxiety and pain in patients with breast and lung cancer. *Oncol Nurs Forum.* 2000;27:67-72.

90. Cassileth BR, Deng GE, Gomez JE, Johnstone PA, Kumar N, Vickers AJ. Complementary therapies and integrative oncology in lung cancer: ACCP evidence-based clinical practice guidelines (2nd edition). *Chest.* 2007;132:340S-354S.

91. Meleger AL, Krivickas LS. Neck and back pain: musculoskeletal disorders. *Neurol Clin.* May 2007;25(2):419-438.

92. Claydon LS, Chesterton LS, Barlas P. Dose-specific effects of transcutaneous electrical nerve stimulation (TENS) on experimental pain: a systematic review. *Clin J Pain.* September 2011;27(7):635-647.

93. Robb K, Oxberry SG, Bennett MI, Johnson MI, Simpson KH, Searle RD. A cochrane systematic review of transcutaneous electrical nerve stimulation for cancer pain. *J Pain Symptom Manage.* 2009 Apr;37(4):746-753.

94. Lee H, Schmidt K, Ernst E. Acupuncture for the relief of cancer-related pain—a systematic review. *Eur J Pain.* 2005;9:437-444.

95. Dawidson I, Angmar-Mansson B, Blom M, Theodorsson E, Lundeberg T. Sensory stimulation (acupuncture) increases the release of vasoactive intestinal polypeptide in the saliva of xerostomia sufferers. *Neuropeptides.* 1998;32:543-548.

96. Wu MT, Hsieh JC, Xiong J, et al. Central nervous pathway for acupuncture stimulation: localization of processing with functional MR imaging of the brain—preliminary experience. *Radiology.* 1999;212:133-141.

97. Manheimer E, White A, Berman B, Forys K, Ernst E. Meta-analysis: acupuncture for low back pain. *Ann Intern Med.* 2005;142:651-663.

98. Ernst E, Pittler MH. The effectiveness of acupuncture in treating acute dental pain: a systematic review. *Br Dent J.* 1998;184:443-447.

99. Melchart D, Linde K, Fischer P, et al. Acupuncture for recurrent headaches: a systematic review of randomized controlled trials. *Cephalalgia.* 1999;19:779-786; discussion 65.

100. Lee A, Done ML. The use of nonpharmacologic techniques to prevent postoperative nausea and vomiting: a meta-analysis. *Anesth Analg.* 1999;88:1362-1369.

101. Paley CA, Johnson MI, Tashani OA, Bagnall AM. Acupuncture for cancer pain in adults. *Cochrane Database Syst Rev.* 2011;(1):CD007753.

102. Hopkins Hollis AS. Acupuncture as a treatment modality for the management of cancer pain: the state of the science. *Oncol Nurs Forum.* 2010;37:E344-E348.

103. Chen ZJ, Guo YP, Wu ZC. Observation on the therapeutic effect of acupuncture at pain points on cancer pain. *Zhongguo Zhen Jiu.* 2008;28:251-253.

104. Alimi D, Rubino C, Pichard-Leandri E, Fermand-Brule S, Dubreuil-Lemaire ML, Hill C. Analgesic effect of auricular acupuncture for cancer pain: a randomized, blinded, controlled trial. *J Clin Oncol.* 2003;21:4120-4126.

105. Dang W, Yang J. Clinical study on acupuncture treatment of stomach carcinoma pain. *J Tradit Chin Med.* 1998;18:31-38.

106. Xia YQ, Zhang D, Yang CX, Xu HL, Li Y, Ma LT. An approach to the effect on tumors of acupuncture in combination with radiotherapy or chemotherapy. *J Tradit Chin Med.* 1986;6:23-26.

107. Jackson E, Kelley M, McNeil P, Meyer E, Schlegel L, Eaton M. Does therapeutic touch help reduce pain and anxiety in patients with cancer? *Clin J Oncol Nurs.* 2008;12:113-120.

108. Wardell DW, Weymouth KF. Review of studies of healing touch. *J Nurs Scholarsh.* 2004;36:147-154.

109. Post-White J, Kinney ME, Savik K, Gau JB, Wilcox C, Lerner I. Therapeutic massage and healing touch improve symptoms in cancer. *Integr Cancer Ther.* 2003;2:332-344.

110. So PS, Jiang Y, Qin Y. Touch therapies for pain relief in adults. *Cochrane Database Syst Rev.* 2008;(4):CD006535.

111. Cook CA, Guerrerio JF, Slater VE. Healing touch and quality of life in women receiving radiation treatment for cancer: a randomized controlled trial. *Altern Ther Health Med.* 2004;10:34-41.

112. Olson K, Hanson J, Michaud M. A phase II trial of Reiki for the management of pain in advanced cancer patients. *J Pain Symptom Manage.* 2003;26:990-997.

113. Tsang KL, Carlson LE, Olson K. Pilot crossover trial of Reiki versus rest for treating cancer-related fatigue. *Integr Cancer Ther.* 2007;6:25-35.

114. Frank LS, Frank JL, March D, Makari-Judson G, Barham RB, Mertens WC. Does therapeutic touch ease the discomfort or distress of patients undergoing stereotactic core breast biopsy? A randomized clinical trial. *Pain Med.* 2007;8:419-424.

115. Hayden JA, van Tulder MW, Malmivaara A, Koes BW. Exercise therapy for treatment of non-specific low back pain. *Cochrane Database Syst Rev.* 20 July 2005;(3):CD000335.

116. Lorig KR, Holman H. Self-management education: history, definition, outcomes, and mechanisms. *Ann Behav Med.* 2003;26:1-7.

117. Lorig KR, Sobel DS, Stewart AL, et al. Evidence suggesting that a chronic disease self-management program can improve health status while reducing hospitalization: a randomized trial. *Med Care.* 1999;37:5-14.

118. Lorig KR, Laurent DD, Deyo RA, Marnell ME, Minor MA, Ritter PL. Can a Back Pain E-mail Discussion Group improve health status and lower health care costs?: a randomized study. *Arch Intern Med.* 2002;162:792-796.

119. Berman RL, Iris MA, Bode R, Drengenberg C. The effectiveness of an online mind–body intervention for older adults with chronic pain. *J Pain.* 2009;10:68-79.

120. Kroenke K, Theobald D, Wu J, et al. Effect of telecare management on pain and depression in patients with cancer: a randomized trial. *JAMA.* 2010;304:163-171.

CHAPTER 4

Interventional Approaches to Pain

Andrew Mannes ■ Philip S. Kim ■ Russell R. Lonser

Interventional and neurosurgical procedures can be utilized to supplement pharmacologic and complementary approaches in the treatment of pain (see Chapters 3 and 4). Pharmacologic therapies are described elsewhere in this text, including the principles of analgesic management using opioid agents and other adjuvant medications. The primary indications for interventional techniques are either for patients whose pain is poorly responsive to systemic analgesic therapies or for patients who suffer from intolerable side effects, in whom efforts to manage adverse effects are unsuccessful including patients experiencing severe dose-limiting side effects that prevent optimal titration to therapeutic levels (e.g., systemic opioids associated with refractory constipation, nausea, vomiting, or sedation).

Patient's response to analgesic medicinal therapies has been best described in the cancer population. The oral administration of analgesics based on recommendations, including those outlined by the World Health Organization, can provide satisfactory relief to many patients. However, poorly relieved pain that is experienced by 5% to 15% (1–3) of the approximately 500,000 patients that die each year from cancer indicates a significant need for additional methods for control of pain, including interventional and neurosurgical procedures, that can offer symptom relief. Aside from optimizing pain control while minimizing side effects, interventional pain therapies can also enhance functional abilities and physical and psychological well-being, enhancing the patient's quality of life (4). It has also been reported that better pain management utilizing interventional techniques may result in increased life. Further, reducing patient visits for symptom management could potentially reduce costs (5).

INITIAL EVALUATION

For the interventionalist, it is important to understand the patient's prognosis, associated comorbidities, as well as the expectations of patient and family. An initial evaluation for interventional pain therapies should ascertain the patient's general medical condition along with the primary disease. A complete history is required that includes a general medical, disease-specific (e.g., patients with oncologic disorders need to be thoroughly evaluated for possible local recurrence or new metastases), psychosocial, and pain histories. The physical examination includes a general medical examination with emphasis on neurologic findings. Examination of the site of pain and surrounding anatomic regions is critical (e.g., if a patient has profound motor and sensory deficits

in a particular region, neurolysis techniques become a more acceptable therapeutic option). Specific pain history includes the following: quality of pain, pain intensity, alleviating/exacerbating factors, temporal characteristics, and duration and associated features (e.g., numbness, weakness, and vasomotor changes). Psychosocial evaluation should assess the presence of psychological symptoms (e.g., anxiety and depression), and psychiatric disorders (e.g., major depression and delirium) should be similarly addressed. The nature and meaning of the presenting pain needs to be distinguished from anxiety and suffering affecting the patient. The ability to cope and the availability of psychosocial support systems need to be assessed and reinforced with proper health and social professionals. A final assessment should determine the patient's expectation of therapeutic interventional options.

Appropriate selection of an intervention is based on therapeutic goals. If the presenting pain is expected to be transient (pain that will be alleviated by primary radiation therapy or chemotherapy, pain that is associated with the treatment of the primary disease, or pain that is), then the intervention should likewise be reversible. However, if the pain is expected to be chronic, a technique that results in more permanent effects is indicated. Life expectancy must be considered when selecting an appropriate intervention. If the patient's life expectancy is short, treatment strategies should strive to minimize the frequency and level of interventions and recovery time and should focus on optimizing a patient's quality of life. A patient with a longer life expectancy may warrant more extensive and expensive interventions (i.e., implantable devices). Certain procedures may not be indicated for patients with longer life expectancy such as neuroablative procedures that are associated with permanent loss of function or a theoretical risk of developing deafferentation pain syndromes.

Once a definitive diagnosis of the cause of the underlying source of pain has been made, a treatment plan should characterize the expected outcome, define contingencies, and plan for reassessment. Longitudinal monitoring of pain and response to interventional therapies is essential and allows implementation of additional options (e.g., complementary therapies, pharmacologic strategies, and behavioral and psychological approaches). This chapter includes some of the frequently utilized procedures in the palliative care pain population (Table 4.1). Not all indications and contraindications are included and consultation with a pain practitioner should be considered before referring the patient for evaluation and treatment.

TABLE 4.1	Comparison of interventional pain procedures			
	Nerve Blocks	**Neurolytic Procedures**	**Neurostimulation**	**Neuraxial Infusion**
Advantages	Ease of performance Useful for diagnostic and therapeutic relief	Ease of performance Provides long-term relief	Nondestructive Reversible	Nondestructive Reversible
Disadvantages	Provides short-term relief	Risk of associated sensory and motor deficits	Requires costly equipment and surgical implantation	Requires costly equipment and possible surgical implantation Requires pharmaceutical and ancillary support

APPROACHES TO INTERVENTIONS

Pharmacologic management of pain can be viewed as a continuum of indirect and direct drug delivery paradigms (4). Indirect drug delivery (i.e., systemic analgesia) refers to the administration of an analgesic into the bloodstream, which is then transported to the receptor site in neural tissue:

1. By systemic absorption
2. By formulation of depot for sustained and continuous release
3. Through the bloodstream

   Direct drug delivery is the administration of an agent to the targeted neural tissue involved in nociception. By delivering directly to the nociceptive pathways, a pronounced analgesic effect at a lower dose with fewer side effects can be achieved. An example of this is comparing equianalgesic morphine doses in the intrathecal, epidural, and intravenous spaces (Table 4.2) (6).

   Interventional pain therapies are often minimally invasive techniques that can be categorized into direct drug delivery, neuroablation, neural blockade, and neurostimulation. Direct drug delivery involves the administration of analgesics, usually opioids and local anesthetics, regional to nociceptive pathways. Other potential agents such as α_2-agonists and calcium channel blockers can be administered. Neuroablation refers to direct chemical, thermal, or surgical destruction of nociceptive pathways. Neurostimulation or neuroaugmentation refers to the application of direct electrical stimulation to inhibit nociceptive transmission. Not all pain, however,

can be adequately addressed using these techniques. In such cases, one can consider consultation with a neurosurgeon about surgical intervention.

Direct Drug Delivery

Neuraxial direct drug delivery involves accessing the epidural or subarachnoid (intrathecal) space by a needle and/or the placement of a continuous infusion system. In general, neuraxial infusion should be considered when severe pain cannot be controlled with systemic drugs and/or because of dose-limiting toxicities. Neuraxial infusions can also be considered when there is an immediate need for using various nonopioid analgesics. Specifically, local anesthetics can have a profound analgesic effect on many intractable opioid-unresponsive pain conditions. Although it is possible to give local anesthetic systemically, higher local concentrations can be achieved, resulting in profound neural blockade through direct drug delivery.

   Neuraxial delivery systems have two components: a subarachnoid or epidural catheter and a delivery mode (e.g., bolus dosing, syringe pump, internal port, or internal or external pump). There are basically five types of neuraxial drug delivery systems, and familiarization with these systems allows the clinician to understand the respective advantages and disadvantages of each (7,8).

   The simplest, least expensive, and least invasive option is a percutaneous catheter, which is typically made of nylon, polyurethane, or polyamide and can be wire reinforced. These catheters are routinely placed in surgical and obstetric

TABLE 4.2	Equianalgesic morphine conversions among routes of administration		
Oral	**Parenteral**	**Epidural**	**Subarachnoid**
300 mg =	100 mg =	10 mg =	1 mg

patients to manage operative and postoperative pain and are designed for short-term use (generally <1 week). But a catheter may be maintained for longer periods without problems and may suffice for the duration of the patient's life. If there is a complication, these catheters can be discontinued by removing the dressing and withdrawing the catheter. Occasionally, these catheters can cause a localized tissue reaction at the site of insertion, can migrate, and are susceptible to accidental displacement.

The next type of drug delivery system uses the same type of catheter as that mentioned in the preceding text, but it is tunneled subcutaneously to decrease the incidence of migration. Placement can be performed in a clinic and requires a small incision with multiple needle insertions. Tunneling the catheter is better suited for the outpatient or the homebound patient.

Implanted catheters with subcutaneous injection site are technologically more advanced and require a minor surgical procedure, resulting in higher costs (for placement). Sterile preparation and the use of fluoroscopy are essential. These systems can be placed in the epidural or intrathecal space. There are two basic designs: exteriorized or completely internalized injection port. In the first design, the proximal catheter is tunneled from the exit site in the back and exteriorized usually along the midaxillary line. This catheter can include an antimicrobial cuff that reduces both infection and catheter migration. In the second design, the port is supported by bone, usually a rib, so as to facilitate needle insertion. It can be used for intermittent bolus dosing or accessed for continuous infusions.

A totally implanted catheter with implanted reservoir and manual pump is being developed by several companies, as well as an implantable patient-activated device. This design allows patient-controlled analgesia by pressing the activation valve and pumping chamber, providing a bolus of medication. Because the entire device is implanted, the reservoir is refilled by inserting a needle into a subcutaneous port in the control pad.

A totally implanted catheter with implanted infusion pump is available in two basic designs. The simpler design is a constant fixed infusion pump in which the dose can be adjusted by a clinician changing the concentration. The second type includes a programmable, peristaltic infusion pump with a drug reservoir, an electronic module, and an antenna allowing reprogramming of drug flow rates. The clinician controls the pump through an external programmer head (such as a pacemaker) to alter the dose, give single doses, or change the continuous infusion rate.

Recently, Medtronic has received U.S. Food and Drug Administration approval for a patient activation device that will allow the patient to receive a medical direct bolus of medication when the device is activated.

Typically, a percutaneous test catheterization of the epidural or intrathecal space would be performed to assess the efficacy and starting doses of medication before implanting a permanent delivery system. There are several approaches to trial the drugs, including bolus dosing, by accessing the intrathecal space with a spinal needle or by placement of a catheter and continuous infusion—either in the epidural or intrathecal space. Ideally, the method utilized for clinical assessment would best emulate the intended route (e.g., a trial with a continuous intrathecal catheter for evaluating future implantable pump placement). Although the complication rate is low, implantable devices can have problems with catheter failure, infection, seroma, wound dehiscence, and catheter tip fibroma formation (9). They also require health-care provider visits for routine refills and adjustment of dosing.

The selection of the appropriate neuraxial drug(s) and delivery system for an individual patient is based on several considerations (7,10):

1. Patient life expectancy
2. Economics and cost-effectiveness
3. Choice of epidural versus subarachnoid route of administration

Patient life expectancy and duration of need are difficult to predict. The more sophisticated implantable systems are expensive devices that require a trial catheter, adjustments of medications, and a surgical procedure for placement. One study by Bedder et al. suggests that an implanted pump system is a more viable financial alternative compared with other drug delivery systems for a period over 3 months (11). The less sophisticated, percutaneous and tunneled catheters are best suited for patients with a limited life expectancy of a few months. Both epidural and subarachnoid drug deliveries can be equally effective. The duration of therapy will usually predict the type of infusion system selected. Catheter obstruction, fibrosis, and loss of analgesic efficacy are well described in long-term epidural drug systems (7). Therefore, intrathecal drug delivery systems are best suited for a protracted duration of therapy (>3 months). A decision-making algorithm for using neuraxial analgesia is shown in Figure 4.1 (12).

Multiple pharmacologic preparations have been administered through the neuraxial drug delivery systems. The gold standard is morphine, which is widely used and successful. When intrathecal morphine provides inadequate relief, other opioids, such as hydromorphone, meperidine, methadone, fentanyl, and sufentanil, have been used. As tolerance develops, one might switch opioids and/or use them in combination with coanalgesics, which include local anesthetics (e.g., tetracaine and bupivacaine), α_2-agonists (e.g., clonidine), and γ-aminobutyric acid (GABA-B) agonists (baclofen). Ziconotide, the first neuronal calcium channel blocker for pain, is the synthetic equivalent of a peptide produced by a snail and has been approved for use in intrathecal pumps for intractable pain not responsive to systemic analgesics including intrathecal morphine (13). Drug selection is based on the patient's pain symptoms using clinical strategies that have been developed (e.g., comprehensive consensus-based guidelines on intrathecal drug delivery systems in the treatment of pain caused by cancer pain updated 2011) (14). The guidelines and algorithms were developed by an expert panel, evaluating existing literature and algorithms for various

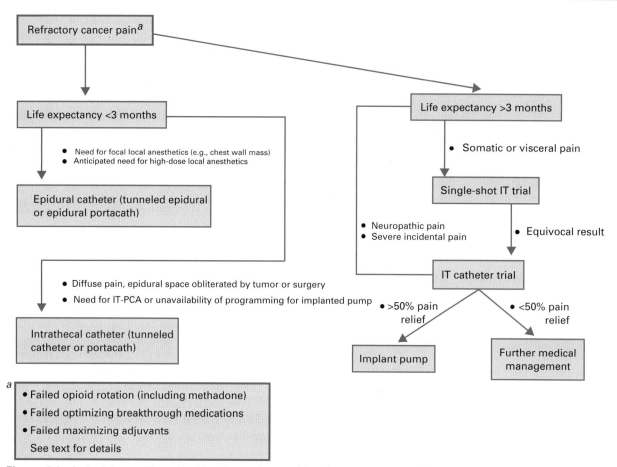

Figure 4.1. A decision-making algorithm for patients with refractory cancer-related pain. IT, intrathecal; IT-PCA, intrathecal patient-controlled analgesia.

intrathecal drugs. The optimal drug dosage, concentration, and issues related to compounding of drugs have been reviewed.

Complications from neuraxial catheter and pump placement may result from anatomic changes, infection, fluid collection, catheter migration, or device failure. Patients with suspected block of the subarachnoid circulation due to tumor extension or subarachnoid hemorrhage/arachnoiditis may have a poor response to the delivery of intrathecal analgesia. Evidence of an obstruction should be sought using magnetic resonance imaging or myelography to determine the level of obstruction. Retesting the efficacy of analgesia by placing the injectant proximal to the obstruction may yield improved analgesic response. Migration or fracture of the catheter should be suspected if the patient reports sudden changes in pain relief or if a fluid collection is seen at the insertion site. Percutaneously placed catheters can be bolused with a test dose of a local anesthetic to assess function. Myelography should be performed with implantable catheters or pumps (through a side port) to determine catheter placement and function when displacement or catheter rupture is suspected.

An infection of the site does not always necessitate immediate removal of a catheter. Superficial infections may only require a course of antibiotics. However, persistent or progressive tissue infection or central nervous system (CNS) involvement necessitates immediate removal of the catheter and/or pump.

A growing body of case reports and studies supports the benefits of direct drug (intrathecal) delivery systems. In a study of 202 patients experiencing refractory cancer pain who were randomized to receive either an implantable drug delivery system or comprehensive medical management (15), the patients receiving implantable intrathecal pump had reported successful pain control with a reduction in common drug toxicities such as fatigue and diminished level of consciousness. Overall, there was an improvement in the quality-of-life measures and survival over the 6 months in the patients receiving implantable intrathecal pump.

Peripheral Nerve/Plexus Drug Delivery

Blockade of peripheral nerves and neural plexi is commonly performed to provide regional anesthesia and analgesia to patients undergoing surgical procedures (15–18). Modified constant infusion systems typically deliver local anesthetics directly to peripheral nerves and neural plexi in patients with inadequate analgesia or intolerable toxicities from systemic medications. Specific localized pain syndromes related to a mononeuropathy, plexopathy, and peripheral neuropathy may benefit from peripheral nerve infusion.

Continuous neural blockade of the brachial plexus is common for postoperative pain. A technique of placing a catheter along the brachial plexus and self-contained infusion system has been described (16,17). A case report describes the successful 2-week management of pain from pancoast syndrome with a brachial plexus infusion system using local anesthetics (19). Other potential areas where neural infusion could be performed include the lumbosacral plexus, paravertebral and selected peripheral nerves, and sympathetic chain.

The current self-contained peripheral nerves/plexi infusion system is a modification of neuraxial infusion systems (16–20). The advantages of this system are the simplicity and the minimal invasiveness of the placement of the system. However, the patient can experience a localized tissue reaction or catheter migration and has a risk of infection for implantations of >1 month's duration. Implantable technology must be improved to provide a completely implanted infusion system for long-term continuous nerve/plexi analgesic infusion.

Neural blockade with longer acting local anesthetics such bupivacaine can provide hours of relief until a more long-term solution can be offered. This window of analgesia can also provide time to titrate systemic medications such as steroids, antidepressants, and anticonvulsants. Many times diagnostic neural blockade will predict the response to neuroablative techniques.

Neuroablation

Neuroablation should be initiated in the following conditions (4):

1. If systemic therapies fail to provide adequate relief and quality of life
2. If neuraxial drug administration fails
3. To accommodate patient preference
4. Early in the natural history of disease (e.g., cancer) in the presence of discrete well-defined pain generators

Contemporary minimally invasive neurolytic techniques can be divided into chemical lysis, cryoneurolysis, and radiofrequency and surgical ablation (21). Chemical neurolysis involves the injection of a destructive chemical such as alcohol or phenol. Historically, other chemicals such as chlorocresol, ammonium salts, and iced and hypertonic saline have been used (21). Ethyl alcohol dehydrates and precipitates neural tissue. Phenol (carbonic acid) denatures neural tissue as well, with an apparently lower incidence of neuritis (21). Radiofrequency neurolysis has numerous advantages compared with chemical neurolysis. Radiofrequency neurolysis involves the placement of insulated needles to localize nociceptive pathways and then pinpoint a heat lesion. The extent of the lesion can be controlled by the size of the probe, duration of application, and the temperature at the tip of the needle. Because a more precise controlled lesion can be performed, radiofrequency lesioning is preferred for cordotomy, rhizotomy, and gangliolysis. The use of pulsed radiofrequency as an alternative to conventional radiofrequency ablation (RFA) techniques is being explored. This technique uses a narrow pulsed current, allowing for cooling time, and a lower tissue temperature (42°C in pulsed radiofrequency vs. 80°C in RFA) with no histologic signs of tissue damage (22). Several studies have reported reversible

antinociceptive effects; therefore, pulsed radiofrequency may be better suited for treating patients with reversible disease or treatment-related pain.

Like radiofrequency neurolysis, cryoneurolysis has an advantage in producing a controlled lesion. Cryoneurolysis is produced by disrupting neuronal transmission by allowing rapid expansion of compressed gas, causing the formation of an "ice ball" at the tip of the needle (21). Nerves encompassed in the frozen tissue develop ice crystals that result in degeneration. However, the architecture of the perineurium and epineurium is not affected, thereby allowing resprouting of the axons without subsequent neuroma formation. The clinical effects are variable and are a function of precise needle tip localization (duration of freezing and lowest temperature achieved). The longevity of the effects needs to be considered when utilizing this technique. If the pain is expected to resolve, the recovery of nerve function would be desirable. However, if the targeted pain is expected to be chronic, relief from symptoms may be short lived. Rarely, peripheral and central nerves can be surgically interrupted. Neurosurgical techniques are included in greater detail in this chapter.

Neurolytic procedures, by definition, often cause irreversible damage to the neurons, but other structures in proximity to the intended site can be damaged because of extension of the therapy or accidental needle migration. Therefore, the resulting effects may include not only the neurons responsible for conveying pain but also lesion neurons that convey touch, proprioception, bladder and bowel control, and motor function. Therefore, these procedures are best performed by trained and experienced practitioners. Although not essential, using local anesthetic blocks is a good trial before implementing an irreversible blockade. It will emulate the level of pain relief that can be provided by the neurolytic procedure while allowing the patient to experience other side effects associated with deafferentation. This includes evaluating the untoward effects such as "numbness" in the affected region that some patients find less desirable than the original pain.

The efferent neuronal pathway can also be a target for interventional therapies. Botulism toxin, a neurotoxin produced by *Clostridium botulinum*, blocks acetylcholine release from nerve terminals, resulting in muscle relaxation. Therapeutic benefit can be achieved by carefully injecting botulinum toxin A into various muscle groups in patients with myofascial pain, migraines, and spastic conditions. However, a *Cochrane Collaboration* review of the use of botulinum toxin A for treating low back pain yielded only low-quality evidence that pain and/or function improved as compared with saline or very low quality as compared with acupuncture or steroid injections (23).

Neurolytic Procedures

Head and Neck Pain

Peripheral neurolysis can be done at various neural structures throughout the body (21,24,25). The head and neck region is richly innervated, and disease resulting in pain in this region (e.g., cancer) is difficult to manage (21). Pain is often aggravated by simple movements related to coughing, swallowing, talking, and eating. The cranial nerves typically affected by neoplastic growth, surgical, and/or radiation therapy are V, VII, IX, and X. Potential problems exist for the pain interventionalist in understanding anatomic distortion due to cancer and its therapies. The avoidance of damage to cranial nerves IX and X is critical for ventilatory and swallowing control.

The cell bodies of the sensory neurons innervating the face, forehead, and upper neck are localized to the trigeminal ganglia (cranial nerve V). The ganglia or branches of the afferent fibers can be selectively targeted by several approaches. Surgical rhizotomies have been supplanted by percutaneous approaches and open surgical microvascular decompression. Radiofrequency thermogangliolysis is the most popularly utilized technique, with over 14,000 cases reported in 33 publications (21). Technically similar to chemical neurolysis, a radiofrequency probe is placed along the divisions of the trigeminal ganglion through the foramen ovale and a brief thermal lesion is performed. In one large series, at 2-year follow-up, 28.3% of patients had recurrence of symptoms after one treatment and 8.3% had recurrence after multiple treatments (26). Trigeminal balloon compression is a surgical approach in which a Fogarty balloon catheter is placed and inflated to perform neurolysis, with reported results being similar to those of radiofrequency neurolysis (27). Microvascular decompression is discussed in the Section Other Neurosurgical Procedures. Eye pain can also be conveyed along the fifth cranial nerve. Pain symptoms may arise from localized pathology or may be referred (e.g., migraine), and patient referral to an ophthalmologist is warranted.

Intractable hiccups (singultus) can be treated with phrenic nerve blocks (21). This is done with fluoroscopic guidance to determine whether one hemidiaphragm is predominant in spasm and should be blocked. If the local anesthetic block is successful, a neurolytic phrenic technique can be done surgically or with RFA (28).

Upper and Lower Extremities

Upper and lower extremity pain can be difficult to treat with interventional neurolytic approaches. The nerves of the brachial and lumbosacral plexi are mainly mixed nerves with motor and sensory components. Difficulties exist in selectively blocking only the sensory components of the nerves and plexi. Subarachnoid and dorsal root neurolysis can be performed with a limited incidence of motor deficits (29). The injection of phenol into the brachial plexus provided four patients with cancer with good to excellent pain relief for 12 weeks (25). Intractable shoulder pain was managed effectively with suprascapular neurolysis using phenol or absolute alcohol (24).

Thorax and Abdomen

Thoracic and abdominal wall pain can be treated with multiple intercostal or paravertebral nerve blocks. If adequate relief is obtained, a percutaneous neurolysis can be performed. Subarachnoid neurolysis can also be performed if the dermatome(s) involved in the pain generator can be identified. Doyle reported a series of 46 hospice patients treated with multiple phenol intercostal blocks (30). The patients received a range of total relief from 1 to 6 weeks (mean, 3 weeks). Peripheral neurolysis of various branches of the lumbosacral plexus (iliohypogastric and ilioinguinal) has been similarly performed for pain in the lower abdomen/pelvic region (31).

Sympathetic Ganglion Neurolytic Blocks

Neuropathic, intra-abdominal, pelvic, and perineal pain can be treated with various sympathetic ganglion neurolytic approaches (32). Unlike the somatic nerves, selective blockade of the sympathetic nervous system will not result in altered motor or sensory function (although other sympathetic-mediated function may be lost).

Celiac plexus and splanchnic blocks are among the frequently utilized neurolytic blocks for neuropathic or cancer pain (33–36). Sympathetic blocks are indicated for treating abdominal and referred back pain secondary to abdominal pathology, especially pancreatic cancer. Pancreatic cancer involving the head of the pancreas is more responsive than that of the tail of the pancreas (37). In addition to providing pain relief, celiac plexus blocks can reduce sympathetic tone, leaving unopposed parasympathetic activity, thereby enhancing gastrointestinal motility—a major benefit for patients with cancer requiring systemic opioids. Serious complications involving the kidney, lung, aorta, and vena cava have been minimized with fluoroscopic or computed tomographic (CT) guidance and modification of the original techniques. A randomized study of early intervention of alcohol versus placebo celiac blocks demonstrated statistically significant pain relief and prolonged survival ranging from 3 to 9 months in alcohol-treated patients (38). A preemptive interventional approach may lead to improved survival rates, but more studies are needed.

An alternative therapy to the celiac axis neurolysis targets the nerves that condense to form the plexus, specifically the greater, lesser, and least splanchnic nerves (derived from the thoracic chain) (32). Neuroablative therapy applied to the splanchnic nerves can achieve the same therapeutic result as celiac plexus neurolysis, although some practitioners think the technique is safer. The lesions must be applied bilaterally, but there is less likelihood for intraperitoneal, bowel, or arterial injections or trauma to these structures. Regardless of the technique, a meta-analysis of the efficacy and safety of celiac plexus neurolysis supports it use in providing long-lasting pain relief (70% to 90% of the patients) with few mild and rare severe adverse side effects (39).

Interventional pain therapies for intractable perineal pain are predisposed to the potential risk of rectal and urinary incontinence. In cases of preexisting incontinence with surgical diversion, a neurolytic subarachnoid saddle block is simple and effective. Other target structures for pelvic and perineal pain include the superior hypogastric plexus and ganglion impar. The superior hypogastric plexus consists of sympathetic and parasympathetic fibers that innervate the pelvis including the vagina, uterus, cervix, testis, ovaries, and bladder (40). The ganglion impar (Walther's ganglion) consists of sympathetic fibers and its blockade can result in relief of burning, urgency, and pain in the perineal region (41). Patients with advanced disease experiencing refractory pain in this region could obtain significant pain relief with a neuroablative procedure.

Sympathetic innervation to the head, neck, and upper extremities can be interrupted with a stellate ganglion block and the lower extremities with a lumbar sympathetic block. An initial injection or series of injections with local anesthetics are useful for diagnosis and possibly for treatment. A successful injection will reduce the patient's pain symptoms and produce evidence of sympathetic blockade (e.g., temperature chance in affected limb) without somatic motor or sensory loss. If symptom relief is reproducible but transient, a trial using a dorsal column stimulator or a neurodestructive procedure using RFA, chemical neurolysis, or surgical procedure can be considered. Early initiation of treatment after an injury or the appearance of symptoms may elicit a better response than that seen with patients who have experienced chronic symptoms.

Other neurolytic approaches may involve interruption of various CNS pathways. Subarachnoid and epidural neurolyses have been reported in various case reports and series (21,42). The disadvantage is the potential spread of these chemicals on other central structures, leading to potential myelopathies. Painful conditions may require multiple-level neurolysis, greatly compounding the probability of serious complications. The use of implantable pumps has reduced the need for this procedure.

Neurostimulation

Neurostimulation is the application of precisely targeted electrical stimulation on nociceptive pathways. Electrical stimulation has a long history in medicine in treating various ailments. Beyond the application of electrodes on the skin such as a transcutaneous electrical nerve stimulation, electrodes have been applied directly to nociceptive pathways.

Spinal cord stimulation (SCS) uses epidural electrodes placed along the dorsal columns to block nociception (43,44). The system entails the surgical placement of epidural electrodes, cables, and radiofrequency transmitter or battery. Minimal discomfort is encountered in the placement of the system and in the postoperative period.

The mechanism of SCS is based on the gate control theory (Melzack and Wall) (43). It postulates that stimulating large nerve fibers (A beta fibers) can inhibit or modulate smaller nerve fibers (A delta or C fibers) transmitting nociceptive input, possibly at the dorsal root or horn of the spinal cord. Strategically placed epidural electrodes stimulate the dorsal columns (A beta fibers) to inhibit or modulate nociceptive input (A delta or C fibers). Ongoing research suggests that SCS may inhibit transmission in the spinothalamic tract, activate central inhibitory mechanisms influencing sympathetic efferent neurons, and release various inhibitory neurotransmitters.

SCS can be applied to treat neuropathic pain conditions including arachnoiditis, complex regional pain syndrome (formerly, reflex sympathetic dystrophy), neuropathies, brachial and lumbosacral plexopathies, radiculopathies, deafferentation syndromes, phantom limb pain, and postherpetic neuralgia (45). Visceral syndromes such as interstitial cystitis, chronic abdominal pain, and chronic pancreatitis have been treated with limited success. SCS for cancer pain is limited to the dynamic nature and progression of neoplasms. SCS may have a role in stable neuropathic cancer pain related to cancer treatments and stable neoplasms.

PERCUTANEOUS VERTERBRAL AUGMENTATION

Percutaneous vertebral augmentation is an image-guided procedure, which may be used to treat pain associated with vertebral compression fractures caused by metastatic tumors or osteoporosis. Vertebroplasty is the injection of poly(methyl methacrylate) into a compressed vertebral body. Most percutaneous vertebral augmentations are performed for osteoporotic compression fractures, but patients with cancer pain can experience significant symptom relief with this procedure. Patients with anterior osteolytic lesions that are not amenable to surgical interventions may be candidates for this less invasive intervention. Contraindications for percutaneous vertebral augmentation include >70% vertebral collapse, epidural disease, asymptomatic stable fractures, or infection (46). However, there is growing evidence that these guidelines may not be absolute contraindications (47).

During vertebroplasty, one or two bone biopsy needles are inserted into the collapsed vertebral body through a small incision in the patient's back and acrylic bone cement is injected through the cannula to stabilize the fracture. Kyphoplasty is done in the same way as vertebroplasty with the inflation of balloon that creates a cavity. In this cavity, cement is placed to stabilize the compression fracture.

The procedure typically requires a local anesthetic; conscious sedation is sometimes helpful, depending on the patient's condition and tolerance for medications that can compound hypotension. For many patients, however, vertebroplasty provides immediate (within 72 hours) and lasting relief from pain. Many patients are able to increase their level of activities within only a few days of the procedure.

Some clinical studies have reported conflicting success utilizing this procedure (48–51). Kyphoplasty has been found to be safe and effective in patients with multiple myeloma in a large patient cohort study (52). These procedures have an extremely low complication rates, including infection, an allergic reaction to methacrylates, pulmonary embolism from intravascular injection, and weakness from displacement of fracture or extravasation of the injection into the intrathecal space.

NEUROSURGICAL PROCEDURES FOR PAIN

Despite optimized medical therapy and the use of interventions, some patients will still not achieve a satisfactory level of symptom control and may require neurosurgical procedures for pain relief. Although these procedures can be quite effective in treating specific cancer pain syndromes, careful patient selection is critical to maximize potential benefit. Neurosurgical treatment of medically refractory cancer pain usually involves the interruption of the specific involved pain–sensory pathways. These interventions most often include cordotomy, myelotomy, and other nervous system ablative procedures.

Cordotomy

Cordotomy is used for patients with unilateral medically intractable cancer pain below the level of C5 (53,54). Cordotomy involves lesioning of the anterior spinothalamic tract of the spinal cord that transmits nociceptive impulses from the contralateral half of the body. Interruption of this tract can be performed by an open operation or percutaneously. Because percutaneous cordotomies can be performed under local anesthesia with minimal morbidity, it has become the preferred technique. Percutaneous cordotomies are performed by placing a needle through the neck contralateral to the pain (because the spinothalamic tract fibers have crossed the spinal cord by this point) at the C1-2 level under CT scan guidance (46). Once the placement of the needle tip in the anterior spinothalamic tracts is confirmed, a permanent thermal lesion is made.

Cordotomy can provide excellent pain relief immediately after the procedure in over 90% of patients. The effectiveness of this operation diminishes with time, and at 1 year after cordotomy 50% to 60% of patients will continue to have adequate pain control. Beyond 1 year, 40% of patients will continue to have adequate analgesia. Complications are rare (usually <5%) and frequently transient. Complications can include ataxia, ipsilateral paresis, bowel/bladder dysfunction, ipsilateral Horner syndrome, sexual dysfunction, respiratory problems (sleep apnea or respiratory failure), and dysesthesias. Because there is a possibility of loss of ipsilateral diaphragmatic function with cordotomy, preoperative pulmonary function studies and dynamic radiographic studies should be performed to assess respiratory and diaphragmatic function. Patients with any pain ipsilateral to cordotomy will often see an exacerbation of this pain (*mirror-image pain*) and may require a second, staged cordotomy on the contralateral side.

Myelotomy

Myelotomy is primarily used for bilateral or midline pain in the lower half of the body. Patients with medically intractable pelvic, lower extremity, visceral, and perineal pain are potential candidates. Classically, myelotomy has been described as incising through the posterior midline of the spinal cord to ventral pia. It is hypothesized that this interrupts the second order crossing spinothalamic pain fibers and has been designed to create a level of analgesia corresponding to the level and extent of interruption. This procedure is typically performed in the thoracolumbar region, and a number of open and closed techniques have been described (54).

Because of the variability in reported techniques, the region treated for relief from pain, and follow-up, it is difficult to draw definitive conclusions about the effectiveness of this technique. Nevertheless, some studies have shown that myelotomy provides pain relief in 80% to 90% of patients immediately after the procedure. Similar to other neurosurgical procedures for pain, the effectiveness of this operation diminishes with time, with reports of variable pain relief at distant time points (approximately 25% to 70% of patients with continued adequate relief). Myelotomy is generally well tolerated with a low rate of morbidity. Complications (approximately 10%) include temporary weakness of the lower extremities, transient loss of pain and temperature sensation, bowel/bladder incontinence, and dysesthesias. Reported mortality rates are generally in the range of 1% to 2%.

OTHER NEUROSURGICAL PROCEDURES

Mesencephalotomy

Candidates for mesencephalotomy include patients with cancer pain of the head and neck or cancer pain of the proximal upper extremity or in those with diaphragmatic paralysis in whom cordotomy may be dangerous. Mesencephalotomy involves stereotactically creating a lesion in the rostral midbrain in structures lying just medial to the lateral spinothalamic tract (55). The results of several small, uncontrolled, retrospective studies suggest that 50% to 75% of patients may have significant pain relief, over both the short term (months) to several years (up to 5 years' follow-up in some studies). Lesions at the level of the superior colliculus are not only more likely to be successful but also more commonly lead to problems such as difficulty with extraocular movements and binocular vision (up to 10%) than do lesions that are placed slightly lower in the midbrain, at the level of the inferior colliculus.

Hypophysectomy

Candidates for hypophysectomy include patients with severe bone pain as a result of metastatic disease (breast or prostate carcinomas). Although both animal studies and clinical work have shown a connection between the pituitary gland and hypothalamus and pain and pain relief, the exact mechanisms remain poorly understood. Several groups in the 1960s and 1970s reported satisfying results with respect to both pain relief and tumor regression in up to 60% of patients treated with total hypophysectomy through a *trans*-sphenoidal approach. Other methods of hypophysectomy, such as direct *trans*-sphenoidal injection of absolute ethanol and Gamma knife radiation, have also been shown to provide moderate or even complete pain relief in most selected patients (56). These results can be difficult to predict, however, and may result from a variety of factors, including endocrine effects due to loss of cortisol, thyroid-stimulating hormone, or growth hormone or due to stimulation of endorphin pathways, activation of stress-analgesic responses, or even a direct neurolytic effect. The natural consequence of the removal of the pituitary is panhypopituitarism, which carries with it significant morbidity. In addition, the need to perform these procedures under general anesthesia in patients who have been medically compromised potentially has led to waning interest in these approaches, except in carefully selected situations.

Microvascular Decompression

Microvascular decompression, an open neurosurgical approach, is based on the theory that aberrant torturous vessels compress the trigeminal nerve root entry zone at the brainstem, causing pain. By surgically placing an Ivalon or Teflon sponge between the artery and nerve, one can alleviate the facial pain. In one study, 90% of patients had sustained pain relief over 5 years and 46% recurrence of pain in 8.5 years (57).

SUMMARY

Whether treating a patient's pain resulting from a life-threatening disease or from a non-malignant source (chronic low back pain), interventional or surgical procedures may dramatically improve a patient's quality of life. Although they provide additional valuable tools when a medicinal or complementary approach fails to provide satisfactory symptom relief, the variability of patient presentation, including progression of disease, results in tremendous unpredictability of the outcome results. Pain may be alleviated in the treated site(s) while other pain elsewhere will not be affected. The distribution of locally administered drug(s) can also be variable, leading to a lessening rather than the complete resolution of the pain symptoms. The duration of the therapeutic effects may be only transient because of incompleteness of the procedure's effects. In rare cases, the intervention may further transiently aggravate or even permanently worsen pain symptoms or other adverse events may further deteriorate the patient's quality of life. Therefore, the risks and benefits must be carefully weighed. Several texts on interventional pain that provide additional information on the indications, procedure, and risks are included in Refs. 58 and 59.

Despite the above cautions, advances in pain interventional techniques continue to improve the therapeutic benefit while reducing the risks. Imaging techniques allow greater visualization and, therefore, facilitate greater ease and precision in needle placement. This provides greater specificity in targeting pain pathways and reduces untoward effects. Further, new therapies that target novel sites are in various stages of clinical development. For example, neurolytic drugs that delete only pain-specific fibers (sparing other afferent and efferent pathways) and a gene therapy approach that target dorsal root ganglia have progressed to clinical testing (60,61).

Finally, more work is needed to validate the use of some, if not most of the many current pain interventions. Although interventional techniques are frequently utilized, many therapies have not undergone rigorous blinded controlled studies to determine efficacy. This is by no means an easy task and represents an ethical dilemma because of the necessity of withholding therapies that could increase suffering in this patient group.

REFERENCES

1. de Leon-Casasola OA. Interventional procedures for cancer pain management: when are they indicated? *Cancer Invest.* 2004;22(4):630-642.
2. Hanks GW, Justins DM. Cancer pain: management. *Lancet.* 1992;339(8800):1031-1036.
3. Meuser T, Pietruck C, Radbruch L, Stute P, Lehmann KA, Grond S. Symptoms during cancer pain treatment following WHO-guidelines: a longitudinal follow-up study of symptom prevalence, severity and etiology. *Pain.* 2001;93(3):247-257.
4. Practice Guidelines for Cancer Pain Management. A report by the American Society of Anesthesiologists Task Force on Pain Management, Cancer Pain Section. *Anesthesiology.* 1996;84(5):1243-1257.
5. Smith TJ, Coyne PJ, Staats PS, et al. An implantable drug delivery system (IDDS) for refractory cancer pain provides sustained pain control, less drug-related toxicity, and possibly better survival compared with comprehensive medical management (CMM). *Ann Oncol.* 2005;16(5):825-833.
6. Ferrante FM. Opioids. In: Ferrante FM, ed. *Postoperative Pain Management.* New York, NY: Churchill Livingston; 1993:161.
7. Ferrante FM. Neuraxial infusion in the management of cancer pain. *Oncology (Williston Park, NY).* 1999;13(5 suppl 2):30-36.
8. Kim PS. Interventional cancer pain therapies. *Semin Oncol.* 2005;32(2):194-199.
9. Yaksh TL, Hassenbusch S, Burchiel K, Hildebrand KR, Page LM, Coffey RJ. Inflammatory masses associated with intrathecal drug infusion: a review of preclinical evidence and human data. *Pain Med.* 2002;3(4):300-312.
10. Mercadante S. Neuraxial techniques for cancer pain: an opinion about unresolved therapeutic dilemmas. *Reg Anesth Pain Med.* 1999;24(1):74-83.
11. Bedder MD, Burchiel K, Larson A. Cost analysis of two implantable narcotic delivery systems. *J Pain Symptom Manage.* 1991;6(6):368-373.
12. Burton AW, Rajagopal A, Shah HN, et al. Epidural and intrathecal analgesia is effective in treating refractory cancer pain. *Pain Med.* 2004;5(3):239-247.
13. Staats PS, Yearwood T, Charapata SG, et al. Intrathecal ziconotide in the treatment of refractory pain in patients with cancer or AIDS: a randomized controlled trial. *JAMA.* 2004;291(1):63-70.
14. Deer TR, Smith HS, Burton AW, et al. Comprehensive consensus based guidelines on intrathecal drug delivery systems in the treatment of pain caused by cancer pain. *Pain Physician.* 2011;14(3):E283-E312.

15. Ripamonti C, Brunelli C. Randomized clinical trial of an implantable drug delivery system compared with comprehensive medical management for refractory cancer pain: impact on pain, drug-related toxicity, and survival. *J Clin Oncol.* 2003;21(14):2801-2802; author reply 2-3.

16. Ilfeld BM, Morey TE, Enneking FK. Continuous infraclavicular perineural infusion with clonidine and ropivacaine compared with ropivacaine alone: a randomized, double-blinded, controlled study. *Anesth Analg.* 2003;97(3):706-712.

17. Ilfeld BM, Morey TE, Wright TW, Chidgey LK, Enneking FK. Continuous interscalene brachial plexus block for postoperative pain control at home: a randomized, double-blinded, placebo-controlled study. *Anesth Analg.* 2003;96(4):1089-1095, table of contents.

18. Klein SM, Greengrass RA, Grant SA, Higgins LD, Nielsen KC, Steele SM. Ambulatory surgery for multi-ligament knee reconstruction with continuous dual catheter peripheral nerve blockade. *Can J Anaesth.* 2001;48(4):375-378.

19. Swerdlow M. Spinal and peripheral neurolysis for managing pancoast syndrome. *Adv Pain Res Ther.* 1982;4:135-143.

20. Ekatodramis G, Borgeat A, Huledal G, Jeppsson L, Westman L, Sjovall J. Continuous interscalene analgesia with ropivacaine 2 mg/ml after major shoulder surgery. *Anesthesiology.* 2003;98(1):143-150.

21. Patt R, Cousins M. *Techniques for Neurolytic Neural Blockade.* Philadelphia, PA: Lippincott Williams & Wilkins; 1998.

22. Cohen SP, Foster A. Pulsed radiofrequency as a treatment for groin pain and orchialgia. *Urology.* 2003;61(3):645.

23. Waseem Z, Boulias C, Gordon A, Ismail F, Sheean G, Furlan AD. Botulinum toxin injections for low-back pain and sciatica. *Cochrane Database Syst Rev (Online)* (1):CD008257.

24. Patt R. *Peripheral Neurolysis.* Philadelphia, PA: JB Lippincott; 1993.

25. Patt RB, Millard R. A role for peripheral neurolysis in the management of intractable cancer pain. *Pain.* 1990;41(suppl 1(0)):S358.

26. Meglio M, Cioni B. Percutaneous procedures for trigeminal neuralgia: microcompression versus radiofrequency thermocoagulation. Personal experience. *Pain.* 1989;38(1):9-16.

27. Mullan S, Lichtor T. Percutaneous microcompression of the trigeminal ganglion for trigeminal neuralgia. *J Neurosurg.* 1983;59(6):1007-1012.

28. Twycross R. *Pain Relief in Advanced Cancer.* Edinburgh: Churchill Livingstone; 1994.

29. Swerdlow M. Subarachnoid and extradural blocks. *Adv Pain Res Ther.* 1979;2:325.

30. Doyle D. Nerve blocks in advanced cancer. *Practitioner.* 1982;226(1365):539, 41-44.

31. Mehta M, Ranger I. Persistent abdominal pain. Treatment by nerve block. *Anaesthesia.* 1971;26(3):330-333.

32. de Leon-Casasola OA. Critical evaluation of chemical neurolysis of the sympathetic axis for cancer pain. *Cancer Control.* 2000;7(2):142-148.

33. Black A, Dwyer B. Coeliac plexus block. *Anaesth Intensive Care.* 1973;1(4):315-318.

34. Chapman C. Issues in designing trials of nonpharmacologic treatments of pain. *Adv Pain Res Ther.* 1991;18:699.

35. Filshie J, Golding S, Robbie DS, Husband JE. Unilateral computerised tomography guided coeliac plexus block: a technique for pain relief. *Anaesthesia.* 1983;38(5):498-503.

36. Gimenez A, Martinez-Noguera A, Donoso L, Catala E, Serra R. Percutaneous neurolysis of the celiac plexus via the anterior approach with sonographic guidance. *AJR Am J Roentgenol.* 1993;161(5):1061-1063.

37. Rykowski JJ, Hilgier M. Efficacy of neurolytic celiac plexus block in varying locations of pancreatic cancer: influence on pain relief. *Anesthesiology.* 2000;92(2):347-354.

38. Lillemoe KD, Cameron JL, Kaufman HS, Yeo CJ, Pitt HA, Sauter PK. Chemical splanchnicectomy in patients with unresectable pancreatic cancer. A prospective randomized trial. *Ann Surg.* 1993;217(5):447-455; discussion 56-57.

39. Eisenberg E, Carr DB, Chalmers TC. Neurolytic celiac plexus block for treatment of cancer pain: a meta-analysis. *Anesth Analg.* 1995;80(2):290-295.

40. Cariati M, De Martini G, Pretolesi F, Roy MT. CT-guided superior hypogastric plexus block. *J Comput Assist Tomogr.* 2002;26(3):428-431.

41. Reig E, Abejon D, del Pozo C, Insausti J, Contreras R. Thermocoagulation of the ganglion impar or ganglion of Walther: description of a modified approach. Preliminary results in chronic, nononcological pain. *Pain Pract.* 2005;5(2):103-110.

42. Wagner KJ, Sprenger T, Pecho C, et al. Risks and complications of epidural neurolysis—a review with case report. *Anasthesiol Intensivmed Notfallmed Schmerzther.* 2006;41(4):213-222.

43. Melzack R, Wall PD. Pain mechanisms: a new theory. *Science.* 1965;150(699):971-979.

44. Tasker R. *Percutaneous Cordotomy: Neurosurgical and Neuroaugmentative Intervention.* Philadelphia, PA: Lippincott; 1993.

45. Tasker R, ed. *Neurostimulation and Percutaneous Neural Destructive Techniques.* Philadelphia, PA: Lippincott Williams & Wilkins; 1998.

46. Jensen M, Kallmes D. Percutaneous vertebroplasty in the treatment of malignant spine disease. *Cancer J.* 2002;8:194-206.

47. Hentschel SJ, Burton AW, Fourney DR, Rhines LD, Mendel E. Percutaneous vertebroplasty and kyphoplasty performed at a cancer center: refuting proposed contraindications. *J Neurosurg Spine.* 2005;2(4):436-440.

48. Buchbinder R, Osborne RH, Ebeling PR, et al. A randomized trial of vertebroplasty for painful osteoporotic vertebral fractures. *N Engl J Med.* 2009;361(6):557-568.

49. Kallmes DF, Comstock BA, Heagerty PJ, et al. A randomized trial of vertebroplasty for osteoporotic spinal fractures. *N Engl J Med.* 2009;361(6):569-579.

50. Klazen CA, Lohle PN, de Vries J, et al. Vertebroplasty versus conservative treatment in acute osteoporotic vertebral compression fractures (Vertos II): an open-label randomised trial. *Lancet.* 2010;376(9746):1085-1092.

51. Wardlaw D, Cummings SR, Van Meirhaeghe J, et al. Efficacy and safety of balloon kyphoplasty compared with non-surgical care for vertebral compression fracture (FREE): a randomised controlled trial. *Lancet.* 2009;373(9668):1016-1024.

52. Huber FX, McArthur N, Tanner M, et al. Kyphoplasty for patients with multiple myeloma is a safe surgical procedure: results from a large patient cohort. *Clin Lymphoma Myeloma.* 2009;9(5):375-380.

53. White JC, Sweet WH. Anterolateral cordotomy: open versus closed comparison of end results. In: Bonica J, Liebeskind JC, Albe-Fessard D, eds. *Advances in Pain Research and Therapy.* New York, NY: Raven Press; 1979;3:911-919.

54. Kanpolat Y, Akyar S, Caglar S, Unlu A, Bilgic S. CT-guided percutaneous selective cordotomy. *Acta Neurochir (Wien).* 1993;123(1-2):92-96.

55. Bosch DA. Stereotactic rostral mesencephalotomy in cancer pain and deafferentation pain. A series of 40 cases with follow-up results. *J Neurosurg.* 1991;75(5):747-751.

56. Hayashi M, Taira T, Chernov M, et al. Gamma knife surgery for cancer pain-pituitary gland-stalk ablation: a multicenter prospective protocol since 2002. *J Neurosurg.* 2002;97(5 suppl):433-437.

57. Loeser J. Tic douloureux and atypical facial pain. In: Wall PD, Melzack R, eds. *Textbook of Pain.* Edinburgh: Churchill Livingston; 1994:688-710.

58. Neural blockade. In: Cousins M, Bridenbaugh P, eds. *Clinical Anesthesia and Management of Pain.* Philadelphia, PA: Lippincott Williams & Wilkins; 1998.

59. Waldman S, Winnie A. *Interventional Pain Management.* Philadelphia, PA: WB Saunders; 2001.

60. Fink DJ, Wechuck J, Mata M, et al. Gene therapy for pain: results of a phase I clinical trial. *Ann Neurol.* 2011;70(2):207-212.

61. Karai L, Brown DC, Mannes AJ, et al. Deletion of vanilloid receptor 1-expressing primary afferent neurons for pain control. *J Clin Invest.* 2004;113(9):1344-1352.

CHAPTER 5

Pathology of Bone Metastases— Implications for Treatment

Patrick W. Mantyh

INTRODUCTION

Similar to cancer itself, the factors that drive cancer pain evolve and change with disease progression. Surgery, radiation, and chemotherapy are used to remove or kill cancer cells and all can induce pain and/or dysfunction of sensory and sympathetic nerve fibers. In cases where the cancer continues to grow or relapse occurs, cancer cells and their associated stromal cells generate an ongoing pain by releasing algogenic substances, including protons, bradykinin, endothelins (ETs), prostaglandins, proteases, and tyrosine kinase activators. With disease progression, tumor growth can directly injure nerve fibers giving rise to a neuropathic pain. Additionally, cancer and associated stromal cells can release growth factors such as nerve growth factor (NGF) that can induce a highly ectopic sprouting and formation of neuroma-like structures by sensory and sympathetic nerve fibers.

This structural reorganization of sensory and sympathetic nerve fibers along with a cellular and neurochemical reorganization in the spinal cord and brain has the potential to drive breakthrough cancer pain. Incorporating this new understanding of the mechanisms that drive cancer pain into new treatments for cancer pain should increase the quality of life and functional status of cancer patients and survivors.

THE CLINICAL PROBLEM

In 2008, over 12 million people were diagnosed with cancer worldwide (excluding non-melanoma skin cancer) and 8 million individuals died from cancer (1). By 2030, the global burden is expected to grow to 21.4 million new cancer cases and 13.2 million cancer deaths simply due to the growth and aging of the population, as well as reductions in childhood mortality and deaths from infectious diseases in developing countries. Cancer incidence rates are stable or slightly falling in developed countries, whereas in developing countries cancer incidence rates are increasing, as smoking, obesity, and increased life expectancy have led to a rapid rise in the incidence of cancer (1–3). Additionally, as the detection and treatment of most cancers have dramatically improved, survival rates have increased so that even patients with metastatic cancer are surviving years to decades beyond their initial diagnosis (4).

Cancer-associated pain is one of the most common presenting symptoms that results in the diagnosis of cancer. While pain can be present at any time during the course of the disease, it generally increases with disease progression so that 75% to 90% of patients with metastatic or advanced stage cancer will experience significant cancer pain (5,6). Mechanisms that drive cancer pain include cancer therapy, factors released from tumors that sensitize or excite primary afferent neurons, tumor-induced nerve injury, and tumor-induced nerve sprouting and neuroma formation (7–10).

In patients with cancer, having surgery or receiving the full dose of radiation or chemotherapy is one of the most significant factors in determining patient survival (7). However, peripheral nerve neurotoxicity and accompanying pain are major side effects of radiation and many of the most commonly used anti-neoplastic agents, including the taxanes (e.g., paclitaxel and docetaxel), vinca alkaloids (e.g., vincristine and vinblastine), platinum-based compounds (e.g., cisplatin and oxaliplatin), and proteasome inhibitors (e.g., bortezomib and disulfiram) (7,11–14). If the chemotherapy-induced peripheral neuropathy becomes severe enough, the oncologist or patient may reduce or cease chemotherapy treatment, which decreases the overall survival rate of the patient and the likelihood that the patient will be disease free.

In cases where the tumor is inoperable or relapse occurs, cancer and associated stromal cells can induce significant pain. This pain can arise from the original site of the cancer (i.e., pancreatic cancer, head and neck cancer, and osteosarcoma) (15–17) or from distant sites (such as bone) where common cancers such as breast, prostate, kidney, and lung avidly metastasize (18). The original presentation of tumor-induced pain is usually described as dull in character, constant in presentation, and gradually increasing in intensity with time (19). If the disease progression continues, a second type of cancer pain known as "breakthrough" or severe "incident pain" can emerge (20). Incident or breakthrough pain, which is defined as a transitory flare of extreme pain superimposed on an otherwise stable pain pattern in patients treated with opioids (21), can occur spontaneously or by the movement or weight bearing of a tumor-bearing organ or tissue (22). Since breakthrough pain is frequently acute and unpredictable in onset, this pain can be severe, debilitating, and difficult to fully control (23,20).

Currently, tumor-induced pain is largely managed with an "analgesic ladder" that was originally promulgated by the World Health Organization in 1986. This ladder begins with a non-steroidal anti-inflammatory drug (NSAID) and if pain worsens the next step is NSAID + a mild opiate and finally when the pain becomes severe, an NSAID + a strong opiate.

In addition to this three-step ladder, other adjuvant therapies including radiation therapy, radioisotopes, nerve block, nerve lesions, antiepileptics (e.g., gabapentin and carbamazepine), antidepressants (e.g., amitriptyline and imipramine), and steroids are commonly employed to control cancer pain (24). It should be stressed that most cancer pain can be controlled if the cancer pain is closely monitored and these therapies are used in a timely and proactive manner. However, all of the above therapies have significant unwanted side effects (25) and closely monitoring and fully controlling cancer pain (especially if breakthrough pain is present) can be very time consuming for the patient, caregiver, and physician (26). Developing new analgesic therapies that are more efficacious and have fewer side effects than current analgesics and incorporating these advances into mainstream cancer therapy will significantly improve the quality of life and functional status of both the patient and the caregiver.

THE TUMOR ENVIRONMENT AND CANCER PAIN

The tumor is composed of not only cancer cells but also tumor-associated stromal cells. In most tumors, stromal cells far outnumber the cancer cells and include endothelial cells, fibroblasts as well as a host of inflammatory and immune cells, including macrophages, mast cells, neutrophils and T lymphocytes (27). Both cancer cells and their associated stromal cells secrete a wide variety of factors (7,27), many of which have been shown to sensitize or directly excite primary afferent neurons (28).

Tumor-Induced Acidosis

The finding that a subpopulation of sensory neurons (Figure 5.1) expressed the transient receptor potential vanilloid 1 (TRPV1, which is also known as the capsaicin receptor) and the acid-sensing ion channel 3 (ASIC3) and that both these channels responded to acidosis was of significant interest to researchers studying cancer pain (28). Thus, cancer cells in general have a lower pH (6.8) than normal cells (pH 7.2) (29). Importantly, many tumors that metastasize to bone induce a marked proliferation and hypertrophy of osteoclasts. Osteoclasts avidly resorb bone by generating a pH of 2 to 4 in their resorption bay, which contributes to the excessive bone resorption that can ultimately lead to fracture of the tumor-bearing bone (30). To test whether TRPV1 channels are expressed by sensory nerve fibers that innervate tumor-bearing tissue and whether a TRPV1 contributed to cancer pain, an in vivo mouse model of bone cancer pain was explored (31). In these studies it was shown that a subpopulation of nerve fibers that innervate the tumor-bearing bone expressed TRPV1, that acute or chronic administration of a TRPV1 antagonist attenuated bone cancer pain, and that disruption of the *TRPV1* gene results in an attenuation of bone cancer pain (31). Furthermore, administration of the TRPV1 antagonist to TRPV1 null animals with bone cancer resulted in no further reduction of pain than what was already present in the TRPV1 null mice (31). To date results from human clinical trials with TRPV1 or ASIC3 channel antagonists have not been reported in cancer pain. However, as discussed below, understanding the role that TRPV1 plays in driving bone cancer pain has provided insight into one mechanism by which therapies that inhibit osteoclasts (including bisphosphonates and denosumab, which is an anti-RANKL [anti-receptor activator of nuclear factor kappa-B ligand] fully humanized monoclonal antibody) are efficacious in reducing bone cancer pain (32–34).

The skeleton is the most common site for distant metastasis of prostate, breast, lung, and renal carcinomas (18). Once tumor cells have metastasized to bone, a cycle of tumor growth, bone destruction, and formation of woven bone begins, which can result in significant pain, skeletal fractures, and hypercalcemia (18). Cancer cells themselves do not destroy bone but rather they and their associated stromal cells express the RANKL which binds to its receptor RANK that is expressed by osteoclasts. The activation of the RANKL/RANK pathway promotes the proliferation and hypertrophy of these bone-destroying osteoclasts (35). Osteoclasts resorb bone by forming a highly acidic resorption "bay" or "pit" between the osteoclast and bone, which can stimulate the TRPV1 or ASIC3 channels and drive bone cancer pain (35). In the last decade, multiple studies have shown that therapies that reduce osteoclast function also significantly reduce bone cancer pain (7,32–34,36,37).

The first and most widely used therapy is the class of compounds known as bisphosphonates that avidly bind to bone. Once the bisphosphonate has bound to bone, osteoclasts that are resorbing bone generally need to actively endocytose the breakdown products of bone at the apical (bone facing) surface and transcytose these products to be released at the distal surface of the osteoclast for disposal by exocytosis (38). However, if a bisphosphonate is tightly bound to the bone that is being resorbed, the bisphosphonate will also be taken up by endocytosis (39). Once internalized, the bisphosphonate interferes either with adenosine triphosphate energy metabolism (non-nitrogen-containing bisphosphonates) or with the mevalonate pathway (nitrogen-containing bisphosphonates), resulting first in osteoclast dysfunction and ultimately in osteoclast apoptosis (39,40). As a significant population of nerve fibers that innervate the bone express TRPV1 (31), one way bisphosphonates appear to relieve bone pain is by decreasing the osteoclast-induced acidosis, which in turn decreases the activation of the ion-sensing TRPV1 or ASIC3 receptors that are expressed by sensory nerve fibers.

Another method that is highly effective in reducing tumor-induced osteoclast bone resorption in both animals and humans is by interfering with the RANKL binding to RANK, which is required for osteoclast proliferation, maturation, and survival (41). Within 2 days of administration of therapies that interfere with RANKL binding to RANK (such as osteoprotegerin or denosumab), there is almost a complete loss of activated osteoclasts, a marked reduction in plasma markers of bone resorption, and a significant attenuation of bone cancer pain (36).

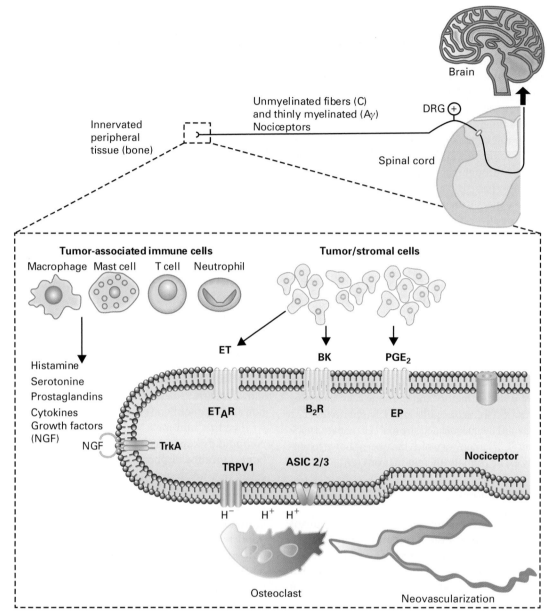

Figure 5.1. Primary afferent sensory nerve fibers and the generation and maintenance of cancer pain. Primary afferent neurons innervating the body have their cell bodies in the dorsal root ganglia (DRG) and transmit sensory information from the periphery to the spinal cord and brain. Unmyelinated C fibers and thinly myelinated Aδ fibers contain small-diameter cell bodies that project centrally to the superficial spinal cord. These fibers are involved in detecting multiple noxious stimuli (chemical, thermal, and mechanical). *Box*. Nociceptors use several different types of receptors to detect and transmit signals about noxious stimuli produced by cancer cells, tumor-associated immune cells, or other aspects of the tumor microenvironment. Multiple factors may contribute to the pain associated with cancer. The transient receptor potential vanilloid receptor 1 (TRPV1) and acid-sensing ion channels (ASICs) detect extracellular protons produced by tumor-induced tissue damage or abnormal osteoclast-mediated bone resorption. Several mechanosensitive ion channels may be involved in detecting high-threshold mechanical stimuli that occur when distal aspects of sensory nerve fibers are distended from mechanical pressure due to the growing tumor or as a result of destabilization or fracture of bone. Tumor cells and associated inflammatory (immune) cells produce a variety of chemical mediators, including prostaglandins (PGE_2), nerve growth factor (NGF), endothelins (ET), bradykinin (BK), and extracellular ATP. Several of these proinflammatory mediators have receptors on peripheral terminals and can directly activate or sensitize nociceptors. NGF, together with its cognate receptor tropomyosin receptor kinase A (TrkA), may serve as a master regulator of bone cancer pain by modulating the sensitivity and increasing the expression of several receptors and ion channels that contribute to the increased excitability of nociceptors in the vicinity of the tumor. Prostaglandin receptor (EP), bradykinin receptor 2 (B_2R), endothelin subtype A receptor (ET_AR).

Tumor-Induced Mechanical Instability of Bone

Therapies that inhibit osteoclast-induced bone resorption also maintain the mechanical strength of bone even though tumor cells are present in the bone. Thus, in addition to acidosis, excessive tumor-induced osteoclast bone resorption destroys bone and leads to mechanical instability and fracture of bone that causes mechanical distortion of the sensory nerve fibers that innervate the bone (42,43). Thus, following significant weakening or fracture due to tumor-induced bone remodeling, there can be significant movement-evoked pain presumably due to mechanical distortion of the mechanosensitive sensory nerve fibers that innervate the bone. Clearly, pain associated with fracture and distortion of the bone is usually attenuated if the bone is stabilized and repositioned into its normal orientation (44). Both osteolytic and osteoblastic tumors induce a loss of the mechanical strength and stability of mineralized bone (45,46), so with significant bone remodeling, bone stress that is normally nontraumatic can now result in bone fracture with resulting distortion and activation of mechanosensitive nerve fibers that innervate the bone. As bisphosphonates and anti-RANKL therapies reduce tumor-induced osteoclast bone remodeling, preserve the mechanical strength of bone, reduce bone fracture, and reduce osteoclast-induced acidosis in both animals and humans, these therapies are now routinely used to prevent cancer-induced bone fractures and manage pain due to cancer metastasis to bone.

Factors Released by Cancer and Associated Stromal Cells that Drive Cancer Pain

One area that has significantly contributed to our understanding of what drives cancer pain is studies examining the factors released by tumor/stromal cells that drive cancer pain and influence disease progression. These factors include bradykinin, cannabinoids (CBs), ETs, interleukin-6, granulocyte–macrophage colony-stimulating factor (GM-CSF), NGF, proteases, and tumor necrosis factor-α (TNF-α).

Recent studies have revealed that the CB system has an important role in modulating cancer pain. It has been reported that the tumor-induced mechanical hyperalgesia in the hindpaw is associated with decreased levels of anandamide (an endogenous agonist of CB-1 and CB-2 receptors) and increased degradation of anandamide in the hindpaw skin ipsilateral to the tumor-bearing paw (47). Furthermore, the injection into the hindpaw of anandamide or an inhibitor of the enzyme that degrades anandamide reduced the tumor-induced hyperalgesia. A recent report also demonstrated that acute and sustained administration of a CB-2 agonist attenuates both spontaneous and evoked pain behaviors in a bone cancer pain model (48). While these studies suggest that the CB system plays a role in driving cancer pain, future clinical studies are warranted to evaluate the analgesic as well as the potential CNS side effects of these drugs.

Human studies have shown that several non-hematopoietic tumors secrete colony-stimulating factors that act on their receptors expressed on myeloid cells, tumor cells, and nerve fibers. For example, it has been reported that the levels of granulocyte colony-stimulating factor (G-CSF) and GM-CSF in the lysates of bone marrow from tumor-bearing mice were significantly increased as compared with the levels in the naive mice (49). Additionally, GM-CSF sensitized the nerves to mechanical stimuli, potentiated the calcitonin gene–related peptide (CGRP) release, and caused sprouting of sensory nerve endings in the skin (49). The actions of these colony-stimulating factors are mediated by the activation of their receptors (G-CSFR and GM-CSFR-α, expressed in the peripheral nerves innervating the tumor-bearing tissue), as the administration of neutralizing antisera against these receptors and the sensory nerve–specific knockdown of GM-CSF receptors reduced the tumor-induced pain behaviors (49). Based on these studies, colony-stimulating factors may be a potential target therapeutic to be exploited in the cancer pain field.

ET antagonists are another group of pharmacologic agents that offer promise in the management of cancer pain and a reduction in disease progression. ETs (ET-1, ET-2, and ET-3) are a family of vasoactive peptides that are expressed at high levels by several types of tumors, including those that arise from the prostate (50,51). Clinical studies have shown a correlation between the severity of the pain and plasma levels of ETs in prostate cancer patients (50). Electrophysiologic studies have shown that ET-1 may directly sensitize or excite C-fiber nociceptors innervating the tumor-bearing tissue through activation of ET_A receptors (52), which are expressed by a subset of small unmyelinated primary afferent neurons (53). Furthermore, direct application of ET to peripheral nerves induces activation of primary afferent fibers and an induction of pain-related behaviors (54,52). These results suggest that ETs play a critical role in tumor-induced thermal and mechanical hyperalgesia. Currently, there are several ongoing human clinical trials examining the effects that ET_A antagonists have on cancer pain and disease progression.

Tumors release a variety of chemical agents that sensitize peripheral afferent neurons, including cytokines. One of the most studied cytokines in the pain field is the proinflammatory and proalgesic cytokine, TNF-α. TNF-α is produced by inflammatory/immune cells, Schwann cells, and by some tumor cells (55). It has been reported that TNF-α levels are significantly increased in tumor microperfusates and tumor site homogenates as compared with the levels from naive mice or contralateral hind limb (56). Furthermore, injection of TNF-α into tumor-bearing mice results in heat and mechanical hyperalgesia, which is blocked by administering the TNF-α antagonist etanercept (57). Another cytokine that has been suggested to be involved in driving cancer pain is the pleiotropic cytokine IL-6. Several studies have shown that the levels of this cytokine are upregulated under various pathologic conditions (58–60) and that the direct injection (intradermal, muscular, and intrathecal) of IL-6 results in mechanical and thermal hyperalgesia (61–63). IL-6 is produced by different inflammatory/immune cells and some tumor cells (59). The actions of IL-6 are mediated by binding to its specific receptor, IL-6R, which exists in both transmembrane and soluble forms (64,60). Binding of IL-6 triggers an association of the IL-6R with the transducer glycoprotein, gp130 (65). Recently, it has been reported that the nociceptor-specific depletion of gp130 resulted in a significant reduction of the heat hyperalgesia induced by the subcutaneous injection of carcinoma cells into the hindpaw without affecting the tumor growth (66). These results suggest that TNF-α or IL-6/gp130 may contribute to cancer pain.

One important concept that has emerged over the last decade is that factors which influence the survival and growth of nerve fibers such as NGF are able to directly activate sensory neurons and that these growth factors can play a key role in the sensitization of nociceptors [see for review Ref. (67)]. For example, NGF can induce a rapid phosphorylation and sensitization of TRPV1 receptors, and the retrograde transport of NGF along with its cognate receptor tropomysin receptor kinase A (TrkA) in an NGF/TrkA complex back to the neuronal cell bodies of the TrkA expressing sensory neuron can induce an increase in the synthesis of the neurotransmitters substance P and CGRP and increased expression of receptors (bradykinin R), channels (P2X3, TRPV1, ASIC3 and sodium channels, transcription factors (ATF-3), and structural molecules (neurofilaments and the sodium channel anchoring molecule p11) (see for review Ref. (67)). Additionally, NGF appears to modulate the trafficking and insertion of sodium channels such as Nav 1.8 (68) and TRPV1 (69) in the sensory neurons, as well as modulating the expression profile of supporting cells in the dorsal root ganglia (DRG) and peripheral nerve, such as non-myelinating Schwann cells and macrophages (70–72).

In light of the potential role that NGF may play in driving bone cancer pain, therapies that block NGF or TrkA have been examined in preclinical models of breast, prostate, and sarcoma bone cancer pain. Interestingly, even though the prostate cancer cells did not express detectable levels of mRNA coding for NGF (73), in all three models of bone cancer pain, administration of anti-NGF therapy (using an antibody that sequesters extracellular NGF) was not only highly efficacious in reducing both early and late-stage bone cancer pain-related behaviors, but this reduction in pain-related behaviors was greater than that achieved with acute administration of 10 mg/kg of morphine sulfate (73,74). If cancer cells do not have to express NGF for anti-NGF to have an analgesic effect, what other tumor-associated cells might be synthesizing and releasing NGF? Previous studies have shown that many tumor-associated stromal cells including macrophages, T lymphocytes, mast cells, and endothelial cells are capable of expressing and releasing NGF (75,67). Thus, therapies that target NGF or its cognate receptor TrkA may be efficacious in attenuating cancer pain not only when the cancer cells express NGF but also in cancers where cancer cells and/or large number of tumor associated stromal cells express and release NGF.

Therapies targeting ET$_A$ receptors, NGF, and TNF-α are currently in human clinical trials in patients with bone cancer pain (www.clinicaltrials.gov). Whether therapies targeting these factors will reach and be successful clinical trials in humans for relieving human cancer pain will largely depend on issues related to safety, efficacy, and effects on tumor growth and metastasis. Choosing which type of cancer pain to target in clinical trials is currently a hit or miss proposition as there are relatively few preclinical models of cancer pain and different types of tumors can have very unique characteristics as shown by chemotherapeutic agents which can be highly effective against one cancer and ineffective in another. Developing a better understanding of what common and what unique factors drive different cancer pains would be of enormous benefit, as it would greatly aid in defining which type of cancer pain will be most likely to respond to targeted analgesic therapies in clinical trials.

Tumor-Induced Nerve Injury and Neuropathic Pain

In the sarcoma and prostate mouse bone cancer pain models and a mouse model of pancreatic cancer pain, as tumor cells invade the normal tissue, the cancer and associated stromal cells come into contact, injure and then destroy the very distal processes of sensory fibers (76). Thus, while sensory fibers appear to have a normal morphology at the leading edge of the tumor, with time the sensory nerve fibers begin to display a discontinuous and fragmented appearance. These data suggest that following initial activation by the tumor cells, the distal processes of the sensory fibers were ultimately injured and destroyed as the invading tumor cells first proliferate and then undergo necrosis as they outgrow the neovascularization that supports them (76). This initial tumor-induced activation and then injury to the sensory nerve fibers is accompanied by an increase in ongoing and movement-evoked pain behaviors. Interestingly, there are several changes in the DRG, including hypertrophy of satellite cells surrounding sensory neuron cell bodies, upregulation of ATF-3, and macrophage infiltration of the DRG, which have also been described in other models of peripheral nerve injury and in other non-cancerous neuropathic pain states (76). These data as well as the fact that a component of bone cancer pain is attenuated by gabapentin (which is approved for the treatment of neuropathic pain) suggest that a component of cancer pain is neuropathic in origin (76).

Tumor-Induced Nerved Sprouting and Neuroma Formation

While tumor-induced injury has been observed in both animals and humans with cancer, an intriguing but largely unexplored mechanism by which cancer pain may be generated is by an active and pathologic tumor-induced sprouting and neuroma formation. Previous studies in humans and experimental animals have shown that inappropriate sprouting and/or neuroma formation can lead to a change in the phenotype of sensory and sympathetic nerve fibers, including an upregulation and inappropriate insertion of sodium channels into the distal tips of injured sensory neurons

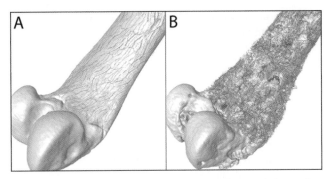

Figure 5.2. Tumor-induced nerve sprouting and formation of neuroma-like structures in bone cancer. Confocal images showing the organization and distribution of sensory nerve fibers that express calcitonin gene-related peptide (CGRP) in the normal (**A**) vs. sarcoma-bearing (**B**) mouse bone. In the normal mouse bone, CGRP $^+$ sensory nerve fibers have a homogeneous "netlike" organization that detects noxious stimuli such as bone fracture. As sarcoma cancer cells invade the periosteum of the bone they induce robust sprouting of CGRP $^+$ sensory fibers and the formation of neuroma-like structure that is never observed in normal bone. Note that in the tumor-bearing femur (**B**), invasion of the cancer cells has induced significant remodeling of the cortical bone. Confocal images from periosteal whole mount preparations were acquired and overlapped on a three-dimensional image of the mouse femur obtained by microcomputed tomography. Images were rendered courtesy of Marvin Landis (University Information Technology Services, University of Arizona).

(77–79). These newly formed sensory nerve fibers (that sprout in response to peripheral nerve injury) exhibit both spontaneous and movement-evoked ectopic discharges, which were accompanied by a pain that was both severe and difficult to manage medically (79–81).

In a mouse model of pancreatic cancer pain (82) and breast (83), prostate (9), and sarcoma (10) models of bone cancer there was first tumor-induced nerve injury and then a subsequent sprouting and formation of neuroma-like structures by sensory and sympathetic nerve fibers (Figure 5.2). To address what might be driving this ectopic sprouting and neuroma formation, anti-NGF therapy was given. It was found that sustained administration of anti-NGF therapy largely blocked the pathologic sprouting of sensory and sympathetic nerve fibers and the formation of neuroma-like structures and significantly inhibited the development of cancer pain in this model (10). Interestingly, injection of canine prostate cancer cells (which do not express detectable levels of mRNA encoding NGF) into the bone of nude mice induces a sprouting of CGRP $^+$ and NF200 $^+$ sensory nerve fibers and TH $^+$ sympathetic nerve fibers and nearly all of these sprouting nerve fibers coexpress TrkA $^+$ (9). What is in some ways impressive about these results is the extent of sprouting, so that even in the bone marrow, which normally receives a very modest innervation by sensory nerve fibers, prostate tumor-associated stromal cells can induce a 10 to 70-fold increase in the density of TrkA $^+$ nerve fibers (9).

Data from these experiments suggested that a significant portion of this ectopic sprouting and neuroma formation is driven by NGF. While it was originally assumed that the majority of the NGF was from tumor cells, another study using a tumor cell that did not express NGF showed exuberant sprouting suggesting that NGF released from tumor-associated stromal cells could drive this ectopic reorganization of sensory and sympathetic nerve fibers. Interestingly, in both the pancreatic (82) and bone models of cancer pain (9,10,83), sprouting and nerve degeneration were not mutually exclusive but rather over a period of weeks to months nerve fibers were first injured, then sprouting occurred and then the nerve fibers reinjured when the tumor became necrotic due to the gradual loss of the vascular supply needed to maintain tumor viability. As damage to even the distal ends of peripheral nerves can induce neuropathic pain, these processes of tumor-induced sprouting and destruction of these newly sprouted sensory and sympathetic fibers have the potential to contribute to both movement-evoked and spontaneous breakthrough cancer pain.

These studies suggest that tyrosine kinase activators, in this case NGF-activating TrkA, can induce a remarkable and active reorganization of sensory and sympathetic nerve fibers that may contribute to an ongoing and breakthrough pain (10). Clearly, other tyrosine kinase activators that induce sensitization in tumor tissues in a manner similar to NGF, such as artemin (84), G-CSF (49), GM-CSF (49), which have been shown to be involved in tumor-induced sensitization, may also play a significant role in promoting tumor-induced sprouting and neuroma formation. Whether a similar sprouting/neuroma formation occurs in painful non-bony cancers has yet to be explored. Previous studies have demonstrated that the activation of tyrosine kinase receptors can induce a sprouting that is both rapid and profuse (85). Importantly, parent tumor cells are constantly proliferating, metastasizing, and undergoing necrosis while the daughter cells are regrowing at new sites. Thus, even if therapies that block NGF or TrkA are given after tumor-induced sprouting and/ or neuroma formation has occurred, NGF and TrkA blocks the nerve sprouting and neuroma formation that occur as the daughter cells proliferate. These results emphasize the evolving nature of cancer pain and suggest that the earlier and more effective the analgesic therapy is commenced, the greater the likelihood of being able to effectively control both early- and late-stage cancer pain.

Central Sensitization in Cancer Pain

The majority of what we know about the mechanisms that generate cancer pain has focused on changes in primary afferent sensory nerve fibers and sympathetic fibers that innervate the tumor-bearing organ. However, several studies have demonstrated that animals with cancer pain also have significant pathologic changes in the CNS that contribute to the generation and maintenance of cancer pain [see for review Ref. (8)]. Thus, it has been reported that in mice with bone cancer pain there are simultaneous changes in the segments of the spinal cord that receive input from nerve fibers that innervate the tumor-bearing tissue. These changes include simultaneous changes in dynorphin, astrocytes, microglia, c-Fos expression, and substance P internalization (86). Other reports have demonstrated that in bone cancer models pain-related behaviors are accompanied by an increased expression of NR2B, an NMDA (N-methyl-D-aspartate) receptor subunit, and interleukin-1β released from glial cells and thought to facilitate pain by enhancing phosphorylation of NMDA receptor NR-1 subunit (87,88). These latter results suggest that chemical mediators released from glial cells may control the amplitude of synaptic responses in animals bearing bone cancer by changing the expression levels of NMDA and AMPA (α-amino-3-hydroxy-5-methyl-4-isoxazolepropionic acid) receptors and their phosphorylation (87,88).

The possibility that cancer pain also involves changes in the CNS is supported by a recent report that used patch-clamp recordings from spinal cord slices with an attached dorsal root, where it was shown that tumor-bearing mice exhibit unique plastic changes in spinal excitatory synaptic transmission mediated through Aδ and C afferent fibers (89). In vivo population studies in rodent model of breast-induced bone cancer pain reveal that in normal animals the proportions of wide dynamic range (WDR) to nociceptive-specific neurons in this lamina lie at 26% WDR to 74% nociceptive-specific, whereas upon establishment of cancer pain, this ratio shifts to 47% WDR to 53% nociceptive-specific. This phenotype shift of the superficial dorsal horn population is accompanied by a WDR hyperexcitabilty to mechanical, thermal, and electrical stimuli in the superficial and deep dorsal horn (90), which correlates with the development of behavioral signs of pain and further suggests an ongoing state of central sensitization that occurs in bone cancer pain.

Other data suggest that in cancer pain central sensitization is not confined to the spinal cord but rather sites including the brain stem, thalamus, amygdala and cerebral cortex that are involved in descending inhibition and facilitation also show clear changes, implying that descending controls also play a role in the maintenance of cancer-induced bone pain (8). Together, these studies suggest that cancer pain not only sensitizes primary afferent neurons, but it induces a significant reorganization within the CNS. Combining preclinical cancer pain studies with brain imaging studies in human cancer pain patients has the potential to not only provide a better understanding of how cancer pain is generated and maintained but also what changes in the processing and perception (i.e., discriminative vs. affective component) of cancer pain occurring in specific areas of the CNS.

CONCLUSIONS

The mechanisms that drive cancer pain appear to evolve and change with disease progression. Cancer cells and their associated stromal cells can generate ongoing and breakthrough pain. Ongoing and breakthrough cancer pain appears to be driven in an additive fashion, first by tumor and stromal cell-releasing factors that sensitize and activate nociceptors, then by injury to sensory nerve fibers, and finally by releasing growth factors that drive ectopic sprouting of nerve fibers and neuroma formation, all of which can contribute to central sensitization. Therapies are now in the clinic or in clinical trials that target specific mechanisms that contribute to cancer pain. This new understanding allows the development of novel mechanism-based therapies that do not have greater efficacy but can attenuate cancer pain without the side effects of currently available analgesics.

REFERENCES

1. American Cancer Society. *Global Cancer Facts & Figures 2nd Edition*. Atlanta: American Cancer Society; 2011.
2. Khan N, Afaq F, Mukhtar H. Lifestyle as risk factor for cancer: evidence from human studies. *Cancer Lett.* 2010;293(2):133-143.
3. Jemal A, Bray F, Center MM, et al. Global cancer statistics. *CA Cancer J Clin.* 2011;61(2):69-90.
4. Jemal A, Siegel R, Xu J, et al. Cancer statistics, 2010. *CA: Cancer J Clin.* 2010;60(5):277-300.
5. van den Beuken-van Everdingen MH, de Rijke JM, Kessels AG, et al. Prevalence of pain in patients with cancer: a systematic review of the past 40 years. *Ann Oncol.* 2007;18(9):1437-1449.
6. Costantini M, Ripamonti C, Beccaro M, et al. Prevalence, distress, management, and relief of pain during the last 3 months of cancer patients' life. Results of an Italian mortality follow-back survey. *Ann Oncol.* 2009;20(4):729-735.
7. Mantyh PW. Cancer pain and its impact on diagnosis, survival and quality of life. *Nat Rev Neurosci.* 2006;7(10):797-809.
8. Gordon-Williams RM, Dickenson AH. Central neuronal mechanisms in cancer-induced bone pain. *Curr Opin Support Palliat Care.* 2007;1(1):6-10.
9. Jimenez-Andrade JM, Bloom AP, Stake JI, et al. Pathological sprouting of adult nociceptors in chronic prostate cancer-induced bone pain. *J Neurosci.* 2010;30(44):14649-14656.
10. Mantyh WG, Jimenez-Andrade JM, Stake JI, et al. Blockade of nerve sprouting and neuroma formation markedly attenuates the development of late stage cancer pain. *Neuroscience.* 2010;171(2):588-598.
11. Quasthoff S, Hartung HP. Chemotherapy-induced peripheral neuropathy. *J Neurol.* 2002;249(1):9-17.
12. Cata JP, Weng HR, Lee BN, et al. Clinical and experimental findings in humans and animals with chemotherapy-induced peripheral neuropathy. *Minerva Anestesiol.* 2006;72(3):151-169.
13. Mielke S, Sparreboom A, Mross K. Peripheral neuropathy: a persisting challenge in paclitaxel-based regimes. *Eur J Cancer.* 2006;42(1):24-30.
14. Bennett GJ. Pathophysiology and animal models of cancer-related painful peripheral neuropathy. *Oncologist.* 2010;15(suppl 2):9-12.
15. Dreghorn CR, Newman RJ, Hardy GJ, et al. Primary tumors of the axial skeleton. Experience of the Leeds Regional Bone Tumor Registry. *Spine (Phila Pa 1976).* 1990;15(2):137-140.
16. Zhu Z, Friess H, Dimola FF, et al. Nerve growth factor expression correlates with perineural invasion and pain in pancreatic cancer. *J Clin Oncol.* 1999;17:2419-2428.
17. Lam DK, Schmidt BL. Orofacial pain onset predicts transition to head and neck cancer. *Pain.* 2011;152(5):1206-1209.

18. Coleman RE. Clinical features of metastatic bone disease and risk of skeletal morbidity. *Clin Cancer Res.* 2006;12(20 Pt 2): 6243s-6249s.

19. Dy SM, Asch SM, Naeim A, et al. Evidence-based standards for cancer pain management. *J Clin Oncol.* 2008;26(23): 3879-3885.

20. Mercadante S. Malignant bone pain: pathophysiology and treatment. *Pain.* 1997;69(1-2):1-18.

21. Casuccio A, Mercadante S, Fulfaro F. Treatment strategies for cancer patients with breakthrough pain. *Expert Opin Pharmacother.* 2009;10(6):947-953.

22. Mercadante S, Villari P, Ferrera P, et al. Optimization of opioid therapy for preventing incident pain associated with bone metastases. *J Pain Symptom Manage.* 2004;28(5):505-510.

23. Coleman RE. Skeletal complications of malignancy. *Cancer.* 1997;80(8 suppl):1588-1594.

24. Desandre PL, Quest TE. Management of cancer-related pain. *Emerg Med Clin North Am.* 2009;27(2):179-194.

25. Montagnini ML, Zaleon CR. Pharmacological management of cancer pain. *J Opioid Manag.* 2009;5(2):89-96.

26. Lossignol DA, Dumitrescu C. Breakthrough pain: progress in management. *Curr Opin Oncol.* 2010;22(4):302-306.

27. Joyce JA, Pollard JW. Microenvironmental regulation of metastasis. *Nat Rev Cancer.* 2009;9(4):239-252.

28. Julius D, Basbaum AI. Molecular mechanisms of nociception. *Nature.* 2001;413(6852):203-210.

29. Griffiths JR. Are cancer cells acidic? *Br J Cancer.* 1991;64:425-427.

30. Clohisy DR, Perkins SL, Ramnaraine ML. Review of cellular mechanisms of tumor osteolysis. *Clin Orthop Rel Res.* 2000;373:104-114.

31. Ghilardi JR, Rohrich H, Lindsay TH, et al. Selective blockade of the capsaicin receptor TRPV1 attenuates bone cancer pain. *J Neurosci.* 2005;25(12):3126-3131.

32. von Moos R, Strasser F, Gillessen S, et al. Metastatic bone pain: treatment options with an emphasis on bisphosphonates. *Support Care Cancer.* 2008;16(10):1105-1115.

33. Stopeck AT, Lipton A, Body JJ, et al. Denosumab compared with zoledronic acid for the treatment of bone metastases in patients with advanced breast cancer: a randomized, double-blind study. *J Clin Oncol.* 2010;28(35):5132-5139.

34. Henry DH, Costa L, Goldwasser F, et al. Randomized, double-blind study of denosumab versus zoledronic acid in the treatment of bone metastases in patients with advanced cancer (excluding breast and prostate cancer) or multiple myeloma. *J Clin Oncol.* 2011;29(9):1125-1132.

35. Clohisy DR, Mantyh PW. Bone cancer pain and the role of RANKL/OPG. *J Musculoskelet Neuronal Interact.* 2004;4(3):293-300.

36. Honore P, Luger NM, Sabino MA, et al. Osteoprotegerin blocks bone cancer-induced skeletal destruction, skeletal pain and pain-related neurochemical reorganization of the spinal cord. *Nat Med.* 2000;6(5):521-528.

37. Lipton A. Emerging role of bisphosphonates in the clinic—antitumor activity and prevention of metastasis to bone. *Cancer Treat Rev.* 2008;34(suppl 1):S25-S30.

38. Stenbeck G. Formation and function of the ruffled border in osteoclasts. *Semin Cell Dev Biol.* 2002;13(4):285-292.

39. Rogers MJ, Gordon S, Benford HL, et al. Cellular and molecular mechanisms of action of bisphosphonates. *Cancer.* 2000;88 (12 suppl):2961-2978.

40. Clezardin P, Ebetino FH, Fournier PG. Bisphosphonates and cancer-induced bone disease: beyond their antiresorptive activity. *Cancer Res.* 2005;65(12):4971-4974.

41. Lipton A, Jun S. RANKL inhibition in the treatment of bone metastases. *Curr Opin Support Palliat Care.* 2008;2(3): 197-203.

42. Yates D, Smith M. Orthopaedic pain after trauma. In: Wall PD, Melzack R, eds. Textbook of pain. New York: Churchill Livingstone: Edinburgh; 1994. pp. 409-421.

43. Jimenez-Andrade JM, Martin CD, Koewler NJ, et al. Nerve growth factor sequestering therapy attenuates non-malignant skeletal pain following fracture. *Pain.* 2007;133(1-3):183-196.

44. Rubert CHR, Malawer M. Orthopedic management of skeletal metastases. In: Body J-J, ed. Tumor bone disease and osteoporosis in cancer patients. New York City: Marcel Dekker; 2000. pp. 305-356.

45. Arrington SA, Schoonmaker JE, Damron TA, et al. Temporal changes in bone mass and mechanical properties in a murine model of tumor osteolysis. *Bone.* 2006;38(3):359-367.

46. Nazarian A, von Stechow D, Zurakowski D, et al. Bone volume fraction explains the variation in strength and stiffness of cancellous bone affected by metastatic cancer and osteoporosis. *Calcif Tissue Int.* 2008;83(6):368-379.

47. Khasabova IA, Khasabov SG, Harding-Rose C, et al. A decrease in anandamide signaling contributes to the maintenance of cutaneous mechanical hyperalgesia in a model of bone cancer pain. *J Neurosci.* 2008;28(44):11141-11152.

48. Lozano-Ondoua AN, Wright C, Vardanyan A, et al. A cannabinoid 2 receptor agonist attenuates bone cancer-induced pain and bone loss. *Life Sci.* 2010;86(17-18):646-653.

49. Schweizerhof M, Stosser S, Kurejova M, et al. Hematopoietic colony-stimulating factors mediate tumor-nerve interactions and bone cancer pain. *Nat Med.* 2009;15(7):802-807.

50. Nelson JB, Hedican SP, George DJ, et al. Identification of endothelin-1 in the pathophysiology of metastatic adenocarcinoma of the prostate. *Nat Med.* 1995;1(9):944-949.

51. Nelson JB, Chan-Tack K, Hedican SP, et al. Endothelin-1 production and decreased endothelin B receptor expression in advanced prostate cancer. *Cancer Res.* 1996;56(4):663-668.

52. Hamamoto DT, Khasabov SG, Cain DM, et al. Tumor-evoked sensitization of C nociceptors: a role for endothelin. *J Neurophysiol.* 2008;100(4):2300-2311.

53. Pomonis JD, Rogers SD, Peters CM, et al. Expression and localization of endothelin receptors: implication for the involvement of peripheral glia in nociception. *J Neurosci.* 2001;21(3):999-1006.

54. Davar G, Hans G, Fareed MU, et al. Behavioral signs of acute pain produced by application of endothelin-1 to rat sciatic nerve. *Neuroreport.* 1998;9(10):2279-2283.

55. Beutler BA. The role of tumor necrosis factor in health and disease. *J Rheumatol Suppl.* 1999;57:16-21.

56. Wacnik PW, Eikmeier LJ, Simone DA, et al. Nociceptive characteristics of tumor necrosis factor-alpha in naive and tumor-bearing mice. *Neuroscience.* 2005;132(2):479-491.

57. Constantin CE, Mair N, Sailer CA, et al. Endogenous tumor necrosis factor alpha (TNFalpha) requires TNF receptor type 2 to generate heat hyperalgesia in a mouse cancer model. *J Neurosci.* 2008;28(19):5072-5081.

58. Smith PC, Hobisch A, Lin DL, et al. Interleukin-6 and prostate cancer progression. *Cytokine Growth Factor Rev.* 2001;12(1):33-40.

59. Nishimoto N, Kishimoto T. Interleukin 6: from bench to bedside. *Nat Clin Pract Rheumatol.* 2006;2(11):619-626.

60. Rose-John S, Scheller J, Elson G, et al. Interleukin-6 biology is coordinated by membrane-bound and soluble receptors: role in inflammation and cancer. *J Leukoc Biol.* 2006;80(2):227-236.

61. Poole S, Cunha FQ, Selkirk S, et al. Cytokine-mediated inflammatory hyperalgesia limited by interleukin-10. *Br J Pharmacol.* 1995;115(4):684-688.

62. DeLeo JA, Colburn RW, Nichols M, et al. Interleukin-6-mediated hyperalgesia/allodynia and increased spinal IL-6 expression in a rat mononeuropathy model. *J Interferon Cytokine Res.* 1996;16(9):695-700.

63. Dina OA, Green PG, Levine JD. Role of interleukin-6 in chronic muscle hyperalgesic priming. *Neuroscience.* 2008;152(2):521-525.

64. Rose-John S, Heinrich PC. Soluble receptors for cytokines and growth factors: generation and biological function. *Biochem J.* 1994;300 (Pt 2):281-290.

65. Taga T, Hibi M, Hirata Y, et al. Interleukin-6 triggers the association of its receptor with a possible signal transducer, gp130. *Cell.* 1989;58(3):573-581.

66. Andratsch M, Mair N, Constantin CE, et al. A key role for gp130 expressed on peripheral sensory nerves in pathological pain. *J Neurosci.* 2009;29(43):13473-13483.

67. Pezet S, McMahon SB. Neurotrophins: mediators and modulators of pain. *Annu Rev Neurosci.* 2006;29:507-538.

68. Gould HJ, 3rd, Gould TN, England JD, et al. A possible role for nerve growth factor in the augmentation of sodium channels in models of chronic pain. *Brain Res.* 2000;854(1-2):19-29.

69. Ji RR, Samad TA, Jin SX, et al. p38 MAPK activation by NGF in primary sensory neurons after inflammation increases TRPV1 levels and maintains heat hyperalgesia. *Neuron.* 2002;36(1):57-68.

70. Heumann R, Korsching S, Bandtlow C, et al. Changes of nerve growth factor synthesis in nonneuronal cells in response to sciatic nerve transection. *J Cell Biol.* 1987;104(6):1623-1631.

71. Heumann R, Lindholm D, Bandtlow C, et al. Differential regulation of mRNA encoding nerve growth factor and its receptor in rat sciatic nerve during development, degeneration, and regeneration: role of macrophages. *Proc Natl Acad Sci USA.* 1987;84(23):8735-8739.

72. Obata K, Tsujino H, Yamanaka H, et al. Expression of neurotrophic factors in the dorsal root ganglion in a rat model of lumbar disc herniation. *Pain.* 2002;99(1-2):121-132.

73. Halvorson KG, Kubota K, Sevcik MA, et al. A blocking antibody to nerve growth factor attenuates skeletal pain induced by prostate tumor cells growing in bone. *Cancer Res.* 2005;65(20):9426-9435.

74. Sevcik MA, Ghilardi JR, Peters CM, et al. Anti-NGF therapy profoundly reduces bone cancer pain and the accompanying increase in markers of peripheral and central sensitization. *Pain.* 2005;115(1-2):128-141.

75. Vega JA, Garcia-Suarez O, Hannestad J, et al. Neurotrophins and the immune system. *J Anat.* 2003;203(1):1-19.

76. Peters CM, Ghilardi JR, Keyser CP, et al. Tumor-induced injury of primary afferent sensory nerve fibers in bone cancer pain. *Exp Neurol.* 2005;193(1):85-100.

77. Devor M, Govrin-Lippmann R, Angelides K. Na+ channel immunolocalization in peripheral mammalian axons and changes following nerve injury and neuroma formation. *J Neurosci.* 1993;13(5):1976-1992.

78. England JD, Happel LT, Kline DG, et al. Sodium channel accumulation in humans with painful neuromas. *Neurology.* 1996;47(1):272-276.

79. Black JA, Nikolajsen L, Kroner K, et al. Multiple sodium channel isoforms and mitogen-activated protein kinases are present in painful human neuromas. *Ann Neurol.* 2008;64(6):644-653.

80. Lindqvist A, Rivero-Melian C, Turan I, et al. Neuropeptide- and tyrosine hydroxylase-immunoreactive nerve fibers in painful Morton's neuromas. *Muscle Nerve.* 2000;23(8):1214-1218.

81. Devor M. Neuropathic pain: what do we do with all these theories? *Acta Anaesthesiol Scand.* 2001;45(9):1121-1127.

82. Lindsay TH, Jonas BM, Sevcik MA, et al. Pancreatic cancer pain and its correlation with changes in tumor vasculature, macrophage infiltration, neuronal innervation, body weight and disease progression. *Pain.* 2005;119(1-3):233-246.

83. Bloom AP, Jimenez-Andrade JM, Taylor RN, et al. Breast cancer-induced bone remodeling, skeletal pain and sprouting of sensory nerve fibers. *J Pain.* 2011;12(6):698-711.

84. Elitt CM, McIlwrath SL, Lawson JJ, et al. Artemin overexpression in skin enhances expression of TRPV1 and TRPA1 in cutaneous sensory neurons and leads to behavioral sensitivity to heat and cold. *J Neurosci.* 2006;26(33):8578-8787.

85. Diamond J, Foerster A, Holmes M, et al. Sensory nerves in adult rats regenerate and restore sensory function to the skin independently of endogenous NGF. *J Neurosci.* 1992;12(4):1467-1476.

86. Schwei MJ, Honore P, Rogers SD, et al. Neurochemical and cellular reorganization of the spinal cord in a murine model of bone cancer pain. *J Neurosci.* 1999;19(24):10886-10897.

87. Zhang RX, Liu B, Li A, et al. Interleukin 1beta facilitates bone cancer pain in rats by enhancing NMDA receptor NR-1 subunit phosphorylation. *Neuroscience.* 2008;154(4):1533-1538.

88. Gu X, Zhang J, Ma Z, et al. The role of N-methyl-d-aspartate receptor subunit NR2B in spinal cord in cancer pain. *Eur J Pain.* 2010;14(5):496-502.

89. Yanagisawa Y, Furue H, Kawamata T, et al. Bone cancer induces a unique central sensitization through synaptic changes in a wide area of the spinal cord. *Mol Pain.* 2010;6:38.

90. Urch CE, Donovan-Rodriguez T, Dickenson AH. Alterations in dorsal horn neurones in a rat model of cancer-induced bone pain. *Pain.* 2003;106(3):347-356.

CHAPTER 6

Pathophysiology of Chemotherapy-Induced Peripheral Neuropathy

Xiao-Min Wang ■ Jane M. Fall-Dickson ■ Tanya J. Lehky

INTRODUCTION

Chemotherapy-induced peripheral neuropathy (CIPN) is a common dose-limiting side effect of taxanes, platinum compounds, vinca alkaloids, epothilones, bortezomib, thalidomide, and lenalidomide. CIPN commonly occurs in 30% to 40% of patients undergoing chemotherapy treatment, ranging from 10% to 90% of patients (1). CIPN is one of the main reasons that patients decide to stop chemotherapy treatment before completion. Early termination of chemotherapy negatively affects patient outcomes because current oncology practice uses more aggressive single agent or combination regimens to decrease the risk of recurrence and improve patient's survival rates (2–4). CIPN remains a challenging treatment sequela for both patients and clinicians. For patients, CIPN can be a life-long burden, particularly for younger cancer survivors. CIPN limits the ability of oncologists to administer the optimal and aggressive regimens that improve cancer survival. Although a variety of neuroprotective approaches have been investigated in both experimental studies and clinical trials, there is no available preventive strategy or effective treatment for chemotherapy-induced neurotoxicity because its etiology has not been fully elucidated. Therefore, defining the mechanisms of CIPN is critical to develop preventive and treatment strategies and to enhance health-related quality of life.

Most chemotherapeutic drugs penetrate the blood–brain barrier poorly, but readily penetrate the blood–nerve barrier (BNB) and bind to the dorsal root ganglia (DRG) and peripheral nerves (5). Experimental studies reveal that chemotherapeutic drugs preferentially accumulate and bind in the DRG cells and peripheral nerves (5). This mechanism of action may be related in part to the relative deficiency and higher permeability of the BNB at the areas of the DRG and nerve terminals (6). Additionally, endoneural compartments have no lymphatic system to remove toxins (7). These factors increase peripheral nerve vulnerabilities to toxicity when compared with the central nervous system. Thus, chemotherapy-induced neurotoxicity mainly targets the peripheral nervous system (PNS) and manifests as distal peripheral neuropathy. Although there are cases of central nervous system toxicity manifested as encephalopathy, these cases are very uncommon and mostly unpredictable (8). For this reason, this chapter mainly focuses on chemotherapy-induced neuropathophysiology in the PNS, focusing on the localized lesions, followed by description of the known mechanisms underlying CIPN.

WHAT IS CIPN?

CIPN is primarily a polyneuropathy, with simultaneous malfunction of many peripheral nerves. The symptoms most commonly associated with CIPN are related to sensory neuropathy. Numbness, burning, tingling, pain, and weakness in the limbs are the most common complaints reported by oncologists. The onset of symptoms can be subacute, such as paclitaxel acute pain syndrome (P-APS) (9), or may gradually progress over time. Initially, patients frequently feel abnormal sensations like tingling, burning pain, or numbness. These symptoms often start symmetrically in the toes and fingers and spread proximally in a "stocking and glove" distribution. Many patients complain of difficulty in walking, dropping things, or feeling as if they are wearing gloves or stockings when they are not. If internal organs are affected, patients may experience diarrhea or constipation, low blood pressure, irregular heartbeat, or difficulty breathing. The incidence and severity of CIPN are influenced by multiple factors, including chemotherapy dose intensity, cumulative dose, duration of infusion, and combination regimen, as well as age, and preexisting conditions, such as diabetes, vitamin B_{12} deficiency, alcohol abuse, and prior chemotherapy exposure. These factors may have a negative effect on the progression of neuropathic symptoms.

CIPN presents with unique clinical characteristics that are different from those seen with peripheral nerve injury in diabetes, metabolic neuropathy, stoke, or trauma. Table 6.1 summarizes the characteristics of peripheral neuropathy induced by the most common chemotherapeutic agents. These features include the following:

1. Unlike neuropathic pain associated with diabetes, which starts in the feet and spreads to the hands over months or years, neuropathic pain caused by chemotherapy often begins in the feet and the hands acutely.
2. Presentation is predominantly dose-dependent sensory symptoms (especially pain) in both frequency and severity, rather than motor symptoms.
3. There exists a length-dependent "dying back" distribution, with the earliest symptoms occurring at fingertips and toes, followed by a progression of symptoms proximally along the limbs as the neuropathy progresses. This pattern of CIPN has been attributed to the fact that the longest fibers have the greatest surface area exposed to CIPN drugs and hence are at risk for greater toxicity.

TABLE 6.1 Characteristics of peripheral neuropathy induced by common chemotherapeutic agents

Anticancer Drugs	Taxanes (Paclitaxel, Docetaxel)	Platinum (Cisplatin, Carboplatin, Oxaliplatin)	Vinca Alkaloids (Vincristine, Vinblastine, Vinorelbine, Vindesine)	Bortezomib	Thalidomide
Treatment	Breast, ovarian, non–small cell lung cancer	Testicular, ovarian, lung, bladder, colorectal cancers	Hematological cancers Pediatric sarcomas	Multiple myeloma	Multiple myeloma
Incidence	30–60% (overall)	30–100% (overall) Early (90%)[a], late (60%)[b]	30–50% (overall)	30–55% (overall) 10–20% (severe)	25–80% (overall) 28% (severe)
Symptoms	Symmetrical painful paresthesias or numbness in a stocking-glove distribution, sensory loss Motor symptoms at high dose	Symmetrical painful paresthesias or numbness in a stocking-glove distribution Early: cold allodynia and hyperalgesia Later: loss of motor function Long-term chronic sensory neuropathy	Symmetrical sensorimotor painful neuropathy: tingling paresthesias, proprioceptive loss, areflexia, and ataxia Constipation Muscle weakness Gait dysfunction	Hallmark: sensory painful neuropathy, resistant to treatment	Symmetrical distal paresthesias, dysesthesias Sensory painful neuropathy Muscle cramps
Main toxic targets	Axons and Schwann cells	Dorsal root ganglia	Axons	Axons	Axon Dorsal root ganglia
Possible mechanisms	Microtubule disruption Mitochondrial dysfunction Neurofilament accumulation DRG damage Damage blood supply to PNS	Bind to DNA adducts →apoptosis Anterograde axonal neuropathy Myelin sheath damage Channelopathy (Na+, Ca2+, K+) Damage blood supply to PNS	Dysfunctions of mitochondria and endoplastic reticulum Microtubule disruption Autoimmune Inflammation	Binds to the proteasome complex, leading to cell cycle interruption and apoptosis Mitochondrial disturbance Microtubule disruption	Antiangiogenesis Direct toxic effects on the DRG Neurotrophin dysregulation

Molecular-genetic profiles	Matrix metalloproteinase-3 and CD163 IL-1, TNF, and CD11b Voltage-dependent calcium channel $\alpha_2\delta$-1 (**dorsal spinal cord**) ITGBL1	TRPM8 Voltage-dependent calcium channel $\alpha_2\delta$-1 (DRG)	TRPM8 ITGBL1, AURKA, MK167	RHOBTB2, CPCT1C ITGBL1, SOX8,
Single-nucleotide polymorphisms	ABCB1	ERCC1, GSTP1, C118T, GSTP1	PARP1, LTA, GLI1 ABCC1, DPYD, *ADRB2,* *CAMKK1, CYP2C9,* *NFATC2, ID3, SLC10A2,* *CYP2C8*	ALOX12, IGF1R, SOD2, MYO5A, MBL2, PPARD, ERCC4, ERCC3	ABCA1, ICAM, PPARD), *SLC12A6,* SERPINB2, SLC12A6, *LIG4,*

DRG, dorsal root ganglia; PNS, peripheral nervous system; IL-1, interleukin 1, TNF, tumor necrosis factor.
[a]Early onset—after first cycle of induction of treatment; [b]Late onset—after two to three cycles of induction treatment.

4. Known onset and extent of neuronal or nerve injury induced by chemotherapeutic drugs provides an opportunity for translational work through both basic and clinical research to test preemptive trials for CIPN.

5. Histological findings have indicated that, unlike painful peripheral neuropathies due to trauma and diabetes, CIPN-related pain occurs in the absence of axonal degeneration in peripheral nerves.

PATHOPHYSIOLOGY OF CIPN

Various CIPN mechanisms have been proposed based on the findings of in vitro and in vivo animal models. However, the pathophysiology of CIPN has not yet been fully established and can vary with different classifications of chemotherapeutic agents. An elucidation of the underlying mechanisms of peripheral neuropathy is imperative to identify potential targets for the prevention and treatment of CIPN. At the histological level, it has been generally accepted that chemotherapeutic drugs commonly induce (1) axonopathy or distal axonal neuropathy, causing a "dying back" axonal degeneration; (2) ganglionopathy, affecting cell bodies in the DRG; and (3) myelinopathy with primary segmental demyelination (10). At the cellular level, chemotherapeutic agents damage microtubules and interfere with microtubule-based axonal transport; interrupt mitochondrial function; or directly target DNA (11). Peripheral nerve degeneration or small fiber neuropathy occurs that leads to sensitization and spontaneous activity of these fibers through an increase in voltage-gated sodium and calcium channels, which then facilitates the release of substance P and glutamate and leads to hyperexcitability of these fibers. Figure 6.1 illustrates the proposed targets of chemotherapy-induced neurotoxicity in the PNS.

Taxane compounds, including paclitaxel and docetaxel, bind to β-tubulin subunits, stabilize polymerization, and interfere with microtubule dynamics. Tubulin is a primary component of microtubules and the basis of cellular cytoskeletal structure. Microtubules are fundamental to axonal transport processes, providing trophic factors and energy for the long axons of peripheral nerves. In vitro, paclitaxel exposure induces marked microtubule aggregation in large myelinated axons (12) and DRG (13), and correspondingly paclitaxel interferes with anterograde axonal transport (14). It has been postulated that taxanes elicit neurotoxic action through interaction with microtubules in the long axons of peripheral nerves, perhaps because microtubules are the key components in axonal transport. Thus, microtubule damage and subsequent dysfunction of axonal transport have long been associated with taxane-induced axonopathy (15).

Vinca alkaloid compounds include vincristine, vinblastine, vinorelbine, vindesine, and vinflunine. Axonal sensorimotor neuropathy induced by vincristine often occurs early during treatment and manifests itself by paresthesias followed by motor weakness. Histological studies show that vincristine causes main lesions of axonal degeneration in both small and large fibers by disorientation of microtubules and disruption

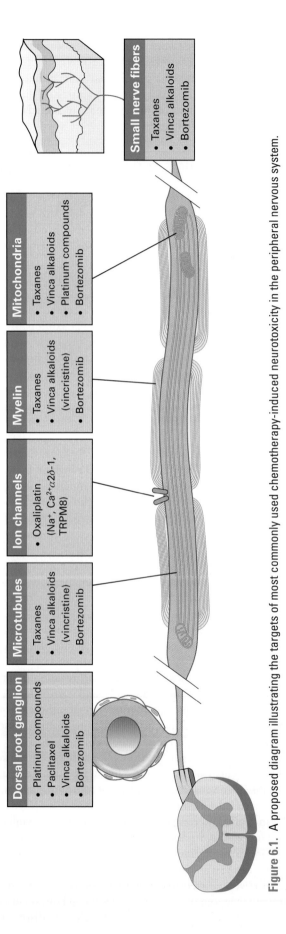

Figure 6.1. A proposed diagram illustrating the targets of most commonly used chemotherapy-induced neurotoxicity in the peripheral nervous system.

of the myelin sheath, leading to a decrease in nerve conduction velocity (16). Vincristine-induced neuropathic pain is characterized by abnormal spontaneous discharges in the A-fiber and C-fiber primary afferent neurons (17), but pain is not a prominent feature of vincristine-induced peripheral neuropathy (18).

Similar to taxanes, vinca alkaloids bind to tubulin and inhibit microtubule dynamics (19). The affinity for tubulin differs among vinca alkaloid compounds (vincristine, vinblastine, vinorelbine, and vinflunine in descending order). For example, vincristine produces significant alterations in axonal cytoskeletal structure, including microtubule disorientation and neurofilament accumulation (20,21), which contribute to interruption of axonal transport (22) and result in Wallerian-like axonal degeneration and axonopathy (20,21,23). In addition, these compounds have also been reported in vitro to produce direct axonal toxicity (24). Both taxanes and vinca alkaloids affect the stability of microtubules and disrupt the axonal transport of growth factors and molecules essential to normal nerve function. However, this does not explain why platinum-based compounds, which induce DNA adducts in the nucleus, also cause the painful sensory neuropathy that taxanes and vinca alkaloid compounds do.

Platinum compounds, including cisplatin, carboplatin, and oxaliplatin, predominantly target and accumulate in the DRG. This preferential accumulation might be partially due to the relative deficiency of the BNB in peripheral nerves, especially in the DRG area, or their high affinity for the DRG cells (25). These compounds form DNA intrastrand adducts and interstrand crosslinks that lead to DNA derangement, morphologic changes, and subsequent apoptosis (26,27). Platinum compounds exert direct damage on neurons and non-neuronal cells in the DRG, and the levels of platinum in DRG of treated patients correlate with the severity of CIPN (11,28–30). Histological study reveals axonal loss associated with a secondary DRG atrophy. Therefore, platinum compound–associated symptoms, such as cisplatin-induced peripheral neuropathy, are described as a primary neuronopathy rather than an axonopathy (31). Additionally, the oxidative stress and mitochondria dysfunction are involved in triggering neuronal apoptosis (32). Cisplatin can also disrupt axonal microtubule growth that may also contribute to the cisplatin-induced peripheral neuropathy (33).

The platinum compounds, specifically cisplatin, share the "coasting" phenomenon in which symptoms and signs often do not start until the end of treatment or continually worsen even after the cessation of treatment (34). This particularly troublesome aspect of cisplatin neurotoxicity prevents timely discontinuation of treatment in most patients with chemotherapy-induced neurotoxicity. Oxaliplatin-induced peripheral neuropathy has a distinctive spectrum of symptoms in addition to chronic presentations. Oxaliplatin also provokes an acute, cold-induced, and transient syndrome characterized by paresthesias in the distal extremities and perioral region that usually appear during infusion or within hours after infusion, and last 1 to 2 days. This acute transient neurotoxicity occurs in nearly all patients (82% to 92% of all neurotoxicity grads) (28). It is thought that the acute form of oxaliplatin toxicity may be associated with transit dysfunction of nodal axonal sodium or potassium channels. More precisely, oxalate, an oxaliplatin metabolite, is thought to be involved in the cold hyperalgesia, due to calcium or magnesium chelation by oxalate released from the drug, which adversely affects ion channels and synaptic transmission (35,36). Additionally, gene expression of transient receptor potential melastatin 8 (TRPM8, a cold thermal sensor channel) is increased in mouse DRG following oxaliplatin treatment, suggesting the mediating effect of TRPM8 on cold allodynia induced by oxaliplatin (37). Alteration of axonal ion channels may be responsible for the immediate neuropathic symptoms following oxaliplatin treatment and, over time, may result in chronic axonal degeneration (38).

Bortezomib, a novel proteasome inhibitor, induces painful sensory neuropathy with moderate or severe neurotoxicity reported in up to 30% of patients. The clinical hallmark of bortezomib-induced CIPN is painful sensory neuropathy that can be severe and resistant to treatment. Similar to other chemotherapeutic agents, bortezomib-induced motor impairment occurs occasionally. Neurophysiologic evaluation reveals a deficit of three major nerve fibers, A-β, A-δ, and C fibers, in patients with bortezomib-induced pain (39). In animal models, short-term treatment with bortezomib causes alteration in both DRG and peripheral nerves (40), whereas long-term treatment with bortezomib induces peripheral nerve axonopathy characterized by small fiber neuropathy (41).

Bortezomib is an inhibitor of proteasomes. The proteasome pathway facilitates the destruction of ubiquitinated protein and is critical for normal cellular activity (42). Bortezomib binds to the proteasome complex, leading to cell cycle interruption and apoptosis. Because of the importance of the proteasome pathway, bortezomib may exert neurotoxicity via multiple mechanisms, such as protein aggregation and cytoskeletal damage in DRG neurons (43), disruption in tubulin polymerization leading to axonal loss (44,45), and mitochondrial disturbance and injury in Schwann cells that lead to demyelination (40). In a preclinical animal model, exposure to bortezomib caused pathological lesions in Schwann cells and myelin with intracytoplasmic vacuolization (40). A more severe demyelination neuropathy has been described with a combination therapy of bortezomib and thalidomide (46). In addition, recent studies also suggest that bortezomib inhibits some cytokines and transcription factors, including nuclear factor-kappa B (NF-κB) (47). The NF-κB cell signaling pathway is involved in the promotion of neuronal survival (48). Thus, bortezomib, interfering with this pathway, leads to cell cycle arrest, apoptosis, and angiogenesis inhibition (49).

As described above, there are several basic mechanisms in which chemotherapeutic agents can cause axonal damage and peripheral neuropathy. Although these mechanisms of chemotherapy-induced neurotoxicity differ among classes of chemotherapeutic agents, all neurotoxic chemotherapeutic agents cause a common sensory disruption leading to painful paresthesias. These mechanisms alone do not explain the development of acutely painful neuropathies that occur even prior to the pathological loss of axons or alterations in the diagnostic testing for neuropathy. Thus, the common sensory disruption induced by these chemotherapeutic agents may result from a shared mechanism that is most probably not associated with their antineoplastic mechanisms. As described below, mitochondrial dysfunction and inflammatory cytokines may be the contributors, and may play a critical role in the common clinical signs and symptoms of CIPN and contribute to chemotherapy-induced painful paresthesias.

MITOCHONDRIAL DYSFUNCTION MAY CONTRIBUTE TO CHEMOTHERAPY-INDUCED PAINFUL PARESTHESIAS

Recent data from clinical and experimental studies indicate that interference with the energy mechanisms of axons through damage to mitochondria may play an important role in chemotherapy-induced neurotoxicity, particularly in the painful sensory disruption. Mitochondrial dysfunction and dysregulation of Ca^{2+} homeostasis have been implicated in chemotherapy-induced neurotoxicity because intracellular Ca^{2+} level plays an essential role in axonal degeneration via initiation of a cascade of damaging cellular processes. Paclitaxel, vincristine, and oxaliplatin cause prominent abnormalities in axonal mitochondria, including swelling (50) and microtubule–mitochondrial aggregation (51). Bortezomib influences mitochondrial and endoplasmic reticulum integrity in animal models, particularly in myelin-producing Schwann cells, which leads to myelin sheath degeneration and myelinopathy (40,44). Recent research has confirmed the presence of defects in mitochondrial respiratory complexes I and II in peripheral nerves taken from rats with painful peripheral neuropathy after treatment with paclitaxel and oxaliplatin-induced (52).

Energy depletion and deficiency led to oxygen consumption and adenosine triphosphate (ATP) product decrease in axons that result in dysfunction of the energy-dependent Na/K-ATP pump. The energy-dependent Na/K-ATP pump is the key component in maintaining the normal membrane resting/action potential. Impaired mitochondrial function causes energy deficit and subsequently results in the abnormal spontaneous discharge of A-fiber and C-fiber that account for the sensation of pain and dysesthesia. In animal models, treatment with acetyl-L-carnitine (ALC), an agent synthesized in the mitochondria and known to improve mitochondrial function (53), decreases the spontaneous discharges of A-fiber and C-fiber and also prevents and reverses chemotherapy-induced painful peripheral neuropathy (17,50,54). In clinical trials, the efficacy of ALC has been demonstrated through reduction in the severity of existing sensory peripheral neuropathy in patients treated with paclitaxel or cisplatin (55). There are currently ongoing randomized, placebo-controlled trials that investigate the intervention effects of ALC on painful peripheral neuropathy induced by paclitaxel or sagopilone in breast or prostate cancer patients (56).

INFLAMMATORY CYTOKINES, A TARGET FOR CIPN

Emerging data in clinical and experimental studies strongly support the critical role of pro-inflammatory cytokines in the development and maintenance of peripheral neuropathic pain (57–60). After intravenous administration of paclitaxel, the neurons and surrounding satellite cells in the DRG and peripheral nerves show notable pathological changes, accompanied by behavioral changes such as allodynia and hyperalgesia. As a better understanding of the molecular mechanisms underlying CIPN emerges, the role of the neuroimmune interaction and the actions of cytokines/chemokines are becoming more appreciated in the context of CIPN. In addition to the entry of immune cells into the PNS, both macrophages and T lymphocytes communicate with neurons and their satellite cells in DRG, as well as Schwann cells. One of the primary mechanisms facilitating neuroimmune communication is the release of cytokines and chemokines. These pathological changes include a massive increase in the number of activated macrophages in DRG and peripheral nerves and an increased expression of activating transcription factor 3 (ATF3) in both neuronal and non-neuronal cells in DRG, peripheral nerves, and Schwann cells. ATF3 is a marker of nerve injury and was observed in neuronal nuclei in DRG of paclitaxel-treated rats (13,61–63). In animal models, the increased ATF3 expression occurred as early as 1 day after paclitaxel infusion, which is the time point patients first report pain in the course of P-APS. Interestingly, it appears that the initial intensity of acute pain in P-APS predicts the severity of symptoms associated with sensory peripheral neuropathy, specifically, the severity of burning and shooting pain at the later phase (9).

Macrophage infiltration in response to chemotherapy-induced injury leads to a subsequent production and secretion of various cytokines (tumor necrosis factor alpha [TNF-α], interleukin [IL]-1β, IL-6, and IL-8), chemokine C-C motif ligand 2 (CCL2) and characteristically heparin binding proteins (CXC family), growth factors, and inflammatory mediators such as bradykinin, prostaglandins, serotonin, and nitric oxide (NO), which are the potential mediators for the development of peripheral neuropathy (64). These molecules promote continued neuroinflammation through recruitment of macrophages (65). TNF-α and IL-1β can directly sensitize nociceptors and increase axonal spontaneous discharges by directly stimulating A-fiber and C-fiber (66). Intrathecal injection of IL-1ra and IL-10 gene therapy suppresses the expression of TNF-α and IL-1β in DRGs and attenuates paclitaxel-induced neuropathic pain in animal experiments (67,68). The antinociceptive effect of IL-10 may be associated with its inhibitory effect on the expression of TNF-α and IL-1β, as well as through inducible NO synthase (69,70). These findings provide evidence that proinflammatory cytokines, chemokines, and their receptors

and signaling pathways are involved in the development of chemotherapy-induced neuropathic pain. Therefore, characterization of cytokine and chemokine expression after chemotherapy might yield a new insight into the development of CIPN and elucidate targets for the development of effective prevention or treatment strategies for CIPN.

As discussed above, the release of proinflammatory cytokines/chemokines by activated macrophages, satellite cells in the DRG, and Schwann cells may be the primary cause of the pain symptom in CIPN, which is an early sign of initial peripheral neuropathy in most cancer patients undergoing chemotherapy treatment. Therefore, targeting the production of proinflammatory cytokines may be a promising therapeutic strategy for prevention or relief of CIPN, especially for the pain symptom. Extracellular matrix metalloproteinases (MMPs) control the integrity of the BNB, myelin protein turnover, and phenotypic remodeling of glia and neurons. The specific role of MMPs in the pathogenesis of painful peripheral neuropathy is believed to relate to their control of cytokine release. Pharmacologic inhibition of MMPs or administration of small interfering RNA for MMPs produced immediate and sustained attenuation of mechanical allodynia (71,72). Treatment with the MMP inhibitor GM6001 or minocycline significantly reduces the mechanical allodynia after nerve injury (72,73). Minocycline, a broad-spectrum tetracycline antibiotic, has been reported to attenuate neuropathic pain (74) by inhibition of MMP3 upregulation, macrophage accumulation and proinflammatory cytokine release in the paclitaxel-treated rats. Treatment with minocycline effectively prevents both taxol-induced mechanical hyperalgesia and intraepidermal nervefiber (IENF) loss in rats (73). Its inhibitory effect on cytokine release has been reported to be associated with its suppression of the NF-κ pathway (75). Therefore, minocycline protects against cytokine-related damage to axons and Schwann cells (76). However, its inhibitory effect seems most effective when treatment begins prior to nerve injury (77) because that minocycline does not reverse existing hypersensitivity after nerve injury (78). Pretreatment with minocycline inhibits macrophage infiltration and activation, suppresses ATF3 expression in DRGs, and partially blocks the loss of intraepidermal nerve fibers (73,79). Therefore, it is not difficult to understand its preventive effect on the mechanical allodynia and hyperalgesia induced by chemotherapeutic drugs (79,80). Minocycline may be a promising drug to prevent the development of CIPN in clinical practice. According to the National Cancer Institute at National Institutes of Health, minocycline is currently under investigation for the prevention or treatment of CIPN.

Biomarkers are generally used in clinical practice as diagnostic and prognostic tools to identify diseases and to monitor disease activity and treatment response. Unfortunately, no biomarkers are currently available to assess the extent of CIPN or to predict outcomes in CIPN. Neurologists mostly rely on clinical examination and electrophysiologic studies as diagnostic criteria for CIPN. But some information cannot be obtained from clinical examination and electrophysiology, especially when nerve damage is restricted to the distal extremities, as is the case with CIPN. Neurophysiologic tests are limited to evaluate large diameter fibers and thus correlate poorly with physical examination or patient reported paresthesias and numbness (81). Changes in neurophysiologic findings likely lag behind the onset of CIPN pathophysiology that leads to symptoms (82). Thus, discovery of cytokines as candidate biomarkers has the potential to predict the onset of CIPN and identify the early damage of axons. Moreover, CIPN presents a unique manifestation of the precise time and extent of neuronal or nerve injury induced by chemotherapy drugs and provides opportunities to conduct preemptive trials in preclinical and clinical setting. If CIPN can be blocked or attenuated by a preemptive therapy, it is more likely that a full and more aggressive chemotherapy regimen can be administered and completed, which will increase the survival rate of patients with cancer and enhance these patients' quality of life.

ACKNOWLEDGMENTS

The authors are thankful to Mary Ryan, MLS, Biomedical Librarian/Informationist, NIH Library, National Institutes of Health, for her critical reading of this manuscript.

REFERENCES

1. Wolf S, Barton D, Kottschade L, Grothey A, Loprinzi C. Chemotherapy-induced peripheral neuropathy: prevention and treatment strategies. *Eur J Cancer.* (Oxford, England: 1990) 2008;44:1507-1515.

2. Cocconi G, Bisagni G, Ceci G, et al. Three new active cisplatin-containing combinations in the neoadjuvant treatment of locally advanced and locally recurrent breast carcinoma: a randomized phase II trial. *Breast Cancer Res Treat.* 1999;56:125-132.

3. Mielke S, Sparreboom A, Mross K. Peripheral neuropathy: a persisting challenge in paclitaxel-based regimes. *Eur J Cancer.* 2006;42:24-30.

4. Pasini F, Durante E, De Manzoni D, Rosti G, Pelosi G. High-dose chemotherapy in small-cell lung cancer. *Anticancer Res.* 2002;22:3465-3472.

5. Cavaletti G, Cavalletti E, Oggioni N, et al. Distribution of paclitaxel within the nervous system of the rat after repeated intravenous administration. *Neurotoxicology.* 2000;21:389-393.

6. Alessandri-Haber N, Dina OA, Yeh JJ, Parada CA, Reichling DB, Levine JD. Transient receptor potential vanilloid 4 is essential in chemotherapy-induced neuropathic pain in the rat. *J Neurosci.* 2004;24:4444-4452.

7. Weimer LH. Medication-induced peripheral neuropathy. *Curr Neurol Neurosci Rep.* 2003;3:86-92.

8. Sioka C, Kyritsis AP. Central and peripheral nervous system toxicity of common chemotherapeutic agents. *Cancer Chemother Pharmacol.* 2009;63:761-767.

9. Loprinzi CL, Reeves BN, Dakhil SR, et al. Natural history of paclitaxel-associated acute pain syndrome: prospective cohort study NCCTG N08C1. *J Clin Oncol.* 2011;29:1472-1478.

10. Argyriou AA, Koltzenburg M, Polychronopoulos P, Papapetropoulos S, Kalofonos HP. Peripheral nerve damage associated with administration of taxanes in patients with cancer. *Crit. Rev. Oncol. Hematol.* 2008;66:218-228.

11. Windebank AJ, Grisold W. Chemotherapy-induced neuropathy. *J Peripher Nerv Syst.* 2008;13:27-46.

12. Cavaletti G, Tredici G, Braga M, Tazzari S. Experimental peripheral neuropathy induced in adult rats by repeated intraperitoneal administration of taxol. *Exp Neurol.* 1995;133:64-72.

13. Jimenez-Andrade JM, Peters CM, Mejia NA, Ghilardi JR, Kuskowski MA, Mantyh PW. Sensory neurons and their supporting cells located in the trigeminal, thoracic and lumbar ganglia differentially express markers of injury following intravenous administration of paclitaxel in the rat. *Neurosci Lett.* 2006;405:62-67.

14. Theiss C, Meller K. Taxol impairs anterograde axonal transport of microinjected horseradish peroxidase in dorsal root ganglia neurons in vitro. *Cell Tissue Res.* 2000;299:213-224.

15. Scuteri A, Nicolini G, Miloso M, et al. Paclitaxel toxicity in post-mitotic dorsal root ganglion (DRG) cells. *Anticancer Res.* 2006;26:1065-1070.

16. Rosenthal S, Kaufman S. Vincristine neurotoxicity. *Ann Intern Med.* 1974;80:733-737.

17. Xiao WH, Bennett GJ. Chemotherapy-evoked neuropathic pain: abnormal spontaneous discharge in A-fiber and C-fiber primary afferent neurons and its suppression by acetyl-L-carnitine. *Pain.* 2008;135:262-270.

18. Casey EB, Jellife AM, Le Quesne PM, Millett YL. Vincristine neuropathy. Clinical and electrophysiological observations. *Brain.* 1973;96:69-86.

19. Leveque D, Jehl F. Molecular pharmacokinetics of catharanthus (vinca) alkaloids. *J Clin Pharmacol.* 2007;47:579-588.

20. Sahenk Z, Brady ST, Mendell JR. Studies on the pathogenesis of vincristine-induced neuropathy. *Muscle Nerve.* 1987;10:80-84.

21. Topp KS, Tanner KD, Levine JD. Damage to the cytoskeleton of large diameter sensory neurons and myelinated axons in vincristine-induced painful peripheral neuropathy in the rat. *J Comp Neurol.* 2000;424:563-576.

22. Macfarlane BV, Wright A, Benson HA. Reversible blockade of retrograde axonal transport in the rat sciatic nerve by vincristine. *J Pharm Pharmacol.* 1997;49:97-101.

23. Tanner KD, Levine JD, Topp KS. Microtubule disorientation and axonal swelling in unmyelinated sensory axons during vincristine-induced painful neuropathy in rat. *J Comp Neurol.* 1998;395:481-492.

24. Silva A, Wang Q, Wang M, Ravula SK, Glass JD. Evidence for direct axonal toxicity in vincristine neuropathy. *J Peripher Nerv Syst.* 2006;11:211-216.

25. Holmes J, Stanko J, Varchenko M, et al. Comparative neurotoxicity of oxaliplatin, cisplatin, and ormaplatin in a Wistar rat model. *Toxicol Sci.* 1998;46:342-351.

26. Cavaletti G, Fabbrica D, Minoia C, Frattola L, Tredici G. Carboplatin toxic effects on the peripheral nervous system of the rat. *Ann Oncol.* 1998;9:443-447.

27. McDonald ES, Windebank AJ. Cisplatin-induced apoptosis of DRG neurons involves bax redistribution and cytochrome c release but not fas receptor signaling. *Neurobiol Dis.* 2002;9:220-233.

28. Wilkes G. Peripheral neuropathy related to chemotherapy. *Semin Oncol Nurs.* 2007;23:162-173.

29. Chaudhry V, Rowinsky EK, Sartorius SE, Donehower RC, Cornblath DR. Peripheral neuropathy from taxol and cisplatin combination chemotherapy: clinical and electrophysiological studies. *Ann Neurol.* 1994;35:304-311.

30. Legha SS. Vincristine neurotoxicity. Pathophysiology and management. *Med Toxicol.* 1986;1:421-427.

31. Walsh TJ, Clark AW, Parhad IM, Green WR. Neurotoxic effects of cisplatin therapy. *Arch Neurol.* 1982;39:719-720.

32. Huff LM, Sackett DL, Poruchynsky MS, Fojo T. Microtubule-disrupting chemotherapeutics result in enhanced proteasome-mediated degradation and disappearance of tubulin in neural cells. *Cancer Res.* 2010;70:5870-5879.

33. Tulub AA, Stefanov VE. Cisplatin stops tubulin assembly into microtubules. A new insight into the mechanism of anti-tumor activity of platinum complexes. *Int J Biol Macromol.* 2001;28:191-198.

34. Hilkens P, Palnting, AST, van der Burg MEL, et al. Clinical course and risk factors of neurotoxicity following cisplatin in an intensive dosing schedule. *Eur J Neurol.* 1994;1(1):45-50.

35. Benoit E, Brienza S, Dubois JM. Oxaliplatin, an anticancer agent that affects both Na+ and K+ channels in frog peripheral myelinated axons. *Gen Physiol Biophys.* 2006;25:263-276.

36. Grolleau F, Gamelin L, Boisdron-Celle M, Lapied B, Pelhate M, Gamelin E. A possible explanation for a neurotoxic effect of the anticancer agent oxaliplatin on neuronal voltage-gated sodium channels. *J Neurophysiol.* 2001;85:2293-2297.

37. Gauchan P, Andoh T, Kato A, Kuraishi Y. Involvement of increased expression of transient receptor potential melastatin 8 in oxaliplatin-induced cold allodynia in mice. *Neurosci Lett.* 2009;458:93-95.

38. Krishnan AV, Goldstein D, Friedlander M, Kiernan MC. Oxaliplatin-induced neurotoxicity and the development of neuropathy. *Muscle Nerve.* 2005;32:51-60.

39. Cata JP, Weng HR, Burton AW, Villareal H, Giralt S, Dougherty PM. Quantitative sensory findings in patients with bortezomib-induced pain. *J Pain.* 2007;8:296-306.

40. Cavaletti G, Gilardini A, Canta A, et al. Bortezomib-induced peripheral neurotoxicity: a neurophysiological and pathological study in the rat. *Exp Neurol.* 2007;204:317-325.

41. Meregalli C, Canta A, Carozzi VA, et al. Bortezomib-induced painful neuropathy in rats: a behavioral, neurophysiological and pathological study in rats. *Eur J Pain.* 2010;14:343-350.

42. Rajkumar SV, Richardson PG, Hideshima T, Anderson KC. Proteasome inhibition as a novel therapeutic target in human cancer. *J Clin Oncol.* 2005;23:630-639.

43. Csizmadia V, Raczynski A, Csizmadia E, Fedyk ER, Rottman J, Alden CL. Effect of an experimental proteasome inhibitor on the cytoskeleton, cytosolic protein turnover, and induction in the neuronal cells in vitro. *Neurotoxicology.* 2008;29:232-243.

44. Filosto M, Rossi G, Pelizzari AM, et al. A high-dose bortezomib neuropathy with sensory ataxia and myelin involvement. *J Neurol Sci.* 2007;263:40-43.

45. Poruchynsky MS, Sackett DL, Robey RW, Ward Y, Annunziata C, Fojo T. Proteasome inhibitors increase tubulin polymerization and stabilization in tissue culture cells: a possible mechanism contributing to peripheral neuropathy and cellular toxicity following proteasome inhibition. *Cell Cycle.* 2008;7:940-949.

46. Chaudhry V, Cornblath DR, Polydefkis M, Ferguson A, Borrello I. Characteristics of bortezomib- and thalidomide-induced peripheral neuropathy. *J Peripher Nerv Syst.* 2008;13:275-282.

47. An J, Sun YP, Adams J, Fisher M, Belldegrun A, Rettig MB. Drug interactions between the proteasome inhibitor bortezomib and cytotoxic chemotherapy, tumor necrosis factor (TNF) alpha, and TNF-related apoptosis-inducing ligand in prostate cancer. *Clin Cancer Res.* 2003;9:4537-4545.

48. Maggirwar SB, Sarmiere PD, Dewhurst S, Freeman RS. Nerve growth factor-dependent activation of NF-kappaB contributes to survival of sympathetic neurons. *J Neurosci.* 1998;18:10356-10365.

49. Balayssac D, Ferrier J, Descoeur J, et al. Chemotherapy-induced peripheral neuropathies: from clinical relevance to preclinical evidence. *Expert Opin Drug Saf.* 2011;10:407-417.

50. Flatters SJ, Bennett GJ. Studies of peripheral sensory nerves in paclitaxel-induced painful peripheral neuropathy: evidence for mitochondrial dysfunction. *Pain.* 2006;122:245-257.

51. Raine CS, Roytta M, Dolich M. Microtubule-mitochondrial associations in regenerating axons after taxol intoxication. *J Neurocytol.* 1987;16:461-468.

52. Zheng H, Xiao WH, Bennett GJ. Functional deficits in peripheral nerve mitochondria in rats with paclitaxel- and oxaliplatin-evoked painful peripheral neuropathy. *Exp Neurol.* 2011;232:154-161.

53. Virmani A, Gaetani F, Binienda Z. Effects of metabolic modifiers such as carnitines, coenzyme Q10, and PUFAs against different forms of neurotoxic insults: metabolic inhibitors, MPTP, and methamphetamine. *Ann N Y Acad Sci.* 2005;1053:183-191.

54. Jin HW, Flatters SJ, Xiao WH, Mulhern HL, Bennett GJ. Prevention of paclitaxel-evoked painful peripheral neuropathy by acetyl-L-carnitine: effects on axonal mitochondria, sensory nerve fiber terminal arbors, and cutaneous Langerhans cells. *Exp Neurol.* 2008;210:229-237.

55. Bianchi G, Vitali G, Caraceni A, et al. Symptomatic and neurophysiological responses of paclitaxel- or cisplatin-induced neuropathy to oral acetyl-L-carnitine. *Eur J Cancer.* 2005;41:1746-1750.

56. Pachman DR, Barton DL, Watson JC, Loprinzi CL. Chemotherapy-induced peripheral neuropathy: prevention and treatment. *Clin Pharmacol Ther.* 2011;90:377-387.

57. Uceyler N, Kafke W, Riediger N, et al. Elevated proinflammatory cytokine expression in affected skin in small fiber neuropathy. *Neurology.* 2010;74:1806-1813.

58. Scholz J, Woolf CJ. The neuropathic pain triad: neurons, immune cells and glia. *Nat Neurosci.* 2007;10:1361-1368.

59. Watkins LR, Maier SF. Beyond neurons: evidence that immune and glial cells contribute to pathological pain states. *Physiol Rev.* 2002;82:981-1011.

60. Mantyh PW. Cancer pain and its impact on diagnosis, survival and quality of life. *Nat Rev Neurosci.* 2006;7:797-809.

61. Peters CM, Jimenez-Andrade JM, Jonas BM, et al. Intravenous paclitaxel administration in the rat induces a peripheral sensory neuropathy characterized by macrophage infiltration and injury to sensory neurons and their supporting cells. *Exp Neurol.* 2007;203:42-54.

62. Peters CM, Jimenez-Andrade JM, Kuskowski MA, Ghilardi JR, Mantyh PW. An evolving cellular pathology occurs in dorsal root ganglia, peripheral nerve and spinal cord following intravenous administration of paclitaxel in the rat. *Brain Res.* 2007;1168:46-59.

63. Nishida K, Kuchiiwa S, Oiso S, et al. Up-regulation of matrix metalloproteinase-3 in the dorsal root ganglion of rats with paclitaxel-induced neuropathy. *Cancer Sci.* 2008;99:1618-1625.

64. Sommer C, Kress M. Recent findings on how proinflammatory cytokines cause pain: peripheral mechanisms in inflammatory and neuropathic hyperalgesia. *Neurosci Lett.* 2004;361:184-187.

65. Tofaris GK, Patterson PH, Jessen KR, Mirsky R. Denervated Schwann cells attract macrophages by secretion of leukemia inhibitory factor (LIF) and monocyte chemoattractant protein-1 in a process regulated by interleukin-6 and LIF. *J Neurosci.* 2002;22:6696-6703.

66. Schafers M, Sorkin L. Effect of cytokines on neuronal excitability. *Neurosci Lett.* 2008;437:188-193.

67. Bethea JR, Nagashima H, Acosta MC, et al. Systemically administered interleukin-10 reduces tumor necrosis factor-alpha production and significantly improves functional recovery following traumatic spinal cord injury in rats. *J Neurotrauma.* 1999;16:851-863.

68. Ledeboer A, Jekich BM, Sloane EM, et al. Intrathecal interleukin-10 gene therapy attenuates paclitaxel-induced mechanical allodynia and proinflammatory cytokine expression in dorsal root ganglia in rats. *Brain Behav Immun.* 2007;21:686-698.

69. Plunkett JA, Yu CG, Easton JM, Bethea JR, Yezierski RP. Effects of interleukin-10 (IL-10) on pain behavior and gene expression following excitotoxic spinal cord injury in the rat. *Exp Neurol.* 2001;168:144-154.

70. Abraham KE, McMillen D, Brewer KL. The effects of endogenous interleukin-10 on gray matter damage and the development of pain behaviors following excitotoxic spinal cord injury in the mouse. *Neuroscience.* 2004;124:945-952.

71. Kawasaki Y, Xu ZZ, Wang X, et al. Distinct roles of matrix metalloproteases in the early- and late-phase development of neuropathic pain. *Nat Med.* 2008;14:331-336.

72. Kobayashi H, Chattopadhyay S, Kato K, et al. MMPs initiate Schwann cell-mediated MBP degradation and mechanical nociception after nerve damage. *Mol Cell Neurosci.* 2008;39:619-627.

73. Boyette-Davis J, Xin W, Zhang H, Dougherty PM. Intraepidermal nerve fiber loss corresponds to the development of Taxol-induced hyperalgesia and can be prevented by treatment with minocycline. *Pain.* 2011;152:308-313.

74. Mika J, Osikowicz M, Makuch W, Przewlocka B. Minocycline and pentoxifylline attenuate allodynia and hyperalgesia and potentiate the effects of morphine in rat and mouse models of neuropathic pain. *Eur J Pharmacol.* 2007;560:142-149.

75. Nikodemova M, Duncan ID, Watters JJ. Minocycline exerts inhibitory effects on multiple mitogen-activated protein kinases and IkappaBalpha degradation in a stimulus-specific manner in microglia. *J Neurochem.* 2006;96:314-323.

76. Keilhoff G, Schild L, Fansa H. Minocycline protects Schwann cells from ischemia-like injury and promotes axonal outgrowth in bioartificial nerve grafts lacking Wallerian degeneration. *Exp Neurol.* 2008;212:189-200.

77. Mika J. Modulation of microglia can attenuate neuropathic pain symptoms and enhance morphine effectiveness. *Pharmacol Rep.* 2008;60:297-307.

78. Raghavendra V, Tanga F, DeLeo JA. Inhibition of microglial activation attenuates the development but not existing hypersensitivity in a rat model of neuropathy. *J Pharmacol Exp Ther.* 2003;306:624-630.

79. Liu CC, Lu N, Cui Y, et al. Prevention of paclitaxel-induced allodynia by minocycline: effect on loss of peripheral nerve fibers and infiltration of macrophages in rats. *Mol Pain.* 2010;6:76.

80. Cata JP, Weng HR, Dougherty PM. The effects of thalidomide and minocycline on taxol-induced hyperalgesia in rats. *Brain Res.* 2008;1229:100-110.

81. Cavaletti G, Marmiroli P. Chemotherapy-induced peripheral neurotoxicity. *Nat Rev Neurol.* 2010;6:657-666.

82. du Bois A, Schlaich M, Luck HJ, et al. Evaluation of neurotoxicity induced by paclitaxel second-line chemotherapy. *Supportive Care Cancer.* 1999;7:354-361.

CHAPTER 7

Cancer-Related Fatigue

Xin-Shelley Wang

INTRODUCTION

Cancer-related fatigue (CRF) is one of the most prevalent symptoms reported by cancer patients and survivors—and one that presents many challenges. Most epidemiologic studies of fatigue indicate that it occurs more frequently and more severely than other symptoms in patients with cancer during the course of their disease and its treatment, regardless of the type of cancer or type of therapy; one 1997 study described the fatigue seen in patients with cancer as "both pervasive and profound" (1). In another study, a significantly greater percentage of cancer patients than healthy individuals reported severe fatigue (rated 7 or higher on a 0 to 10 scale) (2). CRF may persist even among cancer survivors who have no evidence of active disease (3,4).

Such findings evidence the importance of establishing a standardized method for assessing and managing fatigue in routine clinical oncology care (5,6). Efforts to develop educational and research initiatives that would help patients and health care providers better understand fatigue and help clinicians better treat fatigue began about a decade ago; since then, knowledge of CRF has progressed, allowing new hypotheses to be generated for further study. Nonetheless, knowledge about the pathophysiologic mechanisms of CRF is limited, and an effective intervention in oncology patient care has yet to be established.

In this chapter, we define CRF, summarize the available research on clinical factors and underlying mechanisms of CRF, discuss methodological issues in measuring CRF and interpreting fatigue assessment results, and review innovations in CRF intervention.

DEFINING CRF

Although fatigue is reported to be the most common symptom of cancer, definitions of CRF have varied from study to study. However, many definitions of CRF share similar features, describing CRF as physical, subjective, temporal, emotional, cognitive, unusual, and affecting the patient's ability to function. Table 7.1 shows a review of these 7 characteristics of CRF, distilled from 24 definitions considered by the working group "Assessing the Symptoms of Cancer using Patient-Reported Outcomes" (ASCPRO) (7).

ASCPRO defined CRF as the "perception of unusual tiredness that varies in pattern and severity and has a negative impact on ability to function in people who have or have had cancer" (7). Similarly, the well-known and accepted National Comprehensive Cancer Network (NCCN) guidelines on fatigue define CRF as "a persistent subjective sense of tiredness related to cancer or cancer treatment that interferes with usual functioning" (8).

Fatigue could be described clinically with a range of terms, such as weariness, exhaustion, lassitude, weakness, malaise, discomfort, impatience, and the inability to perform aspects of normal functioning. Although patients with CRF use a variety of phrases to describe their fatigue, more often than not they characterize themselves as "suffering" from fatigue. However, the distinction between patient perception of CRF and that of "typical" fatigue remains somewhat vague. CRF may be ever-present or transient (a "fatigue attack," in which its onset is more rapid than that of typical fatigue). CRF also lasts longer, drains more energy, and is more severe and unrelenting than typical fatigue. Because CRF overlaps with multifactorial physical and psychological disorders (e.g., depression), it has been recognized as falling into "muddy water" conceptually. The European Association for Palliative Care has recognized both a physical and a cognitive dimension to fatigue and recommends that screening for fatigue include both a question about weakness to cover the physical dimension and a question about tiredness to cover the cognitive dimension (9).

Data from qualitative studies could help create a simplified approach to understanding CRF. For example, a qualitative study compared the key domains of adaptation for "tired," "fatigued," and "exhausted" in patients with cancer, suggesting that behavioral changes in sleep quality, stamina, cognition, and emotional reactivity may serve as early markers of impending fatigue and that decreased control over body processes and reduced social interaction may be signs that an individual has entered a state of fatigue (10). A recent review and synthesis of qualitative research on CRF between 1996 and 2009 identified concepts and language used by patients to describe CRF (11). In this study, patient quotes suggested that the word "tiredness" does not adequately capture the multidimensional nature of the CRF experience.

TABLE 7.1	Characteristics of fatigue	
Characteristics	**Terms Indicative of the Characteristics**	**% Definitions Including Characteristics**
Subjective	Self-report, self-perception	58
Physical sensation	Severity of sensations, including exhaustion, decreased energy, weakness, malaise, tiredness, lassitude	92
Unusual	Unrelieved by rest, unusual, abnormal, not proportional to activity, unusual need for rest, unpredictable	42
Impact on functioning	Decreased function, decreased capacity for work, decreased quality of life, difficulty completing tasks, poor sleep quality, withdrawal from activities, debilitation	66
Unpleasant emotions	Helplessness, vulnerability, distress, reactivity, impatience, anxiety, emotional numbness, unpleasant experience, emotional lability	54
Decreased cognitive ability	Decreased attention, decreased concentration, decreased motivation, memory deficits, decreased mental capacity, decreased capacity for mental work	46
Temporal variability	Pervasive, chronic, acute, persistent, episodic	58

Reprinted from Barsevick AM, Cleeland CS, Manning DC, et al. ASCPRO recommendations for the assessment of fatigue as an outcome in clinical trials. *J Pain Symptom Manage.* 2010;39(6):1086-1099, © 2010, with permission from Elsevier.

CRF negatively affects a patient's daily functioning and can diminish the quality of life. It can be so overwhelming that patients elect to discontinue treatment, or oncologists may give patients a "chemo holiday" to recover from severe symptom burden. A quantitative study found that CRF-related interference with functioning, as measured by the Brief Fatigue Inventory, helped differentiate fatigue severity levels (2). In this study, an increase in a patient's worst-fatigue rating was associated with an increase in the fatigue's interference with patient function. When the worst fatigue reached 6 or greater on the Brief Fatigue Inventory's 0 to 10 scale, its interference with all aspects of daily life was moderate to severe (4 or higher on the 0 to 10 scale) (12).

CLINICAL FACTORS IN CRF

The NCCN guidelines attribute the causes of CRF to both the cancer and the cancer therapy (8). CRF can occur during any phase of the disease, and it often results from a combination of cancer progression and the body's acute or late response to cancer therapy, plus the impact from other medical and psychological conditions and chronic illness.

Disease-related CRF is often observed in patients newly diagnosed with cancer. Unusual tiredness is frequently the first indicator that something is amiss (13). In a study of elderly patients newly diagnosed with various cancers, higher levels of fatigue were found in patients with late-stage disease

than in patients with early-stage disease and with lung cancer (14). In patients with advanced cancer, tumor progression affects multiple organ systems and causes neurologic and physiologic changes in skeletal muscle that are potentially relevant to CRF.

Cancer therapies, especially chemotherapy, can induce CRF and exacerbate existing CRF (5,15–18). A history of chemotherapy was independently associated with severe CRF in patients with various types of advanced cancer (19). Chemotherapy-related toxicities, such as hematologic, gastrointestinal tract, and neural toxicities, may also increase the CRF severity. For some chemotherapy regimens, CRF is an expected adverse event, and patients receiving such regimens as standard care during acute treatment often accept CRF as the price they must pay to achieve a cure. For patients undergoing maintenance therapy (such as patients with chronic myeloid leukemia receiving long-term imatinib therapy), CRF is often a critical factor in deciding whether or not to withdraw from treatment.

Other cancer therapies, such as surgery, radiotherapy, stem cell transplantation, and immunotherapy, can also induce or exacerbate CRF. Patients with cancer often experience postoperative fatigue immediately after a curative surgical procedure, although increased analgesia has been shown to attenuate immediate postsurgical fatigue (20). Gradual increases in fatigue severity have been observed during radiotherapy or concurrent chemoradiation (5,15–18).

Radiotherapy can induce anemia, diarrhea, anorexia, weight loss, and chronic pain, any of which may be associated with an increase in CRF. When high-dose chemotherapy is paired with stem cell transplantation, patients experience a dip in white blood cell count after the transplant, which has been found to be associated with a peak in fatigue levels (21,22). Biological response modifiers, such as proinflammatory cytokines and hormones, are also known to produce CRF. Administration of interferon (IFN)-α can cause flu-like symptoms and has been shown to produce fatigue in 70% of patients (23). In patients with breast cancer, hormone treatment has been associated with lethargy and lack of energy equivalent in severity to the postradiotherapy fatigue experienced by patients with prostate cancer during hormone treatment (24). In addition, fatigue is one of the most common side effects of many tyrosine kinase inhibitors (25). Even though fatigue is a well-known issue for cancer patients and survivors, CRF was not noted among a list of adverse drug reactions that occurred after initial labels for targeted anticancer agents were approved on the basis of randomized phase III clinical trials (26), and there are no existing data on the impact of CRF-related drug discontinuation on disease control.

Even for cancer survivors who have completed therapy and have no evidence of active disease, CRF can be a persistent and functionally bothersome symptom. A population-based survey of 1-year cancer survivors revealed that fatigue was 1 of 3 most negative symptoms (along with depression and pain) among 67 symptoms affecting health-related quality of life (27). Fatigue is also perceived to be a significant problem in child and young adult cancer survivors. Meeske et al. (28) found that 30% of 161 long-term survivors of acute lymphoblastic leukemia whose cancer was diagnosed before the age of 18 years reported having fatigue and that fatigue was highly associated with depression. In a multicenter study of 1,897 adult long-term survivors of childhood cancer (those who had a cancer diagnosis before age 21 and survived at least 5 years after the diagnosis), the overall prevalence of CRF was 19% among all survivors and 15% among the acute lymphoblastic leukemia survivors, after adjustment for medical and socioeconomic factors, including depression (29). Survivors were significantly more fatigued than their siblings. Survivors with fatigue were also more likely to experience depression than were survivors who did not have fatigue. These findings indicate that long-term follow-up care should include psychological assessments and interventions for childhood cancer survivors at highest risk (30).

Research over the past decade has revealed that acute physiologic conditions (which may or may not be related to cancer or cancer therapy), chronic medical conditions and their treatments (e.g., pain, disturbed sleep, decreased activity levels, infections, anemia, nutritional deficiencies, dehydration, electrolyte disturbances, cardiac deconditioning, pulmonary disorders, neuromuscular disorders, thyroid dysfunction, liver failure, renal insufficiency, and diabetes), psychosocial stress and emotional distress (e.g., anxiety, depression, and environmental reinforcers), and concurrent exposure to sedating medications (e.g., opioids) can also contribute to CRF in patients with cancer, although the exact nature of these influences cannot be determined. In addition, most patients with cancer are of advanced age, increasing the likelihood that they suffer from comorbidities that are also risk factors for CRF.

POTENTIAL UNDERLYING MECHANISMS OF CRF

Several descriptive studies have carefully documented the development of fatigue and how it interacts with potential biological mechanism targets in specific cohorts. However, numerous challenges exist in the translational area of the biomedical sciences for narrowing down host factors related to CRF. Thus, little progress has been made in identifying a biomarker that could serve as an objective measure of fatigue. Few neuroimaging studies have examined CRF expression in the human brain, and animal models representing CRF have not been established. Translational work is needed to find a mechanism-driven intervention for fatigue.

CRF does not develop in all patients at risk for it. Studies of genomic encoding for CRF are now beginning to explore the increased activity of proinflammatory transcription factors as contributors to fatigue in cancer survivors. In a study using genome-wide expression microarrays, Bower et al. (31) reported increased expression of inflammation-related genes, particularly those responsive to the proinflammatory nuclear factor-κB transcription control pathway, together with decreased expression of glucocorticoid-dependent anti-inflammatory genes between breast cancer survivors who had persistent fatigue and nonfatigued controls. However, Reinertsen et al. (32) found no association between persistent fatigue and the expression of either single nucleotide polymorphisms in inflammation-related genes (interleukin [IL]-1β, IL-6, IL-6 receptor, and C-reactive protein genes) or mRNA IL-1β and IL-6 receptor in a large sample of breast cancer survivors, even after excluding depressed individuals.

Patients with cancer—especially those undergoing aggressive therapy, those with advanced disease, and those who have accompanying medical comorbidities or psychological disorders—rarely experience just one severe symptom. CRF often accompanies a cluster of other moderate to severe symptoms, such as pain, distress, poor appetite, drowsiness, and disturbed sleep. In a large case-controlled study of survivors with breast cancer, depression and pain were the strongest predictors of fatigue (3). This suggests that a complex interplay exists between the etiological agent (e.g., cancer treatment, infections, and use of centrally acting drugs) and the patient's susceptibility to fatigue.

However, the lack of clear pathophysiologic explanations hampers our ability to determine whether a constellation of mechanisms causes CRF or whether a centrally mediated disorder characterized by CRF exists. Although the underlying etiology of fatigue is not yet fully understood, several working hypotheses to explain the mechanisms of this complex phenomenon have been suggested. Figure 7.1 presents the proposed etiologies of CRF.

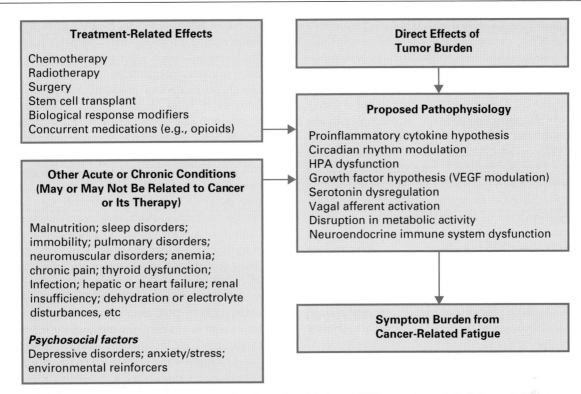

Figure 7.1. Proposed potential etiologies of cancer-related fatigue. VEGF, vascular endothelial growth factor.

The Proinflammatory Cytokine Hypothesis

The proinflammatory cytokine hypothesis, one of the primary proposed explanations of CRF, suggests that dysregulated inflammation and its toxic downstream effects constitute a significant biological basis for CRF and other cancer-related symptoms (13,21,33–37). As a typical nonspecific symptom in patients with cancer, fatigue is similar to certain sickness behaviors observed in animal models in studies of the behavioral effects of cytokine administration (38). Basic research on activation of immune-to-brain communication pathways in response to continued activation of the peripheral immune system indicates that proinflammatory cytokine (mainly IL-1β and tumor necrosis factor [TNF]-α) signaling to the brain leads to an exacerbation of sickness in vulnerable individuals, who develop a constellation of behavioral changes that include fatigue, disturbed sleep, and symptoms of depression (37). Increased expression of positive acute-phase proteins such as C-reactive protein and decreased expression of negative acute-phase proteins such as albumin are also highly correlated with persistent CRF (39). Certain inflammatory biomarkers (IL-6 and TNF-α) were identified in vivo and in vitro (40); these biomarkers are associated with activation of innate immune cells and T-cells (41).

The role of activation of the proinflammatory cytokine network in fatigue and other symptoms has been under investigation since the 1990s, although the relevance of these findings is limited by few translational studies confirming the results. In a quantitative review and meta-analysis of 18 studies, Schubert et al. (42) found that CRF was associated with increased circulating levels of IL-6, IL-1 receptor antagonist, and neopterin. Reductions in fatigue were observed in patients given antagonists of TNF-α as an intervention for improving the tolerability of chemotherapy (43). More recently, clinical studies have indicated that TNF-α signaling plays a role in postchemotherapy fatigue in patients with early-stage breast cancer (44). A temporal association was also found between serum or plasma inflammatory markers induced by aggressive cancer therapy and the development of fatigue and a cluster of other sickness symptoms (pain, disturbed sleep, drowsiness, and poor appetite) that affect physical functioning in patients with cancer (21,45,46). Inflammatory processes associated with tumor growth can cause abnormalities in energy metabolism and inhibit muscle function: Inagaki et al. (47) found that elevated levels of plasma IL-6 were associated with increased levels of fatigue in terminally ill patients with cancer.

The development of a spectrum of symptoms of depression in response to cytokines is well established in both animal models and humans, especially in the context of cytokine immunotherapy (48–51). Current research indicates that proinflammatory cytokines can cause depression in several ways, including glucocorticoid receptor resistance in immunocytes and their cellular targets through the activation of signalling pathways such as p38 mitogen-activated protein kinase and jun-N terminal kinase. This culminates in activation of the tryptophan-degrading enzyme indoleamine 2,3-dioxygenase, which generates neurotoxic metabolites

(52). In cancer patients treated with IFN-α, hypermetabolism in the left putamen and nucleus accumbens, likely related to reduced dopaminergic transmission, was associated with fatigue and lack of energy (53).

Studies of the chronic physical and mental fatigue seen in many neurologic diseases could also help improve understanding of CRF. Such fatigue is not accompanied by the profound weakness and persistent or progressive cognitive decline or failure of peripheral neuromuscular function seen in multiple sclerosis, chronic human immunodeficiency virus infection, or Parkinson's disease. The neuroanatomy of cytokine-induced depression is focused on the brain circuits, with evidence of decreased baseline activity in the frontal and temporal cortex and the insula and increased activity in the cerebellum and subcortical and limbic regions (54). In patients with neurological disorders, including multiple sclerosis, fatigue appears to result from a failure in the integration of limbic input and motor functions within the basal ganglia, affecting the striatal–thalamic–frontal cortical system (55). The origin of fatigue in patients with multiple sclerosis supports the idea that a specific dysfunction or involvement of the basal ganglia might contribute to fatigue (56). To understand the anatomical pathway of fatigue, further investigation into the potential shared mechanisms of and interventions for neurologic disease–associated fatigue and CRF is thus warranted.

Other Hypotheses

Proinflammatory cytokines may act independently to produce CRF or may overlap or work synergistically with such mechanisms as vagal afferent activation, hypothalamic–pituitary–adrenal (HPA) axis disruption, serotonin dysregulation, growth factor activation, and circadian rhythm modulation. These mechanisms may act either directly or indirectly on the brain.

The vagal afferent activation hypothesis posits that cancer and its treatment activate vagal afferent nerves through the peripheral release of neuroactive molecules, resulting in decreased somatic motor output and sustained changes in brain regions associated with fatigue (13,33).

The HPA disruption hypothesis is based on the theory that tumor-related or treatment-related dysregulation of HPA function can lead to endocrine changes that cause or contribute to fatigue (13,33). Fatigue has been linked to reduced HPA axis function and hypocortisolemia in patients with cancer or chronic fatigue syndrome. Reduced levels of cortisol and/or cortisol resistance may allow for increased levels of proinflammatory cytokines.

The serotonin dysregulation hypothesis suggests that cancer or its treatment induces increases in brain serotonin that alter HPA axis functioning and reduce the patient's ability to perform physical activities (33). However, most of these studies have been carried out in the context of endurance training, such that their relevance to CRF is doubtful (57).

The growth factor hypothesis associates treatment-induced fatigue with elevated levels of vascular endothelial growth factor, which stimulates the formation of new blood vessels necessary for tumor growth and metastasis and therefore decreases the blood supply and energy of other organs, including muscles and brain (58).

The circadian rhythm modulation hypothesis focuses on secretion rhythms of the stress hormone cortisol and their relation to rest–activity patterns. Elevated transforming growth factor-α levels have been associated with fatigue (59), flattened circadian rhythms, and loss of appetite in patients with metastatic colorectal cancer. Fatigue has also been associated with alterations in rest–activity cycles, which produce the sleep disruptions commonly seen in patients with cancer. A sleep disorder could cause disturbed arousal mechanisms or, equally plausible, be an indicator of a disorder of arousal. These disorders could be primary or related to metabolic disturbances or the use of centrally acting drugs. However, findings on this topic remain inconclusive. A review of the literature on disturbed circadian rhythms and CRF from 1950 to 2010 found that, although commonalities across studies emerged, the methods for measuring circadian rhythms were inconsistent and that further research with larger sample sizes and more heterogeneous populations (most were focused on patients with breast cancer) is needed (60).

Fundamental disruption in metabolic activity has also been hypothesized as a potential cause of CRF. Cancer and its treatment may disrupt the metabolism of adenosine triphosphate, a major source of energy for skeletal muscle contraction (13,33). Abnormalities in energy metabolism may be related to increased energy need (the hypermetabolic state that can accompany tumor growth, infection, fever, or surgery), decreased substrates (e.g., anemia, hypoxemia of any cause, poor nutrition), or abnormal accumulation of muscle metabolites (e.g., lactate) that impair intermediate metabolism or the normal functioning of muscles. Immobility and lack of exercise may also lead to reduced efficiency of neuromuscular functioning.

Risk factors beyond those involving the neuroendocrine immune system have also been proposed as mechanisms underlying CRF. For example, anemia leads to hypoxia, which can compromise organ function and induce fatigue (61). Longitudinal studies have promoted a better understanding of how CRF fluctuates according to various triggers and critical moderating factors, which should ultimately advance efforts to develop methods of mechanism-driven symptom intervention and prevention.

MEASURING CRF

Even though CRF can cause observable behavioral manifestations and is often accompanied by an objective decrement in performance and by other symptoms, CRF itself is a subjective experience and cannot be directly measured by an observer. Subjective patient reports (patient-reported outcomes) have become the standard method for assessing dimensions of fatigue, as well as its severity and interference with daily activities. The US Food and Drug Administration

(FDA) encourages investigators to use standardized, psychometrically validated patient-reported outcome measures in clinical research for symptom intervention (62). Validated measurement tools are essential for evaluating the treatment and management of CRF and for conducting translational mechanism studies and epidemiologic studies with fatigue as a primary outcome. Even so, patient-reported measures of CRF provide little specific diagnostic information, while objective measures of CRF that are based on physiologic or behavioral markers are frustratingly lacking.

The multifactorial nature of fatigue makes it especially difficult to measure. Even so, although initial efforts to develop a measure of fatigue after World War I were ineffective, it is now widely accepted that a validated fatigue assessment process is possible. Existing validated fatigue measures typically assess severity and the degree to which fatigue interferes with daily life, yet these results should be integrated, on a patient-by-patient basis, with assessments of other factors, such as the quality, temporal pattern, and history of the fatigue and expectations associated with the specific patient's disease phase or treatment status. To be clinically meaningful, a fatigue assessment should also examine the impact of fatigue on physical function, social function, cognition, mood, and other facets of quality of life. The assessment process must give clinical consideration to potential etiologies, such as cancer treatment and current systemic disorders, which should help identify any treatable causes of fatigue.

Selecting an Assessment Tool

Although the FDA has encouraged investigators to use patient-reported outcome measures in their research (62), most fatigue data from clinical studies come from clinician ratings using the National Cancer Institute's Common Terminology Criteria for Adverse Events (NCI CTCAE). Further, no single standardized patient-reported instrument for CRF or other forms of chronic fatigue has been adopted broadly, either in clinical practice or in research. In 2007, Hjollund et al. (63) noted that between 1975 and 2004 more than 250 fatigue assessment tools were developed for use in patients with either cancer or neurologic or systemic disorders; some tools have "crossed over" to be used in additional patient populations. Of these, 150 were used only once. These tools vary in their construction (coverage and structure), frequency of use, recommended frequency of administration, scoring, and psychometric properties. These tools also vary by the type of response collected. For example, with verbal descriptor scales, patients select a category to describe their fatigue, such as "none," "mild," "moderate," or "severe." In visual analog scales, patients mark their fatigue severity along a line. In numerical rating scales, patients rate their fatigue severity on a numbered scale with a verbal anchor at each end (e.g., "no fatigue" and "fatigue as bad as you can imagine").

Tools for measuring persistent fatigue should be both practical and psychometrically sound, should require the rating to occur within a reasonable recall period, should present the instructions in easily understood terms, should incorporate easy-to-use scales and standardized rules for administration and scoring, and should be sensitive enough to detect changes in patient experience. To facilitate cross-cultural validation and comparison, the tool should also be easily translatable into other languages. Most importantly, a good fatigue assessment tool should allow for consistent interpretation of the data.

Although no consensus on the dimensional structure of fatigue has been reached (64), the fatigue assessment tools currently available may be categorized as unidimensional or multidimensional. Quick and easy unidimensional measures used for screening purposes provide such basic information as whether fatigue is present or absent and, if present, its intensity, severity, or impact. Unidimensional measures can be used to determine whether more comprehensive clinical examination is needed and, when used in research or clinical trials, can provide enough data to track changes in fatigue both over time and in response to treatment. Examination of the various facets of fatigue—the mental–cognitive, physical, and emotional domains—requires a multidimensional measure. Because the experience of CRF is subjective and the impact of fatigue on everyday life varies from patient to patient, the information provided by a multidimensional measure can be valuable.

Unidimensional Measures

Using theory-driven exploratory factor analysis to examine a 72-item data bank from a sample of 555 patients with cancer, Lai et al. (65) reported that CRF is sufficiently unidimensional for measurement approaches that require or assume unidimensionality.

Unidimensional measures for CRF can be single-item tools like the widely used NCCN patient-reported fatigue intensity rating (8), which has a 0 to 10 numeric scale, or the NCI CTCAE (version 3.0) (66), which uses a 5-point Likert scale rated by medical staff. Another example is the single-item score given for "fatigue at its worst" on the Brief Fatigue Inventory, which asks patients to rate their level of worst fatigue/tiredness on a 0 to 10 scale during the past 24 hours (2). This item can be used as a rapid screening tool or a continual-monitoring variable in clinical practice (67).

Unidimensional measures for CRF may have multiple items, as do the Brief Fatigue Inventory (2) and the Fatigue Severity Scale (68). Multiple-item unidimensional measures with good reliability can generate usable results even when a small percentage of responses are missing. A unidimensional measure of CRF may also be a validated subscale of a larger quality-of-life measurement tool, such as the 13-item fatigue subscale of the Functional Assessment of Cancer Therapy (69), or 3 items on the European Organization for Research and Treatment of Cancer QLQ-C30 (70).

Multidimensional Measures

Although the psychometric accuracy of unidimensional measures may be satisfactory, unidimensional measures fall short of assessing the full spectrum of CRF (5). Unlike unidimensional measures, multidimensional measures can distinguish physical from mental fatigue and measure responses in dimensions relating to affective functioning and activity. The relatively short and simple Multidimensional Fatigue Inventory (MFI-20) is a commonly used measure of fatigue, and its General Fatigue subscale can serve as a global index of fatigue severity (71). Some multidimensional scales are too long for very ill patients to complete, however, and many of these measures use original phrases or idiomatic expressions that can hinder translation into other languages or cultural settings.

Interpreting Fatigue Assessment Results

As an outcome measure, CRF can be an important component of drug trials and clinical practice. A reduction in CRF could represent reduced treatment toxicity, improved palliation for advanced disease, increased quality assurance and patient satisfaction with medical care, or improved functional and health status for cancer survivors. Thus, accurate interpretation of CRF assessment data is very important, whereas inadequate assessment can be a substantial barrier to good fatigue management in the clinic. Standardized fatigue assessment may expand the attention and resources provided to address this common and debilitating symptom.

One way to begin interpreting fatigue severity is to define levels at which symptoms interfere with physical and affective functioning, especially between cancer patients and healthy individuals. Functional impairment or interference was found to increase as fatigue worsened (12), which is consistent with other pain research findings (72–74). The severity of fatigue may be the most informative indicator of the need for intervention. The boundary between mild–moderate and severe fatigue may be a clinically meaningful indicator for determining whether a fatigue intervention is effective. The best example of fatigue severity delineated by mild–moderate versus severe ratings is the NCCN practice guideline for clinical management of CRF (75).

Tracking changes in self-report over time can introduce response shift, a phenomenon that occurs when patients judge their level of fatigue differently after having experiences that alter their own internal standards, values, or conceptualizations. The possibility of response shift raises methodological concerns, because it can lead to underreporting of fatigue as patients adapt to more severe "normal" levels of fatigue after therapy. For example, response shift occurred in a group of patients receiving radiotherapy who retrospectively minimized their pretreatment fatigue severity compared with their current fatigue levels (76). A meta-analysis of 19 quality-of-life studies revealed response shifts for several measures, with the largest mean effect size of response shift for fatigue (0.32), followed by global quality of life, physical role limitation, psychological well-being, and pain (77).

Studies designed to integrate accumulated dose of cancer therapy with changes in internal standards can explicitly measure response shift effects and account for them to inform the evaluation of treatments or interventions. Importantly, the patient's illness perception, coping skills, and mood may have long-lasting effects on his or her eventual adaptation to chronic fatigue and must be considered in any interpretation of fatigue results.

INTERVENTIONS FOR CRF

A standard intervention for CRF has not yet been established. Current treatments for CRF include individual interventions for various treatable secondary conditions as causes of fatigue (see Figure 7.1). Guidelines for the general supportive care of CRF have been developed by NCCN (78) and the Oncology Nursing Society (79). National clinical practice guidelines (80) and product labeling from the US FDA should direct individualized management of patients with cancer-related or treatment-associated anemia. Open communication between the patient, family, and caregiving team can facilitate better management of CRF and enhance understanding of its effects on daily life (8,9).

A growing number of clinical trials aimed at developing and testing pharmacologic and nonpharmacologic treatments for fatigue have been reported in the past 5 years. Systematic reviews and meta-analyses have analyzed the efficacy of some of the most reported interventions, discussed below. Mitchell and Berger (81) have created a list of interventions for which there is evidence of efficacy in treating CRF, along with interventions whose efficacy has not been established or is supported only by expert opinion. Nonetheless, the generalizability of the CRF intervention studies analyzed remains limited. Improvements in methodological quality and documentation can be gained through more careful study design and adherence to better reporting standards, such as the Consolidated Standard of Reporting Trials(82,83), both of which would provide more accurate data on the efficacy of psychosocial therapy for CRF.

Pharmacologic Treatments

Psychostimulants

In a 2011 meta-analysis of five placebo-controlled trials, it was seen that treatment with psychostimulants caused a small but significant improvement in fatigue (z score, 2.83; $P =$ 0.005) (84). The most studied psychostimulant used to treat CRF is methylphenidate, which works by directly stimulating adrenergic receptors and indirectly causing the release of dopamine and norepinephrine from presynaptic terminals (85). Methylphenidate is generally well tolerated in cancer patients. The data support prescribing 10 to 20 mg daily. Insomnia and agitation are the most common side effects, but these are mostly reversible with discontinuation of the treatment. Close monitoring is recommended, especially for the first few days of treatment. A large placebo effect has been reported in most trials with stimulants; therefore, a clinical trial with a larger sample size would be helpful for making conclusive recommendations for the use of methylphenidate to treat CRF.

Modafinil, another central nervous system stimulant, is used to treat narcolepsy. Fava et al. (86) reported that modafinil is a well-tolerated and potentially effective augmenting agent for patients with fatigue and sleepiness who are partial responders to selective serotonin reuptake inhibitors. In a phase III, randomized, placebo-controlled, double-blind trial, 631 patients undergoing chemotherapy who had severe fatigue at baseline benefited significantly from modafinil (87). It significantly improved daytime sleepiness but had no effect on depression.

Antidepressants

It is not known whether fatigue and depression share pathophysiologic characteristics; however, efforts have been made to treat fatigue with antidepressants in depressed cancer patients. Morrow et al. (88) reported that in a multicenter, double-blind, randomized, placebo-controlled study of paroxetine administered to cancer patients with fatigue who were undergoing chemotherapy, paroxetine produced a significant reduction in depressive symptoms but not in fatigue. Roscoe et al. (89) reported a more favorable outcome from a double-blind placebo-controlled trial.

Nonetheless, patients with sleep difficulties and depression may benefit from antidepressants such as nortriptyline and amitriptyline, which have sedative qualities. In addition, bupropion may benefit patients with CRF because of its ability to increase dopaminergic neurotransmission (90). Further study is needed to determine whether fatigue can be treated effectively with other classes of antidepressants in patients undergoing various modes of cancer therapy.

Corticosteroids

The use of steroids to treat persistent CRF does not appear to be warranted, in part because of concerns about long-term use of steroids and in part because steroids appear to have little effect on fatigue. An analysis of four randomized, placebo-controlled trials indicated that a mean of 8 weeks of progestational steroid therapy (three studies used megestrol acetate and one used medroxyprogesterone acetate) did not reduce fatigue in a group of patients receiving palliative care without chemotherapy (overall z score, 1.06; $P = 0.29$) (91).

Complementary Alternative Therapy

Many patients use herbal and supplemental preparations to cope with CRF. Study participants with unexplained chronic fatigue of unknown etiology lasting for at least 6 months reported that the alternative treatments coenzyme Q10, dehydroepiandrosterone, and ginseng were the most helpful (92). Ginseng is a widely used tonic agent, with a potent smell and aftertaste that are difficult to mask—a challenging impediment to its use in blinded randomized trials (93). Because ginseng is easily acquired at health food stores, patients may not think of it as medication. Research into American ginseng in patients with CRF has indicated that patients receiving the largest doses showed the most improvement in overall energy levels and overall mental, physical, spiritual, and emotional well-being (94,95).

Guarana (*Paullinia cupana*) is a plant native to the Amazon basin with energy-enhancing and tonic properties known to the local people. Dry extract of guarana, at a dose of 75 mg once per day, has been reported to reduce fatigue associated with therapy in breast cancer patients, with no significant side effects and at a relatively low cost (96). These effects are thought to be mainly due to the methylxanthine present in the plant's seeds.

Patients using herbal treatments should exercise caution because of possible profound drug interactions.

Psychological and Activity-Based Interventions

Interest has been growing in the role of cognitive factors (e.g., tendency to perceive catastrophe) and behavioral factors (e.g., physical activity) in exacerbating and prolonging fatigue. A meta-analysis conducted by Schmitz et al. (97) suggested that exercise is an effective way to manage CRF both during and after treatment, although the effect sizes were small. In another summary of 12 randomized, controlled clinical trials, Mustian et al. (98) commented that exercise is safe for and well tolerated by cancer survivors. The Cochrane Collaboration published a meta-analysis of nine studies of the effects of aerobic or resistance exercise on CRF for 452 women receiving adjuvant therapy for breast cancer (99). Although the difference in improvement in patient-reported fatigue between the intervention and control groups was not statistically significant in these patients, exercise appeared to result in improved physical fitness and, as a result, in improved capacity for performing activities of daily life. These studies involved a range of exercise types (walking, cycling, swimming, resistive exercise, and combined exercise), intensity (with most programs at 50% to 90% of the estimated Vo_2 maximum heart rate, from twice a day to two times per week), degree of supervision, and duration (from 2 weeks to 1 year).

A systematic review and meta-analysis of nonpharmacologic therapy in 119 clinical studies with fatigue-related variables as either primary or secondary outcomes found significant and clinically meaningful effect sizes for both psychological interventions (small to moderate effects) and exercise interventions (moderate effects) for fatigue (100). Jacobsen et al. (101) reported only a small overall effect size for 30 randomized controlled trials of nonpharmacologic interventions; 18 psychosocial intervention studies (support group therapy and individual psychotherapy, both of which provided education, coping strategy programs, tailored behavioral interventions, and professionally or self-administered stress management training) had slightly larger effect sizes, but activity-based interventions (home-based and supervised exercise programs) did not significantly improve CRF in 12 studies.

Structured rehabilitation programs have reported significant and sustained improvement in persistent fatigue, especially in cancer survivors. Tailoring the program based on the patient's current level of energy and stage along the treatment trajectory is necessary (102).

Despite methodological limitations for conducting double-blinded trials, preliminary evidence supports the potential effectiveness of integrative approaches in the treatment of fatigue in patients with cancer. A review of mind–body interventions by Kwekkeboom et al. (103) includes such approaches as relaxation, mindfulness-based stress reduction, medical Qigong, massage, healing touch, Reiki, and combined modality interventions such as aromatherapy, lavender foot soak, and reflexology. The interventions analyzed in this review utilized open-label and uncontrolled designs and had small sample sizes, making it difficult to draw firm conclusions about efficacy. However, yoga showed beneficial effects in a randomized study of breast cancer patients undergoing adjuvant radiotherapy (104) and in a study of individuals who did not have unclear thinking along with their fatigue (92). Acupuncture has not been thoroughly studied in patients with CRF, but positive trends in fatigue reduction seen in randomized clinical trials of acupuncture used to treat CRF suggest that the procedure may be an effective way of controlling CRF and other symptoms (105,106).

CONCLUSION

CRF is a common and distressing symptom because it interferes with multiple aspects of daily life. Debilitating fatigue can be produced by cancer or its treatment, especially in patients undergoing active cancer treatment, and it can be a persistent symptom for some survivors who have otherwise been cured of their cancer. The mechanism underlying CRF is poorly understood, and although awareness and study of this symptom have grown in recent years, consistent assessment and effective management of CRF have not been priorities in routine medical practice.

A 2003 National Institutes of Health State-of-the-Science Statement (107) called for additional adequately funded prospective studies of pain, depression, and fatigue—both alone and in combination—which has stimulated tremendous growth in clinical investigations of the effectiveness of interventions for CRF. Improving the understanding of fatigue will require epidemiologic studies and increased reporting of effective therapies. Well-designed clinical trials are needed to evaluate both pharmacologic and nonpharmacologic methods for treating CRF. Education about CRF should be made available to all patients and their caregivers: accurate and age-appropriate information about conditions like CRF alleviates much of the stress and anxiety brought on by poor communication.

Advancing fatigue research and clinical management will also require the measurement of fatigue in a reliable and valid manner that examines widely accepted dimensions, both for screening and for use in clinical trials. Numerous subscales, unidimensional measures, and multidimensional measures exist, and the establishment of a single, standard tool for measuring symptoms was not recommended in the FDA's patient-reported outcomes guidance (62). Rather, clinicians and researchers should consider individual circumstances, good clinical practice, and research goals as guides for choosing the most appropriate fatigue measurement tool.

Effective treatment of the root causes of CRF will require a good understanding of the underlying pathophysiologic mechanisms of CRF, which remain a mystery. The development of mechanism-driven fatigue interventions from physiologic–behavioral fatigue research, implementation of guidelines for experimental designs, and discovery of biomarkers to identify high-risk individuals would provide patients with greater symptom control.

REFERENCES

1. Vogelzang NJ, Breitbart W, Cella D, et al. Patient, caregiver, and oncologist perceptions of cancer-related fatigue: results of a tripart assessment survey. The Fatigue Coalition. *Semin Hematol*. 1997;34:4-12.
2. Mendoza TR, Wang XS, Cleeland CS, et al. The rapid assessment of fatigue severity in cancer patients: use of the Brief Fatigue Inventory. *Cancer*. 1999;85:1186-1196.
3. Bower JE, Ganz PA, Desmond KA, Rowland JH, Meyerowitz BE, Belin TR. Fatigue in breast cancer survivors: occurrence, correlates, and impact on quality of life. *J Clin Oncol*. 2000;18:743-753.
4. Servaes P, Gielissen MF, Verhagen S, Bleijenberg G. The course of severe fatigue in disease-free breast cancer patients: a longitudinal study. *Psychooncology*. 2007;16:787-795.
5. Prue G, Rankin J, Allen J, Gracey J, Cramp F. Cancer-related fatigue: a critical appraisal. *Eur J Cancer*. 2006;42:846-863.
6. Cleeland CS, Mendoza TR, Wang XS, et al. Assessing symptom distress in cancer patients: the M. D. Anderson Symptom Inventory. *Cancer*. 2000;89:1634-1646.
7. Barsevick AM, Cleeland CS, Manning DC, et al. ASCPRO recommendations for the assessment of fatigue as an outcome in clinical trials. *J Pain Symptom Manage*. 2010;39:1086-1099.
8. Mock V, Atkinson A, Barsevick AM, et al. Cancer-related fatigue. Clinical practice guidelines in oncology. *J Natl Compr Canc Netw*. 2007;5:1054-1078.
9. Radbruch L, Strasser F, Elsner F, et al. Fatigue in palliative care patients—an EAPC approach. *Palliat Med*. 2008;22:13-32.
10. Olson K. A new way of thinking about fatigue: a reconceptualization. *Oncol Nurs Forum*. 2007;34:93-99.
11. Scott JA, Lasch KE, Barsevick AM, et al. Patients' experiences with cancer-related fatigue: a review and synthesis of qualitative research. *Oncol Nurs Forum*. 2011;38:E191-E203.
12. Cleeland CS, Wang XS. Measuring and understanding fatigue. *Oncology*. 1999;13:91-97.
13. Wang XS. Pathophysiology of cancer-related fatigue. *Clin J Oncol Nurs*. 2008;12:11-20.
14. Given CW, Given B, Azzouz F, et al. Predictors of pain and fatigue in the year following diagnosis among elderly cancer patients. *J Pain Symptom Manage*. 2001;21:456-466.
15. Wang XS, Fairclough DL, Liao Z, et al. Longitudinal study of the relationship between chemoradiation therapy for non-small-cell lung cancer and patient symptoms. *J Clin Oncol*. 2006;24:4485-4491.
16. Hickok JT, Morrow GR, Roscoe JA, et al. Occurrence, severity, and longitudinal course of twelve common symptoms in 1129 consecutive patients during radiotherapy for cancer. *J Pain Symptom Manage*. 2005;30:433-442.
17. Knobel H, Loge JH, Nordoy T, et al. High level of fatigue in lymphoma patients treated with high dose therapy. *J Pain Symptom Manage*. 2000;19:446-456.

18. Jacobsen PB, Hann DM, Azzarello LM, et al. Fatigue in women receiving adjuvant chemotherapy for breast cancer: characteristics, course, and correlates. *J Pain Symptom Manage.* 1999;18:233-242.

19. Minton O, Strasser F, Radbruch L, et al. Identification of factors associated with fatigue in advanced cancer: a subset analysis of the European Palliative Care Research Collaborative computerized symptom assessment data set. *J Pain Symptom Manage.* 2012;43(2):226-235.

20. Rubin GJ, Hotopf M. Systematic review and meta-analysis of interventions for postoperative fatigue. *Br J Surg.* 2002;89:971-984.

21. Wang XS, Shi Q, Williams LA, et al. Serum interleukin-6 predicts the development of multiple symptoms at nadir of allogeneic hematopoietic stem cell transplantation. *Cancer.* 2008;113:2102-2109.

22. Anderson KO, Giralt SA, Mendoza TR, et al. Symptom burden in patients undergoing autologous stem-cell transplantation. *Bone Marrow Transplant.* 2007;39:759-766.

23. Jones TH, Wadler S, Hupart KH. Endocrine-mediated mechanisms of fatigue during treatment with interferon-alpha. *Semin Oncol.* 1998;25:54-63.

24. Stone P, Hardy J, Huddart R, et al. Fatigue in patients with prostate cancer receiving hormone therapy. *Eur J Cancer.* 2000;36:1134-1141.

25. Guevremont C, Alasker A, Karakiewicz PI. Management of sorafenib, sunitinib, and temsirolimus toxicity in metastatic renal cell carcinoma. *Curr Opin Support Palliat Care.* 2009;3:170-179.

26. Seruga B, Sterling L, Wang L, et al. Reporting of serious adverse drug reactions of targeted anticancer agents in pivotal phase III clinical trials. *J Clin Oncol.* 2011;29:174-185.

27. Shi Q, Smith TG, Michonski JD, et al. Symptom burden in cancer survivors 1 year after diagnosis: a report from the American Cancer Society's studies of cancer survivors. *Cancer.* 2011;117:2779-2790.

28. Meeske KA, Siegel SE, Globe DR, et al. Prevalence and correlates of fatigue in long-term survivors of childhood leukemia. *J Clin Oncol.* 2005;23:5501-5510.

29. Mulrooney DA, Ness KK, Neglia JP, et al. Fatigue and sleep disturbance in adult survivors of childhood cancer: a report from the childhood cancer survivor study (CCSS). *Sleep.* 2008;31:271-281.

30. Zeltzer LK, Recklitis C, Buchbinder D, et al. Psychological status in childhood cancer survivors: a report from the Childhood Cancer Survivor Study. *J Clin Oncol.* 2009;27:2396-2404.

31. Bower JE, Ganz PA, Irwin MR, et al. Fatigue and gene expression in human leukocytes: increased NF-kappaB and decreased glucocorticoid signaling in breast cancer survivors with persistent fatigue. *Brain Behav Immun.* 2011;25:147-150.

32. Reinertsen KV, Grenaker Alnæs GI, Landmark-Høyvik H, et al. Fatigued breast cancer survivors and gene polymorphisms in the inflammatory pathway. *Brain Behav Immun.* 2011;25:1376-1383.

33. Ryan JL, Carroll JK, Ryan EP, et al. Mechanisms of cancer-related fatigue. *Oncologist.* 2007;12:22-34.

34. Cleeland CS, Bennett GJ, Dantzer R, et al. Are the symptoms of cancer and cancer treatment due to a shared biologic mechanism? *Cancer.* 2003;97:2919-2925.

35. Kurzrock R. The role of cytokines in cancer-related fatigue. *Cancer.* 2001;92:1684-1688.

36. Lee BN, Dantzer R, Langley KE, et al. A cytokine-based neuroimmunologic mechanism of cancer-related symptoms. *Neuroimmunomodulation.* 2004;11:279-292.

37. Dantzer R, O'Connor JC, Freund GG, et al. From inflammation to sickness and depression: when the immune system subjugates the brain. *Nat Rev Neurosci.* 2008;9:46-56.

38. Dantzer R, Kelley KW. Twenty years of research on cytokine-induced sickness behavior. *Brain Behav Immun.* 2007;21:153-160.

39. Orre IJ, Murison R, Dahl AA, et al. Levels of circulating interleukin-1 receptor antagonist and C-reactive protein in long-term survivors of testicular cancer with chronic cancer-related fatigue. *Brain Behav Immun.* 2009;23:868-874.

40. Collado-Hidalgo A, Bower JE, Ganz PA, et al. Inflammatory biomarkers for persistent fatigue in breast cancer survivors. *Clin Cancer Res.* 2006;12:2759-2766.

41. Bower JE, Ganz PA, Aziz N, et al. Fatigue and proinflammatory cytokine activity in breast cancer survivors. *Psychosom Med.* 2002;64:604-611.

42. Schubert C, Hong S, Natarajan L, et al. The association between fatigue and inflammatory marker levels in cancer patients: a quantitative review. *Brain Behav Immun.* 2007;21:413-427.

43. Monk JP, Phillips G, Waite R, et al. Assessment of tumor necrosis factor alpha blockade as an intervention to improve tolerability of dose-intensive chemotherapy in cancer patients. *J Clin Oncol.* 2006;24:1852-1859.

44. Bower JE, Ganz PA, Irwin MR, et al. Inflammation and behavioral symptoms after breast cancer treatment: do fatigue, depression, and sleep disturbance share a common underlying mechanism? *J Clin Oncol.* 2011;29:3517-3522.

45. Wang XS, Shi Q, Mao L, Cleeland CS, Liao Z. Association between inflammatory cytokines and the development of multiple symptoms in patients with non-small cell lung cancer undergoing chemoradiation therapy [abstract taken from *J Clin Oncol.* 2008;26]. American Society of Clinical Oncology 44th Annual Meeting; May 30-June 3, 2008; Chicago, IL.

46. Bower JE, Ganz PA, Tao ML, et al. Inflammatory biomarkers and fatigue during radiation therapy for breast and prostate cancer. *Clin Cancer Res.* 2009;15:5534-5540.

47. Inagaki M, Isono M, Okuyama T, et al. Plasma interleukin-6 and fatigue in terminally ill cancer patients. *J Pain Symptom Manage.* 2008;35:153-161.

48. Payne JK, Piper B, Rabinowitz I, et al. Biomarkers, fatigue, sleep, and depressive symptoms in women with breast cancer: a pilot study. *Oncol Nurs Forum.* 2006;33:775-783.

49. Raison CL, Capuron L, Miller AH. Cytokines sing the blues: inflammation and the pathogenesis of depression. *Trends Immunol.* 2006;27:24-31.

50. Dantzer R, Capuron L, Irwin MR, et al. Identification and treatment of symptoms associated with inflammation in medically ill patients. *Psychoneuroendocrinology.* 2008;33:18-29.

51. Miller AH, Ancoli-Israel S, Bower JE, Capuron L, Irwin MR. Neuroendocrine-immune mechanisms of behavioral comorbidities in patients with cancer. *J Clin Oncol.* 2008;26:971-982.

52. Irwin MR, Miller AH. Depressive disorders and immunity: 20 years of progress and discovery. *Brain Behav Immun.* 2007;21:374-383.

53. Capuron L, Pagnoni G, Demetrashvili MF et al. Basal ganglia hypermetabolism and symptoms of fatigue during interferon-alpha therapy. *Neuropsychopharmacology* 2007;32:2384-2392.

54. Fitzgerald PB, Laird AR, Maller J, et al. A meta-analytic study of changes in brain activation in depression. *Hum Brain Mapp.* 2008;29:683-695.

55. Chaudhuri A, Behan PO. Fatigue and basal ganglia. *J Neurol Sci.* 2000;179:34-42.

56. Téllez N, Alonso J, Rio J, et al. The basal ganglia: a substrate for fatigue in multiple sclerosis. *Neuroradiology.* 2008;50:17-23.

57. Davis JM, Bailey SP. Possible mechanisms of central nervous system fatigue during exercise. *Med Sci Sports Exerc.* 1997;29:45-57.

58. Mills PJ, Parker BA, Dimsdale JE, et al. The relationship between fatigue, quality of life and inflammation during anthracycline-based chemotherapy in breast cancer. *Biol Psychol.* 2005;69:85-96.

59. Rich T, Innominato PF, Boerner J, et al. Elevated serum cytokines correlated with altered behavior, serum cortisol rhythm, and dampened 24-hour rest-activity patterns in patients with metastatic colorectal cancer. *Clin Cancer Res.* 2005;11:1757-1764.

60. Payne JK. Altered circadian rhythms and cancer-related fatigue outcomes. *Integr Cancer Ther.* 2011;10(3):221-233.

61. Hurter B, Bush NJ. Cancer-related anemia: clinical review and management update. *Clin J Oncol Nurs.* 2007;11:349-359.

62. US Food and Drug Administration. Guidance for industry. Patient-reported outcome measures: use in medical product development to support labeling claims. http://www fda gov/downloads/Drugs/GuidanceComplianceRegulatoryInformation/Guidances/UCM071975 pdf [serial online]. 2009; Available from: U.S. Department of Health and Human Services. Accessed November 16, 2011.

63. Hjollund NH, Andersen JH, Bech P. Assessment of fatigue in chronic disease: a bibliographic study of fatigue measurement scales. *Health Qual Life Outcomes.* 2007;5:12-16.

64. Jacobsen PB. Assessment of fatigue in cancer patients. *J Natl Cancer Inst Monogr.* 2004;93-97.

65. Lai JS, Crane PK, Cella D. Factor analysis techniques for assessing sufficient unidimensionality of cancer related fatigue. *Qual Life Res.* 2006;15:1179-1190.

66. Basch E, Iasonos A, McDonough T, et al. Patient versus clinician symptom reporting using the National Cancer Institute Common Terminology Criteria for Adverse Events: results of a questionnaire-based study. *Lancet Oncol.* 2006;7:903-909.

67. Escalante CP, Manzullo EF, Lam TP, Ensor JE, Valdres RU, Wang XS. Fatigue and its risk factors in cancer patients who seek emergency care. *J Pain Symptom Manage.* 2008;36:358-366.

68. Krupp LB, LaRocca NG, Muir-Nash J, Steinberg AD. The fatigue severity scale. Application to patients with multiple sclerosis and systemic lupus erythematosus. *Arch Neurol.* 1989;46:1121-1123.

69. Yellen SB, Cella DF, Webster K, Blendowski C, Kaplan E. Measuring fatigue and other anemia-related symptoms with the Functional Assessment of Cancer Therapy (FACT) measurement system. *J Pain Symptom Manage.* 1997;13:63-74.

70. Aaronson NK, Ahmedzai S, Bergman B, et al. The European Organization for Research and Treatment of Cancer QLQ-C30: a quality-of-life instrument for use in international clinical trials in oncology. *J Natl Cancer Inst.* 1993;85:365-376.

71. Smets EMA, Garssen B, Bonke B, De Haes JCJM. The Multidimensional Fatigue Inventory (MFI): psychometric qualities of an instrument to assess fatigue. *J Psychosom Res.* 1995;39:315-325.

72. Serlin RC, Mendoza TR, Nakamura Y, Edwards KR, Cleeland CS. When is cancer pain mild, moderate or severe? Grading pain severity by its interference with function. *Pain.* 1995;61:277-284.

73. Cleeland CS, Ryan KM. Pain assessment: global use of the Brief Pain Inventory. *Ann Acad Med Singapore.* 1994;23:129-138.

74. Cleeland CS, Gonin R, Hatfield AK, et al. Pain and its treatment in outpatients with metastatic cancer. *N Engl J Med.* 1994;330:592-596.

75. National Comprehensive Cancer Network. NCCN clinical practice guidelines in oncology: cancer-related fatigue. http://www.nccn.org/professionals/physician_gls/PDF/fatigue.pdf [serial online]. 2007;V.3.2007. Accessed September 13, 2007.

76. Visser MR, Smets EM, Sprangers MA, de Haes HJ. How response shift may affect the measurement of change in fatigue. *J Pain Symptom Manage.* 2000;20:12-18.

77. Schwartz CE, Bode R, Repucci N, Becker J, Sprangers MA, Fayers PM. The clinical significance of adaptation to changing health: a meta-analysis of response shift. *Qual Life Res.* 2006;15:1533-1550.

78. Mock V, Atkinson A, Barsevick A, et al. NCCN practice guidelines for cancer-related fatigue. *Oncology (Huntington).* 2000;14:151--161.

79. Mitchell SA, Beck SL, Eaton LH. Putting evidence into practice (PEP): fatigue. In: Eaton LH, Tipton JM, eds. *Putting Evidence into Practice: Improving Oncology Patient Outcomes.* 1st ed. Pittsburgh, PA: Oncology Nursing Society; 2009: 149-174.

80. National Comprehensive Cancer Network. NCCN clinical practice guidelines in oncology: cancer- and chemotherapy-induced anemia. http://www nccn org/professionals/physician_gls/PDF/anemia pdf [serial online]. 2012;V.2.2012. Accessed February 16, 2012.

81. Mitchell SA, Berger AM. Fatigue. In: DeVita VT, Lawrence TS, Rosenberg SA, eds. *Cancer: Principles & Practice of Oncology.* 9th ed. Philadelphia, PA: Wolters Kluwer Health/Lippincott Williams & Wilkins; 2011:2387-2392.

82. Moher D, Jones A, Lepage L. Use of the CONSORT statement and quality of reports of randomized trials: a comparative before-and-after evaluation. *JAMA.* 2001;285:1992-1995.

83. Moher D, Schulz KF, Altman D. The CONSORT statement: revised recommendations for improving the quality of reports of parallel-group randomized trials. *JAMA.* 2001;285:1987-1991.

84. Minton O, Richardson A, Sharpe M, Hotopf M, Stone PC. Psychostimulants for the management of cancer-related fatigue: a systematic review and meta-analysis. *J Pain Symptom Manage.* 2011;41:761-767.

85. Breitbart W, Alici Y. Psychostimulants for cancer-related fatigue. *J Natl Compr Canc Netw.* 2010;8:933-942.

86. Fava M, Thase ME, DeBattista C. A multicenter, placebo-controlled study of modafinil augmentation in partial responders to selective serotonin reuptake inhibitors with persistent fatigue and sleepiness. *J Clin Psychiatry.* 2005;66:85-93.

87. Morrow GR, Jean-Pierre P, Roscoe JA, et al. A phase III randomized, placebo-controlled, double-blind trial of a eugeroic agent in 642 cancer patients reporting fatigue during chemotherapy: a URCC CCOP Study [abstract taken from *J Clin Oncol.* 2008;26]. American Society of Clinical Oncology 44th Annual Meeting; May 30-June 3, 2008; Chicago, IL.

88. Morrow GR, Hickok JT, Roscoe JA, et al. Differential effects of paroxetine on fatigue and depression: a randomized, double-blind trial from the University of Rochester Cancer Center Community Clinical Oncology Program. *J Clin Oncol.* 2003;21:4635-4641.

89. Roscoe JA, Morrow GR, Hickok JT, et al. Effect of paroxetine hydrochloride (Paxil) on fatigue and depression in breast

cancer patients receiving chemotherapy. *Breast Cancer Res Treat.* 2005;89:243-249.

90. Moss EL, Simpson JS, Pelletier G, Forsyth P. An open-label study of the effects of bupropion SR on fatigue, depression and quality of life of mixed-site cancer patients and their partners. *Psychooncology.* 2006;15:259-267.

91. Minton O, Richardson A, Sharpe M, Hotopf M, Stone P. A systematic review and meta-analysis of the pharmacological treatment of cancer-related fatigue. *J Natl Cancer Inst.* 2008;100:1155-1166.

92. Bentler SE, Hartz AJ, Kuhn EM. Prospective observational study of treatments for unexplained chronic fatigue. *J Clin Psychiatry.* 2005;66:625-632.

93. Elam JL, Carpenter JS, Shu XO, Boyapati S, Friedmann-Gilchrist J. Methodological issues in the investigation of ginseng as an intervention for fatigue. *Clin Nurse Spec.* 2006;20:183-189.

94. Ginseng may relieve cancer treatment fatigue. *Mayo Clin Health Lett.* 2007;25:4.

95. Barton DL, Soori GS, Bauer B, et al. A pilot, multi-dose, placebo-controlled evaluation of American ginseng (panax quinquefolius) to improve cancer-related fatigue: NCCTG trial N03CA [abstract taken from *J Clin Oncol.* 2007;25]. American Society of Clinical Oncology 43rd Annual Meeting; June 1-5, 2007; Chicago, IL.

96. Campos MP, Hassan BJ, Riechelmann R, Del Giglio A. Cancer-related fatigue: a review. *Rev Assoc Med Bras.* 2011;57: 211-219.

97. Schmitz KH, Holtzman J, Courneya KS, Mâsse LC, Duval S, Kane R. Controlled physical activity trials in cancer survivors: a systematic review and meta-analysis. *Cancer Epidemiol Biomarkers Prev.* 2005;14:1588-1595.

98. Mustian KM, Morrow GR, Carroll JK, Figueroa-Moseley CD, Jean-Pierre P, Williams GC. Integrative nonpharmacologic behavioral interventions for the management of cancer-related fatigue. *Oncologist.* 2007;12:52-67.

99. Markes M, Brockow T, Resch KL. Exercise for women receiving adjuvant therapy for breast cancer. *Cochrane Database Syst Rev.* 2006;(4):CD005001.

100. Kangas M, Bovbjerg DH, Montgomery GH. Cancer-related fatigue: a systematic and meta-analytic review of nonpharmacological therapies for cancer patients. *Psychol Bull.* 2008;134:700-741.

101. Jacobsen PB, Donovan KA, Vadaparampil ST, Small BJ. Systematic review and meta-analysis of psychological and activity-based interventions for cancer-related fatigue. *Health Psychol.* 2007;26:660-667.

102. van Weert E, Hoekstra-Weebers JE, May AM, Korstjens I, Ros WJ, van der Schans CP. The development of an evidence-based physical self-management rehabilitation programme for cancer survivors. *Patient Educ Couns.* 2008;71: 169-190.

103. Kwekkeboom KL, Cherwin CH, Lee JW, Wanta B. Mind-body treatments for the pain-fatigue-sleep disturbance symptom cluster in persons with cancer. *J Pain Symptom Manage.* 2010;39:126-138.

104. Vadiraja SH, Rao MR, Nagendra RH, et al. Effects of yoga on symptom management in breast cancer patients: a randomized controlled trial. *Int J Yoga.* 2009;2:73-79.

105. Balk J, Day R, Rosenzweig M, Beriwal S. Pilot, randomized, modified, double-blind, placebo-controlled trial of acupuncture for cancer-related fatigue. *J Soc Integr Oncol.* 2009; 7:4-11.

106. Molassiotis A, Sylt P, Diggins H. The management of cancer-related fatigue after chemotherapy with acupuncture and acupressure: a randomised controlled trial. *Complement Ther Med.* 2007;15:228-237.

107. Patrick DL, Ferketich SL, Frame PS, et al. National Institutes of Health State-of-the-Science Conference Statement: symptom management in Cancer: pain, depression, and fatigue, July 15-17, 2002. *J Natl Cancer Inst.* 2003;95:1110-1117.

CHAPTER 8

Fever and Sweats

James F. Cleary

TEMPERATURE AND ASSOCIATED SYMPTOMS

Temperature has long been used in clinical medicine and was included in the cardinal signs of inflammation described as "tumor, rubor, dolor, and fever." The measurement of temperature by a thermometer, in the sublingual, subaxillary, or rectal locations, is not a clinical skill practiced regularly by doctors. In most cases, temperature is recorded by other health workers or by patients themselves. Normal body temperature is considered to be 37°C, the average core temperature for an adult population.

Temperature is tightly controlled within a narrow range in each individual. Fever is defined as any elevation in the core body temperature above the normal and results from the upregulation of body temperature. More commonly, a temperature >38°C is considered a clinically significant fever. In oncologic practice and many clinical studies, a significant fever is defined as a single temperature reading >38.5°C or three readings (at least an hour apart) of >38°C. The term *fever* (or pyrexia) *of unknown origin*, FUO (PUO), is used commonly, and often incorrectly, in the daily practice of medicine. An FUO is defined as an illness lasting at least 3 weeks with a fever higher than 38°C on more than one occasion and which lacks a definitive diagnosis after 1 week of evaluation in a hospital (1).

Fever is often accompanied by other symptoms, including sweating and rigors. Sweating, when it accompanies fever, is a cooling response by the body wherein heat is released from the body as it evaporates water on the skin's surface. Rigors and shivering also contribute to temperature control and are rapid muscle spasms designed to increase heat production within the body. For adult humans and most large mammals, shivering is the major means of increased heat production in response to a cold environment. Nonshivering thermogenesis, a process involving heat production in brown adipose tissue, is important in the temperature control of infants.

CONTROL OF TEMPERATURE

It is proposed that core body temperature is controlled by neurologic mechanisms centered in the anterior hypothalamus. The onset of fever in patients results from an elevation of the body's regulated set-point temperature through a resetting of the temperature "gauge" in the hypothalamus (2). This may be caused by various drugs or by endogenous pyrogens. As a result of the reset hypothalamic temperature, the body increases the core body temperature to this new

level (Figure 8.1) through shivering or nonshivering thermogenesis. The continued presence of pyrogen at the hypothalamus results in the maintenance of this higher temperature. Eventually, either as a result of a decrease in the quantity of pyrogen or the administration of an antipyretic, the hypothalamic temperature is reset to a lower or normal level. The core body temperature is therefore lowered through sweating. This control mechanism may be suppressed in patients administered steroids or anti-inflammatory agents. Older patients may not be able to mount the anticipated febrile response.

The endogenous pyrogens that are responsible for the onset of fever are largely derived from monocytes and macrophages. These cells, as a result of challenge by either endotoxin or infective sources, release tumor necrosis factor (TNF) and interleukin (IL)-1β. Their production is part of the complex cascade that results in the stimulation of other cytokines, such as IL-6, IL-8, and changes in prostaglandin metabolism. Serum levels of IL-6 and IL-8 have been found to correlate with core body temperature in patients with febrile neutropenia (3). The ultimate end point of this cascade is the activation of granulocytes, monocytes, and endothelial cells. Although fever appears to be associated with enhanced function of the immune system, it must nonetheless be noted that a direct connection between such phenomena and a beneficial effect of fever on outcome of infections has not been established. Fever, in fact, may be deleterious in the setting of autoimmune disorders or infections (4).

ETIOLOGY OF FEVER IN CANCER PATIENTS

Fever is commonly seen in patients with cancer, even in the absence of infection. The wide range of etiologies of fever in patients with cancer will be considered in relation to the pathophysiology of fever in these patients.

Tumor

Fever associated with tumor is believed to be associated with the release of pyrogens, either directly from a tumor or from tumor stimulation of immunologic mechanisms that cause an elevation in temperature through action on the anterior hypothalamus. The classic association of fever with particular tumor diagnoses relates more to tumors associated with a diagnosis of FUO (Table 8.1). In the combined results of six studies documenting the etiology of FUO, 23% of adults meeting the defined diagnosis were found to have

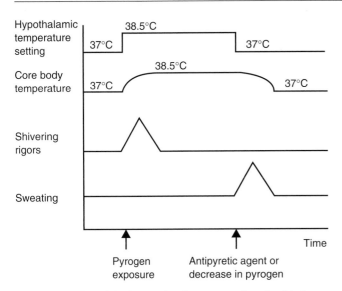

Figure 8.1. Physiologic mechanisms associated with fever and accompanying symptoms. (Adapted from Boulant JA. Thermoregulation. In: Mackowiak P, ed. *Fever: Basic Mechanisms and Management.* New York: Raven Press; 1991: 1–22, with permission.)

malignancy as the cause (8% of children) (5). In another study of 111 elderly (age >65 years) patients with FUO, 26 had associated malignancy, with 15 patients diagnosed with lymphoma and 4 with renal cell carcinoma (6). Almost 7,000 cancer patients with fever were reviewed by Klastersky et al. and only 47 (0.7%) fit the diagnostic criteria for an FUO (7). Twenty-seven of the 47 patients had leukemia or lymphoma, with disease rather than infection being the cause of the fever in only 11. Tumor was responsible for fever in seven patients with widespread metastatic carcinomas; in six of these, large liver metastases were present.

Hodgkin's disease has classically been associated with the Pel-Ebstein fever (Figure 8.2), where a patient experiences 3- to 10-day cycles of fever alternating with periods of normal temperature (8). Although the presence of fever is an important prognostic indicator in patients with Hodgkin's disease, there has been some discussion (9) about the value of Pel-Ebstein fever as a diagnostic tool particularly because the original description of the Pel-Ebstein fever was made in

two patients who were subsequently found, on pathologic review, not to have Hodgkin's disease.

Although classical teaching is that fever is associated with particular tumors, fever also occurs in patients with many of the more common cancers (Table 8.2). Forty-one percent of those who underwent autopsy had evidence of infection as an explanation of their fever (10). The incidence of infection among the autopsied patients was 50% for acute leukemia, 75% for lymphoma, and 80% for chronic lymphocytic leukemia. Infection was only found in a third of those with chronic myeloid leukemia, 17% of those with Hodgkin's disease, and 15% of those with lung cancer.

Infection (Including Neutropenia)

Although infection and fever can be a common presentation in patients with cancer, it is of particular concern in patients with neutropenia. Neutropenia, defined as a peripheral blood neutrophil count of <500/μL, results from either increased destruction or decreased production of white blood cells. Decreased production by the bone marrow may result either from disease involving the marrow or from myelosuppression due to chemotherapy. The cause of fever is not identified in approximately 60% to 70% of patients with neutropenia (11). Risk factors for the development of fever in the setting of neutropenia have been identified and include a rapid decrease in the neutrophil count and a protracted neutropenia of <500 cells/μL or >10 days (12). Twenty percent of patients with 1 week of chemotherapy-induced neutropenia develop a fever and the rate of infection increases with lengthening periods of neutropenia. Other factors that may alter the risk of the patient with neutropenia include phagocyte function, the status of the patient's immune system, and alterations in the physical defense barriers of the body (e.g., mucositis).

Fever and neutropenia in patients with cancer are associated with a high risk of medical complications, with a death rate ranging from 4% to 12%. Twenty-one percent of patients with febrile neutropenia at the Dana Farber Cancer Center developed serious medical complications (13). The investigators identified four risk groups for patients with febrile neutropenia. Group 1 consisted of inpatients at the time of onset of fever; group 2, outpatients who developed significant comorbidity within 24 hours of presentation;

TABLE 8.1	Tumors classically associated with fever
Hodgkin's disease	
Lymphoma	
Leukemia	
Renal cell carcinoma	
Myxoma	
Osteogenic sarcoma	

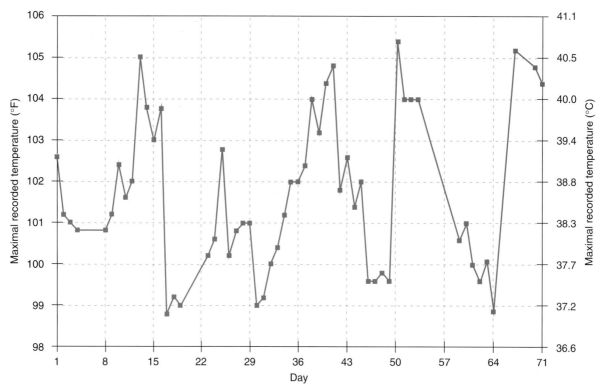

Figure 8.2. A 50-year-old man had fever, night sweats, and nonproductive cough for 10 weeks. He took antipyretic medications during the febrile periods. His wife recorded his temperatures, shown in the preceding text, on 56 of the 71 days. Biopsy of a rapidly enlarging cervical lymph node revealed nodular sclerosing Hodgkin's lymphoma. The patient's fevers and other symptoms promptly disappeared after the first cycle of doxorubicin, bleomycin, vinblastine, and dacarbazine. (From Good GR, Dinubile MJ. Images in clinical medicine. Cyclic fever in Hodgkin's disease (Pel-Ebstein fever). *N Engl J Med*. 1995;332:436, with permission.)

TABLE 8.2	Incidence of fever without evidence of infection at autopsy in patients of different primary tumor types

Primary Site	Number of Patients Observed	Number of Patients with Fever Without Associated Infection	
		Number	%
Stomach	1,498	573	41
Kidney	208	39	19
Colon and rectum	113	75	66
Liver and gallbladder	98	43	44
Uterus	81	19	36
Squamous skin cancer	41	20	49
Esophagus	20	7	35
Breast	48	16	33
Lung	17	8	47
Small bowel	17	1	6
Prostate	11	7	64
Bladder	10	6	60
Bone	10	7	70

From Boggs DR, Frei E. Clinical studies of fever and infection in cancer. *Cancer*. 1960;13:1240–1253, with permission.

TABLE 8.3	Incidence of multiple medical complications and mortality in patients with febrile neutropenia as defined by risk		
Patient Group	**Number of Patients**	**Multiple Complications (%)**	**Deaths (%)**
Group 1	268	51 (19)	25 (9)
Group 2	43	3 (7)	5 (12)
Group 3	29	3 (10)	4 (14)
Group 4	104	0 (0)	0 (0)
All patients	444	57 (13)	34 (8)

Risk groups are defined in text.

From Talcott JA, Siegel RD, Finberg R, et al. Risk assessment in cancer patients with fever and neutropenia: a prospective, two center validation of a prediction rule. *J Clin Oncol.* 1992;10;316–322, with permission.

group 3, outpatients with uncontrolled cancer but without serious concurrent comorbidity; and group 4, outpatients without serious concurrent comorbidity and whose cancer was well controlled. The model was validated in 444 patients with febrile neutropenia, of whom 36% had a significant comorbidity, 27% had serious medical complications, and 8% died. Group 1 had the greatest risk and group 4 had little risk in relation to medical complications and risk (Table 8.3).

An important component of this study was the identification of those patients at low risk for medical complication 24 hours after the onset of fever. Some of these low-risk patients developed medical complications (5%), but these either were transient and asymptomatic or were heralded by at least 7 days of medical deterioration and therefore readily detectable by appropriate follow-up. Two additional risk factors—a latency period of <10 days from the time of chemotherapy administration to the onset of fever and neutropenia and age >40 years—correlated with the occurrence of more frequent complications. Mucositis was associated with decreased risk of medical complications, suggesting that infection associated with mucositis may be responsive to antibiotics. The identification of a causative organism or positive blood cultures was not associated with increased risk. Talcott et al. then conducted a randomized controlled trial with usual care in hospital versus the same antibiotics at home based on these risk factors, but the study was closed early because of accrual difficulties (14). Five outpatients were readmitted to the hospital, but the number of major medical complications was not significantly different in the two arms. No patient died in either of the study arms and patient-reported quality of life was similar on both arms. The authors concluded that it is safe for clinicians to treat rigorously characterized low-risk patients with febrile neutropenia in suitable outpatient settings with appropriate surveillance for an unexpected clinical deterioration.

In a multinational study, a risk index score was developed to "stage" those patients with febrile neutropenia (15). Predictive factors included blood pressure, presence of chronic obstructive pulmonary disease or solid tumor, previous fungal infection in patients with hematologic malignancies, outpatient status, status of hydration, and age in relation to 60 years (Table 8.4) On the validation set, a Multinational Association for Supportive Care in Cancer (MASCC) risk index score ≥21 identified low-risk patients with a positive predictive value of 91%, specificity of 68%, and sensitivity of 71%. The authors went on to test their rules with low-risk patients treated with oral antibiotics after an initial observation period (16). Seventy-nine of 178 patients treated orally were discharged early, with only 3 having to be readmitted, a success rate of 96%.

This tool was further used to assess those deemed to have "apparent clinical stability." However when used in this population, the tool had a low sensitivity in predicting those who may develop complications (17). However, the authors identified risk factors for the development of complications, which included a performance status >1, chronic bronchitis, chronic heart failure, stress hyperglycemia, a low monocyte count (<200 mm^3), and stomatitis (>grade 1). It was suggested that clinicians should be cautious in sending home patients with febrile neutropenia, especially those with the above clinical findings.

On the basis of a number of retrospective studies, similar definitions of low risk have been applied to pediatric patients with fever and neutropenia (18). Low risk included evidence of bone marrow recovery in culture-negative patients who were afebrile for at least 24 hours and who had no other reason to continue intravenous antibiotics in the hospital. The control of any localized infection and the patient's ability to return promptly in the event of fever or other complications were also necessary. In a prospective study of 70 patients who met these criteria and who were discharged home with neutropenia, none were readmitted with fever. Seven patients who were inadvertently discharged without evidence of marrow recovery were readmitted with recurrence of fever. Neutropenic children with positive cultures were also assessed to identify risk factors for bacteremia (19). Of the

TABLE 8.4 Multinational Association for Supportive Care in Cancer scoring index	
Characteristic	**Score**
Burden of illness: no or mild symptoms	5
Burden of illness: moderate symptoms	3
Burden of illness: severe symptoms	0
No hypotension (systolic BP > 90 mmHg)	5
No chronic obstructive pulmonary disease	4
Solid tumor/lymphoma with no previous fungal infection	4
No dehydration	3
Outpatient status (at onset of fever)	3
Age < 60 years	2

Scores ≥21 are at low risk of complications.

Points attributed to the variable "burden of illness" are not cumulative. The maximum theoretical score is therefore 26.

cases of bacteremia, 92.5% occurred in those where cancer was not controlled, were <1 year of age, <10 days past their last chemotherapy, and had no evidence of marrow recovery.

Two studies reported that hypotension and bacteremia in the setting of neutropenia are significant risk factors for prolonged hospitalization (>7 days) and high mortality. Malik et al. (20) reported, from Pakistan, a mortality rate of 82% associated with febrile neutropenia in patients presenting with shock and a study from France reported that patients admitted to an ICU with febrile neutropenia experienced a 54% 30-day mortality, with a higher mortality in those with respiratory and renal failure (21). While a number of clinical characteristics may provide prognostic information regarding the outcomes of hospitalized patients with febrile neutropenia, predictive models are needed to better identify high-risk patients who may benefit from the addition of adjunctive colony-stimulating factors (CSFs).

Organisms (Bacteriology)

A basic understanding of the classification and sensitivities of the different organisms is essential to understand the infection in patients with cancer. Over time there have been changes in the underlying organisms associated with febrile neutropenia as evidenced by progressive studies by the European Organization for Research and Treatment of Cancer (EORTC) (22). Gram-negative organisms were the leading cause of infection in patients with febrile neutropenia, but their incidence decreased from 71% of identified causative organisms during the 1973 to 1978 period to 31% during the 1989 to 1991 period. Infection by one of these gram-negative organisms—*Pseudomonas aeruginosa*—became a driving force in the selection of antibiotics. However, the incidence of pseudomonas infection also decreased as reflected by an incidence of only 0.1% of febrile neutropenic cases at the National Cancer Institute (23).

The incidence of both acute and chronic fungal infections increased, with up to 33% of patients with febrile neutropenia not responding to a week of antibiotic therapy having a systemic fungal (*Candida* or *Aspergillosis*) infection (24).

The incidence of gram-positive organisms increased from 29% during the 1973 to 1978 period to 69% during the 1989 to 1991 period, requiring a review in treatment regimens used in patients with febrile neutropenia. Some of these gram-positive organisms, such as coagulase-negative staphylococci or *Corynebacterium jeikeium*, represent indolent infections that were methicillin resistant and only susceptible to vancomycin, quinupristin–dalfopristin, and linezolid. Other gram-positive bacteria such as *Staphylococcus aureus*, viridans streptococci, and pneumococci may cause fulminant infections with serious complications and possibly death if not treated promptly. Gram-negative bacilli, especially *P. aeruginosa*, *Escherichia coli*, and *Klebsiella* species, remain prominent causes of infection and must be treated with selected antibiotics as recommended by the Guidelines of the Infectious Disease Society of America (IDSA) (25). This was supported by a single cancer center review of the cause of bacterial infections in low-risk, febrile neutropenic patients (26). Among microbiologically documented infections, monomicrobial, gram-positive infections accounted for 49% (with coagulase-negative staphylococci the most frequent); monomicrobial, gram-negative infections accounted for 36% (with *E. coli* the most frequent); and 15% of infections were polymicrobial.

Location

Infections can occur throughout the body and need to be sought carefully through history and examination. Collapse, consolidation, and superimposed infection may develop behind an obstructing bronchial tumor. Aspiration pneumonia may occur in those with esophageal tumor either secondary to an obstruction or as a result of a tracheoesophageal fistula.

The gastrointestinal system is the most common site of indigent organisms that cause infection in patients with neutropenia. *Clostridium difficile* infection may present with fever and diarrhea and must be considered in those who are already taking antibiotics. Fungal and viral infections of the esophagus need to be suspected in those with dysphagia and odynophagia. Anaerobic infections may be a factor in severe mucositis or gingivitis and in those patients with perianal discomfort. Spontaneous bacterial peritonitis may be a cause of fever in patients with ascites. A urinary catheter increases the risk of urinary tract infection as does the presence of urinary obstruction, but the presence of asymptomatic bacteriuria in a catheterized patient without neutropenia is not usually an indication for antibiotic treatment.

Central nervous system infections can be difficult to diagnose and usually require lumbar puncture to confirm. Infection is the most common complication of Ommaya reservoirs, used to administer intraventricular chemotherapy, and is more likely to occur in those with previous radiotherapy or in whom repeated surgical procedures have been necessary (27). Most infections are due to *Staphylococcus epidermidis* and can usually be successfully treated with antibiotics (28).

Particular attention to sites of recent surgery is essential in assessing infection. Surgical collections may include infected hematomas that develop following surgery. The skin is also a common site of infection that may range from infected decubitus ulcers to herpes zoster infections. The use of percutaneous catheters in oncology has created another portal for the introduction of infection in patients with cancer. Of a total of 322 indwelling devices placed in 274 patients with cancer by a single surgeon, device-related sepsis occurred in 28 of 209 patients (13%) with catheters and 6 of 113 patients (5%) with subcutaneous ports (29). Triple lumen catheters were associated with a higher rate of thrombosis but not of infection. The complications of 1,630 venous access devices for long-term use in 1,431 consecutive patients with cancer were reviewed (30). Of the catheters inserted, 341 of 788 (43%) had caused at least one device-related infection compared with 57 of 680 (8%) of the completely implanted ports ($P = 0.001$). The number of infections per 1,000 device days was 2.77 for catheters compared with 0.21 for ports ($P = 0.001$). The predominant organisms isolated in catheter-related bacteremia were gram-negative bacilli (55%) compared with gram-positive cocci (65.5%) in port-related bacteremia. Patients with solid tumors were less likely to have device-related infectious morbidity compared with patients with hematologic cancers. Updates on reducing the risk of infections from intravascular devices have been provided by the Center of Disease Control (CDC) (31).

Transfusion-Related

Blood products, administered extensively to patients with cancer, may be associated with febrile reactions. The incidence of side effects following the administration of over 100,000 units of red blood cells to more than 25,000 patients with cancer over a 4-year period was retrospectively reviewed (32). Of all transfused units, 0.3% had caused a transfusion-associated reaction; 51.3% were febrile nonhemolytic, and 36.7% were allergic urticarial reactions. The incidence of transfusion-related side effects was significantly lower in this study than that reported in the noncancer population. Infection may also be a source of fever in patients receiving blood products. The Canadian Red Cross (33) estimated that the true positive rate of bacterial contamination of platelet concentrate units was between 4.4 and 10.7/10,000 units and recommended screening of all such units. The percentage of those patients developing bacteremia or septicemia from infected units was not discussed. A later report from Canada showed that febrile nonhemolytic transfusion reactions were more likely after platelet than red blood cell transfusions and that prestorage leukoreduction resulted in a significant reduction in their occurrence (34).

Thrombosis

Trousseau's self-diagnosis of gastric cancer on the basis of venous thrombosis is a reminder that patients with cancer are at a particular risk for thrombosis. Deep vein thrombosis may present with fever and, given the uncertainty of clinical diagnosis, investigation may be necessary in the "at-risk" patient. Pelvic thrombophlebitis may sometimes occur after pelvic surgery and, if septic, may manifest with either low-grade or high-grade fever. Pulmonary embolus also needs to be considered in the differential diagnosis of fever in patients with cancer. Of 97 patients with confirmed pulmonary embolus in the Urokinase Pulmonary Embolism Trial, 17 had associated malignancy (35). Of those with confirmed malignancy, 54% had a fever >37.5°C and 19.6% had a fever >38°C. Forty-one percent of the patients with cancer had associated sweating. Fever was a positive indicator of the diagnosis of thrombosis in patients with gynecologic malignancy (36). Pulmonary infarction, with the primary signs of tachypnea, tachycardia, and fever, may be a presentation of pulmonary thrombi. Other thrombotic syndromes, such as cerebral venous thrombosis, although associated with fever, are not common in the setting of malignancy.

Hemorrhage

Gastrointestinal bleeding may present with fever and should be considered in the differential diagnosis of a patient with low-grade fever and sweats. However, in a major review of fever in patients with cancer (10), serious hemorrhage was followed by fever in a minority of cases; the usual sequence has been that of hemorrhage in an already febrile patient.

Drugs

Drug-associated fever is an ill-defined syndrome in which fever is the predominant manifestation of an adverse drug reaction. It is normally a diagnosis of exclusion (37). The drugs commonly associated with fever are antibiotics,

TABLE 8.5	Cytotoxic agents associated with fever after administration
Bleomycin	Mustine
Cisplatin	Mithramycin
Cytarabine	Streptozocin
Cyclophosphamide	Thiotepa
Etoposide	Vinblastine
5-Fluorouracil	Vincristine
Methotrexate	

cardiovascular drugs, central nervous system drugs (e.g., phenytoin), cytotoxics, and immune therapy drugs (either as biologic response modifiers or as growth factors). Antimicrobial agents were responsible for 46 of 148 drug-related fevers in a review (38) of the experience of two hospitals in Texas and the United Kingdom with a mean lag time from initiation of treatment to onset of fever of 21 days (median, 8 days). For 11 cases of cytotoxic-induced fever, the mean lag time was 6 days with a median of 0.5 days. Shaking chills were more common with the administration of cytotoxic-associated drugs than with other drugs.

Cytotoxics

There is a diverse range of cytotoxic drugs whose administration is associated with fever (Table 8.5). The febrile response to bleomycin was described in the original phase I studies (39) and characteristically occurs 3 to 5 hours after injection. It is more common after intravenous than after intramuscular injection and is seen in approximately 25% of patients who were administered the drug. The fever becomes less frequent with repeated injections. An anaphylactic reaction manifested by hyperpyrexia, shock, hypotension, urticaria, and wheezing occurs in 1% of patients administered bleomycin (40). Fever following the administration of cisplatin was also reported in early clinical trials (41). Streptozocin administration may result in fever associated with chills, as can cytarabine and etoposide. Fever can occur after the administration of 5-fluorouracil and high-dose methotrexate. Confusion concerning the etiology of a fever arises more commonly in the situation of intensive chemotherapeutic regimens where patients with neutropenia may be administered cytotoxic agents that cause fever. Awareness of the symptoms produced by the different agents assists in discerning the etiology of the fever.

Antibiotics

Antibiotics commonly associated with fever are penicillins, cephalosporins, and amphotericin. Out of 50 patients who were administered at least 100 mg of amphotericin-B over a minimum of 3 days, fever was experienced by 34% and chills

by 56%, with rates of 2.6 and 3.5 mean episodes per patient per treatment course, respectively (42). In patients who had received 20 mg or more of amphotericin-B per day for at least 10 consecutive days, shivering occurred first at the test dose, with the percentage of patients who shivered increasing with each successive dose and peaking at the fifth therapeutic dose (43). Use of liposomal amphotericin is associated with a lower incidence of fever than amphotericin alone (44).

Opioids

Intravenous injection of morphine is often associated with sweating and vasodilatation, but not necessarily with fever. Fever may occur as a result of the interaction between meperidine (pethidine) and monoamine oxidase inhibitor, which is to be avoided. Drug withdrawal is associated with a syndrome that may include fever and needs to be suspected in febrile patients with cancer in whom opioids have been suddenly stopped. Withdrawal from benzodiazepines, often coadministered with opioids, may also be associated with fever.

Biologic Therapy

Interferons (IFNs) are associated with the development of fever (45). Partially purified IFN administered at low doses, intramuscularly, induces a fever (38°C to 40°C) within 6 hours that persists for approximately 4 to 8 hours. More severe side effects are seen with intravenous and intrathecal administration or in patients older than 65. The use of highly purified recombinant DNA IFN induces similar side effects. IFN at doses of 50 to 120 MU results in a sharp febrile response with severe rigors, peripheral cyanosis, vasoconstriction, nausea and vomiting, severe muscle aches, and headaches. In those patients receiving IFN daily, the febrile response and accompanying symptoms usually decrease in intensity and disappear within 7 to 10 days. Fever, however, persists, with intermittent (nondaily) injections resulting in peaks at 6 to 12 hours, and tends to last longer than the normal 4 to 8 hours. The administration of other biologic factors is associated with the onset of fever (e.g., TNF). Growth factor administration is also associated with the onset of fever, although the incidence following granulocyte colony-stimulating factor (G-CSF) is very low. Fever occurs much more commonly following granulocyte–macrophage colony-stimulating factor (GM-CSF) administration than following G-CSF administration.

Graft-versus-Host Disease

Chronic graft-versus-host disease is very much like a systemic collagen vascular disease and may be associated with infection, with or without the presence of fever. Acute graft-versus-host disease that is associated with fever and infection is also commonly seen.

Radiation-Induced Fever

Patients receiving radiotherapy alone may present with fever a few hours after the initial treatment. Acute radiation pneumonitis may develop 2 to 3 months after completion of radiation therapy. A high spiking fever may be part of the syndrome that consists of a dyspnea and an unproductive cough. Lung biopsy may be necessary to establish the diagnosis. Amifostine, a radiosensitizing agent has been reported to be associated with fever (46).

Other Diseases

Other diseases that may cause fever may coexist in patients with cancer (e.g., systemic lupus erythematosus and rheumatoid arthritis). Careful review of the patient's past medical history and current symptoms is essential.

DIAGNOSIS

The classical teaching that history provides 95% of the diagnosis is certainly true when it comes to the symptoms of fever in patients with cancer. Following the physical examination, the use of diagnostic aids is very much dependent on the relevant history. Although two-thirds of patients with febrile neutropenia do not have an identifiable cause of the fever, culture of relevant body fluids is still essential. However, routine surveillance cultures in patients with neutropenia, before the development of fever, are not cost productive (47). Although a chest x-ray (CXR) may not be an indicator in symptomatic patients presenting with febrile neutropenia (48), a recent CXR may be an important baseline in a patient without respiratory symptoms or signs but who is likely to have a prolonged period of neutropenia.

The diagnosis of fever due to the cancer itself can be confirmed with the use of naproxen (49). Proponents of "the naproxen test" state that it does not result in a decrease in temperature in patients with infection. Successful treatment of "neoplastic" fever was demonstrated in 21 patients with cancer, with 15 responding to a dose of 250 mg/d, whereas others responded following an increase in the dose of naproxen administered. The true sensitivity and specificity of this test are uncertain, but the authors stress that infectious fever and noninfectious fever due to drug toxicity, allergic reaction, and adrenal insufficiency need to be excluded before making the diagnosis of "neoplastic fever."

The use of fluorodeoxyglucose positron emission tomography (FDG-PET) and fluorodeoxyglucose positron emission tomography/computed tomography (FDG-PET/CT) in the assessment of FUO unidentified by conventional workup has been proposed. In a recent systematic review of nine studies, FDG-PET appears to be a sensitive and promising diagnostic tool for the detection of the causes of FUO (50). Positron emission tomography scanning may be considered among the diagnostic tools for patients with FUO in whom conventional diagnostics have been unsuccessful.

TREATMENT

Primary to any treatment of fever in patients with cancer is the treatment of the underlying cause of fever. Antibiotics should not be used to control fever in patients without neutropenia in the absence of evidence of infection, but nonsteroidal anti-inflammatory drugs may be useful in the treatment of fever associated with infection.

Physical cooling (e.g., through sponging) alone is likely to be *uncomfortable* for patients with fever and should be reserved for those in a hot and humid environment that may impede evaporative heat loss or for those with defective heat loss mechanisms (51). Sponging, when it is done, should be with tepid water because the use of cold water will induce shivering, which increases patient discomfort and causes an elevation in temperature (52). Aggressive cooling of critically ill patients through sponging resulted in early closure of a randomized study that studied its effect because of increased mortality in those receiving the aggressive cooling (53).

Agents that lower body temperature (antipyretics) primarily comprise three groups:

1. pure antipyretics that do not work in the absence of pyrogen and do not affect normal temperature at usual therapeutic doses (e.g., acetaminophen);
2. agents that cause hypothermia in afebrile subjects by directly impairing thermoregulatory function; and
3. those that are antipyretic at lower doses and cause hypothermia at higher doses (e.g., chlorpromazine).

Only salicylates, acetaminophen, and ibuprofen have been approved for antipyretic use in the United States, and none of these agents is likely to cause hypothermia in normothermic patients. Aspirin is not recommended for use in children because of the risk of Reye's syndrome, a disease process that results in liver failure (54). Aspirin has been the standard of reference in nearly two-thirds of clinical comparisons of antipyretic activity, but only one comparison of aspirin has been performed in patients with cancer (55). Every patient with low-grade fever received doses of aspirin and placebo in random order. No useful conclusions could be drawn, as the mean reduction in temperature for the patients on 600 mg of aspirin was only 0.3°C, a difference that was not statistically significant from that for the patients on placebo.

In children, acetaminophen has a dose–response effect, with doses of 5, 10, and 20 mg/kg bringing about a reduction in temperature of 0.3, 1.6, and 2.5°C, respectively, after 3 hours (51). Aspirin and acetaminophen appear equally effective at approximately 10 mg/kg. Ibuprofen, 0.5 mg/kg, is about as effective as 10 mg/kg of aspirin and 12.5 mg/kg of acetaminophen and probably lasts longer. Indomethacin has been reported to be more effective than these three compounds in limiting febrile responses to IFN (56), but it is not approved for antipyretic use in the United States. Indomethacin (75 mg), naproxen (500 mg), and diclofenac sodium (75 mg) have been found to be equally effective in the management of paraneoplastic fever (57). Steroids may be useful in treating fever, acting in the same manner as non-steroidal anti-inflammatory drugs. Steroids may be particularly effective in patients who are imminently dying.

Treatment of Infection

The treatment of fever in a non-neutropenic patient with cancer is not, in itself, a "medical emergency." Shock associated with such a patient may well make this an emergency. A thorough review of the history and examination and the performance of appropriate tests should guide both the timing and the type of treatment initiated.

The presence of fever in a patient who is immunocompromised is a medical emergency and empirical therapy should be initiated as soon as possible. Patients at risk for neutropenia should be instructed to record their temperature and to report the presence of fever to healthcare staff. Antibiotic recommendations by The Infectious Diseases Society of America (IDSA) Consensus Statement on Febrile Neutropenia, updated in 2010 (25), should be considered together with more recent studies on the choice of antibiotics in febrile neutropenia. The decision as to which antibiotic regimen to be used rests with individual clinicians and institutions and should take into consideration local experience and infection trends together with the risk assessment of the patient.

For low-risk patients (defined above), the outpatient administration of oral empirical, broad-spectrum antibiotics is now permissible. This has been tested methodically with a series of studies, the first being a randomized, double-blind, placebo-controlled study of oral ciprofloxacin plus amoxicillin–clavulanate versus intravenous ceftazidime in hospitalized neutropenic patients (58). Out of 116 episodes in each group, treatment was successful in 71% of episodes in the oral therapy group and 67% of episodes in the intravenous therapy group. The place of outpatient treatment of low-risk patients with neutropenia was examined at the M.D. Anderson Cancer Center (59). Oral ciprofloxacin combined with clindamycin was as effective in the control of infection as was the combination of intravenous aztreonam and clindamycin. However, the oral regime was associated with increased renal toxicity that resulted in the study's early termination. The authors recommended the development of better outpatient antibiotic regimens and

urged caution as none of their patients had gram-negative bacteremias or pneumonias, a group that may be more difficult to treat.

Outpatient treatment was further studied in Pakistan, where 188 low-risk patients with febrile neutropenia were randomized to receive either inpatient or outpatient oral ofloxacin (60). The same investigators had previously found oral ofloxacin to be as effective for inpatient care as their standard intravenous regimen (61). The patient group consisted of patients with both solid tumors and leukemias and *excluded those in whom the duration of neutropenia was likely to exceed 7 days.* Fever control was the same in both the groups, with 78% of inpatient and 77% of outpatient fevers resolving without modification of the initial treatment. However, 21% of the outpatients required hospitalization. Mortality was 2% in those assigned inpatient treatment and 4% in outpatients, with 1 death occurring outside of the hospital.

Having established a risk identification system for patients with febrile neutropenia (13), Talcott et al. (14) sought to test the hypothesis that clinicians can elect to "treat rigorously characterized low-risk patients with febrile neutropenia in suitable outpatient settings with appropriate surveillance for unexpected clinical deterioration." In 121 febrile neutropenic episodes in 117 patients, patients were randomized to inpatient medical therapy or outpatient care with the same intravenous antibiotics. There was no difference in the major complications between the two groups. Although the study was closed early due to poor accrual, the authors concluded that home-based care was a reasonable approach for the treatment of febrile neutropenia with low-risk characteristics. A further analysis showed significant cost savings with the in-home care ($3,000) without significantly increased indirect costs or caregiver burden (62).

Based on these combined data, the IDSA guidelines (25) conclude that low-risk patients should receive initial oral or intravenous empirical antibiotic doses in a clinical or hospital setting and may be transitioned to outpatient oral or intravenous treatment if they meet specific clinical criteria. Oral agents can be given to those with a good support system at home, with the ability to take oral medications and with an expected short duration of neutropenia. Ciprofloxacin plus amoxicillin–clavulanate in combination is recommended for oral empirical treatment, while other oral regimens, including levofloxacin or ciprofloxacin monotherapy or ciprofloxacin plus clindamycin, have been less well studied but can be used. Low-risk patients, who have started therapy in hospital, may be switched to outpatient antibiotic regimens, but they should be admitted to hospital if fever recurs in 48 hours of discharge.

High-risk patients require hospitalization for intravenous empirical antibiotic therapy; while previous recommendations did not recommend monotherapy, the 2010 guidelines (25) recommended this using either an anti-pseudomonal β-lactam agent, such as cefepime, a carbapenem (meropenem or imipenem–cilastatin), or piperacillin–tazobactam. A meta-analysis has been performed on 13 studies that compared ceftazidime monotherapy with different combination therapies (63). No difference was found in treatment failure, and there was no difference in outcome when febrile and bacteremic episodes were considered independently. Therapy was modified in similar percentages for both monotherapy and combination therapy. In a later multicenter, randomized controlled trial involving the treatment of 876 febrile, neutropenic episodes in 696 patients (64), single-agent ceftazidime was found to be safer than piperacillin and tobramycin combined, with similar effectiveness (62.7% versus 61.1%; $P > 0.2$). Infectious mortality was 6% for ceftazidime and 8% for the combination therapy while 38 episodes of super infection developed in each group. An adverse event occurred in 8% of the episodes treated with ceftazidime compared with 20% of the episodes treated with combination therapy ($P < 0.001$). It is to be noted that 83% of the patients enrolled in the study had leukemia or had undergone transplantation and therefore were often experiencing profound and prolonged neutropenia.

Other antimicrobials (aminoglycosides, fluoroquinolones, and/or vancomycin) may be added to the initial regimen for management of complications (e.g., hypotension and pneumonia) or if antimicrobial resistance is suspected or proven. Without suggestion of these complications or specific clinical indications (e.g., catheter-related infection), the use of vancomycin is not recommended for febrile neutropenia. Modifications to this therapy should be considered for those at risk for antibiotic-resistant organism, with positive blood cultures or clinical instability.

It is essential to continually review a patient's clinical situation and therapy. The consensus panel agreed that from days 2 to 4, a patient with neutropenia who was either afebrile or had continuing fever but with no progression of the infective process could continue on the same antibiotics. Antibiotics should be changed if fever persisted and there was progression of the infective process. Either vancomycin could be added at that stage (if not already in use) or monotherapy in the form of a third-generation cephalosporin could be commenced. If the patient remained both neutropenic and febrile after 4 to 7 days and was unlikely to have white cell recovery in the near future, antifungal therapy should be added (65). Antianaerobic therapy should be considered in patients with persistent fever and severe oral mucositis, necrotizing gingivitis, or perianal tenderness.

The current duration of antibiotic treatment, where patients with febrile neutropenia have been admitted to hospital for antibiotic treatment until their neutropenia resolved, is based on the results of a 1979 study (66). Early stopping of antibiotics at day 7 in 17 patients with resolved fever but persistent neutropenia resulted in the recurrence of fever in 7 patients, of whom 2 died. They considered that therapy could be stopped after 7 days in patients without fever and who were clinically well but with a neutrophil count of <500/μL, provided that the patient was carefully observed, mucous membranes and skin were intact, and no invasive procedure or ablative chemotherapy was imminent, although this was not strongly supported by scientific data.

Other studies have suggested that in patients at lower risk for complications, outpatient treatment and early stopping of antibiotics may be possible. Attempts have been made to shorten hospital stays by discontinuing intravenous antibiotics in blood culture–negative patients who remained clinically stable and afebrile after 48 hours of treatment (67). Thirty patients with febrile neutropenia, identified to have a low complication risk after 48 hours of inpatient intravenous treatment, were continued on the same antibiotics at home until neutropenia resolved (68). Four patients were readmitted with medical complications (hypotension, 3; acute renal failure, 1) and 5 others were readmitted for observation. Overall costs were similar for those treated at home and for those who were medically eligible for home treatment but were treated in the hospital. The higher-than-expected cost of home treatment related to extended periods of neutropenia in these patients. The authors included a retrospective review of 134 admissions for neutropenic fever, where the median duration of intravenous antibiotics decreased significantly from 7 days before institution of such a policy to 5 days (4 to 6) and 4 days (3 to 5) over the next two consecutive 6-month periods with implementation. The median duration of hospital stay decreased from 10 days to 7 days (5 to 8) and 6 days (5 to 7) over the same periods. The authors concluded that intravenous antibiotics might be discontinued in patients who remained afebrile and clinically stable for 48 hours and who had negative blood cultures, resulting in a shorter duration of hospital stays, with the potential for reduction in hospital costs.

Early stopping of antibiotics together with a selective decontamination regimen (neomycin, polymyxin, amphotericin, and pipemidic acid) was prospectively studied in 52 adult patients with hematologic malignancies and a neutrophil count <500/μL (69). Patients experienced 77 febrile episodes while receiving the oral antibiotics and further treatment (either broad-spectrum or disease-specific antibodies) was initiated only if clinical signs or microbiologic culture results indicated an infection. Consequently, antibiotics were adjusted according to culture findings or discontinued if evidence of infection was lacking after 72 to 96 hours. For the 40 episodes without confirmed infection, the median duration of therapy was 3 days (range, 0 to 13 days) and the survival rate 100%, with 15 receiving no additional antibiotics. For the 37 episodes with confirmed infection, the median duration of therapy was 12 days (range, 1 to 49 days, $P < 0.0001$) and the survival rate 85%. Broad-spectrum therapy was only used for the duration of neutropenia in 18% of the treated episodes, and none of the six deaths could be attributed to the withholding or stopping of broad-spectrum therapy. It was concluded that in patients with febrile neutropenia on this selective decontamination regimen, the standard prolonged administration of broad-spectrum antibiotics was not necessary. The authors recommended that systemic antibiotics be discontinued after 3 to 5 days if infection is unlikely, that a narrower antibiotic spectrum be chosen according to the clinical situation, and that empirical antifungal treatment be considered after 7 days for this population. Although very promising, the findings of this study have not been confirmed in randomized clinical trials and have not been supported by the IDSA guidelines (25).

In summary, for patients with fever who continue to have neutropenia for a week or more, broad-spectrum antibiotic therapy for the duration of the neutropenia along with empirical antifungal therapy in those who remain febrile is the current consensus. The use of narrow-spectrum agents or abbreviated courses of antibiotics continues to evolve.

Vascular access devices often create a treatment dilemma in patients with febrile neutropenia. These may be left in place in most patients, even if bacteremia is detected, and managed with antibiotic and local care (70). Catheters should be removed if they are nonpatent, associated with thrombosis, have evidence of septic emboli, or if there is a subcutaneous tunnel infection. Prompt removal of catheters is also indicated with fungemia due to *Candida* spp. and bacteremia due to *Bacillus* spp. or a bacteremia that persists for >48 hours after initiation of appropriate antibiotics.

Antiviral medications may be required in patients with neutropenia as well as in those who are immunocompromised and without neutropenia. However, the empirical use of antiviral drugs in the management of febrile neutropenia in patients without mucosal lesions or evidence of viral disease is not indicated. The recommended dose of acyclovir for the treatment of established herpes infections in the immunocompromised patients ranges from 5 mg/kg q8h i.v. for herpes simplex to 10 to 12 mg/kg q8h i.v. for herpes zoster.

Although popular throughout the 1970s and 1980s, the use of granulocyte infusions has faded, despite evidence of efficacy. In a review (71) of the use of granulocyte transfusions, this decline was related to the administration of ineffective doses of granulocytes. The authors recommended that the physicians assess the outcome of persistent febrile neutropenia in their own institutions and, if poor, the addition of granulocyte transfusions, at therapeutic doses (2 to 3 $\times 10^{10}$ PMN), may be useful along with other changes such as the use of different antibiotics. When 2 of the 10 trials that met the criteria for analysis were excluded because of low granulocyte doses, patients who received granulocyte infusions were less likely to die of infection, but the overall survival was similar. Most of these studies were performed some years ago with the recipients experiencing significant side effects. A randomized study of the safety and effectiveness of granulocytes in resolving infection in people with neutropenia (http://clinicaltrials.gov/show/NCT00627393) opened in 2008 and is still actively enrolling patients.

Hematologic CSFs have been used to "harvest" granulocytes and can also be used to reduce treatment-associated myelosuppression by shortening the duration of neutropenia and by reducing the nadir of neutrophil counts. The role of CSF as "adjuvant" therapy has been the subject of multiple studies. Two meta-analyses of trials of adjunctive CSF therapy for cancer patients with febrile neutropenia have now been reported. These analyses included different patient numbers as a consequence of different search strategies and the inclusion by one analysis of data that were not published in English. Berghmans et al.'s analysis (72), which incorporated 962 patients, detected no advantage for the use of CSF in terms of mortality from febrile neutropenia, with a relative risk of 0.71 (95% CI 0.44 to 1.15). No other analysis of clinical benefit was reported. In a Cochrane systematic review (73) and meta-analysis, which included 1,518 patients from 13 trials, patients randomized to receive CSF experienced less prolonged neutropenia, less prolonged hospitalization, and marginally less infection–related mortality. There was no significant difference in overall mortality and bone and joint pain and arthralgias were more common in CSF-treated patients.

However, concern about their appropriate clinical use led to the continued updating of guidelines from the American Society of Clinical Oncology (ASCO) (74). The Committee did not recommend the general use of CSFs for the treatment of established fever and neutropenia as no evidence has been found to support the routine use of CSFs in patients with febrile neutropenia, although those at particularly high risk may have some benefit. High-risk features include expected prolonged (>10 days) and profound ($<0.1 \times 10^9$/L) neutropenia, age >65 years, uncontrolled primary disease, pneumonia, hypotension and multiorgan dysfunction (sepsis syndrome), invasive fungal infection, or being hospitalized at the time of the development of fever. The Infectious Disease Society of America guidelines have supported the use of CSFs in similar circumstances, referring to the ASCO guidelines (25).

Treatment of Transfusion Reactions

Transfusion reactions can be prevented by the filtration of blood products and also by premedication with an antihistamine. The use of erythropoietin-stimulating agents in anemia associated with malignancy may reduce the need for blood transfusions, thereby avoiding both transfusion reactions and a source of infection. Both the safety in patients with advanced cancer and the cost of such treatment need to be considered carefully (75).

Treatment of Amphotericin-Related Febrile Reaction

For the prevention of amphotericin-related fever and rigors, 12.5 to 25.0 mg of intravenous meperidine (pethidine) is useful. However, slowing the rate of amphotericin infusion may also reduce toxicity. Amphotericin administered over 45 minutes was much more toxic in relation to fever and rigors than the same dose administered over 4 hours (76). Less meperidine was required for the control of symptoms in the 4-hour infusion arm. In another study, no difference in amphotericin induced fever was found between a 45-minute and a 2-hour infusion (77). Liposomal amphotericin reduces the incidence of fever significantly (44).

PROPHYLAXIS

Prophylaxis, either in the form of antibiotics or other supportive treatment, may be useful in the prevention of febrile neutropenia.

Growth Factors

Hematologic CSFs reduce treatment-associated myelosuppression by shortening the duration of neutropenia and by reducing the nadir of neutrophil counts. However, concern about their appropriate clinical use led to the continued updating of guidelines from the American Society of Clinical Oncology (ASCO) (74). Two indications for the prophylactic use of G-CSF administration were addressed—primary CSF use in those receiving their initial chemotherapy and secondary use in those who have previously had chemotherapy-induced neutropenia.

To assess a benefit in primary prevention, the incidence of grade 4 neutropenia following the use of CSF in different randomized treatment protocols was considered. The incidence of neutropenia ranged from 0% in patients with breast cancer receiving the combination of cyclophosphamide, doxorubicin, and 5-fluorouracil to 98% of 102 patients with lung cancer who were administered cyclophosphamide, doxorubicin, and etoposide. G-CSF was found to decrease the incidence of febrile neutropenia significantly, whereas the placebo group had an incidence of neutropenia > 40%. However, in these randomized CSF trials, no difference in infectious mortality, response rates, or survival between CSF-treated and placebo-treated patients was documented. The National Comprehensive Cancer Network (78) has issued guidelines advocating the use of CSFs in patients with a greater than 20% risk of developing febrile neutropenia. This agrees with the ADSA Guideline Committee (25) which recommends that the prophylactic use of myeloid CSFs should be considered for patients in whom the anticipated risk of fever and neutropenia is >20%.

When less myelotoxic chemotherapy is planned, primary administration of CSFs should be reserved for those patients who are at high risk for neutropenic complications because of host-related or disease-related factors. Individual cases should also be considered in patients at higher risk for chemotherapy-induced, infectious complications (e.g., extensive prior chemotherapy). Elderly patients tolerate chemotherapy as well as younger patients do and should not receive CSFs purely on the basis of age.

If a patient has already experienced chemotherapy-induced neutropenia, then CSF can be used if there is proven benefit in maintaining the dose. It is important to remember that there was no difference in infectious mortality, tumor response, or survival for the primary use of CSF. In the absence of a reason to maintain the same dose of chemotherapy, dose reduction should be considered, especially if other toxicities not responsive to CSFs are present.

Therefore, there has been no evidence to recommend the use of CSFs to increase chemotherapy dose intensity outside of the clinical trials addressing this issue. CSFs may be useful for mobilizing peripheral blood stem cells, and they have a benefit in reducing the period of neutropenia in autologous and peripheral blood stem cell transplants. However, there was no indication for their use in patients receiving combined chemotherapy and radiotherapy. When used, the group recommended a G-CSF dose of 5 µg/kg/d (GM-CSF, 250 µg/m ^{2}/d), without dose escalation, administered 24 to 72 hours after chemotherapy until the neutrophil count is >10,000/µL after the neutrophil nadir. These recommendations are also supported by the European Society of Medical Oncology (ESMO). ESMO, however, reported that achieving a target absolute neutrophil count of >10,000/µL was not necessary as long as there was evidence of a sufficient/stable count (79).

The implications, including cost, of the use of G-CSF in the treatment of small cell lung cancer at the University of Indiana were reviewed (80). The overall incidence of neutropenia was 18% in the 137 patients treated with standard chemotherapy and in whom dose reductions were allowed in subsequent courses. The estimated total cost of this treatment was approximated to be $192,000. There would have been more than a sixfold increase in cost ($1,200,000) if primary treatment of all patients with G-CSF had taken place. The cost of the secondary use of G-CSF in those with a previous episode of fever and neutropenia ($272,000) would have been less than twice that of not using growth factors at all. The authors concluded that the routine use of G-CSF in patients with small cell lung cancer treated with standard-dose chemotherapy was expensive and not associated with obvious therapeutic benefits or cost savings. They suggested that careful analysis of the incidence of infectious complications, rather than granulocyte nadir and duration, be performed.

Pegfilgrastim, which is produced by the covalent binding of a 20-kDa polyethylene glycol moiety to the N-terminus of filgrastim, has been shown to have a sustained CSF effect (81). Pegylated agents have longer half-lives, superior physical and thermal stability, greater protection from enzymatic degradation, more stable plasma concentrations, and reduced immunogenicity (82). Pegfilgrastim has largely been used in the prevention of chemotherapy-induced neutropenia. A phase II dose-finding study compared single injections of pegfilgrastim (30, 60, or 100 µg/kg) and daily filgrastim (5 µg/kg) in patients with breast cancer treated with four cycles of doxorubicin and docetaxel. Treatment with both the drugs began 24 hours following the completion of chemotherapy (83). Results demonstrated that a single dose of pegfilgrastim was as effective in supporting neutrophil counts and as safe as daily filgrastim (84). Similarly, two randomized, double-blind, phase III trials in patients with breast cancer treated with myelosuppressive chemotherapy demonstrated that a single dose of pegfilgrastim provided comparable neutrophil support as an average of 11 daily injections of filgrastim (85). Currently, pegfilgrastim is administered once (6 mg), 24 hours following the completion of chemotherapy prior to the development of neutropenia.

Other Prophylactic Measures

Although total protected environments (involving laminar flow, the oral administration of nonabsorbable antibiotic, and cutaneous decontamination) reduce the incidence of infection, their use proved cumbersome and expensive and they have largely been abandoned for those patients for whom the duration of neutropenia is likely to be short (23). Individual components of these regimens, however, continue to be used in many treatment protocols, especially those with anticipated prolonged neutropenia.

Antibiotic Prophylaxis for Patients with Afebrile Neutropenia

The IDSA Guideline Panel (25) recommended that all patients at risk for *Pneumocystis carinii* pneumonitis, regardless of neutropenia, receive prophylaxis with trimethoprim–sulfamethoxazole (TMP–SMX). Because of the concern regarding antibiotic-resistant bacteria resulting from the overuse of antibiotics, there is no consensus to recommend TMP–SMX or quinolones for routine use for all patients with afebrile neutropenia.

The panel reported that the efficacy of prophylaxis with TMP–SMX and quinolones in reducing the number of infectious episodes during neutropenic periods is adequate and would warrant recommendation from the standpoint of efficacy alone. However, concern regarding the emergence of drug-resistant organisms due to extensive antibiotic use, plus the fact that prophylaxis with TMP–SMX or quinolones has not significantly reduced mortality rates, prevented the consensus panel from recommending the routine use of this prophylactic therapy (25). There is a strong evidence that fluoroquinolone prophylaxis decreases the incidence of febrile neutropenia and infection-related mortality in patients receiving chemotherapy for acute leukemia or high-dose chemotherapy, and National Comprehensive Cancer Network guidelines recommended that fluoroquinolone prophylaxis be considered in these patient groups (86). The incidence of these events is that febrile neutropenia reduced in patients receiving cyclical chemotherapy for solid tumors and there is evidence to support the use of this inexpensive and well-tolerated intervention in this group. However, current guidelines (25) advise against prophylaxis in view of concerns regarding antibiotic resistance, but there is no convincing evidence that antibiotic prophylaxis in this group results in a significant increase in colonization or infection with resistant microorganisms (87). Further research is required to demonstrate the clinical significance of antimicrobial resistance associated with antibiotic prophylaxis. This is especially important in the setting of cancer patients at low risk for neutropenic fever, for whom the uncertainties about using prophylaxis are greater and for whom there are least microbiologic surveillance data. There is a continuing need for prospective randomized trials for low-risk patient groups to evaluate the potential strategies for targeting antibiotic prophylaxis to achieve most benefit from least exposure.

Prophylaxis also extends to antiviral medications. Acyclovir use decreases the incidence of herpetic gingivostomatitis in patients with neutropenia, and the administration of acyclovir decreases the incidence of cytomegalovirus pneumonitis in patients who have undergone bone marrow transplant.

ETHICAL CONSIDERATIONS FOR TREATMENT OF INFECTIONS

There is no doubt that if the intention of treatment is to ensure the prolongation of survival, then treatment of the infective episode needs to be initiated. Dilemmas may arise in those patients in whom the intention of treatment is palliation. Antibiotics may make a patient feel more comfortable, but they may also prolong the dying process. A balance between the two should be assessed in each individual patient, including in particular factors such as prognosis and treatment goals.

Even if a patient is nearing death, indications for commencement of antibiotics may include convulsions or mental changes attributed to fever, extreme temperature (>40°C), extreme age (very young and very old), and a past history of adverse reaction to fever, marked subjective discomfort pronounced by patient, a prolonged high fever causing significant hypercatabolic state, and a reduced cardiac or pulmonary function to the extent that further tachycardia or tachypnea may be harmful. Further issues pertaining to this will be discussed in other chapters.

REFERENCES

1. Petersdorf RG, Beeson PB. Fever of unexplained origin: report of 100 cases. *Medicine*. 1961;40:1-29.
2. Boulant JA. Thermoregulation. In: Mackowiak P, ed. *Fever: Basic Mechanisms and Management*. New York: Raven Press; 1991:1-22.
3. Engel A, Kern WV, Murdter G, et al. Kinetics and correlation with body temperature of circulating interleukin-6, interleukin-8, tumor necrosis factor alpha and interleukin-1 beta in patients with fever and neutropenia. *Infection*. 1994;22:160-164.
4. Ashman RB, Mullbacher A. Host damaging immune responses in virus infections. *Surv Immunol Res*. 1984;3:11-15.
5. Greenberg SB, Taber L. Fever of unknown origin. In: Mackowiak P, ed. *Fever: Basic Mechanisms and Management*. New York: Raven Press; 1991:183-195.
6. Esposito AL, Gleckman RA. Fever of unknown origin in the elderly. *J Am Geriatr Soc*. 1978;26:498-505.
7. Klastersky J, Weerts D, Hensgens C, et al. Fever of unexplained origin in patients with cancer. *Eur J Cancer*. 1973;9:649-656.
8. Good GR, Dinubile MJ. Images in clinical medicine. Cyclic fever in Hodgkin's disease (Pel-Ebstein fever). *N Engl J Med*. 1995;332:436.
9. Asher R. *Richard Asher Talking Sense*. London: Pittman Medical; 1972:21-22.
10. Boggs DR, Frei E. Clinical studies of fever and infection in cancer. *Cancer*. 1960;13:1240-1253.
11. Pizzo PA. Evaluation of fever in the patient with cancer. *Eur J Cancer Clin Oncol*. 1989;25:S9-S16.
12. Bodey GP, Buckley M, Sathe YS, et al. Quantitative relationships between circulating leucocytes and infection in patients with acute leukemia. *Ann Intern Med*. 1966;64:328-340.
13. Talcott JA, Siegel RD, Finberg R, et al. Risk assessment in cancer patients with fever and neutropenia: a prospective, two center validation of a prediction rule. *J Clin Oncol*. 1992;10:316-322.
14. Talcott JA, Yeap BY, Clark JA, et al. Safety of early discharge for low-risk patients with febrile neutropenia: a

multicenter randomized controlled trial. *J Clin Oncol.* 2001;29(30):3977-3983.

15. Klastersky J, Paesmans M, Rubenstein EB, et al. The Multinational Association for Supportive Care in Cancer risk index: a multinational scoring system for identifying low-risk febrile neutropenic cancer patients. *J Clin Oncol.* 2000;18(16): 3038-3051.

16. Klastersky J, Paesmans M, Georgala A, et al. Outpatient oral antibiotics for febrile neutropenic cancer patients using a score predictive for complications. *J Clin Oncol.* 2006;24(25):4129-4134.

17. Carmona-Bayonas A, Gómez J, González-Billalabeitia E, et al. Prognostic evaluation of febrile neutropenia in apparently stable adult cancer patients. *Br J Cancer.* 2011;105(5):612-617.

18. Buchanan GR. Approach to treatment of the febrile cancer patient with low-risk neutropenia. *Hematol Oncol Clin North Am.* 1993;7:919-935.

19. Pappo AS, Buchanan GR. Predictors of bacteremia in febrile neutropenic children with cancer [abstract]. *Proc Am Soc Clin Oncol.* 1991;10:331.

20. Malik I, Hussain M, Yousuf H. Clinical characteristics and therapeutic outcome of patients with febrile neutropenia who present in shock: need for better strategies. *J Infect.* 2001;42: 120-125.

21. Darmon M, Azoulay E, Alberti C, et al. Impact of neutropenia duration on short-term mortality in neutropenic critically ill cancer patients. *Intensive Care Med.* 2002;28(12):1775-1780.

22. Klastersky J. Therapy of infections. In: Klastersky J, Schimpff SC, Senn HJ, eds. *Handbook of Supportive Care in Cancer.* New York: Marcel Decker; 1994:1-44.

23. Pizzo PA. Management of fever in patients with cancer and treatment-induced neutropenia. *N Engl J Med.* 1993;328:1323-1332.

24. Pizzo PA, Robichaud KJ, Witebsky FG. Empiric antibiotics and antifungal treatment for cancer patients with prolonged fever and neutropenia. *Am J Med.* 1982;72:101-111.

25. Freifeld AG, Bow EJ, Spekowsitz KA, et al. Clinical practice guideline for the use of antimicrobial agents in neutropenic patients with cancer: 2010 update by the Infectious Diseases Society of America. *Clin Infect. Dis.* 2011;52(4):e56-e93.

26. Kamana M, Escalante C, Mullen CA. Bacterial infections in low-risk, febrile neutropenic patients. *Cancer.* 2005;104(2):422-426.

27. Machado M, Salcman M, Kaplan RS, et al. Expanded role of the cerebrospinal fluid reservoir in neurooncology: indications, causes of revision, and complications. *Neurosurgery.* 1985;17:600-603.

28. Siegal T, Pfeffer MR, Steiner I. Antibiotic therapy for infected Ommaya reservoir systems. *Neurosurgery.* 1988;22:97-100.

29. Eastridge BJ, Lefor AT. Complications of indwelling venous access devices in cancer patients. *J Clin Oncol.* 1995;13:233-238.

30. Groeger JS, Lucas AB, Thaler HT, et al. Infectious morbidity associated with long-term use of venous access devices in patients with cancer. *Ann Intern Med.* 1993;119:1168-1174.

31. O'Grady NP, Alexander M, Burns LA, et al. *Guidelines for the Prevention of Intravascular Catheter-Related Infections.* Center for Disease Control; 2011.

32. Huh YO, Lichtiger B. Transfusion reactions in patients with cancer. *Am J Clin Pathol.* 1987;87:253-257.

33. Blajchman MA. Bacterial contamination of blood products and the value of pretransfusion testing. *Immunol Invest.* 1995;24:163-170.

34. Kleinman S, Chan P, Robillard P. Risks associated with transfusion of cellular blood components in Canada. *Transfus Med Rev.* 2003;17:120-162.

35. Manganelli D, Palla A, Donnamaria V, et al. Clinical features of pulmonary embolus. Doubts and certainties. *Chest.* 1995;107:S25-S32.

36. Santoso JT, Evans L, Lambrecht L, Wan J. Deep venous thrombosis in gynecological oncology: incidence and clinical symptoms study. *Eur J Obstet Gynecol Reprod Biol.* 2009;2:173-176.

37. Mackowiak PA. Drug fever. In: Mackowiak PA, ed. *Fever: Basic Mechanisms and Management.* New York: Raven Press; 1991:255-265.

38. Mackowiak PA, LeMaistre CF. Drug fever: a critical appraisal of conventional concepts. An analysis of 51 episodes diagnosed in two Dallas hospitals and 97 episodes reported in the English literature. *Ann Intern Med.* 1987;106:728-733.

39. Sonntag RW. Bleomycin (NSC-125066): phase I clinical study. *Cancer Chemo Rep.—Part 1* 1972;56:197-205.

40. Ma DD, Isbister JP. Cytotoxic-induced fulminant hyperpyrexia. *Cancer.* 1980;45:2249-2251.

41. Ashford RF, McLachlan A, Nelson I, et al. Pyrexia after cisplatin. *Lancet.* 1980;2:691-692.

42. Clements JS Jr, Peacock JE Jr. Amphotericin B revisited: reassessment of toxicity. *Am J Med.* 1990;88:22N-27N.

43. Carney-Gersten P, Giuffre M, Levy D. Factors related to amphotericin-B-induced rigors (shivering). *Oncol Nurs Forum.* 1991;18:745-750.

44. Walsh TJ, Finberg RW, Arndt C, et al. Liposomal amphotericin B for empirical therapy in patients with persistent fever and neutropenia. *N Engl J Med.* 1999;340:764-771.

45. Quesada JR, Talpaz M, Rios A, et al. Clinical toxicity of interferons in cancer patients: a review. *J Clin Oncol.* 1986;4:234-243.

46. Boehme S, Wilson DB. Amifostine-induced fever: case report and review of the literature. *Pharmacotherapy.* January 2004;24(1):155-158.

47. Kramer BS, Pizzo PA, Robichaud KJ, et al. Role of serial microbiologic surveillance and clinical evaluation in the management of cancer patients with fever and granulocytopenia. *Am J Med.* 1982;72:561-568.

48. Feusner J, Cohen R, O'Leary M, et al. Use of routine chest radiography in the evaluation of fever in neutropenic pediatric oncology patients. *J Clin Oncol.* 1988;6:1699-1702.

49. Chang JC, Gross HM. Neoplastic fever responds to the treatment of an adequate dose of naproxen. *J Clin Oncol.* 1985;3:552-558.

50. Dong MJ, Zhao K, Liu ZF, Wang GL, Yang SY, Zhou GJ. A meta-analysis of the value of fluorodeoxyglucose-PET/PET-CT in the evaluation of fever of unknown origin. *Eur J Radiol.* 2011;80(3):834-844.

51. Clark WG. Antipyretics. In: Mackowiak P, ed. *Fever: Basic Mechanics and Management.* New York: Raven Press; 1991:297-340.

52. Steele RW, Tanaka PT, Lara RP, et al. Evaluation of sponging and of oral antipyretic therapy to reduce fever. *J Pediatr.* 1970;77:824-829.

53. Schulman CI, Namias N, Doherty J, et al. The effect of antipyretic therapy upon outcomes in critically ill patients: a randomized, prospective study. *Surg Infect (Larchmt).* 2005;6(4):369-375.

54. Pinsky PF, Hurwitz ES, Schonberger LB, et al. Reye's syndrome and aspirin. Evidence for a dose response effect. *JAMA.* 1988;260:657-661.

55. Seed JC. A clinical comparison of the antipyretic potency of aspirin and sodium salicylate. *Clin Pharmacol Ther.* 1965;6:354-358.

56. Paolozzi F, Zamkoff K, Doyle M, et al. Phase I trial of recombinant interleukin-2 and recombinant beta-interferon in refractory neoplastic diseases. *J Biol Response Mod.* 1989;8:122-139.

57. Tsavaris N, Zinelis A, Karabelis A, et al. A randomized trial of the effect of three non-steroid anti-inflammatory agents in ameliorating cancer-induced fever. *J Intern Med.* 1990;228:451-455.

58. Freifeld A, Marchigiani D, Walsh T, et al. A double-blind comparison of empirical oral and intravenous antibiotic therapy for low-risk febrile patients with neutropenia during cancer chemotherapy. *N Engl J Med.* 1999;341(5):305-311.

59. Rubenstein EB, Rolston K, Benjamin RS, et al. Outpatient treatment of febrile episodes in low-risk neutropenic patients with cancer. *Cancer.* 1993;71:3640-3646.

60. Malik IA, Khan WA, Karim M, et al. Feasibility of outpatient management of fever in cancer patients with low-risk neutropenia: results of a prospective randomized trial [see comments]. *Am J Med.* 1995;98:224-231.

61. Malik IA, Abbas Z, Karim M. Randomised comparison of oral ofloxacin alone with combination of parenteral antibiotics in neutropenic febrile patients. *Lancet.* 1992;339:1092-1096.

62. Hendricks AM, Loggers ET, Talcott JA. Costs of home versus inpatient treatment for fever and neutropenia: analysis of a multicenter randomized trial. *J Clin Oncol.* 2011;29(30):3984-3989.

63. Sanders JW, Powe NR, Moore RD. Ceftazidime monotherapy for empiric treatment of febrile neutropenic patients: a meta-analysis. *J Infect Dis.* 1991;164:907-916.

64. De Pauw BE, Deresinski SC, Feld R, et al. Ceftazidime compared with piperacillin and tobramycin for the empiric treatment of fever in neutropenic patients with cancer. A multicenter randomized trial. The Intercontinental Antimicrobial Study Group. *Ann Intern Med.* 1994;120:834-844.

65. EORTC International Antimicrobial Therapy Cooperative Group. Empiric antifungal therapy in febrile granulocytopenic patients. *Am J Med.* 1989;86:668-672.

66. Pizzo PA, Robichaud KJ, Gill FA, et al. Duration of empiric antibiotic therapy in granulocytopenic patients with cancer. *Am J Med.* 1979;67:194-200.

67. Tomiak AT, Yau JC, Huan SD, et al. Duration of intravenous antibiotics for patients with neutropenic fever. *Ann Oncol.* 1994;5:441-445.

68. Talcott JA, Whalen A, Clark J, et al. Home antibiotic therapy for low-risk cancer patients with fever and neutropenia: a pilot study of 30 patients based on a validated prediction rule. *J Clin Oncol.* 1994;12:107-114.

69. de Marie S, van den Broek PJ, Willemze R, et al. Strategy for antibiotic therapy in febrile neutropenic patients on selective antibiotic decontamination. *Eur J Clin Microbiol Infect Dis.* 1993;12:897-906.

70. Newman KA, Reed WP, Schimpff SC, et al. Hickman catheters in association with intensive cancer chemotherapy. *Support Care Cancer.* 1993;1:92-97.

71. Strauss RG. Granulocyte transfusion therapy. *Hematol Oncol Clin North Am.* 1994;8:1159-1166.

72. Berghmans T, Paesmans M, Lafitte J, et al. Therapeutic use of granulocyte and granulocyte–macrophage colony-stimulating factors in febrile neutropenic cancer patients. A systematic review of the literature with meta-analysis. *Support Care Cancer.* 2002;10(3):181-188.

73. Clark OAC, Lyman G, Castro AA, Clark LGO, Djulbegovic B. Colony stimulating factors for chemotherapy induced febrile neutropenia. *Cochrane Database Syst Rev.* 2000;(4):CD003039. doi:10.1002/14651858.CD003039.

74. Smith TJ, Khatcheressian J, Lyman GH, et al. 2006 update of recommendations for the use of white blood cell growth factors: an evidence-based clinical practice guideline. *J Clin Oncol.* 2006; 24:3187-3205.

75. Rizzo JD, Brouwers M, Hurley P, et al. American Society of Clinical Oncology–American Society of Hematology clinical practice guideline update on the use of epoetin and darbepoetin in adult patients with cancer. *J Clin Oncol.* 2010;28(33):4996-5010.

76. Ellis ME, al-Hokail AA, Clink HM, et al. Double-blind randomized study of the effect of infusion rates on toxicity of amphotericin B. *Antimicrob Agents Chemother.* 1992;36:172-179.

77. Cleary JD, Weisdorf D, Fletcher CV. Effect of infusion rate on amphotericin B-associated febrile reactions. *Drug Intell Clin Pharm.* 1988;22:769-772.

78. McNeil C. NCCN guidelines advocate wider use of colony-stimulating factor. *J Natl Cancer Inst.* 2005;97(10):710-711.

79. Greil R, Jost LM. ESMO recommendations for the application of hematopoietic growth factors. *Ann Oncol.* 2005;16(S1): i80-i82.

80. Nichols CR, Fox EP, Roth BJ, et al. Incidence of neutropenic fever in patients treated with standard-dose combination chemotherapy for small-cell lung cancer and the cost impact of treatment with granulocyte colony-stimulating factor. *J Clin Oncol.* 1994;12:1245-1250.

81. Biganzoli L, Untch M, Skacel T, et al. Neulasta (pegfilgrastim): a once-per-cycle option for the management of chemotherapy-induced neutropenia. *Semin Oncol.* 2004;31(S8):27-34.

82. Yowell SL, Blackwell S. Novel effects with polyethylene glycol modified pharmaceuticals. *Cancer Treat Rev.* 2002;28(SA):3-6.

83. Holmes FA, Jones SE, O'Shaughnessy J, et al. Comparable efficiency and safety profiles of once-per-cycle pegfilgrastim and daily filgrastim in chemotherapy-induced neutropenia: a multicenter dose-finding study in women with breast cancer. *Ann Oncol.* 2002;13:903-909.

84. Holmes FA, O'Shaughnessy JA, Vukelja S, et al. Blinded, randomized, multicenter study to evaluate single administration pegfilgrastim once per cycle versus daily filgrastim as an adjunct to chemotherapy in patients with high-risk stage II or stage III/IV breast cancer. *J Clin Oncol.* 2002;20: 727-731.

85. Crawford J. Once-per-cycle pegfilgrastim (Neulasta) for the management of chemotherapy-induced neutropenia. *Semin Oncol.* 2003;30(S13):24-30.

86. NCCN Supportive Care Guidelines for Prevention and Treatment of Infection, 2009.

87. Pascoe J, Steven, N. Antibiotics for the prevention of febrile neutropenia. *Curr Opin Hematol.* 2009;16(1):48-52.

CHAPTER 9

Hot Flashes

Kunal C. Kadakia ■ Charles L. Loprinzi

Menopause can be associated with multiple adverse symptoms, including vasomotor instability, urinary incontinence, sexual dysfunction, depression, and insomnia. Vasomotor instability is a constellation of symptoms commonly referred to as *hot flashes*. Although variable, hot flashes are often characterized as a sudden and disturbing sensation of intense warmth perceived mainly in the upper part of the chest. Red blotches can appear on the skin and the increase in skin temperature can lead to profuse diaphoresis. This feeling of intense warmth can be accompanied by palpitations, irritability, and anxiety. Hot flashes usually last a few minutes but can occur for a few seconds or for 10 minutes or longer. The frequency of hot flashes can also be quite variable, ranging from every 20 minutes to once a month. Nearly one-third of women during perimenopause and three-quarters of women during menopause experience hot flashes (1). However, the prevalence of (or reporting of) hot flashes has been noted to be variable among differing cultures and ethnic groups. African American women, cigarette smoking, low socioeconomic status, and obesity are associated with a higher prevalence of hot flashes (2). The majority of women experience hot flashes for 6 months to 2 years, although some women have them for 10 years or longer.

Hot flashes can be more substantial in patients with cancer. In many premenopausal women with breast cancer and other gynecologic malignancies, the precipitation of menopause by oophorectomy, chemotherapy, radiotherapy, or hormonal manipulation can lead to the rapid onset of hot flash symptoms that are more frequent and severe than those associated with natural menopause (3). Other reasons for the high frequency of menopausal symptoms in breast cancer survivors include age at diagnosis (frequently older than 50 years) and the abrupt withdrawal of hormonal therapy.

Hot flashes also affect men undergoing androgen deprivation therapy for prostate cancer. Hot flashes have been reported to occur in up to 70% of men after orchiectomy, 80% of men receiving neoadjuvant hormonal therapy before radical prostatectomy, and 70% to 80% of men receiving long-term androgen deprivation therapy (4–6). Hot flash symptoms can have serious detrimental effects on a patient's work, recreation, sleep, and general perception of quality of life (7).

PATHOPHYSIOLOGY OF HOT FLASHES

The pathophysiology of hot flashes is not entirely understood. The thermoregulatory nucleus in the medial preoptic area of the hypothalamus is felt to regulate the mechanism leading to heat loss during hot flashes. The thermoregulatory nucleus activates perspiration and vasodilatation to keep core body temperature within a tightly regulated range, known as the thermoregulatory zone. In menopausal women with hot flashes, the thermoregulatory zone is shifted downward and is narrower than it is in menopausal women who do not have hot flashes (8). Therefore, in women with hot flashes, small changes in body temperature (as low as 0.01°C) may trigger the mechanisms of heat loss and lead to vasomotor symptoms (9).

The dramatic decreases in sexual hormone levels that occur in menopausal women and in men receiving androgen deprivation therapy are thought to be responsible for lowering and narrowing the thermoregulatory zone. However, sexual hormones have profound effects on multiple neuroendocrine pathways, and the exact mechanisms by which they affect the thermoregulatory zone continue to be elucidated. Since estrogen withdrawal results in decreased central serotonergic activity and since some of the newer antidepressants have been shown to relieve hot flashes in placebo-controlled, randomized clinical trials (*vide infra*), serotonin (5-HT) is thought to play an important role in mediating the thermoregulatory effects of estrogen. In particular, the 5-HT$_{2A}$ receptor has been closely associated with thermoregulation in mammals. Multiple animal and human studies have shown that central expression of the 5-HT$_{2A}$ receptor decreases after estrogen withdrawal and that estrogen treatment reverses this change in estrogen-deficient animals and women (10,11). In addition, tamoxifen has been shown to block the positive effects of estrogen on central 5-HT$_{2A}$ receptor expression in ovariectomized rats (12). Since estrogen withdrawal and tamoxifen treatment result in decreased central expression of 5-HT$_{2A}$ receptors, it is possible that the efficacy of the newer antidepressants against hot flashes is due, at least in part, to their ability to cause a "compensatory" increase in central 5-HT$_{2A}$ signaling (13). Similarly, norepinephrine has also been implicated in the pathophysiology of hot flashes. Estrogen withdrawal leads to increased norepinephrine levels in the hypothalamus, which are thought to contribute to the lowering and narrowing of the thermoregulatory zone as well (8).

Another possible mechanism for hot flashes is endogenous opioid peptide withdrawal. In morphine-dependent rats, abrupt opioid withdrawal was associated with rapid temperature changes, which were eliminated with estrogen administration (14). This theory suggests that estrogen increases central opioid peptide activity, and therefore, estrogen deficiency may be associated with decreased endogenous central opioid activity and subsequent thermoregulatory dysfunction.

The neuroendocrine pathways that govern thermoregulation in mammals are extraordinarily complex and, as yet, incompletely understood. There is a clear need for further research to clarify the pathophysiology of hot flashes and guide the development of more targeted nonhormonal therapeutic options.

TREATMENT OF HOT FLASHES

It is recommended that hot flashes are routinely assessed during clinical encounters in both cancer and noncancer patients as a component of systematic symptom surveys. Assessment of frequency, intensity, duration, and potential triggers of hot flashes may be helpful. Self-directed diaries to record these variables can be used to formulate treatment recommendations. The Hot Flash Related Daily Interference Scale (HFRDIS) is a validated tool utilized in the research setting to monitor hot flash symptomology prior to and following treatment (15). Studies are ongoing regarding devices that measure skin conductance as an objective marker for hot flashes; however, these have not been well validated (16). At this time, patient reports of hot flash experiences are the most reasonable measure.

PHARMACOLOGIC INTERVENTIONS

Hormonal Therapy

Estrogen

Estrogen therapy is the most established effective treatment option for hot flashes and can reduce symptoms by 80% to 90% (17). However, the use of estrogen has become controversial in the last decade, due to evidence of associated long-term health risks including coronary heart disease, cerebrovascular disease, venous thromboembolism, and breast cancer (18,19). The controversy surrounding its effect on breast cancer has been especially influential on clinical practice. The Woman's Health Initiate trial demonstrated a 26% increased risk of breast cancer in females receiving combination hormonal therapy (estrogen plus progestin) (19). The HABITS (hormonal replacement therapy after breast cancer—is it safe?) trial was stopped prematurely after an interim analysis found an increased risk of new breast cancers in breast cancer survivors (HR = 2.4) with the use of combination hormonal therapy after 2 years (20). However, the Stockholm trial found no such risk at a median follow-up of 4 years (21). The major difference in the Stockholm trial was the use of a lower dose of progestin. Several other prospective and retrospective studies suggest that at least some breast cancer survivors (small tumors, negative lymph node status, long disease-free survival, or estrogen receptor–negative tumors) could be safely treated with estrogen replacement (22). Despite these data, the use of estrogen in women with a

history of, or at high risk for, breast cancer remains controversial and is not recommended.

Commonly utilized estrogen formulations include daily oral micronized 17-β-estradiol (1 mg), conjugated equine estrogens (0.625 mg), piperazine estrone sulfate (1.25 mg), and transdermal 17-β-estradiol (50 μg/d). Although the preceding doses are effective, lower doses have also been shown to be efficacious and should be used for the shortest period of time possible. Contraindications to estrogen use include known coronary heart disease, previous venous thromboembolic disease or stroke, active liver disease, history of estrogen-dependent cancer, or those at high risk for these pathologies.

Progesterone Analogs

Progesterone therapy alone is another effective hormonal agent for the treatment of hot flashes. A placebo-controlled, randomized clinical trial of megestrol 40 mg daily in 97 women with a history of breast cancer and 66 men receiving androgen deprivation therapy showed a marked reduction in hot flashes, of 75% to 80%, in the treatment group compared with 20% to 25% in the placebo group (23). Three years after the completion of the trial, one-third of the women who were still taking megestrol reported having less hot flashes than women who had discontinued therapy (24). Similar results were found in another trial utilizing depot intramuscular medroxyprogesterone acetate (DMPA), a progestational agent (25). Most recently, the use of a single intramuscular dose of MPA was better tolerated and more efficacious than venlafaxine at a target dose of 75 mg daily over a 6-week period (26).

Despite the efficacy of progestational agents for the treatment of hot flashes, many physicians are hesitant in using hormonally active agents in patients with a history of breast or prostate cancer. Though there is some evidence that progestational agents are active against breast cancer (27), in vitro data suggest that they can increase epithelial cell proliferation, a potentially undesirable effect in patients with a history of breast cancer (28). In addition, megestrol was reported to increase the prostate-specific antigen level in a patient with prostate cancer (29).

Despite its efficacy, patients need to be counseled before starting a progestational agent if they have a history of breast or prostate cancer. Commonly prescribed regimens include oral megestrol acetate 20 to 40 mg daily, intramuscular DMPA 400 to 500 mg once, or intramuscular DMPA 400 to 500 mg every 2 weeks for three doses. Adverse effects of progestational agents include vaginal bleeding upon discontinuation of the medication, weight gain, bloating, and thromboembolic phenomena.

Nonhormonal Therapy

The reluctance to use hormonal agents in patients with a history of breast cancer provided an impetus for finding nonhormonal agents that could help alleviate hot flashes. The following is a summary of their clinical development and therapeutic yield (Table 9.1).

| TABLE 9.1 | Evidence and adverse effects of beneficial nonestrogenic therapeutics |

	Treatment	Evidence[a]	Adverse Events
Women	Citalopram	Two large RCTs	Constipation, dry mouth, nausea
	Desvenlafaxine	Two large RCTs	Dizziness, nausea, vomiting
	DMPA	One large RCT Three moderate RCTs One small RCT	Bloating, weight gain, thrombogenic
	Escitalopram	One large RCT	Fatigue, headaches, insomnia, nausea
	Gabapentin	Two large RCT Two moderate RCTs	Dizziness, fatigue, somnolence
	Megestrol acetate	Two moderate RCTs	Bloating, weight gain, thrombogenic
	Paroxetine	Two large RCTs	Insomnia, nausea, sexual dysfunction
	Pregabalin	One moderate RCT	Cognitive difficulty, sleepiness, weight gain
	Venlafaxine	Three large RCTs One moderate RCT	Anorexia, dry mouth, insomnia, nausea
Men on ADT	DMPA	One large RCT One small RCT	Bloating, weight gain, thrombogenic
	Gabapentin	One large RCT	Dizziness, fatigue, somnolence
	Megestrol acetate	One moderate RCT	Bloating, weight gain, thrombogenic
	Paroxetine	One pilot study	Insomnia, nausea, sexual dysfunction
	Venlafaxine	One pilot study One large RCT (not placebo-controlled)	Anorexia, dry mouth, insomnia, nausea

Note: See sections on each therapeutic for further details.

[a]Number of participants in study: large: >100; moderate: 50 to 99; and small: <50.

DMPA, depomedroxyprogesterone acetate; RCT, randomized controlled trial; ADT, androgen deprivation therapy.

Newer Antidepressants

In the 1990s, several authors reported reductions in hot flash frequency and severity in postmenopausal women who were taking four of the newer antidepressants for other reasons. Since then, the results of multiple prospective studies of antidepressants for the treatment of hot flashes have been reported. These studies have been reviewed and systematically analyzed in detail elsewhere (30,31). Given the reluctance to use hormonal agents in women with a history of breast cancer, many of these studies were done in this patient population, but some studies have been done in noncancer patients as well as in men with a history of prostate cancer. Self-completed daily hot flash diaries were used to document the frequency and severity of hot flashes in the majority of

these studies. Data on toxicity, quality of life, and mood status were commonly obtained. The main efficacy measures used in most studies were the change from baseline in the weekly average number of daily hot flashes and average hot flash score (defined as the number of mild hot flashes plus twice the number of moderate hot flashes plus three times the number of severe hot flashes plus four times the number of very severe hot flashes during that week).

Venlafaxine. Venlafaxine selectively inhibits serotonin, norepinephrine, and dopamine reuptake, in order of decreasing potency and is referred to as a serotonin norepinephrine reuptake inhibitor (SNRI). In 1998, the efficacy of venlafaxine for the treatment of hot flashes was first supported (32). This pilot study included 23 women with a history of breast cancer and 5 men receiving androgen deprivation therapy for prostate cancer. Patients treated with venlafaxine 12.5 mg twice daily had a greater than 50% reduction in median hot flash scores at 4 weeks. Patients also reported significant improvement in fatigue, sweating, and difficulty sleeping, and, at the completion of the study, 64% of the patients chose to continue venlafaxine.

Subsequently, a placebo-controlled, double-blind, randomized clinical trial was conducted to assess the efficacy and toxicity of venlafaxine in women with hot flashes (33). One-hundred and ninety one women were randomized to placebo or one of three target doses of venlafaxine extended release (ER): 37.5 mg daily, 75 mg daily, or 150 mg daily for 4 weeks. After 4 weeks of treatment, the median frequency of hot flashes decreased by 19%, 30%, 46%, and 58% in women in the four study groups, respectively. Despite improvement in Beck Depression Inventory scores, patients with normal baseline depression scores had a similar reduction in hot flashes to those with higher scores. Dry mouth, nausea, constipation, and decreased appetite were dose-dependent toxicities associated with venlafaxine. Sixty-nine percent of the women were taking tamoxifen and efficacy was similar whether tamoxifen was being used or not.

In another placebo-controlled, double-blind, randomized clinical trial, venlafaxine ER at a target dose of 75 mg daily was found to significantly decrease patient-perceived hot flash scores. This trial included 80 postmenopausal women who were treated for a total of 12 weeks. Despite the improvement in subjective hot flash scores, there were no statistically significant differences between the two groups in hot flash frequency or severity. This is likely because the authors of this study did not collect pretreatment baseline measures for hot flash frequencies or severity (34). Dry mouth, insomnia, and decreased appetite were significantly more common in the venlafaxine group. Mental health and vitality were significantly improved in the venlafaxine group and 93% of women in this group chose to continue venlafaxine at the conclusion of the trial.

Venlafaxine has also been compared with gabapentin and DMPA in two separate clinical trials. To compare venlafaxine and gabapentin, a group-sequential, open-label, randomized, crossover clinical trial of 4 weeks on each therapy was constructed (35). When compared with gabapentin at a target dose of 300 mg three times daily, venlafaxine ER 75 mg daily was found to be as effective in reducing hot flash scores (66% reduction in each group). However, women preferred venlafaxine to gabapentin at the end of the trial period (68% vs. 32%). Clinically, since there were approximately one-third of women in this trial who felt that gabapentin worked better for their hot flashes, this can be tried in those where venlafaxine is not helpful.

When compared with a single intramuscular dose of DMPA 400 mg, venlafaxine ER 75 mg daily was found to be less effective and less well tolerated (26). However, there were significant reductions in hot flash scores in both groups over the 6-week period (79% vs. 55%), respectively.

The efficacy of venlafaxine for the alleviation of hot flashes in men undergoing androgen deprivation therapy was evaluated in two published trials to date. In the first pilot study, 23 men were treated with venlafaxine 12.5 mg twice daily for 4 weeks; however, only 16 completed the study (36). Of these, 10 patients had a greater than 50% reduction in their hot flash scores at the end of the study. Treatment was well tolerated and median weekly hot flash scores decreased by 54%. The average incidence of severe and very severe hot flashes decreased from 2.3 per day at baseline to 0.6 per day at the end of the study. In the second trial, 919 men undergoing androgen deprivation therapy were randomly assigned to either venlafaxine 75 mg daily, oral MPA 20 mg daily, or cyproterone acetate 100 mg daily over a 1-month period (37). In this double-blind trial, the change in median daily hot flash scores between randomization and 1 month was −47%, −84%, and −95%, respectively.

Given available data, venlafaxine is a viable first-line option for the treatment of hot flashes in women and men. Therapy should be initiated with venlafaxine ER 37.5 mg daily and increased to 75 mg daily after 1 week, if tolerated. Common adverse effects include loss of appetite, dry mouth, insomnia, and nausea.

Desvenlafaxine. Desvenlafaxine is a newer SNRI and is the succinate salt form of the major active metabolite of venlafaxine. Desvenlafaxine has been studied in two large, randomized, placebo-controlled, clinical trials involving women without a history of breast cancer (38,39). In both trials, desvenlafaxine was associated with a 60% to 70% reduction in severity and frequency of hot flashes compared with placebo (~50% reduction). Therapy should be initiated at 50 mg daily and increased to 100 mg daily after 3 days if tolerated. The major adverse effect is dose-dependent nausea, vomiting, and dizziness.

Paroxetine. Paroxetine is a selective serotonin reuptake inhibitor (SSRI), with minimal effects on the reuptake of norepinephrine. The efficacy of paroxetine against hot flashes was initially supported in a pilot study in 2000 (40). In this study, women were treated with paroxetine 10 mg daily for 1 week, followed by 20 mg daily for 4 weeks. After 5 weeks of treatment, the mean hot flash frequency decreased by 67%, while the mean hot flash severity score decreased by 75%. There was also a statistically significant, change from baseline, improvement in depression, sleep, anxiety, and quality of life scores.

Given the positive findings, the authors conducted a placebo-controlled, double-blind, randomized clinical trial evaluating paroxetine controlled release (CR) in women suffering from hot flashes (41). One hundred and sixty-five women were randomized to either placebo, paroxetine CR 12.5 mg daily, or paroxetine CR 25 mg daily for 6 weeks. Among the 139 women who completed the trial, the hot flash score had decreased by 62% and 65% in the lower and higher dose paroxetine groups, respectively, compared with a 38% reduction in the placebo group. The mean daily hot flash frequency decreased from 7.1 to 3.8, 6.4 to 3.2, and 6.6 to 4.8 in the three groups, respectively. The improvement in hot flash symptoms was independent of tamoxifen use. Adverse events were reported by 54% of women taking placebo and by 58% of women taking paroxetine. Subsequent to this trial, a placebo-controlled, double-blind, randomized, crossover clinical trial evaluating paroxetine 10 and 20 mg daily was completed (42). In this trial, 151 women were assigned to receive 4 weeks of paroxetine 10 or 20 mg daily followed by placebo or vice versa. Paroxetine 10 mg daily was found to reduce hot flash frequency by 41% compared with 14% with placebo. Paroxetine 20 mg reduced the frequency of hot flashes by 52% compared with 27% with placebo. While doses had relatively similar efficacy, patients taking the 10 mg dose were less likely to discontinue treatment.

Two pilot studies have demonstrated the efficacy of paroxetine for the treatment of hot flashes in men undergoing androgen deprivation therapy. In the first, 26 men were treated with ER paroxetine to a target dose of 37.5 mg daily over 4 weeks (43). Of the 18 patients who completed the study, the median frequency of hot flashes decreased from 6.2 per day at baseline to 2.5 per day and the hot flash scores decreased from 10.6 per day to 3 per day. In the second study, 10 patients treated with paroxetine 10 mg daily had modest improvements in both hot flash frequency (3.5 per day vs. 2 per day) and severity (44).

Paroxetine, thus, is an effective therapeutic option for the treatment of hot flashes in women and possibly in men. Therapy should be initiated at 10 mg daily with no data to support increased dosing leading to significantly improved outcomes. It is not recommended to use paroxetine in women taking tamoxifen due to concern for reducing tamoxifen's effectiveness (*vide infra*). Common adverse effects are dose-dependent and include sexual dysfunction, nausea, and insomnia.

Fluoxetine. Fluoxetine is an SSRI with minimal effects on the reuptake of norepinephrine. The efficacy of fluoxetine for the treatment of hot flashes was first studied in an 8-week, placebo-controlled, double-blind, crossover clinical trial involving women (45). Patients were randomized to fluoxetine 20 mg daily or placebo, and after 4 weeks, were crossed over. By the end of the first treatment period, a non-significant difference was seen in hot flash scores in the fluoxetine arm compared with placebo (50% vs. 36%). However, cross-over analysis demonstrated a significantly greater improvement in hot flash scores with fluoxetine than with placebo. There was no statistically significant difference in adverse events and efficacy was similar whether tamoxifen was being used or not.

The long-term efficacy and toxicity of fluoxetine and citalopram were compared in a placebo-controlled, double-blind, randomized clinical trial (46). One hundred and fifty women with a history of breast cancer were randomized to placebo, fluoxetine, or citalopram over a 9-month period. Fluoxetine and citalopram were started at 10 mg and then increased to 20 mg daily at 1 month and further increased to 30 mg daily at 6 months. There were no statistically significant differences among the three groups with respect to hot flashes at any time during the trial. Discontinuation rates were 40% in the placebo group, 34% in the fluoxetine

group, and 34% in the citalopram group. Baseline information was obtained on the first day of treatment rather than preceding initiation of therapy. This is a possible confounder as previous studies have shown efficacy within 1 day of treatment (30).

Common adverse effects include loss of appetite, nausea, and insomnia. Similar to paroxetine, fluoxetine should not be used in patients receiving tamoxifen (*vide infra*). Given the evidence to date, fluoxetine should not be considered among the current nonhormonal therapies.

Citalopram. Citalopram is a potent and specific SSRI. The efficacy of citalopram for hot flashes was first supported in two small pilot studies. In contrast, a large, placebo-controlled, randomized trial evaluating citalopram and fluoxetine at a target dose of 30 mg daily concluded that neither were effective compared with placebo (46). This trial failed to collect baseline data prior to starting the study drug (see Section Fluoxetine). The most recent double-blind, placebo-controlled, randomized clinical trial evaluated 254 women who were allotted to either placebo or citalopram at target doses of 10, 20, or 30 mg daily over a 6-week period (47). Hot flash frequency decreased by 20%, 46%, 43%, and 50%, respectively. Although reductions in hot flash frequency were relatively similar in all citalopram groups, citalopram 20 mg daily appeared to be more effective than 10 mg daily in regard to beneficial impacts on daily life, including sleep, mood, and enjoyment, as measured by the HFRDIS.

Citalopram is, thus, an effective treatment for women suffering from hot flashes. Therapy should be initiated and continued at 20 mg daily. Common adverse effects include nausea, constipation, and dry mouth. Given the available data, citalopram can be safely utilized in patients receiving tamoxifen (*vide infra*).

Escitalopram. Escitalopram, being the S-enantiomer of racemic citalopram, is also an SSRI. Only one double-blind, placebo-controlled, randomized trial evaluating escitalopram at 10 to 20 mg daily has been published to date (48). Two-hundred and five postmenopausal women without a history of breast cancer were randomized to placebo or escitalopram 10 mg daily for 8 weeks. Escitalopram was found to be modestly more effective than placebo at decreasing the frequency of hot flashes (47% vs. 33%). Adverse events were higher in the placebo group (53% vs. 63%) and only seven patients in the escitalopram arm discontinued therapy due to an adverse event.

Given the available data, escitalopram is a therapeutic option in women suffering from hot flashes. Therapy should be initiated at 10 mg daily and increased to 20 mg daily after 4 weeks if ineffective. Common adverse effects include nausea, headaches, fatigue, and sleeping difficulties.

Sertraline. Sertraline is a potent and specific SSRI. To date, there have been three published trials assessing the efficacy of sertraline in reducing hot flashes with variable results. In the first double-blind, placebo-controlled, randomized, crossover clinical trial, 62 women, with early-stage breast cancer on adjuvant tamoxifen, were randomized to sertraline 50 mg daily or placebo for 6 weeks and then crossed over (49). A non-statistically significant difference was seen between the sertraline and placebo groups (36% vs. 27%). At the end of 12 weeks, 49% of patients preferred the sertraline period, 11% the placebo period, and 41% had no preference. Another double-blind, placebo-controlled, crossover clinical trial involving 102 women without a history of breast cancer were randomized to sertraline 50 mg daily or placebo for 4 weeks and then crossed over after a 1 week washout period (50). Although the hot flash score was significantly better in the sertraline group, no difference was seen in the severity of symptoms between groups. In the most recent double-blind, placebo-controlled, randomized clinical trial, sertraline, 50 to 100 mg daily over a 6-week period, was found to be no more effective than placebo in either hot flash frequency or hot flash scores (51).

Given the available evidence, sertraline has not been found to be consistently helpful in alleviating hot flashes and is not recommended.

Mirtazapine. Mirtazapine has antihistaminic, antiserotonergic, and α_2-blocking activity without any significant effect on the synaptic reuptake of catecholamines. Two pilot studies have been published to date with promising results. In the first study, 22 women were treated with mirtazapine to a target dose of 30 mg daily during a 4-week period (52). The median reduction from baseline in total daily hot flashes and weekly hot flash scores was 53% and 60%, respectively. Patients reported improvements in tension and trouble sleeping as well. In another pilot study, 40 women with a history of breast cancer were treated with mirtazapine 30 mg daily for 3 months (53). Of the 20 women who completed the study, there was a 56% and 62% reduction in hot flash frequency and score, respectively. Of the original 40 patients, 13 patients never started mirtazapine and 7 discontinued therapy due to somnolence.

Given that the only available data are derived from pilot studies, there is insufficient evidence to recommend mirtazapine among other nonhormonal therapies at this time.

Interactions between Tamoxifen and the Newer Antidepressants. Tamoxifen is converted to its active metabolite, endoxifen, by the hepatic enzyme cytochrome P450 2D6 (CYP2D6). It has been hypothesized that patients on tamoxifen with reduced CYP2D6 activity, due to genomic variants or by drugs that inhibit CYP2D6 function, might result in poorer outcomes (54,55). SSRIs are an important class of drugs that inhibit CYP2D6 function. Among the SSRIs, paroxetine, a potent CYP2D6 inhibitor, has been associated with an increased risk of death from breast cancer (54). It is important to bear in mind that there is a gradient of potency for inhibition of CYP2D6 among the SSRIs and SNRIs with paroxetine and fluoxetine having greater inhibitory potential compared with citalopram and venlafaxine. Given currently available data, use of venlafaxine or citalopram should be preferentially considered in patients receiving tamoxifen (56,57).

Antiepileptics

Gabapentin. Gabapentin is a γ-aminobutyric acid (GABA) analog that is used in a variety of neurologic and pain syndromes. The exact mechanism of action is unclear but it is suggested that it reduces noradrenergic hyperactivity. The efficacy of gabapentin for the treatment of hot flashes was first noted serendipitously in a group of six patients at the University of Rochester (58). Since then, four trials as well as a pooled analysis have shown the benefit of gabapentin in reducing hot flashes in women (30). The first placebo-controlled, randomized clinical trial involved 59 postmenopausal women without a history of breast cancer who were treated with either gabapentin 900 mg daily or placebo (59). After 12 weeks of therapy, patients receiving gabapentin had a significantly greater reduction in hot flash frequency compared with placebo (45% vs. 29%). An open-label treatment phase followed during which gabapentin was able to be increased (maximum dose of 2,700 mg daily) and was associated with a greater reduction in hot flash frequency from baseline. Two other placebo-controlled, randomized clinical trials involving a similar population showed comparable reductions in hot flash scores compared with placebo (51% vs. 26% and 71% vs. 54%, respectively) (60,61). Gabapentin (900 mg daily) in breast cancer survivors was also effective at reducing hot flashes (62). A placebo-controlled, randomized clinical trial of gabapentin in men receiving androgen deprivation therapy for prostate cancer showed similar but less robust results (63). In this trial, patients receiving gabapentin 900 mg daily had a statistically significant reduction in hot flash frequency from baseline compared with placebo (46% vs. 22%). However, no statistically significant difference was observed in men taking gabapentin at 300 to 600 mg daily.

Gabapentin, thus, is an effective therapeutic option in the treatment of hot flashes in women and men. Therapy should be initiated at 300 mg daily and titrated up to 300 mg three times daily (900 mg daily), if tolerated. The most common adverse effects of gabapentin are dose-dependent and include dizziness, somnolence, and fatigue.

Pregabalin. Pregabalin is a newer generation GABA analog that appears to be a more potent analgesic than gabapentin. A pilot study, consisting of six patients, demonstrated a reduction in hot flashes by 65% with pregabalin 50 to 150 mg daily (64). This was corroborated by a double-blind, placebo-controlled, randomized clinical trial, involving 163 women who received pregabalin at a target dose of 75 mg twice daily, 150 mg twice daily, or placebo (65). After 6 weeks, hot flash scores decreased by 65%, 71%, and 50%, respectively.

Therefore, pregabalin is an effective therapeutic option in the treatment of hot flashes in women. Therapy should be initiated at 50 mg at bedtime for the first week, then 50 mg twice daily for the second week, then 75 mg twice daily thereafter, if tolerated. Adverse effects are primarily dose-dependent and include cognitive difficulty, dizziness, weight gain, and sleepiness.

Levetiracetam. The mechanism of action of levetiracetam is unknown and is not felt to be related to inhibitory or excitatory neurotransmission. In the only pilot study published to date, 28 women were treated with levetiracetam to a target dose of 2,000 mg daily for a total of 4 weeks (66). Of the 20 women who completed the study, there was a 53% and 57% reduction in hot flash frequency and score, respectively. There is insufficient evidence to recommend levetiracetam among other nonhormonal therapies at this time.

Other Centrally Acting Compounds

Clonidine. Clonidine is a centrally acting α_2-receptor agonist first proposed as a treatment for hot flashes in the 1970s. One purported mechanism of action is that clonidine raises the sweating threshold by reducing norepinephrine release. The efficacy of transdermal clonidine (equivalent to an oral dose of 0.1 mg daily) for the treatment of tamoxifen-induced hot flashes was first shown in a placebo-controlled, randomized clinical trial (67). However, transdermal clonidine was associated with significant adverse effects, including fatigue, dry mouth, and constipation. A similar study in men with post-orchiectomy hot flashes failed to demonstrate a significant decrease in hot flash frequency or severity (68). Another placebo-controlled, randomized clinical trial, involving 194 women with tamoxifen-induced hot flashes, demonstrated a decrease in hot flashes in the clonidine group (0.1 mg orally nightly) compared with the placebo group, after 8 weeks of therapy (38% vs. 24%) (69). Patients in the clonidine group had more adverse effects, especially insomnia. Although clonidine decreases hot flashes, its unfavorable toxicity profile, and the availability of other agents, limits its use.

Methyldopa. Methyldopa is a centrally acting α_2-receptor agonist that has been investigated as a treatment for hot flashes. A 2006 systematic review, including three poor-quality crossover trials, found no difference in frequency of hot flashes in patients receiving methyldopa versus placebo (31). Fatigue, dizziness, and dry mouth occurred more often in the study groups. Due to its limited efficacy and toxicity profile, methyldopa is not recommended as a therapy for hot flashes.

Bellergal. Bellergal Retard is a brand name for a combination product of ergotamine, belladonna alkaloids, and phenobarbital. Although several reports favor its use over placebo, this therapy should not be recommended given marginal reported efficacy, the dose-dependent anticholinergic side effects of belladonna (dizziness, constipation, dry mouth, and blurry vision), and the risk of phenobarbital dependence (70).

Veralipride. Veralipride is a substituted benzamide derivative with antidopaminergic (D_2) properties. There have been two small placebo-controlled reports, suggesting marked improvements in hot flash frequency and severity with the use of veralipride (100 mg daily) (71,72). However, this medication is not approved for use in the United States due to its toxicity profile, which includes mastodynia, galactorrhea, gastrointestinal distress, and tardive dyskinesia.

Complementary and Alternative Therapies

Vitamin E. Based on some case series, vitamin E (α-tocopherol) was first recognized in the 1940s as a treatment for hot flashes. In 1998, a placebo-controlled, randomized, crossover clinical trial involving 120 women demonstrated a marginal benefit with an average of one less hot flash per day with vitamin E (800 IU daily) compared with placebo (73). Side effects were similar in both groups. A subsequent prospective, double-blind, placebo-controlled trial also reported positive results; however, the treatment arms were not randomized (all patients received placebos for 4 weeks followed by a washout period and then 4 weeks of vitamin E) (74). Thus, while there is a suggestion that vitamin E may help decrease hot flashes to some extent, there is not yet convincing proof. Although concerns regarding the carcinogenicity of vitamin E have been raised, a 2008 meta-analysis found no effect on cancer incidence or mortality (75). Thus, vitamin E is a reasonable option to try, albeit it has limited efficacy.

Phytoestrogens and Soy. When compared with the United States, the prevalence of hot flashes is significantly less in Asia. One theory for this difference is the predominance of soy-based dietary intake. Phytoestrogens are classified into three main classes: isoflavones, lignins, and coumestans. These compounds are purported to have both estrogenic and antiestrogenic properties. Isoflavone precursors are found in soy, red clover, alfalfa, and other beans. A 2006 meta-analysis concluded that neither red clover nor soy isoflavone extracts consistently showed a benefit to be considered an effective treatment of hot flashes (31). In addition, there is an ongoing debate over whether soy decreases, or increases, the risk of estrogen-dependent tumors. Lignan precursors are found in seeds (flaxseed), whole grains, millet, fruits, and vegetables. The most recent randomized, clinical trial involving 188 women failed to show a benefit in hot flash scores with a daily flaxseed bar (providing 410 mg of lignins) compared with placebo over a 6-week period (76).

Black Cohosh. Black cohosh (*Cimicifuga racemosa*) is a herbaceous perennial plant native to North America. Although historical trials suggested improvement in vasomotor symptoms in nonmedication-induced menopause (77), more recent trials have not shown similar efficacy. Two placebo-controlled, randomized clinical trials failed to show any evidence that black cohosh was superior to placebo in reducing hot flashes in women (78,79). In 2009, a double-blind, randomized clinical trial compared black cohosh, red clover, conjugated equine estrogens plus MPA, and placebo for the relief of vasomotor symptoms (hot flashes and night sweats) in noncancer patients (80). After 12 months of intervention, the reductions in the number of vasomotor symptoms were as follows: black cohosh (34%), red clover (57%), Conjugated Equine Estrogens(CEE)/MPA (94%), and placebo (63%). It was concluded that black cohosh was no more effective than placebo in reducing vasomotor symptoms. In 2010, a meta-analysis involving noncancer patients concluded that more data regarding effectiveness and safety were needed (81). Although previously suggested to be associated with hepatoxicity, the most recent evidence suggests no such risk (82).

Other Herbal Remedies. Dong quai (*Angelica sinensis*), a Chinese herb purported to treat vasomotor symptoms, does not have established efficacy for the treatment of hot flashes and there is concern regarding safety due to its estrogen-like activity (83). Wild yam (*Dioscorea villosa*) is a natural product that has also been found to be no different than placebo for the treatment of vasomotor instability. Both ginseng (*Panax ginseng*) and evening primrose oil (*Oenothera biennis*) have been found to be ineffective as well. Thus, currently, there is no strong evidence to support the utility of any of these agents for the treatment of hot flashes.

NONPHARMACOLOGIC INTERVENTIONS

Multiple nonpharmacologic interventions have been purported to alleviate hot flashes. These include the use of air conditioners, cold water, special diets, exercise programs, acupuncture, yoga, relaxation techniques, paced respiration, biofeedback, and more. However, none of these have yet shown consistently positive results, and the placebo effect likely plays a significant role in their apparent efficacy. Indeed, placebo-controlled, randomized clinical trials addressing hot flashes have consistently shown a 20% to 50% placebo effect.

Acupuncture

Over the last two decades, multiple trials have explored the efficacy of acupuncture in reducing hot flashes. A meta-analysis including three randomized controlled trials did find a statistical difference favoring acupuncture over sham procedure (84). However, due to a high degree of heterogeneity, the investigators concluded that the evidence was not convincing. Two systematic reviews published in 2009 found no significant difference between acupuncture and sham procedure in women (85,86). Evidence for acupuncture in men with prostate cancer suffering from hot flashes has also been unconvincing (87). In 2010, a randomized, clinical trial including 175 women found that acupuncture plus usual care was more effective than usual care alone (88). Future trials will have to confirm these results prior to establishing the role of acupuncture in the treatment of hot flashes.

Psychoeducational Interventions

Many different modalities of relaxation (i.e., paced breathing and mindfulness-based stress reduction) have been investigated for the treatment of menopausal symptoms. Although small trials have shown positive results, a systematic review from 2008 concluded that further investigation is needed prior to recommending these interventions (89).

Stellate Ganglion Block

This procedure involves injection of an anesthetic next to a nerve group in the neck (stellate ganglion) and has been used for decades to treat chronic pain. Since 2005, one case report and two pilot studies have shown positive results in reducing hot flash severity and frequency (90–92). The mechanism of action is not completely understood but may be associated with the neurological connection of the stellate ganglion to the insular cortex, a structure that is known to play a role in the pathophysiology of hot flashes (93). Further research is needed before this promising therapy can be considered an effective nonpharmacological intervention.

Hypnosis

Hypnosis is one of the many mind–body therapies utilized in both cancer and noncancer supportive care. Two small pilot studies supported that hypnosis could substantially decrease hot flash symptoms by 40% to 70% in women (94,95). In 2008, the first randomized controlled trial of hypnosis was completed and included 60 women who were assigned to receive hypnosis five times a week or no treatment. After 5 weeks, women in the intervention arm had a 68% reduction in hot flash scores compared with baseline (96). Despite its apparent efficacy, further placebo-controlled trials involving hypnosis will need to be completed prior to considering this therapy an effective and safe nonpharmacological intervention.

Breast Cancer versus No Breast Cancer

When nonhormonal therapies were initially shown to be helpful in women with a history of breast cancer, many of whom were taking tamoxifen, the question arose as to whether hot flash treatments would work differently in women with a history of breast cancer and/or taking tamoxifen, versus other women. This question was evaluated, concluding that hot flash treatments did not appear to be different in these different groups of women (97).

RECOMMENDATIONS

It is well known that hot flashes can have serious detrimental effects on quality of life. Clinicians should be aware of the prevalence of hot flashes and the multitude of therapeutic options available. Given the available research to date, a few evidence-based recommendations can be made when evaluating and considering therapy in patients suffering from hot flashes (Table 9.2). It is important to obtain the frequency, intensity, duration, and potential triggers of hot flashes prior to considering pharmacological therapy.

If a patient has mild symptoms that do not interfere with his or her daily activities, a trial of vitamin E 800 IU daily is a reasonable option. Despite the marginal benefit seen over placebo, this readily available and inexpensive therapy may allow a patient to get the well-known placebo

TABLE 9.2	Dosing schedules and expected response of beneficial nonestrogenic therapeutics	
Treatment	**Dosing Schedule**	**Expected HF Reduction (%)[a]**
Citalopram	Initiate and continue at 20 mg daily	50–60
Desvenlafaxine	Initiate at 50 mg daily and increase to goal of 100 mg daily after 3 d	50–60
DMPA	Give 400 mg IM once, can repeat after 3–12 mo, if needed	70–90
Escitalopram	Initiate at 10 mg daily and increase to 20 mg daily after 4 wk if needed	40–50
Gabapentin	Initiate at 300 mg daily and titrate up to 300 mg three times daily if tolerated	50–60
Megestrol acetate	Initiate and continue at 20–40 mg daily	70–90
Paroxetine	Initiate and continue at 10 mg daily	50–60
Pregabalin	Initiate at 50 mg QHS for 1 wk, then 50 mg twice daily for 1 wk, then 75 mg twice daily thereafter	50–60
Vitamin E	Initiate and continue at 800 IU daily	20–30
Venlafaxine	Initiate venlafaxine ER at 37.5 mg daily and increase to 75 mg daily after 1 wk	50–60

See sections on each therapeutic for further details.

[a]Expected percentage reduction is based on HF reduction from patients baseline; placebo effect is ~20% to 50%.

HF, hot flash; DMPA, depomedroxy progesterone acetate; QHS, at bedtime; ADT, androgen deprivation therapy.

effect without associated costs and toxicities of other therapeutic options.

If a patient has more severe symptoms, it is of prime importance to assess the feasibility of hormonal therapy, as hormonal therapy has been shown to have the most significant therapeutic potential. However, if contraindications or patient preferences preclude the use of hormonal therapy, nonhormonal therapy should be considered.

In women, citalopram, venlafaxine, paroxetine, desvenlafaxine, gabapentin, and pregabalin should be considered first-line therapeutics. It is of importance to minimize undesired toxicities by utilizing known side effects to their advantage. For example, in women with a history of depressive symptoms, an antidepressant would be a more reasonable option than gabapentin. Given the randomized trial that compared venlafaxine with gabapentin (35), it seems reasonable to start with an antidepressant first. While good cross-study comparisons have not been completed between the antidepressants, citalopram may be the best tolerated among the antidepressants that appear to work well against hot flashes.

Men undergoing androgen deprivation therapy have been less well studied in clinical trials. Nonetheless, with clonidine appearing to be an exception, it appears that hot flash therapies that work in women usually also work in men (98). Thus, it appears reasonable to try hot flash treatments in men based on what has been learned in women.

REFERENCES

1. Avis NE, Crawford SL, McKinlay SM. Psychosocial, behavioral, and health factors related to menopause symptomatology. *Womens Health.* 1997;3:103-120.
2. Gold EB, Sternfeld B, Kelsey JL, et al. Relation of demographic and lifestyle factors to symptoms in a multi-racial/ethnic population of women 40-55 years of age. *Am J Epidemiol.* 2000;152:463-473.
3. Carpenter JS, Andrykowski MA, Cordova M, et al. Hot flashes in postmenopausal women treated for breast carcinoma: prevalence, severity, correlates, management, and relation to quality of life. *Cancer.* 1998;82:1682-1691.
4. Buchholz NP, Mattarelli G, Buchholz MM. Post-orchiectomy hot flushes. *Eur Urol.* 1994;26:120-122.
5. Schow DA, Renfer LG, Rozanski TA, et al. Prevalence of hot flushes during and after neoadjuvant hormonal therapy for localized prostate cancer. *South Med J.* 1998;91:855-857.
6. Lanfrey P, Mottet N, Dagues F, et al. Hot flashes and hormonal treatment of prostate cancer. *Prog Urol.* 1996;6:17-22.
7. Daly E, Gray A, Barlow D, et al. Measuring the impact of menopausal symptoms on quality of life. *BMJ.* 1993;307:836-840.
8. Freedman RR, Krell W. Reduced thermoregulatory null zone in postmenopausal women with hot flashes. *Am J Obstet Gynecol.* 1999;181:66-70.
9. Freedman RR, Norton D, Woodward S, et al. Core body temperature and circadian rhythm of hot flashes in menopausal women. *J Clin Endocrinol Metab.* 1995;80:2354-2358.

10. Bethea CL, Lu NZ, Gundlah C, et al. Diverse actions of ovarian steroids in the serotonin neural system. *Front Neuroendocrinol.* 2002;23:41-100.

11. Moses-Kolko EL, Berga SL, Greer PJ, et al. Widespread increases of cortical serotonin type 2A receptor availability after hormone therapy in euthymic postmenopausal women. *Fertil Steril.* 2003;80:554-559.

12. Sumner BE, Grant KE, Rosie R, et al. Effects of tamoxifen on serotonin transporter and 5-hydroxytryptamine(2A) receptor binding sites and mRNA levels in the brain of ovariectomized rats with or without acute estradiol replacement. *Brain Res Mol Brain Res.* 1999;73:119-128.

13. Sipe K, Leventhal L, Burroughs K, et al. Serotonin 2A receptors modulate tail-skin temperature in two rodent models of estrogen deficiency-related thermoregulatory dysfunction. *Brain Res.* 2004;1028:191-202.

14. Merchenthaler I, Funkhouser JM, Carver JM, et al. The effect of estrogens and antiestrogens in a rat model for hot flush. *Maturitas.* 1998;30:307-316.

15. Carpenter JS. The Hot Flash Related Daily Interference Scale: a tool for assessing the impact of hot flashes on quality of life following breast cancer. *J Pain Symptom Manage.* 2001;22:979-989.

16. Loprinzi CL, Barton DL. Gadgets for measuring hot flashes: have they become the gold standard? *J Support Oncol.* 2009;7:136-137.

17. Notelovitz M, Lenihan JP, McDermott M, et al. Initial 17beta-estradiol dose for treating vasomotor symptoms. *Obstet Gynecol.* 2000;95:726-731.

18. Estrogen and progestogen use in postmenopausal women: 2010 position statement of The North American Menopause Society. *Menopause.* 2010;17:242-255.

19. Rossouw JE, Anderson GL, Prentice RL, et al. Risks and benefits of estrogen plus progestin in healthy postmenopausal women: principal results From the Women's Health Initiative randomized controlled trial. *JAMA.* 2002;288:321-333.

20. Holmberg L, Iversen OE, Rudenstam CM, et al. Increased risk of recurrence after hormone replacement therapy in breast cancer survivors. *J Natl Cancer Inst.* 2008;100:475-482.

21. von Schoultz E, Rutqvist LE. Menopausal hormone therapy after breast cancer: the Stockholm randomized trial. *J Natl Cancer Inst.* 2005;97:533-535.

22. Col NF, Hirota LK, Orr RK, et al. Hormone replacement therapy after breast cancer: a systematic review and quantitative assessment of risk. *J Clin Oncol.* 2001;19:2357-2363.

23. Loprinzi CL, Michalak JC, Quella SK, et al. Megestrol acetate for the prevention of hot flashes. *N Engl J Med.* 1994;331:347-352.

24. Quella SK, Loprinzi CL, Sloan JA, et al. Long term use of megestrol acetate by cancer survivors for the treatment of hot flashes. *Cancer.* 1998;82:1784-1788.

25. Bertelli G, Venturini M, Del Mastro L, et al. Intramuscular depot medroxyprogesterone versus oral megestrol for the control of postmenopausal hot flashes in breast cancer patients: a randomized study. *Ann Oncol.* 2002;13:883-888.

26. Loprinzi CL, Levitt R, Barton D, et al. Phase III comparison of depomedroxyprogesterone acetate to venlafaxine for managing hot flashes: North Central Cancer Treatment Group Trial N99C7. *J Clin Oncol.* 2006;24:1409-1414.

27. Dixon AR, Jackson L, Chan S, et al. A randomised trial of second-line hormone vs single agent chemotherapy in tamoxifen resistant advanced breast cancer. *Br J Cancer.* 1992;66:402-404.

28. Hofseth LJ, Raafat AM, Osuch JR, et al. Hormone replacement therapy with estrogen or estrogen plus medroxyprogesterone acetate is associated with increased epithelial proliferation in the normal postmenopausal breast. *J Clin Endocrinol Metab.* 1999;84:4559-4565.

29. Sartor O, Eastham JA. Progressive prostate cancer associated with use of megestrol acetate administered for control of hot flashes. *South Med J.* 1999;92:415-416.

30. Loprinzi CL, Sloan J, Stearns V, et al. Newer antidepressants and gabapentin for hot flashes: an individual patient pooled analysis. *J Clin Oncol.* 2009;27:2831-2837.

31. Nelson HD, Vesco KK, Haney E, et al. Nonhormonal therapies for menopausal hot flashes: systematic review and meta-analysis. *JAMA.* 2006;295:2057-2071.

32. Loprinzi CL, Pisansky TM, Fonseca R, et al. Pilot evaluation of venlafaxine hydrochloride for the therapy of hot flashes in cancer survivors. *J Clin Oncol.* 1998;16:2377-2381.

33. Loprinzi CL, Kugler JW, Sloan JA, et al. Venlafaxine in management of hot flashes in survivors of breast cancer: a randomised controlled trial. *Lancet.* 2000;356:2059-2063.

34. Evans ML, Pritts E, Vittinghoff E, et al. Management of postmenopausal hot flushes with venlafaxine hydrochloride: a randomized, controlled trial. *Obstet Gynecol.* 2005;105:161-166.

35. Bordeleau L, Pritchard KI, Loprinzi CL, et al. Multicenter, randomized, cross-over clinical trial of venlafaxine versus gabapentin for the management of hot flashes in breast cancer survivors. *J Clin Oncol.* 2010;28:5147-5152.

36. Quella SK, Loprinzi CL, Sloan J, et al. Pilot evaluation of venlafaxine for the treatment of hot flashes in men undergoing androgen ablation therapy for prostate cancer. *J Urol.* 1999;162:98-102.

37. Irani J, Salomon L, Oba R, et al. Efficacy of venlafaxine, medroxyprogesterone acetate, and cyproterone acetate for the treatment of vasomotor hot flushes in men taking gonadotropin-releasing hormone analogues for prostate cancer: a double-blind, randomised trial. *Lancet Oncol.* 2010;11:147-154.

38. Archer DF, Seidman L, Constantine GD, et al. A double-blind, randomly assigned, placebo-controlled study of desvenlafaxine efficacy and safety for the treatment of vasomotor symptoms associated with menopause. *Am J Obstet Gynecol.* 2009;200:172.e1-172.e10.

39. Speroff L, Gass M, Constantine G, et al. Efficacy and tolerability of desvenlafaxine succinate treatment for menopausal vasomotor symptoms: a randomized controlled trial. *Obstet Gynecol.* 2008;111:77-87.

40. Stearns V, Isaacs C, Rowland J, et al. A pilot trial assessing the efficacy of paroxetine hydrochloride (Paxil) in controlling hot flashes in breast cancer survivors. *Ann Oncol.* 2000;11:17-22.

41. Stearns V, Beebe KL, Iyengar M, et al. Paroxetine controlled release in the treatment of menopausal hot flashes: a randomized controlled trial. *JAMA.* 2003;289:2827-2834.

42. Stearns V, Slack R, Greep N, et al. Paroxetine is an effective treatment for hot flashes: results from a prospective randomized clinical trial. *J Clin Oncol.* 2005;23:6919-6930.

43. Loprinzi CL, Barton DL, Carpenter LA, et al. Pilot evaluation of paroxetine for treating hot flashes in men. *Mayo Clin Proc.* 2004;79:1247-1251.

44. Naoe M, Ogawa Y, Shichijo T, et al. Pilot evaluation of selective serotonin reuptake inhibitor antidepressants in hot flash patients under androgen-deprivation therapy for prostate cancer. *Prostate Cancer Prostatic Dis.* 2006;9:275-278.

45. Loprinzi CL, Sloan JA, Perez EA, et al. Phase III evaluation of fluoxetine for treatment of hot flashes. *J Clin Oncol.* 2002;20:1578-1583.

46. Suvanto-Luukkonen E, Koivunen R, Sundstrom H, et al. Citalopram and fluoxetine in the treatment of postmenopausal symptoms: a prospective, randomized, 9-month, placebo-controlled, double-blind study. *Menopause.* 2005;12:18-26.

47. Barton DL, LaVasseur BI, Sloan JA, et al. Phase III, placebo-controlled trial of three doses of citalopram for the treatment of hot flashes: NCCTG trial N05C9. *J Clin Oncol.* 2010;28:3278-3283.

48. Freeman EW, Guthrie KA, Caan B, et al. Efficacy of escitalopram for hot flashes in healthy menopausal women: a randomized controlled trial. *JAMA.* 2011;305:267-274.

49. Kimmick GG, Lovato J, McQuellon R, et al. Randomized, double-blind, placebo-controlled, crossover study of sertraline (Zoloft) for the treatment of hot flashes in women with early stage breast cancer taking tamoxifen. *Breast J.* 2006;12:114-122.

50. Gordon PR, Kerwin JP, Boesen KG, et al. Sertraline to treat hot flashes: a randomized controlled, double-blind, crossover trial in a general population. *Menopause.* 2006;13:568-575.

51. Grady D, Cohen B, Tice J, et al. Ineffectiveness of sertraline for treatment of menopausal hot flushes: a randomized controlled trial. *Obstet Gynecol.* 2007;109:823-830.

52. Perez DG, Loprinzi CL, Barton DL, et al. Pilot evaluation of mirtazapine for the treatment of hot flashes. *J Support Oncol.* 2004;2:50-56.

53. Biglia N, Kubatzki F, Sgandurra P, et al. Mirtazapine for the treatment of hot flushes in breast cancer survivors: a prospective pilot trial. *Breast J.* 2007;13:490-495.

54. Kelly CM, Juurlink DN, Gomes T, et al. Selective serotonin reuptake inhibitors and breast cancer mortality in women receiving tamoxifen: a population based cohort study. *BMJ.* 2010;340:c693.

55. Kiyotani K, Mushiroda T, Imamura CK, et al. Significant effect of polymorphisms in CYP2D6 and ABCC2 on clinical outcomes of adjuvant tamoxifen therapy for breast cancer patients. *J Clin Oncol.* 2010;28:1287-1293.

56. Desmarais JE, Looper KJ. Interactions between tamoxifen and antidepressants via cytochrome P450 2D6. *J Clin Psychiatry.* 2009;70:1688-1697.

57. Lash TL, Cronin-Fenton D, Ahern TP, et al. Breast cancer recurrence risk related to concurrent use of SSRI antidepressants and tamoxifen. *Acta Oncol.* 2010;49:305-312.

58. Guttuso TJ Jr. Gabapentin's effects on hot flashes and hypothermia. *Neurology.* 2000;54:2161-2163.

59. Guttuso T Jr, Kurlan R, McDermott MP, et al. Gabapentin's effects on hot flashes in postmenopausal women: a randomized controlled trial. *Obstet Gynecol.* 2003;101:337-345.

60. Butt DA, Lock M, Lewis JE, et al. Gabapentin for the treatment of menopausal hot flashes: a randomized controlled trial. *Menopause.* 2008;15:310-318.

61. Reddy SY, Warner H, Guttuso T Jr, et al. Gabapentin, estrogen, and placebo for treating hot flushes: a randomized controlled trial. *Obstet Gynecol.* 2006;108:41-48.

62. Pandya KJ, Morrow GR, Roscoe JA, et al. Gabapentin for hot flashes in 420 women with breast cancer: a randomised double-blind placebo-controlled trial. *Lancet.* 2005;366:818-824.

63. Loprinzi CL, Dueck AC, Khoyratty BS, et al. A phase III randomized, double-blind, placebo-controlled trial of gabapentin in the management of hot flashes in men (N00CB). *Ann Oncol.* 2009;20:542-549.

64. Presant CA, Kelly, C. Palliation of vasomotor instability (hot flashes) using pregabalin. *Community Oncol.* 2007;4:83-84.

65. Loprinzi CL, Qin R, Balcueva EP, et al. Phase III, randomized, double-blind, placebo-controlled evaluation of pregabalin for alleviating hot flashes, N07C1. *J Clin Oncol.* 2010;28:641-647.

66. Thompson S, Bardia A, Tan A, et al. Levetiracetam for the treatment of hot flashes: a phase II study. *Support Care Cancer.* 2008;16:75-82.

67. Goldberg RM, Loprinzi CL, O'Fallon JR, et al. Transdermal clonidine for ameliorating tamoxifen-induced hot flashes. *J Clin Oncol.* 1994;12:155-158.

68. Loprinzi CL, Goldberg RM, O'Fallon JR, et al. Transdermal clonidine for ameliorating post-orchiectomy hot flashes. *J Urol.* 1994;151:634-636.

69. Pandya KJ, Raubertas RF, Flynn PJ, et al. Oral clonidine in postmenopausal patients with breast cancer experiencing tamoxifen-induced hot flashes: a University of Rochester Cancer Center Community Clinical Oncology Program study. *Ann Intern Med.* 2000;132:788-793.

70. Bergmans MG, Merkus JM, Corbey RS, et al. Effect of Bellergal Retard on climacteric complaints: a double-blind, placebo-controlled study. *Maturitas.* 1987;9:227-234.

71. David A, Don R, Tajchner G, et al. Veralipride: alternative antidopaminergic treatment for menopausal symptoms. *Am J Obstet Gynecol.* 1988;158:1107-1115.

72. Melis GB, Gambacciani M, Cagnacci A, et al. Effects of the dopamine antagonist veralipride on hot flushes and luteinizing hormone secretion in postmenopausal women. *Obstet Gynecol.* 1988;72:688-692.

73. Barton DL, Loprinzi CL, Quella SK, et al. Prospective evaluation of vitamin E for hot flashes in breast cancer survivors. *J Clin Oncol.* 1998;16:495-500.

74. Ziaei S, Kazemnejad A, Zareai M. The effect of vitamin E on hot flashes in menopausal women. *Gynecol Obstet Invest.* 2007;64:204-207.

75. Bardia A, Tleyjeh IM, Cerhan JR, et al. Efficacy of antioxidant supplementation in reducing primary cancer incidence and mortality: systematic review and meta-analysis. *Mayo Clin Proc.* 2008;83:23-34.

76. Pruthi S, Qin R, Terstreip SA, et al. A phase III, randomized, placebo-controlled, double-blind trial of flaxseed for the treatment of hot flashes: NCCTG N08C7. *Menopause.* 2012; 19:48-53.

77. Kronenberg F, Fugh-Berman A. Complementary and alternative medicine for menopausal symptoms: a review of randomized, controlled trials. *Ann Intern Med.* 2002;137:805-813.

78. Jacobson JS, Troxel AB, Evans J, et al. Randomized trial of black cohosh for the treatment of hot flashes among women with a history of breast cancer. *J Clin Oncol.* 2001;19:2739-2745.

79. Pockaj BA, Gallagher JG, Loprinzi CL, et al. Phase III double-blind, randomized, placebo-controlled crossover trial of black cohosh in the management of hot flashes: NCCTG trial N01CC1. *J Clin Oncol.* 2006;24:2836-2841.

80. Geller SE, Shulman LP, van Breemen RB, et al. Safety and efficacy of black cohosh and red clover for the management of vasomotor symptoms: a randomized controlled trial. *Menopause.* 2009;16:1156-1166.

81. Shams T, Setia MS, Hemmings R, et al. Efficacy of black cohosh-containing preparations on menopausal symptoms: a meta-analysis. *Altern Ther Health Med.* 2010;16:36-44.

82. Firenzuoli F, Gori L, di Sarsina PR. Black cohosh hepatic safety: follow-up of 107 patients consuming a special cimicifuga racemosa rhizome herbal extract and review of literature. *Evid Based Complement Alternat Med.* 2011;2011:821392.

83. Lau CB, Ho TC, Chan TW, et al. Use of dong quai (*Angelica sinensis*) to treat peri- or postmenopausal symptoms in women with breast cancer: is it appropriate? *Menopause.* 2005;12:734-740.

84. Lee MS, Kim KH, Choi SM, et al. Acupuncture for treating hot flashes in breast cancer patients: a systematic review. *Breast Cancer Res Treat.* 2009;115:497-503.

85. Cho SH, Whang WW. Acupuncture for vasomotor menopausal symptoms: a systematic review. *Menopause.* 2009;16:1065-1073.

86. Lee MS, Shin BC, Ernst E. Acupuncture for treating menopausal hot flushes: a systematic review. *Climacteric.* 2009;12:16-25.

87. Lee MS, Kim KH, Shin BC, et al. Acupuncture for treating hot flushes in men with prostate cancer: a systematic review. *Support Care Cancer.* 2009;17:763-770.

88. Kim KH, Kang KW, Kim DI, et al. Effects of acupuncture on hot flashes in perimenopausal and postmenopausal women—a multicenter randomized clinical trial. *Menopause.* 2010;17:269-280.

89. Tremblay A, Sheeran L, Aranda SK. Psychoeducational interventions to alleviate hot flashes: a systematic review. *Menopause.* 2008;15:193-202.

90. Haest K, Kumar A, Leunen K, et al. Does the stellate ganglion block reduce severe hot flushes and sleep disturbances in breast cancer patients? *Cancer Res.* 2009;69(24 suppl):Abstract 809.

91. Lipov EG, Joshi JR, Sanders S, et al. Effects of stellate-ganglion block on hot flushes and night awakenings in survivors of breast cancer: a pilot study. *Lancet Oncol.* 2008;9:523-532.

92. Pachman DR, Barton D, Carns PE, et al. Pilot evaluation of a stellate ganglion block for the treatment of hot flashes. *Support Care Cancer.* 2011;19:941-947.

93. Lipov E, Kelzenberg BM. Stellate ganglion block (SGB) to treat perimenopausal hot flashes: clinical evidence and neurobiology. *Maturitas.* 2011;69:95-96.

94. Elkins G, Marcus J, Stearns V, et al. Pilot evaluation of hypnosis for the treatment of hot flashes in breast cancer survivors. *Psychooncology.* 2007;16:487-492.

95. Stevenson DW, Delprato DJ. Multiple component self-control program for menopausal hot flashes. *J Behav Ther Exp Psychiatry.* 1983;14:137-140.

96. Elkins G, Marcus J, Stearns V, et al. Randomized trial of a hypnosis intervention for treatment of hot flashes among breast cancer survivors. *J Clin Oncol.* 2008;26:5022-5026.

97. Bardia A, Novotny P, Sloan J, et al. Efficacy of nonestrogenic hot flash therapies among women stratified by breast cancer history and tamoxifen use: a pooled analysis. *Menopause.* 2009;16:477-483.

98. Loprinzi CL, Wolf SL. Hot flushes: mostly sex neutral? *Lancet Oncol.* 2010;11:107-108.

CHAPTER 10

Anorexia/Weight Loss

Egidio Del Fabbro ■ Eduardo Bruera

CACHEXIA

Cancer cachexia is defined as a multifactorial syndrome characterized by involuntary loss of skeletal muscle (with or without fat loss) that leads to progressive, impaired function and cannot be fully reversed by conventional nutritional support (1). Cancer cachexia is common, reported to occur in up to 90% of patients with advanced cancer, and is often accompanied by a pro-inflammatory response and a cluster of symptoms that include fatigue and poor appetite. The clinical implications of cancer cachexia are profound, since weight loss is associated with more chemotherapy-related side effects; fewer completed cycles of chemotherapy; and decreased survival (2,3). Furthermore, severe involuntary weight loss impairs cancer patients' quality of life (QOL) (4) and sense of dignity (5).

EPIDEMIOLOGY

An autopsy series of 816 patients with solid tumors at MD Anderson Cancer Center found that infection was the commonest cause of death, followed by organ failure; however, in 10% of patients no cause could be attributed other than severe emaciation and/or electrolyte imbalance (6). Subsequently, a landmark study by Dewys et al. (3) of more than 3,000 patients reported a shorter median survival in patients with weight loss compared with those without weight loss. Except in patients with pancreatic or gastric cancer, decreased weight correlated with poor performance status and within each performance status category or tumor stage, weight loss was associated with decreased survival. Up to 70% of patients with breast cancer or acute lymphoblastic leukemia had no evidence of weight loss, but about half of prostate cancer, colon cancer, and lung cancer patients experienced weight loss and 85% of gastric and pancreatic patients lost weight (one-third >10%). The study also suggested that any weight loss (0% to 5%) was associated with a poorer prognosis, and the prognostic effect of weight loss was greater in patients with a more favorable prognosis (good performance status or early tumor stage).

A prospective study carried out in 1979 at the National Cancer Institute in Milan of 280 patients with a variety of tumors (7) reported that specific cancers and advanced stage were more likely to be associated with weight loss. Patients with upper gastrointestinal tumors (esophagus and stomach) had significantly decreased weight, serum albumin, and triceps skinfold thickness, and treatment with chemotherapy or radiotherapy was associated with an additional decrease in arm muscle circumference. Malnutrition also became progressively more severe as the disease advanced, except in patients with breast or cervix cancer.

PROGNOSIS

A number of studies have reported that weight loss is associated with a poor prognosis in patients with advanced cancer. A systematic review of prognostic factors in patients with recently diagnosed incurable cancer showed (8) that weight loss, fatigue, anorexia, nausea, dyspnea, pain, multiple comorbidities, and poor performance status were all associated with decreased survival.

In 1,555 consecutive patients with locally advanced or metastatic gastrointestinal carcinomas (esophagus, stomach, pancreas, and colorectal), weight loss at presentation was more common in men than in women and correlated with decreased tumor response, QOL, and performance status (9). Patients with weight loss received lower chemotherapy doses, but they developed more severe dose-limiting toxicity (plantar–palmar syndrome and stomatitis) and received 1 month less treatment. Another prospective study of 770 lung cancer patients found that weight loss was reported by 59%, 58%, and 76% of patients with small cell lung cancer, non–small cell lung cancer (NSCLC), and mesothelioma, respectively (10), and those patients with weight loss had increased treatment toxicity and decreased survival.

MECHANISMS OF CACHEXIA

Starvation versus Cachexia

Unlike starvation, which is characterized by a loss of fat primarily, weight loss due to cachexia is characterized by a loss of both muscle and fat (Table 10.1). Cachexia will occur despite caloric supplementation and can be differentiated from starvation by endocrine abnormalities such as insulin and ghrelin resistance and frequently also by increased

TABLE 10.1 Starvation versus cachexia		
	Starvation	**Cachexia**
Caloric intake	↓↓	↓
Resting energy expenditure	↓	↓↑ or ↔
Body fat	↓↓	↓
Lean body mass	↓	↓↓
Inflammatory markers	↔	↑ or ↔
Insulin	↓	↑

↔, unchanged; ↓, reduced; ↓↓, markedly reduced; ↓↑, increased or reduced; ↑, increased.

resting energy expenditure. Unfortunately, most patients with cancer cachexia will also have a significant component of "starvation" that exacerbates muscle wasting through either a decline in appetite or other symptoms that affect oral intake (e.g., nausea and dysgeusia).

Inflammation

An aberrant pro-inflammatory response as a result of the tumor–host interaction has detrimental effects on cell metabolism, protein synthesis, hormone action, and the autonomic nervous system (ANS). Although increased activity of pro-inflammatory cytokines is proposed as the principle unifying mechanism causing both anorexia (11) and muscle wasting (12), the pathophysiology of cachexia is complex and multifactorial (Figure 10.1), so none of the interrelated mechanisms that contribute to this syndrome should be viewed in isolation. The primary sites of dysregulation are known to be the hypothalamus centrally (producing anorexia) and skeletal muscle and adipose tissue peripherally (increased catabolism and decreased anabolism).

Peripheral

In cancer cachexia, pro-inflammatory cytokines appear to induce muscle wasting by targeting only certain muscle gene products. Skeletal muscle is composed of core myofibrillar proteins, including myosin heavy chain (MyHC), actin, troponin, and tropomyosin. Transcription of the myosin heavy chain gene and many other muscle genes is regulated in part by the nuclear transcription factor MyoD. Myogenic cell cultures and animal models of tumor-induced cachexia indicate that MyHC is a selective target for pro-cachectic inflammatory cytokines (TNF-α and IFN-γ) by inhibiting MyoD and increasing the degradation of MyHC via the ligase-dependent ubiquitin–proteasome pathway (by IL-6) (13). The ubiquitin ligase–dependent proteasome pathway is a major cellular mechanism that degrades proteins and regulates skeletal muscle wasting in cancer and other disease states.

These basic science studies demonstrating the dual requirement of inflammatory cytokines for muscle wasting are supported by recent clinical trials showing interventions (etanercept (14) and infliximab (15)) against a single cytokine (TNF-α) produced no improvement in cachexia-related clinical outcomes.

More recently, animal models indicated that the muscle wasting induced by circulating cytokines may be modulated by genetic ablation of adipose triglyceride lipase (ATL) (16). Animals with and without ATL activity were injected with tumor cells, which resulted in high circulating levels of inflammatory cytokines such as IL-6, TNF-α, and lipid-mobilizing factor (zinc-α$_2$-glycoprotein). However, only the animals with ATL activity experienced adipose tissue wasting and subsequent muscle loss accompanied by an increased expression of the ubiquitin–proteasome pathway. These studies suggest that lipolysis plays an important role in cancer cachexia and that lipases may be important therapeutic targets for the prevention of muscle wasting.

Finally, the identification of specific factors produced by the tumor, e.g., PIF (proteolysis-inducing factor), may be important for future therapeutic targets (17).

Central

Systemic pro-inflammatory cytokines stimulate the production of cytokines within the hypothalamus. Pro-inflammatory cytokines are implicated in causing anorexia by stimulating neural pathways within the arcuate nucleus of the hypothalamus to secrete anorexigenic peptides such as α-melanocyte-stimulating hormone (α-MSH), which is derived from proopiomelanocortin. α-MSH inhibits feeding and increases energy expenditure by activating melanocortin receptors, primarily the type 4 melanocortin receptor (MC4-R). In healthy animals, orally administered selective MC4-R antagonists (18) that penetrate the blood–brain barrier increase food intake, and in mice with C26 adenocarcinoma, selective MC4-R antagonists prevent tumor-induced loss of body weight, fat mass, and lean body mass. Inflammatory cytokines also inhibit the release of orexigenic neuropeptides such as agouti-related protein from another set of neurons within the hypothalamus that stimulate feeding.

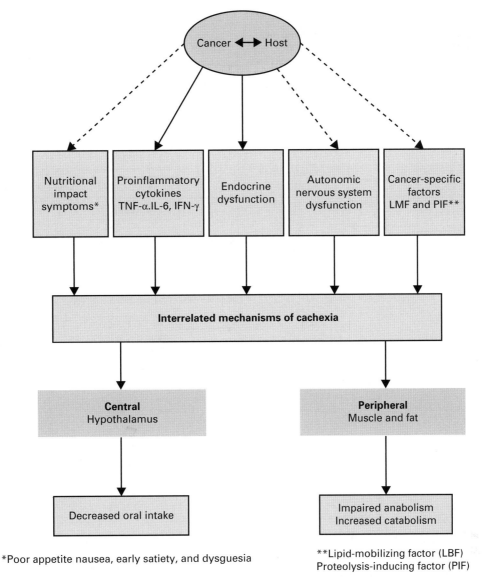

Figure 10.1. Mechanisms of cancer cachexia.

Cytokines also have other central effects that decrease the oral intake indirectly by producing symptoms such as early satiety (via IL-1) and depression (IL-6) (19).

Although animal models have shown a compelling association between pro-inflammatory cytokines and cachexia, the evidence in human studies is less consistent with some studies demonstrating a correlation between serum cytokines and clinical outcomes, e.g., weight loss (20,21) or performance status (22,23), and others showing no significant relationship (24–26). It might be that pro-inflammatory cytokines such as TNF-α act in a paracrine rather than in an endocrine fashion, so that serum levels do not accurately reflect tissue concentrations (27) or that single-nucleotide polymorphisms (28–30) determine an individual's susceptibility to developing cachexia. In addition, as described earlier in this chapter, animal models of cachexia suggest that downstream targets such as ATL may be key determinants of susceptibility to circulating inflammatory cytokines.

Neuroendocrine

The neural pathways within the hypothalamus are also influenced by orexigenic anti-inflammatory hormones such as ghrelin and testosterone. Ghrelin and insulin levels are elevated in patients with cachexia, suggesting resistance to these hormones, possibly mediated by inflammatory cytokines. In addition, the ANS may play a role in producing the syndrome of cachexia. Since many patients with advanced cancer have a dysfunctional ANS (31), other chronic sympathetic activation (32,33) or abnormalities of parasympathetic nerves such as the vagus, which has a role in ghrelin activity (34) and an acute anti-inflammatory effect (35), may amplify the mechanisms causing cachexia (Figure 10.2).

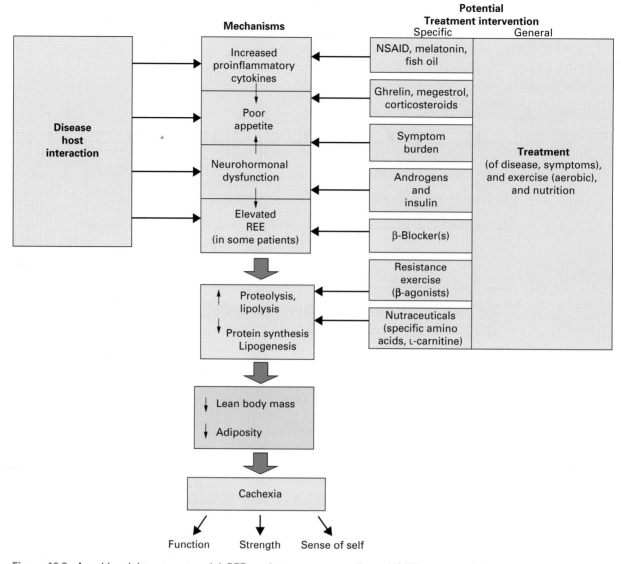

Figure 10.2. A multimodal treatment model. REE, resting energy expenditure; NSAID, non-steroidal anti-inflammatory drug.

DIAGNOSIS OF CACHEXIA

The diagnosis of cachexia is obvious in those patients who present with temporal wasting, anorexia, poor performance status, and a markedly underweight body mass index (BMI). The challenge is to diagnose patients earlier in the disease trajectory so as to initiate effective therapy before cachexia becomes "refractory" to intervention or patients are unable to comply with anti-cachexia treatment because of disease progression, frailty, or delirium. A history of weight loss >5% within the previous 6 months in the absence of simple starvation is most consistently used for the diagnosis of cachexia in clinical trials. The history of weight loss is important to obtain, since an underweight BMI at an initial visit is the exception in most outpatients because of the increased prevalence of obesity in the general population; 95% of patients referred to a cachexia clinic at a comprehensive cancer center

had a normal or even overweight BMI (36) despite having metastatic cancer and a palliative care outpatient center reported marked weight loss in 71% of patients (30% with significant muscle mass reduction) in spite of a normal or increased BMI (37).

CLASSIFICATION

Patients considered for intervention trials should be enrolled at similar points along their illness trajectory. Unfortunately, patients with cachexia may be enrolled in clinical trials at different inception points, making it very difficult to compare outcomes between participants and between clinical trials. Also, many participants in cachexia intervention trials are frail and often unable to complete the full duration of study treatment. To address these challenges a classification of cachexia has been proposed by an International Consensus

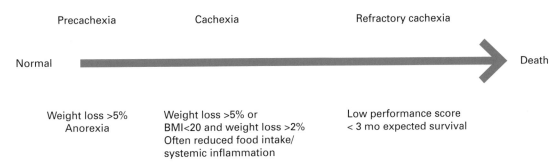

Figure 10.3. Classification of cachexia.

Group that divides the syndrome into cachexia, pre-cachexia, and refractory cachexia (Figure 10.3). Pre-cachexia is characterized by early clinical and metabolic signs (e.g., anorexia, impaired glucose tolerance, or elevated C-reactive protein [CRP]) that may precede an involuntary weight loss of ≤5%. Patients who have >5% loss of body weight over the last 6 months, or a BMI <20 kg/m^2 and ongoing weight loss of >2%, or sarcopenia (skeletal muscle index of males <7.26 kg/m^2 and females <5.45 kg/m^2) and ongoing weight loss of >2% (but have not entered the refractory stage) are classified as having cachexia. The last stage, refractory cachexia, attempts to identify those patients with weight loss that are thought to be "refractory" to anti-cachexia therapy. Patients with cachexia who have a poor performance status (WHO 3 or 4) and a life expectancy of <3 months are placed within this category. In future, criteria need to be determined for patients that will be predictive of resistance to therapeutic interventions.

CLINICAL ASSESSMENT

The clinical assessment includes a careful history that is focused on nutrition (quantity and composition), symptoms contributing to poor oral intake, weight and body composition, a physical examination, and identification of any reversible metabolic abnormalities.

A clinical approach to cachexia in terms of "primary" and "secondary" cachexia is a useful framework for approaching the clinical management of patients with cancer and involuntary weight loss. Primary cachexia denotes the syndrome (discussed earlier in this chapter) that is characterized by muscle loss (with or without loss of fat). Secondary cachexia includes potentially treatable contributors to the weight loss of primary cachexia such as nutritional impact symptoms (NISs) and comorbid metabolic abnormalities (e.g., hypogonadism, thyroid dysfunction, and vitamin B$_{12}$ and vitamin D deficiency). Other causes of weight loss that have a predominant starvation component such as gastrointestinal obstruction may also be included in this category, especially if they respond to endoscopic or surgical treatment (e.g., stent placement or endoscopic dilatation for esophageal obstruction).

Nutritional Impact Symptoms

Advanced cancer patients with cachexia may have multiple concurrent symptoms that compromise oral intake and contribute to nutritional decline (Table 10.2). These NISs have been included in the Patient-Generated Subjective Global Assessment (PG-SGA) of Nutritional Status, a validated screening tool that includes a patient report of weight and weight change, food intake, symptoms, activities, function, and a physician evaluation of the disease and its related nutritional requirements. NISs listed in the PG-SGA include poor appetite, pain, nausea, vomiting, constipation, altered smell and taste, mouth sores, dry mouth, dysphagia, depression, and diarrhea. The NIS section of the PG-SGA questionnaire is completed by patients and it provides the clinician with important information since many NISs can be treated effectively with inexpensive therapies. Although NIS can be assessed without completion of the entire PG-SGA, the screening tool has other advantages in terms of identifying patients at risk for malnutrition and facilitating quantitative outcome data collection for research purposes. The PG-SGA uses a numerical score as well as provides a global rating of well-nourished, moderately, or suspected of being malnourished or severely malnourished. The higher the score, the greater is the risk for malnutrition. A score of ≥9 indicates a critical need for nutrition intervention. Nutrition triage recommendations include patient and family education, symptom management, and nutrition intervention such as additional food, oral nutrition supplements, and enteral or parenteral nutrition (PN). In clinical practice, the scored PG-SGA has been shown to be a quick, valid, and reliable nutrition assessment tool that enables malnourished patients with cancer to be identified and triaged for nutritional support (38) and has been accepted by the Oncology Nutrition Dietetic Practice Group of the American Dietetic Association as the standard for nutrition assessment of patients with cancer. A retrospective study at a comprehensive cancer center found that most patients with involuntary weight loss had three or more uncontrolled NISs Table 10.2 shows the interventions commonly used to treat NIS.

The Edmonton Symptom Assessment Scale is a valid, commonly used questionnaire in cancer patients that can

TABLE 10.2	Findings and interventions for secondary nutritional impact in 151 cancer patients referred to a cachexia clinic		
Nutritional Impact Symptoms	**Number (%)**	**Corresponding Interventions**	**Number (% Treated Among Affected Individuals)**
Early satiety	94 (62%)	Metoclopramide	74 (79%)
Constipation	78 (52%)	Laxatives	68 (87%)
Nausea or vomiting	67 (44%)	Antiemetics (mostly metoclopramide)	54 (81%)
Depressed mood	63 (42%)	Antidepressant (mostly mirtazapine)	51 (81%)
Dysgeusia	42 (28%)	Zinc supplement	20 (48%)
Dysphagia	21 (14%)	GI or speech therapy evaluation	5 (24%)
Dry mouth	14 (9%)	Artificial saliva	2 (14%)
Mucositis	11 (7%)	Opioids and topical mouthwash	3 (27%)
Dental pain	8 (5%)	Dental referral	2 (25%)

GI, gastrointestinal.

From Del Fabbro E, Hui D, Dalal S, et al. Clinical outcomes and contributors to weight loss in a cancer cachexia clinic. *J Palliat Med.* 2011 September;14(9):1004-1008.

identify the presence as well as the severity of some NISs such as nausea, depression, and fatigue, but unfortunately it does not include many other NISs such as early satiety, constipation, and dysgeusia.

Body Composition

Although both muscle and fat are usually depleted in patients with cachexia, the body composition in patients with the same BMI could vary considerably. Most patients reporting weight loss have normal or elevated BMIs and a significant proportion of obese cancer patients (20%) are sarcopenic. Muscle wasting may therefore be underrecognized and masked by adipose tissue. Patients with the combination of sarcopenia and obesity have a worse prognosis and a higher risk of chemotherapy-related adverse effects (39).

The least invasive method to assess body composition is the midarm muscle area which requires measuring the triceps skinfold thickness using calipers (in millimeters) and the midarm circumference (in centimeters) and entering them into the following equation: midarm muscle area = (midarm circumference in centimeters) − π × tricipital skinfold thickness in millimeters)2/(4 × π) − a correction factor of 10 for men and 6.5 for women.

Bioimpedance analysis (BIA) relies on the different electrical properties of fat and muscle (increased water content). The bioimpedance devices are relatively easy to use and not burdensome to patients, but they may provide falsely elevated results of muscle mass when patients have edema. Additional information such as the ratio of resistance and reactance (phase angle) provided by BIA may also be useful for prognostication (40).

Dual-energy X-ray absorptiometry (DEXA) scans are based on the three-component model of body composition. DEXA uses two x-ray energies to measure body fat, muscle, and bone mineral. DEXA is more burdensome to patients (must be in supine position while the image is taken) than BIA and is more expensive. The results may be viewed as whole body estimates of body fat, muscle, and bone mineral as well as regional body estimates.

Computed tomography (CT) scan is expensive and not practical for many palliative care patients with cachexia. However for those patients who are being routinely evaluated for the purpose of restaging and follow-up, CT is useful to distinguish between muscle and adipose tissue (41) and can be used to assess body composition changes longitudinally.

Indirect Calorimetry

Handheld indirect calorimetry (IC) provides more detailed information regarding patients' caloric requirements and identifies the presence of hypermetabolism. Since more than 80% of caloric daily requirements are due to basal energy expenditure (BEE), IC will provide an accurate measured BEE for an individual rather than a "predicted estimate," e.g., by using a formula such as the Harris Benedict Equation (HBE). About half of patients with cachexia will be hypermetabolic (BEE > 110% of predicted). The assessment of BEE by IC allows clinicians to recommend more accurate, individualized daily caloric goals. In addition there is evidence that elevated metabolic rates may be modified pharmacologically, so that IC may be useful in future to determine therapeutic options. Preliminary studies using β-blockers (42) have demonstrated some success in decreasing the resting energy expenditure of hypermetabolic patients and maintaining lean body mass.

When IC is not practical, energy expenditure can be estimated by using equations such as the HBE or a general estimate of 30 to 35 kcal/kg body weight. These estimates should be used with caution since there are inconsistencies and variations in predicted estimates for energy requirements (43).

Harris Benedict Equation (kcal/day):

$$\text{Males} = 66.5 + (13.7 \times W) + (5.0 \times H) - (6.8 \times A)$$

$$\text{Females} = 655 + (9.6 \times W) + (1.7 \times H) - (4.7 \times A)$$

W = usual or adjusted weight in kilograms, H = height in centimeters, and A = age in years.

When using HBE, the total caloric requirements (TCRs) can be estimated by multiplying the BEE by the sum of the stress and activity factors, i.e., TCR = BEE × activity factor × stress factor. The stress factor for cancer is controversial, but depending on the clinical condition of the patient it ranges from 1.1 to 1.3 (44). The activity factors for sedentary patients are usually reported as 1.2.

Laboratory Assessment

Laboratory tests for levels of hormones and vitamins, such as testosterone, thyroid-stimulating hormone, vitamin B_{12}, and vitamin D, may be helpful to identify secondary causes of weight loss or muscle weakness. A retrospective study of patients with cancer referred to a cachexia clinic found that 73% of males were hypogonadic, while 4% of patients were hypothyroid and only 3% were vitamin B_{12} deficient (36). Another study of 100 consecutive patients complaining of moderate fatigue or poor appetite demonstrated a high frequency of low vitamin D levels (70%) (45). Although these vitamin and testosterone deficiencies are associated with muscle weakness and weight loss, their clinical relevance in cancer patients is unclear. Randomized placebo-controlled trials of replacement doses will be required to assess their impact on symptoms, function, and QOL. An elevated serum CRP level is helpful (but not essential) for the diagnosis of cachexia (and pre-cachexia) and useful for directing therapy with an immune modulator (e.g., non-steroidal anti-inflammatory drugs [NSAIDs]). Other laboratory tests that provide indirect evidence of the pro-inflammatory state and metabolic dysregulation include a decreased hemoglobin, elevated white blood cell count, and hypoalbuminemia.

MANAGEMENT

In the past, cachexia was seen as an inevitable consequence of cancer's progression, with no effective therapeutic interventions. While there have been advances in the management of cancer cachexia, with several trials (see Table 10.3) showing improved clinical outcomes including lean body mass, appetite, and function, it must be emphasized that there is still no standard treatment for cachexia. Because the mechanisms of the cachexia syndrome are multifactorial, a comprehensive multidimensional approach using pharmacologic and non-pharmacologic interventions is most likely to be effective in reversing or stabilizing weight loss and muscle wasting (46).

Ideally, treatment should be individualized, taking into account the patients' overall condition, the principal mechanisms of their weight loss, and their goals of care. Although many patients and their families perceive poor appetite as a significant burden, patients with cachexia may have very different priorities and so the therapeutic options may vary quite considerably. For many, maintaining lean body mass and function may be important, while for others the ability to preserve their appetite in order to enjoy meals with family and friends may be the primary goal. Some patients may be very concerned about their body image and the obvious, visible external manifestation of their illness.

Symptom Management

The foundation of cachexia management should begin with the identification and management of NISs contributing to decreased nutritional intake (Table 10.2). Early satiety is the most common gastrointestinal symptom in cachectic patients and can be treated effectively with metoclopramide (10 mg every 4 hours orally) (69). Metoclopramide enables the stomach to accommodate more food and improves motility. Patients should be made aware of the risk for extrapyramidal symptoms (particularly within the first 48 hours), which are usually reversible. Tardive dyskinesia, however, is often irreversible and the duration of treatment and total cumulative dose are associated with an increased risk. Metoclopramide treatment considered beyond 3 months should be discussed with patients regarding the risk versus benefit. Constipation may also contribute to early satiety and can be effectively managed with laxatives.

Depressed mood can also lead to decreased oral intake and should be managed with counseling and antidepressants if indicated. Mirtazapine and olanzapine are useful agents for both depression and nausea (70). Mirtazapine improves gastric accommodation and like metoclopramide has $5HT_4$ agonist activity that promotes gastric (71) emptying and intestinal secretions.

In animal models, orally administered zinc increases appetite and appears to mediate its effects through the vagus to increase expression of orexigenic hypothalamic neuropeptides (72). Zinc supplementation has objectively improved dysgeusia in a study of patients with advanced cancer complaining of taste alteration (73), but it was not effective in another placebo-controlled study (74) when administered prior to radiation therapy. In the absence of other effective agents, a trial of zinc sulfate is warranted in patients with dysgeusia since this supplement has few side effects.

Appetite Stimulation

Progestational agents such as megestrol acetate and medroxyprogesterone have improved appetite, body weight, and other symptoms such as fatigue and nausea. These benefits were confirmed by systematic reviews (75,76) and a Cochrane meta-analysis (64), but unfortunately the weight gain due to progestational agents appears to be predominantly fat or fluid rather than lean body mass.

TABLE 10.3   Review of selected cachexia trials

Author	Intervention	Methodology	Outcome Measured	Intervention Duration	Participants	Relevant Results
Thalidomide						
Davis et al. 2010 (47)	Thalidomide 50 mg for 2 wk, then 100 mg for 2 wk	Phase II dose escalation with 35 patients	Appetite weight	4 wk	Poor appetite and active cancer	Improved appetite and weight
Mantovani et al. 2008 (48)	Multimodal dietary supplement, antioxidants, and thalidomide 200 mg, progestin, L-carnitine, fish oil 2.2 g vs. any single agent	Randomized 332 patients	Appetite, Lean body mass strength, Physical activity PS, REE, Inflammatory cytokines	12 wk	Solid tumors, Weight loss >5%, Expected survival ≥4 mo	Only combination therapy, Improved all outcomes, Lean body mass, Resting energy expenditure, Physical activity, Performance status, IL-6 and TNF-α levels
Gordon et al. 2005 (49)	Thalidomide 200 mg	**RCT of 50 patients, placebo controlled**	Weight, Arm muscle	24 wk	Pancreatic cancer >10% weight loss	Improvement in weight and arm muscle mass compared with placebo
Bruera 1999 (82)	Thalidomide 100 mg qhs	Open-label single-arm, 37 patients	Appetite, Symptoms, Caloric intake	10 d	Metastatic cancer, decreased appetite, and weight loss >5%	Improved caloric intake and trend to better appetite
Melatonin						
Lissoni 2002 (51)	Melatonin 20 mg	**RCT of 1,440 patients, no placebo, unblinded**	Clinical response, Toxicity, Patient reported, Asthenia, Cachexia, Anorexia, Mood	12 mo	Untreatable advanced solid tumors	Cachexia, anorexia, and asthenia better in melatonin group; Assessment tool used to measure symptoms is unclear

Study	Intervention	Design	Outcome measure	Duration	Population	Results
Lissoni et al. 1996 (52)	Melatonin 20 mg	**RCT of 100 patients, no placebo, unblinded**	Prevention of 10% weight loss	12 wk	Metastatic solid tumors	Prevented >10% weight loss and decreased TNF-α levels, but no difference in caloric intake
Fish Oil						
Murphy et al. 2011 (53)	Fish oil 2.2 g	**RCT of 40 patients, no placebo**	Skeletal muscle Total adipose tissue	6 wk	Advanced cancer	Skeletal muscle improved as measured by CT
Ries et al. 2011 (54)	Fish oil/omega-3-FAs (n-3-FA)/EPA	**Systematic review of 38 included studies**	Cachexia	2–8 wk	Advanced cancer	Not enough evidence to support a net benefit of n-3-FA for cachexia in advanced cancer
van der Meij et al. 2010 (55)	Fish oil—enriched supplement	**RCT of 40 patients, placebo controlled**	Weight FFM Energy intake Arm circumference	4 wk	Stage III NSCLC	Improved all outcomes and trend for greater arm circumference
Dewey et al. 2007 (56)	Fish oil (EPA) 1.5–2.2 g	**Systematic review of 5 trials and 587 cancer patients**	Effectiveness and safety of EPA in relieving symptoms associated with cachexia	2–8 wk	Advanced cancer	Insufficient evidence for the use of fish oil (on its own or with other treatments) for weight loss in patients with advanced cancer
Burns et al. 2004 (57)	High-dose fish oil (4.7 g EPA and 2.8 g DHA as part of 8.5 g omega-3 FAs)	Phase II	Weight	>4 wk	Advanced cancer >2% weight loss in 1 mo	Majority did not gain weight and many had GI side effects, but a small subset of patients had weight stabilization or weight gain
NSAIDs						
Madeddu et al. 2011 (58)	Celecoxib plus L-carnitine plus megestrol vs. celecoxib plus L-carnitine	**RCT of 60 patients**	Lean body mass	4 mo	Advanced cancer Weight loss >5% last 6 mo	Non-inferiority of two drug combination vs. three drug combination

(Continued)

TABLE 10.3 **Review of selected cachexia trials** (*Continued*)

Author	Intervention	Methodology	Outcome Measured	Intervention Duration	Participants	Relevant Results
Lai et al. 2008 (59)	Celecoxib vs. placebo	**RCT of 11 patients**	Weight LBM QOL	3 wk	Head and neck or upper GI cancer With >5% weight loss	Celecoxib arm improved in weight and QOL No change in LBM, REE, and CRP
Mantovani et al. 2006 (60)	Antioxidants Medroxyprogesterone Celecoxib Omega-3 supplement	Single arm of 44 patients	Performance status Lean body mass Appetite Resting energy expenditure Pro-inflammatory cytokines Reactive oxygen Species QOL	16 wk	Advanced cancer, solid tumors	LBM, QOL, appetite, and pro-inflammatory cytokines all improved. Grip strength and PS did not
Cerchietti et al. 2004 (61)	Celecoxib plus medroxyprogesterone	Single-arm trial of 15 patients	Symptoms Weight Performance status	4 wk	Lung cancer, weight loss, anorexia, fatigue, performance status ≥2, and ↑ acute phase	Improved body-weight-change rate, nausea, early satiety, fatigue, appetite, and performance status
Mcmillan et al. 1999 (62)	Ibuprofen plus megace vs. megace plus placebo	**Randomized double-blind trial of 73 patients**	Weight QOL Midarm circumference	12 wk	Metastatic GI cancers Weight loss > 5%	Ibuprofen plus Megace more effective regarding weight preservation QOL Midarm circumference CRP levels No change in appetite

Reference	Intervention	Study type	Outcomes	Duration	Population	Results
Lundholm et al. 1994 (33)	Indomethacin or prednisone vs. placebo	Double-blind RCT of 135 patients	Survival Weight Arm circumference	Until death	Solid tumors with some weight loss	Indomethacin = better survival Prednisone showed greater weight gain and arm circumference Both groups maintained performance status better than placebo group
Megestrol						
Lesniak et al. 2008 (63)	Megestrol 160–1,600 mg in comparison with placebo or other drugs	Systematic review and meta-analysis of 30 studies including 5 abstracts	Appetite Weight gain QOL Survival PS	1 wk–2 y	Advanced cancer	Benefits for appetite NNT = 3 as effectively at lowest dose of 160 mg; benefit for weight NNT = 8 at lower dose also
Berenstein and Ortiz 2005 (64)	Megestrol 100–1,600 mg daily compared with placebo or other drugs	Systematic review including 26 RCTs with 4,148 cancer patients	Appetite Weight QOL	10 days–24 wk with a median of 8 wk	Solid and liquid tumors	Increased appetite weight gain compared with placebo Not dose dependent and no better QOL
Pascual Lopez et al. 2004 (65)	Megestrol 160–1,600 mg	Systematic review including 26 trials of 3,887 patients	Appetite Weight QOL	2–24 wk	Solid and liquid tumors	Appetite, weight, and QOL better Not dose dependent >800 vs. <800
Loprinzi et al. 1999 (66)	Megestrol vs. dexamethasone 0.75 mg qid, fluoxymesterone 10 mg orally bid	Randomized double-blind trial of 475 patients into 3 arms	Appetite Weight Adverse effects	4 wk	Cancer, lost 5lbs in 2 mo and PS 2 or better Advanced cancer	Megestrol and dexamethasone better appetite and weight Non-significant trend favoring megestrol More discontinued on Dexamethasone but more Thrombosis on megestrol

(Continued)

TABLE 10.3 Review of selected cachexia trials (*Continued*)

Author	Intervention	Methodology	Outcome Measured	Intervention Duration	Participants	Relevant Results
			Cannabinoids			
Strasser et al. 2006 (67)	Cannabis extract vs. delta-9-tetrahydrocannabinol vs. placebo	Three arms, double-blind RCT of 243 patients	Weight Appetite QOL	6 wk	Advanced cancer with 5% weight loss and PS ≥ 2	No difference in appetite, QOL, or weight
Jatoi et al. 2002 (68)	Megestrol plus dronabinol vs. dronabinol vs. megestrol	Randomized double-blind trial of 469 patients	Appetite Weight	4 wk	Advanced cancer, weight loss 5 lbs in 2 mo	Appetite and weight, QOL better with megace than with dronabinol Impotence worse

PS, pinch strength; REE, resting energy expenditure; RCT, randomized controlled trial; CT, computed tomography; FA, fatty acid; EPA, eicosapentaenoic acid; FFM, fat-free mass; NSCLC, non–small cell lung cancer; DHA, docosahexaenoic acid; GI, gastrointestinal; LBM, lean body mass; QOL, quality of life; CRP, C-reactive protein; NNT, number needed to treat.

The usual starting dose of megestrol acetate is 160 mg/d, titrating up to a maximum of 800 mg/d. Since two systematic reviews (73,74) found that improvement in appetite was not dose dependent (>800 mg vs. <800 mg were compared), it seems prudent to start at low doses and discuss the potential side effects with patients before initiating treatment. Common side effects include hypertension, hyperglycemia, and fluid retention; however, it is the more serious side effects such as thromboembolism, hypogonadism, and hypoadrenalism that often limit the use of these agents. While the risk for thromboembolism appears to be dose dependent, megestrol acetate < 480 mg/d does not appear to increase the incidence of thrombosis compared with placebo. Two studies using doses of 800 mg (33,66,77) reported an increased frequency of thromboembolism ranging from 5% to 9% versus 1% to 2% for placebo. Megestrol should be avoided in patients with a history of deep venous thrombosis, pulmonary embolism, or severe cardiac disease. Patients on megestrol should never discontinue their medication abruptly, as there is a risk of precipitating adrenal insufficiency, and stress dose corticosteroids should be given to those patients admitted for an acute illness. While patients are on megestrol, strong consideration should be given to monitoring testosterone levels, since profound hypogonadism is a common but treatable side effect. Clinical trials using megestrol in combination with other agents have not demonstrated any additive benefits. Large randomized studies comparing megestrol with combination therapy with either fish oil (78) or cannabinoids (68) have shown no greater benefit with combination therapy than with megestrol alone. These trials were of short duration (4 weeks) and outcomes of lean body mass and physical function were not assessed.

Corticosteroids may stimulate appetite, decrease nausea, and improve fatigue in the short term. The effects of corticosteroids on appetite and food intake are usually limited to a couple of weeks, and (79) the side effects such as myopathy, immunosuppression, and hyperglycemia increase dramatically over time. Corticosteroids should therefore be reserved for patients with limited life expectancy (<6 weeks). There is no established dose for corticosteroids, but doses of prednisone ranging from 5 to 40 mg or dexamethasone at an equivalent dosage are effective.

Cannabinoids: Dronabinol, a synthetic cannabinoid, is approved for use in anorexia related to AIDS and chemotherapy-induced nausea and emesis. A large multicenter trial (67) in cancer patients with anorexia showed no benefit of dronabinol or cannabis extract over placebo. Also, the use of dronabinol is limited by central nervous system side effects at higher doses, such as sedation, confusion, and perceptual disturbances. These side effects are especially of concern in advanced cancer patients, as they are at an increased risk for delirium.

Ghrelin and ghrelin agonists are under investigation in human trials after promising preliminary results showed improved appetite and gains in lean body mass. The dominant effect of these agents is likely to be an increased appetite, since ghrelin is the only orexigenic circulating hormone identified in humans. Ghrelin may also have beneficial effects on the immune and cardiovascular systems. The ghrelin mimetic anamorelin has shown benefit in preliminary trials (50) and is currently being tested in a large, multicenter, phase III study.

Immune Modulation

"Sickness behavior" manifested by fatigue and other related symptoms such as poor appetite is likely the result of an aberrant pro-inflammatory response. Therapy with immune modulators may therefore improve multiple symptoms associated with cachexia and advanced cancer. Non-specific immune modulators used in clinical trials for cancer cachexia include fish oil, thalidomide, NSAIDs, and melatonin.

Specific immune modulators such as IL-1 and IL-6 monoclonal antibodies (80) have demonstrated some potential as effective therapies in preliminary studies, but this should be tempered by recent placebo-controlled trials of TNF-α inhibitors, infliximab (15) and etanercept (14), which showed no weight gain or improved appetite in patients with cancer.

Non-steroidal Anti-inflammatory drugs

NSAIDs, including celecoxib, ibuprofen, and indomethacin, have been used in combination with other pharmacologic agents to treat cachexia (see Table 10.3). Indomethacin has been used in several trials, often in combination with β-blockers and nutritional support by the same group of investigators. A double-blind trial of indomethacin (50 mg bid) or prednisone (10 mg bid) versus placebo in 135 patients with solid tumors and weight loss showed improved survival in the group administered with indomethacin (33). The prednisone group demonstrated more weight gain and greater arm circumference. Subsequently, indomethacin along with erythropoietin in selected patients was adopted as standard of care and compared with patients who also received nutritional support (oral or home Parenteral Nutrition). Three hundred and nine patients with cachexia and solid tumors (primarily gastrointestinal) were randomized to this study, and besides an improvement in energy balance, there were no other differences in outcomes after intention-to-treat analysis (81). Most recently this multimodal approach (indomethacin, nutritional support, erythropoietin, and β-blockers in selected patients) was extended to include insulin. The study is discussed in *Hormone Replacement Therapies*.

The only prospective randomized study of an NSAID in combination with a progestin found that ibuprofen (1,200 mg daily in divided doses) and megestrol increased lean body mass and improved QOL compared with megestrol alone (62). Notably, individuals on combination therapy did not appear to be at greater risk for major hemorrhage than those on megestrol alone (800 mg daily). Other preliminary trials combining NSAIDs with progestins (either medroxyprogesterone or megestrol acetate) or with l-carnitine are given in Table 10.3 (60–62).

Thalidomide

As single-agent thalidomide has improved multiple symptoms, including appetite, nausea, and insomnia in patients with advanced cancer (4,82); however, its history of teratogencity and potential for side effects at high doses may limit its clinical use. Esophageal cancer (83) patients given 2 weeks of thalidomide (200 mg/d) experienced transitory somnolence and gained lean body mass loss, while a randomized placebo-controlled trial (49) of 50 patients with pancreatic cancer showed that thalidomide (200 mg/d) was well tolerated and effective at attenuating loss of weight and lean body mass after 4 weeks of therapy. There were no significant differences in QOL, survival, strength, or physical function between thalidomide and placebo. A recent dose escalation study (4) also confirmed the benefits of thalidomide at low doses (see Table 10.3); however, a cautionary randomized controlled study in advanced esophageal cancer using doses of 200 mg daily (84) suggested that the drug was poorly tolerated since only 6 patients given thalidomide and 16 patients given placebo completed the protocol; all withdrawals were due to adverse drug reactions or complications of disease. Thalidomide showed no benefit over placebo.

Melatonin

Melatonin (52) has shown some benefit as a therapy for cachexia and appears to have few adverse effects, even at doses of 20 mg daily, but unfortunately there are no placebo-controlled trials. Patients with metastatic solid tumors randomized to either supportive care alone or melatonin for a period of 3 months had weight loss >10% occur less often in the melatonin group and symptoms of depression and performance status improved from baseline. In a subsequent trial, patients with solid tumors who had received at least one cycle of chemotherapy and no prior biologic therapy were randomized to supportive care alone or supportive care plus 20 mg of melatonin at night (51). Cachexia, weakness, anorexia, and depression occurred more frequently in the group receiving supportive care alone.

Fish Oil

Fish oil has anti-inflammatory and anti-carcinogenic effects (85), and a long-term prospective study indicated that fish and long-chain n-3 fatty acids may decrease the risk of colorectal cancer (86). In patients with advanced pancreatic cancer, a protein-dense oral supplement enriched with n-3 fatty acid eicosapentaenoic acid (EPA) was associated with an encouraging increase in physical activity, despite no gain in weight or lean body mass (87). Unfortunately, the absence of any substantive improvement in appetite or weight has been reported in other randomized controlled trials and in at least two systematic reviews. A randomized placebo-controlled trial of 60 patients with advanced cancer showed no improvement in appetite or weight after 2 weeks and (81) systematic reviews by *Cochrane and the European Palliative Care Research Collaborative* (53,54) concluded that there was insufficient evidence to support the use of oral fish oil (on its own or in the presence of other treatments) in the management of cachexia in patients with advanced cancer (56). Despite these negative studies in patients with advanced cancer, fish oil may prove to be useful in some subsets of patients depending on their tumor type, disease trajectory, or ability to tolerate prolonged anti-cachexia therapy. A recent randomized controlled trial of 40 patients with NSCLC receiving chemotherapy showed gains in weight and skeletal muscle mass in those patients receiving fish oil (53), and an earlier phase II study suggested that higher doses of fish oil may be more effective in certain patients although likely to be limited by an increased frequency of gastrointestinal side effects (57). Finally, an industry-sponsored systematic review suggested that supplementation with 1.5 g daily of EPA and/or docosahexaenoic acid for prolonged periods (8 weeks) in pancreatic and upper digestive tract cancers seemed to be associated with improvements in various clinical, biochemical, and QOL parameters (88).

Hormone Replacement Therapies

Insulin

Cachexia is typically associated with insulin resistance, and so exogenous administration may benefit cachectic individuals. Although insulin decreases appetite centrally, it has peripheral anabolic effects particularly with regard to fat metabolism. A Swedish Group (89) randomized 138 patients with a variety of gastrointestinal malignancies to receive insulin plus supportive care versus supportive care alone. Once daily, long-acting insulin was started at 4 units/d with a stepwise increase of 2 units/wk to a total of 10 to 16 units/d. Supportive care comprised a multimodal regimen of anti-inflammatories (indomethacin), recombinant erythropoietin for prevention of anemia, and specialized nutritional care oral supplements plus home parenteral nutrition (HPN) if intake declined to <80% of expected levels. The addition of insulin to the multimodal regimen did not result in weight gain or improved QOL but did show increased retention of body fat, improved metabolic efficiency during a close to maximum work load, and a survival benefit. The improved survival could be attributed to the anti-lipolytic effect of insulin. However, these results are from a single center and need to be replicated in larger multicenter studies.

Testosterone

Low testosterone is associated with poor appetite (90) in individuals with cancer and poor survival (91) in those with cancer cachexia, but as yet, no randomized testosterone replacement trials have been conducted in patients with cachexia. The development of selective androgen receptor modulators (SARMs) such as ostarine may in theory provide the anabolic effects of testosterone with reduced virilization.

Modulating Elevated Metabolic Rate

β-Blockers improve survival and modulate body composition (92) in individuals with congestive heart failure and they attenuate weight loss in catabolic conditions such as burns

(93). A small study of cachectic patients with solid tumors showed that β-blockers decrease resting energy metabolism (42). Randomized controlled trials are required to determine whether these medications are effective for cancer patients who are hypermetabolic or have increased sympathetic activity.

Exercise

Multiple studies show that exercise attenuates the fatigue experienced by individuals with cancer. Unfortunately, there are no studies evaluating the effect of exercise on appetite, weight, and body mass in patients with advanced cancer. Animal models suggest that high-intensity exercise training increases the life span of tumor-bearing rats, promotes a reduction in tumor mass, and prevents indicators of cachexia such as reduced food intake and weight loss (94).

In non-cancer conditions such as age-related sarcopenia and HIV-related cachexia, resistance exercise in combination with testosterone (95) increases muscle mass (96). Exercise has the potential to be an important component of cachexia therapy by modulating expression of cytokines and acting in concert with anabolic hormones to improve strength and function (97).

Nutrition

Relying on caloric intake alone will not improve lean body mass or function. Nonetheless, patients may overestimate their daily caloric intake and are unable to appreciate the magnitude of the "starvation" component contributing to their cachexia. Nutritionists are able to identify and make recommendations to those patients who have insufficient caloric intake. Although individualized nutritional counseling has not been evaluated in the context of a multimodal strategy, this low-risk intervention is able to improve QOL (98) outcomes and should be used in the comprehensive management of cachectic cancer patients. Nutritional counseling could be helpful in aiding patients and their families understand that a shift to conscious control of eating is necessary.

The addition of specific substrates to the daily diet such as essential and nonessential amino acids as well as branched chain amino acids may be useful, although the evidence is derived mostly from animal models of cachexia and preliminary clinical trials. Systemic carnitine depletion has been described in several diseases and is characterized by fatigue and muscle weakness. l-Carnitine administration to tumor-bearing rats reduces cytokine levels, increases food intake (99), and in cachectic cancer patients, l-carnitine improved lean body mass when used either in combination with celecoxib or as a component of multimodal drug therapy (95).

Parenteral Nutrition

Families and patients may inquire about the value of PN when the enteral route is impossible or ineffective in stabilizing a patients' weight. Health care professionals need to address the concerns in an empathic manner and relay the risks and benefits of such therapy with a clear understanding. In general, patients at the end of life are unlikely to benefit from PN, and systematic reviews (100) as well as guidelines (101) from the American Society for Parenteral and Enteral Nutrition recommend against the routine use of PN in advanced cancer. However, qualitative research (102) suggests that patients and their family might experience social and psychological benefits from HPN treatment. In an earlier study (103), the same group of researchers reported that family members feel powerless and frustrated when facing a loved one's inability to eat. There was also a perception that health care providers neglected nutritional problems. Since patients and family were no longer able to solve the nutritional problems within the family, the offer of HPN was viewed as a "positive" alternative. Counseling patients and their families is especially important to avoid inappropriate use of PN and to prevent any perception of the selective neglect of nutritional issues.

The health care team also needs to be aware that once PN is initiated in the hospital, families may have difficulty accepting the lack of an "alternative" and that withdrawal of PN on discharge could have a considerable psychological impact (104).

In clinical circumstances when the tumor is slow growing and there is mechanical obstruction, PN may be indicated to treat the starvation component of the cachectic patient. However, it should be emphasized that clinical guidelines (105) from the European Association for Palliative Care (EAPC) suggest that PN should be considered only for a small subset of patients with a good performance status who may die of starvation rather than of their cancer. A retrospective review from one center (106) in the United States found that benefits of HPN were confined to a small subset of patients with slow-growing tumors (e.g., carcinoid). Practical guidelines (107) regarding the use of PN are fairly consistent and include the following: PN should be considered if the expected survival of the patient is >3 months and enteral feeding is impossible. Patients must be aware of their diagnosis, desire PN, spend >50% of the time out of bed, and be able to manage intravenous infusions. Patients and family members must be made aware of the potential complications (108) such as sepsis and thrombosis of catheters. As always, the evaluation and treatment of each patient should be individualized, weighing the benefits against potential harm. In addition to the difficult clinical decisions regarding PN, there are reimbursement issues to consider in the United States when a patient is transferred to hospice care. PN might not be covered by health insurance, thereby hindering appropriate transition to hospice care.

Multimodal Interventions

Past efforts to treat cachexia with nutritional or medical interventions may have failed, because they were directed at appetite stimulation alone (usually with a single therapeutic agent) and were not accompanied by therapy to reverse the underlying catabolic process. A more effective approach might be comprehensive multifaceted therapy targeting different pathophysiologic mechanisms simultaneously. More recently, a trial demonstrated that a multimodal strategy is feasible and effective. The large trial of over 330 patients (109) showed that a combination of multiple therapeutic agents (medroxyprogesterone [500 mg/d] or megestrol acetate [320 mg/d], EPA, l-carnitine, and thalidomide) was superior to any single arm. Patients had improved appetite, performance status, spontaneous physical activity, and lean body mass.

A theoretical model of multimodal therapy for cachexia is shown in Figure 10.2. The specific therapies used in combination for cachexia will vary until large trials are able to confirm the efficacy of a particular multimodal intervention. Depending on patient goals, the treatment of cachexia should be modified to target the individual's pathophysiology, since the contribution by the different mechanisms of cachexia to an individual's weight loss may vary. Also, additional clinical and biologic markers are needed to better identify individuals who may respond to specific interventions so that effective individualized therapeutic regimens can be initiated earlier and with fewer unnecessary side effects.

In summary, the evidence for individual pharmacologic interventions (see Table 10.3) remains inconsistent so that no single agent can currently be considered standard of care for cachexia. Symptom management, nutritional counseling, and exercise when feasible should be the foundation of any multimodal treatment of cancer cachexia. Megestrol and corticosteroids have a beneficial effect on appetite, while thalidomide and NSAIDs have demonstrated improvements in outcomes such as lean body mass and function. Other investigational anabolic agents including SARMs, ghrelin, and ghrelin mimetics show promise in preliminary human studies.

CACHEXIA AT THE END OF LIFE

Family members providing care are concerned about nutrition and may perceive the loss of appetite by a loved one as the most burdensome issue at the end of life (110), often more so than pain. For the family, food and eating may be symbolic of nurturing and compassion as well as "not letting go" (111). Although high importance is placed by families on patients' ability to eat and maintain weight, this aspect of care is sometimes neglected by health care providers. Physicians and nurses may not wish to engage in a lengthy discussion about poor appetite and weight loss because of the belief that this is an inevitable outcome of the cancer and no effective therapeutic options are available. Unfortunately, the consequences of avoiding this dialogue could include resentment on the part of families, who might perceive that important aspects of patient care have been neglected. Families in turn may feel frustrated by their failure to increase a patient's oral intake despite the best of efforts. They could also inadvertently worsen symptoms such as early satiety, nausea, abdominal distention, and pain by pressurizing patients to increase their oral intake. Families need to understand that providing more calories or improving oral intake will not reverse cachexia toward the end of life and may in fact cause unnecessary gastrointestinal distress due to bloating, cramping, and nausea. Having to explain this difficult, counterintuitive concept may pose a challenge for many health care providers. Usually, an empathic and straightforward explanation of the widespread, overwhelming nature of the cancer and its effect on muscle and appetite will allay concerns of starvation and reassure families that useful therapy is not being withheld. The body's inability to utilize protein and calories, coupled with the continued breakdown of muscle and fat by tumor products and inflammatory factors, needs to be explained without medical jargon. It helps to remind families that a loved one is not suffering because their calorie intake has declined and that patients almost universally report no hunger at the end of life. To the contrary, aggressive oral feeding as well as tube feeds may exacerbate distressing symptoms such as nausea and increase the risk of aspiration pneumonia.

REFERENCES

1. Fearon K, Strasser F, Anker SD, et al. Definition and classification of cancer cachexia: an international consensus. *Lancet Oncol.* May 2011;12(5):489-495.

2. Bachmann J, Heiligensetzer M, Krakowski-Roosen H, Buchler MW, Friess H, Martignoni ME. Cachexia worsens prognosis in patients with resectable pancreatic cancer. *J Gastrointest Surg.* July 2008;12(7):1193-1201.

3. Dewys WD, Begg C, Lavin PT, et al. Prognostic effect of weight loss prior to chemotherapy in cancer patients. Eastern Cooperative Oncology Group. *Am J Med.* October 1980;69(4):491-497.

4. Davis M, Lasheen W, Walsh D, Mahmoud F, Bicanovsky L, Lagman R. A phase II dose titration study of thalidomide for cancer-associated anorexia. *J Pain Symptom Manage.* Jan 2012;43(1):78-86.

5. Chochinov HM, Hack T, Hassard T, Kristjanson LJ, McClement S, Harlos M. Dignity in the terminally ill: a cross-sectional, cohort study. *Lancet.* December 2002;360(9350):2026-2030.

6. Inagaki J, Rodriguez V, Bodey GP. Proceedings: causes of death in cancer patients. *Cancer.* February 1974;33(2):568-573.

7. Bozzetti F, Migliavacca S, Scotti A, et al. Impact of cancer, type, site, stage and treatment on the nutritional status of patients. *Ann Surg.* August 1982;196(2):170-179.

8. Hauser CA, Stockler MR, Tattersall MH. Prognostic factors in patients with recently diagnosed incurable cancer: a systematic review. *Support Care Cancer.* October 2006;14(10):999-1011.

9. Andreyev HJ, Norman AR, Oates J, Cunningham D. Why do patients with weight loss have a worse outcome when undergoing chemotherapy for gastrointestinal malignancies? *Eur J Cancer.* March 1998;34(4):503-509.

10. Ross PJ, Ashley S, Norton A, et al. Do patients with weight loss have a worse outcome when undergoing chemotherapy for lung cancers? *Br J Cancer.* May 2004;90(10):1905-1911.

11. Braun TP, Marks DL. Pathophysiology and treatment of inflammatory anorexia in chronic disease. *J Cachex Sarcopenia Muscle.* December 2010;1(2):135-145.

12. Acharyya S, Ladner KJ, Nelsen LL, et al. Cancer cachexia is regulated by selective targeting of skeletal muscle gene products. *J Clin Invest.* August 2004;114(3):370-378.

13. Chamberlain JS. Cachexia in cancer—zeroing in on myosin. *N Engl J Med.* November 2004;351(20):2124-2125.

14. Jatoi A, Dakhil SR, Nguyen PL, et al. A placebo-controlled double blind trial of etanercept for the cancer anorexia/weight loss syndrome: results from N00C1 from the North Central Cancer Treatment Group. *Cancer.* September 2007;110(6):1396-1403.

15. Wiedenmann B, Malfertheiner P, Friess H, et al. A multicenter, phase II study of infliximab plus gemcitabine in pancreatic cancer cachexia. *J Support Oncol.* January 2008;6(1):18-25.

16. Das SK, Eder S, Schauer S, et al. Adipose triglyceride lipase contributes to cancer-associated cachexia. *Science.* July 2011;333(6039):233-238.

17. Mirza KA, Wyke SM, Tisdale MJ. Attenuation of muscle atrophy by an N-terminal peptide of the receptor for proteolysis-inducing factor (PIF). *Br J Cancer.* June 2011;105(1):83-88.

18. Weyermann P, Dallmann R, Magyar J, et al. Orally available selective melanocortin-4 receptor antagonists stimulate food intake and reduce cancer-induced cachexia in mice. *PLoS One.* 2009;4(3):e4774.

19. Lutgendorf SK, Weinrib AZ, Penedo F, et al. Interleukin-6, cortisol, and depressive symptoms in ovarian cancer patients. *J Clin Oncol.* October 2008;26(29):4820-4827.

20. Pfitzenmaier J, Vessella R, Higano CS, Noteboom JL, Wallace D, Jr., Corey E. Elevation of cytokine levels in cachectic patients with prostate carcinoma. *Cancer.* March 2003;97(5):1211-1216.

21. Fortunati N, Manti R, Birocco N, et al. Pro-inflammatory cytokines and oxidative stress/antioxidant parameters characterize the bio-humoral profile of early cachexia in lung cancer patients. *Oncol Rep.* December 2007;18(6):1521-1527.

22. Ebrahimi B, Tucker SL, Li D, Abbruzzese JL, Kurzrock R. Cytokines in pancreatic carcinoma: correlation with phenotypic characteristics and prognosis. *Cancer.* December 2004;101(12):2727-2736.

23. Martin F, Santolaria F, Batista N, et al. Cytokine levels (IL-6 and IFN-gamma), acute phase response and nutritional status as prognostic factors in lung cancer. *Cytokine.* January 1999;11(1):80-86.

24. Maltoni M, Fabbri L, Nanni O, et al. Serum levels of tumour necrosis factor alpha and other cytokines do not correlate with weight loss and anorexia in cancer patients. *Support Care Cancer.* March 1997;5(2):130-135.

25. Kayacan O, Karnak D, Beder S, et al. Impact of TNF-alpha and IL-6 levels on development of cachexia in newly diagnosed NSCLC patients. *Am J Clin Oncol.* August 2006;29(4):328-335.

26. Shibata M, Nezu T, Kanou H, et al. Decreased production of interleukin-12 and type 2 immune responses are marked in cachectic patients with colorectal and gastric cancer. *J Clin Gastroenterol.* April 2002;34(4):416-420.

27. Garcia JM, Garcia-Touza M, Hijazi RA, et al. Active ghrelin levels and active to total ghrelin ratio in cancer-induced cachexia. *J Clin Endocrinol Metab.* May 2005;90(5):2920-2926.

28. Song B, Zhang D, Wang S, Zheng H, Wang X. Association of interleukin-8 with cachexia from patients with low-third gastric cancer. *Comp Funct Genomics.* 2009;11:1-6.

29. Inui A. Cancer anorexia–cachexia syndrome: current issues in research and management. *CA Cancer J Clin.* March–April 2002;52(2):72-91.

30. Sun F, Sun Y, Zhang D, Zhang J, Song B, Zheng H. Association of interleukin-10 gene polymorphism with cachexia in

Chinese patients with gastric cancer. *Ann Clin Lab Sci*. Spring 2010;40(2):149-155.

31. Fadul N, Strasser F, Palmer JL, et al. The association between autonomic dysfunction and survival in male patients with advanced cancer: a preliminary report. *J Pain Symptom Manage*. February 2010;39(2):283-290.

32. Straub RH, Cutolo M, Buttgereit F, Pongratz G. Energy regulation and neuroendocrine-immune control in chronic inflammatory diseases. *J Intern Med*. June 2010;267(6):543-560.

33. Lundholm K, Gelin J, Hyltander A, et al. Anti-inflammatory treatment may prolong survival in undernourished patients with metastatic solid tumors. *Cancer Res*. November 1994;54(21):5602-5606.

34. Shrestha YB, Wickwire K, Giraudo SQ. Direct effects of nutrients, acetylcholine, CCK, and insulin on ghrelin release from the isolated stomachs of rats. *Peptides*. June 2009;30(6):1187-1191.

35. Rosas-Ballina M, Tracey KJ. Cholinergic control of inflammation. *J Intern Med*. June 2009;265(6):663-679.

36. Del Fabbro E, Hui D, Dalal S, Dev R, Noorhuddin Z, Bruera E. Clinical outcomes and contributors to weight loss in a cancer cachexia clinic. *J Palliat Med*. September 2011;14(9):1004-1008.

37. Sarhill N, Mahmoud F, Walsh D, et al. Evaluation of nutritional status in advanced metastatic cancer. *Support Care Cancer*. October 2003;11(10):652-659.

38. Bauer J, Capra S, Ferguson M. Use of the scored Patient-Generated Subjective Global Assessment (PG-SGA) as a nutrition assessment tool in patients with cancer. *Eur J Clin Nutr*. August 2002;56(8):779-785.

39. Prado CM, Lieffers JR, McCargar LJ, et al. Prevalence and clinical implications of sarcopenic obesity in patients with solid tumours of the respiratory and gastrointestinal tracts: a population-based study. *Lancet Oncol*. July 2008;9(7):629-635.

40. Crawford GB, Robinson JA, Hunt RW, Piller NB, Esterman A. Estimating survival in patients with cancer receiving palliative care: is analysis of body composition using bioimpedance helpful? *J Palliat Med*. November 2009;12(11):1009-1014.

41. Prado CM, Birdsell LA, Baracos VE. The emerging role of computerized tomography in assessing cancer cachexia. *Curr Opin Support Palliat Care*. December 2009;3(4):269-275.

42. Hyltander A, Daneryd P, Sandstrom R, Korner U, Lundholm K. Beta-adrenoceptor activity and resting energy metabolism in weight losing cancer patients. *Eur J Cancer*. February 2000;36(3):330-334.

43. Reeves MM, Capra S. Predicting energy requirements in the clinical setting: are current methods evidence based? *Nutr Rev*. April 2003;61(4):143-151.

44. Reeves MM, Battistutta D, Capra S, Bauer J, Davies PS. Resting energy expenditure in patients with solid tumors undergoing anticancer therapy. *Nutrition*. June 2006;22(6):609-615.

45. Dev R, Del Fabbro E, Schwartz GG, et al. Preliminary report: vitamin D deficiency in advanced cancer patients with symptoms of fatigue or anorexia. *Oncologist*. 2011;16(11):1637-1641.

46. Del Fabbro E. More is better: a multimodality approach to cancer cachexia. *Oncologist*. 2010;15(2):119-121.

47. Davis M, Lasheen W, Walsh D, Mahmoud F, Bicanovsky L, Lagman R. A phase II dose titration study of thalidomide for cancer-associated anorexia. *J Pain Symptom Manage*. January 2011;43(1):78-86.

48. Mantovani G, Maccio A, Madeddu C, et al. Randomized phase III clinical trial of five different arms of treatment for patients with cancer cachexia: interim results. *Nutrition*. April 2008;24(4):305-313.

49. Gordon JN, Trebble TM, Ellis RD, Duncan HD, Johns T, Goggin PM. Thalidomide in the treatment of cancer cachexia: a randomised placebo controlled trial. *Gut*. April 2005;54(4):540-545.

50. Garcia J, Boccia RV, Graham C, Kumor K, Polvino W. A phase II randomized, placebo-controlled, double-blind study of the efficacy and safety of RC-1291 (RC) for the treatment of cancer cachexia. *J Clin Oncol*. 2007;25(18S):9133.

51. Lissoni P. Is there a role for melatonin in supportive care? *Support Care Cancer*. March 2002;10(2):110-116.

52. Lissoni P, Paolorossi F, Tancini G, et al. Is there a role for melatonin in the treatment of neoplastic cachexia? *Eur J Cancer*. July 1996;32A(8):1340-1343.

53. Murphy RA, Mourtzakis M, Chu QS, Baracos VE, Reiman T, Mazurak VC. Nutritional intervention with fish oil provides a benefit over standard of care for weight and skeletal muscle mass in patients with non small cell lung cancer receiving chemotherapy. *Cancer*. April 2011;117(8):1775-1782.

54. Ries A, Trottenberg P, Elsner F, et al. A systematic review on the role of fish oil for the treatment of cachexia in advanced cancer: an EPCRC cachexia guidelines project. *Palliat Med*. August 2011;1.

55. van der Meij BS, Langius JA, Smit EF, et al. Oral nutritional supplements containing (n-3) polyunsaturated fatty acids affect the nutritional status of patients with stage III non-small cell lung cancer during multimodality treatment. *J Nutr*. October 2012;140(10):1774-1780.

56. Dewey A, Baughan C, Dean T, Higgins B, Johnson I. Eicosapentaenoic acid (EPA, an omega-3 fatty acid from fish oils) for the treatment of cancer cachexia. *Cochrane Database Syst Rev*. 2007;(1):CD004597.

57. Burns CP, Halabi S, Clamon G, et al. Phase II study of high-dose fish oil capsules for patients with cancer-related cachexia. *Cancer*. July 2004;101(2):370-378.

58. Madeddu C, Dessi M, Panzone F, et al. Randomized phase III clinical trial of a combined treatment with carnitine + celecoxib ± megestrol acetate for patients with cancer-related anorexia/cachexia syndrome. *Clin Nutr*. Apr 2012;31(2):176-182.

59. Lai V, George J, Richey L, et al. Results of a pilot study of the effects of celecoxib on cancer cachexia in patients with cancer of the head, neck, and gastrointestinal tract. *Head Neck*. January 2008;30(1):67-74.

60. Mantovani G, Maccio A, Madeddu C, et al. A phase II study with antioxidants, both in the diet and supplemented, pharmaconutritional support, progestagen, and anti-cyclooxygenase-2 showing efficacy and safety in patients with cancer-related anorexia/cachexia and oxidative stress. *Cancer Epidemiol Biomarkers Prev*. May 2006;15(5):1030-1034.

61. Cerchietti LC, Navigante AH, Peluffo GD, et al. Effects of celecoxib, medroxyprogesterone, and dietary intervention on systemic syndromes in patients with advanced lung adenocarcinoma: a pilot study. *J Pain Symptom Manage*. January 2004;27(1):85-95.

62. McMillan DC, Wigmore SJ, Fearon KC, O'Gorman P, Wright CE, McArdle CS. A prospective randomized study of megestrol acetate and ibuprofen in gastrointestinal cancer patients with weight loss. *Br J Cancer*. February 1999;79(3-4):495-500.

63. Lesniak W, Bala M, Jaeschke R, Krzakowski M. Effects of megestrol acetate in patients with cancer anorexia–cachexia syndrome—a systematic review and meta-analysis. *Pol Arch Med Wewn*. November 2008;118(11):636-644.

64. Berenstein EG, Ortiz Z. Megestrol acetate for the treatment of anorexia–cachexia syndrome. *Cochrane Database Syst Rev.* 2005;(2):CD004310.

65. Pascual Lopez A, Roque i Figuls M, Urrutia Cuchi G, et al. Systematic review of megestrol acetate in the treatment of anorexia–cachexia syndrome. *J Pain Symptom Manage.* April 2004;27(4):360-369.

66. Loprinzi CL, Kugler JW, Sloan JA, et al. Randomized comparison of megestrol acetate versus dexamethasone versus fluoxymesterone for the treatment of cancer anorexia/cachexia. *J Clin Oncol.* October 1999;17(10):3299-3306.

67. Strasser F, Luftner D, Possinger K, et al. Comparison of orally administered cannabis extract and delta-9-tetrahydrocannabinol in treating patients with cancer-related anorexia–cachexia syndrome: a multicenter, phase III, randomized, double-blind, placebo-controlled clinical trial from the Cannabis-In-Cachexia-Study-Group. *J Clin Oncol.* July 2006;24(21): 3394-3400.

68. Jatoi A, Windschitl HE, Loprinzi CL, et al. Dronabinol versus megestrol acetate versus combination therapy for cancer-associated anorexia: a North Central Cancer Treatment Group study. *J Clin Oncol.* January 2002;20(2):567-573.

69. Shivshanker K, Bennett RW Jr, Haynie TP. Tumor-associated gastroparesis: correction with metoclopramide. *Am J Surg.* February 1983;145(2):221-225.

70. Kast RE, Foley KF. Cancer chemotherapy and cachexia: mirtazapine and olanzapine are 5-HT3 antagonists with good antinausea effects. *Eur J Cancer Care (Engl).* July 2007;16(4): 351-354.

71. Kim SW, Shin IS, Kim JM, et al. Mirtazapine for severe gastroparesis unresponsive to conventional prokinetic treatment. *Psychosomatics.* September–October 2006;47(5):440-442.

72. Suzuki H, Asakawa A, Li JB, et al. Zinc as an appetite stimulator—the possible role of zinc in the progression of diseases such as cachexia and sarcopenia. *Recent Pat Food Nutr Agric.* 2011; e-pub ahead of print.

73. Ripamonti C, Zecca E, Brunelli C, et al. A randomized, controlled clinical trial to evaluate the effects of zinc sulfate on cancer patients with taste alterations caused by head and neck irradiation. *Cancer.* May 1998;82(10):1938-1945.

74. Halyard MY, Jatoi A, Sloan JA, et al. Does zinc sulfate prevent therapy-induced taste alterations in head and neck cancer patients? Results of phase III double-blind, placebo-controlled trial from the North Central Cancer Treatment Group (N01C4). *Int J Radiat Oncol Biol Phys.* April 2007;67(5):1318-1322.

75. Maltoni M, Nanni O, Scarpi E, Rossi D, Serra P, Amadori D. High-dose progestins for the treatment of cancer anorexia–cachexia syndrome: a systematic review of randomised clinical trials. *Ann Oncol.* March 2001;12(3):289-300.

76. Ruiz-Garcia V, Juan O, Perez Hoyos S, et al. Megestrol acetate: a systematic review usefulness about the weight gain in neoplastic patients with cachexia. *Med Clin (Barc).* July 2002;119(5):166-170.

77. Rowland KM Jr, Loprinzi CL, Shaw EG, et al. Randomized double-blind placebo-controlled trial of cisplatin and etoposide plus megestrol acetate/placebo in extensive-stage small-cell lung cancer: a North Central Cancer Treatment Group study. *J Clin Oncol.* January 1996;14(1):135-141.

78. Jatoi A, Rowland K, Loprinzi CL, et al. An eicosapentaenoic acid supplement versus megestrol acetate versus both for patients with cancer-associated wasting: a North Central Cancer Treatment Group and National Cancer Institute of Canada collaborative effort. *J Clin Oncol.* June 2004;22(12):2469-2476.

79. Popiela T, Lucchi R, Giongo F. Methylprednisolone as palliative therapy for female terminal cancer patients. The Methylprednisolone Female Preterminal Cancer Study Group. *Eur J Cancer Clin Oncol.* December 1989;25(12): 1823-1829.

80. Trikha M, Corringham R, Klein B, Rossi JF. Targeted anti-interleukin-6 monoclonal antibody therapy for cancer: a review of the rationale and clinical evidence. *Clin Cancer Res.* October 2003;9(13):4653-4665.

81. Bruera E, Strasser F, Palmer JL, et al. Effect of fish oil on appetite and other symptoms in patients with advanced cancer and anorexia/cachexia: a double-blind, placebo-controlled study. *J Clin Oncol.* January 2003;21(1):129-134.

82. Bruera E, Neumann CM, Pituskin E, Calder K, Ball G, Hanson J. Thalidomide in patients with cachexia due to terminal cancer: preliminary report. *Ann Oncol.* July 1999;10(7): 857-859.

83. Khan ZH, Simpson EJ, Cole AT, et al. Oesophageal cancer and cachexia: the effect of short-term treatment with thalidomide on weight loss and lean body mass. *Aliment Pharmacol Ther.* March 2003;17(5):677-682.

84. Wilkes EA, Selby AL, Cole AT, Freeman JG, Rennie MJ, Khan ZH. Poor tolerability of thalidomide in end-stage oesophageal cancer. *Eur J Cancer Care* (Engl). September 2011;20(5):593-600.

85. Roynette CE, Calder PC, Dupertuis YM, Pichard C. n-3 polyunsaturated fatty acids and colon cancer prevention. *Clin Nutr.* April 2004;23(2):139-151.

86. Hall MN, Chavarro JE, Lee IM, Willett WC, Ma J. A 22-year prospective study of fish, n-3 fatty acid intake, and colorectal cancer risk in men. *Cancer Epidemiol Biomarkers Prev.* May 2008;17(5):1136-1143.

87. Moses AW, Slater C, Preston T, Barber MD, Fearon KC. Reduced total energy expenditure and physical activity in cachectic patients with pancreatic cancer can be modulated by an energy and protein dense oral supplement enriched with n-3 fatty acids. *Br J Cancer.* March 2004;90(5):996-1002.

88. Colomer R, Moreno-Nogueira JM, Garcia-Luna PP, et al. N-3 fatty acids, cancer and cachexia: a systematic review of the literature. *Br J Nutr.* May 2007;97(5):823-831.

89. Lundholm K, Korner U, Gunnebo L, et al. Insulin treatment in cancer cachexia: effects on survival, metabolism, and physical functioning. *Clin Cancer Res.* May 2007;13(9):2699-2706.

90. Garcia JM, Li H, Mann D, et al. Hypogonadism in male patients with cancer. *Cancer.* June 2006;106(12):2583-2591.

91. Del Fabbro E, Dev R, et al. Vitamin D deficiency in advanced cancer. *Oncologist.* 2011;16(11):1637-1641.

92. Lainscak M, Keber I, Anker SD. Body composition changes in patients with systolic heart failure treated with beta blockers: a pilot study. *Int J Cardiol.* January 2006;106(3):319-322.

93. Herndon DN, Hart DW, Wolf SE, Chinkes DL, Wolfe RR. Reversal of catabolism by beta-blockade after severe burns. *N Engl J Med.* October 2001;345(17):1223-1229.

94. Bacurau AV, Belmonte MA, Navarro F, et al. Effect of a high-intensity exercise training on the metabolism and function of macrophages and lymphocytes of walker 256 tumor bearing rats. *Exp Biol Med (Maywood).* November 2007;232(10): 1289-1299.

95. Lambert CP, Sullivan DH, Freeling SA, Lindquist DM, Evans WJ. Effects of testosterone replacement and/or resistance exercise on the composition of megestrol acetate stimulated weight gain in elderly men: a randomized controlled trial. *J Clin Endocrinol Metab.* May 2002;87(5):2100-2106.

96. Grinspoon S, Corcoran C, Parlman K, et al. Effects of testosterone and progressive resistance training in eugonadal men with AIDS wasting. A randomized, controlled trial. *Ann Intern Med.* September 2000;133(5):348-355.

97. Lewis MI, Fournier M, Storer TW, et al. Skeletal muscle adaptations to testosterone and resistance training in men with COPD. *J Appl Physiol.* October 2007;103(4):1299-1310.

98. Ravasco P, Monteiro Grillo I, Camilo M. Cancer wasting and quality of life react to early individualized nutritional counselling! Clin Nutr. February 2007;26(1):7-15.

99. Laviano A, Molfino A, Seelaender M, et al. Carnitine administration reduces cytokine levels, improves food intake, and ameliorates body composition in tumor-bearing rats. *Cancer Invest.* 2011;29(10):696-700.

100. Klein S, Simes J, Blackburn GL. Total parenteral nutrition and cancer clinical trials. *Cancer.* September 1986;58(6):1378-1386.

101. August DA, Huhmann MB. A.S.P.E.N. clinical guidelines: nutrition support therapy during adult anticancer treatment and in hematopoietic cell transplantation. *JPEN J Parenter Enteral Nutr.* September-October 2009;33(5):472-500.

102. Orrevall Y, Tishelman C, Permert J. Home parenteral nutrition: a qualitative interview study of the experiences of advanced cancer patients and their families. *Clin Nutr.* December 2005;24(6):961-970.

103. Orrevall Y, Tishelman C, Herrington MK, Permert J. The path from oral nutrition to home parenteral nutrition: a qualitative interview study of the experiences of advanced cancer patients and their families. *Clin Nutr.* December 2004;23(6):1280-1287.

104. Strasser F. Eating-related disorders in patients with advanced cancer. *Support Care Cancer.* January 2003;11(1):11-20.

105. Ripamonti C, Twycross R, Baines M, et al. Clinical-practice recommendations for the management of bowel obstruction in patients with end-stage cancer. *Support Care Cancer.* June 2001;9(4):223-233.

106. Hoda D, Jatoi A, Burnes J, Loprinzi C, Kelly D. Should patients with advanced, incurable cancers ever be sent home with total parenteral nutrition? A single institution's 20-year experience. *Cancer.* February 2005;103(4):863-868.

107. McKinlay AW. Nutritional support in patients with advanced cancer: permission to fall out? *Proc Nutr Soc.* August 2004;63(3):431-435.

108. Mullady DK, O'Keefe SJ. Treatment of intestinal failure: home parenteral nutrition. *Nat Clin Pract Gastroenterol Hepatol* September 2006;3(9):492-504.

109. Mantovani G, Maccio A, Madeddu C, et al. Randomized phase III clinical trial of five different arms of treatment in 332 patients with cancer cachexia. *Oncologist.* 2010;15(2):200-211.

110. Suarez-Almazor ME, Newman C, Hanson J, Bruera E. Attitudes of terminally ill cancer patients about euthanasia and assisted suicide: predominance of psychosocial determinants and beliefs over symptom distress and subsequent survival. *J Clin Oncol.* April 2002;20(8):2134-2141.

111. van der Riet P, Good P, Higgins I, Sneesby L. Palliative care professionals' perceptions of nutrition and hydration at the end of life. *Int J Palliat Nurs.* March 2008;14(3):145-151.

CHAPTER 11

Dysphagia/Speech Rehabilitation in Palliative Care

Jeri A. Logemann

The speech–language pathologist is the usual professional to evaluate and treat speech and swallowing disorders at all points in a patient's care, whether at the time of their initial diagnosis or in palliative care (1). There are several populations of individuals with speech and swallowing problems that are frequently cared for in palliative care by speech–language pathologists. These include patients who have been treated for head and neck cancer and patients with degenerative neurologic disease. Patients with degenerative neurologic disease most often are those with Parkinson's disease or with motor neuron disease, particularly amyotrophic lateral sclerosis (ALS). Each of these patient types exhibits different problems in their speech and swallowing and requires a different approach to their speech and swallowing management. There is no single remediation technique that can apply to all patients, as the following case studies of two patients illustrate. Each of these patient types exhibits different speech, voice, and/or swallowing disorders requiring careful assessment and management.

A 56-year-old patient who had undergone chemoradiation for squamous cell carcinoma of the tongue base was treated for postoperative swallowing disorders, which did not improve despite intensive swallowing therapy, practice, and his high motivation. After 6 months of living without oral feeding and dealing with chronic aspiration, the patient requested total laryngectomy. The patient was counseled that after chemoradiation there were many factors that might make it difficult for him to eat well even after a total laryngectomy, which would, however, eliminate aspiration (2). When asked what he meant by "eating," the patient stated that he wanted to take his nutrition by mouth, understanding that it would be unlikely that he could chew and swallow a steak or even mashed potatoes because of his previous chemoradiation. The chemoradiation made generating adequate pressure to push the food through his mouth a problem, especially through the reconstructed pharyngoesophagus. The patient stated that he understood this but did not want to continue non–oral feeding under any circumstance. He was also counseled about voice loss and alternative speech rehabilitation methods were discussed. After the counseling, the total laryngectomy was completed at the patient's request and the patient returned to full oral intake without meat or other difficult to chew and swallow foods. He was able to take soft foods and liquids of all kinds without any aspiration. To this patient, communication was less important than eating, but he received a surgical voice restoration procedure, the tracheoesophageal puncture, and was able to communicate effectively.

The patient developed a recurrence in the pharynx and when in palliative care continued to be able to speak but needed a diet of thinner and thinner foods, as he was unable to generate adequate pressure to swallow anything thicker. Regular swallow reevaluation by the speech–language pathologist, as the patient's function deteriorated, resulted in continued oral feeding until his death.

A second patient, with motor neuron disease, was losing all speech intelligibility and swallowing was worsening. The speech–language pathologist evaluated the patient for a computerized augmentative communication device and found one appropriate for the patient's function of arms and hands. Swallowing was regularly reevaluated to identify safe food consistencies until the time that non–oral feeding was needed. These two patients illustrate the role of the speech–language pathologist in palliative care.

The speech–language pathologist generally approaches the patient in palliative care in the same way as she/he approaches the patient in rehabilitation, beginning by establishing goals to improve or maintain safe and efficient swallow and understandable speech or communication in patients with significant medical problems such as terminal squamous cell cancer of the head and neck or neurologic disease.

PROCESS FOR PALLIATIVE CARE BY THE SPEECH–LANGUAGE PATHOLOGIST

Although there is no single "best swallow technique" or "best choice" of communication procedures or aids for all patients, there is a common process used to define the best swallow or speech/communication techniques for each individual patient. The process includes the following:

1. Counseling to allow the patient, family, and other caregivers to understand the nature of the speech and swallowing problems the patient exhibits and the types of help that can be provided to them
2. Regular reevaluation of function to define changes in functional needs
3. Regular interaction/therapy as needed

FACTORS DETERMINING FUNCTIONAL NEEDS IN SWALLOWING AND COMMUNICATION

There are a number of factors that determine the patient's functional needs in palliative care. These include the etiology and nature of the patient's dysfunction(s), the patient and family's reaction to the idea of therapy/intervention, and the patient's goals for their function. As will be described in further detail later in this chapter, various medical diagnoses and the patient's stage of deterioration result in various speech and swallowing problems that must be managed. In the case of chemoradiation, the patient's exact radiation dose, area radiated, and type of drugs used must be defined and it must be ascertained whether the chemoradiation was concurrent. For surgical procedures, both the extent and location of the resection, the nature of the surgical reconstruction, and location of recurrence of new tumor play major roles in defining the patient's speech and swallowing abilities. Knowledge of the diagnosis is critical to appropriate speech and swallowing management for patients with neurologic disease. Patients with some diagnoses such as Parkinson's disease benefit from active exercise, while others such as those with motor neuron disease will worsen with any active exercise.

Parkinson's Disease

The patient with Parkinson's disease often exhibits worsening speech throughout his/her disease progression, which is usually quite slow and frequently lasts for at least 20 or more years. As the patient begins to have more difficulty being understood, they may benefit from a communication device, which ranges from a communication board, enabling them to point to words or letters to spell words to a computerized system that can be highly sophisticated. If the patient develops dementia, use of some of these instruments may not be possible.

Motor Neuron Disease

The patient with motor neuron disease, most often ALS, may utilize oral speech for a period of a year or more and then generally need some type of more sophisticated communication device. All patients with motor speech disorders require full assessment of their ability to use hand manipulations, typing, and other types of motor movements to control the various devices. There are patients with a diagnosis of ALS who utilize computerized artificial communication systems for years prior to their death.

Partial Laryngectomy

A partial laryngectomy for cancer of the larynx, either a supraglottic (horizontal partial laryngectomy) or a hemilaryngectomy (vertical partial laryngectomy), generally causes some change in voice (hoarseness), as well as potential difficulty in protecting the airway during swallowing (3–5) and sometimes unremitting aspiration. There are a number of rehabilitation procedures involving volitional airway protection for swallowing, which patients can be taught, as well as exercises to improve range of motion of residual structures in the larynx (6–8).

Total Laryngectomy

The patient who receives a total laryngectomy will obviously have no voice source any longer and will need to replace that with an artificial larynx, esophageal speech, or tracheoesophageal puncture (surgical prosthetic) voice restoration (9–11). The latter procedure has become quite popular, as it restores voice rather quickly and the patient does not need to go through the long process of learning esophageal speech. However, to be a good candidate for a tracheoesophageal puncture, the patient must be willing to maintain a small prosthesis in the puncture site and therefore to do more stomal care. If these patients develop a recurrence of their disease, the prosthesis may need to be removed and they may need to utilize an artificial larynx.

Total laryngectomy also creates changes in swallowing, requiring the patient to increase the effort and pressure needed to swallow postoperatively (6,12–14). However, after total laryngectomy the patient should be able to eat a full, normal diet. Few patients experience more significant swallowing problems that are related to a stricture or narrowing in their reconstructed pharyngoesophagus or a flap of "extra" mucosa at the base of the tongue known as a *pseudoepiglottis* (6). With recurrence of disease these problems, particularly cervical esophageal strictures, may recur or worsen.

The involvement of the speech–language pathologist in palliative care is a relatively new development, but it is increasing with some rapidity. In care of patients who are terminally ill, it is important that a team approach be used involving the speech–language pathologist with the gastroenterologist in management of oropharyngeal (speech–language pathologist) and esophageal (gastroenterologist) disorders. In addition, the interaction of speech–language pathologists with the patient's primary care physician and others can facilitate smooth transitions for the patient as their function may worsen. The constant goal is always to maintain optimal function for the patient in terms of communication with staff and family as well as best nutritional intake.

High-Dose Chemoradiation

Concomitant high-dose chemotherapy and radiation therapy now added to the head and neck are often called *organ preservation protocols*. They are designed to preserve the anatomic continuity of the upper aerodigestive tract by curing the patient's disease without the need for surgery and at the same time maintaining function. Recent studies have shown, however, that for some patients, some of the functions of the upper aerodigestive tract are not maintained in these protocols, particularly swallowing ability (15–16). Currently, it appears that the patient with a hypopharyngeal tumor is at the greatest risk for swallowing disorders. The swallowing disorders of these individuals are often severe and prolonged and are sometimes permanent. They include severely restricted laryngeal elevation and often virtually absent pharyngeal wall contraction. Reduced opening of the upper esophageal sphincter is a result of both of these problems. During swallowing, there is little pressure generated on the food to drive it through the pharynx and into the esophagus, leaving most of the food in the pharynx to be aspirated after the swallow. Some patients also develop cervical esophageal strictures, which require repeated dilatation, where possible. Some of these patients require conversion to total laryngectomy in an attempt to eat. However, such conversion may not result in successful return to full oral intake, because total laryngectomy requires generation of even more pressure to drive the bolus through the reconstructed pharyngoesophagus than does normal swallowing. Because these patients already have diminished ability to generate pressure to drive food through the pharynx and, in this case, the pharyngoesophagus, a total laryngectomy will stop chronic aspiration of the patient's own secretions and of food and liquid but may not enable the patient to get adequate nutrition orally.

These swallowing impairments are thought to result from severe fibrosis, particularly in the muscles of the pharynx, which appear to be quite sensitive to radiotherapy. In some cases, this fibrosis continues to worsen over time so that immediately after the completion of their radiotherapy the patient may be able to continue to eat successfully, but a year or two later may be unable to swallow efficiently and safely. If the larynx is in the field of radiotherapy, changes in voice quality may result, most of which are relatively temporary. Ability to articulate speech sounds is relatively unimpaired compared with swallowing function. With any disease recurrence, these problems may worsen significantly and a non–oral feeding may be required.

MANAGEMENT OF TUMORS OF THE HARD AND/OR SOFT PALATE

Generally, the patient who has a tumor of the hard palate, which will be surgically removed, should be seen preoperatively by the maxillofacial prosthodontist and is frequently provided an intraoral obturator prosthesis by the maxillofacial prosthodontist at the time of surgery. In that way, when the patient awakens after surgery, they have a temporary prosthesis in place (17). This prosthesis is then redesigned once the patient's healing is complete, at 2 to 4 or more weeks postoperatively. With this temporary prosthesis in place, the patient's speech and swallowing are often relatively intact.

Resection of the Soft Palate

Surgical removal of part or all of the soft palate often requires another type of intraoral prosthesis, a palatal bulb, which extends posteriorly into the surgical defect. If the palate is only partially resected, fitting the prosthesis can be more difficult than if the entire soft palate is removed. The success of a palatal bulb prosthesis depends upon the ability of the patient's lateral pharyngeal walls to move inward to meet the prosthesis to achieve velopharyngeal closure during speech and swallowing (6,17–19). This can be difficult to design, particularly in patients who also have had or will

have radiotherapy to the pharynx. Radiotherapy damages pharyngeal wall motion. There are patients who are never able to wear a prosthesis successfully to obturate the velopharyngeal port because they have inadequate pharyngeal wall activity. In these patients, the prosthesis may need to be so large that it blocks the passage to the nose completely and is uncomfortable. If the prosthesis is too small, it allows air to pass through the nose, leaving the patient with nasality during speech and leakage of food up the nose during swallowing. Despite the most experienced prosthodontist and speech–language pathologist's input to the design of palatal bulb prosthesis, there is sometimes no ability to achieve an optimum result. The same difficulties occur with attempts at surgical reconstruction of the soft palate. Generally, prosthetics have been more successful than surgical procedures in these patients.

ORAL CANCER SURGICAL PROCEDURES INVOLVING THE TONGUE

In general, the percentage of oral tongue and tongue base that are resected and the nature of the surgical reconstruction used will dictate the extent of the patient's speech and swallowing problems postoperatively (20,21). This is true whether the locus of disease is anterior or posterior. Generally, if the patient undergoes resection of >50% of the tongue, significant speech and swallowing defects will result regardless of the nature of the reconstruction. If disease recurs in the region, the patient's muscle strength in the tongue may be reduced so that they are less intelligible.

ANTERIOR ORAL CAVITY RESECTIONS

Resection of part of the anterior floor of mouth and tongue generally results in changes in speech understandability and swallowing related to reduced range of motion and shaping of the anterior tongue (22–25). The anterior tongue is used to produce speech sounds such as "t," "d," "s," and "z" as well as to lift and contact the food and bring it laterally to the teeth for chewing. After chewing is complete, the anterior tongue also contributes to forming the food into a bolus or ball prior to the start of the swallow. The anterior tongue initiates the oral stage of swallow by propelling the food backward. All of these functions can be affected by resection of the anterior floor of mouth and tongue. If the surgical reconstruction after the resection further inhibits tongue motion, then greater functional deficit can be anticipated. Generally, because of the severity of the cosmetic defect, resection of the anterior portion of the mandible is not done or, if resected, the anterior mandible is immediately reconstructed.

The patient who has undergone resection of the anterior oral cavity may exhibit some delay in triggering the pharyngeal swallow because tongue motion is changed postoperatively and oral tongue motion contributes to the sensory input for triggering the pharyngeal stage of swallowing. These patients need speech and swallowing therapy as soon after surgery as possible, after healing. The motor control of the pharyngeal stage of swallowing is not impaired, unless muscles of the floor of mouth are cut in the anterior resection. The floor of mouth muscles contribute to lifting and pulling the larynx anteriorly and opening the upper esophageal sphincter during swallowing (26,27). Generally, the patient with an anterior oral resection has less functional sequela than the patient with a more posterior oral cavity resection, as described in the subsequent text (28).

POSTERIOR ORAL CAVITY RESECTIONS

The patient who has undergone a posterior oral cavity resection, typically, has both speech and swallowing problems because of the removal of tongue tissue and/or because of the type of reconstruction used. Posterior oral cavity resections usually affect oral aspects of swallowing, including chewing and propulsion of the food toward the back of the mouth, triggering of the pharyngeal stage of swallowing, and the efficiency of the motor aspects of the pharyngeal stage of swallow as well (6,28). These patients can return to intelligible speech and full oral intake with a fairly normal diet if they have some degree of remaining tongue mobility (29,30) and have speech and swallowing therapy and an intraoral prosthesis (a palatal augmentation or reshaping device) designed to reshape the hard palate to interact with the function of the remaining tongue. If the tumor recurs in this site, both speech and swallowing may be negatively affected.

Pharyngeal Wall Resections

The patient who has radiotherapy or surgery to the pharyngeal wall for a pharyngeal tumor, generally, has permanent difficulty generating adequate pressure to propel food efficiently through the pharynx for swallowing posttreatment (6). These individuals can have significant residual food left in the pharynx after the swallow and may aspirate. Postural techniques for swallow may sometimes compensate for pharyngeal resections, which tend to be on one side, whereas radiotherapy generally has bilateral effects. Some of these patients will have dietary restrictions because they have difficulty propelling thicker food through the pharynx, which requires greater pressures.

ASSESSMENT FOR SPEECH AND SWALLOWING

Even patients whose diagnoses fall into the same category as ALS, that is, motor speech disorders, may have very different speech and swallowing disorders requiring very different management. Both are first assessed clinically at bedside to define the disordered aspects of their speech and swallowing ability, largely focusing on oral control. Reliable assessment of the pharynx and larynx at bedside is not possible as neither can be visualized without instrumentation.

The pharyngeal assessment normally utilizes the modified barium swallow (the videofluorographic study of oropharyngeal swallow) and, if needed, followed by the barium swallow

to assess the esophagus. Patients with esophageal disorders should be referred to the gastroenterologist for medication or other assistance. The modified barium swallow should provide the patient and caregivers with a complete description of the abnormalities in their oropharyngeal swallow followed by an assessment of the effectiveness of various treatment techniques that could be appropriate for the patient and be presented to them during the radiographic study. The treatment techniques, therefore, can be assessed for their immediate effectiveness (18,31,32). Most recent data (33) indicate that approximately 50% of patients can be immediately helped by the introduction of treatment strategies that have an immediate effect, including postural changes to redirect the flow of food, as shown in Table 11.1, heightening of sensory stimulation to facilitate oral awareness of food and faster triggering of the pharyngeal swallow, and voluntary maneuvers or controls to change selected aspects of the pharyngeal swallow, including airway entrance closure, vocal fold closure, tongue base movement to increase pressure on the bolus, and the opening of the upper esophageal sphincter. Each of these is shown in Tables 11.2 and 11.3 and their effects defined. The simplest procedures such as postural change and sensory enhancement, as well as dietary changes, are often easiest for the patient in palliative care since swallow maneuvers or voluntary controls require greater energy and effort on the patient's part. Patients in palliative care may not have the strength needed to successfully execute these swallowing controls. Changes in diet such as thickening liquids or adding heightened tastes or avoiding certain foods in terms of consistency may be useful as well, though patients often dislike these interventions. However, patients with motor neuron disease, for example, may actually spontaneously alter their diets to avoid thicker foods that require greater pressure to be swallowed. These patients may also eliminate foods requiring chewing, since they may not be able to lateralize food to the teeth with the tongue and thereby control chewing. There are many commercially available products from a variety of companies that produce nectar-thickened liquids, honey-thickened liquids, pureed foods, etc., which are broadly available to patients.

Swallowing assessment in patients with suspected pharyngeal swallow problems includes a radiographic study of swallowing to define the nature of the patient's swallow physiology and to identify effective strategies to assure safe and efficient oral intake. Often, the effects of these strategies can be assessed during the radiographic study (6,28–32). Some of these therapies such as postural changes can immediately compensate for the patient's swallowing problem, so the patient can continue or restart oral intake (18,32). Sometimes exercise programs can begin to enable the patient to eventually eat without these compensations, but in palliative care patients may be too weak to regularly exercise. Typically, compensatory strategies in the area of swallowing may involve changing head position to alter the direction of the flow of the food through the mouth and pharynx, pre-swallow sensory stimulation to heighten sensory awareness of the food, and voluntary changes in swallowing (maneuvers)

| TABLE 11.1 | Postural techniques generally most appropriate for each swallow disorder and the physiologic/anatomic effect(s) of the posture on pharyngeal dimensions or bolus flow |

Disorder Observed on Fluoroscopy	Posture Applied	Physiologic/Anatomic Effect of Posture
Inefficient oral transit (reduced posterior propulsion of bolus by tongue)	Chin up	Uses gravity to clear oral cavity
Delay in triggering the pharyngeal swallow (bolus past ramus of mandible, but pharyngeal swallow is not triggered)	Chin down	Widens valleculae to prevent bolus entering airway and narrows airway entrance
Reduced tongue base retraction (residue in valleculae)	Chin down	Pushes tongue base backward toward pharyngeal wall
Unilateral laryngeal dysfunction (aspiration during swallow)	Chin down	Places epiglottis in more posterior, protective position
	Head turned to damaged side	Pushes damaged side toward midline
Reduced laryngeal closure (aspiration during the swallow)	Head rotated to damaged side and chin down	Increases vocal fold closure by applying extrinsic pressure and narrows laryngeal entrance. Places epiglottis in more protective position
Reduced pharyngeal contraction (residue spread throughout pharynx)	Lying down on one side	Eliminates gravitational effect on pharyngeal residue
Unilateral pharyngeal paresis (residue on one side of pharynx)	Head rotated to damaged side	Eliminates damaged side from bolus path
Cricopharyngeal dysfunction (residue in pyriform sinuses)	Head rotated	Pulls cricoid cartilage away from posterior pharyngeal wall, reducing resting pressure in cricopharyngeal sphincter

Use of postural techniques is generally the first management procedure evaluated during the radiographic swallow study (modified barium swallow) if a patient regularly gets food or liquid into their airway.

designed to improve selected aspects of the swallow physiology, as well a variety of range of motion exercises (6). The effectiveness of these techniques can be assessed during the radiographic study. Swallowing maneuvers are designed to take voluntary control of selected aspects of the pharyngeal stage of swallow, such as closing the true vocal folds, closing the airway entrance, improving laryngeal elevation and thereby upper sphincter opening into the esophagus, and improving the pressure generated on the bolus (6,8,9,27). Patients are instructed to use these maneuvers or other exercises in practice 5 to 10 times per day for 5 minutes each to improve muscle function. Occasionally, such voluntary controls must be used during each swallow to enable oral intake (34).

INTERVENTIONS FOR SPEECH AND SWALLOWING

Clinicians are always in search of a single set of procedures that will improve both speech and swallowing. There are some types of patients who can successfully use one type of

exercise for both speech and swallowing. Because the nature of the speech and swallowing impairment in the oral cancer patient relates in large part to the reduction in range of motion created by either surgical procedures or radiotherapy, use of range of motion exercises often improves both speech and swallowing. Speech production relies on the ability of the tongue to make complete or near-complete contacts with the palate at various locations. The degree of contact or approximation and the location of this contact or approximation determines the nature of the sound produced. Similarly, during swallowing, the tongue must make complete contact with the hard palate sequentially from front to back to propel the food into the pharynx. Gravity alone will not provide an efficient swallow.

For patients with Parkinson's disease, the Lee Silverman Voice Treatment focusing on increasing vocal loudness has been shown to improve both speech and swallowing (35). Other speech and swallowing interventions are prescribed and conducted as needed for each patient based on their assessment. Throughout the patient's speech and swallowing interventions, the social worker or other psychosocial

TABLE 11.2	Bolus consistencies most appropriate for various swallow problems

Food Consistencies	Disorders for Which These Foods are Most Appropriate
Thin liquids	Reduced tongue base retraction[a]
	Reduced pharyngeal wall contraction[a]
	Reduced laryngeal elevation[a]
	Reduced cricopharyngeal opening
Thickened liquids (nectar and/or honey)	Oral tongue dysfunction[a, b]
	Delayed pharyngeal swallow
Purees and thick foods	Reduced laryngeal closure at the entrance
	Reduced laryngeal closure throughout the larynx
Foods with texture such as yogurt containing small particles of cookie	Sensory dysfunction and poor recognition of food

The patient should be tested radiographically with each bolus type to see what food consistency can be most efficiently and safely swallowed.

[a]All of these disorders affect the generation of pressure to drive the bolus through the oral cavity and/or pharynx. Thinner foods (liquids) require less pressure to swallow.

[b]Must be combined with airway protection techniques such as chin down with head turned posture of a voluntary breath hold when swallowing.

counselor should be providing the patient with needed psychosocial support.

Voice Amplification

As some patients become weaker, or for patients with respiratory disease, voice may become extremely soft. For these patients, a voice amplifier may be most helpful. The level of loudness can be set as needed.

Voice Replacement

The electrolarynx (one type of artificial larynx) can be useful in patients with a very weak voice or extremely poor respiratory support who cannot exhale hard enough to produce voice but who have the ability to articulate. A handheld artificial larynx placed against their neck can transmit sound into the patient's vocal tract. Articulation can be superimposed over this voice source. The speech–language pathologist must train the patient, family, or staff to hold the instrument in the location on the neck that results in best transmission of the sound and clearest speech.

Augmentative/Alternative Communication Devices

The speech–language pathologist will evaluate the patient's need for and ability to use a communication device and identify the best device for the individual patient. Both a voice amplifier and an artificial larynx could be classified as augmentative/alternative devices. The speech–language pathologist then works with the patient to facilitate their learning

to use the instrument. The speech–language pathologist also works with the staff in the palliative care facility to help them know best how to help the patient to use the instrument effectively. Instruments can range from a computer keyboard for typing to such a keyboard with a switch that can be controlled by eyeblinks or eyebrow movements and thereby choose letters to spell words. A website (http://www.cini.org) (36) provides information about the wide range of devices.

THIRD-PARTY REIMBURSEMENT STRATEGIES

Unfortunately, Medicare and other third-party payers may not provide adequate funding for palliative speech/swallowing services. This means that the patient may not be able to receive optimal services for the necessary length of time. Many patients are highly motivated to maintain their function. They are able to follow directions easily, so rehabilitation professionals can provide them with written exercises and videotaped examples of exercise programs and can design other interventions that are as cost effective as possible, for as long as needed by the patient in order to restore optimal function.

In summary, the key to successful palliative care by speech–language pathologists is to begin and maintain ongoing evaluation and treatment planning in a multidisciplinary format that examines the effectiveness of interventions in light of our knowledge of functional effects of the treatments and nature of each patient's potential functional needs (37,38). Speech–language pathologists should be involved from the time the patient in palliative care is identified as exhibiting symptoms of any speech, voice, or swallowing problems.

TABLE 11.3   Immediate effects of treatment

	Treatment Effects Visible During the X-Ray Study of Swallow			Effects Not Immediately Visible on X-Ray
Disorder/(Symptoms)	Posture	Heightened Sensory Stimulation	Swallow Maneuvers	Exercise Programs (Ref. (22))
Reduced lip closure (food lost from mouth)	Chin up	—	—	Lip resistance exercises
Reduced oral tongue range of motion (reduced tongue vertical or lateral motion)	Chin down, then elevated	—	—	Range of motion exercises
Reduced oral tongue strength (increasing residue as food thickens)	Chin up	—	—	Tongue strength and resistance exercises
Pharyngeal delay (bolus passes trigger point but no pharyngeal swallow)	Chin down	Thermal-tactile stimulation	Supraglottic swallow (breath hold)	—
Reduced velopharyngeal closure (nasal regurgitation)	Chin up	—	—	—
Reduced laryngeal elevation (residue on top of larynx, visibly reduced elevation)	Lie down	—	Mendelsohn maneuver (improves laryngeal lifting)[a]	Shaker exercise (strengthens muscles that lift larynx)
Unilateral pharyngeal wall disorder (residue on damaged side, in pyriform sinus)	Head rotation to damaged side	—	Supraglottic swallow (breath hold)	—
Bilateral pharyngeal wall disorder (residue equal in both pyriform sinuses and on both walls)	Lie down	—	Supraglottic swallow (breath hold)	Tongue holding maneuver (strengthens tongue base movement)
Oral and pharyngeal weakness on the same side (residue in mouth and pharynx on same side)	Lean or tilt to strong side	—	—	Range of motion oral and tongue base exercises
Reduced airway entrance closure (penetration)	Chin down and head turned if damage is asymmetrical	—	Super-supraglottic swallow (breath hold while bearing down)[b]	Effortful breath hold
Reduced laryngeal closure (aspiration during swallow)	Chin down and head turned if damage is asymmetrical	—	Super-supraglottic swallow (breath hold while bearing down)[b]	Adduction exercises and effortful breath hold
Reduced tongue base (residue in valleculae)	Chin down	—	Effortful swallow (squeeze hard during swallow)	Tongue base range of motion exercises (yawn, pull tongue straight back, and gargle)

TABLE 11.3	**Immediate effects of treatment** (*Continued*)

	Treatment Effects Visible During the X-Ray Study of Swallow			**Effects Not Immediately Visible on X-Ray**
Disorder/(Symptoms)	**Posture**	**Heightened Sensory Stimulation**	**Swallow Maneuvers**	**Exercise Programs (Ref. (22))**
Reduced cricopharyngeal opening (residue in pyriform sinuses, visible reduced width of opening)	Head rotation to weak side of the pharynx	—	Mendelsohn maneuver (improves laryngeal lifting clearing swallow)[a]	Shaker exercise Mendelsohn maneuver
Be sure to examine the combination of posture and swallow maneuvers where feasible	—	—	—	—

[a]Patient swallows and prolongs laryngeal elevation during the swallow. Source: Logemann JA. *Evaluation and Treatment of Swallowing Disorders.* 2nd ed. Austin, TX: Pro-Ed; 1998.

[b]Holding the breath with effort while swallowing closes the airway at the arytenoids to base of epiglottis.

Logemann JA. *Evaluation and Treatment of Swallowing Disorders.* 2nd ed. Austin, TX: Pro-Ed; 1998.

REFERENCES

1. Eckman S, Roe J. Speech and language therapists in palliative care: what do we have to offer? *Int J Palliat Nurs.* 2005;11(4):179-181.

2. Lazarus CL, Logemann JA, Shi G, et al. Does laryngectomy improve swallowing after chemoradiotherapy? *Arch Otolaryngol Head Neck Surg.* 2002;128:54-57.

3. McConnel FMS, Mendelsohn MS, Logemann JA. Manofluorography of deglutition after supraglottic laryngectomy. *Head Neck Surg.* 1987;9:142-150.

4. Logemann JA, Gibbons P, Rademaker AW, et al. Mechanisms of recovery of swallow after supraglottic laryngectomy. *J Speech Hear Res.* 1994;37:965-974.

5. Rademaker AW, Logemann JA, Pauloski BR, et al. Recovery of postoperative swallowing in patients undergoing partial laryngectomy. *Head Neck.* 1993;15:325-334.

6. Logemann JA. *Evaluation and Treatment of Swallowing Disorders.* 2nd ed. Austin, TX: Pro-Ed; 1998.

7. Griffith J, Lyman JA, Blackhall LJ. Providing palliative care in ambulatory care setting. *Clin J Oncol Nurs.* 2010;14(2):171-175.

8. Ohmae Y, Logemann JA, Kaiser P, et al. Effects of two breath-holding maneuvers on oropharyngeal swallow. *Ann Otol Rhinol Laryngol.* 1996;105:123-131.

9. McConnel FMS, Sisson GA, Logemann JA. Three years experience with a hypopharyngeal pseudoglottis for vocal rehabilitation after total laryngectomy. *Trans Am Acad Ophthal Otolaryngol.* 1976;84:63-67.

10. Singer M, Blom E. An endoscopic technique for restoration of voice after laryngectomy. *Ann Otol Rhinol Laryngol.* 1980;89:529-533.

11. Kearney A. Nontracheoesophageal speech rehabilitation. *Otolaryngol Clin North Am.* 2004;37(3):613-625.

12. McConnel FMS, Hester TR, Mendelsohn MS, et al. Manofluorography of deglutition after total laryngopharyngectomy. *Plast Reconstr Surg.* 1988;81(3):346-351.

13. McConnel FMS, Mendelsohn MS, Logemann, JA. Examination of swallowing after total laryngectomy using manofluorography. *Head Neck Surg.* 1986;9:3-12.

14. Pauloski BR, Blom ED, Logemann JA, et al. Functional outcome after surgery for prevention of pharyngospasms in tracheoesophageal speakers. Part II: swallow characteristics. *Laryngoscope.* 1995;105:1104-1110.

15. Lazarus CL, Logemann J, Pauloski BR, et al. Swallowing disorders in head and neck cancer patients treated with radiotherapy and adjuvant chemotherapy. *Laryngoscope.* 1996;106:1157-1166.

16. Logemann JA, Rademaker AW, Pauloski BR, et al. Site of disease and treatment protocols as correlates of swallowing function in head and neck cancer patients treated with chemoradiation. *Head Neck.* 2006;28(1):64-73.

17. Logemann JA. Speech and swallowing rehabilitation for head and neck tumor patients. In: Myers E, Sten D, eds. *Cancer of the Head and Neck.* 2nd ed. New York: Churchill Livingstone; 1989:1021-1043.

18. Rasley A, Logemann JA, Kahrilas PJ, et al. Prevention of barium aspiration during videofluoroscopic swallowing studies: value of change in posture. *Am J Roentgenol.* 1993;160:1005-1009.

19. Hanson DG, Logemann JA, Hast M. Physiology of pharynx & larynx. In: Meyerhoff WL, Rice DH, eds. *Otolaryngology—Head and Neck Surgery.* Orlando, FL: WB Saunders; 1992: 683-698.

20. McConnel FMS, Logemann JA, Rademaker AW, et al. Surgical variables affecting postoperative swallowing efficiency in oral cancer patients: a pilot study. *Laryngoscope.* 1994;104(1):87-90.

21. Pauloski BR, Logemann JA, Colangelo LA, et al. Surgical variables affecting speech in treated oral/oropharyngeal cancer patients. *Laryngoscope.* 1998;108:908-916.

22. Pauloski BR, Logemann JA, Rademaker A, et al. Speech and swallowing function after anterior tongue and floor of mouth resection with distal flap reconstruction. *J Speech Hear Res.* 1993;36:267-276.

23. Logemann JA, Bytell DE. Swallowing disorders in three types of head and neck surgical patients. *Cancer.* 1979;44:1095-1105.

24. Pauloski BR, Logemann JA, Fox JC, Colangelo LA. Biomechanical analysis of the pharyngeal swallow in postsurgical patients with anterior tongue and floor of mouth resection and distal flap reconstruction. *J Speech Hear Res.* 1995;38:10-123.

25. Logemann J. Articulation management of the oral pharyngeal impaired patient. In: Perkins WH, ed. *Current Therapy for Communication Disorders.* New York: Thieme and Stratton; 1983.

26. Kahrilas PJ, Lin S, Chen J, et al. Oropharyngeal accommodation to swallow volume. *Gastroenterology.* 1996;111:297-306.

27. Kahrilas PJ, Logemann JA, Krugler C, et al. Volitional augmentation of upper esophageal sphincter opening during swallowing. *Am J Physiol.* 1991;260(*Gastrointestinal Physiology* 23):G450-G456.

28. Logemann JA, Pauloski BR, Rademaker AW, et al. Speech and swallow function after tonsil/base of tongue resection with primary closure. *J Speech Hear Res.* 1993;36:918-926.

29. Davis J, Lazarus C, Logemann J, et al. Effect of a maxillary glossectomy prostheses on articulation and swallowing. *J Prosthet Dent.* 1987;57(6):715-719.

30. Wheeler R, Logemann J, Rosen MS. A maxillary reshaping prosthesis: its effectiveness in improving the speech and swallowing of postsurgical oral cancer patients. *J Prosthet Dent.* 1980;43:491-495.

31. Logemann JA. *A Manual for Videofluoroscopic Evaluation of Swallowing.* 2nd ed. Austin, TX: Pro-Ed; 1993.

32. Logemann JA, Rademaker AW, Pauloski BR, et al. Effects of postural change on aspiration in head and neck surgical patients. *Otolaryngol Head Neck Surg.* 1994;110:222-227.

33. Martin-Harris B, Logemann JA, McMahon S, et al. Clinical utility of the modified barium swallow. *Dysphagia.* 2000;15:136-141.

34. Lazarus C, Logemann JA, Gibbons P. Effects of maneuvers on swallowing function in a dysphagic oral cancer patient. *Head Neck.* 1993;15:419-424.

35. El Sharkawi, Ramig L, Logemann JA, et al. Swallowing and voice effects of Lee Silverman Voice Treatment (LSVT®): a pilot study. *J Neurol Neurosurg Psychiatry.* 2002;72:31-36.

36. Communication Independence for the Neurologically Impaired (CINI). A not-for-profit organization disseminating information about available communication technology for people with ALS/MND (Lou Gehrig's disease). Website. www.cini.org. Accessed October 15, 2011.

37. World Health Organization. Palliative care. Update 2011. http://www.who.int/cancer/palliative/en/. Accessed October 15, 2011.

38. Center for Advance Palliative Care. What is palliative care. Updated 2011. http://www.getpalliativecare.org/whatis. Accessed October 15, 2011

Chemotherapy-Related Nausea and Vomiting and Treatment-Related Nausea and Vomiting

Elizabeth Blanchard

The ability of chemotherapy to cause nausea and vomiting is legendary and remains a widespread fear among cancer patients. Indeed, nausea and vomiting related to chemotherapy significantly decreases patient quality of life (1). Over the past two decades, however, prevention of chemotherapy-induced nausea and vomiting (CINV) has improved dramatically. This is largely due to new classes of drugs used in prevention. This has meant improvements in quality of life for cancer patients and likely increased compliance in oncologic treatment. Radiation therapy also carries a risk of nausea and vomiting depending on the anatomic location of therapy, though there is less in the way of randomized data to guide therapy.

SYNDROMES OF CINV

CINV can be described as three distinct syndromes: acute, delayed, and anticipatory nausea and vomiting. Though in clinical practice these syndromes can overlap, the terms are helpful to define and categorize CINV. Acute CINV refers to nausea and vomiting that develops within the first 24 hours after chemotherapy administration, often within a couple of hours for most emetogenic chemotherapy agents. Delayed CINV refers to nausea and vomiting that develops more than 24 hours after chemotherapy and is generally considered to last 3 to 5 days following chemotherapy administration, but can vary, depending on many factors, including control of emesis during the acute period. Delayed emesis is considered not as severe as acute emesis (2), though less well understood and may be underappreciated and undertreated by clinicians. Cisplatin has been the most well studied in defining delayed emesis and is the archetype chemotherapy agent in the investigation of antiemetic agents. Without prophylaxis, more than 90% of patients will have some symptoms of nausea or vomiting in the delayed emesis period. Anticipatory CINV occurs when nausea or emesis is triggered by events or settings of prior chemotherapy such as the sights or smells of the infusion room, chemotherapy equipment, or care providers.

RISK OF CINV

The intrinsic emetogenicity of an individual chemotherapy agent appears to be the most important predictive factor for the development of CINV, though CINV is also influenced by patient characteristics. Such characteristics include gender, age, and history of alcohol consumption (3). In addition, experiencing nausea and vomiting with prior chemotherapy is also a risk factor. Consistently, women are more prone to both nausea and vomiting associated with chemotherapy. Older patients are less likely to experience nausea and vomiting compared with younger patients in some series (4). A history of alcohol consumption is protective against the risk of nausea and vomiting associated with chemotherapy. History of motion sickness and hyperemesis gravidarum are not well-established risk factors for CINV.

The emetogenicity of individual chemotherapy agents depends on the type of chemotherapy, dose and route, and rate of administration. Chemotherapeutic agents are classified by their risk of inducing CINV, and the most commonly used classification is modified from the Hesketh classification, originally described as five levels of emetic risk (5). It has now been modified to four levels: high, moderate, low, or minimal risk of inducing emesis (Table 12.1) (6).

RESEARCH IN PREVENTION OF CINV

The prevention of CINV is an area of very solid and consistent clinical research, which has resulted in the development of guidelines that are evidence based. In the research setting, it is useful to distinguish periods of acute and delayed emesis, as well as overall response. Vomiting is more frequently used as an endpoint, because it is a more consistent measure than nausea, which tends to be more subjective. Visual analogue scales do exist for nausea, which can help patients quantify their symptoms. Another endpoint used to judge the effectiveness of antiemetic therapy is the use of rescue medications as a measure of how well or poorly both nausea and emesis are controlled. Complete response or protection is often defined as no vomiting and no use of rescue medications. Episodes of vomiting and degree of nausea are often captured with the use of a diary or frequent telephone contact.

TABLE 12.1	Classification of emetic risk of intravenous antineoplastic agents

Emetic Risk (Estimated Incidence without Prophylaxis)	Antineoplastic Agents
High (>90%)	Cisplatin
	Mechlorethamine
	Streptozotocin
	Cyclophosphamide ($\geq$1,500 mg/m^2)
	Carmustine
	Dacarbazine
Moderate (30–90%)	Oxaliplatin
	Cytarabine (>1 g/m^2)
	Carboplatin
	Ifosfamide
	Cyclophosphamide (<1,500 mg/m^2)
	Doxorubicin
	Daunorubicin
	Epirubicin
	Idarubicin
	Irinotecan
	Azacitidine
	Bendamustine
	Clofarabine
	Alemtuzumab
Low (10–30%)	Paclitaxel
	Docetaxel
	Mitoxantrone
	Doxorubicin HCl liposome injection
	Ixabepilone
	Topotecan
	Etoposide
	Pemetrexed
	Methotrexate
	Mitomycin
	Gemcitabine
	Cytarabine ($\leq$100 mg/m^2)
	5-Fluorouracil
	Bortezomib
	Cetuximab
	Trastuzumab
	Panitumumab
	Catumaxomab

TABLE 12.1	Classification of emetic risk of intravenous antineoplastic agents (*Continued*)
Emetic Risk (Estimated Incidence without Prophylaxis)	**Antineoplastic Agents**
Minimal (<10%)	Bleomycin
	Busulfan
	2-Chlorodeoxyadenosine
	Fludarabine
	Vinblastine
	Vincristine
	Vinorelbine
	Bevacizumab
	Rituximab

Roila F, Herrstedt J, Aapro M, et al. Guideline update for MASCC and ESMO in the prevention of chemotherapy and radiotherapy-induced nausea and vomiting: results of the Perugia consensus conference. *Ann Oncol.* 2010;21:v232-v243, by permission of Oxford University Press.

PATHOPHYSIOLOGY OF CINV

Nausea and vomiting resulting from chemotherapy involves a complicated and multifaceted physiology. Afferent stimulatory input likely comes from several sources, including vagal afferent nerves in the abdomen. These are known to have a number of receptors on their terminal ends, including 5-hydroxytryptamine-3 ($5\text{-}HT_3$), neurokinin (NK)-1, and cholecystokinin-1. Enteroendocrine cells located within the gastrointestinal tract release neurotransmitters in response to chemotherapy, including 5-HT, substance P, and cholecystokinin, which then bind to the vagal afferent nerves in the abdomen. The so-called chemotherapy trigger zone is also thought to provide afferent input in response to chemotherapy. Anatomically, this is the area postrema where the blood–brain barrier is less restrictive and thus may be an area exposed to chemotherapy or chemotherapy by-products. Input then flows into the central nervous system proper to an area termed the "vomiting center," though it is now more widely believed that this represents a number of separate brain stem areas that are connected to coordinate emesis, including the parvocellular reticular formation, the Botzinger complex, and the nucleus tractus solitarius (7).

Key to the process of emesis is the involvement of a number of neurotransmitters. In CINV, the most important neurotransmitters include dopamine, serotonin ($5\text{-}HT_3$), substance P, and the cannabinoids (8). Dopamine antagonists such as phenothiazines have been used for decades for prevention of CINV, exemplifying the importance of dopamine as an active neurotransmitter. More recently, the importance of 5-HT in CINV has been realized, with the type 3 receptor emerging as the most relevant. This is likely to be mainly at the level of the afferent signals in the gastrointestinal area, though $5\text{-}HT_3$ receptors are found not only in the vagal afferent fibers but also in the area postrema and the nucleus tractus solitarius (8,9).

Substance P is a neuropeptide that also plays an important role in CINV. It belongs to a family of neurotransmitters called tachykinins, which bind to NK receptors. Substance P has an affinity for NK_1 receptors, which are located in the gastrointestinal tract, the area postrema, and the nucleus solitarius—all important areas active in the physiology of emesis (8). It was discovered in the initial animal studies that emesis was prevented by inhibitors of substance P, proving the principle of importance of this neurotransmitter. This occurred with both centrally acting and peripherally acting stimuli (10).

RADIATION THERAPY–INDUCED NAUSEA AND VOMITING

The risk of radiation therapy–induced nausea and vomiting (RINV) is primarily dependent on the area of the body being treated. Depending on the type of radiation, the risk of nausea and vomiting is divided into four categories: high, moderate, low, and minimal (11,12). High risk includes total body irradiation and total nodal irradiation. Moderate risk involves radiation sites in the upper abdomen, half-body irradiation, and upper body irradiation. Low risk includes cranial and craniospinal irradiation as well as head and neck, lower thorax, and pelvis. Minimal risk includes radiation to the extremities and breast.

Animal studies have demonstrated the importance of $5\text{-}HT_3$ in the pathophysiology of RINV, with a better response to inhibition of $5\text{-}HT_3$–mediated pathways than with dopamine pathways (13). It is speculated that the direct toxic effects on areas such as the gastrointestinal tract stimulate afferent fibers and transmit signals to the collective vomiting center. Additional potential stimuli include the tissue breakdown products that occur as a consequence of radiation treatment.

DRUGS USED IN THE PREVENTION OF TREATMENT-RELATED NAUSEA AND VOMITING

The three classes of drugs that have the most relevance in the prevention of treatment-related nausea and vomiting include the 5-HT$_3$ receptor antagonists, the NK$_1$ antagonists, and corticosteroids (Table 12.2). They may be given alone or in combination, depending on the clinical setting. These three classes are now in routine use in the place of dopamine antagonists, which are now mainly used as supplemental medications in cases where standard prophylaxis has not worked.

5-HT$_3$ Antagonists

This class of drugs includes the first-generation agents dolasetron, granisetron, ondansetron, tropisetron, and ramosetron and the second-generation agent palonosetron. They are given as oral, intravenous (IV), and transdermal preparations, with first-generation IV formulations considered equivalent to oral administration (14). Previously, all first-generation agents had been considered to be of equal efficacy and used interchangeably (15), though a meta-analysis (16) has suggested that while ondansetron and granisetron are equivalent, granisetron is more effective than tropisetron. Data for ramosetron and dolasetron

TABLE 12.2	**Doses of commonly used antiemetic agents**	
	Prechemotherapy Dose	
Drug	**Acute Emesis Prophylaxis**	**Delayed Emesis Prophylaxis**
Highest therapeutic index		
Aprepitant	125 mg orally	80 mg orally days 2 and 3
	110 mg IV	
Fosaprepitant	150 mg IV	
Dexamethasone		
With aprepitant	12 mg orally or IV	8 mg days 2–4[a]
Without aprepitant	20 mg orally or IV[a]	8 mg bid days 2–4[a]
	8 mg orally or IV[b]	8 mg days 2 and 3[c]
Ondansetron	24 mg orally[a]; 8 mg orally bid[b]	
	8 mg or 0.15 mg/kg IV	
Granisetron	2 mg orally	
	1 mg or 0.01 mg/kg IV	
Tropisetron	5 mg orally or IV	
Dolasetron	100 mg orally	
	100 mg or 1.8 mg/kg IV	
Palonosetron	0.25 mg IV	
	0.5 mg orally	
Lower therapeutic index		
Prochlorperazine	10 mg orally or IV	—
Dronabinol	5 mg/m² orally	5 mg/m² orally q2–4h PRN
Nabilone	1–2 mg orally	1–2 mg bid or tid PRN
Olanzapine	5 mg orally daily for 2 d preceding chemotherapy; 10 mg on day 1	10 mg days 2–4

IV, intravenously; bid, twice daily; tid, thrice daily.

[a]When used with highly emetic chemotherapy.

[b]When used with moderately emetic chemotherapy.

[c]When used with moderately emetic chemotherapy with potential for delayed emesis.

are more limited. Side effects of 5-HT$_3$ receptor antagonists include constipation, headache, and a transient rise in liver enzymes. The Multinational Association of Supportive Care in Cancer (MASCC)/European Society for Medical Oncology (ESMO) guidelines laid out several principles in regard to 5-HT$_3$ receptor antagonists: the lowest therapeutic dose should be used; the adverse effects of this class are similar among agents; and the use of a single dose prior to chemotherapy remains the optimal integration of this class of medications.

Prior to the development of 5-HT$_3$ receptor antagonists, high-dose metoclopramide was used for both acute and delayed emesis following cisplatin and other high-risk chemotherapy agents. Early studies showed better control of CINV with 5-HT$_3$ receptor antagonists. One series (17) involved 307 patients being treated with cisplatin of at least 100 mg/m^2 for a variety of cancers, though most patients had either lung or head and neck cancer. Patients were randomized to ondansetron at a dose of 0.15 mg/kg every 4 hours for a total of three doses of metoclopramide 2 mg/kg every 2 hours for three doses, then every 3 hours for three additional doses starting 30 minutes before cisplatin administration. Responses were defined as a complete response if the patient experienced no emesis for the first 24 hours of the study, a major response if one to two episodes of emesis occurred, minor response if three to five episodes occurred, and treatment failure if more than five episodes of emesis occurred or if a patient required rescue emetic therapy with PRN medications. The complete response rate was higher in the ondansetron group, with 54% of patients experiencing no vomiting in the first 24 hours after therapy compared with 41% of patients treated with metoclopramide (P = 0.70). In addition, more patients in the metoclopramide arm were considered treatment failures, with 36% in the metoclopramide group compared with 21% in the ondansetron group (P = 0.007). The median time to onset of emesis was 20.5 hours in the ondansetron group compared with 4.3 hours in the metoclopramide group. As expected, global satisfaction with nausea and vomiting control was also higher in the ondansetron group (85% vs. 63%, P = 0.001). Adverse events in the metoclopramide group included acute dystonic reactions in eight patients, versus none in the ondansetron group (P = 0.005). Diarrhea was more common in the metoclopramide group, whereas headache and increased liver function abnormalities were more common in the ondansetron group.

Granisetron has been formulated into a transdermal patch called the granisetron transdermal delivery system (GTDS), which delivers granisetron over a period of 7 days. In a phase III trial (18) of 641 patients designed as a non-inferiority study, the GTDS patch was compared with oral granisetron given at 2 mg/d for 3 to 5 days. All patients were being treated with chemotherapy regimens that contained multiple days of chemotherapy administration involving either highly or moderately emetogenic chemotherapy. The primary endpoint of non-inferiority was met and the

patients' global satisfaction with antiemetic therapy was similar in the two groups. The American Society of Clinical Oncology (ASCO) guidelines on the use of antiemetics suggest consideration for use of the GTDS patch during multiple-day regimens of chemotherapy as an alternative to taking a 5-HT$_3$ receptor antagonist on a daily basis (12).

Palonosetron has a longer half-life than first-generation 5-HT$_3$ antagonists and can be given intravenously or orally. Oral palonosetron at a dose of 0.5 mg was found to be equivalent to IV palonosetron at 0.25 mg (19). Several randomized trials have compared first-generation 5-HT$_3$ antagonists to palonosetron. In one trial of patients receiving highly emetogenic chemotherapy (20), palonosetron was compared with ondansetron given at a dose of 32 mg on the day of chemotherapy. In this trial, steroids for delayed emesis were not consistently given or mandated by trial design. In a post hoc subgroup analysis, patients who did receive steroids had improvements in both acute and delayed emesis in the palonosetron group compared with ondansetron. Palonosetron (21) was also compared with granisetron in patients receiving either cisplatin or combination therapy with doxorubicin or epirubicin and cyclophosphamide. Patients were randomized to either a single dose of palonosetron at 0.75 mg or granisetron 40 µg/kg prior to chemotherapy. All patients received steroids for delayed emesis. Palonosetron was found to be similar in efficacy in the acute phase, with a 75.3% response rate in the palonosetron group compared with 73.3% in the granisetron group. However, palonosetron was found to be superior to granisetron for delayed emesis, with 56.8% of patients in the palonosetron group experiencing a complete response compared with 44.5% (P < 0.0001) of patients treated with granisetron. Overall, 56.8% of patients experienced no vomiting through the acute and delayed phase compared with 44.5% in the granisetron group (P < 0.0001). Complete response was defined as no vomiting or use of rescue medications. In highly emetogenic chemotherapy, palonosetron appears to be more efficacious than first-generation 5-HT$_3$ antagonists, though the antiemetic regimen for highly emetogenic chemotherapy now includes NK$_1$ antagonists, and the comparison of first-generation 5-HT$_3$ antagonists with palonosetron when used with an NK$_1$ antagonist is unknown.

Two large phase III trials (22,23) have compared palonosetron with first-generation 5-HT$_3$ antagonists in moderately emetogenic chemotherapy. These trials were designed as non-inferiority studies and in this setting, palonosetron was found to be non-inferior to the first-generation 5-HT$_3$ antagonist. In one trial comparing dolasetron 100 mg with palonosetron at 0.25 mg, palonosetron was found in post hoc analysis to have a higher rate of complete response in the delayed emesis setting as well as overall. In the other trial, ondansetron given at a dose of 32 mg was found to have a decreased rate of complete response compared with palonosetron 0.25 mg in both acute and delayed emesis as well as overall. This was also a post hoc analysis.

Corticosteroids

Corticosteroids have been an integral part of the prevention and treatment of nausea and vomiting for decades. A large meta-analysis (24) looked at a select group of 32 studies that used dexamethasone as antiemetic prophylaxis in a comparative setting. More than 5,000 patients were included. The analysis concluded that dexamethasone increased the chances of no vomiting in the acute setting by 25% to 30%. It was also found to be superior to metoclopramide, though comparable to a 5-HT$_3$ receptor antagonist in the acute setting. In the delayed setting, dexamethasone also increased the chances of no vomiting by 25% to 30%. In this setting, a trend toward superior efficacy was noted compared with metoclopramide. One trial compared dexamethasone to a 5-HT$_3$ receptor antagonist and found dexamethasone to be more effective in the delayed emesis setting. Steroids are most often used with additional antiemetics for prevention in highly emetogenic and moderately emetogenic chemotherapy or as a single agent for prevention with the use of mildly emetogenic chemotherapy agents.

NK$_1$ Receptor Antagonists

The newest class of drugs to be used in the prevention of CINV are antagonists of the binding of substance P to the NK$_1$ receptor. In an early study with substance P antagonists (25), 159 patients treated with cisplatin of at least 70 mg/m^2 were randomized to one of three groups. All groups were treated with dexamethasone at a dose of 20 mg and granisetron prior to cisplatin. Delayed emesis was given as rescue medication, but not prophylactically and consisted of oral or IV metoclopramide and/or oral dexamethasone. Group one was also given the substance P antagonist L-754,030 at 400 mg on days 2 to 5, group two was given L-754,030 on day 1 only and placebo on days 2 to 5, and group three was given placebo on days 1 to 5 in addition to the standard antiemetic prophylaxis. The groups receiving the L-754,030 had the least amount of vomiting, with 93% reporting no vomiting in group one, 94% in group two, and 67% in group three ($P < 0.001$ for the comparison between groups one and two with group three). Patients randomized to the substance P antagonist also fared better during the delayed emesis phase. In patients receiving daily L-754,030, 52% had no emesis and used no rescue medications, compared with 43% of patients in group two and 16% of patients in group three ($P < 0.001$ for the comparison between groups one and three, $P = 0.003$ for the comparison between groups two and three). Nausea was also measured using a visual analogue scale. Nausea scores were lower in group one compared with group three for days 1 to 5 ($P = 0.003$) and in groups one and two compared with placebo on day 2 ($P = 0.002$ for group one vs. group three, $P = 0.005$ for group two vs. group three). L-754,030 has gone on to further study and is now in routine clinical use under the generic name aprepitant. Aprepitant was the first substance P antagonist to enter clinical use. Casopitant is another NK$_1$ antagonist that has similar efficacy

to aprepitant, but was tested mainly as a single daily dose, ether orally or intravenously. The manufacturer of casopitant has decided not to pursue regulatory approval for this medication (26). An IV formulation, fosaprepitant is also in routine clinical use.

The importance of aprepitant was shown in a phase III trial (27) in patients being treated with high-dose cisplatin. In this trial, more than 500 patients were randomized to either aprepitant plus ondansetron and dexamethasone or ondansetron, dexamethasone, and placebo. All patients received delayed emesis protection with dexamethasone on days 1 through 4; patients in the aprepitant group also received aprepitant on days 2 and 3. The groups receiving aprepitant fared better in all categories. For acute emesis, the complete response rate was 89.2% compared with 78.1% ($P < 0.001$), whereas for delayed emesis, the compete response rate was 75.4% compared with 55.8% ($P < 0.001$). Similarly, the overall complete response rate was 72.7% in the aprepitant group compared with 52.3% in the group that received placebo plus ondansetron and dexamethasone. Another phase III trial originating in Latin America and using similar trial design in patients receiving highly emetogenic chemotherapy showed comparable outcomes (28).

Though cyclophosphamide and doxorubicin (AC) are considered moderately emetogenic chemotherapy agents, the combination is considered more emetogenic than other moderately emetogenic combinations. In breast cancer setting where this combination is used most frequently, aprepitant has been studied in addition to an ondansetron and dexamethasone–containing premedication regimen. In one study (29), aprepitant was used for delayed emesis in the experimental arm, whereas ondansetron was used for delayed emesis in the control arm. During the 5 days studied, the aprepitant-containing regimen was found to offer better protection, with an overall complete response rate of 50.8% compared with 42.5% in the arm treated with ondansetron and dexamethasone alone. The data for the use of aprepitant in other types of moderately emetogenic chemotherapy are not as clear. In a phase III study (30), the addition of aprepitant with different moderately emetogenic chemotherapy regimens including doxorubicin and cyclophosphamide was tested. All patients received ondansetron and dexamethasone. Overall, complete response was better in the aprepitant-containing arm (62.8% vs. 47.1%, $P < 0.01$). However, retrospective analysis considered the doxorubicin/cyclophosphamide-containing regimens separately and found that the aprepitant-containing arms continued to be superior, while complete response rates were similar among other moderately emetogenic regimens regardless of the treatment arm.

Like other chemotherapy side effects, nausea and vomiting can increase with subsequent chemotherapy cycles. There is a suggestion that aprepitant may improve the durability of CINV protection. In one series of approximately 200 patients receiving at least 70 mg/m^2 of cisplatin, patients were given a premedication regimen of ondansetron and dexamethasone on day 1 and dexamethasone on days 2 through 5 and randomized to aprepitant or placebo on days 1 through 3.

Antiemetic protection was recorded through six cycles of chemotherapy. In the first cycle, the complete response rate was 64% in the aprepitant group compared with 49% ($P < 0.05$) in the group treated with ondansetron and dexamethasone alone. By cycle 6, the complete response rate was 59% in the aprepitant-containing group, but had dropped to 34% in the ondansetron and dexamethasone group ($P < 0.05$) (31).

The effectiveness of aprepitant might raise the question of how much additional contribution is being made by including the 5-HT$_3$ receptor antagonist. One series (32) looked at a regimen of aprepitant, dexamethasone, and granisetron compared with aprepitant, dexamethasone, and placebo in more than 300 patients receiving highly emetogenic chemotherapy. The group with all three active drugs fared the best, with an overall complete response rate of 80% compared with 57% in the placebo-containing group ($P < 0.01$).

The dosing and schedule of aprepitant have evolved with the introduction of the IV preparation fosaprepitant. In a non-inferiority study (33), the 3-day oral regimen of aprepitant (125 mg on day 1, 80 mg on days 2 and 3) was compared with a single dose of fosaprepitant of 150 mg. The study included 2,322 patients who were starting treatment with cisplatin at a dose of at least 70 mg/m^2. All patients received dexamethasone for delayed emesis. Similar rates of complete response were seen in both arms, with an overall complete response rate of 71.9% in the fosaprepitant group compared with 72.3% in the aprepitant group. Complete response rates were similar for acute and delayed emesis considered separately, as was the use of rescue medications and nausea.

Side effects of aprepitant are few. Headache and constipation are reported, though in the study that compared aprepitant-containing regimens to those without a 5-HT$_3$ receptor antagonist, no significant difference was noted between the groups (32). Aprepitant is an inhibitor of the cytochrome P450 enzyme CYP3A4, which has implications for interactions with chemotherapy and other medications. Aprepitant decreases the metabolism of dexamethasone and therefore plasma concentrations are higher when given with aprepitant (34). This has led to a reduction in the dose of dexamethasone when it is given with aprepitant from 20 to 12 mg on day 1, and 8 to 4 mg on days 2 and 3. Steroids are not decreased, however, when they are part of an antineoplastic regimen. Aprepitant does not seem to have any clinically meaningful interactions with chemotherapy.

Other Drugs Useful in CINV

Though the mainstay of prevention of CINV includes dexamethasone, 5-HT$_3$ antagonists, and NK$_1$ antagonists, other medications may be useful in cases of intolerance to standard antiemetic therapy or as a supplement when standard preventive regimens fall short. Phenothiazines such as prochlorperazine are often used as single agents to prevent CINV given prior to administration of chemotherapy agents of low emetic risk or as rescue medication for nausea or vomiting that occurs despite prophylaxis. Benzodiazepines are also used for nausea and vomiting that occurs despite prophylaxis,

as well as for anticipatory CINV. Cannabinoids may be useful as supplemental agents when standard antiemetic protection fails. They are considered to have weak antiemetic properties, but can have significant side effects including sedation, dizziness, and dysphoria.

Olanzapine has antagonist properties against multiple pathways relevant to CINV including dopamine and 5-HT$_3$ receptors (35). It has been studied in combination with a 5-HT$_3$ receptor antagonist and was found to control both acute and delayed emesis (36). It has also been compared with aprepitant directly. In a study (37) of patients undergoing treatment with either high-dose cisplatin or the combination of doxorubicin and cyclophosphamide, the combination of aprepitant (days 1 to 3), palonosetron (day 1), and dexamethasone (days 2 to 4) was compared with olanzapine, palonosetron, and dexamethasone. Palonosetron and dexamethasone were dosed similarly in both arms. Olanzapine was given at a dose of 10 mg orally on days 1 to 4. There was an overall complete response rate of 73% in the aprepitant-containing arm compared with 77% in the olanzapine-containing arm, which was not a statistically significant difference. Nausea, however, was better controlled in the olanzapine arm in both the delayed emesis time period and overall, with 69% of patients on the olanzapine arm reporting no nausea compared with 38% in the aprepitant arm for both parameters ($P < 0.01$). ASCO guidelines (12) have called for additional trials before incorporating this drug into routine practice.

MANAGEMENT OF CINV

The goal of antiemetic therapy in treatment-related nausea and vomiting is complete prevention; therefore, a guideline-driven approach to choose the optimal antiemetic regimen for the chemotherapy given is important. The level of emetogenicity is defined by the chemotherapeutic agent of greater emetic risk. It may be useful to provide antiemetics for patients to have at home in case nausea or vomiting occurs despite optimal prophylaxis. Nausea and vomiting in the cancer patient may be complex and difficult to discern, as there are multiple potential causes of emesis in addition to chemotherapy that the practitioner needs to consider, such as constipation, small bowel obstruction or ileus, metabolic disturbances, and occult central nervous system metastases.

Highly Emetogenic Chemotherapy

The optimal preventive regimen in highly emetogenic chemotherapy is an NK$_1$ receptor antagonist, a 5-HT$_3$ receptor antagonist, and dexamethasone (Table 12.3). The ASCO guidelines in their update in 2011 (12) now classify the combination of doxorubicin and cyclophosphamide as highly emetogenic based on the high rate of emesis seen historically. Either a single daily dose of fosaprepitant on day 1 of chemotherapy or a 3-day oral course of aprepitant is considered acceptable. Based on randomized data, any 5-HT$_3$ receptor antagonist is considered acceptable in

TABLE 12.3	Recommended antiemetic therapy for single-day intravenous chemotherapy	
Emetic Risk	**Prevention of Acute Emesis**	**Prevention of Delayed Emesis**
High	5-HT$_3$ receptor antagonists:	Dexamethasone 8 mg oral or IV days 2–4 plus aprepitant 80 mg days 2 and 3 or dexamethasone 8 mg oral or IV alone if fosaprepitant is used
	Granisetron 2 mg oral; 0.01 mg/kg or 1 mg IV	
	Ondansetron 8 mg oral twice daily; 8 mg or 0.15 mg/kg IV	
	Dolasetron 100 mg oral	
	Tropisetron 5 mg oral or IV	
	Ramosetron 0.3 mg IV	
	Palonosetron 0.5 mg oral; 0.25 mg IV	
	Dexamethasone:	
	12 mg oral or IV	
	Aprepitant:	
	125 mg oral	
	or Fosaprepitant:	
	150 mg IV	
Moderate	Palonosetron 0.5 mg oral; 0.25 mg IV	Dexamethasone 8 mg days 2 and 3
	Dexamethasone 12 mg oral or IV	
Low	Dexamethasone 8 mg or Prochlorperazine 10 mg oral or IV	No preventive measures
Minimal	As needed	No preventive measures

this setting. Dexamethasone is recommended for delayed emesis on days 2 to 4.

Moderately Emetogenic Chemotherapy

The optimal preventive regimen for moderately emetogenic chemotherapy is palonosetron on day 1 and dexamethasone on days 1 to 3, based on trials that showed superiority of palonosetron to first-generation 5-HT$_3$ receptor antagonists in this setting (Table 12.3). Delayed emesis is recommended with dexamethasone on days 2 and 3. The utility of dexamethasone for delayed emesis was looked at in a phase III study (38) of patients receiving a variety of moderately emetogenic chemotherapy regimens including AC. There was no difference in complete response rates in the acute phase between the group receiving 1 day of dexamethasone and the 3-day regimen (88.6% vs. 84.3%; $P = 0.262$) or the delayed phase (68.7% vs. 77.7%; $P = 0.116$). There was a preplanned subset analysis of AC chemotherapy versus non-AC regimens. In the non-AC group, there was no difference in the complete response rates between the two treatment groups in either the acute or delayed phases. Dexamethasone continues to be incorporated into ASCO guidelines for delayed emesis until these data can be validated.

Low and Minimal Emetogenic Chemotherapy

The optimal preventive regimen for low-risk emetogenic chemotherapy is single-dose dexamethasone on day 1 prior to administration (Table 12.3) (12). For minimal risk

emetogenic chemotherapy, no prophylaxis is recommended (Table 12.3).

Chemotherapy Given over Multiple Days

The optimal preventive regimen for chemotherapy regimens given over multiple days is more complex, particularly when highly emetogenic chemotherapy is used, and there are little data. One approach is to use a 5-HT$_3$ receptor antagonist daily during chemotherapy followed by dexamethasone for delayed emesis after the chemotherapy is complete (39). The granisetron patch is another option, as its efficacy is designed to last 7 days. The Hoosier Oncology Group incorporated aprepitant daily into a 5-day cisplatin regimen for testicular cancer patients in addition to a 5-HT$_3$ antagonist and dexamethasone. A preliminary report suggests that it is safe and well tolerated (40). ASCO guidelines (12) suggest the use of aprepitant, though acknowledging the paucity of data.

High-Dose Chemotherapy

High-dose chemotherapy in anticipation of transplant also presents a challenge in terms of emesis. Aprepitant-containing regimens have shown efficacy. In one series (41), the addition of aprepitant to ondansetron and dexamethasone resulted in an increase in no emesis in 73.3% of patients in the aprepitant group versus 22.5% in the control arm. In another series (42) of patients with multiple myeloma treated with melphalan in preparation for stem cell transplant, three different schedules of palonosetron were compared in addition to dexamethasone. The arms that contained multiple-day dosing of palonosetron were more effective.

Anticipatory Nausea and Vomiting

Anticipatory nausea and vomiting can be difficult to manage. The best preventative measure is insuring that optimal antiemetic prophylaxis is given, starting with the first cycle of chemotherapy. The incidence of anticipatory nausea and vomiting has decreased as antiemetic therapies have improved. If it does develop, potential options or management includes systemic desensitization, hypnosis, or pharmacologic therapy, though often routinely given antiemetics are not effective. Benzodiazepines and a support group showed benefit in one study (43).

Nausea and Vomiting Despite Prophylaxis

At times, despite guideline-driven prophylaxis, patients develop nausea and vomiting during the course of their cancer treatment. The first step in management is an evaluation of the cause of nausea and vomiting to ensure it represents a failure of antiemetic therapy or is the result of another process. If prophylaxis has failed, the addition of a benzodiazepine may be of use. Olanzapine has also shown early promise and may be added to the prophylaxis regimen. High-dose metoclopramide may also be used in the place of a 5-HT$_3$ receptor antagonist (12).

ORAL CHEMOTHERAPY

Though nausea and vomiting may be a significant risk with oral chemotherapy, it does not follow the same pattern of acute and delayed emesis that IV chemotherapy does, as oral therapies are often given on a continuous basis. The ESMO/MASCC guidelines (11) include oral chemotherapy, though the risks of emesis are not as well established as with IV therapy (see Table 12.4). The ESMO/MASCC guidelines divide agents into similar high, moderate, low, and minimal risk categories. No recommendation was made regarding antiemetic prophylaxis, though it would seem reasonable to use a well-tolerated phenothiazine or 5-HT$_3$ receptor antagonist prophylactically in patients being treated with highly emetogenic oral chemotherapy or for patients in whom nausea or vomiting develops.

RADIATION-INDUCED NAUSEA AND VOMITING

There are less randomized data to base recommendations for RINV compared with CINV. Both ESMO/MASCC (11) and ASCO guidelines (12) recommend the use of a 5-HT$_3$ antagonist with both moderately and highly emetogenic radiation therapy, which includes total body or total nodal irradiation, and moderately emetogenic radiation, which includes the upper abdomen or half-body irradiation (Table 12.5). Dexamethasone is also recommended during fractions 1 to

TABLE 12.4	Antiemetic classification of oral chemotherapy
Degree of Emetogenicity	**Agent**
High (>90%)	Hexamethylmelamine
	Procarbazine
Moderate (30–90%)	Cyclophosphamide
	Temozolomide
	Vinorelbine
	Imatinib
Low (10–30%)	Capecitabine
	Tegafur-uracil
	Fludarabine
	Etoposide
	Sunitinib
	Everolimus
	Lapatinib
	Lenalidomide
	Thalidomide
Minimal (<10%)	Chlorambucil
	Hydroxyurea
	L-Phenylalanine mustard
	6-Thioguanine
	Methotrexate
	Gefitinib
	Erlotinib
	Sorafenib

5 at a dose of 4 mg daily. The addition of dexamethasone is supported by a study of 211 patients undergoing radiation to the upper abdomen (44). In this trial, all patients were treated with a daily prophylactic 5-HT$_3$ receptor antagonist and randomized to dexamethasone 4 mg daily on fractions 1 to 5 or placebo. During the prophylactic period, while dexamethasone was being given, no difference in complete control of emesis, nausea, or the use of rescue medications was noted. However, parameters were looked at over fractions 1 to 15 and improvements in overall nausea were noted, as well as better complete protection from vomiting (23% vs. 12%, $P = 0.02$) and a trend toward less use of rescue medications (71% vs. 82%, $P = 0.09$). For radiation in the low-risk category, a 5-HT$_3$ antagonist is recommended as prophylaxis or rescue medication. For minimal risk, rescue therapy only is recommended, though if used, subsequent prophylaxis is recommended. When treatment involves combined

TABLE 12.5	Recommended antiemetic therapy for radiation-induced nausea and vomiting	

Risk Level	Irradiated Area	Antiemetic Guidelines
High (>90%)	Total body irradiation, total nodal irradiation	Prophylaxis with **5-HT$_3$ receptor antagonists:** Granisetron 2 mg oral; 0.01 mg/kg or 1 mg IV Ondansetron 8 mg oral twice daily; 8 mg or 0.15 mg/kg IV Dolasetron 100 mg oral Tropisetron 5 mg oral or IV Palonosetron 0.5 mg oral; 0.25 mg IV plus **Dexamethasone** 4 mg oral or IV days 1–5
Moderate (60–90%)	Upper abdomen, HBI, UBI	Prophylaxis with **5-HT$_3$ receptor antagonists:** Granisetron 2 mg oral; 0.01 mg/kg or 1 mg IV Ondansetron 8 mg oral twice daily; 8 mg or 0.15 mg/kg IV Dolasetron 100 mg oral Tropisetron 5 mg oral or IV Palonosetron 0.5 mg oral; 0.25 mg IV plus **Dexamethasone** 4 mg oral or IV days 1–5
Low (30–60%)	Cranium, craniospinal, H&N, lower thorax region, pelvis	Prophylaxis or rescue with **5-HT$_3$ receptor antagonists:** Granisetron 2 mg oral; 0.01 mg/kg or 1 mg IV Ondansetron 8 mg oral twice daily; 8 mg or 0.15 mg/kg IV Dolasetron 100 mg oral Tropisetron 5 mg oral or IV Palonosetron 0.5 mg oral; 0.25 mg IV
Minimal (<30%)	Extremities, breast	Rescue with **dopamine receptor antagonists** or **5-HT$_3$ receptor antagonists:** Granisetron 2 mg oral; 0.01 mg/kg or 1 mg IV Ondansetron 8 mg oral twice daily; 8 mg or 0.15 mg/kg IV Dolasetron 100 mg oral Tropisetron 5 mg oral or IV Palonosetron 0.5 mg oral; 0.25 mg IV

HBI, half-body irradiation; UBI, upper body irradiation; H&N, head and neck.

In low or minimal risk situations, if a patient requires rescue antiemetics, therapy should then be used prophylactically for the remainder of treatment.

chemotherapy and radiation, antiemetic prophylaxis is given on the basis of the chemotherapeutic agent unless the risk of emesis is higher from the radiation.

COMPLEMENTARY THERAPIES

In addition to standard pharmacologic therapy to prevent treatment-related nausea and vomiting, alternative therapies and techniques have been studied in addition to or in place of antiemetic therapy. Acupuncture has long been reported to decrease nausea and vomiting, and several studies have investigated its use in treatment-related nausea and vomiting. The P6 acupuncture point, which is located three finger-breadths proximal to the flexor crease of the wrist, is the most commonly used acupuncture point. In a meta-analysis (45) of studies testing acupuncture in CINV, several techniques were investigated including acupuncture (using a needle), electroacupuncture (acupuncture with the addition of an electrical current), noninvasive electrostimulation (using a wrist device without a needle), and acupressure (manual pressure on the acupuncture site). There were mixed results. Overall, acupuncture decreased the rate of vomiting, but many of the studies included did not follow guidelines in terms of antiemetic therapy. In one that did, there was no effect of the acupuncture. While this implies that acupuncture may have an antiemetic effect, how these data should be used in clinical practice is unclear and no major guideline has included acupuncture as a recommended therapy.

Nausea can be a challenging problem both to treat and to study. In one study of 644 patients, those who experienced nausea with prior chemotherapy cycles were randomized to varying doses of ginger or placebo (46). Ginger extract was given for 6 days starting 3 days before chemotherapy. All doses of ginger were found to decrease nausea ($P = 0.003$), with the largest reduction occurring with the lower two doses. This is an intriguing data set that requires validation and further study.

FUTURE DIRECTIONS

Clinical and basic science research in the area of treatment-induced nausea and vomiting continues. Additional research will best define the optimal prophylaxis of moderately emetogenic therapy in both the acute and delayed settings. Current research involves expansion of the various classes of drugs that are in current use for prophylaxis as well as trials of new medications such as olanzapine, whose role continues to evolve. The delivery of antiemetic therapy remains an active area of research, testing newer ways to administer antiemetic therapy such as transdermal methods or as a dissolving tablet. Nausea continues to be a difficult problem for cancer patients and current research is also focusing on this important area. In addition, patient-reported outcomes are more frequently being used in an attempt to more accurately reflect patient's experiences and side effects. As personalized medicine continues to move forward, another active area of research is the influence of genetic makeup on the risk of emesis and degree of protection from particular antiemetic therapies. For example, 5-HT$_3$ receptor antagonists are metabolized by the cytochrome P450 system, of which there are more than 30 types of isoenzymes that participate in metabolism (47).

CONCLUSION

Nausea and vomiting remains a difficult problem and is widely feared by patients receiving cancer treatment. The last several decades have seen tremendous advances with new pharmacologic therapy for the prevention of treatment-related nausea and vomiting. Challenges remain, including nausea, emesis that occurs despite prophylaxis, and adherence to guidelines. Future directions should address quality measures as they relate to appropriate antiemetic prophylaxis and new therapies to improve upon the gains that have been made.

REFERENCES

1. Martin CG, Rubenstein EB, Elting LS, et al. Measuring chemotherapy-induced nausea and emesis. *Cancer.* 2003;98:645-655.
2. Kris MG, Gralla RJ, Clark RA. Incidence, course and severity of delayed nausea and vomiting following the administration of high-dose cisplatin. *J Clin Oncol.* 1985;3:1379-1384.
3. Osoba D, Zee B, Pater J, et al. Determinants of postchemotherapy nausea and vomiting in patients with cancer. *J Clin Oncol.* 1997;15:116-123.
4. Pollera CF, Giannarelli D. Prognostic factors influencing cisplatin-induced emesis. *Cancer.* 1989;64:1117-1122.
5. Hesketh PJ, Kris MJ, Grunberg SM, et al. Proposal for classifying the acute emetogenicity of cancer chemotherapy. *J Clin Oncol.* 1997;15:103-109.
6. Blanchard EM, Hesketh PJ. Management of adverse effects of treatment: nausea and vomiting. In: DeVita VT, et al., eds. *Cancer: Principles and Practice of Oncology.* Philadelphia, PA: Lippincott Williams and Wilkins; 2011:2321-2328.
7. Hesketh PJ. Drug therapy: chemotherapy induced nausea and vomiting. *New Engl J Med.* 2008;358:2482-2494.
8. Hesketh PJ. Understanding the pathobiology of chemotherapy-induced nausea and vomiting. *Oncology.* 2004;18:9-14.
9. Andrews PLR, Sanders GJ. Abdominal afferent neurons: an important target for the treatment of gastrointestinal dysfunction. *Curr Opin Pharmacol.* 2002;2:650-656.
10. Hesketh PJ, van Bells S, Aapro M, et al. Differential involvement of neurotransmitters through the time course of cisplatin-induced emesis as revealed through specific antagonists. *Eur J Cancer.* 2003;39:1074-1080.
11. Roila F, Herrstedt J, Aapro M, et al. Guideline update for MASCC and ESMO in the prevention of chemotherapy- and radiotherapy-induced nausea and vomiting: results of the Perugia consensus conference. *Ann Oncol.* 2010;21:v232-v243.
12. Basch E, Prestrud AA, Hesketh PJ, et al. Antiemetics: American Society of Clinical Oncology clinical practice guideline update. *J Clin Oncol.* 2011;29:published online ahead of print.
13. Miner WD, Sanger GJ, Turner DH. Evidence that 5-hydroxytryptamine3 receptors mediate cytotoxic drug and radiation-evoked emesis. *Br J Cancer.* 1987;56:159-162.
14. Perez EZ, Hesketh P, Sandbach J, et al. Comparison of single dose oral granisetron versus intravenous ondansetron in the prevention of nausea and vomiting induced by moderately emetogenic chemotherapy: a multicenter, double-blind, randomized parallel study. *J Clin Oncol.* 1998;16:754-760.
15. Kris MG, Hesketh PJ, Somerfield MR, et al. American Society of Clinical Oncology guideline for antiemetics in oncology: update 2006. *J Clin Oncol.* 2006;24:2932-2947.
16. Jordan K, Hinke A, Grothey A, et al. A meta-analysis comparing the efficacy of four 5-HT-3 receptor antagonists for acute chemotherapy-induced emesis. *Support Care Cancer.* 2007;15:1023-1033.
17. Hainsworth J, Harvey W, Pendergrass K, et al. A single-blind comparison of intravenous ondansetron, a selective serotonin antagonist, with intravenous metoclopramide in the prevention of nausea and vomiting associated with high-dose cisplatin chemotherapy. *J Clin Oncol.* 1991;9:721-728.
18. Boccia RV, Gordan LN, Clark G, et al. Efficacy and tolerability of transdermal granisetron for the control of chemotherapy-induced nausea and vomiting associated with moderately and highly emetogenic multi-day chemotherapy: a randomized, double blind, phase III study. *Support Care Cancer.* 2011;19:1609-1617.
19. Grunberg S, Voisin E, Zufferli M, Piraccini G. Oral palonosetron is as effective as intravenous palonosetron: a phase 3 dose ranging trial in patients receiving moderately emetogenic chemotherapy. *Eur J Cancer.* 2007;(suppl 5):155.
20. Aapro MS, Grunberg SM, Manikas GM, et al. A phase II double blind, randomized trial of palonosetron compared with ondansetron in preventing chemotherapy-induced nausea and vomiting following highly emetogenic chemotherapy. *Ann Oncol.* 2006;17:1441-1449.
21. Saito M, Aogi K, Sekine I, et al. Palonosetron plus dexamethasone versus granisetron plus dexamethasone for prevention of nausea and vomiting during chemotherapy: a double-blind, double dummy, randomized, comparative phase III trial. *Lancet Oncol.* 2009;10:115-124.

22. Eisenberg P, Figueroa-Vadillo J, Zamora R, et al. Improved prevention of moderately emetogenic chemotherapy-induced nausea and vomiting with palonosetron, a pharmacologically novel 5-HT3 receptor antagonist: results of a phase III, single-dose trial versus dolasetron. *Cancer.* 2003;93:2473-2482.

23. Gralla R, Lichinitser M, Van Der Vegt S, et al. Palonosetron improves prevention of chemotherapy-induced nausea and vomiting following moderately emetogenic chemotherapy: results of a double-blind randomized phase III trial comparing single doses of palonosetron with ondansetron. *Ann Oncol.* 2003;14:1570-1577.

24. Ioannidis JPA, Hesketh PJ, Lau J. Contribution of dexamethasone to control of chemotherapy-induced nausea and vomiting: a meta-analysis of randomized evidence. *J Clin Oncol.* 2000;18:3409-3422.

25. Navari RM, Reinhardt RR, Gralla RJ, et al. Reduction of cisplatin-induced emesis by a selective neurokinin-1-receptor antagonist. *N Engl J Med.* 1999;340:190-195.

26. Grunberg S, Rolski J, Strausz J, et al. Efficacy and safety of casopitant mesylate, a neurokinin-1 (NK1)-antagonist in the prevention of chemotherapy related nausea and vomiting in patients receiving cisplatin based highly emetogenic chemotherapy: a randomized, double-blind placebo-controlled trial. *Lancet Oncol.* 2009;10:549-558.

27. Hesketh PJ, Grunberg SM, Gralla RJ, et al. The oral neurokinin-1 antagonists aprepitant for the prevention of chemotherapy-induced nausea and vomiting: a multinational, randomized, double-blind, placebo-controlled trial in patients receiving high-dose cisplatin—the aprepitant protocol 052 study group. *J Clin Oncol.* 2003;21:4112-4119.

28. Poli-Bigelli S, Rodrigues-Pereira J, Carides AD, et al. Addition of the neurokinin 1 receptor antagonist aprepitant to standard antiemetic therapy improves control of chemotherapy induced nausea and vomiting. *Cancer.* 2003;97:3090-3098.

29. Warr DG, Hesketh PJ, Gralla RJ, et al. Efficacy and tolerability of aprepitant for the prevention of chemotherapy-induced nausea and vomiting in patients with breast cancer after moderately emetogenic chemotherapy. *J Clin Oncol.* 2005;23:2822-2830.

30. Rapoport BL, Jordan K, Boice JA, et al. Aprepitant for the prevention of chemotherapy-induced nausea and vomiting associated with a broad range of moderately emetogenic chemotherapy and tumor types: a randomized, double blind study. *Support Care Cancer.* 2010;18:423-431.

31. de Wit R, Herrstedt J, Rapoport B, et al. Addition of the oral NK1 antagonist aprepitant to standard antiemetics provides protection against nausea and vomiting during multiple cycles of cisplatin-based chemotherapy. *J Clin Oncol.* 2003;21:4105-4111.

32. Campos D, Pereira JR, Reinhardt RR, et al. Prevention of cisplatin-induced emesis by the oral neurokinin-1 antagonist, MK-869, in combination with granisetron and dexamethasone or with dexamethasone alone. *J Clin Oncol.* 2001;19:1759-1767.

33. Grunberg S, Chua D, Maru A, et al. Single dose fosaprepitant for the prevention of chemotherapy-induced nausea and vomiting associated with cisplatin therapy: randomized, double blind study protocol-EASE. *J Clin Oncol.* 2011;29: 1495-1501.

34. McCrea JB, Majumdar AK, Goldberg MR, et al. Effects of the neurokinin 1 antagonist aprepitant on the pharmacokinetics of dexamethasone and methylprednisolone. *Clin Pharmacol Ther.* 2003;74:17-24.

35. Feyer P, Jordan K. Update and new trends in antiemetic therapy: the continuing need for novel therapies. *Ann Oncol.* 2011;22:30-38.

36. Navari RM, Einhorn LH, Passik SD, et al. A phase II trial of olanzapine for the prevention of chemotherapy-induced nausea and vomiting: a Hoosier Oncology Group study. *Support Care Cancer.* 2005;13:529-534.

37. Navari RM, Gray SE, Kerr AC. Olanzapine versus aprepitant for the prevention of chemotherapy induced nausea and vomiting: a randomized phase III trial. *J Support Oncol.* 2011;9:188-195.

38. Celio L, Frustaci S, Denaro A. Palonosetron in combination with 1-day versus 3-day dexamethasone for prevention of nausea and vomiting following moderately emetogenic chemotherapy: a randomized, multicenter, phase III trial. *Support Care Cancer.* 2011;19:1217-1225.

39. Einhorn LH, Rapoport B, Koeller J, et al. Antiemetic therapy for multiple-day chemotherapy and high dose chemotherapy with stem cell transplant: review and consensus statement. *Support Care Cancer.* 2005;13:112-116.

40. Brames M, Johnston E, Nichols C, et al. Phase III study of granisetron+dexamethasone +/- aprepitant in patients with germ cell tumors undergoing 5 day courses of cisplatin based combination: a Hoosier Oncology Group (H.O.G.) study. *Support Care Cancer.* 2009;17:871-872 abstract.

41. Stiff P, Fox-Geiman M, Kiley K, et al. Aprepitant vs. placebo plus oral ondansetron and dexamethasone for the prevention of nausea and vomiting associated with highly emetogenic preparative regimens prior to hematopoietic stem cell transplantation; a prospective, randomized double-blind phase III trial. *Blood (ASH Annu Meet Abstr).* 2009;114:abstract 2267.

42. Giralt S, Mangan K, Maziarz R, et al. Palonosetron (PALO) for prevention of chemotherapy-induced nausea and vomiting (CINV) in patients receiving high-dose melphalan prior to stem cell transplant (SCT). *J Clin Oncol.* 2008;26:531s (suppl; abstract 9617).

43. Razavi D, Delvaux N, Farvacques C, et al. Prevention of adjustment disorders and anticipatory nausea secondary to adjuvant chemotherapy: a double-blind, placebo-controlled study assessing the usefulness of alprazolam. *J Clin Oncol.* 1993;11:1384-1390.

44. Wong RKS, Paul N, Ding K, et al. 5-Hydroxytryptamine-3 receptor antagonist with or without short-course dexamethasone in the prophylaxis of radiation induced emesis: a placebo-controlled randomized trial of the National Cancer Institute of Canada Clinical Trials Group (Sc19). *J Clin Oncol.* 2006;24:3458-3464.

45. Ezzo J, Vickers M, Richardson MA, et al. Acupuncture-point stimulation for chemotherapy-induced nausea and vomiting. *J Clin Oncol.* 2005;23:7188-7198.

46. Ryan JL, Heckler C, Dakhil SR, et al. Ginger for chemotherapy-related nausea in cancer patients: a URCC CCOP randomized, double blind, placebo controlled clinical trial of 644 cancer patients. *J Clin Oncol.* 2009;27:9511 (abstract).

47. Nielson M, Olsen NV. Genetic polymorphisms in the cytochrome P450 system and efficacy of 5-hydroxytryptamine type 3 receptor antagonists for postoperative nausea and vomiting. *Br J Anaesth.* 2008;101:441-445.

CHAPTER 13

Assessment and Management of Chronic Nausea and Vomiting

Jamie H. Von Roenn

INTRODUCTION

Nausea and vomiting are common and distressing symptoms in patients with cancer, occurring in up to 70% of patients with advanced disease and in at least 40% during the last 6 weeks of life (1–3). These symptoms rarely occur in isolation and cause substantial psychological distress for both patients and families. Inadequately treated nausea and vomiting may lead to serious complications, including dehydration, electrolyte disturbances, anorexia, weight loss, and psychological distress, which may exacerbate patient and family concerns about starvation and progressive decline.

Nausea and vomiting, though commonly clustered together, are separate entities. Nausea is a subjective phenomenon often described as the unpleasant sensation of the need to vomit, of feeling "queasy," or "sick in your stomach." It is frequently associated with autonomic symptoms such as cold sweats, pallor, diarrhea, and tachycardia (4). Vomiting is a protective reflex triggered by chemical or physical stimuli, which leads to the expulsion of gastric contents through the mouth and, sometimes, the nose. The vomiting act has two phases, retching and expulsion. Retching is the strong involuntary effort to vomit without bringing anything up. It involves a deep inspiration against a closed glottis. The act of vomiting involves contraction of the abdominal muscles, leading to a pressure differential between the abdominal and thoracic cavities. The stomach and gastric contents are pushed toward the thoracic cavity. The expulsion phase occurs when the upper esophageal sphincter relaxes and the gastric contents are expelled through the mouth. Vomiting occurs as a result of complex muscular and neurophysiologic interactions, which provide the foundation for current pathophysiology-based treatment recommendations. The neural pathways that mediate nausea are not known. The anticipated level of success in controlling vomiting as opposed to nausea may reflect the limited understanding of the pathophysiologic basis of nausea.

ETIOLOGY AND ASSESSMENT OF NAUSEA AND VOMITING

A pathophysiology-based treatment approach is generally recommended for the control of nausea and vomiting (5–12). The effectiveness of this approach relies on the ability to accurately identify the cause of the symptoms. Etiology-based guidelines for the management of nausea and vomiting in hospice patients are moderately effective. In one recent investigation, physicians expressed confidence in their ability to identify a clear etiology of nausea and vomiting 75% of the time (8). As many as a quarter of patients were felt to have multiple causes to explain their symptoms. The most common cause of nausea and vomiting was delayed gastric emptying (44%), followed by "chemical" causes (metabolic, medications, and infection) (33%). Using etiology-based guidelines, nausea was controlled for 44% of patients at 48 hours and for 56% at 1 week. Vomiting was more effectively controlled: 69% of patients had control at 48 hours and 89% at 1 week. These results are consistent with those previously reported (11,12). Careful patient assessment, identification of the source of nausea and vomiting when possible, use of pathophysiology-based guidelines, and clinical judgment underlie effective management of nausea and vomiting in patients with advanced illness (5,8–10).

CLINICAL EVALUATION OF NAUSEA AND VOMITING

Careful clinical evaluation is the first step to ascertain the etiology of nausea and vomiting. Initial assessment begins with a thorough history and physical examination, including a review of recent and current medication use (including supplements and over-the-counter medications), comorbid conditions, associated signs and symptoms, history of the frequency and acuity of nausea and vomiting, the impact of oral intake, and changes in bowel habits. This assessment can focus the diagnostic evaluation and limit the need for biochemical evaluation or radiologic investigations. A simple pneumonic for recalling the potential causes of nausea and vomiting are the 12 Ms. Table 13.1 lists the 12 Ms of nausea and vomiting, many of which can be excluded on the basis of history and physical examination alone.

In patients with advanced cancer, the onset of any new symptom may raise patient and family concern of progressive cancer. Progressive metastatic disease may cause nausea and vomiting based on multiple etiologies. New or recurrent brain metastases may present with nausea and vomiting. Increased intracranial pressure is one of the few causes of vomiting without nausea, classically described as projectile vomiting and associated with an early morning headache. A patient with hydrocephalus secondary to carcinomatous meningitis may present with intractable nausea and vomiting in association with neck stiffness, with or without other signs of central nervous system (CNS) disease, such as diplopia. Nausea and vomiting from CNS metastases is generally not

TABLE 13.1	Common causes of nausea and vomiting
Metastases	Meningeal involvement
Mental anxiety	Movement
Medications	Mucosal irritation
Motility	Mechanical obstruction
Metabolic	Microbes
Myocardial	Maternity

effected by oral intake and has no effect on bowel pattern. Intra-abdominal metastases leading to partial or complete bowel obstruction often presents with continuous nausea, briefly relieved by acute large volume emesis (if the obstruction is in the proximal small bowel). The nausea and vomiting of bowel obstruction is associated with difficulty eating both solids and liquids, and the absence of flatus or bowel movements if the obstruction is complete. These symptoms may be accompanied by colicky abdominal pain. The clinical presentation paints a picture of the etiology of the symptoms. Table 13.2 compares and contrasts the clinical presentation of some of the most common causes of nausea and vomiting in patients with advanced cancer.

Clinical assessment includes a thorough description of the characteristics of the symptoms. Does the nausea occur primarily in the morning or after eating? Is the nausea precipitated by movement? Did it begin after medication changes? A change in dose? Initiation of new over-the-counter medications or supplements? Are the symptoms chronic or acute? Nausea, a subjective symptom, is not always clearly defined by patients. A patient report of anorexia or dyspepsia

may represent low-grade chronic nausea. Are the symptoms constant or intermittent? Are there interventions that have improved the symptoms? Does eating make the symptoms worse? Gastroparesis is associated with significant difficulty with advancing solids, particularly fiber-rich foods, out of the stomach. Are there associated symptoms of abdominal distention and early satiety as might be expected in a patient with increasing intra-abdominal cancer or progressive ascites? Does early satiety occur without significant abdominal distension, which might suggest gastric stasis? Has the patient's bowel pattern changed? Constipation is a potential cause of nausea, especially in patients with decreased ambulation and for those receiving opioids. The frequency and consistency of bowel movements is essential historical information. The presence of delerium raises the suspicion for a metabolic cause of nausea. Comorbid conditions, such as diabetes mellitus, systemic infection, hypothyroidism, acquired immunodeficiency syndrome, or cardiac disease, may lead to nausea and vomiting. A list of current medications may quickly clarify the etiology of a patient's nausea and vomiting. A recent prescription for opioids and rapid titration of the opioid are frequent causes of nausea and vomiting. In the setting of advanced cancer, opioids are the most common cause of medication-related nausea and vomiting, but there are many medications that need to be considered (13) (see Table 13.3).

Physical examination provides diagnostic information and an assessment of the overall status of the patient. The presence of marked muscle wasting, poor performance status, and other hallmarks of very advanced illness may temper a decision for diagnostic studies. Physical examination may identify papilledema or cranial nerve abnormalities that suggest elevated intracranial pressure or meningeal disease, respectively. Examination of the abdomen may identify a succussion splash on auscultation of the epigastric area when the patient moves, suggesting gastroparesis. The presence of

TABLE 13.2	The clinical presentation of nausea and vomiting				
	CNS Disease	**Constipation**	**MBO**	**Metabolic**	**Gastric Stasis**
Timing	Early morning	Daily	↑ with oral intake	Intermittent	Postprandial
Acuity	Acute	Chronic	Chronic	Chronic	Chronic
Frequency	Daily at least	Intermittent	Intermittent	Intermittent	Daily
Associated signs and symptoms	Headache, stiff neck, neurologic abnormalities	Abdominal distension, +/− early satiety, abdominal discomfort	Colicky abdominal pain, distended abdomen	+/− delirium, +/− ↓u/o, +/− sedation	Hiccups, abdominal fullness, +/− reflux, early satiety, ↑ nausea with eating
Eating pattern	No change	↓ intake	↓ intake	No change	↓ intake
Bowels	No change	↓↓ BM	No BM	Varies with etiology	+/− constipation

MBO, malignant bowel obstruction; u/o, —urine output; BM, —bowel movement; +/−, —with or without.

TABLE 13.3	Medications that cause nausea and vomiting
Nonsteroidal anti-inflammatory agents	Opioids
Tramadol	Antibiotics
Selective seratonin reuptake inhibitors	Digitalis
Potassium supplements	Bupropion
Bisphosphonates	

abdominal distention and absent bowel sounds in the setting of vomiting and constipation are highly suggestive of bowel obstruction. Rectal examination can rule out constipation as a cause of nausea. Hepatomegaly and/or ascites are useful clues to explain symptoms of early satiety due to gastric stasis or delayed gastric emptying.

Depending on the goals of care, directed by discussion with the patient and family, a biochemical and radiologic evaluation may be advised. Simple laboratory tests will identify hypercalcemia, hyponatremia, pancreatitis, and liver or renal failure as potential causes of nausea and vomiting. When the clinical picture suggests bowel obstruction, an abdominal x-ray is diagnostic. Imaging of the brain or abdomen is only appropriate, however, if the information will change the treatment plan. For a patient with otherwise well-controlled cancer, and/or a survival measured in months, more extensive evaluation, including radiologic studies (computed tomography of the abdomen or magnetic resonance imaging of the brain) and endoscopy, is frequently recommended.

PATHOPHYSIOLOGY OF NAUSEA AND VOMITING

Once the etiology of nausea and vomiting is ascertained, treatment is directed by the pathway and neurotransmitters triggered by a particular cause. The pathways and neurotransmitters involved in nausea and vomiting are summarized in Figure 13.1 (14–19). The vomiting center is the

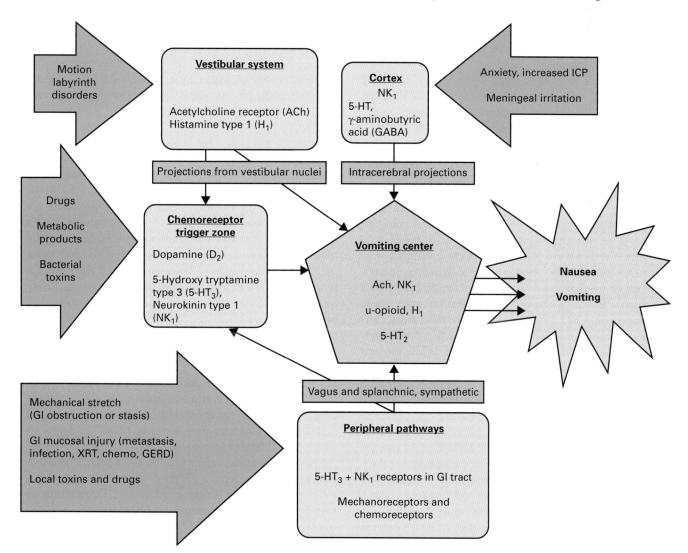

Figure 13.1. The pathways and neurotransmitters involved in nausea and vomiting. (Courtesy of Shannah Moore, MD San Diego Palliative Care Institute.)

final common pathway, likely mediated through substance P, for the generation of the complex patterned response that results in the vomiting reflex. There are four major pathways that provide input to the vomiting center:

1. The chemoreceptor trigger zone (CTZ), a receptor-rich area of the floor of the fourth ventricle, has numerous dopamine (D_2), serotonin (hydroxytryptamine type 3 receptor [5-HT$_3$] and hydroxytryptamine type 4 receptor [5-HT$_4$]), opioid, acetylcholine, and substance P receptors. It is a circumventricular organ, lying outside of the blood–brain barrier, allowing for stimulation by toxins from the blood and cerebral spinal fluid.

2. The vestibular system is rich in histamine (H_1) and muscarinic receptors. Its stimulation of the vomiting center is mediated through labyrinthine inputs via cranial nerve VIII, the vestibulocochlear nerve, which plays a major role in motion sickness.

3. The vagal and enteric nervous system transmits information to the brain regarding the state of the gastrointestinal system. The vagal efferent neurons are located in close proximity to the enterochromaffin cells of the small intestine, the body's primary storage site for serotonin. Distention of the gut or irritation of the mucosal surface leads to activation of 5-HT$_3$ receptors, stimulation of vagal afferents, and an emetic response.

4. The cortex is thought to mediate nausea and vomiting from meningeal irritation, increased intracranial pressure, psychiatric disorders, and unpleasant inputs from the five senses (for example, foul odors).

TREATMENT—NON-PHARMACOLOGIC

Treatment of any symptom can be divided into non-pharmacologic and pharmacologic approaches. Common sense recommendations for patients with nausea and vomiting include a recommendation for frequent small meals, particularly if early satiety plays a role in the patient's symptoms. Avoidance of hot food may be of benefit as it has a stronger aroma than either cold or room temperature foods. Psychiatric techniques to promote relaxation and provide distraction or positive imagery may offer relief from nausea and vomiting, especially for patients with a psychological component to their symptoms (20,21). While medical hypnosis may significantly reduce anticipatory chemotherapy-related nausea and vomiting, there are inadequate data to recommend it in patients with advanced cancer (22,23). Both acupuncture and acupressure have been purported to be of benefit (23). A meta-analysis evaluating the effectiveness of acupuncture and acupressure for control of chemotherapy-induced nausea and vomiting concluded that there is some beneficial effect of acupuncture-point stimulation on acute chemotherapy-induced nausea and vomiting (23,24). A Cochrane Library review of 40 trials assessing the use of acupuncture/acupressure for non–chemotherapy-related nausea and vomiting, mostly comprised studies of healthy adults undergoing elective surgery with general anesthesia, evaluated stimulation of the P6 point (a point on the wrist; it's stimulation prevents nausea and vomiting) versus either a sham or pharmacologic antiemetic treatment (25). Acupressure of the P6 point significantly reduced the incidence of postoperative nausea and vomiting compared with the sham procedure. There are no reliable data demonstrating the relative efficacy of pharmacologic interventions and acupuncture/acupressure for treatment of nausea and vomiting (25). In the palliative care setting, one very small study suggested that acupressure may reduce nausea and vomiting in patients with advanced illness (26).

TREATMENT—PHARMACOLOGIC

The pharmacologic approach to nausea and vomiting in the setting of cancer, unrelated to chemotherapy or radiation therapy, may be based either on a pathophysiologic (etiologic) or an empiric basis. Most palliative care guidelines recommend an etiologic approach although there are limited clinical trial data to support specific recommendations for antiemetics (6). No head-to-head efficacy comparisons between etiologic and empiric-based selection of antiemetics exist (27).

ANTIEMETICS

There are a wide variety of antiemetics available. Table 13.4 summarizes the receptor site of specific activity, dosage, and side effects of commonly used agents.

Dopamine Antagonists

Haloperidol, a butyrophenone antipsychotic, is one of the most potent D_2 receptor antagonists at the CTZ (28–30). In spite of this, no high quality data from randomized trials are available to substantiate its benefit in patients with nausea and vomiting in the advanced disease setting. Substantially lower doses are needed to treat emesis compared with those used for psychiatric illness. Haloperidol has the benefit of a long half-life (16 hours), allowing it to be prescribed only once or twice daily. While there is the potential for sedation or hypotension with its use, this is less of a problem with haloperidol than with the phenothiazines because of haloperidol's weak anticholinergic and α-adrenergic receptor blocking effects.

The most commonly prescribed phenothiazine is prochlorperazine. It not only has activity as a D_2 receptor antagonist but also has antagonist activity at α1-adrenergic, acetylcholine, and histamine receptors (14). The degree to which each of the phenothiazines has antagonist activity at the various receptors predicts the side-effect profile. Blockade of α-adrenergic receptors produces sedation, hypotension, reflex tachycardia, and muscle relaxation. Hypotension is seen primarily with chlorpromazine because of its effect at α-adrenergic receptors while diphenhydramine (a phenothiazine antihistamine may cause xerostomia and sedation due to its activity at the acetylcholine receptor. Sedation and extrapyramidal symptoms are important potential side

| TABLE 13.4 | Antiemetics |

	Receptor Site of Activity	Dosage—Oral	Side Effects	Notes
Dopamine antagonists				
Haloperidol	D_2	1.5–2.5 mg daily	↑ Q-T interval (dose related) Dystonia Dyskinesia Akathesia	– $T_{1/2}$ = 16 h, can be given once or twice daily – Less sedation and hypotension than phenothiazines – Contraindicated in Parkinson's disease
Phenothiazines (prochlorperazine, chlorpromazine)	D_2	Prochlorperazine 5–10 mg every 6–8 h (maximum: 50 mg/d orally)	↑ Q-T interval ↓ salivation ↓ BP Sedation Akithesia	– Glaucoma, epilepsy, and prostate hypertrophy are relative contraindications – Contraindicated in Parkinson's disease
	H_1 ACh Ala	Chlorpromazine 10–25 mg every 4–6 h	Dystonia Dyskinesia	– more sedating than prochlorperazine
Metoclopramide	D_2 5-HT$_3$ (high dose) 5-HT$_4$ (potentiation)	10 mg every 6 h Extended release: 40 mg twice daily	Diarrhea Akithesia Fatigue	– dose must be reduced with renal impairment – Contraindicated in Parkinson's disease
Antihistamines				
Cyclizine	H_1	25–50 mg every 8 h	Sedation	– Cyclizine is least sedating of antihistamines
Diphenhydramine	H_1 ACh	25–50 mg every 6 h	Dry mouth Urinary retention	
Anticholinergics				
Hyoscine (scopolamine)	ACh	0.125–0.25 mg SL or orally every 4 h	Dry mouth Sedation Neurologic toxicity Urinary retention Ileus	– Should not be used in patients with narrow angle glaucoma – Will reverse effect of prokinetic agents
Serotonin Antagonists				
Ondansetron Granisetron and ropistron Palonestron	5-HT$_3$	4–8 mg every 4–8 h	Headache Constipation Fatigue	– Thought to be more effective in combination with dexamethasone

(Continued)

TABLE 13.4	Antiemetics (*Continued*)			
	Receptor Site of Activity	**Dosage—Oral**	**Side Effects**	**Notes**
Other Agents				
Corticosteroids	Unclear	Dexamethasone: 4–8 mg orally each morning	Glucose intolerance Proximal muscle weakness Lymphopenia Fluid retention Osteoporosis Behavioral/ psychiatric toxicity including psychosis Gastric irritation	– Dexamethasone is the drug of choice – Add proton pump inhibitor – Anti-inflammatory effects may provide beneficial effects for other symptoms
Cannabinoids	Unclear	2.5–5 mg orally every 8–12 h	Dysphoria Hallucinations Sedation	– Side effects are dose related – Side effects are increased in the elderly
Olanzapine	Ala D_2 H_1 ACh 5-HT		Sedation Diabetes ↓ Seizure threshold	– Long half-life allows once daily dosing – Limited efficacy data – May ↑ appetite and weight

D_2, dopamine type 2 receptor; H_1, histamine type 1 receptor; Ach, muscarinic acetylcholine receptor; Ala, α1-adrenergic receptor; 5-HT_3, 5-hydroxytryptamine type 3 receptor; 5-HT_4, 5-hydroxytryptamine type 4 receptor.

effects. The latter is less common with prochlorperazine than with other phenothiazines at usual antiemetic doses.

Metoclopramide has broad receptor site activity. As an antiemetic its major effect is through dopamine (D_2) antagonism at the CTZ (9,31). Unlike the phenothiazines, metoclopramide does not have activity as an antipsychotic or tranquilizing agent. It is widely prescribed for its prokinetic effect which is mediated through release of gastrointestinal acetylcholine secondary to activation of gastrointestinal 5-HT_4 receptors. As a prokinetic agent, metoclopramide increases gastric emptying and peristalsis of the duodenum and jejunum. This effect is reversed by anticholinergics. Although there are some conflicting data, a number of small studies concluded that metoclopramide is effective for chronic nausea in patients with cancer (32–36).

A controlled-release preparation (40 mg every 12 hours) has been reported to improve nausea with an improved side-effect profile compared with the short-acting drug (35). The major toxicities of metoclopramide are akithesia, especially in children and young adults, drowsiness, and extrapyramidal side effects. In high doses, metoclopramide has weak 5-HT_3 receptor antagonist activity.

Domperidone and cisapride are D_2 antagonist, prokinetic agents that are no longer available in the United States (37,38). Domperidone has a lower risk of extrapyramidal side effects than metoclopramide but was taken off of the market because of cardiac toxicity. Cisapride, unlike the other prokinetic agents, has activity throughout the gastrointestinal tract. Cardiac arrhythmias with the agent's use led to its withdrawal from the US market.

Antihistamine

Antihistamines have their primary antiemetic effect via H_1 receptors in the vomiting center, on the vestibular nucleus and in the CTZ (39,40). These agents also have variable antimuscarinic activity leading to decreased gastrointestinal mucosal secretory activity, peristalsis, and gut smooth muscle tone. These agents are most commonly prescribed for motion sickness. Cyclizine is the drug of choice for this because it is the least sedating of the antihistamines.

Anticholinergics

Hyoscine (scopalomine) is a muscarinic antagonist (41). It has antisecretory and antiemetic effects. Its two primary uses are for motion sickness and to decrease gastrointestinal secretions in patients with bowel obstruction. The primary side effects are dry mouth, sedation, ileus, urinary retention, and neurologic toxicities (confusion, hallucinations, tremors, acute psychosis, sedation, and dizziness).

In the elderly or in those patients with renal or hepatic dysfunction, neurologic side effects are more common.

Serotonin Antagonists

Serotonin receptors have been demonstrated centrally (vomiting center and CTZ) and peripherally (terminals of vagal afferents in the gut). The body's largest storage site for serotonin is in the enterochromaffin cells of the gut. Local insults to the gut (for example, abdominal irradiation) lead to active secretion of serotonin and stimulation of local vagal 5-HT_3 receptors. The serotonin antagonists block vagal afferent activity.

The 5-HT_3 receptor antagonists have become a mainstay of antiemetic guidelines for chemotherapy-induced nausea and vomiting (42,43). There are multiple agents commercially available with no demonstrated difference in their efficacy or toxicity at the recommended doses (44,45). There is some evidence to support their use for radiation-induced and post-operative nausea though there is limited evidence to support their use for chronic nausea in patients with advanced cancer (6,9,46). One trial reported improved control of emesis with tropisetron in patients with advanced illness, compared with dexamethasone plus chlorpromazine, while another reported ondansetron to be no better than placebo (47,48).

Other Agents

Corticosteroids

Corticosteroids are widely prescribed for nausea and vomiting, both as a single agent (for increased intracranial pressure, for example) and for its synergistic effect with serotonin antagonists (for chemotherapy induced emesis), and additive effect (as a component of combination regimens for malignant bowel obstruction [MBO], for example) (48). The mechanism of antiemetic activity of corticosteroids remains unknown. It has been postulated that corticosteroids reduce the permeability of the blood–brain barrier to emetic toxins, reduce brain stem release of enkephalin, deplete medullary amine γ-aminobutyric acid from medullary antiemetic neurons, and inhibit central prostaglandin synthesis and/or serotonin synthesis and release (49).

Dexamethasone is the recommended steroid of choice because of its limited mineralocorticoid effect and its prolonged half-life, allowing once daily dosing.

Patients with advanced illness may have multiple symptoms palliated by steroids. However, steroids also have significant toxicity. An initial dose of 4 to 8 mg daily is common, followed by a slow taper once symptoms are adequately controlled. The lowest effective dose should be utilized.

Cannabinoids

Synthetic cannabinoids have some antiemetic efficacy, although cannabis may be more effective than its synthetic analogues (50). The mechanism of their antiemetic effect is not clear, but recognition of a brain stem cannabinoid receptor suggests a potential site of activity of these compounds. The μ-opioid receptor may also be involved in the mechanism of action of the synthetic cannabinoids as naloxone reverses some of their antiemetic effect. The limited available data suggest that the synthetic cannabinoids have antiemetic efficacy on a par with prochlorperazine. Central nervous system side effects, including dysphoria, hallucinations, and sedation, limit their usefulness in the elderly.

Olanzapine

Olanzapine, an atypical antipsychotic, has antagonistic activity at a broad array of receptors, including α1, dopamine, histamine, and serotonin (51). Olanzapine is significantly more potent as an antagonist of 5-HT_2 receptors than D_2 receptors, accounting for its relative decrease in extrapyramidal effects compared with typical antipsychotic agents. Olanzapine's antimuscarinic, antihistamine, and α1-receptor antagonism may explain its anticholinergic side effects, the sedation, and orthostatic hypotension, respectively, observed as toxicities. There are relatively little data on the use of olanzapine as an antiemetic (52). The potential for appetite stimulation and weight gain is noteworthy.

Overall Approach

Once an etiology-based drug is selected, it is scheduled around the clock for ongoing nausea and vomiting. If relief is not achieved, the agent is titrated to maximum benefit or toxicity. If the symptoms remain inadequately controlled, a second agent with a different mechanism of action is added. A second agent, which works by blocking the same receptor as the first, is likely to add toxicity without further benefit. The second agent is also titrated to toxicity or control before considering an alternate approach.

An etiologic approach to antiemetic selection promotes a systematic approach to the evaluation and treatment of nausea and vomiting. Examples of common causes of nausea and vomiting in patients with advanced cancer, the responsible receptors, and recommended first-line antiemetics are shown in Table 13.5.

TABLE 13.5	Etiology-based antiemetic selection for common causes of nausea and vomiting		
Etiology	**Mechanism**	**Receptor**	**Recommended Antiemetics**
Opioid induced	Stimulates of CTZ	D_2	Haloperidol, prochlorperazine
	Gastroparesis	D_2, 5-HT$_4$	Metoclopramide, ondansetron
	Sensitize vestibular system	H_1, ACh	Prochlorperazine
	Constipation	H_1, ACh	
Impaired gastric motility	Gastroparesis	D_2	Metoclopramide
CNS metastases	CNS metastases	Stimulates VC and meningeal mechanoreceptors	Dexamethasone
	Increased intracranial pressure; meningeal irritation		
Malignant bowel obstruction	Stimulates CTZ	D_2	Metoclopramide for partial obstruction only
	Stimulates peripheral mechanoreceptors	H_1 ACh	Dexamethasone, octreotide/ anticholinergic

CTZ, chemoreceptor trigger zone; D_2, dopamine type 2 receptor; H_1, histamine type 1 receptor; ACh, acetylcholine receptor; VC, vomiting center; CNS, central nervous system; 5-HT$_4$, 5-hydroxytryptamine type 4 receptor.

OPIOID-INDUCED NAUSEA AND VOMITING

Opioid-induced nausea and vomiting occurs with the initiation of opioids or with dose titration in about 25% of patients (53). The symptoms are generally self-limited, lasting 3 to 5 days, if the opioids are continued, but should be promptly treated to avoid patient discontinuation of effective pain management. The etiology of opioid-induced nausea is multifactorial: reduced gastric motility, direct stimulation of the CTZ, and heightened vestibular sensitivity (54). The patient's associated symptoms may clarify which mechanism is playing the greatest role for an individual and aid in selecting antiemetic therapy. There are multiple antiemetics that are likely to resolve the symptoms and there is no evidence that one agent is of greater benefit than another. Cost and patient comorbidities may lead a clinician to choose one over another. As demonstrated in Table 13.5, opioid-related stimulation of the CTZ is mediated through dopamine receptors. Haloperidol and prochlorperazine each blocks D_2 and are considered first-line agents by many palliative care experts (30) (see Table 13.4 for major antiemetic adverse events and dosing). Metoclopramide blocks D_2 in the CTZ and increases peristalsis through release of gastrointestinal acetylcholine.

Antihistamines and anticholinergics reduce opioid-induced vestibular sensitivity. These agents should be considered in patients whose symptoms are worsened by movement.

A small proportion of people will develop persistent nausea and vomiting with opioids. If around-the-clock antiemetics are ineffective, a change in the opioid prescription may relieve the nausea and vomiting. For patients with well-controlled pain, the opioid dose may be titrated down until control of the nausea and vomiting or inadequate control of the pain. The likelihood of success may be increased by addition of an adjuvant analgesic. Opioid rotation may be considered if nausea and vomiting persists in spite of a reduction in opioid dose. The concept of opioid rotation is based on the variable affinity of different opioids to the opioid receptors. Nausea from one opioid may be relieved by changing to an alternate analgesic. The dose of the new opioid should be based on the degree of pain control, equianalgesic opioid conversion tables, and clinical assessment.

GASTROPARESIS

Gastroparesis is an important cause of nausea and vomiting and may present with associated reflux symptoms, bloating, early satiety, hiccups, and difficulty with oral intake. Gastroparesis may be secondary to a variety of causes. In the general population, diabetes mellitus is a common etiology. Malignant gastroparesis results from both obstructive and nonobstructive causes. It is most common in patients with upper gastrointestinal malignancies (55). It occurs in as many as 60% of patients with pancreatic cancer (56). Medications, such as opioids, may delay gastric emptying and small intestinal motility. Massive ascites, hepatomegaly, and intra-abdominal tumor progression may contribute to decreased gastrointestinal motility. Furthermore, abdominal radiation may lead to decreased tolerance of liquids and solids, though it is unclear whether this is due to decreased gastrointestinal motility.

Prokinetic agents are the treatment of choice for gastroparesis (9,57). These agents stimulate gastric emptying and small intestinal motility through potentiation of the 5-HT$_4$ receptor in the gastrointestinal tract. Metoclopramide sensitizes tissues to the effects of acetylcholine in the gut and blocks dopamine receptors centrally and peripherally to provide its antiemetic effect. Small trials in patients with advanced cancer have demonstrated improvement of gastroparesis-related symptoms from metoclopramide (58). Two randomized trials of controlled-release metoclopramide demonstrated improved symptom control in patients with advanced cancer and gastroparesis-related symptoms when compared with the immediate release formulation (33,34).

Cisapride and domperidone are prokinetic agents that are unavailable in the United States (37,38). While both agents improve gastric motility, each has been associated with unacceptable cardiac toxicity. Tegaserod acts as a partial 5-HT$_4$ agonist and stimulates secretions in the gastrointestinal tract. This agent increases gastric motility but has also been removed from the market in the United States because of cardiac toxicity (59). Erythromycin is a macrolide antibiotic with prokinetic effects. In small studies, it has led to improvement in gastroparesis-related symptoms. A meta-analysis suggested that erythromycin improves gastric motility by about 43%. (60).

MALIGNANT BOWEL OBSTRUCTION

The most common causes of MBO are ovarian cancer and colon cancer (61). All gastrointestinal malignancies are potential causes of bowel obstruction.

MBO presents with slowly progressive abdominal distension, colicky abdominal pain, nausea, vomiting, and changes in bowel habits. The symptoms progress as the obstruction progresses. The clinical characteristics provide clues to the level of obstruction. Large volume, watery, bilious emesis without a foul odor suggests a gastric or upper small intestinal obstruction. The presence of small volume emesis with particulate matter, with or without a foul odor, is suggestive of a distal small bowel or colon obstruction. For patients with advanced illness, surgery is rarely the recommended course of action.

Endoscopically inserted stents for patients with gastric or proximal small bowel obstructions frequently provide rapid relief of nausea and vomiting and allow patients to resume oral intake without significant morbidity (62).

Medical management may control symptoms for patients who are not candidates for stents or surgery. A combination of an antisecretory agent, antiemetic, and analgesics

is recommended (see Chapter 15 for a full discussion of MBO). Hyoscyamine and the somatostatin analog, octreotide, diminish gastrointestinal secretions and decrease nausea and pain by decreasing mucosal distention and peristalsis (62–64). If nausea persists, metoclopramide is recommended for patients with an incomplete obstruction. For patients with a complete obstruction, the prokinetic effect of metoclopramide may lead to colic. A central D$_2$ antagonist is generally recommended in this setting. Abdominal pain is controlled with opioids. Dexamethasone is often added to this treatment combination, though it is unclear whether its benefit is as an antiemetic or anti-inflammatory drug (48). A Cochrane review reported a nonsignificant trend, suggesting that corticosteroids are effective for the treatment of MBO (64).

If medical management is ineffective for the control of the symptoms of MBO, a venting gastrostomy may be placed. It is important that the goals and expectations from this intervention are clearly discussed as it portends a very short survival.

Not infrequently this discussion raises many issues related to nutrition and hydration. Psychoemotional support for the patient and family is an important component of care.

INTRACTABLE NAUSEA AND VOMITING

Despite best efforts, utilizing a mechanism-based approach to nausea with around-the-clock dosing of multiple targeted therapies at appropriate doses, some patients continue to experience nausea and vomiting. There are no clinical trial data to direct treatment. Corticosteroids are often recommended in spite of data to suggest a lack of benefit from steroids added to metoclopramide for patients with advanced cancer and nausea (34). A number of atypical antiemetics are available which may be considered for patients with intractable symptoms. Mirtazapine, an antidepressant, antagonizes the 5-HT$_3$ receptor. Limited clinical data suggest that it may provide some relief of intractable symptoms (65–67). Cannabinoids have been studied primarily for their impact on chemotherapy-induced nausea and vomiting. It has been suggested that the potency of cannabinoids as antiemetics is similar to that of phenothiazines (50). These agents should be used with caution in the elderly because of the potential for hallucinations, dysphoria, and confusion. Olanzapine, an atypical antipsychotic, blocks multiple receptors involved in emetogenesis, including dopamine, acetylcholine, histamine, and serotonin. There are inadequate data to discern its efficacy (51,52). Megestrol acetate, a synthetic progestational agent, used to stimulate appetite in patients with advanced cancer and other advanced illnesses, has been reported to decrease nausea though it is rarely prescribed for this indication (68).

The choice of agents used for patients with intractable symptoms must consider drug–drug interactions, comorbid illness, as well as potential efficacy. The route of administration is another important consideration for this population.

For the patient with refractory nausea and vomiting, the oral route of administration may not be feasible. Many of the common agents are available as rectal suppositories, sublingual formulations, or can be delivered as a subcutaneous infusion or injection.

Treatment of nausea and vomiting based on its presumed etiology may improve symptoms in as many as 90% of patients, though may not be as effective for patients with multiple potential causes of the symptoms (5,11,12). Of note, similar response rates have been found when antiemetics are chosen empirically.

Three randomized studies evaluating an empiric approach to antiemetic selection demonstrated limited benefit from metoclopramide (30% to 40% effective) but significant symptomatic relief from either serotonin or dopamine antagonists (80% to 90% effective) (33,35,47). As many of the currently available antiemetics work at multiple receptor sites, it is not surprising that empirical drug selection is often effective (5).

CONCLUSIONS

Nausea and vomiting are frequent symptoms of cancer and increase in frequency as the disease progresses. Whether one chooses to use an empiric or mechanism-based approach to treatment, it is essential to know the site of action of the prescribed antiemetics. This will allow for the broadest impact on the underlying causes of nausea and vomiting, limit toxicity, and maximize the benefit of treatment.

If symptoms are not adequately controlled with a single, around-the-clock medication, in adequate doses, a second agent should be added and titrated to effect. Further investigation of new agents and of combination therapies are needed to provide maximum relief of nausea and vomiting for patients with advanced illness.

REFERENCES

1. Tranmer JE, Heyland D, Dudgeon D, et al. Measuring the symptom experience of seriously ill cancer and noncancer hospitalized patients near the end of life with the memorial symptom assessment scale. *J Pain Symptom Manage.* 2003;25:420-429.
2. Solano JP, Gomes B, Higginson I. A comparison of symptom prevalence in far advanced cancer, AIDS, heart disease, chronic obstructive pulmonary disease and renal disease. *J Pain Symptom Manage.* 2006;31:58-69.
3. Twycross R, Wilcock A. *Palliative Car Formulary 3.* 3rd ed. Nottingham: Palliativedrugs.com Ltd; 2007.
4. Twycross R, Back I. Nausea and vomiting in advanced cancer. *Eur J Palliative Care.* 1998;5:39-44.
5. Glare PA, Dunwoodie D, Clark K, et al. Treatment of nausea and vomiting in terminally ill cancer patients. *Drugs.* 2008;68 (18):2575-2590.
6. Davis MP, Hallerberg G. A systematic review of the treatment of nausea and/or vomiting in cancer unrelated to chemotherapy or radiation. *J Pain Symptom Manage.* 2010;39:756-766.
7. Harris DG. Nausea and vomiting in advanced cancer. *Br Med Bull.* 2010;96:175-185.
8. Stephenson J, Davies A. An assessment of aetiology-based guidelines for the management of nausea and vomiting in patients with advanced cancer. *Support Care Cancer.* 2006;14: 348-353.
9. Wood GJ, Shega JW, Lynch B, Von Roenn JH. Management of intractable nausea and vomiting in patients at the end of life: "I was feeling nauseous all of the time… nothing was working." *JAMA.* 2007;298 (10):1196-1207.
10. Ang SK, Shoemaker LK, Davis MP. Nausea and vomiting in advanced cancer. American *J Hosp Palliat Med.* 2010;27(3):219-225.
11. Bentley A, Boyd K. Use of clinical pictures in the management of nausea and vomiting: a prospective audit. *Palliat Med.* 2001;15(3):247-253.
12. Lichter I. Results of antiemetic management in terminal illness. *J Palliat Care.* 1993;9(2):19-21.
13. Veehof LJ, Stewart RE, Meyboom-de Jong B, Haaijer-Ruskamp FM. Adverse drug reactions and polypharmacy in the elderly in general practice. *Eur J Clin Pharmacol.* 1999;55(7):533-536.
14. Ison PJ, Peroutka SJ. Neurotransmitter receptor binding studies predict anti-emetic efficacy and side effects. *Cancer Treat Rep.* 1986;70:637-641.
15. Dalal S, Palat G, Bruera E. Chronic nausea and vomiting. In: Berger A, Shuster J, Von Roenn J, eds. *Principles and Practice of Palliative Care and Supportive Oncology.* 3rd ed. Philadelphia, PA: Lippincott Williams & Wilkins;2007:151-162.
16. Borison HL, Wang SC. Physiology and pharmacology of vomiting. *Pharmacol Rev.* 1953;5(2):193-230.
17. Carpenter DO. Neural mechanisms of emesis. *Can J Physiol Pharmacol.* 1990;68(2):230-236.
18. Lang IM. Noxious stimulation of emesis. *Dig Dis Sci.* 1999;44(8) (suppl):58S-63S.
19. Mannix K. Palliation of nausea and vomiting in malignancy. *Clin Med.* 2006;6(2):144-147.
20. Burish TG, Tope DM. Psychological techniques for controlling the adverse side effects of cancer chemotherapy: findings from a decade of research. *J Pain Symptom Manage.* 1992;7(5): 287-301.
21. Morrow GR, Rosenthal SN. Models, mechanisms and management of anticipatory nausea and emesis. *Oncology.* 1996;53(suppl):4-7.
22. Richardson J, Smith JE, McCall G, et al. Hypnosis for nausea and vomiting in cancer chemotherapy: a systematic review of the research evidence. *Eur J Cancer Care.* September 2007;16(5):402-412.
23. Vickers AJ. Can acupuncture have specific effects on health? A systematic review of acupuncture antiemesis trials. *J R Soc Med.* 1996;89(6):303-311.
24. Pan CX, Morrison RS, Ness J, Fugh-Berman A, Leipzig RM. Complementary and alternative medicine in the management of pain, dyspnea, and nausea and vomiting near the end of life: a systematic review. *J Pain Symptom Manage.* 2000;20(5):374-387.
25. Lee A, Done ML. *Stimulation of the Wrist Acupuncture Point P6 for Preventing Postoperative Nausea and Vomiting (Cochrane Review).* The Cochrane Library, Issue 3. Chichester: John Wiley & Sons, Ltd; 2004.
26. Perkins P, Vowler SL. Does acupressure help reduce nausea and vomiting in palliative care patients? Pilot study. *Palliat Med.* 2008;22:193-194.
27. Glare P, Pereira G, Kristjanson LJ, Stockler M, Tattersall M. Systematic review of the efficacy of antiemetics in the treatment

of nausea in patients with far-advanced cancer. *Support Care Cancer.* 2004;12(6):432-440.

28. Hardy JR, O'Shea A, White C, Gilshenan K, Welch L, Douglas C. The efficacy of haloperidol in the management of nausea and vomiting in patients with cancer. *J Pain Symptom Manage.* 2010;40(1):111-116.

29. Perkins P, Dorman S. Haloperidol for the treatment of nausea and vomiting in palliative care patients. *Cochrane Database Syst Rev.* 2009; 2: Art. No.: CD006271. doi:10.1002/14651858.CD006271.pub2.

30. Critchley P, Plach N, Grantham M, et al. Efficacy of haloperidol in the treatment of nausea and vomiting in the palliative patient: a systematic review. *J Pain Symptom Manage.* 2001;22:631-634.

31. Parischa PJ. Prokinetics, antiemetics and agents used in irritable bowel syndrome. In: Hardman JG, Limbird LE, Gilman AG, eds. *Goodman & Gilman's The Pharmacologic Basis of Therapeutics.* 10th ed. New York, NY: McGraw-Hill; 2001:1021-1037.

32. Bruera E, Seifert L, Watanabe S, et al. Chronic nausea in advanced cancer patients: a retrospective assessment of a metoclopramide-based antiemetic regimen. *J Pain Symptom Manage.* 1996;11:147-153.

33. Bruera E, Balzile M, Neumann C, et al. A double-blind, crossover study of controlled-release metoclopramide and placebo for the chronic nausea and dyspepsia of advanced cancer. *J Pain Symptom Manage.* 2000;19:427-435.

34. Bruera E, Moyano JR, Sala R, et al. Dexamethasone in addition to metoclopramide for chronic nausea in patients with advanced cancer: a randomized controlled trial. *J Pain Symptom Manage.* 2004;28(4):381-388.

35. Bruera ED, MacEachern TJ, Spachynski KA, et al. Comparison of the efficacy, safety, and pharmacokinetics of controlled release and immediate release metoclopramide for the management of chronic nausea in patients with advanced cancer. *Cancer.* 1994;74(12):3204-3211.

36. Corli O, Cozzolino A, Battaiotto L. Effectiveness of levosulpiride versus metoclopramide for nausea and vomiting in advanced cancer patients: a double-blind, randomized, crossover study. *J Pain Symptom Manage.* 1995;10(7):521-526.

37. Osborne RJ, Slevin ML, Hunter RW, et al. Cardiotoxicity of intravenous domperidone. *Lancet.* 1985;II:385.

38. McCallum RW, Prakash C, Campoli-Richards DM, et al. Cisapride: a preliminary review of its pharmacodynamic and pharmacokinetic properties, and therapeutic use as a prokinetic agent in gastrointestinal motility disorders. *Drugs.* 1988;36:652-681.

39. Paton DM, Webster DR. Clinical pharmacokinetics of H1-receptor antagonists (the antihistamines). *Clin Pharmacokinet.* 1985;10:477-497.

40. McCawley EL, Kulasavage RJ, Warrington WR, Pasquesi TJ. The intravenous use of diphenhydramine hydrochloride in the control of nausea and vomiting. *Portland Clin Bull.* 1951;5(3):43-48.

41. Golding JF, Stott JR. Comparison of the effects of a selective muscarinic receptor antagonist and hyoscine (scopolamine) on motion sickness, skin conductance and heart rate. *Br J Clin Pharmacol.* 1997;43:633-637.

42. Gregory RE, Ettinger DS. 5-HT3 receptor antagonists for the prevention of chemotherapy-induced nausea and vomiting: a comparison of their pharmacology and clinical efficacy. *Drugs.* 1998;55:173-189.

43. Hesketh PJ, van Belle S, Aapro M, et al. Differential involvement of neurotransmitters through the time course of cisplatin-induced emesis as revealed by therapy with specific receptor antagonists. *Eur J Cancer.* 2003;39:1074-1080.

44. Aapro M. 5-HT(3)-receptor antagonists in the management of nausea and vomiting in cancer and cancer treatment. *Oncology.* 2005;69:97-109.

45. Currow DC, Coughlan M, Fardell B, et al. Use of ondansetron in palliative medicine. *J Pain Symptom Manage.* 1997;13:302-307.

46. Priestman TJ, Roberts JT, Lucraft H, et al. Results of a randomized, double-blind comparative study of ondansetron and metoclopramide in the prevention of nausea and vomiting following high-dose upper abdominal irradiation. *Clin Oncol (R Coll Radiol).* 1990;2(2):71-75.

47. Mystakidou K, Befon S, Liossi C, et al. Comparison of the efficacy and safety of tropisetron, metoclopramide, and chlorpromazine in the treatment of emesis associated with far advanced cancer. *Cancer.* 1998;83:1214-1223.

48. Aapro, MS. Present role of corticosteroids as antiemetics. *Recent Results Cancer Res.* 1991;121:91-100.

49. Malagelada JR, Malagelada C. Nausea and vomiting. In: Feldman M, Friedman LS, Brandt LJ, eds. *Sleisenger & Fordtran's Gastrointestinal and Liver Disease.* 8th ed. Philadelphia, PA: Saunders; 2006:143-158.

50. Doblin RE, Kleiman, MAR. Marijuana as antiemetic medicine: a survey of oncologists' experiences and attitudes. *J Clin Oncol.* 1991;9:1314-1319.

51. Licup N, Baumrucker S. Olanzapine for Nausea and Vomiting. *Am J Hosp Palliat Med.* 2010;27(6):432-434.

52. Passik SD, Navari RM, Jung SH, et al. A phase I trial of olanzapine for the prevention of delayed emesis in cancer patients: a Hoosier Oncology Group study. *Cancer Invest.* 2004;22(3):383-388.

53. Campora E, Merlini L, Pace M, et al. The incidence of narcotic-induced emesis. *J Pain Symptom Manage.* 1991;6(7):428-430.

54. Gutner LB, Gould WJ, Batterman RC. The effects of potent analgesics upon vestibular function. *J Clin Invest.* 1952;31(3):259-266.

55. Schraml FV, Krueger WH. Presentation of gastric carcinoma on a radionuclide gastric-emptying study. *Clin Nucl Med.* 2005;30:574.

56. Barkin JS, Goldberg RI, Sfakianakis GN, Levi J. Pancreatic carcinoma is associated with delayed gastric emptying. *Dig Dis Sci.* 1986;31:265.

57. Bruera E, Catz Z, Hooper R, Lentle B, MacDonald N. Chronic nausea and anorexia in advanced cancer patients: a possible role for autonomic dysfunction. *J Pain Symptom Manage.* 1987;2(1):19-21.

58. Nelson KA, Walsh TD. Metoclopramide in anorexia caused by cancer-associated dyspepsia syndrome (CADS). *J Palliat Care.* 1993;9(2):14-18.

59. Loughlin J, Quinn S, Rinero E, Wong J, et al. Tegaserod and the risk of cardiovascular ischemic events: an observational cohort study. *J Cardiovasc Pharmacol Ther.* 2010;15(2):151-157.

60. Maganti K, Onyemere K, Jones MP. Oral erythromycin and symptomatic relief of gastroparesis: a systematic review. *Am J Gastroenterol.* 2003;98:259.

61. Legendre H, Vanbuyse F, Caroli-Bosc FX, Pector JC. Survival and quality of life after palliative surgery for neoplastic gastrointestinal obstruction. *Eur J Surg Oncol.* 2001;27:364-367.

62. Ripamonti CI, Easson AM, Gerdes H. Management of malignant bowel obstruction. *Eur J Cancer.* 2008;44(8):1105-1115. [review].

63. Ripamonti C, Mercadante S, Groff L, et al. Role of octreotide, scopolamine butylbromide, and hydration in symptom control of patients with inoperable bowel obstruction and nasogastric tubes: a prospective randomized trial. *J Pain Symptom Manage.* 2000;19(1):23-34.

64. Feuer DJ, Broadley KE. Corticosteroids for the resolution of malignant bowel obstruction in advanced gynaecological and gastrointestinal cancer. *Cochrane Database Syst Rev.* 2000;(3):CD001219.

65. Pae CU. Low-dose mirtazapine may be successful treatment option for severe nausea and vomiting. *Prog Neuropsychopharmacol Biol Psychiatry.* 2006;30(6):1143-1145.

66. Thompson DS. Mirtazapine for the treatment of depression and nausea in breast and gynecological oncology. *Psychosomatics.* 2000;41(4):356-359.

67. Kim SW, Shin IS, Kim JM, et al. Mirtazapine for severe gastroparesis unresponsive to conventional prokinetic treatment. *Psychosomatics.* 2006;47(5):440-442.

68. Loprinzi CL, Michalak JC, Schaid DJ, et al. Phase III evaluation of four doses of megestrol acetate as therapy for patients with cancer anorexia and/or cachexia. *J Clin Oncol.* 1993;11:762-767.

CHAPTER 14

Diarrhea, Malabsorption, and Constipation

Sebastiano Mercadante

The pathophysiology of the gastrointestinal (GI) tract leading to changes in normal activity is complex. The GI function is mediated through endocrine, paracrine, and neural forms of cellular communication. The GI tract has its own intrinsic nervous system in the form of myenteric and submucosal plexuses, receiving an extrinsic input from the central nervous system via the autonomic nervous system. Furthermore, the GI tract has its own pacemaker cells, which generate rhythmic electrical activity. Complex communication and coordination are required to produce segmental contraction that serves to produce segmental and peristaltic contractions that mix and move the endoluminal content forward. Many neurotransmitters mediate this communication. Any damage occurring due to different causes in patients with cancer at the different levels of this complex system may result in changes of GI mobility and activity.

DIARRHEA

Diarrhea is generally defined as the frequent passage of loose stools with urgency, commonly more than three unformed stools in 24 hours (1). Diarrhea is a common and significant problem among patients with cancer, occurring in 5% to 10% of patients with advanced disease, and is seen as a major treatment complication in patients receiving chemotherapy, particularly with some agents (2). Women are more likely to have diarrhea than men after excluding gender-specific cancers (3). Diarrhea is also included among the top 10 consequences of adverse drug reactions in hospitalized patients with cancer (4). The consequences of diarrhea can be troublesome and include loss of water, electrolytes, and albumin, failure to reach nutritional goals, declining immune function, and the risk of bedsores or systemic infection. Diarrhea also brings additional work for the nursing staff or family who have to prevent maceration and bedsores. Moreover, losses of comfort and dignity have to be considered. Severe diarrhea, other than being debilitating, is a costly complication of chemotherapy in colorectal cancer (5). The median length of hospital stay due to diarrhea was 8 days, translating to a mean cost of $8,230 per patient (6).

Although a practical definition is lacking, diarrhea is commonly diagnosed when an abnormal increase in daily stool weight, water content, and frequency, whether or not accompanied by urgency, perianal discomfort, or incontinence, is present as a consequence of incomplete absorption of electrolytes and water from luminal content.

Mechanisms

From the physiopathologic point of view, different mechanisms may produce diarrhea, although it is quite difficult in certain clinical conditions to distinguish among mechanisms that frequently overlap.

Osmotic Diarrhea

The ingestion of a poorly absorbable solute modifies the osmolarity of the luminal content and induces osmotic diarrhea. The proximal small bowel is highly permeable to water; sodium and water influx across the duodenum rapidly adjusts the osmolarity of luminal fluid toward that of plasma, secreting water even after the osmolarity values between luminal contents and plasma are similar. On the contrary, the mucosa of the ileum and colon has a low permeability to sodium and solutes. However, there is an efficient active ion transport mechanism that allows the reabsorption of electrolytes and water even against electrochemical gradients.

Excessive doses of laxatives or magnesium-containing antacids commonly result in diarrhea. When large amounts of lactulose, an unabsorbable sugar in the small intestine, are ingested, the protective role of colonic bacteria may be exhausted, producing diarrhea proportional to the osmotic force of the malabsorbed saccharide (7). It is characterized by an osmotic gap in stool analysis equivalent to the concentration of the osmotically active agents in fecal fluid that cause diarrhea. Similarly, carbohydrate malabsorption may induce osmotic diarrhea, which is characterized by a low stool pH, because of the presence of short-chain fatty acids, a high content of carbohydrates, a high stool osmolarity, and flatulence. Moreover, reversible chemotherapy-related hypolactasia and lactose intolerance are not infrequent in patients treated with 5-fluorouracil (5-FU)–based adjuvant chemotherapy for colorectal cancer. Avoidance of lactose during chemotherapy may improve treatment tolerability in these patients (8).

The ingestion of other substances, such as magnesium, sulfate, and poorly absorbed salts may produce osmotic diarrhea. However, there will be a normal pH, unlike in carbohydrate-induced diarrhea. In the perioperative period, massive antibiotic therapy is able to suppress normal colonic metabolism, thereby resulting in diarrhea (7). Osmotic diarrhea commonly subsides as the patient discontinues the poorly absorbable agents.

Secretory Diarrhea

Secretory diarrhea is rarely present as the sole mechanism and is often associated with other mechanisms (7). This kind of diarrhea is associated with an abnormal ion transport in intestinal epithelial cells, with a reduction in absorptive function or increase in the secretion of epithelial cells. Unlike in osmotic diarrhea, the anionic gap is small and eating does not markedly increase stool volume. Moreover, diarrhea usually persists despite fasting.

Many factors may affect ion transport in the epithelial cells of the gut. These include bacterial toxins, intraluminal secretagogues (such as bile acids or laxatives), or circulating secretagogues (such as various hormones, drugs, and poisons). Moreover, other medical problems that compromise regulation of intestinal function or reduce absorptive surface area (by disease or resection) can induce secretory diarrhea (9).

Endocrine tumors may cause diarrhea through the release of secretagogue transmitters (10). Diarrhea is a common manifestation of a carcinoid syndrome, occurring in approximately 70% of patients, and seems to be mediated by the release of serotonin and substance P. In the Zollinger-Ellison syndrome, secretory diarrhea is the consequence of gastric hypersecretion caused by a high concentration of circulating gastrin, overwhelming the intestinal absorptive capacity. In a medullary carcinoma of the thyroid, circulating calcitonin is the major mediator of intestinal secretion (11).

Malabsorption due to different mechanisms may equally produce diarrhea (see Section Malabsorption).

Cancer treatment–related diarrhea is the most known and is caused by chemotherapeutic agents such as fluoropyrimidines, taxanes, capecitabine, and irinotecan (6), and graft-versus-host disease (GVHD) (12) and targeted therapy significantly affect morbidity and mortality. Diarrhea is a significant consequence of colorectal chemotherapy, with most patients experiencing grade 3 or 4 diarrhea (13). Patients who experienced chemotherapy-induced diarrhea underwent changes in their regimen, including dose reductions, delays in therapy, reduction in dose intensity, and discontinuation of therapy (2). These agents cause acute and chronic damage to the intestinal mucosa, necrosis, and extensive inflammation of the bowel wall. Mucosal and submucosal factors, produced directly or indirectly by the inflamed intestine, stimulate secretion of intestinal fluid and electrolytes. Similar anatomic changes have been observed in patients with GVHD-induced diarrhea, as well as with radiation enteritis (14). The toxicity grades of these agents seem to depend on individual genotypes (15); 53% of patients treated with concurrent pelvic radiation therapy and fluorouracil develop diarrhea (16). The severity of diarrhea is correlated with the volume of small bowel receiving at least 15 Gy of radiation (17). Chronic radiation enteritis is less common and is usually associated with radiation doses >45 Gy. In this case, the underlying pathology is an endoarteritis that causes intestinal ischemia (13).

On the other hand, intestinal mucositis also increases the risk of superinfection by opportunistic pathogens such as *Clostridium difficile*, *Clostridium perfringens*, *Bacillus cereus*, *Giardia lamblia*, *Cryptosporidium*, *Salmonella*, *Shigella*, *Campylobacter*, and *Rotavirus*, particularly in patients who may be neutropenic or immunosuppressed. Bacterial enterotoxins or other infective agents induce secretion probably by a local nervous reflex mediated by enteroendocrine cells or inflammation (1). The incidence of *C. difficile*–induced diarrhea is very high—2.2% in patients receiving standard-dose regimens and 20% in patients receiving high-dose regimens (18).

The use of long-term antibiotics is also associated with diarrhea in patients who recently underwent surgery or are immunocompromised. Agents more frequently causing diarrhea include ampicillin, clindamycin, or cephalosporins, because of the disruption of the normal flora and facilitation of the overgrowth of pathogens. *C. difficile*, an anaerobic organism producing an enteric toxin, induces pseudomembranous enterocolitis, which presents as a severe microbial diarrhea. Other infectious agents include *C. perfringens*, *Staphylococcus aureus*, *Klebsiella oxytoca*, *Candida* species, and *Salmonella* species (19).

Diarrhea induced by enteral feeding is via nasogastric tube or gastroenterostomies. It is a common problem that is observable in 10% to 60% of patients. Formula osmolarity, rate of delivery, and contamination are determinants (13). Finally, many drugs may cause diarrhea. Diuretics, caffeine, theophylline, antacids, antibiotics, and poorly absorbable laxative agents and osmotically active solutes, often chronically administered in a palliative care setting, likely produce reflex nervous secretion or directly activate secretory cellular mechanism (1).

Deranged Motility

Deranged motility may reduce the contact time between luminal contents and epithelial cells. This commonly occurs in patients with cancer with postsurgical disorders, such as postgastrectomy dumping syndrome, postvagotomy, ileocecal valve resection, or neoplastic and chronic diseases such as malignant carcinoid syndrome, medullary carcinoma of the thyroid, and diabetes. The mechanism by which diabetic neuropathy causes dysmotility is attributed to a sympathetic denervation of the bowel with a prevalence of cholinergic innervation (19). Similarly, procedures such as celiac plexus block produce a sympathetic denervation of the bowel, which may leave a cholinergic innervation unopposed, leading to an increase in intestinal motility and diarrhea, until adaptation mechanisms develop (13).

Spinal cord damage may reduce intestinal mobility favoring bacterial overgrowth, which induces a deconjugation of bile acids in the small bowel and thereby causes diarrhea and steatorrhea. Diarrhea secondary to dysmotility disorders commonly subsides after a 1 to 2-day fast, determining a small stool volume and an osmolality in the range of 250 to 300 mOsm.

Assessment

The assessment includes a detailed medical history, dietary history, previous surgery, medication review, physical examination, and description of stools. Frequency, amounts, and consistency of the stools should be carefully obtained. When the stools are consistently large, light in color, watery or greasy, free of blood, or contain undigested food particles, the underlying disorder is likely to be in the small bowel or the proximal colon. Indeed, small stool diarrhea, in which frequent but small quantities of feces that are dark in color and often contain mucus or blood pass in spite of a sense of urgency, is associated with a disorder of the left colon or rectum (1,13). Widespread inflammation may simultaneously produce both patterns of diarrhea, confirmed by the passage of nonbloody diarrheal fluid, pus, or exudates. Other useful information includes fecal incontinence, change in stool caliber, rectal bleeding, and small, frequent, but otherwise normal stools.

Timing and spontaneous recovery are also important. Although osmotic diarrhea typically stops or reduces after fasting or stopping the drug previously used, secretory diarrhea persists in spite of fasting. Chemotherapy-induced diarrhea typically occurs 2 to 14 days after therapy. Radiation colitis is probable in patients who have recently received pelvic radiation for malignancies of the urogenital tract and of the prostate.

A physical examination should precede any further investigation. Signs of anemia, fever, postural hypotension, lymphadenopathy, neuropathy, hepatosplenomegaly, ascites, gaseous abdominal distention or lymphadenopathy, reduced anal sphincter tone, a rectal mass or impaction, and deterioration of nutritional status are of paramount importance in defining the type of diarrhea. Some etiologies may have a typical clinical pattern. For example, carbohydrate malabsorption is typically associated with excessive flatus and mushy stools, whereas intermittent diarrhea and constipation are frequent in diabetic neuropathy, as well as in irritable bowel syndrome or subobstructive disorders. Autonomic neuropathy or anal sphincter dysfunction may be characterized by nocturnal diarrhea and fecal soiling. Alternating diarrhea and constipation suggests fixed colonic obstruction. Fecal impaction may cause apparent diarrhea because only liquids pass a partial obstruction. Symptoms of dumping syndrome after gastric surgery, such as early nausea, abdominal distention, weakness, and diarrhea after a meal followed by hypoglycemia, sweating, dizziness, and tachycardia, are typical. Secretory diarrhea combined with upper GI symptoms caused by refractory peptic ulcer disease is suggestive of a gastrin-secreting tumor. High circulating serotonin levels in carcinoid syndrome cause other effects besides diarrhea, including hypotension, sweating, flushing, palpitation, and wheeziness (19). The association of heat intolerance, palpitations, and weight loss suggests possible hyperthyroidism. Intestinal dysmotility or bacterial overgrowth due to diabetes, neoplastic conditions, or postoperative conditions should be suspected, excluding other causes.

Chronic bowel ischemia should be considered in elderly patients with the clinical features of diffuse atherosclerotic disease. Rectal examination and abdominal palpation should be performed to look for fecal masses and to exclude fecal impaction and intestinal obstruction, as well as for perianal fistula or abscess. Rectal involvement is probable in the presence of *tenesmus*, commonly defined as the passing of a little or no stool in spite of a sense of rectal urgency.

Of course, the site of neoplasm and metastases is of paramount importance. An abdominal x-ray will help the diagnosis. The location of the tumor will be verified by computed tomography scan, magnetic resonance imaging, angiography, or laparoscopy.

Laboratory findings should complete the investigation. If feasible, collected diarrhea stool specimen should be submitted for qualitative study. A positive finding in either the stool guaiac or the leukocyte test leads to a suspicion of an exudative mechanism, as in radiation colitis, colonic neoplasm, or infective diarrhea. Stool cultures for bacterial, fungal, and viral pathogens, as well as a formal evaluation of the GI tract, should complete the initial assessment (14). Gram stain of the stool can diagnose the presence of *Staphylococcus*, *Campylobacter*, or *Candida* infection. Multiple stool cultures should be obtained from patients with secretory diarrhea to rule out microorganisms producing enterotoxins that stimulate intestinal secretion. The presence of a microorganism in the stools is diagnostic.

An anionic gap of >50 mmol/L due to a reduction of stool content in sodium and potassium suggests an osmotic diarrhea, whereas lower values (<50 mmol/L) indicate a secretory diarrhea due to active secretion of salts and water.

Treatment

As a general rule, current medication should be revised, considering the use of laxatives, antacids, theophylline preparations, central nervous system drugs, antiarrhythmics, and antibiotics. Dietary advice may be helpful in some circumstances, although difficult to follow by most patients with cancer. A gluten-free diet can reduce abdominal cramping and frequency of bowel movement in the presence of intestinal fermentation with bowel distention. Binders of osmotically active substances (kaolin–pectin) give a thicker consistency to loose stools, producing a viscous, colloidal, and absorbent solution, but their antidiarrheal effectiveness is disputable. Apples without the peel are particularly rich in pectin. Other dietary advices include avoiding cold meals, milk, vegetables rich in fibers, fatty meat, and fish, coffee, and alcohol.

As diarrhea is associated with the occurrence of dehydration, the patient should be rehydrated, possibly by oral solutions containing glucose, electrolytes, and water. However, clinical signs of dehydration, such as orthostatic hypotension, decreased skin turgor, and a dry mouth, suggest the need for intensive hydration through intravenous route, especially in patients suffering from nausea and vomiting in whom oral

TABLE 14.1   Etiology-Based treatment

Etiology	Treatment
All conditions	Dietary advice and adequate hydration
Radiation-induced diarrhea	Hypofractionated–accelerated radiotherapy and amifostine
	Cholestyramine, aspirin, sucralfate, silicate smectite, and steroids
Bacterial overgrowth–related diarrhea	Antibiotics
Antibiotic-associated diarrhea	Discontinuation of antibiotics and start with metronidazole
	Probiotic bacteria
Chemotherapy-induced diarrhea	Alkalization, activated charcoal, loperamide, and octreotide
Hormonal gastrointestinal tumors	Octreotide
Diabetic diarrhea	Clonidine

therapy is ineffective. Patients may experience electrolyte imbalance, particularly hypokalemia (1)

Considering the different mechanisms involved in determining diarrhea in patients with cancer, there are no broadly accepted treatment protocols. Particular strategies have been anecdotally suggested for specific etiologies (Table 14.1). The most common treatment medications and doses used for diarrhea are given in Table 14.2. Cholestyramine, aspirin, and sucralfate have been favorably used in radiation-induced

TABLE 14.2   Treatment medications for diarrhea

Bile acid sequestrant	
Cholestyramine	4–12 g
Antibiotics	
Vancomycin	125–250 mg 8 hourly
Metronidazole	250–500 mg 8 hourly
Mucosal prostaglandin inhibitors	
Aspirin	300 mg 4 hourly
Opioid agents	
Codeine	10–60 mg 4 hourly
Loperamide	4 mg stat, then 2 mg 6 hourly and after each loose
Somatostatin analogs	
Octreotide	0.3–0.6 mg/d (continuous infusion)
	0.1 mg 8 hourly

diarrhea (20). Silicate smectite has proved to be a promising drug in the prophylaxis of radiotherapy-induced diarrhea, particularly in patients with a low, irradiated, small bowel volume (21). From recent investigations, it seems that the best treatment would be prevention. In gynecologic malignancies, prior operation with low pelvic fields and prior operation with small volume were significantly protective factors for overall diarrhea. Conversely, large volume was a significant factor of overall and moderate to severe diarrhea in patients with large-field operations (22). Hypofractionated and accelerated radiotherapy for prostate cancer were supported with a high dose of amifostine (1,000 mg s.c.) daily to protect normal tissues against early and late effects and produced only grade 0 to 1 cystitis or diarrhea (5/7 grade 0) (23). Amifostine reduced the incidence and severity of diarrhea associated with 5-fluorouracil, although its use may be associated with hypotension (24).

Steroids may exert a positive effect on several conditions associated with diarrhea, including secretory diarrhea, intestinal pseudo-obstruction, radiation-induced enteritis, endocrine tumors due to anti-inflammatory effects, and the capability of reducing the release and effect of inflammation mediators and promoting salts and water absorption. They are also included in the pharmacologic approach to GVHD-induced diarrhea (14). Budesonide, a topically active steroid, demonstrated a substantial activity in preventing irinotecan-induced diarrhea (25).

Antibiotics, such as norfloxacin and amoxicillin–clavulanic acid, are effective in the treatment of bacterial overgrowth–related diarrhea (26). On the contrary, antibiotic-associated diarrhea (pseudomembranous enterocolitis) requires the discontinuation of antibiotics and the starting of either metronidazole or vancomycin (27). Bismuth subsalicylate in doses of 30 to 60 mL every 30 minutes for eight doses may bring mild symptomatic relief in patients with acute infectious diarrhea with an unknown effect. Probiotic bacteria (i.e., live bacteria that survive passage through the GI tract) may have beneficial effects on the host (28). Live *Lactobacillus acidophilus* plus *Bifidobacterium bifidum* reduced the incidence of radiation-induced diarrhea and the need for antidiarrheal medication and had a significant benefits on stool consistency (29).

Alkalization of the intestinal tract by oral administration of sodium bicarbonate has been reported to be a promising method for preventing delayed diarrhea, a dose-limiting toxicity in patients receiving chemotherapy with irinotecan, without decreasing the blood levels of irinotecan and its active metabolites, thereby improving the tolerability of long-term chemotherapy without reducing the efficacy (30). An oral adsorbent (2 g Kremezin × three times) has been shown to decrease the number of bowel motions, without decreasing the plasma clearance of irinotecan much (31). Activated charcoal, given the evening before the irinotecan dose and then t.i.d. for 48 hours after the dose, reduced irinotecan-induced diarrhea and optimized its dose intensity, possibly by adsorbing free luminal SN-38, the irinotecan-active moiety that has a direct effect on mucosal topoisomerase-I (32). Broad-spectrum antibiotics may influence the intestinal toxicity of irinotecan. Although neomycin had no effect on the systemic exposure of irinotecan and its major metabolites, it changed fecal β-glucuronidase activity and decreased fecal concentrations of the pharmacologically active metabolite SN-38. It was associated with an improvement in diarrhea and not with hematologic toxicity, suggesting that bacterial β-glucuronidase plays a crucial role in irinotecan-induced diarrhea without affecting enterocyclic and systemic SN-38 levels (33).

Opioids have been traditionally used for their antidiarrheal properties owing to the widespread presence of opioid receptors at different peripheral sites, including smooth muscle, myenteric plexus, and spinal cord. It is well known that their activation increases ileocecal tone and decreases small intestine and colon peristalsis (increasing electrolyte and water absorption). It also impairs the defecation reflex by inhibiting anorectal sphincter relaxation and diminishing anorectal sensitivity to distention. As a consequence, the contact time between the intestinal mucosa and luminal contents is enhanced by the reduction of colonic propulsive activity, resulting in greater fluid absorption (34). Antidiarrheal effects can be obtained by both oral and parenteral opioids. Among opioids, loperamide is more specific because of the prevalent peripheral effect due to the inability to cross the blood–brain barrier. Loperamide shows the highest antidiarrheal/analgesic ratio among the opioid-like agents and is proved to be the drug of choice because of its few adverse effects. The standard dose of loperamide is 4 mg followed by 2 mg after every unformed stool. The dosage is titrated against the effect and higher doses of 2 mg every 2 hours have been recommended (up to 12 mg/d or more) in conjunction with chemotherapeutic agents associated with a high incidence of diarrhea (35). Loperamide–simethicone

combination was significantly more effective than the drugs taken alone in the treatment of acute diarrhea with gas-related abdominal discomfort (36). However, the risk of developing paralytic ileus in the presence of continuous secretion should be considered as a life-threatening complication. Of interest, opioids may paradoxically cause diarrhea secondary to fecal impaction.

Data from several clinical trials suggest that octreotide may be useful in the symptomatic treatment of diarrhea refractory to other medications (34,35). The mechanism by which octreotide produces these beneficial effects is probably multifactorial, as it reduces the secretion of many pancreatic and GI hormones, prolonging intestinal transit time and thereby promoting absorption of electrolytes (37). Octreotide has been found to control diarrhea in several conditions, such as carcinoid tumors, vipoma, gastrinoma, small cell lung cancer, and acquired immunodeficiency syndrome–related diarrhea (38). However, hormonal responses to the somatostatin analog do not always parallel clinical responses, probably because of the effects of cosecreted peptides. A dose–response effect of octreotide has been demonstrated. Octreotide seems to be an effective agent in the management of chemotherapy-related diarrhea and refractory GVHD-associated diarrhea (39,40). Doses of 0.3 to 1.2 mg/d subcutaneously are commonly effective. Octreotide was also effective in the treatment of radiation-induced diarrhea (41).

Long-acting, biodegradable, and microsphere formulation of octreotide for monthly subcutaneous administration (30 mg) has been evaluated for the prophylaxis of diarrhea, speeding the resolution of diarrhea and preventing further episodes during subsequent cycles of chemotherapy (42). A preventive strategy with octreotide long acting release (LAR) as prophylaxis has been proposed for patients with a prior cycle of chemotherapy complicated by persistent diarrhea (36,43). Depot octreotide did not prevent diarrhea during pelvic radiation therapy, underlining the differences between prevention and treatment (16,44).

MALABSORPTION

An ineffective absorption of breakdown products in the small intestine may occur because a disorder interferes either with the digestion of food or directly with the absorption of nutrients. The digestive and absorptive processes are inextricably linked. The series of events include the reduction of particle size, solubilization of hydrophobic lipids, and enzymatic digestion of nutrients to small fragments, absorption of the products of digestion across the intestinal cells, and transport through lymphatics.

Physiopathology of Digestion

The pancreatic secretion of lipase, amylase, and proteases breaks down fat to monoglycerides and fatty acids, carbohydrates to monosaccharides and disaccharides, and proteins to peptides and amino acids. Several processes have been recognized to facilitate the absorption of fat from the aqueous luminal environment. Triglycerides are emulsified together with phospholipids, bile salts, and monoglycerides and diglycerides and dispersed into a variety of phases and particles. Lipid digestion begins in the mouth and in the stomach, active at a low pH, promoting emulsion stability and facilitating the action of pancreatic lipases. Gastric and pyloric motility further promotes emulsification of lipids. This effect is amplified by bile salts and biliary phospholipids, which also influence the absorption of cholesterol and sterol vitamins. Lipolysis to fatty acids and monoglycerides is mediated by pancreatic lipases (34). Protein digestion begins in the stomach. Acid denaturation leads to proteolysis, which is promoted by endopeptidases activated by an acidic environment, cleaving the internal bonds of large proteins to form nonabsorbable peptides. Pancreatic peptidases convert proteins and polypeptides into amino acids and oligopeptides. Hormonal and neural stimulation stimulates the release of proenzymes by the pancreas. Enteropeptidases and trypsin activate a cascade of events that promote the activation of chymotrypsin, elastase, and carboxypeptidases A and B in the duodenum. Digestion of carbohydrates has been described in Section Osmotic Diarrhea.

The hydrolysis of fat, protein, and carbohydrate by pancreatic enzymes, and the solubilization of fat by bile salts, may be altered by several conditions (34,45). In pancreatic carcinoma or following pancreatic resection, decreased pancreatic enzymes and bicarbonate release may limit the digestion of fat and protein leading to pancreatic insufficiency. These disorders may also be associated with malabsorption of fat-soluble vitamins. The Zollinger-Ellison syndrome is characterized by an extreme acid hypersecretion, causing a low luminal pH, which inactivates pancreatic enzymes with consequent fat malabsorption. A decrease in intraluminal bile salts due to disruption of the enterohepatic circulation is also seen in patients with Zollinger-Ellison syndrome. Biliary tract obstruction, terminal ileal resection, or cholestatic liver disease results in decreased formation of bile salts or delivery to the duodenum (46). Many postsurgical disorders have been associated with a marked proliferation of intraluminal microorganisms, including an afferent loop of a Billroth II partial gastrectomy, a surgical blind loop with end-to-side anastomosis, or a recirculating loop with side-to-side anastomosis. The final consequence depends on the extension of resection. With limited small bowel resections, malabsorbed bile acids pass into the colon and increase colon motility, while decreasing water and electrolyte absorption, resulting in diarrhea. In contrast, after massive small bowel resection, the bile acid pool will decrease because of the loss of intestinal bile salts. This phenomenon is associated with a loss of the absorptive intestinal surface and bacterial overgrowth. These processes will result in steatorrhea. Bacterial overgrowth causes catabolism of carbohydrates by gram-negative aerobes, deconjugation of bile salts by anaerobes, and the binding of cobalamin by anaerobes. Other than massive resection involving the ileocecal calve, causes of bacterial overgrowth include obstruction or strictures and autonomic neuropathy (45).

Physiopathology of Absorption

Products of digestion are normally absorbed from the lumen through the enterocyte to appear in the lymphatics or the portal vein. This passage is specific for each digested substance, according to the circumstances. Active transport requires energy to move nutrients against a gradient, whereas passive diffusion allows nutrients to pass according to gradient differentials. Facilitated diffusion is an intermediate mechanism, similar to passive diffusion, but carrier-mediated and subject to competitive inhibition. Endocytosis is a process in which parts of a cell membrane engulf nutrients.

Absorption of monosaccharides occurs predominantly in the proximal small intestine, although not all the dietary carbohydrate is absorbed. The simple diffusion of monosaccharides across membranes is slow, but it is important in the presence of high luminal concentrations of glucose. When luminal concentrations of glucose are low, specific active transport systems, especially through sodium-coupled transporters, mediate efficient transport of these substances. Monosaccharides may also enter enterocytes by facilitated diffusion. However, the uptake may be limited by enzyme activity, for example, lactase. Xylose is not digested and has a low affinity for carriers. Some of the carbohydrates reach the colon and are fermented by bacteria into short-chain fatty acids with the production of gases such as hydrogen and methane. Short-chain fatty acids are subsequently absorbed by colonic epithelial cells.

Fat products rapidly diffuse passively into enterocytes, with the rate of transfer depending on the chain length. Fatty acids and monoglycerides are metabolized into triglycerides and assembled with phospholipids and cholesteryl esters into chylomicrons. Short-chain and medium-chain fatty acids have a less complex absorptive mechanism. They may be absorbed intact by passive diffusion or completely hydrolyzed, but they are not reesterified inside the enterocytes. Lipid absorption is highly efficient; only small amounts of lipids enter the colon. These may be absorbed by the colonic mucosa or undergo bacterial metabolism.

Bile salts are synthesized from cholesterol in the liver, conjugated with amino acids, secreted into the bile, and recycled back to the liver through the portal system. Minimal daily losses are balanced by hepatic synthesis. Passive diffusion and active transport are involved in bile salt transport in the small intestine to limit fecal loss. A certain amount of bile salt in the colonic lumen is essential for normal colonic function. In the colon, bile salts are not absorbed but they stimulate colonic motility and secretion of sodium chloride and water. In contrast, bile salt deficiency may cause constipation (34).

Amino acids are absorbed by enterocytes and oligopeptides are digested by the enterocyte and oligopeptidases and dipeptidases of the brush border. A specific transport mechanism exists for the intracellular transport of amino acids and dipeptides. Protein absorption is efficient and occurs mainly in the jejunum and ileum (47).

Mucosal damage, as observed with radiation enteritis, may impair epithelial cell transport. Other than extensive mucosal damage, lymphatic obstruction and bacterial over-growth are the principal mechanisms of radiation-induced malabsorption (48).

After gastrectomy, low levels of vitamin E and total cholesterol were found as a consequence of loss of passage through the duodenum (49). A large surgical resection of the small intestine reduces the epithelial surface area available for absorption. The extent and specific level of resection are predictive of severe malabsorption and short bowel syndrome. Most patients with short bowel syndrome have either a high jejunostomy with a residual jejunal length <100 cm or a jejunocolic anastomosis. The recovery from massive small bowel resection depends on the adaptive response of the remaining mucosa (47). Resection of >50% of the small intestine still results in significant malabsorption. The inclusion of the distal two-thirds of the ileum and ileocecal sphincter in the resected section increases the risk of malabsorption. Preservation of the ileocecal sphincter is important, because it may prevent small bowel contamination from colonic flora and may increase the transit time of the intraluminal content.

After intestinal resections, increased amount of bile salts reach the colon promoting water and electrolyte secretion, unless liver production compensates the losses as in limited resections. The consequent lack of solubilization of intraluminal fat will worsen the effects of bile salts on the colon mucosa. Enterostomy or intestinal fistulae may also result in a reduced absorption due to the loss of intestinal surface area.

Diabetic neuropathy may result in intestinal dysmotility and bacterial overgrowth and, as a consequence, in malabsorption. Lymphatic transport of chylomicrons and proteins is limited by lymphatic obstruction leading to dilatation and potential rupture of intestinal lymphatic vessels that cause intestinal leakage of proteins, chylomicrons, and small lymphocytes. Localized ileal tumors, diffuse intestinal lymphomas, metastatic carcinoma, and metastatic carcinoid disease may all lead to lymphatic obstruction, fat malabsorption, and protein-losing enteropathy (34).

Assessment

Patients with malabsorption usually lose weight. If fats are not absorbed properly, the stools are light colored, soft, bulky, and foul smelling. Documentation of steatorrhea is the cornerstone of the diagnostic evaluation. Malabsorption can cause deficiencies of all nutrients or proteins, fats, vitamins, or minerals selectively. Certain physical signs are frequently associated with specific deficiency states secondary to malabsorption, such as glossitis in folate or vitamin B_{12} deficiency and hyperkeratosis, ecchymoses, and hematuria due to fat-soluble vitamin deficiency (vitamins A and K). Anemia (chronic blood loss or malabsorption of iron, folate, or vitamin B_{12}), leukocytosis with eosinophilia, low serum levels of albumin, iron, cholesterol, and an extension of the prothrombin time are the most common laboratory findings in malabsorption (34). Impaired absorption of calcium and magnesium may induce weakness, paresthesias, and

tetany. Osteopenia and bone pain, spontaneous fractures, and vertebral collapse may develop from vitamin D and calcium deficiency. Peripheral neuropathy may occur after gastric resection because of vitamin B_{12} deficiency. Weakness, severe weight loss, and fatigue result from caloric deprivation. In pancreatic carcinoma, floating, bulky, and malodorous stools and increased gas production are often associated with anorexia. Steatorrhea, peripheral lymphocytopenia, hypoalbuminemia, chylous ascites, and peripheral edema are the hallmarks of abnormalities of lymphatic transport. Symptoms of dumping syndrome after gastrectomy include early nausea, abdominal distention, weakness, and diarrhea after a meal, followed by hypoglycemia, sweating, dizziness, and tachycardia.

Other symptoms depend on the disorder that is causing the malabsorption. For example, an obstructed bile duct may cause jaundice; poor blood supply to the intestine may cause abdominal pain.

Malabsorption is suspected when an individual loses weight and has diarrhea and nutritional deficiencies despite eating well, although weight loss alone can have other causes in patients with cancer.

Reviewing current drugs is important in the diagnostic evaluation. Colchicine, neomycin, and clindamycin are the most common drugs causing malabsorption, although the pathophysiologic mechanisms are unknown. Dietary phosphate absorption may be limited by the use of aluminum-containing antacids, resulting in hypophosphatemia and hypercalciuria.

Laboratory tests can help confirm the diagnosis. Tests that directly measure fat in stool samples are the most reliable ones for diagnosing malabsorption of fat. Other laboratory tests can detect malabsorption of other specific substances, such as lactose or vitamin B_{12}. Undigested food fragments may mean that food passes through the intestine too rapidly. Such fragments also can indicate an anatomically abnormal intestinal pathway, such as a direct connection between the stomach and the large intestine that bypasses the small intestine. Small intestinal barium x-rays may define anatomic abnormalities after massive resection. Biochemical examination of the fecal material may give information about the origin of a fistula (pancreatic or enteric). Liver function tests and imaging of the liver or biliary tract may demonstrate parenchymal liver disease as a cause of decreased production of bile salts or a biliary tract obstruction (Table 14.3).

Treatment

After assessing the causes of malabsorption, therapy should be directed to correct the deficiencies, including enzyme replacement, bicarbonate supplements, vitamins, calcium, magnesium, and iron. Pancreatic enzyme replacement along with a low-fat, high-protein diet is indicated in the case of malabsorption due to pancreatic insufficiency. The effectiveness of enzyme replacements is variable and, in part, depends on a high enough gastric pH to prevent their degradation in the stomach (50). Large doses of pancreatic extract are required with each meal. Sodium and bicarbonate or anti-H_2

TABLE 14.3	Malabsorption: signs and symptoms

- Steatorrhea
- Weight loss, weakness, and fatigue (caloric deprivation)
- Glossitis (folate or vitamin B_{12} deficiency)
- Hyperkeratosis, ecchymoses, and hematuria (vitamins A and K deficiency)
- Weakness, paresthesias, and tetany (calcium and magnesium deficiencies)
- Early nausea, abdominal distention, weakness, and diarrhea after a meal, followed by hypoglycemia, sweating, dizziness, and tachycardia (after gastric resection)
- Osteopenia and bone pain, spontaneous fractures (vitamin D and calcium deficiencies)
- Chylous ascites—peripheral edema (abnormalities of lymphatic transport)
- Peripheral neuropathy (vitamin B_{12} deficiency)
- Laboratory findings: anemia (iron, folate, or vitamin B_{12} deficiencies), leukocytosis with eosinophilia, peripheral lymphocytopenia, and hypoalbuminemia

inhibitors and hydrogen pump inhibitors are mainly added to raise the duodenal pH.

Fat intake should be strictly limited, especially in short bowel syndrome. Medium-chain triglycerides may be substituted for long-chain triglycerides to improve fat absorption after a small intestinal resection, and they are useful in the presence of lymphatic obstruction because they do not require intestinal lymphatic transport.

For patients with prominent dumping, dietary modification comprising frequent small, dry meals that are high in protein and low in carbohydrates, along with ingestion of substances that prolong the absorption of carbohydrates, such as pectin, may be useful (34).

An aggressive approach should be reserved in the presence of severe malnutrition and dehydration, especially after surgery. Parenteral nutrition is strongly indicated in the immediate postoperative period after massive intestinal resection. The duration of parenteral nutrition is inversely proportional to the length of the remaining intestine. The weaning to oral nutrition depends on several variables, including the preoperative nutritional state, the absorptive deficit, and the tolerance to oral intake. Oral feeding should be started as soon as possible, as adaptation of the remaining bowel to resection is facilitated by the early introduction of oral or enteral nutrients. Moreover, intraluminal nutrients stimulate trophic GI hormones regulating mucosal repair. H_2-blocking agents may also favorably influence the rate of adaptation of the remaining intestine after massive resection, possibly by a mucosal trophic effect improving nutrient absorption. Nutrients requiring minimal digestion for absorption should be chosen, such as commercial preparations containing simple sugars, amino acids, or oligopeptides, as well as medium-chain triglycerides. An excessive osmolar load should be avoided to prevent the occurrence of diarrhea. More complex food should be added gradually.

Vitamin B_{12} replacement is necessary after terminal ileal resection. H_2 blockers are used to treat the transient acid hypersecretion after extensive bowel resection or the acid hypersecretion state in patients with gastrinoma (Zollinger-Ellison syndrome). Hydrogen pump inhibitors produce a greater antisecretory effect than that achieved by H_2-antagonist drugs alone. The use of cholestyramine should be carefully considered. It may be indicated in limited intestinal resections, because it binds bile salts and prevents their irritant effects on the colon. However, in short bowel syndrome after massive intestinal resection, it may reduce the bile salt pool, thereby increasing fat malabsorption. The suggested dose is 4 g three times daily before meals. Aluminum hydroxide exerts similar effects. Colesevelam has also been used for bile acid malabsorption in patients unresponsive to cholestyramine (51).

Antibiotic-associated malnutrition requires discontinuation of any implicated antimicrobial agents. However, if there is stasis with bacterial overgrowth caused by impaired motility or stricture, such as in radiation enteritis or blind loop syndrome, broad-spectrum antibiotics should be administered. A 10-day course of cephalosporin and metronidazole seems to be effective in suppressing the flora and correcting malabsorption. However, cyclic therapy may be needed (39).

In patients affected by malabsorption due to short bowel syndrome, it is useful to reduce the intestinal output or the transit time. Loperamide can delay the transit time or reduce secretions (34). Octreotide has been used because of its ability to reduce gastric, pancreatic, and biliary secretions, as well as intestinal transit time (47). Dosages from 0.2 to 0.6 mg daily have been advocated. It may reduce or shorten the use of parenteral administration in several postoperative conditions, such as enterocutaneous or pancreatic fistulae. Its use in terminally ill patients has been favorably reported (34).

Reversal of a short segment of the bowel or construction of a recirculating loop has been advocated in patients with life-threatening malabsorption and uncontrolled weight loss. However, such operations may have negative consequences, as they can lead to stasis and bacterial overgrowth, further compromising intestinal absorption. More often the benefit is of limited value (34).

CONSTIPATION

In the general population, the prevalence of constipation is significant and increases with age. In advanced cancer patients, the combination of underlying disease and medication often leads to a dramatic increase in occurrence. The range of prevalence in hospitalized patients receiving cancer treatment varies from 70% to 10% and is reported by approximately 50% of hospice patients at admission (52) and 72% of patients receiving oral morphine for cancer pain (53). Moreover, constipation is considered the first cause of adverse drug reactions in hospitalized patients with cancer (4).

In addition to causing discomfort, constipation affects daily living, nutrition intake, and socialization, therefore compromising quality of life. Moreover, synergism of constipation with other abdominal processes such as ascites or tumor may increase pain and can limit diaphragmatic excursion worsening dyspnea. Untreated constipation may progress to obstipation, which may potentially lead to life-threatening complications associated with bowel obstruction (52).

Pathophysiology

There are many, often concomitant, causes of constipation in patients with cancer (Table 14.4). Constipation may be secondary to systemic diseases or those solely afflicting the GI tract. It may be directly due to a cancer or secondary effects of the cancer. Furthermore, a great number of substances are known to cause medication-induced constipation, that is, opioid-induced constipation is caused by the linkage of the opioid-to-opioid receptors in the bowel and the central nervous system (52).

Constipation is frequently noted in patients with various neurologic disorders. A visceral neuropathy seems to be present in most patients with severe slow-transit constipation. Disturbance in the extrinsic nerve supply to the colon has been found in these patients, along with a lack of inhibitory innervation of colonic circular muscle and a diminished release of acetylcholine. Patients with advanced cancer frequently complain of GI symptoms, including anorexia, chronic nausea, and early satiety—a symptom complex often associated with physical signs of an autonomic neuropathy. Autonomic neuropathy may also be manifested as severe constipation, including postural hypotension and resting tachycardia. It is a multifactorial syndrome, and malnutrition, decreased activity, diabetes, and drugs, such as vinca alkaloids, opioids, and tricyclic antidepressants, are all possible causative factors (34).

Diabetic dysmotility has traditionally been thought to reflect a generalized autonomic neuropathy. However, secretions of GI hormones may also be important. Decreased

TABLE 14.4	Causes of constipation in patients with cancer
Neurogenic disorders	
Periphery	
Ganglionopathy	
Autonomic neuropathy	
Central nervous system	
Spinal cord lesions	
Parkinson's disease	
Metabolic and endocrine diseases	
Diabetes	
Uremia	
Hypokalemia	
Hypothyroidism	
Hypercalcemia	
Pheochromocytoma	
Enteric glucagon excess	
Malignancy	
Direct effects	
Cerebral or spinal cord tumors	
Intestinal obstruction	
Hypercalcemia	
Secondary effects	
Inadequate food intake and low-fiber diet	
Poor fluid intake	
Reduced activity	
Previous bowel surgery	
Autonomic neuropathy	
Radiotherapy	
Sedation, low level of consciousness	
Drugs	
Opioids	
Nonsteroidal anti-inflammatory drugs	
Anticholinergics	
Anticonvulsants	
Antidepressants	
Diuretics	
Antacids	
Anti-Parkinson drugs	
Antihypertensive agents	
Vinca alkaloids	

amounts of substance P in the rectal mucosa of constipated patients with diabetes have been thought to contribute to the pathogenesis of diabetic constipation.

Peripheral neuropathy is a common complication of cancer chemotherapy. Patients receiving a high cumulative dose of vincristine or cisplatin seem to be at a significantly elevated risk for the development of long-term side effects (1). These drugs have been shown to cause symptoms of autonomic polyneuropathy with constipation, bladder atony, and hypotension. Whereas many reports describe acute neurologic side effects during therapy, little is known about persistent and late damage to the peripheral nervous system. The long-term neurologic side effects in patients with curable malignancies, such as Hodgkin's disease and testicular cancer, may be particularly troublesome.

Ogilvie's syndrome describes a variety of states with a similar clinical picture due to intrinsic defects in the intestinal smooth muscle, with a massive colonic dilatation in the absence of an obstruction or inflammatory process. Also termed as *pseudo-obstruction*, this syndrome can be categorized into those with myopathic and those with neuropathic features. Several conditions involving the intestinal smooth muscle are associated with colonic pseudo-obstruction, including endocrine and metabolic disorders, neurologic diseases, nonoperative trauma, surgery, nonintestinal inflammatory processes, infections, malignancy, radiation therapy, drugs, and cardiovascular and respiratory diseases. Extensive damage to the submucosal and myenteric nerve plexuses associated with lymphoid infiltrate has been observed as a specific disorder, different from other processes that produce intestinal pseudo-obstruction (52).

Long-term denervation abolishes the normal pelvic floor muscle activity. This neurologic impairment may be produced by nerve damage not only following chemotherapy but also as a consequence of radiotherapy, pelvic surgery, compression, or invasion by neoplastic growth or during prolonged chronic opioid therapy. Loss of the normal rectal muscle tone is also a consequence of prolonged immobility that is often seen in debilitated patients with cancer. Rectal sensation may be reduced and the rectal capacity to distention may be increased after vincristine treatment or as a consequence of neoplastic involvement of the pelvic sacral nerves. The rectosigmoid junction is a key area in the mechanism of constipation. Rectal outlet obstruction and failure of the puborectalis and anal sphincter muscles to relax are frequent findings in patients with neurologic diseases with intractable constipation. Several mechanisms are possible for constipation by outlet obstruction, including a hyperactive rectosigmoid junction, an increased storage capacity of the rectum, spasticity, and hypertonicity of the anal canal with incoordination of the reflex between the rectum and anus. Anismus is a spastic pelvic floor syndrome, recently termed *rectosphincteric dyssynergia* for its similarity with vesicourethral dyssynergia. Similar extrinsic innervation of the bladder and the rectum has been observed, explaining why patients with severe slow-transit constipation often complain of urologic symptoms (52).

The integrity of the spinal cord neurons is essential to maintain normal defecation. In patients with spinal cord lesions above the lumbosacral area, incontinence is controlled but defecation is impaired. This is due to the interruption of the cortical pathways, demonstrating the importance of supraspinal control of distal colonic function and defecation. Moreover, colonic response to a meal is reduced. However, appropriate stimuli may be sufficient to result in an evacuation. In patients with damage to the cauda equina, transit time is prolonged and the recto–anal inhibitory reflex is weaker, offering little protection against fecal incontinence.

In patients with cancer having Parkinson's disease, constipation is probably caused by the degeneration of the autonomic nervous system, particularly the myenteric plexus. Psychiatric and neurologic diseases are frequently associated with colonic dysmotility (54).

A large variety of metabolic disorders predispose to constipation. Of particular relevance to patients with cancer are dehydration, hypercalcemia, hypokalemia, and uremia. Chronic dehydration can also result in dry stools that are difficult to expel. Many drugs induce constipation.

Many drugs with anticholinergic actions, antiemetics, and diuretics induce constipation. Patients treated with carbamazepine may develop severe constipation that is not dose related, but it is refractory to the concomitant use of oral laxatives, necessitating drug discontinuation. Selective 5-HT3-receptor antagonists cause constipation. They antagonize the ability of 5-hydroxytryptamine (5-HT) to evoke cholinergically mediated contractions of the intestinal longitudinal muscle (55).

One of the most striking pharmacologic features of opioids is their ability to cause constipation. Opioids cause constipation by binding to specific opioid receptors in the enteric and central nervous systems. Opioid receptors have been identified on gut smooth muscle, suggesting that there is a local effect of opioid drugs, although central opioid effects cannot be excluded. Opioids affect the intestines by different mechanisms. Opioids augment the tone and nonpropulsive motility of both the ileum and the colon, thereby increasing transit time. Opioids desiccate the intraluminal content, reducing secretion and increasing intestinal fluid absorption, with an indirect mechanism, possibly by tryptaminergic neurons in the myenteric plexus, resulting in the release of noradrenaline, which antagonize the secretory mechanism of the enterocytes, regulated by α_2-adrenoreceptors. Opioids may also suppress the release of the vasointestinal peptide, an inhibitory neurotransmitter. Vasointestinal peptide is a potent colonic secretagogue and an important inhibitor of smooth muscle contraction. Moreover, the prolonged bowel transit on its own may facilitate the increased intestinal absorption of fluid and electrolytes. Opioid use may lead to fecal impaction, spurious diarrhea, and bowel pseudo-obstruction, causing abdominal pain, nausea and vomiting, and interference with drug administration and absorption (56).

Oral morphine invariably causes constipation when used in repeated doses to treat cancer pain. Although other common unwanted effects, such as sedation, nausea, and vomiting, tend to improve with continued use and often resolve completely, opioid-induced constipation does not get better with repeated administration. It is likely that other factors can contribute to slow intestinal transit, such as immobility, concomitant medications, or disease-related factors. The importance of other factors in the development of constipation is demonstrated by the fact that approximately 50% of hospice patients not on opioids required regular oral laxatives.

In a population receiving oral morphine for cancer pain, constipation affected 72% of patients, although an interindividual variation was observed (53). Postoperative pain relief by both parenteral and intraspinal opioids is often associated with adynamic ileus. Gastric emptying and small bowel transit are inhibited. This is an important consideration for patients with cancer undergoing surgical procedures in which the ileus is likely to be a severe problem. Epidural anesthesia with local anesthetics appears to disrupt GI motility less than systemic opioids (52).

Assessment

There are challenges associated with defining constipation in cancer patients. The subjective assessment is often different to the objective view, as assessed by the healthcare professional.

It is of paramount importance to first establish what the patient means by constipation—if the stools are too small, too hard, too difficult to expel, or too infrequent or if the patients have a feeling of incomplete evacuation after defecation. A variety of definitions have been used by patients and healthcare providers—straining, hard stools, the desire but inability to defecate, infrequent stools, and abdominal discomfort. Stool weight and consistency, possible parameters to measure, may be unreliable because of the wide range in healthy subjects (52).

Constipation is commonly defined as a decrease in the frequency of the passage of formed stools and characterized by stools that are hard and difficult to pass (57). A frequency of at least 3 bowel movements/wk is viewed as an objective indicator of normality.

Different tools have been proposed to assess constipation. The Rome II Criteria highlights the physical characteristics of the stool, frequency of bowel movements, and subjective perceptions of distress as important to the definition, as well as component of chronicity, including six elements: straining, hard stool, the sensation of incomplete evacuation, the sensation of anorectal obstruction, fewer than 3 bowel movements/wk, and 2 weeks of ≥2 of these symptoms in 1 year. The development of the bowel function index was based on established criteria of known assessment tool for opioid-induced constipation. This index is a subjective scale assessment, including three simple questions to be rated from 0 to 100 during the last 7 days: ease of defecation, feeling of incomplete bowel evacuation, and personal judgment regarding constipation (58). The Victoria Hospice Bowel Performance scale uses images to describe stool consistency and has been found to be meaningful for patients (59). The Patient Assessment Constipation Symptoms is composed of three domains: abdominal symptoms (4 items), rectal symptoms (3 items), and stool symptoms (5 items) and is validated for opioid-induced constipation (60).

A careful history and physical examination will be helpful. A careful history should be taken regarding the onset of constipation, bowel habits, current bowel performance, and the use of laxatives. Patients who develop progressive constipation in the absence of any clear precipitating cause should be considered for an evaluation that may include determination of electrolytes and renal and hepatic function tests.

Impaction with overflow should be excluded by performing a rectal examination. Therefore, the first step is to completely evacuate the bowel. Multiple oil or saline enemas may be needed. Digital fragmentation is unpleasant, but it may permit most of the fecal impactions in the rectum to be diagnosed. A pseudodiarrhea in the presence of impaired anal sphincter function may be discovered. Gentle digital examination of the rectum may reveal a hard mass, a rectal tumor, rectal ulcers, an anal stenosis, anismus, or a lax anal sphincter. Patients with spinal cord lesions may have reduced sensation, but the anal tone is preserved, whereas patients with sacral nerve root infiltration will have a reduced anal tone. The examination of the abdomen may reveal fecal masses in the left iliac fossa. Fecal masses are usually not tender, are relatively mobile, and can be indented with pressure (52).

An abdominal radiograph may distinguish between constipation and obstruction. Examination after a barium meal may help distinguish between paralytic ileus and mechanical obstruction. Barium studies may help reveal a small intestine motility dysfunction in chronic intestinal pseudo-obstruction. In visceral myopathy, intestinal contractions are infrequent, whereas with a visceral neuropathy, patients tend to have less distension and faster intestinal transit time due to uncoordinated contractions (52).

When constipation is due to ineffective colonic musculature, measurement of colonic transit time may be a useful tool to detect specific areas of the bowel that are not functioning properly. Pieces of radiopaque nasogastric tube are ingested, and the progression of markers along the colon is observed by a daily radiograph until total expulsion. This study may demonstrate a delayed transit in the colon, a long storage of feces in the rectum, or a retrograde movement due to a distal spasm. A radiologic constipation score has been proposed, assessing the amount of stool in each of the four abdominal quadrants (61). Recently, no concordant correlation has been found (62).

Treatment

Recommendations from different expert groups have been reported recently (59,63), confirming the lack of existing scientific evidence and the need for controlled studies in the field. General recommendations suggest that it would be useful to synergize pharmacologic interventions and principal mechanism considered to be responsible for constipation. Thus, an extensive effort should be made to find a specific cause of constipation and then treatment can be directed at that cause.

The management of constipation should be divided into general interventions and therapeutic measures. Etiologic factors, such as physiologic consequences of cancer-associated debility, biochemical abnormalities, including hypercalcemia and hyperkalemia, and drug use, should be identified and reversed wherever possible. An adequate fluid intake is helpful in increasing the stool water content (52).

Fluids, fruit juice, fruit, and bran are all recommended. However, fiber deficiency is unlikely to account for a lower stool weight, and there is no justification for the claim that treatment with bran can return stool output and transit time to normal. In patients with far-advanced cancer, the use of high amounts of fiber is beyond the capacity of most patients. Fiber consumption may decrease fluid intake relatively, thereby paradoxically worsening the situation. Since an unfavorable toilet environment, such as lack of privacy or inappropriate posture, may lead to constipation, patients should be provided privacy and appropriate facilities in the hospital setting.

When irreversible causes of constipation cannot be directly treated, symptomatic relief should be provided. Moreover, in spite of prophylaxis, most of these patients will require chronic laxatives, especially in the advanced stage of their disease or when treated with chronic opioid therapy. It is appropriate to begin prophylactic laxative treatment in patients with risk factors for constipation, including the elderly, those who are bedridden, or those requiring drugs that are known to cause constipation.

In the presence of a low-rectal impaction should be removed manually. Appropriate sedation and analgesics are usually required to make this procedure comfortable. A more proximal mass can be broken by a sigmoidoscope or by delivering a pulsating stream of water against the stool. The use of enemas and rectal interventions is limited to the acute short-term management of more severe episodes. Therapeutic interventions for the management of constipation are based on the administration of laxatives, either orally or rectally. Laxatives will promote active electrolyte secretion, decrease water and electrolyte absorption, increase intraluminal osmolarity, and increase hydrostatic pressure in the gut. Although laxatives can be divided into several groups, no agent acts purely to soften the stool or stimulate peristalsis. Clinical criteria, responsiveness, acceptability, and the patient's preference should guide the selection of the drug. Table 14.5 outlines different medications that are useful in constipation.

Laxatives

According to their modes of action, they are divided into bulk-forming laxatives, osmotic laxatives, stimulant laxatives, lubricating agents, and others. Bulk-forming laxatives are not recommended for use in palliative care patients, since such patients are normally not able to take in the required amount of fluids.

Patients with advanced cancer are likely to have chronic constipation and will need continuous laxative treatment. No data exist to guide the clinician or patient in the optimal choice of laxatives, as there have been no adequate comparative studies of long-term management of opioid-induced constipation. One of the main limitations of such trials is the lack of reliable clinical assessment tools. In a randomized, crossover clinical trial of laxatives in a hospice, lactulose/senna combination produced a significantly greater stool frequency than co-danthramer in patients receiving opioids and reduced the usage of rectal measures, although the penalty for this achievement was an increased likelihood of diarrhea (64). In a comparative study conducted with the objective of determining treatment and cost efficiency for senna and lactulose in patients with terminal cancer treated with opioids, no difference was found in defecation-free intervals or in days with defecation between the laxatives (65). In a recent systematic review, the use of docusate for constipation in palliative care has been found to be based on inadequate experimental evidence (66). In a study of healthy volunteers, in which constipation was induced by loperamide, a combination of stimulant and softening laxatives was most likely to maintain normal bowel function at the lowest dose and least adverse effects. Senna was associated with significantly more adverse effects than the other laxatives (67).

Bulk-forming agents are high-fiber foods containing polysaccharides or cellulose derivatives that are resistant to bacterial breakdown. These agents increase stool bulk and correct its consistency by increasing the mass and the water content of the stool. Evidence of their effect may be observed after 24 hours or more. Their effectiveness and feasibility in the patient with advanced cancer are doubtful, as they require the patients to drink extra fluids to prevent viscous mass formation.

Emollient laxatives are surfactant substances that are not adsorbed in the gut, acting as a detergent and facilitating the mixture of water and fat. They also promote water and electrolyte secretion. Stimulant laxatives are the most commonly used drugs to treat constipation. They are represented by the anthraquinone derivatives, such as senna, cascara, and danthron, and the diphenylmethane derivatives, such as bisacodyl and phenolphthalein. This class of drugs acts at the level of the colon and distal ileum by directly stimulating the myenteric plexus. Senna is converted to an active form by colonic bacteria. As a consequence, its site of action is primarily the colon. An increase in myoelectric colonic activity has been observed after the administration of oral senna. Danthron and the polyphenolic agents bisacodyl and sodium picosulfate undergo glucuronidation and are secreted in the bile (68). The enterohepatic circulation may prolong their effect. Bisacodyl stimulates the mucosal nerve plexus, producing contractions of the entire colon and decreasing water absorption in the small and large intestine. Castor oil is metabolized into ricinoleic acid that has stimulant secretory properties and an effect on glucose absorption.

TABLE 14.5	Laxatives used for constipation		

Class–Drugs–Doses	Onset	Comments
Lubricant laxatives		
Liquid paraffin (10 mL/d)	1–3 d	Paraffin inhalation
Surfactant laxatives		
Docusate (300 mg)	1–3 d	Not together with mineral oil
Bulk-forming agents	2–4 d	
Bran (8 g)		If taken with inadequate amount of water can precipitate fecal impaction in intestinal obstruction
Methylcellulose and ispaghula (4 g)		
Osmotic laxatives	1–2 d	
Lactulose (15 mL b.i.d.)		Dose-related cramps, gaseous distention, and useful in hepatic encephalopathy
Mannitol		
Sorbitol		
Amidotrizoate (50 mL)		
Polyethylene glycol (two sachets daily in water)		High volumes of water needed to be ingested
Anthracenes (6–12 h) 6–12		Colicky pain
Senna (15 mg)		Urine pink discoloration
Dantron (50 mg)		
Polyphenolics (6–12 h)		Colicky pain
Bisacodyl (10 mg)		
Sodium picosulfate (5 mg)		
Opioid antagonists		
Naloxone (dose titration)	1–2 h	Possible withdrawal syndrome
Methylnaltrexone (5 mg)	1–2 h	

All of these drugs may cause severe cramping. The cathartic action occurs within 1 to 3 days. Starting doses proposed are 15 mg of senna daily, 50 mg of danthron daily, or 10 mg of bisacodyl daily. Bisacodyl suppositories promote colonic peristalsis with a short onset due to rapid conversion to its active metabolite by the rectal flora. Docusate, alone or in combination with danthron, is most commonly used at doses of 100 to 300 mg every 8 hours. The effectiveness of docusate has been questioned (52).

Lubricant laxatives are represented by mineral oil. It may be useful in the management of transient acute constipation or fecal impaction, but it has little role in the management of chronic constipation. It lubricates the stool surface. Coated feces may pass more easily and the colonic absorption of water is decreased. It may also decrease the absorption of fat vitamins. Absorption of small amounts may cause foreign body reactions in the bowel lymphoid tissue. Liquid paraffin,

10 mL/d, may be given orally or rectally, with an effect noted in 8 to 24 hours.

Hyperosmotic agents are not broken down or absorbed in the small bowel, drawing fluid into the bowel lumen. They pull water along with luminal contents to keep the stool softer and more voluminous. Lactulose increases fecal weight and frequency, but it may result in bloating, colic, and flatulence due to bacterial metabolization when it reaches the colon. Moreover, it is expensive in comparison with other preparations. The latency of action is 1 to 2 days. Starting doses are 15 to 20 mL twice a day. Orally administered macrogol is not metabolized, and pH value and bowel flora remain unchanged resulting in less gas bloating. Macrogol hydrates hardened stools, increases stool volume, decreases the duration of colon passage, and dilates the bowel wall, which then triggers the defecation reflex. Even when given for some time, the effectiveness of macrogol will not decrease (69).

Amidotrizoate has been found to be highly effective and safe in the treatment of constipation resistant to laxatives in advanced cancer patients, with about half of the patients having a bowel movement after 10 hours (70).

Saline laxatives exert an osmotic effect by increasing the intraluminal volume. They also appear to directly stimulate peristalsis and increase water secretion. The starting dose is 2 to 4 g daily. Magnesium, sulfate, phosphate, and citrate ions are the ingredients in saline laxatives. Saline laxatives usually produce results in a few hours. Their use may lead to electrolyte imbalances with accumulation of magnesium in patients with renal dysfunction or an excessive load of sodium in patients with hypertension. Administered rectally, they stimulate rectal peristalsis within 15 minutes. Repeated use of a phosphate enema may cause hypocalcemia and hyperphosphatemia or rectal gangrene in patients with hemorrhoids. Glycerin can be used rectally as an osmotic and as a lubricant. Magnesium salts tend to cause urgent liquid stools, making them less convenient for many patients, other than leading to toxicity with continuing use, especially in patients with renal insufficiency.

Prokinetic drugs: Metoclopramide given by the subcutaneous route, but not by the oral route, seems to be effective in narcotic bowel syndrome. Effects of metoclopramide are mediated by a central and peripheral antidopaminigeric effect and a stimulation of cholinergic receptors (4). Neostigmine has been proposed for refractory constipation for its cholinergic activity (71).

Opioid Antagonists and Opioid Therapy Modification

Opioid-induced constipation can be severe and refractory to therapy with conventional laxatives. Opioid concentration in the enteric nervous system correlates better with opioid-induced, prolonged, intestinal transit time than concentrations in the central nervous system (72). Naloxone is a competitive antagonist of opioid receptors inside and outside the central nervous system and, after systemic administration, it reverses both centrally and peripherally mediated opioid effects. Naloxone has a low oral bioavailability of <2%. It undergoes extensive hepatic metabolism to form the partly active metabolite 6β-naloxol and glucuronide of naloxone and 6β-naloxol. Oral administration theoretically allows selective blocking of intestinal opioid receptors without blocking the desired opioid effects, as long as hepatic first-pass capacity is not exceeded. The low systemic bioavailability due to marked hepatic first-pass metabolism allows for the low plasma levels and high enteric wall concentration. According to this observation, oral administration of naloxone can reverse opioid-induced constipation, without causing systemic opioid withdrawal in most patients.

Pioneer studies with oral administration of naloxone at a daily dose of approximately 20% of the daily morphine dose demonstrated a clinical laxative effect without antagonizing opioid analgesia (73). Adverse effects of short duration, including yawning, sweating, and shivering, were observed in approximately one-third of patients. Although oral naloxone doses <2 to 4 mg or 10% or less of the morphine dose are mostly ineffective, opioid withdrawal may be present. Reversal of analgesia does not seem to be an early symptom of systemic opioid antagonism. The naloxone dose has been based on the preexisting morphine dose and expressed in percentages of daily morphine. However, the reaction to opioid antagonists seems to be proportional to the degree of opioid tolerance rather than to opioid concentration, and the risk of systemic withdrawal may increase if the same percentage relationship is used in patients with high opioid doses (74).

In recent years, coadministration of slow-release oxycodone and naloxone in a ratio of 2:1 has been found to be associated with a significant improvement in bowel function compared with slow-release oxycodone alone, with no reduction in the analgesic efficacy of naloxone, in a dose range of 20 to 80 mg (75). It is likely that the slow absorption of naloxone avoids possible peaks overlapping the extracting capacity of liver. Studies in cancer patients, where multiple conditions play a role, are lacking, unless an open-label trial with a low number of patients showed an improvement in bowel transit (76).

Methylnaltrexone, the first peripheral opioid receptor antagonist and currently under clinical investigation, has the potential to prevent or treat opioid-induced, peripherally mediated side effects, such as constipation, without interfering with analgesia. Methylnaltrexone is an opioid antagonist that cannot penetrate the blood–brain barrier and has been shown to reverse morphine-induced delay of gastric emptying and intestinal transit time after intravenous infusion in volunteers. Methylnaltrexone, administered every second day for 2 weeks at a dosage of 0.15 mg/kg subcutaneously, produced a faster time to laxation in comparison with placebo, with most patients having a bowel movement within the first 2 hours after administration (77). It has been shown that there is no apparent dose–response above 5 mg (78). Failure rate, observed in about half the patients, may be due to other concomitant causes of constipation and/or to the possible central constipating effect exerted by opioids at level of spinal dorsal horn (79). Methylnaltrexone should be considered a breakthrough medication.

Constipation may require modification of opioid therapy (80). Opioid switching is a strategy for maintaining or improving analgesic quality directed toward decreasing the effects of previous opiates on the GI tract. Present research indicates that there is a relation between the type of opioid and the degree of constipation, that is, treatment with transdermal fentanyl or methadone tends to cause less constipation compared with morphine or hydromorphone. Among opioids, there may be differences in the analgesia/constipation ratio. Clinical studies have revealed that at doses of oral morphine and transdermal fentanyl that yield equivalent pain relief, constipation differs significantly between the two drugs. Although most of the early studies were not randomized, different methodologies were used, and the analysis was performed while switching patients from oral morphine to transdermal fentanyl. More recent trials that are remarkably consistent in that transdermal fentanyl cause less constipation than oral, sustained morphine at the same level of analgesia (52). Differences in pharmacologic profiles, in the affinity to opioid receptor and a higher exposure of opioid-binding receptors in the GI tract following oral administration of morphine compared with transdermal administration of fentanyl, may offer an explanation for the clinically observed variations in the constipation-inducing potentials of equipotent doses of morphine and fentanyl. The lipophilicity profile of fentanyl allows for the ease with which fentanyl penetrates the brain. As less opioid is required to produce a central analgesic effect, less opioid is available in the peripheral circulation to induce constipation. Experimental studies using a castor oil–induced diarrhea model have shown a more favorable analgesia/constipation ratio of subcutaneous fentanyl as compared with oral morphine, although the difference was less pronounced with oral fentanyl. Considerably larger amounts of naloxones were needed to reverse the morphine than the fentanyl-induced antidiarrheal effects (52). Methadone has a high oral bioavailability and a rapid and extensive distribution phase, followed by a slow elimination. The end of the distribution phase is at or below the minimum effective concentration necessary for an effect. This may result in limiting the continuous bathing of intestinal receptors. The high lipophilicity of methadone allows for the maintenance of a low plasma concentration with a relevant clinical effect. Constipation seems to be the symptom that improves the most after opioid switching. This could be simply due to difference in tolerance of different opioids at the level of receptors located in the bowel. Moreover, different reports have shown that methadone therapy may cause less constipation than morphine. In a retrospective analysis, the laxative/opioid dose ratio was lower in patients receiving methadone than in patients on morphine. Moreover, there is a rationale in changing the route of administration. The use of a parenteral administration should also result in a change of the opioid concentration at intestinal receptors. However, in a retrospective study no difference in the doses of laxatives required to maintain regular bowel movements was found between patients receiving oral opioids and those receiving subcutaneous opioids (81).

Therapeutic Strategy

The treatment consists of basic measures and the application of laxatives. Sixty-four percent of patients admitted to a hospice and not receiving opioid analgesia required laxatives, although the doses of laxative required were higher in patients receiving opioids. Although there is no correlation between the dose of opioids and the dose of laxatives, an upward titration of laxatives in parallel with increasing doses of morphine has been observed (52). Approximate equivalents of laxatives and typical requirements of opioid therapy have been proposed, but clearly, there is a large individual patient variation. However, proportionally less laxative is required at a higher opioid dose. Higher doses of danthron were associated with better physical functioning

(but not opioid dose), suggesting that for any given dose of opioid, fitter patients were treated with larger doses of laxatives. However, there was no relationship between opioid dose, bowel activity, and dantron doses. Thus, factors other than opioid dose and physical functioning may be more important in contributing to constipation in this group of patients (82).

In a constipated patient, after excluding bowel obstruction, it is mandatory to promote a bowel movement. Local measures to soften fecal mass are necessary in cases of rectal impaction. The short latency of action of rectal laxatives may be useful to remove hard feces impacted in the rectum. Glycerin suppositories or sorbitol enemas soften the stool by osmosis, also lubricating the rectal wall. Water penetration may be facilitated by a stool softener. Saline enemas cannot be regularly administered and should be used as a last resort if suppositories fail. Any patient requiring an enema should be reevaluated for a possible laxative dose titration. Methylnaltrexone is recommended as a breakthrough medication for patients on opioids who have failed to respond to optimal laxative therapy (59). Such medications should be avoided if a bowel obstruction is suspected. Amidotrizoate is less expensive and may be helpful in all the conditions of constipation resistant to laxatives and may be helpful in patients with bowel subobstruction (70).

Practical and economic consideration may influence the choice of drug for chronic constipation, according to the setting (home, hospital, hospice, or palliative care unit). Laxatives are the mainstay of pharmacologic intervention. Although stimulant agents may cause painful colic, softener drugs may be useful in the presence of a hard stool. Peristaltic stimulants are indicated in patients who are unable to pass soft stool. Senna is the most useful drug in the presence of soft feces in the rectum. All patients who were started on opioid analgesia should have a prophylactic laxative unless a contraindication exists, although periodic laxative-free intervals have been advocated for patients with a relatively long prognosis to avoid tolerance (52).

Laxative dose should usually be titrated according to the response and not according to the dose of opioids. The opioid dose increments do not determine laxative efficacy, indicating that the constipating effect of opioids is not a function of the dose. Combination therapy with different mechanisms may be more useful when higher doses of one laxative are required. In patients suspected of having intestinal obstruction, laxatives with a softening action may be tried. However, treatment should be immediately interrupted when transit stops. Patients with colostomies require the same treatment. Before using stimulating agents, an obstruction should be excluded in the absence of feces in a colostomy. Patients with paraplegia often require regular manual evacuation. Glycerin and bisacodyl suppositories should be given to patients with cauda equina syndrome.

Opioid switching may be indicated in cases in which there are serious therapeutic difficulties in maintaining bowel transit. Some slow-release formulations of opioid antagonist, such as oxycodone–naloxone, may improve the bowel transit. Opioid switching as well as the use of opioid antagonists should be carefully monitored.

REFERENCES

1. Solomon R, Cherny N. Constipation and diarrhea in patients with cancer. *Cancer J.* 2006;12:355-364.
2. Arnold RJ, Gabrail N, Raut M, et al. Clinical implications of chemotherapy-induced diarrhea in patients with cancer. *J Support Oncol.* 2005;3:227-232.
3. Komurcu S, Nelson KA, Walsh D, et al. Gastrointestinal symptoms among inpatients with advanced cancer. *Am J Hosp Palliat Care.* 2002;19:351-355.
4. Lau PM, Stewart K, Dooley M. The ten most common adverse drug reactions (ADRs) in oncology patients: do they matter to you? *Support Care Cancer.* 2004;12:626-633.
5. Dranitsaris G, Maroun J, Shah A. Severe chemotherapy-induced diarrhea in patients with colorectal cancer: a cost of illness analysis. *Support Care Cancer.* 2005;13:318-324.
6. Dranitsaris G, Maroun J, Shah A. Estimating the cost of illness in colorectal cancer patients who were hospitalized for severe chemotherapy-induced diarrhea. *Can J Gastroenterol.* 2005;19:83-87.
7. Clausen MR, Jorgensen J, Mortensen PB. Comparison of diarrhea induced by ingestion of fructooligosaccharide Idolax and disaccharide lactulose: role of osmolarity versus fermentation of malabsorbed carbohydrate. *Dig Dis Sci.* 1998;43:2696-2707.
8. Osterlund P, Ruotsalainen T, Peuhkuri K, et al. Lactose intolerance associated with adjuvant 5-fluorouracil-based chemotherapy for colorectal cancer. *Clin Gastroenterol Hepatol.* 2004;2:696-703.
9. Schiller LR. Secretory diarrhea. *Curr Gastroenterol Rev.* 1999;1:389-397.
10. Jensen RT. Overview of chronic diarrhea caused by functional neuroendocrine neoplasms. *Semin Gastrointest Dis.* 1999;10:156-172.
11. Riley SA, Turnberg LA. Maldigestion and malabsorption. In: Sleisinger MH, Fordtran JE, eds. *Gastrointestinal Disease.* Philadelphia, PA: WB Saunders; 1993:977-1008.
12. Radu B, Allez M, Gornet JM, et al. Chronic diarrhoea after allogenic bone marrow transplantation. *Gut.* 2005;54:161-174.
13. Cherny N. Evaluation and management of treatment-related diarrhea in patients with advanced cancer: a review. *J Pain Symptom manage.* 2008;36:413-423.
14. Kornblau S, Benson AB, Catalano R, et al. Management of cancer treatment-related diarrhea. Issues and therapeutic strategies. *J Pain Symptom Manage.* 2000;19:118-129.
15. Carlini LE, Meropol NJ, Bever J, et al. UGT1A7 and UGT1A9 polymorphisms predict response and toxicity in colorectal cancer patients treated with capecitabine/irinotecan. *Clin Cancer Res.* 2005;11:1226-1236.
16. Martenson J, Halyard M, Sloan J, et al. Phase III, double-blind study of depot octreotide versus placebo in the prevention of acute diarrhea in patients receiving pelvic radiation therapy: results of North Central Cancer Treatment Group N00CA. *J Clin Oncol.* 2008;26:5248-5253.
17. Robertson JM, Sohn M, Yan D. Predicting grade 3 acute diarrhea during radiation therapy for rectal cancer using a cutoff-dose logistic regression normal tissue complication probability model. *Int J Radiat Oncol Biol Phys.* 2010;77:66-72.
18. Hogenauer C, Hammer HF, Krejs GJ, et al. Mechanisms and management of antibiotic-associated diarrhea. *Clin Infect Dis.* 1998;27:702-710.
19. Schiller LR. Diarrhea. *Med Clin North Am.* 2000;84:1259-1274.
20. Martenson JA, Bollinger JW, Sloan JA, et al. Sucralfate in the prevention of treatment-induced diarrhea in patients receiving pelvic radiation therapy: a North Central Cancer Treatment Group phase III double-blind placebo-controlled trial. *J Clin Oncol.* 2000;18:1239-1245.
21. Hombrick J, Frohlich D, Glazel M, et al. Prevention of radiation-induced diarrhea by smectite. Results of a double-blind randomized, placebo-controlled multicenter study. *Strahlenther Onkol.* 2000;17:173-179.
22. Huang EY, Hsu HC, Yang KD, et al. Acute diarrhea during pelvic irradiation: is small-bowel volume effect different in gynecologic patients with prior abdomen operation or not? *Gynecol Oncol.* 2005;97:118-125.
23. Koukourakis MI, Touloupidis S, Manavis J, et al. Conformal hypofractionated and accelerated radiotherapy with cytoprotection (HypoARC) for high risk prostatic carcinoma: rationale, technique and early experience. *Anticancer Res.* 2004;24:3239.
24. Tsavaris N, Kosmas C, Vadiaka M, et al. Amifostine, in a reduced dose, protect against severe diarrhea associated with weekly fluorouracil and folinic acid chemotherapy in advanced colorectal cancer: a pilot study. *J Pain Symptom Manage.* 2003;26:849-854.
25. Karthaus M, Ballo H, Abhenardt W, et al. Prospective, double-blind, placebo-controlled, multicenter, randomized phase III study with orally administered budesonide for prevention of irinotecan (CPT-11)-induced diarrhea in patients with advanced colorectal cancer. *Oncology.* 2005;68:326-332.
26. Attar A, Flourie B, Ranbaud JC, et al. Antibiotic efficacy in small intestinal bacterial overgrowth-related chronic diarrhea: a crossover, randomized trial. *Gastroenterology.* 1999;117:794-797.
27. Gorenek L, Dizer U, Besirbellioglu B, et al. The diagnosis and treatment of *Clostridium difficile* in antibiotic-associated diarrhea. *Hepatogastroenterology.* 1999;46:343-348.
28. Saavedra J. Probiotics and infectious diarrhea. *Am J Gastroenterol.* 2000;95(suppl 1):S16-S18.
29. Chitapanarux I, Chitapanarux T, Traisathit P, et al. Randomized controlled trial of live *Lactobacillus acidophilus* plus *Bifidobacterium bifidum* in prophylaxis of diarrhea during radiotherapy in cervical cancer patients. *Radiat Oncol.* 2010;5:31.
30. Valenti Moreno V, Brunet J, Manzano Alemany H, et al. Prevention of irinotecan associated diarrhea by intestinal alkalization. A pilot study in gastrointestinal cancer patients. *Clin Transl Oncol.* 2006;8:208-212.
31. Maeda Y, Ohune T, Nakamura M, et al. Prevention of irinotecan-induced diarrhoea by oral carbonaceous adsorbent (Kremezin) in cancer patients. *Oncol Rep.* 2004;12:581-585.
32. Michael M, Brittain M, Nagai J, et al. Phase II study of activated charcoal to prevent irinotecan-induced diarrhea. *J Clin Oncol.* 2004;22:4410-4417.
33. Kehrer DF, Sparreboom A, Verweij J, et al. Modulation of irinotecan-induced diarrhea by cotreatment with neomycin in cancer patients. *Clin Cancer Res.* 2001;7:1136-1141.
34. Mercadante S. Diarrhea in terminally ill patients: pathophysiology and treatment. *J Pain Symptom Manage.* 1995;10:298-309.
35. Cascinu S, Bichisao E, Amadori D, et al. High-dose loperamide in the treatment of 5-fluorouracil-induced diarrhea in colorectal cancer patients. *Support Care Cancer.* 2000;8:65-67.
36. Kaplan MA, Prior MJ, Ash RR, et al. Loperamide–simethicone vs. loperamide alone, simethicone alone, and placebo in the treatment of acute diarrhea with gas-related abdominal

discomfort. A randomized controlled trial. *Arch Fam Med.* 1999;8:243-248.

37. Mercadante S. The role of octreotide in palliative care. *J Pain Symptom Manage.* 1994;9:406-411.

38. Cello JP, Grendell JH, Basuk P, et al. Effect of octreotide on refractory AIDS-associated diarrhea: a prospective, multicenter clinical trial. *Ann Intern Med.* 1991;115:705-710.

39. Ippoliti C, Champlin R, Bugazia N. Use of octreotide in the symptomatic management of diarrhea induced by graft-versus-host disease in patients with hematologic malignancies. *J Clin Oncol.* 1997;15:3350-3354.

40. Wasserman EI, Hidalgo M, Hornedo J, et al. Octreotide (SMS 201-995) for hematopoietic support-dependent high-dose chemotherapy (HSD-HDC)-related diarrhea: dose finding study and evaluation of efficacy. *Bone Marrow Transplant.* 1997;20:711-714.

41. Yavuz M, Yavuz A, Aydin F, et al. The efficacy of octreotide in the therapy of acute radiation-induced diarrhea: a randomized controlled study. *Int J Radiat Oncol Biol Phys.* 2002;54:195-202

42. Rosenoff SH. Octreotide LAR resolves severe chemotherapy-induced diarrhoea (CID) and allows continuation of full-dose therapy. *Eur J Cancer Care.* 2004;13:380-383.

43. Anthony L. New strategies for the prevention and reduction of cancer treatment-induced diarrhea. *Semin Oncol Nurs.* 2003;19(suppl 3):17-21.

44. Zacharian B, Gwede C, James J, et al. Octreotide acetate in prevention of chemoradiation-induced diarrhea in anorectal cancer: randomized RTOG trial 0315. *J Natl Cancer Inst.* 2010;102:547-556.

45. Westergaard H, Spady DK. The short bowel syndrome. In: Sleisenger MH, Fordtran JS, eds. *Gastrointestinal Disease.* Philadelphia, PA: WB Saunders; 1993:1249-1256.

46. Ung KA, Kilander AF, Lindgren A, et al. Impact of bile acid malabsorption on steatorrhoea and symptoms in patients with chronic diarrhoea. *Eur J Gastroenterol Hepatol.* 2000;12:541-547.

47. Toskes PP. Malabsorption. In: Wyngaarden JB, Smith LH, Bennett JC, eds. *Cecil Textbook of Medicine.* Philadelphia, PA: WB Saunders; 1992:667-699.

48. Vistad I, Kristensen G, Fossà D, Morkrid L. Intestinal malabsorption in long-term survivors of cervical cancer treated with radiotherapy. *Int J Radiat Oncol Biol Phys.* 2009;73:1141-1147.

49. Rino Y, Suzuki Y, Kuroiva Y et al. Vitamin E malabsorption and neurological consequences after gastrectomy for gastric cancer. *Hepatogastroenterology.* 2007;54:1858-1861.

50. Harewood GC, Murray JA. Approaching the patient with chronic malabsorption syndrome. *Semin Gastrointest Dis.* 1999;10:138-144.

51. Wedlake L, Thomas K, Lalji A, Anagnostopoulos C, Andreyev H. Effectiveness and tolerability of colesevelam hydrochloride for bile-acid malabsorption in patients with cancer: a retrospective chart review and patient questionnaire. *Clin Ther.* 2009;31:2549-2558.

52. Mercadante S. Diarrhea, malabsorption, and constipation. In: Berger A, ShusterJ, and Van Roenn J, eds. *Principles and Practice of Palliative Care and Supportive Oncology.* Philadelphia, PA: Lippincott Williams & Wilkins; 2007:163-176.

53. Droney J, Ross J, Gretton S, Welsh K, Sato H, Riley J. Constipation in cancer patients on morphine. *Support Care Cancer.* 2008;16:453-459.

54. Mercadante S. Nausea and vomiting. In: Voltz R, Bernat J, Borasio G, et al., eds, *Palliative Care in Neurology.* Oxford: Oxford University Press; 2004:210-220.

55. Gershon MD. Review article: serotonin receptors and transporters—roles in normal and abnormal gastrointestinal motility. *Aliment Pharmacol Ther.* 2004;20(suppl 7):3-14.

56. Kurz A, Sessler D. Opioid-induced bowel dysfunction. Pathophysiology and potential new therapies. *Drugs.* 2003;63:649-671.

57. McMillan S. Assessing and managing opiate-induced constipation in adults with cancer. *Cancer Control.* 2004;11(suppl 1): 3-9.

58. Rentz A, Yu R, Muller-Lissner S, Leyendecker P. Validation of the bowel function index to detect clinically meaningful changes in opioid-induced constipation. *J Med Econ.* 2009;12:371-383.

59. Librach S, Bouvette M, De Angelis C, et al. Consensus recommendations for the management of constipation in patients with advanced, progressive illness. *J Pain Symptom Manage.* 2010;40:761-773.

60. Slappendel R, Simpson K, Dubois D, Keininger D. Validation of the PAC-SYM questionnaire for opioid-induced constipation in patients with chronic low back pain. *Eur J Pain.* 2006;10:209-217.

61. Bruera E, Suarez-Almazor M, Velasco A, et al. The assessment of constipation in terminal cancer patients admitted to a palliative care unit: a retrospective review. *J Pain Symptom Manage.* 1994;9:515-519.

62. Nagaviroy K, Yong WC, Fassbender K, Zhu G, Oneschnuk D. Comparison of the constipation assessment scale and plan abdominal radiography in the assessment of constipation in advanced cancer patients. *J Pain Symptom Manage.* 2011; 42:222-228.

63. Larkin PJ, Sykes NP, Centeno C, et al. The management of constipation in palliative care: clinical practice recommendations. *Palliat Med.* 2008;22:796-807.

64. Sykes NP. A clinical comparison of laxatives in a hospice. *Palliat Med.* 1991;5:307-314.

65. Agra Y, Sacristan A, Gonzalez M, et al. Efficacy of senna versus lactulose in terminal cancer patients treated with opioids. *J Pain Symptom Manage.* 1998;15:1-7.

66. Hurdon V, Viola R, Schroder C. How useful is docusate in patients at risk for constipation? A systematic review of the evidence in the chronically ill. *J Pain Symptom Manage.* 2000;19:130-136.

67. Sykes NP. A volunteer model for the comparison of laxatives in opioid-related constipation. *J Pain Symptom Manage.* 1996;11:363-369.

68. Twycross R, McNamara P, Schuijt C, Kamm M, Jordan C. Sodium picosulphate in opioid-induced constipation: results of an open-label, prospective, dose ranging study. *Palliat Med.* 2006;20:419-423.

69. Klaschik E, Nauck F, Ostgathe C. Constipation—modern laxative therapy. *Support Care Cancer.* 2003;11:679-685.

70. Mercadante S, Ferrera P, Casuccio A. Effectiveness and tolerability of amidotrizoate for the treatment of constipation resistant to laxative in advanced cancer patients. *J Pain Symptom Manage.* 2011;41:421-425.

71. Rubiales AS, Hernansanz S, Gutierrez C, Del valle LM, Flores LA. Neostigmine for refractory constipation in advanced cancer patients. *J Pain Symptom Manage.* 1006;32:204-205.

72. Culpepper-Morgan JA, Inturrisi CE, Portenoy RK, et al. Treatment of opioid-induced constipation with oral naloxone: a pilot study. *Clin Pharmacol Ther.* 1992;52:90-95.

73. Sykes NP. An investigation of the ability of oral naloxone to correct opioid-related constipation in patients with advanced cancer. *Palliat Med.* 1996;10:135-144.

74. Meissner W, Schimdt U, Hartmann M, et al. Oral naloxone reverses opioid-associated constipation. *Pain*. 2000;84: 105-109.

75. Meissner W, Leyendecker P, Mueller-Lissner S, et al. A randomized controlled trial with prolonged-release oral oxycodone and naloxone to prevent and reverse opioid-induced constipation. *Eur J Pain*. 2009;13:56-64.

76. Clemens K, Quednau I, Klaschik E. Bowel function during pain therapy with oxycodone/naloxone prolonged-release tablets in patients with advanced cancer. *Clin Pract*. 2011;65:472-478.

77. Thomas J, Karver S, Cooney GA et al. Methylnaltrexone for opioid-induced constipation in advanced illness. *N Eng J Med*. 2008;358:2332-2343.

78. Portenoy RK, Thomas J, Mohel Boatwright M, et al. Subcutaneous methylnaltrexone for the treatment of opioid-induced constipation in patients with advanced illness: a double-blind, randomized, parallel group, dose-range in study. *J Pain Symptom Manage*. 2008;35: 458-468.

79. Berde C, Nurko S. Opioid side effects—mechanism based therapy. *N Engl J Med*. 2008;358:2400-2401.

80. Tamayo AC, Diaz-Zuluaga PA. Management of opioid-induced bowel dysfunction in cancer patients. *Support Care Cancer*. 2004;12:613-618.

81. Mancini I, Bruera E. Constipation in advanced cancer patients. *Support Care Cancer*. 1998;6:356-364.

82. Bennett M, Cresswell H. Factors influencing constipation in advanced cancer patients: a prospective study of opioid dose, dantron dose and physical functioning. *Palliat Med*. 2003;17:418-422.

CHAPTER 15

Bowel Obstruction

Carla I. Ripamonti ■ Hans Gerdes ■ Alexandra M. Easson

DEFINITION AND EPIDEMIOLOGY

Malignant bowel obstruction (MBO) was defined using the following criteria: clinical evidence of bowel obstruction (history/physical/radiologic examination); bowel obstruction beyond the ligament of Treitz, in the setting of a diagnosis of intra-abdominal cancer with incurable disease; or a diagnosis of non–intra-abdominal primary cancer with clear intraperitoneal disease (1,2).

MBO is a common complication in patients with abdominal or pelvic cancers, such as those arising from colon, ovary, and stomach. Bowel obstruction occurs in patients with a diagnosis of advanced primary or metastatic intra-abdominal malignancy such as ovarian cancer (5.5% to 51%) and colorectal cancer (10% to 28%) (3,4). MBO has also been reported in patients with non–intra-abdominal cancers, such as melanoma, breast cancer, and lung cancer (5). The interval from diagnosis of cancer to onset of MBO is significantly longer between intra-abdominal (mean 22.4 months) and extra-abdominal primary tumors (mean 57.5 months) (5–10).

Pancreatic cancer spreads directly to the duodenum or stomach; cancer of the colon spreads to the jejunum and ileum; and prostate and bladder cancers spread to the rectum (11). Tumors at the splenic flexure can cause bowel obstruction in 49% of cases, tumors of right and left colon in 25% of cases, and tumors of the rectum and rectosigmoid junction in 6% of cases (11).

Bowel obstruction may be partial or complete, and at single or multiple sites, the small bowel is more commonly involved than the large bowel (61% vs. 33%) and both are involved in over 20% of the patients. Even in advanced cancer, the obstruction may be due to benign causes such as adhesions, postirradiation bowel damage, inflammatory bowel disease, hernia, or intussusceptions of the bowel. Some reports suggest that a benign cause is responsible for obstruction in about 48% of the patients with colorectal cancer (2,3,11–13).

Cancer patients may develop bowel obstruction at any time in their clinical history: at the time of diagnosis of the malignancy or as part of recurrent disease, sometimes associated with an end-of-life state.

PATHOPHYSIOLOGY

Several physiopathologic mechanisms and causes may be involved in the onset of bowel obstruction and there is variability in both presentation and etiology.

Mechanical obstruction is caused by the following: (1) *extrinsic occlusion of the lumen* due to an enlargement of the primary tumor or recurrence, mesenteric and omental masses, and abdominal or pelvic adhesions (caused by either the tumor or secondary to surgery), postirradiation fibrosis; and postirradiation intestinal damage; (2) *intraluminal occlusion of the lumen* due to neoplastic mass, polypoidal lesions, or annular tumoral dissemination; (3) *intramural occlusion of the lumen* due to intestinal linitis plastica.

Functional obstruction (or adynamic ileus) is caused by intestinal motility disorders consequently to: (1) *tumor infiltration of the mesentery or bowel muscle and nerves (peritoneal carcinomatosis)*, malignant involvement of the celiac plexus; (2) *paraneoplastic neuropathy* in patients with lung cancer; (3) *chronic intestinal pseudo-obstruction* mainly due to diabetes mellitus, previous gastric surgery, and other neurologic disorders; and (4) *paraneoplastic pseudo-obstruction.*

At least four factors occur in bowel obstruction: (1) accumulation of gastric, pancreatic, and biliary secretions that are a potent stimulus for further intestinal secretions; (2) decreased absorption of water and sodium from the intestinal lumen; (3) increased secretion of water and sodium into the lumen as distension increases; and (4) bowel wall edema proximal to the level of the obstruction secondary to inflammation (Figure 15.1). These factors produce a vicious circle of secretion–distension–secretion–motor hyperactivity. Depletion of water and salt in the lumen is considered the most important "toxic factor" in bowel obstruction (11,13).

Clinical and Radiologic Diagnosis

In cancer patients, compression of the bowel lumen develops slowly and often remains partial. Symptoms become more frequent and last longer until near to complete obstruction results. Initial management includes a clinical assessment to rule out acute causes of obstruction and to ensure that the patient does not have a surgical emergency. Gastrointestinal (GI) symptoms such as pain at the tumor site, abdominal cramps, nausea and vomiting, abdominal distension are caused by the sequence of distension–secretion–motor activity of the obstructed bowel. The symptoms occur in different combinations and intensity depending on the site of obstruction (Figure 15.1) (Table 15.1) (9–11,13,14). In order to be able to diagnose the condition in a proper manner, a complete clinical history and a physical examination are mandatory before any investigation is ordered.

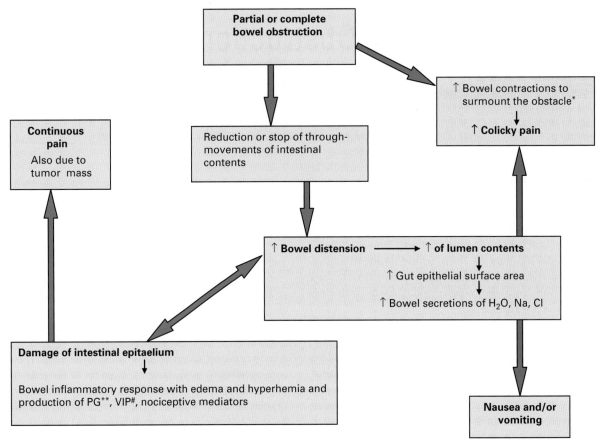

*Mechanical obstruction only, ** Prostaglandins , # Vasoactive intestinal polypeptide

Figure 15.1. Pathophysiology of bowel obstruction.

The symptoms referred to by the patient should be monitored daily. Vomiting can be evaluated in terms of quantity, quality, and number of daily episodes. Other symptoms such as nausea, pain, dry mouth, drowsiness, dyspnea, hunger, and thirst can be assessed by numerical or verbal scales.

Radiologic imaging in the evaluation of patients with the acute abdomen and the confirmation of the diagnosis of MBO have assumed a pivotal role. The preferred radiologic procedure has evolved in recent years, but it varies in different parts of the world according to the local expertise and the availability of each imaging modality.

For decades, plain abdominal radiography taken in the supine and standing positions has been the standard in the initial evaluation of patients with acute abdominal pain or suspected obstruction, but its usefulness in the present era is questionable (Figure 15.2). Plain radiography can document the air-filled dilated loops of bowel, differential air–fluid levels, or both, but the accuracy for localizing the point and cause of obstruction is low. The sensitivity of plain films in making a diagnosis of small bowel obstruction has been reported to be as low as 66% (15). Despite this, it remains an important step in the evaluation of most patients with acute and chronic abdominal symptoms.

Contrast GI series using barium suspensions provide excellent radiologic definition of the mucosal pattern and luminal patency, particularly in the assessment of the stomach and proximal small bowel (Figure 15.3), but more distal points of small bowel obstruction may not be seen as clearly due to the difficulty in the barium reaching this far in the small bowel and the effects of retained luminal fluid. As it is not absorbed, the retention of barium in the lumen, and the inability to subsequently eliminate it in the setting of obstruction, can then interfere with subsequent radiographic studies. For these reasons, barium small bowel series should be used selectively, and preferably, for evaluating more chronic symptoms or for searching the cause of persistent intestinal symptoms when acute obstruction has already been ruled out.

In the evaluation of large bowel obstruction, barium enema provides a quick, accurate, and inexpensive assessment of the location and cause of obstruction. This, however, should be performed with caution to avoid excessive insertion of barium proximal to the point of obstruction, as this can lead to retention of the barium proximal to the obstruction leading to dehydration of the barium and potential impaction. This is especially a problem in patients with incomplete and inoperable large bowel obstruction. Similarly, if large bowel obstruction is suspected on initial plain abdominal X-rays, a small bowel series should not be performed to avoid the barium from

TABLE 15.1	Common symptoms in cancer patients with malignant bowel obstruction			
Vomiting	Intermittent or continuous	It develops early and in great amounts in gastric, duodenum, and small bowel obstruction and develops later in large bowel obstruction	Biliary vomiting is almost odorless and indicates an obstruction in the upper part of the abdomen. The presence of bad smelling and fecaloid vomiting can be the first sign of an ileal or colic obstruction
Nausea	Intermittent or continuous		
Colicky pain	Variable intensity and localization due to distension proximal to the obstruction; secondary to gas and fluid accumulation most of which are produced by the gut	If it is intense, periumbilical, and occurring at brief intervals may be an indication of an obstruction at the jejunum-ileal level. In large bowel obstruction, the pain is less intense, deeper, occurring at longer intervals, and spreads toward the colon wall	An overall acute pain that begins intensely and becomes stronger or a pain that is specifically localized, may be a symptom of a perforation or an ileal or colic strangulation. A pain that increases with palpation may be due to peritoneal irritation or the beginning of a perforation
Continuous pain	Variable intensity and localization	It is due to abdominal distension, tumor mass, and/or hepatomegaly	
Dry mouth		It is due to severe dehydration, metabolic alterations, and above all it is due to the use of drugs with anticholinergic properties and poor mouth care	
Constipation	Intermittent or complete	In case of complete obstruction, there is no evacuation of feces and no flatus	In case of partial obstruction, the symptom is intermittent
Overflow diarrhea		It is the result of bacterial liquefaction of the fecal material	

becoming trapped in the proximal obstructed regions of the colon.

Gastrografin (diatrizoate meglumine) may also be useful in evaluating small and large bowel obstructions (Figure 15.4), but it usually only provides good visualization of proximal small bowel obstruction as the water soluble nature of the Gastrografin will result in it being diluted by the excess fluid retained in the distal small bowel.

Enteroclysis (the small bowel enema) requires the insertion of a long nasoenteric tube, which is manipulated under fluoroscopy guidance beyond the stomach by the radiologist. The contrast is then inserted under pressure resulting in full distension of the loops of small bowel, permitting better assessment of the mucosal pattern and patency, and improving the accuracy of diagnosis in small bowel obstruction. The discomfort associated with the procedure results in the need for it to be done with the use of sedatives. Unfortunately, as it requires radiologists with expertise in the technique, it is not widely available. Transcutaneous ultrasonography has been

used successfully in making the diagnosis of MBO, but it has limited usefulness when bowel loops are filled with air. It is also more operator dependent and is therefore less utilized for this indication in the United States than in Europe.

Although the diagnosis and location of obstruction can, at times, be suggested by the history, physical examination, and plain or contrast radiography, oncology patients often have altered GI motility caused by the use of narcotics and antidiarrheal agents or certain chemotherapeutic agents that can result in a paralytic ileus. This may confuse the initial presentation, resulting in a delay of diagnosis and initiation of treatment. Cross-sectional imaging by computed tomography (CT) scanning (Figure 15.5) or magnetic resonance imaging (MRI) has now been shown to provide superior results in the assessment of abdominal symptoms and in the diagnosis of bowel obstruction. Maglinte et al. (16) advise the initial use of abdominal CT scanning for the evaluation of patients presenting with acute abdominal symptoms that are suggestive of obstruction, but use of enteroclysis or small

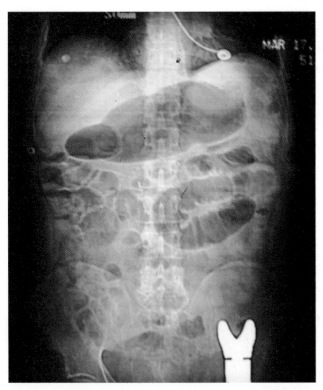

Figure 15.2. Plain abdominal X-ray image of a patient with obstructing metastasis from renal cancer. Dilated small bowel loop seen, but cause or severity not clearly determined. (Image kindly provided by Dr. Mark Gollub, MSKCC.)

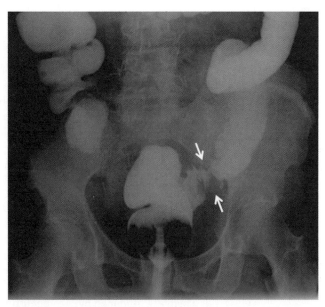

Figure 15.4. Gastrografin enema image of a patient with ovarian cancer causing partial sigmoid colon obstruction, shown between the *arrows*.

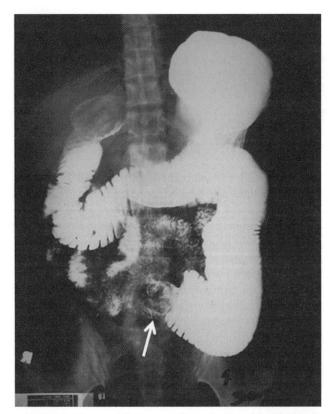

Figure 15.3. Barium gastrointestinal series image demonstrating high-grade, malignant-appearing, small bowel obstruction from a primary jejunal cancer (arrow). (Image kindly provided by Dr. Mark Gollub, MSKCC.)

bowel fluoroscopic GI follow-through examinations for the evaluation of mildly symptomatic patients or those with chronic or intermittent complaints.

Comparative studies have demonstrated superior results with cross-sectional imaging in accurately predicting the cause of symptoms. The diagnostic accuracy for determining the cause of obstruction was reported to be 87% for CT, 23% for ultrasound, and 7% for plain film radiography (17). Newer technology in CT scanning such as spiral and multidetector scanners provides a better global assessment of the abdomen and pelvis and when coupled with multiplanar reconstruction can help focus on the transition point in bowel obstruction, thereby helping determine the site, cause, and severity of obstruction (Figure 15.6) (18). CT scanning also provides a greater appreciation for the integrity of the bowel wall proximal to the obstruction, helping to predict the existence of ischemia, pneumatosis, or early perforation with greater accuracy than other modalities.

A recent report by Angelilli et al. (19) demonstrated a sensitivity, specificity, and accuracy for CT scan of 74%, 100%, and 92%, respectively, in confirming a neoplastic cause of MBO. Multidetector computed tomography scanning has also been shown to be highly accurate in identifying the malignant cause of colonic obstruction and in identifying specific features such as the presence of air–fluid levels in the colonic lumen, mural pneumatosis, and a right colon diameter of >10 cm as poor prognostic features (Figure 15.7) (20). These features help expedite making a decision on management, which can sometimes be critical in the overall prognosis for patients with strangulating bowel obstruction.

MRI may also provide similar diagnostic information, but it is not as widely available as CT scanning and local expertise in its use in the assessment of bowel obstruction is limited. The strength of MRI is the absence of radiation

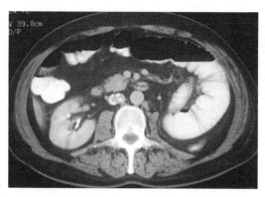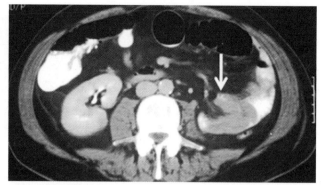

Figure 15.5. **A**: Computed tomography scan image of a patient with malignant bowel obstruction caused by metastasis from renal cancer (same patient as in Figure 15.2) showing the dilated jejunal loop. **B**: Subsequent image showing obstructing mass causing intussusceptions (*arrow*). (Images kindly provided by Dr. Marc Gollub, MSKCC.)

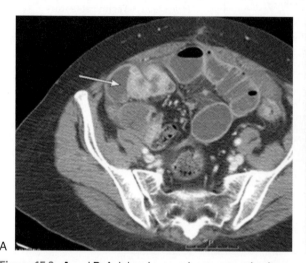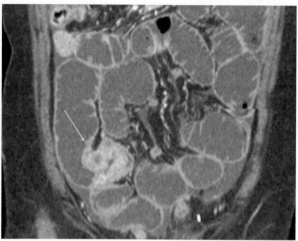

Figure 15.6. **A** and **B**: Axial and coronal reconstruction images of a computed tomography scan in a patient with malignant small bowel obstruction from an ovarian cancer implant (*arrow*). (Images kindly provided by Dr. Mark Gollub, MSKCC.)

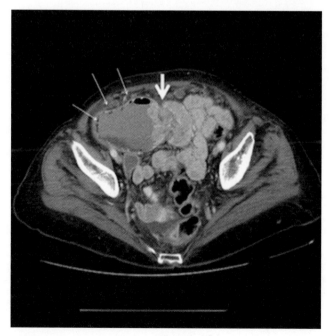

Figure 15.7. Computed tomography scan image of an obstructing small bowel metastasis (*large arrow*) with edema and pneumatosis (*small arrows*) of the jejunal wall. (Image kindly provided by Dr. Mark Gollub, MSKCC.)

exposure, so in the pediatric population, especially in those with chronic or recurrent GI symptoms, such as in patients with inflammatory bowel disease, it is becoming the preferred modality of repeated imaging. The expected results with MRI should be similar to CT scanning, but the data on the sensitivity, specificity, and accuracy are still awaited.

THERAPIES

The management of patients with MBO is one of the greatest challenges for physicians who care for cancer patients. The approach to management of the patient with MBO is completely different in each situation. Although MBO is usually associated with advanced-stage disease when it occurs at the time of initial diagnosis, regardless of the primary site of malignancy, management generally proceeds with curative intent and each patient should be managed according to appropriate principles/guidelines for the underlying malignancy. On the other hand, MBO as part of recurrent disease is often managed with palliative intent; in this context, different factors should be considered to determine the most appropriate treatment.

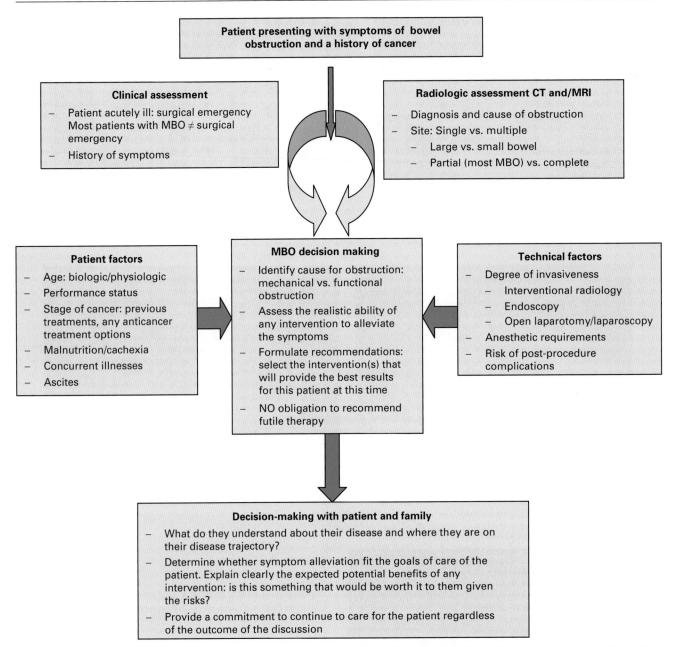

Figure 15.8. Algorithm for assessing and managing a patient with malignant bowel obstruction. MBO, malignant bowel obstruction; CT, computed tomography; MRI, magnetic resonance imaging.

For patients with recurrent disease, MBO generally occurs in a chronic and slow fashion that results in narrowing of the diameter of the small or large bowel (or both simultaneously).

In the face of a clearly incurable situation, significant patient discomfort and suffering must be balanced with the need to simplify the care of those patients with a short time to live. The goal in any decision we make needs to impact the quality of life (QOL) of the affected person in a positive way and each assessment and management needs to be tailored to the specific needs of the patients. Figure 15.8 shows the algorithm for assessing and managing a patient with MBO. The physicians need to consider a series of questions when faced with terminal cancer patients (patients are no longer responsive to specific oncologic therapies) with bowel obstruction:

Is the patient fit for surgery? Is there a place for stenting? Is it necessary to use a venting nasogastric tube (NGT) in inoperable patients? When should a venting gastrostomy be considered? What drugs are indicated for symptom control? What is the proper route for drug administration? What is the role of parenteral hydration and total parenteral nutrition (PN)? Figure 15.8 shows the algorithm for assessing and managing a patient with MBO.

Endoscopic Management of Gastroduodenal and Proximal Jejunal Obstruction

Gastric outlet obstruction (GOO) and small bowel obstruction are very debilitating presentations of malignancy that are commonly seen in patients with pancreatic cancer, distal

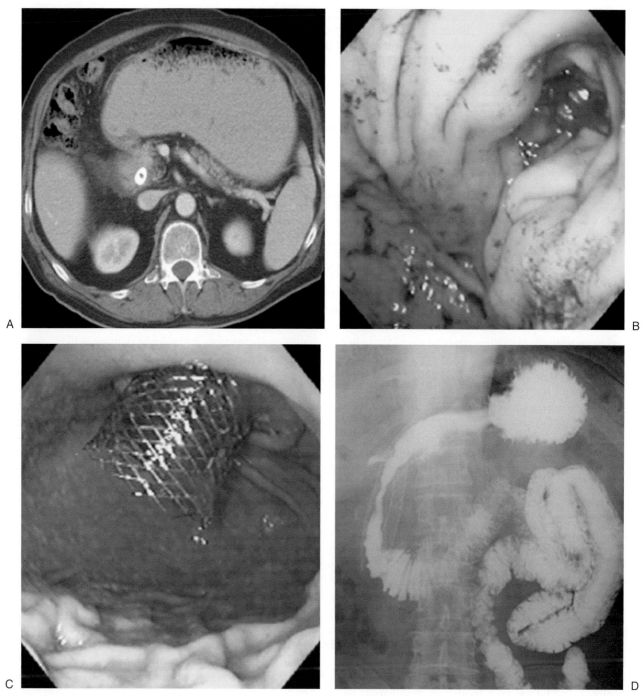

Figure 15.9. Radiographic and endoscopic images of a patient with malignant duodenal obstruction treated with endoscopic stenting. **A**: Computed tomography scan demonstrating dilated stomach and transition point in duodenum. **B**: Endoscopy showing obstructed pylorus. **C**: Endoscopy image after insertion of stent. **D**: Barium gastrointestinal series after stent insertion demonstrating relief of obstruction.

gastric cancer, gall bladder cancer, and cholangiocarcinoma. This can also result from metastases of a variety of extra-abdominal malignancies, such as breast cancer and lung cancer. Although GOO is technically not considered MBO, it will be discussed here as it is a common source of morbidity in cancer patients and is managed in a manner similar to other forms of MBO. Advances in endoscopic techniques have now permitted the treatment of this problem to be readily accomplished with the endoscopic insertion of a

self-expanding metal stent (SEMS) (Figure 15.9) or gastric venting via a percutaneously placed gastrostomy (drainage percutaneous endoscopic gastrostomy [PEG]). These approaches are particularly useful for patients with limited expected survival.

The procedure is easily performed using techniques similar to those used for inserting bile duct stents in patients with obstructive jaundice, but it has still not become widely available except at university or cancer centers with interventional

TABLE 15.2 Summary results from two multicenter studies of endoscopic stent placement for treatment of malignant gastroduodenal obstruction		
	Dorman et al. (23)	**Telford et al. (22)**
Number of cases	606	176
Study design	Pooled analysis	Multicenter study
Technical success	97%	98%
Clinical success	87%	84%
Perforation/bleeding	1.2%	2%
Migration	5%	6%
Re-obstruction	18%	20%

endoscopists. The technical success rates for placement of enteral stents have been reported to be >90% and clinical success for resolution of nausea and vomiting with improved ability to consume food orally is reported over 75% (21–25) (Table 15.2).

In the limited comparative studies published, endoscopic stent placement has been associated with shorter hospital stay and lower periprocedural mortality in patients with GOO secondary to pancreatic cancer (26,27) and with more rapid food intake compared with surgical bypass (26,28). Stent placement has even been shown to be effective in palliating symptoms from obstruction in the setting of limited degrees of peritoneal carcinomatosis (29).

Delayed stent failure can occur, however, from food impaction or re-obstruction caused by tumor ingrowth. Stent migration also can occur, sometimes in association with cancer treatment, if there is reduction in the size of the tumor. In most cases, re-obstruction due to tumor ingrowth can be managed with the placement of a second stent or tumor ablation by Nd:YAG laser or argon plasma coagulator (30). In comparative studies, those managed with stent did just as well initially as patients managed with surgical bypass, but they had a greater need for re-intervention because of delayed stent occlusion (28,31).

The effect of palliative treatments on the patient's QOL in malignant GOO has been limited or absent from most studies (32,33). In a prospective, non-randomized study, Schmidt et al. showed that stent placement was associated with a shorter hospital stay than surgical bypass, but both the procedures were associated with improvements in nausea, vomiting, ability to eat, and several measures of QOL (33). In another prospective study examining QOL in patients with malignant GOO, Mehta et al. randomized 27 patients to receive laparoscopic gastrojejunostomy or endoscopic stent placement for malignant GOO. Stent placement was associated with less pain and shorter hospital stay, with a greater improvement in physical health following stent placement relative to those managed surgically (32).

We presently consider surgical bypass to be the preferred option for patients with a good performance status,

a slowly progressive disease, and a relatively longer life expectancy (>60 days). Furthermore, if the site of obstruction is more distal in the jejunum or if there are multiple sites of obstruction, endoscopic stenting is likely to have a lower rate of technical success, so surgical intervention or drainage gastrostomy should be considered. We estimated that the patients who are best suited for endoscopic stenting are those with a short length of tumor and a single site of obstruction that is located at the pylorus or in the proximal two-thirds of the duodenum, with an intermediate to high performance status and an intermediate life expectancy of >30 days. Patients with a poor performance status, a rapidly progressive disease, an evidence of advanced carcinomatosis with moderate to severe ascites or multiple levels of obstruction on cross-sectional imaging, and a very short life expectancy of <30 days are best served by medical palliation of symptoms or the insertion of a drainage PEG.

Endoscopic Management of Malignant Small Bowel Obstruction

Much of the experience with endoscopic management of small bowel obstruction comes from that which has just been reviewed in the setting of gastroduodenal obstruction above. Most gastroscopes are unable to reach beyond the ligament of Treitz and colonoscopes are unable to reach very far retrograde up into the terminal ileum, so most cases of small bowel obstruction have not been amenable to endoscopic stenting.

The recent development of long enteroscopes that can be advanced far into the small intestine through an overtube, which permits the pleating of the small bowel, has permitted some investigators to report success in stenting areas of the small intestine not previously accessible to standard endoscopes. Most of these reports are anecdotal, but with time, increasing interventional endoscopist experience, and further development of the enteroscopes, stents, and manipulating tools, the ability to treat mid-jejunal and ileal points of malignant obstruction may become more available and such patients will have another option for treatment (34,35). The

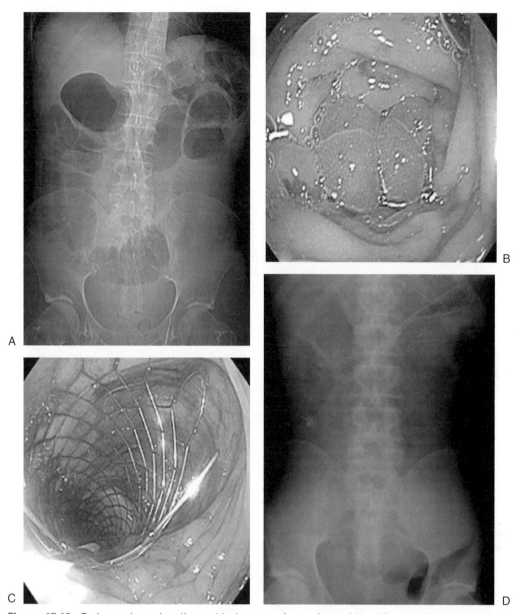

Figure 15.10. Endoscopic and radiographic images of a patient with malignant obstruction of the transverse colon, treated with stent placement. **A**: Abdominal X-ray showing dilated right colon. **B**: Endoscopy image showing obstructed colon. **C**: Endoscopy image after stent insertion. **D**: Abdominal X-ray showing the decompressed right colon, and partially expanded transverse colon stent.

selection of patients appropriate for such interventions will, however, remain challenging.

Endoscopic Management of Malignant Colorectal Obstruction

The endoscopic management of malignant large bowel obstruction has paralleled the experience reported with the treatment of malignant esophageal and gastroduodenal obstruction. Although initially approached with thermal ablative techniques such as Nd:YAG laser, greater success has been noted with the ability to insert SEMS in the colon (Figure 15.10). The technical success rates for insertion of metallic stents have ranged from 80% to 100%, with

clinical improvement in symptoms reported to be in >75% of patients (36–38). Many patients treated with stents have a durable relief of symptoms until death from progression of disease, but as has been seen with the use of stents in other parts of the body, restenosis, usually caused by tumor ingrowth through the interstices of the stent or stent migration, can cause delayed failure. This can usually be managed with insertion of another stent, endoscopic dilation, or laser ablation (36,37,39,40).

Two analyses of pooled data from the multiple reported case series have been published (41,42) (Table 15.3). Both analyses report clinical success rates of 88% and 91%, defined as a resolution of obstructive symptoms following the insertion of stents. The limitations to success are a very proximal

TABLE 15.3	Results of systematic reviews of efficacy and safety of colorectal stenting in the management of acute malignant colorectal obstruction	
	Khot et al. (41)	**Sebastian et al. (42)**
Technical success	551 (92%)	1,198 (94%)
Clinical success	525 (88%)	1,198 (91%)
Palliative success	301/336 (90%)	791 (93%)
Deaths	3 (1%)	7 (0.6%)
Perforation	22 (4%)	45 (3.8%)
Stent migration	54 (10%)	132 (11.8%)
Re-obstruction	53 (10%)	82 (7.3%)

location of obstruction with a higher rate of failure in the proximal colon in some reported series and the ability to traverse a tightly obstructing tumor with the endoscope or a guide wire. A greater success with stenting primary colorectal cancer has been noted, with lesser success for obstruction caused by extrinsic compression from metastatic or locally invasive pelvic tumors such as ovarian cancer, but some good results have also been reported for such patients (40,43,44). Limited data on cost effectiveness of colorectal stenting are available in published reports, with some calculations suggesting a potential reduction of approximately 50% in the estimated cost of palliation for such patients compared with surgical patients. This is predominantly attributed to a reduced hospital stay with stenting (41).

A recent multicenter study was completed demonstrating similar results with a newer generation of nitinol SEMS, the Wallflex (45). This study, like most others, demonstrates the ease of use, high technical and short-term clinical efficacy, and low overall and serious complication rate.

The proper evaluation of the efficacy of palliative treatments requires a careful assessment of the effect of the treatment on symptoms and the QOL and less attention on survival. In one prospective, non-randomized series evaluating the effect of endoscopic stenting and surgical diversion in palliating malignant colorectal obstruction, symptoms improved significantly after either treatments, but were more durable after stenting than after surgery. Although there was a trend toward improved QOL, neither treatment had a significant effect on overall QOL (45). This and other studies demonstrate how difficult it is to actually quantify the benefits of therapeutic interventions in the dying patient.

Drainage Percutaneous Endoscopic Gastrostomy in Bowel Obstruction

Often all efforts to completely reconstitute the patency of the GI tract will fail or be considered inappropriate due to the extent of intraperitoneal disease or the realization of the medical futility of such attempts. In this setting in a patient with intractable nausea and vomiting, the insertion of an NGT will often immediately stop the vomiting, but it may be associated with severe nasopharyngeal discomfort, pain associated with swallowing or coughing, or be cosmetically unacceptable, confining the patient at home.

Gastric venting with PEG tube placement has become widely acceptable, in this setting, for palliation of nausea and vomiting due to GI obstruction in patients with abdominal malignancies (46,47). Drainage PEG tube placement provides a rapid and safe method of achieving symptomatic relief without the risks of a surgical procedure or the discomfort of an NGT.

Clinical guidelines following the early experience with PEG tubes for nutritional support suggested that patients with advanced abdominal malignancies or prior surgery were contraindicated for PEG placement due to the presence of ascites, adhesions, or tumor infiltration of the stomach, but published data have shown that endoscopic PEG placement can be safely performed and can provide meaningful palliation of the severe nausea and vomiting occurring with such irreversible forms of bowel obstruction (47).

In an early series, Campagnutta et al. (46) reported on 34 patients with bowel obstruction from gynecologic malignancies that were palliated with drainage PEG. Using 15 and 20 Fr tubes, 94% had PEGs successfully placed and 84.4% had resolution of symptoms, with return of the ability to consume liquids or soft food for a median of 74 days.

In a retrospective study, 28 Fr PEG tube placement was feasible in 98% of patients with advanced recurrent ovarian cancer, even in patients with tumor encasing the stomach, diffuse carcinomatosis, and ascites (47). This approach has also been used to temporarily palliate symptoms in patients still undergoing systemic anticancer therapy with curative intent. However, for most patients with MBO from advanced peritoneal carcinomatosis, drainage PEG tubes only help reduce some of the symptoms associated with MBO such as nausea and vomiting, but often will require additional treatments to control pain from the distension associated with ascites, direct tumor effect in the abdomen, and elsewhere.

In some cases where the stomach has been partially or completely removed, the insertion of a venting PEG becomes impossible, so a drainage PEJ (jejunostomy) tube can be inserted and serve the same purpose (48).

Surgical Procedures

Surgical interventions, either open or laparoscopically, may benefit select patients with MBO. The best surgical procedure that is most likely to relieve symptoms for the greatest length of time with reasonable operative morbidity is chosen (49).

Complete surgical resection of a tumor is most desirable. However, it is only worthwhile if the entire tumor in that area can be resected with negative margins. The exception can be ovarian or some GI cancers, where intraperitoneal chemotherapy can treat the residual disease after a "debulking" operation of all obvious disease. Otherwise, debulking of a tumor is generally not beneficial, as the tumor will only grow back in the absence of anticancer therapy.

If the tumor cannot be resected, but there is a healthy non-obstructed bowel before and after the site of obstruction, a side-to-side bypass can be performed. This will restore bowel continuity and allow the patients to eat and maintain their nutritional status. In the case of distal obstruction, a stoma can be created out of the most distal unaffected bowel segment. In order to maintain one's nutrition orally, it is necessary to have a minimum of 100 cm of proximal bowel before a stoma, so the length of proximal bowel should be measured prior to creating a proximal stoma. Proximal stomas also have high outputs and may cause significant fluid balance problems.

Finally, in the absence of any other option, a gastrostomy tube may be placed to avoid the need for an NGT. A venting gastrostomy tube may provide significant symptomatic relief for the patients with intractable nausea and vomiting not controlled by antiemetics and may allow discharge from hospital and death at home (50). These tubes can be inserted by endoscopic procedures, by interventional radiology, or by open surgery. They can only be placed if the stomach can be brought up freely to the adjacent abdominal wall that is free of tumor. Ascites is a relative contraindication; however, they may still be successful if the ascites is drained prior and after placement to allow the stomach and abdominal wall to be brought together. Symptomatic relief from an NGT suggests that the tube will be effective to relieve symptoms. However, placement of a percutaneous tube is an invasive procedure and is associated with discomfort, complications, and a failure rate and should be offered only to patients with poorly controlled symptoms on aggressive medications and those who are not imminently dying.

The likelihood of success depends on the location of the bowel obstruction, with large bowel obstruction successfully relieved in 80% of cases versus 25% if both large and small bowels are involved (51). The number of obstructed sites also affects the likelihood of success; a single site of obstruction has a high likelihood of success as compared with multiple sites of obstruction. It is worth emphasizing that MBO from generalized carcinomatosis is a distinct entity that responds poorly, or not at all, to surgical intervention and these patients are not surgical candidates (13,52,53).

Surgical Decision-Making

In addition to the technical factors already described, surgical decision-making must take into account individual patient and disease factors. Performance status remains one of the best predictors of low complication rates and survival (54); patient factors associated with poor surgical outcomes include advanced age (both physiologic and chronologic), poor nutritional status (see below), ascites, concurrent illness and comorbidities, previous and future anticancer treatment, psychological health, and social support (55–57).

Disease factors such as etiology, time from primary presentation, tumor grade, and tumor extent and available anticancer treatment options also affect decision-making. Slow-growing, well-differentiated tumors are more likely to be associated with better outcomes and longer survival. The best predictor of the future is the pace of the disease in the past and its response to treatment prior to the presentation of obstruction, due to the biology and inherent growth characteristics of the tumor. Patients with bulky liver or lung metastatic disease will die much sooner than those with localized pelvic or intraperitoneal disease and are therefore less likely to benefit from surgery.

The selection of patients who will benefit from these procedures is an ongoing challenge and can be done only by individualizing management. Because the management of MBO is rarely an emergency, time can and should be taken into account to come up with an appropriate individualized treatment plan. In the face of an incurable, progressive illness, the balance between honesty and maintaining hope and optimism can be difficult to achieve, but it is necessary to avoid the use of futile treatments and harm to the patient (58). A futile treatment is carried out when it is unlikely to produce the desired benefit (59). It may be easier to offer a treatment just to do something; the more difficult decision may be not to do something when it is not going to help. However, there is little guidance on what should be considered a futile treatment as the definition will vary from patient-to-patient and/or clinician-to-clinician based on previous personal experiences and expectations. Most clinicians agree, however, that palliative surgery in oncology patients should not be offered to meet emotional, existential, and/or psychological needs (60).

An approach to this decision-making can be outlined as follows. The clinician first needs to decide which, if any, treatments are appropriate or feasible. This can only be done through a thorough preoperative evaluation to avoid intraoperative surprises or emergencies. The patient is asked what they understand about where they are on their disease trajectory and what their expectations are. Their current medical condition and expected prognosis are discussed. All treatment options including surgery, interventional radiology, and medications should be discussed; along with the complication rates and the expected success of each intervention. Reasonable treatment goals are set, whether this is continued curative therapy, withdrawal of inappropriate therapies, or vigorous palliative care. The goals addressed include relief of suffering and improvement of QOL and may vary between similar patients as they are based on the patients' perceptions and life experiences. Questions are answered and a plan is developed with the patient. This may take several visits as the patient comes to terms with their disease.

With careful preoperative planning, it is possible to determine before the operation in most cases which option is most likely; however, the final decision must always be made in the operating room. The possibility that no surgical procedure may be possible must also be discussed and the patient and family must be prepared for that option. Finally, there must be a commitment to ongoing care with a clear care plan whatever the outcome of the surgery. Several recent papers from large cancer centers have followed patients prospectively with MBO. Significant symptom relief can be obtained by selecting appropriate patients for either surgery or stenting with minimal procedural mortality (54,57,61,62).

Nutritional Considerations

Any malignancy will influence patients' nutritional status, whether due to the disease itself or due to cancer-related treatments. Nutritional status may be further impaired due to decreased oral intake of patients with MBO, which affects the course of disease and therefore the prognosis of a patient (63).

Cachexia is a catabolic metabolic state that is commonly seen in advanced end-stage cancer, where the patient is metabolically breaking down intrinsic muscle, protein, and fat (64). Cachexia is associated with inflammation, hypercatabolism, hormonal changes, and production of tumor factors. There is no consensus in the literature on how to best diagnose cachexia. It is important to try to distinguish cachexia from malnutrition caused by inadequate oral intake due to MBO. Cachexia is not reversible by increasing nutritional intake, it represents end-stage disease, and therefore interventions to improve oral intake will not be helpful. Unfortunately, in advanced cancer patients, cachexia, MBO, and poor nutritional status are often seen together.

The European Society for Clinical Nutrition and Metabolism (ESPEN) defined severe malnutrition as existing when patients have at least one of the following risk factors: weight loss ≥10% to 15% within 6 months; body mass index ≤18 kg/m², and serum albumin ≤30 g/L (without evidence of renal and/or liver dysfunction) (65).

The use of PN in advanced cancer remains controversial. Recent guidelines by ESPEN were published for the use of PN in patients who will undergo a surgical procedure (65) and for those who will not undergo a surgical intervention (66). For those patients who meet the ESPEN definition for severe malnutrition or undernourishment (body mass index <18.5 to 22 kg/m² depending on age), in whom a surgery is

planned, and who cannot be enterally fed, ESPEN recommends starting PN 7 to 10 days preoperatively to decrease the rate of postoperative infections, length of stay in hospital, and postoperative mortality. Postoperative PN is indicated for malnourished patients who required emergency surgery and therefore could not receive PN preoperatively (65).

For those patients with advanced cancer and poor nutritional status who do not require surgery, PN is considered ineffective if the reason for the poor nutritional status is not located in the GI tract. Also, PN does not have a role as a supplement while patients are on chemotherapy, radiation treatment, or both therapies simultaneously and also are able to receive oral or enteral nutrition adequately (66).

One recently published study evaluated the effectiveness of a home PN program in 38 patients with advanced malignant disease. The most common indication for home PN in this group was MBO. Patients who started on PN with a Karnofsky Performance Status ≥50 did have a longer survival compared with those patients who had a score ≤50 at the time of the beginning of PN (67). There may therefore be a role for PN for select patients with MBO for whom some improvement in QOL and extension of life may be expected.

Pharmacologic Treatment of Symptoms

Symptomatic pharmacologic approach *should* be used in inoperable patients with the following aims: (1) to relieve continuous abdominal pain and intestinal colic, (2) to reduce vomiting to an acceptable level for the patient (e.g., 1 to 2 times in 24 hours) without the use of the NGT, (3) to relieve nausea, (4) to achieve hospital discharge, and (5) to allow for care at home/hospice if otherwise possible (14).

Clinical practice recommendations for the management of MBO in patients with end-stage cancer have been published by the Working Group of the European Association for Palliative Care (13). Intravenous (i.v) or subcutaneous (s.c.) hydration and the use of NGT are most common methods adopted mainly due to vomiting. Although an aggressive volume and electrolyte i.v or s.c resuscitation may be necessary, the volume of fluids administered should be monitored carefully because an overdose will increase bowel secretions and a worsening of the symptoms.

Drug therapy, comprising analgesics, antisecretory drugs, and antiemetics, without the use of an NGT was first described 30 years ago. Several authors have confirmed the efficacy of this approach, and it is successfully used by palliative care centers throughout the world in both inpatients and outpatients (13,68–73).

The drugs of choice may vary between different countries and different centers, based on the clinical experience, drug availability, cost, and fashion. Medication should be tailored to each patient with regard to both the drugs to be administered and the route of administration (Figure 15.11) (13). Dosage and choice of drug should be highly personalized. Most MBO patients are not able to use the oral route and therefore alternative routes should be considered. If a central venous catheter has been previously inserted, this can be used

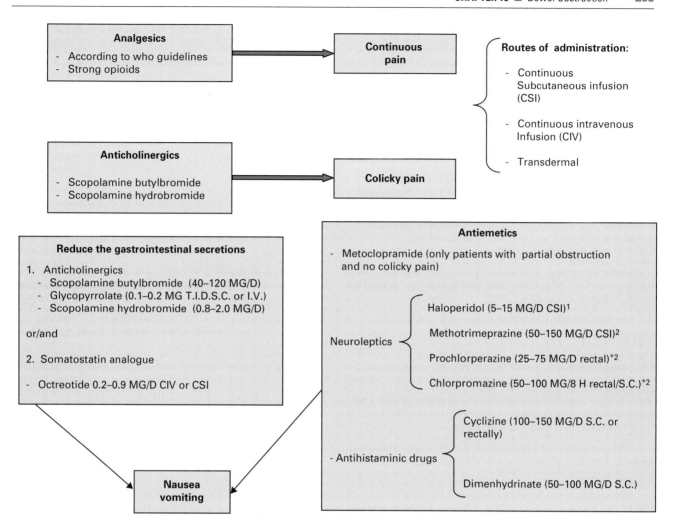

Figure 15.11. Symptomatic pharmacologic approach.

to administer drugs for symptom control. Continuous subcutaneous infusion of drugs using a portable syringe driver allows the parenteral administration of different drug combinations, produces minimal discomfort for the patient, and is easy to use in a home setting. Rectal and sublingual administration can occasionally be used. Finally, some drugs, such as fentanyl and scopolamine, may also be administered by the transdermal route.

Pain

Opioid analgesics, administered according to the World Health Organization (WHO) and European Society of Medical Oncology (ESMO) guidelines (74,75), are the most effective drugs in the management of abdominal, continuous and colicky, pain associated with bowel obstruction. The dose of opioids should be titrated against the effect and most usually be administered parenterally. In patients with subsequent episodes of subacute obstruction to which opioids may negatively contribute, it may be useful to choose the drug on

the basis of presumed selectivity of distribution at the intestinal sites. Morphine tends to accumulate in intestinal tissues, interacting with local opioid receptors. It has been reported that more lipophilic drugs, like methadone and fentanyl, may limit their presence at the opioid intestinal receptors (70,76).

Anticholinergic drugs such as scopolamine butylbromide, scopolamine hydrobromide, or glycopyrrolate can be associated with opioids in the presence of colicky pain if the opioids alone are not effective (13,69–73) (Figure 15.11).

Nausea and Vomiting

Nausea and vomiting can be managed using two different pharmacologic approaches (Figure 15.11):

1. Administration of drugs that reduce GI secretions such as anticholinergics (hyoscine hydrobromide, hyoscine butylbromide, and glycopyrrolate) and/or somatostatin analogues (octreotide) (13,68–73,77,78)
2. Administration of antiemetics acting on the central nervous system, alone or in association with drugs to reduce

GI secretions. Metoclopramide is the drug of choice in functional intestinal obstruction, it is not recommended in the presence of complete bowel obstruction as it may increase nausea, vomiting, and colicky pain. It is a prokinetic acting at the level of acetylcholine and dopamine receptors, thus stimulating the musculature of the GI tract. Other antiemetics are the butyrophenones, antihistaminic–antiemetic, and phenothiazines (prochlorperazine and chlorpromazine (13)) (Figure 15.11). Haloperidol, a dopamine antagonist and a potent suppressor of the chemoreceptor trigger zone, is considered to be the antiemetic drug of first choice when the obstruction is complete. Haloperidol can be combined with scopolamine butylbromide and opioid analgesic in the same syringe.

There are no comparative studies on the efficacy of these different approaches. Generally, physicians are guided by drug availability and costs.

Corticosteroids have also been used because of their anti-inflammatory effect. There is no consensus on which is the most effective steroid in this condition; however, dexamethasone and methylprednisolone are the most commonly used. A systematic review showed a tendency but no definite significant reduction of symptoms in the steroid group compared with the placebo group. In terms of mortality, there are no differences between the groups (79).

The coadministration of octreotide, corticosteroids, and metoclopramide produced a prompt resolution of GI symptoms and recovery of bowel movements within 5 days (68).

Recently, a meta-analysis compared the effectiveness of histamine-2 receptor antagonists and proton pump inhibitors (PPI) in reducing gastric secretions in patients with MBO. It was done based on seven randomized controlled trials. In total, 445 patients were included, of which 223 received ranitidine and 222 different PPI's (omeprazole, lansoprazole, pantoprazole, and rabeprazole). Both drugs were able to reduce the gastric secretions and between them, ranitidine was the most potent (80). Based on this report, we cannot make final conclusions, but these findings represent another tool available in the management of this condition and something that needs further investigation.

Octreotide, a synthetic analogue of somatostatin that has a more potent biologic activity and a longer half-life, has also been used to manage the symptoms of bowel obstruction. It may be administered subcutaneously or intravenously either as a bolus or as a continuous infusion. Somatostatin and its analogues have been shown to inhibit the release and activity of GI hormones, modulate GI function by reducing gastric acid secretion, slow down intestinal motility, decrease bile flow, increase mucous production, and reduce splanchnic blood flow. It reduces GI contents and increases absorption of water and electrolytes at the intracellular level, via cyclic adenosine monophosphate and calcium regulation. The inhibitory effect of octreotide on both peristalsis and GI secretions reduces bowel distension and the secretion of water and sodium by the intestinal epithelium, thereby reducing vomiting and pain. The drug may therefore break the vicious circle represented by secretion, distension, and contractile hyperactivity (81). Additionally, octreotide indirectly inhibits submucosal excitatory nerves, thus reducing spastic activity responsible for colicky pain.

The first prospective open-label study was performed on 14 patients with MBO who received doses of octreotide ranging from 0.3 to 0.6 mg/d after unsuccessful symptom control of nausea and vomiting with haloperidol and chlorpromazine. All the patients had a reduction in nausea and quantity of vomiting at different levels and in two patients the NGT was removed (82).

Many studies, although uncontrolled, strongly support the use of octreotide for reducing GI secretions, nausea, and vomiting in patients with MBO (3,10,11,13,14,83,84). In many cases, the NGT can be removed. Reported effective doses range from 100 to 600 μg/d, either as a continuous infusion or as intermittent subcutaneous boluses. Octreotide has been coadministered with numerous other agents, including morphine, haloperidol, and scopolamine butylbromide.

The combination of the two drugs (octreotide and scopolamine butylbromide) may reduce GI secretions and vomiting whenever the use of one drug alone is ineffective (77,78).

Three randomized trials have compared octreotide with hyoscine butylbromide (77,78,85). In all of these trials, octreotide was superior in the control of symptoms compared with hyoscine butylbromide.

Two randomized, prospective studies were carried out by Ripamonti et al. to compare the antisecretory effects of octreotide (0.3 mg/d) and Scopolamine butylbromide (SB) (60 mg/d) that were administered by continuous subcutaneous infusion for 3 days in 17 patients with inoperable bowel obstruction having an NGT (77) and in 15 patients without NGT (78). In both the studies, half of the patients were cared for at home and the other half were admitted to surgical wards. In both the studies, the hospitalized patients received significantly more parenteral hydration per day (2,000 mL vs. 500 mL) than the patients cared for at home.

In the study of Ripamonti et al. (77), the NGT could be removed in all 10 home care and in 3 hospitalized patients without changing the dosage of the drugs. Octreotide significantly reduced the amount of GI secretions already at T2 ($p = 0.016$) and T3 ($p = 0.020$). Pain relief was obtained in all 17 patients and only 2 patients required an increase in the morphine dose at T1. In the second study (78), octreotide treatment induced a significantly more rapid reduction in the number of daily episodes of vomiting and intensity of nausea when compared with scopolamine butylbromide treatment at the different time intervals examined.

In the third randomized controlled trial, Mystakidou et al. (85) evaluated the efficacy of octreotide in the management of nausea, vomiting, and abdominal pain secondary to MBO in inoperable cancer patients. Sixty-eight terminally ill patients were enrolled and the patients were randomly assigned into two equal groups. One group received scopolamine butylbromide 60 to 80 mg/d and chlorpromazine 15 to 25 mg/d and the comparative group received octreotide 0.6

to 0.8 mg/d and chlorpromazine 15 to 25 mg/d. The drugs were administered via continuous subcutaneous infusion. Patients on octreotide presented significant less intensity of nausea and quantity of vomiting episodes. The survival time ranged from 7 to 61 days (85).

Mercadante et al. (86) studied 15 consecutive advanced cancer patients with inoperable MBO receiving octreotide in combination with metoclopramide, corticosteroids, and an initial bolus of amidotrizoato (a mixture of sodium diatrizoate, meglumine diatrizoate, and a wetting agent [polysorbate 80]). Recovery of bowel transit appeared in 1 to 5 days in 14 of 15 patients till death.

Octreotide is significantly more effective and faster than hyoscine butylbromide in reducing the amount of GI secretions in patients having an NGT and in reducing the intensity of nausea and the number of vomiting episodes in patients without NGT.

Few studies have addressed the use of long-acting octreotide in patients with advanced malignancies who developed MBO at some point during the course of the disease (87,88). The efficacy and safety of octreotide long-acting release (LAR) at a dose of 30 mg on Day 1 and octreotide for 2 weeks were evaluated in a pilot study of 15 patients with advanced ovarian cancer. Of 13 evaluable patients, 3 had a major efficacy to LAR treatment with reduction in GI symptoms, 2 had minor response, 4 had no response, and 4 had progressive symptoms. No significant toxicities were due to LAR (87).

We do think this is an interesting finding, but based on only a small numbers of patients, we are unable to make further conclusions at the present time. It will be interesting to see more research in this area, because this drug might be used potentially in the ambulatory setting. Although octreotide is an expensive therapy, considering the fact that the goal of the treatment is improvement in the QOL of the patient and based on the strong evidence available in the literature that supports a real benefit with the use of this medication, the authors of this chapter consider that octreotide should be part of the treatment once the patient is diagnosed.

REFERENCES

1. Anthony T, Baron T, Mercadante S, et al. Report of the clinical protocol committee: development of randomized trials for malignant bowel obstruction. *J Pain Symptom Manage.* 2007;34:S49-S59.
2. Krouse RS. The international conference on malignant bowel obstruction: a meeting of the minds to advance palliative care research. *J Pain Symptom Manage.* 2007;34:S1-S6.
3. Correa R, Ripamonti CI, Dodge JE, Easson AM. Malignant bowel obstruction. In: Davis M et al. eds. *Supportive Oncology.* Vol 30. 2011;30:326-341.
4. Tunca JC, Buchler DA, Mack EA, Ruzicka FF, Crowley JJ, Carr WF. The management of ovarian-cancer-caused bowel obstruction. *Gynecol Oncol.* 1981;12:186-192.
5. Idelevich E, Kashtan H, Mavor E, Brenner B. Small bowel obstruction caused by secondary tumors. *Surg Oncol.* 2006;15:29-32.
6. Turnbull ADM, Guerra J, Starners HF. Results for surgery for obstructing carcinomatosis of gastrointestinal, pancreatic, or biliary origin. *J Clin Oncol.* 1989;7:381-386.
7. Aabo K, Pedersen H, Bach F, Knudsen J. Surgical management of intestinal obstruction in the late course of malignant disease. *Acta Chir Scand.* 1984;150:173-176.
8. Phillips RKS, Hittinger R, Fry JS, Fielding LP. Malignant large bowel obstruction. *Br J Surg.* 1985;72:296-302.
9. Ripamonti C, De Conno F, Ventafridda V, Rossi B, Baines MJ. Management of bowel obstruction in advanced and terminal cancer patients. *Ann Oncol.* 1993;4:15-21.
10. Ripamonti C, Bruera E. Palliative management of malignant bowel obstruction. *Int J Gynecol Cancer.* 2002;12:135-143.
11. Ripamonti C, Mercadante S. How to use octreotide for malignant bowel obstruction. *J Support Oncol.* 2004;2(4):357-364.
12. Krebs HB, Goplerud DR. Mechanical intestinal obstruction in patients with gynecologic disease: a review of 368 patients. *Am J Obstet Gynecol.* 1987;157:577-583.
13. Ripamonti C, Twycross R, Baines M, et al. Clinical-practice recommendations for the management of bowel obstruction in patients with end-stage cancer. *Support Care Cancer.* 2001;9:223-233.
14. Ripamonti C, Easson A, Gerdes H. Management of malignant bowel obstruction. *Eur J Cancer.* Special Issue on Palliative Care. 2008;44:1105-1115.
15. Shrake PD, Rex DK, Lappas JC, et al. Radiographic evaluation of suspected small-bowel obstruction. *Am J Gastro.* 1991;86:175-178.
16. Maglinte DDT, Balthazar EJ, Kelvin FM, et al. The role of radiology in the diagnosis of small-bowel obstruction. *Am J Radiol.* 1997;168:1171-1180.
17. Suri S, Gupta S, Sudhakar PJ, et al. Comparative evaluation of plain films, ultrasound and CT in the diagnosis of intestinal obstruction. *Acta Radiol.* 1999;40(4):422-428.
18. Caoili EM, Paulson EK. CT of small-bowel obstruction: another perspective using multiplanar reformations. *AJR Am J Roentgenol.* 2000;174:993-998.
19. Angelilli G, Moschetta M, Sabato L, et al. Value of "protruding lips" sign in malignant bowel obstructions. *Eur J Radiol.* 2011;80(3): 681-685.
20. Angelilli G, Moschetta M, Binetti F, et al. Prognostic value of MDCT in malignant large-bowel obstructions. *Radiol Med.* 2010;115:747-757.
21. Lowe AS, Beckett CG, Jowett S, et al. Self-expandable metal stent placement for the palliation of malignant gastroduodenal obstruction: experience in a large, single, UK centre. *Clin Radiol.* 2007;62:738-744.
22. Telford JJ, Carr-Locke DL, Baron TH, et al. Palliation of patients with malignant gastric outlet obstruction with the enteral Wallstent: outcomes from a multicenter study. *Gastrointest Endosc.* 2004;60:916-920.
23. Dormann A, Meisner S, Verin N, et al. Self-expanding metal stents for gastroduodenal malignancies: systematic review of their clinical effectiveness. *Endoscopy.* 2004;36:543-550.
24. Nassif T, Prat F, Meduri B, et al. Endoscopic palliation of malignant gastric outlet obstruction using self-expandable metallic stents: results of a multicenter study. *Endoscopy.* 2003;35:483-489.
25. Costamagna G, Tringali A, Spicak J, et al. Treatment of malignant gastroduodenal obstruction with a nitinol self-expanding metal stent: an international prospective multicentre registry. *Dig Liver Dis.* 2012; 44(1):37-43.

26. Espinel J, Sanz O, Vivas S, et al. Malignant gastrointestinal obstruction: endoscopic stenting versus surgical palliation. *Surg Endosc.* 2006;20:1083-1087.

27. Lillemoe KD, Cameron JL, Hardacre JM, et al. Is prophylactic gastrojejunostomy indicated for unresectable periampullary cancer? A prospective randomized trial. *Ann Surg.* 1999;230:322-328; discussion 328-330.

28. Jeurnink SM, Steyerberg EW, Hof GV, et al. Gastrojejunostomy versus stent placement in patients with malignant gastric outlet obstruction: a comparison in 95 patients. *J Surg Oncol.* 2007;96(5):389-396.

29. Mendelsohn RB, Gerdes H, Markowitz AJ, Dimaio CJ, Schattner MA. Carcinomatosis is not a contraindication to enteral stenting in selected patients with malignant gastric outlet obstruction. *Gastrointest Endosc.* June 2011;73(6):1135-1140; e-pub April 5 2011.

30. Holt AP, Patel M, Ahmed MM. Palliation of patients with malignant gastroduodenal obstruction with self-expanding metallic stents: the treatment of choice? *Gastrointest Endosc.* 2004;60:1010-1017.

31. Wong YT, Brams DM, Munson L, et al. Gastric outlet obstruction secondary to pancreatic cancer: surgical vs endoscopic palliation. *Surg Endosc.* 2002;16:310-312.

32. Mehta S, Hindmarsh A, Cheong E, et al. Prospective randomized trial of laparoscopic gastrojejunostomy versus duodenal stenting for malignant gastric outflow obstruction. *Surg Endosc.* 2006;20:239-242.

33. Schmidt C, Gerdes H, Hawkins W, et al. A prospective observational study examining quality of life in patients with malignant gastric outlet obstruction. *Am J Surg.* 2009;198:92-99.

34. Lennon AM, Chandrasekhara V, Shin EJ, et al. Spiral-enteroscopy-assisted enteral stent placement for palliation of malignant small-bowel obstruction. *Gastrointest Endosc.* 2010;71(2):422-425.

35. Ross AS, Semrad C, Waxman I, et al. Enteral stent placement by double balloon enteroscopy for palliation of malignant small bowel obstruction. *Gastrointest Endosc.* 2006;65(5):835-837.

36. Camunez F, Echenagusia A, Simo G, et al. Malignant colorectal obstruction treated by means of self-expanding metallic stents: effectiveness before surgery and in palliation. *Radiology.* 2000;216:492-497.

37. Law WL, Chu KW, Ho JW, et al. Self-expanding metallic stent in the treatment of colonic obstruction caused by advanced malignancies. *Dis Colon Rectum.* 2000;43:1522-1527.

38. Mainar A, De Gregorio MA, Tejero E, et al. Acute colorectal obstruction: treatment with self-expandable metallic stents before scheduled surgery—results of a multicenter study. *Radiology.* 1999;210:65-69.

39. Nash CL, Markowitz AJ, Schattner M, et al. Colorectal stents for the management of malignant large bowel obstruction. *Gastrointest Endo.* 2002;55:AB216.

40. Pothuri B, Guiguis A, Gerdes H, et al. The use of colorectal stents for palliation of large bowel obstruction due to recurrent gynecologic cancer. *Gynecol Oncol.* 2004;95:513-517.

41. Khot UP, Wenk Lang A, Murali K, et al. Systematic review of the efficacy and safety of colorectal stents. *Br J Surg.* 2002;89:1096-1102.

42. Sebastian S, Johnston S, Geoghegan T, et al. Pooled analysis of the efficacy and safety of self-expanding metal stenting in malignant colorectal obstruction. *Am J Gastro.* 2004;99:2051-2057.

43. Caceres A, Zhou Q, Iasonos A, Gerdes H, Chi DS, Barakat RR. Colorectal stents for palliation of large-bowel obstructions in recurrent gynecologic cancer: an updated series. *Gynecol Oncol.* March 2008;108(3):482-485.

44. Nagula S, Ishil N, Nash C, et al. Quality of life and symptom control after stent placement or surgical palliation of malignant colorectal obstruction. *J Am Coll Surg.* 2010;210:45-53.

45. Meisner S, Gonzalez-Huix F, Vandervoort JG, et al. Self-expandable metal stents for relieving malignant colorectal obstruction: short-term safety and efficacy within 30 days of stent procedure in 447 patients. *Gastro Endo.* 2011;74(4):876-884.

46. Campagnutta E, Cannizzaro R, Gallo A, et al. Palliative treatment of upper intestinal obstruction by gynecological malignancy: the usefulness of percutaneous endoscopic gastrostomy. *Gynecol Oncol.* 1996;62:103-105.

47. Pothuri B, Montemarano M, Gerardi M, et al. Percutaneous endoscopic gastrostomy tube placement in patients with malignant bowel obstruction due to ovarian carcinoma. *Gynecol Oncol.* 2005;96:330-334.

48. Piccinni G, Angrisano A, Testini M, et al. Venting direct percutaneous jejunostomy (DPEJ) for drainage of malignant bowel obstruction in patients operated on for gastric cancer. *Support Care Cancer.* 2005;13:535-539.

49. Krouse RS, McCahill LE, Easson AM, Dunn GP. When the sun can set on an unoperated bowel obstruction: management of malignant bowel obstruction. *J Am Coll Surg.* 2002;195:117-128.

50. Brooksbank M, Game P, Ashby M. Palliative venting gastrostomy in malignant intestinal obstruction. *Palliat Med.* 2002;16:520.

51. Bryan D, Radbod R, Berek J. An analysis of surgical versus chemotherapeutic intervention for the management of intestinal obstruction in advanced ovarian cancer. *Int J Gynecol Cancer.* 2006;16:125-134.

52. Helyer LK, Law CH, Butler M, et al. Surgery as a bridge to palliative chemotherapy in patients with malignant bowel obstruction from colorectal cancer. *Ann Surg Oncol.* 2007;14:1264-1271.

53. Abbas SM, Merrie AE. Resection of peritoneal metastases causing malignant small bowel obstruction. *World J Surg Oncol.* 2007;5:122.

54. Wright FC, Chakraborty A, Helyer L, Moravan V, Selby DJ. Predictors of survival in patients with non-curative stage IV cancer and malignant bowel obstruction. *Surg Oncol.* 2010;101(5):425-429.

55. Weiss SM, Skibber JM, Rosato FE. Bowel obstruction in cancer patients: performance status as a predictor of survival. *J Surg Oncol.* 1984;25:15-17.

56. Medina-Franco H, García-Alvarez MN, Ortiz-López LJ, Cuairán JZ. Predictors of adverse surgical outcome in the management of malignant bowel obstruction. *Rev Invest Clin.* May–June 2008;60(3):212-216.

57. Imai K, Yasuda H, Koda K, et al. An analysis of palliative surgery for the patients with malignant bowel obstruction. *Gan To Kagaku Ryoho.* December 2010;37(suppl 2):264-267.

58. Tattersall MH, Butow PN, Clayton JM. Insights from cancer patient communication research. *Hematol Oncol Clin North Am.* 2002;16:731-743.

59. Schneiderman LJ, Jecker N. Futility in practice. *Arch Intern Med.* February 1993;153(4):437-441.

60. Hofmann B, Håheim LL, Søreide JA. Ethics of palliative surgery in patients with cancer. *Br J Surg.* 2005;92:802-809.

61. Dalal KM, Gollub MJ, Miner TJ, et al. Management of patients with malignant bowel obstruction and stage IV colorectal cancer. *J Palliat Med.* July 2011;14(7):822-828.

62. Chakraborty A, Selby D, Gardiner K, et al. Malignant bowel obstruction: natural history of a heterogeneous patient population followed prospectively over two years. *J Pain Symptom Manage.* 2011;41(2):412-420.

63. Andreyev HJ, Norman AR, Oates J, Cunningham D. Why do patients with weight loss have a worse outcome when undergoing chemotherapy for gastrointestinal malignancies? *Eur J Cancer.* 1998;34(4):503-509.

64. MacDonald N, Easson AM, Mazurak VC, Dunn GP, Baracos VE. Understanding and managing cancer cachexia. *J Am Coll Surg.* July 2003;197(1):143-161.

65. Braga M, Ljungqvist O, Soeters P, Fearon K, Weimann A, Bozzetti F. ESPEN guidelines on parenteral nutrition: surgery. *Clin Nutr.* 2009;28(4):378-386.

66. Bozzetti F, Arends J, Lundholm K, Micklewright A, Zurcher G, Muscaritoli M. ESPEN guidelines on parenteral nutrition: non-surgical oncology. *Clin Nutr.* 2009;28(4):445-454.

67. Soo I, Gramlich L. Use of parenteral nutrition in patients with advanced cancer. *Appl Physiol Nutr Metab.* 2008;33(1):102-106.

68. Porzio G, Aielli F, Verna L, et al. Can malignant bowel obstruction in advanced cancer patients be treated at home? *Support Care Cancer.* 2011;19:431-433.

69. Ventafridda V, Ripamonti C, Caraceni A, et al. The management of inoperable gastrointestinal obstruction in terminal cancer patients. *Tumori.* 1990;76:389-393.

70. Mercadante S. Pain in inoperable bowel obstruction. *Pain Digest.* 1995;5:9-13.

71. De Conno F, Caraceni A, Zecca E, Spoldi E, Ventafridda V. Continuous subcutaneous infusion of hyoscine butylbromide reduces secretions in patients with gastrointestinal obstruction. *J Pain Symptom Manage.* 1991;6:484-486.

72. Fainsinger RL, Spachynski K, Hanson J, et al. Symptom control in terminally ill patients with malignant bowel obstruction. *J Pain Symptom Manage.* 1994;9:12-18.

73. Mercadante S, Sapio M, Serretta R. Treatment of pain in chronic bowel subobstruction with self-administration of methadone. *Support Care Cancer.* 1997;5:327-329.

74. World Health Organization. *Cancer Pain Relief.* 2nd ed. Geneva: WHO; 1996.

75. Ripamonti CI, Bandieri E, Roila F, on behalf of the ESMO Guidelines Working Group. Management of cancer pain: ESMO Clinical Practice Guidelines. *Ann Oncol.* 2011;22(suppl 6):vi69-vi77.

76. Haazen L, Noorduin H, Megens A, Meert T. The constipation-inducing potential of morphine and transdermal fentanyl. *Eur J Pain.* 1999;3(suppl A):9-15.

77. Ripamonti C, Mercadante S, Groff L, Zecca E, De Conno F, Casuccio A. Role of octreotide, scopolamine butylbromide and hydration in symptom control of patients with inoperable bowel obstruction having a nasogastric tube. A prospective, randomized clinical trial. *J Pain Symptom Manage.* 2000;19:23-34.

78. Mercadante S, Ripamonti C, Casuccio A, Zecca E, Groff L. Comparison of octreotide and hyoscine butylbromide in controlling gastrointestinal symptoms due to malignant inoperable bowel obstruction. *Support Care in Cancer.* 2000;8:188-191.

79. Feuer DJ, Broadley KE. Systematic review and meta-analysis of corticosteroids for the resolution of malignant bowel obstruction in advanced gynaecological and gastrointestinal cancers. Systematic Review Steering Committee. *Ann Oncol.* 1999;10:1035-1041.

80. Clark K., Lam L, Currow D. Reducing gastric secretions—a role for histamine 2 antagonists or proton pump inhibitors in malignant bowel obstruction? *Support Care Cancer.* 2009;17(12):1463-1468.

81. Riley J, Fallon MT. Octreotide in terminal malignant obstruction of the gastrointestinal tract. *Eur J Palliative Care.* 1994;1:23-28.

82. Mercadante S, Spoldi E, Caraceni A, Maddaloni S, Simonetti MT. Octreotide in relieving gastrointestinal symptoms due to bowel obstruction. *Palliat Med.* 1993;7:295-299.

83. Shima Y, Ohtsu A, Shirao K, Sasaki Y. Clinical efficacy and safety of octreotide (SMS201-995) in terminally ill Japanese cancer patients with malignant bowel obstruction. *Jpn J Clin Oncol.* 2008;38:354-359.

84. Hisanaga T, Shinjo T, Morita T, et al. Multicenter prospective study on efficacy and safety of octreotide for inoperable malignant bowel obstruction. *Jpn J Clin Oncol.* 2010;40:739-745.

85. Mystakidou K, Tsilika E, Kalaidopoulou O, Chondros K, Georgaki S, Papadimitriou L. Comparison of octreotide administration vs conservative treatment in the management of inoperable bowel obstruction in patients with far advanced cancer: a randomized, double-blind, controlled clinical trial. *Anticancer Res.* 2002;22(2B):1187-1192.

86. Mercadante S, Ferrera P, Villari P, Maeeazzo A. Aggressive pharmacological treatment for reversing bowel obstruction. *J Pain Symptom Manage.* 2004;28:412-416.

87. Matulonis UA, Seiden MV, Roche M, et al. Long-acting octreotide for the treatment and symptomatic relief of bowel obstruction in advanced ovarian cancer. *J Pain Symptom Manage.* 2005;30:563-569.

88. Massacesi C, Galeazzi G. Sustained release octreotide may have a role in the treatment of malignant bowel obstruction. *Palliat Med.* 2006;20:715-716.

CHAPTER 16

Diagnosis and Management of Effusions

Gary T. Buckholz ■ Charles F. von Gunten

DIAGNOSIS AND MANAGEMENT OF ASCITES

Ascites, the accumulation of fluid in the abdomen, is common. Its formation may be a direct result of a malignant process or secondary to liver cirrhosis or other comorbidities. Because the pathophysiology of fluid collection varies, treatment strategies differ. Clinical distinction between the causes of ascites is therefore important.

Of all patients with ascites, approximately 80% have cirrhosis (1). Other causes of nonmalignant ascites include the following: heart failure, 3%; tuberculosis, 2%; nephrogenic ascites related to hemodialysis, 1%; pancreatic disease, 1%; and miscellaneous entities such as hepatic vein thrombosis (Budd-Chiari syndrome), pericardial disease, and the nephrotic syndrome account for approximately 2% (1). Only 10% of patients who have ascites have malignancy as the primary cause (1). In these patients, epithelial malignancies, particularly ovarian, endometrial, breast, colon, gastric, and pancreatic carcinomas, cause over 80% of malignant ascites. The remaining 20% are due to malignancies of unknown origin (2). In one study, Runyon has shown that 53.3% of malignant ascites is associated with peritoneal carcinomatosis, 13.3% is associated with massive liver metastases, 13.3% is associated with peritoneal carcinomatosis and massive liver metastases, 13.3% is associated with hepatocellular carcinoma with portal hypertension, and 6.7% is associated with chylous ascites (3).

In general, the presence of ascites portends a poor prognosis, regardless of the cause. Patients with nonmalignant ascites related to cirrhosis have a survival rate of approximately 50% at 2 years (1). The mean survival in patients with malignant ascites is generally <4 months (4). However, with ascites due to a malignancy that is relatively sensitive to chemotherapy, such as newly diagnosed ovarian cancer or lymphoma, the mean survival may improve significantly (4).

PATHOPHYSIOLOGY

Nonmalignant Ascites

The mechanisms that lead to the development of ascites are many, and controversy still exists regarding which factors are most important. The most common cause of nonmalignant ascites is cirrhosis of the liver. In cirrhotic ascites, abnormal sodium retention is mediated by various hormonal and neural mechanisms, similar to those responsible for excess fluid retention in congestive heart failure (CHF). A hemodynamic state exists where total blood volume is increased, cardiac output is increased, and systemic vascular resistance is low. Studies have implicated nitric oxide as one of the potential mediators of this arterial vasodilation (5). In response, the vasoconstrictors of the renin–angiotensin–aldosterone system and the sympathetic nervous system are activated. Although atrial natriuretic peptide levels are increased, there is reduced renal responsiveness (6). In addition, arginine vasopressin, a potent vasoconstrictor, is activated in a manner independent of the osmotic state (7). The net result is an increase in total body sodium and water. In conjunction with cirrhosis, which has caused increased hepatic venous and lymphatic resistance, severe portal hypertension ensues. The increase in hepatic venous sinusoidal and portal pressures causes the excess fluid volume to localize to the peritoneal cavity secondary to fluid transudation from the splanchnic capillary bed. Ascites accumulation is also exacerbated by diminished intravascular oncotic pressure, resulting from hypoalbuminemia due to decreased synthetic capacity of the cirrhotic liver.

Malignant Ascites

Malignant ascites arises through pathophysiologic mechanisms different from those of nonmalignant ascites. First, in peritoneal carcinomatosis, neovascularization and subsequent "leak" from vessels is thought to play a prime role in ascites development. Researchers have identified a vascular growth and permeability factor that increases fluid leak from peritoneal vasculature; vascular endothelial growth factor (VEGF) is a prime candidate for this activity (8). Compared with cirrhotic ascites, high levels of VEGF are present in malignant ascites from gastric, colon, and ovarian cancers (9). In animal models, inhibiting the tyrosine kinase activity of VEGF receptors reduced ascites formation (10). Matrix metalloproteinases (MMPs) also appear to be involved in this process. Breaking down the extracellular matrix is an important step in neovascularization and metastatic spread. In animal models, MMP inhibitors significantly reduced malignant ascites (11). Second, portal pressures may be raised by direct tumor invasion of the liver with resultant hepatic venous obstruction. The resultant portal hypertension leads to transudation of fluid across the splanchnic bed into the abdominal cavity similar to cirrhotic ascites. A final mechanism of ascites formation is due to lymphatic obstruction, commonly caused by lymphoma, resulting in chylous ascites.

DIAGNOSIS

History

Patients with ascites commonly notice an increase in abdominal girth, a sensation of fullness or bloating, and early satiety. Other useful historical features include recent weight gain and ankle swelling. Patients may describe vague, generalized abdominal discomfort or a feeling of heaviness with ambulation. They may also note indigestion, nausea, and vomiting due to delayed gastric emptying, esophageal reflux symptoms due to increased intra-abdominal pressure, or protrusion of the umbilicus.

Physical Examination

Physical examination for ascites includes inspection for bulging flanks, percussion for flank dullness, a test for shifting dullness, and a test for a fluid wave. Jugular venous distention should also be assessed, as it may indicate a potentially reversible cardiac cause of ascites.

When significant ascites is present, the abdominal flanks bulge due to the weight of abdominal free fluid. The examiner should look for bulging flanks when the patient is supine. The distinction between excess adipose tissue and ascites may be made by percussing the flanks to assess for dullness (Figure 16.1). To detect flank dullness in the supine patient, approximately 1,500 mL of fluid must be present (12).

If dullness to percussion is found, examination for shifting dullness is a useful maneuver. The flank is tapped and a mark is made on the skin at the location where the tone changes. The patient is then turned partially toward the side that has been percussed. If the location of the dullness shifts upward toward the umbilicus, it is further evidence of intra-abdominal ascites (Figure 16.2).

The elicitation of a fluid wave may also help to confirm the diagnosis. The test is performed by having an assistant place the medial edges of both hands firmly down the midline

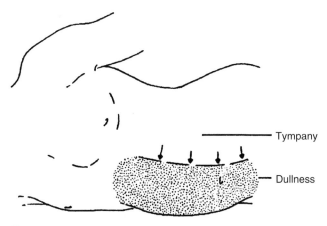

Figure 16.2. Tympany and dullness.

of the abdomen to block transmission of a wave through subcutaneous fat. The examiner places his/her hands on the flanks and then taps one flank sharply while simultaneously using the fingertips of the opposite hand to feel for an impulse transmitted through the ascites to the other flank. This test is 90% specific, but it is only 62% sensitive (13).

Several additional aspects of the physical examination may also be helpful. The liver may be ballotable, if it is enlarged and ascites is present. If ascites is severe, the examiner may discern umbilical, abdominal, or inguinal hernias; scrotal or lower extremity edema; or abdominal wall venous engorgement. The umbilicus may be flattened or slightly protuberant. The puddle sign and auscultatory percussion, the two additional maneuvers that have been described for the physical diagnosis of ascites, are not recommended (13).

Several diagnostic tests may be useful, particularly if the physical examination is equivocal. A plain radiograph of the abdomen may demonstrate a hazy or ground glass pattern. Ultrasonography or computed tomography (CT) of the abdomen readily identifies as little as 100 mL of free fluid. These latter tests are most helpful in making the diagnosis when there is a relatively small amount of fluid or when loculation is present.

Laboratory Abnormalities

A diagnostic paracentesis of 10 to 20 mL of fluid is useful to confirm the presence of ascites. More importantly, it is essential to help determine its cause. Identifying the cause has profound implications for what treatment is attempted.

To perform paracentesis, one of the two locations is chosen. The first is a midline location 2 cm inferior to the umbilicus. This location is over the linea alba, which is typically avascular. The second is a location 2 cm superior and medial to the anterior iliac spine and lateral to the edge of the rectus sheath, avoiding entry into the inferior epigastric artery. Ultrasonography may be performed if the fluid is difficult to obtain, loculation is suspected, or surgical scarring is present. Previous surgery in the area of the procedure

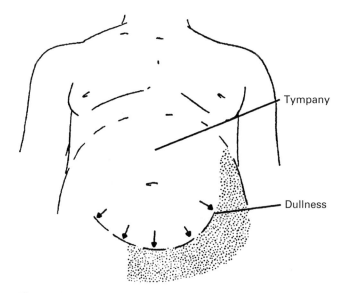

Figure 16.1. Shifting dullness.

increases the possibility that the bowel may be adherent to the abdominal wall.

After careful cleansing and local anesthetizing, a 2″, 20G angiocatheter is attached to a 20-mL syringe. To minimize the risk of fluid leaking after the procedure, the Z technique is performed. The skin is displaced 2 cm relative to the deep fascia. The needle is slowly advanced while a small amount of negative pressure is intermittently applied through the syringe until ascitic fluid is obtained. The intermittent pressure helps to avoid trapping omentum or bowel against the needle tip. After the necessary amount of fluid has been obtained, the needle is withdrawn. The fascial planes overlap to prevent fluid leakage, a common complication with a more direct approach.

The color of the fluid should be noted. A white milky fluid is characteristic of chylous ascites. Bloody fluid is almost always malignant in origin, although it may be due to abdominal tuberculosis. Initial bloody fluid that clears is more likely related to the trauma of the procedure.

The fluid should undergo cytologic analysis, determination of cell counts with a differential, and determination of albumin and total protein concentrations. A Gram's stain with culture can be performed if infection is suspected, but it has a low sensitivity. Inoculation of ascites directly into blood culture bottles increases the sensitivity of detecting infection up to 85% (14). The cell count, particularly the absolute neutrophil count, is useful in the presumptive diagnosis of bacterial peritonitis. If the neutrophil count is >250 cells/mL, bacterial peritonitis is presumed and empiric antibiotics should be started.

Cytology is the most specific test to demonstrate that the ascites is due to malignancy. Cytology is approximately 97% sensitive with peritoneal carcinomatosis (3), but it is not helpful in the detection of other types of malignant ascites such as massive hepatic metastasis or lymphomatous obstruction of lymph vessels. Therefore, the absence of malignant cells does not exclude malignancy as a cause.

In the past, the total protein concentration has been used to classify ascites into the broad categories of exudate (total protein > 25 g/L) and transudate (total protein < 25 g/L). However, this classification system has limitations and sometimes fails to lead to optimal treatment. It has been superseded by the serum-ascites albumin gradient (SAAG). It is defined as the serum albumin concentration minus the ascitic fluid albumin concentration. The SAAG directly correlates with the portal pressure (15). Patients with an SAAG of 1.1 g/dL or more have ascites that is due in part to increased portal pressures, with an accuracy of 97%. Patients with an SAAG <1.1 g/dL do not have portal hypertension, with an accuracy of 97% (16).

The superiority of the SAAG to the exudate/transudate characterization is shown using two examples. Cardiac ascites is associated with portal hypertension and would be expected to be transudative; however, the total protein levels in cardiac ascites are often exudative (16,17). In this example, although total protein is not useful for primary categorization, it may be useful to identify some forms of ascites.

Furthermore, ascites associated with spontaneous bacterial peritonitis (SBP) would be expected to be exudative consistent with an infection. However, SBP almost exclusively develops in low protein content ascites associated with portal hypertension, and total protein levels are typically in the transudative range (16).

MANAGEMENT

Overall goals for patient care should be considered before specific choices for managing ascites are made. The prognosis, expected response to management of the underlying conditions, and preferences for treatment should be established with the patient and family before any treatment plan is instituted. Each ascites treatment modality has associated burdens and benefits that deserve to be considered and discussed.

Whether ascites has a low or a high SAAG is critical in determining the overall management plan. Ascites due to portal hypertension *is* in equilibrium with total body fluid. The most common cause of nonmalignant ascites, cirrhosis, falls within this category. Efforts to restrict salt and to affect fluid balance with diuretics are often successful. Malignant ascites may or may not be responsive to these efforts, depending on its cause. In peritoneal carcinomatosis, the SAAG is low, there is no portal hypertension, and the ascites *is not* in equilibrium with total body fluid (18). Consequently, salt and fluid restriction and diuretics may be of little use. Their injudicious use may result in intravascular volume depletion, diminished renal perfusion, azotemia, hypotension, and fatigue (2). However, there are high SAAG forms of malignant ascites that are responsive to salt restriction and diuretics. For example, in cases of massive hepatic metastasis, portal hypertension is present and salt restriction and diuretics are indicated (18). One exception to this rule is nephrotic syndrome in which the SAAG is low but the ascites is diuretic responsive (19). The total protein is also low (<25 g/L) in nephrotic syndrome and thus is helpful in identifying this form of ascites (see Table 16.1 for a summary).

Interventions for ascites management in the supportive or palliative care setting should generally be reserved for patients who are symptomatic. The following ascites-related symptoms may spur intervention:

■ Dyspnea
■ Fatigue
■ Anorexia or early satiety
■ Nausea/vomiting
■ Pain
■ Diminished exercise tolerance

Dietary Management

The dietary management of ascites with a high SAAG begins with sodium restriction. Patients with cirrhosis may excrete as little as 5 to 10 mEq of sodium/d in their urine. Limiting sodium intake to 88 mmol or 2 g/d (equivalent to 5 g of

TABLE 16.1 Causes of ascites and diuretic responsiveness		
Cause of Ascites	Serum-Ascites Albumin Gradient	Typical Diuretic Response
Cirrhosis	High (≥1.1 g/dL)	Yes
Alcoholic hepatitis	High (≥1.1 g/dL)	Yes
Cardiac ascites	High (≥1.1 g/dL)	Yes
Fulminant hepatic failure	High (≥1.1 g/dL)	Yes
Budd-Chiari syndrome	High (≥1.1 g/dL)	Yes
Portal vein thrombosis	High (≥1.1 g/dL)	Yes
Venoocclusive disease	High (≥1.1 g/dL)	Yes
Acute fatty liver of pregnancy	High (≥1.1 g/dL)	Yes
Myxedema	High (≥1.1 g/dL)	Yes
Tuberculosis (without cirrhosis)	Low (≤1.1 g/dL)	No
Pancreatic ascites (without cirrhosis)	Low (≤1.1 g/dL)	No
Biliary ascites (without cirrhosis)	Low (≤1.1 g/dL)	No
Nephrotic syndrome	Low (≤1.1 g/dL)	Yes
Serositis from connective tissue disease	Low (≤1.1 g/dL)	No
Bowel obstruction/infarction	Low (≤1.1 g/dL)	No
Mixed ascites (i.e., cirrhosis plus infection or cancer)	High (≥1.1 g/dL)	Yes
Peritoneal carcinomatosis	Low (≤1.1 g/dL)	No
Massive hepatic metastasis	High (≥1.1 g/dL)	Yes

sodium chloride/d) is an attainable goal for a motivated patient, but it does make food less palatable. Considering a patient's goals of care, it may be better to liberalize the sodium intake and control ascites through other methods.

Patients are also prone to develop dilutional hyponatremia. The management of this condition has typically been by fluid restriction to 1 L/d. In the patient with advanced disease, when treatment goals are purely palliative, fluid restriction is usually intolerably burdensome. Judicious medical management may be less burdensome. For patients with cirrhotic ascites, serum sodium levels as low as 120 mmol/L are well tolerated and rarely dictate intervention (1).

Pharmacologic Management

For the majority of patients, the pharmacologic management of ascites is palliative. That is, the goal of therapy is to minimize symptoms and optimize quality of life without the expectation that the underlying cause can be reversed.

Systemic chemotherapy may be an effective management strategy for patients with malignant ascites due to a responsive cancer (e.g., lymphoma, breast, or ovarian cancer). In addition to systemic chemotherapy, intraperitoneal chemotherapy is an option. In theory, intraperitoneal chemotherapy can deliver high doses to peritoneal sites with minimal

systemic side effects. In practice, intraperitoneal chemotherapy is often limited by uneven distribution and poor tissue penetration. Hyperthermic intracavitary chemotherapy after surgical debulking may overcome some of these limitations and enhance the cytotoxicity of chemotherapy (20,21). Biologically active agents have also been used intraperitoneally to treat malignant ascites. Early clinical trials have used interferon (IFN)-α, IFN-β, and IFN-γ, tumor necrosis factor, interleukin-2, anti-VEGF antibodies, anti-VEGF receptor antibodies, VEGF receptor tyrosine kinase inhibitors, and metalloproteinase inhibitors. To date, no phase III clinical trials have been performed. Overall, the efficacy and role of intraperitoneal chemotherapeutic and biologic agents in both curative and palliative care remain to be determined.

Diuretic therapy could be useful in patients whose ascites has a high SAAG, as opposed to low SAAG ascites that is typically diuretic unresponsive. As with any drug therapy in the supportive care setting, the patient's symptoms should first be ascertained and the benefit versus the burden of therapy considered. The goal of diuretic therapy is to reduce extravascular fluid accumulation. Diuretic therapy should be directed to achieve a slow and gradual diuresis that does not exceed the capacity for mobilization of ascitic fluid. In the patient with ascites and edema, edema acts as a fluid reservoir to buffer the effects of a rapid contraction of plasma volume. Approximately 1 L/d (net) can safely be diuresed. In patients with ascites but without edema, diuresis may be achieved at the expense of the intravascular volume, leading to symptomatic orthostatic hypotension. In these patients, a more modest goal is to achieve net diuresis of 500 mL/d. Diuretics should not be administered with the goal to render the patient free of edema and ascites. Rather, only enough fluid should be mobilized to promote the patient's comfort. Overly aggressive diuretic therapy for ascites in a patient with high SAAG ascites has been associated with the hepatorenal syndrome and death (22).

For patients with high SAAG ascites in whom diuretics may be helpful, the renin–angiotensin–aldosterone system is activated. Therefore, the initial diuretic of choice for management is one that acts at the distal nephron to block the effect of increased aldosterone activity (23,24). Spironolactone, an aldosterone receptor antagonist, is a first-line therapy. Dosing begins at 100 mg/d and can be titrated up to effect or a maximum of 400 mg/d (Table 16.2). Given spironolactone's long half-life, daily dosing is sufficient. Spironolactone may cause painful gynecomastia (25). Amiloride hydrochloride, 10 mg/d, is an alternative. It acts faster and does not cause gynecomastia. It can be titrated up to a dose of 40 mg/d. Because these diuretics are relatively potassium sparing, patients should be advised not to use salt substitutes, as these are usually preparations of potassium chloride. If patients have a suboptimal response despite maximal use of the distal diuretics, a loop diuretic may be added, beginning at low doses (e.g., furosemide, 40 mg orally daily). There is evidence to support the combined use of a distal tubule diuretic and a loop diuretic at the beginning of therapy (24). This combination may effect a more rapid diuresis while maintaining potassium homeostasis. A ratio of 100 mg of spironolactone to 40 mg of furosemide is recommended as a starting point (1). The ratio can be adjusted to maintain normokalemia. The dosages can be increased in parallel until the goals of therapy have been attained, up to a maximum of spironolactone, 400 mg/d, and furosemide, 160 mg/d, or until therapy is limited by side effects (1). If there is no response to this level of therapy, the ascites is considered refractory to diuretic therapy if the following are true: (a) salt intake is appropriately limited and (b) nonsteroidal anti-inflammatory medications, which can affect glomerular filtration, are not being used.

Aquaretics comprise a new class of agents that can enhance water excretion. There are two types that are in the early stages of clinical evaluation in cirrhotic ascites—κ-opioid agonists and vasopressin receptor antagonists. In advanced cirrhosis, hyponatremia and hypoosmolality are in part due to elevated vasopressin levels that are independent of osmolality. Although the mechanism of action is not clear, κ-opioid agonists can increase free water excretion and raise the plasma sodium concentration (26). Renal V2 vasopressin receptors mediate the insertion of water channels into renal tubules thereby rendering them permeable to water. A specific V2 receptor antagonist has been effective in promoting water excretion and correcting hyponatremia (27). The clinical utility of these agents remains to be established.

In the patient who has limited mobility, urinary tract outflow symptoms such as hesitancy and frequency, poor appetite, and poor oral intake or who has difficulties related to polypharmacy, diuretic therapy may be excessively burdensome. Injudicious diuretic therapy can result in incontinence (with attendant self-esteem and skin care issues), sleep deprivation from frequent urination, fatigue from hyponatremia or hypokalemia, and falls from postural hypotension.

SBP PROPHYLAXIS

Patients with cirrhotic ascites with low protein content are at increased risk for SBP (28). This increased risk may be due to decreased opsonin levels in the ascites (29). Patients with SBP may be asymptomatic or may observe fever, abdominal pain, nausea/vomiting, or mental status changes. Studies have indicated that antibiotic prophylaxis is effective in preventing SBP. Norfloxacin (400 mg/d), ciprofloxacin (750 mg/wk), or one trimethoprim and sulfamethoxazole (Septra DS)/d Monday through Friday as primary prophylaxis significantly decreases the risk of developing SBP (30–32). Liver transplant protocols call for the routine use of SBP prophylaxis (33). Prophylaxis raises the concern of drug-resistant organisms. The long-term clinical significance remains unknown, but after 6 months on once a week ciprofloxacin there was no evidence of resistance (31). The use of prophylaxis in an

TABLE 16.2	Diuretics		
Diuretics	**Major Site of Action**	**Dosage Range (mg/d)**	**Comments**
Spironolactone	Distal tubule	100–400	Long half-life and gynecomastia
Amiloride hydrochloride	Distal tubule	10–40	—
Triamterene	Distal tubule	100–300	—
Furosemide	Loop of Henle	40–160	—
Ethacrynic acid	Loop of Henle	50–200	Can be used for sulfa allergy

individual case is dependent on the overall treatment goals and the disease context.

INVASIVE INTERVENTIONS

Therapeutic Paracentesis

Large-volume therapeutic paracentesis (≥5 L) of high SAAG ascites with concurrent colloid infusion is a simple procedure and is associated with minimal morbidity or mortality (34,35). The symptom response is much faster than when diuretics are used alone. In the patient with refractory ascites, it may be the only therapeutic modality that is effective. In fact, total paracentesis (mean, 10.7 L) associated with colloid infusion has been shown to be safe (36). If the ascites is in equilibrium with the systemic circulation, as is the case with portal hypertension, there is a risk of hemodynamic compromise. Colloid plasma volume expansion (e.g., 6 to 8 g of albumin/L of ascites removed) has been used to avoid this complication; recent meta-analysis suggests it is superior to other approaches to volume expansion (35). However, the choice for albumin infusions should be judicious. Most patients with paracentesis-induced circulatory dysfunction are asymptomatic, though increased renin levels are predictive of worse outcome (37). Albumin is expensive, but it is not known to cause harm. There are no reports of hepatorenal syndrome associated with paracentesis for low SAAG malignant ascites.

Surgical Procedures

Liver transplantation offers cure for a subset of patients with cirrhosis (33) and a subset of patients with small hepatocellular carcinoma (38).

Other surgical techniques offer palliation. Peritoneovenous shunts have been reported for management of malignant and nonmalignant ascites. They are placed surgically during a 30- to 60-minute procedure while the patient is under local anesthesia. Their purpose is to drain ascites from the peritoneal space via a one-way valve into the thoracic venous system. Unfortunately, the rate of complications is high, including shunt occlusion, heart failure due to fluid overload, infection, and disseminated intravascular coagulation. Stanley et al. (39) and Gines et al. (40) compared serial paracentesis with peritoneovenous shunts in patients with cirrhosis. There was no survival improvement but there was a high rate of complications with the peritoneovenous shunts. Similarly, Gough and Balderson (41) compared peritoneovenous shunts with nonoperative management in patients with malignant ascites. They found no difference in survival or quality of life. Thus, although there may be specific cases in which peritoneovenous shunting is advantageous in either nonmalignant or malignant ascites, serial paracentesis remains the first-line therapy.

Externally draining, implanted abdominal catheters may be beneficial for selected patients who require repeated large-volume paracentesis for comfort and whose prognosis warrants a surgical procedure. The catheter is surgically placed in the peritoneal cavity with an external drain, which can be accessed intermittently by physicians, nurses, or even trained family members (42). There are no comparative studies between these implanted catheters and serial paracentesis in patients with cirrhotic or malignant ascites. A study of 17 patients with an implanted catheter and abdominal carcinoma was complicated by 2 cases of cellulitis, 1 case of peritonitis, and 8 cases of asymptomatic culture-positive ascites (43). With no guidance from the literature, use of implanted catheters must be individualized.

The transjugular intrahepatic portosystemic shunt (TIPS) is a procedure performed by interventional radiologists that creates a side-to-side shunt that effectively relieves portal hypertension. The role of TIPS in patients with cirrhosis and refractory ascites remains controversial, potentially due to studies on differing populations. Rössle et al. showed that in comparison with serial large-volume paracentesis, TIPS led to a higher rate of ascites resolution and improved survival without transplantation (44). However, Sanyal et al. found that although TIPS improved ascites control versus paracentesis, there was no improvement in quality of life or survival (45). Given the rate of shunt complications and trend of increased frequency of worse encephalopathy, these authors recommend against TIPS as a first-line therapy. TIPS has also been employed in a few cases of malignant ascites associated with portal hypertension. In two cases of malignant portal and hepatic vein occlusion, TIPS improved ascites and quality of life (46). Whether to pursue any of the above invasive surgical procedures is dependent on the patient's goals and the disease context, and the decision must be individualized.

DIAGNOSIS AND MANAGEMENT OF PLEURAL EFFUSIONS

The pleural space is bordered by the parietal and visceral pleuras. The visceral pleura covers all lung surfaces including the intralobar fissures. The parietal pleura covers the inner surfaces of the thoracic cavity including the mediastinum, diaphragm, and chest wall. Fluid accumulates in this space from systemic capillaries through a pressure gradient and is drained by a network of lymphatics along the diaphragm and parietal pleura to the mediastinal lymph nodes. The pleural space is important as it couples movement of the chest wall with the lungs by creating a vacuum to keep the pleural spaces close and the small amount of fluid collected in this space acts as a lubricant. A pleural effusion is created when a wide range of diseases create excessive fluid collection through a variety of mechanisms.

Pleural effusions are common with approximately 1.5 million cases occurring annually in the United States (47). Internationally, in industrialized countries, the prevalence is thought to be approximately 320 cases per 100,000 people (48). The incidence of pleural effusions between sexes is equal; however, two-thirds of malignant pleural effusions occur in women and are often associated with breast and gynecologic malignancies. Malignant effusions in men are most common in lung cancer. Effusions associated with mesothelioma are more common in men, likely due to occupational exposure. Additionally, effusions associated with chronic pancreatitis and rheumatoid arthritis are more common in men.

It is critical to determine the underlying mechanism and disease process as there are significant prognostic implications. Morbidity and mortality correlate with the underlying disease process. Patients with nonmalignant pleural effusions experience less morbidity and mortality when effusions and causes are recognized and treated promptly. Most parapneumonic effusions or empyemas occur in patients with a predisposition to aspiration and systemic or local immunocompromised status, such as malignancy, chronic lung disease, or diabetes mellitus (49). Empyema has a mortality of up to 20% and is associated with high hospital cost (50,51). Radiologic characteristics (as defined by The American College of Chest Physicians) associated with poor prognosis are effusions that occupy more than 50% of the hemithorax, are loculated, or are associated with a thickened parietal pleura (51).

Approximately, 25% of all pleural effusions identified in the hospital setting are due to malignancy and the finding of a malignant effusion means that the primary tumor is likely not resectable as it implies disseminated disease (52). Median survival depends on the site and stage of the primary tumor (3 to 12 months, with the shortest in lung and the longest in breast primaries) (53). When the effusion is due to malignancy, laboratory work-up of the fluid and the serum also yield helpful prognostic information.

PATHOPHYSIOLOGY

The normal amount of fluid in the pleural space is between 7 and 14 mL (54). Excessive fluid can be created in this space through a variety of mechanisms. Mechanisms that cause an increased hydrostatic pressure gradient generally cause a transudate with low protein content. Transudative mechanisms include the following:

- Increased pulmonary capillary pressure (e.g., CHF)
- Decreased intrapleural pressure (e.g., atelectasis)
- Decreased plasma oncotic pressure causing excess leakage from pulmonary vessels as well as leakage across the diaphragm and pleural membranes (e.g., low albumin)

Mechanisms that increase permeability of the pleural vessels or obstruct lymphatic drainage generally cause an exudate with high protein content. Examples that cause this include malignancy and infection. Distinguishing between a transudate and an exudate is important to establish a working differential diagnosis.

DIAGNOSIS

History

When a pleural effusion is present, history and physical examination can begin to establish the likelihood of transudate versus exudate and what further work-up may be needed (55). It will also be important to establish whether the patient is critically ill, the severity of their symptoms, and their goals of care especially given the invasiveness of further work-up and potential management.

Important components of history include constitutional symptoms such as weight loss, night sweats, and asthenia, which are associated with exudative causes. Cough productive of purulent sputum may suggest an infectious etiology. Patients may have dyspnea with or without orthopnea. Pleural effusions will decrease chest wall compliance, depress the diaphragm, and decrease lung volume resulting in shortness of breath. Dyspnea itself is nonspecific; however, presence of orthopnea may suggest a transudate caused by CHF. If the pleura, ribs, or chest walls are involved (e.g., exudate caused by infection, malignancy, or pulmonary embolism), then pleuritic pain can be a presenting symptom. Patients with pulmonary embolism often have pleuritic pain and the high severity of their dyspnea is often out of proportion to the size of the effusion elicited by examination or imaging. They may also have a history of recent leg swelling. Skin, eye, or joint issues may suggest collagen vascular disease.

Past medical history for chronic or recent illnesses listed in Table 16.3 will be helpful. For example, a recent or recurrent diagnosis of pneumonia may suggest parapneumonic effusion or empyema. A recent history of deep vein thrombosis may suggest pulmonary embolism.

A medication history may reveal medications associated with toxicities that may cause exudative pleural effusions. While this is not a common adverse effect, some of the more common medications where this can be encountered are listed in Table 16.3. An occupational history may elicit asbestos exposure and risk of mesothelioma from occupations such as shipbuilding, electrical work, construction, carpentry, and insulation work.

Physical Examination

Upon examination, it is important to note the presence of labored breathing (use of accessory muscles and/or intercostal retractions in a child or thin adult), tachypnea, and anxiety (potentially caused by dyspnea). With severe effusions, there may be decreased chest wall movement on the affected side. Generally upon auscultation, there are decreased or absent breath sounds over the effusion area and a pleural friction rub may be present. Dullness to percussion over the area of effusion is the most accurate examination finding for diagnosing pleural effusion while the absence of reduced tactile vocal fremitus made pleural effusion less likely (57). Additionally, pleural effusion and ascites together are common in patients with malignant disease (58) and this is associated with spread of malignant disease to the pleura and peritoneum.

Laboratory Abnormalities

If pleural effusion is suspected by history and physical examination, confirmation of the diagnosis can be made by imaging. If at least 200 to 300 mL of fluid is present, an

| TABLE 16.3 | **Unilateral pleural effusions: differential diagnosis of transudates and exudates (52,53,56)** |

Transudative Effusions

Congestive heart failure[a]	Atelectasis[a]
Cirrhosis[a]	Myxedema
Nephrotic syndrome[a]	Pulmonary embolism
Peritoneal dialysis[a]	Urinothorax

Exudative Effusions

Malignancy[a]	*Other inflammatory*
Lung	Pulmonary embolism with infarction[a]
Lymphoma	Dressler's syndrome
Mesothelioma	Asbestosis
Metastatic	Uremia
	Trapped lung
Infectious	Radiation therapy
Parapneumonic[a]	Meigs syndrome
Tuberculous[a]	
Fungal	*Lymphatic disease*
Viral	Chylothorax
Parasitic	Lymphangiomyomatosis
Abdominal abscess	Yellow nail syndrome
Hepatitis	
	Drug induced
Noninfectious gastrointestinal	Drug-induced lupus
Pancreatitis	Nitrofurantoin
Esophageal rupture	Dantrolene
Abdominal surgery	Amiodarone
Variceal sclerotherapy	Methysergide
	Procarbazine
Collagen vascular disease	Practolol
Lupus erythematosus	Bromocriptine
Rheumatoid arthritis	Minoxidil
Wegener's granulomatosis	Bleomycin
Churg-Strauss syndrome	Methotrexate
Familial Mediterranean fever	Mitomycin
Sjogren's syndrome	
Immunoblastic lymphadenopathy	

[a]Common causes of unilateral pleural effusions.

erect posteroanterior chest radiograph may detect effusions with blunting of the costophrenic angles. Pleural thickening can be distinguished from fluid by using the decubitus view, as gravity will pull fluid to the dependent part of the lung. Therefore, decubitus views are more sensitive and can detect as little as 50 mL of fluid (59); however, to attain 100% sensitivity with chest radiographs, the amount of fluid must exceed 500 mL (60). Chest radiographs may also show consolidation, tumor, or pleural calcification.

Ultrasound is very sensitive, as it can also detect fluid levels as little as 50 mL; however, for 100% sensitivity, the amount of fluid must exceed only 100 mL (60). Therefore, ultrasound is more sensitive than radiographs. If available, ultrasound can be helpful to diagnose relatively small or loculated effusions and can be extremely helpful in performing diagnostic or therapeutic thoracentesis with lower complication rates.

While chest radiographs and/or ultrasound are usually the first step(s) and are often sufficient to guide further work-up, CT) of the chest is the best imaging study to see the entire pleural space as well as the pulmonary parenchyma and mediastinum (61). This could be especially helpful if exudative causes are suspected and fluid analysis does not lead to immediate diagnosis.

Between physical examination and imaging, distinguishing between unilateral and bilateral effusions is important. The differential for unilateral effusion is extensive, and is encompassed in Table 16.3. Massive unilateral effusions with near "white-out" are often due to malignancy (62). Bilateral effusions are usually limited to the transudative causes listed in Table 16.3.

A diagnostic thoracentesis can be performed to help narrow the differential diagnosis and determine the specific cause. Relative contraindications include a small volume of fluid, the inability of the patient to cooperate, a bleeding diathesis, a systemic anticoagulation, a mechanical ventilation,

and a cutaneous disease such as herpes zoster at the needle entry site (63).

Since major complication rates of thoracentesis are significant, it is critical to consider the overall context of the individual patient's situation (medical, psychosocial, and spiritual) and their goals of care prior to thoracentesis and other invasive work-up. Major complication rates of thoracentesis done by house officers have ranged from 11.6% to 30.3%, with pneumothorax being the most common complication with 3.9% to 6.1% of patients requiring a chest tube. In addition, up to 14% of diagnostic thoracenteses yielded inadequate fluid for analysis (52). Ultrasound guidance and experienced clinicians decrease the rate of complications. Aside from the goals of care, which may not include invasive tests, if the clinical course is typical and includes pleural effusion, sampling may not be necessary. For example, bilateral pleural effusion consistent with CHF can be observed with ongoing traditional and/or supportive therapies.

If fluid is obtained, the appearance and odor of the fluid may indicate certain illnesses (see Table 16.4 (64)). Most often it is straw yellow in color, which is nonspecific and is caused by many disease states. The pleural fluid should be sent for laboratory analysis and initially include pH, protein, lactate dehydrogenase (LDH), glucose, cytology, Gram stain, and acid-fast bacillus stains with culture and sensitivities. While several techniques have been put forth to help distinguish between transudates and exudates, the Light's criteria have been the gold standard for approximately 40 years (65). The fluid is considered an exudate if one or more of the following criteria are met:

- Ratio of pleural fluid LDH to serum level of LDH is >0.6.
- Pleural fluid level of LDH is >200.
- Ratio of pleural fluid level of protein to serum level of protein is >0.5.

TABLE 16.4 Relationship between pleural fluid appearance and causes (64,56)	
Cause	**Fluid Appearance/Odor**
Pseudochylothorax and chylothorax	Milky white
Urinothorax	Urine
Anaerobic empyema	Putrid
Chylothorax	Bile stained
Aspergillus infection	Black
Empyema	Turbid
Amebic liver abscess	"Anchovy" brown
Esophageal rupture	Food particles
Trauma, pulmonary embolism, benign asbestos-related effusion, pneumonia, malignant neoplasm, after myocardial infarction syndrome	Blood stained

Light's criteria have high sensitivity and specificity for differentiating between transudates and exudates. When used alone these have an accuracy of 96% (66). However, they may lose accuracy for transudates due to CHF after a patient has been diuresed (52). In this scenario, a pleural fluid cholesterol level >55 mg/dL (67,68) and/or serum albumin minus pleural fluid albumin of >1.2 mg/dL (69) may help diagnose an exudate.

A pH <7.2 in infected effusions indicates an empyema that in turn necessitates prompt chest tube drainage. A low pH can also occur in esophageal rupture, rheumatoid arthritis, and malignancy associated with poor outcome. A low pH and a low glucose level are both associated with more extensive pleural involvement with tumor, a higher yield on fluid cytology, decreased success rates of pleural sclerosis, and shorter survival times (52). In one study, mean survival was 2.1 months for low-pH malignant effusions and 9.8 months for normal-pH malignant effusions (70). If malignancy is suspected, cytology is important and positive in 60% of patients with neoplasm. If the first sample is negative, a second sample increases the chance of diagnosing malignancy to about 72% (64,71).

In the rare case that fluid analysis and a CT imaging do not yield a diagnosis, an expanded pleural fluid analysis including polymerase chain reaction for *Streptococcus pneumoniae* and tuberculosis, specific tumor markers, and complement levels (low levels in rheumatoid arthritis and systemic lupus) may help establish a diagnosis (64). Bronchoscopy may be helpful if the patient has parenchymal abnormalities or hemoptysis, but negative fluid cytology (52). Finally, a pleural biopsy (radiologically or with thoracoscopy) can be considered (64).

MANAGEMENT

Management of pleural effusions depends on the underlying illness. Generally, this means that the use of conventional therapies to treat the underlying illness, if possible, will also treat the pleural effusion. For example, once the diagnosis of tuberculous pleural effusion is made, the best way to treat the effusion is to treat the patient appropriately for pulmonary tuberculosis. If a patient has a malignancy that is responsive to chemotherapy, such as breast or small cell lung cancer, then the malignant pleural effusion may resolve with traditional anticancer therapies. Radiation may suffice for the malignant pleural effusion associated with lymphoma.

Patients with empyema or complicated parapneumonic effusion should be managed with antibiotics and prompt drainage of the infected pleural effusion. Some guidelines also add the intrapleural administration of fibrinolytic medications (50,51). However, there is a wide variation in the management and it is questionable that the addition of fibrinolytics change outcomes significantly (72). Video-assisted thoracoscopic surgery (VATS) may be utilized, but it is usually reserved for empyema that is refractory to thoracostomy or fibrinolytic therapy. Further studies are needed to clarify the role of VATS.

Symptomatic management of malignant pleural effusion does not improve survival, and it primarily focuses on the relief of dyspnea. Removal of the fluid by therapeutic thoracentesis can achieve dramatic and prompt relief of dyspnea. However, in nearly 100% of cases the fluid reaccumulates within 30 days (73) and one study showed symptoms recurring within an average of 4.2 days (74). Also, up to 50% of patients may not achieve significant improvement in dyspnea or exercise tolerance secondary to comorbid conditions, general debility from the malignancy, or trapped lung (75). With repeated therapeutic thoracentesis, there is an increased risk of adhesions, loculations, and infection (76). In spite of this, patients who achieve significant symptomatic relief and have a limited prognosis of days to weeks may benefit from repeated thoracentesis. The best volume of pleural fluid to drain while avoiding reexpansion pulmonary edema and maintaining best symptomatic relief is not known; however, 1 to 1.5 L/thoracentesis is recommended (77).

If symptomatic relief is achieved with therapeutic thoracentesis and the patient's prognosis is months to years, they may benefit from chest tube thoracostomy and chemical pleurodesis. It is important to evaluate the patient's goals of care and describe the procedure, which usually requires a hospital stay. A chest catheter is inserted into the pleural space with the patient under local anesthesia or conscious sedation. After drainage of fluid, chemical agents are instilled that cause inflammation with fibrin deposition and adhesion between the layers of pleura. This may produce significant pain and fever. Numerous clinical trials have been performed to help determine the best chemical agent and talc appears to be favored (78,79). Talc may also be instilled via thoracoscopy with insufflation. This is performed by a trained pulmonologist or thoracic surgeon with a flexible pleuroscope. This has a success rate of up to 90% and a recent meta-analysis showed that the relative risk of nonrecurrence of effusion is 1.19 in favor of thoracoscopic pleurodesis compared with tube thoracostomy pleurodesis (79). VATS with talc poudrage has also yielded high success rates; however, it is more invasive and requires surgical expertise and more ancillary and logistical support (75).

If chemical pleurodesis is not recommended, is not within the patient's goals of care, or is not successful, a long-term, indwelling, tunneled pleural catheter may be a good option, particularly if the patient's prognosis is at least many weeks to months. Generally, the procedure is performed under conscious sedation as an outpatient. This allows the fluid to be drained at home with nursing assistance or sometimes the patient or family can be trained to do it as well. Cost effectiveness depends on prognosis, with one study showing an indwelling pleural catheter becoming more cost effective when prognosis was 6 weeks or less (80). Safety, efficacy, and survival appear to be similar between the two therapies (81).

Finally, a pleuroperitoneal shunt where the fluid is manually pumped from the pleural space to the peritoneal cavity can be an option especially in the case where trapped lung makes lung expansion inadequate for pleurodesis.

While this intervention is often successful, shunt clotting, risk of infection, and manual operation are factors that have made this intervention fall out of favor for the majority of patients (75).

REFERENCES

1. Runyon B. Current concepts: care of patients with ascites. *N Engl J Med.* 1994;330(5):337-342.
2. Sharma S, Walsh D. Management of symptomatic malignant ascites with diuretics: two case reports and a review of the literature. *J Pain Symptom Manage.* 1995;10(3):237-242.
3. Runyon B, Hoefs J, Morgan T. Ascitic fluid analysis in malignancy related ascites. *Hepatology.* 1988;8:1104-1109.
4. Garrison R, Kaelin L, Galloway R, et al. Malignant ascites: clinical and experimental observations. *Ann Surg.* 1986; 203: 644-649.
5. Martin P, Gines P, Schrier RW. Nitric oxide as a mediator of hemodynamic abnormalities and sodium and water retention in cirrhosis. *N Engl J Med.* 1998;339(8):533-541.
6. Gines P, Jimenez W, Arroyo V, et al. Atrial natriuretic factor in cirrhosis with ascites; plasma levels, cardiac release and splanchnic extraction. *Hepatology.* 1988;8(3):636-642.
7. Bichet D, Szatalowicz V, Chaimovitz, et al. Role of vasopressin in abnormal water excretion in cirrhotic patients. *Ann Intern Med.* 1982;96:413-417.
8. Senger DR, Galli SJ, Dvorak AM, et al. Tumor cells secrete a vascular permeability factor that promotes accumulation of ascites fluid. *Science.* 1983;219:983-985.
9. Zebrowski BK, Liu W, Ramirez K, et al. Markedly elevated levels of vascular endothelial growth factor in malignant ascites. *Ann Surg Oncol.* 1999;6(4):373-378.
10. Xu L, Yoneda J, Herrera C, et al. Inhibition of malignant ascites and growth of human ovarian carcinoma by oral administration of a potent inhibitor of the vascular endothelial growth factor receptor tyrosine kinases. *Int J Oncol.* 2000;16(3):445-454.
11. Watson SA, Morris TM, Robinson G, et al. Inhibition of organ invasion by the matrix metalloproteinase inhibitor batimastat (BB-94) in two human colon carcinoma metastasis models. *Cancer Res.* 1995;55(16):3629-3633.
12. Cattau EL Jr, Benjamin SB, Knuff TE, et al. The accuracy of the physical exam in the diagnosis of suspected ascites. *JAMA.* 1982;247(8):1164-1166.
13. Williams JW Jr, Simel DI. Does this patient have ascites? How to divine fluid in the abdomen. *JAMA.* 1992;267(19):2645-2648.
14. Runyon BA, Antillon MR, Akriviadis EA, et al. Bedside inoculation of blood culture bottles with ascitic fluid is superior to delayed inoculation in the detection of spontaneous bacterial peritonitis. *J Clin Microbiol.* 1990;28:2811-2812.
15. Hoefs JC. Serum protein concentration and portal pressure determine the ascitic fluid protein concentration in patients with chronic liver disease. *J Lab Clin Med.* 1983;102:260-273.
16. Runyon BA, Montano AA, Akriviadis EA, et al. The serum-ascites albumin gradient is superior to the exudate–transudate concept in the differential diagnosis of ascites. *Ann Intern Med.* 1992;117:215-220.
17. Runyon BA. Cardiac ascites: a characterization. *J Clin Gastroenterol.* 1988;10(4):410-412.
18. Pockros PJ, Esrason KT, Nguyen C, et al. Mobilization of malignant ascites with diuretics is dependent on ascitic fluid characteristics. *Gastroenterology.* 1992;103(4):1302-1306.
19. Ackerman Z. Ascites in nephrotic syndrome: incidence, patients' characteristics, and complications. *J Clin Gastroenterol.* 1996;22:31-34.
20. Loggie BW, Perini M, Fleming RA, et al. Treatment and prevention of malignant ascites associated with disseminated intraperitoneal malignancies by aggressive combined-modality therapy. *Am Surg.* 1997;63(2):137-143.
21. Shen P, Hawksworth J, Lovato J, et al. Cytoreductive surgery and intraperitoneal hyperthermic chemotherapy with mitomycin C for peritoneal carcinomatosis from nonappendiceal colorectal carcinoma. *Ann Surg Oncol.* 2004;11(2):178-186.
22. Roberts LR, Kamath PS. Ascites and hepatorenal syndrome: pathophysiology and management. *Mayo Clin Proc.* 1996;71(9):874-881.
23. Pérez-Ayuso RM, Arroyo V, Planas R, et al. Randomized comparative study of efficacy of furosemide versus spironolactone in nonazotemic cirrhosis with ascites: relationship between the diuretic response and the activity of the renin–aldosterone system. *Gastroenterology.* 1983;84:961-968.
24. Fogel MR, Sawhney VK, Neal EA, et al. Diuresis in the ascitic patient: a randomized controlled trial of three regimens. *J Clin Gastroenterol.* 1981;3(suppl 1):73-80.
25. Mantero F, Lucarelli G. Aldosterone antagonists in hypertension and heart failure. *Ann Endocrinol.* 2000;61(1):52-60.
26. Gadano A, Moreau R, Pessione F, et al. Aquaretic effects of niravoline, a kappa-opioid agonist, in patients with cirrhosis. *J Hepatol.* 2000;32(1):38-42.
27. Wong F, Blei AT, Blendis LM, et al. A vasopressin receptor antagonist (VPA-985) improves serum sodium concentration in patients with hyponatremia: a multicenter, randomized, placebo-controlled trial. *Hepatology.* 2003;37(1):182-191.
28. Runyon BA. Low-protein concentration ascitic fluid is predisposed to spontaneous bacterial peritonitis. *Gastroenterology.* 1986;91(6):1343-1346.
29. Runyon BA. Patients with deficient ascitic fluid opsonic activity are predisposed to spontaneous bacterial peritonitis. *Hepatology.* 1988;8(3):632-635.
30. Grangé JD, Roulot D, Pelletier G, et al. Norfloxacin primary prophylaxis of bacterial infections in cirrhotic patients with ascites: a double-blind randomized trial. *J Hepatol.* 1998;29(3): 430-436.
31. Rolachon A, Cordier L, Bacq Y, et al. Ciprofloxacin and long-term prevention of spontaneous bacterial peritonitis: results of a prospective controlled trial. *Hepatology.* 1995;22:1171-1174.
32. Singh N, Gayowski T, Yu VL, et al. Trimethoprim–sulfamethoxazole for the prevention of spontaneous bacterial peritonitis in cirrhosis: a randomized trial. *Ann Intern Med.* 1995;122(8): 595-598.
33. Saab S, Han SH, Martin P. Liver transplantation: selection, listing criteria, and preoperative management. *Clin Liver Dis.* 2000;4(3):513-532.
34. Ginés P, Arroyo V, Quintero E, et al. Comparison of paracentesis and diuretics in the treatment of cirrhotics with tense ascites: results of a randomized study. *Gastroenterology.* 1987;93(2):234-241.
35. Bernardi M, Caraceni P, Navickis RJ, Wilkes MM. Albumin infusion in patients undergoing large-volume paracentesis: a meta-analysis of randomized trials. *Hepatology.* 2012;55(4): 1172-1181.
36. Tító L, Ginès P, Arroyo V, et al. Total paracentesis associated with intravenous albumin management of patients with cirrhosis and ascites. *Gastroenterology.* 1990;98(1):146-151.

37. Gines A, Fernandez-Esparrach G, Monescillo A, et al. Randomized trial comparing albumin, dextran 70, and polygeline in cirrhotic patients with ascites treated by paracentesis. *Gastroenterology*. 1996:111(4):1002-1010.

38. Llovet JM, Bruix J, Fuster J, et al. Liver transplantation for small hepatocellular carcinoma: the tumor-node-metastasis classification does not have prognostic power. *Hepatology*. 1998;27(6):1572-1577.

39. Stanley MM, Ochi S, Lee KK, et al. Peritoneovenous shunting as compared with medical treatment in patients with alcoholic cirrhosis and massive ascites: Veterans Administration Cooperative Study on Treatment of Alcoholic Cirrhosis with Ascites. *N Engl J Med*. 1989;321(24):1632-1638.

40. Gines P, Arroyo V, Vargas B, et al. Paracentesis with intravenous infusion of albumin as compared with peritoneovenous shunting in cirrhosis with refractory ascites. *N Engl J Med*. 1991;325:829-835.

41. Gough IR, Balderson GA. Malignant ascites: a comparison of peritoneovenous shunting and nonoperative management. *Cancer*. 1993;71(7):2377-2382.

42. Murphy M, Rossi M. Managing ascites via the Tenckhoff catheter. *Med Surg Nurs*. 1995;4:468-471.

43. Belfort MA, Stevens PJ, DeHaek K, et al. A new approach to the management of malignant ascites: a permanently implanted abdominal drain. *Eur J Surg Oncol*. 1990;16(1): 47-53.

44. Rössle M, Ochs A, Gülberg V, et al. A comparison of paracentesis and transjugular intrahepatic portosystemic shunting in patients with ascites. *N Engl J Med*. 2000;342(23):1701-1707.

45. Sanyal A.J, Genning C, Reddy KR, et al. The North American Study for the Treatment of Refractory Ascites. *Gastroenterology*. 2003:124(3):634-641.

46. Burger JA, Ochs A, Wirth K, et al. The transjugular stent implantation for the treatment of malignant portal and hepatic vein obstruction in cancer patients. *Ann Oncol*. 1997;8(2): 200-202.

47. Sahn SA. The value of pleural fluid analysis. *Am J Med Sci*. January 2008;335(1):7-15.

48. Sahn SA. Pleural effusions of extravascular origin. *Clin Chest Med*. June 2006;27(2):285-308.

49. Bartlett JG. Anaerobic bacterial infections of the lung and pleural space. *Clin Infect Dis*. June 1993;16(suppl 4):S248-S255.

50. Colice GL, Curtis A, Deslauriers J, et al. Medical and surgical treatment of parapneumonic effusions : an evidence-based guideline. *Chest*. October 2000;118(4):1158-1171.

51. Davies CW, Gleeson FV, Davies RJ. BTS guidelines for the management of pleural infection. *Thorax*. May 2003;58(suppl 2):ii18-ii28.

52. Bartter T, Santarelli R, Akers SM, Pratter MR. The evaluation of pleural effusion. *Chest*. October 1994;106(4):1209-1214.

53. Rahman NM, Chapman SJ, Davies RJ. Pleural effusion: a structured approach to care. *Br Med Bull*. 2004;72:31-47.

54. Sahn SA. State of the art. The pleura. *Am Rev Respir Dis*. July 1988;138(1):184-234.

55. Scheurich JW, Keuer SP, Graham DY. Pleural effusion: comparison of clinical judgment and Light's criteria in determining the cause. *South Med J*. December 1989;82(12):1487-1491.

56. Maskell NA, Butland RJ. BTS guidelines for the investigation of a unilateral pleural effusion in adults. *Thorax*. May 2003;58(suppl 2):ii8-ii17.

57. Wong CL, Holroyd-Leduc J, Straus SE. Does this patient have a pleural effusion? *JAMA*. January 2009;301(3):309-317.

58. Covey AM. Management of malignant pleural effusions and ascites. *J Support Oncol*. March-April 2005;3(2):169-73, 76.

59. Blackmore CC, Black WC, Dallas RV, Crow HC. Pleural fluid volume estimation: a chest radiograph prediction rule. *Acad Radiol*. February 1996;3(2):103-109.

60. Gryminski J, Krakowka P, Lypacewicz G. The diagnosis of pleural effusion by ultrasonic and radiologic techniques. *Chest*. July 1976;70(1):33-37.

61. McLoud TC, Flower CD. Imaging the pleura: sonography, CT, and MR imaging. *AJR Am J Roentgenol*. June 1991;156(6): 1145-1153.

62. Maher GG, Berger HW. Massive pleural effusion: malignant and nonmalignant causes in 46 patients. *Am Rev Respir Dis*. March 1972;105(3):458-460.

63. Sokolowski JW Jr, Burgher LW, Jones FL Jr, Patterson JR, Selecky PA. Guidelines for thoracentesis and needle biopsy of the pleura. This position paper of the American Thoracic Society was adopted by the ATS Board of Directors, June 1988. *Am Rev Respir Dis*. July 1989;140(1):257-258.

64. McGrath EE, Anderson PB. Diagnosis of pleural effusion: a systematic approach. *Am J Crit Care*. March 2011;20(2):119-127; quiz 28.

65. Light RW, Macgregor MI, Luchsinger PC, Ball WC Jr. Pleural effusions: the diagnostic separation of transudates and exudates. Ann Intern Med. October 1972;77(4):507-513.

66. Romero S, Martinez A, Hernandez L, et al. Light's criteria revisited: consistency and comparison with new proposed alternative criteria for separating pleural transudates from exudates. *Respiration*. 2000;67(1):18-23.

67. Hamm H, Brohan U, Bohmer R, Missmahl HP. Cholesterol in pleural effusions. A diagnostic aid. *Chest*. August 1987;92(2):296-302.

68. Valdes L, Pose A, Suarez J, et al. Cholesterol: a useful parameter for distinguishing between pleural exudates and transudates. *Chest*. May 1991;99(5):1097-1102.

69. Roth BJ, O'Meara TF, Cragun WH. The serum-effusion albumin gradient in the evaluation of pleural effusions. *Chest*. September 1990;98(3):546-549.

70. Sahn SA, Good JT Jr. Pleural fluid pH in malignant effusions. Diagnostic, prognostic, and therapeutic implications. *Ann Intern Med*. March 1988;108(3):345-349.

71. Ryan CJ, Rodgers RF, Unni KK, Hepper NG. The outcome of patients with pleural effusion of indeterminate cause at thoracotomy. *Mayo Clin Proc*. March 1981;56(3):145-149.

72. Schiza S, Siafakas NM. Clinical presentation and management of empyema, lung abscess and pleural effusion. *Curr Opin Pulm Med*. May 2006;12(3):205-211.

73. Antunes G, Neville E, Duffy J, Ali N. BTS guidelines for the management of malignant pleural effusions. Thorax. May 2003;58(suppl 2):ii29-ii38.

74. Rodriguez-Panadero F, Janssen JP, Astoul P. Thoracoscopy: general overview and place in the diagnosis and management of pleural effusion. *Eur Respir J*. August 2006;28(2): 409-422.

75. Musani AI. Treatment options for malignant pleural effusion. *Curr Opin Pulm Med*. July 2009;15(4):380-387.

76. Lombardi G, Zustovich F, Nicoletto MO, Donach M, Artioli G, Pastorelli D. Diagnosis and treatment of malignant pleural

effusion: a systematic literature review and new approaches. *Am J Clin Oncol.* August 2010;33(4):420-423.

77. Antony VB, Loddenkemper R, Astoul P, et al. Management of malignant pleural effusions. *Eur Respir J.* August 2001;18(2):402-419.

78. Tan C, Sedrakyan A, Browne J, Swift S, Treasure T. The evidence on the effectiveness of management for malignant pleural effusion: a systematic review. *Eur J Cardiothorac Surg.* May 2006;29(5):829-838.

79. Shaw P, Agarwal R. Pleurodesis for malignant pleural effusions. *Cochrane Database Syst Rev.* 20041:CD002916.

80. Olden AM, Holloway R. Treatment of malignant pleural effusion: PleuRx catheter or talc pleurodesis? A cost-effectiveness analysis. *J Palliat Med.* January 2010;13(1):59-65.

81. Putnam JB Jr, Light RW, Rodriguez RM, et al. A randomized comparison of indwelling pleural catheter and doxycycline pleurodesis in the management of malignant pleural effusions. Cancer. November 1999;86(10):1992-1999.

CHAPTER 17

Hiccups and Other Gastrointestinal Symptoms

Nabeel Sarhill ■ Fade Mahmoud

Gastrointestinal (GI) symptoms are commonly seen in patients with cancer, regardless of the disease site. These symptoms are experienced during the course of the illness or as a result of therapy. However, it should be remembered that many GI problems seen in patients with cancer are also seen in those without cancer. In fact, some GI symptoms are very common, and although they cause distress, they rarely represent life-threatening pathology. This presents a problem, as patients and physicians face the concern that every new symptom is related to the cancer. This chapter focuses primarily on GI symptoms as they relate to cancer and its treatment, but the reader is reminded that most GI symptoms are not directly due to the cancer.

HICCUPS

Definition/Incidence

Hiccup is a spasmodic, involuntary contraction of the inspiratory (external) intercostal muscles and the diaphragm associated with a strong, sudden inspiration and abrupt glottic closure (1). The medical term for hiccups, singultus, is of Latin origin and means to gasp or sigh. Hiccups were first attributed to phrenic nerve irritation by Shortt in 1833 (2). Hiccups can be classified by their duration as acute (up to 48 hours), persistent or protracted (longer than 48 hours), and intractable (>1 month) (1,2).

Pathophysiology/Etiology

Hiccup is a primitive reflex that contains three parts. The afferent portion consists of branches of the vagus nerve, the phrenic nerve, and the sympathetic chain from T6 to T12. The hiccup center is located in the spinal cord between C3 and C5. The efferent limb is primarily the phrenic nerve with involvement of the efferents to the glottis and accessory muscles of respiration (1).

In addition to the neural pathways, numerous anatomic structures are involved in the mechanism of hiccup (epiglottis, larynx, hyoid muscles, superior constrictor of the pharynx, esophagus, stomach, diaphragm, and exterior intercostal, sternocleidomastoid, anterior serratus, and scalene muscles). Given this extensive list, it is not surprising that hiccup has been associated with many conditions affecting the central nervous system (CNS), thorax, mediastinum, and abdominal viscera, although a cause-and-effect relationship has not always been clear. One report listed over 100 causes, the most common being an overdistended stomach (3). Some cancer-related causes of persistent and intractable hiccups are listed in Table 17.1.

Treatment/Management

Management is usually aimed at inhibiting or interrupting the irritated reflex arc. Nonpharmacologic therapies (4) include the Valsalva maneuver (expiring forcefully against a closed glottis), ocular compression, carotid sinus massage, traction on the tongue, ice water gargles, noxious odors or tastes, breath holding, rebreathing into a paper bag, gagging, drinking from a glass while holding a pencil between the teeth or while bending over head down, taking as many sips of fluid as rapidly as possible without breathing, ingesting granulated sugar, biting a lemon wedge, or inducing emesis. Physical changes that may help stop hiccups include pulling the knees to chest, leaning forward to compress the chest, tapping over the fifth cervical vertebra, or applying ice over the phrenic nerve. Although these measures have not been subjected to controlled clinical trials, most are worth a try. However, many are not practical for these patients, who may be too debilitated to tolerate even simple maneuvers (e.g., holding breath).

Acupuncture may be a clinically useful, safe, and low-cost therapy for persistent hiccups in patients with cancer. In a recent retrospective case series, 16 adult male patients aged 27 to 71 with persistent cancer-related hiccups received one to three acupuncture sessions over a 1- to 7-day period. Thirteen patients experienced complete remission of persistent hiccups ($p < 0.0001$) and three patients experienced decreased hiccups severity. Significant improvement was observed in discomfort ($p < 0.0001$), distress ($p < 0.0001$), and fatigue ($p = 0.0078$) (5).

Many drugs have been used to treat hiccups (Table 17.2). The literature is largely based on case reports and no definitive clinical evidence is available to define the standard treatment. The only medication approved by the US Food and Drug Administration for hiccups is the antipsychotic phenothiazine chlorpromazine (25 to 50 mg through i.v., orally, or rectally three to four times a day) (6). Chlorpromazine is less attractive in patients with cancer due to side effects of hypotension and sedation. Other medical therapies include haloperidol (1 to 5 mg orally three times daily or subcutaneously every 12 hours) (7), nifedipine (10 mg p.o. three times daily) (8), metoclopramide (10 mg p.o. or i.v. every 6 hours) (9), and baclofen (10 to 20 mg p.o. three times a day) (10).

TABLE 17.1 Causes of hiccups in the patient with cancer
Uremia
Alcohol
Hyponatremia, hypokalemia, and hypocalcemia
Fever
Diaphragmatic irritation (diaphragmatic tumors and pericarditis)
Pleuritis
Esophageal obstruction
Pericarditis
Hepatomegaly
Subphrenic abscess
Esophageal cancer
Mediastinal tumors
Herpes zoster
Lung cancer
Gastric distension
Gastric cancer
Pancreatic cancer
Intra-abdominal abscess
Bowel obstruction
Gastrointestinal hemorrhage
Short-acting barbiturates
Dexamethasone
Diazepam and chlordiazepoxide
Infections (meningitis)
Grief reaction
Psychosis

A comprehensive list of the causes of hiccups can be found in Launois S, Bizec JL, Whitelaw WA, et al. Hiccup in adults: an overview. *Eur Respir J.* 1993;6:563-575.

Baclofen should be given with caution to the elderly due to frequent side effects of sedation, insomnia, dizziness, weakness, ataxia, and confusion (10). If hiccups persist, amitriptyline (10 mg three times a day) (11), carbamazepine (200 mg three times a day) (12), diphenylhydantoin (200 mg i.v. and then 100 mg p.o. four times a day) (13), or valproic acid (15 mg/kg/d in divided doses) (14) can be administered. Midazolam has been successfully utilized in patients with terminal hiccups (15). Midazolam infusion may be especially useful if intractable hiccups occur in the setting of refractory terminal delirium or agitation.

Gabapentin, an anticonvulsant, produces blockade of neural calcium channels and increases release of γ-aminobutyric acid (GABA), which may modulate diaphragmatic excitability. Case series have shown gabapentin

(300 mg p.o. three times daily with dose titration) to be effective in intractable hiccups (16). In a retrospective study, 37 (3.9%) of 944 in-hospital patients and 6 (4.5%) of 134 patients observed at home presented with severe chronic hiccups. Gabapentin (300 mg three times a day with dose titration) was effective in these cases. Responses were observed in 32 patients (74.4%) with gabapentin at a dosage of 900 mg/d and in 9 patients (20.93%) at a dosage of 1,200 mg/d (17). Gabapentin is not hepatically metabolized and has a relatively safe side-effect profile making it a potentially useful agent in the advanced cancer setting, especially among patients requiring adjuvant analgesia due to neuropathic cancer pain (18,19). Nebulized lidocaine may be effective via a local anesthetic effect upon irritant sensory afferents and has a much greater safety profile than does the intravenous

TABLE 17.2	**Commonly used drugs in the treatment of hiccups**	

Drug	Dose	Side Effects
Chlorpromazine	25–50 mg i.v. three to four times daily, infused slowly 25–50 mg p.o. three times daily	Sedation, hypotension, and extrapyramidal symptoms
Metoclopramide	10 mg p.o. or i.v. three to four times daily	Extrapyramidal symptoms[a]
Gabapentin	300 mg p.o. three times daily	Drowsiness, headache, fatigue, blurred vision, tremor, anxiety, skin rash, itching, fever, flu-like symptoms, and seizures
Haloperidol	1–5 mg p.o. three times daily or s.c. q12h	Sedation and extrapyramidal symptoms
Baclofen	10–20 mg p.o. three times daily	Sedation, confusion, and less commonly, nausea and fatigue
Nifedipine	10 mg p.o. three times daily	Hypotension, use with caution in patients with coronary artery disease
Amitriptyline	10 mg p.o. three times daily	Cardiac arrhythmias, blurred vision, urinary retention, dry mouth, constipation, and dizziness
Carbamazepine	200 mg three times daily	Dizziness, drowsiness, nausea or vomiting, and low red and white blood cell counts
Diphenylhydantoin	200 mg i.v. once and then 100 mg p.o. four times daily	Enlarged gums, unsteadiness, confusion, lymphadenopathy, fever, muscle pain, skin rash or itching, slurred speech, sore throat, and nervousness or irritability
Valproic acid	15 mg/kg p.o. daily in one to three divided doses	Dizziness, drowsiness, nervousness, upset stomach, vomiting, diarrhea, tremor, sore throat, and drug-induced hepatitis
Ketamine (Ketalar)	0.4 mg/kg (one-fifth of the usual anesthetic dose) i.v.; supplemental dose of one-third to half initial dose may be given for maintenance	Resuscitative equipment should be immediately available during administration of medication
Lidocaine	1 mg/kg i.v. loading dose followed by an infusion of 2 mg/min i.v.	May increase risk of adverse central nervous system and cardiac effects in elderly; high plasma concentrations can cause seizures, heart block, and atrioventricular conduction abnormalities
Ephedrine	25 mg i.m. q6h	Headache, restlessness, anxiety, tremor, weakness, dizziness, confusion, delirium, hallucinations, palpitations, sweating, nausea or vomiting, and urinary retention
		Serious side effects include severe hypertension that may lead to cerebral hemorrhage or cardiac ischemia
Methylphenidate (Ritalin)	5 mg p.o. daily or divided b.i.d.; not to exceed 60 mg/d	Insomnia, anorexia, irritability, nervousness, upset stomach, headaches, dry mouth, blurry vision, nausea, hypersensitivity, palpitations, and cardiac arrhythmias
Other therapies	Behavioral conditioning (including other members of the family unit) Hypnosis Acupuncture Phrenic nerve or diaphragmatic pacing	

[a]More common in younger women.

Adapted from Liu FC, Chen CA, Yang SS, et al. Acupuncture therapy rapidly terminates intractable hiccups complicating acute myocardial infarction. *South Med J.* 2005;98(3):385-387; Schiff E, River Y, Oliven A, et al. Acupuncture therapy for persistent hiccups. *Am J Med Sci.* 2002;323(3):166-168.

route (20). Similarly, nebulized saline solution has been reported by some authors to terminate hiccups in the palliative care setting (21). Efficacy has been claimed for a variety of drugs that have a peripheral action such as atropine, edrophonium, procainamide, and quinidine. Methylphenidate (10 mg p.o. daily) is reported to be effective in the treatment of hiccups (22).

Various invasive methods have been tried. As gastric distension is the most common cause of hiccups in patients with cancer, initial treatment should be aimed at relieving the distension and increasing gastric emptying. The insertion of a nasogastric tube may also serve the purpose by stimulating the pharynx or causing gagging. High-pressure oxygen inhalation has been tried. Percutaneous stimulation of the phrenic nerve has also been reported. Phrenic nerve injection may be a reasonable option for drug refractory hiccups if an experienced practitioner is available. In a case series, 1% lidocaine solution was administered via ultrasonographic guidance to the area of the phrenic nerve to five cancer patients with intractable hiccups. Hiccups ceased in all five patients within 5 minutes. Hiccups did not recur in three patients, and there were no adverse effects (23). A surgical approach consists of an attack on the phrenic nerve (by a crush technique), usually first attempted on the left. Regardless of the treatment, in most cases, hiccups stop because of, or in spite of, therapeutic measures (24,25).

It is important to remember that hiccups in cancer may be extremely distressing and affect the quality of life by interfering with food intake, causing insomnia, or exacerbating pain and other symptoms. For this reason, it may be advisable to pursue diagnosis and treatment more aggressively than in the general population (26).

DYSPEPSIA

Definition/Incidence

Dyspepsia consists of episodic or persistent symptoms that include abdominal pain or discomfort, postprandial fullness, abdominal bloating, belching, early satiety, anorexia,

nausea, vomiting, heartburn, and regurgitation. There is considerable overlap between this constellation of symptoms and those of gastroesophageal reflux disease (GERD), biliary tract disease, irritable bowel syndrome, and chronic pancreatitis. This condition is reported in approximately 25% of the population each year, but most do not seek medical care (27,28).

Pathophysiology/Etiology

Results of upper GI endoscopy in 3,667 general medical patients with dyspepsia were as follows: normal (34%), gastroesophageal reflux (24%), inflammation (20%), ulcer (20%), and cancer (2%) (27). Dyspepsia is divided into two categories: organic dyspepsia and functional dyspepsia. Patients in the first group have anatomical abnormalities (e.g., peptic ulcer disease, GERD, or gastric or esophageal cancer). Patients in the second category have symptoms for which no focal lesion can be found (Table 17.3). Recent studies have shown potential associations between specific pathophysiologic disturbances and functional dyspeptic symptoms. Delayed gastric emptying reported in approximately 30% of patients with functional dyspepsia is associated with postprandial fullness, nausea, and vomiting. Impaired gastric accommodation present in 40% of patients with functional dyspepsia is found to be associated with early satiety. Hypersensitivity to gastric distension is observed in 37% of patients with functional dyspepsia and is associated with postprandial pain, belching, and weight loss. Psychosocial factors have also been identified as pathophysiologic mechanisms (29,30).

Dysmotility-like dyspepsia, or gastroparesis, is commonly seen in patients with cancer due to autonomic nervous system dysfunction or use of anticholinergic drugs or opioids. It is associated with symptoms like bloating, abdominal distension, flatulence, and prominent nausea. Patients with this condition tend to have premature satiety with resultant epigastric heaviness or fullness even after the consumption of small meals (31). The diagnosis of paraneoplastic dyspepsia requires a high index of clinical suspicion.

TABLE 17.3	Classification of nonulcer dyspepsia by symptom type and their treatments
Classification	**Symptoms**	**Treatment**
Reflux-like	Heartburn and regurgitation without esophagitis	Antacid, H_2-blocker, and proton pump inhibitor
Ulcer-like	Epigastric pain relieved by food and antacids, relapse, and remission, without ulcer	As above
Dysmotility-like	Abdominal bloating, distension, early satiety, nausea, and vomiting	Prokinetic agent and antiflatulence agent
Nonspecific	Symptoms do not fall into one of the three categories in the preceding text	Start simple: antacid and antiflatulence agent (simethicone)

A panel of serologic tests for paraneoplastic autoantibodies, scintigraphic gastric emptying, and esophageal manometry are useful as first-line screening tests. Nuclear scintigraphy is considered the gold standard for diagnosing and quantifying delayed gastric emptying. Seropositivity for type 1 antineuronal nuclear antibody, Purkinje cell cytoplasmic antibody, or N-type calcium channel–binding antibodies has been detected in patients with paraneoplastic gastroparesis, but its diagnostic value is under investigation (32).

Recent studies have linked gastroparesis to disruption of the interstitial cells of Cajal (ICC). These are fibroblast-like cells, which have been identified in the gut by electron microscopy and by immunohistochemistry for Kit protein. By generating electrical slow waves, the ICC are intercalated between the intramural neurons and the effector smooth muscular cells to form a gastroenteric pacemaker system. It has been recently found that the loss of ICC causes dysmotility-like symptoms in vivo. A loss of these cells has been detected in patients with paraneoplastic gastroparesis (33).

Other causes of cancer-induced dyspepsia include gastric cancer or lymphoma, gastritis secondary to radiotherapy/chemotherapy, gastric compression secondary to intra-abdominal tumor, hepatomegaly, splenomegaly, ascites, or gastric outlet obstruction due to tumor. Medications that have been associated with dyspepsia include acarbose, alcohol, alendronate, codeine, iron, metformin, nonsteroidal anti-inflammatory drugs, erythromycin, potassium, corticosteroids, and theophylline. Dosage reduction or discontinuation of the offending agent may relieve dyspepsia.

Management/Treatment

The management of organic dyspepsia should be directed at the cause. Treatment may be based on previous history (e.g., obstructing lesion responding to primary tumor treatment) or recent endoscopy findings. In functional dyspepsia, treatment should be based on symptoms (Table 17.3). Nutrition support in gastroparesis begins with encouraging smaller volume, low-fat, low-fiber meals and, if necessary, liquid caloric supplements. Metoclopramide is now the prokinetic drug of choice (34). Controlled-release metoclopramide (20 to 80 mg q12h) is effective in ameliorating symptoms of the cancer-induced dyspepsia such as nausea, vomiting, loss of appetite, and bloating (35).

Moreover, subcutaneous administration of metoclopramide is an important method, allowing for continued guaranteed absorption. Low-dosage erythromycin also has a prokinetic role, either alone or in combination with metoclopramide. Domperidone, a centrally acting antiemetic and prokinetic, is not available in US markets. Antiemetics should be used for nausea, which is a very severe debilitating symptom. There should be a low threshold for placing a jejunal feeding tube either by laparoscopy or by mini-laparotomy. Parenteral nutrition should be used only briefly during hospitalization and not encouraged or sustained in an outpatient. Most excitingly, the era of gastric electrical stimulation has arrived for patients not responding to standard medical

therapy. The dramatic decrease in nausea and vomiting, as well as a sustained evidence of improved quality of life, gastric emptying, nutritional status, and decreased hospitalizations by this device, is documented by a long-term follow-up of more than a year (36). Gastric pacemaker has been studied in patients with diabetes-induced gastroparesis but not in cancer. Further research is needed in patients with cancer-induced gastroparesis (37,38).

HEARTBURN

Definition/Incidence

Heartburn is the most common GI complaint in the western population; 33% to 44% of the population complain of heartburn at least monthly and 7% to 13% may have it daily (39). Heartburn is a retrosternal burning sensation that usually radiates proximally from the xiphoid process to the neck. It is caused by the reflux of the gastric content into the esophagus. GERD occurs when the amount of gastric content that refluxes into the esophagus exceeds the normal limit, causing symptoms with or without esophagitis. Although there is no clear evidence that GERD is more common in those with cancer, certain conditions in this population may increase their risk, such as intra-abdominal lesions, which increase pressure on the stomach. In addition to the typical symptoms (heartburn, regurgitation, and dysphagia), abnormal reflux can cause atypical symptoms such as coughing, chest pain, and wheezing and also damage to the lungs (pneumonia, asthma, and idiopathic pulmonary fibrosis), vocal cords (laryngitis and cancer), ear (otitis media), and teeth (enamel decay). Approximately 50% of the patients with reflux develop esophagitis, which is classified on the basis of severity.

Pathophysiology/Etiology

The most important pathophysiologic factor in GERD is frequent transient relaxation of the lower esophageal sphincter (LES). Other factors include anatomic disruption of the LES as in hiatal hernia, transient increase in intra-abdominal pressure, abnormal esophageal peristalsis with impaired clearance of acid, and gastroparesis.

A number of foods, drugs, and neurohumoral factors reduce basal LES pressure, making patients prone to gastroesophageal reflux and heartburn (Table 17.4). Avoiding these foods and medications often constitutes the initial treatment of GERD. Some common agents that increase LES pressure include a protein meal, bethanechol, metoclopramide, and α-adrenergic agonists.

Heartburn is most frequently noted within 1 hour of eating, particularly after the largest meal of the day. Wine drinkers may have heartburn after hearty consumption of red wine but not after white wine. Lying down, especially after a late meal, causes heartburn within 1 to 2 hours; in contrast to peptic ulcer disease, heartburn does not awaken the person in the early morning. Heartburn may be accompanied by

| TABLE 17.4 | **Aggravating factors for heartburn** |

Low LES Pressure	Direct Mucosal Irritant	Increased Intra-abdominal Pressure	Others
Certain foods	Certain foods	Bending over	Supine position
Fats	Citrus products	Lifting	Lying on right side
Sugars	Tomato-based products	Straining at stool	Red wine
Chocolate	Spicy foods	Exercise	Emotions
Onions	Coffee		
Coffee	Medications		
Alcohol	Aspirin		
Cigarettes	Nonsteroidal anti-inflammatory drug		
Medications	Tetracycline		
Progesterone	Quinidine sulfate		
Theophylline	Potassium chloride tablets		
Anticholinergic agents	Iron salts		
Adrenergic agonists			
Adrenergic antagonists			
Diazepam			
Estrogens			
Mint, anise, and dill			
Benzodiazepines			
Meperidine hydrochloride			
Nitrates			
Calcium channel blockers			

LES, lower esophageal sphincter.

regurgitation, a bitter acidic fluid in the mouth that is common at night or when the patient bends over. The regurgitated material comes from the stomach and is yellow or green in color, suggesting the presence of bile. It is important to distinguish regurgitation from vomiting. The absence of nausea, retching, and abdominal contractions suggests regurgitation rather than vomiting. Furthermore, the regurgitation of bland material is atypical for acid reflux disease and suggests the presence of an esophageal motility disorder (i.e., achalasia) or delayed gastric emptying.

Many disorders cause epigastric or substernal pain similar to heartburn, making it important to determine the cause in each patient. Causes include collagen vascular disorders, scleroderma, mixed connective tissue disorders, raised intra-abdominal pressure, gastroparesis, nasogastric tube, prolonged recumbent position, persistent vomiting, pregnancy, hypothyroidism, Zollinger-Ellison syndrome, medications, and some surgical procedures (e.g., myotomy and esophagogastrectomy).

Treatment/Management

Treatment is a stepwise approach. The goal is to control symptoms, to heal esophagitis, and to prevent recurrent esophagitis or complications. The treatment is based on lifestyle modification and control of gastric acid secretion. Lifestyle modification includes losing weight and avoiding precipitating factors such as chocolate, spicy food, alcohol, citrus juice, and tomato-based products. The patient is asked to eat several small meals during the day and avoid large ones and elevate the head of the bed. Antacids are effective in mild symptoms if given after each meal and at bedtime. More aggressive therapy includes H_2-receptor blockers, sucralfate, or omeprazole. Metoclopramide works very well in GERD among patients with cancer who commonly have gastroparesis. It increases the LES pressure and enhances gastric emptying. Long-term therapy is usually necessary. Approximately 80% of patients have a recurrent but nonprogressive GERD that is controlled with medications. In 20% of patients, the disease is progressive and severe complications may occur, such as strictures or Barrett's esophagus. Laparoscopic fundoplication or other palliative procedures should be considered and discussed with patients having cancer. Over the last decade, a new noninvasive endoscopic technique, called *Enteryx*, has been developed to treat GERD (40). This procedure involves the injection of a compound called *ethylene polyvinyl alcohol* into the LES, just within the stomach. The injection is administered with guidance from real-time x-ray. The compound is in liquid form outside the body, but when it comes in contact with the tissues inside the body, it turns into an expanding, spongy material. The procedure may cause a sore throat or chest pain. Although this treatment resulted in a highly significant improvement at 6 and 12 months, longer follow-up is needed to better assess the duration of efficacy of these positive effects.

EARLY SATIETY

Definition/Incidence

Early satiety is the desire to eat combined with an inability to consume more than an unusually small amount of food. This is in contrast to anorexia, in which there is a reduced desire to eat. Early satiety should be distinguished not only from anorexia but also from nausea, bloating, postprandial filling, pyrosis, food aversion, and dyspepsia. However, all of these symptoms may be due to the same physiologic abnormality—delayed gastric emptying. Patients generally do not report this symptom unless questioned. The incidence of cancer-related early satiety varies from 13% to 62% depending on the study and population being evaluated (41–43).

Pathophysiology/Etiology

Satiety results from overlapping stimuli from the CNS and the GI tract affecting food intake. The nutrients ingested and peptide hormones (insulin, glucagon, and norepinephrine-stimulating α_2-adrenergic receptors in the medial hypothalamus), along with serotonin and dopaminergic-α-adrenergic receptors in the lateral hypothalamus, all affect satiety. Cholecystokinin may have primary effects on satiety. Exogenous administration of peptides like cholecystokinin and bombesin affect satiety both centrally and peripherally and inhibit feeding activity in animals.

Early satiety may be due to tumor encroachment on the GI tract, inappropriate satiety signals from oropharyngeal receptors, hyperglycemia, or gastric muscle atrophy. Another important cause appears to be reduced upper GI motility due to autonomic nervous system dysfunction, possibly a paraneoplastic syndrome (44). Tumor type and previous chemotherapy treatment have not been shown to affect the incidence of early satiety in cancer. However, patients with taste aversions appear to have a higher incidence of early satiety than those without (45).

Treatment/Management

It is important to determine if early satiety is the reported symptom. If bloating, pyrosis, anorexia, or nausea not due to gastric status is present, it should be treated appropriately. If there is pressure on the stomach ("squashed stomach"), it should be reduced if possible, although in many cases it is not. Problems such as ascites may be amenable to paracentesis, which can provide temporary relief. Those with gastroduodenal ulcers should be treated with appropriate therapy (H_2-blocker, proton pump inhibitor, and antibiotics). In patients with cicatrization at the pyloric outlet, balloon dilatation may afford relief for variable periods.

Patients with early satiety should be instructed to eat frequent, small meals, with the bulk of their daily intake consumed early, as gastric stasis increases as the day progresses. They should also be instructed to eat sitting up and avoid liquids at mealtimes, as liquids promote gastric distension and a sense of fullness. Prokinetic agents (e.g., metoclopramide and domperidone) may be of particular use. The rationale for prokinetic agent use in early satiety is based on the assumption that the symptom(s) is due to delayed gastric emptying. Metoclopramide is the drug of choice in the United States (34). It is a dopamine antagonist that increases LES pressure and enhances gastric antral contractility. It is generally well-tolerated orally, but extrapyramidal reactions, which appear to be more common in young women, do occur; insomnia (often noted to be "jumpy legs" on further questioning) and sedation have also been reported. Metoclopramide, 10 mg three times daily orally, is an effective treatment for many and enhances food intake. The central effects of metoclopramide may have a direct effect on anorexia to improve appetite in addition to the peripheral effects on gastric contractility. The other prokinetic agents, cisapride and domperidone, are not available in the United States. Cisapride has been removed from the market due to drug interactions causing cardiac abnormalities. Domperidone, also a dopamine antagonist, does not cross the blood–brain barrier, and hence its side-effect profile is superior to metoclopramide; unfortunately, it has not yet been approved in the United States. Erythromycin is another prokinetic agent, but it is less useful in cancer-related gastroparesis as it causes gastric dumping, which is useful in acute gastric stasis (e.g., diabetic gastroparesis). Treatments for early satiety, dyspepsia, and heartburn are listed in Table 17.5.

GI HEMORRHAGE

Definition/Incidence

GI bleeding may originate at any site from the mouth to the anus. It can be occult or overt, with varying degrees of severity. A careful history and physical examination often suggest the site as well as the cause of the bleeding. Although controversial, most agree that 20% loss of circulating volume produces hemodynamic changes and >30% produces shock with organ damage. In the debilitated patient with cancer,

TABLE 17.5	Treatment of dyspepsia, heartburn, and early satiety
Dyspepsia	1. Antacids (aluminum hydroxide, magnesium hydroxide, and simethicone): 10–20 mL or 2–4 tablets p.o. four to six times daily between meals and at bedtime
	2. Treat *Helicobacter pylori*
	3. Treat peptic ulcer disease with proton pump inhibitors
	4. Prokinetic drug:
	Metoclopramide: 10 mg p.o. or i.v. three to four times daily
	Controlled-release metoclopramide: 20–80 mg p.o. q12h
	Domperidone: 10–20 mg p.o. three to four times daily, 15–30 min before meals (not available in the United States)
	Cisapride: 5–20 mg p.o. four times daily at least 15 min before meals and at bedtime (not available in the United States)
	Erythromycin: 30–50 mg/kg p.o. daily in two to four divided doses; maximum 2 g daily
Early satiety	1. Eat frequent, small meals, with the bulk of their daily intake consumed early
	2. Eat sitting up and avoid liquids at mealtimes
	3. Prokinetic drug (e.g., metoclopramide, domperidone, and erythromycin) (see preceding text for doses)
Heartburn	1. Lifestyle modification:
	Weight loss
	Avoid chocolate, spicy food, alcohol, citrus juice, and tomato-based products
	Eat several small meals during the day
	Elevate the head of the bed
	2. Antacids (aluminum hydroxide, magnesium hydroxide, and simethicone): 10–20 mL or 2–4 tablets p.o. four to six times daily between meals and at bedtime
	3. H_2-receptor antagonist: Cimetidine 300 mg p.o. four times daily or 800 mg p.o. at bedtime or 400 mg p.o. twice daily for up to 8 wk
	i.m., i.v.: 300 mg every 6 h
	Ranitidine 150 mg twice daily or 300 mg once daily at bedtime
	4. Proton pump inhibitors: omeprazole 20 mg p.o. daily

the ability to tolerate a GI hemorrhage is compromised and these signs and symptoms may occur with far less blood loss.

The overall incidence of acute upper GI hemorrhage is 100 hospitalizations per 100,000 adults per year (46). In a study of over 15 million people, there was an overall mortality rate of 14% (47). However, in patients younger than 60 without malignancy or organ failure, the mortality was only 0.6%. In 800 admissions to a palliative home care program, the incidence of GI bleeding was 2.3%; those with liver cancer or hepatic metastases were at higher risk (48).

Pathophysiology/Etiology

GI bleeding can be multifactorial, and one should not assume that a tumor is the source of bleeding. In a general population of 2,225 patients, duodenal ulcer (24%), gastric erosions (23%), and gastric ulcer (21%) accounted for most of the upper GI bleeding (49). In cancer, gastritis (36%), peptic or stress ulceration (26%), and tumor necrosis (23%) are the most common causes. *Candida* esophagitis, particularly during chemotherapy administration, Mallory-Weiss mucosal tears with significant bleeding in the setting of thrombocytopenia (50), and inflammatory conditions (e.g., radiation therapy) are less common (51). In the general population, 43% of lower GI bleeding is due to diverticulosis (52). Massive lower GI bleeding can be a late complication of the high-dose radiation therapy used for treatment of GI, gynecologic, or genitourinary cancer.

Other causes of bleeding in patients with cancer include thrombocytopenia and coagulopathies secondary to the disease or the treatment. Aggressive chemotherapy may cause stress-related ulceration of the mucosa or suppress bone marrow production. The incidence of GI perforation after chemotherapy is 10%, most of whom are patients with lymphoma. GI lymphomas are more common sources of tumor bleeding than other intra-abdominal malignancies. Bleeding is the presenting symptom in 15% to 28% of patients, but only 3% to 4% have perforation (53). Hemorrhage has been reported in 27% of those receiving chemotherapy for unresected lymphoma. Resection before treatment may reduce the bleeding and perforation by 50%. Cytosine arabinoside can cause bowel necrosis, and hepatic arterial infusion of fluorodeoxyuridine may cause upper GI toxicity, resulting in gastritis and peptic ulcers. The initiation of chemotherapy has been reported to trigger or accelerate disseminated intravascular coagulation in lymphoma, presumably due to release of thromboplastin-like or other clot-promoting agents (53).

Medications may be responsible for GI bleeding. Drugs usually implicated are corticosteroids, nonsteroidal anti-inflammatory drugs, and aspirin (54). Cephalosporins, streptomycin, isoniazid, penicillin, β-lactam, and amphotericin B may cause bleeding due to their ability to inhibit clotting factor or impair platelet function.

Upper GI Bleeding—Diagnostic Evaluation

Hematemesis is the vomiting of blood, either bright red or dark, with a "coffee grounds" appearance. Melena is foul smelling stool with a coal black, sticky, tar-like appearance. Hematemesis and melena indicate that the bleeding may be from the nasopharynx, esophagus, stomach, duodenum, or, rarely, the proximal jejunum. Endoscopy is used to evaluate upper GI bleeding. Hemodynamically unstable patients should undergo emergent endoscopy, as they may benefit from both diagnosis and therapy (e.g., ligation for variceal bleeding).

Lower GI Bleeding—Diagnostic Evaluation

Hematochezia is the passage of red blood from the anus. Blood from the distal colon, rectum, or anus is fresh and usually bright red, whereas blood from the proximal colon is likely to be darker. Bleeding from the cecum or ascending colon may appear black, but it is not as shiny or tar-like as in melena. Early colonoscopy for the detection of lower lesions may be the first diagnostic step (55). However, when the bleeding is significant it is often difficult to identify the source. A technetium 99–labeled red cell scan may identify the general location of bleeding; however, results are variable. If the source remains unknown, the next step is typically angiography. It can detect the bleeding site as well as allow treatment with intra-arterial infusion of vasopressin or embolization (56).

Treatment/Management

General

It is important to understand the status of the primary disease, the expected survival, and the potential for cure in patients with GI hemorrhage. If the long-term survival rate is poor, patients should not be subjected to unnecessary tests and procedures in their final days. The goal is to determine the source of the hemorrhage, stop the bleeding, and prevent recurrence. A quick assessment of the hemodynamic status including vital signs and postural blood pressure should be started. A sudden increase in pulse or postural hypotension may be the first indication of bleeding. The hematocrit should follow; however, it may take hours to equilibrate. Packed red blood cells should be transfused until the hematocrit is >25%. A coagulopathy should initially be corrected with four units of fresh frozen plasma; thrombocytopenia <50,000/mm^3 requires platelet transfusions.

Upper GI Bleeding Treatment

To prevent stress ulceration and recurrent bleeding several medications are now available, although there is no evidence of their benefit in the immediate posttreatment period (Table 17.6) (57). Endotracheal intubation to prevent aspiration may be necessary in massive upper GI bleeding. Supportive measures with antacids, H$_2$-receptor blockers, and blood products control the bleeding in 60% of patients with gastritis or ulceration. Endoscopic control using Bipolar system of electrocoagulation (BICAP),

TABLE 17.6 Drugs used to prevent recurrent upper gastrointestinal bleeding	
Drug	**Dose**
Antacid	Two tablespoons of high potency liquid, after meals (heartburn)
H$_2$-blocker	Ranitidine hydrochloride, 150 mg p.o. twice daily
	Famotidine, 40 mg, at bedtime
	Nizatidine, 150 mg, at bedtime (duodenal)/150 mg p.o. b.i.d. (gastric ulcer)
Proton pump inhibitor	Omeprazole, 20 mg p.o. daily
Sucralfate	1 g twice daily
Prokinetic	Metoclopramide, 5–15 mg p.o. four times daily

yttrium–aluminum–garnet laser, and other modalities may provide temporary control of bleeding ulceration or tumors. If medical management fails, surgery should be considered. The decision to operate should also be based on the patient's potential quality of life and disease prognosis, as surgery is associated with high morbidity and mortality (58).

Variceal bleeding may be treated with endoscopic sclerotherapy or variceal ligation. Medical management is less effective, but octreotide acetate, a long-acting synthetic analog of somatostatin (50 to 100-μg i.v. bolus followed by an infusion at 25 to 50 μg/h) may reduce portal hypertension in acute variceal hemorrhage. Balloon tamponade may temporize bleeding until more definitive therapy is begun. However, it is associated with a high rate of complications and mortality. Splenorenal and portosystemic shunts control variceal bleeding in a very select group of patients (59).

Lower GI Bleeding—Treatment

For lower GI bleeding, colonoscopy, radionuclide imaging, or mesenteric angiography may be required to identify the source. However, it may be difficult to determine the source due to significant bleeding when performing colonoscopy. If the bleeding rate is >1 mL/min, selective mesenteric arteriography is the best procedure to localize the source. When it is not possible to localize the source, subtotal colectomy should be performed. In poor-risk patients, therapy with selective infusion of vasopressin or embolization of the bleeding vessel can be performed, but there is a risk of bowel infarction (60).

The Dying Patient

GI hemorrhage may be a terminal event in advanced cancer, and the family and professional team should be prepared as this can be a very distressing time. Bleeding may occur very rapidly, and the patient will die immediately of asphyxiation (upper GI bleed) or a precipitous drop in blood pressure resulting in cardiac arrest due to massive lower GI bleed. GI hemorrhage prevented a peaceful death in 2% of patients in a study of 200 hospice patients (61). The key to successful symptom management in the final days, particularly in the home, is preparation. It is important to have a plan to control these symptoms. Neuroleptics are the drugs of choice to sedate patients who have catastrophic bleeds (e.g., chlorpromazine, 25 mg i.v. slow push or 50 mg p.r.n. can be given). Benzodiazepines may increase anxiety (62), and unless the patient is having pain, opioids should not be given, as they may cause restlessness, diaphoresis, and hallucinations (63). It is helpful to have dark sheets and towels available to camouflage the bleeding. Although symptoms can be managed well in most, poor preparation precludes a comfortable death.

BILIARY OBSTRUCTION

Definition/Incidence

Biliary obstruction is the blockage of the flow of bile resulting in increased pressure in the biliary system. Malignant obstruction can occur anywhere in the biliary tree, but it most often affects the extrahepatic biliary tree or liver hilum. Its incidence in malignant disease varies depending on the etiology and the stage of disease. Extrahepatic biliary obstruction is common in carcinoma of the head of the pancreas. Less common tumors are in the ampulla, bile duct, gall bladder, or liver. Cholangiocarcinoma, metastatic tumor, or enlarged lymphatic nodes are other causes of biliary obstruction (64).

Pathophysiology/Etiology

Normally, the hepatocyte secretes bile. Blocking the flow raises pressure in the biliary system rendering the hepatocyte unable to secrete more. The pressure needed to stop secretion is 300 mmHg of H_2O, but there is evidence of cholestasis with lesser pressure. A neural or hormonal mechanism may be responsible for cholestasis before the necessary biliary pressure is reached.

Treatment/Management

Patients usually present in the advanced stage of the disease and surgical resection is rarely possible. Patients with symptomatic biliary obstruction should be evaluated for some type of biliary bypass procedure (65). Although survival is often limited, the symptoms, particularly pruritus, are quite distressing and less amenable to other treatments. Open surgical procedures have not been shown to prolong survival and are associated with greater morbidity and mortality than endoscopically placed stents (66). Unless the patient is moribund, a stenting procedure should be considered, as it may offer dramatic relief.

Stent placement with biliary drainage results in decreased serum bilirubin, and symptoms of pruritus usually resolve within 24 to 48 hours. The duration of palliation afforded by stenting depends on the underlying disease and the type of stent used to relieve the obstruction (67).

There are two types of endoscopically placed stents: self-expanding metallic stents (SEMSs) and plastic stents. The major drawback of plastic stents is occlusion with a bacterial biofilm. This results in occlusion and recurrence of jaundice and requires one or more stent changes in 30% to 60% of patients. In randomized trials comparing plastic stents with SEMS in malignant bile duct occlusion, SEMS provided longer patency rates but had no survival advantage. In a three-arm study comparing plastic stent left in place until dysfunction occurred versus plastic stent routinely changed every 3 months versus SEMS, an initial success rate of 97% was obtained. The plastic stent not routinely changed had the poorest complication-free survival rate. The SEMSs were the most cost-effective when life expectancy was >6 months (68,69). Endoscopic ultrasound-guided biliary drainage (EUSBD) has been shown to be effective for palliation of biliary obstruction and a viable alternative to percutaneous transhepatic cholangiography in patients in whom Endoscopic retrograde cholangiopancreatography (ERCP) has been unsuccessful. A case series of eight patients presented with biliary obstruction from inoperable pancreatic cancer or cholangiocarcinoma underwent transduodenal

EUSBD after a failed ERCP. EUS was used to access the common bile duct from the duodenum after which a guidewire was advanced upward toward the liver hilum. The metal stent was then advanced into the biliary tree. Technical success (correct stent placement) and clinical success (a 50% decrease in serum bilirubin level within 2 weeks after the stent placement) were achieved in all eight patients. No stent malfunction or occlusion was observed. Complications included one case of duodenal perforation, which required surgery, and one case of self-limiting abdominal pain (70).

The method to control symptoms that are associated with biliary obstruction depends on the performance status of the patient, tumor type, and local professional expertise. It is important to remember that patients may appear gravely ill due to infection and obstruction, yet may improve dramatically with antibiotics and a procedure to relieve the obstruction.

HEPATIC FAILURE

Definition/Incidence

Hepatic failure is the severe inability of the liver to function normally, as evidenced by jaundice and abnormal plasma levels of ammonia, bilirubin, alkaline phosphatase, glutamic oxaloacetic transaminase, lactic dehydrogenase, and reversal of the albumin/globulin ratio. It quickly leads to failure of other organs. The hallmark of acute hepatic failure is hepatic encephalopathy and coagulopathy (71).

Pathophysiology/Etiology

Most hepatic failure, regardless of cause, results from massive coagulative necrosis of hepatocytes. Viral hepatitis accounts for approximately 70%, and drug ingestion (primarily acetaminophen) accounts for most of the remaining 30%. Malignant causes are associated with metastatic gastric carcinoma, carcinoid, breast cancer, small cell lung cancer, melanoma, leukemia, and lymphoma. Hepatic failure may be the presenting sign of malignancy in some cases (72). Sinusoidal obstruction with subsequent ischemia has been reported in metastatic liver disease. Occlusion of hepatic venous outflow may occur in the setting of intensive chemotherapy or bone marrow transplantation or recrudescence of hepatitis B virus after treatment.

Clinical Manifestations

Regardless of the cause, hepatic failure begins with nausea and malaise. It proceeds to accumulation of ammonia as a result of diminished urea formation, hepatic encephalopathy, cerebral edema, prolonged prothrombin time, rapidly rising bilirubin, metabolic changes, GI bleeding, sepsis, respiratory failure, renal failure, and cardiovascular collapse (73).

Hepatic Encephalopathy

Hepatic encephalopathy is a complex neuropsychiatric syndrome characterized by cognitive changes, fluctuating neurologic signs, and electroencephalographic changes. In severe cases, irreversible coma and death occur (74). It results from severe hepatocellular dysfunction or intrahepatic and extrahepatic shunting of portal venous blood into the systemic circulation bypassing the liver. Toxic substances are not detoxified by the liver; this leads to metabolic abnormalities in the CNS. Most patients have elevated blood ammonia levels (75). Cognitive changes are due to excessive concentrations of GABA. The role of endogenous benzodiazepine agonists is unclear, but these may contribute to hepatic encephalopathy. A partial response has been observed in some after the administration of a benzodiazepine antagonist (flumazenil) (76). The most common predisposing factor is GI bleeding, which leads to an increase in ammonia production. Hypokalemic alkalosis, hypoxia, CNS-depressing drugs (e.g., barbiturates and benzodiazepines), and acute infection may also trigger hepatic encephalopathy (77).

Reversal of the sleep/wake cycle is among the earliest signs of encephalopathy. Mood disturbances, confusion, alterations in personality, deterioration in self-care and handwriting, and daytime somnolence are also seen. The diagnosis of hepatic encephalopathy is usually one of exclusion (78). There are no diagnostic liver function test abnormalities, although an elevated serum ammonia level is highly suggestive of the diagnosis (78). It is sometimes difficult to distinguish hepatic encephalopathy from other forms of delirium.

Portal Hypertension

Tumor burden may compress the hepatic blood vessels; this can result in portal hypertension, which causes collateral vessels in the esophagus and the stomach to become enlarged and tortuous (varices). Bleeding of the varices is likely, because the liver is unable to synthesize vitamin K and clotting factors. Procedures to reduce the pressure include a portal–systemic shunt, and β-adrenergic blockade (e.g., propranolol hydrochloride), if not contraindicated (79).

Spontaneous Bacterial Peritonitis

Spontaneous bacterial peritonitis occurs with ascites without an obvious primary source of infection. The ascitic fluid has low concentrations of opsonic proteins, which normally provide protection against bacteria. Paracentesis reveals cloudy fluid with a white cell count of >500 cells/μL (>250 polymorphonuclear leukocytes). Common isolates are *Escherichia coli*, pneumococci, and, to a lesser extent, anaerobes. Empirical therapy with intravenous cefotaxime sodium (2 g every 8 hours for at least 5 days) and an aminoglycoside should be initiated if clinically appropriate (78).

Hepatorenal Syndrome

Hepatorenal syndrome is a disorder characterized by worsening azotemia, oliguria, hyponatremia, low urinary sodium, and hypotension, with structurally intact kidneys. It is diagnosed only in the absence of identifiable causes of renal dysfunction. Treatment is usually ineffective. Some patients with hypotension and decreased plasma volume may respond to volume expansion, but care must be taken to rehydrate slowly to avoid variceal bleeding (80).

TABLE 17.7	Adverse prognostic indicators in hepatic failure
Indicator	**Value**
Age	<10 y, >40 y
Cause	Idiosyncratic drug reaction, halothane, non-A, non-B hepatitis
Jaundice	>7 d before onset of encephalopathy
Bilirubin	>300 µmol/L (18 mg/dL)
Prothrombin time	>100 s
Factor V level	<20%
Clinical status	Respiratory failure
	Rapid reduction in liver size
	Coma

Treatment/Management

Whenever possible, the inciting agent should be treated or eliminated. There is little role for liver transplant in the patient with cancer. For most, treatment of the underlying disease provides the best method to reverse the process of hepatic failure. It may be useful to review adverse prognostic indicators in hepatic encephalopathy (Table 17.7) before embarking on intensive, supportive therapy in those who survive.

Stenting biliary obstructions may provide relief from jaundice and pruritus. Paracentesis helps control symptomatic ascites. Neuropsychiatric symptoms are distressing and should be controlled with appropriate medications. Flumazenil, a short-acting benzodiazepine antagonist, may have a role in the management of hepatic encephalopathy (74). Reducing oral protein intake in advanced cancer is rarely necessary. Administering lactulose, a nonabsorbable laxative sugar, may help. The initial dose is 30 to 50 mL every hour until diarrhea occurs; thereafter the dose is adjusted (15 to 30 mL three times daily) so that the patient has two to four soft stools daily (78).

In the terminal state, it may be appropriate to allow a deteriorating level of consciousness to progress and to forgo treatment. The neuropsychiatric symptoms are controlled with neuroleptics (if hallucinating, chlorpromazine 50 to 200 mg every 2 to 3 hours) or with diazepam (if agitated). The goal is to relieve distress without concern for the adverse effect of major tranquilizers on the mental status.

TENESMUS

Definition/Incidence

Tenesmus is a painful spasm of the anal sphincter with a sensation of the urgent need to defecate, with involuntary straining, but with little bowel movement if any. Patients complain of an abnormally frequent desire to defecate and a sensation that evacuation is incomplete. Rectal pain is not commonly caused by organic lesions, which more frequently result in tenesmus. It is a distressing, difficult to control problem. In the patient with cancer, it occurs most commonly in cancer of the rectum or after pelvic radiation.

Pathophysiology/Etiology

Tenesmus is thought to be a motility disorder of the rectum, with decreased compliance and high-amplitude pressure waves in the rectal wall. This results in an increased sensitivity to distension of the rectum. Rectal causes of tenesmus include impacted feces, carcinoma, rectal prolapse, rectal polyps, adenoma, hemorrhoids, fissure, proctitis, foreign body, and abscess. Infectious causes include *Shigella*, *Campylobacter*, and *Clostridium difficile*.

In the patient with rectal cancer, tenesmus is usually an ominous sign indicating circumferential growth or ulceration involving the sphincter muscle. Tenesmus typically occurs in the morning on waking and subsides as the day progresses. Accompanying perineal or buttock pain suggests involvement of the sacral nerve plexus. Patients presenting with this symptom complex are unlikely to be candidates for sphincter-saving procedures. Tenesmus can also be caused by damage from radiation therapy (acute and late effects) for rectal cancer or other pelvic structures (e.g., cervix, prostate, bladder, and testes).

Treatment/Management

Treatment is based on the cause and is variably effective. Infectious causes should be treated with appropriate antibiotics. Radiation-induced tenesmus is a difficult problem. Symptoms usually resolve spontaneously within 2 to 6 months (81). Tenesmus and rectal bleeding have been treated with oral sulfasalazine combined with steroid enemas or sucralfate enemas (2 g in 20 mL of tap water) (82).

Curative intent pelvic exenteration effectively controlled pain and tenesmus in 89% and palliative intent in 67% of patients with rectal cancer (83). However, this is a procedure associated with significant morbidity and should not be performed for the sole purpose of controlling pain. Radiotherapy may also provide symptomatic relief, but the primary purpose is to control the disease; and it may be most useful in those who have not received chemotherapy (84). Metal expandable stents have been used successfully and are associated with little morbidity, but these may migrate (85). Lumbar sympathectomy produced complete relief of tenesmus in 10 of 12 patients with cancers in the pelvic region. Duration of relief was 3 days to 7 months (mean, 53 days). In this small series, the only complication was transient hypotension responding to intravenous fluids (86); however, mild, reversible bruising and stiffness at the needle insertion site often occur. Up to 20% of patients have limb pain, which develops after a 10- to 14-day latent period and spontaneously resolves after a few weeks. Major neurologic deficits are uncommon when lumbar sympathectomy is performed by experienced pain practitioners, making it one of the most important treatment modes currently available.

A general treatment plan should include a laxative and stool softener unless diarrhea is the prominent symptom, in which case an obstructing lesion should be ruled out. Care should be taken when prescribing roughage in those with previous radiation, as the bowel/rectal wall can be traumatized. Dexamethasone (4 to 16 mg daily) may provide some relief through its anti-inflammatory actions. The calcium channel antagonist nifedipine (10 to 20 mg two to three times daily) may help to relieve spasms. Epidural opioids and local anesthetics may also be helpful. Systemic opioids should be tried, but these are less effective, as in other forms of neuropathic pain. Traditional neuropathic pain treatment such as tricyclic antidepressants (e.g., amitriptyline hydrochloride) should be used with caution, as one of the main side effects is constipation.

CONCLUSIONS

GI symptoms are so common in the general, healthy population that it may be more difficult to evaluate them in those with cancer. Common symptoms may be disease-related or a comorbidity unrelated to the cancer. Both may represent potentially life-threatening problems, and yet the decision to treat may not be clear if based on management guidelines for the general population. Decisions regarding treatment must be evaluated with an understanding of the goals of therapy, potential quality of life, and life expectancy. Consultation with GI specialists and ongoing communication with the patient and family help to provide the framework in which to make these often difficult decisions.

REFERENCES

1. Askenasy JJM. About the mechanism of hiccup. *Eur Neurol.* 1992;32:159-163.
2. Marinella MA. Diagnosis and management of hiccups in the patient with advanced cancer. *J Support Oncol.* July-August 2009;7(4):122-127, 130.
3. Lewis JH. Hiccups: causes and cures. *J Clin Gastroenterol.* 1985;7:539-552.
4. Launois S, Bizec JL, Whitelaw WA, et al. Hiccup in adults: an overview. *Eur Respir J.* 1993;6:563-575.
5. Ge AX, Ryan ME, Giaccone G, Hughes MS, Pavletic SZ. Acupuncture treatment for persistent hiccups in patients with cancer. *J Altern Complement Med.* July 2010;16(7):811-816.
6. Friedgood CE, Ripstein CB. Chlorpromazine (thorazine) in the treatment of intractable hiccups. *JAMA.* 1955;157:309-310.
7. Ives TJ, Flemming MF, Weart CW, et al. Treatment of intractable hiccup with intramuscular haloperidol. *Am J Psychiatry.* 1985;142:1368-1369.
8. Lipps DC, Jabbari B, Mitchel MH, et al. Nifedipine for intractable hiccups. *Neurology.* 1990;40:531-532.
9. Madanagopolan N. Metoclopramide in hiccup. *Curr Med Res Opin.* 1975;3:371-374.
10. Walker P, Watanabe S, Bruera E. Baclofen, a treatment for chronic hiccup. *J Pain Symptom Manage.* 1998;16:125-132.
11. Parvin R, Milo R, Klein C, et al. Amitriptyline for intractable hiccup. *Am J Gastroenterol.* 1988;63:1007-1008.
12. McFarling DA, Susac JO. Carbamazepine for hiccoughs. *JAMA.* 1974;230:962.
13. Petroski D, Patel AN. Diphenylhydantoin for intractable hiccups. *Lancet.* 1974;1:739.
14. Jacobson PL, Messenheimer JA, Farmer TW. Treatment of intractable hiccups with valproic acid. *Neurology.* 1981;31:1458-1460.
15. Moro C, Sironi P, Berardi E, Beretta G, Labianca R. Midazolam for long-term treatment of intractable hiccup. *J Pain Symptom Manage.* March 2005;29(3):221-223.
16. Alonso-Navarro H, Rubio L, Jiménez-Jiménez FJ. Refractory hiccup: successful treatment with gabapentin. *Clin Neuropharmacol.* May-June 2007;30(3):186-187.
17. Porzio G, Aielli F, Verna L, Aloisi P, Galletti B, Ficorella C. Gabapentin in the treatment of hiccups in patients with advanced cancer: a 5-year experience. *Clin Neuropharmacol.* July 2010;33(4):179-180.
18. Porzio G, Aielli F, Narducci F, et al. Hiccup in patients with advanced cancer successfully treated with gabapentin: report of three cases. *N Z Med J.* 2003;116(1182):U605.
19. Hernandez JL, Pajaron M, Garcia-Regata O, et al. Gabapentin for intractable hiccup. *Am J Med.* 2004;117(4):279-281.
20. Neeno TA, Rosenow EC 3rd. Intractable hiccups. Consider nebulized lidocaine. *Chest.* October 1996;110(4):1129-1130.
21. De Ruysscher D, Spaas P, Specenier P. Treatment of intractable hiccup in a terminal cancer patient with nebulized saline. *Palliat Med.* April 1996;10(2):166-167.
22. Marechal R, Berghmans T, Sculier P. Successful treatment of intractable hiccup with methylphenidate in a lung cancer patient. *Support Care Cancer.* 2003;11(2):126.
23. Calvo E, Fernandez-Torre F, Brugarolas A. Cervical phrenic nerve block for intractable hiccups in cancer patients. *JNCI J Natl Cancer Inst.* 2002;94(15):1175-1176.
24. Aravot DJ, Wright G, Rees A, et al. Non-invasive phrenic nerve stimulation for intractable hiccups. *Lancet.* 1989;2:1047.
25. Salem MR. Treatment of hiccups by pharyngeal stimulation in anesthetized and conscious subjects. *JAMA.* 1967;202:126-130.
26. Smith HS, Busracamwongs A. Management of hiccups in the palliative care population. *Am J Hosp Palliat Care.* 2003;20(2):149-154.

27. Heading RC. Definitions of dyspepsia. *Scand J Gastroenterol.* 1991;26(suppl 182):1-6.

28. Ofman JJ, Etchason J, Fullerton S, et al. Management strategies for *Helicobacter pylori* seropositive patients with dyspepsia: clinical and economic consequences. *Ann Intern Med.* 1997;126:280-291.

29. Tack J, Lee KJ. Pathophysiology and treatment of functional dyspepsia. *J Clin Gastroenterol.* 2005;39(5 suppl):S211-S216.

30. Fisher RS, Parkman HP. Management of nonulcer dyspepsia. *N Engl J Med.* 1998;339:1376-1381.

31. Talley NJ. Nonulcer dyspepsia: current approaches to diagnosis and management. *Am Fam Physician.* 1993;47:1407-1416.

32. Lee HR, Lennon VA, Camilleri M, et al. Paraneoplastic gastrointestinal motor dysfunction: clinical and laboratory characteristics. *Am J Gastroenterol.* 2001;96(2):373-379.

33. Pardi DS, Miller SM, Miller DL, et al. Paraneoplastic dysmotility: loss of interstitial cells of Cajal. *Am J Gastroenterol.* 2002;97(7):1828-1833.

34. Nelson KA, Walsh TD. The use of metoclopramide in anorexia due to the cancer-associated dyspepsia syndrome (CADS). *J Palliat Care.* 1993;9:14-18.

35. Wilson J, Plourde JY, Marshall D, et al. Long-term safety and clinical effectiveness of controlled-release metoclopramide in cancer-associated dyspepsia syndrome: a multicenter evaluation. *J Palliat Care.* 2002;18(2):84-91.

36. McCallum RW, George SJ. Gastric dysmotility and gastroparesis. *Curr Treat Options Gastroenterol.* 2001;4(2):179-191.

37. Forster J, Sarosiek I, Delcore R, et al. Gastric pacing is a new surgical treatment for gastroparesis. *Am J Surg.* 2001;182(6):676-681.

38. Abell T, Lou J, Tabbaa M, et al. Gastric electrical stimulation for gastroparesis improves nutritional parameters at short, intermediate, and long-term follow-up. *JPEN J Parenter Enteral Nutr.* 2003;27(4):277-281.

39. Nebel OT, Fornes MF, Castell DO. Symptomatic gastroesophageal reflux: incidence and precipitating factors. *Dig Dis Sci.* 1976;21:953-964.

40. Johnson DA, Ganz R, Aisenberg J, et al. Endoscopic implantation of Enteryx for treatment of GERD: 12-month results of a prospective, multicenter trial. *Am J Gastroenterol.* 2003;98(9):1921-1930.

41. Donnelly S, Walsh D. The symptom of advanced cancer. *Semin Oncol.* 1995;22(2 suppl 3):67-72.

42. Dunlop GM. A study of the relative frequency and importance of gastrointestinal symptoms, and weakness in patients with far advanced cancer. *Palliat Med.* 1989;4:37-43.

43. Armes PJ, Plant HJ, Allbright A, et al. A study to investigate the incidence of early satiety in patients with advanced cancer. *Br J Cancer.* 1992;65:481-484.

44. Nelson KA, Walsh DT, Sheehan FG, et al. Assessment of upper gastrointestinal motility in the cancer-associated dyspepsia syndrome. *J Palliat Care.* 1993;9(1):27-31.

45. Neilson SS, Theologides A, Vickers ZM. Influence of food odors on food aversions and preferences in patients with cancer. *Am J Clin Nutr.* 1980;33:2253-2261.

46. Longstreth GF. Epidemiology for hospitalization for acute upper gastrointestinal hemorrhage: a population based study. *Am J Gastroenterol.* 1995;90:206-210.

47. Rockall TA, Logan RFA, Devlin HB, et al. Incidence of and mortality from acute upper gastrointestinal haemorrhage in the United Kingdom. *BMJ.* 1995;311:222.

48. Mercadante S, Baressi L, Casuccio A, et al. Gastrointestinal bleeding in advanced cancer patients. *J Pain Symptom Manage.* 2000;19:160-162.

49. Silverstein FE, Gilbert DA, Tedesco FJ. The national ASGE survey on upper gastrointestinal bleeding. *Gastrointest Endosc.* 1981;27:73.

50. Spencer GD, Hackman RC, McDonald GB, et al. A prospective study of unexplained nausea and vomiting after marrow transplantation. *Transplantation.* 1986;42:602-607.

51. Kemeny MM, Brennan MF. The surgical complications of chemotherapy in the cancer patient. *Curr Probl Surg.* 1987;24:613-675.

52. Boley SJ, DiBiase A, Brandt LJ, et al. Lower intestinal bleeding in the elderly. *Am J Surg.* 1979;137:57.

53. Weingrad DN, Decosse JJ, Sherlock P, et al. Primary gastrointestinal lymphoma. *Cancer.* 1982;49:1258-1265.

54. Gabriel SE, Jaakkimaenen L, Bombardier C. Risk for serious gastrointestinal complications related to the use of nonsteroidal anti-inflammatory drugs: a meta-analysis. *Ann Intern Med.* 1991;115:787-797.

55. Jensen DM, Machicado GA. Diagnosis and treatment of severe hematochezia. The role of urgent colonoscopy after purge. *Gastroenterology.* 1988;95:1569-1574.

56. Nusbaum M, Baum S. Radiographic demonstration of unknown sites of gastrointestinal bleeding. *Surg Forum.* 1963;14:374-375.

57. Lind T, Aadland E, Eriksson S, et al. Beneficial effects of I.V. omeprazole in patients with peptic ulcer bleeding. *Gastroenterology.* 1995;108:A150.

58. Cotlon RB, Rosenberg MT, Waldram RPL, et al. Early endoscopy of esophagus, stomach, and duodenal bulb in patients with hematemesis and melena. *BMJ.* 1973;2:505-509.

59. Graham D, Smith JL. The course of patients after variceal hemorrhage. *Gastroenterology.* 1981;80:800-809.

60. Jensen DM. Current management of severe lower gastrointestinal tract bleeding. *Gastrointest Endosc.* 1995;41:171-173.

61. Lichter I, Hunt E. The last 48 hours of life. *J Palliat Care.* 1990;6:7-15.

62. Breitbart W, Marotta R, Platt M, et al. A double-blind trial of haloperidol, chlorpromazine, and lorazepam in the treatment of delirium in hospitalized AIDS patients. *Am J Psychiatry.* 1996;153:231-237.

63. Crain SM, Shen F. Opioids can evoke direct receptor-mediated excitatory effects in sensory neurons. *Trends Pharmacol Sci.* 1990;11:77-81.

64. Stellato TA, Zollinger RM, Shuck JM. Metastatic malignant biliary obstruction. *Am Surg.* 1989;157:381-385.

65. Bear HD, Turner MA, Parker GA, et al. Treatment of biliary obstruction caused by metastatic cancer. *Am J Surg.* 1989;157:381-385.

66. Smith AC, Dowsett JF, Russell RCG, et al. Randomized trial of endoscopic stenting versus surgical bypass in malignant low bile duct obstruction. *Lancet.* 1994;334:1655-1660.

67. Earnshaw JJ, Hayter JP, Teasdale C, et al. Should endoscopic stenting be the initial treatment of malignant biliary obstruction? *Ann R Coll Surg Engl.* 1992;74:338-341.

68. Wagner HJ, Knyrim K, Vakil N, et al. Polyethylene endoprostheses versus metal stents in the palliative treatment of malignant hilar obstruction. A prospective and randomized trial. *Endoscopy.* 1993;25:213-218.

69. Schmassmann A, von Gunten E, Knuchel J, et al. Wall stents versus plastic stents in malignant biliary obstruction: effects of

stent patency of the first and second stent on patient compliance and survival. *Am J Gastroenterol.* 1996;91:654-659.

70. Siddiqui AA, Sreenarasimhaiah J, Lara LF, Harford W, Lee C, Eloubeidi MA. Endoscopic ultrasound-guided transduodenal placement of a fully covered metal stent for palliative biliary drainage in patients with malignant biliary obstruction. Surg Endosc. February 2011;25(2):549-555; e-pub ahead of print July 15 2010.

71. O'Grady JG, Schalm SW, Williams R. Acute liver failure: redefining the syndromes. *Lancet.* 1993;342:273-275.

72. McGuire BM, Cherwitz DL, Rabe KM, et al. Small cell carcinoma of the lung manifesting as acute hepatic failure. *Mayo Clin Proc.* 1997;72:133-139.

73. Fingerote RJ. Fulminant hepatic failure. *Am J Gastroenterol.* 1993;88:1000-1010.

74. Butterworth RF. Pathogenesis and treatment of portal-systemic encephalopathy: an update. *Dig Dis Sci.* 1992;37:321-340.

75. Lockwood AH. Hepatic encephalopathy. *Neurol Clin.* 2002;20:241-246.

76. Howard CD, Seifert CF. Flumazenil in the treatment of hepatic encephalopathy. *Ann Pharmacother.* 1993;27:46-48.

77. Hoyumpa AM, Desmond PV, Avant GR, et al. Clinical conference: hepatic encephalopathy. *Gastroenterology.* 1979;78:184.

78. Hoofnagle JH, Carithers RL, Shapiro C, et al. Fulminant hepatic failure: summary of a workshop. *Hepatology.* 1995;21:240.

79. D'Amico G, Pagliaco L, Bosch J. The treatment of portal hypertension: a meta-analysis review. *Hepatology.* 1995;22: 332-354.

80. Wilkinson SP, Portmann B, Hurst D, et al. Pathogenesis of renal failure in cirrhosis and fulminant hepatic failure. *Postgrad Med J.* 1975;51:503.

81. Sedwick DM, Howard GC, Ferguson A. Pathogenesis of acute radiation injury to the rectum. A prospective study in patients. *Int J Colorectal Dis.* 1994;9:23-30.

82. Regnard CFB. Control of bleeding in advanced cancer. *Lancet.* 1991;337:974.

83. Yeung RS, Moffat FL, Falk RE. Pelvic exenteration for recurrent and extensive primary colorectal adenocarcinoma. *Cancer.* 1993;72:1853-1858.

84. Midgley R, Kerr D. Colorectal cancer. *Lancet.* 1999;353:391-399.

85. Rey JF, Romanczyk T, Graff M. Metal stents for palliation of rectal carcinoma: a preliminary report on 12 patients. *Endoscopy.* 1995;27:501-504.

86. Bristow A, Foster JMG. Lumbar sympathectomy in the management of rectal tenesmoid pain. *Ann R Coll Surg Engl.* 1988;70:38-39.

CHAPTER 18

Biology of Treatment-Induced Mucositis

Rachel J. Gibson ■ Joanne M. Bowen ■ Emma H. Bateman ■ Dorothy M. K. Keefe

INTRODUCTION

This chapter is dedicated to exploring the biology of treatment-induced alimentary tract (AT) mucositis. AT mucositis is a significant complication in the clinical oncology setting. It occurs in a large percentage of patients undergoing cytotoxic chemotherapy and radiotherapy. One of the key problems with AT mucositis is that the underlying mechanisms behind its development are not entirely understood, making it extremely difficult to develop effective interventions. Animal models have provided a detailed and important source of knowledge when sampling from patients is unavailable or interventions are yet to be fully tested. This chapter focuses on how animal models have been used to facilitate our understanding of the mechanisms of AT mucositis.

PATHOBIOLOGY OF AT MUCOSITIS

AT mucositis is an extremely common toxicity occurring after chemotherapy and radiotherapy for cancer (1). AT mucositis occurs in approximately 40% of patients after standard doses of chemotherapy and in up to 100% of patients undergoing high-dose chemotherapy and hematopoietic stem cell transplantation, or radiation for head and neck cancer (2–4), affecting over 2 million people worldwide each year. As the name suggests, AT mucositis can occur anywhere along the alimentary canal and is associated with many symptoms, of which significant pain, ulceration, abdominal bloating, nausea and vomiting, diarrhea, and constipation are a few (5–7).

The potentially severe nature of AT mucositis can have some further devastating effects, including a reduction or cessation of treatment (which may decrease the chance for remission or cure) and increased stays in hospitals, leading to increased costs of treatment and use of opioids for pain management (2–4). In addition to the economic costs associated with AT mucositis, there is also a significant impact on the quality of life of cancer patients, with increased morbidity and mortality (8). The potential market for management interventions in mucositis is between $1 and 2 billion annually, with a number of new agents in the development pipeline looking to capitalize on this unmet need.

Historically, mucositis has been separated into oral mucositis and intestinal mucositis, both mechanistically and for applied interventions. In addition, a number of overlapping terms have been used clinically, including stomatitis, gastrointestinal toxicity, radiation esophagitis, radiation enteritis, radiation proctitis, and the radiation gastrointestinal syndrome. This lack of consistent terminology, for the underlying issue of regimen-related mucosal damage (mucositis), acts as a barrier for research and knowledge advancement. The prevailing consensus is that changes affecting the oral cavity and throat are considered oral mucositis, while changes arising lower in the digestive tract are grouped as gastrointestinal mucositis, which can include esophageal, gastric, and small and large bowel injury. A further level of contention is that gastrointestinal toxicity is sometimes cited as inclusive of the oral cavity, but not always. The concept of alimentary mucositis is relatively new and accommodates regional differences in presentation and diagnosis in an aim to facilitate a unified approach to research, each region then being a subset.

AT MUCOSITIS IN HUMANS

AT mucositis is a field that has rapidly evolved over the last 15 years. There have been exciting and significant advances leading from basic clinical science questions to conducting whole-genome microarray experiments and developing complex algorithms to uncover toxicity clustering. The first step in the AT mucositis matrix started with relatively simple investigations of pathology and malabsorption following radiation or chemotherapy in cancer patients (9,10). One example of an early study investigating the severity and time course of changes in patients' intestinal permeability following high-dose chemotherapy and autologous blood stem cell transplantation will be discussed here (11). Briefly, this study recruited 35 patients and determined the maximum sugar permeability occurring in the small intestine 14 days after the start of chemotherapy. Levels returned to normal 7 weeks after chemotherapy (11). Furthermore, this abnormality was found to correlate with the time frame that the patients suffered from other gastrointestinal symptoms including anorexia and nausea (11). This study offered the first insight into intestinal damage after chemotherapy in patients. It led to further questions about the mechanisms by which chemotherapy damages the small intestine and led to further, more detailed clinical studies.

A second study assessed the frequency, duration, and severity of both oral and gastrointestinal symptoms following chemotherapy. Sixty patients with a variety of malignancies were recruited to this study, including newly diagnosed patients, patients undergoing high-dose chemotherapy, and patients undergoing autologous peripheral blood stem cell transplantation (12). Patients underwent a variety of tests, including questionnaires and noninvasive nutritional assessments and the intestinal sugar permeability tests, as well as invasive blood testing for serum endotoxin. A small number of patients also underwent a series of breath tests before and after chemotherapy (12). Findings indicated that patients experienced gastrointestinal symptoms 3 to 10 days after chemotherapy commenced, with these returning to normal by day 28. In contrast to this, patients did not experience oral symptoms until day 7 after chemotherapy, remaining until day 14 before returning to normal by day 28 (12). These findings led to a third patient-based study, aimed at assessing small intestinal mucosal histology following chemotherapy. Twenty-three patients with a variety of malignancies were recruited to the study and underwent an endoscopy with duodenal biopsy before, and at varying time points after, chemotherapy. Biopsies were assessed using a variety of techniques including the apoptosis-specific assay Terminal deoxynucleotidyl transferase dUTP nick end labelling (TUNEL), enterocyte height, and transmission electron microscopy (13). Findings indicated a sevenfold increase in apoptosis in intestinal crypts 1 day after chemotherapy, followed by a reduction in intestinal morphometry 3 days after chemotherapy. Values had returned to normal by 16 days after chemotherapy (13). These findings are similar to the histopathological changes identified by Trier and Browning during acute phase intestinal injury induced by abdominal radiation, which described reduced mitosis, decreased thickness of the mucosa, and fragments of disintegrating epithelial cells (14).

A further clinical study was conducted and aimed to determine whether apoptosis also occurred in the oral mucosa following chemotherapy (14). Twenty patients with a variety of malignancies were recruited and each underwent a buccal punch biopsy prior to, and at varying time points after, chemotherapy. Biopsies were assessed using the TUNEL assay and transmission electron microscopy. Apoptosis increased in the basal layer of the buccal mucosa in the first 3 days following chemotherapy and had not returned to normal levels by 11 days after treatment. Apoptosis was accompanied by significant ultrastructural changes (14).

Each of these clinical studies clearly indicated that cancer chemotherapy causes significant damage to the AT. While each study answered a specific question, it also led to many questions that needed answers. However, in order to fully understand the mechanisms of how this damage occurs, an appropriate animal model needed to be developed. While it was possible to perform upper gastrointestinal endoscopy and biopsy in a small number of patients, more detailed investigations were required. These simply would not have been possible without the development and use of animal models.

HISTORICAL PATHOPHYSIOLOGY OF AT MUCOSITIS

AT mucositis as a field has rapidly evolved over the last decade. In 1998, Sonis first proposed that oral mucositis followed a distinct cascade of phases, namely the inflammatory/

vascular; the epithelial; the ulcerative/bacteriological; and the healing phase (8). Briefly, it was initially thought that in the first inflammatory phase, following the administration of cytotoxic therapy, various proinflammatory cytokines were released from the epithelial tissues, leading to local tissue damage. This phase was postulated to occur early, within 24 hours after cytotoxic treatment. The second epithelial phase was thought to occur between 4 and 5 days following treatment. Cytotoxic agents were thought to directly inhibit deoxyribonucleic acid (DNA) replication and mucosal cellular reproduction, ultimately leading to a decrease in basal epithelial proliferation (8,15). Consequently, as not all cytotoxic drugs affect DNA synthesis (8), it was thought that there would be a higher probability that patients on particular treatment regimes would be more susceptible to oral mucositis than others. Evidence supporting this notion came from studies in children, known to have a high basal cell proliferation. These children were three times more likely to develop oral mucositis than older adults, who have a slower basal cell proliferation (16). The reduction in cellular proliferation of the oral mucosa was thought to cause mucosal atrophy, with breakdown of collagen and frank mucosal ulceration, marking the beginning of the ulcerative and bacteriological third phase. Clinically, this was the most symptomatic phase for patients and presented approximately 1 week following treatment (8). The fourth and final healing phase referred to the mucosa resuming normal basal cell proliferation and differentiation as well as controlling the oral bacterial flora. The length of this final phase was thought to be related to the duration of the condition; however, it most probably did not relate to the intensity. Additionally, anything that adversely affected wound healing would also affect this final phase (8).

CURRENT HYPOTHESIS FOR THE PATHOBIOLOGY OF AT MUCOSITIS

In 2004, it was recognized that AT mucositis was more than just an epithelial process, prompting a revision of the four-phase model to the current overlapping five-phase model (Figure 18.1). The phases were renamed as follows: 1, initiation; 2, primary damage response; 3, signal amplification; 4, ulceration; and 5, healing (17,18). In this updated model, initiation occurs immediately following exposure to cytotoxic therapy, with both DNA and non-DNA damage occurring, resulting in the generation of reactive oxygen species (ROS) and clonogenic cell death. Clonogenic cell death in the small intestine has been shown to occur within 4 hours following irradiation (19). This leads to the second phase of primary damage response. In this phase, nuclear factor kappa B (NFκB) has been shown to be a key transcription factor that is "turned on" in response to DNA damage and ROS, leading to a cascade of downstream genes including proinflammatory cytokines interleukin (IL)-1β, IL-6, and tumor necrosis factor (TNF). Radiation at physiological doses has been shown to induce both NFκB and another transcription factor, p53, in cells (20), indicating that these stress-responsive factors

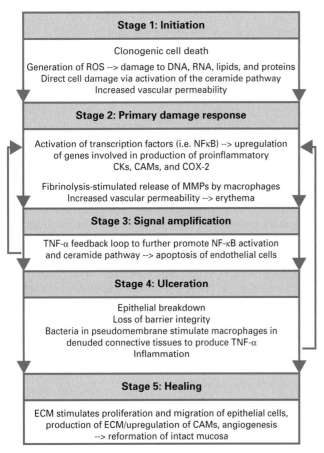

Figure 18.1. Overlapping five-phase model of AT mucositis. ROS, reactive oxygen species; NFκB, nuclear factor kappa B; CKs, cytokines; CAMs, cell adhesion molecules; COX-2, cyclooxygenase-2; MMPs, matrix metalloproteinases; TNF-α, tumor necrosis factor alpha; ECM, extracellular matrix.

are important in mucositis development. Chemotherapy treatment has shown to increase the transcription factor AP1 (21), and this family of transcription factors is known to induce damage in all cells within the mucosa and submucosa (18). In addition, increased expression of IL-1β and TNF has been detected in the submucosal cells of hamsters following acute targeted radiation (22). In the same experiment, interference with TNF-α reduced mucositis, indicating that the cytokine signaling that is set up relatively early on plays a key role in development of injury. In the third phase of signal amplification, the proinflammatory cytokines that were upregulated earlier begin to amplify the original signal and positively feed back on NFκB, thus causing further amplification. In addition, biologically active proteins including but not limited to mitogen-activated protein kinase, cyclooxygenase-2, and matrix metalloproteinases (MMPs) 1 and 3 are activated (17,18,23–25). MMPs are destructive to the basement membrane and potentially stimulate further destructive signals. Collectively, all of these processes lead to the fourth clinically relevant ulcerative phase that can be observed macroscopically. This culminates in the loss of epithelial tissue and ultimate breach of the mucosal barrier.

Patients experience significant pain and there can also be concomitant microbial colonization, leading to increased risk of sepsis. Cell-wall products from colonizing bacteria are likely to penetrate into the submucosa, where they activate infiltrating mononuclear cells to produce and release additional proinflammatory cytokines, further amplifying inflammation (25). In the final phase, healing occurs once the insult has been removed, mediated by signaling from the extracellular matrix and mesenchyme. Interestingly, the time frame varies between individuals (17,18).

Importantly, with the development of this updated five-phase pathophysiology model, it was recognized that these "phases" occur not only in the oral mucosa but also along the entire alimentary canal. Keefe (26) proposed that these mechanisms could, and indeed should, be similar to any region of the AT, as it has the same embryological route of development involving all three germ layers of the developing embryo. The specialized differences in local function along the tract offer an explanation for why different regions are more susceptible to "early" mucositis and others are more susceptible to "late" mucositis (1,26). However, the true extent of the complexity of alimentary mucositis is still unknown, with the timing and sequence of injury events just one of a number of key issues that are not fully understood. The key underlying challenge to understanding mechanisms is the relative difficulty and invasiveness in obtaining samples from sites within the AT. Therefore, in order to obtain longitudinal data from multiple sites, animal models are necessary.

ANIMAL MODELS OF AT MUCOSITIS

Animal models of AT mucositis have provided extensive information on mechanisms. The development of appropriate animal models allows scientists to ask highly specific questions about any region of the AT. Moreover, responses to questions can be measured by only changing one variable at a time. Another key advantage of animal models is the highly homogeneous population, which reduces variability between animals, ensuring an accurate reflection of the damage that is occurring within the AT. Over the last several decades, there has been an increase in both the variety and complexity of these animal models, from basic survival endpoints to examining specialized biomarkers of damage. There have been too many experiments to name them all and their authors; however, a brief summary of the history of animal models of AT mucositis is given in Figure 18.2. It is important to recognize that animal models are highly dynamic, moving between injury-inducing agents and combinations of therapies over time. Below we have described several of the most frequently published models.

ORAL MUCOSITIS ANIMAL MODELS

Wolfgang Dorr and colleagues (27–31) developed a radiation mouse model in the early 1990s (Figure 18.2), which involves irradiating the tongue and snout. This animal

Dorr and colleagues
- Established early 1990s
- Fractionated radiotherapy to tongue and snout
- Model used to assess mucosal response to RT, CT, and targeted therapies and combinations thereof
- Also used to assess effects of agents such as amifostine and palifermin on mucosal damage

Sonis and colleagues
- Established early 1990s; in male Golden Syrian hamster
- Model uses buccal cheek pouches to asess mucosal response to therapy (5-FU plus mechanical irritation of the mucosa)
- Model allowed for development of five-phase model of mucositis (Figure 18.1)
- Also used to assess effects of agents such as EGF, TGF-β, IL-11, velafermin, and palifermin on mucosal damage

Keefe and colleagues
- Established mid-1990s; in Dark Agouti rat
- Isogenic tumor allows for assessment of tumor protection with potential anti-mucotoxic agents
- Model used to assess AT mucositis in response to CT and fractionated RT

Hauer-Jensen and colleagues
- Established early 1990s; in Sprague-Dawley rat
- Model for accelerated fractionated RT on small intestine — by attaching intestinal loop to scrotum following bilateral orchidectomy

Keefe and colleagues
- Established mid-2000s; in albino Wistar rat
- Model assesses toxicity of certain TKIs on AT mucosa following CT

Figure 18.2. Animal models of AT mucositis. AT, alimentary tract; RT, radiotherapy; CT, chemotherapy; 5-FU, 5-fluorouracil; EGF, epithelial growth factor; TGF-β, transformation growth factor beta; IL, interleukin; TKIs, tyrosine kinase inhibitors.

model results in mucosal ulceration within the treatment field of the lower tongue surface, corresponding to confluent mucositis or grade 3 of the classification of the Radiation Therapy Oncology Group/European Organization for Research and Treatment of Cancer. The mouse radiation model accurately assesses mucosal response to treatment and has been used to test a variety of agents, including keratinocyte growth factor (palifermin) (29,30,32–34), sodium selenite (35), and amifostine (36). In addition, it has been used to investigate the effects of combining targeted therapy, with an epidermal growth factor (EGF) receptor tyrosine kinase inhibitor (TKI), and radiation on the mucosal response (37), which is extremely important in the new era of combination therapies. The evolution of this model has also seen it being used extensively to investigate the effects of combined chemotherapy and radiotherapy (32,38). In addition, it has enabled detailed studies to be conducted comparing effects of single-dose and fractionated radiotherapy on the head (34,39–42).

The second model that has significantly advanced the understanding of the mechanisms of oral mucositis is the hamster model, which was first described in 1990 (43) (Figure 18.2). This model of AT mucositis uses male golden Syrian hamsters, as unlike other rodents, they have a buccal cheek pouch that is susceptible to chemotherapy when scratched. Mucositis is induced by the administration of 5-fluorouracil at 60 mg/kg on three days (days 0, 5, and 10). The buccal pouch mucosa is superficially irritated (mechanically scratched) on days 1, 2, and 3, resulting in mucositis in most of the animals (43). The publication of this model revolutionized research into chemotherapy-induced mucositis. However, perhaps more importantly, the development of this model allowed for the current working five-phase hypothesis of mucositis (Figure 18.1) to be developed (17,18). In addition, this model has been used to test many agents, including EGF (44), transforming growth factor beta (45), IL-11 (22,46,47), keratinocyte growth factor (palifermin), velafermin (fibroblast growth factor 20, FGF-20) (48,49), among others (50).

GASTROINTESTINAL MUCOSITIS ANIMAL MODELS

The DAMA (*D*ark *A*gouti Rat *M*ammary *A*denocarcinoma) Model of AT Mucositis

The development of the DAMA model of AT mucositis occurred in the mid-1990s (12) (Figure 18.2). Unlike other previously described animal models, this model is unique as it is capable of modeling the changes that occur in the human AT distal to the mouth following insult with chemotherapy (13). An important advantage that the DAMA model has over the other models is the isogenic tumor that allows simultaneous assessment of tumor protection, a major concern with any potential anti-mucotoxin under development. There is excellent homogeneity between all animals in tumor growth and response to chemotherapy. This model has been used extensively to determine mechanisms underlying AT following a variety of different chemotherapeutic agents (21,51–61). More recently, the DAMA model of AT mucositis has been modified to study fractionated radiotherapy. In a small pilot study, a 6-week fractionated radiotherapy course (total 45 Gy/18 fractions/6 weeks treating at a radiation dose of 2.5 Gy/fraction) (62) was given to DA rats and the resulting subacute and acute injury profile determined. Fractionated radiotherapy induced gut changes from as early as week 1 (i.e., 7.5 Gy), with severe injury seen in the small intestine at later time points (62). Furthermore, many of the changes that were induced by fractionated radiotherapy were identical to those induced by chemotherapy (62), adding considerable weight to the current five-phase AT mucositis hypothesis (17,18).

MUCOSITIS MODEL FOR NATURAL THERAPIES

A variation of the DA rat mucositis model has also been used to study natural-based anti-mucotoxic agents (63). By administering methotrexate three times daily, AT damage and bacterial translocation can be induced and studied in this non–tumor-bearing model (63–66). Using this model, investigators have extensively studied the mechanisms of action of the potential mucotoxic agent, whey-derived growth factor extract (67–69), a by-product of cheese production (63,68,69). In addition, this model has also been used to investigate the mechanisms of damage following abdominal radiation in the DA rat (70–72). Rats receive a single 10 Gy dose of radiation to the abdomen, inducing significant AT radiation enteritis. A variety of markers including growth curves, intestinal weight, and mucosal morphometry can then be investigated 4 days later (70–72).

FRACTIONATED RADIOTHERAPY MODEL OF ACUTE AND CHRONIC MUCOSAL INJURY

Hauer-Jensen and colleagues (73) have developed another animal model detailing accelerated fractionation on radiation injury of the small intestine (Figure 18.2). This model allows investigation of both acute radiation AT damage at 2 weeks and chronic radiation AT damage at 26 weeks following completion of treatment. This animal model is unique in that a segment of small intestine is transposed and fixed to the scrotum following bilateral orchidectomy. This intestinal loop can then be subjected to repeated irradiation at varying time points and Gy (73). By using this model, scientists have been able to demonstrate that the changes occurring in the acute phase of damage are associated with the severity of damage seen long term (73,74).

TARGETED THERAPIES MODEL OF AT MUCOSITIS

The newest area of development for investigating AT toxicities following cytotoxic therapy is in the field of small molecule TKIs. A new animal model of lapatinib-induced diarrhea and mucosal injury has been developed using Albino Wistar rats to study mechanisms and potential interventions (75) (Figure 18.2). This model capitalizes on the appropriate drug metabolic enzyme profile of the Wistar rats for investigating TKIs, which are metabolized predominantly through the CYP3A4 pathway. Briefly, animals can be administered with daily oral lapatinib for 4 weeks, with or without concurrent weekly chemotherapy, and changes along the length of the AT can be assessed. Emerging findings from this new model indicate that intervention agents that protect the local small intestinal mucosa could prove effective in preventing TKI-induced diarrhea.

SUCCESSES AND FAILURES OF TRANSLATED AGENTS

Anti-mucotoxic agents progress from discovery, to animal models, to clinical trials in the hope of being the next palifermin, the first and only agent currently approved for the prevention of oral mucositis. In animal models, palifermin was shown to protect against mucositis by improving weight loss and crypt survival (76), protecting the oral mucosa (30,33,34), and reducing diarrhea and mortality (77). In the clinical setting, studies have consistently shown benefit in patients receiving palifermin, with less severe and shorter duration oral mucositis (78,79). Palifermin is used clinically for patients receiving hematopoietic stem cell transplantation for hematological malignancies, and more recently, it has been investigated in head and neck cancer (80) and sarcoma patients (81), with generally positive results. However, palifermin has yet to be approved for standard multi-cycle chemotherapy and may possibly be limited by oral mucosal thickening.

Many other agents have progressed from animal models of mucositis to early clinical trials, with varying degrees of success. Just to name a few, these include VSL#3 (82), IL-11 (83), low-level lasers (84,85), amifostine (86,87), glutamine (88,89), and various herbal-based agents. While many are still under further investigation, a number of agents have failed at the clinical trial level by not adequately reaching clinical endpoints. One example is velafermin, a recombinant human FGF-20 that did not reach its primary endpoint (reduced incidence of severe oral mucositis) in the phase II dose-confirmatory trial of hematologic cancer patients receiving autologous stem cell transplantation. This highlights the issue of success in animal models not always translating to the clinic, which may be due to a variety of issues of which a few are outlined below.

DIFFICULTIES OF ANIMAL MODELS IN AT MUCOSITIS RESEARCH

Animal models have played fundamental roles in furthering our understanding of AT mucositis. However, it would be naïve to suggest that animal models provide all of the answers for the clinical setting. Each model has its own series of difficulties and limitations. The hamster model has the confounding issue of wound healing, as although hamsters have cheek pouches and AT mucositis can be induced by following chemotherapy (43) or radiotherapy (22), the cheek pouch needs to be "mechanically" scratched or irritated in order to induce the ulcerative lesions. In humans, however, the oral mucosa does not need to be "mechanically" scratched in order to induce ulcerative lesions, and so this model is not exactly the same as the clinical setting. Additionally, this irritation may also result in wound healing mechanisms being initiated. Difficulties also arise in the DAMA model of AT mucositis. In the rat, visible oral mucositis does not occur due to the highly keratinized nature of the epithelium. This makes it difficult to successfully investigate oral mucositis using this model. Furthermore, squamous epithelium is present within the rat stomach, which can lead to reduction in oral intake when keratinocyte growth factor, a stimulator of epithelial growth, is used. Rats do not have an emetogenic reflex, and since some vomiting is a manifestation of mucosal injury, this is a disadvantage. However, it is possible to use pica as an indirect marker for nausea (90).

In all animal models, dose and scheduling issues of the cytotoxic agents are also important. The doses used in most animal models do not always translate into humans, as there may be species differences in susceptibility to different agents. The route of administration of chemotherapy has important implications for drug metabolism. In the DAMA model of AT mucositis, intravenous administration of cytotoxic agents is extremely difficult, with administration into the tail vein especially difficult due to the skin pigmentation. This means that investigation into AT mucositis induced by drugs administered via this route is not often undertaken. Although all chemotherapeutic drugs cause damage (91–94), the underlying mechanisms behind how they do this may be different. Furthermore, the traditional mg/kg dosing of rodents is not often used in humans, where (for reasons that are not always logical) body surface area dosing is most commonly used. This highlights that despite similarities, animal models are never identical to humans, and there will always be issues with translation from animal to human research.

Other contributing factors also cause difficulties in animal research. These include stresses in the animals from isolation due to experimental procedures, the need to anesthetize animals on a regular basis and the effect that this has on mucosal homeostasis, and the efficacy of any investigative drugs on tumor load. Toxicities associated with cancer treatment include those that are localized or regional (ulcers, xerostomia, abdominal pain, and malabsorption) and those that are more generalized or systemic (fatigue, lack of appetite, nausea, and cognitive impairment) (95). The recent realization of concurrent tissue-based and systemic toxicities has resulted in the new paradigm of toxicity clustering (96). Interestingly, the proof of principle testing for this new way of thinking was carried out in cancer patients (96). Translational research in the laboratory using animal testing is now occurring, in order to examine in greater detail some of the initial findings. Looking at multiple toxicities in combination will add new knowledge in the area as well as uncover new challenges in applying the models.

Another important issue with the use of animal modes is strain and sex differences in metabolic enzyme profiles for xenobiotics, particularly CYP family members (97,98). Differences in the metabolic enzyme profiles can lead to a profound impact on drug clearance and therefore toxicity of agents at equivalent doses. Careful consideration of the animal model and the drugs to be administered is paramount for a successful animal trial.

SUMMARY

To summarize, AT mucositis is an extremely common side effect following cancer chemotherapy and radiotherapy occurring in a large percentage of patients. This chapter has described the use of a variety of different animal models currently in use to investigate the clinical problem of AT mucositis. The strong relationship between animal investigation and translation to the clinical setting has provided a unique opportunity to conduct effective research in what continues to be a major problem. With continuing dedication to research and drug development in this area, alleviating mucositis by using anti-mucotoxins may lead to increased maximum tolerated doses of chemotherapy or radiotherapy and improve the quality of life for cancer patients both during and after treatment. This is extremely important, as mucositis is expected to increase due to the aging population and the introduction of more targeted therapy agents that have significant oral and gastrointestinal complications. Research needs to continue to focus on developing anti-mucotoxins that are both effective and safe. Identification of therapeutic targets and development of these novel agents require well-validated and clinically relevant animal models to be employed. The future will see more anti-mucotoxic agents reach clinical trials in a broader range of therapeutic settings, in particular targeted therapies and multimodality regimens.

REFERENCES

1. Sonis ST, Elting LS, Keefe D, et al. Perspectives on cancer therapy-induced mucosal injury: pathogenesis, measurement, epidemiology, and consequences for patients. *Cancer.* 2004;100(9 suppl):1995-2025.
2. Elting LS, Cooksley C, Chambers M, Cantor SB, Manzullo E, Rubenstein EB. The burdens of cancer therapy. Clinical and economic outcomes of chemotherapy-induced mucositis. *Cancer.* 2003;98(7):1531-1539.
3. Elting LS, Cooksley CD, Chambers MS, Garden AS. Risk, outcomes, and costs of radiation-induced oral mucositis among patients with head-and-neck malignancies. *Int J Radiat Oncol Biol Phys.* 2007;68(4):1110-1120.
4. Keefe DMK. Mucositis management in patients with cancer. *Support Cancer Ther.* 2006;3(3):154-157.
5. Bowen JM, Gibson RJ, Keefe DMK, Cummins AG. Cytotoxic chemotherapy increases proapoptotic Bax and Bak expression in crypts of the rat and human small intestine. *Pathology.* 2005;37(1):56-62.
6. Gibson RJ, Keefe DMK. Cancer chemotherapy-induced diarrhoea and constipation: mechanisms of damage and prevention strategies. *Support Care Cancer.* 2006;14(9):890-900.
7. Keefe DMK, Gibson RJ, Hauer-Jensen M. Gastrointestinal mucositis. *Semin Oncol Nurs.* 2004;20(1):38-47.
8. Sonis ST. Mucositis as a biological process: a new hypothesis for the development of chemotherapy-induced stomatotoxicity. *Oral Oncol.* 1998;34(1):39-43.
9. Shaw MT, Spector MH, Ladman AJ. Effects of cancer, radiotherapy and cytotoxic drugs on intestinal structure and function. *Cancer Treat Rev.* 1979;6(3):141-151.
10. Trier JS, Browning TH. Morphologic response of the mucosa of human small intestine to x-ray exposure. *J Clin Invest.* 1966;45(2):194-204.
11. Keefe DMK, Cummins AG, Dale BM, Kotasek D, Robb TA, Sage RE. Effect of high-dose chemotherapy on intestinal permeability in humans. *Clin Sci.* 1997;92(4):385-389.
12. Keefe DMK. *The Effect of Cytotoxic Chemotherapy on the Mucosa of the Small Intestine* [dissertation]. Adelaide: Department of Medicine, University of Adelaide; 1998.
13. Keefe DMK, Brealey J, Goland GJ, Cummins AG. Chemotherapy for cancer causes apoptosis that precedes hypoplasia in crypts of the small intestine in humans. *Gut.* 2000;47(5):632-637.

14. Gibson RJ, Cummins AG, Bowen JM, Logan RM, Healey T, Keefe DMK. Apoptosis occurs early in the basal layer of the oral mucosa following cancer chemotherapy. *Asia-Pac J Clin Oncol.* 2006;2(1):39-49.

15. Wilkes JD. Prevention and treatment of oral mucositis following cancer chemotherapy. *Semin Oncol.* 1998;25:538-551.

16. Sonis A, Sonis S. Oral complications of cancer chemotherapy in pediatric patients. *J Pedod.* 1979;3(2):122-128.

17. Sonis ST. A biological approach to mucositis. *J Support Oncol.* 2004;2(1):21-32; discussion 35-36.

18. Sonis ST. The pathobiology of mucositis. *Nat Rev Cancer.* 2004;4(4):277-284.

19. Marshman E, Ottewell PD, Potten CS, Watson AJ. Caspase activation during spontaneous and radiation-induced apoptosis in the murine intestine. *J Pathol.* 2001;195(3):285-292.

20. Criswell T, Leskov K, Miyamoto S, Luo G, Boothman DA. Transcription factors activated in mammalian cells after clinically relevant doses of ionizing radiation. *Oncogene.* 2003;22(37):5813-5827.

21. Bowen JM, Gibson RJ, Tsykin A, Stringer AM, Logan RM, Keefe DMK. Gene expression analysis of multiple gastrointestinal regions reveals activation of common cell regulatory pathways following cytotoxic chemotherapy. *Int J Cancer.* 2007;121(8):1847-1856.

22. Sonis ST, Peterson RL, Edwards LJ, et al. Defining mechanisms of action of interleukin-11 on the progression of radiation-induced oral mucositis in hamsters. *Oral Oncol.* 2000;36(4):373-381.

23. Sonis ST. The biologic role for nuclear factor-kappaB in disease and its potential involvement in mucosal injury associated with anti-neoplastic therapy. *Crit Rev Oral Biol Med.* 2002;13(5):380-389.

24. Al-Dasooqi N, Gibson RJ, Bowen JM, Logan RM, Stringer AM, Keefe DMK. Matrix metalloproteinases are possible mediators for the development of alimentary tract mucositis in the dark agouti rat. *Exp Biol Med (Maywood).* 2010;235(10):1244-1256.

25. Engels-Deutsch M, Pini A, Yamashita Y, et al. Insertional inactivation of pac and rmlB genes reduces the release of tumor necrosis factor alpha, interleukin-6, and interleukin-8 induced by *Streptococcus mutans* in monocytic, dental pulp, and periodontal ligament cells. *Infect Immun.* 2003;71(9):5169-5177.

26. Keefe DMK. Gastrointestinal mucositis: a new biological model. *Support Care Cancer.* 2004;12(1):6-9.

27. Dorr W, Baumann M, Herrmann T. Radiation-induced lung damage: a challenge for radiation biology, experimental and clinical radiotherapy. *Int J Radiat Biol.* 2000;76(4):443-446.

28. Dorr W, Hamilton CS, Boyd T, Reed B, Denham JW. Radiation-induced changes in cellularity and proliferation in human oral mucosa. *Int J Radiat Oncol Biol Phys.* 2002;52(4):911-917.

29. Dorr W, Reichel S, Spekl K. Effects of keratinocyte growth factor (palifermin) administration protocols on oral mucositis (mouse) induced by fractionated irradiation. *Radiother Oncol.* 2005;75(1):99-105.

30. Dorr W, Spekl K, Farrell CL. Amelioration of acute oral mucositis by keratinocyte growth factor: fractionated irradiation. *Int J Radiat Oncol Biol Phys.* 2002;54(1):245-251.

31. Dorr W, Spekl K, Martin M. Radiation-induced mucositis in mice: strain differences. *Cell Prolif.* 2002;35(suppl 1):60-67.

32. Dorr W, Heider K, Spekl K. Reduction of oral mucositis by palifermin (rHuKGF): dose-effect of rHuKGF. *Int J Radiat Biol.* 2005;81(8):557-565.

33. Dorr W, Noack R, Spekl K, Farrell CL. Modification of oral mucositis by keratinocyte growth factor: single radiation exposure. *Int J Radiat Biol.* 2001;77(3):341-347.

34. Dorr W, Spekl K, Farrell CL. The effect of keratinocyte growth factor on healing of manifest radiation ulcers in mouse tongue epithelium. *Cell Prolif.* 2002;35(suppl 1):86-92.

35. Gehrisch A, Dorr W. Effects of systemic or topical administration of sodium selenite on early radiation effects in mouse oral mucosa. *Strahlenther Onkol.* 2007;183(1):36-42.

36. Fleischer G, Dorr W. Amelioration of early radiation effects in oral mucosa (mouse) by intravenous or subcutaneous administration of amifostine. *Strahlenther Onkol.* 2006;182(10):567-575.

37. Fehrmann A, Dorr W. Effect of EGFR-inhibition on the radiation response of oral mucosa: experimental studies in mouse tongue epithelium. *Int J Radiat Biol.* 2005;81(6):437-443.

38. Dorr W, Hirler E, Honig M. Response of mouse tongue epithelium to single doses of bleomycin and radiation. *Radiother Oncol.* 1993;27(3):237-244.

39. Kilic Y, Rajewski K, Dorr W. Effect of post-exposure administration of keratinocyte growth factor (Palifermin) on radiation effects in oral mucosa in mice. *Radiat Environ Biophys.* 2007;46(1):13-19.

40. Haagen J, Krohn H, Rollig S, Schmidt M, Wolfram K, Dorr W. Effect of selective inhibitors of inflammation on oral mucositis: preclinical studies. *Radiother Oncol.* 2009;92(3):472-476.

41. Dorr W, Schlichting S, Bray MA, Flockhart IR, Hopewell JW. Effects of dexpanthenol with or without Aloe vera extract on radiation-induced oral mucositis: preclinical studies. *Int J Radiat Biol.* 2005;81(3):243-250.

42. Pabst S, Spekl K, Dorr W. Changes in the effect of dose fractionation during daily fractionated irradiation: studies in mouse oral mucosa. *Int J Radiat Oncol Biol Phys.* 2004;58(2):485-492.

43. Sonis ST, Tracey C, Shklar G, Jenson J, Florine D. An animal model for mucositis induced by cancer chemotherapy. *Oral Surg Oral Med Oral Pathol.* 1990;69(4):437-443.

44. Sonis ST, Costa JW Jr, Evitts SM, Lindquist LE, Nicolson M. Effect of epidermal growth factor on ulcerative mucositis in hamsters that receive cancer chemotherapy. *Oral Surg Oral Med Oral Pathol.* 1992;74(6):749-755.

45. Sonis ST, Van Vugt AG, Brien JP, et al. Transforming growth factor-beta 3 mediated modulation of cell cycling and attenuation of 5-fluorouracil induced oral mucositis. *Oral Oncol.* 1997;33(1):47-54.

46. Sonis S, Edwards L, Lucey C. The biological basis for the attenuation of mucositis: the example of interleukin-11. *Leukemia.* 1999;13(6):831-834.

47. Sonis ST, Van Vugt AG, McDonald J, et al. Mitigating effects of interleukin 11 on consecutive courses of 5-fluorouracil-induced ulcerative mucositis in hamsters. *Cytokine.* 1997;9(8):605-612.

48. Ara G, Watkins BA, Zhong H, et al. Velafermin (rhFGF-20) reduces the severity and duration of hamster cheek pouch mucositis induced by fractionated radiation. *Int J Radiat Biol.* 2008;84(5):401-412.

49. Alvarez E, Fey EG, Valax P, et al. Preclinical characterization of CG53135 (FGF-20) in radiation and concomitant chemotherapy/radiation-induced oral mucositis. *Clin Cancer Res.* 2003;9:3454-3461.

50. Loury D, Embree JR, Steinberg DA, Sonis ST, Fiddes JC. Effect of local application of the antimicrobial peptide IB-367 on the incidence and severity of oral mucositis in hamsters. *Oral Surg Oral Med Oral Pathol Oral Radiol Endod.* 1999;87(5):544-551.

51. Bowen JM, Gibson RJ, Cummins AG, Keefe DMK. Intestinal mucositis: the role of the Bcl-2 family, p53 and caspases in chemotherapy-induced damage. *Support Care Cancer.* 2006;14(7):713-731

52. Bowen JM, Gibson RJ, Tsykin A, Cummins AG, Keefe DMK. Irinotecan changes gene expression profiles in the small intestine of the rat with breast cancer. *Cancer Chemother Pharmacol.* 2007;59:337-348.

53. Bowen JM, Gibson RJ, Stringer AM, et al. Role of p53 in irinotecan-induced intestinal cell death and mucosal damage. *Anticancer Drugs.* 2007;18(2):197-210.

54. Gibson RJ, Bowen JM, Alvarez E, Finnie JW, Keefe DMK. Establishment of a single dose irinotecan model of gastrointestinal mucositis. *Chemotherapy.* 2007;53:360-369.

55. Gibson RJ, Bowen JM, Cummins AG, Keefe DMK. Relationship between dose of methotrexate, apoptosis, p53/p21 expression and intestinal crypt proliferation in the rat. *Clin Exp Med.* 2005;4(4):188-195.

56. Gibson RJ, Bowen JM, Inglis MR, Cummins AG, Keefe DMK. Irinotecan causes severe small intestinal damage, as well as colonic damage, in the rat with implanted breast cancer. *J Gastroenterol Hepatol.* 2003;18(9):1095-1100.

57. Stringer AM, Gibson RJ, Bowen JM, Keefe DMK. Chemotherapy-induced modifications to gastrointestinal microflora: evidence and implications of change. *Curr Drug Metab.* 2009;10(1):79-83.

58. Stringer AM, Gibson RJ, Bowen JM, et al. Irinotecan-induced mucositis manifesting as diarrhoea corresponds with an amended intestinal flora and mucin profile. *Int J Exp Pathol.* 2009;90(5):489-499.

59. Stringer AM, Gibson RJ, Bowen JM, Logan RM, Yeoh AS, Keefe DMK. Chemotherapy-induced mucositis: the role of gastrointestinal microflora and mucins in the luminal environment. *J Support Oncol.* 2007;5(6):259-267.

60. Stringer AM, Gibson RJ, Logan RM, et al. Chemotherapy-induced diarrhea is associated with changes in the luminal environment in the DA rat. *Exp Biol Med (Maywood).* 2007;232(1):96-106.

61. Stringer AM, Gibson RJ, Logan RM, et al. Irinotecan-induced mucositis is associated with changes in intestinal mucins. *Cancer Chemother Pharmacol.* 2009;64(1):123-132.

62. Yeoh AS, Gibson RJ, Yeoh EE, et al. A novel animal model to investigate fractionated radiotherapy-induced alimentary mucositis: the role of apoptosis, p53, nuclear factor-kappaB, COX-1, and COX-2. *Mol Cancer Ther.* 2007;6(8):2319-2327.

63. Howarth G, Francis GL, Cool JC, Xu X, Byard RW, Read LC. Milk growth factors enriched from cheese whey ameliorate intestinal damage by methotrexate when administered orally to rats. *J Nutr.* 1996;126(10):2519-2530.

64. Howarth GS, Cool JC, Bourne AJ, Ballard FJ, Read LC. Insulin-like growth factor-I (IGF-I) stimulates regrowth of the damaged intestine in rats, when administered following, but not concurrent with, methotrexate. *Growth Factors.* 1998;15(4):279-292.

65. Xian CJ, Couper R, Howarth GS, Read LC, Kallincos NC. Increased expression of HGF and c-met in rat small intestine during recovery from methotrexate-induced mucositis. *Br J Cancer.* 2000;82(4):945-952.

66. Xian CJ, Howarth GS, Mardell CE, et al. Temporal changes in TFF3 expression and jejunal morphology during methotrexate-induced damage and repair. *Am J Physiol.* 1999;277(4 pt 1):G785-G795.

67. Howarth GS, Francis GL, Cool JC, Xu X, Byard RW, Read LC. Milk growth factors enriched from cheese whey ameliorate intestinal damage by methotrexate when administered orally to rats. *J Nutr.* 1996;126(10):2519-2530.

68. Clarke JM, Butler R, Howarth GS, Read LC, Regester GO. Exposure of oral mucosa to bioactive milk factors reduces severity of chemotherapy-induced mucositis in the hamster. *Oral Oncol.* 2002;38:478-485.

69. Tran CD, Howarth GS, Coyle P, Philcox JC, Rofe AM, Butler RN. Dietary supplementation with zinc and a growth factor extract derived from bovine cheese whey improves methotrexate-damaged rat intestine. *Am J Clin Nutr.* 2003;77(5):1296-1303.

70. Fraser R, Frisby C, Blackshaw LA, Schirmer M, Howarth G, Yeoh E. Small intestinal dysmotility following abdominal irradiation in the rat small intestine. *Neurogastroenterol Motil.* 1998;10(5):413-419.

71. Fraser R, Frisby C, Schirmer M, et al. Divergence of mucosal and motor effects of insulin-like growth factor (IGF)-I and LR3IGF-I on rat isolated ileum following abdominal irradiation. *J Gastroenterol Hepatol.* 2000;15(10):1132-1137.

72. Howarth GS, Fraser R, Frisby CL, Schirmer MB, Yeoh EK. Effects of insulin-like growth factor-I administration on radiation enteritis in rats. *Scand J Gastroenterol.* 1997;32(11):1118-1124.

73. Hauer-Jensen M, Poulakos L, Osborne JW. Effects of accelerated fractionation on radiation injury of the small intestine: a new rat model. *Int J Radiat Oncol Biol Phys.* 1988;14(6):1205-1212.

74. Hauer-Jensen M. Late radiation injury of the small intestine. Clinical, pathophysiologic and radiobiologic aspects. A review. *Acta Oncol.* 1990;29(4):401-415.

75. Bowen JM, Darby J, Plews E, Stringer AM, Boyle F, Keefe DMK. Characterisation of EGF receptor tyrosine kinase inhibitor-induced diarrhoea. Multinational Association for Supportive Care in Cancer (MASCC) Symposium; Vancouver; June 24-26 2010.

76. Farrell CL, Bready JV, Rex KL, et al. Keratinocyte growth factor protects mice from chemotherapy and radiation-induced gastrointestinal injury and mortality. *Cancer Res.* 1998;58(5):933-939.

77. Gibson RJ, Bowen JM, Keefe DMK. Palifermin reduces diarrhea and increases survival following irinotecan treatment in tumor-bearing DA rats. *Int J Cancer.* 2005;116(3):464-470.

78. Meropol NJ, Somer RA, Gutheil J, et al. Randomized phase I trial of recombinant keratinocyte growth factor plus chemotherapy: potential role as a mucosal protectant. *J Clin Oncol.* 2003;21(8):1452-1458.

79. Speilberger RT, Stiff P, Bensinger W, et al. Palifermin for oral mucositis after intensive therapy for hematological malignancies. *N Engl J Med.* 2004;351:2590-2598.

80. Brizel DM, Murphy BA, Rosenthal DI, et al. Phase II study of palifermin and concurrent chemoradiation in head and neck squamous cell carcinoma. *J Clin Oncol.* 2008;26(15):2489-2496.

81. Vadhan-Raj S, Trent J, Patel S, et al. Single-dose palifermin prevents severe oral mucositis during multicycle chemotherapy in patients with cancer: a randomized trial. *Ann Intern Med.* 2010;153(6):358-367.

82. Delia P, Sansotta G, Donato V, et al. Prevention of radiation-induced diarrhea with the use of VSL#3, a new high-potency probiotic preparation. *Am J Gastroenterol.* 2002;97(8):2150-2152.

83. Tepler I, Elias L, Smith JW 2nd, et al. A randomized placebo-controlled trial of recombinant human interleukin-11 in cancer patients with severe thrombocytopenia due to chemotherapy. *Blood.* 1996;87(9):3607-3614.

84. Schubert MM, Eduardo FP, Guthrie KA, et al. A phase III randomized double-blind placebo-controlled clinical trial to

determine the efficacy of low level laser therapy for the prevention of oral mucositis in patients undergoing hematopoietic cell transplantation. *Support Care Cancer.* 2007;15(10):1145-1154.

85. Zanin T, Zanin F, Carvalhosa AA, et al. Use of 660-nm diode laser in the prevention and treatment of human oral mucositis induced by radiotherapy and chemotherapy. *Photomed Laser Surg.* 2010;28(2):233-237.

86. Anne PR. Phase II trial of subcutaneous amifostine in patients undergoing radiation therapy for head and neck cancer. *Semin Oncol.* 2002;29(6 suppl 19):80-83.

87. Law A, Kennedy T, Pellitteri P, Wood C, Christie D, Yumen O. Efficacy and safety of subcutaneous amifostine in minimizing radiation-induced toxicities in patients receiving combined-modality treatment for squamous cell carcinoma of the head and neck. *Int J Radiat Oncol Biol Phys.* 2007;69(5):1361-1368.

88. Klimberg VS, Nwokedi E, Hutchins LF, et al. Glutamine facilitates chemotherapy while reducing toxicity. *JPEN J Parenter Enteral Nutr.* 1992;16(6 suppl):83S-87S.

89. Rubio IT, Cao Y, Hutchins LF, Westbrook KC, Klimberg VS. Effect of glutamine on methotrexate efficacy and toxicity. *Ann Surg.* 1998;227(5):772-778; discussion 778-780.

90. Vera G, Chiarlone A, Martin MI, Abalo R. Altered feeding behaviour induced by long-term cisplatin in rats. *Auton Neurosci.* 2006;126-127:81-92.

91. Ijiri K, Potten CS. Response of intestinal cells of differing topographical and hierarchical status to ten cytotoxic drugs and five sources of radiation. *Br J Cancer.* 1983;47(2):175-185.

92. Ijiri K, Potten CS. Radiation-hypersensitive cells in small intestinal crypts; their relationships to clonogenic cells. *Br J Cancer Suppl.* 1986;7:20-22.

93. Ijiri K, Potten CS. Further studies on the response of intestinal crypt cells of different hierarchical status to eighteen different cytotoxic agents. *Br J Cancer.* 1987;55(2):113-123.

94. Ijiri K, Potten CS. The circadian rhythm for the number and sensitivity of radiation-induced apoptosis in the crypts of mouse small intestine. *Int J Radiat Biol.* 1990;58(1):165-175.

95. Sonis S, Haddad R, Posner M, et al. Gene expression changes in peripheral blood cells provide insight into the biological mechanisms associated with regimen-related toxicities in patients being treated for head and neck cancers. *Oral Oncol.* 2007;43(3):289-300.

96. Bert B, Fink H, Sohr R, Rex A. Different effects of diazepam in Fischer rats and two stocks of Wistar rats in tests of anxiety. *Pharmacol Biochem Behav.* 2001;70(2-3):411-420.

97. Kawase A, Fujii A, Negoro M, et al. Differences in cytochrome P450 and nuclear receptor mRNA levels in liver and small intestines between SD and DA rats. *Drug Metab Pharmacokinet.* 2008;23(3):196-206.

98. Staack RF, Paul LD, Springer D, Kraemer T, Maurer HH. Cytochrome P450 dependent metabolism of the new designer drug 1-(3-trifluoromethylphenyl)piperazine (TFMPP). In vivo studies in Wistar and Dark Agouti rats as well as in vitro studies in human liver microsomes. *Biochem Pharmacol.* 2004;67(2):235-244.

CHAPTER 19

Oral Manifestations and Complications of Cancer Therapy

Eliezer Soto ■ Jane M. Fall-Dickson ■ Ann M. Berger

The effectiveness of cancer therapies designed to improve cure rates and/or to extend survival time, including chemotherapy (CT), radiation therapy (RT), and conditioning regimens used in the hematopoietic stem cell transplantation (HSCT) setting, is tempered by side effects that may become intolerable and/or life-threatening. Oral complications are one such side effect and include CT- and RT-related oral mucositis and associated oropharyngeal pain, xerostomia, and oral infection, and oral chronic graft-versus-host disease (cGVHD). The pathogenesis of and management strategies for these oral complications, and future clinical research directions, are presented in this chapter.

ORAL MUCOSITIS

Oral mucositis is an inflammation of the mucous membranes of the oral cavity and oropharynx characterized by tissue erythema, edema, and atrophy, often progressing to ulceration (1). The clinical significance of CT- and RT-related oral mucositis as a dose- and treatment-limiting side effect is well appreciated (2). It is a painful and debilitating side effect that not only interferes with further treatment options but also causes a significant impairment in patient's quality of life and functional status (3,4).

The frequency and severity of oral mucositis are influenced by numerous patient- and treatment-related risk factors (Table 19.1) (5,6). Risk factors for CT-related oral mucositis are complex, and study results have been conflicting throughout the years. For example, although younger patients are considered at increased risk for oral mucositis, and women have been reported to have more severe oral mucositis more frequently than men, Driezen (7) reported no age or gender risk factors for development of this oral condition. Children are three times more likely than adults to develop oral mucositis because of a higher proliferating fraction of basal cells. Results from a sample of 332 ambulatory CT patients showed no significant differences in CT-induced oral mucositis incidence between outpatients who wore dental appliances, previously had oral lesions, used diverse oral hygiene and oral care practices, and had a history of smoking and those patients who did not (6). Conflicting study results may be related to lack of defined risk factors for subjects entering clinical trials (5).

Although the full spectrum of treatment-related risk factors for oral mucositis is not defined, known risk factors include continuous CT infusion therapy for breast and colon cancer (5-fluorouracil [5-FU] and leucovorin); administration of selected anthracyclines, alkylating agents, taxanes, vinca alkaloids, antimetabolites, and antitumor antibiotics; myeloablative conditioning regimens for HSCT (e.g., high-dose melphalan or carmustine, etoposide, cytarabine, and melphalan [BEAM]) (8–10); and RT to the head and neck. Individual drug metabolism affects oral mucositis incidence and severity, as seen with patients who are unable to adequately metabolize certain CT.

CT-INDUCED ORAL MUCOSITIS

Approximately 40% of CT patients develop oral mucositis (11), and approximately half of these patients develop severe, painful lesions requiring parenteral analgesia that may lead to treatment modification (12). Higher oral mucositis incidence rates of 60% are seen in the HSCT setting, with reported incidence rates of up to 78% for ulcerative oral mucositis (13). Oral mucositis is also a risk factor for infections, which may be life-threatening in neutropenic patients. Oral infections, such as herpes simplex virus (HSV) in particular, may increase oral mucositis severity. There is a four times greater relative risk of septicemia in patients with oral mucositis and oral infections when compared with patients without oral mucositis. This greater risk is due to mucosal barrier injury, which allows pathogen entry into the peripheral circulation.

The relationship between severe oral mucositis and clinical outcomes in patients receiving conditioning CT for HSCT has been analyzed in several studies (14,16). McCann et al. (15) performed an observational study in 197 patients with multiple myeloma (MM) or non-Hodgkin's lymphoma (NHL) undergoing either high-dose melphalan or BEAM CT, respectively. Parameters such as duration of pain score ≥4, opioid use, dysphagia score ≥4, total parenteral nutrition (TPN) use, incidence and/or duration of fever and infection, and duration of antibiotic use increased gradiently with maximum grade of oral mucositis. The presence of severe oral mucositis (World Health Organization [WHO] grades 3 and 4) increased the duration of TPN use by 2.7 days, opioids by 4.6 days, and antibiotics by 2.4 days, prolonging hospital stay by 2.3 days in MM patients, but not in NHL patients.

Oral mucositis presents with asymptomatic erythema and progresses from solitary, white, elevated desquamative patches that are slightly painful to large, contiguous, pseudomembranous, painful lesions. Histopathologically, edema of the rete pegs and vascular changes are observed. Typical oral sequelae of CT agents include epithelial hyperplasia,

TABLE 19.1	Cancer treatment- and patient-related risk factors for oral mucositis

Patient-Related

Age older than 65 y or younger than 20 y

Gender

Inadequate oral health and hygiene practices

Periodontal diseases

Microbial flora

Chronic low-grade mouth infections

Salivary gland secretory dysfunction

Herpes simplex virus infection

Inborn inability to metabolize chemotherapeutic agents effectively

Inadequate nutritional status

Exposure to oral stressors, including alcohol and smoking

Ill-fitting dental prostheses

Treatment-Related

Radiation therapy: dose; schedule

Chemotherapy: agent; dose; schedule

Myelosuppression

Neutropenia

Immunosuppression

Reduced secretory immunoglobulin A

Inadequate oral care during treatment

Infections of bacterial, viral, fungal origin

Use of antidepressants, opiates, antihypertensives, antihistamines, diuretics, and sedatives

Impairment of renal and/or hepatic function

Protein or calorie malnutrition and dehydration

Xerostomia

Source: Adapted from Barasch A, Peterson DE. Risk factors for ulcerative mucositis in cancer patients: unanswered questions. *Oral Oncol.* 2003;39:91–100; Dodd MJ, Miaskowski C, Shiba GH, et al. Risk factors for CT-induced oral mucositis: dental appliances, oral hygiene, previous oral lesion, and a history of smoking. *Cancer Invest.* 1999;17:278–284.

collagen and glandular degeneration and epithelial dysplasia, atrophy, and localized or diffuse mucosal ulceration. Nonkeratinized mucosal areas are most affected, including the labial, buccal, and soft palate mucosa; the floor of the mouth; and the ventral surface of the tongue. The loss of basement membrane epithelial cells exposes the underlying connective, innervated tissue stroma, which contributes to more severe oropharyngeal pain.

RADIATION-INDUCED STOMATITIS

Oral mucositis is virtually universal when RT targets the oropharyngeal area, with the severity dependent on the type of ionizing radiation, volume of irradiated tissue, daily and cumulative dose, and duration of RT. Oral mucositis is a dose- and rate-limiting toxicity of RT for head and neck cancer and of hyperfractionated RT and CT. Radiation interacts directly with DNA, leading to chromosome and cellular mitotic apparatus damage. Atrophic changes in the oral epithelium usually occur at total doses of 160 to 220 Gy, administered at a rate of 20 Gy/d (17). Doses higher than 600 Gy or concomitant CT place the patient at risk for permanent salivary gland changes (17,18). The addition of total-body irradiation to the HSCT treatment regimen increases oral mucositis severity through both direct mucosal damage and xerostomia.

CT-induced dental effects occur when the glands are within the treatment field and depend more on these effects than on direct irradiation of the teeth. Teeth in the irradiated field may be desensitized, leading to asymptomatic early caries. Therefore, daily fluoride application is necessary. Health care costs associated with oral mucositis in head and neck cancer patients are significant (19,20). In a prospective, longitudinal, multicenter study with 75 patients with head and neck cancer receiving RT with or without CT (20), 76% reported severe mouth and throat pain necessitating an increased number of visits to health care providers, 51% needed a feeding tube, and 37% were hospitalized with a mean stay of 4.9 days. These complications are directly correlated with a significant increase in resource use and excess costs.

RT-RELATED COMPLICATIONS

Long-term effects of head and neck RT include soft tissue fibrosis, obliterative endoarteritis, trismus, nonhealing or slow-healing mucosal ulcerations, and slow-healing dental extraction sites. RT-induced fibrotic changes may occur in the masticatory muscles and/or the temporal mandibular joint up to 1 year post-therapy, becoming more serious over time. Early phases of fibrogenesis following RT may be viewed through a wound healing model that is characterized by upregulation of tumor necrosis factor-alpha (TNFα) and other proinflammatory cytokines (21). However, as this radiation fibrogenic process continues over time, it functions as a nonhealing wound (21).

Osteoradionecrosis (ORN) is a relatively uncommon condition related to hypocellularity, hypovascularity, and tissue ischemia. Higher incidences are seen after total doses to the bone exceed 65 Gy (22). ORN is usually related to trauma such as dental extraction and may lead to pathologic fracture, infection of surrounding soft tissues, and severe pain. Most studies have reported ORN following tooth extractions that were not timed to allow adequate extraction site healing for 10 to 14 days before the start of RT. Osteonecrosis of the jaw bone has been strongly associated with the use of bisphosphonate therapy that is prescribed to treat malignancy-related hypercalcemia, bone metastasis, and metabolic bone diseases (23,24).

Oral candidiasis is a common acute and long-term oral sequela of head and neck RT. These candida lesions frequently present as angular cheilitis and may appear as white and removable, chronic hyperplastic (nonremovable) or chronic erythematous (diffuse patchy erythema).

CHRONIC GVHD ORAL MANIFESTATIONS

Patients who have undergone allogeneic HSCT frequently develop GVHD, an alloimmune condition derived from an immune attack mediated by donor T cells recognizing antigens expressed on normal tissues. GVHD occurs following allogeneic HSCT because of disparities in minor histocompatibility antigens between donor and recipient, inherited independently of human leukocyte antigen genes (25). Acute GVHD has been classified historically as

beginning within the first 100 days after allogeneic HSCT. Chronic GVHD may begin as early as 70 days or as late as 15 months after allogeneic transplant. Increased incidence of cGVHD may be related to the changing patterns of allogeneic HSCT.

The importance of oral cGVHD was recognized by the National Institutes of Health (NIH) Consensus Development Project on Criteria for Clinical Trials in cGVHD (26). Consensus documents have been published, including response criteria guidelines to measure clinical progression over time. The Schubert Oral Mucositis Rating Scale (OMRS) was validated under the auspices of this NIH Consensus Development Project (26). Treister et al. (27) analyzed inter- and intraobserver variability in the component and composite scores using the NIH oral cGVHD Activity Assessment Instrument. Twenty-four clinicians from six major HSCT centers scored high-quality intraoral photographs of 12 patients, followed by a second evaluation 1 week later. Although mean interrater reliability was poor to moderate and unacceptable for the clinical trial setting, greater concordance among the oral medicine experts, high intrarater reliability, and participant feedback suggest that formal training may decrease variability.

Approximately 80% of patients with extensive cGVHD have some type of oral involvement (28) that is a major contributing factor to the morbidity seen with allogeneic HSCT. Although oral lesions are most common in patients with extensive cGVHD, patients may also present with limited disease involving only the oral cavity. Oral cGVHD presents with tissue atrophy and erythema, lichenoid changes (hyperkeratotic striae, patches, plaques, and papules), and pseudomembranous ulcerations occurring typically on buccal and labial mucosa and the lateral tongue, angular stomatitis, and xerostomia (28). Treister et al. (29) correlated the distribution, type, and extent of lesions with patient-reported pain and discomfort. Almost all (93%) of ulcerations, 72% of erythematous lesions, and 76% of reticular lesions occurred on the buccal and labial mucosa and tongue. Ulcerations in the soft palate were uncommon and associated with increased pain. There was a statistically significant inverse relationship between the overall presence of ulceration and time since HSCT. Functional impact was significantly observed as restriction of oral intake due to discomfort. Decreased oral intake related to oral pain leads to serious clinical problems of weight loss and malnutrition.

Although oral cGHVD is one of the major long-term complications after allogenic HSCT, little is known about its pathogenesis. Imanguli et al. (30) have proposed a new pathogenic model of cGVHD in which production of type I interferon by plasmacytoid dendritic cells plays a central role in the initiation and continuation of cGVHD. Fall-Dickson et al. (31) have analyzed the relationship among clinical characteristics of oral cGVHD and related oral pain and dryness, salivary proinflammatory cytokine interleukin 6 (IL-6) and IL-Iα concentrations, and health-related quality of life. Salivary IL-6 was associated with oral cGVHD severity, oral ulceration, and erythema, suggesting its use as a potential biomarker of active oral cGVHD.

STRATEGIES FOR PREVENTION AND TREATMENT OF ORAL COMPLICATIONS

Pretherapy Dental Evaluation and Intervention

Oral/dental stabilization prior to CT and RT is critically important to avoid serious sequelae and requires an experienced dental team and informed patients working together to provide adequate cleaning, eliminate sites of oral infection and trauma, and promote appropriate oral hygiene (32). Many health care institution–specific policies and preventive approaches exist for oral care for CT and RT patients.

Patients scheduled for CT and/or head and neck RT should receive dental screening at least 2 weeks before therapy starts to allow for proper healing of extraction sites, recovery of soft tissue manipulations, and restoration of teeth. These activities promote optimal mucosal health before, during, and following cancer treatment. Oral hygiene is one of the most important screening areas for all patients, regardless of the type of cancer treatment modality. The initial dental appointment includes examination of the patient's dentition for carious lesions and defective restorations that may irritate the oral mucosa and necessitate replacement. The periodontium and pulp vitality must be evaluated. Periodontal status assessment includes measurement of pocket depth and assessment of furcation involvement. Denture fit assessment avoids ill-fitting dentures that may cause irritation of irradiated tissue and potential ulceration to underlying bone (33).

A panoramic radiograph combined with intraoral radiographs as needed is necessary to detect periodontal disease, periapical infections, cyst, third-molar pathology, unerupted or partially erupted teeth, and residual root tips. Significant oral/dental problems that should be addressed before cancer treatment begins include inappropriate oral hygiene, periapical pathology, third-molar pathology, periodontal disease, defective restorations, dental caries, orthodontic appliances, and ill-fitting prostheses. Bacterial load should be reduced prior to cancer treatment via root planning, scaling, and prophylaxis, excluding visible tumor located at the site of anticipated dental manipulation. Comprehensive evaluation also includes assessment of the oral mucosa and the alveolar process to prepare for possible future prosthetic intervention and to assess for ulcerations, fibromas, irritation, hyperplasia, bony spicules, and tori. The decision to extract asymptomatic teeth prior to the commencement of RT is related to several important factors, including radiation exposure, type, portal field, fractionization, and total dosage in addition to tumor prognosis, and expediency of control of the cancer (34). Lack of patient motivation regarding appropriate oral hygiene practices should lead to a decision to extract questionable teeth prior to RT. Teeth that are class II or III mobility without use as abutment teeth for prosthetic retention should also be considered for extraction before RT. Extractions of residual root tips and impacted teeth should be performed atraumatically. Alveolectomy and primary wound closure eliminate sharp ridges and bone spicules that could project to the overlying soft tissues. This is important for prosthetic consideration because negligible bone remodeling is predicted after RT.

Communication between the dentist, patient, and radiation therapist is important for successful healthy maintenance of the oral cavity. Patients are very susceptible to dental caries at the cervical areas of all teeth after RT to the head and neck region. Therefore, patient education is important regarding effective daily plaque removal through use of floss, a soft toothbrush, and fluoridated toothpaste at least three to four times a day. Patient and family education and counseling within the context of patient motivation are necessary to promote successful outcomes of preventive strategies. Patients often receive their cancer treatment in the ambulatory setting and need specific written instructions for appropriate use of oral care agents and instruments for effective daily plaque removal, use of prescribed fluoride treatments, and reportable oral observations and symptoms.

Assessment of the Oral Mucosa

Consistent and frequent oral cavity assessment is needed to assess clinical signs before, during, and after the treatment time course. An adequately intense white light is needed to visualize all soft and hard tissues and dentition. All assessors should have an appropriate knowledge base regarding clinical signs and symptoms of oral complications and the predicted negative sequelae. No standard grading system for severity of oral complications of cancer treatment exists. Numerous available oral complications' grading tools are based on two or more clinical parameters combined with functional status, such as eating ability. One commonly used tool is the National Cancer Institute Common Terminology Criteria for Adverse Events v3.0, which includes both descriptive terminology and a severity grading scale for each reportable adverse event (35). Other frequently used oral mucosal assessment tools are discussed in the subsequent text.

Oral Assessment Guide

The Oral Assessment Guide (OAG) (36) is a concise clinical tool to record oral cavity changes related to cancer therapy using eight assessment categories (voice, swallowing, lips, tongue, saliva, mucous membranes, gingiva, and teeth/dentures), each rated on three levels of descriptors: 1 = normal findings; 2 = mild alterations; and 3 = definitely compromised. The overall oral assessment score is the summation of the subscale score with a possible range of 8 to 24. Content-related validity, construct validity, clinical utility, and a high, trained nurse–nurse interrater reliability ($r = 0.912$) have been reported (36). The OAG has been used frequently to assess the efficacy of oral care protocols, to compare methods designed to determine the nature and prevalence of stomatitis, and to describe the incidence and severity of stomatitis.

World Health Organization Index

The WHO Index gives an overall rating of stomatitis and has frequently been used as a general comparison index to other oral assessment scales (37). The WHO Index is scaled as follows: grade 0 = no change; grade 1 = soreness, erythema; grade 2 = erythema, ulcers, can eat solids; and grade 3 = ulcers, requires liquid diet only; and grade 4 = alimentation not possible. Limitations of this instrument are the lack of reliability and validity data and also the tool's inability to capture the variety of oral changes that are observed with cancer treatment (37).

Oral Mucositis Rating Scale

The OMRS was developed as "… a research tool for the comprehensive measurement of a broad range of oral tissue changes associated with cancer therapy" (38). The OMRS was originally tested in 60 patients who were 180 to 500 days post peripheral blood stem cell transplantation (PBSCT), to examine the relationship between oral abnormalities and cGVHD (38). Findings demonstrated that oral manifestations and related sequelae most strongly associated with cGVHD included atrophy and erythema, lichenoid lesions located on the buccal and labial mucosa, and oral pain.

The item pool consists of 91 items covering 13 areas of the mouth that are assessed for several types of changes in 7 anatomic areas: lips; labial and buccal mucosa; tongue; floor of mouth; palate; and attached gingiva. Each site is divided into upper and lower (lips and labial mucosa), right and left (buccal mucosa), dorsal, ventral, and lateral (tongue), and hard and soft (palate). Descriptive categories are atrophy, pseudomembrane, erythema, hyperkeratosis, lichenoid, ulceration, and edema. Erythema, atrophy, hyperkeratosis, lichenoid, and edema are scored using scales of 0 to 3 (0 = normal/no change, 1 = mild change, 2 = moderate change, and 3 = severe change). Ulceration and pseudomembrane are rated by estimated surface area involved (0 = none, 1 = >0 but ≤1 cm², 2 = >1 cm² but ≤2 cm², and 3 = >2 cm²). The total possible score is the sum of all item scores with a possible range of 0 to 273. The OMRS has shown clinical and research utility (38).

Oral Mucositis Index

The Oral Mucositis Index (OMI) was developed from the finalized OMRS. A downsized 20-item version of the OMI (OMI-20) was developed and validated through a consensus panel of bone marrow transplant (BMT) oral complication specialists in the United States (39). The OMI-20 consists of nine items measuring erythema, nine items measuring ulceration, one atrophy item, and one edema item; all scored from 0 = none to 3 = severe, summed for a possible range of 0 to 60. The two sets of nine items measuring erythema and ulceration may be summed to produce subscale scores ranging from 0 to 27. The OMI-20 has demonstrated internal consistency, test–retest, and inter-rater reliability through evaluation in a sample of 133 adult PBSCT/BMT patients (39).

Oral Mucositis Assessment Scale

The Oral Mucositis Assessment Scale (OMAS) was developed as a scoring system for evaluating the anatomic extent and severity of stomatitis in clinical research studies by a team of oral medicine specialists, dentists, dental hygienists, oncologists, and oncology nurses from the United States, Canada, and Europe (40,41). Oral cavity regions assessed are lip (upper and lower), cheek (right and left), right and lateral tongue, left ventral and lateral tongue, floor of mouth, soft palate/fauces, and hard palate (40). Erythema is rated on a scale of 0 to 2 (0 = none, 1 = not severe, and 2 = severe) and ulceration/pseudomembrane is a combined category rated on scores based on the estimated surface area involved (0 = no lesion, 1 = <1 cm², 2 = 1 to 3 cm², and 3 = >3 cm²) and summed giving a possible score range of 0 to 45 (34,42). Validity and reliability have been demonstrated for the OMAS through clinical research studies (41,43).

Treatment Strategies

The optimal treatment strategies for oral complications and related sequelae are unknown. Treatment strategies for oral mucositis and related oropharyngeal pain are mainly empirical, and testing is needed in the randomized controlled clinical trial setting. Zlotolow and Berger (44) presented a comprehensive review of clinical research regarding treatment strategies for oral complications of cancer strategies. Conflicting study results may be related to inappropriate design issues, use of limited oral assessment instruments unable to capture variations in oral cavity changes, and incorrect timing and dose of interventions. The only standard forms of care are pretreatment oral/dental stabilization, saline mouthwashes, and oropharyngeal pain management (45).

The need for standardized treatment for oral mucositis was appreciated by the Mucositis Study Section of the Multinational Association of Supportive Care in Cancer and the International Society for Oral Oncology through their formulation of the "Updated Clinical Practice Guidelines for the Prevention and Treatment of Mucositis" (46). The original guidelines published in 2004 were based on a comprehensive review of more than 8,000 English language publications (1966 to 2001). The most recent guidelines published in 2007 included 622 articles (2002 to 2005) (Table 19.2). Publications regarding alimentary tract mucositis were rated using criteria for level of evidence and quality of research design (47).

A standardized approach for the prevention and treatment of CT- and RT-induced oral mucositis is essential. The prophylactic measures usually used for the prevention of oral mucositis include chlorhexidine gluconate, ice-cold water, saline rinses, sodium bicarbonate rinses, acyclovir, and amphotericin B. Regimens used commonly for the treatment of oral mucositis and related pain include a local anesthetic such as lidocaine or dyclonine hydrochloride, magnesium-based antacids, diphenhydramine hydrochloride, nystatin, or sucralfate. These agents are used either alone or in various combinations as a mouthwash formulation. Oral and parenteral opiates are used to relieve oral mucositis–related pain.

TABLE 19.2	Guidelines for the care of patients with oral mucositis

Foundations of Care

A multidisciplinary development and evaluation of oral care protocols and patient and staff education in the use of such protocols are needed to reduce the severity of oral mucositis from chemotherapy and/or radiation therapy. As part of the protocol, it would be necessary to use a soft toothbrush that is replaced on a regular basis. Elements of good clinical practice should include the use of validated tools to regularly assess oral pain and oral cavity health. The inclusion of dental professionals is vital throughout the treatment and follow-up phases.

Patient-controlled analgesia with morphine is recommended as the treatment of choice for oral mucositis–related pain in patients undergoing HSCT. Regular oral pain assessment using validated instruments for self-reporting is essential.

Radiation Therapy—Prevention

Sucralfate should not be used for the prevention of radiation-induced oral mucositis.

Antimicrobial lozenges should not be used for the prevention of radiation-induced oral mucositis.

The use of midline radiation blocks and three-dimensional radiation treatment was recommended to reduce mucosal injury.[a]

Benzydamine was recommended for the prevention of radiation-induced mucositis in patients with head and neck cancer receiving moderate-dose radiation therapy.[a]

Chlorhexidine was not recommended to prevent oral mucositis in patients with solid tumors of the head and neck who are undergoing radiotherapy.[a]

Standard-Dose Chemotherapy Prevention

Patients receiving bolus 5-FU chemotherapy should undergo 30 min of oral cryotherapy to prevent oral mucositis.[a]

Acyclovir and its analogs should not be used routinely to prevent mucositis.[a]

Standard-Dose Chemotherapy Treatment

Chlorhexidine should not be used to treat established oral mucositis.[a]

High-Dose Chemotherapy with or without Total-Body Irradiation Plus Hematopoietic Cell Transplantation Prevention

In patients with hematological malignancies receiving high-dose chemotherapy and total-body irradiation with autologous stem cell transplant, the panel recommends the use of keratinocyte growth factor-1 (Palifermin) in a dose of 60 μg/kg/d for 3 d prior to conditioning treatment and for 3 d posttransplant for the prevention of oral mucositis.

Cryotherapy should be used to prevent oral mucositis in patients receiving high-dose melphalan.

The use of pentoxifylline was not recommended to prevent mucositis in patients undergoing HSCT.[a]

Granulocyte–macrophage colony-stimulating factor mouthwashes should not be used for the prevention of oral mucositis in patients undergoing HSCT.

Low-level laser therapy requires expensive equipment and specialized training. Because of interoperator variability, clinical trials are difficult to conduct, and their results are difficult to compare. However, for centers able to support the necessary technology and training, laser therapy should be used to attempt to reduce the incidence of oral mucositis and its associated pain in patients receiving high-dose chemotherapy or chemoradiotherapy before HSCT.[a]

HSCT, hematopoietic stem cell transplantation; 5-FU, 5-fluorouracil.

[a]No change from previous guidelines.

Source: Adapted from Keefe DM, Schubert MM, Elting LS, et al. Mucositis Study Section of the Multinational Association of Supportive Care in Cancer and the International Society for Oral Oncology. Updated clinical practice guidelines for the prevention and treatment of mucositis. *Cancer.* 2007;109:820–831.

BIOLOGICAL RESPONSE MODIFIERS

Epidermal Growth Factors

Studies on epidermal growth factor (EGF) as a potential treatment option for CT- and RT-induced oral mucositis have reported conflicting data. EGF may function as a marker of mucosal damage and could potentially facilitate the healing process (48). In a phase I trial conducted by Girdler et al. (49), EGF mouthwash was used by patients treated with CT, who had a delayed onset and reduction in severity of recurrent ulcerations. However, no statistically significantly difference was seen in resolution of established ulcers. A recent double-blind, placebo-controlled, prospective phase II study reported a potential benefit from EGF oral spray in the management of oral mucositis in patients undergoing RT for head and neck cancer. In this study, 113 subjects were randomized into one of four arms: EGF treatment groups (10-, 50-, and 100-µg/mL doses twice) and placebo. The 50-µg/mL dose was the most efficacious for the treatment of oral mucositis (50). Further randomized controlled trials are needed to confirm these results.

Hematopoietic Growth Factors

Hematologic growth factors are currently the standard treatment for patients who are treated with high-dose CT because of their well-established efficacy to decrease the duration of CT-induced neutropenia. In vitro studies have demonstrated that EGF is present in saliva and has the ability to affect growth, cell migration, and repair mechanisms (51). The development of increased oral toxicity or mucosal repair may be dependent on the timing of EGF administration in relation to CT treatment (52). Gabrilove et al. (53) reported from a sample of 27 patients with bladder cancer who received escalating doses of granulocyte colony-stimulating factor (G-CSF) during treatment with methotrexate, vinblastine, doxorubicin, and cisplatin. The patients received the G-CSF during the first of two cycles of CT. Although significantly less oral mucositis was seen during the first cycle with G-CSF, the positive results may have been biased related to possible cumulative chemotherapeutic toxicity with resultant increase in oral mucositis severity. Conversely, Bronchud et al. (54) reported from a study of 17 patients with breast or ovarian carcinoma treated with escalating doses of doxorubicin with G-CSF that G-CSF did not prevent severe oral mucositis. A third study was conducted comparing clinical outcomes in a sample of 55 adult patients who received CT for NHL and G-CSF with clinical outcomes in 39 patients who received CT alone. Patients who did not receive G-CSF had neutropenia as the primary cause of treatment delay, when compared with those patients who received G-CSF and experienced oral mucositis as the main cause of treatment delay (55). Granulocyte–macrophage colony-stimulating factor (GM-CSF) has demonstrated conflicting results in patients receiving diverse cancer treatments (56–59). A randomized controlled phase III trial conducted by Masucci et al. (57) analyzed the efficacy of GM-CSF in head and neck cancer patients with RT-induced oral mucositis. A significant reduction in oral mucositis severity was observed in the GM-CSF treatment group. Conversely, results from a Radiation Therapy Oncology Group–sponsored double-blind, placebo-controlled, randomized study ($N = 121$) to analyze efficacy and safety of GM-CSF for reducing severity and duration of oral mucositis and related pain in head and neck cancer patients receiving RT (59) showed that GM-CSF had no significant effect on the severity or duration of oral mucositis. The use of CSFs in the treatment of oral mucositis remains investigational.

Keratinocyte Growth Factors

Recently, palifermin, which is a recombinant human keratinocyte growth factor and member of fibroblast growth factor (FGF) family, has shown efficacy in the reduction of oral mucosal injury related to cytotoxic therapy (60). Spielberger et al. (60) reported from a double-blind study that compared the effect of palifermin with a placebo for the development of oral mucositis in 212 subjects with hematologic cancers. Palifermin or placebo was administered intravenously for 3 consecutive days immediately before initiating conditioning therapy. This conditioning therapy used fractionated total-body radiation plus high-dose CT. When compared with placebo, the palifermin group experienced significant reductions in grade 4 oral mucositis, soreness of the mouth and throat, use of opioid analgesics, and the incidence of total parenteral nutrition use. Luthi et al. (61) reported lower grade 3 or 4 oral mucositis in 34 patients who received melphalan or BEAM with HSCT and were treated with palifermin (0.06 mg/kg) injections 3 days before conditioning CT and 3 days following HSCT as compared with controls. Nasilowska-Adamska et al. (62) found that palifermin 60 µg/kg/d for 3 consecutive days before and after conditioning therapy for HSCT significantly reduced the incidence, severity, and duration of oral mucositis in a sample of 106 subjects. In a subsequent study (63), 53 patients with hematological diseases treated with the same regimen also showed a significant reduction in incidence and median duration of oral mucositis, decreased incidence of opiates use and total parenteral nutrition, as well as less prevalence of acute GVHD.

Palifermin has also been studied in patients with solid tumors. In a randomized controlled trial conducted by Rosen et al. (64), 64 patients with metastatic colorectal cancer receiving 5-FU and leucovorin were randomized to receive palifermin (40 µg/kg) for 3 consecutive days before each of two cycles of CT. The incidence of oral mucositis WHO grade 2 or higher was significantly lower and patients reported less severe symptoms in the treatment arm. Brizel et al. (65) compared palifermin (60 µg/kg) versus placebo in patients with locally advanced head and neck cancer treated with chemoradiation. Patients were submitted to two types of RT, standard (total dose of 70 Gy delivered in 2-Gy daily fractions) and hyperfractionated (total dose of 72 Gy delivered in 1.25-Gy fractions twice a day for 7 weeks), and CT including cisplatin (20 mg/m² for 4 days) and continuous infusion of 5-FU (1,000 mg/m²/d for 4 days on weeks 1 and 5 of RT). Palifermin was well tolerated and decreased oral mucositis, dysphagia, and xerostomia in patients treated with hyperfractionated RT but not standard RT. However, palifermin did not reduce the morbidity of concurrent chemoradiotherapy.

Velafermin, another member of the FGF family, is a recombinant human FGF that has been shown to induce proliferation of cell lines from epithelial and mesenchymal origin and decrease tissue inflammation and degeneration as well as luminal blood loss, colonic edema, inflammation, and epithelial loss in animal models (66). Several phase I trials have shown excellent safety profiles. Schuster et al. (67) evaluated the safety and tolerability of velafermin in patients undergoing high-dose CT and autologous HSCT. It was administered in 30 patients 24 hours after stem cell infusion at doses of 0.03, 0.1, or 0.33 mg/kg. Velafermin was well tolerated at doses up to 0.2 mg/kg with the most common side effects being diarrhea, fatigue, pyrexia, vomiting, and nausea. Further clinical trials are needed to confirm its efficacy.

Antimicrobials

Antimicrobial approaches have included systemic agents such as antibiotics, antivirals (acyclovir, valacyclovir, and ganciclovir), and the antifungal agent, fluconazole. Donnelly et al. (68) evaluated the evidence regarding the role of infection in the pathophysiology of oral mucositis via a comprehensive review of 31 prospective randomized trials. The authors concluded that there was no clear pattern of patient type, cancer treatment, or type of antimicrobial agent used and that there was a lack of consistent oral mucositis assessment.

Oral candidiasis is a common acute and chronic oral sequela of head and neck RT, with lesions presenting as removable (whitish) chronic or hyperplastic (nonremovable) and chronic erythematous (diffused as patchy erythema) and frequently appearing as angular cheilitis (first signs or symptoms). Treatment approaches for oral candidiasis include Mycostatin (troches), nystatin (liquid or ointment), and clotrimazole. Pseudomembranous candidiasis is successfully treated topically. Chronic candidiasis usually requires much longer treatment, and it may be necessary to use oral ketoconazole, fluconazole, or intravenous amphotericin B.

Acyclovir prophylaxis is the currently accepted treatment for HSV and cytomegalovirus seropositive HSCT patients. A randomized controlled clinical trial conducted in HSCT patients compared fluconazole with placebo. Results showed that fluconazole prevented systemic fungal infections (7% fluconazole vs. 18% placebo) and significantly reduced the incidence of mucosal infection and oropharyngeal colonization by *Candida albicans* (69).

Conflicting reports have been published regarding the use of chlorhexidine mouthwash for alleviating oral mucositis and reducing oral colonization by Gram-positive, Gram-negative, and *Candida* species in patients receiving CT, RT, or HSCT. The majority of studies have not demonstrated the efficacy of chlorhexidine mouthwash for oral mucositis reduction in patients receiving intensive CT (70). The potential benefit of chlorhexidine may be related to a reduction of caries, dental plaques, gingivitis, oropharyngeal candidiasis, and bacterial colonization. Dodd et al. (71) tested the efficacy of the PRO-SELF Mouth Aware (PSMA) program in conjunction with randomization to one of two mouthwashes (0.12% chlorhexidine or sterile water) for the prevention of CT-related oral mucositis in 222 patients. Although chlorhexidine was found to be no more effective than water regarding oral mucositis incidence, days to onset, and severity, the PSMA program appeared to reduce oral mucositis incidence (71). A double-blind, placebo-controlled, randomized study

of chlorhexidine prophylaxis for 5-FU–based CT-induced oral mucositis in patients with gastrointestinal (GI) malignancies conducted by Sorensen et al. (72) suggested a role for chlorhexidine in the prevention of oral mucositis. Two hundred and twenty-five patients were randomized to chlorhexidine mouth rinse three times a day for 3 weeks versus placebo or cryotherapy with ice 45 minutes during CT. The frequency and duration of oral mucositis were significantly improved in the chlorhexidine and cryotherapy arms.

Sutherland and Browman (73) reviewed 59 studies assessing prophylaxis of RT-induced oral mucositis in head and neck cancer patients. Interventions chosen based on the biological etiology of oral mucositis were effective. A study by Spijkervet et al. (74) evaluated the efficacy of lozenges containing polymyxin E_2 2 mg, tobramycin 1.8 mg, and amphotericin B 10 mg (PTA) taken four times daily for the oropharyngeal flora related to oral mucositis. These researchers compared 15 patients receiving RT using PTA and two other groups of 15 patients each, one of which was using 0.1% chlorhexidine and the other was using placebo. Results showed that the selectively decontaminated group had significantly reduced severity and oral mucositis extent when compared with the chlorhexidine and placebo groups.

Cryotherapy

Cryotherapy administered as ice chips and flavored ice popsicles has been used to prevent oral mucositis. Efficacy of cryotherapy for the reduction of 5-FU–induced oral mucositis severity was demonstrated through a North Central Cancer Treatment Group (NCCTG) and Mayo Clinic–sponsored controlled randomized trial (75). A subsequent study with a sample of 178 patients who were randomized to receive 30 versus 60 minutes of oral cryotherapy reported similar severity of oral mucositis in both groups (76). The study recommended the use of 30 minutes of oral cryotherapy prior to bolus administration of 5-FU–based CT. Additional studies have confirmed these results (77,78). Cryotherapy used to induce vasoconstriction should be considered for patients receiving 5-FU or melphalan (79) when these agents are administered during short infusion times.

Pain relief with intravenous opiates has become a common practice for patients with CT- and RT-induced oral mucositis. Cryotherapy is an important adjuvant technique to opiate analgesia. A randomized controlled trial conducted by Svanberg et al. (80) demonstrated that this technique may alleviate the development of oral mucositis and oral pain, resulting in a reduction in the number of days and total dose of intravenous opiates in patients treated with autologous BMT.

Laser

Several studies have confirmed the effectiveness of low-energy laser for prevention and treatment of CT- or RT-induced oral mucositis (81–86). A preliminary study was conducted in a sample of 36 patients with diverse cancers and CT regimens; 16 patients were treated with laser and 20 patients served as controls (87). Results demonstrated reduced oral mucositis duration from a mean of 19.3 days in the control arm to 8.1 days in the treatment arm (87). A recent phase III double-blind, placebo-controlled randomized study compared two different low-level GaA1As diode lasers (650 and 780 nm) to prevent oral mucositis in HSCT patients treated with either CT or chemoradiotherapy (84). Seventy patients were randomized into treatment with 650 nm laser, 780 nm laser, or placebo. Low-level laser therapy was more effective in decreasing oral mucositis and related oral pain, was safe, and had no side effects. The efficacy of low-energy He/Ne laser was studied in a sample of 30 and 24 patients in two randomized controlled clinical trials (82,88). Low-energy He/Ne laser demonstrated a reduction in the severity and duration of oral mucositis.

Miscellaneous Agents

In animal models, Chung et al. (89) investigated the efficacy of phenylbutyrate, a histone deacetylase (HDAC) inhibitor, for the management of CT- and RT-induced oral mucositis. Carcinogenesis or oral mucositis was induced in hamsters using radiation or 7, 12-dimethylbenz(a)anthracene (DMBA). Phenylbutyrate promoted DNA repair and survival in normal cells after RT. The reduction in oral tumor incidence, burden, and progression correlated with the suppression of oncomiRs and Rad51 overexpression, the upregulation of differentiation markers, and the decrease of intracellular HDAC activity and oxidative stress during DMBA-induced oral carcinogenesis. Mangoni et al. (90) analyzed the protective efficacy of a new heparan mimetic biopolymer, RGTA-OTR4131, alone or with amifostine, in the management of oral mucositis and evaluated its effects on tumor growth in vitro and in vivo. A single dose of 16.5 Gy was delivered to the snout of mice and the effects of OTR4131 were analyzed by macroscopic scoring and histology. OTR4131 was well tolerated and was found to reduce RT-induced oral mucositis without affecting tumor sensitivity to RT. These results need to be confirmed in clinical trials.

Several studies have been published on different herbal and complementary therapies for the management of CT- and RT-induced oral mucositis (91–93). Payayor, *Clinacanthus nutans*, a herb commonly used as a medicinal product in Southeast Asia, has been shown to have good potential for effective oral mucositis treatment. A prospective, randomized clinical trial conducted by Putwatana et al. (91) explored the efficacy of glycerin payayor solution in the prevention and relief of RT-induced oral mucositis versus benzydamine. The average time to onset of oral mucositis was significantly longer, and oral mucositis severity and related pain score were lower than the benzydamine arm. Manuka, *Leptospermum*, and kanuka, *Kunzea ericoides*, are essential oils indigenous to New Zealand that have been used for medicinal purposes for many years. They are known to have antibacterial, antifungal, anti-inflammatory, and analgesic actions. Maddocks-Jennings et al. (92) reported in a small placebo-controlled, randomized study, a significant delay in oral mucositis and a significant decrease

in related oral pain and other symptoms in patients treated with manuka and kanuka versus placebo. Further clinical trials are needed to confirm these results.

RADIOPROTECTORS

Vitamins and Other Antioxidants

Vitamin E has been tested in CT-induced oral mucositis because it can stabilize cellular membranes and may improve herpetic gingivitis, possibly through antioxidant activity. Wadleigh et al. (93) demonstrated the efficacy of vitamin E in 18 CT patients who were randomized to receive topical vitamin E or placebo. Statistically significant results showed that six of nine patients in the vitamin E group had complete oral mucositis resolution within 4 days of starting therapy, when compared with the placebo group, in which only one of nine had oral mucositis resolution during the 5-day study period (93).

Other antioxidants that have been tested for efficacy with oral mucositis include vitamin C and glutathione. Azelastine hydrochloride has shown efficacy in the treatment of aphthous ulcers in Behçet's disease. Osaki et al. (94) reported findings from a study with a sample of 63 patients with head and neck cancer who were treated with chemoradiation. Twenty-six patients received regimen 1 (vitamins C and E and glutathione) and 37 patients received regimen 2 (regimen 1 plus azelastine). Results showed that in the azelastine arm, 21 patients remained at grade 1 or 2 oral mucositis, 6 patients had grade 3 oral mucositis, and 10 patients had grade 4 oral mucositis. In the control group, grade 3 or 4 oral mucositis was observed in more than half the subjects. Azelastine suppressed neutrophil respiratory burst both in vivo and in vitro and also showed cytokine release suppression from lymphocytes. Azelastine may be useful to prevent CT-induced oral mucositis (94). Polaprezinc (zinc L-carnosine), a zinc-containing molecule used for the therapy of gastric ulcer, has been shown to inhibit the induction of TNFα. Watanabe et al. (95) investigated the effect of polaprezinc on CT- and RT-induced oral mucositis, pain, xerostomia, and taste disturbance in patients with head and neck cancer. Thirty-one patients were randomly assigned to polaprezinc or azulene solution as a control for 3 minutes, four times daily until the end of the therapy. There was a markedly decrease in the incidence of oral mucositis, pain, xerostomia, taste disturbance, and analgesic requirement as well as a significant increase in food intake in the polaprezinc group.

Amifostine

Amifostine, a thiol compound, is a selective cytoprotective agent that has been approved by the US Food and Drug Administration for salivary gland protection in patients receiving RT. In animal models, it has been shown to protect various tissues such as mucosa, lung, renal, and bone marrow from alkylating agents without altering tumor activity. A retrospective study conducted by Kouloulias et al. (96) reported reduced severity of oral and esophageal toxicity.

One hundred and seventy-seven patients with diverse tumor types were treated with amifostine before RT. Based on a meta-analysis, including patients receiving amifostine before RT, there is a significant reduction in oral mucositis severity at doses above 300 mg/m² (97).

A multicenter, open-label, randomized controlled trial analyzed the use of amifostine in MM patients receiving conditioning CT with melphalan prior to autologous HSCT (98). Ninety patients were randomized to receive or not receive amifostine (910 mg/m²). The use of amifostine was associated with a reduction in the median grade and the frequency of severe (WHO grade 3 or 4) oral mucositis. However, there was no reduction in parenteral nutrition and analgesics use and no significant difference between the median progression-free or overall survival times.

Glutamine

Glutamine is an amino acid, immunomodulator, and mucosal protective agent that has been studied in multiple clinical trials with conflicting results. An extensive literature review performed by Savarese et al. (99) reported that glutamine supplementation may have an impact in incidence and severity of anthracycline-associated oral mucositis. A randomized, double-blind, placebo-controlled trial on glutamine supplementation in patients undergoing autologous HSCT reported an increase in severe oral mucositis and opiate use and prolonged hospital stay (100). Another randomized controlled study compared oral glutamine supplementation (30 g/d) versus placebo in 58 HSCT patients. There was no difference in the length of hospitalization, nutrition, severity of oral mucositis, engraftment time, survival, relapse, and severity of diarrhea among both groups (101).

Other clinical trials have reported more promising data on the use of glutamine (102,103). In a double-blind, randomized, placebo-controlled trial of oral glutamine for the prevention of oral mucositis in children undergoing HSCT, 120 patients were randomized to receive glutamine or glycine twice a day until 28 days post transplant. The glutamine group showed a significant reduction in days of intravenous opiate use and total parenteral nutrition, but no difference in toxicity was observed between the two groups (104).

A phase III study of topical AES-14, which is a novel drug system designed to concentrate delivery of L-glutamine to oral mucosa for ulceration treatment, was conducted with 121 patients at risk for oral mucositis (105). Subjects were randomized to either AES-14 or placebo and received protocol treatment from day 1 of CT until 2 weeks following the last CT dose or oral mucositis resolution. Results showed a potential 20% reduction of moderate-to-severe oral mucositis in the AES-14 group and a 10% increase in grade 0 oral mucositis.

Anti-inflammatory Agents

Prostaglandins are a family of naturally occurring eicosanoids, some of which have shown cytoprotective activity. Topical dinoprostone was administered four times daily in a nonblinded study to 10 patients with oral carcinomas, who were receiving 5-FU and mitomycin with concomitant RT (106). The control group used 14 patients who were receiving identical treatment. Eight of the 10 patients who received dinoprostone were evaluable, and no patient developed severe oral mucositis when compared with six episodes in the control arm. A second pilot study was conducted with 15 patients who received RT to the head and neck, showing that an inflammatory reaction was detected in only 5 patients in the vicinity of their tumor when treated with topically applied prostaglandin E₂ (PGE₂), and that no patients developed any bullous or desquamating inflammatory lesions (107). A double-blind, placebo-controlled study of PGE₂ in 60 patients undergoing BMT revealed no significant differences in the incidence, severity, or duration of oral mucositis. The incidence of HSV was higher in those on the PGE₂ arm. There was an increase in oral mucositis severity in those patients who developed HSV (108).

Benzydamine is a nonsteroidal anti-inflammatory drug with reported analgesic, anesthetic, and antimicrobial properties without activity on arachidonic acid metabolism. It has been shown to reduce the severity of oral mucositis and associated pain in patients undergoing RT. Epstein and Stevenson-Moore (109) reported in a double-blind, placebo-controlled trial that benzydamine produced statistically significant relief of pain from RT-induced oral mucositis and a reduction in both the total area and the size of ulceration. Positive responses to benzydamine have been reported in at least three other studies (110–112). In a small prospective, double-blind, randomized study comparing the efficacy of chlorhexidine gluconate and benzydamine hydrochloride oral rinse in patients with head and neck cancer to prevent and treat RT-induced oropharyngeal mucositis, a trend emerged showing a decrease in mucositis, oropharyngeal pain, and dysphagia in those receiving benzydamine (113).

Current evidence does not support the use of systemic steroids to reduce the frequency or severity of oral mucositis (114).

Treatment for Oral cGVHD

Almost all patients with extensive cGVHD require systemic immunosuppressive therapy. Therefore, there is a critical need for adjuvant therapies that are both efficacious and avoid the long-term consequences of these corticosteroid therapies. In general, advances in the treatment of cGVHD have been modest, and no standard therapy exists for cGVHD that fails to respond to initial therapy or recurs. Imanguli et al. (115) presented a comprehensive review of available therapies for cGVHD of the oral mucosa. Pharmacotherapy for oral cGVHD may be oral, topical, or injectable. The most common systemic therapy is corticosteroids with or without cyclosporine. Other agents such as tacrolimus, sirolimus, pentostatin, mycophenolate mofetil, and hydroxychloroquine have been used as salvage treatment (115). Emerging systemic therapies include monoclonal antibodies such as infliximab, etanercept, daclizumab, and rituximab (115–116). Extracorporeal photophoresis that separates patient's mononuclear cells through apheresis and exposes them to ultraviolet light A has shown promise.

Topical and local therapy for oral cGVHD offer several advantages over systemic therapy, including fewer side effects. There is no optimal therapy for oral cGVHD. Most trials have been open label with very small sample sizes. Patients with symptomatic disease that is limited to the oral cavity have been found to benefit from topical steroids such as dexamethasone elixir (0.5 mg/5 mL) and budesonide rinse (3 mg/10 mL) (30,116). Dexamethasone elixir has shown efficacy when used as a mouth rinse (10 mL) for 2 to 3 minutes at least four times daily (31,118). Topical steroids such as Lidex have also been tried. Clobetasol 0.05% is a topical high-potency steroid that has been administered four times daily for 2 to 3 weeks depending on the severity of the ulcerative oral cGVHD to decrease inflammation and oral pain. If local steroids alone are not adequate to control oral disease, then topical cyclosporine (119) or topical tacrolimus may be tried (31,120,121). Intraoral psoralen plus ultraviolet A irradiation may be appropriate based on the patient's condition (37,115). These treatments need evaluation in further randomized controlled clinical trials.

SYMPTOM MANAGEMENT

Oropharyngeal Pain

Oral mucositis is the principal etiology of most pain experienced during the 3-week post-BMT time period. This multidimensional oral pain is often described as the most unforgettable ordeal of BMT. McGuire et al. (15) reported in a sample of autologous and allogeneic BMT patients that oral pain was detected before observed stomatitis, that pain intensity did not correlate directly with the extent of mucosal injury, and that some patients reported limited or no pain after BMT. Overall pain ratings paralleling oral tissue changes during 2 weeks after BMT have also been reported. A descriptive, correlational, cross-sectional study of women with breast cancer undergoing autologous HSCT conducted by Fall-Dickson et al. (122) showed a significant positive correlation between oral pain and oral mucositis severity. However, this oral pain was more complex than a direct correlation with the amount of tissue damage, which is consistent with previous reports.

The sensory dimension of oral mucositis–related pain reported with general mucosal inflammation and breakdown ranges from mild discomfort to severe and debilitating pain requiring the use of opioid analgesics (123). Immunocompromised cancer patients with HSV infections have larger, more painful lesions when compared with non-cancer patients. Oral pain is associated strongly with cGVHD and has been described as severe, burning, and irritating, with dryness and loss of taste also reported. Oral mucositis–related oral pain reported with CT is usually of less than 3-month duration, contrasting with the usually chronic oral pain accompanying oral cGVHD.

Research has demonstrated conflicting results regarding the association between age and pain perception and intra-ethnic differences in pain perception. Gender differences have been reported for pain. For example, female subjects in a study testing capsaicin efficacy for oral mucositis–related pain reported higher pain levels. Managing pain is critical to avoid suffering and psychological distress (124). Adequate assessment of this oral pain experience requires a comprehensive pain assessment tool such as the Painometer (Dola Health Systems, Baltimore, MD) (125), which assesses the overall intensity, sensory, and affective dimensions of pain.

Sucralfate

Sucralfate is an aluminum salt of a sulfated disaccharide that has shown efficacy in the treatment of GI ulcerations and has been tested as a mouthwash for the prevention and treatment of oral mucositis. Sucralfate creates a protective barrier at the ulcer site via the formation of an ionic bond to proteins. Additional evidence suggests an increase in the local production of PGE_2 that leads to an increase in mucosal blood flow, mucus production, mitotic activity, and surface migration of cells.

Study results with sucralfate are conflicting. A phase III study was conducted by the NCCTG to compare sucralfate suspension versus placebo for 5-FU–related oral mucositis. Results demonstrated that in the 50 patients who experienced oral mucositis, not only did the sucralfate suspension provide no beneficial reduction in 5-FU–induced oral mucositis severity or duration but also that the sucralfate group had considerable additional GI toxicity (126). Additionally, no efficacy was demonstrated for a sucralfate mouthwash for prevention and treatment of 5-FU–induced oral mucositis in a randomized controlled clinical trial with 81 patients with colorectal cancer who received either sucralfate suspension or placebo four times daily during their first cycle of 5-FU and leucovorin (127). Sucralfate has also been tested in the head and neck RT population. A prospective, double-blind study compared the effectiveness of sucralfate suspension with a formulation of diphenhydramine hydrochloride syrup plus kaolin–pectin for RT-induced oral mucositis. Data regarding oral pain, efficacy of mouth rinses, weight change, and interruption of therapy were collected daily, and oral mucositis grade was collected weekly. Results showed no statistically significant differences between the two groups. In a study designed to compare outcomes in 21 patients who received standard oral care with 24 patients who received sucralfate suspension four times daily, the sucralfate group showed a significant difference in mucosal edema, oral pain, dysphagia, and weight loss (128). Conversely, a double-blind, placebo-controlled study with sucralfate in 33 patients who received RT to the head and neck demonstrated no statistically significant differences in oral mucositis (129). However, the sucralfate group did experience less oral pain and required a later start of topical and systemic analgesics throughout RT (129). Dodd et al. (130) used a pilot randomized controlled clinical trial to evaluate the efficacy of a micronized sucralfate mouthwash compared with a salt and soda mouthwash in 30 patients receiving RT. All patients also used the PSMA, which is a systematic oral hygiene program. Results demonstrated no significant difference in efficacy between the two groups.

Gelclair

Gelclair (Sinclair Pharmaceuticals, Surrey, England, UK) is a concentrated, bioadherent gel that has received US Food and Drug Administration approval as a 510(k) medical device indicated for the management of oral mucositis–related oral pain. Gelclair adheres to the oral surface, creating a protective barrier for irritated tissue and sensitized nociceptors. The safety and efficacy have been evaluated in small clinical trials with mixed results. Innocenti et al. (131) reported a 92% decrease in oral pain from baseline 5 to 7 hours after Gelclair administration in patients with oral mucositis, severe diffuse oral aphthous lesions, and post oral surgery pain. More than half of these patients reported that the maximum effect of Gelclair lasted longer than 3 hours, and 87% of patients reported overall improvements from baseline for pain with swallowing food, liquids, and saliva following 1 week of treatment. DeCordi et al. (51) reported from a clinical study in which Gelclair was administered to patients with oral mucositis three times daily before meals as a 2- to 3-minute swish and spit for 3 to 10 days. Significant improvements were reported from baseline for pain, oral mucositis severity, and function. No adverse effects were reported during either trial and patients reported that the taste, smell, texture, and use of Gelclair were acceptable. Conversely, Barber et al. (132) conducted a prospective, randomized controlled trial comparing Gelclair versus standard therapy with sucralfate and mucaine in patients with RT-induced oral mucositis. This study did not show any significant difference between both therapies regarding general pain. Gelclair can be an important adjuvant to opiate therapy in the management of oral mucositis–related oral pain. However, more randomized controlled trials are needed to further support its use in the clinical setting.

Anesthetic Cocktails

Anesthetic cocktails, composed of agents such as viscous lidocaine or dyclonine hydrochloride, have been used with some success for oral mucositis–related oral pain but provide only temporary pain relief. Also, these agents may alter taste perception that may decrease oral intake. Other analgesics and mucosal-coating agents used for pain control include kaolin–pectin, diphenhydramine, Orabase, and Oratect Gel. Hospital-based pharmacies commonly formulate and dispense topical mixtures containing an analgesic, an anti-inflammatory agent, and a coating agent for use as an oral comfort measure for patients during cancer treatment. One large clinical research center uses a topical formulation that contains lidocaine viscous 2% (40 mL), diphenhydramine 12.5 mg/5 mL (40 mL), and Maalox 10 mg (40 mL) and

prescribes its use every 3 to 4 hours as needed. Testing these various topical formulations through randomized controlled clinical trials is needed.

Doxepin

Doxepin is a tricyclic antidepressant that has been used for many years in the management of patients with chronic benign or malignant pain. Its topical application is prescribed for the management of pruritus and neuropathic pain. Pilot studies on topical doxepin rinse in patient with oral mucositis pain have shown adequate analgesia for up to 4 hours after application (133,134). Epstein et al. (135) assessed the effectiveness of oral doxepin rinse for oral mucositis–related oral pain in head and neck cancer patients in the RT or HSCT setting. Nine subjects rinsed with doxepin (5 mL) three to six times per day during a week and returned for a follow-up visit. Oral mucositis was scored using the OMAS and oral pain was assessed using a Visual Analog Scale (VAS). There was a statistically significant reduction in VAS scores for 2 hours following doxepin rinse at the initial visit and also over a 1-week period showing that repeated dosing continues to bring significant pain relief. Further randomized controlled trials are needed to confirm these results.

Opioids

Severe oral mucositis–related oropharyngeal pain may interfere with hydration and nutritional intake and affect the quality of life. Management of this oropharyngeal pain may require use of opioids, often administered at high doses by patient-controlled analgesia pumps. Other routes of administration are oral, transmucosal, transdermal, and parenteral. The efficacy of oral transmucosal fentanyl citrate was compared with morphine sulfate immediate release in a randomized, controlled clinical trial for the treatment of breakthrough cancer pain in 134 adult ambulatory cancer patients (136). Study results showed that oral transmucosal fentanyl was more effective than morphine sulfate immediate release in treating breakthrough pain. Darwish et al. (137) conducted a phase I, open-label study to investigate the absorption profile of fentanyl buccal tablets in patients with or without oral mucositis. Sixteen patients (50% with oral mucositis) received a single 200-μg dose of fentanyl buccal tablet, which was well tolerated and showed a similar absorption profile within both groups. Transdermal fentanyl has also shown to be an effective, convenient, and well-tolerated treatment in patients with oral mucositis pain in the RT and the HSCT setting (138,139).

Topical morphine for stomatitis-related pain was evaluated in a sample of 26 patients following chemoradiation for head and neck cancer (139). Subjects were randomized to morphine mouthwash (1 mL 2% morphine solution) or magic mouthwash (equal parts of lidocaine, diphenhydramine, and magnesium aluminum hydroxide). Patients in the morphine group demonstrated both significantly shorter duration and lower intensity of oral pain than the magic mouthwash group. Swisher et al. (140) described an oral mucositis pain management algorithm to promote symptom management for HSCT patients who are transitioning from inpatient to ambulatory care. A key component of this successful program was the availability of a multidisciplinary team who could respond to the report of oral pain. At present, no standard treatment has been defined for the prevention or treatment of oral mucositis–related oral pain; thus, it is essential to continue studies of the treatments already available and to develop promising new approaches. Other agents that are currently under investigation or have shown some potential in the management of oral mucositis–related oral pain are sublingual methadone, transdermal buprenorphine, and ketamine mouthwash (141–143).

Xerostomia

Xerostomia experienced by patients receiving head and neck RT is a major sequela, with severity dependent on the radiation dosage and location, and volume of exposed salivary glands. Significant xerostomia has not been shown as a sequela in patients treated with CT alone. Patients who have undergone HSCT may also develop xerostomia as a late oral complication. Brand et al. (144) reported in a cross-sectional study of patients with history of autologous and/or allogeneic HSCT that these patients have significantly higher levels of xerostomia than comparison group of age- and sex-matched individuals. The severity of xerostomia was not significantly associated with RT given before HSCT or the type of stem cell transplantation. The degree of xerostomia is reported subjectively by both patients and clinicians and can affect oral comfort, fit of prostheses, speech, and swallowing. Xerostomia-associated enzymes contribute to the growth of caries (decay)-producing organisms, and the decrease in quantity and quality of saliva may be very harmful to dentition. Oral hygiene regimens that include the use of water/saline and daily fluoride application along with brushing teeth at least three times daily may reduce colonization and proliferation of oral pathogens.

Treatment guidelines for the management of xerostomia have been designed to increase patient's comfort (145). Sialagogues have been investigated as stimulants for the residual salivary parenchyma (pilocarpine, 5- and 10-mg doses), and subjective improvement has been reported in some patients (146). However, extreme caution with the use of pilocarpine is warranted because of reported side effects of glaucoma and cardiac problems. A randomized, controlled trial tested the efficacy of amifostine in a sample of 315 patients with head and neck cancer (147). The subjects received standard fractionated radiation with or without amifostine, administered at 200 mg/m^2 as a 3-minute intravenous infusion 15 to 30 minutes before each fraction of radiation. Patient eligibility criteria required that the radiation field encompassed at least 75% of both parotid glands. The Radiation Therapy Oncology Group Acute and Late Morbidity Score and Criteria was used to rate the severity of xerostomia. The incidence of grade 2 or higher acute xerostomia (90 days from the start of radiotherapy) and late xerostomia (9 to 12 months after radiotherapy) was significantly reduced in patients receiving amifostine. Whole saliva collection 1 year following RT showed that in the amifostine group, more subjects produced 0.1 g of saliva (72% vs. 49%), and that the median saliva production was greater (0.26 vs. 0.1 g). Stimulated saliva collections showed no difference between the treatment arms. Supporting these improvements in saliva production were the patient's reports of oral dryness. Artificial saliva, which usually uses carboxymethylcellulose as a base, has not demonstrated increased oral cavity comfort. Patients have reported subjective improvement in comfort levels through the frequent use of sugarless gum, mints, or candies.

CONCLUSION

Oral complications of cancer treatment are experienced by a large percentage of oncology patients, are biologically complex and often challenging to treat, and lead to a cascade of negative sequelae. Oncology treatment protocols continue to be designed to examine the effect of dose-intensive treatments on clinical and survival outcomes. These treatment outcomes are compromised when dose reduction or treatment cessation is necessary because of treatment-related oral complications. Although there exist numerous recommendations for prevention and treatment of oral complications and related negative sequelae, there remains a critical need to evaluate these interventions in the randomized controlled clinical trial setting using valid and reliable mucositis assessment tools to both advance the science of oral toxicities and to improve patient care. This clinical research requires a multidisciplinary team dedicated to both testing innovative treatment approaches and implementing appropriate findings through evidence-based practice.

REFERENCES

1. Raber-Durlacher JE, Elad S, Barasch A. Oral mucositis. *Oral Oncol*. 2010;46:452-456.
2. National Institutes of Health Consensus Development Panel. Consensus statement: oral complications of cancer therapies. *NCI Monogr*. 1989;9:3.
3. Cheng KK, Leung SF, Liang RH, Tai JW, Yeung RM, Thompson DR. Severe oral mucositis associated with cancer therapy: impact on oral functional status and quality of life. *Support Care Cancer*. 2009;18:1477-1485.
4. Elting LS, Keefe DM, Sonis ST, et al. Patient-reported measurements of oral mucositis in head and neck cancer patients treated with radiotherapy with or without chemotherapy. *Cancer*. 2008;113:2704-2713.
5. Barasch A, Peterson DE. Risk factors for ulcerative mucositis in cancer patients: unanswered questions. *Oral Oncol*. 2003;39:91-100.
6. Dodd MJ, Miaskowski C, Shiba GH, et al. Risk factors for CT-induced oral mucositis: dental appliances, oral hygiene, previous oral lesion, and a history of smoking. *Cancer Invest*. 1999;17:278-284.

7. Driezen S. Description and incidence of oral complications. *NCI Monogr.* 1990;9:11-15.

8. Grazziutti ML, Dong L, Miceli MH, et al. Oral mucositis in myeloma patients undergoing melphalan-based autologous stem cell transplantation: incidence, risk factors and a severity predictive model. *Bone Marrow Transplant.* 2006;38:501-506.

9. Vokurka S, Steinerova K, Karas M, Koza V. Characteristics and risk factors of oral mucositis after allogenic stem cell transplantation with FLU/MEL conditioning regimen in context with BU/CY2. *Bone Marrow Transplant.* 2009;44:601-605.

10. Blijlevens N, Schwenkglenks M, Bacon P, et al. Prospective oral mucositis audit: oral mucositis in patients receiving high-dose melphalan or BEAM conditioning chemotherapy—European Blood and Marrow Transplantation Mucositis Advisory Group. *J Clin Oncol.* 2008;26:1519-1525.

11. Sonis ST. Oral complications of cancer therapy. In: DeVita VT, Hellman S, Rosenberg SA, eds. *Cancer: Principles and Practice of Oncology.* 4th ed. Philadelphia, PA: JB Lippincott; 1993:2385.

12. Sonis ST. Mucositis as a biological process: a new hypothesis for the development of CT-induced stomatotoxicity. *Oral Oncol.* 1998;34:39-43.

13. Woo SB, Sonis ST, Monopoli MM, Sonis AL. A longitudinal study of oral ulcerative mucositis in bone marrow transplant recipients. *Cancer.* 1993;72:1612-1617.

14. McGuire DB, Altomonte V, Peterson DE, Wingard JR, Jones RJ, Grochow LB. Patterns of mucositis and pain in patients receiving preparative chemotherapy and bone marrow transplantation. *Oncol Nurs Forum.* 1993;20:1493-1502.

15. McCann S, Schwenkglenks M, Bacon P, et al.; EBMT Mucositis Advisory Group. The Prospective Oral Mucositis Audit: relationship of severe oral mucositis with clinical and medical resource use outcomes in patients receiving high-dose melphalan or BEAM-conditioning chemotherapy and autologous SCT. *Bone Marrow Transplant.* 2009;43:141-147.

16. Vera-Llonch M, Oster G, Ford CM, Lu J, Sonis S. Oral mucositis and outcomes of allogeneic hematopoietic stem-cell transplantation in patients with hematologic malignancies. *Support Care Cancer.* 2007;15:491-496.

17. Shih A, Miaskowshi C, Dodd MJ, Stotts NA, MacPhail L. Mechanisms for radiation-induced oral mucositis and the consequences. *Cancer Nurs.* 2003;26:222-229.

18. Vera-Llonch M, Oster G, Hagiwara M, Sonis S. Oral mucositis in patients undergoing radiation treatment for head and neck carcinoma: risk factors and clinical consequences. *Cancer.* 2006;106:329-336.

19. Elting LS, Cooksley CD, Chambers MS, Garden AS. Risk outcomes, and costs of radiation-induced oral mucositis among patients with head-and-neck malignancies. *Int J Radiat Oncol Biol Phys.* 2007;68:1110-1120.

20. Murphy BA, Beaumont JL, Isitt J, et al. Mucositis-related morbidity and resource utilization in head and neck cancer patients receiving radiation therapy with or without chemotherapy. *J Pain Symptom Manage.* 2009;38:522-532.

21. Bentzen, SM. Preventing or reducing late side effects of RT: radiobiology meets molecular pathology. *Nat Rev Cancer.* 2006;6:702-713.

22. Vissink A, Jansma J, Spijkervet FK, Burlage FR, Coppes RP. Oral sequelae of head and neck radiotherapy. *Crit Rev Oral Biol Med.* 2003;14:199-212.

23. Merigo E, Manfredi M, Meleti M, Corradi D, Vescovi P. Jaw bone necrosis without previous dental extractions associated with the use of biphosphonates (pamidronate and zolendronate): a four-case report. *J Oral Path Med.* 2005;34:613-617.

24. Ruggiero SL, Mehrotra B, Rosenberg TJ, Engroff SL. Osteonecrosis of the jaws associated with the use of biphosphonates: a review of 63 cases. *J Oral Maxillofac Surg.* 2004;62:527-534.

25. Lazarus HM, Vogelsang GB, Rowe JM. Prevention and treatment of acute graft-versus-host disease: the old and the new. A report from the Eastern Cooperative Oncology Group (ECOG). *Bone Marrow Transplant.* 1997;19:577-600.

26. Pavletic SZ, Martin P, Lee SJ, et al. Measuring therapeutic response in chronic graft-versus-host-disease: National Institutes of Health Consensus Development Project on criteria for clinical trials in chronic graft-versus-host disease: IV. Response criteria working group report. *Biol Blood Marrow Transplant.* 2006;12:252-266.

27. Treister NS, Stevenson K, Kim H, Woo SB, Soiffer R, Cutler C. Oral chronic graft-versus-host disease scoring using the NIH Consensus Criteria. *Biol Blood Marrow Transplant.* 2010;16:108-114.

28. Lloid ME. Oral medicine concerns of the BMT patient. In: Buchsel PC, Whedon, MB, eds. *Bone Marrow Transplantation: Administrative and Clinical Strategies.* Boston, MA: Jones and Bartlett Publishers; 1995:257.

29. Treister NS, Cook EF, Antin J, Lee SJ, Soiffer R, Woo SB. Clinical evaluation of oral chronic graft-versus-host disease. *Biol Blood Marrow Transplant.* 2008;14:110-115.

30. Imanguli MM, Swaim WD, League SC, Gress RE, Pavletic SZ, Hakim FT. Increased T-bet+ cytotoxic effectors and type I interferon-mediated processes in chronic graft-versus-host disease of the oral mucosa. *Blood.* 2009;113:3620-3630.

31. Fall-Dickson JM, Mitchell SA, Marden S, et al. Oral symptom intensity, health-related quality of life, and correlative salivary cytokines in adult survivors of hematopoietic stem cell transplantation with oral chronic graft-versus-host disease. *Biol Blood Marrow Transplant.* 2010;16:948-956.

32. Berger AM, Kilroy, TJ. Oral complications. In: DeVita VT, Hellman S, Rosenberg SA, eds. *Cancer: Principles and Practice of Oncology.* 6th ed. Philadelphia, PA: JB Lippincott; 1997:2714.

33. Beumer J, Curtis, T, Morris LR. Radiation complications in edentulous patients. *J Prosthet Dent.* 1976;36:193-203.

34. Beumer J, Zlotow I, Curtis T. Rehabilitation. In: Silverman S, ed. *Oral Cancer.* New York, NY: American Cancer Society; 1990.

35. US Department of Health and Human Services. *Cancer Therapy Evaluation Program, Common Terminology Criteria for Adverse Events, Version 3.0.* Washington, DC: US Department of Health and Human Services, National Cancer Institute; June 10, 2003.

36. Eilers J, Berger AM, Petersen MC. Development, testing, and application of the oral assessment guide. *Oncol Nurs Forum.* 1988;15:325-330.

37. World Health Organization. *WHO Handbook for Reporting Results of Cancer Treatment.* Offset publication No. 48. Geneva: World Health Organization; 1979:15.

38. Schubert MM, Williams BE, Lloid ME, Donaldson G, Chapko MK. Clinical scale for the rating of oral mucosal changes associated with bone marrow transplantation. Development of an oral mucositis index. *Cancer.* 1992;69:2469-2477.

39. McGuire DB, Peterson DE, Muller S, Owen DC, Slemmons MF, Schubert MM. The 20 item oral mucositis index: reliability and validity in bone marrow and stem cell transplant patients. *Cancer Invest.* 2002;20:893-903.

40. Sonis ST, Eilers JP, Epstein JB, et al. for the Mucositis Study Group. Validation of a new scoring system for the assessment of clinical trial research of oral mucositis induced by radiation or CT. *Cancer.* 1999;85:2103-2113.

41. Sonis ST, Oster G, Fuchs H, et al. Oral mucositis and the clinical and economic outcomes of hematopoietic stem-cell transplantation. *J Clin Oncol.* 2001;19:2201-2205.

42. Schweiger JW. Oral complications following RT: a five year retrospective report. *J Prosthet Dent.* 1987;58:78-82.

43. Elad S, Ackerstein A, Bitan M, et al. A prospective, double-blind phase two study evaluating the safety and efficacy of a topical histamine gel for the prophylaxis of oral mucositis in patients post hematopoietic stem cell transplantation. *Bone Marrow Transplant.* 2006;37:757-762.

44. Zlotolow IM, Berger AM. Oral manifestations of cancer therapy. In: Berger AM, Portnoy RK, Weissman DE, eds. *Principles and Practice of Palliative Care and Supportive Oncology.* Philadelphia, PA: Lippincott Williams & Wilkins; 2002:282.

45. Biron P, Sebban C, Gourmet R, Chvetzoff G, Philip I, Blay JY. Research controversies in management of oral mucositis. *Support Care Cancer.* 2000;8:68-71.

46. Keefe DM, Schubert MM, Elting LS, et al. Updated clinical practice guidelines for the prevention and treatment of mucositis. *Cancer.* 2007;109:820-831.

47. Somerfield M, Padberg J, Pfister D, et al: ASCO clinical practice guidelines: Process, progress, pitfalls, and prospects. *Classic Papers Curr Comments.* 2000;4:881-886.

48. Hong JP, Lee SW, Song SY, et al. Recombinant human epidermal growth factor treatment of radiation-induced severe oral mucositis in patients with head and neck malignancies. *Eur J Cancer Care.* 2009;18:636-641.

49. Girdler NM, Mcgurk M, Aqual S, Prince M. The effect of epidermal growth factor mouthwash on cytotoxic-induced oral ulceration: a phase I clinical trial. *Am J Clin Oncol.* 1995;18:403-406.

50. Wu HG, Song SY, Kim YS, et al. Therapeutic effect of recombinant human epidermal growth factor (RhEGF) on mucositis in patients undergoing radiotherapy, with or without chemotherapy, for head and neck cancer: a double-blind, placebo-controlled prospective phase 2 multi-institutional clinical trial. *Cancer.* 2009;115:3699-3708.

51. DeCordi SD, Giorgutti E, Martina S, et al. Gelclair: potentially an efficacious treatment for CT-induced mucositis. Proceedings from the Italian Anti-tumor League III Congress of Professional Oncology Nurses; October 10-12, 2001; Congliano, Italy [abstract].

52. Sonis ST, Costa JW Jr, Evitts SM, Lindquist LE, Nicolson M. Effect of epidermal growth factor on ulcerative mucositis in hamsters that receive cancer CT. *Oral Surg Oral Med Oral Pathol.* 1992;74:749-755.

53. Gabrilove JL, Jakubowski A, Scher H, et al. Effect of granulocyte colony-stimulating factor on neutropenia and associated morbidity due to CT for transitional-cell carcinoma of the urothelium. *N Engl J Med.* 1988;318:1414-1422.

54. Bronchud MH, Howell A, Crowther D, Hopwood P, Souza L, Dexter TM. The use of granulocyte colony-stimulating factor to increase the intensity of treatment with doxorubicin in patients with advanced breast and ovarian cancer. *Br J Cancer.* 1989;60:121-125.

55. Pettengell R, Gurney H, Radford JA, et al. Granulocyte colony-stimulating factor to prevent dose-limiting neutropenia in non-Hodgkin's lymphoma: a randomized controlled trial. *Blood.* 1992;80:1430-1436.

56. Saarilahti K, Kajanti M, Joensuu T, Kouri M, Joensuu H. Comparison of granulocyte-macrophage colony-stimulating factor and sucralfate mouthwashes in the prevention of radiation-induced mucositis: a double-blind prospective randomized phase III study. *Int J Radiat Oncol Biol Phys.* 2002;2:479-485.

57. Masucci B, Broman P, Kelly C, et al. Therapeutic efficacy by recombinant human granulocyte/monocyte-colony stimulating factor on mucositis occurring in patients with oral and oropharynx tumors treated with curative radiotherapy: a multicenter open randomized phase III study. *Med Oncol.* 2005;22:247-256.

58. Mcaleese JJ, Bishop KM, A'Hern R, Henk JM. Randomized phase II study of GM-CSF to reduce mucositis caused by accelerated radiotherapy of laryngeal cancer. *Br J Radiol.* 2006;79:608-613.

59. Ryu JK, Swann S, LeVeque F, et al. The impact of concurrent granulocyte macrophage-colony stimulating factor on radiation-induced mucositis in head and neck cancer patients: a double-blind placebo-controlled prospective phase III study by Radiation Therapy Oncology Group 9901. *Int J Radiat Oncol Biol Phys.* 2007;67:643-650.

60. Spielberger R, Stiff P, Bensinger W, et al. Palifermin for oral mucositis after intensive therapy for hematologic cancers. *N Engl J Med.* 2004;351:2590-2598.

61. Luthi F, Berwert L, Frosasard V. Prevention of oral mucositis with palifermin in patients treated with high-dose CT and autologous stem cell transplantation: a single center experience. *Blood.* 2006;108:843.

62. Nasilowska-Adamska B, Rzepecki P, Manko J, et al. The significance of palifermin (Kepivance) in reduction of oral mucositis (OM) incidence and acute graft versus host disease (aGVHD) in a patient with hematological disease undergoing HSCT. *Blood.* 2006;108:840.

63. Nasilowska-Adamska B, Rzepecki P, Manko J, et al. The influence of palifermin (Kepivance) on oral mucositis and acute graft versus host disease in patients with hematological diseases undergoing hematopoietic stem cell transplantation. *Bone Marrow Transplant.* 2007;40:983-988.

64. Rosen LS, Abdi E, David ID, et al. Palifermin reduces the incidence of oral mucositis in patients with metastatic colorectal cancer treated with fluorouracil-based chemotherapy. *J Clin Oncol.* 2006;24:5194-5200.

65. Brizel DM, Murphy BA, Rosenthal DI, et al. Phase II study of palifermin and concurrent chemoradiation in head and neck squamous cell carcinoma. *J Clin Oncol.* 2008;26:2489-2496.

66. Jeffers M, McDonald EF, Chillakuru RA, et al. A novel human fibroblast growth factor treats experimental intestinal inflammation. *Gastroenterology.* 2002;123:1151-1162.

67. Schuster MW, Shore TB, Harpel JG, et al. Safety and tolerability of velafermin (CG53135-05) in patients receiving high-dose chemotherapy and autologous peripheral blood stem cell transplant. *Support Care Cancer.* 2008;16:477-483.

68. Donnelly JP, Bellm LA, Epstein JB, Sonis ST, Symonds RP. Antimicrobial therapy to prevent or treat oral mucositis. *Lancet Infect Dis.* 2003;3:405-412.

69. Slavin MA, Osborne B, Adams R, et al. Efficacy and safety of fluconazole prophylaxis for fungal infections after marrow transplantation—a prospective, randomized, double-blind study. *J Infect Dis.* 1995;171:1545-1552.

70. Wahlin BY. Effects of chlorhexidine mouthrinse on oral health in patients with acute leukemia. *Oral Surg Oral Med Oral Pathol.* 1989;68:279-287.

71. Dodd MJ, Larson PL, Dibble SL, et al. Randomized clinical trial of chlorhexidine versus placebo for prevention of oral mucositis in patients receiving CT. *Oncol Nurs Forum.* 1996;23:921-927.

72. Sorensen JB, Skovsgaard T, Bork E, Damstrup L, Ingeberg S. Double-blind, placebo-controlled, randomized study of chlorhexidine prophylaxis for 5-fluorouracil-based chemotherapy-induced oralmucositis with nonblinded randomized

comparison to oral cooling (cryotherapy) in gastrointestinal malignancies. *Cancer.* 2008;112:1600-1606.

73. Sutherland SE, Browman GP. Prophylaxis of oral mucositis in irradiated head-and-neck cancer patients: a proposed classification scheme of interventions and meta-analysis of randomized controlled trials. *Int J Radiat Oncol Biol Phys.* 2001;4:917-930.

74. Spijkervet FK, Van Saene HK, Van Saene JJ, et al. Effect of selective elimination of the oral flora on mucositis in irradiated head and neck cancer patients. *J Surg Oncol.* 1991;46:167-173.

75. Mahoud DJ, Dose AM, Loprinzi CL, et al. Inhibition of fluorouracil-induced stomatitis by oral cryotherapy. *J Clin Oncol.* 1991;9:449-452.

76. Rocke LK, Loprinzi CL, Lee JK, et al. A randomized clinical trial of two different durations of oral cryotherapy for prevention of 5-FU-related stomatitis. *Cancer.* 1993;72(7):2234-2238.

77. Cascinu S, Fedeli A, Fedeli SL, Catalano G. Oral cooling (cryotherapy), an effective treatment for the prevention of 5-FU-induced stomatitis. *Oral Oncol Eur J Cancer.* 1994;30(4):234-236.

78. Papadeas E, Naxakis S, Riga M, Kalofonos C. Prevention of 5-fluorouracil-related stomatitis by oral cryotherapy: a randomized controlled study. *Eur J Oncol Nurs.* 2007;11:60-65.

79. Lilleby K, Garcia P, Gooley T, et al. A prospective, randomized study of cryotherapy during administration of high-dose melphalan to decrease the severity and duration of oral mucositis in patients with multiple myeloma undergoing autologous peripheral blood stem cell transplantation. *Bone Marrow Transplant.* 2006;37:1031-1035.

80. Svanberg A, Birgegård G, Öhrn K. Oral cryotherapy reduces mucositis and opioid use after myeloablative therapy: a randomized controlled trial. *Support Care Cancer.* 2007;15:1155-1161.

81. Bensadoun RJ, Ciais G. Radiation- and chemotherapy-induced mucositis in oncology: results of multicenter phase III studies. *J Oral Laser Appl.* 2002;2:115.

82. Bensadoun RJ, Ciais G, Schubert MM, et al. Low-energy He/Ne laser in the prevention of radiation-induced mucositis. A multicenter phase III randomized study in patients with head and neck cancer. *Support Care Cancer.* 1999;7:244-252.

83. Cowen D, Tardieu C, Schubert M, et al. Low energy helium-neon laser in the prevention of oral mucositis in patients undergoing bone-marrow transplant: results of a double blind randomized trial. *Int J Radiat Oncol Biol Phys.* 1997;38:697-703.

84. Schubert MM, Eduardo FP, Guthrie KA, et al. A phase III randomized double-blind placebo-controlled clinical trial to determine the efficacy of low level laser therapy for the prevention of oral mucositis in patients undergoing hematopoietic cell transplantation. *Support Care Cancer.* 2007;15:1145-1154.

85. Genot-Klastersky MT, Klastersky J, Awada F, et al. The use of lower-energy laser (LEL) for the prevention of chemotherapy-and/or radiotherapy-induced oral mucositis in cancer patients: results from two prospective studies. *Support Care Cancer.* 2008;16:1381-1387.

86. Zanin T, Zanin F, Carvalhosa AA, et al. Use of 660-nm diode laser in the prevention and treatment of human oral mucositis induced by radiotherapy and chemotherapy. *Photomed Laser Surg.* 2010;26:233-237.

87. Pourreau-Schneider N, Soudry M, Franquin JC, et al. Soft-laser therapy for iatrogenic mucositis in cancer patients receiving high-dose fluorouracil: a preliminary report. *J Natl Cancer Inst.* 1992;84:358-359.

88. Arora H, Pai KM, Maiya A, Vidyasagar MS, Rajeev A. Efficacy of He-Ne laser in the prevention and treatment of radiotherapy-induced oral mucositis in oral cancer patients. *Oral Surg Oral Med Oral Pathol Oral Radiol Endod.* 2008;105:180-186.

89. Chung YL, Lee MY, Pui NN. Epigenetic therapy using the histone deacetylase inhibitor for increasing therapeutic gain in oral cancer: prevention of radiation-induced oral mucositis and inhibition of chemical-induced oral carcinogenesis. *Carcinogenesis.* 2009;30:1387-1397.

90. Mangoni M, Yue X, Morin C, et al. Differential effect triggered by a heparin mimetic of the RGTA family preventing oral mucositis without tumor protection. *Int J Radiat Oncol Biol Phys.* 2009;74:1242-1250.

91. Putwatana P, Sanmanowong P, Oonprasertpong L, Junda T, Pitiporn S, Narkwong L. Relief of radiation-induced oral mucositis in head and neck cancer. *Cancer Nurs.* 2009;32:82-87.

92. Maddocks-Jennings W, Wilkinson JM, Cavanagh HM, Shillington D. Evaluating the effects of the essential oils *Leptospermum scoparium* (manuka) and *Kunzea ericoides* (kanuka) on radiotherapy induced mucositis: a randomized, placebo controlled feasibility study. *Eur J Oncol Nurs.* 2009;13:87-93.

93. Wadleigh RG, Redman RS, Graham ML, Krasnow SH, Anderson A, Cohen MH. Vitamin E in the treatment of chemo-induced mucositis. *Am J Med.* 1992;92:481-484.

94. Osaki T, Ueta E, Yoneda K, Hirota J, Yamamoto T. Prophylaxis of oral mucositis associated with chemoradiotherapy for oral carcinoma by Azelastine hydrochloride (azelastine) with other antioxidants. *Head Neck.* 1994;16:331-339.

95. Watanabe T, Ishihara M, Matsuura K, Mizuta K, Itoh Y. Polaprezinc prevents oral mucositis associated with radiochemotherapy in patients with head and neck cancer. *Int J Cancer.* 2010;127:1984-1990.

96. Kouloulias V, Kouvaris JR, Kokakis JD, et al. Impact on cytoprotective efficacy of intermediate interval between amifostine administration and radiotherapy: a retrospective analysis. *Int J Radiat Oncol Biol Phys.* 2004;59:1148-1156.

97. Sasse AD, Clark LG, Sasse EC, Clark OA. Amifostine reduces side effects and improves complete response rate during radiotherapy: results of a meta-analysis. *Int J Radiat Oncol Biol Phys.* 2006;64:784-791.

98. Spencer A, Horvath N, Gibson J, et al. Prospective randomised trial of amifostine cytoprotection in myeloma patients undergoing high-dose melphalan conditioned autologous stem cell transplantation. *Bone Marrow Transplant.* 2005;35:971-977.

99. Savarese DM, Savy G, Vahdat L, Wischmeyer PE, Corey B. Prevention of chemotherapy and radiation toxicity with glutamine. *Cancer Treat Rev.* 2003;29:501-513.

100. Pytlik R, Benes P, Patorkova M, et al. Standardized parenteral alanyl-glutamine dipeptide supplementation is not beneficial in autologous transplant patients: a randomized, double-blind, placebo-controlled study. *Bone Marrow Transplant.* 2002;30:953-961.

101. Coughlin-Dickson TM, Wong RM, Negrin RS, et al. Effects of oral glutamine supplementation during bone marrow transplantation. *J Parent Ent Nutr.* 2000;24:61-66.

102. Anderson PM, Ramsey NK, Shy Xo, et al. Effect of low-dose oral glutamine on painful stomatitis during bone marrow transplantation. *Bone Marrow Transplant.* 1998;22:339-344.

103. Peterson DE, Jones JB, Pettit RG. Randomized, placebo-controlled trial of Saforis for prevention and treatment of oral mucositis in breast cancer patients receiving anthracycline-based chemotherapy. *Cancer.* 2007;109:322-331.

104. Aquino VM, Harvey AR, Garvin JH, et al. A double-blind randomized placebo-controlled study of oral glutamine in the prevention of mucositis in children undergoing hematopoietic stem cell transplantation: a pediatric blood and marrow transplant consortium study. *Bone Marrow Transplant.* 2005;36:611-616.

105. Peterson D, Petit G. Phase III study: AES-14 in CT patients at risk for mucositis. *Proc Am Soc Clin Oncol.* 2003;22:725.

106. Porteder H, Rausch E, Kment G, Watzek G, Matejka M, Sinzinger H. Local prostaglandin E2 in patients with oral malignancies undergoing chemo and radiotherapy. *J Craniomaxillofac Surg.* 1988;16:371-374.

107. Matejka M, Nell A, Kment G, et al. Local benefit of prostaglandin E2 in radioCT-induced oral mucositis. *Br J Oral Maxillofac Surg.* 1990;28:89-91.

108. Labar B, Mrsic M, Pavleric A, et al. Prostaglandin E2 for prophylaxis of oral mucositis following BMT. *Bone Marrow Transplant.* 1993;11:379-382.

109. Epstein JB, Stevenson-Moore P. Benzydamine hydrochloride in prevention and management of pain in mucositis associated with RT. *Oral Surg Oral Med Oral Pathol.* 1986;62:145-148.

110. Epstein JB, Stevenson-Moore P, Jackson S, Mohamed JH, Spinelli JJ. Prevention of oral mucositis in RT: a controlled study with benzydamine hydrochloride rinse. *Int J Radiat Oncol Biol Phys.* 1989;16:1571-1575.

111. Lever SA, Dupuis LL, Chan HS. Comparative evaluation of benzydamine oral rinse in children with antineoplastic-induced stomatitis. *Drug Intell Clin Pharmacol.* 1987;21:359-361.

112. Epstein JB, Silverman S, Paggiarino DA, et al. Benzydamine HCl for prophylaxis of radiation-induced oral mucositis: results from a multicenter, randomized, double-blind, placebo-controlled clinical trial. *Cancer.* 2001;92:875-885.

113. Cheng KK, Yuen JK. A pilot study of chlorhexidine and benzydamine oral rinse for the prevention and treatment of irradiation mucositis in patients with head and neck cancer. *Cancer Nurs.* 2006;29:423-30.

114. Leborgne JH, Leborgne F, Zubizarreta E, Ortega B, Mezzera J. Corticosteroids and radiation mucositis in head and neck cancer: a double-blind placebo-controlled randomized trial. *Radiother Oncol.* 1998;47:145-148.

115. Imanguli M, Pavletic SZ, Guadagnini JP, Brahim JS, Atkinson JC. Chronic graft versus host disease of oral mucosa: review of available therapies. *Oral Surg Oral Med Oral Pathol Oral Radiol Endodontol.* 2006;101:175-183.

116. Zaja F, Bacigalupo A, Patriarca F, et al. Treatment of refractory chronic GVHD with rituximab: a GITMO study. *Bone Marrow Transplant.* 2007;40:273-277.

117. Sari I, Altuntas F, Kocyigit I, et al. The effect of budesonide mouthwash on oral chronic graft versus host disease. *Am J Hematol.* 2007;82:349-356.

118. Wolff D, Anders V, Corio R, et al. Oral PUVA and topical steroids for treatment of oral manifestations of chronic graft-vs-host disease. *Photodermatol Photoimmunol Photomed.* 2004;20:184-190.

119. Epstein JB, Reece DE. Topical cyclosporine A for treatment of oral chronic graft-versus-host disease. *Bone Marrow Transplant.* 1994;13:81-86.

120. Eckardt A, Starke O, Stadler M, Reuter C, Hertenstein B. Severe oral chronic graft-versus-host disease following allogenic bone marrow transplantation: highly effective treatment with topical tacrolimus. *Oral Oncol.* 2004;40:811-814.

121. Albert MH, Becker B, Schuster FR, et al. Oral graft vs host disease in children: treatment with topical tacrolimus ointment. *Pediatr Transplant.* 2007;11:306-311.

122. Fall-Dickson JM, Mock V, Berk RA, Grimm PM, Davidson N, Gaston-Johansson F. Stomatitis-related pain in women with breast cancer undergoing autologous hematopoietic stem cell transplant. *Cancer Nurs.* 2008;31:452-561.

123. Schubert MM, Sullivan KM, Morton TH, et al. Oral manifestations of chronic graft-versus-host disease. *Arch Intern Med.* 1984;144:1591-1595.

124. Vogelsang GB. How I treat chronic graft-versus-host-disease. *Blood.* 2001;97:1196-1201.

125. Gaston-Johansson F. Measurement of pain: the psychometric properties of the Pain-O-Meter, a simple, inexpensive pain assessment tool that could change health care practices. *J Pain Symptom Manage.* 1996;12:172-181.

126. Loprinzi CL, Ghosh C, Camoriani J, et al. Phase III controlled evaluation of sucralfate to alleviate stomatitis in patients receiving fluorouracil-based CT. *J Clin Oncol.* 1997;15:1235-1238.

127. Nottage M, McLachlan S-A, Brittain M-A, et al. Sucralfate mouthwash for prevention and treatment of 5-FU-induced mucositis: a randomized, placebo-controlled trial. *Support Care Cancer.* 2003;11:41-47.

128. Scherlacher A, Beaufort-Spontin E. Radiotherapy of head-neck neoplasms: prevention of inflammation of the mucosa by sucralfate treatment. *HNO.* 1990;38:24-28.

129. Epstein JB, Wong FLW. The efficacy of sucralfate suspension in the prevention of oral mucositis due to RT. *Int J Radiat Oncol Biol Phys.* 1994;28:693-698.

130. Dodd MJ, Miaskowski C, Greenspan D. Radiation-induced mucositis: a randomized clinical trial of micronized sucralfate versus salt & soda mouthwashes. *Cancer Invest.* 2003;21:21-33.

131. Innocenti M, Moscatelli G, Lopez S. Efficacy of Gelclair in reducing pain in palliative care patients with oral lesions. Preliminary findings from an open pilot study. *J Pain Symptom Manage.* 2001;24:456-457.

132. Barber C, Powell R, Ellis A, Hewett J. Comparing pain control and ability to eat and drink with standard therapy vs Gelclair: a preliminary, double centre, randomised controlled trial on patients with radiotherapy-induced oral mucositis. *Support Care Cancer.* 2007;15:427-440.

133. Epstein JB, Truelove EL, Oien H, Allison C, Le ND, Epstein MS. Oral topical doxepin rinse: analgesic effect in patients with oral mucosal pain due to cancer or cancer therapy. *Oral Oncol.* 2001;37:632-637.

134. Epstein JD, Epstein JB, Epstein MS, Oien H, Truelove EL. Oral topical doxepin rinse: analgesic effect and duration of pain reduction in patients with oral mucositis due to cancer therapy. *Anesth Analg.* 2006;103:465-470.

135. Epstein JB, Epstein JD, Epstein MS, Oien H, Truelove EL. Doxepin rinse for management of mucositis pain in patients with *cancer*: one week follow-up of tropical therapy. *Spec Care Dentist.* 2008;28:73-77.

136. Coluzzi PH, Schwartzberg L, Conroy JD, et al. Breakthrough cancer pain: a randomized trial comparing oral transmucosal fentanyl (OTFC) and morphine sulfate immediate release (MSIR). *Pain.* 2001;91:123-130.

137. Darwish M, Kirby M, Robertson P, Tracewell W, Jiang JG. Absorption of fentanyl from fentanyl buccal tablet in cancer patients with or without oral mucositis. *Clin Drug Invest.* 2007;27:605-611.

138. Kim JG, Sohn SK, Kim DH, et al. Effectiveness of transdermal fentanyl patch for treatment of acute pain due to oral mucositis in patients receiving stem cell transplantation. *Transplant Proc.* 2005;37:4488-4891.

139. Cerchietti LC, Navigante AH, Bonomi MR, et al. Effect of topical morphine for mucositis-associated pain following concomitant chemoradiotherapy for head and neck cancer. *Cancer.* 2002;95:2230-2236.

140. Swisher ME, Scheidler VR, Kennedy MJ. A mucositis pain management algorithm: a creative strategy to enhance the transition to ambulatory care. *Oncol Nurs Forum.* 1998.

141. Gupta A, Duckles B, Giordano J. Use of sublingual methadone for treating pain of chemotherapy-induced oral mucositis. *J Opioid Manage.* 2010;6:67-69.

142. Joseph-Ryan A, Lin F, Samady R. Ketamine mouthwash for mucositis pain. *J Palliat Med.* 2009;12:989-991.

143. Huscher A, De Stefani A, Smussi I, et al. Transdermal buprenorphine for oropharyngeal mucositis-associated pain in patients treated with radiotherapy for head and neck cancer. *J Palliat Med.* 2010;13:357-358.

144. Brand HS, Bots CP, Raber-Durlacher JE. Xerostomia and chronic oral complications among patients treated with haematopoietic stem cell transplantation. *Br Dent J.* 2009;207:428-429.

145. Atkinson JC, Grisius M, Massey W. Salivary hypofunction and Xerostomia: diagnosis and treatment. *Dent Clin North Am.* 2005;49:309-326.

146. Agha-Hosseini F, Mirzaii-Dizgah I, Ghavamzadeh L, Ghavamzadeh A, Tohidast-Acrad Z. Effect of pilocarpine hydrochloride on unstimulated whole saliva flow rate and composition in patients with chronic graft-versus-host disease (cGVHD). *Bone Marrow Transplant.* 2007;39:431-434.

147. Brizel DM, Wasserman TH, Strnad V, et al. Final report of a phase III randomized trial of amifostine as a radioprotectant in head and neck cancer. Proceedings of the American Society for Therapeutic Radiology and Oncology 41st Annual Meeting, International Journal of Radiation Oncology Biology Physics; October 31-November 4, 1999; San Antonio, TX [abstract].

CHAPTER 20

Approach to Liver Metastases in Palliative Oncology

Vaibhav Sahai ■ Mary F. Mulcahy

BURDEN OF DISEASE

The liver is the most common site of distant metastases in patients with gastrointestinal cancers (1). Patients with liver metastases may be asymptomatic or present with a range of symptoms depending on the volume of tumor, distribution of metastases, or type of primary carcinoma. Symptoms related to tumor burden may range from vague abdominal discomfort, fever, night sweats, pruritus, anorexia, and early satiety to severe localized pain and signs of liver failure such as ascites, jaundice, encephalopathy, and coagulopathy. Patients with extensive neuroendocrine metastases may experience the classic findings of flushing, wheezing, and diarrhea, as well as symptoms related to carcinoid heart disease. The presence of liver metastases confers a poor prognosis and for most patients represents incurable disease.

Outcomes of medical and/or surgical treatments have been expressed primarily in terms of response rates and disease-free survival, progression-free survival, and overall survival (OS). However, more important but less acknowledged additional measures of outcome are quality-adjusted life years and health-related quality of life (HRQoL) (2,3). These measures have primarily been used by health economists and rarely applied in oncologic clinical trials, even though the value-based HRQoL approach is conceptually similar to the index approach advocated by clinimetrics (4–6). The inclusion of quality of life measures is necessary to discern the overall impact of therapy in clinical trials and for effective communication with patients alongside response and survival outcomes (6).

Colorectal cancer is the third leading cause of cancer in the United States and the third highest in cancer-related deaths every year. It is estimated that approximately 143,460 new cases of colorectal cancer will be diagnosed in the United States in 2012 (7) and that 40% of these patients will develop liver metastasis (8). For many patients, involvement of the liver is the primary determinant of long-term survival. Surgery provides an opportunity for long-term survival (9,10), with an estimated OS of 30% at 5 years (11) and 22% to 23% at 10 years (12) for those that are amenable to surgical resection. Surgical resection is possible for only 15% to 25% of patients with metastatic colon cancer, limited to patients with liver-only metastatic disease that is resectable while leaving adequate liver mass (13). Alternative methods of controlling liver-only metastases are being pursued in an attempt to improve overall outcomes.

Neuroendocrine tumor (NET) presents with disseminated metastatic disease in a large proportion of patients with hepatic metastases present in 60% to 80% of patients (14–16). Patients with metastatic NETs have a 5-year survival rate of 22% (17), and less than 10% of patients have surgically resectable disease (18). The liver metastases usually lead to symptoms through mass effect or release of biologically active polypeptides or amines, which may cause a wide range and multitude of symptoms. The management of NETs with liver metastases is mainly focused on palliation of symptoms and prevention of future complications from the disease (19) as the disease course is usually protracted.

Therapeutic modalities are available for the management of liver metastasis when curative surgical resection is not an option. We can broadly divide them into five categories: 1) medical therapy to control symptoms and cancer, 2) palliative surgical debulking, 3) nonsurgical liver-directed therapy, 4) combination therapies, and 5) nonsurgical management of biliary obstruction. Nonsurgical liver-directed therapy includes local tumor ablative techniques (microwave ablation, radiofrequency ablation [RFA], laser photocoagulation, cryoablation) and transarterial therapy (bland transarterial embolization [TAE], transarterial chemoembolization [TACE], transarterial radioembolization, and hepatic artery infusion [HAI]).

EVALUATION

A detailed history and physical examination is the cornerstone of the evaluation of any oncologic patient. Characteristics to consider when evaluating a patient for liver-directed therapy include prior therapy received, subsequent therapy that may be available, underlying liver disease not related to the malignancy, and the goals of therapy. The goal of liver-directed therapy may be to downsize a tumor to allow for surgical resection, control the disease to improve survival, or treat symptoms related to the tumor burden. Laboratory studies evaluate liver function with regard to synthetic function and signs of portal hypertension and biliary obstruction. Depending on the distribution of disease to be treated, patients must have an adequate albumin, prothrombin time, platelet count, bilirubin, and alkaline phosphatase. Imaging modalities need to evaluate the number, size, and distribution of the metastatic lesions; the patency of the biliary tract; hepatic and portal venous systems; and the presence or absence of cirrhosis, ascites, and extrahepatic disease. High-quality imaging is paramount to decide what can technically be done and what might benefit the patient. This may consist of magnetic resonance imaging or triphasic liver computed tomography, with or without an ultrasound to evaluate evidence of vascular invasion. In the absence of extrahepatic disease, cirrhosis, and portal hypertension, ablative techniques may be limited by location of the tumor and the number and size of the metastases. Tumor adjacent to the gallbladder, main bile ducts, or vena cava may not be amenable to RFA. Intra-arterial embolic therapy is limited to patients without portal vein invasion, as discussed below.

MANAGEMENT

Medical

Systemic Therapy

Systemic chemotherapy is usually the mainstay of therapy for patients with colorectal or other primary cancers and liver metastasis who are not candidates for surgical resection. The chemotherapy indications, response rates, effect on OS, and adverse effects should be appropriately discussed with the patient prior to initiation of therapy. A detailed review of chemotherapy for metastatic cancer is beyond the scope of this chapter; however, some landmark studies comparing chemotherapy to best supportive care are discussed below.

A phase III study randomized patients with metastatic colorectal cancer to irinotecan plus supportive care versus supportive care alone. Improvements in global quality of life score (47.57 vs. 38.47, respectively; $P = 0.009$), survival without weight loss, survival without performance status deterioration, and pain-free survival were observed in the group treated with irinotecan. An improvement in OS (9.2 vs. 6.5 months, respectively; $P = 0.0001$) was also noted (20). Another phase III study randomized patients with metastatic colorectal cancer after progression on 5-fluorouracil to irinotecan versus continuous infusional 5-fluorouracil. An improvement in progression-free survival was observed in the group treated with irinotecan (4.2 vs. 2.9 months, respectively; $P = 0.03$). No improvement in quality of life score (53.90 vs. 53.0, respectively; $P = 0.69$) was noted but trends in symptom-free survival, pain-free survival, time to performance status deterioration, and loss of body weight were noted, along with a significant improvement in OS (10.8 vs. 8.5 months, respectively; $P = 0.035$) (21). More recently, an open-label, randomized trial of panitumumab plus best supportive care versus best supportive care showed improved median progression-free survival (8.0 vs. 7.3 weeks, respectively; hazard ratio [HR] 0.54, 95% CI = 0.44-0.66; $P < 0.0001$) and response outcome (10% vs. 0%, respectively; $P < 0.0001$) for those treated with panitumumab (22).

Systemic chemotherapy for metastatic NET has a limited role in view of the modest response and significant toxicity. Recently, a phase III randomized placebo-controlled study of sunitinib showed improved median progression-free survival (11.4 vs. 5.5 months, respectively; HR 0.42, 95% CI = 0.26–0.66; $P < 0.001$) and response rate (9.3% vs. 0%, respectively; $P = 0.007$) in patients with advanced pancreatic NETs treated with sunitinib (23). Another phase III randomized placebo-controlled study of everolimus showed improved median

progression-free survival (11.0 vs. 4.6 months, respectively; HR 0.35, 95% CI = 0.27–0.45; $P < 0.001$) and response rate (5% vs. 2%, respectively) in patients with advanced pancreatic NETs treated with everolimus (24). Some of the emerging therapies include radionuclides, such as I-131-mIBG and Lu-111-Octreotide.

A large proportion of gastrohepatic NETs secrete biologically active peptides or amines, which may lead to a wide range of symptoms depending on the primary NET. Somatostatin analogues have been the mainstay of treatment for these symptoms. It can be delivered in a depot formulation once a month, with the dose tailored to control the patient's symptoms. Until recently, the ability of these somatostatin analogs to control the growth of the well-differentiated metastatic midgut NETs was a matter of debate. A placebo-controlled, double blind, phase IIIB study in patients with metastatic midgut NETs showed that octreotide LAR significantly prolonged time to tumor progression compared with placebo (14.3 vs. 6.0 months, respectively; HR 0.34, 95% CI = 0.20-0.59; $P = 0.000072$) for both metabolically active and inactive NETs (25).

Symptom Management

Pruritus is a complex process that involves stimulation of free nerve endings found superficially in skin. Many chemicals are pruritogenic, including bilirubin, histamine, opioids, serotonin, and cytokines. In patients with hyperbilirubinemia, treatment involves topical and systemic antihistamines, cholestyramine, corticosteroids, local anesthetics, calcineurin inhibitors, or methods to substitute another sensation for itch, which may include a combination of cooling, heating, scratching, or application of a moisturizing lotion. Cholestyramine is a non-absorbable, anion exchange resin that can bind bile acids in the intestinal lumen, thus depleting serum bile salt pool. Cholestyramine has also been shown to be useful in other conditions, such as polycythemia rubra and uremia and, therefore, likely blocks absorption of other compounds (26). However, cholestyramine is not universally effective and associated gastrointestinal side effects can cause intolerance (27). Interestingly, rifampin at 10 mg/kg oral daily has been shown to lower intra-hepatocyte bile salt concentration by competing for uptake, with subjective improvement in pruritus (26). Other agents used for moderate-severe pruritus are opioid antagonists, such as naltrexone. Its use is based on the hypothesis that there is a higher level of endogenous opioids in patients with cholestasis, and use of an opioid antagonist will reduce the central neurotransmission of pruritic signals. Up to 50 mg oral dose once daily resulted in a significant improvement in itching and sleep in patients with pruritus resistant to cholestyramine. Nausea may be limited by using an initial dose of naltrexone 25 mg once daily, followed by subsequent titration. Caution must be exercised when used in conjunction with opioids for pain management, as the effects may be contradictory.

Patients may experience liver-related abdominal discomfort due to ascites or more severe abdominal pain as a result of stretching of the liver capsule due to liver metastases. Opioids are the mainstay of treatment, even in patients with moderate liver impairment. Concern about side effects of opioids, such as sedation, constipation, confusion, or even hesitation from caregivers, may limit titration for effective palliation. Corticosteroids provide effective adjuvant pain relief by decreasing inflammation and edema. They may also improve appetite and ameliorate constitutional symptoms of fatigue, fever, and night sweats. Extensive liver metastasis can replace most of the liver parenchyma and lead to signs and symptoms of liver failure, such as coagulopathy, encephalopathy, and hypoalbuminemia, and require appropriate medical management for this terminal stage of disease.

Palliative Surgical Resection

Surgical resection may employ hemihepatectomy, segmentectomy, or wedge resection of the metastasis. Surgical resection may provide an opportunity for long-term survival in patients with liver-only metastases from colorectal carcinoma (9,10). However, as mentioned before, only 15% to 25% patients are eligible (13). Contraindications for liver resection, mostly based on a large retrospective multi-institutional review (28), include patients with more than three lesions, bilobar distribution of metastases, portal lymph node or extrahepatic metastases, or inability to achieve 1 cm surgical margins. However, with major technical advances in surgical procedures, the associated morbidity and mortality has improved (29). As a result, surgical and medical oncologists are pushing the envelope and exploring the role of cytoreduction in non-curative patient populations (30). Palliative liver resection is occasionally offered to patients to debulk biochemically active NETs or bypass biliary obstruction. However, debulking or cytoreduction for non-biochemically active cancers, such as colorectal cancers, may not translate into improvement in OS. Some of the newer advances in surgery include sequential hepatic resection (31) and portal vein embolization (32) to allow for hypertrophy of healthy liver parenchyma and permit an aggressive surgery. A combination of liver-directed therapy and systemic chemotherapy (33) has also been used as a "neoadjuvant" approach prior to surgical resection.

Nonsurgical Liver-Directed Therapy

Liver-directed therapy, compared with surgical approaches, is less limited by patient comorbidities and lesion characteristics and, therefore, presents a palliative management option for those not eligible for surgical resection or systemic chemotherapy. Over the past few decades, transcatheter intra-arterial and ablative therapies have been utilized in patients with liver metastases to prolong survival and/or improve quality of life. Liver-directed therapy may provide symptom relief, especially in patients with functional neuroendocrine carcinoma with liver metastasis. Many of the constraints for surgical resection (inadequate liver functional reserve, extrahepatic disease, lesion characteristics, multiple bilobar lesions, or patient comorbidities) are less constraining for nonsurgical liver-directed therapy. However, selection of patients is of major importance to limit toxicity, side effects,

and premature death as well as cost to the patient and the health-care system.

Nonsurgical liver-directed therapy includes local tumor ablation (microwave or RFA, laser photocoagulation, cryo-ablation) and transarterial therapy (bland TAE, TACE, transarterial radioembolization, and HAI) (see Table 20.1).

Since the integration of liver-directed therapy into routine clinical practice, major improvements in catheter, device, and imaging technology have translated into improved outcomes for patients with metastatic lesions to the liver. Unfortunately, there are no standardized treatment protocols for liver-directed therapy, especially when delivered in combination with systemic chemotherapy.

Transarterial Therapy

Secondary liver tumors derive their blood supply from the hepatic artery (34) while the normal liver parenchyma obtains at least 50% of the oxygen supply from the portal system (35). This makes the hepatic artery a promising conduit for intra-arterial techniques. Despite the addition of these increasingly popular nonsurgical therapies to the armamentarium, there are limited data describing outcomes, quality of life measures, and OS compared with surgical metastasectomy.

TACE or Hepatic Artery Chemoembolization. Chemoembolization involves intra-arterial delivery of chemotherapy followed by embolization of the vascular supply to the tumor, resulting in selective ischemia and enhanced chemotherapeutic effect on the lesion. Chemotherapy given via the hepatic artery achieves a 10 times greater intra-tumoral concentration than when delivered via the portal vein (36). Diagnostic angiography of the celiac and mesenteric arteries is performed by the interventional radiologist prior to TACE to evaluate the hepatic arterial anatomy and extrahepatic perfusion. Extrahepatic delivery of chemotherapy can lead to a multitude of adverse effects that can be controlled, or limited, with coil embolization of aberrant vessels or distal catheter placement (37). In most institutions, TACE requires a 1- to 3-day hospital stay for each treatment. The chemotherapy to be infused is suspended in an emulsion with lipiodol (an iodized oil), which is selectively retained by the tumor (39). The lipiodol acts as both a vehicle for the cytotoxic drugs and an agent for vessel occlusion to reduce systemic toxicity. After infusion of this viscous chemotherapeutic mixture, embolization of the arterial blood supply to the tumor is completed using embolic agents, including but not limited to gelatin sponge particles, polyvinyl alcohol particles, or hydrophilic, polyacrylamide microporous beads, known as microspheres (38,39). TACE is typically delivered as a series of treatments, with the number determined by the tumor burden and localization, as well as patient tolerance.

TACE is not usually recommended for patients with portal vein thrombosis and must be used with caution in patients with higher degrees of portal hypertension. It is contraindicated in patients with significant aberrant perfusion that

TABLE 20.1 **Liver-directed therapies**

Type of Procedure	Description of Procedure	Contraindications	Adverse Effects
Radioembolization	Intra-arterial catheter-directed administration of polymer, resin, or glass microspheres, incorporating radioisotopes into the hepatic artery directly targeting the tumor, which leads to local radiotherapeutic effect	Allergy to contrast, uncorrectable bleeding diathesis, vascular abnormalities, portal vein thrombosis without hepatopetal flow, renal insufficiency, severe liver dysfunction, pulmonary insufficiency, or pregnancy	Acute hepatitis, pancreatitis, gastritis, or ulceration, radiation pneumonitis, acute cholecystitis, vague abdominal pain, nausea/vomiting
Transarterial chemoembolization (TACE)	Intra-arterial catheter-directed administration of chemotherapeutic agent/s into the hepatic artery directly targeting the tumor, with embolization of the vascular supply to the tumor resulting in selective ischemia and therefore enhanced chemotherapeutic effect on the metastasis	Allergy to contrast, uncorrectable bleeding diathesis, vascular abnormalities, portal vein thrombosis without hepatopetal flow, renal insufficiency, severe liver dysfunction, pulmonary insufficiency, or pregnancy	Post-embolization syndrome (nausea, vomiting, fever, abdominal pain with transaminitis, liver abscess, acute liver failure, acute cholecystitis, biliary duct injury, renal dysfunction, gastrointestinal bleed, cardiac toxicity
Transarterial embolization	Intra-arterial catheter-directed administration of an embolic agent such as lipiodol, polyvinyl alcohol, angiostat, or gel foam, which results in devascularization and consequent ischemic injury to the lesion	Similar to TACE	Similar to TACE
Radiofrequency ablation	Percutaneous, laparoscopic, or intra-operative insertion of a conductive probe or electrode into the tumor through imaging guidance following which high-frequency alternating current is transmitted to the immediate tissue, which leads to a calorific effect and coagulative necrosis of the tumor and its surrounding microvasculature	Tumor volume >50% of liver or significant impairment of hepatic function, lesions near hilum, vessels, or capsule	Biliary leakage, stricture, hemorrhage, thrombosis, abscess, pleural effusion, damage to vascular system, colon perforation, post-ablation syndrome (fever, chills, nausea, vomiting, malaise, abdominal pain)
Cryoablation	Percutaneous, laparoscopic, or intra-operative insertion of a conductive probe or electrode into the tumor following which rapid freezing process leads to local tissue destruction over multiple freeze–thaw cycles	Tumor volume >50% of liver or significant impairment of hepatic function, extrahepatic disease, or lesions greater than 10 cm in diameter	Biliary leakage, stricture, hemorrhage, "cryoshock phenomenon," abscess, or damage to the vascular system
Hepatic arterial infusion	Transcutaneously placed hepatic arterial catheter-directed administration of chemotherapeutic agent/s directly targeting the tumor	Unable to undergo surgical placement of catheter or with hepatic arterial anatomy suitable for pump placement. Portal vein thrombosis, more than 70% liver replacement by tumor, or significant impairment of hepatic function	Hepatic misperfusion, thrombosis of the hepatic artery, and catheter dislodgement or chemotherapy-related complications including biliary sclerosis specifically with fluorodeoxyuridine therapy. Transaminitis and gastrointestinal toxicity secondary to extrahepatic perfusion

could lead to extrahepatic distribution, bleeding diathesis, greater than 75% hepatic parenchymal involvement, severe liver dysfunction, pregnancy, severe cardiac abnormalities or contraindication to the angiographic or selective visceral catheterization (37).

In addition to tumor destruction, TACE may also cause liver decompensation (40). Approximately 80% of patients develop a post-embolization syndrome characterized by transient abdominal pain, fever, nausea, and vomiting. This is usually self-limited and typically resolves in 7 to 10 days. Serious complications may also occur; a 30-day mortality of 4.3% has been reported, primarily due to hepatic failure or infection (41). After hospital discharge, patients may require 2 to 3 weeks of convalescence prior to the next treatment.

The effect of TACE on survival is difficult to assess due to the variability of techniques, chemotherapy and embolic agents utilized, and retreatment schedules. A prospective study of 463 patients with hepatic metastases from metastatic colorectal cancer by Vogl et al. (39) showed that the median survival was 14 months from date of TACE compared with 7 to 8 months for untreated patients (42). In another prospective non-randomized study by Sanz-Altamira et al. (43), 40 patients underwent TACE and had a median OS of 10 months (see Table 20.2).

TAE or Hepatic Arterial Embolization. The hepatic arterial supply to the tumor is embolized via materials such as lipiodol, polyvinyl alcohol, angiostat, or gel foam, which results in devascularization and consequent ischemic injury to the lesion. Patient selection and adverse effects are similar to those observed with TACE. Similar to TACE, diagnostic angiography of celiac and mesenteric arteries is performed by the interventional radiologist to evaluate the hepatic arterial anatomy.

Randomized controlled trials and other retrospective studies comparing TAE with TACE have demonstrated no advantage of one technique over the other in patients with metastasis from colorectal cancer (58,59) as well as NET (41,60,61) (see Table 20.3).

Transarterial Radioembolization. Radioembolization involves the intra-arterial delivery of either glass or resin microspheres containing radioisotopes into the tumor to produce a local radiotherapeutic effect. There are two different radioisotopes containing commercial microspheres: TheraSphere (MDS Nordion, Canada) which consists of non-biodegradable glass microspheres and SIR-Spheres (Sirtex, USA) which consists of biocompatible polymer microspheres. Yttrium-90 (Y-90), a radioisotope, is an integral constituent of these spheres. Yttrium is a pure beta-emitter and has a physical half-life of 64.2 hours (2.68 days) and decays to stable zirconium-90. The average energy of the beta emissions from Y-90 is 0.9367 MeV. The average tissue range of the radiation is 2.5 mm, with a maximum range less than 1 cm. The microspheres are unable to traverse the tumor microvasculature and exert a local radiotherapeutic effect with relatively limited concurrent injury to the surrounding normal tissue.

Diagnostic angiography is performed by the interventional radiologist to evaluate the hepatic arterial anatomy. Technetium-99m macroaggregated albumin (Tc-99 MAA) hepatic arterial perfusion scintigraphy is completed prior to the procedure to detect shunting of blood to the lungs or gastrointestinal tract. Radioembolization is contraindicated if there is excessive shunting that cannot be corrected by angiographic techniques or if the shunting of blood to lungs results in delivery of greater than 16.6 mCi of radiation to the lungs. To avoid reflux of microspheres into the gastric vasculature, the gastroduodenal artery may be occluded by coil embolization techniques or the catheter advanced beyond the gastroduodenal artery at the time of infusion of the radiomicrospheres.

Radioembolization is contraindicated in patients in whom hepatic artery catheterization is contraindicated, such as those patients with vascular abnormalities, uncorrectable bleeding diathesis, uncorrectable allergy to contrast dye, as well as portal vein thrombosis without hepatopetal flow, or patients with renal insufficiency that cannot undergo treatment using alternatives to iodinated contrast media (CO_2, gadolinium). The procedure is also contraindicated in patients with severe liver dysfunction, pulmonary insufficiency, or pregnancy (66). Clinical trials have excluded patients with elevated bilirubin, except when the tumor can be isolated from a vascular standpoint.

Radioembolization has been shown to cause abdominal pain, nausea, vomiting, ulceration, and bleeding from introduction of microspheres into the gastrointestinal microvasculature (67). Pulmonary vascular shunting can cause pulmonary edema and fibrosis or radiation pneumonitis, which may be irreversible (67). Radiation pneumonitis has been seen in patients with shunting that has resulted in doses greater than 30 Gy delivered to the lungs in a single treatment. A significant deposition of radiomicrospheres can occur in the lungs in patients with arteriovenous malformations that allow the particles to pass directly from the arterial circulation to the venous system without being trapped in the hepatic capillary bed. Radioembolization may also lead to transient fever and abdominal discomfort for a few hours immediately following the procedure. However, typically the side effects experienced with radioembolization are of lower intensity compared with TACE or TAE, with post-embolization syndrome rarely reported (66). Also, radioembolization is an outpatient procedure compared with TAE or TACE, which necessitates 24 to 72 hours hospitalization for post-radioembolization syndrome. However, an evaluation of reimbursement, cost, and profit comparing TACE versus radioembolization showed that the cost for radioembolization was substantially higher (36).

Radioembolization is recognized as a treatment option by the National Comprehensive Cancer Network for metastatic NET. Although the data are limited, recent studies have shown radiologic response between 39% and 64% (68–72) (see Table 20.4).

TABLE 20.2 Outcome comparison with transarterial chemoembolization

Study	Indication	N	Chemotherapy	Radiologic Response % (CR+PR)	Median Overall Survival (months)
Hepatic metastasis from colorectal carcinoma					
Albert et al. (44)	Salvage	121	Mitomycin C cisplatin, doxorubicin	2	9
Vogl et al. (39)	Salvage	243	Mitomycin C	13.6	14
	Salvage	153	Mitomycin C, gemcitabine	11.1	13.9
	Salvage	67	Mitomycin C, irinotecan	19.4	14
Voigt et al. (45)	Salvage	11	Mitomycin, oxaliplatin, IFN-α2b, dexamethasone, 5-FU, folinic acid	33	Not reported
Tellez et al. (46)	Salvage	30	Mitomycin, cisplatin, doxorubicin	63	8.6
Sanz-Altamira et al. (43)	Salvage	40	5-FU, mitomycin	22.8	10
Lang et al. (47)	Not reported	46	Doxorubicin	Not reported	23
Hepatic metastasis from neuroendocrine carcinoma					
Dong et al. (48)	Salvage	123	Doxorubicin or streptozocin	62	39.6
de Baere (49)	Not reported	20	Doxorubicin eluting beads	80	Not reached
Marrache et al. (50)	Salvage	80	Doxorubicin or streptozocin	37	61
Fiorentini et al. (51)	Salvage	10	Lipiodol, mitomycin, cisplatin, epirubicin	70	22
Kress et al. (52)	Salvage	26	Doxorubicin	7	53.5
Gupta et al. (53)	Salvage	31	Cisplatin, vinblastine, floxuridine, doxorubicin, mitomycin, or their combination	44.4	Not reported
Roche et al. (54)	Salvage	14	Doxorubicin	43	Not reported
Desai et al. (55)	Not reported	34	Adriamycin, mitomycin	32.3	Mean OS 8 mo
Dominguez et al. (56)	Salvage	15	Streptozocin	53	Not reported
Kim et al. (57)	Salvage	30	Cisplatin, doxorubicin	37	15

CR, complete response; PR, partial response; IFN, interferon; 5-FU, 5-fluorouracil; OS, overall survival.

| TABLE 20.3 | Outcome comparison of hepatic arterial embolization | | | | |

Study	Indication	N	Device	Radiologic Response % (CR+PR)	Median Overall Survival (months)
Hepatic metastasis from neuroendocrine carcinoma					
Ruutiainen et al. (60)	Salvage	23	Polyvinyl alcohol particles with or without addition of iodized oil	50	39
Strosberg et al. (62)	Salvage (except n = 25 for cytoreduction)	84	Polyvinyl alcohol or microspheres	48	36
Gupta et al. (61)	Salvage in carcinoid tumors	42	Polyvinyl alcohol particles or gelfoam powder	81	33.2
	Salvage in islet cell carcinomas	32		25	18.2
Loewe et al. (63)	Salvage	23	N-butyl-2-cyanoacrylate and ethiodized oil	72.7	69
Eriksson et al. (64)	Salvage in carcinoid tumors	29	Gelfoam powder mixed with iodinated contrast	38	80
	Salvage in islet cell carcinomas	12		17	20
Wangberg et al. (65)	Palliation after surgical cytoreduction	40	Gelfoam powder mixed with iodinated contrast	42.5	Not reported

CR, complete response; PR, partial response.

Hepatic Arterial Infusion. HAI is transarterial delivery of chemotherapy to the liver, to achieve higher drug concentration at the tumor site and limit systemic toxicity. 5-Fluorouracil and fluorodeoxyuridine (FUDR) are the drugs most commonly used for liver metastases from colorectal cancer. Hepatic drug uptake and metabolism is a saturable process, the capacity of which is exceeded at higher drug delivery rates. Continuous HAI is regarded as the most efficacious means of drug delivery to achieve maximal local effect (82). Furthermore, since both these drugs are cell cycle dependent, continuous infusion leads to greater cell damage and apoptosis.

Placement of a percutaneous catheter, either angiographically or more commonly via either laparoscopy or laparotomy, is required. The catheter is connected to either a bedside infusion pump or an implantable subcutaneous pump, which allows for ambulation. Patients appropriate for HAI include those able to undergo surgical placement of the catheter and hepatic arterial anatomy suitable for pump placement. Contraindications include portal vein thrombosis, more than 70% liver replacement by tumor, or significant impairment of hepatic function (83).

Adverse effects include those related to device placement and chemotherapy-related complications. Device-related complications, albeit rare, may include perioperative mortality, hematomas, infections, hepatic misperfusion, thrombosis of the hepatic artery, and catheter dislodgement. Chemotherapy-related complications include biliary sclerosis specifically with FUDR therapy, transaminitis, and gastrointestinal toxicity secondary to extrahepatic perfusion.

Martin et al. randomized 74 patients with hepatic metastases from colorectal carcinoma to either HAI (FUDR) or systemic chemotherapy (5-fluorouracil) and no crossover was allowed. Although the overall response rate (48% vs. 21%) and time to hepatic progression (15.7 vs. 6.0 months) were significantly better for the HAI arm, neither the OS (12.6 vs. 10.5 months) nor the progression-free survival (6.0 vs. 5.0 months) was significantly different between the two arms (84). Kemeny et al. also randomized 162 patients with hepatic metastases from colorectal carcinoma to either systemic chemotherapy (FUDR) or HAI (FUDR). Patients on HAI arm had significantly higher overall response (50% vs. 20%; P = 0.001), and the median time to discontinuation of therapy was 9 months in the HAI arm and 5 months in the systemic arm (P = 0.016). Again, the median OS between the two arms was not significant (17 vs. 12 months). However, 60% of the patients who received systemic FUDR had crossed over at the

TABLE 20.4 Outcome comparison with radioembolization

Study	Indication	N	Device	Radiologic Response % (CR+PR)	Median Overall Survival (months)
Hepatic metastasis from colorectal carcinoma					
Cianni et al. (73)	Salvage	41	Y-90	46.3	11.8
Hong et al. (74)	Salvage	15	Y-90	Not reported	6.9
Sato et al. (75)	Salvage	51	Y-90	Not reported	15.2
Kennedy et al. (67)	Salvage	208	Y-90	35.5	4.5–10.5[a]
Murthy et al. (76)	Salvage	12	Y-90 with adjuvant chemotherapy (n = 2)	0	4.5
Lewandoski et al. (77)	Salvage in 24 patients	27	Y-90	35	9.4
Lim et al. (78)	Salvage	30	Y-90	33	Not reported
Andrews et al. (79)	Salvage	17	Y-90	29.4	15
Hepatic metastasis from neuroendocrine carcinoma					
Memon et al. (72)	Salvage	40	Y-90	64	34.4
Saxena et al. (71)	Salvage	48	Y-90	54	35
Rhee et al. (68)	Salvage	42	Y-90 glass	54	22
			Y-90 resin	50	28
Kennedy et al. (69)	Salvage	148	Y-90	63	70
Sato et al. (75)	Salvage	19	Y-90	Not reported	25.9
Murthy et al. (80)	Salvage	8	Y-90	12	14
McStay et al. (81)	Salvage	23	Y-90-DOTA-lanreotide	16	15

CR, complete response; PR, partial response.

[a]10.5 mo in patients with response and 4.5 mo in patients without response to Y-90.

time of progression to receive HAI, and the crossover group had median OS of 9.5 months versus 3.4 months for the non-crossover group (85). However, this could also be attributed to a favorable selection of patients undergoing crossover. Hohn et al. also randomized 143 patients with hepatic metastases from colorectal carcinoma to either HAI (FUDR) or systemic chemotherapy (FUDR). The authors also noted significant improvement in overall response rate (42% vs. 10%; $P = 0.0001$) and time to progression (396 vs. 201 days; $P = 0.009$), with no significant improvement in median OS (503 vs. 484 days) (86). Rougier et al. randomized 166 patients with hepatic metastases from colorectal carcinoma to either HAI or no HAI. A significant improvement was observed in the survival rate for the patients assigned to the HAI group ($P < 0.02$), with a 1-year survival rate of 64% versus 44% in the control group. However, 30% and 50% of patients received systemic chemotherapy (5-fluorouracil) in HAI versus no HAI arm, respectively (87). Allen-Mersh et al. randomized 100 patients to either HAI (FUDR) or conventional symptom palliation and noted significant improvement in median OS (405 vs. 226 days; $P = 0.03$) as well as physical symptoms ($P = 0.04$), anxiety ($P = 0.04$), and depression ($P = 0.04$) in the HAI arm (88).

Ablative Techniques

Radiofrequency Ablation. RFA involves insertion of a conductive probe or electrode into the tumor through imaging guidance following which high-frequency alternating current is transmitted to the immediate tissue (89). The catheter placement can be performed percutaneously, laparoscopically, or intra-operatively, individualizing the approach based on the location of the lesion, its relation to the vessels, and technical expertise of the surgeon. The radiofrequency waves lead to a calorific effect and coagulative necrosis of the tumor and its surrounding microvasculature (90). The amount of local tissue damage correlates with the impedance of the tissue and its distance from the electrode (91).

The treatment strategy depends on patient comorbidities, number and distribution of lesions, and presence of cirrhosis. Complete tumor ablation can be achieved for tumors less than 5 cm in diameter and have 1 cm distance to allow for coagulative necrosis (91–93). RFA for lesions near the hilum is not advocated since the biliary structures in the area are at a significant risk for stricture and subsequent stenosis from thermal damage (94). Similarly, RFA of lesions near the capsule should be avoided because of the risk of perforation or thermal injury to intestines. Target tumors that are adjacent to major hepatic vessels are at risk for incomplete thermal necrosis due to a cooling effect of the blood flow known as a heat sink effect (95).

RFA is considered a generally safe procedure with a low mortality rate (0% to 2%) and a low major complication rate. The adverse effects localized to the procedural site include abscess, hemorrhage, biliary leakage or stricture (96), liver failure, and subcapsular hematoma. Other side effects that have been reported include vascular thrombosis (97), pleural effusion, damage to the vascular system, wound infection, and colon perforation. Around 30% to 40% of patients may

also experience a self-limited post-ablation syndrome, characterized by fever, chills, malaise, pain, nausea, and vomiting, which generally occurs between days 3 and 8 after the procedure (98).

There are no published randomized controlled trials of RFA for hepatic metastasis from colorectal cancers. The American Society of Clinical Oncology in 2009 completed a clinical review of the literature of RFA for hepatic metastasis from colorectal cancer (98). The report concluded that the data were insufficient to formulate a practice guideline. A clinical evidence review report noted a wide variability in the 5-year survival rate (14% to 55%) and local recurrence rate (3.6% to 60%) among the published studies, likely secondary to procedural expertise, institutional volume, and patient or tumor selection criteria. A phase II trial with a primary objective to exclude a 30-month OS rate ≤ 38% with RFA plus systemic chemotherapy (Fleming Design) was presented at the ASCO 2010 annual meeting. Although the primary endpoint was met, the study design did not allow a formal comparison between treatment arms. Longer follow-up was needed to assess OS and the benefit of adding RFA to systemic chemotherapy (99). A single-arm prospective study of 63 patients with unresectable hepatic disease from carcinoid or islet cell tumors treated with ultrasound-guided laparoscopic RFA ablation demonstrated a median OS of 3.9 years (100) (see Table 20.5).

Cryoablation. Cryoablation delivers argon or liquid nitrogen directly to the liver tumor through a cryoprobe under ultrasound guidance. The catheter can be inserted percutaneously, laparoscopically, or intra-operatively. The rapid freezing process leads to local tissue destruction over multiple freeze–thaw cycles. However, malignant cells may be more resistant to cryoablation than to hyperthermia (114). The technique can be utilized for inoperable disease but is more commonly employed as a complement to surgical resection.

Patient exclusion criteria include tumor volume greater than 50% of the liver, extrahepatic disease, and lesions greater than 10 cm in diameter (115). It may be suitable for ablation adjoining major intrahepatic branches of portal or hepatic veins, hepatic artery, or inferior vena cava, depending on operator expertise, since the warm blood flow protects the vessel wall (115).

As with other ablation techniques, abscess, biliary leakage, and stricture and hemorrhage are potential complications. Coagulopathy and thrombocytopenia have been reported as well (116). A cryotherapy-induced systemic inflammatory response can also lead to disseminated intravascular coagulation, renal failure, hepatic failure, and adult respiratory distress syndrome through massive cytokine release, described as "cryoshock phenomenon" (117).

Korpan et al. prospectively randomized 123 patients with hepatic metastasis (primary colorectal cancer in 66.6%) to either cryogenic surgery (cryoablation, cryoresection, or cryodestruction) or conventional surgery. The 5-year OS rate was 44% after cryogenic surgery versus 36% after conventional surgery but was not statistically significant (118). As mentioned

| TABLE 20.5 Outcome comparison of radiofrequency and cryoablation |

Study	Indication	N	Technique	Survival Rate(s) (%)	Median Overall Survival (months)
Hepatic metastasis from colorectal carcinoma					
Veltri et al. (101)	Salvage	122	Percutaneous RFA (89%) Open RFA (11%)	1, 3, and 5-y survival was 79%, 38%, and 22%, respectively	31.5
Sorensen et al. (102)	Salvage	102	Percutaneous RFA (86%) Open RFA (14%)	1, 2, 3, and 4-y survival was 87%, 62%, 46%, and 26%, respectively	32
Suppiah et al. (103)	Salvage	30	Percutaneous RFA	Not reported	23.2
Machi et al. (104)	Salvage	100	Percutaneous (41.8%) Laparoscopic (15.8%) Open (42.4%)	1, 3, 4, and 5-y survival was 90%, 42%, 31%, and 31%, respectively	28
Jakobs et al. (105)	Salvage	68	Percutaneous RFA	1, 2, and 3-y survival was 96%, 71%, and 68%, respectively	Not reached
Gillams et al. (106)	Salvage	167	Percutaneous RFA	1, 3, and 5-y survival was 71%, 21%, and 14%, respectively	22
Lencioni et al. (107)	Salvage	423	Percutaneous RFA	1, 2, 3, 4, and 5-y survival was 86%, 63%, 47%, 29%, and 24%, respectively	Not reached
Abdalla et al. (108)	Salvage	57	Open RFA	3 and 4-y survival was 37% and 22%, respectively	Not reported
Solbiati et al. (109)	Salvage	117	Percutaneous RFA	1, 2, and 3-y survival was 93%, 69%, and 46%, respectively	36
Hepatic metastasis from neuroendocrine carcinoma					
Akyildiz et al. (110)	Salvage	89	Laparoscopic RFA	5-y survival was 57%	72
Mazzaglia et al. (100)	Salvage	63	Laparoscopic RFA	1, 2, and 5-y survival was 91%, 77%, and 48%, respectively	46.8
Bilchik et al. (111)	Salvage	19	Open cryoablation	1-y survival was 80%	>49
Cozzi et al. (112)	Salvage	6	Open cryoablation	Survival was 100% after median follow-up of 2 y	Not reached
Shapiro et al. (113)	Salvage	5	Open cryoablation	1, 2, and 2.5-y survival was 60%, 40%, and 20%, respectively	Not reported

RFA, radiofrequency ablation.

before, cryoablation has been more commonly employed as a complement to primary surgical resection for either inadequate resection margins or lesions in the remaining lobe of the liver, thus offering the possibility of increasing the proportion of patients with potentially curative treatment (119). In a prospective study of 415 patients with hepatic metastasis from colorectal carcinoma, 291 underwent resection only and 124 underwent combined resection and cryotherapy. However, the authors reported no significant difference in OS between the two groups (120). Only a few studies have reported the use of cryosurgery or cryoablation for patients not amenable to surgical resection or with progressive disease unresponsive to previous therapies. In patients with hepatic metastases from NET, especially with functional tumors, use of cryoablation has resulted in significant alleviation from disabling symptoms from hormonal secretion (111–113).

A few studies have compared RFA with cryoablation in patients with unresectable primary or secondary hepatic malignancies. Pearson et al. published a prospective nonrandomized analysis of 146 patients who received either RFA ($n = 92$) or cryoablation ($n = 54$) and reported increased frequency of complication rate (3.3% vs. 40.7%; $P < 0.001$) and early local recurrences (2.2% vs. 13.6%; $P < 0.01$) with cryoablation (121). A similar result was reported by Bilchik et al. ($n = 308$) (122) and Adam et al. ($n = 68$) (123). RFA may be a preferred approach for patients with unresectable hepatic metastases (124); however, the data are sparse and there are no randomized studies comparing the two modalities (see Table 20.5).

Other Ablative Therapies. Other ablative therapies are being used and investigated, such as laser-induced thermotherapy (LITT), percutaneous ethanol injection (PEI), and microwave coagulation therapy. LITT is an ablation technique using laser light produced by Nd:YAG delivered through a quartz fiber optic with a diameter of 400 mm with diffuse light emission. The laser light is converted to heat in the target area, resulting in coagulative necrosis (125,126). Microwave coagulation therapy involves needle electrode insertion via either percutaneous or laparoscopic approach usually for tumors less than 30 mm (127). PEI is also a safe and minimally invasive technique in which ethanol acts by diffusion within the cells, causing immediate dehydration with coagulative necrosis followed by fibrosis. Although its effectiveness in hepatocellular carcinoma has been shown, its role in hepatic metastases is unclear (127). The advantages of these techniques include their minimally invasive character, lack of short-term and long-term morbidity, and short hospital stay (125,127). However, large patient databases with prospective, comparative, and preferably randomized studies are lacking.

Combination Therapies

Regional treatment of hepatic metastases with either ablative or intra-arterial techniques has been extensively employed, with goals of symptom palliation and/or improvement in OS, either before or after systemic chemotherapy. There is clearly a need to further enhance the improvement in the disease-free survival and OS, and therefore, it is only logical to combine the systemic chemotherapy with different types of liver-directed therapy for both palliation and first-line treatment.

Kemeny et al. randomized 156 patients with liver-only metastases from colorectal carcinoma to either systemic chemotherapy (5-fluorouracil) or HAI (FUDR) plus intravenous 5-fluorouracil after metastasectomy. OS at 2 years was 86% in the combination group and 72% in the systemic therapy alone group ($P = 0.03$) (128). More recently, Alberts et al. reported the results of a phase II intergroup trial in which 55 patients with liver-only metastases from colorectal carcinoma received HAI (FUDR) alternating with systemic chemotherapy (capecitabine and oxaliplatin) after metastasectomy. Overall, 88% of evaluable patients were alive at 2 years and median disease-free survival was 32.7 months (129). Based on the results of this trial, an attempt was made to randomize patients to receive systemic chemotherapy (capecitabine and oxaliplatin) with or without HAI (FUDR) in the NSABP C-09 phase III trial. However, the trial was closed early due to difficulty in adequate accrual of patients and marked decline in the use of HAI in the United States (129).

Van Hazel et al. conducted a randomized phase II trial in 21 patients with previously untreated advanced colorectal liver metastases, with or without extrahepatic disease, who received systemic chemotherapy (5-fluorouracil plus leucovorin) with or without radioembolization with Y-90. Both time to progression (18.6 vs. 3.6 months; $P < 0.0005$) and median survival (29.4 vs. 12.8 months; $P = 0.02$) were significantly longer for combination therapy. However, there was no difference in quality of life over a 3-month period between the two treatments when rated by patients ($P = 0.96$) or physicians ($P = 0.98$) (130). Gray et al. randomized 74 patients with unresectable liver metastases from colorectal carcinoma to either HAI (FUDR) or HAI plus radioembolization with Y-90. The authors reported a significant improvement in response rate (44% vs. 17.6%; $P = 0.01$), median time to progression (15.9 vs. 9.7 months; $P = 0.001$), no increase in grade 3 to 4 treatment-related toxicity and no loss of quality of life for patients receiving combination therapy (131) (see Table 20.6).

Hepatic resection remains the gold standard for the treatment of hepatic metastases from colorectal carcinoma; however, majority of the patients are not good surgical candidates and liver-directed therapies have been increasingly used in recent years and have emerged as a viable option for palliative therapy by alleviation of pain, hormonal symptoms from certain malignancies, and decrease in tumor burden. The range of options is fairly wide, with several patient and procedural variables to be considered prior to recommendation, and the choice is not always easy, especially with a dearth of randomized data comparing the different techniques.

TABLE 20.6   Outcome comparison for combination therapy

Study	Indication	N	Device	Response Rate % (CR+PR)	P value	Median Overall Survival (months)	P value
Hepatic metastasis from colorectal carcinoma							
Hazel et al. (130), phase II	First line	11	5-FU/LV+ Y-90	10	<0.001	29.4	0.02
		10	5-FU/LV	0		12.8	
Gray et al. (131), phase III	First or second line	36	HAI (FUDR) + Y-90	44	0.01	23.5	0.18
		34	HAI (FUDR)	17.6		18.4	
Murthy et al. (132), retrospective	Salvage	10	Y-90 + cetuximab or bevacizumab or chemotherapy	0	NA	Not reached	NA
Stubbs et al. (133), prospective	Salvage	80	HAI (5-FU) + Y-90	Not reported	Not reported	12.62	0.002
		20	Y-90	Not reported		2.63	
Hepatic metastasis from neuroendocrine carcinoma							
King et al. (70), prospective	Salvage	34	HAI (5-FU) + Y-90	50	NA	29.4	NA
Christante et al. (134), retrospective	Salvage	74	HAI (5-FU) followed by TACE (cisplatin, doxorubicin, mitomycin C)	58	NA	39	NA
Drougas et al. (135), retrospective	Salvage	15	HAI (5-FU) followed by TACE (cisplatin, doxorubicin, mitomycin C)	8	NA	16	NA

CR, complete response; PR, partial response; FUDR, fluorodeoxyuridine; NA, not applicable; TACE, transarterial chemoembolization; HAI, hepatic arterial infusion; 5-FU, 5-fluorouracil; LV, leucovorin.

Management of Biliary Obstruction

Malignant intrahepatic and extrahepatic biliary obstruction may arise from intrinsic obstruction or extrinsic compression from liver metastases or lymphadenopathy. Jaundice may be the presenting symptom of an underlying cancer. Symptoms of obstructive jaundice, such as fatigue, pruritus, nausea, loss of appetite, dark urine, and light stools, can adversely impact the quality of life. In these patients, palliative management may significantly improve patient symptoms, quality of life, and even psychosocial outcomes.

Approaches for the treatment of biliary obstruction include endoscopic retrograde cholangiopancreatography (ERCP)–guided stent placement, percutaneous transhepatic cholangiopancreatography (PTC) with catheter placement, and surgical bypass.

ERCP-guided biliary stent placement for strictures or other areas of narrowing is the mainstay of palliative management of malignant biliary obstruction. Metal stents are preferred over plastic stents since the patency of metal stents (111 to 273 days) is longer than plastic stents (62 to 165 days) with similar rates of success and complications (136), especially in palliative management when frequent re-intervention is not optimal. There are a multitude of biliary metal stents, but definitive data favoring covered or uncovered stents are lacking (137).

PTC is an interventional radiologic procedure that uses fluoroscopic guidance to percutaneously proceed through the liver parenchyma, identify the level and cause of biliary obstruction, and placement of an internal or external catheter for drainage. PTC is performed when ERCP is unsuccessful, usually due to abnormal biliary anatomy or distortion due to tumor compression.

Stenting techniques are effective in the short term with a risk of occlusion and cholangitis and may require further intervention via either repeat ERCP or PTC. Surgical bypass (hepaticojejunostomy or cholecystojejunostomy) carries an appreciable risk of postoperative morbidity and mortality up to 24% in some trials (138).

In a 2007 meta-analysis, 24 studies containing 2,436 patients with malignant biliary obstruction, deemed unsuitable for curative surgical treatment, were reviewed. Three trials compared surgery with ERCP-guided plastic stent deployment. There were no significant differences in technical or therapeutic success, but the relative risk of complications was significantly reduced in those receiving stents compared with surgery ($P = 0.0007$), with the 30-day mortality trend in favor of stenting (138).

Adverse effects with stent deployment include concern for re-occlusion, increased propensity for migration, and an increased risk of cholecystitis or even pancreatitis. The most common complications with PTC placement are cholangitis (6.5% to 22%), cholecystitis (1.9% to 12%), and liver abscess (0.3% to 0.5%) (139). Potential complications with surgical bypass include anastomotic leakage, hemorrhage, abdominal abscess, wound infection, renal failure, pancreatitis, and enterocutaneous fistula (140,141).

REFERENCES

1. Liu LX, Zhang WH, Jiang HC. Current treatment for liver metastases from colorectal cancer. *World J Gastroenterol.* 2003;9(2):193-200.
2. Byrne C, Griffin A, Blazeby J, Conroy T, Efficace F. Health-related quality of life as a valid outcome in the treatment of advanced colorectal cancer. *Eur J Surg Oncol.* 2007;33(suppl 2): S95-S104.
3. Gall CA, Weller D, Esterman A, et al. Patient satisfaction and health-related quality of life after treatment for colon cancer. *Dis Colon Rectum.* 2007;50(6):801-809.
4. Wright JG, Feinstein AR. A comparative contrast of clinimetric and psychometric methods for constructing indexes and rating scales. *J Clin Epidemiol.* 1992;45(11):1201-1218.
5. Feinstein AR. An additional basic science for clinical medicine: IV. The development of clinimetrics. *Ann Intern Med.* 1983;99(6):843-848.
6. Wiering B, Oyen WJ, Adang EM, et al. Long-term global quality of life in patients treated for colorectal liver metastases. *Br J Surg.* 2011;98(4):565-571; discussion 571-572.
7. Siegel R, Naishadham D, Jemal A. Cancer statistics, 2012. *CA Cancer J Clin.* 2012;62(1):10-29.
8. Greenway B. Hepatic metastases from colorectal cancer: resection or not. *Br J Surg.* 1988;75(6):513-519.
9. Ballantyne GH, Quin J. Surgical treatment of liver metastases in patients with colorectal cancer. *Cancer.* 1993;71(12 suppl):4252-4266.
10. de Jong MC, Pulitano C, Ribero D, et al. Rates and patterns of recurrence following curative intent surgery for colorectal liver metastasis: an international multi-institutional analysis of 1669 patients. *Ann Surg.* 2009;250(3):440-448.
11. Fong Y, Salo J. Surgical therapy of hepatic colorectal metastasis. *Semin Oncol.* 1999;26(5):514-523.
12. McLoughlin JM, Jensen EH, Malafa M. Resection of colorectal liver metastases: current perspectives. *Cancer Control.* 2006;13(1):32-41.
13. Fusai G, Davidson BR. Management of colorectal liver metastases. *Colorectal Dis.* 2003;5(1):2-23.
14. Hellman P, Lundstrom T, Ohrvall U, et al. Effect of surgery on the outcome of midgut carcinoid disease with lymph node and liver metastases. *World J Surg.* 2002;26(8):991-997.
15. Makridis C, Rastad J, Oberg K, Akerstrom G. Progression of metastases and symptom improvement from laparotomy in midgut carcinoid tumors. *World J Surg.* 1996;20(7):900-906; discussion 907.
16. Soreide O, Berstad T, Bakka A, et al. Surgical treatment as a principle in patients with advanced abdominal carcinoid tumors. *Surgery.* 1992;111(1):48-54.
17. Modlin IM, Sandor A. An analysis of 8305 cases of carcinoid tumors. *Cancer.* 1997;79(4):813-829.
18. Sacks D, Marinelli DL, Martin LG, Spies JB. General principles for evaluation of new interventional technologies and devices. *J Vasc Interv Radiol.* 2003;14(9 pt 2):S391-S394.
19. Chambers AJ, Pasieka JL, Dixon E, Rorstad O. The palliative benefit of aggressive surgical intervention for both hepatic and mesenteric metastases from neuroendocrine tumors. *Surgery.* 2008;144(4):645-651; discussion 651-653.
20. Cunningham D, Pyrhonen S, James RD, et al. Randomised trial of irinotecan plus supportive care versus supportive care alone after fluorouracil failure for patients with metastatic colorectal cancer. *Lancet.* 1998;352(9138):1413-1418.

21. Rougier P, Van Cutsem E, Bajetta E, et al. Randomised trial of irinotecan versus fluorouracil by continuous infusion after fluorouracil failure in patients with metastatic colorectal cancer. *Lancet*. 1998;352(9138):1407-1412.

22. Van Cutsem E, Peeters M, Siena S, et al. Open-label phase III trial of panitumumab plus best supportive care compared with best supportive care alone in patients with chemotherapy-refractory metastatic colorectal cancer. *J Clin Oncol*. 2007;25(13):1658-1664.

23. Raymond E, Dahan L, Raoul JL, et al. Sunitinib malate for the treatment of pancreatic neuroendocrine tumors. *N Engl J Med*. 2011;364(6):501-513.

24. Yao JC, Shah MH, Ito T, et al. Everolimus for advanced pancreatic neuroendocrine tumors. *N Engl J Med*. 2011;364(6):514-523.

25. Rinke A, Muller HH, Schade-Brittinger C, et al. Placebo-controlled, double-blind, prospective, randomized study on the effect of octreotide LAR in the control of tumor growth in patients with metastatic neuroendocrine midgut tumors: a report from the PROMID Study Group. *J Clin Oncol*. 2009;27(28):4656-4663.

26. Khandelwal M, Malet PF. Pruritus associated with cholestasis. A review of pathogenesis and management. *Dig Dis Sci*. 1994;39(1):1-8.

27. Bergasa NV. The pruritus of cholestasis. *J Hepatol*. 2005;43(6): 1078-1088.

28. Hughes KS, Simon R, Songhorabodi S, et al. Resection of the liver for colorectal carcinoma metastases: a multi-institutional study of patterns of recurrence. *Surgery*. 1986;100(2):278-284.

29. Choti MA, Sitzmann JV, Tiburi MF, et al. Trends in long-term survival following liver resection for hepatic colorectal metastases. *Ann Surg*. 2002;235(6):759-766.

30. Tanabe KK. Palliative liver resections. *J Surg Oncol*. 2002;80(2): 69-71.

31. Adam R, Laurent A, Azoulay D, Castaing D, Bismuth H. Two-stage hepatectomy: a planned strategy to treat irresectable liver tumors. *Ann Surg*. 2000;232(6):777-785.

32. Azoulay D, Castaing D, Smail A, et al. Resection of nonresectable liver metastases from colorectal cancer after percutaneous portal vein embolization. *Ann Surg*. 2000;231(4):480-486.

33. Bismuth H, Adam R, Levi F, et al. Resection of nonresectable liver metastases from colorectal cancer after neoadjuvant chemotherapy. *Ann Surg*. 1996;224(4):509-520; discussion 520-522.

34. Breedis C, Young G. The blood supply of neoplasms in the liver. *Am J Pathol*. 1954;30(5):969-977.

35. Schenk WG, Jr., Mc DJ, Mc DK, Drapanas T. Direct measurement of hepatic blood flow in surgical patients: with related observations on hepatic flow dynamics in experimental animals. *Ann Surg*. 1962;156:463-471.

36. Whitney R, Valek V, Fages JF, et al. Transarterial chemoembolization and selective internal radiation for the treatment of patients with metastatic neuroendocrine tumors: a comparison of efficacy and cost. *Oncologist*. 2011;16(5):594-601.

37. Martin RC, Joshi J, Robbins K, et al. Transarterial chemoembolization of metastatic colorectal carcinoma with drug-eluting beads, irinotecan (DEBIRI): multi-institutional registry. *J Oncol*. 2009;2009:539795.

38. Coldwell DM, Stokes KR, Yakes WF. Embolotherapy: agents, clinical applications, and techniques. *Radiographics*. 1994;14(3):623-643; quiz 645-646.

39. Vogl TJ, Gruber T, Balzer JO, et al. Repeated transarterial chemoembolization in the treatment of liver metastases of colorectal cancer: prospective study. *Radiology*. 2009;250(1):281-289.

40. Uchida M, Kohno H, Kubota H, et al. Role of preoperative transcatheter arterial oily chemoembolization for resectable hepatocellular carcinoma. *World J Surg*. 1996;20(3):326-331.

41. Ho AS, Picus J, Darcy MD, et al. Long-term outcome after chemoembolization and embolization of hepatic metastatic lesions from neuroendocrine tumors. *AJR Am J Roentgenol*. 2007;188(5):1201-1207.

42. Vogl TJ, Mack MG, Balzer JO, et al. Liver metastases: neoadjuvant downsizing with transarterial chemoembolization before laser-induced thermotherapy. *Radiology*. 2003;229(2): 457-464.

43. Sanz-Altamira PM, Spence LD, Huberman MS, et al. Selective chemoembolization in the management of hepatic metastases in refractory colorectal carcinoma: a phase II trial. *Dis Colon Rectum*. 1997;40(7):770-775.

44. Albert M, Kiefer MV, Sun W, et al. Chemoembolization of colorectal liver metastases with cisplatin, doxorubicin, mitomycin C, ethiodol, and polyvinyl alcohol. *Cancer*. 2011;117(2): 343-352.

45. Voigt W, Behrmann C, Schlueter A, et al. A new chemoembolization protocol in refractory liver metastasis of colorectal cancer—a feasibility study. *Onkologie*. 2002;25(2):158-164.

46. Tellez C, Benson AB, 3rd, Lyster MT, et al. Phase II trial of chemoembolization for the treatment of metastatic colorectal carcinoma to the liver and review of the literature. *Cancer*. 1998;82(7):1250-1259.

47. Lang EK, Brown CL Jr. Colorectal metastases to the liver: selective chemoembolization. *Radiology*. 1993;189(2):417-422.

48. Dong XD, Carr BI. Hepatic artery chemoembolization for the treatment of liver metastases from neuroendocrine tumors: a long-term follow-up in 123 patients. *Med Oncol*. 2011;28(suppl 1): S286-S290.

49. de Baere T, Deschamps F, Teriitheau C, et al. Transarterial chemoembolization of liver metastases from well differentiated gastroenteropancreatic endocrine tumors with doxorubicin-eluting beads: preliminary results. *J Vasc Interv Radiol*. 2008;19(6):855-861.

50. Marrache F, Vullierme MP, Roy C, et al. Arterial phase enhancement and body mass index are predictors of response to chemoembolisation for liver metastases of endocrine tumours. *Br J Cancer*. 2007;96(1):49-55.

51. Fiorentini G, Rossi S, Bonechi F, et al. Intra-arterial hepatic chemoembolization in liver metastases from neuroendocrine tumors: a phase II study. *J Chemother*. 2004;16(3):293-297.

52. Kress O, Wagner HJ, Wied M, et al. Transarterial chemoembolization of advanced liver metastases of neuroendocrine tumors—a retrospective single-center analysis. *Digestion*. 2003;68(2-3):94-101.

53. Gupta S, Yao JC, Ahrar K, et al. Hepatic artery embolization and chemoembolization for treatment of patients with metastatic carcinoid tumors: the M.D. Anderson experience. *Cancer J*. 2003;9(4):261-267.

54. Roche A, Girish BV, de Baere T, et al. Trans-catheter arterial chemoembolization as first-line treatment for hepatic metastases from endocrine tumors. *Eur Radiol*. 2003;13(1):136-140.

55. Desai DC, O'Dorisio TM, Schirmer WJ, et al. Serum pancreastatin levels predict response to hepatic artery chemoembolization and somatostatin analogue therapy in metastatic neuroendocrine tumors. *Regul Pept*. 2001;96(3):113-117.

56. Dominguez S, Denys A, Madeira I, et al. Hepatic arterial chemoembolization with streptozotocin in patients with metastatic digestive endocrine tumours. *Eur J Gastroenterol Hepatol*. 2000;12(2):151-157.

57. Kim YH, Ajani JA, Carrasco CH, et al. Selective hepatic arterial chemoembolization for liver metastases in patients with carcinoid tumor or islet cell carcinoma. *Cancer Invest*. 1999;17(7):474-478.

58. Salman HS, Cynamon J, Jagust M, et al. Randomized phase II trial of embolization therapy versus chemoembolization therapy in previously treated patients with colorectal carcinoma metastatic to the liver. *Clin Colorectal Cancer*. 2002;2(3):173-179.

59. Martinelli DJ, Wadler S, Bakal CW, et al. Utility of embolization or chemoembolization as second-line treatment in patients with advanced or recurrent colorectal carcinoma. *Cancer*. 1994;74(6):1706-1712.

60. Ruutiainen AT, Soulen MC, Tuite CM, et al. Chemoembolization and bland embolization of neuroendocrine tumor metastases to the liver. *J Vasc Interv Radiol*. 2007;18(7):847-855.

61. Gupta S, Johnson MM, Murthy R, et al. Hepatic arterial embolization and chemoembolization for the treatment of patients with metastatic neuroendocrine tumors: variables affecting response rates and survival. *Cancer*. 2005;104(8):1590-1602.

62. Strosberg JR, Choi J, Cantor AB, Kvols LK. Selective hepatic artery embolization for treatment of patients with metastatic carcinoid and pancreatic endocrine tumors. *Cancer Control*. 2006;13(1):72-78.

63. Loewe C, Schindl M, Cejna M, et al. Permanent transarterial embolization of neuroendocrine metastases of the liver using cyanoacrylate and lipiodol: assessment of mid- and long-term results. *AJR Am J Roentgenol*. 2003;180(5):1379-1384.

64. Eriksson BK, Larsson EG, Skogseid BM, et al. Liver embolizations of patients with malignant neuroendocrine gastrointestinal tumors. *Cancer*. 1998;83(11):2293-2301.

65. Wangberg B, Westberg G, Tylen U, et al. Survival of patients with disseminated midgut carcinoid tumors after aggressive tumor reduction. *World J Surg*. 1996;20(7):892-899; discussion 899.

66. Coldwell D, Sangro B, Wasan H, Salem R, Kennedy A. General selection criteria of patients for radioembolization of liver tumors: an international working group report. *Am J Clin Oncol*. 2011;34(3):337-341.

67. Kennedy AS, Coldwell D, Nutting C, et al. Resin 90Y-microsphere brachytherapy for unresectable colorectal liver metastases: modern USA experience. *Int J Radiat Oncol Biol Phys*. 2006;65(2):412-425.

68. Rhee TK, Lewandowski RJ, Liu DM, et al. 90Y radioembolization for metastatic neuroendocrine liver tumors: preliminary results from a multi-institutional experience. *Ann Surg*. 2008;247(6):1029-1035.

69. Kennedy AS, Dezarn WA, McNeillie P, et al. Radioembolization for unresectable neuroendocrine hepatic metastases using resin 90Y-microspheres: early results in 148 patients. *Am J Clin Oncol*. 2008;31(3):271-279.

70. King J, Quinn R, Glenn DM, et al. Radioembolization with selective internal radiation microspheres for neuroendocrine liver metastases. *Cancer*. 2008;113(5):921-929.

71. Saxena A, Chua TC, Bester L, Kokandi A, Morris DL. Factors predicting response and survival after yttrium-90 radioembolization of unresectable neuroendocrine tumor liver metastases: a critical appraisal of 48 cases. *Ann Surg*. 2010;251(5):910-916.

72. Memon K, Lewandowski RJ, Mulcahy MF, et al. Radioembolization for neuroendocrine liver metastases: safety, imaging, and long-term outcomes. *Int J Radiat Oncol Biol Phys*. 2012;83(3):887-894.

73. Cianni R, Urigo C, Notarianni E, et al. Selective internal radiation therapy with SIR-spheres for the treatment of unresectable colorectal hepatic metastases. *Cardiovasc Intervent Radiol*. 2009;32(6):1179-1186.

74. Hong K, McBride JD, Georgiades CS, et al. Salvage therapy for liver-dominant colorectal metastatic adenocarcinoma: comparison between transcatheter arterial chemoembolization versus yttrium-90 radioembolization. *J Vasc Interv Radiol*. 2009;20(3):360-367.

75. Sato KT, Lewandowski RJ, Mulcahy MF, et al. Unresectable chemorefractory liver metastases: radioembolization with 90Y microspheres—safety, efficacy, and survival. *Radiology*. 2008;247(2):507-515.

76. Murthy R, Xiong H, Nunez R, et al. Yttrium 90 resin microspheres for the treatment of unresectable colorectal hepatic metastases after failure of multiple chemotherapy regimens: preliminary results. *J Vasc Interv Radiol*. 2005;16(7):937-945.

77. Lewandowski RJ, Thurston KG, Goin JE, et al. 90Y microsphere (TheraSphere) treatment for unresectable colorectal cancer metastases of the liver: response to treatment at targeted doses of 135-150 Gy as measured by [18F]fluorodeoxyglucose positron emission tomography and computed tomographic imaging. *J Vasc Interv Radiol*. 2005;16(12):1641-1651.

78. Lim L, Gibbs P, Yip D, et al. Prospective study of treatment with selective internal radiation therapy spheres in patients with unresectable primary or secondary hepatic malignancies. *Intern Med J*. 2005;35(4):222-227.

79. Andrews JC, Walker SC, Ackermann RJ, et al. Hepatic radioembolization with yttrium-90 containing glass microspheres: preliminary results and clinical follow-up. *J Nucl Med*. 1994;35(10):1637-1644.

80. Murthy R, Kamat P, Nunez R, et al. Yttrium-90 microsphere radioembolotherapy of hepatic metastatic neuroendocrine carcinomas after hepatic arterial embolization. *J Vasc Interv Radiol*. 2008;19(1):145-151.

81. McStay MK, Maudgil D, Williams M, et al. Large-volume liver metastases from neuroendocrine tumors: hepatic intraarterial 90Y-DOTA-lanreotide as effective palliative therapy. *Radiology*. 2005;237(2):718-726.

82. de Takats PG, Kerr DJ. Is intra-arterial chemotherapy worthwhile in the treatment of patients with unresectable hepatic colorectal cancer metastases?: Arbiter. *Eur J Cancer*. 1996;32(13):2201-2205.

83. Balch CM, Urist MM, Soong SJ, McGregor M. A prospective phase II clinical trial of continuous FUDR regional chemotherapy for colorectal metastases to the liver using a totally implantable drug infusion pump. *Ann Surg*. 1983;198(5):567-573.

84. Martin JK, Jr., O'Connell MJ, Wieand HS, et al. Intra-arterial floxuridine vs systemic fluorouracil for hepatic metastases from colorectal cancer. A randomized trial. *Arch Surg*. 1990;125(8):1022-1027.

85. Kemeny N, Daly J, Reichman B, et al. Intrahepatic or systemic infusion of fluorodeoxyuridine in patients with liver metastases from colorectal carcinoma. A randomized trial. *Ann Intern Med*. 1987;107(4):459-465.

86. Hohn DC, Stagg RJ, Friedman MA, et al. A randomized trial of continuous intravenous versus hepatic intraarterial floxuridine in patients with colorectal cancer metastatic to the liver: the Northern California Oncology Group trial. *J Clin Oncol*. 1989;7(11):1646-1654.

87. Rougier P, Laplanche A, Huguier M, et al. Hepatic arterial infusion of floxuridine in patients with liver metastases from colorectal carcinoma: long-term results of a prospective randomized trial. *J Clin Oncol*. 1992;10(7):1112-1118.

88. Allen-Mersh TG, Earlam S, Fordy C, Abrams K, Houghton J. Quality of life and survival with continuous hepatic-artery floxuridine infusion for colorectal liver metastases. *Lancet*. 1994;344(8932):1255-1260.

89. Otto G, Duber C, Hoppe-Lotichius M, et al. Radiofrequency ablation as first-line treatment in patients with early colorectal liver metastases amenable to surgery. *Ann Surg*. 2010;251(5):796-803.

90. Lencioni R, Cioni D, Donati F, Bartolozzi C. Combination of interventional therapies in hepatocellular carcinoma. *Hepatogastroenterology*. 2001;48(37):8-14.

91. Timmerman RD, Bizekis CS, Pass HI, et al. Local surgical, ablative, and radiation treatment of metastases. *CA Cancer J Clin*. 2009;59(3):145-170.

92. Solbiati L, Goldberg SN, Ierace T, et al. Hepatic metastases: percutaneous radio-frequency ablation with cooled-tip electrodes. *Radiology*. 1997;205(2):367-373.

93. Lubienski A. Radiofrequency ablation in metastatic disease. *Recent Results Cancer Res*. 2005;165:268-276.

94. Curley SA, Izzo F, Delrio P, et al. Radiofrequency ablation of unresectable primary and metastatic hepatic malignancies: results in 123 patients. *Ann Surg*. 1999;230(1):1-8.

95. Gleisner AL, Choti MA, Assumpcao L, et al. Colorectal liver metastases: recurrence and survival following hepatic resection, radiofrequency ablation, and combined resection-radiofrequency ablation. *Arch Surg*. 2008;143(12):1204-1212.

96. Garrean S, Hering J, Saied A, Helton WS, Espat NJ. Radiofrequency ablation of primary and metastatic liver tumors: a critical review of the literature. *Am J Surg*. 2008;195(4):508-520.

97. Weber SM, Lee FT Jr. Expanded treatment of hepatic tumors with radiofrequency ablation and cryoablation. *Oncology (Williston Park)*. 2005;19(11 suppl 4):27-32.

98. Wong SL, Mangu PB, Choti MA, et al. American Society of Clinical Oncology 2009 clinical evidence review on radiofrequency ablation of hepatic metastases from colorectal cancer. *J Clin Oncol*. 2010;28(3):493-508.

99. T. Ruers CJP, F. van Coevorden, I. Borel Rinkes, et al. Final results of the EORTC intergroup randomized study 40004 (CLOCC) evaluating the benefit of radiofrequency ablation (RFA) combined with chemotherapy for unresectable colorectal liver metastases (CRC LM), in *2010 ASCO Annual Meeting 2010*. *J Clin Oncol*. 2010;28(suppl; abstr 3526):15s.

100. Mazzaglia PJ, Berber E, Milas M, Siperstein AE. Laparoscopic radiofrequency ablation of neuroendocrine liver metastases: a 10-year experience evaluating predictors of survival. *Surgery*. 2007;142(1):10-19.

101. Veltri A, Sacchetto P, Tosetti I, et al. Radiofrequency ablation of colorectal liver metastases: small size favorably predicts technique effectiveness and survival. *Cardiovasc Intervent Radiol*. 2008;31(5):948-956.

102. Sorensen SM, Mortensen FV, Nielsen DT. Radiofrequency ablation of colorectal liver metastases: long-term survival. *Acta Radiol*. 2007;48(3):253-258.

103. Suppiah A, White TJ, Roy-Choudhury SH, et al. Long-term results of percutaneous radiofrequency ablation of unresectable colorectal hepatic metastases: final outcomes. *Dig Surg*. 2007;24(5):358-360.

104. Machi J, Oishi AJ, Sumida K, et al. Long-term outcome of radiofrequency ablation for unresectable liver metastases from colorectal cancer: evaluation of prognostic factors and effectiveness in first- and second-line management. *Cancer J*. 2006;12(4):318-326.

105. Jakobs TF, Hoffmann RT, Trumm C, Reiser MF, Helmberger TK. Radiofrequency ablation of colorectal liver metastases: mid-term results in 68 patients. *Anticancer Res*. 2006;26(1B):671-680.

106. Gillams AR, Lees WR. Radio-frequency ablation of colorectal liver metastases in 167 patients. *Eur Radiol*. 2004;14(12):2261-2267.

107. Lencioni R, Crocetti L, Cioni D, Della Pina C, Bartolozzi C. Percutaneous radiofrequency ablation of hepatic colorectal metastases: technique, indications, results, and new promises. *Invest Radiol*. 2004;39(11):689-697.

108. Abdalla EK, Vauthey JN, Ellis LM, et al. Recurrence and outcomes following hepatic resection, radiofrequency ablation, and combined resection/ablation for colorectal liver metastases. *Ann Surg*. 2004;239(6):818-825; discussion 825-827.

109. Solbiati L, Livraghi T, Goldberg SN, et al. Percutaneous radio-frequency ablation of hepatic metastases from colorectal cancer: long-term results in 117 patients. *Radiology*. 2001;221(1):159-166.

110. Akyildiz HY, Mitchell J, Milas M, Siperstein A, Berber E. Laparoscopic radiofrequency thermal ablation of neuroendocrine hepatic metastases: long-term follow-up. *Surgery*. 2010;148(6):1288-1293; discussion 1293.

111. Bilchik AJ, Sarantou T, Foshag LJ, Giuliano AE, Ramming KP. Cryosurgical palliation of metastatic neuroendocrine tumors resistant to conventional therapy. *Surgery*. 1997;122(6):1040-1047; discussion 1047-1048.

112. Cozzi PJ, Englund R, Morris DL. Cryotherapy treatment of patients with hepatic metastases from neuroendocrine tumors. *Cancer*. 1995;76(3):501-509.

113. Shapiro RS, Shafir M, Sung M, Warner R, Glajchen N. Cryotherapy of metastatic carcinoid tumors. *Abdom Imaging*. 1998;23(3):314-317.

114. Curley SA. Radiofrequency ablation of malignant liver tumors. *The Oncologist*. 2001;6(1):14-23.

115. Kulaylat MN, Gibbs JF. Thermoablation of colorectal liver metastasis. *J Surg Oncol*. 2010;101(8):699-705.

116. Seifert JK, Cozzi PJ, Morris DL. Cryotherapy for neuroendocrine liver metastases. *Semin Surg Oncol*. 1998;14(2):175-183.

117. Seifert JK, Morris DL. World survey on the complications of hepatic and prostate cryotherapy. *World J Surg*. 1999;23(2):109-113; discussion 113-114.

118. Korpan NN. Hepatic cryosurgery for liver metastases. Long-term follow-up. *Ann Surg*. 1997;225(2):193-201.

119. Finlay IG, Seifert JK, Stewart GJ, Morris DL. Resection with cryotherapy of colorectal hepatic metastases has the same survival as hepatic resection alone. *Eur J Surg Oncol*. 2000;26(3):199-202.

120. Niu R, Yan TD, Zhu JC, et al. Recurrence and survival outcomes after hepatic resection with or without cryotherapy for liver metastases from colorectal carcinoma. *Ann Surg Oncol*. 2007;14(7):2078-2087.

121. Pearson AS, Izzo F, Fleming RY, et al. Intraoperative radiofrequency ablation or cryoablation for hepatic malignancies. *Am J Surg*. 1999;178(6):592-599.

122. Bilchik AJ, Wood TF, Allegra D, et al. Cryosurgical ablation and radiofrequency ablation for unresectable hepatic malignant neoplasms: a proposed algorithm. *Arch Surg*. 2000;135(6):657-662; discussion 662-664.

123. Adam R, Hagopian EJ, Linhares M, et al. A comparison of percutaneous cryosurgery and percutaneous radiofrequency for unresectable hepatic malignancies. *Arch Surg*. 2002;137(12):1332-1339; discussion 1340.

124. de Jong KP. Freeze or fry—cryoablation or radiofrequency ablation in liver surgery? *Nat Clin Pract Gastroenterol Hepatol*. 2007;4(9):472-473.

125. Vogl TJ, Mack MG, Straub R, Roggan A, Felix R. Magnetic resonance imaging-guided abdominal interventional radiology: laser-induced thermotherapy of liver metastases. *Endoscopy*. 1997;29(6):577-583.

126. Vogl TJ, Muller PK, Hammerstingl R, et al. Malignant liver tumors treated with MR imaging-guided laser-induced thermotherapy: technique and prospective results. *Radiology*. 1995;196(1):257-265.

127. Qian J. Interventional therapies of unresectable liver metastases. *J Cancer Res Clin Oncol.* 2011;137(12):1763-1772.

128. Kemeny N, Huang Y, Cohen AM, et al. Hepatic arterial infusion of chemotherapy after resection of hepatic metastases from colorectal cancer. *N Engl J Med.* 1999;341(27):2039-2048.

129. Alberts SR, Roh MS, Mahoney MR, et al. Alternating systemic and hepatic artery infusion therapy for resected liver metastases from colorectal cancer: a North Central Cancer Treatment Group (NCCTG)/National Surgical Adjuvant Breast and Bowel Project (NSABP) phase II intergroup trial, N9945/CI-66. *J Clin Oncol.* 2010;28(5):853-858.

130. Van Hazel G, Blackwell A, Anderson J, et al. Randomised phase 2 trial of SIR-Spheres plus fluorouracil/leucovorin chemotherapy versus fluorouracil/leucovorin chemotherapy alone in advanced colorectal cancer. *J Surg Oncol.* 2004;88(2):78-85.

131. Gray B, Van Hazel G, Hope M, et al. Randomised trial of SIR-Spheres plus chemotherapy vs. chemotherapy alone for treating patients with liver metastases from primary large bowel cancer. *Ann Oncol.* 2001;12(12):1711-1720.

132. Murthy R, Xiong H, Nunez R, et al. Hepatic yttrium-90 radioembolotherapy in metastatic colorectal cancer treated with cetuximab or bevacizumab. *J Vasc Interv Radiol.* 2007;18(12):1588-1591.

133. Stubbs RS, O'Brien I, Correia MM. Selective internal radiation therapy with 90Y microspheres for colorectal liver metastases: single-centre experience with 100 patients. *ANZ J Surg.* 2006;76(8):696-703.

134. Christante D, Pommier S, Givi B, Pommier R. Hepatic artery chemoinfusion with chemoembolization for neuroendocrine cancer with progressive hepatic metastases despite octreotide therapy. *Surgery.* 2008;144(6):885-893; discussion 893-894.

135. Drougas JG, Anthony LB, Blair TK, et al. Hepatic artery chemoembolization for management of patients with advanced metastatic carcinoid tumors. *Am J Surg.* 1998;175(5):408-412.

136. Moss AC, Morris E, Leyden J, MacMathuna P. Do the benefits of metal stents justify the costs? A systematic review and meta-analysis of trials comparing endoscopic stents for malignant biliary obstruction. *Eur J Gastroenterol Hepatol.* 2007;19(12):1119-1124.

137. Chu D, Adler DG. Malignant biliary tract obstruction: evaluation and therapy. *J Natl Compr Canc Netw.* 2010;8(9):1033-1044.

138. Moss AC, Morris E, Leyden J, MacMathuna P. Malignant distal biliary obstruction: a systematic review and meta-analysis of endoscopic and surgical bypass results. *Cancer Treat Rev.* 2007;33(2):213-221.

139. Li Sol Y, Kim CW, Jeon UB, et al. Early infectious complications of percutaneous metallic stent insertion for malignant biliary obstruction. *AJR Am J Roentgenol.* 2010;194(1):261-265.

140. Jarnagin WR, Burke E, Powers C, Fong Y, Blumgart LH. Intrahepatic biliary enteric bypass provides effective palliation in selected patients with malignant obstruction at the hepatic duct confluence. *Am J Surg.* 1998;175(6):453-460.

141. Kuhlmann KF, van Poll D, de Castro SM, et al. Initial and long-term outcome after palliative surgical drainage of 269 patients with malignant biliary obstruction. *Eur J Surg Oncol.* 2007;33(6):757-762.

CHAPTER 21

Palliative Endoscopic Procedures

Jörg Albert

PALLIATIVE ENDOSCOPIC PROCEDURES

Interventional endoscopy has evolved into a major instrument for treating patients who suffer from gastrointestinal tumors and to relieve severe ailments such as dysphagia, ileus, intestinal bleeding, icterus, sepsis, and pain. Mainstays in the development of the endoscopic armamentarium were the development of endoscopy-based antitumor therapies, the advances in the construction of self-expanding metal stents (SEMSs), the rapid evolution of interventional endoscopic ultrasound techniques, and the increasing use of combining percutaneous and luminal (endoscopic) treatment approaches ("Rendez-vous" technique).

An important endoscopic task is palliative care of intestinal obstruction in advanced abdominal or pelvic tumors. There has been a significant shift from noncurative surgical management to endoscopic treatment in intestinal obstruction in the last few years, and a detailed overview on the indications, endoscopic technique, and outcome of the management of intestinal obstruction is therefore provided. Specific endoscopic treatment approaches are available to stop bleeding from intestinal tumors, to treat cancer with local ablation techniques (e.g., bile duct cancer and photodynamic therapy [PDT]), to manage biliary obstruction, and to alleviate pain in pancreatic cancer by endoscopic ultrasonography (EUS)-guided lysis of the celiac plexus. These subjects are therefore separately discussed. Moreover, there is a concise overview given on enteral nutrition support and on treating infectious complications by endoscopic means.

ENDOSCOPIC MANAGEMENT OF INTESTINAL OBSTRUCTION

Intestinal obstruction is a severe complication of intra-abdominal and pelvic malignancies. The incidence of bowel occlusion is not exactly known but is frequent in advanced tumor stages and occurs in 6% to about 50% of patients with ovarian cancer (1–3) and in 10% to about 30% of patients with colorectal cancer (1). Related symptoms significantly compromise the quality of life of the patient, and clinical management may be a challenge. Etiology of bowel obstruction is heterogenous, though, and may be benign in up to 40% of cases. Extrinsic (abdominal mass, intestinal or peritoneal carcinomatosis, fibrosis, adhesions, and radiation enteritis) and intrinsic lesions (malignant polyp and fibrosis) are involved, and mechanical obstruction must be discerned from paralytic ileus (Table 21.1). Risk factors for intestinal obstruction are advanced tumor stage, residual primary tumor,

and presence of intestinal carcinomatosis. Symptoms at primary presentation are indicative of the site of the obstruction: dysphagia is caused by oropharyngeal or esophageal lesions or may be of functional origin, whereas mechanical ileus is the sequel of intestinal obstruction and results in colicky pain, abdominal distension, vomiting, dehydration, and, potentially, hypovolemic shock. Immediate diagnostic clarification is mandatory to avoid aggravation of symptoms. Plain abdominal radiography may demonstrate fluid levels. Water-soluble oral contrast can help define the extension and the site of the obstruction. Abdominal computed tomography is useful to locate the exact site of obstruction and to further characterize the reason for it. Endoscopy helps to locate a stenosis and biopsies can determine its etiology.

Antiemetics, steroids, and octreotide are used to relieve symptoms, and metoclopramide is helpful for functional obstruction (1,4). A nasogastric tube is a temporary measure in patients unresponsive to medical treatment, whereas a percutaneous gastrostomy may be placed for permanent gastric decompression. Surgical interventions with bypass procedures and/or segmental bowel resection are associated with significant morbidity, a complication rate of 37% to 64%, and in-hospital mortality of 10% to 30% or greater (2,3,5–7) (Table 21.2). The major underlying value of an operative intervention may be primarily to identify a benign etiology of obstruction in selected cases and only secondarily to alleviate the consequences of carcinomatosis (1). Candidates for surgery must present with a good clinical performance status to achieve acceptable outcomes (9).

Recent advances in SEMS technology have significantly widened their indications for patients with intestinal obstructions. Nitinol, a melt of nickel and titanium, is the primary metal used for SEMS construction. Shape memory, elasticity, maximum expansion force at body temperature, and application with relatively small delivery devices that allow for TTS ("through-the-scope") insertion are characteristics that favor the use of this material. Other substances presently in use include stainless steel and plastics. The covering of SEMS may be made of various materials, including silicone, polyurethane, and expanded polytetrafluoroethylene. The cover may extend over the entire length of the stent (fully covered SEMS) or leave small areas at the ends uncovered (partly covered SEMS).

Sites of obstruction can often be bridged in the upper gastrointestinal tract, the proximal small bowel, and the colon with SEMS, though there are some practical caveats. Importantly, combination of OTW ("over-the-wire") and TTS techniques minimizes the risk of intraprocedural perforation

TABLE 21.1	**Etiology of malignant intestinal obstruction and motility disorders in palliative medicine**

Mechanical Obstruction	Paralytic Ileus	Secondary Etiology for Ileus
Intraluminal occlusion due to neoplastic mass	Peritoneal carcinomatosis	Motility disorder caused by drugs such as • Opioids • Anticholinergics • Antidepressants • Others
Extraluminal neoplasia (mesenteric, omental, abdominal, and pelvic mass) with extrinsic occlusion of the bowel lumen	Paraneoplastic neuropathy or chronic intestinal pseudo-obstruction	Dehydration
Linitis plastica	Neoplastic infiltration of the celiac plexus	Fecal impaction
Postradiation fibrosis/strictures	—	—

in the duodenum, small bowel, and colon. Fluoroscopy is essential to provide secure access beyond the stenosis in case it cannot be traversed endoscopically. In this situation, carefully placing a hydrophilic guidewire through a catheter after contrast injection enables the visualization of the stenosis. The guidewire will transverse the tumor in almost all cases, even if small-caliber endoscopes are not able to pass the obstruction. Moreover, the air column seen with fluoroscopy on the opposite side of the tumor (stenosis) indicates the direction in which to advance the guidewire (Fig. 21.1).

Stent retrieval is rarely necessary in malignant obstruction. Removal may be accomplished with oral or aboral retraction, stent turnover in the stomach, extraction by covering of an overtube, untying the stent by extracting the thread (in case of knotted SEMS from one thread of metal), inversion of the stent (invert from distal to proximal), excavating or trimming the stent by welding it or destroying it in

corpora. While fully covered SEMSs are often easily extracted, removal of noncovered stents is difficult particularly after the elapse of a long time from stent placement (more than several months) or if tumor ingrowth, scarring or granulation tissue provoke stent closure at the stent endings. Granulation tissues can sometimes be removed by inserting a second, fully covered stent within the partially or noncovered stent, for example, in esophageal or in biliary SEMS (10) (Fig. 21.2).

Patients with multiple consecutive strictures—for example, in peritoneal carcinomatosis—may be poor candidates for SEMS placement. Moreover, patients with a short life expectancy, for example, less than 4 weeks, should probably not be considered as candidates. Careful patient selection is of high importance. Endoscopic tumor destruction (argon plasma coagulation [APC], ethanol injection, Nd–YAG laser, and mechanical debulking) is infrequently performed because repeated sessions are usually necessary with a negative effect

TABLE 21.2	**In-hospital mortality and benefit from palliative surgery for bowel obstruction in patients with advanced, nonresectable intra-abdominal cancer**

Author	Year	Indication for Surgery	N	In-Hospital Mortality (%)	Benefit Short-Term Relief of Obstruction	Long-Term Relief of Obstruction (%)
Turnbull et al. (8)	1989	Colon and gastric cancer	89	13	81% (colon) 52.6% (gastric)	46
Rubin et al. (2)	1989	Ovarian cancer	54	7	79.6%	63
Lund et al. (3)	1989	Ovarian cancer	25	—	—	32
Butler et al. (6)	1991	Various	25	38	64%	—
Lau and Lorentz (7)	1993	Nonresectable colorectal cancer	30	17	—	63
Woolfson et al. (5)	1997	Abdominal cancer	32	22	—	52

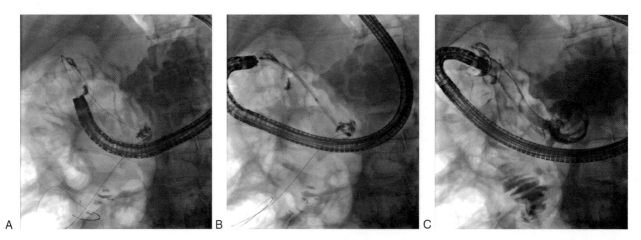

Figure 21.1. Endoscopic placement of a duodenal SEMS in a patient with a symptomatic malignant obstruction of the duodenum: traversing the stenosis with a guidewire (**A**) and TTS placement of the SEMS while the endoscope allows for control of the proximal site of the stenosis (**B**). Optimal outflow of contrast from the SEMS to the small bowel (**C**).

on quality of life because of repeated hospitalizations for a patient with limited life expectancy. Moreover, risk of perforation with these procedures is at least 10% (11), and these are, therefore, reserved for patients with obstructions not amenable to other therapies.

Esophageal Obstruction

The indications for endoscopic therapy for advanced esophageal or mediastinal tumor are relief of dysphagia, maintenance of nutrition, or sealing of a tracheo-esophageal fistula.

Immediate success after SEMS placement for these symptoms is as high as 95%, but long-term stent dysfunction occurs in about 20% to 30% of patients (12,13). At present, noncovered, partially covered, and fully covered SEMSs are all in use (14). Covered or partially covered SEMS may be preferred over noncovered stents because tumor ingrowth is prevented by the stent cover, but dislocation of these stents may be somewhat more frequent (15). When compared to SEMSs, self-expandable plastic stents (SEPSs) provide equal improvement of dysphagia due to tumor stenosis, but stent migration is more common with SEPS (16).

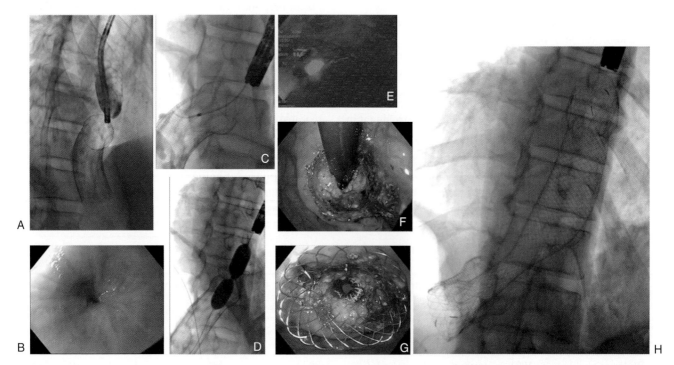

Figure 21.2. Re-administration of a patient to the hospital 15 months after SEMS placement at the distal esophagus for metastasized adenocarcinoma of the cardia: complete obstruction of the proximal part of the SEMS is observed (**A, B**), putatively provoked by the stent itself that has partially dislodged to the stomach and tumor recurrence. Re-opening the access to the SEMS with a stiff catheter (**C**), balloon dilation over the guidewire (**D**), trimming of the nonremovable but aborally dislocated stent with use of argon plasma coagulation (**E, F**), and re-insertion of a second stent (**G, H**) to re-establish oral nutrition intake.

| TABLE 21.3 Complications of SEMS placement in the esophagus for malignant disease ||
Short-Term Complication	Long-Term Complication
Mediastinal pain (more common in patients already complaining of pain)	Reflux and aspiration (e.g., in stents that pass the cardia)
Aspiration (both intraprocedural and postprocedure)	Fistula (e.g., esophago-bronchial fistula)
Migration	Migration
Tracheal compression	Overgrowth (benign/malignant)
—	Bleeding (e.g., caused by erosions of the stent endings)

SEMS, self-expanding metal stents.

The use of a covered SEMS for the treatment of esophageo-bronchial fistulae improves survival. Palliation of malignant fistula is accomplished with an esophageal stent implantation or with parallel (esophagus plus airway) SEMS insertions. In some cases, dual stents provide improved palliation and safety. Particular attention must be paid to potential tracheal compression secondary to esophageal stents. The stent may, depending on the model, have a pronounced radial expansion force and thereby compress the surrounding tissue, including the trachea (Table 21.3). Additional endoscopic treatment options to relieve malignant dysphagia are local tumor ablation using APC, high dose rate brachytherapy, PDT, and a combination of these therapies (17) or in combination with chemoradiation (18).

Gastric Outlet Obstruction

Palliation of malignant gastroduodenal obstruction is as successful with SEMS placement as with gastroenterostomy. While long-term success might favor gastroenterostomy, complication rates are lower with SEMS placement (19,20). Gastroenterostomy may be preferred in some patients with a longer anticipated survival and performed during abdominal exploration for potentially curative resection. SEMS is preferred for patients with poor performance status and if curative surgery is not an option at diagnosis (21). The technical success rate of SEMS in this setting is higher than 90% and the clinical success rate is at least 75% in most studies (22). Device-related adverse events include stent occlusion or malfunction in 9% of patients and perforation in 5% (23). Solid food intake can generally be resumed in more than 50% of patients, and 75% benefited from significant improvement in nutritional status in a multicenter study. The shorter time from stent implantation to initiation of oral intake, low morbidity, and a brief hospital stay favor SEMS over surgical gastroenterostomy (24). The implanted stent should be non-shortening, with maximum flexibility and sufficient radial expansion accompanied by minor axial straightening force (22).

Duodenal tumor as a cause of stenosis has a high frequency of concomitant biliary obstruction, for example, in patients with cancer of the pancreatic head. In these cases,

insertion of a biliary SEMS together with a duodenal SEMS is often most appropriate. The optimal procedure depends on the timing and the sequence of occurrence of the biliary and duodenal stenosis. In most cases, biliary obstruction precedes duodenal occlusion and a biliary SEMS is inserted first to accomplish biliary drainage. Only if a duodenal obstruction occurs some time later is a duodenal stent needed. In this case, the duodenal stent may come close to the biliary SEMS and it may need to be trimmed if the tumor involves the complete descending duodenum (D2) and a trans-papillary stent is envisaged. When biliary and duodenal obstruction occur simultaneously, biliary SEMS insertion and immediate duodenal stent placement is preferred. With an exclusive endoscopic approach, the duodenoscope is placed in the descending duodenum opposite the papilla after complete deployment of the duodenal stent. Now, the mesh of the duodenal SEMS is manipulated at the site of the major papilla (by means of APC or with dilation catheters) and biliary cannulation is attempted to insert the biliary SEMS. This technique is likewise useful in a third, less frequent scenario, when a biliary stenosis develops sometime after duodenal stenosis.

If an endoscopic biliary access is not obtained, a percutaneous SEMS insertion is needed, sometimes combined with endoscopic visualization or the Rendez-vous technique to adjust the exact placement at the level of the duodenal wall. The combination of endoscopic and percutaneous procedures offers a high potential for success, even in technically challenging situations.

Small Bowel Obstruction

New endoscopes and balloon enteroscopy technique enable ordinary endoscopic access to distal portions of the small bowel. TTS placement is limited, though, by the small working channel of balloon enteroscopes (2.8 or 2.2 mm). OTW placement of an SEMS in the distal small intestine is technically feasible but cumbersome and maybe associated with increased risk of perforation. Most importantly, though, it must be clarified that if the patient's symptoms are due to multiple consecutive stenosis of the small bowel, as with peritoneal carcinomatosis, this can rarely be helped with endoscopic stenting. Percutaneous gastrostomy tube placement for decompression and drainage of gastric and enteral secretions is often the best option for these patients.

Colonic Obstruction

Endoscopic palliation of advanced stage colon cancer has been performed for over 20 years. It has found a widened application in the last few years with the development of new SEMS (Table 21.4). There are two clinical settings in which SEMS placement is appropriate. The first is for palliation, that is, diffuse metastasis or advanced comorbidity forecloses curative surgical resection of the tumor. In this situation, endoscopic SEMS is equally successful in the short term and long term as palliative surgery, if failure of stent patency is re-treated endoscopically with stent-in-stent placement (37,38). Moreover, SEMS insertion seems equally effective and less costly than surgery in patients with metastatic colon cancer (42). In the second setting, potentially curative resection of the tumor is envisaged in a patient with acute colonic obstruction. In this setting, "bridge-to-surgery" by inserting SEMS and providing relief of the obstruction may avoid colostomy and facilitate a safe single-stage surgery (43,44) (Table 21.5). Successful treatment of the bowel obstruction by inserting an SEMS avoids emergency surgery and significantly reduces the hospital stay (31). This may be particularly important for elderly patients; the mortality with initial SEMS insertion is significantly lower (3%) than with emergency resection (19%) in patients with acute colon obstruction from tumor (50).

With some SEMS models, complications have been reported with stent placement in the right side of the colon or in the colonic flexures (33), but improvements in the stent design have reduced the complication rate (27). Minimal axial straightening of the stent, in combination with sufficient radial expansion force, seems essential for the optimal risk–benefit balance of SEMS insertion for colorectal cancer. Ideally, the stent should align exactly with the configuration of the organ, have no tendency to migrate, and prevent ingrowth.

There are two meta-analyses, from 2004 and 2002, that review the results of endoscopic palliation of colorectal cancer by SEMS placement. Technical success was reported to be 94% ($n = 1198$) or 92% ($n = 598$) for SEMS insertion for palliation. The use of SEMS placement as a "bridge-to-surgery" was found to have a clinical success rate of 85% to 91%. Perforations occurred in 3.7% or 4% of cases and reported procedure-related mortality was 0.58% and 1%, respectively (43,58). The management of extrinsic blockage of the colon with SEMS is less frequently successful and might be as low as 20% (30,39). Chemotherapy with bevacizumab in colorectal cancer patients with SEMS in situ has been suggested to increase the risk of perforation (28), though this has not been confirmed in other studies. Low rectal obstruction is difficult to treat with SEMS placement, and debulking procedures using APC, laser, or snare resection may be utilized

but are rarely necessary when radiochemotherapy is available (Fig. 21.3).

ENTERAL DECOMPRESSION IN THE PALLIATIVE PATIENT

Enteral decompression is needed in those patients in whom passage of intestinal contents cannot be reconstituted with endoscopic or surgical means and intestinal fluids are not transported via naturalis (Fig. 21.4).

Percutaneous endoscopic gastrostomy (PEG) tube placement is performed by the conventional pull-through technique or with use of gastropexy with catheters ranging from 15 to 24 Fr (59,60). The gastropexy technique is preferred in patients with ascites or peritoneal carcinomatosis because of compromised establishment of the cutano-gastric fistula. Symptomatic relief of nausea and vomiting is achieved in most patients with this technique. Moreover, in low intestinal obstruction or paralytic ileus, percutaneous endoscopic cecostomy tubes can be used to decompress malignant and functional bowel disorders with acceptable morbidity and mortality (61).

MANAGEMENT OF BILIARY OBSTRUCTION AND BILIARY LEAKAGE

To relieve biliary obstruction from neoplastic disease, surgical, endoscopic, and percutaneous approaches are available. For curative treatment, surgical options are the first choice for removal of the tumor and reconstitution of bile flow. Many patients are nonsurgical candidates, though, with unresectable disease or severe comorbidity. In these cases, the choice of endoscopic versus percutaneous drainage depends on the location and extent of the obstructing lesion and the expertise of the clinician. Endoscopic retrograde cholangiography (ERC) has replaced percutaneous transhepatic cholangio drainage as the initial procedure for drainage of distal bile duct obstructions because of its lower complication rate. ERC is generally the first procedure for the treatment of hilar bile duct carcinoma in many institutions (62) (Fig. 21.4). Moreover, EUS, by providing access to the left liver lobe from the stomach or duodenum, can help circumvent biliary obstruction with drainage into the intestinal cavities (63).

Recent studies, formerly routine, challenge the use of preoperative biliary drainage for periampullary tumors. Increased complication rates were reported from preoperative biliary drainage in patients undergoing surgery for cancer of the pancreatic head in a randomized nonblinded study (64). This led to changes in the approach to operable patients: Patients without signs of cholangitis, with planned surgery within 7 to 10 days, and a bilirubin of <250 μmol/L (15 mg/dL) are directly referred to surgery if no neoadjuvant treatment is envisaged. The relatively high rate of endoscopic complications observed in this study might be significantly decreased with the use of covered SEMS in the preoperative setting (65). In palliative patients, biliary decompression relieves the associated symptoms of jaundice, nausea,

TABLE 21.4 Outcome of SEMS implantation in obstructing colorectal cancer

Author	Year	Study	N	Technical Success (%)	Perforation (%)	All Complications (%)
Garcia-Cano et al. (25)	2006	Retrospective	40	95	0	19
Song (26)	2007	Retrospective	151	96	10.6	30.4
van Hooft et al. (27)	2008	Randomized; surgery vs. SEMS	11	90	54	100
Cennamo et al. (28)	2009	Retrospective	28	100	7.1	—
Dronamraju et al. (29)	2009	Retrospective; right-sided CRC	16	88	0	6
Keswani et al. (30)	2009	Retrospective	34	94	0	8.8
Vemulapalli et al. (31)	2009	Retrospective, comparative	53	94	0	—
Al Samaraee et al. (32)	2009	Retrospective	38	92	2	29
Fernandez-Esparrach et al. (33)	2010	Retrospective	47	94	7	45
Jung et al. (34)	2010	Retrospective	39	100	2.5	12.8
Small et al. (35)	2010	Retrospective	168	96	9	24.4
Suh et al. (36)	2010	Retrospective	55	98.2	1.8	30.9
Nagula et al. (37)	2010	Prospective	16	100	0	—
Lee et al. (38)	2011	Retrospective, comparative	71	95.8	0	15.5
Luigiano et al. (39)	2011	Retrospective	39	92	5	26
Manes et al. (40)	2011	Retrospective	201	91.5	5.9	11.9
Meisner et al. (41)	2011	Prospective/registry	447	94.8	3.9	8

SEMS, self-expanding metal stent; CRC, colorectal cancer.

TABLE 21.5 Outcome and benefit from emergency surgery or SEMS implantation in acute obstructing colorectal cancer

Author	Year	Study	Localization of the Tumor	Procedure	N	Associated In-Hospital Mortality (%)	Relief of Obstruction (Clinical Success) (%)
Lau et al. (45)	1995	Retrospective	Left colon	Emergency surgery	35	11	100
Repici et al. (46)	2007	Prospective, multicenter	Colon	SEMS	45	0	81
Dastur et al. (47)	2008	Retrospective, comparative	Left colon	Emergency surgery	23	13	—
				SEMS	19	5	84
Repici et al. (46)	2008	Retrospective	Colon	SEMS	36	0	81
Repici et al (48)	2008	Prospective	Colon	SEMS	42	0	95
Brehant et al. (49)	2009	Prospective	Colon	SEMS	30	0	76.6
Guo et al. (50)	2011	Retrospective, comparative	Left colon	Emergency surgery	58	19	100
				SEMS	34	3	91
Jimenez-Perez (51)	2011	Retrospective	Left Colon	SEMS	182	0.5	94
Driest et al. (52)	2011	Retrospective	Colon	SEMS	45	2	87
White et al. (53)	2011	Retrospective, comparative	Left colon	Emergency surgery	26	7.7	73
				SEMS	30	6	90
Lee et al. (54)	2010	Retrospective	Colon	SEMS	46	2	84.8
Pirlet et al. (55)	2011	Multicenter prospective, randomized	Left colon	Emergency surgery	30	3	100
				SEMS	30	10	40
Iversen et al. (56)	2011	Retrospective	Colon	SEMS	34	2.9	88
Park et al. (57)	2011	Retrospective	Colon	SEMS	103	0	96–100

SEMS, self-expanding metal stent.

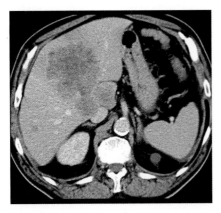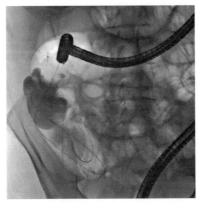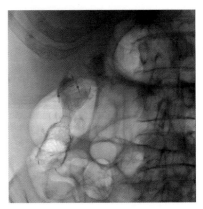

Figure 21.3. Adenocarcinoma of the ascending colon with liver metastasis. Complete obstruction of the colon and SEMS insertion.

and pruritus. If an endoscopic approach fails, percutaneous puncture of the biliary system or EUS-guided transgastric or trans-duodenal drainage is available. Combining the procedures further increases the success rate.

SEMSs are replacing plastic endoprostheses for malignant biliary drainage because of the prolonged patency time and reduced complication rate of the former (66) (Table 21.6). Fully covered SEMSs were developed with hopes of further prolonging patency time but this has not been seen (68). No significant differences detected in patient survival time or complication rate has been detected with covered versus uncovered stents. However, covered stents migrated significantly more often than uncovered stents, and tumor ingrowth was more frequent with uncovered stents (71). No difference in the incidence of pancreatitis or chole-cystitis was observed in a large multicenter study (71). When SEMSs become occluded, covered stents are removed and replaced, while noncovered SEMSs are bridged with insertion of plastic endoprosthesis (72) or another metal stent ("stent-in-stent") (73).

Palliative intraductal tumor treatment of adenocarcinoma or advanced adenoma has been improved with the use of new cholangioscopy techniques, and tumor ablation with advanced pancreatic cancer has been performed under direct visualization in selected cases (74).

PALLIATIVE TREATMENT OF GASTROINTESTINAL TUMOR BLEEDING

Gastrointestinal bleeding from tumors is managed with endoscopic techniques similar to those utilized for malignant bleeding. Injection therapies (e.g., epinephrine and fibrin glue), hemoclip application, and thermo-coagulation techniques are available (75). There are some limitations inherent in endoscopic treatment of bleeding tumors. Large targets are not amenable to endoscopic clip therapy, and bleeding from an arterial vessel larger than 2 mm in diameter may be difficult to stop endoscopically (76). Size limitations may be partially overcome with the OTS clip, a clip that grasps deeply with a clasp of 10 to 14 mm (77). Diffuse tumor bleeding can be controlled with APC or

thermocoagulation (heater probe and bipolar coagulation). Spraying histoacryl (tissue adhesive glue) on a bleeding tumor also helps to stop bleeding (78). In selected patients with stenotic tumors in the intestines, SEMS placement may significantly diminish bleeding. Tumor-associated hemobilia can be reduced by placement of covered or non-covered biliary SEMS. In all patients, coagulation disorders must be treated and platelets should be transfused to reverse the effect of thrombocyte aggregation inhibitors. Alternative or complimentary therapies include angiography with deposition of coils into the bleeding vessel or local radiotherapy to control bleeding if palliative surgery is not indicated.

ENDOSCOPIC PAIN RELIEF IN PANCREATIC CANCER

Pain can be a severe and difficult to treat problem for patients with pancreatic cancer, significantly decreasing the quality of life. Pancreatic cancer or metastasis to regional lymph nodes may infiltrate or stretch nerve fibers of the organ or infiltrate the celiac plexus, thereby exciting neuropathic pain. Classically, this pain is located in the epigastric area with radiation to the back. Options for pain management include medications such as nonsteroidal anti-inflammatory drugs, acetaminophen, opioids, radiation therapy, chemotherapy, and celiac plexus neurolysis (CPN). Increasingly, CPN is used early in the course of the pancreatic cancer for pain management. CPN can be performed percutaneously or endoscopically. The stomach is in direct proximity to the target structures. The EUS-guided injection technique has a shorter distance to cross than with percutaneous techniques for plexus lysis. A local anesthetic and pure alcohol are injected directly into or near the celiac ganglia to destroy the nerve fibers and inhibit pain signaling through afferent nerves. CPN differs from celiac plexus blockage (CPB), in that a glucocorticoid, such as triamcinolon, is used instead of ethanol for the latter. The rational for CPB is not to destroy, but to attenuate, the plexus neural activity. EUS-guided CPN was introduced in the 1990s (79) and has been widely applied in some centers (80).

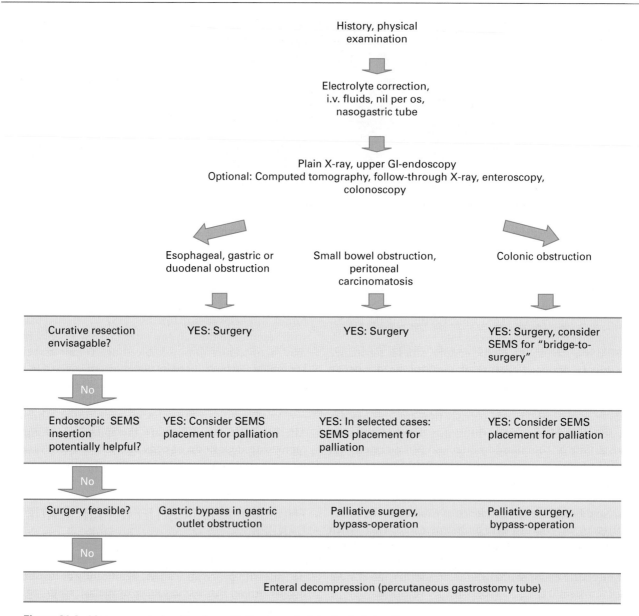

Figure 21.4. Management algorithm for palliation in gastrointestinal obstruction.

CPN provides long-term benefit in 70% to 90% of patients with pancreatic cancer pain with few side effects (10%). In a meta-analysis of eight studies ($n = 283$) of CPN, a success rate of 80.1% (95% CI, 74.4–85.2) was reported with a complication rate of 1.6% to 8%. Reported complications include diarrhea, hypotension, and abscess (81). Others have reported slightly lower success rate of 72% (82). With expansion of the region of injection of the plexus to around the superior mesenteric artery, the success of CPN has been further improved (83).

ENDOSCOPIC THERAPY FOR INFECTIOUS COMPLICATIONS IN TUMOR PATIENTS

Infectious complications in patients with cancer are treatment related and unrelated. Some infections are best treated with an endoscopic approach. A liver abscess may be treated with external drainage (most cases) or drainage via the papilla is preferable if the bile ducts are connected to the abscess. Endoscopic drainage is also an option for patients with infected necrosis after ablation of liver neoplasm, particularly with advanced tumor. Internal drainage avoids the long-term application of stigmatizing percutaneous drains in patients with limited survival. Similarly, intra-abdominal fluid collections and abscesses may be accessible to endoscopic drainage approaches in specialized centers. Endoscopic ultrasound is often useful to direct the insertion route of draining catheters.

ENTERAL NUTRITION SUPPORT IN THE PALLIATIVE PATIENT

Enteral nutrition is considered within the context of the overall goals of care and patient prognosis. Decisions about nutrition and hydration are among the most challenging and emotionally and ethically difficult issues in the end of life

TABLE 21.6	Outcome of SEMS placement for distal neoplastic biliary obstruction

	Year	*n*	Type of SEMS	Study	Stent Failure (%)	Mean Patency (Months)
Ahmad et al. (67)	2002	40	Wallstent	Retrospective	—	8.4 (Wallstent) 3.6 (diamond)
Yoon et al. (68)	2006	77	Covered and noncovered Wallstent	Retrospective	—	13,3 (covered) 10,6 (non-covered)
Soderlund and Linder (69)	2006	100	Metal (Wallstent) vs. plastic stent	Randomized	41% (plastic) 18% (metal)	1.8 (plastic) 3.6 (metal)
Yoon et al. (66)	2009	112	Covered or uncovered Wallstent vs. plastic stent	Retrospective	—	9.2 (metal) 4.4 (plastic)
Loew et al. (70)	2009	241	Zilver (Cook) vs. Wallstent (Boston)	Randomized, multicenter	39% (Zilver 6 mm) 24% (Zilver 10 mm) 21% (Wallstent 10 mm)	4.7 (Zilver 6 mm) 6.2 (Zilver 10 mm) 6.2 (Wallstent 10 mm)
Kullman et al. (71)	2010	400	Wallstent	Prospective, multicenter	—	—

SEMS, self-expanding metal stents.

care. Endoscopy plays a minor role for patients at this critical part of their lives, providing technical assistance to the patient who is unable to eat because of dysphagia, constricting tumors, or swallowing disorders. The decision-making process, indications for enteral nutrition and its application, and an appraisal of the patients' living situation and personal goals are the most important aspects in managing enteral nutrition for patients with very advanced cancer. Most often, these issues are considered before transferring a patient to the endoscopy ward to place a gastrostomy. Critical personal assessment of the patients' situation and close cooperation with the referring doctors, with inclusion of the palliative care team in some cases, is appropriate before placing a gastrostomy. Written informed consent from the patient or his substitute should be obtained at least one day before the intervention.

The indications for enteral nutrition support are impaired ingestion, inability to consume adequate nutrition orally, and impaired digestion, absorption, and metabolism. Advantages of enteral over parenteral nutrition include preserved gut integrity, decreased likelihood of bacterial translocation, and preserved immunologic function of the gut. Complications associated with the insertion procedure include infection, perforation, bleeding, and sedation-related complications. Tube migration or obstruction, risk of bacterial contamination, aspiration, diarrhea, and metabolic complications or hyperhydration are reported late complications. Complications are by far outbalanced by advantages of enteral nutrient application in most cases. Nutritional support may be delivered via placement of a nasogastric or nasojejunal feeding tube for short-term nutrition or by placing

a catheter percutaneously through the abdominal wall into the stomach or the small bowel (PEG or percutaneous endoscopic jejunostomy [PEJ]). Nasogastric tubes may dislodge and are uncomfortable. PEG/PEJ is usually used for patients who require medium- to long-term feeding. Gastrostomy tubes are usually placed endoscopically (PEG); alternative methods are surgical- or radiologically controlled introducer techniques.

A significant benefit of PEG over a nasogastric tube has not been demonstrated and there is a significant mortality/morbidity from PEG insertion itself (84). However, patients generally prefer a PEG to a nasogastric tube for prolonged nutrition for reasons of comfort. A prerequisite is a functioning GI tract. If the gut works, it should be used!

PEG or PEJ is done in the pull-through or direct puncturing technique with endoscopic control of needle insertion percutaneously into the stomach. With PEG, the safety of anterior stomach wall fixation is ensured by the inner and outer bumpers that fix the stomach to the abdominal wall. Gastropexy allows for suturing the stomach to the abdominal wall and thus expands indications to patients with (minor) ascites and peritoneal carcinomatosis. Care must prevail to avoid perforation or puncturing of the small bowel, colon, liver, or spleen. For patients with gastric outlet obstruction, either direct placement of a PEJ or of a PEG with a jejunal limb is required to avoid reflux of nutritional fluids. The direct puncturing technique avoids the risk of puncturing of abdominal wall metastasis (about 1%) and should be considered in all patients with any tumor visualized during endoscopic access (e.g., mouth, pharynx, and esophagus) (85).

TARGETED PALLIATIVE TUMOR TREATMENT WITH USE OF ENDOSCOPY

For targeted, noncurative treatment of endoscopically attainable tumors, ablative therapies and transport of antitumor agents via endoscopy have been used clinically. At present, data from only a few controlled studies of endoscopic techniques, such as PDT for cholangiocarcinoma, have been published. Other therapies, such as the use of EUS to deliver intratumoral therapy, are the subject of current research.

PDT uses a photosensitizer that accumulates in highly proliferating tissue, for example, tumors. The photosensitizer is activated by light of a specific wavelength and reactive oxygen species are generated to induce selective tumor cell death. The light fiber is inserted into the affected intestinal organ by endoscopic means. Several photosensitizers have been used for the treatment of advanced cholangiocarcinoma. Porfimer sodium (Photofrin) is the most widely used agent. Survival was significantly increased with PDT in comparison to simple biliary drainage ("stenting") in randomized controlled trials (RCT) and non-RCT. Photosensitivity is the most common adverse event that is associated with PDT. Actinic dermatitis is reported in 0% to 16% of patients. Skin protection from solar irradiation is necessary for at least 4 weeks after treatment for all patients exposed to PDT. Radiofrequency ablation (RFA) for cholangiocarcinoma has only recently become available for treating advanced cholangiocarcinoma (86). Presently, there are no data available to testify to the comparison of PDT to RFA.

Early investigations of EUS-guided delivery of antitumor agents (e.g., ablation of insulinoma with ethanol, EUS-guided ablation of pancreatic cystic tumors, and local immunotherapy in advanced pancreatic carcinoma) are promising and under study. Application of local ablation therapies such as laser, microwave, cryotherapy, and radiofrequency is also in experimental use and is awaited for the clinical field (87).

REFERENCES

1. Feuer DJ, Broadley KE. Systematic review and meta-analysis of corticosteroids for the resolution of malignant bowel obstruction in advanced gynaecological and gastrointestinal cancers. Systematic Review Steering Committee. *Ann Oncol.* 1999;10:1035-1041.
2. Rubin SC, Hoskins WJ, Benjamin I, Lewis JLJ. Palliative surgery for intestinal obstruction in advanced ovarian cancer. *Gynecol Oncol.* 1989;34:16-19.
3. Lund B, Hansen M, Lundvall F, Nielsen NC, Sorensen BL, Hansen HH. Intestinal obstruction in patients with advanced carcinoma of the ovaries treated with combination chemotherapy. *Surg Gynecol Obstet.* 1989;169:213-218.
4. Ripamonti C, Mercadante S, Groff L, Zecca E, De Conno F, Casuccio A. Role of octreotide, scopolamine butylbromide, and hydration in symptom control of patients with inoperable bowel obstruction and nasogastric tubes: a prospective randomized trial. *J Pain Symptom Manage.* 2000;19:23-34.
5. Woolfson RG, Jennings K, Whalen GF. Management of bowel obstruction in patients with abdominal cancer. *Arch Surg.* 1997;132:1093-1097.
6. Butler JA, Cameron BL, Morrow M, Kahng K, Tom J. Small bowel obstruction in patients with a prior history of cancer. *Am J Surg.* 1991;162:624-628.
7. Lau PW, Lorentz TG. Results of surgery for malignant bowel obstruction in advanced, unresectable, recurrent colorectal cancer. *Dis Colon Rectum.* 1993;36:61-64.
8. Turnbull AD, Guerra J, Starnes HF. Results of surgery for obstructing carcinomatosis of gastrointestinal, pancreatic, or biliary origin. *J Clin Oncol.* 1989;7:381-386.
9. Ripamonti C, Twycross R, Baines M, et al. Clinical-practice recommendations for the management of bowel obstruction in patients with end-stage cancer. *Support Care Cancer.* 2001;9:223-233.
10. Arias Dachary FJ, Chioccioli C, Deprez PH. Application of the "covered-stent-in-uncovered-stent" technique for easy and safe removal of embedded biliary uncovered SEMS with tissue ingrowth. *Endoscopy.* 2010;42(suppl 2):E304-E305.
11. Carazzone A, Bonavina L, Segalin A, Ceriani C, Peracchia A. Endoscopic palliation of oesophageal cancer: results of a prospective comparison of Nd:YAG laser and ethanol injection. *Eur J Surg.* 1999;165:351-356.
12. Van Heel NCM, Haringsma J, Spaander MCW, Didden P, Bruno MJ, Kuipers EJ. Esophageal stents for the palliation of malignant dysphagia and fistula recurrence after esophagectomy. *Gastrointest Endosc.* 2010;72:249-254.
13. White RE, Parker RK, Fitzwater JW, Kasepoi Z, Topazian M. Stents as sole therapy for oesophageal cancer: a prospective analysis of outcomes after placement. *Lancet Oncol.* 2009;10:240-246.
14. van Heel NCM, Haringsma J, Spaander MCW, Bruno MJ, Kuipers EJ. Esophageal stents for the relief of malignant dysphagia due to extrinsic compression. *Endoscopy.* 2010;42:536-540.
15. Vakil N, Morris AI, Marcon N, et al. A prospective, randomized, controlled trial of covered expandable metal stents in the palliation of malignant esophageal obstruction at the gastroesophageal junction. *Am J Gastroenterol.* 2001;96:1791-1796.
16. Conio M, Repici A, Battaglia G, et al. A randomized prospective comparison of self-expandable plastic stents and partially covered self-expandable metal stents in the palliation of malignant esophageal dysphagia. *Am J Gastroenterol.* 2007;102:2667-2677.
17. Rupinski M, Zagorowicz E, Regula J, et al. Randomized comparison of three palliative regimens including brachytherapy, photodynamic therapy, and APC in patients with malignant dysphagia (CONSORT 1a) (revised II). *Am J Gastroenterol.* 2011;106:1612-1620.
18. Yano T, Muto M, Minashi K, et al. Long-term results of salvage photodynamic therapy for patients with local failure after chemoradiotherapy for esophageal squamous cell carcinoma. *Endoscopy.* 2011;43:657-663.
19. Mehta S, Hindmarsh A, Cheong E, et al. Prospective randomized trial of laparoscopic gastrojejunostomy versus duodenal stenting for malignant gastric outflow obstruction. *Surg Endosc.* 2006;20:239-242.
20. Jeurnink SM, van Eijck CHJ, Steyerberg EW, Kuipers EJ, Siersema PD. Stent versus gastrojejunostomy for the palliation of gastric outlet obstruction: a systematic review. *BMC Gastroenterol.* 2007;7:18.
21. Rudolph HU, Post S, Schluter M, Seitz U, Soehendra N, Kahler G. Malignant gastroduodenal obstruction: retrospective comparison of endoscopic and surgical palliative therapy. *Scand J Gastroenterol.* 2011;46:583-590.

22. van Hooft JE, van Montfoort ML, Jeurnink SM, et al. Safety and efficacy of a new non-foreshortening nitinol stent in malignant gastric outlet obstruction (DUONITI study): a prospective, multicenter study. *Endoscopy.* 2011;43:671-675.

23. Piesman M, Kozarek RA, Brandabur JJ, et al. Improved oral intake after palliative duodenal stenting for malignant obstruction: a prospective multicenter clinical trial. *Am J Gastroenterol.* 2009;104:2404-2411.

24. Hosono S, Ohtani H, Arimoto Y, Kanamiya Y. Endoscopic stenting versus surgical gastroenterostomy for palliation of malignant gastroduodenal obstruction: a meta-analysis. *J Gastroenterol.* 2007;42:283-290.

25. Garcia-Cano J, Sanchez-Manjavacas N, Gomez Ruiz CJ, et al. Insercion endoscopica de protesis metalicas autoexpandibles en obstrucciones tumorales del colon. *Gastroenterol Hepatol.* 2006;29:610-615.

26. Song H, Kim JH, Shin JH, et al. A dual-design expandable colorectal stent for malignant colorectal obstruction: results of a multicenter study. *Endoscopy.* 2007;39:448-454.

27. van Hooft JE, Fockens P, Marinelli AW, et al. Early closure of a multicenter randomized clinical trial of endoscopic stenting versus surgery for stage IV left-sided colorectal cancer. *Endoscopy.* 2008;40:184-191.

28. Cennamo V, Fuccio L, Mutri V, et al. Does stent placement for advanced colon cancer increase the risk of perforation during bevacizumab-based therapy? *Clin Gastroenterol Hepatol.* 2009;7:1174-1176.

29. Dronamraju SS, Ramamurthy S, Kelly SB, Hayat M. Role of self-expanding metallic stents in the management of malignant obstruction of the proximal colon. *Dis Colon Rectum.* 2009;52:1657-1661.

30. Keswani RN, Azar RR, Edmundowicz SA, et al. Stenting for malignant colonic obstruction: a comparison of efficacy and complications in colonic versus extracolonic malignancy. *Gastrointest Endosc.* 2009;69:675-680.

31. Vemulapalli R, Lara LF, Sreenarasimhaiah J, Harford WV, Siddiqui AA. A comparison of palliative stenting or emergent surgery for obstructing incurable colon cancer. *Dig Dis Sci.* 2010; 55:1732-1737.

32. Al Samaraee A, Fasih T, Hayat M. Use of self-expandable stents for obstructive distal and proximal large bowel cancer: a retrospective study in a single centre. *J Gastrointest Cancer.* 2010; 41:43-46.

33. Fernandez-Esparrach G, Bordas JM, Giraldez MD, et al. Severe complications limit long-term clinical success of self-expanding metal stents in patients with obstructive colorectal cancer. *Am J Gastroenterol.* 2010;105:1087-1093.

34. Jung MK, Park SY, Jeon SW, et al. Factors associated with the long-term outcome of a self-expandable colon stent used for palliation of malignant colorectal obstruction. *Surg Endosc.* 2010;24:525-530.

35. Small AJ, Coelho-Prabhu N, Baron TH. Endoscopic placement of self-expandable metal stents for malignant colonic obstruction: long-term outcomes and complication factors. *Gastrointest Endosc.* 2010;71:560-572.

36. Suh JP, Kim SW, Cho YK, et al. Effectiveness of stent placement for palliative treatment in malignant colorectal obstruction and predictive factors for stent occlusion. *Surg Endosc.* 2010;24:400-406.

37. Nagula S, Ishill N, Nash C, et al. Quality of life and symptom control after stent placement or surgical palliation of malignant colorectal obstruction. *J Am Coll Surg.* 2010;210:45-53.

38. Lee HJ, Hong SP, Cheon JH, et al. Long-term outcome of palliative therapy for malignant colorectal obstruction in patients with unresectable metastatic colorectal cancers: endoscopic stenting versus surgery. *Gastrointest Endosc.* 2011;73:535-542.

39. Luigiano C, Ferrara F, Fabbri C, et al. Through-the-scope large diameter self-expanding metal stent placement as a safe and effective technique for palliation of malignant colorectal obstruction: a single center experience with a long-term follow-up. *Scand J Gastroenterol.* 2011;46:591-596.

40. Manes G, de Bellis M, Fuccio L, et al. Endoscopic palliation in patients with incurable malignant colorectal obstruction by means of self-expanding metal stent: analysis of results and predictors of outcomes in a large multicenter series. *Arch Surg.* 2011;146:1157-1162.

41. Meisner S, Gonzalez-Huix F, Vandervoort JG, et al. Self-expandable metal stents for relieving malignant colorectal obstruction: short-term safety and efficacy within 30 days of stent procedure in 447 patients. *Gastrointest Endosc.* 2011;74:876-884.

42. Siddiqui A, Khandelwal N, Anthony T, Huerta S. Colonic stent versus surgery for the management of acute malignant colonic obstruction: a decision analysis. *Aliment Pharmacol Ther.* 2007;26:1379-1386.

43. Sebastian S, Johnston S, Geoghegan T, Torreggiani W, Buckley M. Pooled analysis of the efficacy and safety of self-expanding metal stenting in malignant colorectal obstruction. *Am J Gastroenterol.* 2004;99:2051-2057.

44. Zhang Y, Shi J, Shi B, Song C, Xie W, Chen Y. Self-expanding metallic stent as a bridge to surgery versus emergency surgery for obstructive colorectal cancer: a meta-analysis. *Surg Endosc.* 2012; 26:110-119.

45. Lau PW, Lo CY, Law WL. The role of one-stage surgery in acute left-sided colonic obstruction. *Am J Surg.* 1995;169:406-409.

46. Repici A, Fregonese D, Costamagna G, et al. Ultraflex precision colonic stent placement for palliation of malignant colonic obstruction: a prospective multicenter study. *Gastrointest Endosc.* 2007;66:920-927.

47. Dastur JK, Forshaw MJ, Modarai B, Solkar MM, Raymond T, Parker MC. Comparison of short-and long-term outcomes following either insertion of self-expanding metallic stents or emergency surgery in malignant large bowel obstruction. *Tech Coloproctol.* 2008;12:51-55.

48. Repici A, De Caro G, Luigiano C, et al. WallFlex colonic stent placement for management of malignant colonic obstruction: a prospective study at two centers. *Gastrointest Endosc.* 2008;67:77-84.

49. Brehant O, Fuks D, Bartoli E, Yzet T, Verhaeghe P, Regimbeau JM. Elective (planned) 0colectomy in patients with colorectal obstruction after placement of a self-expanding metallic stent as a bridge to surgery: the results of a prospective study. *Colorectal Dis.* 2009;11:178-183.

50. Guo M, Feng Y, Zheng Q, et al. Comparison of self-expanding metal stents and urgent surgery for left-sided malignant colonic obstruction in elderly patients. *Dig Dis Sci.* 2011;56:2706-2710.

51. Jimenez-Perez J, Casellas J, Garcia-Cano J, et al. Colonic stenting as a bridge to surgery in malignant large-bowel obstruction: a report from two large multinational registries. *Am J Gastroenterol.* 2011;106:2174-2180.

52. Driest JJ, Zwaving HH, Ledeboer M, et al. Low morbidity and mortality after stenting for malignant bowel obstruction. *Dig Surg.* 2011;28:367-371.

53. White SI, Abdool SI, Frenkiel B, Braun WV. Management of malignant left-sided large bowel obstruction: a comparison between colonic stents and surgery. *ANZ J Surg.* 2011;81:257-260.

54. Lee JH, Ross WA, Davila R, et al. Self-expandable metal stents (SEMS) can serve as a bridge to surgery or as a definitive therapy in patients with an advanced stage of cancer: clinical experience of a tertiary cancer center. *Dig Dis Sci.* 2010;55:3530-3536.

55. Pirlet IA, Slim K, Kwiatkowski F, Michot F, Millat BL. Emergency preoperative stenting versus surgery for acute left-sided malignant colonic obstruction: a multicenter randomized controlled trial. *Surg Endosc.* 2011;25:1814-1821.

56. Iversen LH, Kratmann M, Boje M, Laurberg S. Self-expanding metallic stents as bridge to surgery in obstructing colorectal cancer. *Br J Surg.* 2011;98:275-281.

57. Park JK, Lee MS, Ko BM, et al. Outcome of palliative self-expanding metal stent placement in malignant colorectal obstruction according to stent type and manufacturer. *Surg Endosc.* 2011;25:1293-1299.

58. Khot UP, Lang AW, Murali K, Parker MC. Systematic review of the efficacy and safety of colorectal stents. *Br J Surg.* 2002;89:1096-1102.

59. Herman LL, Hoskins WJ, Shike M. Percutaneous endoscopic gastrostomy for decompression of the stomach and small bowel. *Gastrointest Endosc.* 1992;38:314-318.

60. Pothuri B, Montemarano M, Gerardi M, et al. Percutaneous endoscopic gastrostomy tube placement in patients with malignant bowel obstruction due to ovarian carcinoma. *Gynecol Oncol.* 2005;96:330-334.

61. Holm AN, Baron TH. Palliative use of percutaneous endoscopic gastrostomy and percutaneous endoscopic cecostomy tubes. *Gastrointest Endosc Clin N Am.* 2007;17:795-803.

62. Speer AG, Cotton PB, Russell RC, et al. Randomised trial of endoscopic versus percutaneous stent insertion in malignant obstructive jaundice. *Lancet.* 1987;2:57-62.

63. Will U, Thieme A, Fueldner F, Gerlach R, Wanzar I, Meyer F. Treatment of biliary obstruction in selected patients by endoscopic ultrasonography (EUS)-guided transluminal biliary drainage. *Endoscopy.* 2007;39:292-295.

64. van der Gaag NA, Rauws EAJ, van Eijck CHJ, et al. Preoperative biliary drainage for cancer of the head of the pancreas. *N Engl J Med.* 2010;362:129-137.

65. Decker C, Christein JD, Phadnis MA, Wilcox CM, Varadarajulu S. Biliary metal stents are superior to plastic stents for preoperative biliary decompression in pancreatic cancer. *Surg Endosc.* 2011;25:2364-2367.

66. Yoon WJ, Ryu JK, Yang KY, et al. A comparison of metal and plastic stents for the relief of jaundice in unresectable malignant biliary obstruction in Korea: an emphasis on cost-effectiveness in a country with a low ERCP cost. *Gastrointest Endosc.* 2009;70:284-289.

67. Ahmad J, Siqueira E, Martin J, Slivka A. Effectiveness of the ultraflex diamond stent for the palliation of malignant biliary obstruction. *Endoscopy.* 2002;34:793-796.

68. Yoon WJ, Lee JK, Lee KH, et al. A comparison of covered and uncovered Wallstents for the management of distal malignant biliary obstruction. *Gastrointest Endosc.* 2006;63:996-1000.

69. Soderlund C, Linder S. Covered metal versus plastic stents for malignant common bile duct stenosis: a prospective, randomized, controlled trial. *Gastrointest Endosc.* 2006;63:986-995.

70. Loew BJ, Howell DA, Sanders MK, et al. Comparative performance of uncoated, self-expanding metal biliary stents of different designs in 2 diameters: final results of an international multicenter, randomized, controlled trial. *Gastrointest Endosc.* 2009;70:445-453.

71. Kullman E, Frozanpor F, Soderlund C, et al. Covered versus uncovered self-expandable nitinol stents in the palliative treatment of malignant distal biliary obstruction: results from a randomized, multicenter study. *Gastrointest Endosc.* 2010;72:915-923.

72. Tham TC, Carr-Locke DL, Vandervoort J, et al. Management of occluded biliary Wallstents. *Gut.* 1998;42:703-707.

73. Bueno JT, Gerdes H, Kurtz RC. Endoscopic management of occluded biliary Wallstents: a cancer center experience. *Gastrointest Endosc.* 2003;58:879-884.

74. Albert JG, Friedrich-Rust M, Elhendawy M, Trojan J, Zeuzem S, Sarrazin C. Peroral cholangioscopy for diagnosis and therapy of biliary tract disease using an ultra-slim gastroscope. *Endoscopy.* 2011;43:1004-1009.

75. Barkun AN, Bardou M, Kuipers EJ, et al. International consensus recommendations on the management of patients with nonvariceal upper gastrointestinal bleeding. *Ann Intern Med.* 2010;152:101-113.

76. Kaltenbach T, Friedland S, Barro J, Soetikno R. Clipping for upper gastrointestinal bleeding. *Am J Gastroenterol.* 2006;101:915-918.

77. Albert JG, Friedrich-Rust M, Woeste G, et al. Benefit of a clipping device in use in intestinal bleeding and intestinal leakage. *Gastrointest Endosc.* 2011;74:389-397.

78. Prachayakul V, Aswakul P, Kachinthorn U. Spraying N-butyl-2-cyanoacrylate (Histoacryl) as a rescue therapy for gastrointestinal malignant tumor bleeding after failed conventional therapy. *Endoscopy.* 2011;43(suppl 2):E227-E228.

79. Wiersema MJ, Wiersema LM. Endosonography-guided celiac plexus neurolysis. *Gastrointest Endosc.* 1996;44:656-662.

80. O'Toole T, Schmulewitz N. Complication rates of EUS-guided celiac plexus blockade and neurolysis: results of a large case series. *Endoscopy.* 2009;41:593-597.

81. Puli SR, Reddy JBK, Bechtold ML, Antillon MR, Brugge WR. EUS-guided celiac plexus neurolysis for pain due to chronic pancreatitis or pancreatic cancer pain: a meta-analysis and systematic review. *Dig Dis Sci.* 2009;54:2330-2337.

82. Kaufman M, Singh G, Das S, et al. Efficacy of endoscopic ultrasound-guided celiac plexus block and celiac plexus neurolysis for managing abdominal pain associated with chronic pancreatitis and pancreatic cancer. *J Clin Gastroenterol.* 2010;44:127-134.

83. Sakamoto H, Kitano M, Kamata K, et al. EUS-guided broad plexus neurolysis over the superior mesenteric artery using a 25-gauge needle. *AJG.* September 2010; doi:10.1038/ajg.2010.339.

84. Dennis MS, Lewis SC, Warlow C. Effect of timing and method of enteral tube feeding for dysphagic stroke patients (FOOD): a multicentre randomised controlled trial. *Lancet.* 2005;365:764-772.

85. Cruz I, Mamel JJ, Brady PG, Cass-Garcia M. Incidence of abdominal wall metastasis complicating PEG tube placement in untreated head and neck cancer. *Gastrointest Endosc.* 2005;62:708-711;quiz 752, 753.

86. Monga A, Gupta R, Ramchandani M, Rao GV, Santosh D, Reddy DN. Endoscopic radiofrequency ablation of cholangiocarcinoma: new palliative treatment modality (with videos). *Gastrointest Endosc.* 2011;74:935-937.

87. Seo DW. EUS-guided antitumor therapy for pancreatic tumors. *Gut Liver.* 2010;4(suppl 1):S76-S81.

88. Ortner MEJ, Caca K, Berr F, et al. Successful photodynamic therapy for nonresectable cholangiocarcinoma: a randomized prospective study. *Gastroenterology.* 2003;125:1355-1363.

89. Witzigmann H, Berr F, Ringel U, et al. Surgical and palliative management and outcome in 184 patients with hilar cholangiocarcinoma: palliative photodynamic therapy plus stenting is comparable to r1/r2 resection. *Ann Surg.* 2006;244:230-239.

90. Zoepf T, Jakobs R, Arnold JC, Apel D, Riemann JF. Palliation of nonresectable bile duct cancer: improved survival after photodynamic therapy. *Am J Gastroenterol.* 2005;100:2426-2430.

91. Kahaleh M, Mishra R, Shami VM, et al. Unresectable cholangiocarcinoma: comparison of survival in biliary stenting alone versus stenting with photodynamic therapy. *Clin Gastroenterol Hepatol.* 2008;6:290-297.

92. Matull W, Dhar DK, Ayaru L, et al. R0 but not R1/R2 resection is associated with better survival than palliative photodynamic therapy in biliary tract cancer. *Liver Int.* 2011;31:99-107.

CHAPTER 22

Palliative Interventional Radiologic Procedures

Thomas J. Vogl ■ Michael K. Eichler ■ Stefan G. Zangos ■ Parviz Farshid

SUMMARY

Especially in the last few years, image-guided minimally invasive procedures have been used with the aim of tumor destruction instead of invasive treatment in patients with unresectable cancer. Management methods with palliative effect include locoregional intra-arterial therapies such as vascular access, management of vascular and nonvascular complications, and approach to the malignant fluid collection. Many patients benefit from the palliative roles of these interventions. These techniques, compared with other treatment options, have some advantages, including symptomatic relief, local anesthesia, short hospital stay, and low postsurgical discomfort.

In this chapter, the authors describe the principle, indications, contraindications, and impact of these therapeutic techniques.

PALLIATIVE INTERVENTIONAL TECHNIQUES: A WIDE SPECTRUM

Palliative interventional oncological methods in patients with cancer are associated with locoregional therapies such as vascular access, management of vascular and nonvascular complications, and approach to the malignant peritoneal and pleural fluid. Interventional procedures with palliative effects are demonstrated in Table 22.1.

LOCOREGIONAL CANCER THERAPY

Locoregional cancer therapies include several techniques that have started with chemoembolization and have been improved by novel systems with the use of drug-eluting beads (DEBs) and radioembolization with yttrium 90. In the last three decades, several minimally invasive locoregional treatments termed new ablation techniques have been used, including thermal ablation, such as radiofrequency ablation (RFA), microwave ablation (MWA), laser-induced thermotherapy (LITT), and cryoablation, and chemical ablation such as ethanol or acetic acid ablation therapy. Isolated or in combination, these techniques have already shown that they can improve patient survival and/or provide acceptable palliation (1).

Embolization therapies, including transarterial chemoembolization (TACE), bland embolization, and radioembolization, have been improved as alternatives to other treatment options such as systemic chemotherapy. In TACE, a solution of chemotherapy suspended in lipiodol, an oily contrast medium selectively retained within the tumor, is injected into the feeding arteries directly supplying the tumor (2).

Chemoembolization is indicated for palliative treatment of unresectable primary or secondary hepatic lesions and reduction of pain. This technique is also used in pulmonary cancer (transpulmonary chemoembolization [TPCE]) and as a novel approach to pulmonary malignant mesothelioma. It is useful for reducing tumor size or decreasing local tumor progression.

In neoadjuvant indication, this treatment aims at reducing the tumor to make an operation possible. In palliative indication, it is performed for pain relief and reducing symptoms, or simply for increased survival time (1–3). During TACE, the arterial system is accessed using the Seldinger technique and a catheter is advanced in the aorta. First, selective vascular trunk should be performed with late-phase imaging of the portal venous anatomy. Once the arterial anatomy is clearly understood, a catheter is advanced superselectively into the artery. Small vessels and branches that cannot be accessed with a standard angiographic catheter can be catheterized with a variety of microcatheters designed for chemoembolization. The choice of the catheter/guide wire combination is usually related to the preference of the interventionist. The end point of the TACE procedure is visualization of the complete blockage of the tumor-feeding branch (3). Palliative indications of TACE include treatment of hormone-producing tumors and reduction of shunt volumes in hemangioendothelioma. TACE has no indication if more than 75% of the liver is involved by tumor and also when there is significant portal hypertension, liver insufficiency, occlusion of the portal vein, or hepatorenal syndrome (3). The most common anticancer drugs are doxorubicin, mitomycin, cisplatin, and mixtures. Lipiodol (iodized oil) is an oily contrast medium that persists more selectively in tumor nodules for a few weeks up to some months when injected into the artery (4). Gelfoam is the most commonly used embolizing agent. This only occludes the artery temporarily with recanalization taking place within 2 weeks (5), achieving more distal obstruction because of a smaller particle size (50 to 250 μm in diameter). The main complication of TACE is the postembolization syndrome (PES). PES is characterized by nausea, vomiting, abdominal pain, and fever occurring in 2% to 7% of patients after the procedure, although PES is a self-limited event that can be managed supportively (6).

Bland embolization is a technique that is performed by injecting an embolic agent and radioembolization with yttrium 90 microspheres into the feeding arteries. Embolic

TABLE 22.1	Applications and methods of palliative interventional oncology
Application	**Method**
Local–regional cancer therapy	Transarterial chemoembolization Drug-eluting bead embolization Transarterial radioembolization Radiofrequency ablation Microwave ablation Cryoablation Chemical ablation—ethanol, acetic acid
Management of vascular complication	Superior vena cava syndrome Arterial obstruction secondary to tumor compression or invasion Hemorrhage secondary to tumor invasion IVC filters for venous thromboembolic complications
Management of nonvascular complications	Biliary drainage and stenting Urinary track drainage and stenting
Management of vascular access	Central venous ports Tunneled central venous catheters PICCS
Management of malignant pleural and peritoneal fluid	Tunneled drainage catheters Decompression

beads preloaded with a chemotherapeutic agent or "DEBs" are new delivery systems. In 2009, Paul et al. reviewed related results and reported that embolization for splenic tumors is an unexplored area with no articles to date discussing its efficacy. Small and large bowel tumors are rarely treated with embolization, and if so, embolization is primarily used prior to operative resection or in cases of tumor-induced gastrointestinal hemorrhage. Embolization of pancreatic insulinoma and carcinoma has been described. In the adrenals, embolization is primarily used for preoperative debulking or for symptomatic relief from hyperfunctioning tumors. Embolization for renal cell carcinoma and angiomyelolipoma is mainly used in the preoperative setting to reduce blood flow prior to surgical resection. The embolization agents used were predominantly permanent, including alcohol, particles, and coils. They suggested that catheter-directed embolization is an important technique in the treatment of non-liver mesenteric tumors, primarily in the setting of nonoperable neoplasms, preoperative tumor control, or tumor hemorrhage (7).

Similar to TACE, **radioembolization** is a palliative treatment; however, during this procedure, radioactive microspheres (isotope yttrium 90) are used instead of chemotherapeutic drugs. Due to fewer side effects and positive response in patients who have received surgical tumor resection or transplantation, this technique may be a good minimally invasive treatment option (8).

Palliative Impact of Locoregional Cancer Therapies

Chemoembolization for Patients with Hepatocellular Carcinoma (HCC)

Although TACE is widely used as a palliative treatment of unresectable hepatic tumor, its role should be further

clarified. Table 22.2 demonstrates the impact of palliative TACE in patients with HCC.

O'Suilleabhain et al. (13) evaluated the long-term survival of TACE in patients with unresectable HCC and suggested that this technique has a palliative effect because a cure for unresectable HCC may only rarely be possible with TACE. They documented 25 5-year survivors (8%) among a cohort study of 320 patients treated with TACE.

TACE for Patients with HCC Using DEBs

DEB has been used in patients with hepatocellular carcinoma. In 2009, Reyes et al. (16) showed overall survival (OS) rates in 20 patients at 1 and 2 years of 65% and 55%, respectively; the median OS was 26 months. In 2010, Malagari et al. compared DEB chemoembolization with bland embolization in patients with HCC who were child A or B showing that stable disease at 12 months was statistically higher in the DEB chemoembolization group. Progression of disease developed in 48.6% in the DEB chemoembolization group and 78.4% in the bland group. However, there was no difference in survival within 1 year between the two groups (17). In 2010, Dhanasekaran et al. evaluated 71 patients who had received chemoembolization with DEB or conventional chemoembolization. Median survival times from the first therapy were 403 and 114 days, respectively. In Child-Pugh classes A and B, survival time from the first therapy between the two groups was 641 versus 323 days (18). In 2010, Scartozzi et al. evaluated traditional chemoembolization and DEB chemoembolization in 150 patients. Median OS times were 46 and 19 months, respectively. Time to progression was 30 months versus 16 months (19). In 2009, Lammer et al. evaluated conventional TACE ($n = 108$) with chemoembolization with embolic beads preloaded with doxorubicin

| TABLE 22.2 | Survival indexes in patients with hepatocellular carcinoma who have received transarterial chemoembolization as a palliative treatment | | | | | |

Authors	No. of Patients	Median Survival (Months)	Survival Rates (%)			
			1 Year	2 Years	3 Years	5 Years
Kalva et al. (9)	54	14.8	59	32	—	—
Jin et al. (10)	58	22	94	84	73	—
Huang et al. (11)	26	9.13	42	—	13	7
Llovet et al. (12)	112	9	96	77	47	—
O'Suilleabhain et al. (13)	320	—	31	—	11	8
Lo et al. (14)	79	—	57	31	26	—
Ernst et al. (15)	160	—	Ok I: 58.89 Ok II: 19.48	28.68	11.39	—

(DEB chemoembolization) ($n = 93$). The DEB chemoembolization group showed higher rates of complete response, objective response, and disease control compared with the conventional chemoembolization group (27% vs. 22%, 52% vs. 44%, and 63% vs. 52%, respectively). These differences were not statistically significant (20).

TACE for Patients with Liver Metastases

TACE represents a safe palliative treatment for patients with unresectable liver metastases. The results of TACE depend on primary cancer, size, and vascularization of the hepatic tumors (21).

Neuroendocrine Tumors Using TACE

Ho et al. (2007) evaluated clinical response for 27 patients with hepatic metastatic lesions from neuroendocrine tumors who underwent hepatic artery chemoembolization or hepatic artery embolization (HAE) because of symptoms. This group consisted of 25 patients with hormonal symptoms and 4 with pain secondary to capsular distention. Twenty-one (78%) of the evaluated patients reported relief of symptoms after the initial cycle of treatment. When evaluated according to the tumor type, 78% of carcinoid patients and 75% of islet cell patients had relief of the presenting symptoms (22).

Eighty percent of carcinoid patients treated for hormonal symptoms had subjective relief of hormonal symptoms after one cycle of therapy. Sixty-six percent of carcinoid patients treated for symptoms related to tumor bulk reported relief of pain. Among patients with islet cell tumors, 66% of patients treated for hormonal symptoms had relief of symptoms. Reduction of the presenting symptoms was achieved in a similar manner in patients with and without extrahepatic disease. Thirteen of 16 patients with extrahepatic disease and 7 of 9 patients with no sign of extrahepatic disease experienced relief of symptoms after one cycle of hepatic artery chemoembolization or HAE (22).

Colorectal cancer (CRC) Using Conventional TACE

In 2011, Albert et al. reported in 121 patients with metastatic CRC a median survival time of 9 months from chemoembolization. The 1-, 2-, and 5-year survival rates were 94%, 74%, and 13%, respectively (23). In 2009, Vogl et al. evaluated 463 patients with colorectal liver metastases with primarily palliative indication for chemoembolization. Results showed a median survival time of 14 months from the start of chemoembolization (24).

CRC Using DEB Chemoembolization

In 2010, Martin et al. documented in 55 patients with CRC liver metastases an OS of 19 months and progression-free survival (PFS) of 11 months using DEB chemoembolization (25).

Malignant Melanoma

In 2010, Schuster et al. evaluated 25 patients with liver metastases from melanoma using TACE and found no grade IV toxicity or catheter-associated complications. The median PFS was 3 months and median OS was 5 months. The 1-year survival rate was 15% (26). In 2009, Gupta et al. (27) reported in 105 patients a median OS and PFS of 6.7 and 3.8 months, respectively. Sharma et al. reported in 20 patients with stage IV melanoma mean and median OS of 334 ± 71 and 271 days, respectively. Sixty-five percent of patients had progression of the disease (28).

Transpulmonary Chemoembolization

TPCE for the palliative treatment of unresectable lung tumors has been used with acceptable outcome. Early use of this method results in a reduction in tumor volume and alleviation of patient symptoms. After superselective catheterization, cytotoxic agents are administered, and the pulmonary arterial supply of the tumor is occluded by injection of microspheres and ethiodized oil. Emerging data suggest that this approach is well tolerated (29).

Vogl et al. evaluated tumor response after treating unresectable lung metastases with TPCE in palliative intention. Fifty-two patients suffering from 106 unresectable lung metastases were treated with 2 to 10 TPCE sessions. Metastases originated from primaries, including colorectal carcinoma ($n = 20$), breast cancer ($n = 6$), renal cellular carcinoma ($n = 5$), thyroid cancer ($n = 4$), cholangiocellular carcinoma ($n = 2$), leiomyosarcoma ($n = 2$), and others ($n = 13$). All patients tolerated the treatment well without major side effects or complications. In 24%, moderate to high lipiodol uptake was found, while 75% of the tumors showed a low uptake. Partial response was achieved in 16 cases, stable disease in 11 cases, and progressive disease in 25 cases; mean and median survival was documented at 17 and 21.1 months, retrospectively (30).

Impact of Radioembolization

Several studies have demonstrated that radioembolization is a safe and effective palliative procedure in patients with unresectable liver metastases and helps slow down the growth of the disease and alleviate symptoms (8,31–35). In 2011, Sangro et al. reported that radioembolization results in average disease control rates above 80% and is usually very well tolerated. Main complications do not result from the microembolic effect, even in patients with portal vein occlusion, but rather from an excessive irradiation of nontarget tissues including the liver. When compared with the standard of care for the intermediate and advanced stages (transarterial embolization and sorafenib), radioembolization consistently provides similar survival rates as hormone and chemotherapy (35). In 2009, Vente et al. showed in a meta-analysis on tumor response and survival using 30 articles on 1,217 patients who underwent ^{90}Y radioembolization that the proportion of "any response" (AR) for HCC and liver metastatic CRC combined varied between 29% and 100% with a median value of 82%. Treatment with glass microspheres showed a lower response than treatment with resin microspheres. They found that complications have been reported when microspheres were inadvertently deposited in excessive amounts in organs other than the liver. For HCC, response was 89% for resin microspheres and 78% for glass microspheres. For CRC liver metastases in a salvage setting, response was 79% for radioembolization combined with 5-fluorouracil/leucovorin (5-FU/LV), and 79% when combined with 5-FU/LV/oxaliplatin or 5-FU/LV/irinotecan, and in a first-line setting 91% and 91%, respectively. In patients with liver metastases from CRC, the tumor response of radioembolization is high, with AR rates of approximately 80% in a salvage setting (36).

For HCC, median survival from treatment was from 7.1 to 21.0 months and from diagnosis or recurrence was 9.4 to 24.0 months. For liver metastases from CRC, median survival after ^{90}Y-RE, irrespective of differences in determinants (microspheres type, chemotherapy protocol, and

stage: salvage or first line), was 6.7 to 17.0 months and from diagnosis of liver metastases from CRC it ranged from 10.8 to 29.4 months (36).

Ablation Therapy

Percutaneous imaging-guided ablative therapies using thermal energy sources such as radiofrequency (RF), microwave (MW), laser, and high-intensity focused sonography have been used as minimally invasive strategies for the treatment of focal malignant diseases (37,38). Thermal ablation therapies have been defined well by Târcoveanu et al. These techniques are used to destroy the malignant cells by heat in a minimally invasive approach without damaging normal tissue. Electromagnetic energy has been used in the form of both RF and MW; photocoagulation uses intense pulses of light produced by a laser as the energy source; high-intensity focused sonography uses sound energy to produce heat; and injection of heated fluids, including saline, ethanol, and contrast material, has been used to induce coagulation by direct thermal contact. In nonresectable hepatic tumors, palliative treatment using focal necrosis by hyperthermia appears as a valuable alternative. These methods of treatment can be performed by percutaneous, laparoscopic, or open approach. The key element in the management of the malignant tumors of the liver is the cooperation between surgeon, intensive care physician, oncologist, and specialist in interventional radiology in order to discuss the indication of therapy (39).

In 2011, Pathak et al. reviewed ablative therapies in CRC liver metastases and showed that cryotherapy (26 studies) had a local recurrence rate of 12% to 39%, with mean 1-, 3-, and 5-year survival rates of 84%, 37%, and 17%, respectively. The major complication rate ranged from 7% to 66%. MWA (13 studies) had a local recurrence rate between 5% and 13% with mean 1-, 3-, and 5-year survival rates of 73%, 30% and 16%, respectively, and a major complication rate ranging from 3% to 16%. RFA (36 studies) had a local recurrence rate of 10% to 31%, with mean 1-, 3-, and 5-year survival rates of 85%, 36%, and 24%, respectively, with major complication rate ranging from 0% to 33% (40). In 2010, Bhardwaj et al. (41) summarized major studies in ablation technologies and presented them in a way that makes comparison between the major modalities easier.

Radiofrequency Ablation

RFA involves insertion of an electrode via skin or intraoperation into a lesion under imaging guidance. Heat created by RF energy leads to coagulative necrosis. Lung tumors that are difficult to reach may require repeated RFA treatments. The most commonly reported complications of RFA are pneumothorax and bleeding (42,43). RFA appears to be effective for rapid tumor reduction and palliation. The combination therapy of this technique can offer new treatment strategies for an improvement of the patient's quality of life and more effective palliative medicine (44).

RFA is a tool that can potentially palliate intractable cancer pain. The scope of cancer pain ranges from minor discomfort relieved with mild pain medication to unrelenting suffering for the patient, poorly controlled by conventional means. In 2006, Jindal et al. (45) presented a case in which RFA provided pain relief in a patient with metastatic prostate cancer with pelvic pain uncontrolled by conventional methods, and when combined with celiac ganglion block and splanchnic nerve block it has been used for visceral pain relief. Several studies reported the feasibility and effect of RFA therapy for the treatment of lung masses in patients with non–small cell lung cancer (NSCLC) or lung metastases but only few studies are related to long-term outcomes in patients with primary and secondary pulmonary tumors. Palliative RFA may be indicated for large tumors (46–48). In 2008, Lencioni (47) reported in 106 patients with NSCLC OS at 1 and 2 years of 70% and 48%, respectively. In 2004, Belfiore et al. evaluated palliative computed tomography (CT)-guided RFA in 33 patients with unresectable primary pulmonary malignancies. Clinical improvement in pretreatment symptoms was observed in 12 of 29 patients seen at 6-month follow-up (49). External beam irradiation is the palliative treatment of choice for osteolytic bone metastases, but additional radiation should not be offered for recurrent sessions. RFA is another alternative for palliating pain from bone metastases. Belfiore et al. evaluated the clinical efficacy of RFA with respect to pain relief in patients with refractory bone metastases or patients who are ineligible to conventional treatments. Immediate pain relief after treatment was experienced by 9 of 12 patients; however, in 2 cases pain recurred within the first week. Long-lasting palliation was obtained in 7 of 12 patients (50). In 2008, Hoffmann et al. evaluated the feasibility and effectiveness of combining RFA and osteoplasty for pain reduction in the treatment of painful osteolytic metastases. Technical success and pain relief was achieved in all patients (51). However, ablation therapy as a palliative treatment for bone tumor management and

indications has been described with a management algorithm by Gangi et al. in 2007 (52) (Fig. 22.1).

These techniques either alone or combined with percutaneous cementoplasty and embolization can be used as treatment options for bone tumors (51,52).

RFA for pancreatic cancer seems to be an attractive palliative treatment option. Only one retrospective comparative study has demonstrated survival benefit for patients with locally advanced pancreatic cancer. In two retrospective studies, the same survival benefit was not demonstrated for patients with metastatic disease (stage IV). If the results are similar in larger and nonconsecutive studies, RFA could then be considered part of a multimodal therapeutic approach for inoperable, locally advanced nonmetastatic pancreatic cancer (53). In 2010, Girelli et al. (54), based on results in 50 patients with locally advanced pancreatic cancer, showed that RFA is feasible and relatively well tolerated, with a 24% abdominal complication rate. Among these patients, 6% showed surgery-related complications. Reduction of RFA temperature from 105°C to 90°C resulted in a significant reduction in complications (10 vs. 2 of 25 patients; $P = 0.028$). Median postoperative hospital stay was 10 (range 7 to 31) days. RFA of renal tumors is a promising investigational palliative alternative. In 2003, Rohde et al. (55) reported that in four patients with renal cancer RFA was found to be favorable for palliative treatment (low performance status and surgical preconditions) and in connection with immunochemotherapy. RFA has a good palliative efficacy in patients with partial or total nephrectomy (56,57). Guidelines on thyroid cancer from the National Comprehensive Cancer Network, 2010 (58), state that distant metastases from recurrent or persistent medullary thyroid carcinoma that are causing symptoms could be considered for palliative resection, RFA, or other regional treatment. In 2011, Kuenzli et al. reviewed RFA of liver tumors. They concluded that over the past decade, RFA

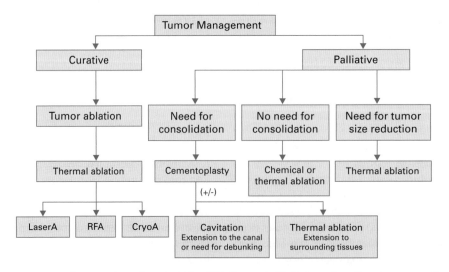

Figure 22.1. Tumor management therapeutic option algorithm (52): thermal ablation can be offered as a curative treatment option in bone tumor. This technique also plays a palliative role regarding consolidation or tumor size reduction. For nonsurgical spinal tumors extending toward the canal with rupture of the posterior wall and epidural extension, percutaneous tumor decompression utilizing radiofrequency ionization is the best technique. After tumor decompression, the cavity created can be filled with cement.

has evolved into an important therapeutic tool for the treatment of nonresectable primary and secondary liver tumors. The clinical benefit of RFA is represented in several clinical studies. They underline the safety and feasibility of this new and modern concept in treating liver tumors. RFA has proven its clinical impact not only in HCC but also in metastatic disease such as CRC. Due to the increasing numbers of HCC and CRC, RFA might play an even more important role in the future. They suggested that the refinement of RFA technology is as important as data evaluation of prospective randomized trials that will help define guidelines for good clinical practice in RFA application in the future. Therefore, the combination of hepatic resection and RFA extends the feasibility of open surgical procedures in patients with extensive tumors (59).

Microwave Ablation

MWA is a well-established and safe local ablative method for liver tumors and locally advanced pancreatic cancer. In 2007, Lygidakis et al. reported that in 15 patients with pancreatic cancer, MWA was as an effective therapy which was feasible and safe with acceptable minor complication rates in a locally advanced pancreatic tumor and could be used as part of a palliative or multimodality treatment. All patients had close follow-up and the longest surviving patient had a follow-up of 22 months (60). The safety and efficacy of retroperitoneoscopic MWA in the treatment of renal hamartoma were evaluated by Guan et al. in 2010 (61), and a total of 16 cases of renal hamartoma were treated with retroperitoneoscopic MWA. Liang et al. evaluated the palliative effect of MWA in 75 patients with liver metastases. The median survival time was 22.1 months and disease-free survival rate was 35%. Cumulative survival was 91% at 1 year decreasing to 29% at 5 years (62). In 2009, Li et al. evaluated the long-term effect and related factors in 334 patients with menorrhagia treated by microwave endometrial ablation. Menstruation reduction rate was 41.6%; in 71.1% of the cases who previously had dysmenorrhea a reduction in pelvic pain was documented and the success rate was 91.9% (63).

Laser-Induced Thermotherapy

Laser-induced interstitial thermotherapy (LITT) is among the relatively new percutaneous ablation techniques that have proved effective. Laser coagulation is accomplished using neodymium–yttrium aluminum garnet laser light with a wavelength of 1,064 nm. The light is delivered through 400-mm-long fibers terminated by a specially developed diffuser that emits laser light to an effective distance of 12 to 15 mm. Cooling the surface of the laser applicator improves the radial temperature distribution, shifting the maximum possible amount of heat energy into deeper tissue layers at the same time avoiding carbonization and thus allowing the use of higher laser power of up to 35 W. These parameters result in a more homogeneous tissue penetration of laser radiation. The laser systems are fully compatible with

magnetic resonance imaging (MRI) units (64). Laser applicator systems can be placed at the desired position under CT fluoroscopy guidance. The multiapplication technique involves the treatment of one lesion with multiple (up to five) laser applicators simultaneously. It is also possible to treat more than one lesion in the same session. Then the patients are transferred to a 0.5-T closed MRI unit. Laser ablation is performed under near real-time magnetic resonance (MR) in transverse section and parallel to the laser applicators repeated every minute for monitoring of thermal ablation. Following the first laser cycle, the laser fiber can be retracted by a distance of 2 cm and a second laser cycle can be performed to enlarge the area of coagulation necrosis. Necrosis manifests as progressively deepening T1 hypointensity. After the procedure, the puncture tract is closed with fibrin glue (64). Alternatively, puncture, applicator positioning, and laser ablation monitoring can all be performed in an open MRI unit. The entire LITT treatment can be tolerated under local anesthesia using 20 to 30 mL of 1% lidocaine and analgesics and sedation. The mean duration of ablation is 20 minutes (range: 2 to 55 min.). Besides, the pull back and repositioning of the laser fiber is calculated on the basis of signal change because the heat deposition in the tissue cannot be predicted, which means that a certain amount of energy can result in different volumes of coagulation necrosis in different settings (64). The indications for percutaneous ablation of liver metastases using LITT are recurrent metastases after partial hepatectomy or segmentectomy, bilobar metastases, locally unresectable lesions, general contraindications for surgery, or refusal of surgery (65,66). LITT is not feasible in patients with more than five lesions, lesions larger than 5 cm in greatest diameter, or extrahepatic metastases (65). Some other possible contraindications are poor coagulability, liver insufficiency, and contraindications for MRI (66). Although the intention for LITT was originally palliative, its favorable survival rates are comparable with those obtained with surgical resection of liver metastases showing at the same time lower morbidity and mortality rates (65–67). Surgery can be combined with LITT in the same treatment plan by using LITT to complement less radical operations like segmentectomy or localized resection instead of lobectomy. These data suggest that in the next few years, the indication for LITT and combined LITT and TACE approach can include more patients with liver metastases, including surgical candidates with no more than five metastases with a maximum diameter of 5 cm. By applying LITT rather than surgery in these patients, minimum healthy liver tissue would be sacrificed and more hepatic reserve salvaged. Keeping in mind the possibility of recurrence of metastases, this approach gives the patients a better prospect (Fig. 22.2).

In 2011, Sercarz et al. reported palliative treatment for 106 patients with recurrent head and neck tumors using LITT. The best results were seen in oral cavity tumors with a mean survival of 29.1 months, when compared with neck tumors (mean 14.4 ± 6.9 months; range 7.5 to 20.7 months, with a 95% confidence interval). Further analysis showed that clinical factors such as gender, smoking, and alcohol use

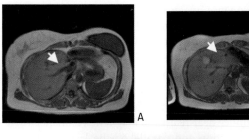

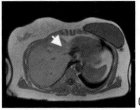

Figure 22.2. T1 weighted MR images in a 53-year-old female patient with liver metastases from breast cancer using laser-induced thermotherapy: (**A**) before, (**B**) the day after intervention, and (**C**) 6 months after using LITT.

were no indicators of poor prognosis, whereas neck disease and tumor stage at first treatment were relevant factors (68). In liver tumors, percutaneous MR-guided LITT achieves a local tumor control rate of 98.7% at 3 months post-therapy and 97.3% at 6 months with metastases smaller than 5 cm in diameter. The mean survival rate for 1,259 patients with 3,440 metastases treated with 14,694 laser applications at the institute (calculated with the Kaplan–Meier method) was 4.4 years and median survival was 3.00 years. No statistically significant difference in survival rates was observed in patients with liver metastases from CRC versus metastases from other primary tumors. The rate of clinically relevant side effects and complications requiring secondary treatment was 2.2%. The clinical use of MR-guided LITT (size < 5 cm, number < 5) is justified in patients with liver metastases of CRC and/or breast cancer if the inclusion criteria are carefully observed. Further indications for MR-guided LITT include recurrent cancer lesions in the head and neck, lung metastases, and bone and soft tissue lesions (69).

Vogl et al. evaluated local tumor control and survival data for MRI-guided LITT of 603 patients with colorectal liver metastases. The indications included recurrent liver metastases after partial liver resection in 37.6% of study patients, metastases in both liver lobes in 32.5%, locally nonresectable lesions in 11.3%, general contraindications for surgery in 4.6%, and refusal to undergo surgical resection in 13.9%. Local recurrence rate at 6-month follow-up was 1.9% for metastases up to 2 cm in diameter, 2.4% for metastases 2.1 to 3.0 cm in diameter, 1.2% for metastases 3.1 to 4.0 cm in diameter, and 4.4% for metastases larger than 4 cm in diameter. The mean survival rate for all treated patients, with calculation started on the date of diagnosis of the metastases (which were treated with LITT) was 4.4 years (1-year survival, 94%; 2-year survival, 77%; 3-year survival, 56%; 5-year survival, 37%). Median survival was 3.5 years. Mean survival after the first LITT treatment was 3.8 years. Median survival was 2.9

years. They suggested that MRI-guided LITT yields high local tumor control and survival rates in well-selected patients with limited liver metastases of colorectal carcinoma (67).

Vogl et al. also presented that LITT of primary and secondary lung tumors analyzing indications and technical concepts. Thirty patients with lung metastases of different primary tumors ($n = 24$) as well as localized lung tumors ($n = 6$) were prospectively treated in 41 sessions using LITT. An MR-compatible puncture system was used with direct puncture technique. The puncture was performed via CT guidance in care vision technique. Eight patients were thermoablated using MR tomographical monitoring and 22 patients using CT monitoring. Local therapy effects, tumor control rate, side effects, complications, and survival were evaluated. In 74% of cases (28/38 lesions) of 24 patients with lung metastases and in all cases of the 6 patients with lung carcinoma, a complete local ablation was achieved. The complication rate (pneumothorax) was 9.8%. One patient with bronchial carcinoma had to be thoracotomized and resected. Ninety-three percent of the patients are still alive. They suggested that Percutaneous LITT of lung tumors permits a complete ablation of lung metastases and lung carcinomas with a low complication rate. Indications for the procedure were defined for patients with no more than five metastases up to 3 cm in size (70).

Cryotherapy Ablation

This technique has been used for local pain control and hemostasis in cancer. Kariappa SM and Morris DL in 2006 evaluated the effect of cryotherapy on 146 patients with unresectable colorectal liver metastases with or without resection for colorectal metastases. At 1, 2, 3, 4, and 5 years, survival rates were 89%, 65%, 41%, 24%, and 19%, respectively (71). In 2003, Yan et al. showed that the number of lesions clearly must be of some importance; however, in the select group of patients with no extrahepatic disease in whom a complete destruction of all liver lesions was achieved, the number of hepatic lesions was not prognostic (72). In 2001, Gruenberger et al. performed cryotherapy in order to treat an involved or close (<1 cm) edge of resection margins for colorectal liver metastases in 110 patients. At a median follow-up of 70.43 months, 49 patients (66%) had liver recurrence, with only 8 patients with local edge recurrence following edge cryotherapy (73). Cryoablation has been used with acceptable palliative outcomes in patients with renal cancer (Tables 22.3 and 22.4).

Chemical Ablation

During chemical ablation, a toxic substance, such as ethanol or acetic acid, is injected into a tumor resulting in subsequent death of the cells. Chemical ablation has been used extensively in the treatment of primary liver cancer and is especially effective for small tumors with a well-defined capsule. In these patients, 5-year survival rates are comparable to those of surgical resection (75). Chemical ablation of the gallbladder is effective in patients at high risk of complications after surgery (76).

| TABLE 22.3 | Survival indexes for cryotherapy alone compared with cryotherapy combined with liver resection (72) | | | | | | |

Operation Type	Number of Patients	Survival Rate (%)					
		1 Year	2 Years	3 Years	4 Years	5 Years	
Cryotherapy alone	92	85	57	32	21	13	
Cryotherapy and liver resection	80	85	66	42	19	19	
Number of cryotreated lesions							
1–2	97	87	61	38	21	17	
3–6	66	85	62	33	17	11	
7–9	9	67	44	33	33	22	

MANAGEMENT OF NONVASCULAR COMPLICATION

Nonvascular complications in the term of postoperative extravascular mass and fluid collection can be treated by interventional radiological procedures. For example, despite medical and surgical advances, nonvascular complications remain common post renal transplantation, occurring in 12% to 20% of patients (77,78). In 2009, Hedegard et al. explained that a thorough understanding of how the complications impair allograft function and survival is essential for adequate treatment. Interventional radiology plays an invaluable role in the postoperative management of renal transplantation and related complications (79).

Catheter placement for drainage of fluid collections and percutaneous image guide excision of mass can relieve pain and facilitate postoperative healing.

MANAGEMENT OF VASCULAR COMPLICATION

Interventional radiological management of vascular complication includes the management of patients with superior vena cava (SVC) syndrome, arterial obstruction secondary to tumor compression or invasion, hemorrhage secondary to tumor invasion, and IVC filters for venous thromboembolic complications.

Superior Vena Cava Syndrome

SVC syndrome is a syndrome with SVC obstruction that can be caused by extrinsic compression, tumor invasion, thrombosis or venous insufficiency return secondary to intra-atrial or intraluminal diseases. Most patients presenting with SVC syndrome secondary to malignant neoplasms are treated without surgery, through radiotherapy, chemotherapy, or the use of intraluminal stents. When the etiology of SVC syndrome is benign, it can be treated with clinical measures (anticoagulation, raising the head, etc.) or, in refractory cases, with angioplasty, stents, or surgery (80). About 46% to 70% of patients with bronchogenic carcinoma respond to radiotherapy (or to chemotherapy and radiotherapy combined) and experience relief from their symptoms within the first 2 weeks of treatment. This improvement can be attributed to vena cava permeability being re-established or to the enhancement of the collateral veins. In general, the reduced venous distention and subjective improvement of symptoms do not occur until 3 to 7 days after the initiation of treatment (81). Catheter-directed thrombolysis has been used as the primary therapy for acute presentation. Kee et al. evaluated 59 patients with SVC syndrome and reported that the technical success was achieved in 56 of 59 (95%) patients. Among 42 patients with underlying malignancy, primary clinical patency was achieved in 33 (79%) patients and secondary clinical patency in 39 (93%) patients. Among 13 patients with benign disease, primary clinical patency was achieved in 10 (77%)

| TABLE 22.4 | Comparison of the relevant literature comparing kidney radiofrequency ablation and cryotherapy (74) | | | |

Modality	Number of Patients	Follow-Up (Mo)	Recurrence Rate (%)	Complications (%)
Radiofrequency	277	10	7.9	13.9
Cryoablation	326	30.8	4.6	10.6

patients and secondary clinical patency in 11 (85%) patients. Four patients were lost to follow-up. Periprocedural mortality and morbidity rates were 3% (2 of 59 patients) and 10% (6 of 59 patients), respectively (82).

In addition to symptom relief, thrombolysis is also beneficial in uncovering the morphology of the lesions and permits optimum angioplasty or stenting (83). For endovascular intervention, stenting is used in addition to angioplasty because angioplasty alone is associated with early restenosis caused by the fibrous, elastic nature of many venous lesions (84). There are some case reports of SVC perforation causing cardiac tamponade during balloon dilatation of the SVC (84).

Arterial Obstruction Secondary to Tumor

Arterial obstruction can be caused by embolus, thrombosis, and trauma in the acute form and by thrombosis, compression, and invasion of benign and malignant tumors and chronic inflammatory tissue or its products during chronic process (85,86).

Inferior Vena Cava Filters

Anticoagulant therapy is the treatment of choice for patients with venous thromboembolism. Patients who have contraindication to anticoagulant therapy may receive good response from an inferior vena cava (IVC) filter (87). Lorch et al. reported that well-founded concerns over the long-term complications of permanent IVC filters, particularly in younger patients in need of Pulmonary embolism (PE) prophylaxis with a temporary contraindication to anticoagulation, have led to the development of temporary and retrievable filters. Temporary filters remain attached to an accessible transcutaneous catheter or wire (88). In 2002, Asch suggested that the time limit of retrievability is in part dependent on the rate of endothelialization of the device, which typically occurs within 2 weeks. However, differences in design may extend the time period in which the filter may be safely retrieved, as has been documented with the recovery filter (89). Certain circumstances preclude the placement of a filter in the infrarenal IVC. This includes thrombus extending into the infrarenal IVC, renal vein thrombosis, or pregnancy. The safety of suprarenal placement of IVC filters is well documented, with no reported instances of renal dysfunction and no differences in the rates of filter migration, recurrent PE, or caval thrombosis (90).

MANAGEMENT OF VASCULAR ACCESS

Vascular access is an important challenge in patients with fistulas, catheters, or grafts for urologists. If postoperative fistula, infected and thrombotic catheter, vascular stenosis, or thrombosis in grafts occur, vascular access has many benefits in terms of interventional diagnosis and emergency management by interventional procedures (91–96). These analyses highlight the importance of practice patterns

in affecting fistula use and contributed to the 2001 Kidney Disease Outcomes Quality Initiative (K/DOQI) Vascular Access guidelines (96).

MANAGEMENT OF MALIGNANT PLEURAL AND PERITONEAL FLUID

Pleural effusion and ascites are common in terminal stage malignancies (97). Fluid sequestration significantly compromises the patient's quality of life. Malignancies of breasts, lungs, ovaries, and lymphomas cause about 75% of all malignant pleural effusions. Ascites results from multiple mechanisms, including vascular permeability changes, peritoneal carcinomatosis, lymph drainage obstruction, hepatic congestion due to tumor infiltration, or neoplastic production of oxidative fluid (98). Ascites may develop in various circumstances though seen mainly in cirrhosis and peritoneal carcinomatosis (99).

Dyspnea is the most common presenting symptom in patients with malignant effusions. Because of the advanced stage of their primary disease, many patients also present with generalized symptoms such as weight loss, anorexia, and malaise. Chest pain, commonly seen in mesothelioma, is typically localized to the side of the effusion and is described as dull and aching rather than pleuritic. A history of hemoptysis in the presence of a pleural effusion is highly suggestive of bronchogenic carcinoma. Other clinically relevant findings may include cachexia and adenopathy (100).

The aim of treatment is to improve the quality of life by decreasing these symptoms. There are several attitudes to manage pleural and abdominal intracavitary refractory effusions in end-stage patients. This procedure greatly reduced the high infection rate (64%) encountered with conventional open chest tubes. Patients' tolerance was excellent and maintenance minimal (101). The goal of treatment is the safe and effective palliation of symptoms with minimal inconvenience to the patient. Malignant fluid collections in the chest and abdomen are amenable to percutaneous management with either intermittent thoracentesis or paracentesis or by placement of temporary or permanent drainage catheters. Repeated pleural aspiration in relapsed cases may be complicated by pneumothorax, bleeding, infection, and spleen or liver laceration (100). Pleurodesis, by minithoracotomy or thoracoscopy, is favored in patients with limited survival (102). In chronic and medical therapy–resistant cases, ascites recirculation with peritoneovenous or intrahepatic portosystemic shunts are treatment options (103). Thoracentesis is typically the first step in the management of a newly diagnosed pleural effusion. In a symptomatic patient, the presence of an effusion can be confirmed with a chest radiograph, and a lateral decubitus film can demonstrate whether the pleural fluid is free-flowing or loculated. Depending on the size and nature of the effusion, a thoracentesis may be performed with or without sonographic guidance (104). Ultrasound-guided thoracentesis can be performed from a posterior intercostal approach with the patient seated or from a midaxillary approach with the patient in a supine, slightly oblique position (105). If two thoracenteses fail to diagnose the etiology of the effusion, a thoracoscopy should be performed (106).

Quality of life of patients with malignant effusions should be evaluated with regard to those symptoms that are related to the effusion itself. Ideally, therapy should minimize discomfort, as well as limit hospitalization time, in these patients with an often limited life span. However, an important aspect in any treatment is prevention of reoccurrence of the symptomatic effusion. Finally, pain relief is another important quality-of-life issue, which must be addressed. This is particularly true for patients with mesothelioma, whose primary complaint is often pain instead of dyspnea (100).

Nontunneled Drainage Catheters

Nontunneled abdominal drainage catheters are associated with an infection rate as high as 35%, tube blockage in up to 30%, and leakage in 20%. Due to the high complication rate, nontunneled drainage catheters are often not considered for the management of malignant ascites; however, two studies suggest that nontunneled catheters may be useful in patients with short life expectancies. In one series of 45 catheters, the mean time for symptomatic infection was 42 days (107); another study of 21 patients reported a mean life span of 6.8 weeks following nontunneled catheter placement with no symptomatic bacterial peritonitis observed (108). The catheters were tolerated well by patients in both studies.

Tunneled Drainage Catheters

Several different types of tunneled drainage catheters, including peritoneal catheters and PleurX catheters, are used for the treatment of malignant ascites that allow external drainage of ascitic fluid. Peritoneovenous shunts and subcutaneous venous access ports are for internal device. Successful placement of cuffed peritoneal dialysis catheters in interventional radiology has been well described (109).

Survival rates for peritoneal catheters have proven to be at least equal to those placed surgically; complication rates are slightly lower and patient recovery time is shorter (110).

The PleurX catheter is a cuffed, silastic tunneled catheter specifically designed for the use in malignant pleural effusion, but it can also be applied to the management of malignant ascites (111).

Treatment of pleural effusion with possible drawback should be followed by hospital staying. Alternatively, a tunneled pleural catheter permits long-term drainage as an outpatient, cost-effectively controlling the effusion and related symptoms in over 80% to 90% of patients. Other advantages are the ability to treat trapped lungs and large locules. Spontaneous pleurodesis may occur in over 40% of patients, and the catheter can be used to administer sclerosant or antineoplastic agents. Complications tend to be minor and easily managed. A tunneled pleura catheter may used in outpatients with malignant pleural effusion (112).

The use of implanted subcutaneous ports for the management of both cirrhotic and malignant ascites has been described (102,113). Rosenblum et al. placed 28 peritoneal ports in 27 patients, 22 of whom had refractory malignant ascites. The long-term patency rate was 100%, and the long-term clinical success rate was 96%. One minor immediate complication, a small hematoma, and two major delayed complications, persistent leakage from the port site and bacterial peritonitis, occurred (102).

Transjugular Intrahepatic Portosystemic Shunt (TIPS)

Refractory ascites after extensive primary or metstastatic hepatic diseases is common. The presence of liver lesions may be as a relative contraindication to placement of TIPS. Wallace in 2003 retrospectively reviewed nine patients, seven with primary hepatic malignancy and two with metastatic disease, using TIPS which was created safely with no immediate procedural complications and comparable outcomes to nontumor patients with the same Child-Pugh classification (114).

CONCLUSION

Over the last three decades, image-guided interventions have used for palliative treatments in cancer patients. These methods can relieve pain and reduce size-, location-, and invasion-related symptoms. However, minimally invasive image-guided interventions with acceptable impacts have an important role in the multidisciplinary management of patients with cancer.

REFERENCES

1. Guimaraes M, Uflacker R. Locoregional therapy for hepatocellular carcinoma. *Clin Liver Dis.* 2011;15(2):395-421.
2. Bruix J, Sherman M. Practice Guidelines Committee, American Association for the Study of Liver Diseases. Management of hepatocellular carcinoma. *Hepatology.* 2005;42(5):1208-1236.
3. Nakai M, Sato M, Kawai N, et al. Hepatocellular carcinoma: involvement of the internal mammary artery. *Radiology.* 2001;219:147-152.
4. Favoulet P, Cercueil JP, Faure P, et al. Increased cytotoxicity and stability of Lipiodol–pirarubicin emulsion compared to classical doxorubicin-Lipiodol: potential advantage for chemoembolization of unresectable hepatocellular carcinoma. *Anticancer Drugs.* 2001;12:801-806.
5. Coldwell DM, Stokes KR, Yakes WF. Embolotherapy: agents, clinical applications, and techniques. *Radiographics.* 1994;14:623-643.
6. Soulen MC. Image-guided therapy of hepatic malignancies. *Appl Radiol.* 2000;29:21-22.
7. Thacker PG, Friese JL, Loe M, et al. Embolization of non-liver visceral tumors. *Semin Intervent Radiol.* 2009;26(3): 262-269.
8. Carr BI, Kondragunta V, Buch SC, Branch RA. Therapeutic equivalence in survival for hepatic arterial chemoembolization

and yttrium 90 microsphere treatments in unresectable hepatocellular carcinoma: a two-cohort study. *Cancer.* 2010;116(5):1305-1314.

9. Kalva SP, Iqbal SI, et al. Transarterial chemoembolization with doxorubicin-eluting microspheres for inoperable hepatocellular carcinoma. *Gastrointest Cancer Res.* 2011;4(1):2-8.

10. Jin X, Shi XJ, Wang MQ, et al. Experience of the treatment following downstaging of larger hepatocellular carcinomas by transcatheter hepaticarterial chemoembolization in 58 patients. 2011;91(14):950-955.

11. Huang YH, Wu JC, Chen SC, et al. Survival benefit of transcatheter arterial chemoembolization in patients with hepatocellular carcinoma larger than 10 cm in diameter. *Aliment Pharmacol Ther.* 2006;23(1):129-135.

12. Llovet JM, Bruix J. Systematic review of randomized trials for unresectable hepatocellular carcinoma: chemoembolization improves survival. *Hepatology.* 2003;37:429-442.

13. O'Suilleabhain CB, Poon RT, Yong JK, et al. Factors predictive of 5-year survival after transarterial chemoembolization for inoperable hepatocellular carcinoma. *Br J Surg.* 2003;90:325-331.

14. Lo CM, Ngan H, Tso WK, et al. Randomized controlled trial of transarterial lipiodol chemoembolization for unresectable hepatocellular carcinoma. *Hepatology.* 2002;35:1164-1171.

15. Ernst O, Sergent G, Mizrahi D, et el. Treatment of hepatocellular carcinoma by transcatheter arterial chemoembolization: comparison of planned periodic chemoembolization and chemoembolization based on tumor response. *AJR Am J Roentgenol.* 1999;172(1):59-64.

16. Reyes DK, Vossen JA, Kamel IR, et al. Single-center phase II trial of transarterial chemoembolization with drug-eluting beads for patients with unresectable hepatocellular carcinoma: initial experience in the United States. *Cancer J.* 2009;15(6):526-532.

17. Malagari K, Pomoni M, Kelekis A, et al. Prospective randomized comparison of chemoembolization with doxorubicin-eluting beads and bland embolization with BeadBlock for hepatocellular carcinoma. *Cardiovasc Intervent Radiol.* 2010;33(3):541-551; e-pub November 24, 2009.

18. Dhanasekaran R, Kooby DA, Staley CA, et al. Comparison of conventional transarterial chemoembolization (TACE) and chemoembolization with doxorubicin drug eluting beads (DEB) for unresectable hepatocellular carcinoma (HCC). *J Surg Oncol.* 2010;101(6):476-480.

19. Scartozzi M, Baroni GS, Faloppi L, et al. Transarterial chemoembolization (TACE), with either lipiodol (traditional TACE) or drug-eluting microspheres (precision TACE, pTACE) in the treatment of hepatocellular carcinoma: efficacy and safety results from a large mono-institutional analysis. *J Exp Clin Cancer Res.* 2010;29:164.

20. Lammer J, Malagari K, Vogl T, et al. Prospective randomized study of doxorubicin-eluting-bead embolization in the treatment of hepatocellular carcinoma: results of the PRECISION V study. *Cardiovasc Intervent Radiol.* 2009;33(1):41-52.

21. Zangos S, Mack MG, Straub R, et al. Transarterial chemoembolization (TACE) of liver metastases. A palliative therapeutic approach. *Radiologe.* 2001;41(1):84-90.

22. Ho AS, Picus J, Darcy MD, et al. Long-term outcome after chemoembolization and embolization of hepatic metastatic lesions from neuroendocrine tumors. *AJR Am J Roentgenol.* 2007;188(5):1201-1207.

23. Albert M, Kiefer MV, Sun W, et al. Chemoembolization of colorectal liver metastases with cisplatin, doxorubicin,

24. Vogl TJ, Gruber T, Balzer JO, et al. Repeated transarterial chemoembolization in the treatment of liver metastases of colorectal cancer: prospective study. *Radiology.* 2009;250(1):281-289.

mitomycin C, ethiodol, and polyvinyl alcohol. *Cancer.* 2011;117(2):343-352. doi:10.1002/cncr.25387.

25. Martin RC, Joshi J, Robbins K, et al. Hepatic intra-arterial injection of drug-eluting bead, irinotecan (DEBIRI) in unresectable colorectal liver metastases refractory to systemic chemotherapy: results of multi-institutional study. *Ann Surg Oncol.* 2010;18(1):192-198.

26. Schuster R, Lindner M, Wacker F, et al. Transarterial chemoembolization of liver metastases from uveal melanoma after failure of systemic therapy: toxicity and outcome. *Melanoma Res.* 2010;20(3):191-196.

27. Gupta S, Bedikian AY, Ahrar J, et al. Hepatic artery chemoembolization in patients with ocular melanoma metastatic to the liver: response, survival, and prognostic factors. *Am J Clin Oncol.* 2009;33(5):474-480.

28. Sharma KV, Gould JE, Harbour JW, et al. Hepatic arterial chemoembolization for management of metastatic melanoma. *AJR Am J Roentgenol.* 2008;190(1):99-104.

29. Lindemayr S, Lehnert T, Korkusuz H, et al. Transpulmonary chemoembolization: a novel approach for the treatment of unresectable lung tumors. *Tech Vasc Interv Radiol.* 2007;10(2):114-119.

30. Vogl TJ, Lehnert T, Zangos S, et al. Transpulmonary chemoembolization (TPCE) as a treatment for unresectable lung metastases. *Eur Radiol.* 2008;18(11):2449-2455.

31. Cao CQ, Yan TD, Bester L, et al. Radioembolization with yttrium microspheres for neuroendocrine tumour liver metastases. *Br J Surg.* 2010;97(4):537-543.

32. Cianni R, Urigo C, Notarianni E, et al. Radioembolisation using yttrium 90 (Y-90) in patients affected by unresectable hepatic metastases. *Radiol Med.* 2010;115(4):619-633.

33. Atassi B, Bangash AK, Lewandowski RJ, et al. Biliary sequelae following radioembolization with Yttrium-90 microspheres. *J Vasc Interv Radiol.* 2008;19(5):691-697.

34. Kennedy AS, McNeillie P, Dezarn WA, et al. Treatment parameters and outcome in 680 treatments of internal radiation with resin 90Y-microspheres for unresectable hepatic tumors. *Int J Radiat Oncol Biol Phys.* 2009;74(5):1494-1500.

35. Sangro B, Iñarrairaegui M, Bilbao JI. Radioembolization for hepatocellular carcinoma. *J Hepatol.* 2011;56(2):464-473.

36. Vente MA, Wondergem M, van der Tweel I, et al. Yttrium-90 microsphere radioembolization for the treatment of liver malignancies: a structured meta-analysis. *Eur Radiol.* 2009;19(4):951-959.

37. Goldberg SN, Livraghi T, Solbiati L, Gazelle GS. In situ ablation of focal hepatic neoplasms. In: Gazelle GS, Saini S, Mueller PR, eds. *Hepatobiliary and Pancreatic Radiology: Imaging and Intervention.* New York, NY: Thieme; 1997:470-502.

38. De Sanctis JT, Goldberg SN, Mueller PR. Percutaneous treatment of hepatic neoplasms: a review of current techniques. *Cardiovasc Intervent Radiol.* 1998;21:273-296.

39. Târcoveanu E, Zugun F, Mehier H, et al. Palliative therapy for malignant hepatic tumors with hyperthermia. *Rev Med Chir Soc Med Nat Iasi.* 2005;109(3):516-527.

40. Pathak S, Jones R, Tang JM, Ablative therapies for colorectal liver metastases (CRLM): a systematic review. *Colorectal Dis.* 2011;13(9):e252-265.

41. Bhardwaj N, Strickland AD, Ahmad F, et al. Liver ablation techniques: a review. *Surg Endosc.* 2010;24(2):254-265.

42. Arenberg D, Pickens A. Metastatic malignant tumors. In: Mason RJ, Murry JF, Courtney V, Nadel JA, eds. *Murray and Nadel's Textbook of Respiratory Medicine.* 5th ed. St Louis, MO: W.B. Saunders Company; 2010:chap 49.

43. Lee JM, Jin GY, Goldberg SN, et al. Percutaneous radiofrequency ablation for inoperable non–small cell lung cancer and metastases: preliminary report. *Radiology.* 2004;230(1):125-134.

44. Takizawa K, Ogawa Y, Yoshimatsu M, et al. Oncology IVR—application to palliative medicine. *Nihon Rinsho.* 2011;69(2):350-356.

45. Jindal G, Friedman M, Locklin J, Wood BJ. Palliative radiofrequency ablation for recurrent prostate cancer. *Cardiovasc Intervent Radiol.* 2006;29(3):482-485.

46. Matsuoka T, Okuma T. CT-guided radiofrequency ablation for lung cancer. *IJO Clin Oncol.* 2007;12(2):71-78.

47. Lencioni R, Crocetti L, Cioni R, et al. Response to radiofrequency ablation of pulmonary tumours: a prospective, intention-to-treat, multicentre clinical trial (the RAPTURE study). *Lancet Oncol.* 2008;9(7):621-628.

48. National Institute for Health and Clinical Excellence (NICE). *Percutaneous Radiofrequency Ablation for Primary and Secondary Lung Cancers.* London, UK: NICE; 2006. *Interventional Procedure Guidance;* vol. 182.

49. Belfiore G, Moggio G, Tedeschi E. CT-guided radiofrequency ablation: a potential complementary therapy for patients with unresectable primary lung cancer—a preliminary report of 33 patients. *AJR Am J Roentgenol.* 2004;183(4):1003-1011.

50. Belfiore G, Tedeschi E, Ronza FM, et al. Radiofrequency ablation of bone metastases induces long-lasting palliation in patients with untreatable cancer. *Singapore Med J.* 2008;49(7):565-570.

51. Hoffmann RT, Jakobs TF, Trumm C, et al. Radiofrequency ablation in combination with osteoplasty in the treatment of painful metastatic bone disease. *J Vasc Interv Radiol.* 2008;19(3):419-425.

52. Gangi A, Alizadeh H, Wong L, et al. Osteoid osteoma: percutaneous laser ablation and follow-up in 114 patients. *Radiology.* 2007;242:293-301.

53. Pezzilli R, Ricci C, Casadei R, et al. Radiofrequency ablation of pancreatic cancer: a new attractive approach or another unsuccessful technique for the treatment of pancreatic adenocarcinoma? A systematic review. *Cancer Ther.* 2008;6:741-744.

54. Girelli R, Frigerio I, Salvia R, et al. Feasibility and safety of radiofrequency ablation for locally advanced pancreatic cancer. *Br J Surg.* 2010;97(2):220-225.

55. Rohde D, Albers C, Mahnken A, Tacke J. Regional thermoablation of local or metastatic renal cell carcinoma. *Oncol Rep.* 2003;10(3):753-757.

56. Janzen N, Zisman A, Pantuck AJ, et al. Minimally invasive ablative approaches in the treatment of renal cell carcinoma. *Curr Urol Rep.* 2002;3(1):13-20.

57. Wood BJ, Ramkaransingh JR, Fojo T, et al. Percutaneous tumor ablation with radiofrequency. *Cancer.* 2002;94(2):443-451.

58. National Comprehensive Cancer Network (NCCN). *Thyroid Carcinoma.* Fort Washington, PA: NCCN; 2010. NCCN Clinical Practice Guidelines in Oncology v.1.2010.

59. Künzli BM, Abitabile P, Maurer CA. Radiofrequency ablation of liver tumors: actual limitations and potential solutions in the future. *World J Hepatol.* 2011;3(1):8-14.

60. Lygidakis NJ, Sharma SK, Papastratis P. Microwave ablation in locally advanced pancreatic carcinoma–a new look. *Hepatogastroenterology.* 2007;54(77):1305-1310.

61. Guan W, Bai J, Hu Z, et al. Retroperitoneoscopic microwave ablation of renal hamartoma: middle-term results. *J Huazhong Univ Sci Technol.* 2010;30(5):669-671.

62. Liang P, Dong B, Yu X, et al. Prognostic factors for percutaneous microwave coagulation therapy of hepatic metastases. *Am J Roentgenol.* 2003;181:1319-1325.

63. Li L, Luo XP, Deng QD, et al. Clinical analysis on long term effect of microwave endometrial ablation in treatment of menorrhagia. *Zhonghua Fu Chan Ke Za Zhi.* 2009;44(11):816-820.

64. Vogl TJ, Straub R, Eichler K, et al. Malignant liver tumors treated with MR imaging–guided laser-induced thermotherapy: experience with complications in 899 patients (2,520 lesions). *Radiology.* 2002;225:367-377.

65. Vogl TJ, Straub R, Eichler K, et al. Colorectal carcinoma metastases in liver: laser-induced interstitial thermotherapy—local tumor control rate and survival data. *Radiology.* 2004; 230(2):450-458.

66. Germer CT, Buhr HJ, Isbert C. Nonoperative ablation for liver metastases. Possibilities and limitations as a curative treatment. *Chirurg.* 2005;76(6):552-554, 556-563.

67. Mensel B, Weigel C, Heidecke CD, et al. Laser-induced thermotherapy (LITT) of tumors of the liver in central location: results and complications. *Fortschr Röntgenstr.* 2005;177:1267-1275.

68. Sercarz JA, Bublik M, Joo J, et al. Outcomes of laser thermal therapy for recurrent head and neck cancer. *Otolaryngol Head Neck Surg.* 2010;142(3):344-350.

69. Vogl TJ, Straub R, Zangos S, et al. MR-guided laser-induced thermotherapy (LITT) of liver tumours: experimental and clinical data. *Int J Hyperthermia.* 2004;20(7):713-724.

70. Vogl TJ, Fieguth HG, Eichler K, et al. Laser-induced thermotherapy of lung metastases and primary lung tumors. *Radiologe.* 2004;44(7):693-699.

71. Kariappa SM, Morris DL. Cryotherapy, a mature ablation technique. *HPB (Oxford).* 2006;8(3):179-181.

72. Yan DB, Clingan P, Morris DL. Hepatic cryotherapy and regional chemotherapy with or without resection for liver metastases from colorectal carcinoma: how many are too many? *Cancer.* 2003;98:320-330.

73. Gruenberger T, Jourdan JL, Zhao J, et al. Reduction in recurrence for involved or inadequate margins with edge cryotherapy after liver resection for colorectal metastases. *Arch Surg.* 2001;136:1154-1157.

74. Weld KJ, Landman J. Comparison of cryoablation, radiofrequency ablation and high-intensity focused ultrasound for treating small renal tumors. *BJU Int.* 2005;9(6):1224-1229.

75. Livraghi T. Radiofrequency ablation, PEIT, and TACE for hepatocellular carcinoma. *J Hepatobiliary Pancreat Surg.* 2003;10:67-76.

76. Lee TH, Park S-H, Kim SP, et al. Chemical ablation of the gallbladder using alcohol in cholecystitis after palliative biliary stenting. *World J Gastroenterol.* 2009;15(16):2041-2043.

77. Kobayashi K, Censullo ML, Rossman LL, et al. Interventional radiologic management of renal transplant dysfunction: indications, limitations and technical considerations. *Radiographics.* 2007;27:1109-1130.

78. Orons PD, Zajko AB. Angiography and interventional aspects of renal transplantation. *Radiol Clin North Am.* 1995;33:461-471.

79. Hedegard W, Saad WE, Davies MG. Management of vascular and nonvascular complications after renal transplantation. *Tech Vasc Interv Radiol.* 2009;12(4):240-262.

80. Cirino LMI, Coelho RF, Dias Da Rocha I. Treatment of superior vena cava syndrome. *J Bras Pneumol.* 2005;31(6):540-550.

81. Armstrong BA, Perez CA, Simpson JR, Hederman MA. Role of irradiation in the management of superior vena cava syndrome. *Int J Radiat Oncol Biol Phys.* 1987;13(4):531-539.

82. Kee ST, Kinoshita L, Razavi MK, et al. Superior vena cava syndrome: treatment with catheter-directed thrombolysis and endovascular stent placement. *Radiology.* 1998;206:187-193.

83. Bauset R. Pacemaker-induced superior vena cava syndrome: a case report and review of management strategy. *Can J Cardiol.* 2002;18:1229-1232.

84. Brown KT, Getrajdman GI. Balloon dilation of the superior vena cava (SVC) resulting in SVC rupture and pericardial tamponade: a case report and brief review. *Cardiovasc Intervent Radiol.* 2005;28:372-376.

85. Balzer JO, Khan V, Thalhammer A, et al. Below the knee PTA in critical limb ischemia results after 12 months: single center experience. *Eur J Radiol.* 2010;75(1):37-42; e-pub May 13, 2010.

86. Grimm J, Müller-Hülsbeck S, Jahnke T. Randomized study to compare PTA alone versus PTA with Palmaz stent placement for femoropopliteal lesions. *J Vasc Interv Radiol.* 2001;12(8):935-941.

87. Büller HR, Agnelli G, Hull RD, et al. Antithrombotic therapy for venous thromboembolic disease: the seventh ACCP conference on antithrombotic and thrombolytic therapy. *Chest.* 2004;126:401S-428S.

88. Lorch H, Welger D, Wagner V, et al. Current practice of temporary vena cava filter insertion: a multicenter registry. *J Vasc Interv Radiol.* 2000;11(1):83-88.

89. Asch MR. Initial experience in humans with a new retrievable inferior vena cava filter. *Radiology.* 2002;225(3):835-844.

90. Greenfield LJ, Proctor MC. Suprarenal filter placement. *J Vasc Surg.* 1998;28(3):432-438.

91. Allon M, Robbin ML. Increasing arteriovenous fistulas in hemodialysis patients: problems and solutions. *Kidney Int.* 2002;62:1109-1124.

92. Allon M, Lockhart ME, Lilly RZ, et al. Effect of preoperative sonographic mapping on vascular access outcomes in hemodialysis patients. *Kidney Int.* 2001;60:2013-2020.

93. Dixon BS, Novak L, Fangman J. Hemodialysis vascular access survival: the upper arm native arteriovenous fistula. *Am J Kidney Dis.* 2002;39:92-101.

94. Oliver MJ, McCann RL, Indridason OS. Comparison of transposed brachiobasilic fistulas to upper arm grafts and brachiocephalic fistulas. *Kidney Int.* 2001;60:1532-1539.

95. Rocco MV, Bleyer AJ, Burkart JM. Utilization of inpatient and outpatient resources for the management of hemodialysis access complications. *Am J Kidney Dis.* 1996;28:250-256.

96. McCarley P, Wingard RL, Shyr Y, et al. Vascular access blood flow monitoring reduces access morbidity and costs. *Kidney Int.* 2001;60:1164-1172.

97. Bennett R, Maskell N. Management of malignant pleural effusions. *Curr Opin Pulm Med.* 2005;11:296-300.

98. Brooks RA, Herzog TJ. Long-term semi-permanent catheter use for the palliation of malignant ascites. *Gynecol Oncol.* 2006;101:360-362.

99. Rosenblum DI, Geisinger MA, Newman JS, et al. Use of subcutaneous venous access ports to treat refractory ascites. *J Vasc Interv Radiol.* 2001;12:1343-1346.

100. Antony VB, Loddenkemper R, Astoul P, et al. Management of malignant pleural effusions. *Eur Respir J.* 2001;18:402-419.

101. Driesen P, Boutin C, Viallat JR, Astoul PH, Vialette JP, Pasquier J. Implantable access system for prolonged intrapleural immunotherapy. *Eur Respir J.* 1994;7:1889-1892.

102. Antunes G, Neville E. Management of malignant pleural effusions. *Thorax.* 2000;55:981-983.

103. Ferral H, Bjarnason H, Wegryn SA, et al. Refractory ascites: early experience in treatment with transjugular intrahepatic portosystemic shunt. *Radiology.* 1993;189:795-801.

104. Stokes, LS. Percutaneous management of malignant fluid collections. *Semin Interv Radiol.* 2007;24(4):398-408.

105. Erasmus JJ, Goodman Philip C, Patz EF Jr. Management of malignant pleural effusions and pneumothorax. *Radiol Clin North Am.* 2000;38:375-383.

106. Neragi-Miandoab S. Malignant pleural effusion, current and evolving approaches for its diagnosis and management. *Lung Cancer.* 2006;54:1-9.

107. Lee A, Lau TN, Yeong KY. Indwelling catheters for the management of malignant ascites. *Support Care Cancer.* 2000;8:493-499.

108. Sartori S, Nielsen I, Trevisani L, et al. Sonographically guided peritoneal catheter placement in the palliation of malignant ascites in end-stage malignancies. *AJR Am J Roentgenol.* 2002;179:1618-1620.

109. Savader SJ. Percutaneous radiologic placement of peritoneal dialysis catheters. *J Vasc Interv Radiol.* 1999;10:249-256.

110. Georgiades CS, Geschwind JF. Percutaneous peritoneal dialysis catheter placement for the management of end-stage renal disease: technique and comparison with the surgical approach. *Tech Vasc Interv Radiol.* 2002;5: 103-107.

111. Rosenberg S, Courtney A, Nemcek AA, Omary RA. Comparison of percutaneous management techniques for recurrent malignant ascites. *J Vasc Interv Radiol.* 2004;15:1129-1131.

112. Pollak JS. Malignant pleural effusions: treatment with tunneled long-term drainage catheters. *Curr Opin Pulm Med.* 2002;8(4):302-307.

113. Savin MA, Kirsch MJ, Romano WJ, et al. Peritoneal ports for treatment of intractable ascites. *J Vasc Interv Radiol.* 2005;16:363-368.

114. Wallace M, Swaim M. Transjugular intrahepatic portosystemic shunts through hepatic neoplasms. *J Vasc Interv Radiol.* 2003;14:501-507.

CHAPTER **23** # Pruritus

Christopher B. Yelverton ■ Laura McGevna

Like the sensation of pain, pruritus (itching) can diminish the quality of life in patients with cancer. Because of the distress pruritus may cause, the cancer clinician should be aware of its importance and management. Pruritus in patients with cancer may be attributable to a primary skin disease, a coexisting medical condition, a medication, or the cancer itself. Indeed, to quote Krajnik and Zylicz, "There is no one cure for all pruritic symptoms. Better understanding of mechanisms of pruritus may help develop better treatments" (1). A number of notable articles, chapters, and texts on itch have been published by leading authorities (1–13). This chapter focuses on pruritus in patients with cancer and reviews its etiology, diagnosis, and management. Readers should bear in mind that patients with cancer can be affected by the same pruritic conditions that those without cancer may acquire, in addition to cancer and cancer treatment–associated conditions.

PRURITUS SENSATIONS

In simplest terms, *pruritus* is the sensation that provokes scratching. Chronic itch can be mild or intractable—a persistent itch state in which the cause cannot be removed or treated and the cure has not been found in the domains of accepted medical practice (14). Like the sensation of pain, objective analysis cannot easily confirm the presence or severity of pruritus. Nevertheless, patients are generally thought to be reliable in their assessment of pruritus severity. Scratch marks (*excoriations*), skin thickening (*lichenification*), and visible cutaneous disease often support patients' subjective complaints.

Patients may complain of burning, stinging, tingling, tickling, or a crawling sensation in addition to, or in lieu of, classic itch. These symptoms are closely related to pruritus, have similar pathogenic mechanisms, and are treated identically. Bernhard (15) summarized this notion by stating, "one man's itch is another man's tickle ... and one man's stinging itch is another man's pain." For most people, itch is readily distinguished from pain, and many patients with severe pruritus would be happy to have pain instead (16). Perhaps more important still, there is new evidence to suggest that itch may not only degrade quality of life but may also actually impact survival. Pruritus in dialysis patients is associated with a 17% higher mortality, though this may be associated with poor sleep quality (16). Gobbi et al. (17) reported that severe pruritus in Hodgkin's disease predicts a poor prognosis.

Pruritus is a distinct, complex sensation that may be considered a primary sensory modality (10). A recently published position paper from the International Forum for the Study of Itch reclassified itch into several overlapping categories so that diagnosis and treatment of this ubiquitous but elusive condition might be optimized (18). They proposed three groups of conditions: pruritus on inflamed skin (Group I), pruritus on non-inflamed skin (Group II), and pruritus presenting with severe secondary skin changes (Group III). Underlying disease, which may be present in one or more groups and may drive the itch sensation, is then defined as a dermatologic disease, a systemic disease, a neurologic disease or, least commonly, a psychiatric disease.

Though there are new data emerging on the origin and propagators of itch in each group or subtype, it is known that at least a portion of the cutaneous itch response is carried by unique sensory histamine–sensitive but mechano-insensitive C fibers (19). These unmyelinated fibers carry sensations to the spinothalamic tract, where they are relayed to the thalamus and subthalamus. Experimental injection of histamine into the skin induces itch or pain. This histamine-induced pruritus may be suppressed by systemic antihistamine administration (20). In spite of the nearly identical histologic characteristics of itch fibers and pain receptors, the two entities may be distinguished electrophysiologically. Nevertheless, the means by which they exert their phenotypic responses may show considerable commonality. For instance, just as sensitization of nerve endings is a known mechanism for chronic pain, patients with chronic itch have demonstrated an increase in skin innervation and may also show central sensitization of itch-signaling spinal neurons (21,22).

Because many patients with pruritus show no signs of histamine release (e.g., cutaneous wheal and flare) and because this pathway cannot explain itch caused by mechanical properties, it is now a well-accepted tenet that other elements (e.g., cytokines and neuropeptides) cause a substantial portion of pruritus. The failure of many pruritic conditions to improve with antihistamines supports this theory and furthermore suggests that histamine may in fact be only a minor pruritus mediator (23,24). In the last several years, there have been landmark developments in this field. It is understood that pruritus may be caused by opiates, serotonin, other neuropeptides, prostaglandins, kinins, proteases, and physical stimuli (10). Tumor necrosis factor-α (TNF-α), though it may not have a direct pruritogenic effect, is elevated in many diseases that are characteristically associated with itch (2). Similarly, a vanilloid receptor, TRPV1, showed increased expression in patients with prurigo nodularis (25). Protease-activated receptor 2 (PAR-2), a specific receptor on primary afferent nerves that is activated by tryptase, was recently found to be elevated in patients with atopic dermatitis (26). Each of these agents may induce pruritus primarily or act through secondary mediators.

Since the 1950s, a plant containing the protease mucunanin was known to cause itch without the characteristically associated flare, an erythematous reaction that is transmitted by mechano-insensitive C fibers (27). Recent evidence revealed that mucunanin induces itch by activating a group of "polymodal" C fibers that respond to mechanical stimuli instead of histamine, a distinctly different population of C fibers than those activated by histamine but with the same end result of itch (28,29). The role of this alternate pathway is yet to be fully understood, though it is thought that "polymodal" C fibers are the most frequent type of afferent C fibers in human skin nerves (30). These advances in our understanding of the propagators of itch proffer hope for potential treatment to those afflicted.

The sensation of pruritus may also arise within the central nervous system (CNS). Systemic opioids induce pruritus, and the opioid antagonists, including naloxone hydrochloride, naltrexone hydrochloride, and nalmefene (which has been withdrawn from the market in the United States), decrease the pruritus of cholestatic and other liver diseases (31–34). Exogenous opioids administered in small quantities to spinal levels in spinal anesthesia relieve pain and can stimulate itching (35). Plasma from patients with cholestatic itching leads to scratching behavior in murine models; this scratching is abolished by administering the opioid receptor antagonist naloxone hydrochloride (36). Itch may also occur paroxysmally after CNS insult or with phantom limb itch as seen after mastectomy (37–39).

DERMATOLOGIC DISEASES AND PRURITUS

Many skin diseases may contribute to the sensation of pruritus. Dry skin, or *xerosis*, is commonly seen in patients with cancer who have generalized wasting or have undergone chemotherapy or radiation therapy. Xerosis makes the skin more susceptible to irritation from environmental assault (40).

Many other diseases may present with pruritus, including scabies, atopic dermatitis, dermatitis herpetiformis, bullous pemphigoid, miliaria, pediculosis, and urticaria (41). These cutaneous diseases are often readily diagnosed by careful clinical examination. Signs of dermatologic diseases may be remarkably subtle or nonspecific in any given patient, particularly in the immunocompromised host. There is no substitute for an excellent physical examination of the skin surface (42–48).

PRURITUS AND MALIGNANCY

Pruritus may be associated with virtually any malignancy (Table 23.1) (5,17,49–63). Some neoplasms, particularly hematologic malignancies, are more frequently associated with pruritus, among them being polycythemia and Hodgkin's disease. Cutaneous T–cell lymphoma, peripheral T–cell lymphoma, and other cutaneous lymphomas are notoriously pruritic. Though it has not been fully investigated, endogenous opioids may play a role in lymphoma-induced pruritus as evidenced by the efficacy of butorphanol, a κ-agonist and μ-antagonist, in treating non-Hodgkin's lymphoma pruritus (64). Furthermore, cytokines such as interleukin (IL)-6 and IL-8, which are suspect in End Stage Renal Disease (ESRD) associated pruritus, have been found to be closely related to the pathophysiology of lymphoma, and therefore may play a role in lymphoma-induced itch as well (14,65,66). Neurokinin-1, a neuropeptide, is suspected to contribute to itch in patients with malignancy as well. The dominant ligand for neurokinin-1 is substance P, and an increase in the number of neurokinin-1 receptors has been found on keratinocytes in patients with chronic pruritus (67–69).

Pruritus may be a presenting symptom in both solid and hematologic cancers (70,71). Pruritus may also be a sign of malignant physical obstruction of the biliary system from either a primary or metastatic tumor (61). In solid tumors, pruritus is thought to be due, at least in part, to a local immune phenomenon and may be generalized or localized, such as with scrotal itch in the setting of prostate cancer (72).

PRURITUS AND NONMALIGNANT INTERNAL DISEASES

Patients with cancer are not exempt from having concurrent medical conditions. There is no question that other internal diseases may be associated with pruritus (Table 23.1). Pruritus has been reported to herald the onset of thyroid disease (73), renal insufficiency (74), liver disease (75), iron deficiency (76), diabetes mellitus (77), paraproteinemia (78), Sjögren's syndrome (79), and other conditions. True mechanisms of pruritus induction in most of these diseases are poorly understood. It has been postulated that renal disease may induce a metastatic calcification, hyperphosphatemia, xerosis, mast cell proliferation, and other changes that might be associated with pruritus.

CANCER THERAPY

Pruritus may be the result of a chemotherapy reaction, radiation therapy, or medications used for symptom management. Pruritus has been reported as an adverse reaction to chemotherapeutic agents, including those listed in Table 23.2 (67,80–86). Adverse effects of some of the chemotherapeutic agents may include anemia and other metabolic disturbances, which could also lead to pruritus. New combinations of chemotherapeutic agents in ever-increasing dosage regimens will undoubtedly be associated with increased cutaneous toxicity.

TABLE 23.1	Systemic conditions reported to be associated with generalized pruritus

Organ Systems and Etiologies	Example
Autoimmune	Sjögren's syndrome Progressive systemic sclerosis Lupus erythematosus Sicca syndrome
Endocrine	Hyperthyroidism Hypothyroidism Parathyroid disease
Central nervous system	Cerebrovascular accident Delusions of parasitosis Depression Multiple sclerosis Neurodermatitis Psychosis Syrinx Brain tumor
Hematopoietic	Paraproteinemia Iron deficiency anemia Mastocytosis
Liver malignancy	Primary biliary cirrhosis Extrahepatic biliary obstruction Hepatitis Breast carcinoma Carcinoid syndrome Cutaneous T–cell lymphoma Gastrointestinal tract cancers: tongue, stomach, and colon Hodgkin's disease Insulinoma Leukemia Lung cancer Multiple myeloma Non-Hodgkin's lymphoma Polycythemia vera Prostatic carcinoma Thyroid carcinoma Uterine carcinoma
Iatrogenic	Drug ingestion Drug-induced cholestasis Injection site reaction
Infectious	Human immunodeficiency virus Parasitic diseases Scabies Syphilis
Renal	Chronic renal insufficiency and renal failure Dialysis dermatosis

For instance, a new generation of epidermal growth factor receptor (EGFR) inhibitors has become available for treating patients with various forms of cancer, but some with considerable dermatologic sequelae including debilitating pruritus, which is thought to be due in part to an accumulation of mast cells in lesional skin of patients treated with the drug (87). Pruritus may be caused by opioids, particularly injectable opioids used for pain control. Additionally, pruritus

TABLE 23.2	Antitumor agents associated with pruritus

Interferon-α

Bacille Calmette-Guérin

Bleomycin sulfate

Carboplatin

Carmustine

Chlorambucil

Cisplatin

Cyclophosphamide

Cytosine arabinoside and daunomycin

Daunomycin

Docetaxel

Doxorubicin

Gemcitabine hydrochloride

Hydroxyurea

Imatinib

Interleukin-2 with levamisole hydrochloride or interferon-α

L-Asparaginase

Mechlorethamine hydrochloride

Megestrol acetate

Methotrexate

Mitomycin

Oxaliplatin

Paclitaxel

Procarbazine hydrochloride

EGFR inhibitors (e.g., erlotinib)

EGFR, epidermal growth factor receptor.

may be caused by other chemicals that may be used in the preparation of medications and medication administration tools (88).

Acute radiodermatitis may cause erythema and pruritus. Additionally, chronic radiodermatitis can be associated with severe xerosis, skin thinning, and ease of irritation. Total body electron beam radiation may make the entire skin surface dry and pruritic.

All clinicians managing patients with cancer are familiar with the typical morbilliform drug rash that may result from the use of supportive agents. Similar to this eruption is the engraftment phenomenon in bone marrow transplant recipients; however, many pruritogenic drugs do not induce any rash. As stated, opiates may induce pruritus

through central nervous mechanisms. Others, such as estrogens or ketoconazole, may precipitate cholestasis and therefore induce pruritus. It is noteworthy that placebo agents may induce pruritus in as many as 5% of the people treated. More than 100 medications are reported to cause pruritus without a rash (81). Careful review of the medication history and simplification of the drug regimen is essential.

NEUROPSYCHIATRIC DISEASE AND PRURITUS

Calnan and O'Neill (89) found that in most patients with a chief complaint of generalized pruritus, the itch began at a time of emotional stress. Edwards et al. (90) later reported that a high level of psychological stress enhances a person's ability to perceive intense itch stimuli. In patients with cancer, psychological stress, depression, anxiety, and organic brain diseases undoubtedly contribute to cutaneous diseases (91–93). Recognition of neuropsychiatric disease may lead to better control.

EVALUATION OF THE PRURITIC PATIENT

Obtaining a focused history, a directed review of symptoms, and a focused clinical examination may lead to a clinical diagnosis. The physician should first probe for likely pharmaceutical agents that could exacerbate pruritus. A temporal history of therapeutic agent initiation within 2 weeks of the onset of pruritus may be helpful. Other historic points of value include an abnormal or excessive bathing history, others in the family or household with similar problems, and symptoms of neuropsychiatric disease. Complete dermatologic clinical examination quickly excludes urticaria, scabies, and a host of other dermatologic diagnoses.

Some patients with long-standing, generalized pruritus may require further evaluation. For practicing dermatologic clinicians, further investigation may be warranted. This evaluation should include a careful history, physical examination, and appropriate, limited, screening laboratory tests. Extensive, undirected evaluation of these patients rarely leads to a specific attributable cause (94).

There is neither a single list nor are there specific guidelines for tests that must be performed in any individual patient. Scabies preparations, fungal examinations, and skin biopsies may be needed to diagnose specific dermatologic diseases.

TREATMENT

Treating pruritus in the patient with cancer can take many forms. In general, the primary approaches to management should involve removal of the cause of itch, if possible, in conjunction with control of symptoms. Although there are some specific issues to consider in this population, most of the management is similar to other forms of itch. It is important to devote adequate time to a given therapy to obtain optimum results. Unfortunately, there are very few guidelines regarding the appropriate duration of therapy for chronic pruritus.

Topical Treatment

Ideally, particularly in localized itch, the physician would choose the single topical medication that corrects the underlying condition. Although this scenario occasionally occurs (e.g., permethrin for scabies infestation), symptomatic treatment is less specific. Therefore, the clinician must use all diagnostic skills to provide the patient with reasonable relief. Table 23.3 presents the advantages and disadvantages of several different topical agents.

One of the most important aspects of skin therapy that must be addressed is hydration and lubrication of the skin surface (40,95). A simple but sometimes effective therapeutic approach is to apply emollients (lotions, creams, and ointments) on the dry skin twice daily. Emollients with camphor and menthol (e.g., Sarna lotion), phenol, pramoxine, or benzocaine (Lanacane) may provide relief. Camphor, phenol, menthol, pramoxine, and benzocaine have local anesthetic effects (12). Age-old remedies such as cool compresses (application of a wet washcloth for 20 min) and shake lotions (calamine) may prove to be highly efficacious.

Topical corticosteroids may be useful as adjunctive agents for pruritus control. When used properly, they should be prescribed in amounts necessary to cover the affected skin. Table 23.4 provides prescribing quantity information. Although any topical corticosteroid may be useful in a given patient, for widespread pruritus, hydrocortisone (1% or 2.5%) or triamcinolone (0.1%) preparations are generally effective. Because of the relatively thin skin of some cancer patients, long-term use of halogenated corticosteroids should be approached with great caution. Overuse of corticosteroids in unsupervised or overzealous patients is a common cause of dermatologic iatrogenic disease (96). Even when topical corticosteroids are required, the use of emollients remains indicated (97,98).

Topical tacrolimus (Protopic) 0.1% ointment is also an effective anti-inflammatory product for itching. It may cause some short-term burning and stinging on topical application, but it can be used for long periods of time on any skin site without risk of atrophy (99,100). Pimecrolimus (Elidel) cream is also safe and effective for long-term use, but it is less effective than tacrolimus. Like tacrolimus, pimecrolimus causes no long-term atrophy, and neither agent suppresses systemic immune function.

Capsaicin cream (Zostrix) is of limited help in select patients with a wide range of inflammatory and noninflammatory dermatoses (101–103). Topical capsaicin should be applied three times daily and may be used indefinitely. Its application requires careful patient instruction, as it often initially produces significant burning or stinging sensations or superficial burns. In many cases, after 1 or more weeks, the burning sensation diminishes and relief from pruritus follows. Capsaicin is not appropriate for generalized pruritus.

Other agents have modest topical efficacy in relieving pruritus. The eutectic mixture of local anesthetics lidocaine and prilocaine has been demonstrated to be helpful in experimentally induced pruritus (104) and may prove useful in recalcitrant pruritic conditions. However, it is likely to offer no additional advantages over other anesthetics mentioned. Topical doxepin hydrochloride (Zonalon), an antidepressant and antihistamine, is a noncorticosteroid pruritus medication with modest demonstrated efficacy (105). Topical doxepin hydrochloride may cause sedation and is particularly likely to cause allergic contact dermatitis. Clinicians should be aware that all topical agents have sensitizing potential and may induce allergic contact dermatitis.

Systemic Treatment

In patients with pruritus that interferes with sleep or pruritus that may have a significant neuropsychiatric component, oral antipruritic agents may prove to be important in symptomatic relief (Table 23.5). Antihistamines, such as hydroxyzine (Atarax) and diphenhydramine hydrochloride (Benadryl), are not only occasionally antipruritic but also have important CNS effects. In a review of the pharmacologic control of pruritus nearly two decades ago, Winkelmann (114) stated that the most effective antihistamines have CNS effects. Moreover, ensuring adequate sedation can be important now, as there is good evidence that pruritus disturbs normal sleep (120). However, some patients, especially the elderly, may have increased sensitivity to antihistamines, and memory impairment or impaired psychomotor function may result from their administration (3,4). Cetirizine hydrochloride (Zyrtec) is an antihistamine that is less sedating than hydroxyzine, but more sedating than the typically nonsedating antihistamines (e.g., desloratadine and fexofenadine hydrochloride). There are conflicting data on the antipruritic efficacy of terfenadine and acrivastine in atopic dermatitis (24,121). Doxepin hydrochloride, a tricyclic antidepressant with antihistamine activity (115), may be an effective agent for the treatment of refractory pruritus, but in vivo it has similar efficacy in suppressing histamine to hydroxyzine.

Although they may be useful agents in the treatment of urticaria, nonsedating antihistamines have limited application in nonurticarial conditions. Moreover, the role of histamine in itch mediation in patients with cancer is even more questionable. Burtin et al. (122) found a decreased skin response to histamine injection in patients with cancer. They postulated that the presence of a tumor mimics the effects of general administration of histamine H_1-antagonists on the skin response to histamine.

Systemic corticosteroids for pruritus are often highly effective, but their use can present certain difficulties. All oncologic practitioners are aware that chronic pathologic states, including hypertension, diabetes, fluid retention, and osteoporosis, may all be exacerbated by intramuscular or oral corticosteroids. Systemic corticosteroids are particularly effective for brief periods for morbilliform drug eruptions and allergic or irritant contact dermatitis. Further prolonged use may induce adverse sequelae.

TABLE 23.3	Advantages and disadvantages of topical agents		
Topical Agent	**Examples**	**Advantages**	**Disadvantages**
Emollients and moisturizers	Petrolatum Moisturizing lotions	Inexpensive and reduces irritant dermatitis	May be too greasy and insufficient in inflammatory diseases
Corticosteroids	Hydrocortisone Desonide Triamcinolone Fluocinonide Clobetasol	Effective for inflammatory dermatoses and mainstay of topical therapy	May cause atrophy, sensitivity, and adrenal suppression
Topical calcineurin inhibitors	Tacrolimus Pimecrolimus	Effective for inflammatory dermatoses and no atrophy	May cause itch or burn on application
Anesthetics	Camphor Pramoxine Benzocaine Prilocaine (EMLA) Menthol	Excellent pruritus relief and no atrophy or adrenal suppression	Potentially sensitizing and short-transient activity
Antihistamines	Diphenhydramine hydrochloride Doxepin hydrochloride	Modest relief and no atrophy or adrenal suppression	Potentially sedating and sensitizing
Cooling agents	Calamine Alcohol	May be soothing and cooling	Calamine leaves visible film Alcohol dries the skin
Miscellaneous	Coal tar Capsaicin	Coal tar is anti-inflammatory in nature Capsaicin works differently than other agents	Tar is not elegant and stains Capsaicin often burns

EMLA, eutectic mixture of topical anesthetics.

TABLE 23.4	**Amounts of topical agent prescribing information**		
Location	**One Application (g)**	**Twice Daily for 1 wk[a]**	**Twice Daily for 1 mo[a]**
Hands, scalp, genitalia, or face	2	30 g (1 oz)	120 g (4 oz)
Upper extremity or one side of trunk	3	45 g (1.5 oz)	180 g (6 oz)
One lower extremity	4	60 g (2 oz)	240 g (8 oz)
Entire body	30–60	540 g (1 lb)	2,700 g (5 lb)

[a]Although the twice-daily dosing of topical agents is appropriate for many patients, clinicians employ these agents from daily to four times daily.

A variety of other systemic agents have been used with some effect in specific disease states (Table 23.5). Activated charcoal (108), naloxone hydrochloride (31,32), naltrexone hydrochloride (34), and cholestyramine (109), for instance, have been demonstrated to be effective in the treatment of pruritus of biliary cirrhosis. However, the use of opioid antagonists may be inappropriate in certain populations, especially when optimizing end-of-life care. Rifampin may be effective in the treatment of pruritus of primary biliary cirrhosis (109,110). Aspirin occasionally exacerbates pruritus, but it

TABLE 23.5	**Systemic or physical pruritus treatment modality for specific conditions**	
Drug or Modality	**Dosage Range**	**Reference**
Ultraviolet B phototherapy	N/A	(74,106,107)
Activated charcoal	50 g every 4 h	(108)
Rifampin	300 mg b.i.d	(109,110)
Ondansetron	8 mg t.i.d	(110,111)
Cholestyramine	4–6 g t.i.d with meals	(109)
Nalmefene	2–10 mg b.i.d	(33,34)
Naltrexone	25–50 mg daily	
Prednisone	5–60 mg daily	(7–10,12,13)
Phototherapy	N/A	(106,107,112)
Thalidomide	100–300 mg daily	(113)
Antihistamines		(13,114)
Cetirizine	10–20 mg daily	
Chlorpheniramine	4–12 mg q8-12h	
Desloratadine	50–10 mg daily	
Diphenhydramine	25–50 mg q6-8h	
Fexofenadine	60–180 mg daily	
Hydroxyzine	10–100 mg q6h	
Loratadine	10–20 mg daily	
Doxepin	10–150 mg qhs	(115)
Paroxetine	10–50 mg daily	(116)
Gabapentin	300–1,500 mg daily	
Aspirin	81–325 mg daily	(60)
Mirtazapine	15 mg qhs	(117,118,119)

N/A, not applicable.

has been reported to be helpful in the treatment of pruritus associated with polycythemia rubra vera (60). Interferon-α has been used with some success in intractable pruritic conditions, especially polycythemia vera (62,63), but its cost and side effects demand careful consideration. Another confounding factor is that 30% of patients receiving interferon-α, in one published melanoma study, experienced pruritus that is thought to be associated with the treatment (123). Thalidomide, a teratogenic anti-inflammatory agent, has gained attention due to its occasionally remarkable success in treating intractable pruritus when skin inflammation is present (113,117). More recently, Levêque reported success that has since been reproduced with treatment of EGFR inhibitor–induced pruritus with the antiemetic, neurokinin-1 receptor antagonist, and aprepitant (124). Finally, gabapentin has achieved modest success in the treatment of pruritus in conditions such as brachioradial pruritus (117,125).

The serotonin agents, paroxetine hydrochloride (116) and ondansetron (111), have shown some effect with intractable pruritus, but their effects may be short-lived (1,117). However, a recent advance in the treatment of refractory pruritus was found with the antidepressant drug, mirtazapine, with a favorable safety profile compared with other antidepressants (117–119).

The reader should always bear in mind that if a patient obtains relief with any given medication, the medication cannot always take credit. In a classic study, Epstein and Pinski (126) found that placebo therapy provides pruritus relief with a surprisingly high success rate.

Physical Treatment Modalities

Ultraviolet A (UVA), ultraviolet B (UVB), and psoralen photochemotherapy have been successfully employed in a wide range of pruritic disorders, from atopic dermatitis to renal disease (74,106,112). Because of its high degree of efficacy, UVB is often considered the treatment of choice for uremic pruritus. UV doses are usually administered three times weekly and UV doses are progressively increased until erythema is attained, then the therapy is individually adjusted to accommodate the patients' photosensitivity (107). To attain symptomatic relief, 20 to 30 treatments may be necessary; occasionally, weekly maintenance therapy is continued. As with all other therapies, patients are known to fail phototherapy. Transcutaneous electrical nerve stimulation is another modality that has been described to offer some relief to patients suffering from generalized itch associated with hematologic malignancies (127).

CONCLUSIONS

Pruritus in patients with cancer is common and provides a diagnostic and therapeutic challenge for the physician. Evaluation may be limited to obtaining an excellent history and physical examination. Alternatively, an exhaustive search for systemic disease may occasionally be indicated. The physician should address the therapeutic intervention to correct the underlying cutaneous disease. Systemic antipruritics are often beneficial and well tolerated, but they have well-known side effects. Above all, diagnosis and therapy should be individualized for the patient.

REFERENCES

1. Krajnik M, Zylicz Z. Understanding pruritus in systemic disease. *J Pain Symptom Manage.* 2001;21:151-168.
2. Lober CW. Pruritus and malignancy. *Clin Dermatol.* 1993;11:125-128.
3. Higgins EM, du Vivier AW. Cutaneous manifestations of malignant disease. *Br J Hosp Med.* 1992;48:552-554.
4. De Conno F, Ventafridda V, Saita I. Skin problems in advanced and terminal cancer patients. *J Pain Symptom Manage.* 1991;6:247-256.
5. Rosenberg FW. Cutaneous manifestations of internal malignancy. *Cutis.* 1977;20:227-234.
6. Campbell J. Management of pruritus in the cancer patient. *Oncol Nurs Forum.* 1981;8:40-41.
7. Bernhard JD. Clinical aspects of pruritus. In: Fitzpatrick TB, Eisen AZ, Wolff K, et al., eds. *Dermatology in General Medicine.* 3rd ed. New York, NY: McGraw-Hill; 1987:78-90.
8. Weisshaar E, Kucenic MJ, Fleischer AB Jr. Pruritus, a review. *Acta Derm Venereol.* 2003;83(suppl 212):5-31.
9. Winkelmann RK. Pruritus. *Semin Dermatol.* 1988;7:233-235.
10. Denman ST. A review of pruritus. *J Am Acad Dermatol.* 1986;14:375-392.
11. Dangel RB. Pruritus and cancer. *Oncol Nurs Forum.* 1986;13:17-21.
12. Gatti S, Serri F. *Pruritus in Clinical Medicine.* New York, NY: McGraw-Hill; 1991.
13. Fleischer AB Jr. *The Management of Itching Diseases.* New York, NY: Parthenon Publishers; 2000.
14. Wang H, Yosipovitch G. New insights into the pathophysiology and treatment of chronic itch in patients with end stage renal disease, chronic liver disease and lymphoma. *Int J Dermatol.* 2010;49:1-11.
15. Bernhard JD. Itches, pains, and other strange sensations. *Curr Chall in Dermatol.* 1991:1-10.
16. Pisoni RL, Wikstrom B, Elder SJ, et al. Pruritus in haemodialysis patients: international results from the Dialysis Outcomes and Practice Patterns Study (DOPPS). *Nephrol Dial Transplant.* 2006;21:3495-3505.
17. Gobbi PG, Attardo-Parrinello G, Lattanzio G, et al. Severe pruritus should be a B-symptom in Hodgkin's disease. *Cancer.* 1983;51:1934-1936.
18. Ständer S, Weisshaar E, Mettang T, et al. Clinical classification of itch: a position paper of the International Forum for the Study of Itch. *Acta Derm Venereol.* 2007;87:291-294.
19. Schmelz M, Schmidt R, Bickel A, et al. Specific C-receptors for itch in human skin. *J Neurosci.* 1997;17:8003-8008.
20. Arnold AJ, Simpson JG, Jones HE, et al. Suppression of histamine-induced pruritus by hydroxyzine and various neuroleptics. *J Am Acad Dermatol.* 1979;1:509-512.
21. Yosipovitch G, Carstens E, McGlone F. Chronic itch and chronic pain: analogous mechanisms. *Pain.* 2007;131:4-7.
22. Toyoda M, Nakamura M, Makino T, et al. Nerve growth factor and substance P are useful plasma markers of disease activity in atopic dermatitis. *Br J Dermatol.* 2002;147:71-9.
23. Krause L, Shuster S. Mechanism of action of antipruritic drugs. *BMJ.* 1983;287:1199-1200.

24. Berth-Jones J, Graham-Brown RAC. Failure of terfenadine in relieving the pruritus of atopic dermatitis. *Br J Dermatol.* 1989;121:635-637.

25. Stander S, Moormann C, Schumacher M, et al. Expression of vanilloid receptor subtype 1 in cutaneous sensory nerve fibers, mast cells, and epithelial cells of appendage structures. *Exp Dermatol.* 2004;13:129-139.

26. Steinhoff M, Neisius U, Ikoma A, et al. Proteinase-activated receptor-2 mediates itch: a novel pathway for pruritus in human skin. *J Neurosci.* 2003;23:6176-6180.

27. Schmelz M, Michael K, Weidner C, et al. Which nerve fibers mediate the axon reflex flare in human skin? *Neuroreport.* 2000;11:645-648.

28. Davidson S, Zhang X, Yoon CH, et al. The itch producing agents histamine and cowhage activate separate populations of primate spinothalamic tract neurons. *J Neurosci.* 2007;27:10007-10014.

29. Namer B, Carr R, Johanek LM, et al. Separate peripheral pathways for pruritus in man. *J Neurophysiol.* 2008;100:2062-2069.

30. Schmidt R, Schmelz, Forster C, et al. Novel classes of responsive and non-responsive C nociceptors in human skin. *J Neurosci.* 1995;15:333-341.

31. Bernstein JE, Swift RM, Soltani K, et al. Antipruritic effect of the opiate antagonist, naloxone hydrochloride. *J Invest Dermatol.* 1982;78:82-83.

32. Bernstein JE, Swift R. Relief of intractable pruritus with naloxone. *Arch Dermatol.* 1979;115:1366-1367.

33. Bergasa NV, Alling DW, Talbot TL, et al. Oral nalmefene therapy reduces scratching activity due to the pruritus of cholestasis: a controlled study. *J Am Acad Dermatol.* 1999;41:431-434.

34. Terra SG, Tsunoda SM. Opioid antagonists in the treatment of pruritus from cholestatic liver disease. *Ann Pharmacother.* 1998;32:1228-1230.

35. Fischer HB, Scott PV. Spinal opiate analgesia and facial pruritus. *Anaesthesia.* 1982;37:777-778.

36. Bergasa NV, Thomas DA, Vergalla J, et al. Plasma from patients with the pruritus of cholestasis induces opioid receptor–mediated scratching in monkeys. *Life Sci.* 1993;53:1253-1257.

37. King CA, Huff FJ, Jorizzo JL. Unilateral neurogenic pruritus: paroxysmal itching associated with central nervous system lesions. *Ann Intern Med.* 1982;97:222-223.

38. Bernhard JD. Phantom itch, pseudophantom itch, and senile pruritus. *Int J Dermatol.* 1992;33:856-857.

39. Lierman LM. Phantom breast experiences after mastectomy. *Oncol Nurs Forum.* 1988;15:41-44.

40. Hunnuksela A, Kinnunen T. Moisturizers prevent irritant dermatitis. *Acta Derm Venereol.* 1992;72:42-44.

41. Gilchrest BA. *Skin and Aging Processes.* Boca Raton, FL: CRC Press; 1984.

42. Beare JM. Generalized pruritus: a study of 43 cases. *Clin Exp Dermatol.* 1976;1:343-352.

43. Botero F. Pruritus as a manifestation of systemic disorders. *Cutis.* 1978;21:873-880.

44. Gilchrest BA. Pruritus: pathogenesis, therapy and significance in systemic disease states. *Arch Intern Med.* 1982;142:101-105.

45. Camp R. Generalized pruritus and its management. *Clin Exp Dermatol.* 1982;7:557-563.

46. Kantor GR, Lookingbill DP. Generalized pruritus and systemic disease. *J Am Acad Dermatol.* 1983;9:375-382.

47. Champion RH. Generalized pruritus. *BMJ.* 1984;289:751-773.

48. Kantor GR. Evaluation and treatment of generalized pruritus. *Cleve Clin J Med.* 1990;57:521-526.

49. Cormia FE. Pruritus, an uncommon but important symptom of systemic carcinoma. *Arch Dermatol.* 1965;92:36-39.

50. Erskine JG, Rowan RM, Alexander JO, et al. Pruritus as a manifestation of myelomatosis. *BMJ.* 1977;1:687-688.

51. Mengel CE. Cutaneous manifestations of the malignant carcinoid syndrome: severe pruritus and orange blotches. *Ann Intern Med.* 1963;58:989-993.

52. Beeaff DE. Pruritus as a sign of systemic disease, report of metastatic small cell carcinoma. *Ariz Med.* 1980;37:831-833.

53. Thomas S, Harrington CT. Intractable pruritus as the presenting symptom of carcinoma of the bronchus: a case report and review of the literature. *Clin Exp Dermatol.* 1983;8:459-461.

54. Shoenfeld Y, Weinburger A, Ben-Bassat M, et al. Generalized pruritus in metastatic adenocarcinoma of the stomach. *Dermatology.* 1977;155:122-124.

55. Degos R, Civatte J, Blanchet P, et al. Prurit, seule manifestation pendant 5 ans d'une maladie de Hodgkin. *Ann Med Interne (Paris).* 1973;124:235-238.

56. Alexander LL. Pruritus and Hodgkin's disease. *JAMA.* 1979;241:2598-2599.

57. Bluefarb SM. *Cutaneous Manifestations of Malignant Lymphomas.* Springfield, IL: Charles C Thomas Publisher; 1959.

58. Stock H. Cutaneous paraneoplastic syndromes. *Med Klin.* 1976;71:356-372.

59. Curth HO. A spectrum of organ systems that respond to the presence of cancer: how and why the skin reacts. *Ann N Y Acad Sci.* 1974;230:435-442.

60. Fjellner B, Hägermark O. Pruritus in polycythemia: treatment with aspirin and possibility of platelet involvement. *Acta Derm Venereol.* 1979;61:505-512.

61. Ballinger AB, McHugh M, Catnach SM, et al. Symptom relief and quality of life after stenting for malignant bile duct obstruction. *Gut.* 1994;35:467-470.

62. de Wolf JT, Hendriks DW, Egger RC, et al. Alpha-interferon for intractable pruritus in polycythemia rubra vera. *Lancet.* 1991;337:241.

63. Flecknoe-Brown S. Relief of itch associated with myeloproliferative disease by alpha interferon. *Aust N Z J Med.* 1991;21:81.

64. Dawn AG, Yospiovitch G. Butorphanol for the treatment of intractable pruritus. *J Am Acad Dermatol.* 2006;54:527-531.

65. Biggar RJ, Johasen JS, Smedby KE, et al. Serum YKL-40 and interleukin 6 levels in Hodgkin lymphoma. *Clin Cancer Res.* 2008;14:6974-6978.

66. Lee HL, Eom HS, Yun T, et al. Serum and urine levels of interleukin-8 in patients with non-Hodgkin's lymphoma. *Cytokine.* 2008;43:71-75.

67. Vincenzi B, Tonini G, Santini D. Aprepitant for erlotinib-induced pruritus. *N Engl J Med.* 2010;363:397-8.

68. Sankhala KK, Pandya DM, Sarantopoulos J, et al. Prevention of chemotherapy induced nausea and vomiting: a focus on aprepitant. *Expert Opin Drug Metab Toxicol.* 2009;5:1607-1614.

69. Curran MP, Robinson DM. Aprepitant: a review of its use in the prevention of nausea and vomiting. *Drugs.* 2009;69:1853-1878.

70. Johnson RE, Kanigsberg ND, Jimenez CL. Localized pruritus: a presenting symptom of a spinal cord tumor in a child with features of neurofibromatosis. *J Am Acad Dermatol.* 2000;43(5 Pt 2): 958-961.

71. King NK, Siriwardana HP, Coyne JD, et al. Intractable pruritus associated with insulinoma in the absence of multiple endocrine neoplasia: a novel paraneoplastic phenomenon. *Scand J Gastroenterol.* 2003;38(6):678-680.

72. Seccareccia D, Gebara N. Pruritus in palliative care. *Can Fam Physician.* September 2011;57:1010-1013.

73. Barnes HM, Sarkany I, Calnan CD. Pruritus and thyrotoxicosis. *Trans St. Johns Hosp Dermatol Soc.* 1974;60:59-62.

74. Gilchrest BA, Rowe JW, Brown RS, et al. Ultraviolet phototherapy of uremic pruritus with ultraviolet light therapy: long term results and possible mechanisms of action. *Ann Intern Med.* 1979;91:17-21.

75. Sherlock S, Scheyer PJ. The presentation and diagnosis of 100 patients with primary biliary cirrhosis. *N Engl J Med.* 1973;289:674-678.

76. Lewiecki EM, Rahman F. Pruritus: a manifestation of iron deficiency. *JAMA.* 1976;236:2319-2320.

77. Stawiski MA, Vorhees JJ. Cutaneous signs of diabetes mellitus. *Cutis.* 1976;18:415-421.

78. Zelicovici Z, Lahav M, Cahane P, et al. Pruritus as a possible early sign of paraproteinemia. *Isr J Med Sci.* 1969;5:1079-1081.

79. Feuerman EJ. Sjögren's syndrome presenting as recalcitrant generalized pruritus. *Dermatologica.* 1968;137:74-86.

80. Breathnach SM, Hinter H. *Adverse Reactions and the Skin.* Oxford, UK: Blackwell Science; 1992:281-304.

81. Bork C. *Cutaneous Side Effects of Drugs.* Philadelphia, PA: WB Saunders; 1988.

82. Call TG, Creagan ET, Frytak S, et al. Phase I trial of combined recombinant interleukin-2 with levamisole in patients with advanced malignant disease. *Am J Clin Oncol.* 1994;17:344-347.

83. Hortobagyi GN, Richman SP, Dandridge K, et al. Immunotherapy with BCG administered by scarification: standardization of reactions and management of side effects. *Cancer.* 1978;42:2293-2303.

84. Ogilvie GK, Richardson RC, Curtis CR, et al. Acute and short-term toxicoses associated with the administration of doxorubicin to dogs with malignant tumors. *J Am Vet Med Assoc.* 1989;195:1584-1587.

85. Valeyrie L, Bastuji-Garin S, Revuz J, et al. Adverse cutaneous reactions to imatinib (STI571) in Philadelphia chromosome-positive leukemias: a prospective study of 54 patients. *J Am Acad Dermatol.* 2003;48(2):201-206.

86. Bhargava P, Gammon D, McCormick MJ. Hypersensitivity and idiosyncratic reactions to oxaliplatin. *Cancer.* 2004;100(1):211-212.

87. Gerber PA, Buhren BA, Cevikbas F, et al. Preliminary evidence for a role of mast cells in epidermal growth factor receptor inhibitor-induced pruritus. *J Am Acad Dermatol.* 2010;63:163-165.

88. Georgieva J, Steinhoff M, Orfanos CE, et al. Ethylene-oxide-induced pruritus associated with extracorporeal photochemotherapy. *Transfusion.* 2004;44(10):1532-1533.

89. Calnan CD, O'Neill D. Itching in tension states. *Br J Dermatol.* 1952;64:274-280.

90. Edwards AE, Shellow WV, Wright ET, et al. Pruritic skin disease, psychological stress, and the itch sensation. *Arch Dermatol.* 1976;112:339-343.

91. Musaph H. Psychodynamics in itching states. *Int J Psychoanal.* 1968;49:336-340.

92. Whitlock FA. Pruritus generalized and localised. In: Whitlock FA, ed. *Psychophysiological Aspects of Skin Disease.* London: WB Saunders; 1976:110-129.

93. Sheehan-Dare RA, Henderson MJ, Cotterill JA. Anxiety and depression in patients with chronic urticaria and generalized pruritus. *Br J Dermatol.* 1990;123:769-774.

94. Fleischer AB Jr. Pruritus in the elderly: management by senior dermatologists. *J Am Acad Dermatol.* 1993;28:603-609.

95. Ghiadially R, Halkier-Sorensen L, Elias PM. Effects of petrolatum on stratum corneum structure and function. *J Am Acad Dermatol.* 1992;26:387-396.

96. Fransway AF, Winkelmann RK. Treatment of pruritus. *Semin Dermatol.* 1988;7:310-325.

97. Watsky KL, Freije L, Leneveu MC, et al. Water-in-oil emollients as steroid sparing adjunctive therapy in the treatment of psoriasis. *Cutis.* 1992;50:383-386.

98. Ronayne C, Bray G, Robertson G. The use of aqueous cream to relieve pruritus in patients with liver disease. *Br J Nurs.* 1993;2:527-528.

99. Fleischer AB Jr. Treatment of atopic dermatitis: role of tacrolimus ointment as a topical noncorticosteroidal therapy. *J Allergy Clin Immunol.* 1999;104:126-130.

100. Kang S, Lucky AW, Pariser D, et al. Long-term safety and efficacy of tacrolimus ointment for the treatment of atopic dermatitis in children. *J Am Acad Dermatol.* 2001;44(suppl 1):S58-S64.

101. Breneman DL, Cardone JS, Blumsack RF, et al. Topical capsaicin for hemodialysis-related pruritus. *J Am Acad Dermatol.* 1992;26:91-94.

102. Leibsohn E. Treatment of notalgia paresthetica with capsaicin. *Cutis.* 1992;49:335-336.

103. Fusco GM, Giacovazzo M. Peppers and pain: the promise of capsaicin. *Drugs.* 1997;53(6):909-914.

104. Shuttleworth D, Hill S, Marks R, et al. Relief of experimentally induced pruritus with a novel mixture of local anesthetic agents. *Br J Dermatol.* 1988;119:535-540.

105. Drake L, Breneman D, Greene S, et al. Effects of topical doxepin 5% cream on pruritic eczema. *J Invest Dermatol.* 1992;98:605.

106. Morison WL, Parrish J, Fitzpartick TB. Oral psoralen photochemotherapy of atopic eczema. *Br J Dermatol.* 1978;98(1):25-30.

107. Zanolli MD, Feldman SR, Clark AR, et al. *Phototherapy and Psoriasis Treatment Protocols.* New York, NY: Parthenon Publishers; 2000.

108. Pederson JA, Matter BJ, Czerwinski AW, et al. Relief of idiopathic generalized pruritus in dialysis patients treated with activated oral charcoal. *Ann Intern Med.* 1980;93:446-448.

109. Ghent CN, Carruthers SG. Treatment of pruritus in primary biliary cirrhosis with rifampin. Results of a double-blind, crossover, randomized trial. *Gastroenterology.* 1988;94:488-493.

110. Bergasa NV. The pruritus of cholestasis. *Semin Dermatol.* 1995;14:302-312.

111. Muller C, Pongratz S, Pidlich J, et al. Treatment of pruritus in chronic liver disease with the 5-hydroxytryptamine receptor type 3 antagonist ondansetron: a randomized, placebo-controlled, double-blind cross-over trial. *Eur J Gastroenterol Hepatol.* 1998;10:865-870.

112. Jekler J, Larko O. UVA solarium versus UVB phototherapy of atopic dermatitis: a paired-comparison study. *Br J Dermatol.* 1991;125:569-572.

113. Calabrese L, Fleischer AB. Thalidomide: current and potential clinical applications. *Am J Med.* 2000;108(6):487-495.

114. Winkelmann RK. Pharmacologic control of pruritus. *Med Clin North Am.* 1982;66:1119-1133.

115. Richelson B. Tricyclic antidepressants block H1 receptors of mouse neuroblastoma cells. *Nature.* 1978;274:176-177.

116. Zylicz Z, Smits C, Krajnik M. Paroxetine for pruritus in advanced cancer. *J Pain Symptom Manage.* 1998;16:121-124.

117. Summey BT, Yosipovitch G. Pharmacologic advances in the systemic treatment of itch. *Dermatol Ther.* 2005;18:328-332.

118. Davis MP, Frandsen JL, Walsh D, et al. Mirtazapine for pruritus. *J Pain Symptom Manage.* 2003;25:288-291.

119. Hundley JL, Yosipovitch G. Mirtazapine for reducing nocturnal itch in patients with chronic pruritus: a pilot study. *J Am Acad Dermatol.* 2004;50:889-891.

120. Aoki T, Kushimoto H, Hishikawa Y, et al. Nocturnal scratching and its relationship to the disturbed sleep of itchy subjects. *Clin Exp Dermatol.* 1991;16:268-272.

121. Doherty V, Sylvester DGH, Kennedy CTC, et al. Treatment of atopic eczema with antihistamines with a low sedative profile. *BMJ.* 1989;298:96.

122. Burtin C, Noirot C, Giroux C, et al. Decreased skin response to intradermal histamine in cancer patients. *J Allergy Clin Immunol.* 1986;78:83-89.

123. Guillot B, Blazquez L, Bessis D, et al. A prospective study of cutaneous adverse events induced by low-dose alpha-interferon treatment for malignant melanoma. *Dermatology.* 2004;208(1):49-54.

124. Levêque D. Aprepitant for erlotinib-induced pruritus. *N Engl J Med.* 2010;363:1680-1681.

125. Winhoven SM, Coulson IH, Bottomley WW. Brachioradial pruritus: response to treatment with gabapentin. *Br J Dermatol.* 2004;150:786.

126. Epstein E, Pinski JB. A blind study. *Arch Dermatol.* 1964;89:548-549.

127. Tinegate H, McLelland J. Transcutaneous electrical nerve stimulation may improve pruritus associated with haematological disorders. *Clin Lab Haematol.* 2002;24(6):389-390.

CHAPTER 24

Treatment of Tumor-Related Skin Disorders

Shali Zhang ■ John A. Carucci

Cutaneous manifestations of internal malignancies are broad and varied. As the number of patients diagnosed with cancer continues to rise, a concomitant increase in tumor-related skin disorders (TRSDs) can be expected. Management of these conditions, which can be challenging, is essential to the patient's overall sense of comfort and well-being. In some cases, diagnosis of TRSDs may even permit early detection of occult malignancy. In this chapter, tumor-associated skin conditions are reviewed with respect to their presentation and commonly associated malignancies (Table 24.1). Potential management strategies are also discussed.

TRSDs are divided into two groups:

1. Generalized eruptions associated with internal malignancy.
2. Cancer-related genodermatoses.

Emphasis is placed on the more common examples of these uncommon conditions.

GENERALIZED ERUPTIONS ASSOCIATED WITH INTERNAL MALIGNANCY

Pruritus

Pruritus, or itch, is a common, nonspecific complaint in the elderly that is often secondary to abnormally dry skin (Fig. 24.1B). However, chronic, intractable pruritus accompanied by severe excoriations may be an indicator of internal malignancy (1). This type of pruritus is most frequently encountered in patients with Hodgkin's lymphoma but may be observed with any internal malignancy (2). There are often no true primary lesions on examination, but secondary changes including excoriations and subsequent lichenification and pigmentary alterations can be significant (Fig. 24.1A). Pruritus has been reported in up to 25% of patients with Hodgkin's lymphoma and is classically described as intense and burning. It may be an indicator of less favorable prognosis when associated with fever or weight loss (1,2).

Pruritus may also be a sign of cholestatic liver disease, renal disease, human immunodeficiency virus disease, thyrotoxicosis, or diabetes (1). Infestation with scabies should also be considered in the differential diagnosis. In contrast to the localized nature of nonmalignant pruritus, malignancy-associated pruritus tends to be generalized.

Intractable pruritus is best evaluated by a dermatologist, who can distinguish primary pruritus from pruritus secondary to another cutaneous condition. Workup should include a thorough history and physical examination with baseline evaluation of complete blood count (CBC), liver function tests (LFTs), and a chest x-ray. Skin biopsy of primary lesions, if present, may determine the cause of the pruritus. In addition, age-appropriate and symptom-directed cancer screening should be performed. Symptomatic treatment options include oral antihistamines (especially, sedating antihistamines), topical corticosteroids, and ultraviolet light therapy (Table 24.2). Zylicz et al. (3) have reported successful treatment of pruritus associated with cholestasis in disseminated cancer using buprenorphine with low-dose naloxone. The antipruritic effects of paroxetine (4) and mirtazapine (5) have also been documented. More recently, Goncalves et al. (6) have reported that thalidomide alleviated refractory pruritus associated with Hodgkin's lymphoma. However, malignancy-associated pruritus only definitively resolves with successful treatment of the underlying cancer (7,8).

Sign of Leser-Trélat

The sign of Leser-Trélat is the sudden increase in the number or size of seborrheic keratoses (SKs) in association with internal malignancy. It has been most commonly associated with gastric carcinomas (9) but has been documented in lymphoid malignancies as well (10). Although the sign has been attributed separately to Edmund Leser and Ulysse Trélat (11,12), it is now believed that both individuals were actually observing cherry hemangiomas. In fact, it was Hollander who first recognized the association between internal cancer and SKs in 1900 (13). While the pathogenesis of Leser-Trélat remains unclear, evidence suggests that increases in tumor-derived growth factors may play a role (14).

On physical examination, SKs are waxy, hyperpigmented papules or plaques (Fig. 24.2) that appear to be "stuck on" and look as though they might be easily peeled away from the surface of the skin. Even though the lesions in Leser-Trélat frequently affect the back, chest, and extremities, the face and groin may also be involved (12). SKs are extremely common in older individuals and represent no danger to patients. However, pruritus may be a prominent feature in some cases. The differential diagnosis includes benign, premalignant, and malignant lesions, including lentigines, nevi, actinic keratoses, atypical nevi, pigmented Bowen's disease, and melanoma. Diagnosis can be confirmed by simple skin biopsy performed by a dermatologist.

It must be emphasized that although SKs are common, the sudden eruption of numerous lesions or their

TABLE 24.1 Tumor-associated skin disorders		
Tumor-Associated Disorder	**Major Features**	**Commonly Associated Cancer**
Pruritus	Secondary excoriation, lichenification and hyperpigmentation	Hodgkin's lymphoma
Leser-Trélat	Eruptive seborrheic keratosis	Gastric adenocarcinoma
Erythema gyratum repens	Scaly, expanding erythematous "wood grain" pattern on trunk and extremities	Lung cancer
Hypertrichosis lanuginosa acquisita	Downy facial hair growth	Lung cancer, colorectal carcinoma
Necrolytic migratory erythema	Blistering, erythematous rash with stomatitis	Glucagonoma
Paraneoplastic pemphigus	Stomatitis, mucocutaneous ulcerations and polymorphous skin lesions	Non-Hodgkin's lymphoma, chronic lymphocytic leukemia
Bazex syndrome	Psoriasiform lesions of ears and acral sites with nail dystrophy	Aerodigestive tract carcinoma
Acanthosis nigricans	Velvety hyperpigmentation of intertriginous regions	Gastric adenocarcinoma
Dermatomyositis	Proximal myopathy, heliotrope rash, Gottron's papules	Ovarian carcinoma
Sweet's syndrome	Painful, erythematous plaques with blisters, pyrexia, and neutrophilia	Leukemia, colorectal carcinoma
Muir-Torre syndrome	Sebaceous adenomas and keratoacanthomas	Colorectal carcinoma
Cowden syndrome	Multiple hamartomas	Breast carcinoma, thyroid carcinoma
Multiple endocrine neoplasia	Lip, tongue, oral neuromas	Pheochromocytoma, thyroid carcinoma
Peutz-Jeghers syndrome	Mucocutaneous pigmentation	Colonic adenoma

appearance before the third decade is unusual and should prompt further investigation. A workup consists of a complete history and physical examination, routine blood studies (CBC and LFTs), chest x-ray, mammogram and Pap smear for women, and prostate-specific antigen (PSA) for men. Endoscopic evaluation of the gastrointestinal tract should also be considered, along with any symptom-directed diagnostic studies. In one instance, Vielhauer et al. (9) reported the diagnosis of occult renal cell carcinoma in a patient with Leser-Trélat. Curative nephrectomy was performed as a result of early diagnosis.

Of note, the presence of SKs itself is not dangerous to the patient and reassurance of this is necessary. However, if desired, skin lesions that are particularly irritating or cosmetically bothersome may be removed by curettage under local anesthesia with little risk of scarring. Other treatment methods include cryosurgery with liquid nitrogen and chemical cauterization with topical application of 70% trichloroacetic acid.

Erythema Gyratum Repens

Erythema gyratum repens is part of the group of gyrate erythemas (15) that share similar morphologic characteristics. These are reactive, inflammatory dermatoses that appear "figurate," "polycyclic," and "serpiginous" (16). Gammel (17) first described erythema gyratum repens in 1952, in association with breast carcinoma. Since that time, the overwhelming instances of cases have been associated with internal malignancies (18).

The rash of erythema gyratum repens is quite distinct from that of other gyrate erythemas. On clinical examination, multiple serpiginous, erythematous bands take on a "wood grain" appearance (Fig. 24.3) and are seen covering the trunk and proximal extremities (19). There is usually scaling associated with the lesions and patients may complain of pruritus. Lesions may be indurated and are likely to migrate over the course of hours. Unlike the characteristic clinical picture, histopathologic findings are nonspecific and may include hyperkeratosis, acanthosis, spongiosis, and

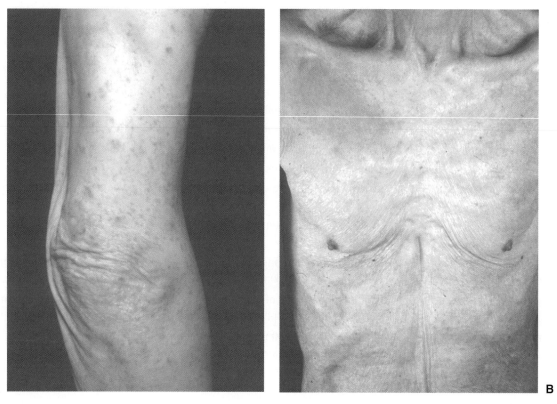

A   B

Figure 24.1. **(A)** Pruritus in Hodgkin's disease. **(B)** Pruritus associated with xerosis (NYU Langone Medical Center, Ronald O. Perelman Department of Dermatology slide collection).

TABLE 24.2	Select symptomatic treatment of pruritus
Medication	**Notes**
Antihistamines • Hydroxyzine • H₁ Antagonists	• Reduces itching by reducing skin inflammation. • Sedating antihistamine is antipruritic partly due to its soporific effects.
Topical corticosteroids • Triamcinolone • Clobetasol	• Reduces itching by controlling the inflammatory response. • Risk of skin atrophy. Avoid using for prolonged periods.
Ultraviolet light therapy (UVA and UVB)	• Nonpharmacologic treatment option. Can be used in patients with contraindications to systemic agents. • Adverse side effects include erythema, burning, photoaging, and potential increased risk of skin cancers.
Antidepressants (SSRIs and SNRIs) • Paroxetine • Mirtazapine	• SNRIs and SSRIs are indicated in paraneoplastic pruritus. • Mirtazapine may cause increased appetite and weight gain.
Tricyclic antidepressants • Doxepin • Amitriptyline	• Doxepin treats depression and anxiety at high doses and has antipruritic effects at lower concentrations.
Opioid receptor antagonists • Naltrexone • Buprenorphine	• Considered in patients refractory to regular antipruritic therapy. • Common side effects may include dizziness, nausea, vomiting, headache, drowsiness, and dry mouth.

UVA, ultraviolet light A; UVB, ultraviolet light B; SSRIs, serotonin reuptake inhibitors; SNRIs, selective norepinephrine reuptake inhibitors.

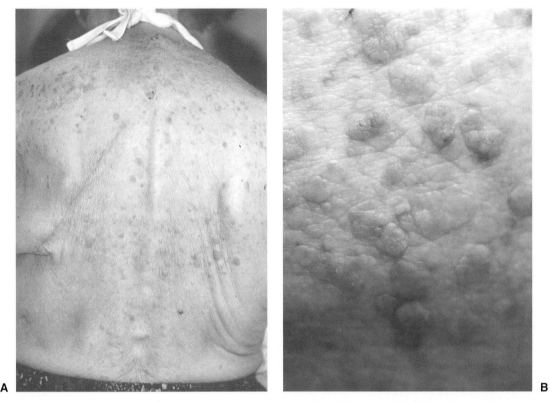

Figure 24.2. **(A)** Leser-Trélat associated with lung cancer—note pneumonectomy scar. **(B)** Close-up view of seborrheic keratoses in Leser-Trélat (Yale Department of Dermatology Residents' slide collection).

a superficial perivascular lymphohistiocytic infiltrate (15). Because deposits of immunoglobulin (Ig)G and C3 have been found at the basement membrane of lesional skin, erythema gyratum repens is thought to be mediated by an immune response to the presence of tumor antigens (20).

On suspicion of erythema gyratum repens, dermatologic consultation is required for confirmation. Because of the likelihood of association with internal malignancy, an extensive search for malignancy is indicated. Standard screening

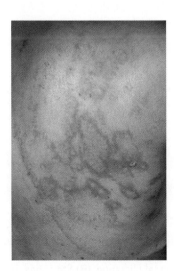

Figure 24.3. Erythema gyratum repens (NYU Langone Medical Center, Ronald O. Perelman Department of Dermatology slide collection).

laboratory and imaging studies should be performed with special attention toward ruling out cancer of the lung (18,19), with which the rash is most commonly associated (21). Erythema gyratum has also been reported with esophageal (10) breast and renal cancer (22). In rare cases, it has even been found in the absence of malignancy (23). However, the cutaneous eruption may precede the onset of malignancy, so it is important to repeat screening tests periodically.

The most effective treatment of cutaneous lesions is therapy targeting the underlying tumor (19). Skin manifestations may resolve after removal of localized tumors but can persist until death in widespread disease. Associated pruritus and inflammation can be treated with oral antihistamines and mid-potency topical corticosteroids (Table 24.2).

Hypertrichosis Lanuginosa Acquisita

Hypertrichosis lanuginosa acquisita (HLA), also referred to as malignant down, is characterized by the growth of fine, non–pigmented hair that occurs primarily on the face (10). It is most commonly associated with small cell and non–small cell carcinoma of the lung (24) and colorectal cancer (25) but has also been reported with carcinomas of the kidney (26), pancreas (27), breast (28), and metastatic melanoma (29). Furthermore, HLA has been associated with other conditions including shock, thyrotoxicosis, and porphyria and ingestion of drugs including cyclosporine, streptomycin, phenytoin, spironolactone, diazoxide, minoxidil, interferons, and corticosteroids (10,16).

In malignancies, HLA frequently appears after the tumor has already metastasized and its presence usually implies poor prognosis with a survival time of less than 2 years (10). However, lanugo hair growth can appear before the tumor is diagnosed (28). Thus, for patients presenting with HLA, blood examination, chest x-ray, and colonoscopy are advised (30).

The most effective treatment for HLA is successful removal of the underlying tumor. Cosmetic management may be attempted through electrolysis, depilatories, or shaving. Because the hairs are not pigmented, treatment with hair removal laser would likely be unsuccessful because lasers target melanin in the hair follicle. Treatment with eflornithine HCl cream (13.9%) applied to the affected area twice daily may be effective. This agent inhibits ornithine decarboxylase, a key hair cycle enzyme, and may result in noticeably diminished hair growth (31).

Necrolytic Migratory Erythema

Necrolytic migratory erythema (NME) is present in almost 70% of patients with glucagonoma (32), a condition caused by a rare neuroendocrine tumor of pancreatic islet α-cells (33). The eruption begins as an erythematous patch involving the groin and spreads to the buttocks, perineum, thighs, and lower extremities (Fig. 24.4).

The erythematous areas eventually undergo scaling and blister formation. Erosions with superficial crusting occur subsequent to the rupture of blisters and healing with induration and pigmentary change follows over the course of several weeks. This may follow a relapsing and remitting course and may be associated with stomatitis. The differential diagnosis includes intertrigo, superficial candidiasis,

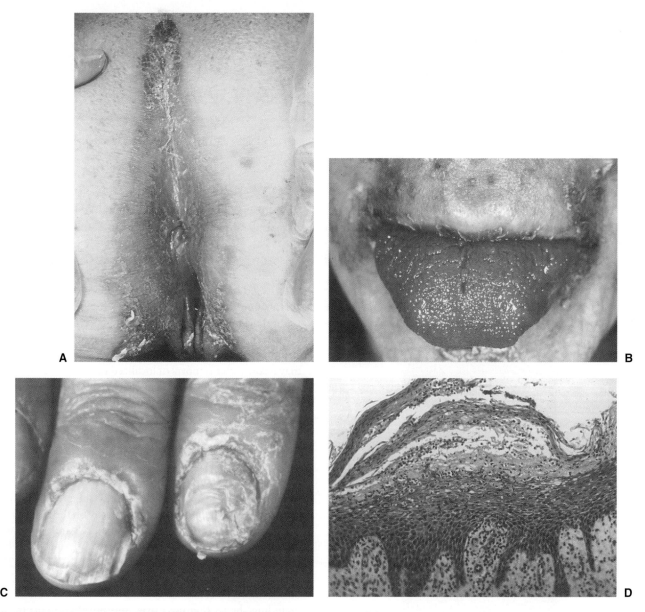

Figure 24.4. Necrolytic migratory erythema in the glucagonoma syndrome. **(A)** Perianal blistering. **(B)** Stomatitis. **(C)** Characteristic periungual involvement. **(D)** Histologic findings include superficial epidermal necrosis and dyskeratotic cells (NYU Langone Medical Center, Ronald O. Perelman Department of Dermatology slide collection).

bullous drug eruption, and pemphigus (21,33). Histologic findings include dyskeratotic epidermal cells with superficial epidermal necrosis (Fig. 24.4D) (33). The diagnostic features include elevated plasma glucagon levels. Dermatologic consultation should be sought to confirm the diagnosis as well as to rule out other skin disorders that may mimic NME.

As with other paraneoplastic syndromes, effective tumor therapy results in the improvement of cutaneous symptoms (32). Unfortunately, patients with NME may have metastatic disease at presentation. There have been reports of successful treatment of cutaneous symptoms using the somatostatin analog octreotide. Poggi et al. (34) reported complete resolution of skin lesions with octreotide after surgery and radiotherapy in a patient with hepatic metastases. Resolution may be noted as early as one week after beginning therapy, but resistance can develop. While waiting for response, denuded areas should be gently cleansed twice daily, covered with a bland emollient, and dressed with a nonstick bandage. Appropriate monitoring for secondary infection is indicated and is especially important in the hospitalized patient.

NME has also been reported in a patient with myelodysplastic syndrome without glucagonoma or evidence of pancreatic disease (35). Recently, NME was diagnosed in a patient with glucagon cell adenomatosis (36).

Paraneoplastic Pemphigus

Paraneoplastic pemphigus (PNP) is a potentially life-threatening, immunologically mediated blistering disorder of the skin (37) that can occur in the context of certain hematologic malignancies. PNP is characterized by severe stomatitis, painful oral ulcers, and skin lesions with variable morphology (Fig. 24.5) (38–40). Though most commonly seen with non-Hodgkin's lymphoma and chronic lymphocytic leukemia

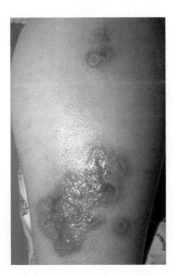

Figure 24.5. Paraneoplastic pemphigus. Although paraneoplastic pemphigus commonly affects the oral mucosa, other areas may present with superficial blisters as seen in this patient (NYU Langone Medical Center, Ronald O. Perelman Department of Dermatology slide collection).

(39), PNP has also been associated with spindle cell sarcoma, Waldenstrom's macroglobulinemia, thymoma (malignant and benign), Castleman's tumor, and pancreatic carcinoma (40).

The pathogenesis of PNP centers on production of autoantibodies that attack components of the hemidesmosome and desmosome that function to link the epidermal cells to their basement membrane and to one another (39). These pathogenic autoantibodies recognize desmoglein 1, desmoglein 3, hemidesmosomal BP230 (BPAg1) antigen, and the plakin proteins (41). Targeting such components weakens the scaffolding system of the skin and renders the epidermal cells more susceptible to shearing forces, causing formation of blisters. These blisters rupture and result in erosive stomatitis, ulceration of the oral mucosa, and cutaneous erosions that are seen on physical examination (39,40).

Microscopically, findings can be varied (39,40). A perilesional biopsy will show suprabasilar acantholysis of oral epithelium or skin epidermis. Necrotic keratinocytes along with a scant lymphocytic infiltrate may be observed. Direct immunofluorescence studies may demonstrate deposition of IgG and C3 on epidermal surfaces and variably along the basement membrane (42). Indirect immunofluorescence studies will show the presence of antibodies that recognize antigens on monkey esophagus as well as transitional epithelium from rat bladder (42). Immunoprecipitation studies will demonstrate the presence of autoantibodies to desmogleins 1 and 3, desmoplakins, or BPAg1. Because of the complex nature of the disease and its diagnosis and a reported mortality rate of up to 90% (43), the consideration of PNP demands consultation with a dermatologist.

Unfortunately, treatment of PNP can be difficult. Topical corticosteroids are considered first-line therapy but they have been mostly unrewarding; though, some patients may experience relief with the application of high-potency steroid gels to affected oral mucosa on a twice-daily basis. Resolution of ulcers has been obtained with administration of the potent immunosuppressive drug cyclosporine (39). However, cyclosporine is not without risk of significant side effects, including hypertension and renal toxicity, and should only be administered by physicians who are familiar with its use and side-effects. Williams et al. (44) have reported successful treatment of skin and oral lesions in a patient with PNP using another potent immunosuppressive agent, mycophenolate mofetil. This drug also has serious potential side effects, including bone marrow suppression. More recently, Nanda et al. (45) reported that intravenous Ig was successful in reducing the severity of cutaneous lesions when used with steroids. Other options include high-dose cyclophosphamide without stem cell rescue and monoclonal antibodies to CD20 (Rituximab) (46).

Bazex Syndrome

Bazex syndrome or acrokeratosis paraneoplastica refers to a cutaneous syndrome of psoriasiform lesions on the ears, fingers, and toes (Fig. 24.6), with associated nail changes that

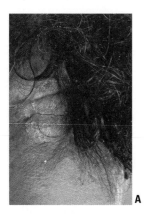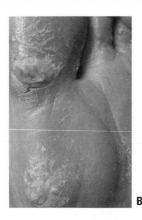

Figure 24.6. Bazex syndrome. **(A)** Psoriasiform dermatitis. **(B)** Foot involvement (NYU Langone Medical Center, Ronald O. Perelman Department of Dermatology slide collection).

occur in the context of an internal malignancy (47). Bazex et al. (48) initially described this in association with carcinoma of the piriform sinus. Subsequent reports have described associations primarily with cancers of the aerodigestive tract and carcinomas metastatic to lymph nodes. In addition, Bazex syndrome has been reported with colon (49), bladder (50), and neuroendocrine cancer (51) and primary cutaneous squamous cell carcinoma (SCC) (52).

The syndrome typically precedes the diagnosis of malignancy (53) and may evolve through three stages (47). In the initial stage, there is vesicle formation with thickening of the periungual skin, subungual hyperkeratosis, and nail dystrophy. Erythematous, scaled plaques develop on the ears, fingers, and toes. The lesions characteristically affect the dorsal aspects of the digits and the helices of the ears. This stage can last anywhere between 2 and 12 months. The second stage ensues if the tumor remains undiagnosed and untreated and is characterized by progression of skin lesions that are usually refractory to local therapy. With progression, violaceous color changes are noted on the palms and soles. If the tumor remains unrecognized, the third stage of Bazex is characterized by the spread of skin lesions to the trunk, extremities, and scalp.

Histopathologic analysis may reveal foci epidermal cytoplasmic eosinophilia and vacuolization of keratinocytes with pyknosis of their nuclei. A perivascular mixed cell infiltrate may be present in the superficial dermis (47). In one report of Bazex syndrome associated with SCC of the tonsil, direct immunofluorescence studies showed deposition of IgA, IgM, IgG, and C3 on the basement membrane (54), supporting an immunologically mediated pathogenic mechanism. While the etiology of Bazex syndrome is currently unknown, genetic susceptibility may also play a role as HLA types A2 and B8 have been reported in several cases (55,56).

Since the most commonly associated malignancy are SCC of the aerodigestive track, inquiries into risk factors including tobacco use, alcohol consumption, and family history should be made. The physical examination should include a thorough inspection of the head and neck (53).

The skin lesions of Bazex syndrome are generally resistant to topical therapy, but treatment of the underlying tumor can result in resolution of cutaneous symptoms (57). For instance, Hara et al. (52) reported resolution of cutaneous manifestations of Bazex syndrome after the excision of a primary cutaneous SCC of the lower extremity.

Acanthosis Nigricans

Acanthosis nigricans is a reactive skin condition that has been associated with a number of internal cancers, as well as endocrinopathies resulting in hyperinsulinemia and insulin resistance (58). The pathogenesis may lie in the similarity of insulin and insulin-like growth factor. Binding of insulin-like growth factor receptors by insulin or by tumor-derived growth factors may result in cellular growth and subsequent development of characteristic clinical findings.

Malignancy-associated acanthosis nigricans typically has a more striking presentation than that associated with obesity or insulin resistance. Patients tend to be older and generally nonobese (59). On physical examination, velvet-like, hyperpigmented plaques are seen on intertriginous areas such as the neck, axilla, inframammary folds, and groin (Fig. 24.7) (60), but florid lesions may develop in unusual locations as well (59). There may also be mucosal thickening (61), and prominent sole and palm involvement. Such observations in tandem with extensive or rapidly progressive lesions should raise the suspicion for malignancy. Microscopic examination will show hyperkeratosis and papillomatosis without epidermal hyperplasia or excess melanin deposition.

Acanthosis nigricans is most frequently associated with adenocarcinoma of the stomach (62) but may be associated with almost any internal cancer, including hepatocellular carcinoma (63) and adenocarcinomas of the lung (64), kidney (65), and ovary (66). Interestingly, the coexistence of acanthosis nigricans and Leser-Trélat was reported in a patient with advanced gastric adenocarcinoma (14). In this case, appearance of both conditions preceded other manifestations

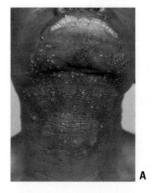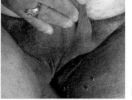

Figure 24.7. Acanthosis nigricans, characterized by velvety, hyperpigmented plaques involving intertriginous areas. **(A)** Acanthosis nigricans of the neck. **(B)** Acanthosis nigricans of the groin (NYU Langone Medical Center, Ronald O. Perelman Department of Dermatology slide collection).

of the malignancy by six months. In patients presenting with acanthosis nigricans, a complete medical history should be elicited with particular attention to the age of onset, family history, medication use (i.e., steroids), and signs and symptoms of hyperinsulinemia and hyperandrogenism (59). An appropriate laboratory panel includes fasting glucose and insulin levels to rule out obesity-related acanthosis nigricans (59). In patients who have been ruled out for insulin resistance and where an underlying malignancy is suspected, screening tests for common gastrointestinal cancers should be considered. Unfortunately, treatment is difficult even with successful treatment of the underlying cancer. However, certain palliative modalities may be beneficial for patients with extensive involvement or pruritus, including psoralen and ultraviolet light A treatment, radiotherapy, chemotherapy, and retinoids (67).

Dermatomyositis

Dermatomyositis (DM) is characterized by proximal muscle weakness in conjunction with characteristic cutaneous findings and may occur in adults in association with any internal cancer (68). The proximal muscle weakness manifests with the inability to perform daily activities such as combing hair, putting on or removing a shirt or a coat, and rising from a seated position. Cutaneous findings usually involve the periorbital area, chest, back, and fingers.

Cutaneous examination frequently reveals a heliotrope rash, Gottron's papules, and poikiloderma in a shawl-like distribution (Fig. 24.8) (68). The heliotrope rash is characterized by an erythematous dermatitis involving the periorbital areas of the face. Gottron's papules are characteristic raised lesions present on the extensor aspects of the fingers. The shawl sign refers to poikiloderma (blotchy erythema with telangiectasias, atrophy, and hypopigmentation), involving the upper chest, shoulders, and upper back.

Skin biopsy is remarkable for superficial and deep perivascular infiltrate, and there may be basement membrane thickening as in lupus (68). Laboratory values of creatine phosphokinase (CPK) and aldolase are elevated in DM. Anti-Jo-1 and antinuclear antibodies may also be present (68). The combination of the characteristic cutaneous findings, proximal muscle weakness, and elevated CPK and aldolase values are diagnostic.

DM may be associated with any malignancy, particularly ovarian cancer (69). This is supported by the findings of Cherin et al. (69), who reported ovarian cancer in 21% of female patients over age 40 with DM. This represents a significant increase over the percentage of ovarian carcinoma in the general population (~1%). DM has also been reported with B-cell lymphoma (70), thymoma (71), colon cancer (72), and metastatic melanoma (73).

Any adult patient with newly diagnosed DM must be evaluated for the presence of an internal malignancy with particular attention to gynecologic cancers. A thorough history and physical with breast, rectal, and pelvic examinations should be performed. Age- and gender-appropriate cancer screening tests such as mammography and colonoscopy are also a valuable part of the workup (28). Additional tests such as CBC, erythrocyte sedimentation rate, serum chemistry, serum CA-125 and CA 19-9, PSA, and stool for occult blood may also be useful (74). Limited radiological evaluation with computed tomography (CT) scans of chest, abdomen, and pelvis is recommended in select high-risk patients (74). Pelvic and transvaginal ultrasounds for women presenting with DM should be considered.

Treatment of DM is directed at improving muscle strength and resolving cutaneous disease. The cutaneous manifestations usually respond to the same agents used to treat the myositis. Systemic glucocorticoids, topical steroids, and steroid-sparing methotrexate and azathioprine have all been beneficial (75). Additionally, sunscreen, protective clothing, and avoidance of sunlight are essential (76) as rashes in DM are photosensitive. In patients with extensive cutaneous disease, antimalarial drug hydroxychloroquine and quinacrine may be used alone or in combination (75). For skin lesions refractory to all other therapy, topical tacrolimus may be effective (76). If pruritus is a significant

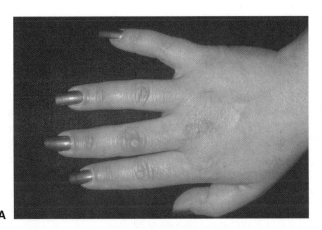
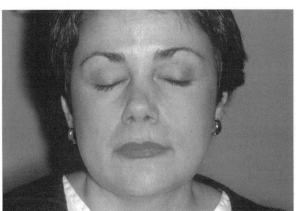

A   **B**

Figure 24.8. Dermatomyositis. (**A**) Gottron's papule. (**B**) Characteristic heliotrope rash (Yale Department of Dermatology Resident slide collection).

complaint, antihistamines such as hydroxyzine, and systemic antidepressants such as doxepin, and amitriptyline can all be used for symptomatic relief (76) (Table 24.2).

Sweet's Syndrome

Acute febrile neutrophilic dermatosis was first described by Dr. Robert Sweet (77,78) in 1964. It is characterized by a combination of acute onset of fever, anemia, neutrophilia, and characteristic skin lesions (10,79,80). The cutaneous lesions can be described as well-demarcated, erythematous to violaceous plaques with blisters that involve the face, neck, chest, and extremities (Fig. 24.9). The plaques may be tender or described as having a burning sensation and are usually not pruritic. There is often extensive edema in the dermis. Oral lesions, initially pseudovesicular, may ulcerate and lesions on the lower extremities can resemble erythema nodosum (81). In addition to the cutaneous lesions, involvement of the eyes, joints, and oral mucosa as well as involvement of the lung, liver, kidney, and central nervous system has been described (80).

Sweet's syndrome occurs in the context of hematopoietic tumors, especially leukemia, and has been reported with solid malignant tumors (82). It has also been reported with chronic inflammatory disorders (83) and, in rare cases, with pregnancy (84). In one review of 249 cases, it was reported that Sweet's syndrome was associated with hematologic malignancies in 40% of cases and with solid tumors in 7% of cases (79). In a study of cases of Sweet's syndrome associated with solid tumors (82), the most commonly associated malignancies were genitourinary carcinomas (37%), breast carcinomas (23%), and cancers of the gastrointestinal tract (17%). The pathogenesis of paraneoplastic Sweet's syndrome remains unclear, though it is postulated to be a hypersensitivity reaction involving cytokines in response to a tumor antigen.

The mainstay treatment of Sweet's syndrome is corticosteroids (81). Symptoms usually resolve rapidly in response to oral prednisone or intravenous methylprednisolone in refractory cases. Intralesional corticosteroid injections and high-potency topical corticosteroids (clobetasol propionate 0.05%) can also be effective. Alternative first-line treatments include potassium iodide and colchicine. The successful use of indomethacin, dapsone, clofazimine, and cyclosporine has also been reported (81).

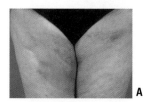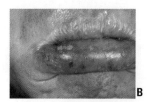

Figure 24.9. Sweet's syndrome. (**A**) An indurated plaque in a patient with Sweet's syndrome. (**B**) Involvement of oral mucosa (NYU Langone Medical Center, Ronald O. Perelman Department of Dermatology slide collection).

CANCER-RELATED GENODERMATOSES

Muir-Torre Syndrome

The Muir-Torre syndrome (MTS) was first described by Muir et al. in 1967 (85), and by Torre in 1968 (86), who noted an association of sebaceous adenomas of the skin with internal cancers. These malignancies are most commonly low-grade colorectal carcinomas, followed by tumors of the urogenital system (endometrium, ovary, bladder, kidney, and ureter) (87). MTS is transmitted in an autosomal dominant manner (88) and is known to result from defects in mismatch repair genes (89). The skin lesions most often associated with MTS are sebaceous adenomas, sebaceous epitheliomas, sebaceous carcinomas, and keratoacanthomas (KAs) (88).

On physical examination, sebaceous adenomas appear as flesh- to yellow-colored papules, usually measuring <5 mm. They are commonly located on the face but can occur anywhere. Sebaceous epitheliomas can take on a cystic appearance, whereas sebaceous carcinomas typically appear as a papule on the eyelid and can be overlooked in the early stages. Sebaceous carcinomas are common on the eyelid but may appear as cystic lesions on the extremities (Fig. 24.10). KAs are benign keratinocyte tumors that are a subtype of SCC and usually occur as a rapidly growing dome-shaped nodule with a keratinaceous central core.

The treatment of choice for sebaceous carcinoma and KA-like SCC on the face is Mohs micrographic surgery (MMS) (90). MMS offers the highest rate of cure and the advantage of tissue conservation due to superior margin control. Sebaceous epitheliomas can be excised with clear margins, whereas sebaceous adenomas can be removed by tangential (shave) excision. Incomplete removal is likely to result in local recurrence.

Management of MTS must proceed beyond treatment of the primary skin lesions and should include a collaboration of dermatologists, gastroenterologists, geneticists, oncologists, and surgeons. Since MTS is inherited in an autosomal dominant manner, appropriate cancer screening must be performed on patients and their family members (88).

Cowden Syndrome

Cowden syndrome, also known as multiple hamartoma syndrome, is characterized by small benign growths on the skin and mucous membranes. While this autosomal dominant condition results in primarily facial and oral lesions, hamartomatous neoplasms in bones and the gastrointestinal and genitourinary tracts can also occur (53). Interestingly, people with Cowden syndrome are at an increased risk for visceral malignancies of the breast, uterus, and thyroid (91). Although Cowden syndrome is relatively rare, as only approximately 100 cases have been reported so far, it may be more common than originally thought (92). About 80% of people with Cowden syndrome is thought to have inherited mutations of the *PTEN* tumor suppressor gene (93).

The usual age of presentation is between 20 and 40 years, and the primary mucocutaneous manifestations include facial

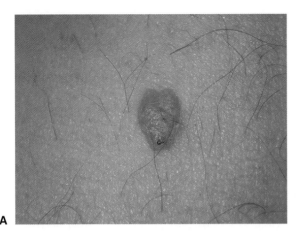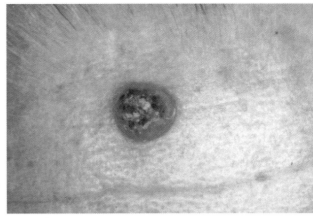

A   B

Figure 24.10. Muir-Torre syndrome. **(A)** Sebaceous carcinomas as shown here are seen in Muir-Torre syndrome (photo by John Carucci). **(B)** Keratoacanthomas may be associated with Muir-Torre syndrome.

trichilemmomas and oral papillomas (92). Trichilemmomas appear as tan to yellow verrucous papules on the center of the face (Fig. 24.11). Oral papillomas give a cobblestone appearance to the tongue and oral mucosa (91). There may be associated acral keratotic papules on the hands and wrists and translucent punctate keratoses on the palms and soles.

When Cowden syndrome is suspected, dermatologic consultation is required for confirmation. Appropriate cancer screening should be performed for breast and thyroid carcinomas (94). Trichilemmomas are benign lesions; however, trichilemmomal carcinoma has been reported in Cowden syndrome (95). Treatment of skin lesions may be attempted by laser ablation, dermabrasion, or shave excision. Oral retinoids such as acitretin have also been proposed but were found to be only transiently efficacious with recurrence of mucocutaneous lesions upon drug withdrawal (96). Because inactivating mutations in the *PTEN* allow for unrestrained Akt and downstream mTOR signaling, sirolimus, an inhibitor of mTOR, has garnered interest. Currently, the National Institute of Health is conducting a phase II study evaluating sirolimus in the treatment of Cowden disease (97).

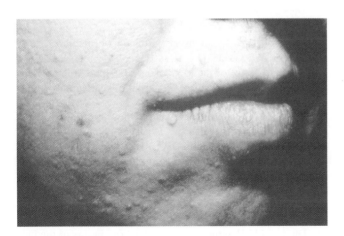

Figure 24.11. Cowden syndrome. Perioral trichilemmomas are characteristic in Cowden syndrome (Yale Department of Dermatology Residents' slide collection).

Multiple Endocrine Neoplasia

Multiple endocrine neoplasia (MEN) IIb is also known as multiple mucosal neuroma syndrome (98). It is due to a mutation in the *RET* proto-oncogene, located on chromosome 10q11.2, which is thought to affect neural crest development (99). Although inherited in an autosomal dominant manner, it can also occur sporadically in up to 50% of cases (98). Patients usually present early; the appearance of mucosal lesions may precede development of internal cancers by 10 years.

Mucocutaneous signs include neuromas on the tongue, lips, and oral mucosa. These appear as papules or nodules and may involve the palatal, nasal, and laryngeal mucosa (98). Patients with MEN IIb typically exhibit a marfanoid habitus. Associated internal cancers include pheochromocytoma and medullary carcinoma of the thyroid. Gastrointestinal neuromas may lead to diarrhea, constipation, and megacolon.

If MEN is suspected, consultation with a dermatologist and geneticist is indicated. Patients and family members need to be evaluated for internal malignancies, and workup should include urine catecholamine level, thyroid scan, thyroid function tests, and CT scan of the abdomen. Because of the hereditary nature and high penetrance of *MEN IIb 2, RET* molecular genetic testing is considered in individuals with clinical diagnosis. Treatment of neuromas by excision often results in recurrence.

Peutz-Jeghers Syndrome

Peutz-Jeghers syndrome (PJS) or periorificial lentiginosis is characterized by perioral skin lesions in association with colonic polyps that have malignant potential (100,101). It can be inherited in an autosomal dominant manner or may occur sporadically (100,101). The pigmented lesions appear around the mouth during the first few years of life and precede the development of colonic polyps by at least 10 years in most cases (100). PJS is associated with the loss

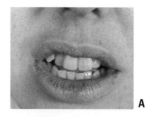 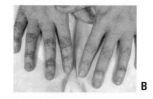

Figure 24.12. **(A)** Peutz-Jeghers syndrome periorificial lentiginosis in a patient with Peutz-Jeghers syndrome. **(B)** Involvement of digits (NYU Langone Medical Center, Ronald O. Perelman Department of Dermatology slide collection).

of heterozygosity or somatic mutations at the LKB1 locus, suggesting that the serine/threonine kinase LKB1 acts as a tumor suppressor (101–103). Genetic testing is widely available, and current techniques can detect LKB1 germ line mutation in approximately 80% of clinically affected PJS families (104).

The cutaneous lesions are pigmented macules usually measuring between 2 and 5 mm (100). They are uniformly brown to black in color, symmetrical, and occur in the perioral area, buccal mucosa, palms, soles, and digits (Fig. 24.12).

When PJS is suspected, consultation with a dermatologist and a gastroenterologist is indicated. PJS is associated with hamartomas of the colon, which have the potential to develop into adenocarcinoma. While colorectal cancers are most frequently reported, there is also increased risk of breast, ovarian, small bowel, gastric, and pancreatic carcinoma (105). According to a recent meta-analysis, the lifetime cumulative cancer risk for a person with PJS can approach 93% (105,106). Thus, adequate periodic screening is essential for patients with PJS.

Lentigines, which may be a source of significant distress, can be successfully treated with the Q-switched alexandrite lasers without recurrences or scars (107).

CONCLUSION

The skin can play an important role in the detection of internal malignancies. Tumor-associated skin disorders may appear in many forms with varying degrees of severity. In select cases, prompt diagnosis and effective management can lead to early detection of cancer and alter prognosis. Since skin abnormalities may be the presenting sign of an occult malignancy, it is essential that any suspected case be evaluated by a dermatologist. Individuals presenting with these cutaneous paraneoplastic syndromes should have a thorough workup for the associated malignancy. Symptomatic relief should be provided. Often, only treatment of the underlying disease permits complete resolution of its cutaneous manifestations.

REFERENCES

1. Duncan WC, Fenske NA. Cutaneous signs of internal disease in the elderly. *Geriatrics.* 1990;45:24-30.
2. Cavalli F. Rare syndromes in Hodgkin's disease. *Ann Oncol.* 1998;9(suppl 5):S109-S113.
3. Zylicz Z, Stork N, Krajnik M. Severe pruritus of cholestasis in disseminated cancer: developing a rational treatment strategy. A case report. *J Pain Symptom Manage.* 2005;29:100-103.
4. Zylicz Z, Smits C, Krajnik M. Paroxetine for pruritus in advanced cancer. *J Pain Symptom Manage.* 1998;16:121-124.
5. Davis MP, Frandsen JL, Walsh D, et al. Mirtazapine for pruritus. *J Pain Symptom Manage.* 2003;25:288-291.
6. Goncalves F. Thalidomide for the control of severe paraneoplastic pruritus associated with Hodgkin's disease. *Am J Hosp Palliat Care.* 2010;27:486-487.
7. Cormia FE. Pruritus, an uncommon but important symptom of systemic carcinoma. *Arch Dermatol.* 1965;92:36-39.
8. Fleischer AB Jr. Pruritus in the elderly. *Adv Dermatol.* 1995;10:41-59; discussion 60.
9. Vielhauer V, Herzinger T, Korting HC. The sign of Leser-Trélat: a paraneoplastic cutaneous syndrome that facilitates early diagnosis of occult cancer. *Eur J Med Res.* 2000;5:512-516.
10. Kurzrock R, Cohen PR. Cutaneous paraneoplastic syndromes in solid tumors. *Am J Med.* 1995;99:662-671.
11. Leser E. Ueber ein die krebskranheit beim Menschen haufig begleitendes. noch wenig gekanntes symptom. *Munch Med Wochenschr.* 1901;51:2035-2036.
12. Schwartz RA. Sign of Leser-Trélat. *J Am Acad Dermatol.* 1996;35:88-95.
13. Hollander E. Beitrage zur fruhdiagnose des darmcarcinomas (hereditatsverhaltnisse und hautveranderungen). *Dtsch Med Wochenschr.* 1900;26:483-485.
14. Yeh JS, Munn SE, Plunkett TA, et al. Coexistence of acanthosis nigricans and the sign of Leser-Trélat in a patient with gastric adenocarcinoma: a case report and literature review. *J Am Acad Dermatol.* 2000;42:357-362.
15. White JW Jr. Gyrate erythema. *Dermatol Clin.* 1985;3:129-139.
16. Kurzrock R, Cohen PR. Erythema gyratum repens. *JAMA.* 1995;273:594.
17. Gammel JA. Erythema gyratum repens; skin manifestations in patient with carcinoma of breast. *AMA Arch Derm Syphilol.* 1952;66:494-505.
18. Boyd AS, Neldner KH. Erythema gyratum repens without underlying disease. *J Am Acad Dermatol.* 1993;28:132.
19. Boyd AS, Neldner KH, Menter A. Erythema gyratum repens: a paraneoplastic eruption. *J Am Acad Dermatol.* 1992;26:757-762.
20. Holt PJ, Davies MG. Erythema gyratum repens—an immunologically mediated dermatosis? *Br J Dermatol.* 1977;96:343-347.
21. Olsen TG, Milroy SK, Jones-Olsen S. Erythema gyratum repens with associated squamous cell carcinoma of the lung. *Cutis.* 1984;34:351-353, 355.
22. Kwatra A, McDonald RE, Corriere JN Jr. Erythema gyratum repens in association with renal cell carcinoma. *J Urol.* 1998;159:2077.
23. Kawakami T, Saito R. Erythema gyratum repens unassociated with underlying malignancy. *J Dermatol.* 1995;22:587-589.
24. Knowling MA, Meakin JW, Hradsky NS, Pringle JF. Hypertrichosis lanuginosa acquisita associated with adenocarcinoma of the lung. *Can Med Assoc J.* 1982;126:1308-1310.
25. Brinkmann J, Breier B, Goos M. Hypertrichosis lanuginosa acquisita in ulcerative colitis with colon cancer. *Hautarzt.* 1992;43:714-716.
26. Duncan LE, Hemming JD. Renal cell carcinoma of the kidney and hypertrichosis lanuginosa acquisita. *Br J Urol.* 1994;74:678-679.

27. McLean DI, Macaulay JC. Hypertrichosis lanuginosa acquisita associated with pancreatic carcinoma. *Br J Dermatol.* 1977;96:313-316.

28. Levine D, Miller S, Al-Dawsari N, et al. Paraneoplastic dermatoses associated with gynecologic and breast malignancies. *Obstet Gynecol Surv.* 2010;65:455-461.

29. Begany A, Nagy-Vezekenyi K. Hypertrichosis lanuginosa acquisita. *Acta Derm Venereol.* 1992;72:18-19.

30. Cohen PR, Kurzrock R. Mucocutaneous paraneoplastic syndromes. *Semin Oncol.* 1997;24:334-359.

31. Hickman JG, Huber F, Palmisano M. Human dermal safety studies with eflornithine HCl 13.9% cream (Vaniqa), a novel treatment for excessive facial hair. *Curr Med Res Opin.* 2001;16:235-244.

32. Shi W, Liao W, Mei X, et al. Necrolytic migratory erythema associated with glucagonoma syndrome. *J Clin Oncol.* 2010;28:e329-e331.

33. Shyr YM, Su CH, Lee CH, et al. Glucagonoma syndrome: a case report. *Zhonghua Yi Xue Za Zhi (Taipei).* 1999;62:639-643.

34. Poggi G, Villani L, Bernardo G. Multimodality treatment of unresectable hepatic metastases from pancreatic glucagonoma. *Rare Tumors.* 2009;1:e6.

35. Technau K, Renkl A, Norgauer J, Ziemer M. Necrolytic migratory erythema with myelodysplastic syndrome without glucagonoma. *Eur J Dermatol.* 2005;15:110-112.

36. Otto AI, Marschalko M, Zalatnai A, et al. Glucagon cell adenomatosis: a new entity associated with necrolytic migratory erythema and glucagonoma syndrome. *J Am Acad Dermatol.* 2011;65:458-459.

37. Camisa C, Warner M. Treatment of pemphigus. *Dermatol Nurs.* 1998;10:115-118, 123-131.

38. Allen CM, Camisa C. Paraneoplastic pemphigus: a review of the literature. *Oral Dis.* 2000;6:208-214.

39. Anhalt GJ. Paraneoplastic pemphigus. *Adv Dermatol.* 1997;12:77-96; discussion 97.

40. Sklavounou A, Laskaris G. Paraneoplastic pemphigus: a review. *Oral Oncol.* 1998;34:437-440.

41. Anhalt GJ. Making sense of antigens and antibodies in pemphigus. *J Am Acad Dermatol.* 1999;40:763-766.

42. Morrison LH. When to request immunofluorescence: practical hints. *Semin Cutan Med Surg.* 1999;18:36-42.

43. Nguyen VT, Ndoye A, Bassler KD, et al. Classification, clinical manifestations, and immunopathological mechanisms of the epithelial variant of paraneoplastic autoimmune multiorgan syndrome: a reappraisal of paraneoplastic pemphigus. *Arch Dermatol.* 2001;137:193-206.

44. Williams JV, Marks JG Jr, Billingsley EM. Use of mycophenolate mofetil in the treatment of paraneoplastic pemphigus. *Br J Dermatol.* 2000;142:506-508.

45. Nanda M, Nanda A, Al-Sabah H, et al. Paraneoplastic pemphigus in association with B-cell lymphocytic leukemia and hepatitis C: favorable response to intravenous immunoglobulins and prednisolone. *Int J Dermatol.* 2007;46:767-769.

46. Wade MS, Black MM. Paraneoplastic pemphigus: a brief update. *Australas J Dermatol.* 2005;46:1-8; quiz 9-10.

47. Bolognia JL. Bazex syndrome: acrokeratosis paraneoplastica. *Semin Dermatol.* 1995;14:84-89.

48. Bazex A, Salvador R, Dupre A. Syndrome para-neoplastique a type d'hyperatose des extremites. Guerison apres le traitement de l'epithelioma larynge. *Bull Soc Fr Dermatol Syphiligr.* 1965;72:182.

49. Hsu YS, Lien GS, Lai HH, et al. Acrokeratosis paraneoplastica (Bazex syndrome) with adenocarcinoma of the colon:

50. Arregui MA, Raton JA, Landa N, et al. Bazex's syndrome (acrokeratosis paraneoplastica)—first case report of association with a bladder carcinoma. *Clin Exp Dermatol.* 1993;18:445-448.

51. Halpern SM, O'Donnell LJ, Makunura CN. Acrokeratosis paraneoplastica of Bazex in association with a metastatic neuroendocrine tumour. *J R Soc Med.* 1995;88:353P-354P.

52. Hara M, Hunayama M, Aiba S, et al. Acrokeratosis paraneoplastica (Bazex syndrome) associated with primary cutaneous squamous cell carcinoma of the lower leg, vitiligo and alopecia areata. *Br J Dermatol.* 1995;133:121-124.

53. Abreu Velez AM, Howard MS. Diagnosis and treatment of cutaneous paraneoplastic disorders. *Dermatol Ther.* 2010;23:662-675.

54. Pecora AL, Landsman L, Imgrund SP, Lambert WC. Acrokeratosis paraneoplastica (Bazex' syndrome). Report of a case and review of the literature. *Arch Dermatol.* 1983;119:820-826.

55. Sarkar B, Knecht R, Sarkar C, Weidauer H. Bazex syndrome (acrokeratosis paraneoplastica). *Eur Arch Otorhinolaryngol.* 1998;255:205-210.

56. Jacobsen FK, Abildtrup N, Laursen SO, et al. Acrokeratosis paraneoplastica (Bazex' syndrome). *Arch Dermatol.* 1984;120:502-504.

57. Wareing MJ, Vaughan-Jones SA, McGibbon DH. Acrokeratosis paraneoplastica: Bazex syndrome. *J Laryngol Otol.* 1996;110:899-900.

58. Kihiczak NI, Leevy CB, Krysicki MM, et al. Cutaneous signs of selected systemic diseases. *J Med.* 1999;30:3-12.

59. Owen C. *Cutaneous Manifestations of Internal Malignancy.* Waltham, MA; UpToDate 2012.

60. Matsuoka LY, Wortsman J, Goldman J. Acanthosis nigricans. *Clin Dermatol.* 1993;11:21-25.

61. Ramirez-Amador V, Esquivel-Pedraza L, Caballero-Mendoza E, et al. Oral manifestations as a hallmark of malignant acanthosis nigricans. *J Oral Pathol Med.* 1999;28:278-281.

62. Fukushima H, Fukushima M, Mizokami M, et al. Case report of an advanced gastric cancer associated with diffused protruded lesions at the angles of the mouth, oral cavity and esophagus. *Kurume Med J.* 1991;38:123-127.

63. Kaminska-Winciorek G, Brzezinska-Wcislo L, Lis-Swiety A, Krauze E. Paraneoplastic type of acanthosis nigricans in patient with hepatocellular carcinoma. *Adv Med Sci.* 2007;52:254-256.

64. Serap D, Ozlem S, Melike Y, et al. Acanthosis nigricans in a patient with lung cancer: a case report. *Case Rep Med.* 2010; 2010:pii: 412159.

65. Moscardi JL, Macedo NA, Espasandin JA, Pineyro MI. Malignant acanthosis nigricans associated with a renal tumor. *Int J Dermatol.* 1993;32:893-894.

66. Oh CW, Yoon J, Kim CY. Malignant acanthosis nigricans associated with ovarian cancer. *Case Rep Dermatol.* 2010;2:103-109.

67. Moore RL, Devere TS. Epidermal manifestations of internal malignancy. *Dermatol Clin.* 2008;26:17-29, vii.

68. Callen JP. Dermatomyositis. *Lancet.* 2000;355:53-57.

69. Cherin P, Piette JC, Herson S, et al. Dermatomyositis and ovarian cancer: a report of 7 cases and literature review. *J Rheumatol.* 1993;20:1897-1899.

70. Anzai S, Katagiri K, Sato T, Takayasu S. Dermatomyositis associated with primary intramuscular B cell lymphoma. *J Dermatol.* 1997;24:649-653.

71. Nagasawa K. Thymoma-associated dermatomyositis and polymyositis. *Intern Med.* 1999;38:81-82.

report of a case and review of the literature. *J Gastroenterol.* 2000;35:460-464.

72. Nyui S, Osanai H, Ohba S, et al. Relapse of colon cancer followed by polymyositis: report of a case and review of the literature. *Surg Today*. 1997;27:559-562.

73. Shorr AF, Yacavone M, Seguin S, et al. Dermatomyositis and malignant melanoma. *Am J Med Sci*. 1997;313:249-251.

74. Miller ML. *Malignancy in dermatomyositis and polymyositis*. In: UpToDate, Basow, DS (Ed), UpToDate, Waltham, MA, 2012.

75. Miller ML, Rudnicki SA. Initial treatment of dermatomyositis and polymyositis in adults. In: Basow DS, ed. Waltham, MA; UpToDate 2012.

76. Vleugels R, Callen JP. Dermatomyositis: current and future therapies. *Expert Rev Dermatol*. 2009;4:581.

77. Sweet RD. Further observations on acute febrile neutrophilic dermatosis. *Br J Dermatol*. 1968;80:800-805.

78. Sweet RD. Acute febrile neutrophilic dermatosis—1978. *Br J Dermatol*. 1979;100:93-99.

79. Burrall B. Sweet's syndrome (acute febrile neutrophilic dermatosis). *Dermatol Online J*. 1999;5:8.

80. Chan HL, Lee YS, Kuo TT. Sweet's syndrome: clinicopathologic study of eleven cases. *Int J Dermatol*. 1994;33:425-432.

81. Cohen PR. Neutrophilic dermatoses: a review of current treatment options. *Am J Clin Dermatol*. 2009;10:301-312.

82. Cohen PR, Holder WR, Tucker SB, et al. Sweet syndrome in patients with solid tumors. *Cancer*. 1993;72:2723-2731.

83. Cohen PR, Kurzrock R. Sweet's syndrome: a neutrophilic dermatosis classically associated with acute onset and fever. *Clin Dermatol*. 2000;18:265-282.

84. Satra K, Zalka A, Cohen PR, Grossman ME. Sweet's syndrome and pregnancy. *J Am Acad Dermatol*. 1994;30:297-300.

85. Muir EG, Bell AJ, Barlow KA. Multiple primary carcinomata of the colon, duodenum, and larynx associated with keratoacanthomata of the face. *Br J Surg*. 1967;54:191-195.

86. Torre D. Multiple sebaceous tumors. *Arch Dermatol*. 1968;98:549-551.

87. Ponti G, Ponz de Leon M. Muir-Torre syndrome. *Lancet Oncol*. 2005;6:980-987.

88. Schwartz RA, Torre DP. The Muir-Torre syndrome: a 25-year retrospect. *J Am Acad Dermatol*. 1995;33:90-104.

89. Bapat B, Xia L, Madlensky L, et al. The genetic basis of Muir-Torre syndrome includes the hMLH1 locus. *Am J Hum Genet*. 1996;59:736-739.

90. Leslie DF, Greenway HT. Mohs micrographic surgery for skin cancer. *Australas J Dermatol*. 1991;32:159-164.

91. Mallory SB. Cowden syndrome (multiple hamartoma syndrome). *Dermatol Clin*. 1995;13:27-31.

92. Longy M, Lacombe D. Cowden disease. Report of a family and review. *Ann Genet*. 1996;39:35-42.

93. Celebi JT, Ping XL, Zhang H, et al. Germline PTEN mutations in three families with Cowden syndrome. *Exp Dermatol*. 2000;9:152-156.

94. Kacem M, Zili J, Zakhama A, et al. Multinodular goiter and parotid carcinoma: a new case of Cowden's disease. *Ann Endocrinol (Paris)*. 2000;61:159-163.

95. O'Hare AM, Cooper PH, Parlette HL 3rd. Trichilemmomal carcinoma in a patient with Cowden's disease (multiple hamartoma syndrome). *J Am Acad Dermatol*. 1997;36:1021-1023.

96. Masmoudi A, Chermi ZM, Marrekchi S, et al. Cowden syndrome. *J Dermatol Case Rep*. 2011;5:8-13.

97. National Cancer Institute (NCI) at National Institute of Health. A pilot study of sirolimus in subjects with Cowden syndrome or other syndromes characterized by germline mutations in PTEN. In: ClinicalTrials.gov [Internet]. Bethesda, MD: National Library of Medicine (US) [cited 2011 Oct). Available from: http://clinicaltrials.gov/ct2/show/NCT00971789 NLM Identifier: NCT00971789.

98. Holloway KB, Flowers FP. Multiple endocrine neoplasia 2B (MEN 2B)/MEN 3. *Dermatol Clin*. 1995;13:99-103.

99. Goodfellow PJ, Wells SA Jr. RET gene and its implications for cancer. *J Natl Cancer Inst*. 1995;87:1515-1523.

100. McGarrity TJ, Kulin HE, Zaino RJ. Peutz-Jeghers syndrome. *Am J Gastroenterol*. 2000;95:596-604.

101. Miyaki M. Peutz-Jeghers syndrome. *Nihon Rinsho*. 2000;58:1400-1404.

102. Hezel AF, Bardeesy N. LKB1; linking cell structure and tumor suppression. *Oncogene*. 2008;27:6908-6919.

103. Marignani PA. LKB1, the multitasking tumour suppressor kinase. *J Clin Pathol*. 2005;58:15-19.

104. Volikos E, Robinson J, Aittomaki K, et al. LKB1 exonic and whole gene deletions are a common cause of Peutz-Jeghers syndrome. *J Med Genet*. 2006;43:e18.

105. van Lier MG, Wagner A, Mathus-Vliegen EM, et al. High cancer risk in Peutz-Jeghers syndrome: a systematic review and surveillance recommendations. *Am J Gastroenterol*. 2010;105:1258-1264; author reply 1265.

106. Giardiello FM, Brensinger JD, Tersmette AC, et al. Very high risk of cancer in familial Peutz-Jeghers syndrome. *Gastroenterology*. 2000;119:1447-1453.

107. Xi Z, Hui Q, Zhong L. Q-switched alexandrite laser treatment of oral labial lentigines in Chinese subjects with Peutz-Jeghers syndrome. *Dermatol Surg*. 2009;35:1084-1088.

CHAPTER 25

Dermatologic Adverse Events during Treatment

Alyx C. Rosen ■ Yevgeniy Balagula ■ Shari B. Goldfarb ■ Mario E. Lacouture

INTRODUCTION

Chemotherapy and radiation have been standard anticancer treatment regimens for decades, and the advent of newer targeted agents has revolutionized the management of patients with various malignancies. However, these anticancer therapies are all associated with a wide range of cutaneous adverse events (AEs) that affect the skin, hair, and nails. The more conventional cytotoxic chemotherapies and radiation cause side effects such as alopecia, stomatitis, and radiation dermatitis, which are well documented. Similarly, the novel targeted therapies have been associated with recently described, specific dermatologic conditions that affect the majority of patients. Regardless of the anticancer therapy involved, these dermatologic AEs can cause significant discomfort to patients and impair their ability to function independently. The inability to care for themselves, along with the physical discomfort, may dramatically diminish patients' quality of life (QoL). For example, the rash to epidermal growth factor receptor (EGFR) inhibitors can necessitate a dose modification or treatment interruption by 36% and 72% of health care providers, respectively, which may negatively affect the clinical outcome (1). The etiology of each dermatologic AE is highly dependent on the type of anticancer therapy or the specific target molecule in the case of targeted therapies. While the pathomechanism of each dermatologic AE has not been elucidated, much work is being done to understand these processes and identify mechanism-based treatment strategies. This chapter will introduce practitioners to the grading scale, basic pathophysiology, clinical appearance, and management of the most common skin, hair, and nail AEs in oncology.

GRADING OF DERMATOLOGIC ADVERSE EVENTS

An AE is any unfavorable and unintended sign, symptom, or disease temporally associated with the use of a medical device, drug, or procedure that may or may not be considered related to such intervention. As patients frequently experience AEs with anticancer therapies, monitoring for their occurrence is an important part of their medical care. AEs are most commonly measured by the National Cancer Institute's Common Terminology Criteria for Adverse Events (NCI-CTCAE) (Table 25.1), a descriptive classification along with a severity grading scale of side effects from anticancer therapies. The NCI-CTCAE version 4.0 is the current version in use, which was updated from previous versions to reflect improvements in treatment-related AEs and severity descriptions.

EFFECT OF DERMATOLOGIC ADVERSE EVENTS ON PATIENT'S QUALITY OF LIFE

While anticancer therapies can lead to improved progression-free survival and overall survival rates, the resultant dermatologic AEs can significantly impact patients' QoL. Certain protocols require that patients receive treatment for extended periods of time making knowledge and treatment of these skin conditions of even greater import. Finally, correlations have linked the severity of cetuximab-induced rash with the extent of tumor response (2). While this has not yet been proven for the other EGFR inhibitors, it emphasizes the importance of proper management of the rash and other skin AEs to minimize patient morbidity and prevent treatment interruption. Various dermatologic QoL scales, including the Skindex-16 questionnaire, have allowed health care professionals treating patients on anticancer therapies to measure how much patients are bothered by their skin conditions. The Skindex-16 is a validated, 16-item, skin-related QoL instrument that is broken down into three domains: symptoms, emotions, and functions. The resultant significant physical and psychosocial discomfort might lead to interruption or dose modification of anticancer agents. Therefore, physicians must be able to recognize and manage cutaneous reactions so that patients can receive these potentially life-prolonging therapies (3).

ADVERSE EVENTS OF THE SKIN—RASH

Papulopustular Rash

Papulopustular rash is the most common dermatologic AE occurring in patients treated with EGFR inhibitors. The incidence varies depending on the specific EGFR inhibitor. The incidences of all-grade rash from single-agent erlotinib and cetuximab previously are reported as 75.2% and 88.2%, respectively (4–6). The risk of all-grade rash for vandetanib is 46.1% (7). While the rates of rash are similar for patients treated with erlotinib or cetuximab monotherapy, they are substantially higher than those found in patients treated with single-agent vandetanib.

The etiology of the papulopustular rash is likely a result of inhibition of EGFR, as this has been described for erlotinib, cetuximab, and panitumumab, three EGFR inhibitors (8). EGFR is crucial for the normal physiologic activities of the epidermis, and in the skin, EGFR is predominately localized to undifferentiated, actively proliferating basal and suprabasal keratinocytes (9,10). The formation of the characteristic

TABLE 25.1   Common terminology criteria for adverse events version 4.0—selected skin and subcutaneous tissue disorders

AE Term	Grade 1	Grade 2	Grade 3	Grade 4	Grade 5
Alopecia	Hair loss of <50% of normal for that individual that is not obvious from a distance but only on close inspection; a different hair style may be required to cover the hair loss, but it does not require a wig to camouflage	Hair loss of ≥50% normal for that individual that is readily apparent to others; a wig is necessary to completely camouflage the hair loss; associated with psychosocial impact			
Dry skin	Covering <10% BSA and no associated erythema or pruritus	Covering 10–30% BSA and associated with erythema or pruritus; limit instrumental ADL	Covering >30% BSA and associated with pruritus; limiting self-care ADL		
Hypertrichosis	Increase in length, thickness, or density of hair that the patient is either able to camouflage by periodic shaving or removal of hairs or is not concerned enough about the overgrowth to use any form of hair removal	Increase in length, thickness, or density of hair at least on the usual exposed areas of the body that requires shaving or use of hair removal to camouflage; associated with psychosocial impact			
Mucositis	Asymptomatic or mild symptoms; intervention not indicated	Moderate pain; not interfering with oral intake; modified diet indicated	Severe pain; interfering with oral intake	Life-threatening consequences; urgent intervention indicated	Death
Palmar-plantar erythrodysesthesia syndrome	Minimal skin changes or dermatitis (e.g., erythema, edema, and hyperkeratosis) without pain	Skin changes (e.g., peeling, blisters, bleeding, edema, and hyperkeratosis) with pain; limiting instrumental ADL	Severe skin changes with pain; limiting self-care ADL		
Papulopustular rash	Papules and/or pustules covering <10% BSA, which may or may not be associated with symptoms of pruritus or tenderness	Papules and/or pustules covering 10–30% BSA, which may or may not be associated with symptoms of pruritus or tenderness; associated with psychosocial impact; limiting instrumental ADL	Papules and/or pustules covering >30% BSA, which may or may not be associated with symptoms of pruritus or tenderness; limiting self-care ADL; associated with local superinfection with oral antibiotics indicated	Papules and/or pustules covering any % BSA, which may or may not be associated with symptoms of pruritus or tenderness and IV antibiotics indicated; life-threatening consequences	Death

AE	Grade 1	Grade 2	Grade 3	Grade 4
Paronychia	Nail fold edema or erythema; disruption of the cuticle	Localized or oral intervention indicated; edema or erythema with pain; associated discharge or nail plate separation; limiting instrumental ADL	Surgical intervention or IV antibiotics indicated; limiting self-care ADL	
Pruritus	Mild or localized; topical intervention indicated	Intense or widespread; intermittent; skin changes from scratching; oral intervention indicated; limiting instrumental ADL	Intense or widespread; constant; limiting self-care ADL or sleep; oral corticosteroid or immunosuppressive therapy indicated	
Radiation dermatitis	Faint erythema or dry desquamation	Moderate to brisk erythema; patchy moist desquamation, mostly confined to skin folds and creases; moderate edema	Moist desquamation in areas other than skin folds and creases; bleeding induced by minor trauma or abrasion	Life-threatening consequences; skin necrosis or ulceration of full thickness dermis; spontaneous bleeding from involved site; skin graft indicated
Rash maculopapular	Macules/papules covering <10% BSA with or without symptoms (e.g., pruritus, burning, and tightness)	Macules/papules covering 10–30% BSA with or without symptoms; limiting instrumental ADL	Macules/papules covering >30% BSA with or without symptoms; limiting self-care ADL	

AE, adverse event; BSA, body surface area; ADL, activities of daily living.

EGFR inhibitor papulopustular rash is believed to be the result of direct EGFR inhibition and induction of an inflammatory response secondary to follicular obstruction (11). This leads to increased apoptosis that can typically be detected between days 4 and 12, which is the time of onset of rash in 45% to 100% of patients (12). The rash is characterized by erythematous papules and/or pustules affecting the seborrheic-rich areas, including the face, specifically the cheeks, nose, forehead, chin, perioral regions, and the scalp and upper trunk (13) (Fig. 25.1). Other physical symptoms often associated with the papulopustular rash include pain, pruritus, burning, and irritation in up to 62% of patients, all of which negatively impact a patient's QoL (14,15).

The guidelines for prevention and treatment of papulopustular rash and most dermatologic AEs to anticancer therapies are developed from expert opinion and evidence-based recommendations (Fig. 25.2). Prophylactic topical therapy includes hydrocortisone 1% cream, moisturizers, doxycycline or minocycline, and broad-spectrum sunblock with sun protection factor (SPF) of at least 15 applied twice daily and every 2 hours when outdoors for the first 6 weeks of EGFR inhibitor treatment (16) (Table 25.2). Sun exposure can exacerbate the papulopustular rash and also lead to severe photosensitivity reactions. Minocycline 100 mg and doxycycycline 200mg daily have been shown in randomized

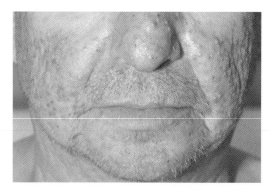

Figure 25.1. EGFR inhibitor–induced papulopustular (acneiform) rash on the face.

trials to reduce the number of lesions during the first 8 weeks of treatment (16–18). Dose modification or discontinuation is only recommended for severe skin reaction (grade ≥3). Bacterial and viral cultures should be obtained if infection is suspected, and patients should be treated for the skin reaction with hydrocortisone 2.5% cream, minocycline 100 mg *or* doxycycline 100 mg twice daily, and prednisone 0.5 mg/kg for 5 days (2,19). Grade 4 skin reactions may require treatment in specialized burn care units.

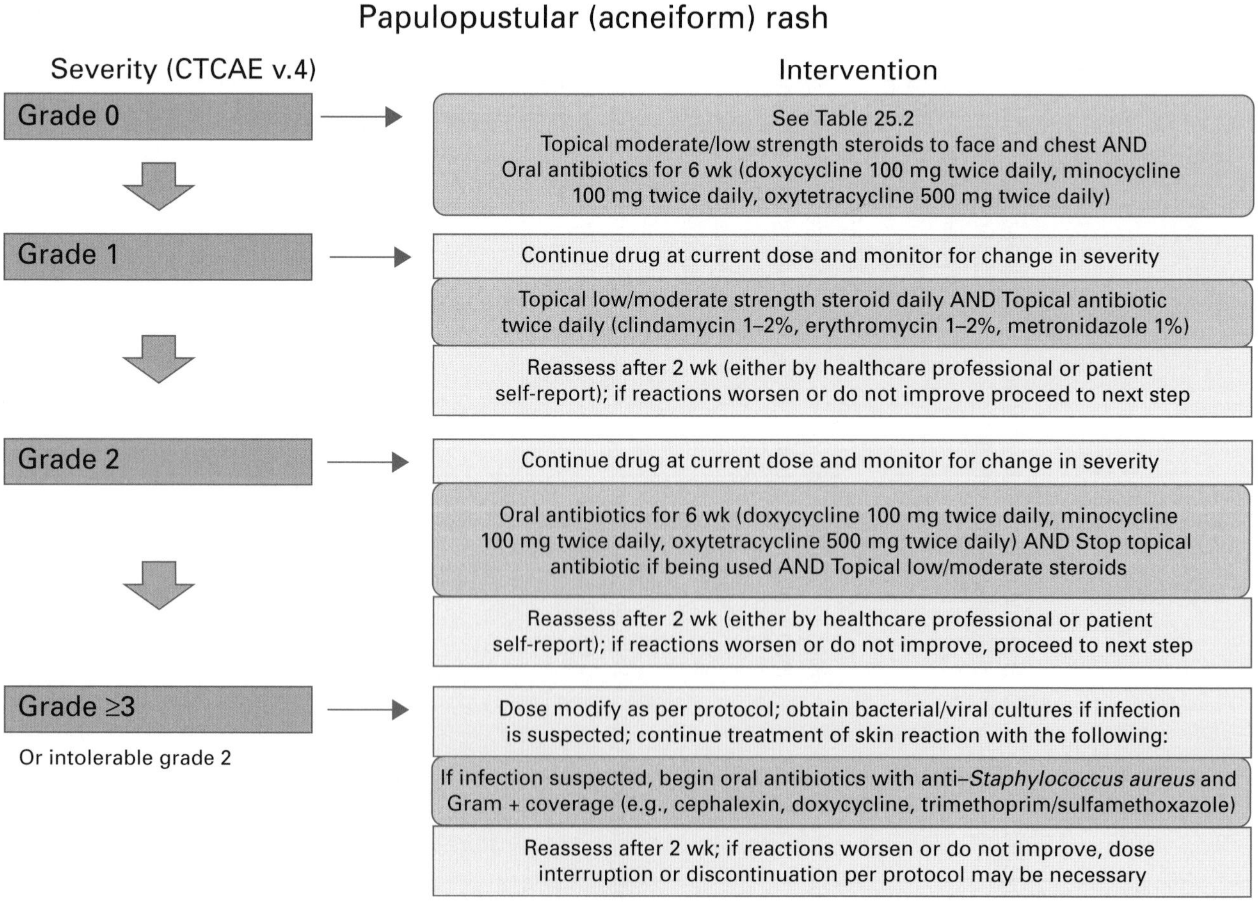

Papulopustular (acneiform) rash

Severity (CTCAE v.4)	Intervention
Grade 0	See Table 25.2 Topical moderate/low strength steroids to face and chest AND Oral antibiotics for 6 wk (doxycycline 100 mg twice daily, minocycline 100 mg twice daily, oxytetracycline 500 mg twice daily)
Grade 1	Continue drug at current dose and monitor for change in severity
	Topical low/moderate strength steroid daily AND Topical antibiotic twice daily (clindamycin 1–2%, erythromycin 1–2%, metronidazole 1%)
	Reassess after 2 wk (either by healthcare professional or patient self-report); if reactions worsen or do not improve proceed to next step
Grade 2	Continue drug at current dose and monitor for change in severity
	Oral antibiotics for 6 wk (doxycycline 100 mg twice daily, minocycline 100 mg twice daily, oxytetracycline 500 mg twice daily) AND Stop topical antibiotic if being used AND Topical low/moderate steroids
	Reassess after 2 wk (either by healthcare professional or patient self-report); if reactions worsen or do not improve, proceed to next step
Grade ≥3 Or intolerable grade 2	Dose modify as per protocol; obtain bacterial/viral cultures if infection is suspected; continue treatment of skin reaction with the following:
	If infection suspected, begin oral antibiotics with anti–*Staphylococcus aureus* and Gram + coverage (e.g., cephalexin, doxycycline, trimethoprim/sulfamethoxazole)
	Reassess after 2 wk; if reactions worsen or do not improve, dose interruption or discontinuation per protocol may be necessary

Figure 25.2. Algorithm for the management of papulopustular (acneiform) rash. (Adapted from Balagula E, Lacouture ME. Dermatologic toxicities. In: Olver IN, ed. *The MASCC Textbook of Cancer Supportive Care and Survivorship*. New York, NY: Springer; 2011:361–380.)

Hand–Foot Syndrome (HFS)

HFS encompasses reactions related to different groups of anticancer therapies. Conventional chemotherapies, including antimetabolites and anthracyclines, produce the reaction known as palmoplantar erythrodysesthesia (PPE) or HFS, while the multikinase inhibitors (MKIs) are associated with a distinct hand–foot skin reaction (HFSR). Hand–foot reactions may also be seen in patients treated with taxanes; however, in this section we will focus on the former two. HFS from conventional chemotherapies occurs frequently in patients treated with capecitabine, 5-fluorouracil (particularly with continuous infusion), doxorubicin or PEGylated doxorubicin (PLD), cytarabine, methotrexate, and docetaxel. HFS is a condition associated with pain, swelling, numbness, tingling, or redness of the hands or feet (20), with progression to blistering and skin desquamation. The predilection for the palms and soles is thought to be due to drug transport to the skin's surface via the vasculature and high proliferation of keratinocytes (21,22). Patients are instructed to avoid warm water bathing, tight restrictive clothing or shoes, and vigorous activities such as running (Table 25.2). Pharmacologic agents have some benefit in the prevention of HFS. The COX-2 inhibitor, celecoxib, at a dose of 200 mg/m^2 twice daily, has been shown to reduce the incidence of overall and high-grade HFS from capecitabine-based chemotherapy (23). Pyridoxine (vitamin B$_6$) has demonstrated negative results in patients treated with PLD, capecitabine, and continuous 5-fluorouracil infusion (24–26). Symptomatic management may include topical moisturizers/keratolytics for low-grade HFS and topical high-potency steroid creams and oral analgesics such as nonsteroidal anti-inflammatory drugs or narcotics for higher grades of HFS. Some patients with HFS from doxorubicin benefit from oral dexamethasone therapy for CTCAE grades ≥2.

HFSR is the most common dose-limiting side effect of the targeted MKIs sorafenib and sunitinib. These two drugs have become first-line therapy for advanced renal cell carcinoma; however, their use in multiple clinical trials is limited by severe and debilitating HFSR. Clinically, patients with HFSR present within the first 2 to 4 weeks of treatment with tender, scaly lesions with surrounding erythema localized to areas of pressure or friction including the tips of fingers and toes, heels, and metatarsophalangeal joints (27). Lesions progress to thickened, hyperkeratotic, painful skin that impairs function and movement (27) (Fig. 25.3). The condition appears to be dose-dependent and typically subsides within several weeks after treatment discontinuation (20). The incidence of all-grade HFSR from sorafenib and sunitinib is 33.8% and 18.9%, respectively (28,29). A newer MKI, pazopanib, shares a similar spectrum of target receptors to sorafenib and sunitinib but is associated with a much lower incidence of HRSF with an all-grade incidence of 4.5% (30). HFSR differs both clinically and mechanistically from classical HFS. One study failed to show any significant levels of sorafenib in the sweat collected from patients' palms (31). HFSR may be the result of the combined inhibition of vascular endothelial growth factor receptor and platelet-derived growth factor receptor that potentially prevents proper functioning of vascular repair mechanisms leading to drug leakage from capillaries damaged by subclinical trauma (27,31). Preventative measures are similar to those implemented for HFS and are most important during the first 2 to 4 weeks of treatment (Table 25.2). They include the avoidance of vigorous activity and tight-fitting

TABLE 25.2	Preventative strategies for dermatologic toxicities of targeted anticancer therapies		
Papulopustular Rash	**Hand–Foot Syndrome/Hand–Foot Skin Reaction**	**Xerosis/Pruritus**	**Nail/Periungual Toxicities**
Broad-spectrum (UVA/UVB) sunscreen with SPF ≥ 15	Wear thick cotton gloves/socks and shoes with padded insoles	Minimize the frequency and duration of hot showers or baths	Avoid wearing tight-fitting shoes
Physical blockers (zinc oxide, titanium dioxide)	Avoid trauma/friction to hands/feet	Use lukewarm water to shower and wash dishes	Keep nails short
Limit excessive sun exposure	Avoid hot water when bathing or dish washing	Eliminate the use of alcohol-containing products	Avoid hot water when bathing or dish washing
Alcohol-free emollients to moisturize dry skin twice a day	Moisturize with creams containing keratolytics (ammonium lactate or urea)	Alcohol-free emollients to moisturize dry skin twice a day	Moisturize periungual areas

UVA, ultraviolet light A; UVB, ultraviolet light B; SPF, sun protection factor.

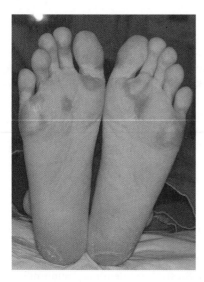

Figure 25.3. Multikinase inhibitor–induced hand–foot skin reaction.

shoes. Gel soles and hand gloves are also recommended to protect the skin's integrity and prevent microinjuries at the fingertips and toes that exacerbate HFSR (32). Urea 10% was shown to decrease HFSR severity by sorafenib (33). Treatment recommendations are based on the CTCAE v4.0 grades for PPE (Fig. 25.4).

Maculopapular Rash

Most maculopapular eruptions are characterized by blanching uniform erythematous patches and plaques that are often pruritic and may cause desquamation. The rash subsides within 2 weeks of stopping the offending drug. Associated chemotherapeutic agents include cytarabine, docetaxel, paclitaxel, cladribine, gemcitabine, premetrexed, liposomal doxorubicin, topotecan, imatinib, and dasatinib (34,35). However, many non-anticancer drugs can lead to a similar cutaneous reaction. Thus, a thorough medication analysis is necessary to help discern the culprit drug. The mainstay of treatment includes topical/oral corticosteroids and antihistamines. Severe reactions can be managed with corticosteroid, antihistamine, and acetaminophen premedication (36).

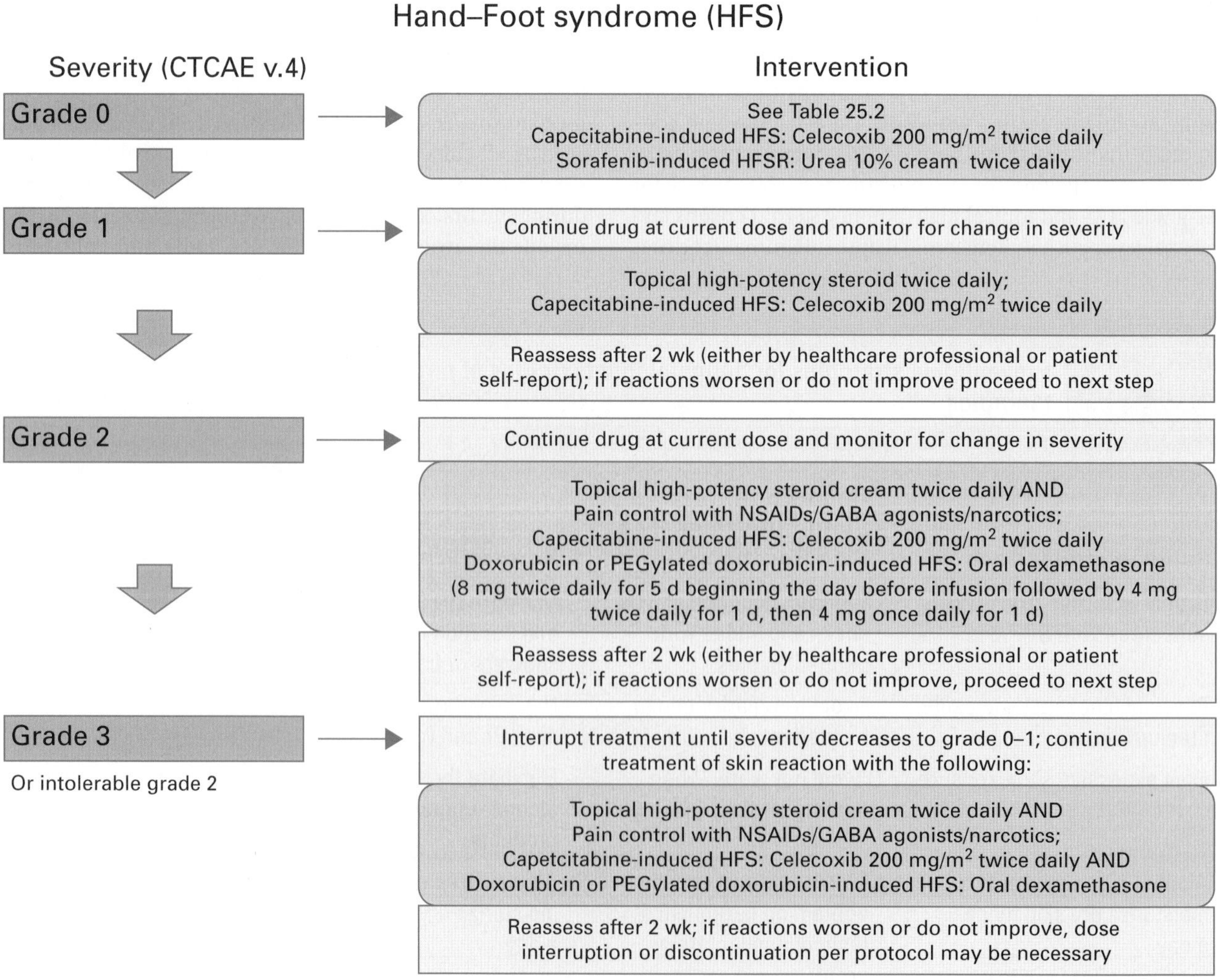

Hand–Foot syndrome (HFS)

Severity (CTCAE v.4) | **Intervention**

Grade 0 →
See Table 25.2
Capecitabine-induced HFS: Celecoxib 200 mg/m² twice daily
Sorafenib-induced HFSR: Urea 10% cream twice daily

Grade 1 →
Continue drug at current dose and monitor for change in severity

Topical high-potency steroid twice daily;
Capecitabine-induced HFS: Celecoxib 200 mg/m² twice daily

Reassess after 2 wk (either by healthcare professional or patient self-report); if reactions worsen or do not improve proceed to next step

Grade 2 →
Continue drug at current dose and monitor for change in severity

Topical high-potency steroid cream twice daily AND
Pain control with NSAIDs/GABA agonists/narcotics;
Capecitabine-induced HFS: Celecoxib 200 mg/m² twice daily
Doxorubicin or PEGylated doxorubicin-induced HFS: Oral dexamethasone
(8 mg twice daily for 5 d beginning the day before infusion followed by 4 mg twice daily for 1 d, then 4 mg once daily for 1 d)

Reassess after 2 wk (either by healthcare professional or patient self-report); if reactions worsen or do not improve, proceed to next step

Grade 3
Or intolerable grade 2 →
Interrupt treatment until severity decreases to grade 0–1; continue treatment of skin reaction with the following:

Topical high-potency steroid cream twice daily AND
Pain control with NSAIDs/GABA agonists/narcotics;
Capetcitabine-induced HFS: Celecoxib 200 mg/m² twice daily AND
Doxorubicin or PEGylated doxorubicin-induced HFS: Oral dexamethasone

Reassess after 2 wk; if reactions worsen or do not improve, dose interruption or discontinuation per protocol may be necessary

Figure 25.4. Algorithm for the management of hand–foot syndrome. (Adapted from Balagula E, Lacouture ME. Dermatologic toxicities. In: Olver IN, ed. *The MASCC Textbook of Cancer Supportive Care and Survivorship.* New York, NY: Springer; 2011:361–380.)

Epidermal Necrolysis: Stevens Johnson Syndrome (SJS)/Toxic Epidermal Necrolysis (TEN)

SJS and TEN are severe and potentially fatal reactions characterized by the involvement of the skin and mucous membranes. Together they represent distinct entities along a spectrum of a single disease, epidermal necrolysis (37). Reactions typically occur within 8 weeks of starting the drug. There is often a prodromal period with flu-like symptoms followed by the onset of the rash. The initial lesions appear symmetrically on the face, upper trunk, and extremities as erythematous dusky-red macules with coalescence, flaccid blister formation, and progression to full-thickness epidermal necrosis resulting in dermal–epidermal detachment. The oral, ocular, and genital mucosae are involved in more than 90% of patients (38,39). Drug exposures are considered the most important etiologic factor and are estimated to cause up to 80% of all SJS and TEN cases. However, the association between SJS/TEN and anticancer therapies, including conventional cytotoxic and novel targeted agents, has not been clearly established (40–42). A literature search conducted in 2009 found only 20 reports of SJS and 22 reports of TEN associated with anticancer drugs. The drugs associated with greater than one case of SJS included imatinib, docetaxel, methotrexate, and bleomycin. Chlorambucil was associated with three cases of TEN, while aldesleukin, cytarabine, gemcitabine, methotrexate, and thalidomide were each associated with two cases of TEN (43). Although the incidences of SJS and TEN are rare, the life threatening nature and need for immediate supportive care requires that all oncologists and dermatologists become aware of the anticancer therapies that are associated with these reactions (43). Management strategies depend on the case severity but include supportive care, systemic steroids, intravenous immunoglobulin therapy, and/or systemic antibiotics.

Intertrigo-Like Rash

Intertrigo-like rash is characterized by erythematous patches that may be painful or pruritic. It typically appears over skin folds, including the axillae, inframammary, and groin regions (19) (Fig. 25.5), as well as areas of pressure or microtrauma, such as the posterior elbow, wrist folds, or the belt region (44). Intertrigo-like rash is a common side effect of PLD, an encapsulated form of doxorubicin in liposomes. PLD allows for better directed drug delivery to target tissues while reducing toxicities to healthy tissues including the myocardium and bone marrow. The mainstay of treatment for intertrigo-like rash involves topical antibacterials and topical corticosteroids. Topical silver sulfadiazine and low-potency topical steroids should be used for lower grade rashes. If candidal intertrigo is suspected, the administration of oral antifungal or a combined topical steroid and antibiotic plus antifungal agent, such as nystatin or an azole cream, should be prescribed (44).

Radiation Dermatitis

Dermatitis occurs in the majority of patients receiving radiotherapy. It results from direct injury to epidermal basal cells and can be seen within the first few weeks of radiation treatment. Mild symptoms include erythema, pruritus, edema, and dry desquamation. Lesions may progress to blisters with moist desquamation. Grade 4 radiation dermatitis, characterized by skin necrosis or ulceration of full thickness dermis, is rare, while impetiginization of open wounds is common. Late side effects of radiation therapy, occurring between 6 months to 10 years later, include hyperpigmentation, telangiectasias, hair loss, or fibrosis of the underlying skin (45). Only rarely do patients develop primary, radiation-induced neoplasms, most commonly basal cell carcinomas. Several factors increase a patient's risk for severe radiation dermatitis. These include poor skin care and hygiene (especially in the irradiated areas), obesity, large breasts (for women with breast cancer), and chemotherapy at the same time or within 1 week (45). The addition of EGFR inhibitors to chemoradiation therapy protocols is associated with an increased risk of high-grade (grade ≥3) radiation dermatitis (46). Cetuximab plus radiotherapy is a standard treatment approach for patients with locally advanced squamous cell carcinoma of the head and neck. Clinical evidence now shows that the skin reactions seen with cetuximab plus radiotherapy are different from those seen with radiotherapy alone. Lesions appear earlier (within the first or second week), resolve rapidly, and do not cause scarring (47). The interaction between radiotherapy and concurrent administration of cetuximab also leads to the production of inflammatory exudate that dries and rapidly forms crusts. These crusts may inhibit proper wound healing, bleed easily, or harbor bacteria increasing the risk of superinfections (47).

The most important step in preventing radiation dermatitis is cleaning and drying the skin in the irradiation field prior to radiation therapy sessions, even when ulcerated. Patients should avoid using any topical products (i.e., ointments, emollients, creams, etc.) during the 4 hours prior to treatment (16). High-potency topical corticosteroids, such as mometasone, methylprednisolone, beclomethasone, and betamethasone creams, have demonstrated benefit in reducing symptoms when applied once daily from the onset and up to 3 weeks after completing radiation therapy (16,48). If infection is suspected, bacterial, viral, and fungal cultures should be obtained. Patients are also directed to apply topical antibiotics to the areas of skin breakdown only, and systemic antibiotics should be prescribed appropriately based on the culture results. A detailed algorithm for the management of radiation dermatitis can be found in Figure 25.6.

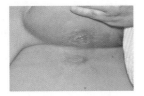

Figure 25.5. Intertriginous rash to doxorubicin.

Radiation dermatitis

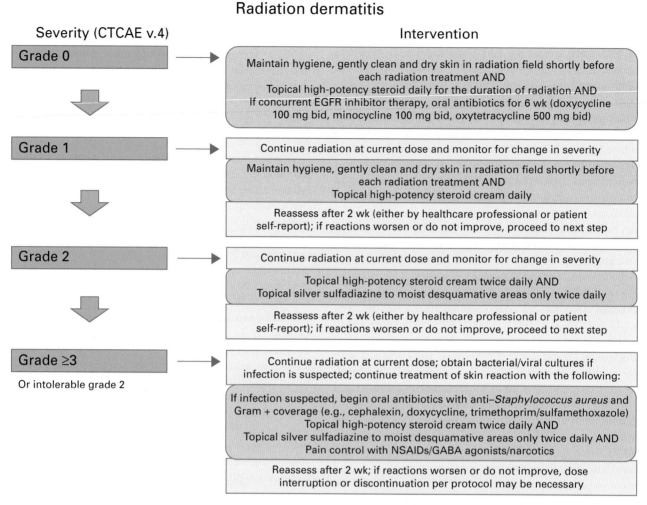

Severity (CTCAE v.4)

Grade 0 → Maintain hygiene, gently clean and dry skin in radiation field shortly before each radiation treatment AND
Topical high-potency steroid daily for the duration of radiation AND
If concurrent EGFR inhibitor therapy, oral antibiotics for 6 wk (doxycycline 100 mg bid, minocycline 100 mg bid, oxytetracycline 500 mg bid)

Grade 1 → Continue radiation at current dose and monitor for change in severity

Maintain hygiene, gently clean and dry skin in radiation field shortly before each radiation treatment AND
Topical high-potency steroid cream daily

Reassess after 2 wk (either by healthcare professional or patient self-report); if reactions worsen or do not improve, proceed to next step

Grade 2 → Continue radiation at current dose and monitor for change in severity

Topical high-potency steroid cream twice daily AND
Topical silver sulfadiazine to moist desquamative areas only twice daily

Reassess after 2 wk (either by healthcare professional or patient self-report); if reactions worsen or do not improve, proceed to next step

Grade ≥3
Or intolerable grade 2
→ Continue radiation at current dose; obtain bacterial/viral cultures if infection is suspected; continue treatment of skin reaction with the following:

If infection suspected, begin oral antibiotics with anti–*Staphylococcus aureus* and Gram + coverage (e.g., cephalexin, doxycycline, trimethoprim/sulfamethoxazole)
Topical high-potency steroid cream twice daily AND
Topical silver sulfadiazine to moist desquamative areas only twice daily AND
Pain control with NSAIDs/GABA agonists/narcotics

Reassess after 2 wk; if reactions worsen or do not improve, dose interruption or discontinuation per protocol may be necessary

Intervention

Figure 25.6. Algorithm for the management of radiation dermatitis. (Adapted from Balagula E, Lacouture ME. Dermatologic toxicities. In: Olver IN, ed. *The MASCC Textbook of Cancer Supportive Care and Survivorship.* New York, NY: Springer; 2011:361–380.)

ADVERSE EVENTS OF THE SKIN—NON-RASH

Xerosis, Pruritus, and Fissures

Xerosis (skin dryness) is a late reaction seen with cetuximab and other EGFR inhibitors as well as the MKIs sorafenib and sunitinib. Gefitinib can also cause xerosis of the face and distal fingers or toes (49). It commonly occurs following the appearance of the papulopustular rash (PPR) and is frequently reported with pruritus (50). Up to 100% of patients treated with EGFR inhibitors for more than 6 months develop xerosis (51). EGFR inhibitor induced xerosis stems from the disruption of epidermal homeostasis and of the normal architecture of stratum corneum, the most superficial layer of the epidermis. In addition to abnormal keratinocyte life cycle, the loss of the skin's water-retention capabilities contributes to the development of xerosis (52). Xerosis appears as scaling or even fine desquamation. Pruritus associated with xerosis can lead to widespread excoriations and an increased risk of secondary skin infections, in particular *Staphylococcus aureus*. Extreme dryness

of the hands and feet can lead to fissures or tiny cracks on the fingertips, toes, and dorsal aspects of interphalangeal joints, which can be extremely painful and bleed (Fig. 25.7).

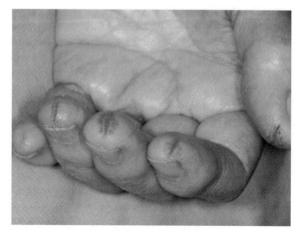

Figure 25.7. EGFR inhibitor–induced fissures on the fingertips of a patient.

Preventative measures include minimizing exposure to hot water during bathing or dish washing and using alcohol-free emollients to moisturize the skin (Table 25.2) (16). In terms of management for xerosis, patients are directed to pat dry their skin after showering and apply moisturizing cream or ointment to the face and body. Severe cases, in which the skin becomes painful and red (xerotic dermatitis), may require topical steroids. If infection is suspected, bacterial, viral, and fungal cultures should be obtained to determine the culprit and drug sensitivities for appropriate management. Pruritus should be managed initially with topical antipruritics and cold compresses on the body. For cases of generalized pruritus, nonsedating oral antihistamines during the day can improve function and sedating systemic antihistamines can improve sleep in the evening. Fissures are best prevented by wearing protective footwear and avoiding friction with fingertips, toes, and heals (16). Thick moisturizers or zinc oxide (13% to 40%) creams, bleach soaks that prevent infection, liquid cyanoacrylate glue that helps seal the cracks, hydrocolloid dressing, and steroid tape have all been recommended for the treatment of fissures (16,50,53). See Figures 25.8 and 25.9 for detailed algorithms for the management of xerosis and pruritus.

Nail Changes

Anticancer agents can cause a wide range of nail toxicities. They can damage the nail bed and cause onycholysis or subungual hemorrhage, or cause inflammation of the proximal nail folds, also known as paronychia. Additional nail changes include nail ridging, brittleness, and alterations in pigmentation (54).

Paronychia

All patients who receive treatment with EGFR inhibitors are at risk for developing nail changes. Paronychia are characterized by painful erythema, edema, and tenderness of the nail folds (Fig. 25.10). With increased severity, painful pyogenic granuloma–like lesions may develop, which bleed with minimal trauma and mimic ingrown nails in patients with no preceding history of ingrown nails. Any and multiple fingers may be affected with a predilection for the great toes and thumbs (55). Paronychia present after 4 to 8 weeks or as late as 6 months after therapy initiation (54). Lesions may fluctuate while on treatment with an EGFR inhibitor and typically resolve with discontinuation, though lesions may last up to

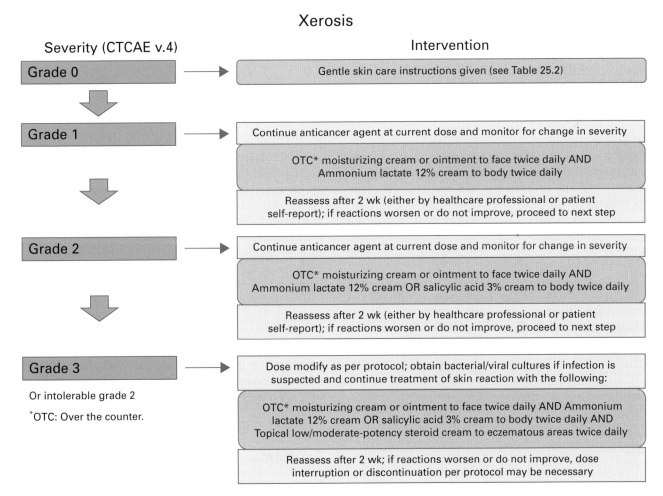

Figure 25.8. Algorithm for the management of xerosis. OTC, over the counter. (Adapted from Balagula E, Lacouture ME. Dermatologic toxicities. In: Olver IN, ed. *The MASCC Textbook of Cancer Supportive Care and Survivorship.* New York, NY: Springer; 2011:361–380.)

Pruritus

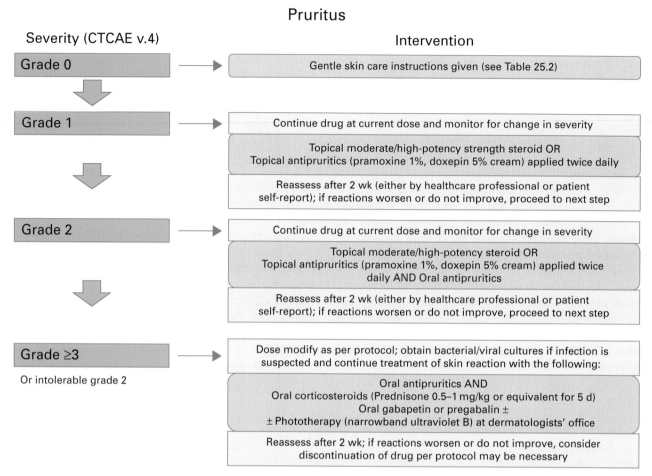

Figure 25.9. Algorithm for the management of pruritus. (Adapted from Balagula E, Lacouture ME. Dermatologic toxicities. In: Olver IN, ed. *The MASCC Textbook of Cancer Supportive Care and Survivorship.* New York, NY: Springer; 2011:361–380.)

several months before complete resolution. Panitumumab-treated patients experience the greatest incidence of all-grade (26.5%) paronychia in comparison to the other EGFR inhibitors. Infection is not the primary event in paronychia development but identification of microorganisms in lesions is common. Gram-positive organisms are isolated in 72% of cases with *Staphylococcal aureus*, corynebacteria, streptococcal,

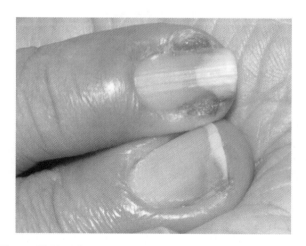

Figure 25.10. EGFR inhibitor–induced paronychia.

and enterococcal species identified most frequently. Gram-negative organisms occur in up to 23% of infected paronychia cases (56). Management strategies are aimed at minimizing periungual trauma, preventing superinfection, and eliminating excessive granulation tissue. Various treatment approaches are utilized, including lifestyle modification such as avoiding wearing tight-fitting shoes, keeping nails short, avoiding exposure to harsh, irritative chemicals, and minimizing frequent hand washing. Treatments may include topical emollients, topical antibiotics, vinegar soaks, high-potency topical steroids, and silver nitrate cauterization (53). Biotin is effective for treating brittle nails and is beneficial for this patient population as well (57). Oral doxycycline 100 mg twice daily has also been shown benefit, possibly due to its anti-inflammatory properties (58). Surgical management with nail plate avulsion for nonresponsive paronychia may be required (Fig. 25.11) (16).

Onycholysis

Taxanes, including docetaxel and paclitaxel, are the most common class of cancer chemotherapeutics that lead to nail toxicities. Onycholysis, which occurs with toxicity to the nail

Paronychia

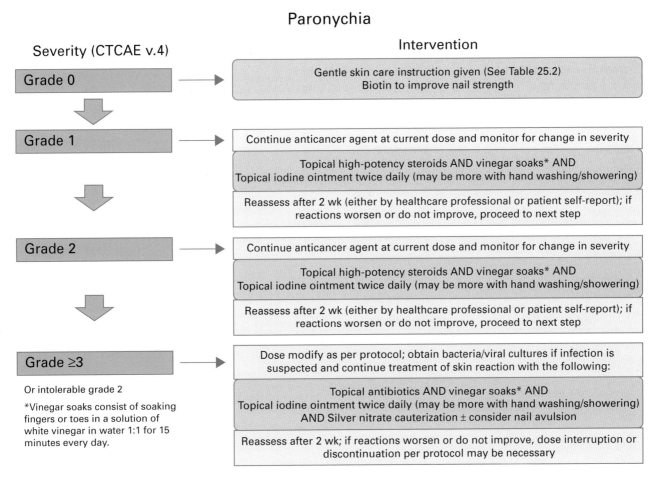

Figure 25.11. Algorithm for the management of paronychia. (Adapted from Balagula E, Lacouture ME. Dermatologic toxicities. In: Olver IN, ed. *The MASCC Textbook of Cancer Supportive Care and Survivorship.* New York, NY: Springer; 2011:361–380.)

bed epithelium and results in separation of the nail plate from the nail bed, is a common nail toxicity associated with this class of drugs (49) (Fig. 25.12). Aside from taxanes, bleomycin, capecitabine, doxorubicin, etoposide, 5-fluoruracil, and methotrexate have also been reported to cause onycholysis.

Prevention and management of onycholysis is similar to paronychia and includes keeping nails short, applying topical antimicrobial solutions, and avoiding contact irritants.

HAIR CHANGES

Alopecia

Chemotherapy-induced alopecia (CIA) is a prevalent toxicity among cancer patients associated with multiple chemotoxic agents (Table 25.3). In general, the incidence and severity of CIA are variable depending on the chemotherapeutic agent. Taxanes (paclitaxel), topoisomerase inhibitors (doxorubicin), alkylators (cyclophosphamide), and antimetabolites can lead to CIA in >80%, 60% to 100%, >60%, and 10% to 50% of cases, respectively (59). However, the degree of alopecia from a given agent varies depending on the dose, duration of treatment, frequency of treatment, and method of administration. For example, intermittent intravenous administration of high-dose chemotherapy is often associated with a higher incidence of complete alopecia than lower doses with either weekly intravenous administration or oral administration. Additionally, it may even be difficult to accurately

Figure 25.12. Taxane-induced onycholysis.

TABLE 25.3 Cytotoxic agents and hair loss		
Cytostatic agents that do cause hair loss	**Cytotoxic agents that sometimes cause hair loss**	**Cytotoxic agents that rarely cause hair loss**
Adriamycin	Amsacrine	Methotrexate
Daunorubicin	Cytarabine	Carmustine
Etoposide	Bleomycin	Mitroxantrone
Irinotecan	Busulfan	Mitomycin C
Epirubicin	5-Fluorouracil	Carboplatin
Docetaxel	Vincristine	Cisplatin
Paclitaxel	Vinblastine	Procarbazine
Ifosfamide	Lomustine	6-Marcaptopurine
Vindesine	Thiotepa	Streptozotocin
Topotecan	Gemcitabine	Fludarabine
Cyclophosphamide (IV)	Vinorelbine	Raltritrexate
	Cyclophosphamide (PO)	Capecitabine
	Eribulin	
	Ixabepilone	

Adapted from Ralph Trueb MD. Chemotherapy-induced alopecia. *Semin Cutan Med Surg.* 2009.

predict the rate of hair loss for individual patients on the same chemotherapy regimen.

While chemotherapy attacks rapidly dividing tumor cells, it also effects rapidly dividing bulb matrix cells of the hair follicles during anagen, the active phase of hair growth (60). Chemotherapy-induced anagen effluvium is one of the major forms, and the most commonly known form, of CIA. Abrupt cessation of mitotic activity leads to weakening of the hair shaft and impaired anchoring such that scalp hairs fall out spontaneously or they are facilitated by mild force such as hair combing. Because up to 90% of scalp hairs are in anagen at a given time, acute disruption leads to profuse hair loss that typically begins within days to weeks and peaks at 1 to 2 months following chemotherapy initiation (60,61) (Fig. 25.13). Eyebrows, eyelashes, beard, axillary, and pubic hair have a lower percentage of anagen hairs but may also be affected by chemotherapy, especially at higher doses. New hair growth typically occurs once the biologic effect of the treatment process is removed and may present with a different texture or color. Chemotherapeutic agents commonly associated with anagen effluvium include cyclophosphamide, etoposide, topotecan, and paclitaxel (62).

Telogen is the resting phase of hair follicles during which reversible hair loss (telogen effluvium) takes place. Telogen effluvium occurs as a normal process in individuals not on chemotherapy as well as in patients on chemotherapy. It occurs due to abnormal hair cycling and excessive loss of telogen hair. Increased shedding diffusely throughout the scalp can be seen 3 to 4 months after drug exposure; however, rarely does it affect >50% of scalp hair (59). Telogen effluvium during chemotherapy is characterized more so by thinning or a decrease in hair density than baldness (62). As with anagen effluvium, resolution of CIA occurs once the medication is stopped, typically after a delay of 3 to 6 months (61).

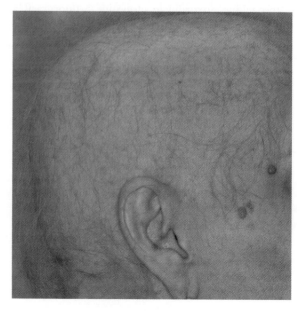

Figure 25.13. Chemotherapy-induced alopecia.

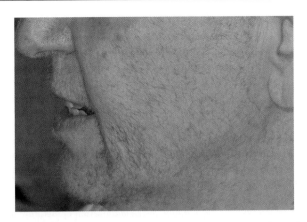

Figure 25.14. Hypertrichosis on the face of a patient from the EGFR inhibitor cetuximab.

Telogen effluvium is frequently associated with methotrexate, 5-fluoruracil, and retinoid (62).

CIA has been a documented traumatic aspect of chemotherapy for over 50 years since the introduction of anticancer therapy, yet no completely effective means of prevention or treatment have been established. The most well-known preventative measure for CIA is scalp cooling either via a cooling cap or with continuous cold air/liquid. The idea is that by cooling the scalp during chemotherapy infusions there is diminished blood flow to the scalp causing diminished drug delivery (59). However, this intervention is advised against in patients with hematologic malignancies since two case reports demonstrated patients with mycosis fungoides and acute myeloblastic leukemia who developed scalp metastases after using a cooling cap during chemotherapy (63,64). During chemotherapy, if alopecia occurs, camouflaging with wigs, head scarves, or hats/turbans is a common approach. Oncologists can provide prescriptions for wigs, which are then often paid for by insurance companies. Cotton head scarves are preferred to polyester or nylon, which may slip off of the patient's scalp (65). Finally, the most notable treatment for acceleration of hair regrowth following chemotherapy is 2% topical minoxidil. In a double-blind, randomized trial, patients who applied 1 mL of 2% topical minoxidil solution to their scalps twice a day throughout chemotherapy and up to 4 months post-chemotherapy experienced hair regrowth on average of 50.2 days sooner than patients in the placebo group (66).

Other Hair Changes

Alopecia is a common side effect of the more conventional cytotoxic chemotherapies. However, with the advent of novel targeted therapies, including EGFR inhibitors, other hair changes have been observed. These include trichomegaly and curling of the eyebrows and eyelashes, hypertrichosis and hirsutism of the face and female lip (Fig. 25.14), and curlier, finer, and more brittle hair on the scalp and extremities after prolonged treatment (51). In men, fewer shavings of the beard may be seen. Although these hair changes are seen less frequently than other common EGFR inhibitor

cutaneous AEs, occurring in only 5% to 6% of patients (2), they may be associated with significant psychosocial discomfort. Additionally, longer curlier eyelashes can cause visual impairment and if growing on the inferior edge of the eyelid (trichiasis) they can result in corneal abrasion or scarring. Regular eyelash trimming or even electrolysis may be necessary (20). Wax depilation, threading, laser, or bleaching of undesired facial hair offers good cosmetic results.

ACKNOWLEDGMENTS

The author Mario E. Lacouture was supported by a Career Development Award from the Dermatology Foundation.

REFERENCES

1. Boone SL, Rademaker A, Liu D, Pfeiffer C, Mauro DJ, Lacouture ME. Impact and management of skin toxicity associated with anti-epidermal growth factor receptor therapy: survey results. *Oncology.* 2007;72(3-4):152-159. doi:10.1159/000112795.
2. Lynch TJ Jr, Kim ES, Eaby B, Garey J, West DP, Lacouture ME. Epidermal growth factor receptor inhibitor-associated cutaneous toxicities: an evolving paradigm in clinical management. *Oncologist.* 2007;12(5):610-621. doi:12/5/610 [pii] 10.1634/theoncologist.12-5-610.
3. Hackbarth M, Haas N, Fotopoulou C, Lichtenegger W, Sehouli J. Chemotherapy-induced dermatological toxicity: frequencies and impact on quality of life in women's cancers. Results of a prospective study. *Support Care Cancer.* 2008;16(3):267-273. doi:10.1007/s00520-007-0318-8.
4. Balagula Y, Wu S, Su X, Lacouture ME. The effect of cytotoxic chemotherapy on the risk of high-grade acneiform rash to cetuximab in cancer patients: a meta-analysis. *Ann Oncol.* 2011. doi:10.1093/annonc/mdr016.
5. Jia Y, Lacouture ME, Su X, Wu S. Risk of skin rash associated with erlotinib in cancer patients: a meta-analysis. *J Support Oncol.* 2009;7(6):211-217.
6. Su X, Lacouture ME, Jia Y, Wu S. Risk of high-grade skin rash in cancer patients treated with cetuximab—an antibody against epidermal growth factor receptor: systemic review and meta-analysis. *Oncology.* 2009;77(2):124-133. doi:10.1159/000229752.
7. Rosen AC, et al. *Risk of rash in cancer patients treated with vandetanib: systematic review and meta-analysis.* J Clin Endocrinol Metab, 2012. 97(4): p.1125-33.
8. Morabito A, Piccirillo MC, Costanzo R, et al. Vandetanib: an overview of its clinical development in NSCLC and other tumors. *Drugs Today (Barc).* 2010;46(9):683-698. doi:1516989 [pii] 10.1358/dot.2010.46.9.1516989.
9. Fuchs E, Raghavan S. Getting under the skin of epidermal morphogenesis. *Nat Rev Genet.* 2002;3(3):199-209. doi:10.1038/nrg758 [pii] nrg758.
10. Nanney LB, Stoscheck CM, King LE Jr, Underwood RA, Holbrook KA. Immunolocalization of epidermal growth factor receptors in normal developing human skin. *J Invest Dermatol.* 1990;94(6):742-748.
11. Perez-Soler R, Delord JP, Halpern A, et al. HER1/EGFR inhibitor-associated rash: future directions for management and investigation outcomes from the HER1/EGFR inhibitor rash management forum. *Oncologist.* 2005;10(5):345-356. doi:10/5/345 [pii] 10.1634/theoncologist.10-5-345.

12. Lacouture ME. Mechanisms of cutaneous toxicities to EGFR inhibitors. *Nat Rev Cancer.* 2006;6(10):803-812. doi:nrc1970 [pii] 10.1038/nrc1970.

13. Agero AL, Dusza SW, Benvenuto-Andrade C, Busam KJ, Myskowski P, Halpern AC. Dermatologic side effects associated with the epidermal growth factor receptor inhibitors. *J Am Acad Dermatol.* 2006;55(4):657-670. doi:S0190-9622(05)03240-8 [pii] 10.1016/j.jaad.2005.10.010.

14. Li T, Perez-Soler R. Skin toxicities associated with epidermal growth factor receptor inhibitors. *Target Oncol.* 2009;4(2):107-119. doi:10.1007/s11523-009-0114-0.

15. Wagner LI, Lacouture ME. Dermatologic toxicities associated with EGFR inhibitors: the clinical psychologist's perspective. Impact on health-related quality of life and implications for clinical management of psychological sequelae. *Oncology (Williston Park).* 2007;21(11 suppl 5):34-36.

16. Lacouture ME, Anadkat MJ, Bensadoun RJ, et al. Clinical practice guidelines for the prevention and treatment of EGFR inhibitor-associated dermatologic toxicities. *Support Care Cancer.* 2011;19(8):1079-1095. doi:10.1007/s00520-011-1197-6.

17. Lacouture ME, Mitchell EP, Piperdi B, et al. Skin toxicity evaluation protocol with panitumumab (STEPP), a phase II, open-label, randomized trial evaluating the impact of a pre-Emptive Skin treatment regimen on skin toxicities and quality of life in patients with metastatic colorectal cancer. *J Clin Oncol.* 2010;28(8):1351-1357. doi:JCO.2008.21.7828 [pii]10.1200/JCO.2008.21.7828.

18. Scope A, Agero AL, Dusza SW, et al. Randomized double-blind trial of prophylactic oral minocycline and topical tazarotene for cetuximab-associated acne-like eruption. *J Clin Oncol.* 2007;25(34):5390-5396. doi:25/34/5390 [pii] 10.1200/JCO.2007.12.6987.

19. Balagula E, Lacouture ME. Dermatologic toxicities. In: Olver IN, ed. *The MASCC Textbook of Cancer Supportive Care and Survivorship.* New York, NY: Springer; 2011:361-380.

20. Lacouture ME, Boerner SA, Lorusso PM. Non-rash skin toxicities associated with novel targeted therapies. *Clin Lung Cancer.* 2006;8(suppl 1):S36-S42.

21. Jacobi U, Waibler E, Schulze P, et al. Release of doxorubicin in sweat: first step to induce the palmar-plantar erythrodysesthesia syndrome? *Ann Oncol.* 2005;16(7):1210-1211. doi:10.1093/annonc/mdi204.

22. Martschick A, Sehouli J, Patzelt A, et al. The pathogenetic mechanism of anthracycline-induced palmar-plantar erythrodysesthesia. *Anticancer Res.* 2009;29(6):2307-2313.

23. Zhang R-X, Wu X-J, Lu S-X, Pan Z-Z, Wan D-S, Chen G. The effect of COX-2 inhibitor on capecitabine-induced hand–foot syndrome in patients with stage II/III colorectal cancer: a phase II randomized prospective study. *J Cancer Res Clin Oncol.* 2011;137(6):953-957. doi:10.1007/s00432-010-0958-9.

24. Jeung HC, Chung HC. Is pyridoxine helpful in preventing palmar-plantar erythrodysesthesia associated with capecitabine? *Asia Pac J Clin Oncol.* 2010;6(3):141-143. doi:10.1111/j.1743-7563.2010.01326.x.

25. Fabian CJ, Molina R, Slavik M, Dahlberg S, Giri S, Stephens R. Pyridoxine therapy for palmar-plantar erythrodysesthesia associated with continuous 5-fluorouracil infusion. *Invest New Drugs.* 1990;8(1):57-63.

26. Lorusso D, Di Stefano A, Carone V, Fagotti A, Pisconti S, Scambia G. Pegylated liposomal doxorubicin-related palmar-plantar erythrodysesthesia ("hand-foot" syndrome). *Ann Oncol.* 2007;18(7):1159-1164. doi:10.1093/annonc/mdl477.

27. Lacouture ME, Wu S, Robert C, et al. Evolving strategies for the management of hand-foot skin reaction associated with the multitargeted kinase inhibitors sorafenib and sunitinib. *Oncologist.* 2008;13(9):1001-1011. doi:10.1634/theoncologist.2008-0131.

28. Chu D, et al. *Risk of hand-foot skin reaction with sorafenib: a systematic review and meta-analysis.* Acta Oncol, 2008. 47(2): p. 176-86.

29. Chu D, et al. *Risk of hand-foot skin reaction with the multitargeted kinase inhibitor sunitinib in patients with renal cell and non-renal cell carcinoma: a meta-analysis.* Clin Genitourin Cancer, 2009. 7(1): p. 11-9.

30. Balagula Y, et al. *The risk of hand foot skin reaction to pazopanib, a novel multikinase inhibitor: a systematic review of literature and meta-analysis.* Invest New Drugs, 2012. 30(4): p. 1773-81.

31. Jain L, Gardner ER, Figg WD, Chernick MS, Kong HH. Lack of association between excretion of sorafenib in sweat and hand-foot skin reaction. *Pharmacotherapy.* 2010;30(1):52-56. doi:10.1592/phco.30.1.52.

32. Boone SL, Jameson G, Von Hoff D, Lacouture ME. Blackberry-induced hand-foot skin reaction to sunitinib. *Invest New Drugs.* 2009;27(4):389-390. doi:10.1007/s10637-008-9196-2.

33. http://www.asco.org/ASCOv2/Meetings/Abstracts?&vmview=abst_detail_view&confID=114&abstractID=97226

34. Heidary N, Naik H, Burgin S. Chemotherapeutic agents and the skin: an update. *J Am Acad Dermatol.* 2008;58(4):545-570. doi:10.1016/j.jaad.2008.01.001.

35. Newman M, Balagula E, Lacouture ME. Management of treatment-related dermatologic adverse effects. In: Mellar Davis, Petra Feyer, Petra Ortner, Camilla Zimmermann, ed. *Supportive Oncology.* Saint Louis, MO: W.B. Saunders; 2011:115-120.

36. Agha R, Kinahan K, Bennett CL, Lacouture ME. Dermatologic challenges in cancer patients and survivors. *Oncology (Williston Park).* 2007;21(12):1462-1472; discussion 73, 76, 81 passim.

37. Bastuji-Garin S, Rzany B, Stern RS, Shear NH, Naldi L, Roujeau JC. Clinical classification of cases of toxic epidermal necrolysis, Stevens-Johnson syndrome, and erythema multiforme. *Arch Dermatol.* 1993;129(1):92-96.

38. French LE. Toxic epidermal necrolysis and Stevens Johnson syndrome: our current understanding. *Allergol Int.* 2006;55(1):9-16. doi:10.2332/allergolint.55.9.

39. Hazin R, Ibrahimi OA, Hazin MI, Kimyai-Asadi A. Stevens-Johnson syndrome: pathogenesis, diagnosis, and management. *Ann Med.* 2008;40(2):129-138. doi:10.1080/07853890701753664.

40. Borchers AT, Lee JL, Naguwa SM, Cheema GS, Gershwin ME. Stevens-Johnson syndrome and toxic epidermal necrolysis. *Autoimmun Rev.* 2008;7(8):598-605. doi:S1568-9972(08)00094-3 [pii] 10.1016/j.autrev.2008.06.004.

41. Lyell A. Toxic epidermal necrolysis (the scalded skin syndrome): a reappraisal. *Br J Dermatol.* 1979;100(1):69-86.

42. Stern RS, Chan HL. Usefulness of case report literature in determining drugs responsible for toxic epidermal necrolysis. *J Am Acad Dermatol.* 1989;21(2 Pt 1):317-322.

43. Sorrell J, West DP, Bennett CL, Raisch DW, Lacouture ME. Life-threatening dermatologic toxicities to cancer drug therapy: an assessment of the published peer-reviewed literature. *J Clin Oncol.* 2009;27(suppl; abstr e20592).

44. Sanchez Henarejos P, Ros Martinez S, Marin Zafra GR, Alonso Romero JL, Navarrete Montoya A. Intertrigo-like eruption caused by pegylated liposomal doxorubicin (PLD). *Clin Transl Oncol.* 2009;11(7):486-487.

45. Berkey FJ. *Managing the adverse effects of radiation therapy.* Am Fam Physician, 2010. 82(4): p. 381-388, 394.

46. Tejwani A, Wu S, Jia Y, Agulnik M, Millender L, Lacouture ME. Increased risk of high-grade dermatologic toxicities with radiation plus epidermal growth factor receptor inhibitor therapy. *Cancer.* 2009;115(6):1286-1299. doi:10.1002/cncr.24120.

47. Bernier J, Russi EG, Homey B, et al. Management of radiation dermatitis in patients receiving cetuximab and radiotherapy for locally advanced squamous cell carcinoma of the head and neck: proposals for a revised grading system and consensus management guidelines. *Ann Oncol.* 2011;22(10):2191-2200. doi:10.1093/annonc/mdr139.

48. Miller RC, Schwartz DJ, Sloan JA, et al. Mometasone furoate effect on acute skin toxicity in breast cancer patients receiving radiotherapy: a phase III double-blind, randomized trial from the North Central Cancer Treatment Group N06C4. *Int J Radiat Oncol Biol Phys.* 2011;79(5):1460-1466. doi:10.1016/j.ijrobp.2010.01.031.

49. Wyatt AJ, Leonard GD, Sachs DL. Cutaneous reactions to chemotherapy and their management. *Am J Clin Dermatol.* 2006;7(1):45-63. doi:715 [pii].

50. Balagula Y, Lacouture ME, Cotliar JA. Dermatologic toxicities of targeted anticancer therapies. *J Support Oncol.* 2010;8(4):149-161

51. Osio A, Mateus C, Soria JC, et al. Cutaneous side-effects in patients on long-term treatment with epidermal growth factor receptor inhibitors. *Br J Dermatol.* 2009;161(3):515-521. doi:10.1111/j.1365-2133.2009.09214.x.

52. Han SS, Lee M, Park GH, et al. Investigation of papulopustular eruptions caused by cetuximab treatment shows altered differentiation markers and increases in inflammatory cytokines. *Br J Dermatol.* 2010;162(2):371-379. doi:BJD9536 [pii] 10.1111/j.1365-2133.2009.09536.x.

53. Quitkin HM, Rosenwasser MP, and Strauch RJ. The efficacy of silver nitrate cauterization for pyogenic granuloma of the hand. *J Hand Surg Am,* 2003. 28(3): p. 435-8.

54. Gilbar P, Hain A, Peereboom VM. Nail toxicity induced by cancer chemotherapy. *J Oncol Pharm Pract.* 2009;15(3):143-155. doi:10.1177/1078155208100450.

55. Fox LP. Nail toxicity associated with epidermal growth factor receptor inhibitor therapy. *J Am Acad Dermatol.* 2007;56(3):460-465. doi:10.1016/j.jaad.2006.09.013.

56. Eames T, Grabein B, Kroth J, Wollenberg A. Microbiological analysis of epidermal growth factor receptor inhibitor therapy-associated paronychia. *J Eur Acad Dermatol Venereol.* 2010;24(8):958-960. doi:JDV3516 [pii] 10.1111/j.1468-3083.2009.03516.x.

57. Floersheim GL. Treatment of brittle fingernails with biotin. *Z Hautkr.* 1989;64(1):41-48.

58. Suh K-Y, Kindler HL, Medenica M, Lacouture M. Doxycycline for the treatment of paronychia induced by the epidermal growth factor receptor cetuximab. *Br J Dermatol.* 2005;154. doi:10.1111/j.1365-2133.2005.07010.x.

59. Trueb RM. Chemotherapy-induced alopecia. *Semin Cutan Med Surg.* 2009;28(1):11-14. doi:10.1016/j.sder.2008.12.001.

60. Trueb RM. Chemotherapy-induced anagen effluvium: diffuse or patterned? *Dermatology.* 2007;215(1):1-2. doi:10.1159/000102025.

61. Wang J, Lu Z, Au JL. Protection against chemotherapy-induced alopecia. *Pharm Res.* 2006;23(11):2505-2514. doi:10.1007/s11095-006-9105-3.

62. Olsen EA. Chemotherapy-induced alopecia: overview and methodology for characterizing hair changes and regrowth. In: Olver IN, ed. *The MASCC Textbook of Cancer Supportive Care and Survivorship* New York, NY: Springer; 2011:381-386.

63. Forsberg SA. Scalp cooling therapy and cytotoxic treatment. *Lancet.* 2001;357(9262):1134.

64. Witman G, Cadman E, Chen M. Misuse of scalp hypothermia. *Cancer Treat Rep.* 1981;65(5-6):507-508.

65. Yeager CE, Olsen EA. Treatment of chemotherapy-induced alopecia. *Dermatol Ther.* 2011;24(4):432-442. doi:10.1111/j.1529-8019.2011.01430.x.

66. Duvic M, Lemak NA, Valero V, et al. A randomized trial of minoxidil in chemotherapy-induced alopecia. *J Am Acad Dermatol.* 1996;35(1):74-78. doi:S0190-9622(96)90500-9 [pii] 10.1016/S0190-9622(96)90500-9.

CHAPTER 26

Management of Pressure Ulcers and Fungating Wounds

Frank D. Ferris ■ Susan K. Bodtke

S kin is one of the vital human organs. It has a highly developed physiology and several essential functions in the regulation of homeostasis and immunity.

Provides protection. Skin surrounds virtually our entire bodies. It is the outer layer of the structures that hold us intact and give shape to our bodies. It also provides protection and a cushion when objects hit our bodies.

Senses environment. Skin is highly innervated. It helps sense the environment and avoid injury. When skin is "wounded" and becomes inflamed or infected, the resulting inflammatory response can sensitize nociceptors, lead to recruitment of additional neurons, and increase neuronal firing of each involved neuron. Patients frequently experience increasing pain associated with the wound and the inflamed structures, that is, hyperalgesia and allodynia (1). Although opioid receptors are not present in normal skin, within minutes to hours of inflammation, they may appear in peripheral sensory nerves (2).

Maintains fluid balance. Skin has a highly developed system of pores that help to control fluid balance. The pores open and close to regulate evaporation and transcutaneous perspiration.

Controls body temperature. Skin also participates in the regulation of body temperature by releasing fluids on the surface as perspiration or sweat to evaporate and cool down the body.

Controls infection. Intact skin presents a physical barrier to infections and immunologic barrier to infections. When skin is "wounded," this barrier is broken and bacteria and other infective agents can colonize or infect the wound and the surrounding tissues and sometimes lead to systemic infections or even sepsis. Wound infections can secrete pathogens that inhibit epithelial cell mitosis and delay granulation and wound healing.

Creates body image. Skin is the most visible organ. Its presence creates a bodily image of who we are. Disfigurement due to wounds may have profound consequences on an individual's body image and the way others respond to her/him. If it is bad enough, the patient may want to withdraw, family members and friends may not want to look at the patient, and healthcare workers may not want to provide care. At a time when the patient may need more support than ever, she/he may be abandoned by family members and caregivers.

Creates body smells. Skin secretes a number of fluids and substance that have associated smells. Over time, many people develop attractions to each other based on familiar scents. If those scents change or become overwhelmed by odors from putrefying tissues or infections, the effect may be repulsive and lead to isolation and abandonment.

There are multiple potential events that can damage skin integrity and/or function acutely or chronically. For patients with advanced cancer, particularly the elderly, pressure and fungating tumor masses are the most common causes of chronic wounds to the skin and the tissues that lie below it, that is, subcutaneous fat, muscles, bone, tendons, nerves, and blood vessels.

When patients with cancer experience chronic wounds, not only do they suffer from the underlying cancer and their wounds, but their whole being is affected by the multiple physical, psychological, social, spiritual, practical, loss, and end-of-life issues that are frequently associated with wounds. To be effective, care of such patients must be consistent with their goals of care and treatment priorities and must manage the whole "wounded" person, not just the "hole" (3,4).

PRESSURE ULCERS

Pressure or decubitus ulcers are encountered frequently in patients with cancer, particularly those who are debilitated by their illness or by treatment (5,6).

The microarterioles that supply blood to the skin run through the subcutaneous fat. In the face of mild pressure, the fat normally cushions and redistributes the pressure. However, when the pressure increases above the capillary filling pressure, the microarterioles close for as long as the pressure is present and the oxygen tension falls in the downstream tissues. Normal skin can withstand 30 to 60 minutes of poor perfusion but not longer. When the pressure and hypoxia are sustained, ischemia and necrosis can develop relatively rapidly (7,8).

In both general hospital and long-term care, pressure ulcers occur in up to 28% of patients (9). One study of 980 home hospice patients found that 10% of patients developed ulcers during the study period (10).

Pressure points, for example, sacrum, heels, and elbows, are at particular risk for the development of ischemia and pressure ulcers. Thin patients with cachexia who lack subcutaneous fat are even more susceptible. When they are weak, fatigued, and unable to move around by themselves, the risk of developing one or more pressure ulcers is very high. Shear, friction, prolonged presence of moisture associated with incontinence, age-related changes in skin, and poor nutrition further compound the risk (11).

Pressure ulcers most often develop at body sites where the pressure is highest. In supine patients, 60% of pressure ulcers occur in the sacrum, and the greater trochanter and heel account for a further 15%. In patients who are constantly sitting, the ischial tuberosities are more susceptible (4).

MALIGNANT ULCERS

Malignant wounds occur in up to 10% of patients with advanced or metastatic cancer, usually in the last 6 months of life (12). They can evolve from a primary tumor of skin or an invasive underlying mass, a recurrence along a surgical suture line, or a metastasis. They can be both erosive ulcers and/or expanding nodules. If many nodules confluence, the result can be a cauliflower-like wound. They are most commonly associated with cancers that start in the breast, particularly when they reoccur locally (50% or more). Other common sites include the head and neck (up to 30%) and axilla or groin (approximately 5%) (13–15).

Although a tumor initially stimulates neovascularization, a rapidly growing tumor can outstrip its available blood supply and necrose centrally. When the process involves the skin, it frequently becomes friable and produces significant exudate; becomes malodorous as the tissue putrefies and/or becomes infected with anaerobes; and frequently bleeds.

ASSESSMENT

In any patient with cancer who has developed a wound, or is at risk of developing one, start with a comprehensive assessment of the patient's illness context, risk of developing a pressure ulcer, wound, surrounding skin, blood supply, and frequently associated issues, for example, pain, odor, or "woundedness."

Illness Context

Assess the context of the patient's illness, including her/his cancer type, stage, and prognosis; functional status, for example, Karnofsky or Palliative Performance Scale; nutritional, fluid, and cognitive status; decision-making capacity; and goals of care (Table 26.1).

Pressure Ulcer Risk

The risk of developing a pressure ulcer increases as cancer advances, particularly when patients are debilitated (16). Periodically assess every patient's risk using either a Braden (17) (http://www.bradenscale.com/) or a Norton (18) risk assessment tool. Both tools examine the most significant risk factors for developing a pressure ulcer including sensory

TABLE 26.1	Context assessment
Issue	**Examples**
Cancer type, stage, prognosis	Stage IV breast cancer with metastases to liver, lungs, bone; prognosis 1–2 mo
Comorbidities	Rheumatoid arthritis
	Autoimmune disorders, for example, systemic lupus, vasculitis
Functional status, for example, KPS or PPS	KPS or PPS = 50%
Nutritional/fluid status	Appetite, for example, anorectic
	Degree of cachexia, for example, 20-lb weight loss, albumin 2.1 g/dL
	Mild dehydration with orthostatic hypotension and 1+ pitting ankle edema
Cognitive status	Alert, oriented ×3, normal mini-mental status
Decision-making capacity	Has capacity
Medications that could delay healing	Steroids
	Nonsteroidal anti-inflammatory drugs
	Immunosuppressive medications
Goals of care	Maintain function
	Minimize symptoms
	Interact clearly with family and friends

KPS, Karnofsky performance scale; PPS, palliative performance scale.

TABLE 26.2	Braden pressure ulcer risk assessment			Score
Sensory perception	Completely limited	Very limited	Slightly limited	No impairment
Moisture	Constantly moist	Very moist	Occasionally moist	Rarely moist
Activity	Bedfast	Chairfast	Walks occasionally	Walks frequently
Mobility	Completely immobile	Very limited	Slightly limited	Walks frequently
Nutrition	Very poor	Probably inadequate	Adequate	Excellent
Friction, shear	Problem	Potential problem	No apparent problem	
			Total score:	

>16 = not at risk of developing pressure ulcers; 15–16 = low risk; 13–14 = moderate risk; ≤12 high risk.

perception, moisture, activity, mobility, nutrition, and friction/shear (Table 26.2, a simplification of the Braden Pressure Ulcer Risk Assessment tool—for complete details, refer to the original tool).

Once a wound develops, assess the following:

1. *The wound*, including the type (etiology), location (Fig. 26.1), duration, description of the structure and base/surface, dimensions—best to document with a labeled photograph or diagram (Fig. 26.2), exudate, and bleeding (Table 26.3). Observe old dressings for strikethrough (i.e., drainage on the outside of an old dressing) and then remove the dressing slowly, starting from the edges. If dressings adhere to the wound surface, moisten them with normal saline or water to reduce adherence and facilitate removal. If you can anticipate that there will be pain or if there is any pain during the removal process, before continuing start on preemptive anesthesia/analgesia until the patient is comfortable (discussed later in this chapter).
2. *The surrounding skin*, including contamination, maceration, signs of infection, and edema (Table 26.4).
3. *The blood supply*, particularly in lower extremity wounds (Table 26.5).
4. *The frequently associated issues*, for example, odor, pain, "woundedness," anxiety, and depression (Table 26.6).

STAGING

Pressure Ulcers

To help determine the management plan, the National Pressure Ulcer Advisory Panel/Agency for Health Care Policy and Research (NPUAP/AHCPR) developed a system that is widely used to stage pressure ulcers (20).

- *Suspected Deep Tissue Injury.* Purple or maroon localized area of discolored intact skin or blood-filled blister due to damage of underlying soft tissue from pressure and/or shear. The area may be preceded by tissue that is painful, firm, mushy, boggy, warmer or cooler as compared with the adjacent tissue. Evolution to a stage III or IV may be rapid.
- *Stage I.* The heralding lesion of skin ulceration is non-blanchable erythema of intact skin usually over a bony prominence. In darker skin, the erythema may appear as persistent blue or purplish discoloration.
- *Stage II.* Partial thickness skin loss involving epidermis, dermis, or both. The ulcer is superficial and looks like an abrasion, a shallow crater, or an open or ruptured blister.
- *Stage III.* Full thickness skin loss involving subcutaneous tissue. The ulcer may extend down to, but not through, the underlying fascia. The ulcer looks like a deep crater, with or without undermining or tunneling of adjacent tissue (i.e., skin that overhangs wound edges).
- *Stage IV.* The ulcer is deep enough to include necrosis and damage to underlying muscle, bone, and/or other supporting structures such as the tendon or joint capsule. Undermining of adjacent skin and sinus tracts or fistula is often present.
- Unstageable, depth unknown.

Monitoring wound progress over time can be accomplished with the Pressure Ulcer Scale for Healing tool, a validated scale that gives a score based on wound size, amount of exudate, and tissue type (21).

Malignant Wounds

There is no specific staging system for malignant wounds.

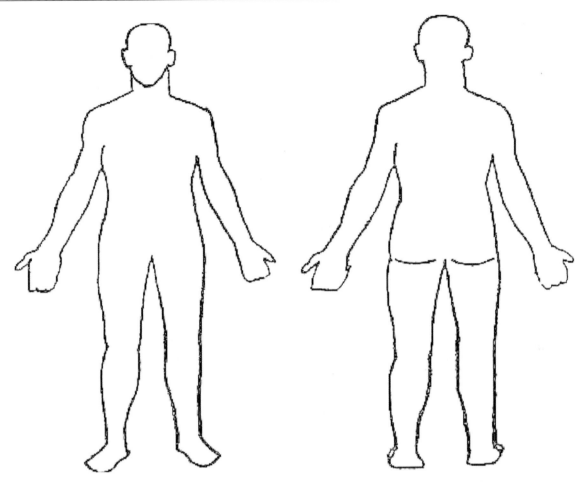

Figure 26.1. Wound location. Mark the location of each wound on the body diagrams. Label sites as A, B, C, D.

MANAGEMENT

If patients who are at risk of developing a pressure ulcer, or those who are in the process of developing one, are caught early and appropriate prevention and treatment initiated, progression can be arrested and significant morbidity preempted.

Interdisciplinary

Wound care always involves an interdisciplinary team that includes a nurse and physician at a minimum and may include an enterostomal therapist who is an expert in wound care, a pharmacist, a social worker, a chaplain, a physiotherapist, and a dietitian, especially when the patient's issues are more complex.

Establish Goals of Care

To develop an effective plan of care, start with effective communication with the patient or her/his surrogate decision maker about the context of the patient's illness, the patient's personal goals of care, and possible therapeutic options including their benefits and risks of harm and burden. Carefully guide a decision-making and treatment-planning process that involves the patient, her/his family, and caregivers.

For patients with pressure ulcers, if the blood supply to the surrounding tissues is adequate (i.e., dorsalis pedis and/or posterior tibial pulses are palpable or ankle brachial index (ABI) >0.5 or toe arterial pressure >40 mm Hg), it may be possible to heal the wound. For many patients with advanced cancer and a short prognosis, it is unrealistic to strive to heal a pressure ulcer. For such patients, it is much more appropriate to focus on stabilizing the wound, relieving interface pressure to prevent further progression, and managing associated symptoms.

For patients with malignant wounds, if it is not possible to treat the underlying cancer, it will not be possible to heal a malignant wound.

PRESSURE ULCERS—WHEN THE GOAL IS TO HEAL

When the goal is to heal a pressure ulcer, management involves conventional wound care strategies (22,23).

1. Optimize nutritional status.
2. Start by reducing the interface pressure.
3. Prepare the wound bed. Cleanse, debride when there is necrotic tissue or slough with preemptive anesthesia/analgesia, and control infection and bleeding (24–27).

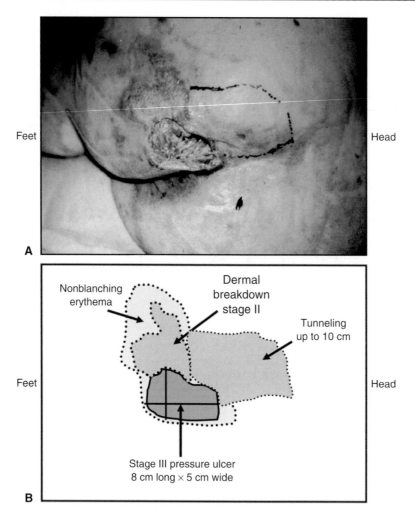

Figure 26.2. Description of a sacral pressure ulcer. Photograph or trace the circumference of the wound and damage to surrounding skin onto a transparency or plastic page protector, including areas of tracking or tunneling (indicating measurements, usually in centimeters). Use plastic wrap next to the skin to avoid bacterial or body fluid contamination.

4. Dress the wound to promote moist interactive wound healing. If there is a risk of significant shearing, tearing, or regular contamination with exudate, urine, or stool that could cause maceration, protect surrounding skin.
5. Pack all dead spaces to keep them open and draining.
6. Layer dressings.
7. Finally, manage all associated issues, including pain, odors, and the patient's "woundedness."

Fluids, Electrolytes, and Nutrition

Patients may be able to tolerate frequent small meals or between-meal supplements, particularly if the diet is liberalized and accommodates personal food preferences. Enforcing dietary restrictions such as sodium restrictions may not be appropriate.

- Calories: provide 30 to 35 kcal/kg/d
- Hydration: ensure adequate electrolyte-containing fluid intake noting that hypervolemia can delay healing. Strive for euvolemia
- Protein: daily allowance of up to 1.5 g/kg/d may delay onset of pressure ulcers and promote healing

- Vitamins: deficiency of vitamin C and zinc can delay healing, but there is little evidence to support routine supplementation. If diet is poor in fruits and vegetables and deficiency suspected or confirmed, offer a mineral and vitamin supplement.

Reduce Interface Pressure

Continuous pressure, particularly over bony prominences, increases the risk of ischemia, skin breakdown, and pain (11). Pressure ulcers can develop within hours if the patient is not moved and circulation remains compromised.

Pressure at an interface is the force per unit area that acts perpendicularly between the body and the support surface. This parameter is affected by the stiffness of the support surface, the composition of the body tissue, and the geometry of the body being supported (16).

- Pressure reduction is a therapeutic strategy to reduce the interface pressure, not necessarily below capillary-closing pressure.
- Pressure relief is a therapeutic strategy to reduce the interface pressure below capillary-closing pressure (28,29).

TABLE 26.3	**Wound assessment**
	Examples
Type of wound (etiology)	Pressure, malignant cavitating or fungating, chemotherapy extravasation, radiation reaction, diabetic, neurotrophic, arterial, venous, acute surgical, acute trauma
Location	Precise location, ideally placing the wound on a body diagram (Fig. 22.1)
Duration	How long the patient has had it
Description of pressure ulcer	Nonblanching erythema of dermis, no breakdown or disruption of epidermis Dermal breakdown Cavity with breakdown extending to subcutaneous fat, muscle, bone
Description of malignant fungating wound	Nodular, cauliflower, cavitating Percent necrosis
Base/surface	Color, for example, black if eschar, red if granulation tissue, or yellow if fibrous tissue or slough Friability, for example, tissue breaking down on contact Exposed structures, for example, tendon, nerve, major blood vessel
Dimensions (Fig. 22.1)	Greatest vertical (head to toe) and horizontal dimensions at right angles Greatest depth of open wound using a probe, or height of a raised fungating wound Depth of any tracks (e.g., overhanging skin) or tunnels that extend underneath the skin through soft tissue and either dead end (e.g., sinus tracts) or open onto the skin in another location (e.g., fistula)
Exudate	Color, for example, serous, sanguineous, serosanguineous Purulence Volume, for example, none, mild, moderate, copious
Bleeding	Oozing or frank bleeding
Strikethrough, that is, drainage on the outside of an old dressing	Color, for example, serous, sanguineous, serosanguineous Purulence Volume, for example, spotting, soaked

In patients with advanced cancer, particularly those who are debilitated, and patients with wounds, implement as many strategies to reduce, if not relieve, the interface pressure as much as possible, including repositioning, turning, massaging, supporting, protecting, and avoiding rolling and bunching of bedsheets and dressings.

Position

To minimize sacral pressure in patients who are bedridden, keep the head of the bed as low as possible, ideally at <30°. Raise it only for short periods of social interaction or use foam wedges to support the patient. Avoid resting one limb on another. Use a

pillow or another cushioning support to keep legs apart. Protect bony prominences with hydrocolloid dressings.

Turn

When a patient is unable to move by herself/himself, turn the patient from side to side every 1.5 to 2 hours. In addition to reducing pressure, this helps to relieve joint position fatigue in immobilized patients. Use a careful "log-roll" technique to distribute forces evenly across the patient's body and minimize pain on movement. Use a draw sheet to reduce shearing forces that could lead to skin tears. If turning is painful, turn the patient less frequently and/or place the patient on

TABLE 26.4	Surrounding skin assessment
Contamination	Urine, stool
Maceration due to excess moisture	White hyperkeratosis
	Wet surface
Signs of infection	Erythema, warmth, tenderness
Edema	Type, for example, pitting, nonpitting
	Volume, for example, mild, moderate, severe

a pressure-reducing surface, for example, air mattress or airbed. As patients approach death, the need for turning lessens as the risk of skin breakdown becomes less important.

Massage

Massage intermittently to stimulate circulation, shift edema, spread out moisturizing lotions, and provide comfort. This is particularly helpful in dependent areas subject to increased pressure, before and after turning. Avoid massaging skin that is erythematous or broken down.

Support

Therapeutic support surfaces that reduce or relieve pressure include specialty mattresses/beds, chairs, wheelchairs, and positioning devices.

Foam Pads

Simple foam pads are often ineffective. If they are used, they may need to be layered so that they are at least 6″ to 8″ thick. If the pressure has been reduced adequately, when a hand is

placed under a pad at the lowest point of the patient's body, for example, under the buttocks, there will be at least 1″ of noncompressed foam between the hand and the patient.

Three groups of mattresses/beds have demonstrated efficacy:

- *Group 1.* Air or water mattress overlays reduce pressure. If employed early enough in any patient who is bed-bound, has limited mobility, or is cachectic, they will help prevent pressure ulcers.
- *Group 2.* Low-air-loss beds are used for any patient who is at high risk of developing a pressure ulcer or for a patient who has developed an ulcer already and the goal is to prevent worsening and/or promote healing.
- *Group 3.* Air-fluidized beds are reserved for patients who need pressure relief. However, patients frequently describe them as overly confining (even "coffin-like"). They are also very expensive.

Cushions

For chairs and wheelchairs, there are a number of pressure-reducing cushions. For chairfast patients who need to use a chair or a wheelchair for a prolonged time, it may be more

TABLE 26.5	Blood supply assessment of extremities		
Dorsalis pedis or posterior tibial pulses	If palpable, systolic pressure is ≈80 mm Hg or greater and perfusion is adequate to facilitate healing.		
Doppler ABI = ankle systolic pressure/ brachial systolic pressure (19) (e.g., 80 mm Hg/100 mm Hg = 0.8)	**ABI**	**Toe Arterial Pressure (mm Hg)**	**Risk of Not Healing**
	>0.8	55	Low
	>0.6	>40	Moderate (adequate perfusion)
	>0.4	>20	High (inadequate perfusion)
	<0.4	<20	Severe
Transcutaneous partial oxygen saturation	>30% indicates adequate perfusion		
Toe arterial pressures (photoplethysmography)	>40 mm Hg indicates adequate perfusion		

ABI, ankle brachial index.

TABLE 26.6	Associated issues
Odor	Fruity or foul smelling
	Just under dressing or throughout the room
Pain (describe for each major site)	Location
	Type, for example, nociceptive, neuropathic, mixed
	Temporal profile, for example, constant, breakthrough, intermittent acute
	Severity, for example, 3/10 on a visual analogue scale
	Effect of medications (benefit and adverse effects, e.g., drowsiness, nausea, constipation)
Anxiety	See Chapter 40
Depression	See Chapter 40
"Woundedness"	Psychological state
	Body image
	Fear

effective to have them assessed professionally for customized pressure-reducing cushions. Never use round cushions commonly called *donuts*. They redistribute pressure without relieving it.

Protect

Protect thin, fragile skin from friction, moisture, and shear to minimize the risk of skin tears. This is particularly important in cachectic patients who have lost the elasticity and resilience effect previously provided by their collagen and subcutaneous fat. Zinc oxide cream or paste can protect the skin from moisture and shearing forces. Thin films will reduce shearing forces. Hydrocolloid dressings will add a cushioning effect.

Caution

Be sure that bedsheets do not wrinkle and dressings do not ripple under the patient, as both will produce new pressure points that could lead to ulceration if sustained, particularly in patients with cachexia.

Cleanse

Prepare the wound bed by cleansing and rinsing away exudate, slough, and debris. Although it may be acceptable to use relatively cytotoxic fluids to clean intact skin, for example, hydrogen peroxide, povidone iodine, or sodium hypochlorite, avoid using them in the wound. Although they decrease bacterial burden, they will be cytotoxic to granulation tissue and delay healing (30).

When choosing a wound cleanser, a useful rule of thumb is "don't put anything into the wound that you wouldn't put into your eye." Unpreserved normal (physiologic) saline or sterile water are the preferred wound cleansers. Although both can be purchased commercially, saline can also be prepared on the stove-top at home. Mix two teaspoons (10 ml) salt in four cups (1 qt or L) water; boil on the stove 3 to 20 minutes; cool to room temperature; do not store more than 72 hours. Alternately, use a commercially available wound cleanser with as little cytotoxicity as possible.

Cleanse the wound gently to avoid flushing away migrating epithelial cells or damaging normal tissues using one of the following four techniques:

1. Soak or compress the wound with a saline-moistened gauze.
2. Gently pour the cleanser over the wound.
3. Irrigate the wound with a piston or bulb syringe that delivers 5 to 8 pounds per square inch (PSI) pressure or, to remove slough or eschar, irrigate with an 18G to 20G Angiocath on a 30 to 60 ml syringe held 4″ to 6″ from the wound, which delivers 5 to 15 PSI pressure.
4. Use a commercial spray wound cleanser with a predetermined PSI pressure. If there is any pain, stop cleansing, start on preemptive anesthesia/analgesia until the patient is comfortable, and then continue cleansing.

Maintain good hygiene on surrounding skin using unpreserved normal saline or sterile water, or with a more cytotoxic fluid or commercially available skin cleanser.

Debride

Necrotic tissue (eschar or slough) and contaminated and foreign material can delay wound healing and harbor infections. Optimal wound healing will not occur until these are removed. If there is significant necrotic tissue or slough, and the blood supply to the surround tissue is adequate for healing to occur, that is, ABI > 0.5, after cleansing the wound to remove debris, debride as much of the necrotic and contaminated tissue as possible and expose dead spaces. Where possible, debride down to a bleeding base. This converts a chronic wound into an acute wound and decreases surface bacterial burden.

Choose from the available debridement techniques, for example, surgical/sharp, autolytic, enzymatic/chemical, mechanical, or larval, on the basis of a thorough assessment of wound and the goals of care for the patient (Table 26.7). If there is associated gangrene, delay debridement until a line of demarcation between healthy and necrotic tissue develops. Avoid blood vessels, nerves, tendons, or other underlying structures. If using surgical or mechanical debridement, instigate preemptive anesthesia/analgesia beforehand.

Control Infection

All wounds are colonized by bacteria, fungi, and other infective agents, but this does not mean they are infected. *Staphylococcus epidermidis* and *Corynebacterium* are the most common colonizers of wounds. *Proteus*, *Klebsiella*, *Pseudomonas*, and *Candida* commonly infect wounds, particularly when there is recurring contamination with urine or feces or immunocompromise.

If present in sufficient quantities, the wound and the surrounding tissue may become infected. Healing can be delayed significantly. Purulent exudates, pain, and/or foul odors may be the first signs of local infection. If the odor is fruity and the wound has a greenish tinge, the wound is likely infected with pseudomonal organisms. If the odor is foul/putrid, it is likely infected with anaerobic bacteria.

If the goal is to heal the wound, establishing when a wound has become infected to the point that the bacterial burden impacts healing can be difficult. A careful swab technique to obtain meaningful samples is most important to gain useful cultures. First, cleanse the wound with normal saline or water, remove all debris and superficial organisms as they are not significant pathogens in wound infections and need to be washed off before culturing. Then swab healthy-appearing granulation tissue in a zigzag pattern, gently rotating the tip of the swab, obtaining specimens for both aerobic and anaerobic cultures. If the wound is dry, premoisten the tip of the swab with a little culture media. If, after culturing swab samples, the cause remains elusive, consider culturing a biopsy from the wound bed.

If the infection is superficial, cleanse the wound with saline or water and apply a topical antibiotic with each change of dressing (Table 26.8) (36). If there is infection in the surrounding tissues or if wound healing is delayed, add a systemic antibiotic until the infection is cleared. If there is obvious candidal growth or a lot of crusting, mix a topical antifungal, for example, ketoconazole, with the topical antibiotic or alternate them. If the ulcer probes to bone, suspect osteomyelitis and consider 4 to 6 weeks of systemic antibiotics.

Honey and yogurt may also be very effective topical antibacterials, even when they are diluted (37). Use only honey that has been irradiated to ensure that it is free of clostridium spores.

Control Bleeding

Bleeding is much more of a problem in malignant wounds than in pressure ulcers. If dressings adhere to the wound surface, moisten the dressing with normal saline or water to reduce adherence and facilitate removal. If uncontrolled bleeding occurs in a pressure ulcer, management strategies are the same as those for malignant wounds (see the Section Malignant Wounds).

Dress the Wound and Surrounding Tissue

This section aims to present the principles and suggest a strategy for dressing chronic wounds, not recommend specific dressings. Any reference to commercial products is only to illustrate a point, not to recommend particular products. Contact manufacturers for detailed information about their products and how to use them.

If healing is the goal of pressure ulcer management, the epithelial cells and fibroblasts that must proliferate to form granulation tissue and fill in the wound require a moist environment that is rich in oxygen and the nutrients necessary to sustain their replication and migration. At the same time, the environment must protect the wound, control excessive exudate, and minimize exposure to infective microorganisms that can inhibit healing. By contrast, a dry environment is conducive to necrosis and eschar, and not to healing.

There are seven classes of dressing: foams, alginates, hydrogels, hydrocolloids, films, gauze, and nonstick dressings (Table 26.9). They are distinguished by their absorbency, wear time, and occlusiveness. Within each class, specific products also vary by size, user friendliness, cost/accessibility, adhesive used, and impact on the wound margin and surrounding skin. As studies of different types of moist wound dressings showed no difference in pressure ulcer healing outcomes, use clinical judgment to select a type of dressing most appropriate for a given wound (38,39).

To hold dressings in place, there are a wide range of tapes and stocking products that use varying adhesives and may result in different hypersensitivity reactions.

Dressing Strategy

If healing is the goal, use a dressing strategy that enables the following:

1. *Keep the wound bed continuously moist.* A dry wound needs to have moisture given to it through a hypotonic gel (donates water). If there is excessive wet exudates, a hypertonic gel, alginate, or foam will remove fluids from the wound.
2. *Control exudate.* This should be done without desiccating the wound bed. Wound exudates can be substantial, especially from stage IV pressure ulcers and malignant wounds. When there are copious exudates, consider uncontrolled edema or increased bacterial burden or infection as possible causes (40).

Both foams and alginates can absorb fluids that are many times heavier and effectively remove copious exudates

TABLE 26.7	Debridement techniques

Technique	Mechanism	Precautions	Comments
Surgical/sharp	Use of curved scissors, curette, or scalpel	Make sure there is adequate blood supply for healing to occur: ABI > 0.5 Toe pressure >40 mm Hg Transcutaneous oxygen saturation >30%	Fastest, most effective technique for large areas of necrosis, a high degree of contamination, or frank infection Requires a skilled clinician Manage procedural pain with preemptive anesthesia (e.g., topical lidocaine cream or spray, EMLA)
Autolytic	Use of moist interactive dressings (e.g., hydrogels, hydrocolloids, alginates, films) to liquefy necrotic tissue	Remove as much loose debris as possible when changing dressings (usually q24–48h initially)	Gentlest technique. Results should be seen within 72 h Occlusive dressings facilitate autolysis by maintaining a moist environment Monitor for overhydration and infection
Enzymic/chemical	Use of collagenase or papain to digest damaged collagen, but not newly formed granulation tissue	Bacterial infection and bacteremia can occur. Detergents, bleach, hexachlorophene, and heavy metals (e.g., silver, mercury) may inactivate enzymes	Faster than autolytic debridement (31). To facilitate the process, score eschar without causing bleeding Do not use on normal or granulation tissue. Enzymes do not facilitate the granulation and re-epithelialization phases of wound care. They may damage normal tissues
Mechanical	Use of gentle irrigation to remove necrotic tissue. Use an 18–20G Angiocath on a 30–60 ml syringe to keep pressure under 15 PSI	Excessive force may flush away migrating epithelial cells or damage normal tissue	Saline wet-to-dry gauze dressings, irrigation, and whirlpool therapy are alternate mechanical debriding techniques. The latter is not recommended as it may cause pain or bleeding and damage normal or granulation tissue that sticks to the dry gauze when the dressing is removed
Larval	Use of larvae to consume necrotic tissue (32–35)	Use larvae cultured for this purpose Enclose them within the wound. Monitor their activity closely. Remove them between 48 and 72 h	Relatively rapid technique to debride large volumes of necrotic tissue May be offensive to patients, families, or staff Generally painless

ABI, ankle brachial index; EMLA, eutectic mixture of long-acting anesthetics; PSI, pounds per square inch.

| TABLE 26.8 | Common topical antibacterial agents |

Agent	Staphylococcus aureus	MRSA	Streptococcus	Pseudomonas	Anaerobes	Comments
Cadexomer iodine dressing	√	√	√	√	√	Microspheres of starch cross-linked with ether bridges and iodine
						Absorbs up to seven times its weight in moisture
						Slowly releases iodine for antibacterial action without being cytotoxic to epithelial cells
						Caution with thyroid disease, iodine allergy
Ionized silver dressings	√	√	√	√	√	Slowly releases silver
						Decreases surface friability
						Must be used with sterile water, not saline (which precipitates the silver as inactive silver chloride)
Fusidic acid cream/ointment	√	—	√	—	—	Lanolin in ointment base may act as a sensitizer
Gentamicin cream/ointment	√	—	√	√	—	—
Metronidazole gel/cream	—	—	—	—	√	Good penetration and wound deodorizer
Polymyxin B sulfate—bacitracin zinc	√	√	√	√	√	Broad spectrum; low cost
Polymyxin B sulfate—bacitracin zinc—neomycin	√	√	√	√	√	Neomycin is a potent sensitizer; may cross-sensitize to other aminoglycosides
Silver sulfadiazine	√	—	√	√	—	Do not use in sulfa-sensitive individuals

MRSA, methicillin-resistant *Staphylococcus aureus*; √, use.

TABLE 26.9 **Dressings**

Class	Absorbency	Wear time	Types	Comments
1. Foams	4+/4	24 h–7 d	Mesh sponges	Ideal for copious exudate May macerate surrounding skin Either protect the surrounding skin with petrolatum or zinc oxide ointment or cut the foam to the inside dimensions of the wound and wick the exudate to secondary dressings
2. Alginates	3+/4	12–48 or more hours	Sheets, ribbons, or ropes	Seaweed derivative Hemostatic Rope wicks vertically—ideal for packing tracks and tunnels Convert to gel on contact with fluid; can wash off in the shower
3. Hydrogels	Variable, depending on the tonicity of the gel	24–72 h	Several different bases used in different products, for example, hydrocolloid, propylene glycol, sodium chloride	Facilitate autolytic debridement Use to hydrate
4. Hydrocolloids	Minimal 1–2+/4	24–48 h for debridement 3–7 d for protection	Millimeter-thick pads consisting of a membrane or other backing with a hydrophilic layer (e.g., gelatin, pectin) and a hydrophobic layer (e.g., carboxymethylcellulose) Gelatin layer liquefies on contact with fluids, minimizing trauma on removal Usually self-adhesive	Facilitate autolytic debridement Protect bony prominences and areas of potential skin breakdown Occlusive barrier for fluids (e.g., urine, feces) and for showering and swimming Occasional allergies to adhesives Must avoid leakage channels, which can introduce bacteria, and rippling, which can result in new pressure points

(Continued)

TABLE 26.9 Dressings (Continued)			
Class	**Absorbency**	**Wear time**	**Types**	**Comments**
5. Transparent films/membranes	None	Up to 7 d	Both adhesive and nonadhesive films	Protect fragile skin from shearing and tearing
				Permit visualization
				Oxygen permeable
				Facilitate re-epithelialization
				Avoid leakage channels, which can introduce bacteria
				Barrier for showering and swimming
6. Gauze	Variable 1–2+/4	Variable, depending on strikethrough Up to 7 d	Pads, tapes, nets	Ideal outer dressings Hold dressing in place Cosmetic
7. Nonstick	None	Up to 7 d	Petroleum-coated pads, inert pads, inert mesh	Facilitate nonadherence
8. Silicone mesh	None	Indefinite	—	Apply as a second skin. Can use topical treatments over mesh

from the environment of the wound. By wicking the exudate away from the wound and surrounding skin, the risk of infection and maceration is minimized. By containing the fluid within the dressing, it will not drip onto clothes and bedsheets and it will be more cosmetically pleasing for everyone. Change dressings once strikethrough is present, that is, leakage through to the outside of the dressing.

3. *Keep surrounding skin dry.* In addition to cleansing surrounding skin, zinc oxide or barrier creams or sprays may help protect the skin from prolonged contact or contamination with fluids, for example, exudates, urine, or feces. Some sprays may also increase adherence of adjacent dressing. When the risk is expected to be ongoing, thin film or hydrocolloid dressings placed around the wound with a cutout for the wound dressings can provide further protection (41).

4. *Eliminate dead space.* Loosely fill all cavities with nonadherent dressing materials, for example, alginates or hydrogel-soaked gauze.

5. *Consider caregiver time, skill, and burden.* Wound care can be burdensome. Do not create a plan that is not physically or financially possible for the patient and caregivers to adhere to.

6. *Monitor dressings applied near the anus.* Dressings close to the anus/perineum tend to move and bunch up under the tremendous friction and shearing forces in the sacral area.

7. *Dress in layers.* As no single dressing will meet all these criteria, use a layered approach for dressing a wound. The primary or first layer goes next to the surface of the wound. It can include a hydrogel, an antibiotic, and/or thromboplastin. Subsequent layers rest one on top of the other. Finally, the top or outer layer typically holds the dressing in place and serves as the "aesthetic" covering. There is no minimum or maximum number of layers. Build the best possible combination for the patient's situation on the basis of your clinical judgment.

Although dressing changes may be initially needed once or even twice daily to control infections and remove copious exudate, as the exudate and infection settle and the wound stabilizes, the frequency of dressing changes may be reduced (even to once or twice per week).

Examples

The dressing of stages I to IV pressure ulcers varies considerably. The following examples illustrate the range of strategies that are possible.

Stage I and II Pressure Ulcers

Dry stage I and II pressure ulcers are typically dressed with a transparent film placed directly on the surface of the wound to protect it from contact or irritation. It forms a semiocclusive barrier to the environment. A film dressing is typically changed every 3 to 5 days (42). Exercise caution when removing it. A strong adhesive can easily lead to tearing of fragile skin. If you are having difficulties removing the dressing, use an adhesive remover to facilitate the process.

When there is limited exudate, a hydrocolloid placed directly on the wound will more effectively absorb the exudate. It forms an occlusive barrier and a moist internal environment to facilitate autolysis and healing. If there is mild necrosis, use a two-layered approach:

1. *Primary dressing (next to the wound).* Apply hydrogel to stimulate autolysis.
2. *Second dressing.* Place a hydrocolloid to form an occlusive barrier and facilitate autolysis and healing.

Hydrocolloid dressings are typically changed every 3 to 7 days or sooner if leakage occurs. Exercise caution when removing them. Their strong adhesive can easily lead to tearing of fragile skin. If you are having difficulties removing the dressing, use an adhesive remover to facilitate the process.

Stage III and IV Pressure Ulcers

Stage III and IV pressure ulcers are often much more complex to dress, depending on their configuration and the involvement of surrounding tissues. As an example, for a newly diagnosed dry stage IV pressure ulcer with tunneling that is infected, has a foul odor, and is somewhat friable and oozing blood, use a four-layered approach:

1. *Primary layer (next to the wound).* Isotonic hydrogel with an antimicrobial against anaerobes, for example, metronidazole.
2. *Second layer.* Alginate for its bacteriostatic properties, ease of conforming to the structure of the wound, and tendency to turn to gel on contact with fluids, thereby minimizing trauma to the wound surface and washing off easily.
3. *Third layer.* Cotton gauze or an abdominal pad to contain and protect the underlying dressing.
4. *Fourth (outer) layer.* Tape to hold the outer dressing layer in place.

For a particularly friable, bleeding wound, the layering might start with an inert nonadherent mesh dressing placed on the surface of the wound to protect the surface from trauma during repeated dressing changes.

Adjuvant Therapies

In addition to standard wound preparation and dressing strategies, for more challenging wounds, there are a number of adjunctive therapies that could help stimulate the granulation process, for example, vacuum-assisted closure (VAC) therapy (see http://www.kci1.com/35.asp), warm-up therapy, and electrostimulation. You can read more about these therapies online, or in Krasner's *Chronic Wound Care III* textbook (4).

PRESSURE ULCERS—WHEN THE GOAL IS TO STABILIZE

When the goal is not to heal a pressure ulcer, the plan of care is based on the assessment of the wound and the surrounding tissues.

Assess and stage the pressure ulcer as discussed earlier.

Management

Reduce Interface Pressure

Always reduce the interface pressure using the techniques described earlier. This will minimize the risk of further progression of the existing pressure ulcers and reduce the risk that new ulcers will develop.

Cleanse, Debride, Dress

Dry Wounds. If the wound is covered with a dry eschar and there is no sign of pain, odor, or infection in the wound, the eschar, or the surrounding tissues, leave the wound alone. The dry eschar may be the most effective barrier against infections. Cleansing or debriding will only soften and ultimately remove the eschar, exposing the underlying tissues to an increased risk of infection and creating the need for routine dressing changes. To reduce bacterial burden, intermittently paint the eschar and the surrounding tissues with an aseptic iodine solution and let it air-dry. While it is contraindicated for healing wounds, the cytotoxicity of iodine can minimize the risk of infection and the need for a more complex wound management strategy (25).

If the wound needs to be covered to protect it, or for aesthetic reasons, cover it with a nonstick, nonocclusive dressing.

Wet Wound. If the wound is open, wet, or infected in the wound bed or surrounding tissues, pursue a conservative wound management strategy to stabilize the wound; control infection, exudate, odors and bleeding; and maintain the best possible body image.

MALIGNANT WOUNDS

The management of malignant wounds is basically the same as for advanced pressure ulcers (12–15,43,44).

For some patients, antineoplastic treatments may offer significant palliation of the symptoms associated with a malignant wound. Radiation therapy may decrease bleeding, pain, and exudate. Chemotherapy or hormonal therapy may even promote wound healing in patients with responsive disease.

Assessment, Staging

Use the same assessment tool (Table 26.1). There is no specific staging system for malignant wounds.

Management

Establish Goals of Care

Ensure that everyone is clear about the goals of care. If there exists chemotherapy or radiation therapy that could treat the underlying cancer and cause it to shrink or disappear, it may be possible to heal the malignant wound. Otherwise, if there is no effective therapy for the underlying disease, there will be no possibility for the wound to heal. Focus goals on stabilizing the wound; controlling infection, exudate, odors, and bleeding; and maintaining the best possible body image.

Reduce Interface Pressure

To minimize the risk of developing or extending any pressure ulcers, particularly in cachectic, debilitated patients with cancer who are chairfast or bedridden, reduce the interface pressure as much as possible by repositioning, turning, massaging, supporting on pressure-reducing surfaces, protecting, and avoiding rolling and bunching of bedsheets and dressings as outlined earlier.

Cleanse

To remove necrotic debris and exudate, flush gently with normal saline or water at low pressures, as underlying necrotic tissue may be friable and bleed easily. Avoid cytotoxic wound cleansers.

Maintain good hygiene on surrounding skin using unpreserved normal saline or sterile water, or with a more cytotoxic fluid or commercially available skin cleanser.

Debride

Debride using autolysis or a very gentle surgical/sharp technique. Cautiously remove as much of the putrefying necrotic tissue that may be infected as possible, particularly if there is an associated foul odor. Use caution when approaching the tumor surface that may be friable, painful, and bleed easily, particularly if there is a lot of neovascularization close to the surface.

Control Infection

Most frequently, anaerobes infect the necrotic tissues and slough associated with a malignant wound and produce a foul/putrid odor and a purulent exudate. If the infection is superficial, cleanse the wound with normal saline or water, debride cautiously, and apply a topical antibiotic with each dressing change (Table 26.8) (36). Metronidazole and silver sulfadiazine are the preferred antimicrobials to control anaerobic infections in tumors. They will usually control superficial infections within 5 to 7 days. If the infection is deep into the tumor or invades surrounding tissues, add systemic metronidazole 250 to 500 mg p.o. or i.v. q8h until the infection clears. Caution patients not to drink alcohol while receiving metronidazole. If there is obvious candidal growth or a lot of crusting, mix a topical antifungal, for example, ketoconazole, with the topical antibiotic or alternate them.

Control Bleeding

Bleeding is a common problem in malignant wounds. As tumors outgrow their blood supply, their surfaces become friable, coagulation is frequently impaired, and they become predisposed to oozing from microvascular fragmentation or frank bleeding if a small or large blood vessel is involved.

Dressings may adhere to the wound and tear the surface when the dressing is removed. For this reason, saline wet-to-dry gauze dressings are contraindicated in the management of malignant wounds. If dressings adhere to the wound surface, moisten them with normal saline or water to reduce adherence and facilitate removal. Remove each dressing slowly, starting from the edges. If you can anticipate that there will be pain or if there is any pain during the removal process, before continuing start on preemptive anesthesia/analgesia until the patient is comfortable (discussed later in this chapter).

When wound surfaces are particularly friable, apply an inert, nonstick, nonabsorbent silicone mesh, for example, Mepitel, as the first dressing layer. This does not need to be removed, and other dressings can be changed routinely with much less risk of tissue disruption and bleeding.

If oozing is significant, during each dressing change apply 5 to 10 ml of low-dose topical thromboplastin as a spray across the wound surface to stimulate coagulation (the 100 or 1,000 units/ml solution is as effective as higher concentration solutions and is less expensive). A 0.5% to 1% silver nitrate solution may be equally effective. Antifibrinolytics, such as topical aminocaproic acid, are occasionally used, although their role is not clear because fibrinolysis is not a major mechanism in wound bleeding.

Other hemostatic agents include Mohs paste (zinc chloride paste) which can be dabbed over large areas. Tranexamic acid 500 mg in 10 ml can be applied to gauze pad and used to apply gentle pressure to the bleeding wound. This can be reapplied three times a day if needed.

Alginate dressings are hemostatic and can be left in place as the primary dressing layer for several days. They turn to jelly on absorbing fluids from the wound and are easily washed off, even in the shower, with minimal trauma to the wound surface. Hemostatic surgical sponges may be equally effective.

A short course of high dose per fraction palliative radiation therapy (typically 250 to 800 cGy/fraction/d) will sclerose most vessels and stop bleeding from a malignant wound in just a few days (45).

For frank bleeding, try silver nitrate sticks and electrocautery and/or apply gentle pressure for 10 to 15 minutes. Interventional radiology may be able to stop bleeding from a larger blood vessel by sclerosing it.

In all situations where bleeding is a significant risk, discuss the situation with the patient, family, and caregivers and decide on how and in what setting everyone will cope with a major catastrophic bleed. If bleeding occurs uncontrollably, dark towels lessen the sight of blood and reduce anxiety of the family, caregiver, and staff. If the patient is aware and distressed by the protracted bleeding, sedation with a rapid-acting benzodiazepine (e.g., midazolam or lorazepam) may be warranted.

Dress the Wound and Surrounding Tissues

Follow the same dressing principles outlined in the preceding text for pressure ulcers. Layer the dressings in a manner similar to the approach used for a stage III or IV pressure ulcer.

1. Keep the malignant wound continuously moist. Do not let a necrotic wound surface dry out. It will be much more susceptible to cracking, bleeding, and infection with anaerobes and candida.
2. Control exudate in a manner similar to pressure ulcers. When there are copious exudates (e.g., malignant fistulae from the gastrointestinal tract), stomal appliances or suction devices such as VAC therapy may be needed to cope with the volume (see http://www.kci1.com/35.asp).
3. Keep surrounding skin dry in a manner similar to pressure ulcers.
4. Eliminate dead space by filling it with nonadherent dressing materials.
5. Consider caregiver time, skill, and burden. Care for a malignant wound with copious exudate or bleeding can be burdensome and psychologically difficult, particularly when the wound is in the head and neck area. Health-care professionals and family caregivers will need a lot of skill building and support to ensure that they adhere to the plan of care effectively.
6. Monitor dressings applied near the anus. They tend to move and bunch up under the tremendous friction and shearing forces in the sacral area.
7. Dress in layers. Use the same layered technique as for advanced pressure ulcers. Hydrogels and alginates are ideal for friable malignant wounds as they liquefy when they absorb fluids and can be washed off easily, even in the shower. Alginates are also hemostatic and conform easily to the many crevices and contours of a malignant wound. Other nonstick dressing, for example, Telfa, will protect and minimize the trauma to a dry malignant wound when the dressing is changed. Ensure that the outer layer is fashioned to optimize the aesthetics for the patient and the family.

ASSOCIATE ISSUES

Odor

Odor emanating from wounds is caused by putrefying tissue and/or infection. When the odor is fruity and there is a green tinge on the wound surface, it is likely emanating from a pseudomonas infection. When the odor is foul/putrid, it is caused by an anaerobic infection in necrotic tissue.

Foul odor can be very distressing to the patient, family, and caregivers. It can lead to embarrassment, depression, and social isolation (46).

Odor management includes the following:

1. *Debride putrefying tissues.* Cleanse the wound carefully to remove any purulent exudate and then debride as much of the necrotic tissue as possible. Treat odorous dressings as biologically contaminated waste. Place them in a plastic puncture-resistant bag and close it securely. Double bag the waste and place in a tightly sealed trash container for pickup and disposal.
2. *Control infection.* If "healing" is not the goal of wound care, cytotoxic cleansers can be used to kill bacteria. Iodine will help keep the wound clean, although some patients find it irritating and painful. For pseudomonas, 0.0025% acetic acid may help inhibit the organism's growth in addition to a topical and/or systemic antibiotic (Table 26.8).

   If there is superficial anaerobic infection, topical treatment with metronidazole or silver sulfadiazine may be sufficient. If there is a deeper tissue infection, add systemic metronidazole 250 to 500 mg p.o./i.v. q8h until the infection resolves.

3. *Modify the environment.* There are multiple environmental changes that will help patients and families cope with foul odors, including the following:

   a. *Ventilate adequately.* Open windows to allow fresh air into the environment. Run a fan on a low speed so that it circulates air around the room without chilling the patient.

   b. *Absorb odors.* Place inexpensive kitty litter or activated charcoal in a flat container with a large surface area under the patient's bed. As long as the air in the room is circulating freely, odors will diminish rapidly. Alternately, burn a flame, for example, a candle, to combust the chemicals causing the odor.

      For particularly odorous wounds, place an occlusive dressing that contains charcoal or a disposable diaper over the wound to contain the odor.

   c. *Alternate odors.* Introduce an alternate odor that is tolerable to the patient and family, for example, aromatherapy, coffee, vanilla, or vinegar. Avoid commercial fragrances and perfumes as many are not tolerated by patients with advanced cancer.

Pain

Pressure ulcers and malignant wounds are often painful unless the patient is paraplegic or has an altered sensorium (47–50). The pain can be constant with or without breakthrough pain, or acute. Constant pain can be the result of a local tissue reaction, underlying cancer, infection, the products of inflammation, or increased pressure at a bony prominence. Intermittent acute pain occurs with specific procedures, for example, debridement. Cyclic acute pain occurs with recurring dressing changes (51–53).

To appropriately treat wound-related pain, it is important to know if the pain is nociceptive in origin, that is, the result of normal nociception and nerve function, neuropathic in origin, that is, the result of abnormal nerve function, or mixed.

Pain management follows standard pain management principles:

1. *Treat the underlying cause.* Where possible treat the cancer, control infections, heal the wound, and/or move the patient to a pressure-reducing or relieving surface.

2. *For constant pain.* Provide oral analgesics around the clock. If pain is nociceptive in origin, particularly if it is associated with inflammation, it will likely respond to a nonsteroidal anti-inflammatory drug (NSAID) and/or an opioid analgesic dosed once every half-life. If the pain is neuropathic in origin, a tricyclic analgesic or an anticonvulsant may be needed as an effective coanalgesic.

   For breakthrough pain, provide 10% of the total 24-hour oral dose of opioid every 1 hour as needed.

   Early evidence suggests that topical opioids mixed into a hydrogel, for example, morphine 0.1% to 0.5%, and

placed against the wound surface in the primary dressing layer may reduce constant wound pain (54,55).

   Please note that if "healing" is the goal of wound care, NSAIDs may interfere with angiogenesis and delay wound healing (56).

3. *For both intermittent and cyclic acute pain.* Provide preemptive anesthesia and/or analgesia. Ensure that the pharmacokinetics of the medication closely follow the temporal profile of the pain.

During debridement, acute intermittent pain will likely last only as long as the procedure. If there is an eschar to debride, score it, then apply EMLA (eutectic mixture of long-acting anesthetics) "like icing on a cake" 30 to 60 minutes before the procedure, and cover it with an occlusive film. If there is slough and debris to be removed, apply a 2% to 4% lidocaine solution to the open wound. If there is likely to be pain at the periphery of the wound, inject s.c. lidocaine (and/or epinephrine to minimize bleeding) into the surrounding tissues and leave it for 5 to 10 minutes before commencing debridement.

Similarly, during dressing changes, acute cyclic pain will likely last only as long as the procedure (57,58). As the edges of the dressing are being slowly removed, moisten the wound and the dressing with a 2% to 4% solution of lidocaine. Allow enough time for the patient to be comfortable.

Careful selection of dressings to minimize tissue adherence, for example, hydrogels, alginates, and nonstick dressings, will minimize pain during dressing changes. If pain persists, consider reducing the frequency of dressing changes.

If local anesthesia is insufficient, try a very short acting opioid, for example, systemic fentanyl or inhaled nitrous oxide (59).

SUMMARY

Chronic wounds are relatively common in patients with advanced cancer. After doing a comprehensive, whole person assessment, consider what the goals of care and treatment plan for the wound will be in light of the context of the patient's underlying cancer (and other comorbidities). Always use therapies that aim to reduce the risk of developing pressure ulcers. Once a pressure ulcer develops, if the goal is to heal it, follow the conventional wound healing strategies outlined in the text. If the goal is to stabilize, but not heal either a pressure ulcer or a malignant wound, the management will depend on whether the wound is dry or wet. Leave dry, noninfected wounds alone. For wet wounds, use relatively conservative wound cleansing, debridement, and dressing strategies to control infection and odor and minimize bleeding and pain.

Patients living with chronic wounds are inevitably "wounded" far beyond their physical wound. They live from day to day knowing that someone will be putting her/his hands into their body for daily dressing changes. Exudates, bleeding, and odors are embarrassing and distressing. Emotions frequently run high. Anxiety and depression are common, particularly in the face of multiple unexpected losses. Changes in intimacy, relationships, and finances can be dramatic and even lead to social isolation. Questions of meaning, value, purpose in life, "why me," and so on, all surface. To successfully manage these patients, interdisciplinary care must focus on the whole "wounded" person, not just the "hole."

REFERENCES

1. Pain Terminology. International Association for the Study of Pain. http://www.iasp-pain.org/Content/NavigationMenu/GeneralResourceLinks/PainDefinitions/default.htm. Accessed October 10, 2011.

2. Hassan AH, Ableitner A, Stein C, et al. Inflammation of the rat paw enhances axonal transport of opioid receptors in the sciatic nerve and increases their density in the inflamed tissue. *Neuroscience.* 1993;55(1):185-195. PMID: 7688879.

3. Alvarez OM, Meehan M, Ennis W, et al. Chronic wounds: palliative management for the frail population. *Wounds.* 2002;14(suppl 8):13-18. http://www.woundsresearch.com/issue/13. Accessed October 10, 2011.

4. Krasner DL, Rodeheaver GT, Sibbald RG, eds. *Chronic Wound Care: A Clinical Source Book for Healthcare Professionals.* 3rd ed. Wayne, PA: HMP Communications; 2001.

5. Walker P. *Update on Pressure Ulcers. Principles & Practice of Supportive Oncology Updates.* Vol. 3. No. 6. 2nd ed. New York, NY: Lippincott Williams & Wilkins; 2000:1-11.

6. Brem H, Lyder C. Protocol for the successful treatment of pressure ulcers. *Am J Surg.* 2004;188(suppl 1A):9-17. Review.

7. Leigh I, Bennett G. Pressure ulcers: prevalence, etiology, and treatment modalities, a review. *Am J Surg.* 1994;167:25S-30S.

8. Eachempati SR, Hydo LJ, Barie PS. Factors influencing the development of decubitus ulcers in critically ill surgical patients. *Crit Care Med.* 2001;29(9):1678-1682.

9. Cuddigan J, Berlowitz DR, Ayello EA. Pressure ulcers in America: prevalence, incidence and implications for the future: an executive summary of the National Pressure Ulcer Advisory Panel Monograph. *Adv Skin Wound Care.* 2001;14:208-215.

10. Reifsnyder J, Magee H. Development of pressure ulcers in patients receiving home hospice care. *Wounds.* 2005;17:74-79.

11. Walker P. The pathophysiology and management of pressure ulcers. In: Portenoy RK, Bruera E, eds. *Topics in Palliative Care.* Vol. 3. New York, NY: Oxford University Press; 1998:253-270.

12. Haisfield-Wolfe ME, Rund C. Malignant cutaneous wounds: a management protocol. *Ostomy Wound Manage.* 1997;43:56-66.

13. Naylor W. Malignant wounds: aetiology and principles of management. *Nurs Stand.* 2002;16:45-56.

14. Collier M. The assessment of patients with malignant fungating wounds—a holistic approach: part 1. *Nurs Times.* 1997;93(49):1-4.

15. Wilkes L, White K, Smeal T, et al. Malignant wound management: what dressings do nurses use? *J Wound Care.* 2002;10:65-69.

16. Agency for Health Care Policy and Research. *Pressure Ulcers in Adults Prediction and Prevention, Clinical Guideline No. 3.* Rockville, MD: AHCPR; 1992. http://www.ncbi.nlm.nih.gov/books/NBK63854/. Accessed October 10, 2011.

17. Bergstrom N, Braden BJ, Laguzza A, et al. The Braden scale for predicting pressure ulcer sore risk. *Nurs Res.* 1987;36:205-210.

18. Norton D, McLaren R, Exton-Smith AN. *An Investigation of Geriatric Nursing Problems in Hospitals.* London: National Corporation for the Care of Old People; 1962.

19. Sykes MT, Godsey JB. Vascular evaluation of the diabetic foot. *Clin Podiatr Med Surg.* 1998;15(1):49-83.

20. Updated Pressure Ulcer Staging System Revised February 2007. http://www.npuap.org/pr2.htm. See also NPUAP at http://www.npuap.org/. Accessed October 10, 2011.

21. Pressure Ulcer Scale for Healing (PUSH) v 3.0. National Pressure Ulcer Advisory Panel 2007. http://www.npuap.org/PDF/push3.pdf. Accessed October 10, 2011.

22. Armstrong DG, Meyr AJ. Basic principles of wound management. UpToDate. http://www.uptodate.com/contents/basic-principles-of-wound-management. Accessed July 17, 2012.

23. Dorner B, Posthauer ME, Thomas D. The role of nutrition in pressure ulcer prevention and treatment: National Pressure Ulcer Advisory Panel White Paper 2009. http://www.npuap.org/Nutrition%20White%20Paper%20Website%20Version.pdf. Accessed October 10, 2011.

24. Walker P. Management of pressure ulcers. *Oncology (Williston Park).* 2001;15(11):1499-1508, 1511.

25. Sibbald RG, Williamson D, Orsted HL, et al. Preparing the wound bed–debridement, bacterial balance, and moisture balance. *Ostomy Wound Manage.* 2000;46(11):14-22, 24-28, 30-35.

26. Krasner DL. How to prepare the wound bed. *Ostomy Wound Manage.* 2001;47(4):59-61.

27. Vowden K, Vowden P. Wound bed preparation. World Wide Wounds, March 2002. http://www.worldwidewounds.com/2002/april/Vowden/Wound-Bed-Preparation.html. Accessed October 10, 2011.

28. Bergstrom N, Bennett MA, Carlson CE, et al. *Pressure Ulcer Treatment. Clinical Practice Guideline. Quick Reference Guide for Clinicians, No. 15.* Rockville, MD: U.S. Department of Health and Human Services, Public Health Service, Agency for Health Care Policy and Research, AHCPR Pub. No. 95-0653; December 1994.

29. Maklebust J, Sieggreen M. *Pressure Ulcers: Guidelines for Prevention and Nursing Management.* 2nd ed. Springhouse, PA: Springhouse Corporation; 1996.

30. Rodeheaver GT. Wound cleansing, wound irrigation, wound disinfection. In: Krasner DL, Rodeheaver GT, Sibbald RG, eds. *Chronic Wound Care: A Clinical Source Book for Healthcare Professionals.* 3rd ed. Wayne, PA: HMP Communications; 2001:369-383.

31. Boxer AM, Gottesman N, Bernstein H, et al. Debridement of dermal ulcers and decubiti with collagenase. *Geriatrics.* 1968;24:75-86.

32. Thomas S, Andrews A, Jones M, et al. Maggots are useful in treating infected or necrotic wounds. *BMJ.* 1999;318(7186):807-808.

33. Jones M. Larval therapy. *Nurs Stand.* 2000;14:47-51.

34. Bonn D. Maggot therapy: an alternative for wound infection. *Lancet.* 2000;356(9236):1174.

35. Sherman R. Maggot debridement therapy (MDT). http://medicaledu.com/maggots.htm. Accessed October 10, 2011.

36. Spann CT, Tutrone WD, Weinberg JM, et al. Topical antibacterial agents for wound care: a primer. *Dermatol Surg.* 2003;29(6):620-626.

37. Molan PC. Re-introducing honey in the management of wounds and ulcers—theory and practice. *Ostomy Wound Manage.* 2002;48(11):28-40.

38. Ovington LG. Dressings and adjunctive therapies: AHCPR guidelines revisited. *Ostomy Wound Manage.* 1999;45(suppl 1A):94S-106S.

39. Ovington L, Peirce B. Wound dressings: form, function, feasibility, and facts. In: Krasner DL, Rodeheaver GT, Sibbald RG,

eds. *Chronic Wound Care: A Clinical Sourcebook for Healthcare Professionals.* 3rd ed. Wayne, PA: HMP Communications; 2001;311-319.

40. Cutting KF. Wound exudate: composition and functions. *Br J Community Nurs.* 2003;8(suppl 9):4-9.

41. White RJ, Cutting KF. Interventions to avoid maceration of the skin and wound bed. *Br J Nurs.* 2003;12(20):1186-1201.

42. Wooten MK. Long-term care in geriatrics: management of chronic wounds in the elderly. *Clin Fam Pract.* 2001;3:599-626.

43. Barton P, Parslow N. Malignant wounds: holistic assessment and management. In: Krasner DL, Rodeheaver GT, Sibbald RG, eds. *Chronic Wound Care: A Clinical Sourcebook for Healthcare Professionals.* 3rd ed. Wayne, PA: HMP Communications; 2001:699-710.

44. Grocott P. The palliative management of fungating malignant wounds. *J Wound Care.* 2000;9(1):4-9.

45. Ferris FD, Bezjak A, Rosenthal SG. The palliative uses of radiation therapy in surgical oncology patients. *Surg Oncol Clin N Am.* 2001;10(1):185-201.

46. Piggin C. Malodorous fungating wounds: uncertain concepts underlying the management of social isolation. *Int J Palliat Nurs.* 2003;9(5):216-221.

47. Krasner D. Using a gentler hand: reflections on patients with pressure ulcers who experience pain. *Ostomy Wound Manage.* 1996;42(3):20-22.

48. Reddy M, Keast D, Fowler E, et al. Pain in pressure ulcers. *Ostomy Wound Manage.* 2003;49(suppl 4):30-35.

49. Popescu A, Salcido RS. Wound pain: a challenge for the patient and the wound care specialist. *Adv Skin Wound Care.* 2004;17(1):14-20.

50. Naylor W. Assessment and management of pain in fungating wounds. *Br J Nurs.* 2001;10(suppl 22):S33-S36.

51. Moffatt C, Briggs M, Hollinworth H, et al. *Pain at Wound Dressing Changes. EWMA Position Document.* London: Medical Education Partnership.

52. Reddy M, Kohr R, Queen D, et al. Practical treatment of wound pain and trauma: a patient-centered approach. An overview. *Ostomy Wound Manage.* 2003;49(suppl 4):2-15.

53. Krasner D. The chronic wound pain experience: a conceptual model. *Ostomy Wound Manage.* 1995;41(3):20-25.

54. Twillman RK, Long TD, Cathers TA, et al. Treatment of painful skin ulcers with topical opioids. *J Pain Symptom Manage.* 1999;17(4):288-292.

55. Zeppetella G, Paul J, Ribeiro MD. Analgesic efficacy of morphine applied topically to painful ulcers. *J Pain Symptom Manage.* 2003;25(6):555-558.

56. Jones MK, Wang H, Peskar BM, et al. Inhibition of angiogenesis by nonsteroidal anti-inflammatory drugs: insight into mechanisms and implications for cancer growth and ulcer healing. *Nat Med.* 1999;5(12):1418-1423.

57. Briggs M, Ferris FD, Glynn C, et al. World Union of Wound Healing Societies Expert Working Group. Assessing pain at wound dressing-related procedures. *Nurs Times.* 2004;100(46):56-57.

58. Kammerlander G, Eberlein T. Nurses' views about pain and trauma at dressing changes: a central European perspective. *J Wound Care.* 2002;11(2):76-79.

59. Parlow JL, Milne B, Tod DA, et al. Self-administered nitrous oxide for the management of incident pain in terminally ill patients: a blinded case series. *Palliat Med.* 2005;19(1):3-8.

CHAPTER 27

Lymphedema

Vaughan L. Keeley

Lymphedema can occur as an aftermath of cancer treatment or it can be a feature of advanced disease. Lymphedema of the arm is a fairly common sequel to treatment for breast cancer, and leg edema may be present in patients with advanced pelvic cancers.

The approaches to management of these two groups may be different. In the former, "supportive" treatment would aim to minimize the edema and enable the patient, with successfully treated cancer, to live as normally as possible with the problem. Methods of preventing the development of lymphedema in this group are also being investigated. In the latter, a "palliative" approach would aim to alleviate symptoms as much as possible while ensuring that any burden of treatment would be outweighed by the benefits. Edema in patients with advanced cancer may be only one of a number of problems that is experienced and would therefore need to be considered in this context.

PATHOPHYSIOLOGY

Lymphedema is defined as the accumulation of a relatively protein-rich fluid in the interstitial space of tissues due to a low-output failure of the lymphatic system, that is, lymph transport is reduced (1).

Lymphedema is usually classified into "primary," which defines a group of lymphedemas arising from a congenital lymphatic dysplasia, and "secondary," in which extrinsic factors damage the lymphatics. Lymphedema associated with cancer and its treatment is therefore "secondary lymphedema."

However, the formation of edema in patients with advanced cancer is usually more complex than this. It is helpful, therefore, to consider the mechanisms of edema formation. Edema is the accumulation of excessive fluid in the interstitial space and results from an imbalance between the formation and drainage of interstitial fluid.

The Formation of Edema

Fluid enters the interstitial space by capillary filtration. The amount of filtrate is determined by the "Starling" forces acting across the capillary wall. These are the hydrostatic pressure gradient, which tends to push fluid from the capillary into the interstitial space, and the colloid osmotic pressure gradient due to plasma proteins that are retained in the capillary which tends to draw water from the interstitial space into

the capillary. The volume of filtrate will also be determined by the permeability of the capillary wall.

In the past, it was felt that this process occurred largely in the arterial end of the capillary and a degree of reabsorption occurred at the venous end of the capillary. However, current thinking suggests that once fluid reaches the interstitial space its route of exit is through the freely permeable initial lymphatic capillary, that is, lymphatic drainage (2). Therefore, edema occurs whenever capillary filtration exceeds lymphatic drainage.

Table 27.1 shows the changes in capillary filtration and lymphatic drainage in a variety of chronic edemas.

In venous edema, for example, in chronic venous insufficiency of the leg, capillary filtration is raised because of increased hydrostatic pressure in the capillaries, but this results in increased lymphatic drainage due to the spare capacity of the lymphatic system to transport fluid. When this capacity is exceeded, then edema occurs (high-output failure of the lymphatics). If high-output failure of the lymphatic system persists, then there is a gradual deterioration in lymphatic transport capacity and worsening edema develops. This situation is often called *edema of mixed etiology*, that is, mixed venous and lymphatic.

In patients with reduced mobility, particularly those who spend a lot of time sitting in a chair, so-called dependency edema can occur. This is, again, a mixture of lymphatic and venous edema. Poor mobility means that the usual muscle pump that aids both venous and lymphatic drainage is impaired, and therefore, capillary filtration is increased and lymphatic drainage is reduced.

In patients with hypoalbuminemia, the colloid osmotic pressure in the plasma is reduced, and therefore, capillary filtration is increased, and edema can occur if lymphatic drainage is unable to cope with this.

Post-cancer Treatment Edema

It has long been assumed that axillary lymphadenectomy carried out as part of the surgical treatment for breast cancer has led to lymphedema of the arm in some women because of simple damage to the lymphatics. The addition of radiotherapy to the axilla may increase the damage to the lymphatics. However, in recent years, it has become clear that this is perhaps too simplistic a view of the etiology of the edema. Studies have shown that, contrary to predictions, lymph flow is increased in both the "at-risk" and contralateral arm in women who go on to develop lymphedema compared with

TABLE	27.1	Chronic edemas		

Type	Pathology	Capillary Filtration	Lymphatic Drainage
Primary lymphedema	Lymphatic dysplasia	Normal	↓
Secondary lymphedema	Lymphatic damage	Probably normal	↓
Venous edema	High-output failure	↑↑	Initial ↑ then ↓
Lymphovenous edema	Reduced venous and lymphatic drainage	↑↑	↓
Advanced cancer	Lymphatic obstruction, venous obstruction, hypoalbuminemia, immobility	↑↑	↓

those who do not. (3). This suggests that there is a constitutional tendency to lymphedema in some women possibly as a result of raised capillary filtration and lymphatic drainage (high-output failure) (4).

Similar mechanisms may contribute to the formation of edema in people who have had groin lymph node dissections for the treatment of tumors such as melanomas of the leg.

Edema in Advanced Cancer

In patients with advanced cancer, the edema is usually of complex etiology (Table 27.2). A patient may have lymphatic obstruction due to metastatic disease in the lymph nodes or due to previous treatment. There may be extrinsic venous compression causing venous hypertension or even venous thrombosis. In advanced disease, hypoalbuminemia is common, and finally, in association with the cachexia of advanced disease, weakness and immobility may result. These factors will lead to increased capillary filtration and reduced lymphatic drainage. This situation is often seen in patients with advanced pelvic malignancies.

INCIDENCE

The literature is not clear about the precise incidence of lymphedema following treatment for cancer (5). Difficulties arise because of a lack of agreement about the definition of the degree of swelling that constitutes lymphedema, the

TABLE	27.2	Causes of edema in advanced cancer

General

- Cardiac failure (which may be secondary to or exacerbated by anemia)
- Hypoalbuminemia
- Late-stage chronic renal failure
- Drugs:
  Nonsteroidal anti-inflammatory drugs and corticosteroids (salt and water retention)
  Calcium channel blockers (vasodilation and impaired lymphatic pump)
- Malignant ascites

Local

- Lymphatic obstruction/damage
  Due to surgery/radiotherapy, metastatic tumor in lymph nodes or skin lymphatics, and recurrent infections
- Venous obstruction
  E.g., deep vein thrombosis, superior vena caval obstruction, inferior vena caval obstruction, extrinsic venous compression by tumor, and thrombophlebitis migrans
- Lymphovenous edema
  Due to immobility and dependency or localized weakness due to neurologic deficit

different ways in which measurements are made and variation in the duration of follow-up.

Cancer treatment–related lymphedema is most commonly seen in patients who have been treated for breast cancer, gynecologic cancers, urologic cancers, and head and neck cancer and those who have had groin dissections for treatment for malignant melanoma.

Breast Cancer–Related Lymphedema (BCRL)

BCRL is the type that has been studied most, but even in this group there remain a number of uncertainties about the true incidence and etiology (5). The prevalence of edema in women who have received conventional treatment for breast cancer is reported to be around 25% to 28% (6), although in some reports the figure is as low as 6% (7). This "conventional" treatment usually involves axillary node sampling in which it is intended to remove a sample of four nodes for staging purposes. Removal of the tumor itself is usually by mastectomy or wide local excision together with postoperative radiotherapy in some instances. It has been argued that with the use of sentinel node biopsy, the incidence of lymphedema may be reduced to approximately 3% in those who have sentinel node biopsy alone (8) but is increased if women have to undergo axillary node clearance subsequently.

Studies have shown that the incidence of BCRL is dependent upon the definition of what constitutes lymphedema, e.g., a difference of >200 mL volume, >10% volume, or >2 cm circumference between the two arms (or from preoperative measurements) (9). Nevertheless, the 10% volume difference definition is frequently used in research studies.

Some of the variations in the results reported may relate to different lengths of follow-up as well as measurement techniques. There is a well-recognized pattern of delay in the onset of swelling which may occur several years after the primary treatment, even in the absence of recurrence of cancer.

The literature is also not consistent in terms of the risk factors identified for the development of lymphedema following treatment of breast cancer, but some of the common factors that emerge include (5) the following:

- Radiotherapy
- The extent of axillary node dissection
- Combined axillary surgery and radiotherapy
- Obesity
- Surgical wound infection
- Tumor stage
- Extent of surgery

Attempts have therefore been made to reduce the incidence of BCRL by modifications of surgical and radiotherapy techniques. The following factors should help with this (10):

- Wide local excision rather than mastectomy
- Sentinel node biopsy rather than axillary node sampling
- Avoidance of axillary radiotherapy following axillary node clearance

- Modification of radiotherapy techniques
- Avoidance of arm infections and inflammation

Because of the often-delayed appearance of lymphedema following treatment, it will take some time to determine whether any of these changes will bring about the desired reduction in incidence.

Gynecologic Cancer

The prevalence of lower limb lymphedema after treatment for gynecologic cancers depends upon the type of cancer and surgery carried out. Nevertheless, one study has shown an overall prevalence of 18% in women treated for all gynecologic cancers (11). In 16% of these women the edema developed between 1 and 5 years following treatment. The prevalence was 47% in women treated for vulval cancer with lymphadenectomy and radiotherapy. However, other studies of vulval cancer have shown a range of between 9% (12) and 70% (13).

Urologic Cancers

There is very little evidence in the literature concerning the incidence of lymphedema of the legs and genitalia following treatment for urologic cancers. The incidence does seem to vary according to the type and location of a tumor and may be up to 50% in advanced stages of penile cancer or following its treatment (14).

Groin Dissection

Again, the literature shows a varied incidence. In one study of groin dissection for malignant melanoma, soft tissue sarcoma, and squamous cell carcinoma, the overall incidence of mild to moderate lymphedema was 21% (15). Sentinel node biopsy in the management of melanomas of the leg has been advocated to reduce the incidence of posttreatment lymphedema.

Other studies have shown the incidence of measurable lymphedema after groin dissection to be >80% after 5 years (16).

Head and Neck Cancer

Lymphedema of the face and submental region can occur following treatment for head and neck cancer. This treatment may involve bilateral lymph node dissections of the neck and postoperative radiotherapy, but there is little evidence in the literature to show how common the problem is.

Incidence of Edema in Advanced Cancer

Edema is a common problem in advanced cancer although, as described in the preceding text, its etiology can be complex. Studies have shown that edema occurs in 20% to 33% of patients with advanced disease (17, 18) and is associated with a poor prognosis (18).

CLINICAL FEATURES

Lymphedema due to Cancer Treatments

Symptoms and Signs

Lymphedema is often described as a firm nonpitting edema. However, in the early stages of its development, the swelling may be soft and "pit" easily on pressure. As the condition progresses, the edema becomes firmer because of the development of fibrosis and fatty tissue within the subcutaneous space.

The development of typical skin changes in lymphedema also takes a variable amount of time and seems to be more prominent in leg edema than in arm edema.

These changes include the following:

- An increase in skin thickness
- Hyperkeratosis: a buildup of horny scale on the skin surface
- A deepening of skin creases, especially round the ankle and base of toes (Figure 27.1)
- A warty appearance to the skin as hyperkeratosis worsens
- Lymphangiectasia: small blisters due to dilated lymph vessels. These may burst and cause significant leakage (lymphorrhea). These are said to occur particularly following radiotherapy, which causes fibrosis and obstruction of the deep collecting lymphatics.

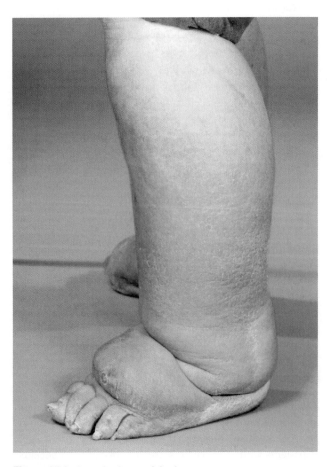

Figure 27.1. Lymphedema of the leg.

- Papillomatosis: with papules consisting of dilated skin lymphatics surrounded by rigid fibrous tissue which may give a "cobblestone" appearance to areas of skin, particularly on the legs

The physical sign, Stemmer's sign, is the inability to pick up a fold of skin at the base of the second toe and its presence is said to be diagnostic of lymphedema (19).

Pain may be a feature of lymphedema. In one study of various types of lymphedema, 57% of patients reported pain, while 32% described "tightness." Patients with active cancer were more likely to report both tightness and pain (20). Four types of pain were described: tissue pressure, muscle stretch, neurologic, and inflammation. Neurologic pain tended to occur in patients with advanced cancer. When lymphedema first appears, particularly if the swelling develops quickly, pain may occur which subsequently subsides.

In the early stages of the development of lymphedema, limb function and mobility may be normal, but as swelling develops, particularly around the joints, mobility is reduced and this may in turn exacerbate the swelling due to the reduced action of the muscle pump on lymphatic drainage. As a result, the limb can become increasingly heavy and cause further pain and discomfort at the shoulder or hip in the case of arm and leg edema, respectively.

Lymphedema after Breast Cancer Treatment

Patients may often develop symptoms before any objective evidence of lymphedema (21). These symptoms may include a feeling of fullness, tightness, or heaviness of the arm, shoulder, or chest, and an altered mobility of the shoulder. Associated with arm swelling, there may be truncal edema and an asymmetric increase in the subcutaneous fatty tissues.

Some patients may develop symptoms shortly after the initial treatment, and it may be that these are transient changes that will resolve. However, it is not clear whether these will predispose to subsequent development of more persistent lymphedema (21).

In women who have had treatment for breast cancer and who develop edema of the arm, it is important to consider whether there may be recurrence of the breast cancer or whether the edema has developed because of an acute deep vein thrombosis (DVT).

Psychosocial Aspects

Lymphedema, especially following cancer treatment, can be associated with a significant psychological morbidity (22). These may relate to issues of altered body image, disability, and the fear of cancer recurrence. The development of arm swelling can be particularly distressing for women who have had to cope with surgery, radiotherapy, and chemotherapy for breast cancer, and their consequences. To have undergone all these treatments and then be left with persistent arm edema as a constant reminder of previous breast cancer can be traumatic.

Complications

The most common complications of lymphedema are as follows:

- Cellulitis
- Lymphorrhea
- DVT
- New malignancies, especially lymphangiosarcoma

Cellulitis

In lymphedematous limbs, there is an altered local immune response (23). This leads to a predisposition to developing infections and new malignancies in the affected area. The most important infection is cellulitis, which can not only be very unpleasant for the sufferer but may also lead to further damage to the lymphatic system and worsening edema, particularly if the cellulitis is recurrent.

Cellulitis in lymphedema is generally believed to be due to infection by β-hemolytic streptococci, although sometimes other bacteria such as staphylococci may be involved.

The usual clinical picture is the development of a flu-like illness with fever, muscular aches, and sometimes headache and vomiting. This is followed by the appearance of red inflamed painful tender areas in the skin of the lymphedematous limb. The skin changes can be very variable ranging from the whole limb being extremely inflamed to a relatively mild patchy rash.

Proving bacterial infection in all cases is difficult. This has led to the idea that some of these episodes are not necessarily infective, and the term *acute inflammatory episodes* or *secondary acute inflammation* has been derived (24) to describe them.

Sometimes it is clear that bacterial infection has entered the tissues through cuts, broken skin, and ruptured lymphangiectasia or papillomas. In the feet, the skin between the toes may be cracked because of tinea pedis infections, to which people with lymphedema are predisposed.

A particular feature of lymphedema is the predisposition to recurrent episodes of cellulitis, which may not only be unpleasant in themselves but may lead to worsening edema, due to damage to the lymphatics.

Lymphorrhea

This is the leakage of lymph through the skin at sites of laceration or ruptured cutaneous lymph blisters (lymphangiectasia). This can be particularly distressing if it affects the legs, as large volumes of fluid can leak out. There is an associated increased risk of infection.

Deep Vein Thrombosis

Patients with lymphedema are at risk for DVT in the affected limb, particularly if the limb is very edematous and immobile or if there is an associated abnormality of venous flow because of treatment for malignancy. A DVT can occur even when a patient is wearing a compression garment as treatment for their lymphedema.

Malignancy

Although rare, malignancies can arise in the skin of affected limbs. The most important of these is lymphangiosarcoma (25). The term *Stewart-Treves syndrome* is used to describe its occurrence in postmastectomy lymphedema. In this situation, the incidence is <0.45% and the mean time from the surgery to onset is approximately 10 years.

Lymphangiosarcoma presents as single or multiple bluish-red nodules in the skin, which spread rapidly locally often forming satellite lesions that may become confluent and ulcerate. Unfortunately, the prognosis is poor with a median survival of <3 years.

Edema of Advanced Cancer

Symptoms and Signs

The general symptoms and signs of edema in advanced cancer may be similar to those described in the previous section. However, as the etiology is often more complex, the clinical picture may also vary (Table 27.2). Pure lymphedema is probably unusual in advanced disease, and if it does occur, because of the short prognosis there is usually no time for the more chronic skin changes to develop. Therefore, edema in advanced cancer is often very soft and pitting. The skin can look stretched and shiny rather than thickened as in chronic lymphedema.

Pain is more likely to be a problem in patients with advanced cancer, particularly neuropathic pain resulting from nerve compression or destruction by tumor. This is often severe with tingling, burning, or stabbing features and altered sensation in the area of the pain. Light touch might be more painful than deep pressure (touch-evoked allodynia).

Patients may also be more prone to infections due to poor skin condition (often fragile, thin, and dry), skin tumors, ulceration, and reduced resistance to infection because of treatment or as a feature of advanced disease.

Ulceration of the skin is generally uncommon in pure lymphedema in comparison with venous disease but can occur in patients with edema in advanced malignancy. There can be significant associated lymphorrhea that can cause distress to patients. Superimposed infection by anaerobic bacteria can lead to unpleasant malodorous discharge and increased pain.

Immobility may be worse in patients with advanced malignancy because of generalized weakness or local nerve injury caused by tumor, such as brachial plexus infiltration in breast cancer.

The psychosocial aspects of edema in these situations are often greater, with patients having to cope with progressive disease and impending death, as well as the problems of lymphedema described in the preceding text.

Specific Situations

Locally Advanced Breast Cancer

In locally advanced breast cancer, a particularly severe and intractable type of edema can develop. In this situation, the deep lymphatic drainage of the arm may have already been

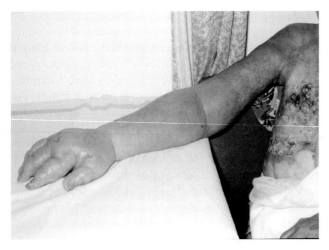

Figure 27.2. Lymphedema of the arm in locally advanced breast cancer.

damaged by surgery and radiotherapy, but this can be worsened by the recurrence of disease in axillary lymph nodes and the development of metastatic disease in the skin of the upper arm and chest wall with infiltration of the skin lymphatics. The arm can become extremely swollen. The problem may be exacerbated by brachial plexopathy, resulting in immobility of the arm and DVT because of extrinsic venous compression by tumor. In the latter, distended collateral veins may be seen around the shoulder.

The arm can become very heavy, swollen, painful, and dysfunctional. Blisters are common and breakdown of the skin may lead to ulceration and persistent lymphorrhea. The hand and fingers may swell to such an extent as to give the appearance of "a boxing glove" (Figure 27.2).

Advanced Pelvic Malignant Disease

Patients with advanced cancers of the uterus, ovary, prostate, bladder, or rectum may have gross edema of the legs and trunk, often of mixed etiology as follows:

- Lymphatic obstruction from metastatic disease in lymph nodes
- Extrinsic venous compression
- Inferior vena caval obstruction (IVCO)
- DVT
- Hypoalbuminemia
- Fluid-retaining drugs
- Ascites

Ascites

Malignant ascites is common in advanced ovarian, colorectal, gastric, pancreatic, and uterine cancers and is associated with a poor prognosis (median survival, 2 to 3 months) (26). Leg edema is often associated with ascites.

Hypoalbuminemia

Hypoalbuminemia is common in advanced cancer because of the cachexia–anorexia syndrome, which causes a reduction in hepatic protein synthesis (27). Hypoalbuminemia may

cause edema on its own but is usually seen in the context of other factors as described in the preceding text.

Superior Vena Caval Obstruction (SVCO)

SVCO is usually seen in patients with extrinsic compression of the vena cava by metastases in the upper mediastinal lymph nodes. It is particularly common in lung cancer. The features may develop very quickly perhaps because of secondary venous thrombosis. The most common presenting symptoms are as follows:

- Dyspnea
- Neck and facial swelling
- Trunk and arm swelling
- A sensation of choking
- A feeling of fullness in the head
- Headache

On examination, the following may be present:

- Thoracic vein distension
- Neck vein distension
- Facial edema
- Tachypnea
- Facial plethora
- Cyanosis
- Arm edema

The condition can be very distressing for patients and, if untreated, may lead to death.

Inferior Vena Caval Obstruction

IVCO usually occurs because of extrinsic compression by retroperitoneal lymphadenopathy or hepatomegaly due to metastatic disease. Patients develop edema of the legs, abdomen, and genitalia, and if the obstruction is above the level of the hepatic veins, ascites may occur as well. Dilated collateral veins are often seen on the abdominal wall.

Complications

Although the complications of edema in advanced cancer may be similar to those of lymphedema described in the preceding text, patients with advanced disease are particularly prone to venous thrombosis due to the increased coagulability of their blood. They are also more prone to lymphorrhea and infections, but the short prognosis means that the development of lymphangiosarcomas is not an issue.

DIFFERENTIAL DIAGNOSIS AND INVESTIGATIONS

In patients with cancer treatment–related lymphedema, the diagnosis is usually based on the clinical history and examination. However, the possibility of DVT or recurrence of malignant disease does need to be borne in mind.

In patients with advanced malignancy, elucidating potentially reversible contributory factors is an important part of the management of edema (Table 27.2).

Investigations

Specific investigations may include the following:

- Computed tomography scan/magnetic resonance imaging/ultrasound scan to look for recurrent disease
- Full blood count to look for anemia
- Echocardiogram/chest x-ray/brain natriuretic peptide/electrocardiogram to look for evidence of heart failure
- Serum albumin to detect hypoalbuminemia
- Plasma urea and creatinine to look for evidence of renal failure

Deep Vein Thrombosis

In the United Kingdom, current diagnostic practice for DVT relies on the use of an algorithm based on signs and symptoms (Well's score (28)—see Table 27.3) together with D-dimer levels in the blood and an ultrasound examination of the leg to assess deep vein blood flow. Unfortunately, in patients with advanced malignancy the level of D-dimers may be elevated in the absence of DVT, so this element of the assessment may not be particularly helpful.

A "Well's score" of 2 or higher indicates that the probability of DVT is "likely"; a score of <2 indicates the probability of DVT is "unlikely." In patients with symptoms in both legs, the more symptomatic leg is used.

DVT can be ruled out in a patient who is scored in the "unlikely" category and who has a negative D-dimer test (28). In those with positive D-dimers, a Well's score in the "likely" category, further investigation with ultrasound imaging of the leg is recommended.

Lymphoscintigraphy

Lymphoscintigraphy is a specific examination for lymphedema. A subcutaneous injection of a radioactively labeled macromolecule, for example, ^{99m}Tc-labeled protein or colloid, is used. This is taken up by the lymphatics, which can then be detected using an external gamma camera. Although this is a useful technique in the assessment of patients with lymphedema in general, its place in patients who have cancer-related lymphedema is limited. However, practice does vary around the world. In the United Kingdom, lymphoscintigraphy is rarely done in this situation, as it is felt it is unlikely to affect management, and the diagnosis is usually clear on clinical grounds. However, in other countries, isotope lymphoscintigraphy is more commonly performed (29).

MANAGEMENT

Prevention of BCRL

There is increased interest in the prevention and early detection of BCRL. It is generally felt that treating any lymphedema in its early stages with complex decongestive therapy (CDT) is more effective than when fibrosis and adipose tissue have become dominant features of the swelling in later stages. Therefore, early detection has advantages. Preoperative limb volume and bioimpedance measurements are advocated (30), but the threshold of change at which intervention is needed is not yet clear. Wearing a compression sleeve daily for a month when the limb volume has increased by 3% has been shown to reduce swelling

---

TABLE 27.3   Well's score

Clinical Model for Predicting the Pretest Probability of Deep Vein Thrombosis

Clinical Characteristics	Score
Active cancer (patient receiving treatment for cancer within the previous 6 mo or currently receiving palliative treatment)	1
Paralysis, paresis, or recent plaster immobilization of the lower extremities	1
Recently bedridden for 3 d or more or major surgery within the previous 12 wk requiring general or regional anesthesia	1
Localized tenderness along the distribution of the deep venous system	1
Entire leg swollen	1
Calf swelling at least 3 cm larger than that on the asymptomatic side (measured 10 cm below tibial tuberosity)	1
Pitting edema confined to the symptomatic leg	1
Collateral superficial veins (nonvaricose)	1
Previously documented deep vein thrombosis	1
Alternative diagnosis at least as likely as deep vein thrombosis	−2

TABLE 27.4	Recommendations to prevent lymphedema after breast cancer treatment

- Avoid injuries including cuts and abrasions, for example, wear gloves when gardening
- Use a thimble when sewing
- Use an oven glove when cooking
- Take care when ironing
- Avoid tight clothing, including tight bra straps
- Avoid irritating cosmetics/soaps
- Avoid sunburn
- Avoid insect bites/cat scratches
- Use an electric razor for shaving
- Avoid obesity
- Avoid injections or venipuncture in the "at-risk" arm
- Avoid blood pressure measurement in the "at-risk" arm
- Seek medical advice if "at-risk" arm becomes inflamed or swollen

and possibly prevent the full development of BCRL in one uncontrolled study (30). However, it is possible that such mild increase in limb volume may resolve spontaneously in many women (31). Further research should clarify the situation.

Other studies have shown that manual lymphatic drainage (MLD) (see below) does not prevent lymphedema (32) but exercise programs may help (33, 34).

In addition, it seems reasonable for patients to take sensible precautions to minimize the risk of infection or overload of the lymphatics that may cause further damage to lymph vessels and precipitate overt edema (35). Examples of these are given in Tables 27.4 and 27.5.

Management of Treatment-Related Edema

The mainstay of cancer treatment–related edema is a combination of physical treatments which together are known as *decongestive lymphatic therapy* (DLT) (36). Other terminology is used to describe similar combinations of treatment, for example, CDT.

The treatment comprises four elements:

- Compression
- Skin care
- Exercise
- Massage: simple lymphatic drainage (SLD) or MLD

TABLE 27.5	Recommendations to patients at risk for developing leg lymphedema

- Avoid standing for several hours
- Maintain skin hygiene especially feet
- Avoid tight shoes, socks, other clothing
- Avoid walking barefoot outdoors
- Avoid irritating cosmetics or soaps
- Avoid injections in the "at-risk" limb
- Avoid insect bites/cat scratches/cuts/injuries
- Treat fungal infections, for example, tinea pedis, early
- Avoid sunburn
- Avoid surgery, for example, for varicose veins, if possible
- Avoid obesity
- Use an electric razor for shaving
- Seek medical advice if "at-risk" leg becomes inflamed or swollen

Compression is carried out either in the form of a specific multilayer lymphedema bandage (MLLB) or elastic compression garments.

Skin care typically involves the use of a moisturizing cream such as aqueous cream, but also looks at ways of protecting the skin such as avoiding cuts and abrasions, avoiding sun burn, avoiding venipuncture, intravenous infusions, and treating conditions such as eczema. It is often also recommended to avoid having blood pressure measured in the lymphedematous arm. The aim of these recommendations is to improve the skin condition and reduce the likelihood of infections.

Exercise encourages lymphatic drainage but some patients may require specific physiotherapy/exercises to improve function if joints have become stiff.

MLD is a type of gentle skin massage applied by trained therapists, which is designed to improve lymph drainage. SLD is based on the principles of MLD, but is carried out by the patient themselves or by a carer.

MLD is said to stimulate contraction of the lymph collectors and enhance protein resorption. The massage technique is designed to improve drainage from congested areas. It includes breathing exercises to improve thoracic duct drainage and gentle superficial massage working distal to proximal, for example, commencing on the trunk, then the proximal part of the limb, and then the distal area, to encourage proximal flow. There are a number of different "schools" of MLD, for example, Vodder, Leduc, Földi and Casley-Smith. Although slightly different techniques are employed, the basic principles are shared by all schools (37).

For patients with moderate to severe edema, an intensive phase of treatment over a period of approximately 2 weeks involving compression bandaging (with or without MLD) to reduce the swelling and improve the shape of the limb is carried out. Patients who have associated truncal edema usually require MLD together with compression bandaging. This intensive phase of treatment is followed by the application of compression garments, that is, an elastic stocking or arm sleeve, which is then worn daily indefinitely.

Some patients require repeated courses of bandaging treatment over a period of time. Other patients with more mild edema may be managed with skin care and compression garments alone.

Patients with "mid-line" edema, that is, truncal, breast, genital, or head and neck edema, are best treated with MLD and SLD as these are not areas to which compression garments can be easily applied. Specialist garments for these areas, however, are available and may be helpful in some situations. Adhesive skin tapes (e.g., Kinesiotape) may also be useful in "mid-line" edema.

Evidence for Effectiveness of Treatments

There is little robust evidence in the literature to validate the individual components of these treatment regimes (38). Nevertheless, the combination of physical treatments has been shown to produce a sustained improvement in limb volume and a reduction in the incidence of episodes of cellulitis (39).

Other treatments that have been used include pneumatic compression pumps. A variety of these devises is available, ranging from single-chambered sleeves providing intermittent compression to a limb, to multichambered devices (e.g., 5 to 10 chambers) that produce an intermittent sequential (peristaltic) compression massaging fluid from the distal to the proximal part of the limb (40).

There has been renewed interest in the use of intermittent pneumatic compression (IPC) in treating lymphedema (41), with the development of more sophisticated devices which produce a massage-like effect rather than simply compressing. IPC is increasingly being used as part of a multimodal management regimen.

Surgery for cancer-related lymphedema is not routinely carried out. Liposuction has been used for patients with severe BCRL where adipose tissue and fibrosis predominate in the swelling (42). However, although the reduction in limb volume is good with this technique, patients have to wear compression hosiery 24 hours per day indefinitely following surgery.

In some reports lymphovenous anastomosis in the axilla is being used to prevent BCRL (43) and lymph node transplantation to facilitate regrowth of surgically damaged lymphatics is being developed (44).

Drug treatments for lymphedema are generally disappointing. Diuretics seem to have no role in the treatment of pure lymphedema, although they can be helpful if fluid retention is present as well.

Some advocate the use of benzopyrones such as oxerutins or coumarin. However, their evidence for effectiveness is inconsistent in the literature, and coumarin has significant hepatotoxicity (45, 46).

Treatment of Infection

Local fungal infections such as tinea pedis are treated with topical antifungals such as Terbinafine cream. Fungal nail infections are more difficult to eradicate and may require treatment with oral Terbinafine.

Treatment of cellulitis is aimed at β-hemolytic streptococci and depending upon the severity of the problem may be managed at home with oral antibiotics, but may require admission to hospital for intravenous therapy (Table 27.6) (47).

Bed rest and elevation of the lymphedematous limb is part of the management. Compression garments are not worn until they can be tolerated comfortably.

If intravenous antibiotics are required, then flucloxacillin 2 g 6 hourly may be used. If there is no response after 48 hours to this management, then clindamycin 600 mg 6 hourly i.v. could be substituted. Once the patient's condition begins to improve, a switch can be made to oral antibiotics.

In patients who develop recurrent cellulitis, that is, who have two or more attacks of cellulitis per year, prophylactic antibiotics should be considered if reduction in limb volume by treatment and improvement of skin condition has failed

TABLE 27.6	Oral antibiotics for the treatment of cellulitis

1. Amoxycillin 500 mg t.i.d. for at least 14 d

2. Flucloxacillin 500 mg q.i.d. if evidence of staphylococcal infections, e.g., folliculitis

3. Clindamycin 300 mg q.i.d. to be substituted for the amoxycillin if there is a poor response to oral antibiotics after 48 h. This is recommended for patients who are allergic to penicillin as the first-line treatment

to reduce the incidence of infection. A suggested antibiotic regimen is phenoxymethylpenicillin 500 mg daily. The duration of prophylaxis is dependent on individual circumstances, but patients in whom attempts to withdraw it have resulted in recurrence of cellulitis may need this therapy life-long.

Management of Patients with Advanced Cancer

The general principles of management are as for patients with lymphedema caused by cancer treatment, but they may have to be modified in the light of circumstances (48). In view of the complex etiology, it is helpful to identify potentially reversible factors as described in the preceding text and treat these accordingly, for example, blood transfusion for anemia.

When uncontrolled tumor is the main cause of the edema, this is unlikely to respond very well to treatment and an emphasis should be based on enhancing the patient's quality of life, respecting their choices and priorities and providing psychological support to the patient and the family. It is important that any burden of treatment should not exceed the benefit gained.

Skin Care

Skin care remains important in advanced disease, and the avoidance of trauma is particularly relevant. The shearing forces when putting on and taking off a compression garment may cause damage to the skin, and a light support bandage may be more appropriate in these circumstances. Where there is skin breakdown, nonadherent dressings may have to be applied. Occasionally, hemostatic dressings may be needed to control bleeding (e.g., calcium alginate) or topical epinephrine solution 1 in 1,000 (1 mg in 1 mL) used when dressings are changed.

Fungating Lesions

Fungating lesions, for example, on the chest wall or upper arm, in locally advanced breast cancer may become malodorous because of superadded anaerobic bacterial infection. Topical metronidazole 0.8% gel daily or oral metronidazole

400 mg b.i.d. for 2 weeks is often helpful. Topical metronidazole is relatively free from adverse effects but sometimes it is difficult to apply the gel to deeper crevices, and in some situations in which there is profuse discharge the gel is flushed away or diluted, thereby making it less effective. In these circumstances, oral metronidazole may be helpful.

Support and Positioning

In very ill patients, support and positioning of swollen limbs using pillows, and so on may relieve discomfort. It is important to try to avoid the use of an arm sling for people with arm edema, as this may cause pooling of fluid of the elbow and stiffness of the elbow joint (49). However, in some patients with severe arm edema and weakness from brachial plexopathy, a sling that can take the weight away from the shoulders and distribute it across the back may help with comfort and improve steadiness on movement (e.g., Lancaster sling).

Exercise

Exercises need to be adjusted to the patients' abilities and condition. Passive movements may be helpful to reduce stiffness and discomfort, but more active exercise regimes are usually inappropriate.

Massage

The presence of active cancer is often considered to be a contraindication to massage techniques such as MLD and SLD. It is argued that stimulation of lymph flow around the site of a tumor may lead to metastasis (50). There is no evidence either way to support or refute this in the literature, but in the presence of advanced metastatic disease the potential benefits of massage, particularly for truncal edema, outweigh any risk of inducing further metastatic spread. It is important that the patient makes an informed choice in this situation.

Compression

The aim of management in advanced cancer is often to relieve discomfort rather than to aggressively try to reduce limb volume. The skin may be too fragile to tolerate significant compression and therefore modifications of bandaging techniques to provide support from light bandages or from low compression garments are often needed. Shaped Tubigrip is a useful alternative to compression garments. In all circumstances, the skin condition needs to be checked regularly, particularly if there is impaired skin sensation, to confirm that the bandage or garment is not causing additional problems (51).

Lymphorrhea is helped by bandaging. A sterile pad or gauze is used to absorb the lymph and the gentle pressure applied by bandage often stops lymphorrhea in 24 to 48 hours. Sometimes, however, the bandage may need changing several times a day initially because of the rapid leakage of lymph.

In certain circumstances, compression bandaging may increase the amount of fluid leakage. For example, in patients with fungating breast tumors in the axilla or chest wall, the application of a bandage to the ipsilateral swollen arm may result in an increased discharge from the lesion. This is believed to be due to the increased flow of lymph through "open" lymphatics near the skin surface.

Compression bandaging, particularly of the legs, should be avoided in patients with acute heart failure, which may be contributing to their edema in advanced disease, and also in those with acute DVT. Because of the multifactorial nature of the edema, those with bilateral leg swelling, genital, and truncal edema often do not tolerate compression bandaging of the legs. This may be ineffective or simply push fluid onto the abdominal wall and genital areas making the edema there worse.

Appliances to Aid Mobility and Function

Various aids that may help with walking, dressing, use of swollen hands and arms, and so on may be provided by an occupational therapist.

Drug Treatments

Corticosteroids

Systemic corticosteroids are often used for a variety of symptoms in advanced cancer. They work by reducing inflammation and peritumour edema and thereby can relieve pressure on neighboring structures such as lymphatics, veins, and nerves. They can therefore have a role in reducing pain and swelling.

Dexamethasone is commonly used as a starting dose of 8 to 16 mg daily. This is usually given as a trial for 1 week to determine whether it is effective. If the drug is ineffective, it is discontinued at this stage. If it is effective, then the dose

is gradually reduced until the lowest level that relieves the symptoms is reached. This usually takes a period of weeks, over which time adverse effects such as fluid retention, gastrointestinal disturbance, weight gain, proximal myopathy, diabetes, and psychosis may develop. Should these occur, the balance of benefit versus the side effects of the drugs should be reviewed with the patient and a decision made whether to continue or gradually withdraw the treatment.

Diuretics

Diuretics may be helpful in the management of edema of advanced cancer if fluid retention, for example, due to drugs, or heart failure is present. Furosemide is commonly used and the dose adjusted according to effect.

Analgesics

Pain associated with edema in advanced cancer may respond to opioid analgesics, but if neuropathic pain is present other approaches such as the use of amitriptyline or one of the anticonvulsant drugs such as gabapentin may be helpful (see Chapter 2).

Treatment of Specific Potentially Reversible Factors

Potentially reversible factors should be treated in the light of a patient's general condition. Aggressive invasive treatment may not be appropriate in patients with a very short prognosis. A detailed description of all the treatment regimes is beyond the scope of this chapter, but a brief summary is given in Table 27.7.

The management of DVT with anticoagulants in patients with advanced cancer is not easy (53). The presence

TABLE 27.7	Treatment of potentially reversible factors in advanced cancer
Condition	**Treatment**
Anemia	Blood transfusion
Heart failure	Diuretics, digoxin, angiotensin-converting enzyme inhibitors
Fluid-retaining drugs	Withdraw if possible or use diuretics
Hypoalbuminemia	Treatment generally unrewarding
Malignant ascites	Paracentesis Diuretic therapy, for example, with spironolactone with or without furosemide Anticancer therapy, for example, in ovarian cancer
Superior vena caval obstruction	Metal stent (52) High-dose corticosteroids plus radiotherapy Chemotherapy
Inferior vena caval obstruction	Corticosteroids Metal stent
Deep vein thrombosis	Anticoagulation with low-molecular-weight heparin or warfarin

of existing bleeding from tumors such as fungating breast lesions would represent a contraindication. Although patients with advanced cancer are more prone to thrombosis, they are also more prone to hemorrhage if anticoagulated with warfarin. Drug interactions between warfarin and other medications that the person may be taking are common. Furthermore, patients who are anticoagulated to a "routine" level with warfarin, that is, international normalized ratio = 2–2.5, may still develop further thromboembolic events. Anticoagulation to a higher level is sometimes used but has an associated increased risk of bleeding. Low-molecular-weight heparins, for example, enoxaparin, may be a more appropriate alternative but are more expensive and require daily subcutaneous injections. The likely risks and benefits of anticoagulation should be considered and an informed decision made with the patient.

Needle Drainage of Edema in Advanced Disease

There has been renewed interest in needle drainage of severe edema in advanced cancer where other techniques have failed to bring about sufficient improvement (54). Case reports suggest that this can relieve symptoms in patients nearing the end of life. Concerns about causing cellulitis by this technique have not been confirmed in these reports to date.

CONCLUSIONS

The management of cancer treatment–related lymphedema is not curative but can help control the significant symptoms experienced by patients. The situation in patients with edema in advanced cancer is different and the treatment is more "palliative" in nature.

It is important to assess patients in the light of the above and decide, with patients, the most appropriate treatment. In all situations, the balance of benefit versus burden should be weighed up.

In recognition of increased interest in this topic the International Lymphoedema Framework has recently produced a "position document" on lymphedema in advanced cancer and edema at the end of life (55).

REFERENCES

1. Consensus Document of the International Society of Lymphology Executive Committee. The diagnosis and treatment of peripheral lymphedema. *Lymphology.* 1995;28:113-117.
2. Levick J, McHale N. The physiology of lymph production and propulsion. In: Browse N, Burnand K, Mortimer P, eds. *Diseases of the Lymphatics.* London: Arnold; 2003:44-64.
3. Stanton AWB, Modi S, Bennett Britton TM, et al. Lymphatic drainage in the muscle and sucutis of the arm after breast cancer treatment. *Breast Cancer Res Treat.* 2009;117(3):549-557
4. Finegold DN, Schacht V, Kimak MA, et al. HGF and MET mutations in primary and secondary lymphoedema. *Lymph. Res. Biol.* 2008;6:65-68
5. Williams AF, Franks PJ, Moffat CJ. Lymphoedema: estimating the size of the problem. *Palliat Med.* 2005;19:300-313.
6. Logan V. Incidence and prevalence of lymphoedema: a literature review. *J Clin Nurs.* 1995;4:213-219.
7. Petrek JA, Heelan MC. Incidence of breast carcinoma-related lymphoedema. *Cancer.* 1998;83:2776-2781.
8. Sener SF, Winchester DJ, Martz CH, et al. Lymphoedema after sentinel lymphadenectomy for breast carcinoma. *Cancer.* 2001;92:748-752.
9. Armer JM, Stewart BR. Post-breast cancer lymphedema: incidence increases from 12 to 30 to 60 months. *Lymphology.* 2010;43:118-127.
10. Meek AG. Breast radiotherapy and lymphoedema. *Cancer.* 1998;83:2788-2797.
11. Ryan M, Stainton MC, Slaytor EK, et al. Aetiology and prevalence of lower limb lymphoedema following treatment for gynaecological cancer. *Aust N Z J Obstet Gynaecol.* 2003;43:148-151.
12. Van der Velden J, Ansink A. Primary groin irradiation vs primary groin surgery for early vulval cancer (Cochrane Review). In: *The Cochrane Library.* No. 3. Chichester: John Wiley and Sons; 2004.
13. Stehman FB, Bundy BN, Thomas G, et al. Groin dissection versus groin radiation in carcinoma of the vulva: a gynaecologic oncology group study. *Int J Radiat Oncol Biol Phys.* 1992;24:389-396.
14. Okeke AA, Bates DO, Gillatt DO. Lymphoedema in urological cancers. *Eur Urol.* 2004;45:18-25.
15. Karakousis CP, Heisler MA, Moore RH. Lymphoedema after groin dissection. *Am J Surg.* 1983;145:205-208.
16. Papachristou D, Fortner JT. Comparison of lymphoedema following incontinuity and discontinuity groin dissection. *Ann Surg.* 1997;185:13-16.
17. Teunissen SCCM, Wesker W, Kruitwagen C, et al. Symptom prevalence in patients with incurable cancer: a systematic review. *J Pain Symptom Manage.* 2007;34(1):94-104.
18. Morita T, Tsunoda J, Inone S, et al. The palliative prognostic index: a scoring system for survival prediction of terminally ill cancer patients. *Support Care Cancer.* 1999;7:128-133.
19. Stemmer R. Ein klinisches Zeichen zur Früh-und differential-diagnose des Lymphödems. *VASA.* 1976;5:261-262.
20. Badger CM, Mortimer PS, Regnard CFB, et al. Pain in the chronically swollen limb. *Prog Lymphol.* 1998;11:243-246.
21. Rockson SG, Miller LT, Senie R, et al. Diagnosis and management of lymphoedema. *Cancer.* 1998;83:2882-2885.
22. Tobin MB, Lacey HJ, Meyer L, et al. Psychological morbidity of breast cancer-related arm swelling. *Cancer.* 1993;72:3248-3252.
23. Mallon E, Powell S, Mortimer P, et al. Evidence of altered cell mediated immunity in post-mastectomy lymphoedema. *Br J Dermatol.* 1997;137:928-933.
24. Casley-Smith JR, Földi M, Ryan TJ, et al. Summary of the 10th international congress of Lymphology working group discussions and recommendations. *Lymphology.* 1985;18:175-180.
25. Mulvenna PM, Gillham L, Regnard CFB. Lymphangiosarcomata—experience in a lymphoedema clinic. *Palliat Med.* 1995;9:55-59.
26. DeSimone GG. Treatment of malignant ascites. *Prog Palliat Care.* 1999;7:10-16.
27. Strasser F Hanks G, Cherny N. et al. The pathophysiology of anorexia/cachexia syndrome. In: Doyle D, et al., eds. *Oxford Textbook of Palliative Medicine*, 3rd ed. Oxford: Oxford University Press; 2004:520-533.
28. Wells PS, Anderson DR, Rodger M, et al. Evaluation of D-dimer in the diagnosis of suspected deep-vein thrombosis. *N Engl J Med.* 2003;349:1227-1235.

29. Keeley V. The role of lymphoscintigraphy in the management of chronic oedema. *J Lymphoedema.* 2006;1(1):42-57.

30. Stout Gergich N, Pfalzer L, McGarvey C, et al. Pre-operative assessment enables the early diagnosis and successful treatment of lymphedema. *Cancer.* 2008;112:2809-2818.

31. Taghian A, Skolny MN, Miller CL, et al. Defining a threshold for intervention in breast cancer-related lymphedema. Is 3% volume change too low? Proceedings of 23rd International Congress of Lymphology. 2011; Malmo, Sweden (in press).

32. Devoogdt N, Christiaens MR, Geraerts I, et al. Effect of manual lymph drainage in addition to guidelines and exercise therapy on arm lymphoedema related to breast cancer: randomized controlled trial. *BMJ.* 2011;343: d5326.

33. Box RC, Reul-Hirche HM, Bullock-Saxton JE, Furnival CM. Physiotherapy after breast cancer surgery: results of a randomized controlled study to minimize lymphoedema. *Breast Cancer Res Treat.* 2002;75(1):51-64.

34. Torres Lacomba M, Yuste Sanchez MJ, Zapico Coni A, et al. Effectiveness of early physiotherapy to prevent lymphoedema after surgery for breast cancer: randomized, single blinded, clinical trial. *BMJ.* 2010: 340:b5396.

35. Földi E, Földi M. Lymphostatic diseases. In: Földi M, Földi E, Kubik S, eds. *Textbook of Lymphology.* Munich: Urban & Fischer; 2003:275-279:chap 5.

36. Lymphoedema Framework. *Best Practice for the Management of Lymphoedema. International Consensus.* London: MEP Ltd; 2006.

37. Jenns K. Management strategies. In: Twycross R, Jenns K, Todd J, eds. *Lymphoedema.* Oxford: Radcliffe Medical Press; 2000:108:chap 7.

38. Preston NJ, Seers K, Mortimer PS. Physical therapies for reducing and controlling lymphoedema of the limbs. *Cochrane Database Syst Rev.* 2004;Issue 4:Art No. CD003141.

39. Ko DSC, Lerner R, Klose G, et al. Effective treatment of lymphoedema of the extremities. *Arch Surg.* 1998;133:452-458.

40. Bray T, Barnett J. Pneumatic compression therapy. In: Twycross R, Jenns K, Todd J, eds. *Lymphoedema.* Oxford: Radcliffe Medical Press; 2000:236-243:chap 4.

41. Wilburn O, Wilburn P, Rockson SG. A pilot prospective evaluation of a novel alternative for maintenance therapy of breast cancer-associated lymphoedema. *BMC Cancer.* 2006; 6:84.

42. Brorson H, Svensson H. Liposuction combined with controlled compression therapy reduces arm lymphoedema more effectively than controlled compression therapy alone. *Plast Reconstr Surg.* 1998;102:1058-1067.

43. Bococardo F, Casabona F, De Cian F, et al. Lymphoedema microsurgical preventive healing approach: a new technique for primary prevention of arm lymphoedema after mastectomy. *Ann Surg Oncol.* 2009;16(3):703-708.

44. Lahteenvuo M, Honkonen K, Tervala T, et al. Growth factor therapy and autologous lymph node transfer in lymphedema. *Circulation.* 2011;123(6):613-620.

45. Casley-Smith JR, Morgan RG, Piller NB. Treatment of lymphoedema of the arms and legs with 5,6 benzo-(alpha)-pyrone. *N Engl J Med.* 1993;329:1158-1163.

46. Loprinzi CL, Kugler JW, Sloan JA, et al. Lack of effect of coumarin in women with lymphedema after treatment for breast cancer. *N Engl J Med.* 1999;340:346-350.

47. BLS/LSN Consensus Guidelines on the Management of Cellulitis in Lymphoedema. www.thebls.com

48. Towers A, Hodgson P, Shay C, Keeley V. Care of palliative patients with cancer-related lymphoedema. *J Lymphoedema.* 2010;5(1):72-80.

49. Badger C. Lymphoedema: management of patients with advanced cancer. *Prof Nurse.* 1987;2:100-102.

50. Wittlinger H, Wittlinger G. Absolute contraindications. In: *Textbook of Dr Vodder's Manual Lymph Drainage Vol 1 Basic Course.* 5th ed. Brussels: Haug International; 1995:74.

51. Crooks S, Locke J, Walker J, Keeley V. Palliative bandaging in breast cancer related arm oedema. *J Lymphoedema.* 2007;2(1):50-54.

52. NICE Guidance. *Stent Placement for Vena Caval Obstruction. Interventional Procedure Guidance 79.* London: National Institute for Clinical Excellence; 2004.

53. Johnson MJ, Sherry K. How do palliative physicians manage venous thromboembolism. *Palliat Med.* 1997;11:46-48.

54. Clein LJ, Pugachev E. Reduction of edema of lower extremities by subcutaneous controlled drainage: eight cases. *Ann J Hospice Palliat Med.* 2004;21:228-232.

55. International Lymphoedema Framework. Position Document. The management of lymphoedema in advanced cancer and oedema at the end of life. 2010. www.lympho.org.

CHAPTER 28

Principles of Fistula and Stoma Management

Paula Erwin-Toth ■ Linda J. Stricker

Fistula formation in people with cancer is not an uncommon complication. Predisposing factors relate fistula formation to the type and extent of the malignancy, comorbid conditions, immunosuppression, and radiation-related damage to tissues and vessels (1–3).

Patients presenting with a variety of pelvic and abdominal cancers undergo fecal or urinary diversions as part of the surgical management plan. Procedures are performed with the intent of primary intervention for curative resection, extensive but resectable malignancy, or as palliation to relieve an obstruction (4,5). Other types of stomas seen in cancer management include esophagostomy, tracheostomy, and gastrostomy (5,6).

Managing fistulae and ostomies during palliative care should focus on maintaining or restoring skin integrity, containing effluent, patient comfort including odor control, and supportive interventions compatible with the patient plan of care (1–3,7,8).

FISTULA MANAGEMENT

Patients presenting with a fistula face immeasurable physical, psychological, social, and financial challenges (1,2). Adding this burden to a poor prognosis is a terrible blow. The goals of management include identifying and treating sepsis, stabilizing fluid and electrolyte balance, nutritional support, quantification of effluent, containment of fistula output, protection of perifistular skin, odor containment, and patient comfort (1,2,9). Even in patients without a terminal disease, mortality rates associated with an enterocutaneous fistula (ECF) range from 5% to 15% (3,10).

Fistula management is rarely a straightforward process. For patients in palliative care, it is even less so (5). Optimizing the physiologic state may not be compatible with the palliative plan of care and the right to self-determination. Patients and families need to understand how decisions will affect the relative success of fistula management (8).

A fistula is an abnormal communication from one epithelial surface to another epithelial surface (1,2,11). This includes internal connections from one organ to another organ or from an organ to the surface of the skin (1,2,11). A fistula, following the path of least resistance, develops at the site of a previous drain or incision, at the site of active disease, proximal to a distal obstruction, or in association with an anastomotic leak, tissue ischemia, an infectious process, or an abscess (1,3,9,11,12).

Signs of an impending fistula include localized erythema and pain with increasing discomfort, leukocytosis (which may not be evident with immunosuppressed patients), fever, fluid and electrolyte imbalances, altered mental state, and general malaise. The specific name of the fistula is according to origin to exit points (1,2,8).

MEDICAL MANAGEMENT

Medical management for a patient with a fistula centers on controlling sepsis, stabilizing fluids and electrolytes, and optimizing nutritional status (1–3,9,12,13). Radiography will identify the origin of fistulae, and computerized tomography (CT) scan will aid in making the diagnosis (9). In some cases, interventional radiology will use CT-guided assistance to drain an abscess and place a catheter to facilitate resolution (9). Depending on the type and extent of the fistula, intravenous fluids, antibiotic therapy, and enteral or parenteral nutritional support are considered in the management plan. Conservative therapy may elicit spontaneous closure of a fistula but only under optimum conditions (1,2,14). Once epithelialization (also known as stomatization) of a fistula tract has occurred, it will not close without surgical intervention (1,9,15). The difficulty arises in determining the role, if any, these interventions play in palliative care (5,8).

Medical management of fistulae has the primary goal of spontaneous closure. Using conservative methods such as nutritional management, fluid and electrolyte balance, and containment provides options for care. In cases where fistulae output is high, using medications (see Table 28.1) such as H_2 antagonists, somatostatin-14, or octreotide to decrease secretions combined with placing the patient NPO with nutritional support can create an environment for spontaneous closure (2,16). Prolonged bowel rest can result in atrophy of the intestinal villa, so use of this strategy is carefully monitored and should be time limited based on patient response (1,2,16).

TOPICAL MANAGEMENT

Topical management of fistulae is an applied science. Combining the fundamentals of wound and ostomy management in unique ways will achieve a plan of care to manage an individual situation. The goals of topical therapy in fistula care include containing effluent to quantify and control odor, facilitate comfort, assist in pain management, and restore and maintain integrity of the perifistular skin (1–3,7,8). Wound, ostomy, continence (WOC) nurses can

TABLE 28.1	Medications for decreasing secretions in fistulas when output is high
Histamine Receptor Antagonists (H2)	**Cimetidine**
	Acts to reduce gastric secretions by decreasing histamine's affect on H2 receptors in gastric cells
	No effect on spontaneous fistula closure, but does reduce gastric output to improve management (2)
Somatostatin-14	**Hormone naturally produced by pancreas** **Octreotide/synthetic form of somatostatin**
	Decreases intestinal output
	Has a short half-life (1–3 min)
	Slows gastric and gastrointestinal motility
	Improves fluid and electrolyte absorption
	Synthetic form is best when used with total parenteral administration (TPN)
	Octreotide has longer half-life (2 h)
	Octreotide administration is every 8 h by subcutaneous injection
	Monitor fistula output for decreased output; discontinue if no response (9)

be a tremendous asset in developing a plan of care for the patient with a fistula (10,16,17,21).

NEGATIVE PRESSURE WOUND THERAPY

Selective use of negative pressure wound therapy (NPWT) in patients with an ECF promotes closure in a nonepithelialized ECF and helps to manage effluent (1,2,14,15,18,19). It is essential for the clinician to follow the manufacturer's guidelines because NPWT systems on the market are not all approved for this use. Application of a contact layer to the base of the wound, protection of perifistular skin, and use of low suction is the standard approach in carefully selected patients (1,2,14,15).

ADDITIONAL TOPICAL THERAPIES

A myriad of wound, ostomy, and draining wound/fistula products may be useful in assisting the clinician in achieving the goals of topical therapy. Use of pouches, solid wafer skin barriers, topical wound dressings, catheter holders, and odor controlling agents may be appropriate (1,2,7,10,11,20). Creative combinations of these products significantly improve the quality of life for a patient with a fistula (8). Determining which combinations of product to use in a given situation requires a careful analysis of the skin planes adjacent to the fistulae (1,2,21). Elevating the head of the patient's bed moves the person to a seated position and exposes any skin folds, creases, and scars evened out for effective pouching (1,2,21).

A holistic approach to the care of these individuals is important. Many patients require one or more people to assist with care, and because of changes in the fistula size and configuration, frequent modifications of the plan are common (1,7,8,11). Financial considerations are significant. Establishment of a set protocol and expected wear time are useful in determining anticipated costs. Involvement of a care manager, social services, and financial specialist will support the patient and family to maximize reimbursement for supplies (7,11,22). For example, a large, single-use fistula pouch alone may cost $70 for each pouch. A vaginal cone to assist in managing a vaginal fistula located high in the vaginal vault may cost as much as $140. Accessory products, frequently needed to improve the efficacy of these devices, further escalate costs. Many insurance policies, including CMS may not readily cover fistula supplies. A detailed letter of medical necessity from a licensed care provider will define the cost benefit of product used and provide a compelling argument to the insurance provider.

An effective and economical approach to fistula care is a plan that includes pouching. The main goals of topical fistula management are realized when an effective and predictable pouch seal is achieved (1,2,8,20,21). If the fistula is not too large, a standard ostomy pouch can provide a secure, straightforward, and cost-effective option (1,7,8,10). Unlike pouching a stoma, managing a fistula with a pouch usually requires several additional steps beyond sizing and application of the pouch. The aperture of an ostomy pouch is sized to one-eighth inch larger than the base of the stoma, but the opening for a fistula may need to extend beyond the margins of the opening to a more even skin surface (7,8,10,20). This leaves the potential for skin exposed to chemical erosion from fistula effluent. Protect exposed skin with skin barrier pastes and powders, and fill uneven skin creases

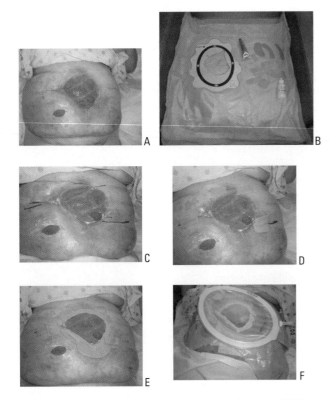

Figure 28.1. **(A–F)** Female patient with a high output ECF in an abdominal wound with a nonfunctioning ileostomy in the right lower quadrant. Steps of pouching application are shown.

with skin barrier (wafers, paste, strips, washers, or rings) to even out the skin contours before the pouch is applied (1,2,7,8,10,20). A standard wear time for an ostomy pouch over a conventional stoma is 3 to 5 days but a 24-hour wear time is a more reasonable expectation over a fistula. Additional days of wearing time are ideal but not always possible. Depending on the amount and consistency of the output, a drainable or urinary pouch will be used. For copious drainage, connection to constant drainage or use of suction to collect the effluent is helpful (3,14,16). See Figure 28.1A–F and Table 28.2.

Application of the more complex fistula management systems can challenge even the most experienced clinician. Patients and caregivers can find the care especially daunting; education requires time, patience, and follow-up. Discharge criteria include caregiver ability to achieve a consistent seal and acquire the supplies at home (11). Even if home health care is included, routine care of the fistula generally lies with the family. Rarely can a patient manage a complex fistula care autonomously.

OSTOMY CARE

The palliative care patient with an ostomy requires special considerations to maintain a secure pouch seal, maintain or restore peristomal skin integrity, and conserve energy with the application and removal process (1,5,7,8,10,20).

The patient with an established ostomy usually has a preferred stoma management method. However, changes in body contour, stoma size, abdominal firmness, skin changes, anemia, and tendency toward mucosal bleeding may necessitate recommendation of a new pouching system (7,8,10).

Fecal diversions are usually best managed with a drainable pouching system (23). In some cases, use of a closed end pouch with a descending or sigmoid colostomy with thick stool and once or twice daily function may be an option. For patients using colostomy irrigation as a management method, it may be best to discontinue this practice. The potential for fatigue and anemia is increased and subsequent ischemia can predispose the patient to colon perforation even with the use of an irrigation cone (24). Rigid catheters used by some patients in past years to irrigate also increase the risk for perforation and should not be used under any circumstances. Increasing fluids and use of stool softeners will ease the transition from irrigation to spontaneous evacuation of the colon (24).

Patients with ileostomies and urostomies benefit from the use of extended wear barriers (23). However, skin changes in the palliative care patient could make removal of these more aggressive barriers a problem. Using skin sealants and adhesive removers assists with removal but in many cases a standard wear carboxymethylcellulose barrier may be the best choice (20,23).

Selection of a one piece or two piece systems, flat or convex, regular or extended wear drainable pouch with a clip or integrated closure, or urostomy drain spout is guided by the WOC nurse (23). Size of the pouch opening is usually one-eighth inch larger than the base of the stoma. If mucosal bleeding is a concern, enlarging the aperture by another one-eighth inch decreases mucosal trauma and bleeding (5,22).

Efforts made to simplify the pouching procedure will minimize fatigue and ease the process for the patient and caregiver (5,8,11). Establishing a predictable wear time is essential and adds continuity to the plan of care. A pouch should not be left on until it leaks because undermining of the seal can leave the skin exposed to damage from effluent (20,22).

Urinary or fecal diversions not only result in an alteration in elimination but also can cause a profound impact on body image (22,23). Ostomy surgeries performed as part of a cancer surgery is a constant reminder of disease for some patients (5,8). Counseling focused on encouraging the patient to verbalize feelings and concerns will provide important clues that individualize the plan to address those issues (5,8).

Advances in the manufacturing of ostomy pouches offer secure, odor proof, and discreet care for the person with an ostomy (20,22). Even with modern technology nothing promotes effective ostomy management like a well-sited, well-constructed stoma (20–23). Consultation with a WOC nurse preoperatively, postoperatively, and after discharge provides the patient and family specialized ostomy care teaching, counseling, and follow-up.

TABLE 28.2	Common peristomal skin conditions (20)	
Conditions	**Characteristics**	**Treatment**
Folliculitis	Traumatic removal of hair during pouch change results in inflammation and infection of hair follicles. Lesions are painful and moist.	Topical antimicrobial powder, cover large lesions with non-adherent dressing. Once healed, carefully shave area. Use of adhesive remover and sealant is advised after lesions healed.
Candidiasis	Warm, moist environment creates an environment for growth of *Candida albicans*. Generally diffuse red patches with characteristic advancing border and satellite lesions. Severe itching common.	Topical antifungal powder. Assess system for leakage or undermining of seal. Refit pouching system as appropriate.
Irritant dermatitis	Chemical destruction of the skin caused by topical products or leakage. Area appears red, moist, and painful. May be localized to a specific area of pouch undermining or leakage.	Review product usage and techniques to determine cause. Correct/revise pouching system.
Pseudoverrucous lesions (formerly called PEH)	Overgrowth of tissue caused by overexposure to moisture. Appears as raised, moist lesions with a wart-like appearance. Lesions are painful.	Assess equipment for proper aperture and fit. Resize as needed. In severe cases, sharp debridement of the tissue may be required.
Mechanical trauma	External item or force causing damage to the stoma and/or skin from pressure, laceration, friction, or shear.	Assess equipment and technique. Modify to prevent re-injury.
Allergic contact dermatitis	Allergic response generated by patient sensitivity to a particular product. Skin appears red, swollen, eroded, weepy, or bleeding. Generally corresponds to the exposed area.	Remove the allergen, avoid other irritants, and protect the skin. Patch test with other products as needed. Refer to dermatologist for multiple allergies.
Peristomal abscess	One or more open, painful lesions surrounded by a halo of redness. Not uncommon in patients with active Crohn's disease in the distal bowel.	Unroofing of ulcer by surgeon. Management depends on size. Review options, including non-adherent dressings, hydrogel, astringent solution, calcium alginate, hydrofiber, or hydrocolloid wafer. A non-adherent pouching system can be fashioned with a one-piece pouch with belt tabs, an extra gasket and a solid skin barrier wafer.
Pyoderma gangrenosum	Associated with inflammatory bowel diseases, arthritis, leukemia, polycythemia vera, and multiple myeloma. Red open lesions become raised with irregular purplish margins.	Systemic treatment of underlying disease, local ulcer treatment by unroofing the area is generally not advised. Intralesional and systemic steroid therapy may be prescribed. Topical therapy and pouching same as with an abscess.

(Continued)

TABLE 28.2   Common peristomal skin conditions (20)   (Continued)

Conditions	Characteristics	Treatment
Radiation injury	Red, thinned skin. Easily traumatized by removal of skin adhesives.	Gently cleanse skin with cool water. Use a skin barrier that is easy to remove. Be cautious in use of solvents or skin sealants due to frequent sensitivities and risk of chemical trauma.
Caput medusae (peristomal varices)	In patients with portal (liver) hypertension, the pressure at the portal systemic shunt in the mucocutaneous junction increases, creating venous engorgement. With trauma, profuse bleeding can occur.	Apply pressure and/or use hemostatic agents, for example, silver nitrate. Cautery or surgical ligation may be necessary. Remove pouch carefully. Avoid aggressive skin barriers and skin sealants. If stoma is relocated varices will eventually recur around the new stoma unless underlying liver disease is treated (e.g., liver transplant).
Necrosis/ischemia	Dark red to black mucosa may appear dry, mottled. Stoma may be firm or flaccid. Ischemia usually noticeable within 12–24 h; can be evident up to 3–5 d post-op. Results from: a. Excessive tension on the mesentery with resultant compromise to arterial inflow, venous outflow, or both. Can be a result of abdominal distension, obesity, excessive edema. b. Interruption of blood supply to the stoma, for example, embolus, clot. c. Excessive devascularization d. Narrowly spaced sutures; sutures tied snugly around stoma, or continuous constricting sutures.	Distal necrosis: if superficial, conservative management—tissue allowed to demarcate, slough • Stoma will then be flush or slightly retracted; stenosis may occur Necrosis extending below fascial level • Run risk of perforation and subsequent peritonitis • Notify surgeon immediately • Mucocutaneous separation develops • Usually requires re-operation with construction of new stoma Intervention • Ongoing mucosal assessment • Prompt notification of surgeon of mucosal changes • Utilization of clear pouches in postoperative period, proper sizing of equipment, frequent pouch changes. • Odor control as tissue sloughs. • Psychological support to patient and family.

Mucocutaneous Separation	Separation of the suture line at the junction of the stomal mucosa and skin. Maybe superficial or deep; may be partial or circumferential.	Interventions: a. Gently probe with swab to determine depth, undermining. b. Irrigate with normal saline to clean. c. If deep: use rope packing, for example, hypertonic saline rope. A two-piece system may be beneficial. d. Shallow wounds: use powder or granules to fill defect, then cover and pouch. e. If separation is draining large amount of fluid, it may need to be included in pouch opening. f. If peritoneal contamination is a concern, the surgeon may resuture stoma to skin, either locally or under anesthesia.
Bleeding	Portal hypertension (caput medusae). Due to underlying liver disease. A-V shunt formation can lead to profuse bleeding at a mucocutaneous junction. Trauma Results from improperly sized or applied pouching systems; incorrect shaving techniques, forceful irrigation; sports-related injuries. Disease process/medication Underlying blood dyscrasias; anticoagulant therapy.	Avoid trauma to area. Gentle technique when applying and removing products. If bleeding occurs apply pressure and seek medical attention. Cautery or ligation may be needed. Revise equipment and technique. Avoid re-injury If bleeding continues seek medical assistance. Avoid trauma to area. Gentle technique when applying and removing products. If bleeding occurs apply pressure and seek medical attention.

Prolapse	Telescoping of bowel through the stoma	Interventions
		• Surgery
		• Conservative management
		    Reduce prolapse
		    Use of binder or prolapse belt to keep reduced
		• Modify pouching system as needed to avoid trauma to bowel mucosa.

Retraction	Stoma resting at or below skin level. Can be due to weight changes. Recession may be indicative of recurrent Crohn's disease due to scarring and contracting of bowel.	Modify pouching system; maintain seal between pouch and skin without undermining a. Use of convexity b. Accessory products Surgery as needed.

(Continued)

TABLE 28.2 Common peristomal skin conditions (20) *(Continued)*

Conditions	Characteristics	Treatment
Parastomal hernia	Most common with colostomies; appears as a bulge around the stoma; the bulge represents loops of the intestine that protrude through the fascial defect around the stoma and into the subcutaneous tissue. Results from • Stoma placed outside of rectus muscle • Increased intra-abdominal pressure with lifting and straining • Defect in abdominal musculature loss of muscle tone (as with weight gain or aging) • Excessively large fascial defect • Placement of stoma in midline incision • Wound infection	Avoid colostomy irrigations. If hernia can be reduced apply hernia belt/binder. If obstructed or incarcerated seek immediate medical care.
Food bolus obstruction	Most common with ileostomies. Results from ingestion of high-fiber foods such as nuts, popcorn, string vegetables, oranges, or fruit peels (insoluble fibers) Symptoms: severe cramping, abdominal pain, nausea, vomiting, cessation of stomal output or watery, odorous output, high-pitched tinkling bowel sounds, stomal edema Occur usually just proximal to stoma. Teach prevention: limited intake of high-fiber food, especially insoluble fibers, chew food well, adequate fluid intake.	Home-relief measures. a. Warm bath. b. Peristomal massage and knee-chest position to attempt to dislodge mass. c. If stoma is swollen, remove pouch and replace with one that has a larger aperture. d. If able to tolerate fluids and is passing stool, avoid solid foods and increase intake of fluids to help replace electrolytes. e. If vomiting or not passing stool, or both, take nothing by mouth. Physician should be notified. f. Physician is notified: 1. Stool output stops. 2. Symptoms persist with use of conservative measures for 24 h. 3. Cannot tolerate fluids. Ileal lavage may be necessary to relieve food bolus obstruction

CONCLUSION

Care of palliative care patients presenting with fistulae or ostomies can be challenging for the patient, family, and health-care team. A systematic, multidisciplinary approach with collaboration of a WOC nurse can support the plan of care and improve the patient's quality of life (5).

REFERENCES

1. Erwin-Toth P, Stricker L. Drain, tube, & fistula management. In: Baranoski S, Ayello E, eds. *Wound Care Essentials: Practice Principles.* 3rd ed. Philadelphia, PA: Wolters Kluwer Health/ Lippincott Williams & Wilkins; 2012;19:477-490.

2. Bryant R, Rolstad B. Management of draining wounds & fistulas. In: Bryant R, Nix D, eds. *Acute & Chronic Wounds: Current Management Concepts.* 4th ed. St. Louis, MO: Mosby/Elsevier; 2012;490-516.

3. Martinez A, Ferron G, Le Gal M, Torrent J, Capdet J, Querleu D. Management of ileocutaneous fistulae using TNP after surgery for abdominal malignancy. *J Wound Care.* 2009;18(7):282-288.

4. Beitz J. Gastrointestinal etiologies leading to a fecal diversion. In: Colwell J, Goldberg M, Carmel J, eds. *Fecal & Urinary Diversions: Management Principles.* St. Louis, MO: Mosby/ Elsevier; 2004;136-162.

5. Floruta C, Berschorner J, Hull T. Gastrointestinal cancers: medical management. In: Colwell J, Goldberg M, Carmel J. eds. *Fecal & Urinary Diversions: Management Principles.* St. Louis, MO: Mosby/Elsevier; 2004;102-125.

6. Carmel J, Scardillo J. Tube management. In: Colwell J, Goldberg M, Carmel J, eds. *Fecal & Urinary Diversions: Management Principles.* St. Louis, MO: Mosby/Elsevier; 2004;351-380.

7. Cobb A, Knaggs E. The nursing management of enterocutaneous fistulae: a challenge for all. *Wound Care.* 2003;8:S32-S38.

8. Phillips J, Walton M. Caring for patients with enterocutaneous fistula. *Br J Nurs.* 1993;2(9):496-500.

9. Schecter WP, Hirshberg A, Chang DS, et al. Enteric fistulas: principles of management. *J Am Coll Surg.* 2009;209(4):484-491.

10. Brindle C, Blankenship J. Management complex abdominal wounds with small bowel fistulae. *J WOCN.* 2009;36(4):396-403.

11. Slater R. Supporting patients with enterocutaneous fistula: from hospital to home. *Br J Community Nurs.* 2011;16(2):66-73.

12. Mawdsley J, Hollington P, Bassett P, et al. An analysis of predictive factors for healing and mortality in patients with enterocutaneous fistula. *Aliment Pharmacol Ther.* 2008;28:1111-1121.

13. Austin T. Nutrition management of enterocutaneous fistula. *Support Line.* 2006;28(6):10–16.

14. Bovill E, Banwell P, Teot L, et al. Topical negative pressure wound therapy: a review of its role and guidelines for its use in the management of acute wounds. *Int Wound J.* 2008;5(4):511-529.

15. Schein M. What's new in postoperative enterocutaneous fistula. *World J Surg.* 2008;32:336-338.

16. Kordasiewicz L. Abdominal wound with a fistula and large amount of drainage status after incarcerated hernia. *J WOCN.* 2004;31(3):150-153.

17. Davis M, Dere K, Hadley G. Options for managing an open wound with draining enterocutaneous fistula. *J WOCN.* 2000;27(2):118-123.

18. Wainstein D, Fernandez E, Gonzales D, et al. Treatment of high-output enterocutaneous fistula with a vacuum-compaction device. *World J Surg.* 2008;32:430-435.

19. Gunn LA, Follmar KE, Wong MS, Lettieri SC, Levin LS, Erdmann D. Management of enterocutaneous fistulas using negative-pressure dressings. *Ann Plast Surg.* 2006;57(6):621-625.

20. Erwin-Toth P, Stricker L, van Rijswijk L. Peristomal skin complications. *Am J Nurs.* 2010;110(2):43-48.

21. Geiger-Jones E, Harbit M. Management of an ileostomy and mucous fistula located in a dehisced wound in a patient with morbid obesity. *J WOCN.* 2003;30(6):351-356.

22. Skovgaard R, Keiding H. A cost-effectiveness analysis of fistula treatment in the abdominal region using a new integrated fistula and wound management system. *J WOCN.* 2008;35(6):592-592.

23. Colwell J. Principles of stoma management. In: Colwell J, Goldberg M, Carmel J, eds. *Fecal & Urinary Diversions: Management Principles.* St. Louis, MO: Mosby/Elsevier; 2004;240-262.

24. Carmel J, Goldberg M. Pre-operative & post-operative management. In: Colwell J, Goldberg M, Carmel J, eds. *Fecal & Urinary Diversions: Management Principles.* St. Louis, MO: Mosby/ Elsevier; 2004;207-239.

CHAPTER **29** # Dyspnea in the Cancer Patient

Deborah Dudgeon

INTRODUCTION

Dyspnea, an unpleasant awareness of breathing, is a very common symptom that is often unrecognized in people with cancer. It is a complex and distressing symptom that can impact people's daily functioning (1) and result in impaired quality of life (2,3), social isolation (4), and prompt terminal sedation (5). Patients with breathlessness are more likely to visit the emergency department (6) and die in the hospital than at home (7).

Despite the fact that breathlessness is very common in people with cancer (8–13), it is often not well controlled. Studies show that unlike pain that is usually improved with current interventions, the intensity of dyspnea is not impacted (14,15). Higginson and McCarthy (14) found that in a group of terminally ill cancer patients cared for at home, pain scores decreased but there was no change in dyspnea scores over time. In a convenience sample of patients admitted to an acute care palliative care unit, Dudgeon et al. (15) also found that for patients who had scores >50 mm on a 100-mm visual analog scale after 7 days of intervention, the median score for breathlessness remained at 50 mm while pain decreased to 30 mm. A recent study found that 27% and 39% of cancer outpatients with moderate to severe pain and dyspnea, respectively, had no evidence of a comprehensive assessment (16).

To optimally manage this distressing symptom, it is necessary to have an understanding of its prevalence and impact; the multidimensional nature of the symptom; the underlying pathophysiology and associated factors; components of a thorough assessment; the clinical syndromes common in cancer patients; and the indications and limitations of current therapeutic approaches.

PREVALENCE

In a large, geographically based cohort with a full scope of cancer diagnoses, over one-half of the patients reported shortness of breath, with half of them having scores on the Edmonton Symptom Assessment System (ESAS) in the moderate to severe range (13). In another study of an outpatient general population, 46% reported breathlessness with only 15% describing the intensity as moderate to severe (8).

The differences in intensity may be related to cancer type and/or proximity to death. The first study found that patients with lung cancer had higher intensity scores than other diagnoses and patients with lung cancer composed 19% of the patients as opposed to 4% in the second study. Seow et al. found that patients with lung cancer had 50% greater chance of reporting moderate to severe breathlessness and that the intensity of dyspnea increased over the last 6 months of life (17). Muers and Round found breathlessness to be present at diagnosis in 60% of 298 patients with non–small cell lung cancer and in nearly 90% just prior to death (10). In a radiation oncology community setting, Lutz et al. found that 73% of patients with locally advanced lung cancer presented with breathlessness and the severity was worse in the group that survived <3 months (18). Two studies examined the trajectory of breathlessness in patients with advanced cancer (11,12). In a study of 5,386 cancer patients, Currow et al. showed that the intensity of breathlessness and the prevalence of severe breathlessness increased as death approached, with a significant increase in the rate of change between 3 and 10 days before death (11). Bausewein et al. prospectively followed the intensity of breathlessness in 49 advanced cancer patients and found that breathlessness increased over time and there were 4 different trajectories for individual patients, with fluctuating breathlessness being the most common (12).

IMPACT OF DYSPNEA

Breathlessness is one of the most distressing symptoms for patients (3) and can severely impair their quality of life. In a study of 70 patients with advanced cancer, Reddy et al. identified that patients experienced 2 types of dyspnea: continuous and breakthrough. The majority of patients had breakthrough dyspnea alone (61%), with 39% experiencing constant dyspnea and 20% also having episodes of breakthrough breathlessness (2). Breakthrough dyspnea occurred on an average five to six times a day with a median intensity of 5/10 on ESAS. The median intensity of breathlessness in patients with constant dyspnea was 7/10. Those who experienced continuous dyspnea had a worse quality of life than those with breakthrough dyspnea only, with significant differences in their general activity, mood, walking ability, normal work, and enjoyment of life (2). In a study of late-stage cancer patients, Roberts et al. (1) found that various activities intensified dyspnea for patients: climbing stairs—95.6%, walking slowly—47.8%, getting dressed—52.2%, talking or eating—56.5%, and at rest—26.1% (1). This study showed that the patients decreased their activity to whatever degree would relieve their breathlessness. Sixty-two percent of the patients with dyspnea had been short of breath for >3 months and most had received no assistance from nurses or physicians, leaving them to cope in isolation. Other studies of patients with lung cancer showed that 97% had decreased their activities, 80% had socially isolated themselves from friends and family (4), 36% were housebound, and 10% largely chair bound because of their breathlessness (19). In a study of terminally ill cancer patients, the willingness to live was directly related to the intensity of breathlessness (20). Uncontrolled dyspnea prompted terminal sedation in 25% to 53% of patients requiring sedation for uncontrolled symptoms (5).

MULTIDIMENSIONAL NATURE OF DYSPNEA

Dyspnea is a complex subjective experience that depends on the integration of respiratory afferent activity, respiratory motor drive, affective state, attention, experience, and learning (21).

Ventilation results from activation of the respiratory motor drive that is generated in the brainstem respiratory neural network. Receptors in the upper airway, lower airway, lung parenchyma and respiratory muscles, and peripheral and central chemoreceptors provide sensory input to the brainstem respiratory network as well as to higher brain centers (somatosensory and association cortices) (see Fig. 29.1).

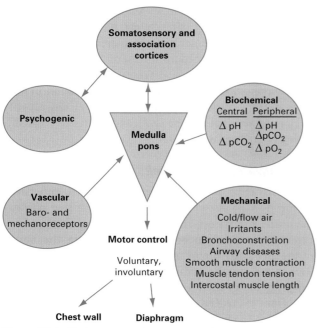

Figure 29.1. Brainstem respiratory network.

Normally breathing is not uncomfortable, but if the magnitude of the stimulus from one or more of these sensory afferents is great enough then changes in breathing effort are perceived. Attention, experience/learning, and the person's affective state further modulate respiratory sensation and perception (21). Recent brain imaging studies suggest that the unpleasantness of dyspnea is processed cortically in the anterior insula and amygdala areas of the brain (22). These neural networks for processing dyspnea are shared with other unpleasant sensations such as pain (23).

Abernethy and Wheeler proposed a new conceptual model of breathlessness that they named "Total Dyspnea" (24). This model of Total Dyspnea encompasses four domains: physical, psychological, interpersonal, and existential that contribute to a patient's distress and suffering. They suggest that "Total Dyspnea" provides a more comprehensive, integrated, conceptual framework to help clinicians understand breathlessness and the suffering of patients and families.

FACTORS ASSOCIATED WITH DYSPNEA IN THE CANCER PATIENT

A number of authors have examined the factors that are associated with dyspnea in patients with cancer (Table 29.1) (2,8,9,25–31). In two different studies, investigators found that dyspnea in cancer patients had diverse etiologies, commonly with more than one factor contributing to the breathlessness (26,31). In another study, the presence and intensity of dyspnea were strongly related to the number of risk factors a patient had (8). Primary or metastatic involvement of the lung or pleura with cancer was associated with the presence of dyspnea in most studies (2,8,9,25,26,31). In a study of 923 cancer outpatients, Dudgeon et al. found that the risk factors significantly related to the presence of dyspnea were a history of smoking, asthma, or chronic obstructive pulmonary disease (COPD), lung irradiation, or a history of exposure to asbestos, coal dust, cotton dust, or grain dust (8). They also found that the intensity of shortness of breath was significantly associated with the presence of hilar, mediastinal, and rib metastases; and surprisingly, the presence of mediastinal or hilar metastases was associated with a higher intensity of dyspnea than was the presence of lung metastases (8).

The general debility of terminal cancer (9), respiratory muscle weakness (26–28), and the presence of the hyperventilation syndrome (25) have been associated with the presence of dyspnea in cancer patients. Interestingly, the presence or severity of dyspnea could not be predicted by the level of oxygen saturation, air flow obstruction, or the type or severity of abnormal spirometry (26–28).

The intensity of fatigue, sleep, anxiety, depression, and sense of well-being were significantly associated with ESAS shortness of breath scores in univariate analyses in a prospective observational study of 70 cancer patients with dyspnea (2). In multivariate analyses, ESAS dyspnea was

TABLE 29.1	**Factors associated with dyspnea in cancer patients**

A. Dyspnea Due Directly to Cancer

- Lung involvement (primary or metastatic)
- Pleural involvement (primary or metastatic)
- Hilar or mediastinal metastases
- Rib metastases

B. Dyspnea Due Indirectly to Cancer

- General debility
- Fatigue
- Respiratory muscle weakness

C. Dyspnea Due to Cancer Treatment

- Lung included in the radiation field

D. Dyspnea Unrelated to Cancer

- History of smoking
- Chronic obstructive pulmonary disease
- Asthma
- History of exposure to: asbestos, coal dust, cotton dust, and grain dust
- Anxiety
- Depression
- Poor sleep

associated with fatigue, forced expiratory volume in 1 minute (FEV_1), pain, and depression.

In another study of 171 consecutive outpatients with lung cancer, psychological distress, the presence of organic causes, cough, and pain were significantly correlated with total dyspnea as measured by the Cancer Dyspnea Scale (30). In this study, heart rate significantly correlated with the "sense of effort" subscale, and psychological distress and pain significantly correlated with the "sense of anxiety" factor.

Anxiety is significantly correlated with the intensity of dyspnea in a number of studies in cancer patients (2,25–28,30). These correlations are significant ($p = 0.03$–0.001) but low ($r = 0.26$–0.32), with anxiety explaining only 9% of the variance in the intensity of dyspnea. Tanaka et al. also found significant correlations with the intensity of dyspnea and depression scores as measured by the Hospital Anxiety and Depression Scale (HADS) (30). When they combined the HADS anxiety and depression scores the correlation coefficient was $r = 0.63$ ($p < 0.01$), explaining 36% of variance in the intensity of dyspnea. Reddy et al. found HADS depression, but not anxiety, to be significantly correlated in univariate and multivariate analyses with the Oxygen Cost Diagram,

an instrument that evaluates the effect of shortness of breath on the person's activities of daily living (2).

PATHOPHYSIOLOGY

The pathophysiologic mechanisms of dyspnea can be categorized as increased ventilatory demand, impaired mechanical responses, or a combination of these two mechanisms. Spirometry and other pulmonary function tests (PFTs) are useful in determining the underlying etiology of dyspnea. Table 29.2 outlines the pathophysiologic mechanisms of dyspnea with the potential clinical causes in a person with cancer.

Increased Ventilatory Demand

The brainstem respiratory neural network will activate the respiratory motor drive and ventilation if there is an increase in physiologic dead space in the lung, hypoxia from any cause, severe deconditioning with early and accelerated rise in blood lactate levels, changes in V_{CO_2} or arterial P_{CO_2} set points, and psychological causes such as anxiety and depression. Increased physiologic dead space can occur as a result of thromboemboli, tumor emboli, vascular obstruction, or chemo- or radiation acute or chronic pneumonitis.

When dyspnea is secondary to an increased ventilatory demand spirometry is usually normal.

Impaired Mechanical Responses

Impaired mechanical responses result in restrictive or obstructive ventilatory deficits or a combination of both.

Restrictive Ventilatory Deficit

A restrictive ventilatory deficit results from decreased distensibility of the lung parenchyma, pleura, or chest wall; from reduced movement of the diaphragm; or from a reduction in the maximum force exerted by the respiratory muscles. The principal diagnostic features of a restrictive ventilatory deficit are a concurrent reduction in both FEV_1 and vital capacity (FVC), decreased total lung capacity (TLC) and residual volume (RV), and often decreased diffusing capacity as well.

Obstructive Ventilatory Deficit

An obstructive ventilatory deficit refers to impedance to the flow of air within the lung. Progressive narrowing of the airways can result from structural changes from external compression or obstruction within the lumen of the airway by tumor, mucus, inflammation, or edema. Bronchoconstriction, a functional change which causes narrowing of the airways, results from increased bronchomotor tone from the release of histamine, leukotrienes, and other mediators. The hallmarks of an obstructive ventilatory deficit are a reduced FEV_1/FVC and an increased TLC, RV, and functional residual capacity.

TABLE 29.2	Pathophysiologic and clinical mechanisms of dyspnea in the cancer patient

A. Impaired Mechanical Response

(a) Restrictive ventilatory deficit

  (i) Pleural or parenchymal disease

  • Primary or metastatic

  • Pleural effusion

  (ii) Reduced movement of diaphragm

  • Ascites

  • Hepatomegaly

  (iii) Reduced chest wall compliance

  • Pain

  • Hilar/mediastinal involvement

  • Chest wall invasion with tumor

  • Deconditioning

  • Neuromuscular

  • Neurohumoral

  (iv) Respiratory muscle weakness

  • Phrenic nerve paralysis

  • Cachexia

  • Electrolyte abnormalities

  • Steroid use

  • Deconditioning

(b) Obstructive ventilatory deficit

  (i) Tumor obstruction

  (ii) Asthma

  (iii) COPD

(c) Mixed Obstructive/Restrictive Disease (any combination of factors)

B. Increased Ventilatory Demand

(a) Increased physiologic dead space

  (i) Thromboemboli

  (ii) Tumor emboli

  (iii) Vascular obstruction

  (iv) Radiation pneumonitis

  (v) Chemotherapy-induced pneumonitis

(b) Severe deconditioning

(c) Hypoxemia—Anemia

(d) Change in V_{CO_2} or arterial P_{CO_2} set point

(e) Increased neural reflex activity

(f) Psychological causes

  - Anxiety

  - Depression

COPD, chronic obstructive pulmonary disease.

Modified from Booth S, Dudgeon D. *Dyspnea in advanced disease: a guide to clinical management.* New York, NY: Oxford University Press, 2006.

MULTIDIMENSIONAL ASSESSMENT OF DYSPNEA

As dyspnea is a complex subjective experience a comprehensive assessment requires a qualitative appraisal, clinical assessment, and measurement of the different factors that impact on the perception of breathlessness and the effects of shortness of breath on the individual.

Qualitative Aspects of Dyspnea

The majority of scientists studying dyspnea accept that dyspnea is not a single sensation (32). They have found that there are a variety of sensations of breathing discomfort that differ in the quality of the experience, the stimuli that evoke them, and the afferent pathways (32). In COPD patients, there are at least four different "qualities" of uncomfortable breathing sensations: air hunger, work, unsatisfied inspiration, and tightness (21). In a study of 131 patients with primary or secondary lung cancer, Wilcock et al. found that there were clusters of words that were associated with the underlying cause of breathlessness (collapse, metastases, and pleural thickening) but that the overlap in the clusters between groups was too great to be useful in differential diagnosis (33).

Others suggest that to adequately characterize dyspnea, measurement of both the sensory intensity and affective intensity or unpleasantness of dyspnea is necessary. There is growing evidence to support that there are different/separate dimensions of sensory intensity and affective intensity or unpleasantness and that the ratio of sensory intensity to affective rating varies among subjects (32). In addition, there is cognitive evaluation and an emotional response to the sensation that will be affected by the person's life experiences and personal situation and perhaps personality (32). There is great variation in the "dyspnea" experienced by different patients with similar disease states. Lansing et al. (32) suggest that knowing whether a therapy works by decreasing intensity or reducing the affective response can help determine which patients are most likely to benefit. Better measurement/assessment could provide a more sophisticated assessment of how potential therapies work and lead to appropriate choice of treatments for individuals in whom affect is a major component of respiratory discomfort.

Clinical Assessment

Clinical assessments are usually directed to determine the underlying pathophysiology and appropriate treatments and to evaluate response to therapy.

History

As in all areas of medicine, a thorough history is central to determining the underlying etiology of a person's breathlessness. This should include its temporal onset (acute or chronic), whether it is affected by positions, qualities, associated symptoms, precipitating and relieving events or activities, and response to medications. A past history of smoking, underlying lung or cardiac disease, concurrent medical conditions, allergy history, and details of previous medications or treatments should be elicited (34,35).

The initial approach to assessment and possible treatment is greatly affected by whether the breathlessness is an acute, subacute, or chronic problem (36). The differential diagnosis of acute shortness of breath is relatively narrow: pneumonia, pulmonary embolism, congestive heart failure, or myocardial infarction. This knowledge should guide further questioning, the physical examination and possible investigations. In the setting of advanced disease, it is important to determine if the breathlessness is related to the underlying disease and potentially irreversible or whether it is completely unrelated and potentially curable.

To determine if dyspnea is present, it is important to ask more than the question, "Are you short of breath?". Patients universally respond to breathlessness by decreasing their activity. It is therefore helpful to ask about shortness of breath in relation to activities such as "walking at the same speed as someone of your age," "stopping to catch your breath when walking upstairs," or "eating." It is also important to quantify the amount of exercise, or lack of, that is needed for the person to become breathless, as this will provide a baseline for comparison to assess progression or improvement (37).

It can be helpful in establishing a diagnosis to inquire in which position dyspnea occurs (37). Positional dyspnea common in cancer patients includes orthopnea (difficulty in breathing while lying flat) with superior vena cava syndrome, pericardial effusion; platypnea (difficulty in breathing while sitting up and relieved by lying flat) is rare, but it occurs status post-pneumonectomy; and trepopnea (when patients are more comfortable breathing while lying on one side) occurs in people with a large pleural effusion (37).

Physical Examination

A careful physical examination focused on possible underlying causes of dyspnea should be performed. Particular attention should be directed to identify signs that are associated with the clinical syndromes identified in the history or common in people with cancer (see Table 29.3).

It is important to recognize that dyspnea, like pain, is a subjective experience that may not be evident to an observer. Tachypnea, a rapid respiratory rate, is not dyspnea. Medical personnel must learn to ask and accept the patient's assessments, often without measurable physical correlates. When patients say that they are having discomfort with breathing, we must believe they are dyspneic. In a study of patients with COPD with high, medium, and low levels of breathlessness, Gift et al. (38) found that there were no significant differences in respiratory rate, depth of respiration, or peak expiratory flow rates at the three levels of dyspnea. There was, however, a significant difference in the use of accessory muscles between patients with high and low levels of dyspnea suggesting that the extent of use of accessory muscles is a physical finding that is helpful when assessing the intensity of breathlessness.

Laboratory Evaluation

There are a number of tests that can help determine the etiology of a person's dyspnea, but the choice of the appropriate diagnostic tests should be guided by the stage of the disease, the prognosis, the risk/benefit ratios of any proposed tests or interventions, and the desires of the patient and family.

Possible blood tests include a hemoglobin, white blood cell count and differential, and serum calcium, potassium, magnesium, and phosphate.

If appropriate, radiologic examinations may include a chest radiograph, ventilation/perfusion scan, computed tomography (CT) scan, CT angiogram, magnetic resonance imaging, or an echocardiogram.

A pulse oximeter measures oxygen saturation noninvasively. At high saturations pulse oximeters are reasonably accurate ($+/- 3\%$), but less accurate below saturations of about 80% (39). Measures of oxygen saturation while walking are helpful in unmasking hypoxia with exercise. It should be remembered that oxygen saturation does not indicate whether the person has adequate ventilation. A person who is retaining carbon dioxide can have normal or near-normal oxygen saturations, so arterial blood gas analysis should be considered in situations where information about not only

TABLE 29.3	Causes of dyspnea in cancer patients

A. Dyspnea Due Directly to Cancer

- Lung involvement (primary or metastatic)
- Lymphangitic carcinomatosis
- Intrinsic or extrinsic airway obstruction by tumor
- Pleural effusion
- Pericardial effusion
- Ascites
- Hepatomegaly
- Phrenic nerve paralysis
- Tumor microemboli
- Pulmonary leukostasis
- Superior vena cava syndrome

B. Dyspnea Due Indirectly to Cancer

- Cachexia
- Na, K, Mg, PO_4 abnormalities
- Anemia
- Pneumonia
- Pulmonary aspiration
- Pulmonary emboli
- Neurologic paraneoplastic syndromes

C. Dyspnea Due to Cancer Treatment

- Surgery
- Radiation pneumonitis/fibrosis
- Chemotherapy-induced pulmonary disease
- Chemotherapy-induced cardiomyopathy
- Radiation-induced pericardial disease

D. Dyspnea Unrelated to Cancer

- Chronic obstructive pulmonary disease
- Asthma
- Congestive heart failure
- Interstitial lung disease
- Pneumothorax
- Anxiety
- Chest wall deformity
- Obesity
- Neuromuscular disorders
- Pulmonary vascular disease

Modified from Dudgeon D, Rosenthal S. Management of dyspnea and cough in patients with cancer. In: Cherny NI, Foley KM, eds. *Hematology/Oncology Clinics of North America: Pain and Palliative Care*, Vol. 10(1). Philadelphia, PA: W.B. Saunders Co.; 1996:157–171.

oxygenation (Po_2) but also ventilation (Pco_2) and/or acid–base balance (pH) would be helpful (39).

Lung function tests vary from simple spirometry with handheld electronic devices to more complicated tests that require sophisticated equipment in a lung function laboratory. Standardized PFTs are helpful to determine the underlying diagnosis, its severity, and response to treatment. Two basic patterns of disorder are demonstrated with spirometry: obstructive and restrictive (see Table 29.1). Results of PFTs do not necessarily reflect the intensity of a person's dyspnea (40). Maximum inspiratory and expiratory measurements are helpful in assessing respiratory muscle strength, but they are dependent on patient effort. Unlike others (26,27), Bruera et al. (28) found that in cancer patients with moderate to severe dyspnea, multivariate analysis showed that maximum inspiratory pressure (PImax) ($p = 0.02$) was an independent correlate of the intensity of dyspnea.

Exercise testing with increasing workloads on either a cycle ergometer or treadmill is performed to identify a cardiac or respiratory cause for exercise limitation, quantify functional disability, and assess the response to treatment (39). Simpler measures of exercise capacity include the 6- or 12-minute walking test and the shuttle walking test. The walking tests correlate with measures of both dyspnea and exercise capacity (38). The shuttle walking test was validated in comparison with the treadmill exercise test (41) and is a reproducible test of functional capacity in ambulatory advanced cancer patients (42).

MEASUREMENT

Measurement instruments bring objectivity and precision to the evaluation of clinical assessments or interventions and to research questions. Which instrument is appropriate depends on the question, the setting, the acuity of the symptom, the functional status of the patient, and what dimensions you wish to examine. Most of the measurement instruments for breathlessness were developed for use in patients with COPD, only a few have been validated in patients with cancer (see Table 29.4).

Unidimensional Instruments

Three types of unidimensional scales are commonly used to measure breathlessness: Visual Analog Scale (VAS), Numerical Rating Scale (NRS), and the Modified Borg Scale (43). Unidimensional scales are self-administered and quick to complete. They can measure breathlessness in general or in relation to exercise. The VAS and NRS are anchored by words such as "no breathlessness" or "worst possible breathlessness." These scales can be used as an initial assessment to monitor progress and to evaluate effectiveness of treatment in an individual patient (44). Magnitude estimation scales use a ratio scaling technique that measures the relationship between the intensity of a physical stimulus and its perceived magnitude (45,46). This type of scale allows

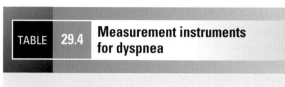

A. Unidimensional
- Visual Analog Scales
- Numerical Rating Scales

B. Magnitude Estimation Scales
- Modified Borg Scale
- Oxygen Cost Diagram

C. Multidimensional Assessment Instruments
- Dyspnea Assessment Questionnaire
- Cancer Dyspnea Scale

D. Quality of Life Instruments
- The Lung Cancer Symptom Scale
- The European Organization for Research and Treatment Quality of Life Questionnaire and Lung Cancer Module
- The Functional Assessment of Cancer Therapy—Lung Cancer Quality of Life Instrument

comparisons within individuals and across population groups (47). The Borg scale (48) and Oxygen Cost Diagram (49) are examples.

Multidimensional Assessment Instruments

The Dyspnea Assessment Questionnaire (DAQ) (25) and the Cancer Dyspnea Scale (CDS) (50) are examples of scales developed to assess the multidimensional nature of dyspnea in cancer patients. The DAQ measures both qualitative and quantitative components of breathlessness (25). The CDS measures three factors: sense of effort, sense of anxiety, and sense of discomfort (50).

Quality of Life Instruments

Measurement of quality of life attempts to provide standardized estimates of the *overall* impact on the individual. The Lung Cancer Symptom Scale (LCSS) (51,52) has six items that measure major symptoms of people with lung cancer and three related to symptomatic distress, activity status, and overall quality of life. The European Organization for Research and Treatment Quality of Life Questionnaire and Lung Cancer Module assesses the physical, emotional, social, and cognitive dimension of the person's life (53,54). The Functional Assessment of Cancer Therapy—Lung Cancer Quality of Life Instrument measures five dimension of quality of life: physical, social and family, emotional well-being, and functional well-being, and relationship with physician (55).

CAUSES AND MANAGEMENT OF DYSPNEA

The causes of dyspnea in the cancer patient fall into four clinical categories: direct tumor effects, indirect tumor effects, treatment-related causes, and problems unrelated to the cancer (Table 29.2).

Direct Tumor Effects

The causes of dyspnea due directly to cancer include parenchymal involvement by tumor (primary or metastatic), lymphangitic carcinomatosis, extrinsic or intrinsic obstruction of airways by tumor, pleural tumor, pleural effusion, pericardial effusion, ascites, hepatomegaly, phrenic nerve paralysis, superior vena cava obstruction, multiple tumor microemboli, and pulmonary leukostasis.

If the tumor is the cause of the shortness of breath, then chemotherapy, external beam radiation, brachytherapy, or surgery should be considered if appropriate to the stage of disease and the overall condition and wishes of the patient. Chapter 30 address management of airway obstruction, pleural and pericardial effusions, and superior vena cava obstruction.

Dyspnea Due to Cancer Treatment

Dyspnea can result from surgery, radiation therapy, and/or systemic therapy. The management of toxicity related to radiation and systemic therapy is discussed in Chapter 32.

Surgery

Pneumonectomy or lobectomy can result in shortness of breath in patients with preexisting impairment of pulmonary function. In a study examining the long-term effects, 5 or more years, after pneumonectomy for lung cancer, Deslauriers et al. found that 37% had moderate to severe dyspnea (56).

Dyspnea Indirectly Due to Cancer

Dyspnea can result from indirect consequences of the cancer such as malnutrition, mineral and electrolyte deficiencies, infection, anemia, pulmonary emboli, aspiration, neurologic paraneoplastic syndromes, and severe deconditioning. These underlying causes of dyspnea should be treated if appropriate to the person's stage of disease, prognosis, and wishes.

Muscle Weakness

Studies demonstrate that there is an association between dyspnea and respiratory (26–28,57) and generalized (9,58) muscle weakness in the advanced cancer patient. Both generalized and ventilatory muscle weaknesses can result from severe deconditioning but other factors that can affect muscle function are hypocalcemia, hypokalemia, hypomagnesemia, severe hypophosphatemia, malnutrition, and possibly the cancer or its treatment (59,60). There is evidence that pulmonary rehabilitation programs improve dyspnea and functional capacity in patients who participate preoperatively, during aggressive chemotherapy and/or radiation treatments (61), or in the palliative phase of their illness (62). Although there are no studies in cancer patients, there is evidence in COPD patients that refeeding and anabolic steroids improve exercise tolerance (63–65).

Infection

Patients with cancer are at an increased risk for pneumonia due to immunosuppression from the disease or its treatment and also from the tumor causing mucosal erosion or an abscess, fistula, or obstruction.

Pulmonary Emboli

Cancer patients have a fourfold to sevenfold higher risk of developing a venous thromboembolism than patients without cancer. The risk depends on the extent and type of tumor with pancreatic, brain, myeloproliferative, and gastric cancers at the highest risk. Surgery, chemotherapy, radiation therapy, growth factors, immobility, and the presence of central venous catheters increase the risk of a pulmonary embolism for patients (66). Typically, patients with acute pulmonary embolic disease describe a single or multiple episodes of acute shortness of breath. Less commonly, multiple small emboli produce pulmonary hypertension with no history of acute episodes (67). It is possible that an episode of acute shortness of breath just prior to death is a result of a large pulmonary embolus. Chapter 32 addresses this issue.

Dyspnea Unrelated to the Cancer

Risk factors for dyspnea unrelated to cancer include preexisting COPD, cardiovascular disease, asthma, interstitial lung disease, pneumothorax, anxiety, chest wall deformity, obesity, neuromuscular disorders, and pulmonary vascular disease.

PHARMACOLOGIC MANAGEMENT

Opioids

There are three systematic reviews that examined the effectiveness of oral or parenteral opioids for the management of dyspnea, two for palliation in cancer patients (68,69) and one in all patient groups (70).

In the *Cochrane Review* (70), the authors identified 18 randomized double-blind, controlled trials comparing the use of any opioid drug against placebo for the treatment of breathlessness in patients with any illness (only two studies conducted with cancer patients met the inclusion criteria for review [one parenteral and one nebulized]). There

was statistically strong evidence for a small effect of oral and parenteral opioids for the treatment of breathlessness in the studies (71–78) involving the non-nebulized route of administration (70).

Opioid receptors are located throughout the respiratory tract and it is hypothesized that if the receptors are interrupted directly, lower doses, with fewer systemic side effects, would be required to control breathlessness (79). The *Cochrane Review* (70) identified nine randomized double-blind, controlled trials comparing the use of nebulized opioids or placebo for the control of breathlessness (80–88). One of these trials (82) included only cancer patients. The authors concluded that there was no evidence that nebulized opioids were more effective than nebulized saline in relieving breathlessness (70).

There are eight randomized trials that include only cancer patients (69,77,82,89–93). Two placebo-controlled crossover trials (77,89) showed that a single bolus dose of morphine significantly improved dyspnea.

Allard et al. (90) studied the effectiveness of supplemental doses of opioids, equivalent to 25% or 50% of their regular 4-hourly dose of opioids, to improve breathlessness in terminally ill cancer patients. They found significant decrements relative to baseline for mean dyspnea ($p < 0.0001$) and respiratory frequency ($p = 0.004$) in all patients. They concluded that a 25% dose of the 4-hourly opioid was sufficient to improve dyspnea.

One randomized, 2-day, crossover study of only 11 patients of the planned 100 compared subcutaneous versus nebulized morphine (93). Both treatments improved dyspnea 1 hour posttreatment with no differences between the effect of the two treatments, but the sample size was not large enough to make meaningful conclusions.

A double-blind, randomized, crossover, controlled trial of 20 cancer patients comparing the effects of nebulized hydromorphone, systemic hydromorphone, and nebulized saline for the relief of acute episodic breathlessness showed that all treatments resulted in statistically significant improvements in breathlessness (92). Only the nebulized hydromorphone resulted in what was considered a clinically significant change (1 cm VAS). The authors, however, suggested that nebulized saline provided significant relief of incident breathlessness that was not significantly different from the effect of opioids.

Sedatives and Tranquilizers

Chlorpromazine decreases breathlessness without affecting ventilation or producing sedation in healthy subjects (94). There are conflicting results from trials studying the effectiveness of promethazine, a phenothiazine antiemetic, in reducing dyspnea (94–96). In an open-labeled trial McIver et al. found chlorpromazine effective for relief of dyspnea in advanced cancer (97).

In a double-blind, placebo-controlled, randomized trial, Light et al. studied the effectiveness of morphine alone, morphine and promethazine, and morphine and pro-chlorperazine for the treatment of breathlessness in COPD patients (74). The combination of morphine and promethazine significantly improved exercise tolerance without worsening dyspnea compared with placebo, morphine alone, or the combination of morphine and prochlorperazine (74). Ventafridda et al. have also found the combination of morphine and chlorpromazine to be effective (98). In their systematic review, Viola et al. suggested that phenothiazines could be used as an alternative when systemic opioids could not be used or in addition to systemic opioids (68).

In a *Cochrane Review*, Simon et al. examined the efficacy of benzodiazepines for the relief of breathlessness in patients with advanced disease (99). They identified 7 studies including 200 participants with advanced cancer and COPD. Analysis of the seven studies, and meta-analysis of six, did not show a significant beneficial effect of benzodiazepines for relief of breathlessness in patients with advanced COPD and cancer. No significant effect on prevention of breakthrough dyspnea in cancer patients was found. They observed that there was a slight but nonsignificant trend toward a beneficial effect. They suggested that benzodiazepines could be considered as second-line or third-line options in an individual therapeutic trial if opioids and nonpharmacologic agents had failed.

Navigante et al. (91) in a single-blinded 2-day study compared subcutaneous morphine with subcutaneous midazolam or a combination of both morphine and midazolam to alleviate severe dyspnea in terminally ill cancer patients. Significant improvements in dyspnea intensity occurred in all three arms. Significantly, more patients in the combined group reported relief of dyspnea at 24 and 48 hours and had less episodes of breakthrough dyspnea than the other groups.

Navigante et al. (100) randomized 63 ambulatory advanced cancer patients to receive oral morphine or oral midazolam using a fast drug titration followed by an ambulatory 5-day period. During the titration period, all patients had their dyspnea improve by at least 50%. On the second day, dyspnea intensity decreased in both the morphine and midazolam groups and on subsequent days maintained this level or continued to drop. During the ambulatory phase, midazolam was superior to morphine in controlling baseline and breakthrough dyspnea.

Oxygen

Oxygen in the hypoxic patient with COPD is associated with improved survival, quality of life, and neuropsychologic functioning (101). The benefits in cancer patients are unfortunately less clear. In a systematic review and meta-analysis of all randomized controlled studies on the use of oxygen for the relief of dyspnea in chronic terminal illness, Cranston et al. identified 4 papers involving a total of 97 patients with cancer (102). Two studies of a total of 52 participants at rest who received 4 to 5 L/min of oxygen for up to 15 minutes resulted in a reduction of shortness of breath

over the baseline (77,103). The meta-analysis, however, failed to show a significant improvement in their dyspnea when oxygen inhalation was compared with air inhalation. The change in dyspnea with oxygen inhalation was inconsistent and appeared to be independent of resting hypoxia (102). The meta-analysis showed that participants appeared to perceive an improvement in their dyspnea at rest and during exercise. In the two studies that examined the effect of oxygen inhalation during exercise, oxygen did neither appear to reduce exercise-induced dyspnea nor increase the distance walked (102).

In another systematic review and meta-analysis, Uronis et al. identified five randomized controlled trials comparing oxygen and air in people with cancer who were mildly hypoxemic or nonhypoxemic (104). One hundred and thirty-four people were included in the analysis. Oxygen did not improve dyspnea and only two or four studies detected a statistically significant individual preference for oxygen. In a large cohort study of 1,239 patients, most of whom had cancer and were prescribed oxygen, approximately one-third had an improvement in their breathlessness. It was not possible to predict the responders from demographic factors, baseline breathlessness, or underlying diagnosis (105). Despite the lack of clear evidence of benefit some terminally ill patients reported a marked improvement in both their breathlessness and quality of life with supplemental oxygen and, therefore, most palliative care physicians would suggest a therapeutic trial.

NONPHARMACOLOGIC MANAGEMENT

A *Cochrane Review* by Bausewein et al. identified 47 studies that tested a variety of interventions mostly in COPD patients. The interventions with the highest strength of evidence were all conducted in COPD patients and included neuromuscular electrical stimulation, chest wall vibration, walking aids, and breathing training (106).

Numerous small studies in healthy males (107) and patients with COPD have demonstrated that a fan directed against the cheek improved breathlessness (107,108) and improved exercise time (109,110). Galbraith et al. examined the effectiveness of a handheld fan to reduce the sensation of breathlessness in 50 patients, 11 with primary or secondary lung cancer (111). They found that a fan directed at the face for 5 minutes significantly reduced the score on the VAS breathless scale more than if it was directed at the leg (111).

GUIDES TO MORE PRACTICE

Cancer Care Ontario's web site (112) has a number of useful tools to help clinicians manage dyspnea effectively. In their web site under CCO Toolbox, there is a section called Symptom Management Tools. These include a Dyspnea Algorithm (Fig. 29.2), Pocket Guide, Guide to Practice, Video Series on Managing Shortness of Breath, and iPhone and Windows Phone7 apps.

A

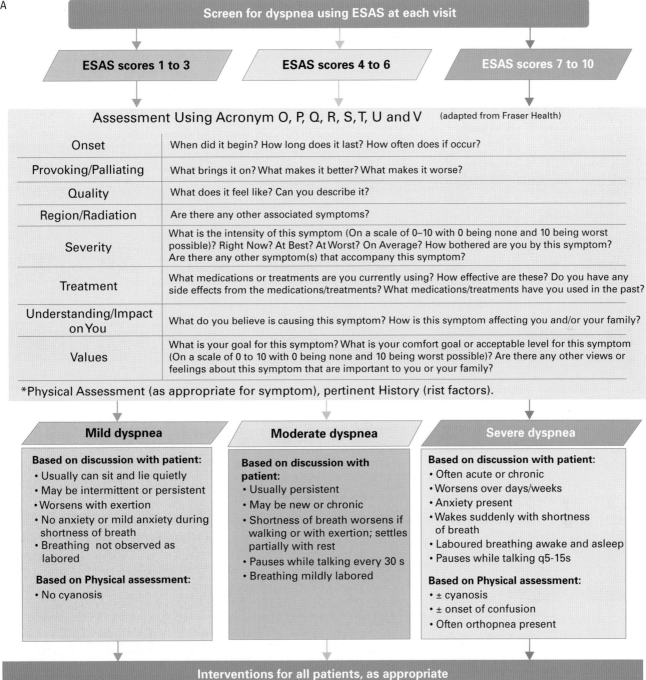

Screen for dyspnea using ESAS at each visit

| ESAS scores 1 to 3 | ESAS scores 4 to 6 | ESAS scores 7 to 10 |

Assessment Using Acronym O, P, Q, R, S, T, U and V   (adapted from Fraser Health)

Onset	When did it begin? How long does it last? How often does if occur?
Provoking/Palliating	What brings it on? What makes it better? What makes it worse?
Quality	What does it feel like? Can you describe it?
Region/Radiation	Are there any other associated symptoms?
Severity	What is the intensity of this symptom (On a scale of 0–10 with 0 being none and 10 being worst possible)? Right Now? At Best? At Worst? On Average? How bothered are you by this symptom? Are there any other symptom(s) that accompany this symptom?
Treatment	What medications or treatments are you currently using? How effective are these? Do you have any side effects from the medications/treatments? What medications/treatments have you used in the past?
Understanding/Impact on You	What do you believe is causing this symptom? How is this symptom affecting you and/or your family?
Values	What is your goal for this symptom? What is your comfort goal or acceptable level for this symptom (On a scale of 0 to 10 with 0 being none and 10 being worst possible)? Are there any other views or feelings about this symptom that are important to you or your family?

*Physical Assessment (as appropriate for symptom), pertinent History (rist factors).

Mild dyspnea

Based on discussion with patient:
- Usually can sit and lie quietly
- May be intermittent or persistent
- Worsens with exertion
- No anxiety or mild anxiety during shortness of breath
- Breathing not observed as labored

Based on Physical assessment:
- No cyanosis

Moderate dyspnea

Based on discussion with patient:
- Usually persistent
- May be new or chronic
- Shortness of breath worsens if walking or with exertion; settles partially with rest
- Pauses while talking every 30 s
- Breathing mildly labored

Severe dyspnea

Based on discussion with patient:
- Often acute or chronic
- Worsens over days/weeks
- Anxiety present
- Wakes suddenly with shortness of breath
- Laboured breathing awake and asleep
- Pauses while talking q5-15s

Based on Physical assessment:
- ± cyanosis
- ± onset of confusion
- Often orthopnea present

Interventions for all patients, as appropriate

Cognitive Behavioral Interventions
- Provide information and support for management of breathlessness, instructions for breathing control, relaxation, distraction techniques, and breathing exercises
- Provide goal setting to enhance breathing and relaxation techniques, enable participation in social activities, and develop coping skills
- Identify early signs of problems that need medical or pharmacotheraphy intervention

Positioning
- Suggest positions that maximize respiratory function while reducing physical effort.

Breathing
- Provide ambient air flow on face & cool facial temperatures (use window, fan, or nasal prongs)
- Increasing chest expansion can make the most of one's lung capacity and increase oxygen delivery.
- Consider referral to a respiratory therapist, physiotherapist, or nurse with expertise in managing dyspnea
- Assess the need for oxygen
- Assess breath lessness—what improves and what hinders

Supportive Counseling
- The meaning of symptoms cannot be separated from the symptom experience. In order to relieve suffering and provide good symptom support, the health care professional must explore the meaning of the symptom to the patient.

Figure 29.2. Dyspnea algorithm. ESAS, Edmonton Symptom Assessment System; PPS, Palliative Performance Scale; CCO, Cancer Care Ontario.

B

Dyspnea in Adults with Cancer: Care Map

| **Mild Dyspnea** Care pathway 1 | **Moderate Dyspnea** Care pathway 2 | **Severe Dyspnea** Care pathway 3 |

PHARMACOLOGIC

- Supplemental oxygen is recommended for hypoxic patients experiencing dyspnea.

- Supplemental oxygen is <u>not</u> recommended for nonhypoxic, dyspneic patients.

- Systemic opioids, by the oral or parenteral routes, can be used to manage dyspnea in advanced cancer patients.

PHARMACOLOGIC

For Patients with PPS 100%–10%:

Non Opioids
- May use benzodiazepines for anxiety.
- There is no evidence for the use of systemic corticosteroids.

Systemic Opioids

For opioid-native patients:
- Morphine (or equivalent dose of alternate immediate-release opioid) 5 mg po q4th regularly and 2.5 mg po q2h prn for breakthrough dyspnea.
- If the oral route is not available or reliable, morphine 3 mg subcut q4h regularly and 1.5 mg subcut q1h prn for breakthrough dyspnea.

For patients already taking systemic opioids:
- Increase the patient's regular dose by 25%, guided by the total breakthrough doses used in the previous 24 h.
- The breakthrough dose is 10% of the total 24-h regular opioid dose, using the same opioid by the same route.
  - Oral breakthrough doses q2 h as needed.
  - Subcutaneous breakthrough doses q1h as needed, due to more rapid peak effect.
- Do not use nebulized opioids, nebulized furosemide, nebulized lidocaine, or benzodiazepines.

NON-PHARMACOLOGIC

- Attend to the meaning of the symptom (or attend to fear/anxiety).
- If dyspnea is acute or there is an unexpected change, further assessment may be required to identify potentially treatable causes.

PHARMACOLOGIC

For Patients with PPS 100%–10%:
Systemic Opioids

For opioid-naïve patients:
- Give a subcut bolus of morphine 2.5 mg (or an equivalent dose of an alternate opioid).
  - If tolerated, repeat dose every 30 min if needed.
  - Consider doubling dose if two doses fail to produce an adequater reduction in dyspnea and are tolerated.
  - Monitor the patient's respiratory rate closely, since the time to peak effect of a subcut dose of morphine may be longer than 30 min.
- If intravenous access is available, consider giving an IV bolus of morphine 2.5 mg (or an equivalent dose of an alternate opioid) to achieve a more rapid effect.
  - If tolerated, repeat dose every 30 min if needed.
  - Consider doubling dose if two doses fail to produce an adequate reduction in dyspnea and are tolerated.
  - Monitor the patient's respiratory rate closely, since IV boluses of morphine result in faster and higher peak effects.
- Start a regular dose of an immediate-release opioid, guided by the bolus doses used.
  - For the breakthrough opioid dose, consider using the subcut route initially for severe dyspnea until the symptom comes under control.

For patients already taking systemic opioids:
- Follow the same suggestions as above for opioid naïve patients, with the following changes.
  - Give a subcut bolus of the patient's current opioid, using a dose equal to 10% of the regular, 24-h, parenteral-dose-equivalent of the patient's current opioid (a parenteral dose is equivalent to half the oral dose).
  - Consider giving an IV bolus of the patient's current opioid, using a dose equal to 10% of the regular, 24-h, parenteral-dose-equivalent of the patient's current opioid.
  - Increase the regular opioid dose by 25%, guided by the bolus doses used.

Psychoactive medications
- Consider a trial of chlorpromazine or methotrimeprazine, if severe dyspnea persists despite other therapies.
- Methotrimeprazine 2.5–10 mg po or subcut q6-8h regularly or as needed.
- Chlorpromazine 7.5–25 mg po or IV q6-8h regularly or as needed.
- Consider benzodiazepine for coexisting anxiety.

For Patients with PPS 100%–20%:
- If patient has or may have COPD, consider a 5-d trial of a corticosteroid
  - Dexamethasone 8 mg/d po or subcut or IV
  - Prednisone 50 mg/d po
  - Discontinue corticosteroid if there is no obvious benefit after 5 d.
- If the patient does not have COPD, but has known or suspected lung involvement by the cancer, weight the risks before commencing a 5-d trial.
  - Other potential benefits, such as for appetite stimulation or pain management, may justify a 5-d trial of a corticosteroid.
- Do not start prophylactic gastric mucosal protection therapy during a 5-d trial of a corticosteroid, but consider such therapy if the corticosteroid is continued past the trial.
- Prochlorperazine is not recommended as a therapy for managing dyspnea.
- No comparative trials are available to support or refute the use of other phenothiazines, such as chlorpromazine and methotrimeprazine, however oral promethazine may be used as a second-line agent if systemic opioids cannot be used or in addition to systemic opioids.

For Patients with PPS 30%–10%:
- Consider a trial of chlorpromazine or methotrimeprazine, if dyspnea persists despite other therapies.
  - Methotrimeprazine 2.5–10 mg po or subcut q6-8h regularly or as needed.
  - Chlorpromazine 7.5–25 mg po q6-8h regularly or as needed
- Anxiety, nausea, or agitation, may justify a trial of chlorpromazine or methotrimeprazine.

Follow-Up and Ongoing Monitoring
If dyspnea remains unrelieved despite the approaches outlined above, request the assistance of a palliative care consultation team.

For full references and more information please refer to *CCO's Symptom Management Guide-to-Practice: Dyspnea* document.

Disclaimer: Care has been taken by Cancer Care Ontario's Algorithm Development group in the preparation of the information contained in this Guide-to-Practice document. Nonetheless, any person seeking to apply or consult the Guide-to-Practice document is expected to use independent clinical judgement and skills in the context of individual clinical circumstances or seek out the supervision of a qualified specialist clinician. CCO makes no representation or warranties of any kind whatsoever regarding their content or use or application and disclaims any responsibility for their application or use in any way.

Figure 29.2. *(Continued)*

SUMMARY

Dyspnea is a very common symptom in patients with cancer. Despite breathlessness' profound effect on people's quality of life, it is often unrecognized and therefore people often receive little assistance in managing this distressing symptom. Effective management requires an understanding of its prevalence and impact; the multidimensional nature of the symptom; the underlying pathophysiology and associated factors; components of a thorough assessment; the clinical syndromes common in cancer patients; and the indications and limitations of current therapeutic approaches. More research is necessary to further optimize the available treatment options.

REFERENCES

1. Roberts DK, Thorne SE, Pearson C. The experience of dyspnea in late-stage cancer. Patients' and nurses' perspectives. *Cancer Nurs.* 1993;16(4):310-320.
2. Reddy SK, Parsons HA, Elsayem A, Palmer JL, Bruera E. Characteristics and correlates of dyspnea in patients with advanced cancer. *J Palliat Med.* 2009;12(1):29-35.
3. Tishelman C, Petersson L-M, Degner LF, Sprangers MAG. Symptom prevalence, intensity, and distress in patients with inoperable lung cancer in relation to time of death. *J Clin Oncol.* 2007;25(34):5381-5389.
4. Brown ML, Carrieri V, Janson-Bjerklie S, Dodd MJ. Lung cancer and dyspnea: the patient's perception. *Oncol Nurs Forum.* 1986;13(5):19-24.
5. Fainsinger R, Waller A, Bercovici M, et al. A multicentre international study of sedation for uncontrolled symptoms in terminally ill patients. *Palliat Med.* 2000;14(4):257-265.
6. Barbera L, Taylor C, Dudgeon D. Why do patients with cancer visit the emergency department near the end of life? *CMAJ.* 2010;182(6):563-568.
7. Edmonds P, Higginson I, Altmann D, Sen-Gupta G, McDonnell M. Is the presence of dyspnea a risk factor for morbidity in cancer patients? *J Pain Symptom Manage.* 2000;19(1):15-22.
8. Dudgeon DJ, Kristjanson L, Sloan JA, Lertzman M, Clement K. Dyspnea in cancer patients: prevalence and associated factors. *J Pain Symptom Manage.* 2001;21(2):95-102.
9. Reuben DB, Mor V. Dyspnea in terminally ill cancer patients. *Chest.* 1986;89:234-236.
10. Muers MF, Round CE. Palliation of symptoms in non-small cell lung cancer: a study by the Yorkshire Regional Cancer Organisation Thoracic Group. *Thorax.* 1993;48:339-343.
11. Currow D, Davidson PM, Agar MR, et al. Do the trajectories of dyspnea differ in prevalence and intensity by diagnosis at the end of life? A consecutive cohort study. *J Pain Symptom Manage.* 2010;39(4):680-690.
12. Bausewein C, Booth S, Gysels M, Kulkarni AG, Haberland B, Higginson IJ. Individual breathlessness trajectories do not match summary trajectories in advanced cancer and chronic obstructive pulmonary disease: results from a longitudinal study. *Palliat Med.* 2010;24(8):777-786.
13. Barbera L, Hsien S, Howell D, et al. Symptom burden and performance status in a population-based cohort of ambulatory cancer patients. *Cancer.* 2010;116(24):5767-5776.
14. Higginson I, McCarthy M. Measuring symptoms in terminal cancer: are pain and dyspnoea controlled? *J Royal Soc Med.* 1989;82:264-267.
15. Dudgeon D, Harlos M, Clinch JJ. The Edmonton Symptom Assessment Scale (ESAS) as an audit tool. *J Palliat Care.* 1999;15(3):14-19.
16. Dudgeon D, King S, Hughes E, et al. Improving the quality of care and decreasing the morbidity of patients with lung cancer through routine symptom screening. *Am Soc Clin Oncol.* May 2008;26(suppl):abstr 9621.
17. Seow H, Barbera L, Sutradhar R, et al. Trajectory of performance status and symptom scores for patients with cancer during the last six months of life. *J Clin Oncol.* 2011;29(9):1151-1158.
18. Lutz S, Norrell R, Bertucio C, et al. Symptom frequency and severity in patients with metastatic or locally recurrent lung cancer: a prospective study using the Lung Cancer Symptom Scale in a community hospital. *J Palliat Med.* 2001;4(2):157-165.
19. Gore JM, Brophy CJ, Greenstone MA. How well do we care for patients with end stage chronic obstructive pulmonary disease (COPD)? A comparison of palliative care and quality of life in COPD and lung cancer. *Thorax.* 2000;55:1000-1006.
20. Chochinov MH, Tataryn D, Clinch JJ, Dudgeon D. Will to live in the terminally ill. *Lancet.* 1999;354(9181):816-819.
21. O'Donnell DE, Banzett RB, Carrieri-Kohlman V, et al. Pathophysiology of dyspnea in chronic obstructive pulmonary disease. A roundtable. *Proc Am Thoracic Soc.* 2007;4:145-168.
22. von Leupoldt, A, Sommer T, Kegat S, et al. The unpleasantness of perceived dyspnea is processed in the anterior insula and amygdala. *Am J Respir Crit Care Med.* 2008;177(9):1026-1032.
23. Peiffer C. Dyspnea and emotion: what can we learn from functional brain imaging? *Am J Respir Crit Care Med.* 2008;177:937-939.
24. Abernethy AP, Wheeler JL. Total dyspnoea. *Curr Opin Support Palliat Care.* 2008;2:110-113.
25. Heyse-Moore LH. *On Dyspnoea in Advanced Cancer.* Southampton: Southampton University; 1993.
26. Dudgeon D, Lertzman M. Dyspnea in the advanced cancer patient. *J Pain Symptom Manage.* 1998;16(4):212-219.
27. Dudgeon DJ, Lertzman M, Askew GR. Physiological changes and clinical correlations of dyspnea in cancer outpatients. *J Pain Symptom Manage.* 2001;21(5):373-379.
28. Bruera E, Schmitz B, Pither J, Neumann CM, Hanson J. The frequency and correlates of dyspnea in patients with advanced cancer. *J Pain Symptom Manage.* 2000;19(5):357-362.
29. Dudgeon DJ, Webb KA, O'Donnell DE. Unexplained dyspnea and exercise intolerance in patients with cancer: physiological correlates. *Am Soc Clin Oncol.* 2001;20:303b.
30. Tanaka K, Akechi T, Okuyama T, Nishiwaki Y, Uchitomi Y. Factors correlated with dyspnea in advanced lung cancer patients: organic causes and what else? *J Pain Symptom Manage.* 2002;23(6):490-500.
31. Escalante CP, Martin CG, Elting LS, et al. Dyspnea in cancer patients. Etiology, resource utilization, and survival—implications in a managed care world. *Cancer.* 1996;78(6):1314-1319.
32. Lansing RW, Gracely RH, Banzett RB. The multiple dimensions of dyspnea: review and hypotheses. *Respir Physiol Neurobiol.* 2009;167(1):53-60.
33. Wilcock A, Crosby V, Hughes AC, Fielding K, Corcoran R, Tattersfield AE. Descriptors of breathlessness in patients with cancer and other cardiorespiratory diseases. *J Pain Symptom Manage.* 2002;23(3):182-189.

34. Silvestri GA, Mahler DA. Evaluation of dyspnea in the elderly patient. *Clin Chest Med.* 1993;14(3):393-404.

35. Ferrin MS, Tino G. Acute dyspnea. *Am Assoc Crit Care Nurs Clin Issues.* 1997;8(3):398-410.

36. Man GCW, Hsu K, Sproule BJ. Effect of alprazolam on exercise and dyspnea in patients with chronic obstructive pulmonary disease. *Chest.* 1986;90(6):832-836.

37. Swartz MH. *Textbook of Physical Diagnosis: History and Examination.* 4th ed. Philadelphia, PA: W.B. Saunders Company; 2002.

38. Gift AG, Plaut SM, Jacox A. Psychologic and physiologic factors related to dyspnea in subjects with chronic obstructive pulmonary disease. *Heart Lung.* 1986;15:595-601.

39. Hancox B, Whyte K. *McGraw-Hill's Pocket Guide to Lung Function Tests.* Roseville, NSW: McGraw-Hill, 2001.

40. Heyse-Moore LH, Beynon T, Ross V. Does spirometry predict dyspnoea in advanced cancer? *Palliat Med.* 2000;14(3):189-195.

41. Singh SJ, Morgan MD, Hardman AE, Rowe C, Bardsley PA. Comparison of oxygen uptake during a conventional treadmill test and the shuttle walking test in chronic airflow limitation. *Eur Respir J.* 1994;7(11):2016-2020.

42. Booth S, Adams L. The shuttle walking test: a reproducible method for evaluating the impact of shortness of breath on functional capacity in patients with advanced cancer. *Thorax.* 2001;56(2):146-150.

43. Bausewein C, Farquhar M, Booth S, Gysels M, Higginson IJ. Measurement of breathlessness in advanced disease: a systematic review. *Respir Med.* 2006;101:399-410.

44. Gift AG. Clinical measurement of dyspnea. *Dimens Crit Care Nurs.* 1989;8(4):210-216.

45. Wilcock A, Corcoran R, Tattersfield AE. Safety and efficacy of nebulized lignocaine in patients with cancer and breathlessness. *Palliat Med.* 1994;8:35-38.

46. van der Molen, B. Dyspnoea: a study of measurement instruments for the assessment of dyspnoea and their application for patients with advanced cancer. *J Adv Nurs.* 1995;22:948-956.

47. Killian KJ. Assessment of dyspnoea. *Eur Respir J.* 1988;1(3):195-197.

48. Borg GAV. Psychophysical basis of perceived exertion. *Med Sci Sports Exerc.* 1982;14(5):377-381.

49. McGavin CR, Artvinli M, Naoe H, McHardy G. Dyspnoea, disability and distance walked: comparison of estimates of exercise performance in respiratory disease. *Br Med J.* 1978;2:241-243.

50. Tanaka K, Akechi T, Okuyama T, Nishiwaki Y, Uchitomi Y. Development and validation of the cancer dyspnoea scale: a multidimensional, brief, self-rating scale. *Br J Cancer.* 2000;82(4):800-805.

51. Hollen PJ, Gralla RJ, Kris MG, Potanovich LM. Quality of life assessment in individuals with lung cancer: testing the Lung Cancer Symptom Scale (LCSS). *Eur J Cancer.* 1993;29A:S51-S58.

52. Hollen PJ, Gralla RJ. Comparison of instruments for measuring quality of life in patients with lung cancer. *Sem Oncol.* 1996;23(2 suppl 5):31-40.

53. Aaronson NK, Ahmedzai S, Bergman B. The European Organization for Research and Treatment of Cancer QLQ-C30: a quality-of-life instrument for use in international clinical trials in oncology. *J Natl Cancer Inst.* 1993;85:365-376.

54. Bergman B, Aaronson NK, Ahmedzai S. The EORTC QLQ-LC13: a modular supplement to the EORTC core Quality of Life Questionnaire (QLQ-C30) for use in lung cancer clinical trials. *Eur J Cancer.* 1994;30A:635-642.

55. Cella DF, Bonomi AE, Lloyd SR, Tulsky DS, Kaplan E, Bonomi P. Reliability and validity of the Functional Assessment of Cancer Therapy-Lung (FACT-L) quality of life instrument. *Lung Cancer.* 1995;12:199-220.

56. Deslauriers J, Ugalde P, Miro S, et al. Adjustments in cardiorespiratory function after pneumonectomy: results of the pneumonectomy project. *J Thoracic Cardiovasc Surg.* 2010;141(1):7-15.

57. Travers J, Dudgeon D, Amjadi K, et al. Mechanisms of exertional dyspnea in patients with cancer. *J Appl Physiol.* 2007;104(1):57-66.

58. Dudgeon, DJ, O'Donnell DE, Day A, Webb KA, McBride I, Dillon K. Mechanisms of exertional dyspnea in patients with cancer: a case-matched control study. *J Palliat Care.* 2002;18(3), 207.

59. Lewis MI, Belman MJ. Nutrition and the respiratory muscles. *Clin Chest Med.* 1988;9(2):337-347.

60. Rochester DF, Arora NS. Respiratory muscle failure. *Med Clin North Am.* 1983;67(3):573-597.

61. Shannon VR. Role of pulmonary rehabilitation in the management of patients with lung cancer. *Curr Opin Pulm Med.* 2010;16(4):334-339.

62. Oldervoll LM, Loge JH, Paltiel H, et al. The effect of a physical exercise program in palliative care: a phase II study. *J Pain Symptom Manage.* 2006;31(5):421-430.

63. Whittaker JS, Ryan CF, Buckley PA, Road JD. The effects of refeeding on peripheral and respiratory muscle function in malnourished chronic obstructive pulmonary disease patients. *Am Rev Respir Dis.* 1990;142:283-288.

64. O'Donnell DE, McGuire M, Samis L, Webb KA. The impact of exercise reconditioning on breathlessness in severe chronic airflow limitation. *Am J Respir Crit Care Med.* 1995;152:2005-2013.

65. Schols AM, Soeters PB, Mostert R, Pluymers RJ, Wouters EF. Physiologic effects of nutritional support and anabolic steroids in patients with chronic obstructive pulmonary disease. A placebo-controlled randomized trial. *Am J Respir Crit Care Med.* 1995;152(4:1):1268-1274.

66. Streiff MB. Anticoagulation in the management of venous thromboembolism in the cancer patient. *J Thromb Thrombolysis.* 2011;31(3):282-294.

67. Scully RE, Mark EJ, McNeely WF, McNeely BU. Case record of the Massachusetts General Hospital (Case 30-1987). *N Engl J Med.* 1987;317(4):225-235.

68. Viola R, Kiteley C, Lloyd NS, Mackay JA, Wilson J, Wong RKS. The management of dyspnea in cancer patients: a systematic review. *Support Care Cancer.* 2008;16:329-337.

69. Ben-Aharon I, Gafter-Gvili A, Leibovici L, Stemmer SM. Interventions for alleviating cancer-related dyspnea: a systematic review. *J Clin Oncol.* 2008;26(14):2396-2404.

70. Jennings AL, Davies A, Higgins JPT, Broadley K. *Opioids for the Palliation of Breathlessness in Terminal Illness (Cochrane Review). The Cochrane Library [4].* Oxford: Update Software; 2001.

71. Woodcock AA, Johnson MA, Geddes DM. Breathlessness, alcohol and opiates. *N Engl J Med.* 1982;306:1363-1364.

72. Woodcock AA, Gross ER, Gellert A, Shah S, Johnson M, Geddes DM. Effects of dihydrocodeine, alcohol, and caffeine on breathlessness and exercise tolerance in patients with chronic obstructive lung disease and normal blood gases. *N Engl J Med.* 1981;305(27):1611-1616.

73. Poole PJ, Veale AG, Black PN. The effect of sustained-release morphine on breathlessness and quality of life in severe chronic

obstructive pulmonary disease. *Am J Respir Crit Care Med.* 1998;157(6 Pt 1):1877-1880.

74. Light RW, Stansbury DW, Webster JS. Effect of 30 mg of morphine alone or with promethazine or prochlorperazine on the exercise capacity of patients With COPD. *Chest.* 1996;109(4):975-981.

75. Johnson MA, Woodcock AA, Geddes DM. Dihydrocodeine for breathlessness in "pink puffers." *Br Med J.* 1983;286:675-677.

76. Eiser N, Denman WT, West C, Luce P. Oral diamorphine: lack of effect on dyspnoea and exercise tolerance in the "pink puffer" syndrome. *Eur Respir J.* 1991;4(8):926-931.

77. Bruera E, MacEachern T, Ripamonti C, Hanson J. Subcutaneous morphine for dyspnea in cancer patients. *Ann Intern Med.* 1993;119(9):906-907.

78. Chua TP, Harrington D, Ponikowski P, Webb-Peploe K, Poole-Wilson PA, Coats AJ. Effects of dihydrocodeine on chemosensitivity and exercise tolerance in patients with chronic heart failure. *J Am Coll Cardiol.* 1997;29(1):147-152.

79. Zebraski SE, Kochenash SM, Raffa RB. Lung opioid receptors: pharmacology and possible target for nebulized morphine in dyspnea. *Life Sci.* 2000;66(23):2221-2231.

80. Beauford W, Saylor TT, Stansbury DW, Avalos K, Light RW. Effects of nebulized morphine sulfate on the exercise tolerance of the ventilatory limited COPD patient. *Chest.* 1993;104(1):175-178.

81. Davis CL, Hodder C, Love S, Shah R, Slevin M, Wedzicha J. Effect of nebulised morphine and morphine 6-glucuronide on exercise endurance in patients with chronic obstructive pulmonary disease. *Thorax.* 1994;49:393P.

82. Davis CL, Penn K, A'Hern R, Daniels J, Slevin M. Single dose randomised controlled trial of nebulised morphine in patients with cancer related breathlessness. *Palliat Med.* 1996;10(1), 64-65.

83. Harris-Eze AO, Sridhar G, Clemens RE, Zintel TA, Gallagher CG, Marciniuk DD. Low-dose nebulized morphine does not improve exercise in interstitial lung disease. *Am J Respir Crit Care Med.* 1995;152:1940-1945.

84. Jankelson D, Hosseini K, Mather LE, Seale JP, Young IH. Lack of effect of high doses of inhaled morphine on exercise endurance in chronic obstructive pulmonary disease. *Eur Respir J.* 1997;10(10):2270-2274.

85. Leung R, Hill P, Burdon JGW. Effect of inhaled morphine on the development of breathlessness during exercise in patients with chronic lung disease. *Thorax.* 1996;51(6):596-600.

86. Masood AR, Reed JW, Thomas SHL. Lack of effect of inhaled morphine on exercise-induced breathlessness in chronic obstructive pulmonary disease. *Thorax.* 1995;50(6):629-634.

87. Noseda A, Carpiaux JP, Markstein C, Meyvaert A, de Maertelaer V. Disabling dyspnoea in patients with advanced disease: lack of effect of nebulized morphine. *Eur Respir J.* 1997;10(5):1079-1083.

88. Young IH, Daviskas E, Keena VA. Effect of low dose nebulised morphine on exercise endurance in patients with chronic lung disease. *Thorax.* 1989;44:387-390.

89. Mazzocato C, Buclin T, Rapin CH. The effects of morphine on dyspnea and ventilatory function in elderly patients with advanced cancer: a randomized double-blind controlled trial. *Ann Oncol.* 1999;10(12):1511-1514.

90. Allard P, Lamontagne C, Bernard P, Tremblay C. How effective are supplementary doses of opioids for dyspnea in terminally ill cancer patients? A randomized continuous sequential clinical trial. *J Pain Symptom Manage.* 1999;17(4):256-265.

91. Navigante AH, Cerchietti LCA, Castro MA, Lutteral MA, Cabalar ME. Midazolam as adjunct therapy to morphine in the alleviation of severe dyspnea perception in patients with advanced cancer. *J Pain Symptom Manage.* 2006;31(1):38-47.

92. Charles MA, Reymond L, Israel F. Relief of incident dyspnea in palliative cancer patients: a pilot, randomized, controlled trial comparing nebulized hydromorphone, systemic hydromorphone, and nebulized saline. *J Pain Symptom Manage.* 2008;36(1):29-38.

93. Bruera E, Sala R, Spruyt O, Palmer JL, Zhang T, Willey J. Nebulized versus subcutaneous morphine for patients with cancer dyspnea: a preliminary study. *J Pain Symptom Manage.* 2005;29(6):613-618.

94. O'Neill PA, Morton PB, Stark RD. Chlorpromazine—a specific effect on breathlessness? *Br J Clin Pharmacol.* 1985;19:793-797.

95. Woodcock AA, Gross ER, Geddes DM. Drug treatment of breathlessness: contrasting effects of diazepam and promethazine in pink puffers. *Brit Med J.* 1981;283:343-346.

96. Rice KL, Kronenberg RS, Hedemark LL, Niewoehner DE. Effects of chronic administration of codeine and promethazine on breathlessness and exercise tolerance in patients with chronic airflow obstruction. *Br J Dis Chest.* 1987;81:287-292.

97. McIver B, Walsh D, Nelson K. The use of chlorpromazine for symptom control in dying cancer patients. *J Pain Symptom Manage.* 1994;9(5):341-345.

98. Ventafridda V, Spoldi E, De Conno F. Control of dyspnea in advanced cancer patients. *Chest.* 1990;98:1544-1545.

99. Simon ST, Higginson IJ, Booth S, Harding R, Bausewein C. *Benzodiazepines for the Relief of Breathlessness in Advanced Malignant and Non-malignant Diseases in Adults (Review).* Cochrane Pain, Palliative and Supportive Care Group: Canada: John Wiley & Sons Ltd; 2011.

100. Navigante AH, Castro MA, Cerchietti LC. Morphine versus midazolam as upfront therapy to control dyspnea perception in cancer patients while its underlying cause is sought or treated. *J Pain Symptom Manage.* 2010;39(5):820-830.

101. Philip J, Gold M, Milner A, Di Iulio J, Miller B, Spruyt O. A randomized, double-blind, crossover trial of the effect of oxygen on dyspnea in patients with advanced cancer. *J Pain Symptom Manage.* 2006;32(6):541-550.

102. Cranston JM, Crockett A, Currow D. Oxygen therapy for dyspnoea in adults (review). *Cochrane Libr.* 2008;3(4):1-54.

103. Booth S, Kelly M, Cox NP, Adams L, Guz A. Does oxygen help dyspnea in patients with cancer? *Am J Respir Crit Care Med.* 1996;153:1515-1518.

104. Uronis H, Abernethy AP. Oxygen for relief of dyspnea: what is the evidence? *Curr Opin Support Palliat Care.* 2008;2(2):89-94.

105. Currow DC, Agar M, Smith J, Abernethy, AP. Does palliative home oxygen improve dyspnoea? A consecutive cohort study. *Palliat Med.* 2009;23(4):309-316.

106. Bausewein C, Booth S, Higginson GM. *Non-pharmacological Interventions for Breathlessness in Advanced Stages of Malignant and Non-malignant Diseases (Review).* Cochrane Pain, Palliative and Supportive Care Group: Canada: John Wiley & Sons Ltd; 2008.

107. Schwartzstein RM, Lahive K, Pope A, Weinberger SE, Weiss JW. Cold facial stimulation reduces breathlessness induced in normal subjects. *Am Rev Respir Dis.* 1987;136:58-61.

108. Baltzan, M, Alter A, Rotaple M, Kamel H, Wolkove N. Fan to palliate exercise-induced dyspnea with severe COPD. *Am J Respir Crit Care Med.* 2000;161(suppl 3):A59.

109. Marchetti N, Travaline JM, Criner JL. Air current applied to the face of COPD patients enhances leg ergometry performance. *Am J Respir Crit Care Med.* 2004:169: A773.

110. Spence DP, Graham DR, Ahmed J, Rees K, Pearson MG, Calverley PM. Does cold air affect exercise capacity and dyspnoea in stable COPD? *Chest.* 1993;103:693-696.

111. Galbraith S, Fagan P, Perkins P, Lynch A, Booth S. Does the use of a handheld fan improve chronic dyspnea? A randomized, controlled, crossover trial. *J Pain Symptom Manage.* 2009;39(5):831-838.

112. Cancer Care Ontario. Symptom Management Tools [Internet]. https://www.cancercare.on.ca/toolbox/symptools/. Toronto: Cancer Care Ontario; 2010.

CHAPTER 30

Hemoptysis, Airway Obstruction, Bronchospasm, Cough, and Pulmonary Complications/ Symptoms of Cancer and Its Treatment

Jaya Vijayan ■ J. Hunter Groninger

INTRODUCTION

Complications from malignancies abound in and around the pulmonary tree and chest cavity. Excepting primary brain malignancies, any cancer has the capacity to wreak havoc in vital organs and circulatory structures as well as potential spaces. For most of these malignancies, complications in the chest cavity or pulmonary tree suggest advanced, incurable disease. From the perspective of supportive oncology and/or palliative care, the clinical approach to the patient with such complications should reflect both evaluation of disease-modifying treatment options and management of symptom burden, always considering the patient's goals of care. Finally, many of the complications described here correlate with worsened functional status and prognosis and can lead directly to death. In addition to a comprehensive approach to managing these clinical situations, the supportive oncology or palliative care expert should always be prepared to counsel patients and families and to provide best end-of-life care when other interventions fail.

This chapter provides an overview of more common complications arising in the chest cavity in patients with malignancies and corresponding management strategies. It also broaches more common symptoms arising in the pulmonary system (of note, a most common symptom, dyspnea, is discussed elsewhere in this text). Finally, we summarize discussion points regarding noninvasive positive pressure ventilation (NIPPV), a treatment option that may often be overlooked, particularly in the palliative care setting. Although by no means exhaustive, this chapter should provide a sense of the breadth and depth to which malignancy can affect these critical organ systems and anatomy.

PLEURAL EFFUSIONS

Incidence

Malignant pleural effusions are a significant clinical problem in the management of the cancer patient. In any given general hospital patient population, up to 60% of all pleural effusions are malignant, the highest incidence seen in patients over 50 years old (1–4). In up to 50% of patients, it is the initial manifestation of cancer (4,5) but eventually, about half of all patients with disseminated cancer develop a malignant pleural effusion (4). Table 30.1 lists the frequency of the various tumor types that are associated with malignant pleural effusions.

Diagnosis

The approach to the diagnosis and subsequent treatment of a patient with a suspected malignant pleural effusion is shown in Figure 30.1. Initial screening begins with the posterior–anterior chest radiograph with decubitus views. Blunting of the costophrenic angle may suggest 175 to 500 mL of free fluid; a decubitus view may show as little as 100 mL (6). Computed tomography (CT) scans may be especially necessary if the hemithorax is opaque on chest radiograph, when a mesothelioma is suspected, or when the underlying primary tumor is unknown. Occasionally, chest ultrasonography can be employed to differentiate pleural fluid and pleural thickening (7), but this modality is more commonly used to localize smaller effusions en route to diagnostic or therapeutic thoracentesis (8).

If the patient is symptomatic, enough fluid should be drained by thoracentesis to relieve symptoms. Rapid removal of a large amount of fluid (especially over 1,500 mL) may result in life-threatening re-expansion pulmonary edema (9). A malignant effusion is frequently hemorrhagic (erythrocyte count >100,000/mm³), but this is nonspecific and occurs in only one-third of cases (5). Elevated levels of lactate dehydrogenase (LDH) or protein in the fluid, and ratios of fluid to concurrent serum levels of LDH and protein, distinguish transudate from an exudate (10). If findings suggest transudate, malignancy may be essentially excluded. However, an exudate with a negative cytology result necessitates a second diagnostic thoracentesis with cytology to improve sensitivity by another 10% (3). Cytology remains the cornerstone to diagnosing a malignant pleural effusion, although important variables contribute to its efficacy: tumor type, cytopathologist experience, and the volume of fluid sent for cytologic analysis (11). With

TABLE 30.1	Tumor causes of malignant pleural effusions from collected series

Tumor Type	Incidence (%)
Lung	35
Breast	23
Lymphoma/leukemia	10
Adenocarcinoma (unknown primary)	12
Reproductive tract	6
Gastrointestinal tract	5
Genitourinary tract	3
Primary unknown	3
Other cancers	5

From Hausheer FH, Yarbro JW. Diagnosis and treatment of malignant pleural effusion. *Semin Oncol.* 1985;12:54–75, with permission.

some cell types, such as Hodgkin's disease, the rate of positive cytology results may prove as low as 23%, while with others, such as breast or lung cancer, remain as high as 73% (3).

When two exudative pleural fluid cytology results are negative for malignancy in the face of high clinical suspicion for malignancy, most clinicians move to video-assisted thoracoscopy surgery (VATS), which permits visually directed pleural biopsy and direct therapeutic intervention including lysis of adhesions, mechanical or chemical pleurodesis, or pleurectomy (12).

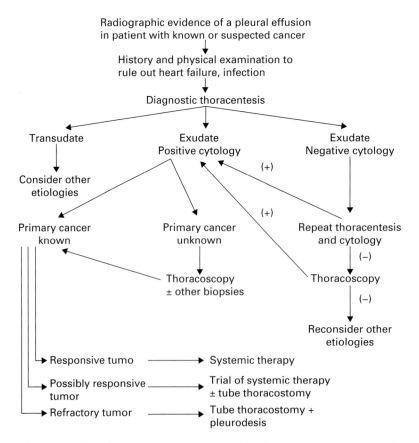

Figure 30.1. Approach to the diagnosis and treatment of malignant pleural effusions. +, study result is positive; –, study result is negative. (From Ruckdeschel JC. Management of malignant pleural effusion: an overview. *Semin Oncol.* 1988;15:24–28, with permission.)

Prognosis

Most patients with malignant pleural effusions have an incurable disease. Treatment should be targeted to the most effective palliation for maximal, comfortable time outside the hospital. For all patients, the overall mean survival time is 3 to 6 months. In general, mortality in the setting of this complication is high: from 54% at 1 month to 84% at 6 months (13–15).

Management

Management of Underlying Malignancy

Whenever indicated, a therapeutic thoracentesis should be followed by appropriate disease-modifying therapies such as systemic chemotherapy or hormonal therapy (16,17). If the malignancy is resistant to systemic therapies, then tube thoracostomy followed by intrapleural therapy may be appropriate, if the patient has a reasonable life expectancy. If the patient's performance status is poor, simple prolonged drainage by an indwelling catheter may be more appropriate.

Management of Fluid Accumulation

While thoracentesis relieves symptoms briefly, fluid usually re-accumulates quickly—in up to 97% of patients by 1 month (18). Tube thoracostomy demonstrates a role in draining the pleural cavity and maintaining opposition of the pleural surfaces when a therapeutic agent is infused into the chest cavity for sclerotherapy.

Soft silastic indwelling catheters, often placed under local anesthesia, allow patient or caregiver to periodically drain the pleural space for symptomatic relief. When employed more than 6 weeks, these catheters facilitate spontaneous pleurodesis between 40% and 46% of the time (19–21).

Fibrinolytic Agents. Intrapleural instillation of a fibrinolytic agent such as urokinase may help to break up more gelatinous or fibrous fluid accumulations (22,23).

Pleurodesis. Drainage of the pleural space with re-expansion of the lung, followed by instillation of a chemical agent into the pleural cavity, remains the most common management strategy for malignant pleural effusions. The mechanism of this intervention, called *pleural sclerotherapy* or *pleurodesis*, is considered to be creation of an inflammatory pleuritis between visceral and parietal pleuras that facilitates more permanent closing of the potential space. A table of available agents used for pleurodesis is given in Table 30.2.

Pleuroperitoneal Shunt. Internal drainage of the malignant effusion into the abdomen using an implanted, valved, manually operated pump is occasionally an option in compliant, well-motivated patients with good performance status who have a trapped lung and an intractable effusion (5,17,24).

Recurrent Effusions. A common frustrating problem remains the refractory pleural effusion in which the first attempt at pleural sclerotherapy has failed. At times, a second tube thoracostomy, followed by intrapleural sclerotherapy, is

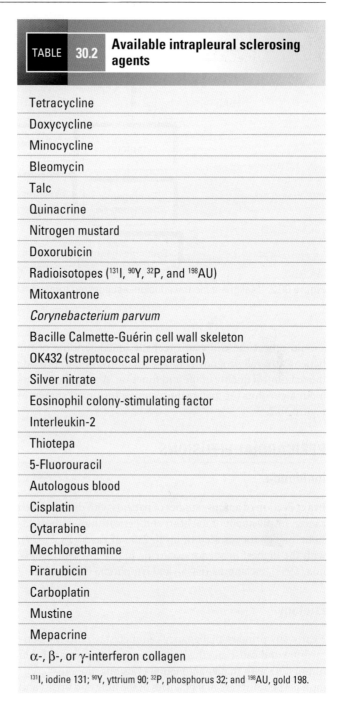

TABLE 30.2	Available intrapleural sclerosing agents
Tetracycline
Doxycycline
Minocycline
Bleomycin
Talc
Quinacrine
Nitrogen mustard
Doxorubicin
Radioisotopes (^{131}I, ^{90}Y, ^{32}P, and ^{198}AU)
Mitoxantrone
Corynebacterium parvum
Bacille Calmette-Guérin cell wall skeleton
OK432 (streptococcal preparation)
Silver nitrate
Eosinophil colony-stimulating factor
Interleukin-2
Thiotepa
5-Fluorouracil
Autologous blood
Cisplatin
Cytarabine
Mechlorethamine
Pirarubicin
Carboplatin
Mustine
Mepacrine
α-, β-, or γ-interferon collagen

^{131}I, iodine 131; ^{90}Y, yttrium 90; ^{32}P, phosphorus 32; and ^{198}AU, gold 198.

attempted, usually employing a different agent. If this second attempt fails, and if the patient had a good performance status and a reasonable estimated life span, then VATS talc poudrage may be considered. In many instances, the placement of a silastic catheter with prolonged external drainage has become the treatment of choice.

Summary

Patients with malignant pleural effusions generally have terminal disease with a very limited life span—often just a few months at best. Choice to pursue disease-modifying therapy

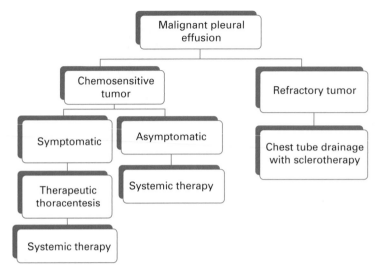

Figure 30.2. Malignant pleural effusion—suggested treatment algorithm.

should reflect the clinician's realistic understanding of the patient's overall prognosis along with motivation to provide the maximum quality of life and function. A suggested treatment algorithm for malignant pleural effusions is shown in Figure 30.2.

PERICARDIAL EFFUSIONS

Incidence

In a collection of autopsy studies of patients with disseminated cancer, involvement of the heart and pericardium with metastatic malignancy is seen in up to 21% of cases (24,25–29), with the highest incidence occurring in patients with leukemia (69%), melanoma (64%), and lymphoma (24%) (29).

Etiology

Nearly any primary malignancy can metastasize to the pericardium and cause an effusion (29) excepting primary brain tumors. As with malignant pleural effusions, the most common perpetrators are malignancies of the lung and breast and lymphoma or leukemia; together these account for almost 75% of all pericardial malignant events (30). Elucidating the cause of such an effusion is critically important, since approximately 40% of patients with an underlying cancer have a nonmalignant etiology (31).

Pathophysiology

The increase in pericardial fluid, threatening to cause tamponade, typically results from obstruction of the mediastinal lymphatic system, especially by cancers that commonly involve the mediastinal lymph nodes (26). With slow accumulation of fluid, the pericardium can distend to contain up to 2 L. Rapid accumulation does not allow such tissue distension and hemodynamic compromise may occur with

as little an accumulation as 200 mL (32). The critical outcome is impaired diastolic filling of the right side of the heart. *Cardiac tamponade* occurs when accumulating pericardial contents overwhelm compensatory mechanisms leading to hemodynamic instability (33).

Clinical Presentation

The most common presenting symptom is dyspnea on exertion, which may progress to dyspnea at rest as cardiac function becomes compromised (26,31,33). Other common symptoms include chest pain or heaviness (63%), cough (30% to 43%), and weakness or fatigue (26%) (29). Less common symptoms include peripheral edema, low-grade fever, dizziness, nausea, diaphoresis, and peripheral venous constriction.

On examination, the classic signs associated with cardiac tamponade are often referred to as *Beck's triad*: faint heart sounds, hypotension, and venous distention (33). Hypotension may be found in over 60% of patients, elevated venous pressure is seen in 50% to 60%, and resting tachycardia occurs in up to 90% (26). A central venous pressure >15 mm Hg along with hypotension is highly suggestive of tamponade. The pathophysiologic effects of cardiac tamponade tend to exaggerate the normal fall in systolic blood pressure (usually <10 mm Hg) and stroke volume that occur with inspiration, a phenomenon termed *pulsus paradoxus*. Other signs, less frequent, that may be present include a narrowed pulse pressure, a visible increase in venous pressure on inspiration (Kussmaul's sign), hepatomegaly, hepatojugular reflux, peripheral edema, cyanosis, pericardial friction rub, arrhythmias, cold clammy extremities, low-grade fever, and ascites.

Diagnosis

Radiographic

In any patient with cancer, a change in the size and contour of the heart in the setting of clear lung fields on a standard chest x-ray should provoke consideration of a pericardial effusion. The cardiac silhouette might resemble the so-called water-bottle heart with bulging of the normal contours. However, a normal-size heart shadow does not exclude the presence of a pericardial effusion or even a life-threatening tamponade. A chest CT scan is more sensitive and may suggest a malignant pericardial process if the effusion has a high density, there is pericardial thickening, masses are contiguous with the pericardium, or there is an obliteration of the tissue planes between the mass and the heart (26).

A more invasive diagnostic procedure is right heart catheterization. The findings from this procedure in true tamponade are depressed cardiac output and the equalization of diastolic pressures in all heart chambers (33).

Electrocardiography (ECG)

ECG changes—including sinus tachycardia, atrial and ventricular arrhythmias, low-voltage QRS, and diffuse nonspecific ST- and T-wave abnormalities—may reflect presence of an effusion. Electrical alternans (alternating large and small P wave and QRS complexes) is occasionally seen and generally resolves immediately with drainage of the effusion (27,33).

Echocardiography

Echocardiography may detect as little as 15 mL of fluid as well as identifying myocardial masses and even loculations of fluid.

Pericardial Fluid Examination

Percutaneous, ultrasound-guided pericardiocentesis can safely be performed in patients with larger effusions (>1 cm anterior clear space on echocardiogram), yielding fluid sample for examination in approximately 90% of patients and temporary tamponade relief (26,34). In a malignant effusion, the result of cytology will be positive for malignant cells in 65% to 90% of cases (35). False-negative cytologic results can frequently be seen with lymphoma and mesothelioma. Negative cytology alone does not exclude neoplastic pericarditis, and it may be necessary to obtain pericardial tissue for histology if clinical suspicion remains high.

Differential Diagnosis of Pericardial Effusion

Up to 40% of patients with a symptomatic pericardial effusion and cancer will have a benign etiology of the effusion (31). Generally, the pericardial fluid analysis together with the patient's history will exclude most of the potential diagnoses and will pinpoint the actual cause of the effusion.

Prognosis

Quality of life and functional status depend largely on malignancy cell type and stage. In general terms, prognosis is limited at best; for example, after surgical drainage of an effusion, patients with breast cancer have a mean survival of 8 to 18 months (36,37), patients with lymphoma have a mean survival of 10 months (36), and patients with lung cancer have a mean survival of 3 to 5 months (38,36).

Management

Pericardiocentesis

This is the initial procedure of choice in the emergency management of life-threatening tamponade. When combined with echocardiography the success rate in obtaining fluid for diagnosis and relieving symptoms rises to almost 97% with a decrease in the complication rate to 2.4% (26,37). Most (39% to 56%) malignant effusions will recur even after single or repeated taps (26,37). During initial drainage, insertion of a small pigtail catheter into the pericardial space can facilitate intermittent drainage over several days (26).

Intrapericardial Sclerosis

The logic extension of pericardiocentesis with catheter drainage is injection of a sclerosing agent into the pericardium through the indwelling catheter to prevent a recurrence of the effusion, much like that practiced with malignant pleural effusions. Agents used in small studies include tetracycline, doxycycline, minocycline, bleomycin, and talc.

Radiotherapy

External beam radiotherapy has been advocated for a variety of tumors with cardiac and pericardial involvement (39). Generally, this strategy is reserved for radiotherapy-naïve patients with radiosensitive tumors (26).

Surgical Approaches

The most popular approach to surgical treatment of a malignant pericardial effusion is the *subxiphoid pericardiectomy* (i.e., "pericardial window"), which offers the distinct advantages of very low mortality (1% or less), 1% major morbidity, and 100% immediate efficacy in relieving tamponade. The long-term effusion recurrence rate is low (3% to 7%) (26,40–43). Diagnostic accuracy approaches 100% because fluid and pericardial tissue are both removed and sent for pathologic evaluation. If necessary, a *left anterior thoracotomy* for pericardiectomy has a low morbidity and mortality and allows examination and biopsy of the contents of the left pleural cavity if desired. More extensively, the *median sternotomy with pericardiectomy* gives very wide exposure to most of the pericardium. Alternatively, the advent of *VATS* has allowed a minimally invasive approach to pericardiectomy; one series of 28 patients demonstrated 100% long-term success, no significant morbidity, and 0% mortality (44). Finally, more novel attempts to maximize fluid drainage while minimizing surgical risks include the pericardioperitoneal shunt (45) and the percutaneous balloon pericardiotomy (46).

Summary

Malignant pericardial effusion is not uncommon in advanced cancers, especially with cancers of the lung and breast and with leukemia or lymphoma. In general, these patients have incurable disease. Nonetheless, most patients with symptomatic effusions deserve treatment evaluation, as they may respond rapidly to pericardial decompression. Therapy must

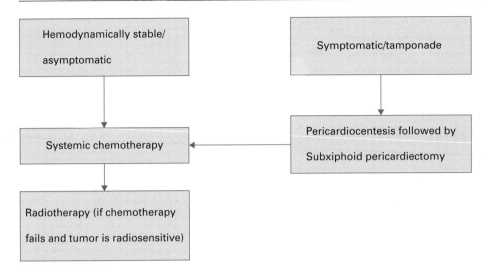

Figure 30.3. Malignant pericardial effusion treatment algorithm for patients with chemosensitive tumor.

be individualized, taking into consideration tumor cell type and sensitivity to disease-modifying therapies, patient performance status and prognosis, and presence/absence of pericardial tamponade, leading to some meaningful period of palliation. A suggested treatment algorithm for patients with chemosensitive tumor is shown in Figure 30.3.

SUPERIOR VENA CAVA SYNDROME

Primary or metastatic tumors can cause superior vena cava (SVC) obstruction, also known as *SVC syndrome* (47). Cancers classically associated with SVC syndrome include lung cancer (particularly right-sided), breast cancer, primary mediastinal lymphoma, lymphoblastic lymphoma, thymoma, and germ cell tumors (either primary or metastatic to mediastinum).

Presentation

The extent of obstruction and acuity of development dictate the patient's presentation. Blockage is better tolerated when there has been time for collateral veins to develop in adjacent venous systems like the azygos and internal mammary, a process that usually takes weeks. The veins on the patient's chest wall may be visibly distended. Edema in the arms, facial plethora (not necessarily unilateral), chemosis, and periorbital edema may also occur. Stridor is an alarming sign that edema is narrowing the luminal diameter of the pharynx and larynx. Hoarseness and dysphagia can result from edema around the airway and digestive tract. Presyncope or syncope is more common early on, when cardiac output declines without compensation. Headaches stem from distension of cerebral vessels against the dura, but confusion may indicate cerebral edema. All of these symptoms may be more noticeable when the patient is supine.

Diagnosis

Radiographic imaging is crucial to diagnosis and treatment planning. While the gold standard for localizing obstruction remains selective venography, multidetector CT and magnetic resonance imaging (MRI) are usually preferable for their noninvasiveness, easier availability, and decreased contrast load.

Treatment

SVC syndrome requires prompt recognition and treatment, but the clinical course typically permits completion of appropriate diagnostic studies before definitive therapy begins (48). Patients who have neurologic symptoms or airway compromise merit immediate treatment. *Endovascular stenting* is the treatment of choice and generally relieves symptoms more quickly than chemoradiation (49). *Chemotherapy* may be the only necessary treatment in patients presenting nonemergently with small cell lung cancer, lymphoma, or germ cell tumors. Changes in the SVC lumen following mediastinal *radiation* may be disproportionately small relative to the magnitude of symptom improvement. Cases of catheter-related thrombosis have been successfully treated with instillation of *thrombolytics* into the device (50), but fibrinolytic therapy should be administered carefully in cases in which brain metastases have been diagnosed or not excluded.

TRACHEOBRONCHIAL OBSTRUCTION

Tracheobronchial obstruction may be intrinsic or extrinsic in etiology. *Intrinsic* obstruction is usually caused by primary lung malignancies or from metastases arising from the airway epithelium (most commonly renal cell, colon, rectum, cervical, breast carcinomas, and malignant melanomas) (51,52). *Extrinsic* obstruction occurs when the airways are surrounded by solid tumor or are encased by enlarged lymph nodes. This scenario usually results from locally advanced disease arising from lung, esophagus, thyroid, or lymphoma. Table 30.3 lists the common etiologies of airway obstruction.

Clinical Presentation

Patients with proximal airway obstruction usually present with dyspnea, hemoptysis, wheezing, or stridor and sometimes with pneumonia or atelectasis. Distal airway

TABLE 30.3	Etiologies of airway obstruction

Intrinsic Obstruction

Malignant

- ■ Primary tumors
  - ● Tracheal
    - – Squamous carcinoma
    - – Adenoid cystic carcinoma
  - ● Bronchogenic
  - ● Squamous
  - ● Adenocarcinoma
  - ● Small cell
  - ● Mixed morphology
- ■ Metastatic
  - ● Breast cancer
  - ● Melanoma
  - ● Larynx
  - ● Esophagus
  - ● Renal cell
  - ● Colon

Extrinsic Obstruction

- ● Rectal
- ● Cervical
- ● Kaposi sarcoma (rarely obstructing)

Benign

- ● Papillomas
- ● Chondromas
- ● Hamartoma
- ● Lipoma
- ● Leiomyoma
- ● Granular cell myoblastoma
- ● Granuloma 2 retained foreign body
- ● Hemangiomas
- ● Postintubation strictures

Low-grade Malignancy

- ● Carcinoid

Malignant

- ● Lung
- ● Lymphoma
- ● Esophageal
- ● Thyroid

Benign

- ● Fungal infection
- ● Reactive lymphadenopathy
- ● Bronchomalacia
- ● Mediastinal fibrosis
- ● Vascular compression
- ● Goiter

obstruction, on the other hand, tends to present with obstructive pneumonitis (53).

Evaluation

A grossly abnormal radiograph with a large central parenchymal mass or mediastinal mass/adenopathy causing tracheal narrowing or deviation raises concern for airway patency. Often, abnormalities become more evident on the lateral x-ray view.

CT scan of the neck and chest better defines airway anatomy (51,53). In medically stable patients, pulmonary function testing (including spirometry and flow-volume loops) may be an inexpensive and noninvasive method to identify upper airway obstruction. Often, such testing can determine if the obstructing lesion is intrinsic or extrinsic. A more complete evaluation, with potential for tissue biopsy includes direct visualization with laryngoscopy or bronchoscopy.

Management

Patients who have airway obstruction because of primary tracheal or laryngeal malignancies or benign strictures/lesions should be referred to the appropriate specialist (otolaryngologist, oncologist, and/or radiation oncologist) for evaluation toward definitive therapy. Palliative therapeutic options (Table 30.4) for airway management in patients who are not candidates for definitive therapeutic procedures include airway stents, laser therapy, brachytherapy, photodynamic therapy (PDT), and tracheostomy. Patients with obstructions either laryngeal or especially high in the tracheobronchial tree may require tracheostomy to maintain airway patency.

Management of Intrinsic Obstruction

Any palliative therapy necessitates an adequate diameter for passage of a bronchoscope while maintaining adequate oxygenation and ventilation. For large exophytic intraluminal masses, *rigid bronchoscopy* can be used selectively to "core out" the obstructing tumor (51,54,55). In one series (55), 51 of 56 patients had significant improvement in airway obstruction after bronchoscopic "core out," and only 2 patients required a repeat procedure.

Another option for palliative resection of intrinsic obstructing lesions of the large airways is *laser endobronchial resection* (53). Success rates are quite substantial and most patients demonstrate relief of symptoms and/or re-expansion of the obstructed lung. In one study, it was found to be a fair alternative to tracheostomy (56).

Bronchoscopic brachytherapy involves the placement of a radiation source in close proximity to an endobronchial tumor. This therapy can improve symptoms of dyspnea and hemoptysis in approximately 90% of patients with stable airway disease (57).

PDT is another option for the obstructed airway secondary to a malignant lesion. Studies have found PDT to be effective in treating endobronchial tumor (58,59). Complications

TABLE 30.4 Treatment options for central obstructing malignant airway lesions	
Intrinsic	**Extrinsic**
External beam radiation	External beam radiation
Mechanical "core out"	Stent
Laser therapy	
Brachytherapy	
Cryotherapy	
Photodynamic therapy	
Stent	

Combination of treatment plans often necessary.

from PDT can include airway edema and mucous plugging with atelectasis.

Freezing endoluminal tumor through *cryotherapy* is another option to palliate airway obstruction. A major drawback to cryotherapy is its lack of immediate tumor response (55,60).

Management of Extrinsic Obstruction

Over the last two decades, insertion of airway stents to maintain airway patency has gained popularity as an effective palliative treatment for extrinsic compression. Their most impressive benefit is the immediate palliation of airway obstruction on placement of the stent. Figure 30.4 gives an algorithm for the management of central airway obstruction.

STRIDOR

Stridor is loud, harsh breathing, noticed particularly on inspiration, generated from obstructed airflow in the upper airway and large intrathoracic central airways. Treatment depends on the location of the obstruction and its etiology. When evaluating a patient presenting with stridor, it is useful to consider the airway as three zones (60–62): the *supraglottic zone* (nose, oral cavity, pharynx, and supraglottic larynx), the *extrathoracic tracheal zone* (glottis and subglottis), and the *intrathoracic tracheal zone*. Stridor originating from the

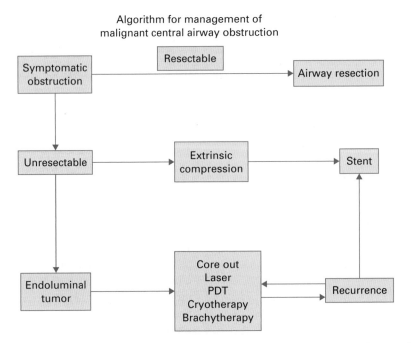

Figure 30.4. Algorithm for the management of central airway obstruction. PDT, photodynamic therapy. (Adapted from Wood D. Management of malignant tracheobronchial obstruction. *Surg Clin North Am.* 2002;82(3):640:figure 6.)

TABLE	30.5	**Causes of stridor**

Infection
  Tracheitis: bacterial or viral
  Epiglottitis
  Abscess: peritonsillar or retropharyngeal
  Viral laryngotracheobronchitis

Neoplasm
  See Table 30.3

Congenital
  Laryngomalacia
  Tracheomalacia/tracheal stenosis
  Vocal cord cysts/paralysis
  Webs

Trauma
  Facial
  Ingestion
  Inhalation injury

Postintubation
  Airway fracture
  Postsurgical

Neurologic
  Central nervous system malformation
  Hypoxic encephalopathy

Other
  Foreign bodies (airway and esophageal)
  Psychogenic
  Exercise

supraglottic zone tends to occur on inspiration. Lesions in the extrathoracic tracheal zone tend to produce biphasic stridor (on both inspiration and expiration). Stridor from the intrathoracic tracheal zone may be more expiratory, often mistook for wheezing in distal airways. Some causes of stridor are listed in Table 30.5.

Evaluation

If a patient presents in severe respiratory distress with inadequate oxygenation or ventilation, establishment of an airway comes first. In the stable patient, a brief history may help determine the cause. Gradual onset of symptoms over weeks or months, especially if accompanied by constitutional symptoms, may suggest neoplasm. Stridor manifesting over hours to days, especially in a febrile patient, is suspicious for an infectious etiology (e.g., epiglottis, croup, or abscess). A history of previous prolonged or traumatic intubation may suggest subglottic stenosis (63).

Physical examination demonstrates loud, noisy breathing. Respiratory rate, depth of respiration, use of accessory muscles of respiration, level of alertness, and evidence of cyanosis should be evaluated. Intense pain or inability to handle oral secretions may suggest peritonsillar abscess,

retropharyngeal hematoma or abscess, epiglottis, or foreign body. Crepitation on airway palpation suggests subcutaneous emphysema. A displaced trachea or firm mass could indicate tumor or goiter. Lymphadenopathy may suggest neoplasm.

Radiologic studies of the neck and chest can be obtained, but CT scans will provide more definitive anatomic information. Spirometry with flow-volume loops may be beneficial in evaluation of stridor.

Management

Stridor secondary to infectious etiologies requires treatment with appropriate antimicrobial therapy. Several pharmacologic therapies are available to stabilize the stridorous patient who is clinically decompensating. *Heliox*, a mixture of helium and oxygen available in different proportions, has been useful in improving oxygenation, ventilation, and decreasing work of breathing in patients with stridor from various etiologies (64–68), including status asthmaticus, postextubation edema, and extrinsic compression from tumor. Although somewhat nonspecific, *corticosteroids* administered intravenously can be beneficial. *Racemic epinephrine* may be used especially for postextubation stridor (69).

Although no specific trials comment on this, in more extreme cases, NIPPV may decrease the work of breathing and overcome large airway obstruction, although currently no studies have evaluated the efficacy of this therapy. Finally, endotracheal intubation or tracheostomy must be considered in appropriate clinical situations.

BRONCHOSPASM

Bronchospasm, defined as abnormal narrowing of the airways, is usually episodic and can occur in a variety of pulmonary disorders. Patients complain of dyspnea, wheezing, chest tightness, or pressure, although occasionally cough is the only symptom. Exacerbation of symptoms may frequently occur in the early hours of the morning, when the bronchial tone is normally increased. Auscultation of the chest reveals wheezing, usually with prolonged expiration.

Evaluation

An individual patient may suffer from multiple etiologies of bronchospasm. The differential diagnosis includes asthma, chronic obstructive pulmonary disease (COPD), upper/large airway obstruction (see Section Tracheobronchial Obstruction) congestive heart failure, gastroesophageal reflux disease (GERD), bronchiectasis, bronchiolitis (infectious or inflammatory, medication induced), lymphangitic tumor spread, or rarely pulmonary embolism.

Chest radiographs may demonstrate bronchial wall thickening, flattened diaphragms, and increased retrosteral air space, consistent with hyper-expansion and air trapping and would support the diagnosis of asthma or COPD. A chest radiograph with no change from the patient's baseline film or with atelectasis or small pleural effusion should alert the clinician to possible pulmonary embolism.

Therapy

Relief of bronchospasm is aimed at dilation of distal airways and reduced inflammation. Many pharmacologic agents are available to treat bronchospasm (Table 30.6).

TABLE 30.6	Therapy for bronchospasm		
Medications			
β-agonists			
Albuterol (Proventil and Ventolin)	MDI	Two to three puffs up to q.i.d.	
	Neb	0.5–0.75 mL in 2.5-mL saline q.i.d.	
Levalbuterol (Xopenex)	MDI	One to two puffs q.i.d.	
Pirbuterol	MDI	Two to three puffs q.i.d.	
Anticholinergics			
Ipratropium bromide (Atrovent)	MDI	Two puffs up to q.i.d.	
	Neb	500 µg in 2.5-mL saline t.i.d. to q.i.d.	
Tiotropium (Spiriva)	DPI	18 µg or one capsule once daily	
Nonsteroidal anti-inflammatory			
Cromolyn sodium (Intal)	MDI	Two to four puffs b.i.d. to q.i.d.	
	Neb	1–2 mL (10–20 mg) b.i.d. to q.i.d.	
Nedocromil sodium (Tilade)	MDI	Two puffs b.i.d. to q.i.d.	
Long-acting β-agonist			
Formoterol (Foradil)	DPI	12 µg b.i.d.	
Salmeterol (Serevent)	DPI	50 µg b.i.d.	
Inhaled corticosteroids			
Beclomethasone (QVAR)	MDI	40, 80 µg one to two inhalations b.i.d.	
Budesonide (Pulmicort)	Neb	0.25–0.50 mg b.i.d.	
	DPI	Two to four inhalations b.i.d.	
Flunisolide (Aerobid)	MDI	Two to four inhalations b.i.d.	
Fluticasone (Flovent)	DPI	44, 110, 220 µg strengths, one to two inhalations b.i.d.	
Mometasone (Asmanex)	Spray DPI	One to two inhalations b.i.d.	
Triamcinolone (Azmacort)	MDI	Two to four puffs t.i.d. to q.i.d.	
Combination medications			
Advair (Fluticasone/Salmeterol)	DPI	100/50, 250/50, 500/50	
		One inhalation b.i.d.	
Combivent (Albuterol/Ipratropium)	MDI	One to two inhalations q.i.d.	
		3 mL q.i.d.	
Leukotriene receptor antagonists			
Montelukast (Singulair)	Oral	10 mg daily	
Zafirlukast (Accolate)	Oral	20 mg b.i.d.	
Zileuton (Zyflo)	Oral	600 mg up to q.i.d. monitor LFTs	

MDI, metered-dose inhaler; Neb, through nebulizer; DPI, dry powder inhaler; LFTs, liver function tests.

β-*agonists* promote airway smooth muscle relaxation, increase mucociliary clearance, and increase the secretion of electrolytes by the airways. Side effects include tremor, tachycardia, palpitations, hypokalemia, and hyperglycemia. In general, to prevent tachyphylaxis, patients are advised not to use β-agonists more than four to five times a day.

Anticholinergic agents act by decreasing the parasympathetic bronchoconstriction of the airways. Ipratropium bromide and new dry powder tiotropium are the anticholinergic agents available for inhalational use in the United States. Because of studies showing that ipratropium bromide may be more effective than β-agonists in promoting bronchodilation in patients with COPD, it is now the first agent used in maintenance therapy in COPD with persistent airway obstruction (70–72).

Corticosteroids are widely used in the treatment of bronchospasm (73). Even patients with mild to moderate symptoms may benefit from inhaled corticosteroids. Patients should be cautioned that these medications must be used regularly and may take weeks for therapeutic effect and should always be combined with a short-acting agent for breakthrough relief. Patients with more serious symptoms or those in respiratory distress may require systemic corticosteroids. Besides corticosteroids, other pharmacologic *anti-inflammatory agents* may be employed to stem the inflammatory pathways leading to bronchospasm. Cromolyn sulfate and nedocromil sodium appear to work as mast cell stabilizers. Leukotriene receptor antagonists work to block additional components of inflammation and allow mild bronchodilation (73,74).

HEMOPTYSIS

Hemoptysis, the expectoration of blood originating in the lung, can range in presentation from blood-tinged sputum to massive hemoptysis (defined as blood loss of 400 to 600 mL/d). While massive hemoptysis occurs in fewer than 5% of cases, it carries a mortality rate of up to 85% if surgical intervention is not possible (75,76). Given such stakes, management of hemoptysis necessitates careful consideration of etiology and severity in the context of the patient's functional status and goals. Table 30.7 lists the causes of hemoptysis.

Diagnosis

A diagnosis of hemoptysis rests on localization of bleeding to the lower respiratory tract. Nasopharyngeal, laryngeal, or gastrointestinal tract bleeding may be difficult to clinically distinguish from frank hemoptysis. Bleeding from these sources may result in bloody cough, which can be misinterpreted as hemoptysis. A thorough examination of the nasopharynx, larynx, and upper gastrointestinal tract should be included in evaluation.

The next step is bleeding site localization within the pulmonary tree. A chest x-ray is often helpful in revealing a tumor or abscess. Bronchoscopy may allow direct visualization of the source or lung segment and allows tissue sampling for cytologic, histologic, and microbiologic testing (77,78). CT remains superior to bronchoscopy in identifying bronchiectasis, lung abscess, aspergilloma, and distal parenchymal abnormalities.

Management

The severity of hemoptysis determines the pace of workup and management. In a review of one decade experience at an academic medical center, the general mortality rate was 9% if blood loss was <1,000 mL/24 h, but it was 58% if the blood loss was >1,000 mL/24 h (75). Here, a malignant cause for hemoptysis >1,000 mL/24 h increased the mortality rate to 80%.

Bronchoscopy

If bronchoscopy identifies the site of bleeding, concomitant local therapies may be employed. A pulmonary tamponade balloon can be inflated in the segmental bronchus leading to the site of bleeding, allowing time for stabilization of the patient and potentially more definitive therapy (79). Bleeding from visible lesions in the trachea and proximal bronchi can be coagulated with a laser.

Radiotherapy

External beam radiation for 6 to 7 weeks is usually employed to attempt a cure for inoperable non–small cell carcinoma. In the palliative setting, therapy is delivered in the shortest time possible, with lower doses to achieve symptom relief while minimizing side effects. *Endobronchial brachytherapy* with ^{192}Ir is another alternative, alone or in combination with bronchoscopic laser therapy. In recent years, high dose rates have been favored to decrease the time of treatment and permit outpatient rather than inpatient therapy. Potential complications of brachytherapy include mucositis, fistula formation, and fatal hemoptysis (80).

Angiographic and Surgical Intervention

After angiographic identification of the vessels in question, a variety of agents (e.g., Gelfoam, polyvinyl alcohol particles, and metallic coils) can be injected selectively to stem bleeding. Reported success rates vary between 75% and 90%, with a re-bleeding rate of 15% to 30% (81). The definitive therapy for massive hemoptysis is resection of the diseased portion of the lung, but this intervention depends on specific anatomy and residual lung function.

Other Modalities

Other modalities can be used to manage hemoptysis of varying degrees, including neodymium yttrium aluminum garnet

TABLE 30.7	Causes of hemoptysis

Pulmonary	**Traumatic**
Bronchitis	Blunt/penetrating chest injury
Bronchiectasis	Ruptured bronchus
Pulmonary embolism	**Systemic Disease**
Cystic fibrosis	Goodpasture's syndrome
Infectious	Vasculitis
Lung abscess	Systemic lupus erythematosus
Mycetoma	**Drugs/Toxins**
Necrotizing pneumonia	Aspirin
Viral	Anticoagulation
Fungal	Penicillamine
Parasitic	Solvents
Septic embolism	Crack cocaine
Cardiac	**Drugs/Toxins**
Mitral stenosis	Aspirin
Congestive heart failure	Anticoagulation
Neoplastic	Penicillamine
Bronchogenic carcinoma	Solvents
Bronchial adenoma	Crack cocaine
Endobronchial hamartoma	**Miscellaneous**
Metastatic disease	Foreign body
Tracheal tumors	Endometriosis
Hematologic	Broncholithiasis
Coagulopathy	Cryptogenic hemoptysis
Platelet dysfunction	**Iatrogenic**
Thrombocytopenia	Lung biopsy
Disseminated intravascular coagulation	Pulmonary artery catheterization
Vascular	Lymphangiography
Pulmonary hypertension	Transtracheal aspirate
Arteriovenous malformation	
Aortic aneurysm	

Modified from Cahill BC, Ingbar DH. Massive hemoptysis: assessment and management. *Clin Chest Med.* 1994;15:147. with permission.

(Nd:YAG) laser photocoagulation, electrocautery, cryotherapy, argon plasma coagulation, and PDT.

Exsanguination and End-of-Life Care

If oxygenation is compromised or the patient continues to bleed vigorously, intubation may become necessary. In such extreme situations, goals of care need to be clarified up front. The decision to intubate a patient with a terminal illness may be challenging. If bleeding can be localized and controlled quickly, a short period of ventilator support may be quite reasonable if it allows for improved quality of life. This may be unlikely for a patient in the later stages of a terminal illness, especially in the setting of massive hemoptysis. In the setting of fatal hemoptysis, exsanguination usually occurs within seconds to minutes with rapid loss of consciousness. In such situations, intravenous opiates and benzodiazepines can be administered to control dyspnea and anxiety. Attention and emotional support need to be paid to family members as well. While use of continuous oral suction and judicious placement of dark towels or blankets may help obscure the blood loss, many family members may be disturbed by frank gross blood loss associated with exsanguination.

BRONCHORREA/SECRETIONS

Bronchial secretion is observed in 44% of terminally ill cancer patients and can cause significant distress for both patients and family members.

Etiology

Primary lung cancer, pneumonia, and dysphagia are significantly associated with development of bronchial secretion (82). The hypothesized pathophysiology is the inability to expectorate the products in the respiratory system. Classical "death rattle" (type I) corresponds to a combined syndrome of aspiration due to dysphagia and expectoration inability. Theoretically, this is caused by aspiration of saliva related to terminal consciousness disturbance and/or neurologic complications and anti-muscarinic medications are assumed to be effective when the products are saliva. "Pseudo" death rattle (type II) is a syndrome of inability to expectorate increased pulmonary secretion from tumor, infection, edema, and bleeding. This type does not always occur near death, and anti-muscarinic medications are assumed to be less effective.

Clinical Presentation

Bronchial secretion is defined as sounds audible at the bedside produced by movement of secretions in the hypopharynx or the bronchial tree in association with respiration. Morita et al., as part of a prospective observational study to investigate the incidence and underlying etiologies of bronchial secretion, proposed criteria for classifying the severity: inaudible (*Grade 0*), audible only very close to the patient (*Grade 1*), clearly audible at the end of the bed in a quiet room (*Grade 2*), and clearly audible at about 6 meters or at the door of the room (*Grade 3*) (82). Bronchial secretion is regarded as present when patients have a score of Grade 1 or higher.

Treatment

Treatment of bronchorrhea in palliative care is limited by a lack of clinical trials. Anti-muscarinic medications are used for as many as 73% of patients with bronchial secretions with 79% effectiveness, but 10% of all dying patients have refractory secretion or receive palliative sedation therapy (82). A 2010 *Cochrane Review* of four studies comparing atropine, glycopyrrolate, hyoscine butylbromide, and scopolamine (hyoscine hydrobromide) found no conclusive evidence of one drug being superior to another (83).

COUGH

Etiology

A protective, complicated reflex that helps clear the airways of foreign material or excessive secretions; cough is common in patients with advanced malignancy. Etiologies may stem from the malignancy—such as endobronchial tumor burden, pericardial disease, vocal cord paralysis, or aspiration—or from its treatment—such as radiation pneumonitis or chemotherapy-induced interstitial lung disease (84). Additionally, patients with underlying cancer may have all the same causes of cough found in the general population; the most common etiologies of chronic cough remain upper airway cough syndrome (previously known as postnasal drip syndrome), asthma, and GERD (85,86).

A detailed history and physical examination are important to determine the cause of chronic cough (87). Chest radiographs should be obtained early in the evaluation of cough (88). In patients who chronically produce sputum or in whom there is a suspicion of interstitial lung disease, a high-resolution chest CT scan may be helpful. Notably, among patients with interstitial lung disease, up to 10% to 15% have a normal chest radiograph.

If evaluation points toward sinus etiology, radiographs and CT scans may be indicated. Some experts recommend a trial of antihistamine decongestants before pursuing sinus radiographic studies (89). Spirometry, before and after inhaled bronchodilators and methacholine challenge, helps to evaluate for asthma or chronic obstructive lung disease. Barium esophagography or 24-hour esophageal pH monitoring can be used to evaluate for GERD. Finally, bronchoscopy may be considered to evaluate for occult foreign body aspiration or small endobronchial lesions, although studies have found this to be of low yield (85).

Management

Treatment of cough is most successful when tailored to a specific etiology (asthma, GERD, upper airway cough syndrome, etc.). In patients for whom no cause is found for their cough or it is due to airway involvement with tumor, empiric pharmacologic therapy with a β_2-adrenergic agonist or corticosteroid is reasonable.

Opiates continue to be used as effective antitussives (90,91). To date, there is no evidence of superiority of one opiate over another for this indication. Codeine, 15 to 30 mg every 4 to 6 hours, is a reasonable starting dose, with titration upward to control symptoms if the side effects are tolerable.

TABLE 30.8	Helpful phrases to use in communicating with family about the goals of care using noninvasive positive pressure ventilation	
	Primary Goals of Care	**Potentially Helpful Phrases to Clarify Goals with Family and/or Patient**
Category 1	Restore health; will use intubation if necessary and indicated	We can use the mask (NIPPV) to try to get him over this without having to put the breathing tube in his throat. If this does not improve things or is too uncomfortable for him, we will use the breathing tube.
Category 2	Restore health without using endotracheal intubation and without causing unacceptable discomfort	We can use the mask (NIPPV) to try to get him over this. He has been very clear that he does not want the breathing tube, so if the mask does not improve things or is too uncomfortable for him, we will plan to stop using it and focus on keeping him comfortable. In this situation, it would mean that he would likely die, although we would make it as comfortable as possible for him.
Category 3	Maximize comfort while minimizing adverse effects of opiates	It may be reasonable to try the mask (NIPPV) to see if it makes him more comfortable. We know that it would not fix the underlying problem, but it might improve his breathing temporarily. If it does not make him more comfortable, we will stop it and try something else so his death will be as comfortable as possible.

NIPPV, noninvasive positive pressure ventilation.

Adapted from Curtis JR, Cook DJ, Sinuff T, et al. Noninvasive positive pressure ventilation in critical and palliative care settings: understanding the goals of therapy. *Crit Care Med*. March 2007;35(3):932-939.

Non-narcotic cough preparations, including guaifenesin, dextromethorphan, and benzonatate may be tried, although studies show them to be only weakly beneficial. Studies of over-the-counter antitussive preparations demonstrate wide variability in efficacy (91–93).

Lidocaine appears to have an antitussive effect when inhaled through a nebulizer, likely acting on afferent C fibers in the larynx and trachea (90,84). When administered, patients should be cautioned regarding anesthesia of the oropharynx and larynx and potential buccal injury or aspiration. There are currently no specific guidelines for this therapy.

Noninvasive Positive Pressure Ventilation

NIPPV can be used to palliate dyspnea in terminally ill patients. The cost and experience needed to initiate NIPPV limit its use mostly to the hospital setting, although it can be used at home or a hospice facility provided adequate nursing, respiratory therapy, and physician support are available to employ it safely. Continuing NIPPV for palliation in patient and families who are already comfortable managing home NIPPV (e.g., for COPD or amyotrophic lateral sclerosis) can be practical in the home or hospice facility setting, as long

as it is consistent with care goals (94). A shared approach between the patient, family, and clinician exchanging clinical information and patient preferences is important for decision-making. Table 30.8 lists some helpful phrases to use in communicating with the patient and family about the goals of care using NIPPV.

Monitoring of pulse oximetry and arterial blood gases are not needed for patients using NIPPV only for symptom control. Rather, the effect of NIPPV should be assessed based on subjective improvement of dyspnea and decrease in respiratory rate. For a more detailed discussion on the practical aspects and settings of NIPPV, please see Chapter on *Palliative Care in the ICU*.

NIPPV should be discontinued if it does not provide relief from dyspnea within an hour of the maximally tolerated setting, once a patient is no longer alert, or at any point when it is no longer meeting a patient's goals. If the patient does not tolerate the mask, or feels claustrophobic, a small dose of a benzodiazepine can be administered to alleviate anxiety. If the patient is still uncomfortable, then NIPPV should be stopped; after revisiting goals of care, other symptom management avenues may be pursued (94).

REFERENCES

1. Light RW, MacGregor MI, Luchsinger PC, et al. Pleural effusions: the diagnostic separation of transudates and exudates. *Ann Intern Med.* 1972;77:507-513.

2. Tinney WS, Olsen AM. The significance of fluid in the pleural space: a study of 274 cases. *J Thorac Surg.* 1945;14:248-252.

3. Hausheer FH, Yarbro JW. Diagnosis and treatment of malignant pleural effusion. *Semin Oncol.* 1985;12:54-75.

4. Matthay RA, Coppage L, Shaw C, et al. Malignancies metastatic to the pleura. *Invest Radiol.* 1990;25:601-619.

5. Fenton KN, Richardson JD. Diagnosis and management of malignant pleural effusions. *Am J Surg.* 1995;170:69-74.

6. Woodring JH. Recognition of a pleural effusion on supine radiographs: how much fluid is required? *Am J Roentgenol.* 1984;142:59-64.

7. Doust BD, Baum JK, Maklad NF, et al. Ultrasonic evaluation of pleural opacities. *Radiology.* 1975;114:135-140.

8. Ravin CE. Thoracentesis of loculated pleural effusions using grey scale ultrasonic guidance. *Chest.* 1977;71:666-668.

9. Ratliff JL, Chavez CM, Jamchuk A, et al. Re-expansion pulmonary edema. *Chest.* 1973;64:654-656.

10. Health and Public Policy Committee, American College of Physicians. Diagnostic thoracentesis and pleural biopsy in pleural effusions. *Ann Intern Med.* 1985;103:799-802.

11. Leff A, Hopewell PC, Costello J. Pleural effusion from malignancy. *Ann Intern Med.* 1978;88:532-537.

12. LoCicero J III. Thoracoscopic management of malignant pleural effusion. *Ann Thorac Surg.* 1993;56:641-643.

13. Chernow B, Sahn SA. Carcinomatous involvement of the pleura. *Am J Med.* 1977;63:695-702.

14. Roy RH, Can DT, Payne WS. The problem of chylothorax. *Mayo Clin Proc.* 1967;42:457-467.

15. Van de Molengraft FJJM, Vooijs GP. Survival of patients with malignancy-associated effusions. *Acta Cytol.* 1989;33:911-916.

16. Ruckdeschel JC. Management of malignant pleural effusion: an overview. *Semin Oncol.* 1988;15:24-28.

17. Olopade OI, Ultmann JE. Malignant effusions. *CA Cancer J Clin.* 1991;41:166-179.

18. Anderson CB, Philpott GW, Ferguson TB. The treatment of malignant pleural effusions. *Cancer.* 1974;33:916-922.

19. Patz EF Jr, McAdams HP, Erasmus JJ, et al. Sclerotherapy for malignant pleural effusions: a prospective randomized trial of bleomycin vs doxycycline with small bore catheter drainage. *Chest.* 1998;113(5):1305-1311.

20. Pollak JS, Burdge CM, Rosenblatt M, et al. Treatment of malignant pleural effusions with tunneled long-term drainage catheters. *J Vasc Interv Radiol.* 2001;12(2):201-208.

21. Putnam JB Jr, Light RW, Rodriguez RM, et al. A randomized comparison of indwelling pleural catheter and doxycycline pleurodesis in the management of malignant pleural effusions. *Cancer.* 1999;86(10):1992-1999.

22. Robinson LA, Fleming WH, Galbraith TA. Intrapleural doxycycline control of malignant pleural effusions. *Ann Thorac Surg.* 1993;55:1115-1122.

23. Robinson LA, Moulton AL, Fleming WH, et al. Intrapleural fibrinolytic treatment of multiloculated thoracic empyemas. *Ann Thorac Surg.* 1994;57:803-814.

24. Pass HI. Treatment of malignant pleural and pericardial effusions. In: DeVita VT Jr, Hellman S, Rosenberg SA, eds. *Cancer: Principles and Practice of Oncology.* 4th ed. Philadelphia, PA: JB Lippincott Co; 1993:2246-2255.

25. Hawkins JW, Vacek JL. What constitutes definitive therapy of malignant pericardial effusion? "Medical" versus surgical treatment. *Am Heart J.* 1989;118:428-432.

26. Theologides A. Neoplastic cardiac tamponade. *Semin Oncol.* 1978;5:181-192.

27. Thurber DL, Edwards JE, Achor RWP. Secondary malignant tumors of the pericardium. *Circulation.* 1962;26:228-241.

28. Lokich JJ. The management of malignant pericardial effusions. *JAMA.* 1973;224:1401-1404.

29. Buzaid AC, Garewal HS, Greenberg BR. Managing malignant pericardial effusion. *West J Med.* 1989;150:174-179.

30. Spodick DH. Macrophysiology, microphysiology, and anatomy of the pericardium: a synopsis. *Am Heart J.* 1992;124:1046-1051.

31. Posner MR, Cohen GI, Skarin AT. Pericardial disease in patients with cancer—the differentiation of malignant from idiopathic and radiation-induced pericarditis. *Am J Med.* 1981;71:407-413.

32. Spodick DH. The normal and diseased pericardium: current concepts of pericardial physiology, diagnosis and treatment. *J Am Coll Cardiol.* 1983;1:240-251.

33. Beck CS. Acute and chronic compression of the heart. *Am Heart J.* 1937;14:515-525.

34. Eisenberg MJ, Oken NK, Guerrero S, et al. Prognostic value of echocardiography in hospitalized patients with pericardial effusion. *Am J Cardiol.* 1992;70:934-939.

35. Reyes VC, Strinden C, Banerji M. The role of cytology in neoplastic cardiac tamponade. *Acta Cytol.* 1982;26:299-302.

36. Miller JI Jr. Surgical management of pericardial disease. In: Schlant RC, Alexander RW, O'Roiurke RA, et al., eds. *The Heart, Arteries and Veins.* 8th ed. New York, NY: McGraw-Hill; 1994:1675-1680.

37. Press OW, Livingston R. Management of malignant pericardial effusion and tamponade. *JAMA.* 1987;257:1088-1092.

38. Palatianos GM, Thurer RJ, Pompeo MQ, et al. Clinical experience with subxiphoid drainage of pericardial effusions. *Ann Thorac Surg.* 1989;48:381-385.

39. Cham WC, Freiman AH, Carstens HB, et al. Radiation therapy of cardiac and pericardial metastases. *Radiology.* 1975;114:701-704.

40. Sanchez-Armegol A, Rodriguez-Panadero F. Survival and talc pleurodesis in metastatic pleural carcinoma, revisited. *Chest.* 1993;104:1482-1485.

41. Ruckdeschel JC, Chang P, Martin RG, et al. Radiation-related pericardial effusions in patients with Hodgkin's disease. *Medicine (Baltimore).* 1975;54:245-270.

42. Zwischenberger JB, Bradford DW. Management of malignant pericardial effusion. In: Pass HI, Mitchell JB, Johnson DH, et al., eds. *Lung Cancer: Principles and Practice.* Philadelphia, PA: Lippincott–Raven; 1996:655-662.

43. Moores DWO, Allen KB, Faber LP, et al. Subxiphoid pericardial drainage for pericardial tamponade. *J Thorac Cardiovasc Surg.* 1995;109:546-552.

44. Liu H-P, Chang C-H, Lin PJ, et al. Thoracoscopic management of effusive pericardial disease: indications and technique. *Ann Thorac Surg.* 1994;58:1695-1697.

45. Wang N, Feikes JR, Mogensen T, et al. Pericardioperitoneal shunt: an alternative treatment for malignant pericardial effusion. *Ann Thorac Surg.* 1994;57:289-292.

46. Ziskind AA, Pearce AC, Lemmon CC, et al. Percutaneous balloon pericardiotomy for the treatment of cardiac tamponade and large pericardial effusions: description of techniques and report of first 50 cases. *J Am Coll Cardiol.* 1993;21:1-5.

47. Lewis MA, Hendrickson AW, Moynihan TJ. Oncologic emergencies: pathophysiology, presentation, diagnosis, and treatment. *Cancer J Clin.* 2011;61:287-314

48. Schraufnagel DE, Hill R, Leech JA, Pare JA. Superior vena caval obstruction. Is it a medical emergency? *Am J Med.* 1981;70:1169-1174.

49. Ganeshan A, Hon LQ, Warakaulle DR, Morgan R, Uberoi R. Superior vena caval stenting for SVC obstruction: current status. *Eur J Radiol.* 2009;71:343-349.

50. Guijarro EJF, Anton RF, Colmenarejo RA, et al. Superior vena cava syndrome with central venous catheter for chemotherapy treated successfully with fibrinolysis. *Clin Transl Oncol.* 2007;9:198-200.

51. Wood D. Management of malignant tracheobronchial obstruction. *Surg Clin North Am.* 2002;82:621-642.

52. Braman SS, Whitcomb ME. Endobronchial metastasis. *Arch Intern Med.* 1995;135:543.

53. Chen K, Vawn J, Wenker O. Malignant airway obstruction: recognition and management. *J Emerg Med.* 1998;16(1):83-92.

54. Mathisen DJ. Surgical management of tracheobronchial disease. *Clin Chest Med.* 1992;13:151.

55. Mathisen DJ, Grillo HC. Endoscopic relief of malignant airway obstruction. *Ann Thorac Surg.* 1989;48:469.

56. Paleri V, Stafford FW, Sammut MS. Laser debulking in malignant upper airway obstruction. *Head & Neck.* 2005;27: 296-301.

57. Marsh BR. Bronchoscopic brachytherapy. *Laryngoscope.* 1989;99:1.

58. Diaz-Jimenez J, Martinez-Ballaren J, Llunell A, et al. Efficacy and safety of photodynamic therapy versus Nd-YAG laser resection in NSCLC with airway obstruction. *Eur Respir J.* 1999;14:800-855.

59. McCaughan J, Williams T. Photodynamic therapy for endobronchial malignant disease: a prospective fourteen year study. *J Thorac Cardiovasc Surg.* 1997;114:940-946.

60. Lee P, Temm M, Chhajed P. Advances in bronchoscopy—therapeutic bronchoscopy. *JAPI.* 2004;52:905-914.

61. Santamaria JP, Schafermeyer R. Stridor: a review. *Pediatr Emerg Care.* 1992;8:229.

62. Stool SE. Stridor. *Int Anesthesiol Clin.* 1988;26:19.

63. O'Hollaren MT, Everts EC. Evaluating the patient with stridor. *Ann Allergy.* 1991;67:301.

64. Curtis JL, Mahlmeister M, Fink JB, et al. Helium–oxygen gas therapy use and availability for the emergency treatment of inoperable airway obstruction. *Chest.* 1986;90:455.

65. Orr JB. Helium–oxygen gas mixtures in the management of patients with airway obstruction. *Ear Nose Throat J.* 1988;67:866.

66. Skrinskas GJ, Hyland RH, Hutcheon MA. Using helium–oxygen mixtures in the management of acute airway obstruction. *Can Med Assoc J.* 1983;R8:555.

67. Gluck E, Onorato DJ, Castriotta R. Helium–oxygen mixtures in intubated patients with status asthmaticus and respiratory acidosis. *Chest.* 1990;98:693.

68. Gupta V, Cheifetz I. Heliox administration in the pediatric intensive care unit: an evidence-based review. *Pediatr Crit Care Med.* 2005;6:204.

69. Schmitt G, Hall R, Wood LDH. Management of the ventilated patient. In: Murray JF, Nadel JA, eds. *Textbook of Respiratory Medicine.* Philadelphia, PA: WB Saunders; 1992.

70. Tashkin DP, Ashutosh K, Bleecker ER, et al. Comparison of the anticholinergic bronchodilator ipratropium bromide with metaproterenol in chronic obstructive pulmonary disease. *Am J Med.* 1986;81:81.

71. Marlin GE, Bush DE, Berent N. Comparison of ipratropium bromide and fenoterol in asthma and chronic bronchitis. *Br J Clin Pharmacol.* 1978;6:547.

72. Braun SR, Levy SF. Comparison of ipratropium bromide and albuterol in chronic obstructive lung disease: a three-center study. *Am J Med.* 1991;91(4):S28-32.

73. National Asthma Education and Prevention Program. *Expert Panel Report 2.* Bethesda, MD: National Institute of Health, Publication No. 97-405; April 1997.

74. Kamada AK, Szefler SJ, Martin RJ, et al. Issues in the use of inhaled glucocorticoids. *Am J RespirCrit Care Med.* 1996;153:1739-1748.

75. Corey R, Hla KM. Major and massive hemoptysis: reassessment of conservative management. *Am J Med Sci.* 1987;294:301-309.

76. Thompson AB, Teschler H, Rennard SI. Pathogenesis, evaluation, and therapy for massive hemoptysis. *Clin Chest Med.* 1992;13:69-82.

77. Set PA, Flower CDR, Smith IE, et al. Hemoptysis: comparative study of the role of CT and fiberoptic bronchoscopy. *Radiology.* 1993;189:677-680.

78. McGuinness G, Beacher JR, Harkin TJ, et al. Hemoptysis: prospective high-resolution CT/bronchoscopic correlation. *Chest.* 1994;105:1155-1162.

79. Saw EC, Gottlieb LS, Yokayama T, et al. Flexible fiberoptic bronchoscopy and endobronchial tamponade in the management of massive hemoptysis. *Chest.* 1976;70:589-591.

80. Khanavkar B, Stern P, Alberti W, et al. Complications associated with brachytherapy alone or with laser in lung cancer. *Chest.* 1991;99:1062-1065.

81. Menchini L, Remy-Jardin M, Faivre JB, et al. Cryptogenic haemoptysis in smokers: angiography and results of embolisation in 35 patients. *Eur Respir J.* 2009;34(5):1031

82. Morita T, Hyodo I, Yoshimi T, et al. Incidence and underlying etiologies of bronchial secretion in terminally ill cancer patients: a multicenter, prospective, observational study. *J Pain Symp Manage.* June 2004;27(6):533-539.

83. Wee B, Hillier R. Interventions for noisy breathing in patients near to death. *Cochrane Database Syst Rev.* 2008 Jan 23;(1): CD005177.

84. Cowcher K, Hank GW. Long-term management of respiratory symptoms in advanced cancer. *J Pain Symptom Manage.* 1990;5:320.

85. Poe RH, Israel RH, Utell MJ, et al. Chronic cough: bronchoscopy or pulmonary function testing? *Am Rev Respir Dis.* 1982;126:160.

86. Irwin RS, Curley FJ, French CL. Chronic cough. *Am Rev Respir Dis.* 1990;141:640.

87. Shuttair MF, Braun SR. Contemporary management of chronic persistent cough. *Mo Med.* 1992;89:795.

88. Irwin RS, Curley FJ. The treatment of cough. A comprehensive review. *Chest.* 1991;99:1477.

89. Pratter MR, Bartter T, Akers S, et al. An algorithmic approach to chronic cough. *Ann Intern Med.* 1993;119:977.

90. Fuller RW, Jackson DM. Physiology and treatment of cough. *Thorax.* 1990;45:425.

91. Irwin RS, Curley FJ, Bennett FM. Appropriate use of antitussives and protussives. A practical review. *Drugs.* 1993;46:80.

92. Irwin RS, Baumann MN, Bolser DC, et al. Diagnosis and management of cough: ACCP evidence-based clinical practice guidelines. *Chest.* 2006;129:1S-292S.

93. Smith MB, Feldman W. Over-the-counter cold medications. A critical review of clinical trials between 1950 and 1991. *JAMA.* 1993;269:2258.

94. Yeow ME, Szmuilowicz E. Practical aspects of using noninvasive positive pressure ventilation at the end of life #231. *J Palliat Med.* September 2010;13(9):1150-1151.

CHAPTER 31

Prevention, Assessment, and Management of Treatment-Induced Cardiac Disease in Cancer Patients

David A. Slosky

INTRODUCTION

During the last 30 years, the development of effective detection and treatment strategies for many malignancies has led to a significant population of cancer survivors (1,2). It is estimated that approximately 60% of adults newly diagnosed with cancer will survive for 5 or more years beyond the time of diagnosis. The National Cancer Institute and the Centers for Disease Control and Prevention estimate that there are more than 12 million cancer survivors in the United States (1). The impact of cancer and cancer treatment on the health of a survivor is substantial. Effects include organ damage and functional disabilities that occur as a consequence of the disease and/or the treatments. In addition, there are numerous psychosocial issues that confront adult cancer survivors. The recognition of these effects is increasing and there is accumulating evidence available to guide the physician caring for these people. The effects have become more common with the increased use of complex, intensive multi-agent and multi-modality cancer interventions. As a consequence of improved survival in cancer patients, they are reaching an age where cardiovascular disease is manifest. There is an increase in cardiovascular events including myocardial ischemia, myocardial infarction, hypertension, pericardial effusion, congestive heart failure, stroke, and depression. Long-term cancer survivors are at risk for a variety of cardiac effects.

The care of a patient with cardiovascular disease is a challenging and complex process. Caring for a patient with a malignancy multiplies these complexities and requires strong collaboration and evidence-based decisions. As the complexity of cancer therapeutics continues to rise and specialized molecular targets of cancer growth are targeted, collaborative management of multiple comorbidities will be required. These treatments may have important adverse effects on the cardiovascular system. It then becomes imperative for cardiovascular specialists to have an understanding of the prevention, identification, and treatment of cardiac disease in cancer patients in order to provide optimal care and outcomes. Today's oncologists must be fully aware of cardiovascular risks to avoid or prevent adverse cardiovascular effects.

Management of hypertension, coronary artery disease (CAD), the surgical patient with cancer, metastatic pericardial effusion, and valvular or structural heart disease; recognition of behavioral effects of a cancer with an emphasis on

depression; and end of life decisions all require an organized, multidisciplinary approach to provide the best care and optimize outcomes while maintaining a high quality of life. This chapter will attempt to elucidate these challenges and provide a framework to approach these issues.

Chemotherapy-induced cardiovascular toxicity traditionally has included cardiomyopathy with or without overt congestive heart failure, endothelial dysfunction, and arrhythmias. Doxorubicin-induced cardiomyopathy is the most studied form of chemotherapy-induced cardiotoxicity.

Radiotherapy-induced cardiotoxicity is a significant issue that is under-recognized and may lead to CAD, valvular heart disease, chronic pericardial disease, arrhythmias, conduction system disease, and carotid artery stenosis. Cancer patients represent a rapidly expanding patient population at risk for premature cardiovascular disease. This growth leads to an increase in cardiovascular-related mortality and potentially may offset the advancements in cancer survival.

Chemotherapeutic Agents Associated with Cardiovascular Toxicity

Anthracyclines: The original anthracycline was isolated from the bacteria *Streptomyces peucetius* and was subsequently named daunorubicin. Adriamycin was developed as a derivative and later designated as doxorubicin. This agent serves as one of the gold standards of oncologic treatment, particularly because of its broad spectrum of activity.

The mechanism of oncologic action for anthracyclines has not been fully defined. There appear to be multiple mechanisms that play a role in tumor destruction. These include inhibition of DNA and RNA synthesis (3). There may also be an interaction with topoisomerase II and direct reaction with the cellular membrane, which leads to alteration of function (4). Anthracyclines have been shown to induce breaks in double-stranded DNA and free radical formation. This can lead to intracellular accumulation of mutated or oxidatively modified proteins, which can lead to endoplasmic reticulum stress. This reaction may induce activation of the cascade of caspases, which leads to apoptosis (cell death). It has been established that anthracyclines can induce myocyte injury via the induction of autophagy. This is an evolutionary mechanism in which damaged proteins and organelles are removed and recycled. This process supports cell survival during stress; however, within the context of disease and treatment, autophagy promotes cell death (5).

Doxorubicin and other anthracyclines generally lead to irreversible cardiotoxicity. This toxicity is related to cumulative lifetime total dose; however, using cardiac biomarkers and sophisticated imaging techniques, left ventricular (LV) dysfunction may be detected before clinical manifestations are apparent. Early animal studies with anthracyclines demonstrated cardiotoxicity, which was later confirmed in clinical trials. Von Hoff and colleagues defined a curve plotting the probability of developing congestive heart failure as a function of the cumulative dose in approximately 4,000 patients who had received the drug on a 3-week administration schedule (6,7). Dosing guidelines emerged from these studies, which demonstrated that a cumulative dose of approximately 550 mg/m² correlated with a likelihood of congestive heart failure in approximately 5% of patients. Subsequent information suggests the dose at which one sees toxicity is lower and likely cumulative. The toxicity associated with anthracyclines is variable in individual patients. There have been a number of investigations into this phenomenon; however, there are no current screening or predictive tools to determine which patients will develop cardiac dysfunction. There are studies to identify cardiac biomarkers such as brain natriuretic peptide (BNP) and troponin in the early detection of cardiac toxicity; however, the data require further validation (8,9). The only test that has been shown to be sufficiently sensitive to detect early cardiotoxicity is a cardiac biopsy.

Unfortunately, the examination is expensive and confers risk to the patient such as cardiac perforation and tamponade. Therefore, there is a need for noninvasive techniques to identify cardiotoxicity. The focus of identification of cardiotoxicity from anthracyclines has shifted to prevention and protection. The first goal of cardioprotection is to allow the cancer therapy to be administered with maximum effectiveness with a minimum of cardiotoxicity. A second goal is to preserve the structural and functional integrity of the heart so that there is sufficient reserve when exposed to additional stressors later in life. These include additional chemotherapy exposure, radiation, hypertension, valvular heart disease, and ischemic heart disease. The assumption should be made that anthracycline toxicity begins with the first exposure and that each subsequent dose is additive. There are multiple modalities that have evolved for cardioprotection. These include dose limitation, schedule modification, innovative delivery systems, analogues, and chemical cardioprotection.

A number of pharmacologic agents for cardioprotection have been explored, which include Coenzyme Q10, N-acetylcysteine, calcium channel blockers, and alpha tocopherol.

Dexrazoxane is the singular compound that has shown efficacy in reducing doxorubicin cardiotoxicity. This compound belongs to a class of agents called bisdioxopiperazines which, when hydrolyzed, yield a compound that is similar to ethylenediaminetetra acetic acid, a metal ion chelating agent. It is postulated that dexrazoxane may enter the cell by diffusion and chelate free iron or iron bound to iron–anthracycline complexes, thereby reducing oxygen radical production (10,11). Preclinical studies of dexrazoxane suggested reduced cardiotoxicity in a number of different models and set the stage for human studies to protect patients from anthracycline toxicity. Two large multicenter trials were conducted by Swain et al. (12). These studies were performed to evaluate the ability of dexrazoxane to confer cardioprotection in patients with metastatic breast cancer who were anthracycline naïve. From these trials, one can conclude that dexrazoxane is cardioprotective for patients who receive it from the initiation of chemotherapy onward. A concern that dexrazoxane may interfere with tumor response has been raised and remains a source of controversy. Though the trial data by Swain may inform how anthracyclines are used, these findings are not conclusive. Additional studies are needed to define the role of this drug in cancer patients receiving anthracyclines. Currently, the drug is not approved for early use by the FDA in adults (13).

Doxorubicin affects the heart in a number of different ways (14,15). Cardiotoxicity has been categorized as early and late forms. Early toxicity occurs with or follows infusion within hours or days. Late toxicity is seen weeks, months, or years following the administration of the drug and primarily manifests as cardiac dysfunction (16,17). Early toxicity is more common in the elderly and may manifest as transient electrocardiographic (ECG) changes in the ST segment with T-wave changes (18). The patient may also experience atrial or ventricular ectopy (19,20). There is an association between early cardiotoxicity and the use of large single doses of doxorubicin.

Clinical Recognition of Doxorubicin-Associated Cardiotoxicity

Congestive heart failure is generally a progressive process with a preclinical course. Patients with doxorubicin-induced cardiomyopathy may not experience symptoms until the cardiac damage is established. Manifestations may include tachycardia or a slow return of the heart rate to baseline after minimal activity, which indicates limited cardiac reserve. Another symptom that is common is dyspnea while performing activities that did not previously elicit this symptom. This is another indicator of diminished cardiac reserve. The patient may also complain of difficulty with climbing stairs or fatigue that is out of proportion to the activity level. As cardiac dysfunction progresses, the patient may experience resting dyspnea, nocturnal dyspnea, weight gain, fluid retention, and a diastolic gallop (S3). Modalities such as transthoracic echocardiography (TTE) and radionuclide assessment of LV function (multigated acquisition [MUGA]) have traditionally been used to evaluate LV function. Small changes in noninvasive measurements may indicate early toxicity. Cardiac ultrasound has an advantage in that there is no radiation exposure and is less costly. Valve integrity and wall thickness may also be evaluated. There is evidence that a difference of 2% in the mean LV ejection fraction is significant. It is important to emphasize that measurement of the ejection fraction is a snapshot in time. Factors that may have an influence on cardiac function include changes in sympathetic and parasympathetic tone, heart rate variability, metabolic changes, anemia, hormonal variation, nutritional state, pharmacologic interventions, and analgesic medications.

Risk Factors for Doxorubicin Cardiotoxicity

Factors that are associated with increased risk include nonanthracycline anticancer therapies such as radiation to the heart, extremes of age, and preexisting heart disease (Table 31.1). Significant data related to susceptibility to cardiovascular injury have evolved from the study of children with cancer enrolled in protocols in which they received anthracycline-based therapy for hematologic malignancies such as leukemia, lymphoma, and sarcomas. In a study of pediatric cancer survivors compared with their siblings, 14,358 patients followed for up to 30 years after their cancer diagnosis were three times more likely to experience a chronic cardiovascular event (1).

Management of Patients Receiving Anthracyclines

Noninvasive testing using echocardiography or nuclear imaging should be used to assess LV function at baseline. Subsequent evaluation may vary according to the dose of anthracycline used and the clinical symptoms of the patient. If patients receive 300 to 450 mg/m^2 and are asymptomatic with no clinical signs of cardiac dysfunction, then one might consider the assessment of LV function, troponin, and BNP every one to two cycles. An echocardiogram approximately 3 to 4 months after completion of therapy is reasonable, as is a follow-up study annually for 5 years and then every 2 to 3 years. There is no ideal algorithm to avoid

anthracycline-induced cardiac dysfunction. However, the goal is to maximize survival and minimize mortality from cancer and the cardiotoxicity of cancer therapy. Therefore, the oncologic benefit is weighed against the cardiotoxic risks. Clinical judgment is critical and is as important as algorithms in the decision-making process.

Treatment of Established Doxorubicin-Associated Cardiac Dysfunction

The principles of intervention for patients who have experienced anthracycline cardiotoxicity include amelioration of additional cardiac damage, optimization of cardiac reserve, symptom reduction, reduction of workload, improvement of cardiac output, facilitation of cellular regeneration, and possible organ transplantation. It is critical to consider avoidance of additional exposure to anthracycline if cardiotoxicity exists. There is no evidence that a change to a different form of anthracycline is of benefit. This could result in additional damage to the myocardium. It is important to be sure that the patient's symptoms are due to LV dysfunction and not due to other causes. Symptoms of cardiac dysfunction are many times nonspecific and may be related to other conditions such as pulmonary infiltrates, metastatic disease progression, endocrine abnormalities, infections, deconditioning, neurologic conditions, and anemia.

Modalities available for patients who have experienced anthracycline-associated heart failure include mitigation of additional injury, optimization of cardiac reserve, pharmacologic intervention to reduce workload and increase cardiac output, and possible organ transplantation. After withdrawal of the agent and the patient's symptoms have been treated, the physician should follow standard guidelines for the treatment of heart failure that have been well publicized by the American Heart Association (AHA) and the American College of Cardiology (ACC). Angiotensin-converting enzyme (ACE) inhibitors and beta-adrenergic blocking drugs have been shown to improve symptoms and prolong survival in patients with congestive heart failure. There is limited information and there are no large clinical trials to suggest that the cancer patient should receive different therapy.

Commonly used agents include enalapril, carvedilol, and metoprolol. The drugs should be administered at low dosage levels and titrated according to the patient's clinical response including blood pressure since these agents may lead to hypotension. This is particularly important in the cancer patient who is receiving therapy and may be volume depleted. Patients with advanced heart failure should be managed by an experienced team of cardiologists. These patients may require intravenous inotropic agents, LV assist devices, biventricular pacing, and implantable cardioverter defibrillators. The need for heart transplantation in the cancer patient with advanced heart failure is rare; however, the indications are expanding (21).

The potential cardiotoxicity of selected nonanthracycline chemotherapy drugs is summarized in Table 31.2.

TABLE 31.1	Anthracycline Cardiotoxicity (Risk Factors)

Pediatric age group

Advanced age

Prior anthracycline exposure

Radiation exposure with cardiac exposure

Hypertension

Cardiomyopathy

Valvular heart disease

Exposure to other chemotherapeutic agents

Trastuzumab

Cyclophosphamide

TABLE 31.2	**Cardiotoxicity of selected nonanthracycline cancer chemotherapy agents**
Drug/Therapy	**Comments and Potential Associated Cardiovascular Toxicities**
Trastuzumab	Potential for transient cardiac dysfunction, heart failure (22–24)
Sunitinib	Hypertension
Androgen deprivation therapy	Accelerated atherosclerosis, metabolic syndrome, myocardial infarction, cardiac death
Antimetabolites	
Fluorouracil	Angina, myocardial infarction, arrhythmias, acute pulmonary edema, pericarditis; resulting from coronary vasospasm, myocarditis, and thrombogenesis (25–30)
Capecitabine	Similar to fluorouracil
Fludarabine	Hypotension, chest pain; risk of severe cardiotoxicity in combination with melphalan (31)
Methotrexate	No definite cardiotoxicity
Cytarabine	Pericarditis, pericardial effusion, tamponade
Microtubule-Targeting Agents	
Vinca alkaloids	Hypertension, myocardial ischemia or infarction, vaso-occlusive events
Paclitaxel	Bradycardia, heart block; low incidence of cardiotoxicity unless concomitant or previous exposure to anthracyclines
Ifosfamide	Arrhythmias, ST-T segment changes, heart failure (generally reversible)
Cisplatin	Sustained ventricular tachycardia, bradycardia, ST-T segment changes, bundle branch block, ischemic events, hypertension (32,33)
Thalidomide	Bradycardia
Monoclonal Antibodies	
Trastuzumab	(see section on anthracyclines)
Rituximab	Arrhythmias, angina; long-term toxicity has not been reported
Bevacizumab	Angina, myocardial infarction, heart failure, hypertension, thromboembolic events, left ventricular dysfunction; increased risk if used after anthracycline exposure or in patients older than 65 (34,35)
Alemtuzumab	Arrhythmias, heart failure
Cetuximab	Cardiac events when combined with fluorouracil
Topoisomerase Inhibitors	
Etoposide	Myocardial infarction, vasospastic angina (based on case reports only) (36,37)
Biologic Response Modifiers	
Interferon alpha	Myocardial ischemia or infarction, arrhythmias; prolonged administration is associated with cardiomyopathy (38–42)
Interleukin 2	Arrhythmias, hypotension, and capillary leak syndrome; hypotension and capillary leak syndrome, if present, usually peaks at 4 h after infusion and responds to fluid resuscitation and vasopressors, though systemic resistance may not return to normal for up to 6 d (43)
Differentiation Agents	
All-trans retinoic acid	Pericardial effusion, myocardial ischemia, or infarction
Multitargeted Tyrosine Kinase Inhibitors	
Lapatinib	Left ventricular dysfunction in 1.6%; 2.2% and 1.7% if previously treated with anthracycline or trastuzumab, respectively (44)
Sorafenib and sunitinib	Heart failure; cardiac injury usually reversible but a history of coronary artery disease or hypertension increases risk of cardiotoxicity (45–48)
Sorafenib	Myocardial ischemia or infarction in 2.9% (49)
Imatinib	Small risk of cardiomyopathy (50)
Nilotinib	QT interval prolongation
Dasatinib	Angina, pericardial effusion, left ventricular dysfunction, and heart failure (51)

ARRHYTHMIAS

A number of arrhythmias are associated with cancer patients and particularly with antineoplastic agents. Below is a brief listing of the complications that may occur. In most instances, treatment may continue with careful monitoring. In a minority of cases, the patient may require a temporary and/or permanent pacer to allow cancer therapy to continue.

QT INTERVAL PROLONGATION

The QT interval is an ECG measure of ventricular repolarization. Abnormalities of repolarization may lead to an increased risk of ventricular arrhythmias. Cancer patients have a tendency for QT prolongation, with an incidence of 16% to 36% of baseline ECG abnormalities. In addition, cancer patients have many comorbidities such as structural heart disease, coronary heart disease, hepatic and renal dysfunction, as well as concomitant medications that are known to prolong the QT interval. These include antiemetics, antifungals, quinolone, and mycin antibiotics. This is coupled with electrolyte abnormalities and dehydration in cancer patients who commonly experience nausea, vomiting, and diarrhea (52,53). Please refer Table 31.3 for a list of common agents associated with QT interval prolongation.

HYPERTENSION

There is a significant interest in hypertension in patients with malignancy. This focus has surged due to the increased prevalence of hypertension related to the use of angiogenesis inhibitors in targeted cancer therapy, although it has been described with more traditional therapies. Hypertension is common and may be a preexisting condition exacerbated by these therapies. In fact, it is the most common reported comorbid condition in cancer registries and may affect prognosis (54,55). It is important that hypertension be diagnosed and managed effectively to reduce the complications known to exist and to reduce cardiotoxicity from cancer therapy. Table 31.4 lists the agents most commonly associated with hypertension in patients with cancer.

TABLE 31.3	Drugs associated with QT interval prolongation
Cardiac	Noncardiac
Amiodarone	Arsenic trioxide
Disopyramide	Dasatinib
Dofetilide	Lapatinib
Ibutilide	Nilotinib
Procainamide	Tacrolimus
Quinidine	Tamoxifen
Sotalol	Venlafaxine
	Vorinostat

TABLE 31.4	Chemotherapeutic agents associated with hypertension
Bevacizumab (monoclonal antibody tyrosine kinase inhibitor)
Sorafenib (small-molecule tyrosine kinase inhibitor)
Sunitinib (small-molecule tyrosine kinase inhibitor)

The imperative in the treatment of hypertension in any population is to reduce morbidity and mortality and reduce the incidence of target organ damage, for example, myocardial ischemia, infarction, stroke, and renal failure. The treatment modalities are those recommended by the guidelines developed by the joint national committee of the National Institutes of Health (JNC7) (56). The choice of an antihypertensive agent should take into consideration the mechanism and pathophysiology of the blood pressure elevation, the potential drug–drug interactions, and indications or contraindications for particular agents, that is, ACE inhibitors or beta blockers for heart failure. Patients with hypertension associated with anti-angiogenic agents such as bevacizumab, sorafenib, and sunitinib may require multiple antihypertensive medications. The patient will need to be monitored carefully during therapy and appropriate adjustments made as the blood pressure may vary. There may be significant drug–drug interactions with sorafenib, which is metabolized by the cytochrome P450 system (CYP3A4) in the liver. Drugs such as verapamil and diltiazem are inhibitors of the CYP3A4 isoenzyme and may lead to increased sorafenib levels.

There are data to suggest an association between cancer treatment response and the development of hypertension (57). In addition, the patient may need long-term monitoring as a function of continuation or cessation of the cancer therapy. The mechanism of hypertension in this setting in not well understood and continues to be a subject of investigation. Some theories that have been proposed include endothelial dysfunction with a reduction in nitric oxide availability; increased vascular and renal endothelin production; increased vascular tone; density reduction of microvessels; and renal thrombotic microangiopathy with functional and structural changes in the glomerulus leading to proteinuria and hypertension (12,58).

RADIATION

Radiation-induced vasculopathy has been associated with the treatment of a number of malignancies including lymphoma, breast cancer, head and neck cancer, and thoracic tumors. Interestingly, the incidence of ischemic heart disease and stroke does not increase until years after treatment (59–61). Intravascular radiation therapy (brachytherapy) has been used for the prevention of restenosis after coronary intervention. This technique has been limited by late restenosis and vascular occlusion and currently has limited utility for patients with CAD. In addition, surgical wounds within previously irradiated tissues are prone to vascular alterations associated with increased incidence of microvascular occlusion and delayed wound healing (61). The adverse effects of radiation on tissues can be acute, usually occurring within 4 to 6 weeks after exposure, and late effects that may manifest months to years after irradiation. These effects indicate an ongoing, progressive process. The evidence for late adverse effects is primarily derived from epidemiological studies. Most experimental studies have focused on the acute effects in cell culture experiments. Radiation sensitivity of the vasculature has been linked to endothelial dysfunction, activation of which may lead to atherosclerosis and a prothrombotic state (62–66). Martin et al. (67) recently reported sustained inflammation due to NF-kB activation in human irradiated arteries which may explain cardiovascular disease years after radiation.

The clinical consequences of radiation injury to the blood vessels are significant. The relative risk of suffering an adverse cardiovascular event (e.g., myocardial infarction) related to radiation injury ranges from approximately 1.5- to 4-fold. This risk is further amplified in the presence of traditional cardiovascular risk factors. Most cardiac events occur more than 10 years after completing radiotherapy; therefore, the proof of causality is complicated. It is estimated that 50 million cancer survivors worldwide have received radiation therapy as a component of their therapy (67–73). Therefore, clinicians must be aware of the potential cardiovascular risk and manage the risk factors appropriately. Additional research is needed to determine the clinical significance of these findings and assess the efficacy of current and emerging therapy on these processes. Current approaches including risk factor modification, medical therapy, and traditional revascularization procedures remain the mainstay of intervention at the present time.

ISCHEMIC HEART DISEASE AND CANCER

Chronic ischemic heart disease is primarily due to obstruction of the coronary arteries, which is a consequence of atherosclerosis. The pathogenesis of atherosclerosis is multifactorial and is related to the accumulation of lipid-laden plaque within the coronary arteries. The importance of ischemic heart disease is a consequence of the epidemic manifestations of the disease.

CAD leads to more deaths, disability, and economic loss in developed nations than any other disease. Each year, there are more than 200,000 adverse events in the millions of people who are afflicted by the disease. The economic costs are extraordinary and are in the multibillion dollar range, which entails health expenditures and loss of productivity. The patient with cancer and the patient with ischemic heart disease represent two groups with diseases that compound the above effects by severalfold.

There is a tremendous focus on the primary prevention of CAD, with emphasis on behavioral and environmental changes that reduce the risk of adverse events in patients at risk for CAD. The primary goal is to prevent atherosclerosis and ultimately thrombosis that leads to myocardial infarction. Preventive measures should be directed at the establishment of healthy lifestyles as early in life as possible. The initial approach should include identification of the high-risk patient and implementation of a successful preventative program.

The history and physical examination including a detailed family history are critical to this process. The patients should be screened for hypertension and hyperlipidemia. There are significant data that the pharmacologic control of hypertension and hyperlipidemia is an effective way of preventing adverse cardiac events such as stroke and myocardial infarction. Timely recognition and treatment of hypertension becomes extremely important in the cancer patient who is receiving targeted therapy with vascular endothelial growth factor inhibitors. These agents lead to an increase in the incidence of hypertension. The National Cholesterol Education Program (NCEP) has published updated guidelines for the diagnosis and treatment of patients with hyperlipidemia. Additional interventions include the appropriate diagnosis and treatment of diabetes, smoking cessation, a reduction in saturated fat with adoption of a Mediterranean-type diet, weight control, and an increase in physical activity.

The diagnosis of coronary disease includes a history and physical examination, an electrocardiogram, and a chest x-ray. Additional modalities for evaluation of the coronary patient include standard exercise ECG (exercise stress test). Adjunctive imaging has taken a significant place in the evaluation since this increases the sensitivity and specificity of detection of disease. This includes myocardial perfusion imaging with radioisotopes, contrast echocardiography, and magnetic resonance (MR) perfusion imaging. Tests that allow evaluation of LV function include TTE which is noninvasive, does not expose the patient to radiation, and is relatively inexpensive. Multigated radionuclide ventriculography (MUGA) is also an option. This technique is less dependent on technical issues such as patient obesity and there is no significant intra-observer variation. It does involve low-level radiation, which is an ongoing issue with cancer patients who have multiple scans that are a part of their surveillance. MR imaging may also be used for LV function analysis. This does not involve radiation; however, it is currently more expensive than echocardiography or radionuclide imaging.

The treatment of CAD has as its foundation behavioral and environmental interventions, pharmacologic therapy, myocardial revascularization, transplantation, and stem cell therapy. Among the agents commonly used are beta-adrenoceptor blocking agents, nitrates (short and long acting), lipid-lowering agents, calcium channel antagonists, and late sodium (Na) channel antagonists. Revascularization procedures include percutaneous transluminal coronary angioplasty, intracoronary stenting with bare metal or drug-eluting stents, coronary artery bypass surgery, and hybrid procedures. Many patients with CAD and/or cancer also have arrhythmias that require pharmacologic intervention and possible ablative procedures. The decisions for implementation of these should be a collaborative one among the cardiologist, the oncologist, and the surgeon.

The patient with CAD may be asymptomatic or present with clinical symptoms of ischemia. This can manifest as stable angina or acute coronary syndrome (ACS). This syndrome is subcategorized as unstable angina, non–ST segment elevation myocardial infarction, and ST segment elevation myocardial infarction. The clinical presentation of patients with cancer and ACS is the same as patients in the non-cancer population. However, there is always considerable discussion about management, especially when they have hematologic abnormalities such as thrombocytopenia. It is well known that patients who have survived cancer are at risk for CAD (73–75). The pathophysiology of ACS involves unstable atherosclerotic plaques, inflammation, platelet aggregation, and thrombosis. Individuals with cancer are also prothrombotic and may involve some of the same mechanisms including platelet activation, aggregation, and an increase in procoagulant factors (76). The AHA/ACA guidelines recommend antiplatelet agents in ACA, specifically, the use of aspirin (ASA). However, a traditional contraindication has been thrombocytopenia. As with many guidelines, they are developed based on trials with specific patient demographics, that is, a normal platelet count. Also, the major clinical trials of ACS and antithrombotic therapy have excluded patients with cancer. Sarkiss et al. demonstrated that in cancer patients with ACS and thrombocytopenia, those who did not receive ASA had a 7-day survival rate of 6% compared with 90% in those who received ASA. There were no severe bleeding complications. Patients with a platelet count (>100 cells k/μL) who received ASA had a 7-day survival of 88% compared with 45% in those who did not receive ASA (77).

Additional issues of importance are related to the deployment of stents and the decision for a bare metal stent compared with a drug-eluting stent. This becomes important when considering the duration of recommended dual antiplatelet therapy in cancer patients who may be receiving additional chemotherapy and are subject to bleeding risk.

PREOPERATIVE ASSESSMENT OF THE CANCER PATIENT WITH HEART DISEASE FOR NONCARDIAC SURGERY

Preoperative assessment of the cancer patient with heart disease is vital to a successful outcome after noncardiac surgery. Most clinicians feel that detailed assessment and management and appropriate interventions will lead to a successful outcome. This is particularly important since there are significant changes in physiologic functions for these patients in the operating room and postoperatively. The primary goal of a collaborative effort among the anesthesiologist, cardiologist, and surgeon is to reduce or eliminate perioperative complications.

The initial step in this process involves assessment by the anesthesiologist in a preoperative clinic before the procedure. This encounter should bring the patient's medical record together and lead to clearance or additional investigation and clearance by other specialists. The physician will examine the patient's comorbidities and attempt modification or evaluation so that a treatment plan is developed. This may require consultation from other specialties. The American Society of Anesthesiologists has developed and updated a classification system that is widely used for risk stratification (Table 31.5). There is general consensus that previous treatment for malignancy (chemotherapy, radiotherapy, and surgery) may affect the patient's subsequent response to anesthesia and surgery. In addition, many tumors are associated with physiologic disturbances. They may have secretory properties, paraneoplastic syndromes, and endocrine effects. The clinical manifestations may include bronchospasm, fever secondary to cytokine release, hypotension, hypertension, hypercalcemia, and hypermetabolic syndromes.

The cardiologist will be involved in these patients because they have existing coronary, valvular, or structural heart disease. In addition, they have been treated for their cancer with potentially cardiotoxic chemotherapy and radiotherapy. The cardiologist must account for these factors and their interaction with the individual with heart disease. The ACC/AHA has developed guidelines that are periodically updated and may be viewed on the ACC web site (79,80). These guidelines have been endorsed by the

TABLE 31.5	American Society of Anesthesiologist physical status classification
P1	Normal healthy patient
P2	Patient with mild systemic disease without functional impairment
P3	Patient with severe systemic disease and functional impairment
P4	Patient with severe systemic disease that is a threat to life
P5	Patient who is moribund and not expected to live more than 24 h with or without the surgery
P6	Patient who is brain-dead and is an organ donor

American Society of Anesthesiologists. *ASA Physical Status Classification System.* Available at http://www.asahq.org/clinical/physicalstatus.htm.

Society of Cardiovascular Anesthesiologists (81). Despite the availability of guidelines, the ultimate evaluation of the patient with cancer and heart disease is the responsibility of the consultant asked to evaluate the patient in collaboration with the care team. In particular, the cardiologist has a number of tools available for the risk stratification process. In addition to the history, physical examination, ECG, and risk factor assessment, there are a number of adjunctive techniques that are available.

These include stress testing with or without adjunctive imaging, echocardiography, coronary angiography, percutaneous or surgical intervention, and meticulous medical therapy and careful monitoring. A risk assessment paradigm is displayed in Table 31.6.

The highest risk patients are those with congestive heart failure, unstable angina, significant arrhythmias, and recent myocardial infarction. One must also consider the type and length of surgery, mode of anesthesia, expected blood loss, and fluid balance issues.

In summary, the preoperative evaluation of the cancer patient, particularly if they have heart disease, must take into account the type of cancer, the type of heart disease and the current level of activity, previous chemotherapy, radiation exposure, and comorbid conditions. There is significant consideration that the proposed procedure may be a part of a continuum of therapy and there must be collaboration to achieve the best outcome in the short and long term. Ultimately, the goal is to achieve the best outcome with the lowest risk (81).

TABLE 31.6	Preoperative risk assessment in cancer patients

High Risk

Decompensated congestive heart failure
Acute coronary syndrome
Large area of ischemia on noninvasive testing
High-degree atrioventricular block
Supraventricular tachycardia with an
    uncontrolled rate
Complex ventricular ectopy
Severe valvular heart disease

Intermediate Risk

Stable coronary artery disease
Compensated congestive heart failure
Prior myocardial infarction
Chronic kidney disease
History of cardiotoxic therapy
Diabetes mellitus

Low Risk

Advanced age (>70 years)
Poor hypertension control
Abnormal electrocardiography
History of stroke

SUMMARY

Today's oncologists must be fully aware of cardiovascular risks to avoid or prevent adverse cardiovascular effects, and cardiologists must be ready to assist oncologists by performing evaluations relevant to the choice of therapy. There is a need for cooperation between these two areas and for the development of a novel discipline. High-quality care for patients with cancer and cardiovascular disease requires the coordination of multiple disciplines. The rigor of involving multiple disciplines continues to evolve. The coordination of patient care with the goal of optimizing outcomes is built around communication. This includes personal relationships with the various providers, multidisciplinary conferences, multidisciplinary care clinics, development of oncology multispecialty groups, development of guideline-based care, and a central society for the development of research and clinical guideline development.

Cardiology-Oncology or onco-cardiology is a term that has been developed to describe a new field of integrative medicine between specialists in cardiovascular disease and oncology. This evolving specialty involves evaluation and treatment of the cardiotoxic effects of chemotherapy, radiation therapy, thrombosis, hypertension, congestive heart failure, coronary heart disease, and the new field of targeted therapy. The care of these patients requires an extensive network of collaboration and communication throughout the course of their illness, including end of life decisions. The care of a patient with heart disease and cancer is immensely challenging. A delicate balance exists to manage multiple diseases in order to achieve an ideal outcome for the individual patient. The goal of this collaboration is to improve the outcomes and quality of life of patients with heart disease and cancer.

REFERENCES

1. Krischer JP, Epstein S, Cuthbertson DD, et al. Clinical cardiotoxicity following anthracycline treatment for childhood cancer: The Pediatric Oncology Group experience. *J Clin Oncol.* 1997;15:1544-1552.
2. van Dalen EC, van der Pal HJ, Bakker PJ, et al. Cumulative incidence and risk factors of mitoxantrone induced cardiotoxicity in children: a systematic review. *Eur J Cancer.* 2004;40:643-652.
3. Chairs J. Biophysical chemistry of the daunomycin-DNA interaction. *Biophys Chem.* 1990;35:191-202.
4. Tritton TR. Immobilized doxorubicin: a tool for separating cell surface from intracellular drug mechanism. *Fed Proc.* 1983;42:184-289.
5. Zhu H, Tannous P, Johnstone JL, et al. Cardiac autophagy is a maladaptive response to hemodynamic stress. *J Clin Invest.* 2007;117(7):1782-1793.
6. von Hoff D, Rozencwieg M, Layard M, et al. Daunomycin-induced cardiotoxicity in children and adults: a review of 110 cases. *Am J Med.* 1977;62:200-208.
7. von Hoff D, Rozenzweig M, Layard M, et al. Risk factors for doxorubicin-induced congestive heart failure. *Ann Intern Med.* 1979;91:710-717.
8. Cardinale D, Sandri MT, Colombo A, et al. Prognostic value of troponin I in cardiac risk stratification of cancer

patients undergoing high-dose chemotherapy. *Circulation.* 2004;109(22):2749-2754.

9. Lenihan DJ, Massey MR, Baysinger KB, et al. Superior detection of cardiotoxicity during chemotherapy using biomarkers. *J Card Fail.* 2007;13(6 suppl):S151.

10. Helmann K. Overview and historical developments of dexrazoxane. *Semin Oncol.* 1998;25(suppl 10):48-54.

11. Hasinoff BB. Chemistry of dexrazoxane and analogues. *Semin Oncol.* 1998;25(suppl 10):3-9.

12. Swain S, Whaley PS, Gerber MC, et al. Cardioprotection with dexrazoxane for doxorubicin-containing therapy for advanced breast cancer. *J Clin Oncol.* 1997;15:1318-1332.

13. Swain S, Whaley F, Gerber M, et al. Delayed administration of dexrazoxane provides cardioprotection for patients with advanced breast cancer treated with doxorubicin-containing chemotherapy. *J Clin Oncol.* 1997;15:1333-1340.

14. Minow R, Benjamin R, Lee E, Gottlieb J. Adriamycin cardiomyopathy—risk factors. *Cancer.* 1977;39:1397-1402.

15. Singal P, Iliskovic N. Doxorubicin-induced cardiomyopathy. *N Engl J Med.* 1998;339:900-905.

16. Ali M, Ewer M. *Cancer and the Cardiopulmonary System.* New York, NY: Raven Press; 1984.

17. Bristow M, Mason J, Billingham M, Daniels J. Doxorubicin cardiomyopathy: evaluation by phonocardiography, endomyocardial biopsy, and cardiac catheterization. *Ann Intern Med.* 1978;88:168-175.

18. Lefrak E, Pitha J, Rosenheim S, Gottlieb J. A clinico-pathologic analysis of adriamycin cardiotoxicity. *Cancer.* 1973;32:302-314.

19. Signori E, Guevarra D. Evaluation of cardiac arrhythmias by 24-hour Holter monitoring during adriamycin administration (abstract). *Proc Am Assoc Cancer Res.* 1981;22:355.

20. Wortman J, Lucas V, Shuster E, et al. Sudden death during doxorubicin administration. *Cancer.* 1979;44:1588-1591.

21. Armitage JM, Kormor R, Griffith B, et al. Heart transplantation in patients with malignant disease. *J Heart Transplant.* 1990;9:627-629.

22. Slamon DJ, Leyland-Jones B, Shak S, et al. Use of chemotherapy plus a monoclonal antibody against HER2 for metastatic breast cancer that over-expresses HER2. *N Engl J Med.* 2001;344(11):783-792.

23. Ewer MS, Vooletich MT, Durand JB, et al. Reversibility of trastuzumab-related cardiotoxicity: new insights based on clinical course and response to medical treatment. *J Clin Oncol.* 2005;23(31):7820-7826.

24. Sawyer DB, Zuppinger C, Miller TA, Eppenberger HM, Suter TM. Modulation of anthracycline-induced myofibrillar disarray in rat ventricular myocytes by neuregulin-1beta and anti-erbB2: potential mechanism for trastuzumab induced cardiotoxicity. *Circulation.* 2002;105(13):1551-1554.

25. Anand AJ. Fluorouracil cardiotoxicity. *Ann Pharmacother.* 1994;28:374.

26. Akhtar SS, Salim KP, Bano ZA. Symptomatic cardiotoxicity with high dose 5-fluorouracil infusion: a prospective study. *Oncology.* 1993;50:441.

27. Saif MW, Szabo E, Grem J, Hamilton M. The clinical syndrome of 5-fluorouracil cardiotoxicity (abstract). *Proc Am Soc Clin Oncol.* 2001;20:404a.

28. de Forni M, Malet-Martino MC, Jaillais P, et al. Cardiotoxicity of high dose infusion fluorouracil: a prospective clinical study. *J Clin Oncol.* 1992;10:1795.

29. Labianca R, Beretta G, Clerici M, et al. Cardiac toxicity of 5-fluorouracil: a study on 1083 patients. *Tumori.* 1982;68:505.

30. Wacker A, Lersch C, Scherpinski U, et al. High incidence of angina pectoris in patients treated with 5-fluorouracil. A planned surveillance study with 102 patients. *Oncology.* 2003;65:108.

31. Gutheil J, Finucane D. Antimetabolites. In: Perry MD, ed. *The Chemotherapy Sourcebook.* 3rd ed. Philadelphia, PA: Lippincott, Williams & Wilkins; 2001:208.

32. Geerts WH, Bergqvist D, Pineo GF, et al. Prevention of venous thromboembolism. *Chest.* 2008;133(suppl):381S-453S.

33. Lyman GH, Khorana AA, Falanga A, et al. American Society of Clinical Oncology guideline. *J Clin Oncol.* 2007;25:5490-5505.

34. Miller KD, Chap LI, Holmes FA, et al. Randomized phase III trial of capecitabine compared with bevacizumab plus capecitabine in patients with previously treated metastatic breast cancer. *J Clin Oncol.* 2005;23:792.

35. Percy Ivy S, Chen H. IND safety report: cardiac events. May 20, 2005 (letter).

36. Schwarzer S, Eber B, Greinix H, Lind P. Non-Q-wave myocardial infarction associated with bleomycin and etoposide chemotherapy. *Eur Heart J.* 1991;12:748.

37. Yano S, Shimada K. Vasospastic angina after chemotherapy with carboplatin and etoposide in a patient with lung cancer. *Jpn Circ J.* 1996;60:185.

38. Sonnenblick M, Rosin A. Cardiotoxicity of interferon. A review of 44 cases. *Chest.* 1991;99:557.

39. Martino S, Ratanatharathorn V, Karanes C, et al. Reversible arrhythmias observed in patients treated with recombinant alpha 2 interferon. *J Cancer Res Clin Oncol.* 1987;113:376.

40. Friess GG, Brown TD, Wrenn RC. Cardiovascular rhythm effects of gamma recombinant DNA interferon. *Invest New Drugs.* 1989;7:275.

41. Budd GT, Bukowski RM, Miketo L, et al. Phase-I trial of Ultrapure™ human leukocyte interferon in human malignancy. *Cancer Chemother Pharmacol.* 1984;12:39.

42. Grunberg SM, Kempf RA, Itri LM, et al. Phase II study of recombinant alpha interferon in the treatment of advanced non-small cell lung carcinoma. *Cancer Treat Rep.* 1985;69:1031.

43. White RL Jr, Schwartzentruber DJ, Guleria A, et al. Cardiopulmonary toxicity of treatment with high dose interleukin-2 in 199 consecutive patients with metastatic melanoma or renal cell carcinoma. *Cancer.* 1994;74:3212.

44. Perez EA, Koehler M, Byrne J, et al. Cardiac safety of lapatinib: pooled analysis of 3689 patients enrolled in clinical trials. *Mayo Clin Proc.* 2008;83:679.

45. Chu TF, Rupnick A, Kerkela R, et al. Cardiotoxicity associated with tyrosine kinase inhibitor sunitinib. *Lancet.* 2007;370:2011.

46. Khakoo AY, Kassiotis CM, Tannir N, et al. Heart failure associated with sunitinib maleate: a multitargeted receptor tyrosine kinase inhibitor. *Cancer.* 2008;112:2500.

47. Telli M, Witteles RM, Fisher GA, Srinivas JS. Cardiotoxicity associated with sunitinib maleate (abstract). 2008 ASCO GU Cancers Symposium, San Francisco, California.

48. Motzer RJ, Hutson TE, Tomczak P, et al. Sunitinib versus interferon alfa in metastatic renal-cell carcinoma. *N Engl J Med.* 2007;356:115.

49. Clinical trial and prescribing information at fda.gov (December 23, 2005).

50. Verweij J, Casali PG, Kotasek D, et al. Imatinib does not induce cardiac left ventricular failure in GI stromal tumor patients. Analysis of EORTC-ISG-AGITG study 62005. *Eur J Cancer.* 2007;43:974.

51. Bristol-Myers Squibb Company: Dasatinib prescribing information. Princeton, NJ; 2006.

52. Yusuf SW, Razeghi P, Yeh ET. The diagnosis and management of cardiovascular disease in cancer patients. *Curr Probl Cardiol.* 2008;33:163-196.

53. Strevel EL, Ing DJ, Siu LL. Molecularly targeted oncology therapeutics and prolongation of the QT interval. *J Clin Oncol.* 2007;25:3362-3371.

54. Jain M, Townsend RR. Chemotherapy agents and hypertension: a focus on angiogenesis blockade. *Curr Hypertens Rep.* 2007;9:320-328.

55. Ray A, Ray S, Koner BC. Hypertension, cancer and angiogenesis relevant epidemiological and pharmacological aspects. *Indian J Pharmacol.* 2004;36:341-347.

56. Chobanian AV, Bakris GL, Black HR, et al. Seventh report of the Joint National Committee on Prevention, Detection, Evaluation, and Treatment of High Blood Pressure. *Hypertension.* 2003;42:1206-1252.

57. Rixe O, Bolleont B, Izzedine H. Hypertension as a predictive factor of sunitinib activity. *Ann Oncol.* 2007;18:1117.

58. Eremina V, Jefferson JA, Kowalewska J, et al. VEGF inhibition and renal thrombotic microangiopathy. *N Engl J Med.* 2008;358(11):1129-1136.

59. Early Breast Cancer Trialists Collaborative Group. Favourable and unfavourable effects on long-term survival of radiotherapy for early breast cancer: an overview of the randomised trials. *Lancet.* 2000;355:1757-1770.

60. Early Breast Cancer Trialists Collaborative Group. Effects of radiotherapy and of differences in the extent of surgery for early breast cancer on local recurrence and 15-year survival: an overview of the randomised trials. *Lancet.* 2005;366:2087-2106.

61. Rutqvist LE, Rose C, Cavallin-Stahl E. A systematic overview of radiation therapy effects in breast cancer. *Acta Oncol.* 2003;42:532-545.

62. Fisher B, Constantino J, Redmond C, et al. Lumpectomy compared with lumpectomy and radiation for the treatment of intraductal breast cancer. *N Engl J Med.* 1993;328:1581-1586.

63. Fisher B, Dignam J, Wolmark N, et al. Lumpectomy and radiation therapy for the treatment of intraductal breast cancer: findings from National Surgical Adjuvant Breast and Bowel Project B-17. *J Clin Oncol.* 1998;16:441-452.

64. Taylor CW, Nisbet A, McGale P, Darby SC. Cardiac exposures in breast cancer radiotherapy: 1950s-1990s. *Int J Radiat Oncol Biol Phys.* 2007;69:1484-1495.

65. Taylor CW, Poval JM, McGale P, et al. Cardiac dose from tangential breast cancer therapy in the year 2006. *Int J Radiat Oncol Biol Phys.* 2008;72:501-507.

66. Gyenes G, Fofwander T, Carlens P, Glas U, Rutqvist LE. Myocardial damage in breast cancer patients treated with adjuvant radiotherapy: a prospective study. *Int J Radiat Oncol Biol Phys.* 1996;36:899-905.

67. Halle M, Gabrielsen A, Paulsson-Berne G, et al. Sustained inflammation due to nuclear factor-kappa B activation in irradiated human arteries. *J Am Coll Cardiol.* March 2010;55(12):1227-1239.

68. Rutqvist LE, Johansson H. Mortality by laterality of the primary tumour among 55,000 breast cancer patients from the Swedish Cancer Registry. *Br J Cancer.* 1990;61:866-868.

69. Rubino C, de Vathaire F, Diallo I, Shamsaldin A, Le MG. Increased risk of second cancers following breast cancer: role of the initial treatment. *Breast Cancer Res Treat.* 2000;61: 183-195.

70. Cepi, DC. http://www.cepidc.vesinet.inserm.fr/inserm/html/pages/dictionnaire_variables_fr.htm. Accessed July 2010.

71. Darby SC, McGale P, Taylor CW, Petro R. Long term mortality from heart disease and lung cancer after radiotherapy for early breast cancer: prospective cohort study of about 30,000 women in US SEER cancer registries. *Lancet Oncol.* 2005;6: 557-565.

72. Taylor CW, McGale P, Darby SC. Cardiac risks of breast-cancer radiotherapy: a contemporary view. *Clin Oncol (R Coll Radiol).* 2006;18:236-246.

73. Paszat LF, Mackillop WJ, Groome PA, et al. Mortality from myocardial infarction after adjuvant radiotherapy for breast cancer in surveillance, epidemiology, and end-results cancer registries. *J Clin Oncol.* 1998;16:2625-2631.

74. Hull MCD, Morris CG, Pepine CJ, Mendenhall NP. Valvular dysfunction and carotid, subclavian, and coronary artery disease in survivors of Hodgkin lymphoma treated with radiation therapy. *JAMA.* 2003;290:2831-2837.

75. Harris EE, Correa C, Hwang WT, et al. Late cardiac mortality and morbidity in early-stage breast cancer patients after breast-conservation treatment. *J Clin Oncol.* 2006;24:4100-4106.

76. McClure MW, Berkowitz SD, Sparapani R, et al. Clinical significance of thrombocytopenia during a non-ST-elevation acute coronary syndrome. The platelet glycoprotein IIb/IIIa in unstable angina: receptor suppression using integrilin therapy (PURSUIT) trial experience. *Circulation.* 1999;99:2892-2900.

77. Sarkiss MG, Yusuf SW, Warneke CL, et al. Impact of aspirin therapy in cancer patients with thrombocytopenia and acute coronary syndromes. *Cancer.* 2007;109(3):621-627.

78. Eagle KA, Berger PB, Calkins H, et al. ACC/AHA guideline update for perioperative cardiovascular evaluation for non-cardiac surgery-executive summary. *Circulation.* 2002;105: 1257-1267.

79. Eagle K, Berger P, Calukins H, et al. ACC/AHA guideline update for perioperative cardiovascular evaluation for non-cardiac surgery-executive summary. *J Am Coll Cardiol.* 2002;39: 543-553.

80. Eagle K, Berger PB, Calkins H, et al. ACC/AHA guideline update for perioperative cardiovascular evaluation for non-cardiac surgery-executive summary. *Anesth Analg.* 2002:94: 1052-1064.

81. Ewer MS. Specialists must communicate in complex cases. *Int Med World Rep.* 2001;16(5):17.

CHAPTER 32

Management of Hypercoagulable States and Coagulopathy

Jenny Petkova ■ Thomas J. Raife ■ Kenneth D. Friedman

Hemostasis is carefully balanced: hemostatic plugs form at inappropriate openings in the vascular network, but thrombus extension is limited, so the remainder of the vascular highway remains fluid. Many disease processes can undermine this wondrous balance, either by stimulating inappropriate occlusion of intact blood vessels or by failure of hemostatic plug formation at sites of vascular wall breakdown. This chapter reviews clinical approaches to both pathologic thrombosis and failure of hemostasis, with an eye toward practical measures in a palliative care setting.

THROMBOTIC DISORDERS

Thrombosis can be considered a pathologic clot formation, occurring either in an inappropriate location or to an inappropriate extent. This review mainly focuses on venous thromboembolic (VTE) disease. Risk factors for the development of thrombosis are many, and the prevalence of thrombosis increases with age and the severity of predisposing conditions. A high proportion of hospice patients are on warfarin sodium, reflecting the high rate of thrombotic complications in this patient population (1). The presenting symptoms of some arterial and most venous thrombotic events are vague. A high index of suspicion and specific testing for confirmation are required. Therapeutic intervention is undertaken with an understanding of the opposing risks of thrombotic progression on the one hand and the hemorrhagic potential of anticoagulation on the other. Studies of the value of various diagnostic protocols, the efficacy and safety of specific interventions, and the risk of bleeding or recurrent thrombosis have led to the development of clinical pathways for diagnosis and have defined "acceptable" rates for complications such as bleeding and recurrent thrombosis. However, these studies have largely been conducted in patients with expected survival of 3 months or longer, and the principles defined in them may not fully translate to the palliative care setting (2,3). The palliative care physician must integrate acute care principles with specific end-of-life goals and expectations to arrive at an appropriate palliative care plan for thrombosis.

Mechanism Underlying Thrombotic Risk

Cancer is a well-established risk factor for VTE. Thrombosis is a major cause of morbidity in patients with neoplastic disease and is reported to be clinically evident in 11% to 15% of patients being treated for malignancy. The risk of thrombosis increases with disease progression. One study of hospice patients with cancer revealed a 50% prevalence of thrombosis, often associated with poor mobility and low albumin level (4). Thrombosis has been observed in up to 50% of patients with cancer at autopsy (2,3). The most thrombogenic tumors include ovarian, brain, pancreatic, gastric, and colorectal neoplasms. Breast carcinoma has a relatively low risk, but the risk rises with certain hormonal manipulations (5).

The three sides of Virchow's triad—stasis, hypercoagulability, and vessel wall dysfunction—all play a role in the pathogenesis of cancer-related thrombosis. Prolonged immobilization due to pain and poor performance status and external vascular wall pressure by tumor contribute to venostasis. Vessel wall injury can be caused by direct infiltration by tumor, central venous catheters, or chemotherapy-related vascular damage. Hypercoagulability has been attributed to the aberrant expression of tissue factor by tumors or reactive endothelium, tumor-derived procoagulant factors that can activate factor X on malignant cells, dysfunctional prothrombotic hematopoietic clones, hyperviscosity, and inflammatory mechanisms (6,7). Inactivation of the tumor suppressor genes Pten and p53 and activation of K-ras have been associated with increased expression of tissue factor (8,9), while induction of the oncogene MET has been associated with disseminated intravascular coagulation (DIC) in human liver carcinoma (10). Proinflammatory cytokines such as tumor necrosis factor-α and interleukin-1β induce expression of tissue factor on endothelial cells (11). These mechanisms may explain why patients with cancer are at increased risk for the development of DIC, which sometimes presents as localized thrombosis. Finally, a host of chemotherapeutic drugs and hormonal manipulations add to thrombotic risk (5).

Many other advanced comorbid conditions, present in cancer patients, are complicated by thrombosis. The incidence of stroke and venous thrombosis is as high as 4% in severe heart failure (12). Hepatic dysfunction increases the risk of thrombosis in part through decreased hepatic clearance of activated coagulation factors (13).

Although most thrombotic events that complicate the care of cancer patients are venous, arterial thrombosis is also a potential problem. Arterial events are generally attributed to atherosclerotic disease, with formation of platelet–fibrin thrombi. Hypotension may worsen the progression of vascular ischemia in the face of preexisting arterial disease. Polycythemia vera and essential thrombocythemia are the predisposing factors in both arterial and venous thrombosis (9). Finally, embolic venous thrombi may cross into the arterial circulation through cardiac shunts and present as "paradoxical" arterial emboli in patients with patent foramen ovale.

Evaluation of the Patient with Venous Thrombosis

The presenting signs and symptoms of VTE are often non-specific, and the problem may be particularly pronounced in the palliative care setting. Alternative causes of extremity swelling include nonthrombotic vascular obstruction, heart failure, renal insufficiency, hypoalbuminemia, lymphatic obstruction, neurologic factors, and hypothyroidism. Similarly, the sensation of breathlessness may stem from anxiety, cardiac failure, tumor invasion, infection, and obstructive pulmonary disease. Conversely, edema in unusual sites may indicate venous thrombosis in palliative care patients. Upper extremity edema may be due to axillary or mediastinal metastasis, catheter-related thrombosis, or venous thrombosis. Hepatic vein thrombosis may present as worsening hepatic failure or sudden onset of ascites (2). Detection of VTE disease is important because it can be successfully treated. Treatment not only reduces the risk of fatal pulmonary embolism (PE) but can also reduce leg pain, immobility, and symptoms of breathlessness (14). Bilateral asymmetric leg edema was the most common presenting finding in one study of hospice patients with advanced cancer who later developed VTE (14). Investigation of symptoms consistent with thrombosis is strongly recommended in patients in whom antithrombotic therapy may be considered.

Noninvasive studies are the diagnostic tools of choice, because contrast venography and conventional pulmonary angiography (the reference standards) are inconvenient, costly, and associated with substantial morbidity. Quantitation of fibrin D-dimer (the plasmin-derived degradation product of cross-linked fibrin clot) may be insufficient for exclusion of VTE in patients with cancer (15). Although one study observed a satisfactory negative predictive value in patients with cancer (16), another study reported that the negative predictive value of the SimpliRED bedside D-dimer test was only 79% in patients with cancer versus 97% in a more general population of ambulatory patients (17,18).

Clinical approaches that include noninvasive imaging studies are recommended for the evaluation of suspected VTE (19,20). Compression ultrasonography may be the best study for the diagnosis of proximal deep vein thrombosis (DVT) in the terminal patient. It is simple, highly accurate, and fast when done by experienced personnel. The sensitivity for proximal leg DVT is reported at over 97%, with specificity reported at 92% to 100%. Compression ultrasonography is significantly less useful in the evaluation of thrombosis below the knee (2,20).

Helical computed tomographic (helical CT) pulmonary angiography has replaced lung scintigraphy (also known as *ventilation/perfusion scan*) as the diagnostic procedure of choice for noninvasive evaluation of patients with suspected PE. Helical CT scan has a high sensitivity for detection of PE in central pulmonary vessels (sensitivity and positive predictive value approach 95%). Advances using multidetector CT scan have improved visualization of subsegmental pulmonary vessels (21), and clinical trial evidence supports the safety of withholding anticoagulation therapy based on a negative helical CT scan study (22). CT scan is also useful for uncovering alternative sources of pulmonary symptoms in patients with advanced disease, because the images provide details of lung parenchyma, mediastinum, and pleura. Concerns about CT scan include the requirement for intravenous injection of a significant iodine-contrast dye load, the high cost of the study, lingering questions regarding sensitivity for detection of embolism in subsegmental pulmonary arteries, and the occasional misinterpretation of studies (23).

Utilization of these diagnostic techniques in the palliative care setting has not been extensively evaluated. An early survey of palliative care physicians in the United Kingdom revealed that only 60% to 80% of responding physicians would use tests to confirm a clinically suspected VTE (24). One palliative care group's protocol is to establish the degree of clinical suspicion, and if high, to obtain leg ultrasonography. When PE is suspected and the leg ultrasound is inconclusive, helical CT scan was obtained. Pulmonary scintigraphy was reserved for patients in whom dye load was contraindicated (25).

Treatment of the Patient with Venous Thrombosis

The American College of Chest Physicians periodically updates its recommendations for the management of VTE in the nonpalliative care setting (26). The goals of treatment of VTE are to prevent death from progressive PE and to minimize the postphlebitic symptoms of pain, swelling, and dyspnea. Thrombolytic therapy is usually considered overly aggressive in the palliative care setting. Anticoagulation is the mainstay of therapy and is instituted immediately to inhibit new clot formation while intrinsic fibrinolytic mechanisms reopen obstructed blood vessels. Anticoagulation is then continued on a long-term basis to prevent recurrent thrombosis. In a general population of patients, the duration of anticoagulation therapy is stratified according to the patient's risk of recurrence (26).

The main complication of anticoagulation therapy is hemorrhage, and assessment of the risks of hemorrhage should be undertaken before instituting anticoagulation (Table 32.1). Absolute contraindications include significant active bleeding or severe bleeding tendency. Relative contraindications include recent bleeding, recent surgery, moderate to severe bleeding tendency, thrombocytopenia, active peptic ulcer disease, uncontrolled hypertension, and severe renal or liver disease. Central nervous system hemorrhage is a particular concern in patients with metastatic cancer in the brain, especially from melanoma, choriocarcinoma, or renal cell carcinoma. However, several authors advocate the safety of anticoagulation in the setting of nonhemorrhagic metastatic disease to the central nervous system when close control of anticoagulation is maintained (27–29). When hemorrhagic risk contraindicates

TABLE 32.1	Contraindications and relative risk factors for hemorrhagic complications of anticoagulant therapy

Contraindications

Significant active bleeding (gastrointestinal or elsewhere)

Recent major surgery or central nervous system procedure

Severe bleeding tendency

Factors Conferring Increased Bleeding Risk

Preexisting abnormality of hemostasis

    Thrombocytopenia

    Concomitant use of platelet-inhibiting drugs

    Coagulopathy

Recent hemorrhagic episode

Recent major surgery

Comorbid disease states

    Advanced disease

    Active peptic ulcer disease

    Uncontrolled hypertension

    Severe renal or hepatic disease

Central nervous system metastasis

Heavy ethanol use

Advanced age

anticoagulation therapy or anticoagulation has been proved to be insufficient to prevent thrombotic progression, inferior vena cava (IVC) filter devices can be inserted to preserve lung function and prevent death due to acute PE (27,29).

Heparin drugs have been the mainstay of initial anticoagulation therapy, owing to their immediate onset of action (30). Their anticoagulant effect is achieved by promoting the inhibitory activity of antithrombin and inhibiting factor Xa. Heparin drugs have been subdivided into unfractionated heparin (UFH), low-molecular-weight heparin (LMWH) derived by depolymerization of UFH, and synthetic pentasaccharides (fondaparinux).

LMWH preparations offer several important pharmacologic advantages over UFH (29,30) and have become the primary medication used for initial management of VTE disease. Many large clinical trials have demonstrated that LMWH is equivalent in safety and efficacy to UFH in the management of acute VTE and that it is safe for use in outpatient community–based care (31). A meta-analysis of randomized trials revealed that LMWH is more effective and safer than UFH, and furthermore, long-term LMWH is superior to warfarin in patients with cancer (29,32). Similar to UFH, LMWH is a parenteral medication, but depolymerization results in a longer half-life, greater bioavailability, and more predictable pharmacodynamics. For the average patient with VTE, these

pharmacologic advantages translate into weight-adjusted dosing once or twice daily without a requirement for laboratory monitoring. These advantages also render LMWH an appropriate agent for outpatient use. Other potential advantages include reduced risks for the development of osteoporosis (33), and heparin-induced thrombocytopenia (HIT) (34). The main disadvantages of LMWH are increased cost and a more prolonged anticoagulant effect that is less reversible with protamine sulfate. While the parenteral (subcutaneous) route of administration would appear to be a disadvantage, LMWH is generally well accepted in patients that are educated as to why their physician is recommending this approach. This was even shown to hold true in a palliative care setting (32). Among patients with cancer, one study found a trend toward increased thrombus recurrence with once-daily dosing of enoxaparin compared with twice-daily dosing (35); however, the potential benefit of twice-daily dosing must be balanced against inconvenience and cost when considering the care of patients in a palliative care setting. Multiple LMWH preparations are available and the dosing schedules for each were largely empirically determined. The dosing schedule should appropriately match the LMWH preparation being used. Because LMWH is cleared by the kidney, in patients with renal insufficiency (creatinine greater than 2 mg/dL or estimated creatinine clearance of under 30 mL/min) use of UFH or dose modification of LMWH with monitoring of levels is advisable. Although target levels of LMWH have not been established through therapeutic trials, a target peak level of 0.6 to 1.0 antifactor Xa units per mL measured 3 to 4 hours after subcutaneous administration of LMWH has been recommended (36). Dose escalation should be considered in cancer patients who experience progressive thrombotic complications (29,37).

UFH may still be used for the initial management of VTE in some patients. Its main advantages are low cost, short half-life, and reversibility by administration of protamine sulfate. The main disadvantages of UFH are its wide dose–response variability, narrow therapeutic window, and the need for parenteral administration. Other complications include the rare but serious immunologic condition HIT (38) and the risk of osteoporosis with very long term heparin therapy (33). While UFH is often given by continuous infusion (39), outpatient subcutaneous administration every 12 hours has also been used. The therapeutic dose is determined empirically. Algorithms for prescriptive dose adjustment are based on frequent monitoring of anticoagulant effect (30). The sensitivity of the activated partial thromboplastin time (aPTT) to heparin effect varies widely between laboratories; it is advisable to consult the local laboratory to learn the recommended therapeutic range. Alternatively, direct heparin assessment by "antifactor Xa" assays can be requested (therapeutic range: 0.35 to 0.70 U/mL) (36).

Synthetic pentasaccharide anticoagulant, fondaparinux, is also approved for initial treatment of VTE, with randomized trials demonstrating non-inferiority to LMWH and UFH (36). Like LMWH, fondaparinux requires subcutaneous administration and is cleared by the kidney. Potential advantages include a longer half-life (17 to 21 hours) allowing once-daily administration, and emerging experience suggests a potential use in patients with a history of HIT.

After achieving initial anticoagulation, long-term anticoagulation (secondary prophylaxis) is undertaken to prevent recurrence of VTE. Oral vitamin K antagonists (e.g., warfarin) are frequently chosen for this phase of care (26,36), but LMWH should be considered in some settings (see subsequent text). Vitamin K antagonists inhibit hepatic synthesis of multiple coagulation factors. The onset of oral anticoagulant effect is delayed until previously synthesized coagulation factors are cleared. Therefore, "loading" doses do not overcome the long half-life of circulating clotting factors. Because of this delay, heparin drugs are usually used concurrently with initial oral anticoagulation to provide protection before the onset of oral anticoagulation effect. Current recommendations suggest that heparin drugs be maintained for at least 5 days and continued for 2 days after laboratory studies confirm that adequate oral anticoagulation has been established.

Management of oral warfarin anticoagulation is complex due to the narrow therapeutic window, multiple drug interactions, inter-individual differences in hepatic metabolism, and the shifting intensity of anticoagulation due to changes in diet (26). The therapeutic intensity of oral anticoagulation requires laboratory monitoring. A prothrombin time (PT)–based international normalized ratio (INR) target of 2.5 is suggested in most settings, but a higher target of 3.0 is suggested for patients with many types of mechanical heart valves (40). The typical initial dose of warfarin sodium is 5 mg/d in acute care patients, but initial doses may need to be lower in chronically ill patients, patients with poor nutrition, patients on medications that are known to increase oral anticoagulant effect, and in the elderly. Owing to individual variation in anticoagulant effect, ongoing monitoring of individual patient response and dose adjustment are required. Initially, INR monitoring and dose adjustment are performed daily, with monitoring intervals lengthened as the dose requirement is empirically established. Weekly evaluation may be prudent for at least the first 6 to 12 weeks of therapy, the time when the highest rate of hemorrhage occurs (41). In general patient populations, the risk of bleeding with INRs in the therapeutic range is between 2% and 3%, but patients with cancer are at increased risk for bleeding complications (2). Adverse events may be avoided through more frequent monitoring (42). Outcome data are scant in the palliative care literature. In this setting, oral anticoagulation may be more problematic owing to changes in diet, gastrointestinal (GI) or hepatic disturbances, changes in medications, the need to discontinue anticoagulation to accomplish invasive interventions without untoward risk of bleeding, and the burden imposed by laboratory monitoring. One small hospice audit revealed a high incidence of oral anticoagulation–related hemorrhagic events and found that external bleeding was quite distressing to the patients and their caregivers (1,43). Tight INR control was somewhat helpful, but required frequent INR monitoring (averaging once every 2.4 days), adding a considerable burden to dying patients.

Management of a patient with an INR above the target value requires consideration of the degree of INR elevation and patient's intrinsic risk of hemorrhage (Table 32.2). In patients who are not bleeding, dose adjustments may be sufficient. Low-dose oral vitamin K_1 can be used to shorten the time required for reestablishing the target INR level (44). In a bleeding patient, in addition to considering the use of intravenous vitamin K supplementation, coagulation factor replacement in the form of prothrombin complex concentrate (PCC) or fresh frozen plasma (FFP) transfusion speeds up correction of the INR (26,45). PCCs are preferred over FFP because the smaller volume load allows more rapid and complete factor replacement and there is reduced risk of allergic complications (26); however, the complexity and expense of these measures should be carefully considered in the palliative care setting.

LMWH has also been evaluated for the long-term anticoagulation of patients. LMWH offers two advantages. The first is improved efficacy of LMWH over oral anticoagulation in patients with cancer. In such patients, the annual rate of recurrent thrombosis while on oral anticoagulation is much higher than in other populations and may be as high as 27% (46). In two randomized trials, assignment to long-term LMWH rather than oral anticoagulation was shown to reduce the rate of recurrent VTE by half without an increase in major bleeding events (29,47). The second advantage is the simplicity of the use of LMWH, including the absence of laboratory monitoring requirements and dietary or drug interactions, which offers significant advantages for the terminally ill patient. The recommended dose is generally similar to that used during initial anticoagulation therapy, and once-daily dosing may be sufficient for long-term secondary prophylaxis (36).

Two new oral direct-acting anticoagulant medications have been recently approved. Rivaroxaban is an inhibitor of factor X and dabigatran is a direct thrombin inhibitor. Both drugs are approved for thromboembolic stroke prevention in patients with non-valvular atrial fibrillation. These agents have also been demonstrated to have efficacy in the treatment and prevention of recurrence of VTE (37). They have the advantage of the oral route without the inconvenience of frequent INR monitoring associated with warfarin. Their disadvantages include the lack of reversing therapy in case of bleeding, their relatively higher cost compared with vitamin K antagonists, and the need for dose adjustment in patients with renal insufficiency (37).

Duration of anticoagulation is determined by the risk of recurrence (36). Three to 6 months of anticoagulation is recommended for the general patient with a reversible short-term risk factor, a minimum of 3 months for the patient with idiopathic VTE, and 12 months to an indefinite period for the patient with a significant long-term risk factor. In terminally ill patients with persistent risk factors (such as cancer or immobility), the decision to continue anticoagulation should be regularly revisited because it is unclear at

TABLE 32.2	Guidelines for reversal of warfarin sodium anticoagulation

INR	Urgency of Reversal	Recommendation
<5.0	1–2 d	Decrease or discontinue warfarin sodium until INR improves
	12–24 h	Discontinue warfarin sodium
		Consider vitamin K_1: 2.5 mg orally
	As soon as possible	Discontinue warfarin sodium
		Vitamin K_1: 5–10 mg i.v.[a]
		Fresh frozen plasma (at least 15 mL/kg)
5.0–9.0	1–3 d	Discontinue warfarin sodium until INR improves
	12–24 h	Discontinue warfarin sodium
		Vitamin K_1: 2.5–5.0 mg orally or 2.0–4.0 mg subcutaneously
	As soon as possible	Discontinue warfarin sodium
		Vitamin K_1: 10 mg i.v.[a]
		Fresh frozen plasma (at least 15 mL/kg)
		Consider prothrombin complex concentrate or recombinant factor VIIa for life-threatening bleeds
>9.0	1–3 d	Discontinue warfarin sodium
		Vitamin K_1: 2.5–5.0 mg orally or subcutaneously
	12–24 h	Discontinue warfarin sodium
		Vitamin K_1: 2.5–5.0 mg orally or 10 mg subcutaneously
		Consider fresh frozen plasma (at least 15 mL/kg)
	As soon as possible	Discontinue warfarin sodium
		Vitamin K_1: 10 mg i.v.,[a] consider repeat doses
		Fresh frozen plasma (at least 15 mL/kg)
		Consider prothrombin complex concentrate or recombinant factor VIIa for life-threatening bleeds

INR, international normalized ratio.

[a]i.v. Vitamin K_1 should be administered slowly; rare anaphylactic reactions have occurred.

Modified from Pineo GF, Hull RD. The use of heparin, low-molecular-weight heparin, and oral anticoagulants in the management of thromboembolic disease. In: Portenoy R, Bruera E, eds. *Topics in Palliative Care*. Vol 4. New York, NY: Oxford University Press; 2000:185,201–205, with permission.

what point the reduction in risk of thrombotic recurrence justifies the logistical burden of anticoagulant therapy and the ongoing risk of hemorrhage. While continuing antithrombotic therapy is controversial when patients transition to a palliative care phase, precedent exists (32,48). A patient's prothrombotic risk is presumed to increase with disease progression. Case series document systemic VTE recurrence in palliative care patients in whom antithrombotic therapy was discontinued. Furthermore, administration of LMWH was considered acceptable from both nursing and patient perspectives (32). Palliative care practitioners should

attempt to balance the morbidity of recurrent VTE with that of continuing anticoagulation. However, if the patient declines therapy, has low palliative performance status, or experiences adverse events, discontinuation of anticoagulant medication is reasonable (2,32,49).

Recurrence of venous thrombosis in the face of anticoagulation appears to be a particular problem in patients with cancer or the antiphospholipid antibody syndrome (29,50). A patient who develops thrombosis with a subtherapeutic INR may be retreated with UFH or LMWH for 5 to 7 days and then continued on oral anticoagulation with the usual target INR of 2.5. For the patient who is already in the therapeutic INR range at the time of thrombosis, possible measures include aiming for a higher INR of 3 to 4.5 (and accepting the higher risk of bleeding events), switching to long-term LMWH, or considering adding an IVC filter (29). For a patient with recurrent VTE while on LMWH, escalating the dose of LMWH by 20% to 30% can be an effective strategy. This approach, however, can be associated with the increased risk of bleeding (38).

An IVC filter is not an alternative to anticoagulation, but placement of a filter may prolong life by prevention of acute PE. IVC filters reduce the short-term risk of PE, but they do so at the expense of increased risk of progressive leg thrombosis and postphlebitic syndrome (45,51). Placement of an IVC filter should be reserved for patients with active bleeding or a high risk of bleeding, or for patients who develop recurrent thrombosis despite anticoagulant therapy. In the latter setting, concurrent anticoagulation should also be considered; thrombotic complications occurred in 2% to 30% of patients with cancer who had a filter placed (45). Because of the expense and morbidity associated with IVC filters, their use in the palliative care setting should be carefully considered.

The role of primary VTE prophylaxis in the care of oncology patients is currently under evaluation. A predictive model for chemotherapy-associated thrombosis has identified five independent risk factors for developing symptomatic VTE during the first four cycles of therapy—site of cancer, prechemotherapy platelet count, hemoglobin level and/or use of erythropoiesis-stimulating agents, prechemotherapy white cell count, and body mass index (52). This model can identify patients with 7% short risk of symptomatic VTE who may benefit from primary thromboprophylaxis. A recent meta-analysis concluded that LMWH improves the overall survival in cancer patients even in those with advanced disease with no increase in major bleeding (53). Although the risk–benefit ratio of thromboprophylaxis in hospitalized oncology patients has not been extensively evaluated, both American College of Chest Physicians and American Society of Clinical Oncology recommend thromboprophylaxis in this patient population (54,55). However, at this time, the data remain limited and VTE prophylaxis therapy is rarely maintained in palliative care units (49). While this may be explained by the need to balance the benefits of controlling symptoms with the risks and inconvenience of the use of anticoagulant drugs in a palliative setting, one should be mindful that VTE is twice as frequent in palliative care cancer patients when compared with a general cancer population and that symptomatic VTE is a frequent cause of admission to inpatient palliative care units (49).

Catheter-Related Thromboses

Eliminating venipuncture clearly increases a patient's comfort level. As a result, central venous catheters are commonly used in patients with cancer and other chronic illness for administration of medications, transfusions, and laboratory monitoring. These devices are associated with a number of complications, including increased risk of infection and thrombosis (56). Thrombus may obstruct a line tip, form a sleeve around the intravascular portion of the catheter, or obstruct the veins of the arm, neck, or mediastinum.

Intraluminal catheter obstruction is common, but low-dose thrombolytic therapy, instilled as a single dose (or occasionally as repeated doses), is usually effective in opening a tip thrombosis. Streptokinase, urokinase, and tissue plasminogen activator have been used for this purpose (56). The inability to draw from a line (the so-called ball-valve effect) may be due to obstruction, but venography reveals that approximately 40% of these problems are attributable to nonthrombotic, local mechanical effects.

Vein thrombosis is a common complication of central lines. The incidence of venous thrombosis is unclear, ranging from 12% to 74% of lines; however, most thrombotic episodes are asymptomatic. Symptoms of central vein thrombosis may be nonspecific, including arm, neck, or head swelling, headache, arm pain or numbness, prominent surface venous pattern of the arm, or erythema. Owing to the smaller size of the upper extremity veins, symptomatic PE is a rare complication (56). Objective imaging is necessary to confirm the diagnosis. Although anatomic limitations reduce the sensitivity of sonography to only 54% to 100%, the high specificity of sonography (estimated at 94% to 100%) makes a positive study useful (57). Repeated ultrasound, spiral CT scan, or contrast venography may be useful in some patients.

Optimal therapy of central vein thrombosis is uncertain because comparative prospective trials have not been performed. Catheter removal should be considered if the line is nonfunctional, but anticoagulation without line removal is acceptable in patients in whom continued use of the line is desired. Currently, anticoagulation therapy is modeled from studies of DVT of the leg. Initial management using an immediate-acting anticoagulant such as LMWH is followed by longer term oral anticoagulation or continued LMWH (56). Superior vena cava filters have rarely been placed in patients in whom anticoagulation is not an option (45). While older open-label prospective randomized studies suggested a utility of prophylaxis with very-low-dose (1 mg/d) warfarin sodium or daily subcutaneous dalteparin 2,500 IU, these data have been called into question by the more recent studies (56,55). Given the risk of excessive oral anticoagulation in patients with anorexia and the inconvenience of prophylactic LMWH, prophylaxis against thrombosis is not recommended for patients with central venous catheters (56,55).

HEMORRHAGIC DISORDERS

Bleeding occurs in up to 10% of patients with advanced cancer (46). When visible, and especially when massive, it can cause considerable anxiety for the patient, family, and health care providers (6). It may present as simple bruising or petechiae on the skin or as blood loss from mucosal or tumor surfaces. Bleeding may lead to debilitation from

TABLE 32.3	Mechanisms of hemorrhagic risk

Loss of Vascular Integrity
   Tumor surface bleeding
   Tumor erosion into a major vessel
   Mucositis (stress, drug-related, acid peptic disease, chemotherapy-induced, and radiation therapy–induced)

Platelet Defects
   Thrombocytopenia
      Marrow proliferative failure (myelophthisis, drug-induced, radiation therapy–induced, viral, and vitamin deficiency)
      Accelerated platelet clearance (disseminated intravascular coagulation, sepsis, immunologic, and hypersplenism)
      Platelet function defects (drug-induced, uremic, and paraprotein effect)

Coagulation Defects
   Vitamin K deficiency (decreased intake or bowel flora production, malabsorption, and oral anticoagulant–induced)
   Liver disease
   Disseminated intravascular coagulation
   Accelerated fibrinolysis
   Coagulation inhibitors (heparin drugs and autoimmune)

anemia and serve as a reminder of the uncontrolled and progressive course of illness. Patients may be unsettled by specific complications associated with bleeding in certain locations, such as chronic cough or dyspnea related to pulmonary bleeding. In addition, episodic low-volume bleeding may herald a more catastrophic hemorrhagic event. The clinical approach to these situations requires a balanced consideration of the underlying causes of bleeding (Table 32.3), the available therapeutic modalities, and the patient's palliative care goals.

Mechanisms of Hemorrhagic Risk

Vascular Integrity

The loss of vascular wall integrity underlies all bleeding events. Multiple factors conspire to destroy vascular integrity in the terminally ill patient. Local tumor invasion in the GI tract is associated with 12% to 17% of cases of GI hemorrhage in patients with cancer (58). Chest wall breast carcinoma, endobronchial lung cancer, and locally invasive head and neck or cervical cancer can all cause local hemorrhage. Mucositis may be induced by nonsteroidal anti-inflammatory drugs, stress, peptic ulcer disease, local infection, or as a result of chemotherapy or radiation treatment. Finally,

primary vascular defects may be involved, as in amyloidosis or vitamin C deficiency.

Platelet Function

Failure of hemostatic mechanisms may allow minor defects of vascular integrity to become manifest. Many factors can result in thrombocytopenia or diminished platelet function. Platelet counts above 50,000 per mm^3 are generally well tolerated in the absence of trauma (59), and significant risk of spontaneous hemorrhage is rare in clinically stable patients until counts fall below 10,000 per mm^3 (59).

Failure of marrow production is a very common mechanism of thrombocytopenia. Extensive marrow replacement by tumor (myelophthisis) occurs early in leukemia but is a sign of advanced metastatic disease in solid tumors. Peripheral blood abnormalities that are supportive of a diagnosis of myelophthisis include pancytopenia and the presence of circulating neutrophil precursors, nucleated red blood cells, and "teardrop" red cells. Marrow failure is an anticipated complication of many antineoplastic drugs and may complicate radiation therapy. Other causes of marrow failure include vitamin deficiency (B$_{12}$ or folate), hypothyroidism, viral infections, and adverse medication effects. If required, marrow failure can be confirmed by bone marrow biopsy. Platelet-selective cytopenias and disorders characterized by shortened platelet survival are characteristic of some drug-induced complications. Infection, DIC, hypersplenism, and autoimmune phenomena are among the potential underlying mechanisms of thrombocytopenia. The approach to diagnosis and treatment of thrombocytopenia in the palliative care setting requires judgment as to potential benefits in relation to the discomfort, cost, and risk to the patient.

Medication-related inhibition of platelet function should be considered in the bleeding patient because adjusting medications may be a relatively simple means of restoring platelet function in some patients in the palliative care setting (60). Aspirin and most nonsteroidal anti-inflammatory drugs exert antiplatelet effect due to cyclo-oxygenase inhibition. In addition, these agents increase the risk of gastric erosion and bleeding. Continued use of antiplatelet agents (such as clopidogrel) in a patient with vascular disease should be questioned if the patient develops significant bleeding complications.

Coagulation Defects

Abnormalities of the coagulation mechanism such as vitamin K deficiency, hepatic disease, and DIC should be considered in a palliative care patient with bleeding (61).

Vitamin K is a fat-soluble factor required for hepatic synthesis of multiple coagulation proteins. Oral anticoagulants produce their effect through inhibition of vitamin K metabolism. Nutritional deficiency of vitamin K occurs when there is impairment of either dietary intake or bowel flora synthesis of vitamin K. Disruption of both mechanisms is common (60). In addition, malabsorption disorders such as bowel resection/bypass and biliary obstruction and the use of cholestyramine may undermine fat-soluble vitamin absorption.

Supportive laboratory evidence includes a prolonged PT with a normal or less prolonged aPTT and normal fibrinogen and platelet levels. The PT should correct after 1:1 mixing with normal plasma, and the abnormalities should improve with vitamin K_1 administration.

Liver dysfunction contributes to bleeding in a variety of ways. The liver produces most coagulation proteins and is a reservoir for vitamin K. In addition to impaired synthetic capacity from parenchymal liver disease, liver dysfunction may cause portal hypertension with resulting thrombocytopenia from hypersplenism and GI bleeding due to esophageal or rectal varices. Owing to its short half-life, factor VII levels fall early in the course of liver disease, resulting in prolongation of the PT, which should correct in a 1:1 mix with normal plasma. Mildly elevated fibrin degradation products may reflect defective hepatic clearance. The aPTT is typically less prolonged than the PT, and levels of fibrinogen and platelets are variable. Other clinical or biochemical evidence should support the diagnosis of hepatic disease. In the patient with severe liver disease, responsiveness to vitamin K_1 administration is generally limited.

DIC is a secondary coagulation disturbance associated with many disorders. Frequently, DIC is associated with cancer. Other causes include trauma, burns, sepsis, and prolonged circulatory insufficiency. DIC is characterized by the activation of both procoagulant and fibrinolytic pathways. Activation of these pathways results in consumption of platelets and coagulation factors, intravascular deposition of fibrin, simultaneous release of fibrin degradation products, and destabilization of hemostatic plugs (62). The thrombotic spectrum of DIC includes large vessel thrombosis and microvascular thrombosis with multiorgan failure. The hemorrhagic spectrum ranges from asymptomatic laboratory abnormalities to increased bruising, reoccurrence of bleeding at sites of prior trauma, or even spontaneous mucosal bleeding. The diagnosis of DIC rests on clinical suspicion supported by laboratory abnormalities, including prolonged PT and aPTT, decreased fibrinogen and platelets, and a positive test for fibrin split products or D-dimer.

Clinical Approaches to the Bleeding Patient

The cause and severity of bleeding define the spectrum of available interventions. The patient's anticipated life expectancy, quality of life, care setting, and palliative care goals may narrow the spectrum. The potential benefits of intervention (Table 32.4) must be weighed against the consequences. In addition to general supportive measures, the care plan may entail avoidance of interventions that increase bleeding risk, local measures to treat bleeding, and systemic interventions to improve hemostasis.

General Supportive Measures

It is helpful to identify patients who are at particular risk for massive bleeding. Tumors likely to present bleeding problems include fungating tumors of the head and neck, gynecologic tumors, and tumors close to major vessels. Patients

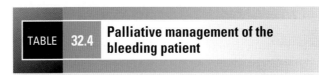

TABLE 32.4	Palliative management of the bleeding patient

General Supportive Measures
Identify the patient at risk
Establish open communication of issues of care
Generate care plan
   Consider measures for catastrophic bleeding
   Use of sedatives (midazolam hydrochloride)
   Revisit as required by patient course

Local Measures
Packing
Compressive dressings and postures
Topical hemostatics (collagen, thrombin, fibrin gel, and antifibrinolytics)
Topical astringents or vasoconstrictors (silver nitrate, alum, formaldehyde, cocaine, and epinephrine)

Special Techniques
Endoscopic interventions (cauterization, sclerosis, and ligation)
Interventional radiology (vascular embolization)
Palliative radiotherapy
Palliative surgery (vascular ligation)

Systemic Interventions
Discontinue antiplatelet and antithrombotic medications
Vitamin K administration
Antifibrinolytic medication (tranexamic acid and ε-aminocaproic acid)
Transfusion support
   Platelets or plasma for hemostatic support
   Red cells for symptomatic anemia
Desmopressin
Somatostatin analogs (octreotide acetate)

Modified from Gagnon B, Mancini I, Pereira J, et al. Palliative management of bleeding events in advanced cancer patients. *J Palliat Care.* 1998;14:50–54.

on antithrombotic therapy and those with severe liver disease or marrow failure are also at increased risk for hemorrhage. Massive bleeding can be extremely distressing to patients and caregivers alike (63). Panic responses and calls to emergency medical personnel may result in the initiation of inappropriate interventions. If a risk of catastrophic bleeding exists, sensitive anticipatory conversations involving the entire care provision team serve to empower caregivers to act compassionately and appropriately if massive bleeding develops (46,63,64). Patients with hematemesis should be placed in the left lateral position to reduce respiratory compromise. The use of dark-colored towels and basins helps make blood loss less evident and reduces anxiety associated with bleeding. It may be helpful to have prefilled syringes containing sedative medication (e.g., 2.5 to 5 mg of midazolam hydrochloride) available for subcutaneous or intravenous administration in the event of catastrophic hemorrhage (64). Finally, terminal bleed events remain vivid in the nurses' memory, and a structured debriefing session should be offered to all affected staff after such an incident (63).

Local Measures

Local interventions to control hemorrhage include compression dressings, application of materials to improve hemostasis, and special procedures to occlude bleeding vessels (46). Packing is useful in areas such as the nose, rectum, or vagina. Pressure through the use of balloon catheters or posturing is of additional benefit in areas of small capillary or venous bleeding. Choice of topical agents to further improve hemostasis is generally based on local factors, cost, and individual considerations. Topical cocaine has been used with nasal packing. Acetone may similarly improve the efficacy of vaginal packing. Purified gelatin in the form of compressed packed foam (Gelfoam), sterile sponge dressings, or sterile powdered bovine-derived collagen provides surfaces for formation of a hemostatic clot. Bovine thrombin can be applied topically in powder form to dressings or directly onto oozing surfaces. It can also be used in solution to moisten dressings (65). Topical fibrin sealant derived from human plasma can be applied directly to bleeding surfaces (66). Hematuria should be evaluated to exclude reversible causes such as infection. Aluminum astringents, such as 1% alum solution, have been applied in the form of continuous bladder irrigation. Aluminum hydroxide complexed with sulfated sucrose (sucralfate) is an active ulcer healing drug, which has been used successfully for the control of esophagitis, rectal bleeding, or vaginal bleeding; 1 g of sucralfate tablet dispersed in water-soluble gel (e.g., K-Y jelly) can be applied to bleeding sites once or twice daily. Cauterizing and vasoconstrictive agents are alternative approaches for controlling hemorrhage. Formaldehyde solutions have been used to control hematuria (67) and may control bleeding associated with radiation proctitis (68). However, special precautions, including management of pain and prevention of damage to adjacent structures, must be considered when using formaldehyde-based therapy. Silver nitrate cauterization is commonly used for nasal bleeding. Epinephrine (as a 0.002% solution) may be used to induce vasoconstriction. Epinephrine use in combination with lidocaine is discouraged (46), but if combination medication is used, the lidocaine doses should not exceed 7 mg/kg (65).

Special Techniques

Specific local interventions include endoscopic or intravascular application of hemostatic measures and use of radiotherapy to induce vascular sclerosis. The spectrum of endoscopic procedures includes cauterization and electrically induced coagulation, application of sclerosing agents and ligation of esophageal varices, and topical or injection application of hemostatic agents (46). In addition to inconvenience, the risks of endoscopic procedures include worsened bleeding through physical trauma and perforation of viscera.

In a subset of patients, vascular embolization performed by interventional radiology has been used for a variety of bleeding indications (61,45). This is especially important to consider in patients with head and neck tumors where there is a risk of carotid artery rupture. The unpredictable evolution of hemorrhagic episodes is particularly alarming to patients with these tumors (69). Percutaneous endovascular procedures entail minimal discomfort and allow rapid recovery, ideal for a palliative setting. Embolic particles include metal coils, polyvinyl alcohol spheres, and gelatin sponges. The technique is restricted to vascular beds in which catheters can be easily guided. Vascular access is usually obtained through an axillary or femoral approach, the blood vessels supplying the bleeding area are identified angiographically, and then the hemostatic agent is inserted into the vessel. Embolization therapy is well established in the treatment of head and neck, pelvic, GI, and pulmonary neoplasm–associated bleeding. Complications include the need for mild sedation during the procedure, embolization of vascular beds not affected by tumor, bleeding at the site of vascular access, and a "postembolization" syndrome characterized by discomfort, malaise, and low-grade fever after vascular occlusion of a large tumor mass. Symptoms may persist for 2 to 7 days (45). Palliative radiation therapy may be used to control hemorrhage from head and neck, gynecologic, GI, bladder, and other tumors (61). The optimal method of treatment remains controversial. Prior therapy in the same radiation field increases the risk of adverse events and limits the utility of this approach in some patients. (For further discussion of this area, see Chapter 49.)

Systemic Interventions

Systemic interventions include augmentation of platelet or coagulation mechanisms and inhibition of fibrinolytic mechanisms. Alternatively, some medications may improve vascular or other responses to bleeding. Red blood cell transfusion may palliate the symptoms of anemia.

In the bleeding patient with a platelet count under 50,000 per mm³, platelet transfusion may temporarily help control bleeding. Prophylactic platelet transfusions are used in the care of patients with marrow failure and severe thrombocytopenia. The use of a 10,000 per mm³ threshold for prophylaxis appears to have a similar safety for a 20,000 per mm³ threshold (59); however, bleeding may occur with platelet counts over 20,000 per mm³ when associated with vascular and anatomic abnormalities (70). Platelet transfusion therapy is complicated by the short survival of transfused platelets. Although the mean platelet life span is 9.5 days in normal individuals, platelet survival may be less than 3 days in patients with stable platelet counts near 20,000 per mm³ owing to marrow hypoplasia (71). In the palliative care setting, marrow failure is often a chronic problem and a single platelet transfusion is unlikely to raise the platelet count for more than a few days.

The limited role and complications associated with platelet transfusions should be discussed with the patient by the care providing team to arrive at an appropriate care plan. Prophylactic platelet transfusion (or trial of growth factors such as romiplostim and eltrombopag) is generally not warranted in a palliative care setting (2). However, palliation with limited platelet transfusions may be considered when symptoms of bleeding are distressing, such as painful hematomas, headache, disturbed vision due to recent hemorrhage, and continuous oral, GI, or genitourinary tract bleeding (72). (For more extensive comments, see Chapter 6.)

The treatment of coagulopathy should be based on the underlying mechanism, the extent of coagulation disturbance, and the urgency for correction of the defect. Vitamin K deficiency and oral anticoagulation effect usually respond to vitamin K_1 within 24 hours. Vitamin K_1 is available as 5-mg oral tablets; parenteral administration might be considered in patients in whom malabsorption is a factor. Chronic administration (such as 5 mg twice per week) may be required to maintain the effect. Intravenous infusion of vitamin K_1 is generally discouraged because of rare reports of anaphylactoid reactions, but this route is justified in urgent settings, and infusion rates of under 1 mg/min may decrease the risk of such reactions (26,46). For rapid correction of the coagulopathy of vitamin K deficiency, transfusion of FFP has been a mainstay of therapy (60), but if available, PCC is a preferred product. FFP may also provide temporary improvement for bleeding in patients with liver disease or malignancy-associated DIC. Although FFP contains all necessary coagulation proteins, transfusion of FFP may be considered excessive in the palliative care setting. In DIC, some recommendations have been made for the use of heparin to control thrombin-generated consumption of platelets and coagulation factors, but its use in this setting remains controversial (60,62).

Desmopressin is an analog of the posterior pituitary hormone vasopressin. 1-Deamino-[8-D-arginine] vasopressin (DDAVP) has been used extensively in the management of patients with mild deficiency of coagulation factor VIII (mild hemophilia A) or von Willebrand factor (type I von Willebrand disease) because levels of these proteins rise approximately two- to threefold after administration of this agent (73). DDAVP has also been used successfully in patients with acquired defects of platelet function resulting from uremia, cirrhosis, and aspirin. It has also proved useful for the management of variceal bleeding, possibly due to splanchnic vasoconstriction and decreasing portal pressures. DDAVP is administered as either an intravenous infusion (0.3 to 0.4 µg/kg over 20 minutes) or through nasal inhalation (a single 150-µg application for weight under 50 kg and two applications for patients of larger weight). Common side effects include mild facial flushing and headache. Water retention with hyponatremia can occur owing to the potent antidiuretic effect of desmopressin. Excessive administration of fluids should be avoided.

Antifibrinolytic agents prevent clot lysis by blocking the binding sites of plasmin and its activators in plasma or saliva. Among these agents, tranexamic acid is 10 times more potent than ε-aminocaproic acid and has a longer half-life (73). These drugs are rapidly absorbed from the GI tract and excreted in the urine, and both have dose-related nausea, vomiting, and diarrhea as the main toxicities. A dose of tranexamic acid of 1.5 g, followed up by 1 g three times per day, or ε-aminocaproic acid started at 5 g, followed up by 1 g four times per day, was used in one palliative care study (74). Fourteen of 16 patients had cessation of tumor-associated bleeding, with most having a complete control of hemorrhage within 4 days. Treatment was continued for up to 54 days and bleeding was not reported after cessation of the therapy. Topical administration of these agents was described in this study and in several case series of oral surgery (57). Although antifibrinolytic agents have been used in patients with thrombocytopenic bleeding, results of studies have not been consistent. One placebo-controlled trial did not demonstrate benefit in a population of patients with aplastic anemia or myelodysplasia, but two small studies with aminocaproic acid showed some effect on control of hemorrhage (74). Antifibrinolytic therapy is generally avoided in the treatment of upper urinary tract hemorrhage as ureteral clots may obstruct urinary flow. Systemic antifibrinolytic therapy increases the risk of thrombosis and should be used very cautiously in DIC.

Systemic interventions are occasionally used to alter the physiologic responses to bleeding. An example is the use of the somatostatin analog, octreotide acetate, in patients with GI bleeding (61). Although mostly used in the treatment of acute upper GI bleeding, at least one successful use in a palliative care setting is reported (64). It was suggested that octreotide acetate results in decreased splanchnic blood flow, reduced venous pressures, cytoprotection, and suppression of gastric acid secretion. The recommended dose was 50 to 100 µg administered subcutaneously every 12 hours and increased according to the clinical response to a maximum of 600 µg/d. Continuous infusion by either intravenous or subcutaneous route is a possible alternative (63). Adverse effects are dose dependent and include nausea, abdominal discomfort, and diarrhea.

Massive or ongoing bleeding will exacerbate anemia in chronically ill patients. Anemia may present as poor tolerance to exercise or chronic fatigue. Arbitrary thresholds for transfusion support often fail to take into account the particular situation of a patient, and anemia is often better tolerated by younger individuals and patients without comorbidities of cardiopulmonary or vascular diseases. Decisions regarding either indirect support of red cell production with growth factors (such as erythropoietin) or direct transfusion of red blood cells should be consistent with the goals of care for the patient. Response to growth factors is generally slow, and a trial of transfusion may be more appropriate. If within a day or two of transfusion there is no improvement in fatigue, dyspnea, or associated symptoms, further transfusion will probably be unhelpful (2).

REFERENCES

1. Johnson MJ. Problems of anticoagulation within a palliative care setting: an audit of hospice patients taking warfarin. *Palliat Med.* 1997;11:306-312.

2. Davis MP. Hematology in palliative medicine. *Am J Hosp Palliat Med.* 2004;21:445-454.

3. Kirkova J, Fainsinger RL. Thrombosis and anticoagulation in palliative care: an evolving clinical challenge. *J Palliat Care.* 2004;2:101-104.

4. Johnson MG, Sproule MW, Paul J. The prevalence and associated variables of deep venous thrombosis in patients with advanced cancer. *Clin Oncol.* 1999;11:105-110.

5. Linenberger ML, Wittkowsky AK. Thromboembolic complications of malignancy: risks. *Oncology.* 2005;19:853-861.

6. Dicato M, Ries F, Duhem C. Bleeding and coagulation problems. In: Klastersky J, Schimpf J, Senn H-J, eds. *Handbook of Supportive Care in Cancer.* New York, NY: Marcel Dekker Inc; 1995;63-98.

7. Gordon S. Cancer cell procoagulants and their implications. *Hematol Oncol Clin North Am.* 1992;6:1359-1374.

8. Rong Y, Post DE, Pieper RO, et al. PTEN and hypoxia regulate tissue factor expression and plasma coagulation by glioblastoma. *Cancer Res.* 2005;65(4):1406-1413.

9. Yu JL, May L, Lhotak V, et al. Oncogenic events regulate tissue factor expression in colorectal cancer cells: implications for tumor progression and angiogenesis. *Blood.* 2005;105(4):1734-1741.

10. Boccaccio C, Sabatino G, Medico E, et al. The MET oncogene drives a genetic programme linking cancer to haemostasis. *Nature.* 2005;434:396-400.

11. Bevilacqua MP, Pober JS, Majeau GR, et al. Recombinant tumor necrosis factor induces procoagulant activity in cultured human vascular endothelium: characterization and comparison with the actions of interleukin-1. *Proc Natl Acad Sci USA.* 1996;83:4533-4537.

12. Lip GY, Gibb CR. Does heart failure confer a hypercoagulable state? Virchow's triad revisited. *J Am Coll Cardiol.* 1999;33:1424-1426.

13. Lisman T, Porte RJ. Rebalanced hemostasis inpatients with liver disease: evidence and clinical consequences. *Blood.* 2010;116:878-885.

14. Kirkova J, Oneschuk D, Hanson J. Deep vein thrombosis (DVT) in advanced cancer patients with lower extremity edema referred for assessment. *Am J Hosp Palliat Med.* 2005;22:145-149.

15. Gomes MP, Deitcher SR. Diagnosis of venous thromboembolic disease in cancer patients. *Oncology.* 2003;17:126-135.

16. ten Wolde M, Kraaijenhagen RA, Prins MH, et al. The clinical usefulness of D-dimer testing in cancer patients with suspected deep venous thrombosis. *Arch Intern Med.* 2002;162:1880-1884.

17. Lee AYY, Julian JA, Levine MN, et al. Clinical utility of a rapid whole-blood D-dimer assay in patients with cancer who present with suspected acute deep venous thrombosis. *Ann Intern Med.* 1999;131:417-423.

18. Wells PJ, Brill-Edwards P, Stevens P, et al. A novel and rapid whole-blood assay for D-dimer in patients with clinically suspected deep vein thrombosis. *Circulation.* 1995;91:2184-2187.

19. Lee AYY. Treatment of venous thromboembolism in cancer patients. *Thromb Res.* 2001;102:V195-V208.

20. Perrier A, Desmarais S, Miron M-J, et al. Non-invasive diagnosis of venous thromboembolism in outpatients. *Lancet.* 1999;353:190-195.

21. Russo V, Piva T, Lovato L, et al. Multidetector CT: a new gold standard in the diagnosis of pulmonary embolism? State of the art and diagnostic algorithms. *Radiol Med.* 2005;109: 49-61.

22. Moore LK, Jackson WL, Shorr AF, et al. Meta-analysis: outcomes in patients with suspected pulmonary embolism managed with computed tomographic pulmonary angiography. *Ann Intern Med.* 2005;141:866-874.

23. Rathbun SW, Raskob GE, Whitsett TL. Sensitivity and specificity of helical computed tomography in the diagnosis of pulmonary embolism: a systematic review. *Ann Intern Med.* 2000;132:227-232.

24. Johnson MJ, Sherry K. How do palliative care physicians manage venous thromboembolism? *Palliat Med.* 1997;11:462-468.

25. Merminod T, Zulian GB. Diagnosis of venous thromboembolism in cancer patients receiving palliative care. *J Pain Symptom Manage.* 2000;19:238-239.

26. Kearon C, Akl EA, Comerota AJ, et al. Antithrombotic therapy for VTE disease: Antithrombotic Therapy and prevention of thrombosis, 9th ed: American College of Chest Physicians evidence-based clinical practice guideline. *Chest* 2012;141: e419S-e494S.

27. Ihnat DM, Mills JL, Hughes JD, et al. Treatment of patients with venous thromboembolism and malignant disease: should vena cava filter placement be routine? *J Vasc Surg.* 1998;28:800-807.

28. Batchelor TT, Byrne TN. Supportive care of brain tumor patients. *Hematol Oncol Clin North Am.* 2006;20(6):1337-1361.

29. Lee AY. Thrombosis in cancer: an update on prevention, treatment, and survival benefits of anticoagulants. *Hematology Am Soc Hematol Educ Program.* 2010;2010:144-149.

30. Hirsh J, Bauer KA, Donait MB, Gould M, Samama MM, Weitz JI. Parenteral anticoagulants: American College of Chest Physicians evidence-based clinical practice guidelines (8th ed.). *Chest.* 2008;133:160S-198S.

31. Wells PJ, Kovacs MJ, Bormanis J, et al. Expanded eligibility for outpatient treatment of deep venous thrombosis and pulmonary embolism with low-molecular-weight heparin. *Arch Intern Med.* 1998;158:2001-2003.

32. Tran QN. Role of palliative low-molecular-weight heparin for treating venous thromboembolism in patients with advanced cancer. *Am J Hosp Palliat Care.* 2010;27(6):416-419;. e-pub ahead of print March 2, 2010.

33. Monreal M, Lafoz E, Olive A, et al. Comparison of subcutaneous unfractionated heparin with a low molecular weight heparin (Fragmin) in patients with venous thromboembolism and contraindications to coumarin. *Thromb Haemost.* 1994;71:7-11.

34. Warkentin TE, Levine MN, Hirsh J, et al. Heparin-induced thrombocytopenia in patients treated with low-molecular-weight heparin or unfractionated heparin. *N Engl J Med.* 1995;332:1330-1335.

35. Merli G, Spiro TE, Olsson C-G, et al. Subcutaneous enoxaparin once or twice daily compared with intravenous unfractionated heparin for treatment of venous thromboembolic disease. *Ann Intern Med.* 2001;134:191-202.

36. Kearon C, Kahn SR, Agnelli G, Goldhaber S, Raskob GE, Comerota AJ; American College of Chest Physicians. Antithrombotic therapy for venous thromboembolic disease: American College of Chest Physicians evidence-based clinical practice guidelines (8th ed.). *Chest.* 2008;133 (6 suppl):454S-545S.

37. Eriksson BI, Quinlan DJ, Eikelboom W. Novel oral factor Xa and thrombin inhibitors in management of thromboembolism. *Ann Rev Med.* 2011;62:41-57.

38. Carrier M, Le Gal G, Cho R, et al. Dose escalation of low molecular weight heparin to manage recurrent venous thromboembolic events despite systemic anticoagulation in cancer patients. *J Thromb Haemost.* 2009;7:760-765.

39. Warkentin TE, Greinacker A, Koster A, Lincoff AM. Treatment and prevention of heparin-induced thrombocytopenia: American College of Physicians evidence-based clinical practice guidelines (8th ed.). *Chest.* 2008;133(6 suppl):181S-453S.

40. Pineo GF, Hull RD. The use of heparin, low molecular weight heparin, and oral anticoagulants in the management of thromboembolic disease. In: Portenoy R, Bruera E, eds. *Topics in Palliative Care.* Vol 4. New York, NY: Oxford University Press; 2000;185-205.

41. Salem DN, O'Gara PT, Madias C, Pauker SG; American College of Chest Physicians. Valvular and structural heart disease: American College of Chest Physicians evidence-based clinical practice guidelines (8th ed.). *Chest.* 2008;133 (6 suppl):593S-629S.

42. Fihn SD, McDonell M, Martin D, et al. Risk factors for complications of chronic anticoagulation. *Ann Intern Med.* 1993;118:511-520.

43. Prandoni P. Antithrombotic strategies in patients with cancer. *Thromb Haemost.* 1997;78:141-144.

44. Johnson MJ. Problems of anticoagulation within a palliative care setting—correction. *Palliat Med.* 1998;12:463.

45. J Hague, R Tippett. Endovascular techniques in palliative care. *Clin Oncol.* 2010;22(9):771-780.

46. Pereira J, Phan T. Management of bleeding in patients with advanced cancer. *Oncologist.* 2004;9:561-570.

47. Lee AYY, Levine MN. Venous thromboembolism and cancer: risks and outcomes. *Circulation.* 2003;107:117-121.

48. Noble S. The challenges of managing cancer related venous thromboembolism in the palliative care setting. *Postgrad Med J.* 2007;83(985): 671-674.

49. Soto-Cárdenas MJ, Pelayo-García G, Rodríguez-Camacho A, Segura-Fernández E, Mogollo-Galván A, Giron-Gonzalez JA. Venous thromboembolism in patients with advanced cancer under palliative care: additional risk factors, primary/secondary prophylaxis and complications observed under normal clinical practice. *Palliat Med.* 2008;22(8):965-968.

50. Khamashta MA, Cuadrado MJ, Mujic F, et al. The management of thrombosis in antiphospholipid-antibody syndrome. *N Engl J Med.* 1995;332:993-997.

51. Decousus H, Leizorovicz A, Parent F, et al. A clinical trial of vena caval filters in the prevention of pulmonary embolism in patients with proximal deep-vein thrombosis. *N Engl J Med.* 1998;338:409-415.

52. Khorana AA, Kuderer NM, Culakova E, Lyman GH, Francis CW. Development and validation of a predictive model for chemotherapy-associated thrombosis. *Blood.* 2008;111(10):4902-4907.

53. Lazo-Langner A, Goss GD, Spaans JN, Rodger MA. The effect of low-molecular-weight heparin on cancer survival. A systematic review and meta-analysis of randomized trials. *J Thromb Haemost.* 2007;5(4):729-737.

54. Lyman GH, Khorana AA, Falanga A, et al. American Society of Clinical Oncology guideline: recommendations for venous thromboembolism prophylaxis and treatment in patients with cancer. *J Clin Oncol.* 2007;25:5490-5505.

55. Geerts WH, Bergqvist D, Pineo GF, et al. Prevention of venous thromboembolism: American College of Chest Physicians evidence-based clinical practice guidelines (8th ed.). *Chest.* 2008;133:381S-453S.

56. Rosovsky RP, Kuter DJ. Catheter-related thrombosis in cancer patients: pathophysiology, diagnosis, and management. *Hematol Oncol Clin North Am.* 2005;19:183-202.

57. Mustafa BO, Rathbun SW, Whitsett TL, et al. Sensitivity and specificity of ultrasonography in the diagnosis of upper extremity deep vein thrombosis: a systematic review. *Arch Intern Med.* 2002;162:401-404.

58. Schnoll-Sussman F, Kurtz RC. Gastrointestinal emergencies in the critically ill cancer patient. *Semin Oncol.* 2000;27:270-283.

59. Slichter SJ. Relationship between platelet count and bleeding risk in thrombocytopenic patients. *Transfus Med Rev.* 2005;18:153-167.

60. Raife TJ, Rosenfeld SB, Lentz SR. Bleeding from acquired coagulation defects and antithrombotic therapy. In: Simon TL, Dzik WH, Snyder EL, et al., eds. *Rossi's Principles of Transfusion Medicine.* 3rd ed. Philadelphia, PA: Lippincott Williams & Wilkins; 2002;399-414.

61. Pereira J, Mancini I, Bruera E. The management of bleeding in advanced cancer patients. In: Portenoy R, Bruera E, eds. *Topics in Palliative Care.* Vol 4. New York, NY: Oxford University Press; 2000;163-183.

62. Levi M, Toh CH, Thachil J, Watson HG. Guidelines for the diagnosis and management of disseminated intravascular coagulation. British Committee for Standards in Haematology. *Br J Haematol.* 2009;145:24-33.

63. Harris DG, Flowers S, Noble SIR. Nurses' views of the coping and support mechanisms experienced in managing terminal haemorrhage. *Int J Palliat Nurs.* 2011;17(1):7-13.

64. Gagnon B, Mancini I, Pereira J, et al. Palliative management of bleeding events in advanced cancer patients. *J Palliat Care.* 1998;14:50-54.

65. McEvoy GK. *AHFS Drug Information 2004.* Bethesda, MD: American Society of Health-System Pharmacists Inc; 2004.

66. Mankad PS. The role of fibrin sealants in surgery. *Am J Surg.* 2001;182:21S-28S.

67. White RD, Sawczuk I. Hematuria. In: Walsh TD, ed. *Symptom Control.* Cambridge, MA: Blackwell Scientific Publications; 1989;229-233.

68. Roche B, Chautems R, Marti MC. Application of formaldehyde for treatment of hemorrhagic radiation-induced proctitis. *World J Surg.* 1996;20:1092-1094.

69. García-Egido AA, Payares-Herrera MC. Managing hemorrhages in patients with head and neck carcinomas: a descriptive study of six years of admissions to an internal medicine/ palliative care unit. *J Palliat Med.* 2011;14(2):124-125.

70. Bernstein SH, Vose JM, Tricot G, et al. A multicenter study of platelet recovery and utilization in patients after myeloablative therapy and hematopoietic stem cell transplantation. *Blood.* 1998;91:3509-3527.

71. Hanson SR, Slichter SJ. Platelet kinetics in patients with bone marrow hypoplasia: evidence for a fixed platelet requirement. *Blood.* 1985;66:1105-1109.

72. Lassauniere JM, Bertolino M, Hunault M, et al. Platelet transfusion in advanced hematologic malignancy: a position paper. *J Palliat Care.* 1996;12:38-42.

73. Mannucci PM. Hemostatic drugs. *N Engl J Med.* 1998;339: 245-253.

74. Dean A, Tuffin P. Fibrinolytic inhibitors for cancer-associated bleeding problems. *J Pain Symptom Manage.* 1997;13:20-24.

CHAPTER 33

Urologic Issues in Palliative Care

Eric A. Singer ■ Faisal Ahmed ■ Compton J. Benjamin ■ Adam R. Metwalli ■ Peter A. Pinto

INTRODUCTION

Urologic malignancies account for more than 40% of all new cancer diagnoses and 15% of all cancer deaths in the United States (1). In addition to these primary sites of disease, metastases from other malignancies and the side effects of the surgery, radiation, and chemotherapy used to treat them can all deleteriously impact the genitourinary system. This chapter will review many of the most common urologic issues cancer patients experience and provide a schema for their evaluation and management.

It is our belief that palliative care and supportive oncology should be incorporated into the treatment plan early, if not from the time of diagnosis, for many patients. The work of the American Urological Association's web-based ethics curriculum, American College of Surgeons' ethics curriculum and guide to surgical palliative care, and Northwestern University's Education in Palliative and End-of-Life Care program has increased surgeon awareness regarding the importance of interventions that are designed to improve patients' quality of life (QOL) even though they may not prolong survival (2–4). However, two recent publications have shown that early supportive oncology involvement improves QOL, which is not surprising, but that structured palliative care in addition to routine cancer treatment can actually improve survival when compared with standard oncologic therapy alone, which will certainly stimulate further research on the possible synergy between curative and supportive care (5–6).

SURGICAL PALLIATIVE CARE

Just as palliative care has evolved in scope and practice within the field of internal medicine, the concept of surgical palliative care has matured along with it (7). The definition of surgical palliative care can now be understood as any procedure whose primary intent is to improve QOL or mitigate symptoms caused by advanced disease (2). The efficacy of surgical palliation should be evaluated by the magnitude and duration of improvement in patient-reported symptoms (2).

The American College of Surgeons has outlined three key components that must be addressed prior to undertaking a palliative intervention. These include (i) understanding the patient's symptoms and goals of care, (ii) estimating the likely impact the proposed intervention will have on the

patient's symptoms, and (iii) the patient's prognosis and trajectory of disease (2). While not an exhaustive list, using these points to frame discussions with patients and their families about potential procedures/surgery can help develop realistic expectations, respect patient autonomy, and avoid the harms of unnecessary surgery (7,8). Another specific issue that should be discussed prior to palliative surgery is whether an advance directive such as a do-not-resuscitate (DNR) order has been completed, and how it should be handled during the perioperative period (9).

The American Society of Anesthesiologists, American College of Surgeons, and the Association of Operating Room Nurses have stated that it is inappropriate to automatically discontinue a patient's DNR order upon entry into the operating room (9). Instead, they advocate for "required reconsideration" when a patient with a DNR needs a surgical intervention. This allows the patient, surgeon, and anesthesiologist to review the goals of care and proposed treatment plan in order to determine the best course of action. The DNR order may then be maintained, suspended, or revised during the perioperative period. Advance directives are reviewed in detail in Chapter 57 of this textbook.

URINARY OBSTRUCTION

Obstruction of the urinary tract can occur due to a wide range of pathophysiology. It can be chronic resulting in the slow deterioration of renal function, but it can also be acute resulting in significant discomfort and life-threatening illness. Common causes of upper urinary obstruction include kidney and ureteral stones, strictures of the ureter, and extrinsic compression of the ureter from abdominal or retroperitoneal masses. Lower urinary tract obstruction may be due to benign prostatic obstruction, bladder stones, urethral strictures, and extrinsic compression from pelvic masses. Naturally, upper urinary tract obstruction has a different evaluation and treatment algorithm compared with lower urinary tract obstruction.

The etiology of obstruction may be secondary to prior disease treatment, the consequence of progressive disease, or even age-related pathophysiology unrelated to the primary diagnosis. Keeping these factors in mind, treatment plans should be individualized for each patient after taking into consideration life expectancy, anesthesia risk, and social support

TABLE 33.1	Management options for urinary tract obstruction
Upper Tract	**Lower Tract**
Steroid therapy (retroperitoneal fibrosis)	α-Blockers (e.g., doxazosin and tamsulosin)
Internal ureteral stent (various types)	5-α-Reductase inhibitors (e.g., finasteride)
Percutaneous nephrostomy tube	Clean intermittent catheterization
Surgical urinary diversion	Indwelling urethral catheter
	Suprapubic catheter
	Transurethral surgery (e.g., TURP and PVP)

TURP, transurethral resection of the prostate; PVP, photovaporization of the prostate.

systems. As with any medical workup, the first step is still a detailed history and physical examination to assess the possible location(s) and acuity of the obstruction. The treatment of urinary tract obstruction is variable, and the treatment of choice may change as the patient's goals of care evolve (Table 33.1).

Upper Urinary Tract Obstruction

Acute obstruction of the upper urinary tract typically presents with classic symptoms such as flank pain, dysuria, and hematuria. These symptoms can be elicited by intrinsic and extrinsic obstructive processes. Intrinsic obstruction can be caused by urinary stones, blood clots, and strictures, whereas extrinsic obstruction can occur when any abdominal or pelvic structure compresses the ureter or renal pelvis. Common causes of extrinsic obstruction include tumors, fibrosis, and enlarged lymph nodes.

Imaging is a mainstay in the evaluation of upper tract obstruction. Dilatation of the renal pelvis/ureters and intrarenal stones can be visualized very well on ultrasound; however, identifying the cause of obstruction below the renal pelvis may be difficult because the entire length of the ureter may not be well visualized with ultrasound alone. The quality of the images is also dependent on patient's body habitus as well as the skill of the technician. Abdominal x-ray without the use of intravenous contrast has virtually no value in evaluating upper urinary tract obstruction. An intravenous pyelogram (IVP), which consists of serial abdominal x-rays shot in a timed fashion after the injection of intravenous contrast, helps delineate the renal shadow and the drainage patterns of the ureters. The IVP was the standard radiologic evaluation for the upper urinary tract until recently but has been supplanted by computed tomography (CT) urogram or CT-IVP due to increased sensitivity as well as additional anatomic information provided by the CT images.

A CT urogram consisting of a non-contrast CT scan followed by a CT scan with intravenous contrast in three phases (arterial, venous, and delayed) is now considered the standard of care by most urologists. Urolithiasis and renal masses are readily identified and characterized, a basic assessment of renal function can be done, and filling defects within the renal pelvis and ureters can be seen. The primary limitation of CT urography in this patient population is the prevalence of renal insufficiency/failure, which often precludes the use of intravenous contrast.

Magnetic resonance imaging (MRI) delineates soft tissue better than CT but tends to be used more as a secondary test to clarify questions posed by the original scan (10). MRI is the study of choice when evaluating for tumor involvement in the renal vein or vena cava (11). Magnetic resonance urography (MRU) also allows for visualization of all anatomic components of the urinary tract using heavily T2-weighted sequences or gadolinium-enhanced T1 images. Since there is no ionizing radiation, it is especially useful for pediatric and/or pregnant patients. However, there are a few disadvantages to MRU that keep it from being a first-line test. MRU is still limited in its ability to visualize stones; compared with CT the availability of the test itself is limited; the time needed to perform an MRU is significantly longer than a CT urogram (30 to 60 minutes versus 10 to 15 minutes, respectively) (10).

After obtaining a detailed history, general lab work (serum chemistries and urine analysis), and appropriate imaging, urologic consultation may be needed for a more in-depth evaluation and treatment plan. More invasive evaluation with cystoscopy/ureteroscopy may be warranted if a questionable filling defect were to be seen on delayed CT images for example.

Non-surgical Treatment

The treatment of extrinsic compression of the upper urinary tract will vary depending on the etiology, symptoms, and the effect on renal function. If caused by extrinsic compression from malignancy, the primary goal is to treat the underlying disease when possible. Obstruction due to a primary genitourinary malignancy may be treated with either local surgical treatment or systemic therapy, depending on the stage of disease. Obstruction caused by iatrogenic injury or treatment side effect can be temporized with a percutaneous nephrostomy tube or ureteral stent until the inciting factor resolves or definitive surgical treatment/repair is safe to attempt.

Surgical Treatment

Internal ureteral stenting has long been a mainstay for the treatment of upper tract obstruction. Urinary stents are not permanent; and, if left in too long, stents may become encrusted and eventually fail. Traditionally, urologists have recommended replacing stents every 3 to 6 months. It is preferred to place ureteral stents endoscopically in a retrograde fashion in the operating room under general anesthesia. Chung et al. described their 15-year experience with internal ureteral stents for management of extrinsic obstruction and showed a 40.6% failure rate within the first 11 months. Predictors of stent failure include a diagnosis of cancer (regardless of type), baseline creatinine more than 1.3 mg/dL, and post-stenting radiation or chemotherapy (12).

The Resonance metallic ureteral stent (Cook Medical, Bloomington, IN, USA) is a stent designed for the long-term management of extrinsic ureteral obstruction and may remain in place up to 12 months. The metal stent has greater tensile strength than plastic stents and does not compress as readily. Liatsikos et al. performed a prospective study of 50 patients, consisting of both malignant extrinsic obstruction and intrinsic stricture disease, and patients with malignant extrinsic obstruction showed patency rates of 100% with a mean follow-up time of 8.5 months, while patients with intrinsic stricture disease had a patency rate of 44%. Failure was noted within the first 2 weeks in the latter group (13).

Thermo-expandable stents such as the Memokath (PNN Medical, Denmark) have also been developed as an alternative solution for the long-term management of ureteric obstruction. Agrawal et al. performed a prospective study on 55 patients, a mix of malignant extrinsic compression and intrinsic stricture disease, who had a Memokath placed with a mean follow-up of 16 months (range 4 to 98). Fourteen patients required reinsertion over a mean of 7.1 months for migration, encrustation, stricture progression, or incorrect length. The remaining patients maintained their stents between 8 and 12 months and then they were routinely replaced (14). Like the Resonance and Memokath stents, many new innovations in ureteral stents are in development, but the long-term efficacy of all stents is not well defined and more data are needed.

Percutaneous nephrostomy tubes drain urine directly from the kidney through the patient's back and into an external collection device. These tubes are often placed under local anesthesia with sedation by an interventional radiologist under ultrasound guidance, with fluoroscopy, or CT guidance for the most difficult cases. However, patients will be required to be prone for the procedure which may be difficult in elderly and obese patients and those with respiratory compromise. Like ureteral stents, nephrostomy tubes should be exchanged every 3 to 6 months. The advent of external/internal drainage systems (nephroureteral stents) have allowed for temporary nephrostomy tube placement with the ability to later convert to anterogradely placed internal ureteral stents.

In acute obstruction with clinical signs of sepsis (e.g., fever, tachycardia, and hypotension), percutaneous nephrostomy tube placement is the recommended intervention. Retrograde instrumentation with cystoscopy and ureteral stent placement in the setting of an active infection puts patients at significant risk for urosepsis, which can be life-threatening (15). Other times, nephrostomy tubes are used as a last resort after failure of attempts to place a ureteral stent endoscopically. Ku et al. described a recent retrospective analysis of complications in 148 patients with malignant extrinsic ureteral obstruction who underwent either nephrostomy tube or ureteral stent placement. The study noted no significant differences in fevers, acute pyelonephritis, or catheter-related complications between the two groups (15). When considering primary palliative treatment for obstruction, the risks of anesthesia and the procedure itself as well as the impact of the nephrostomy tube/stent on QOL must be discussed with the patient or his/her health care proxy.

Given the fact that nephrostomy tubes involve direct puncture of the kidney, there is a small risk of bleeding, which is not seen in ureteral stenting. A review of a single-center experience with 500 percutaneous nephrostomy tube placements revealed a major complication rate of 0.45% and a minor complication rate of 14.2% (16). Major complication was defined as gross hematuria and hemodynamic instability requiring surgical intervention and/or blood transfusion. Minor complications were tube complications (e.g., dislodgement and kinking) or gross hematuria for greater than 48 hours without clinical symptoms. Given the risk of bleeding, an anti-coagulated or thrombocytopenic patient is rarely a candidate for immediate diversion with a percutaneous nephrostomy tube.

There are not many studies comparing QOL after nephrostomy tube placement and after ureteral stenting. The percentage of patients describing their stents as "terrible" or having a "serious impact on daily life" is as high as 66% in some QOL studies (17). QOL studies using standardized methods for nephrostomy tubes are few. Of the studies that do exist, the most common complaints involve tube dislodgement, urine leakage around tube, and skin excoriation at the tube exit site (17). Although hard to objectively measure, the concept of extra medical devices (e.g., nephrostomy with external drainage bag) is anecdotally always a concern to patients and their caregivers. Ultimately, the decision for ureteral stent versus percutaneous nephrostomy will be unique to each patient.

In general, surgical treatments for obstructive uropathy in a palliative care setting are temporizing measures and aggressive surgical approaches are generally not indicated. However, advanced prostate and/or bladder cancer can cause obstruction due to local tumor extension occluding the distal ureters. In cases where it is difficult to pass internal stents, in percutaneous nephrostomy tube failure, or in QOL choice by the patient, pelvic exenteration can be considered. Palliative exenteration is a poorly studied area, but several small series have reported 5-year life expectancy ranging from 25% to 40% in well-selected metastasis-free patients (18). Select palliative exenteration patients show life expectancy ranging from 18 to 24 months with improved QOL (18). Given the morbidity of any exenterative surgery, it is important to ensure that the patient has a good estimated life expectancy. In addition, patients should be counseled extensively on the long recovery process, high likelihood of perioperative complications, and no guarantee of extending life or improving QOL.

Lower Urinary Tract Obstruction

Stones in the lower urinary tract are far more common in men due to prostatic outlet obstruction leading to elevated residual urine in the bladder, although women can also develop them. Advanced prostate cancer can cause bladder outlet obstruction as well, regardless of the actual overall size of the prostate. Transitional cell tumors of the bladder can obstruct outflow as well. Urethral stricture disease is more common in patients who have had long-term urinary catheters, recurrent cystoscopy, sexually transmitted infections, or pelvic trauma.

The male lower urinary tract is generally defined as the bladder, bladder neck, prostatic urethra, and the penile urethra. A detailed medical history, including past surgeries, plus a validated questionnaire (e.g., International Prostate System Score) will be the basis for evaluating obstruction of the lower urinary tract. While always recommended, a digital rectal examination (DRE) assessment of "prostate size" does not always correlate with symptoms of obstruction. "Small" prostates on DRE can still cause significant obstruction due to anatomic variations such as an enlarged prostatic median lobe, which can act as a ball valve causing outlet obstruction.

The female lower urinary tract has a much shorter urethra due to the lack of a prostate; consequently, lower urinary tract obstruction in females is far less common. Extrinsic compression of the bladder from pelvic malignancies and pelvic organ prolapse can cause dysfunctional voiding such as incomplete emptying, urinary frequency and urgency, and incontinence. Iatrogenic causes such as pelvic/vaginal/urologic surgery in the past can also cause lower urinary tract obstruction, which reinforces the need for a detailed history. Therefore, a pelvic speculum examination is a key component to the physical assessment. Abdominal ultrasound is a safe and effective way of evaluating lower urinary tract obstruction. Using ultrasonography, a post-void residual can be calculated and larger bladder stones can be imaged. Urinalysis can also help rule out the presence of infection, which in itself can exacerbate symptoms of lower urinary tract obstruction. A serum creatinine will also help assess overall renal function, which can dictate the type and timing of treatment. These basic evaluations should be completed prior to urologic consultation for urinary obstruction.

Non-surgical Treatment

Benign prostatic hyperplasia (BPH) will affect many men as they age. Maximal medical therapy, as defined in the Medical Therapy of Prostatic Symptoms trial, found significant improvement in American Urological Association symptom scores when patients were given a combination of α-blockade (doxazosin) and 5-α-reductase inhibitor (finasteride) together compared with either drug alone. The study was double blinded with a mean follow-up of 4.5 years and involved 3,047 patients (19). If a patient is assessed by DRE or ultrasound and is found to have a prostate larger than 30 g, combination therapy with an α-blocker and 5-α-reductase inhibitor (e.g., finasteride and dutasteride) can be instituted (20). It should be noted that the effects of α-blockers are often appreciated within several days, whereas 5-α-reductase inhibitors take months to improve urinary symptoms. Additionally, 5-α-reductase inhibitors decrease serum prostate-specific antigen (PSA) values, and the use of this medication must be taken into account for men undergoing prostate cancer screening, although screening may no longer be appropriate for many men in the palliative care/supportive oncology population (21).

Although medical therapy significantly improves the voiding function of many patients, its effects are limited. Many patients with voiding difficulties are older and may have baseline mobility issues. This may be especially true of patients with advanced malignancy who have decreased performance status and spend considerable time in bed. Normal voiding function is difficult to achieve in a recumbent position.

When manual dexterity is preserved, clean intermittent catheterization (CIC) is a reasonable option. First described by Lapides et al. (22) in 1971, CIC education and training allows patients to empty their bladder on a schedule. This is still the simplest form of intervention for outlet obstruction. The key caveat is that patients are required to have the mental and manual dexterity to be able to do this for themselves or they should have a reliable caregiver assume this responsibility.

When a patient is not a candidate for CIC, an indwelling urinary catheter is a very common intervention for lower urinary tract obstruction. A semi-permanent catheter creates a pathway for bacteria to enter the urinary tract; therefore, bacteriuria is a common problem in chronically catheterized patients. If asymptomatic, treatment for bacteriuria is usually discouraged to avoid the creation of drug-resistant organisms (23). Indwelling catheters should routinely be changed every 10 to 12 weeks (23). Oftentimes, the immobilized patient may benefit most from an endoscopically placed suprapubic catheter. By removing the catheter from the urethra, the risk of urethral erosion or stricture is decreased and general comfort is improved.

Surgical Treatment

Surgical approaches to bladder outlet obstruction have become varied over the years but the gold standard is still the traditional electrosurgical transurethral resection of the prostate (TURP). Although the approach is endoscopic, a TURP is not without morbidity. Irrigation solutions such as glycine or mannitol were used in the past putting patients at risk for dilutional hyponatremia (TUR-syndrome) if too much fluid was absorbed through open venous sinuses during resection. Today, most cases are done using a bipolar resectoscope and normal saline, but a patient can still become fluid overloaded from the absorption of irrigant (24). As with any surgical procedure, anesthesia risk and blood loss are always concerns as well. Caution still needs to be used when considering TURP for patients with significant cardiopulmonary history.

Specific to the palliative care setting, the concept of the "channel TURP" has become more popular. Rather than subjecting patients to complete resection, which increases the risk of morbidity, the goal of the "channel TURP" is to remove enough tissue to allow successful bladder emptying while minimizing the amount of time spent under anesthesia and the amount of fluid absorbed by the patient during the procedure. Patients with significant comorbidities or even with prostate cancer that may be invading the bladder can be considered candidates for a channel TURP. Marszalek et al. (25) described a rate of 25% repeat TURP, 11% requiring permanent catheters, and 10% with some incontinence in a series of 89 prostate cancer patients who underwent a "channel TURP."

Laser photovaporization of the prostate (PVP) is one of the newer tools at the disposal of urologists for managing benign prostatic hyperplasia (BPH). The "greenlight laser" (AMS Medical Systems) energy is selectively absorbed within tissue by hemoglobin. This selective absorption improves the hemostatic effect of the laser while vaporizing prostatic tissue. Multiple studies have shown that the PVP compares favorably with the TURP with significantly less blood loss and shorter catheterization time (26).

The improvement in blood loss has led many urologists to expand the indications of PVP use. With many older patients on oral anticoagulant or antiplatelet therapy, PVP is being used to relieve bladder outlet obstruction in patients who are not candidates for TURP due to increased risk of bleeding. Woo and Hossack recently described their experience with PVP in 43 men who were on Coumadin during their procedure. No patient needed a blood transfusion and only six (14%) patients required a catheter for more than 24 hours (27). In the palliative care and supportive oncology population, PVP is a reasonable option to consider in patients who may have more significant medical comorbidities or require long-term thromboprophylaxis due to blood clots associated with malignancy.

HEMATURIA

While there are many benign causes of hematuria, including glomerulonephritis, cystitis, renal trauma, BPH, kidney, ureteral and bladder stones, radiation cystitis, and bacterial and viral infections, hematuria, whether gross or microscopic, may also be an indicator of a malignant process within the urinary collecting system. Therefore, a thorough investigation of the entire upper and lower urinary tract should always be considered. The two most common tests used for the detection of blood in the urine are the urine dipstick and microscopy. Urine dipsticks can have false-positive reactions in the presence of hemoglobin or myoglobin; consequently, when a dipstick is positive, microscopy is usually necessary to verify the presence of red blood cells (RBCs) and assess RBC morphology.

Once hematuria is confirmed, then a urine culture should be done to eliminate infection as the etiology of bleeding. In the absence of infection or after resolution of infection, a second positive urinalysis/microscopy would indicate the need for a complete urinary tract evaluation (28). If an MRI urogram or CT urogram is performed adequately, then the evaluation is complete after cystoscopy. However, if an ultrasound or cross-sectional imaging with incomplete or absent delayed phase images of the upper urinary tract is used for evaluation, then cystoscopy with bilateral retrograde pyelograms is indicated.

Gross hematuria refers to the presence of blood in the urine that can be seen with the unaided eye. It is important to confirm the presence of RBCs once dark urine is seen. There are multiple other potential causes of discoloration within a urine specimen. Some of the more common causes of discolored urine include concentrated urine and systemic administration of flutamide, phenazopyridine, sulfasalazine, phenolphthalein (seen with the use of some over-the-counter laxatives), nitrofurantoin, metronidazole, methylene blue, bilirubinuria, and vitamin B complex. When a patient presents with a history of gross hematuria and no evidence of infection, the hematuria workup may be done without confirmatory testing of the urine. Anticoagulated patients with hematuria should not be excluded from the workup since the anticoagulation may unmask a previously unidentified lesion in as many as 25% of patients (29).

Causes of asymptomatic microscopic hematuria (Table 33.2) range from minor, clinically insignificant findings that require no intervention to lesions that could be life threatening. When presented with a patient with asymptomatic hematuria, it is important to distinguish whether the bleeding originates from the lower urinary tract (urethra/prostate/bladder) or the upper urinary tract (ureters/kidneys). Often the history and physical examination may identify the location of the hematuria.

The appropriate evaluation (Figure 33.1) includes a history and physical examination, laboratory analysis of the urine, upper tract evaluation of the ureters and kidney with a CT, lower tract evaluation by cystoscopy, and urine cytology. A flexible cystoscopy can be performed in the office by most urologists. With a thorough cystoscopy, the urethra, prostate, bladder, and ureteral orifices can be carefully examined and the source of bleeding often identified. Observation of the ureteral orifices may demonstrate bloody efflux from one side, further aiding in the identification of the laterality of an upper urinary tract source. In patients with microscopic hematuria, as many as 16% will have a malignancy identified through this evaluation and 3% of patients with a negative hematuria evaluation will have a malignancy found on a subsequent workup (31). Lateralizing hematuria requires a retrograde pyelogram or delayed imaging with CT to properly visualize the ureters. The finding of a filling defect may necessitate ureteroscopy and fulguration, biopsy, or resection, as well as the treatment of non-malignant causes of upper tract hematuria.

TABLE 33.2	Causes of hematuria

Glomerular Causes

Primary glomerulonephritis
  Focal glomerular sclerosis
  IgA nephropathy
  Membranoproliferative glomerulonephritis
  Postinfectious glomerulonephritis
  Rapidly progressive glomerulonephritis
Secondary glomerulonephritis renal tumors
  Cryoglobulinemia
  Hemolytic-uremic syndrome
  Medication-induced nephritis
  Systemic lupus erythematosus
  Thrombotic thrombocytopenic purpura
  Vasculitis
Hereditary
  Alport's syndrome
  Fabry's disease
  Thin glomerular basement membrane disease

Renal Causes

Arteriovenous malformations/fistulas
Infarct
Medullary sponge kidney
Papillary necrosis
Polycystic kidney disease
Renal trauma
Renal tumors
Renal vein thrombosis

Extrarenal Causes

Benign prostatic enlargement
Calculus disease
Cyclophosphamide cystitis
Foreign body
Indwelling ureteral stent
Indwelling urethral catheter
Lower urinary tract infection
Radiation cystitis
Trauma to ureter, bladder, urethra
Tumor of ureter, bladder, prostate, urethra

When symptomatic, lower urinary tract bleeding may present with dysuria, frequency, urgency, lower abdominal pain, and urinary retention. As the symptoms can sometimes be severe, it is important to treat them while awaiting results from the urine tests. When lateralizing hematuria is found on cystoscopy, one should begin with a radiographic study. Retrograde pyelography or delayed imaging of an abdominal CT scan with oral and IV contrast may be sufficient to identify filling defects and masses in the ureters and kidneys.

Symptomatic upper tract hematuria usually presents with lateralizing flank or abdominal pain caused by obstruction, or if brisk bleeding from the upper tract is present, the patient may also have lower urinary tract symptoms and urinary retention secondary to clots.

Management of Lower Urinary Tract Hematuria

The initial management of all hematuria is dependent on the patient's hemodynamic stability. When hemodynamically unstable, the patient should be aggressively hydrated, transfused, and coagulopathies reversed as needed. Once stabilized, the source of bleeding can be found and treated. If the patient is stable and bleeding is not profuse, the patient may be allowed to hydrate themselves to dilute the blood in their urine and should limit physical exertion as that may exacerbate bleeding. A careful medication review for non-steroidal anti-inflammatory drugs, aspirin, antiplatelet agents, low-molecular weight heparins, warfarin, and other drugs that can potentiate bleeding is also critical. These should not be stopped until the reason for their use and the risk of withdrawing them have been carefully determined. A summary of management of gross hematuria is shown in Table 33.3.

When lower urinary tract obstruction secondary to clots occurs, a large-bore three-way catheter should be placed and the bladder aggressively hand irrigated to remove all clot. Once the clots are removed, continuous bladder irrigation (CBI) may be initiated in order to prevent further clot formation. Alternatively, the patient may be observed without CBI if the resulting urine is clear, indicating that the bleeding was self-limited. Should persistent catheter obstruction occur due to recurrent or persistent clots, a Couvelaire catheter can be used as these catheters have a larger channel through which to hand irrigate out large volumes of clots and are therefore less likely to obstruct. If these measures fail, then the patient may be taken to the operating room for clot evacuation and resection or fulguration of the bleeding source.

Once the conservative treatment of hematuria fails, there are several adjunctive treatments that may be used for protracted bleeding in the bladder. If the bleeding is from the prostate, placing a Foley catheter with a 30 cc balloon on gentle traction may be sufficient to tamponade the bleeding. Alternatively, 5-α-reductase inhibitors have been used and have been shown to be effective in reducing bleeding (32). For severe cases of prostatic bleeding, transurethral fulguration or resection of the prostate can be effective in halting the bleeding. ϵ-Aminocaproic acid, an inhibitor of fibrinolytic enzymes like plasmin, can be given intravenously at a loading dose of 5 g followed by hourly doses of 1.00 to 1.25 g. Once the patient responds, usually within 6 to 8 hours, the drug can be dosed and administered orally. Alternatively, ϵ-aminocaproic acid can be given intravesically as 200 mg/L of normal saline solution through CBI, which is continued for 24 hours after the bleeding has stopped. This approach has an observed resolution of hematuria in 91% of the cases (33). It should be employed with great caution since an increase in thromboembolic events

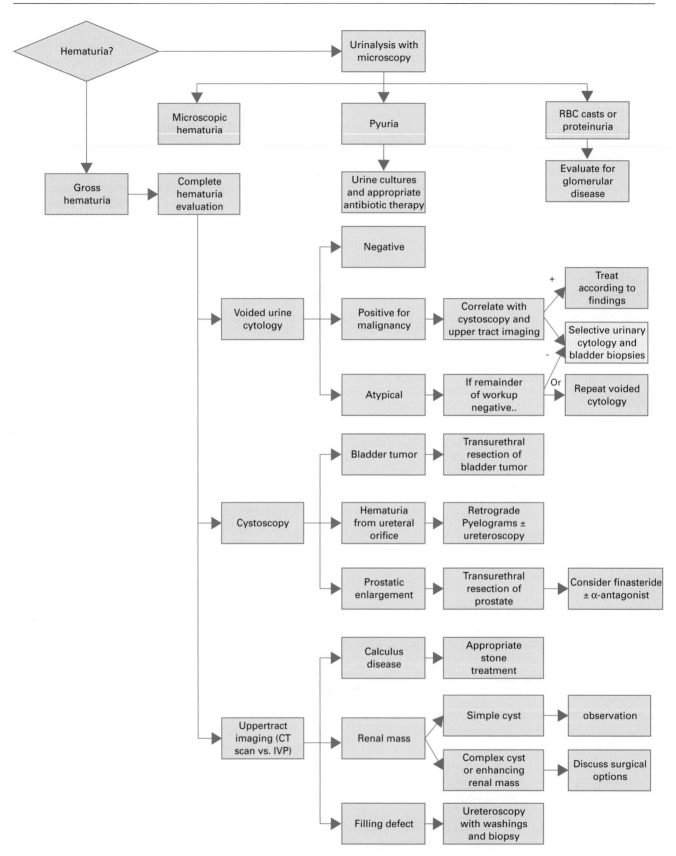

Figure 33.1. Evaluation and management of hematuria. CT, computed tomography; IVP, intravenous pyelogram. Reproduced from Kunkle et al. with permission (30).

TABLE 33.3	Management of gross hematuria

History and physical examination

Hydrate and transfuse as necessary to stabilize hemodynamics

Stop anticoagulants as necessary

If no clot retention, patient may potentially avoid having catheter placed

Three-way Foley catheter with hand irrigation +/– continuous bladder irrigation

Cystoscopy and clot evacuation +/– fulguration

Lower urinary tract bleeding

Prostate-related bleeding

   Traction on Foley catheter

   Continuous bladder irrigation

   Prostate fulguration or resection

   5-α-Reductase inhibitor may be used

Bladder-related bleeding

   Three-way Foley catheter and hand irrigation

   Continuous bladder irrigation

   Cystoscopy and clot evacuation +/– fulguration (resection as necessary)

   Intravesical agents

      Hyperbaric oxygen (best for hemorrhagic cystitis and radiation cystitis)

      May require up to 60 treatments

      70–80% improvement or resolution of bleeding

   Aminocaproic acid (0.1% intravesical)—inhibits plasmin. Contraindicated in patients with DIC

   May be given IV, PO, or intravesically

   Patient will need clot evacuation before treatment

Alum (1%)

   Promotes clotting in bladder

   Bladder should be free of clot before using

   Patient should be monitored for aluminum toxicity

   Contraindicated in patients with renal compromise

Silver nitrate (0.5–1%) precipitates protein and induces clotting

   Kept in bladder for 15 min

Formalin (1% intravesical)

   Needs cystogram to determine reflux

   Painful; anesthesia needed

   Resolution within 48 h

   Bladder function impaired after treatment

Transurethral resection and/or fulguration

   Best for discreet bleeding/bladder mass

Embolization—may manage or stop bleeding

Percutaneous nephrostomy—may divert urine and allow bleeding to tamponade

Cystectomy—for intractable bleeding

Upper tract–related bleeding

   Kidney bleeding may be embolized if discreet or vascular source of bleeding found

   Ureteral stent may allow urine to pass source of obstruction

   Ureteroscopy for identification and possible treatment of upper tract bleeding

   Percutaneous nephrostomy may allow bypass of urine into the bladder

   Nephrectomy may be required for intractable bleeding from kidney

DIC, disseminated intravascular coagulation.

has been observed and the formation of large intravesical clots is a risk when ε-aminocaproic acid is used (34).

Other intravesical agents commonly used are alum, silver nitrate, and formalin. Alum precipitates proteins and may quickly stop bleeding by forming clots at the source of bleeding. It is important to minimize clot formation in the bladder when using alum as it also forms large amorphous clots that are difficult to remove even endoscopically (35). Serum aluminum levels should be monitored in patients with renal insufficiency, as high levels may cause encephalopathy secondary to acute neurotoxicity. Treatment of acute systemic aluminum toxicity involves chelation with deferoxamine (36). An intravesical solution of 0.5% to 1.0% silver nitrate causes chemical coagulation at the bleeding sites but may also cause renal failure in patients with reflux, necessitating a pre-treatment cystogram to assess for the presence of vesicoureteral reflux (37). Formalin can also be used in cases of severe, intractable hematuria.

It permanently precipitates the bladder proteins as well as proteins in the small vessels of the bladder. This may cause fibrosis, and in some cases a small-capacity bladder. It may cause severe renal injury in patients with vesicoureteral reflux, so pre-treatment cystogram is again mandatory (38). Intravesical formalin is painful and requires general anesthesia to administer. Selective embolization of vesicle arteries by interventional radiology has been used with success in patients with severe intractable bleeding that was refractory to most other treatments (35). Hyperbaric oxygen has been used for hemorrhagic cystitis with an observed 82% response rate. However, as many as 60 treatments may be needed before the desired effect is seen and this therapy is not widely available at most institutions (39). In severe cases of hematuria originating from the bladder, a cystectomy may be necessary to stop bleeding.

Radiation cystitis is seen in as many as 8% of patients who have received radiation therapy for prostate cancer.

TABLE 33.4	Common side effects associated with androgen deprivation therapy

Early Onset	Later Onset
Hot flushes	Osteopenia/osteoporosis
Fatigue	Weight gain from increased adiposity
Erectile dysfunction/diminished libido	Loss of muscle mass
Mildly decreased cognition/memory	Elevation of serum cholesterol
QT prolongation/cardiac arrhythmia	Increased insulin resistance

The management of radiation cystitis may involve many of the treatments discussed above, as it is often recurrent and refractory. Similarly, treatment with chemotherapeutic agents such as cyclophosphamide and iphosphamide may result in hemorrhagic cystitis, a problem that may be avoided if pretreated with Mesna during chemotherapy. Careful surveillance for the presence of malignancy should be done in these patients as the bleeding may represent a secondary malignancy. Treatment of radiation cystitis and hemorrhagic cystitis secondary to chemotherapeutic agents should follow the previously described guidelines for the treatment of hematuria, being as conservative as possible yet aggressive enough to prevent clot retention and further discomfort. Hyperbaric treatment of recurrent radiation cystitis works by increasing oxygenation of the bladder mucosa and may also cause vasoconstriction, resulting in decreased hematuria and healing (39).

Management of Upper Urinary Tract Hematuria

The management of upper tract bleeding is similar to that of the lower tract bleeding. Conservative measures should be used whenever possible. However, when signs of obstruction are present, a percutaneous nephrostomy may be needed to divert the urine or a ureteral stent may be placed from below to allow drainage past the obstruction. In addition, ε-aminocaproic acid may be used for intractable bleeding; but, again, it should be used with caution as noted previously (40). Biopsy and fulguration of the area of bleeding through endoscopic means may be diagnostic as well as therapeutic. Pseudoaneurysms, arteriovenous malformations, and renal masses may be treated by embolization with good effect after identification by an arteriogram. Total nephrectomy may be needed in extreme cases.

ANDROGEN DEPRIVATION THERAPY (ADT)

Adenocarcinoma of the prostate is the most common cancer in males and has an age-dependent incidence. Some autopsy series indicate that 60% to 80% of men in their eighties will have detectable prostate cancer (41–43). Given the multiple comorbidities found in older patients, this malignancy is often managed with watchful waiting or ADT alone as the

likelihood of death resulting from prostate cancer is often quite low in this patient population (44).

Long-term treatment with ADT is associated with a variety of metabolic complications. Well-known complications of ADT include weight gain, loss of muscle mass, fatigue, decreased libido, erectile dysfunction (ED), and hot flushes. However, longer term therapy can result in more serious complications that are less well known (Table 33.4). In addition, the short- and long-term cardiovascular impact of ADT has been characterized more clearly recently and has been shown to contribute to the small but significant rate of cardiovascular mortality associated with ADT. In the setting of palliative care and supportive oncology, the impact of ADT can be quite significant and deserves careful evaluation in every patient in order to appropriately manage side effects, prevent avoidable long-term complications, and, perhaps most important, confirm the need for continued use.

Palliative Benefits of ADT

The use of ADT in advanced prostate cancer has been practiced since the seminal article by Huggins and Hodges (45) demonstrated the link between prostate cancer and androgen in 1941. The clinical benefits were widely known but had not been well quantified until the publication of the Medical Research Council randomized trial of early versus delayed ADT in locally advanced or asymptomatic metastatic disease (46). This landmark study demonstrated statistically significant improvements in pathological fractures, spinal cord compression, and ureteral obstruction favoring early initiation of ADT. This study also demonstrated a survival advantage for early treatment which was a contrary finding to the previously published Veterans Administration Cooperative Urological Research Group (VACURG) trial (47). The VACURG trial was essentially a comparison of early versus delayed ADT but it did not include the evaluation of any palliative endpoints.

The duration of therapy for most patients with metastatic disease ranges from 14 to 20 months and patients often receive continued ADT with standard luteinizing hormone–releasing hormone (LHRH) agonists or gonadotrophin-releasing hormone (GnRH) antagonists during chemotherapy even after the disease has progressed to endocrine refractory state (48,49). Thus, the long-term impact of ADT in advanced prostate cancer patients becomes increasingly relevant in the management of these patients as the disease continues to progress.

A related issue in ADT is the method by which castrate levels of testosterone are achieved (Table 33.5). The original standard treatment was bilateral simple orchiectomy. Over time, chemical castration has become the standard treatment with LHRH agonists, GnRH antagonists, and oral steroidal and non-steroidal antiandrogens (NSAAs). Studies have shown that patients prefer chemical castration over surgical castration because it is less disfiguring and can be reversed (50). The available data suggest that chemical castration is equivalent to surgical castration with respect to disease control (51,52). More recently, some data have emerged suggesting that lower testosterone levels than are typically achieved by LHRH agonists may have added benefit (53). This may explain the benefits of secondary hormonal ablative therapies such as ketoconazole which ablate not only gonadal androgens but also adrenal androgen synthesis (54,55). To that end, new agents have been developed and recently approved that more selectively target the adrenal androgen synthesis pathways (56). As such, the clinical application of these new therapies will undoubtedly prolong the duration of ADT for advanced prostate cancer patients. Consequently, the long-term impact of this therapy may potentially become even more of a clinical management dilemma as these patients live longer with the disease.

Early-Onset Adverse Effects of ADT

The most common side effect of ADT is hot flushes, which occur in as many as 80% of treated men and often significantly affect their QOL (57). This side effect is exceedingly common and bothersome but does not, by itself, have any long-term or compounded deleterious impact. A randomized controlled trial of megestrol in breast cancer and prostate cancer patients being treated with ADT showed a significant reduction in hot flushes but this is not commonly used among urologists due to concerns about impact on therapeutic efficacy since PSA levels sometimes actually increase when megestrol is added to ADT (58,59). A few small trials have evaluated antidepressant medications (selective serotonin reuptake inhibitors) for the treatment of hot flushes resulting from ADT but these data are not strong and this practice has not been widely adopted to treat this side effect (60,61).

Diminished libido is a common early-onset adverse effect of ADT. Testosterone is critical in the maintenance of a healthy libido, so the ablation of androgen production logically results in a marked decrease in sexual interest and sexual function in men treated with ADT (62). The Prostate Cancer Outcomes Study showed an increase in men reporting a total lack of sexual interest to 60% after surgical or medical castration. The incidence of severe ED was reported in over 70% of men in these groups, and the cessation of sexual activity was reported in over 80% of men (63). Of course, phosphodiesterase inhibitors (PDEi) can be used to treat ED in men who maintain sexual interest, but if the ED is secondary to diminished libido then PDEi therapy is unlikely to be successful. There are no data systematically evaluating these medications or other ED treatments in this clinical situation.

The impact of ADT on cognition and mood has recently become an area of intense study as conflicting evidence has emerged. A randomized study of men with prostate cancer who were treated with ADT compared with men who were observed demonstrated decreased attention span and memory in the patients on ADT (64). However, other studies have shown little or no deleterious impact of ADT with decreases occurring only in selected cognitive and memory domains and, in fact, subjects demonstrated some improvement in object recall (65,66). These data indicate that the effects of ADT are as much physical as cognitive with slowing of reaction times and visuomotor responses as well as decreased performance on vigilance and attention testing.

The impact of ADT on memory has been purported to result from decreased estradiol rather than decreased testosterone (67). In a study by Salminen and colleagues, cognitive decreases were significantly associated with low estradiol rather than low testosterone, and the negatively affected domains included reduced speed of number recognition and decreased visual memory of figures. However, verbal fluency actually improved over the year-long evaluation. The magnitude of the decrease of estradiol dictated the extent of the changes in cognition. Conversely, Almeida and colleagues followed patients treated with ADT for 9 months and evaluated them eight times over a 1-year period and their results revealed a paradoxical increase in verbal memory and visual memory using the Cambridge Examination for Mental Disorders of the Elderly-Cognitive Battery (CAMCO-G) (68). Given the frequency of the evaluations, this study has been criticized because patients are likely to improve over time if administered the same examination repetitively (69).

Clearly, this area of research into the cognitive impact of ADT is still evolving and the data as a whole are limited largely by small sample sizes and some conflicting results. An overall review of the available literature demonstrated that between 47% and 69% of men treated with ADT demonstrated decreased function in at least one cognitive parameter evaluated and that the affected domains were typically visuospatial capability as well as higher order cognitive skills such as problem solving, abstract concept initiation, cognitive flexibility, and self-regulation required for functional independence and social integration (69,70). Thus, the impact of ADT on cognition is subtle and the effects are not global in elderly patients. Furthermore, the impact of confounding factors such as depression has not been adequately addressed yet. Unlike the treatment for standard age-related hypogonadism, testosterone replacement is at best highly controversial and generally regarded as absolutely contraindicated in the setting of advanced prostate cancer.

TABLE 33.5   Methods to achieve androgen suppression

Method	Products	Mechanism of Action	Route of Administration	Effect on Hypothalamic–Pituitary–Gonadal Axis	Advantages	Disadvantages
Simple orchiectomy	N/A	Removal of majority of testosterone-producing tissue	Trans-scrotal surgery	↓ Testosterone ↓ Estrogens ↑ LH ↑ LHRH	Single treatment, low morbidity, inexpensive	Irreversible, psychological impact of castration
Estrogens	DES	Feedback inhibition of LH production	Oral	↓ Testosterone ↑ Estrogens ↓ LH ↓ LHRH	Inexpensive, avoids loss of bone mineral density	Increased risk of thromboembolic events, gynecomastia
LHRH agonists	Leuprolide, goserelin, triptorelin	Feedback inhibition of LHRH production	Injections or implants (subcutaneous or intramuscular)	↓ Testosterone ↓ Estrogens ↓ LH ↑ LHRH	Effective reversible testosterone suppression, longer acting depot formulation (3, 4, 6, and 12 mo)	Multiple repeat injections, expensive, induces initial testosterone surge
LHRH antagonists	Degarelix	Feedback inhibition of LHRH production	Injection (subcutaneous)	↓ Testosterone ↓ Estrogens ↓ LH ↓ LHRH	Immediate reversible testosterone suppression, no surge or flare phenomena	Multiple repeat injections required, expensive, only 1 mo depot available currently
NSAAs	Bicalutamide flutamide, nilutamide	Competitive blockade of testosterone receptor binding	Oral	↑ Testosterone ↑ Estrogens ↔ LH ↔ LHRH	Preserves libido and erectile function, preserves bone density, may prevent flare phenomenon when used in combination with LHRH agonist	Not proven equally effective as monotherapy, gynecomastia, expensive

Class	Agent	Mechanism	Route	Hormonal effects	Advantages	Comments
SAAs	Cyproterone acetate	Competitive blockade of testosterone receptor binding	Oral	↑Testosterone ↑Estrogens ↔LH ↔LHRH	Preserves libido and erectile function, preserves bone density, may prevent flare phenomenon when used in combination with LHRH agonist	Increased cardiovascular risk, may not be as effective as NSAAs, gynecomastia, expensive, not available in the USA
General adrenal androgen ablation	Ketoconazole	Non-specific blockade of androgen biosynthesis in the testis and adrenal via p450 enzymes	Oral	↓Testosterone ↓Estrogens ↑LH ↑LHRH	May be effective in patients who fail initial ADT, inexpensive, can reverse DIC associated with disseminated prostate cancer	Requires oral corticosteroids to prevent adrenal crisis
Selective adrenal androgen ablation	Abiraterone	Inhibition of CYP17A1 enzyme which converts pregnenolone and progesterone to androgen precursors	Oral	↓Testosterone ↓Estrogens ↑LH ↑LHRH	Reduces tissue and serum testosterone levels to nearly undetectable levels, shows activity in patients who have failed ADT and chemotherapy	Newly approved by the FDA, approved for use after chemotherapy, also used with corticosteroids although this may not be physiologically necessary

LH, luteinizing hormone; LHRH, luteinizing hormone—releasing hormone; DES, diethylsilbestrol; NSAA, non-steroidal antiandrogen; SAA, steroidal antiandrogen; ADT, androgen deprivation therapy; DIC, disseminated intravascular coagulation; FDA, Food and Drug Administration.

Later-Onset Adverse Effects of ADT

The long-term use of ADT results in significant decreases in bone mineral density (BMD) compared with men not receiving ADT. The data from a number of prospective trials have demonstrated that this loss of BMD is substantially greater than that seen in menopausal women (71). The cumulative loss of BMD over the first year of therapy is so significant that men receiving ADT are at higher risk for skeletal fractures. This risk appears to increase in proportion with the number of doses of ADT received (72). The loss of BMD can be treated with bisphosphonate therapy, which prevents additional bone loss but has not been demonstrated to prevent fractures. The Food and Drug Administration recently approved the use of denosumab, a monoclonal antibody against RANK (receptor activator of nuclear factor κ-B) ligand, which has been shown in prospective randomized trials to prevent not only loss of BMD but also skeletal-related events compared with intravenous bisphosphonate therapy (73,74). The National Osteoporosis Foundation recommends pre-treatment assessment of osteoporotic fracture risk using the World Health Organization Fracture Risk Assessment (FRAX) calculator. The FRAX score includes risk factors such as family history of osteoporosis, smoking, glucocorticoid use, low vitamin D levels, low body weight, and history of prior fractures. This calculator has been shown to identify more men at high risk for skeletal-related events than traditional assessments that rely primarily on DEXA (dual energy x-ray absorptiometry) scan results (75).

Cardiovascular Impact of ADT

The use of ADT in advanced prostate cancer has been the standard of care for many years, and the primacy of cardiovascular mortality among causes of death in the United States has long been known (76–79). However, ADT has recently been associated with an increased risk of coronary artery disease, myocardial infarction, and sudden cardiac death (80). A SEER (Surveillance, Epidemiology, and End Results) database analysis also revealed that men who were treated with ADT had a 20% increased risk of cardiovascular morbidity (81). In fact, cardiovascular mortality is the most common noncancer cause of death for men with prostate cancer (82,83).

The adverse impact of hypogonadal levels of testosterone on coronary artery disease may be due to increased arterial rigidity (84). Testosterone replacement therapy has been shown to improve the symptoms of acute angina pectoris as well as have beneficial effects on myocardial infarction (85). Other studies have shown that testosterone supplementation has beneficial effect on exercise-induced cardiac ischemia (86,87). Given the anabolic characteristics of testosterone and the predominantly muscular composition of the heart, it logically stands to reason that ADT may result in some measure of cardiac dysfunction.

Most recently, a population-based analysis of patients with newly diagnosed prostate cancer registered in the United

Kingdom's General Practice Research Database revealed an increased risk of cerebrovascular accidents (CVAs) and transient ischemic attacks (TIAs) for patients treated with ADT (88). This database study included 15,375 men who received ADT during the follow-up period of 3 years, and preexisting cardiovascular risk factors at baseline did not alter the correlation between ADT and CVA/TIA risk. Interestingly, patients under 65 or older than 75 years of age appeared to be at a higher risk for CVA/TIA than the intermediate cohort of 65 to 75 years old. These data are similar to the findings of two previously published studies evaluating the risk of ADT and CVA (89,90). However, two other reports suggest that the association between ADT and CVA is weak or non-existent. A published study from the Longitudinal Health Insurance Database in Taiwan did not demonstrate any increased risk of CVA in patients with prostate cancer treated with ADT (91). This study may be limited by smaller numbers ($n = 365$) compared with the larger database analyses but the 1.7% difference found between the groups in this analysis is not likely to be clinically significant regardless of the power of the study. The other report suggesting no correlation between ADT and CVA did not suffer from a small sample size ($n = 19,079$), but this evaluation of the Ontario Cancer Registry may have had a selection bias that could have influenced the findings (88,92,93).

The available data suggest that ADT may have an impact on cardiovascular and cerebrovascular function, but it is evident that the degree of impact is yet to be clearly defined. Furthermore, the physiological mechanisms for this increased risk are also unclear, so the appropriate tests to identify patients at high risk for these life-threatening outcomes have not been identified nor have the appropriate preventive measures been definitively elucidated.

Metabolic Impact of ADT

Recent research has revealed that hypogonadal levels of testosterone leads to a metabolic syndrome characterized by increasing insulin resistance (94,95). This phenomenon appears to occur peripherally rather than as a direct effect on the islet cells of the pancreas. Other associated metabolic abnormalities include hypertriglyceridemia, hypercholesterolemia, hypertension, and obesity. The definition for classic metabolic syndrome includes any three of the following diagnostic findings: blood pressure ≥ 130/85 mm Hg, waist circumference > 102 cm, triglycerides ≥ 150 mg/100 mL, high-density lipoproteins < 40 mg/100 mL, and fasting glucose ≥ 110 mg/100 mL (96). Given the association of many of these criteria with advancing age in Western society, many men with prostate cancer may meet the definition of classic metabolic syndrome prior to starting ADT. However, these criteria can be markedly worsened by the initiation of ADT. In addition, the metabolic syndrome associated with ADT has some distinct differences relative to the definition of classic metabolic syndrome. Table 33.6 outlines the criteria for diagnosing ADT-induced metabolic syndrome in men in comparison to the findings of classic metabolic syndrome.

TABLE 33.6	Characteristics of ADT-induced metabolic syndrome compared to classic metabolic syndrome	
	ADT-Induced Metabolic Syndrome	**Classic Metabolic Syndrome**
Blood pressure	↔	↑
Waist circumference	↑	↑
Ratio of waist–hip measurements	↔	↑
Triglycerides	↑	↑
High-density lipoprotein	↓	↑
Fasting glucose	↑	↑
Fat accumulation	Truncal, subcutaneous	Internal, visceral

Interestingly, men who are already taking cholesterol-lowering medications such as statins still demonstrate negative changes in their lipid profiles after starting ADT (97). Other studies have demonstrated that ADT worsens insulin resistance, which has been correlated with cardiovascular mortality (81).

Therefore, in this patient population with many preexisting comorbidities that may be exacerbated by the initiation of ADT, it is imperative to establish a baseline for these parameters prior to starting ADT, and continuous regular monitoring of these factors over time is important to detect and treat the onset of ADT-induced metabolic syndrome. Furthermore, a recently completed randomized controlled trial demonstrated significant improvements in abdominal girth measurements, weight, body mass index, and systolic blood pressure for men treated with ADT who were concomitantly started on an exercise program compared with men who received ADT alone (98). Therefore, several parameters that define metabolic syndrome can be influenced by lifestyle changes that incorporate regular physical activity.

QOL Impact of ADT

The general perception among urologists regarding how patients tolerate ADT is that it minimally impacts QOL for most patients. However, when this issue was studied, the data suggest that patients on ADT have statistically significantly decreased physical function and general health (99). In this evaluation of 96 men, there were no significant differences between men on ADT for less than 6 months and those on ADT for longer than 6 months. There were no differences between men on ADT and healthy controls with respect to the mental health component, but men on ADT scored significantly lower in physical functioning and general health. Total testosterone was significantly associated the physical health component with lower testosterone levels corresponding with lower physical health component scores, whereas pre-existing comorbidities understandably correlated inversely

with physical health component summary score. These data are somewhat in contrast with other data which suggest that ADT has negative effect not only on physical functioning but also on emotional and overall QOL measures as well. In men with locally advanced prostate cancer, ADT was shown to lower overall QOL scores and increase emotional distress compared with delayed treatment (100).

An earlier evaluation of the QOL effect of ADT enrolled over 700 patients with advanced prostate cancer in a QOL survey protocol that was administered at 1, 3, and 6 months after ADT was started (101). The comparison groups were ADT with simple orchiectomy plus flutamide, an NSAA, or placebo. Response rates were in excess of 80% for the entire study, and interestingly, the expected difference in body image between the two groups was not noted despite higher incidence of gynecomastia in the flutamide group. In general, the addition of flutamide produced a negative QOL difference between the groups with respect to treatment-specific symptoms such as diarrhea as well as physical and emotional functioning. These data indicate that the QOL impact of combined androgen blockade, whether it is with LHRH agonist and NSAA or with orchiectomy and NSAA, has a greater impact on QOL than monotherapy. Therefore, it is important not only to discuss the potential impact of ADT on QOL with patients but also to note that the different types of ADT may have different impacts on QOL.

ERECTILE DYSFUNCTION

The issue of sexual function in elderly men was not a major focus of urologists and gerontologists until the last four or five decades when men began living substantially longer. Even after the average life expectancy exceeded 70 years, a common misperception was that ED was part of the normal aging process. As a result, very little effort was expended on characterizing and treating sexual dysfunction in geriatric populations. However, with the advent of geriatric medicine as a specific discipline and with improvements in overall medical care, the performance status and physiologic condition of many elder men have improved and a greater proportion of elderly men desire continued sexual activity throughout their life span. Furthermore, the proportion of men older than 65 years of age is expected to more than double by 2025 (102). As a result, more interest and resources are being focused on the prevention and treatment of ED in the elderly. The classic definition of ED is persistent and recurrent difficulty to achieve and/or maintain an erection adequate for the completion of intercourse (103).

ED is not a single complaint but is a spectrum of dysfunctions that can be somewhat difficult to quantify. The Massachusetts Male Aging Study provided data on the effect of advancing age on sexual function as well as other health-related QOL measures. In this report, ED was characterized as minimal, moderate, or complete, and the prevalence of ED varied dramatically depending on the definition. For all three degrees of ED, the prevalence was over 50% for the entire cohort of men (aged 40 to 70) but the prevalence of complete ED was only 5% in the youngest group and 15% in the oldest set, indicating that the incidence and prevalence of severe ED are far less common than lesser degrees (104).

Diagnosing ED

Given the multifactorial nature of ED (Table 33.7), a broad evaluation of a patient presenting with ED is mandatory. A complete medical, sexual, and psychosocial history should be obtained in order to identify the specific erectile problem (i.e., difficulty maintaining an erection vs. difficulty achieving an erection vs. lack of interest in sex) as well as recognize reversible contributing comorbidities such as metabolic syndrome, hypogonadism, diabetes, or obesity. In addition, it is very important that the patient clearly expresses his expectations and values so that a satisfactory, patient-centered treatment plan can be implemented.

A complete medication list is critical to the assessment of ED because many commonly used drugs can cause or worsen ED. Furthermore, drug interactions between commonly used cardiac medications and ED medications can be life threatening. Specifically, nitrate-based medications such as nitroglycerine or isosorbide dinitrate are specifically contraindicated with the use of phosphodiesterase 5 inhibitors (PDE5i) due to a resulting severe refractory hypotension that is extremely difficult to treat (105). While this class of interactions is well known, many others are less well known, which emphasizes the importance of a complete and thorough documentation of all medications (prescription and over-the-counter), supplements, and herbal preparations being used. In addition, the presence of antidepressants may contribute to complaints of anorgasmia, whereas new prescriptions or increases in antihypertensive medications may unmask or exacerbate subclinical ED.

A detailed sexual history should include information about the onset of ED, alleviating and aggravating factors as well as emotional and physical status of the patient, the patient's sexual partner(s), and the exact complaint. The patient should clearly describe the physical factors associated with ED, including presence or absence of nocturnal erections, rigidity of erections, and differences in erections with sexual arousal, masturbation, and nocturnal erections. The

TABLE 33.7	Common risk factors for erectile dysfunction and atherosclerosis
Erectile Dysfunction	**Atherosclerosis**
Hypogonadism	Hypertension
Diabetes mellitus	Diabetes mellitus
Atherosclerosis/hyperlipidemia	Hyperlipidemia *(elevated triglycerides and low-density lipoproteins)*
Obesity	Obesity
Advanced age	Advanced age *(>45 y of age)*
Cigarette smoking/alcohol use	Cigarette smoking
Physical deconditioning	Physical deconditioning
Depression	Family history *(father or brother diagnosed younger than 55 y)*
Medications/drugs	Low high-density lipoproteins
Spinal cord injury	Gender *(male > female)*
Prostate surgery	Erectile dysfunction

interpersonal impact of ED is significant and this information should be obtained not only from the patient but also from the patient's sexual partner, as sexual satisfaction of both parties is often an important factor in seeking medical advice. Furthermore, the perception of the contributing factors may differ substantially between the patient and his partner. Consequently, open dialogue between the patient and his partner is an important part of the diagnosis and treatment of ED, and it is the role of the treating physician to facilitate that aspect as well.

In order to quantify baseline erectile function as well as to assess the efficacy of any treatments, standardized measurement tools such as the Sexual Health Inventory for Men are extremely helpful for the physician and the patient. The questionnaire is a useful adjunct to a thorough history but it does not provide enough detail to be the sole evaluation initially or in follow-up.

The typical portions of a complete history have significance in the evaluation of ED, in particular, the past surgical history can be extremely informative given the prevalence of prostate interventions among elderly men. ED can be a side effect after prostatectomy performed for prostate cancer but ED can also develop after multiple prostate biopsies intended to diagnose prostate cancer (106–108). Furthermore, surgeries for benign prostate disease such as TURP may also be associated with ED as well (109).

The performance of a complete physical examination is important in the evaluation of ED, but it rarely reveals the cause of ED. Rather the physical examination often provides a myriad of clues, suggesting the contributing medical disorders that manifest as ED. The general evaluation must include cardiovascular, neurologic, and metabolic assessments with particular focus on the genitourinary examination. Careful inspection for secondary sex characteristics and testicular size may suggest the presence of hypogonadism. Physical examination may reveal genital abnormalities both physical (i.e., Peyronie's disease) and neurologic (i.e., decreased penile sensation or 'absent bulbocavernosal reflex) that may be the primary cause of the ED.

Laboratory evaluation must include fasting glucose, lipid profile, and hormonal levels in order to identify the presence of androgen deficiency, metabolic syndrome, or diabetes. There is virtually no role for imaging modalities in the initial evaluation of ED. A penile duplex ultrasound to evaluate cavernosal blood flow is a useful study but is typically utilized by specialists after initial treatments are unsuccessful. More invasive studies such as infusion cavernosometry, arteriography, and neurophysiologic testing are rarely indicated in the geriatric population.

Medical Treatment of ED

Detailed counseling of patients is necessary not only to educate the patient and his partner as to the cause of the ED but also to establish realistic expectations with respect to the effectiveness of any treatment program. For example, in most elderly patients, ED is due to a constellation of contributing comorbidities and, therefore, the patient needs to be clearly informed that oral medical therapy may improve the symptom of ED somewhat but that oral medications are unlikely to produce the rigid erections of his youth. In addition, the physician should address other forms of sexual activity that do not rely upon penetrative sexual intercourse in the context of both partners' sexual satisfaction and the limitations of the patient's overall physical condition. This portion of the counseling may be uncomfortable for the physician and the patient but, given the link between sexual satisfaction and mental health, if the patient can accept the fact that sexual satisfaction can be achieved with alternative forms of intimacy, then improvements in overall mental health may occur as well (110). A detailed discussion of the various treatments for ED should be undertaken and the choice of treatment should be made by the patient in conjunction with his partner. Table 33.8 outlines the pharmacologic and mechanical treatment choices for patients with ED. In addition, continued observation should be offered as an option and the patient should be informed that spontaneous remission of ED does occur in a small percentage of patients who are followed expectantly without intervention (111).

Lifestyle modification can have beneficial effects on ED and patients should be strongly encouraged to implement durable changes to not only improve their erections but also lower their risk of cardiovascular disease in the future. The addition of statin medication has been shown to improve ED and should be considered for men with elevated cholesterol and ED. Many antihypertensive medications may induce or exacerbate ED and consideration of changing types of medications may improve ED. Specifically, thiazide diuretics as well as α- and β-blockers have been implicated in the worsening of ED. While depression can cause ED, tricyclic antidepressants can also induce diminished libido and orgasmic dysfunction in addition to classic ED (112,113). Thus, a discussion with the prescribing physician about a change in the class of drug may be helpful in improving ED in a patient on these medications. For example, calcium channel blockers, angiotensin receptor blockers, and angiotensin-converting enzyme inhibitors may improve ED while maintaining hypertensive control. Alternatively, changing from a non-specific α-blocker to a subtype-specific α-blocker such as doxazosin or tamsulosin may minimize the ED-inducing potential of α-blockade for the treatment of hypertension or benign prostatic hyperplasia. Finally, polypharmacy is a major problem among the geriatric population, and a review of medications with the intent of discontinuing non-essential medications may have broadly beneficial effects over and above any improvement in ED that may result.

Pharmacotherapy for ED has improved recently with the development of selective PDE5i. These drugs are analogs of cyclic guanosine monophosphate (cGMP) that competitively bind to the PDE5 enzyme. This slows the degradation of cGMP, thereby prolonging smooth muscle relaxation in the cavernous arteries (114). While these medications have been wildly successful physiologically and commercially, their mechanism of action is dependent upon endogenous production of nitric oxide (NO) which is impaired not only by

TABLE 33.8 Erectile dysfunction treatment options

Category	Products	Mechanism of Action	Route of Administration	Advantages	Disadvantages
Phosphodiesterase 5 inhibitors	Sildenafil Vardenafil Tadalafil	Inhibits degradation of cGMP, promoting smooth muscle relaxation and penile blood flow	Oral	Oral administration, effective, available on demand	Expensive, headaches, facial flushing, nasal congestion, myalgia, back pain, visual changes, requires intact neurovascular pathways
Injectable medication	Caverject Tri-Mix	Vasodilatation of cavernous arteries	Injection	Immediate onset, not dependent on intact nerve function	Injection into penis difficult for patients psychologically, local pain or bruising/hematoma at injection site, expensive, not spontaneous
Transurethral medication	MUSE	Vasodilatation of cavernous arteries through absorption of medication	Intraurethral suppository	Immediate onset, not dependent on intact nerve function, no injection/needles	Urethral burning or discomfort, expensive, variable absorption, not spontaneous
External mechanical	Vacuum erection device, Actis band	Negative pressure draws venous blood into corpora cavernosa, restriction band prevents outflow	External application of device	No medication interactions, not dependent on intact nerve function, no refractory period	Cumbersome equipment, not spontaneous, low rate of continued usage over time
Internal mechanical	Penile prosthesis	Surgically implanted device that can achieve rigidity through inflation or malleable rods	Surgical implantation of device	Erection on demand, very high satisfaction rate, not dependent on intact nerves	Surgical intervention, expensive, irreversible, risk of infection of prosthetic materials requiring explantation

cGMP, cyclic guanosine monophosphate.

advancing age but also by the numerous comorbidities discussed previously. As such, these medications demonstrate decreasing efficacy with increasing age (114). However, due to their relative ease of use and demonstrable clinical safety, these medications are unquestionably the first-line treatment option for men in whom no contraindication exists (115).

Patient education is critical to the successful use of PDE5i medications because sexual stimulation is absolutely required and the efficacy may be affected by factors such as alcohol and food consumption. The success rates with these medications are in excess of 60% for first-time users applying on-demand therapeutic regimens; and up to 50% of non-responders can be converted to responders with adequate counseling of the patient and his partner (116,117). In men for whom episodic dosing is ineffective, a low-dose daily regimen may be beneficial (118,119). And for men with clinical hypogonadism and no contraindication to testosterone supplementation, the effectiveness of PDE5i therapy may be improved with concomitant testosterone replacement because this enhances endogenous NO production (120). The side effects for this class of medication include facial flushing, headaches, nasal congestion, muscle aches, and back pain. Visual changes may occur frequently as well due to the presence of phosphodiesterase 6 in the retina.

Apomorphine SL is a sublingual preparation of a nonselective dopamine agonist and acts centrally to promote erectogenic signals. This is absorbed quickly and the majority of patients are able to achieve erections in 20 minutes. Common side effects are headache, nausea, and dizziness and these are so frequent that clinical utility of this compound is limited. The advantage of this therapy is that no interaction with nitrates exists, so apomorphine is considered frontline oral therapy in patients who are healthy enough for sexual activity but take nitrates for chest pain or hypertension (121).

Prior to the advent of PDE5i therapy, vasoactive compounds were the primary medical therapy for ED; these medications are now the primary non-surgical treatment options for patients in whom PDE5i therapy fails or is contraindicated. The efficacy and safety profiles of these agents are excellent and the onset of action is rapid. Prostaglandin E1 (PGE1) and papaverine induce vasodilatation as a result of cGMP- and cyclic adenosine monophosphate (cAMP)-mediated arterial smooth muscle relaxation. The other medication commonly used is phentolamine, which blocks sympathetic vasoconstriction signals. Endogenous NO production does not affect the efficacy of these medications, which is why these drugs are effective in men for whom PDE5i medications are unsuccessful. Each of these medications can be administered via intracavernosal injection and PGE1 can also be given as an intraurethral suppository. The duration of erection is dose dependent but the onset of erection is typically within a few minutes. Priapism, defined as an erection lasting longer than 4 hours, is a significant side effect and requires immediate medical attention to prevent penile fibrosis. Injection site reactions such as pain or bruising are common and penile fibrosis may develop over time with prolonged use. Intraurethral suppositories of PGE1

may also cause hypotension, dizziness, syncope, urethrodynia, and genital irritation in the partner. Satisfaction rates for this therapy are very high but a bleeding disorder and a history of priapism are relative contraindications for use.

The vacuum erection device (VED) is a mechanical apparatus designed to create negative pressure within a cylinder placed around the penis. This negative pressure draws venous blood into the corpora cavernosa, resulting in the passive generation of an erection. A constriction band is placed around the penile shaft at the penopubic junction to prevent outflow and allow maintenance of the erection. This mechanism is extremely effective with usable erections in nearly 9 out of 10 men, but it is cumbersome and produces an erection that many patients find unnatural (117). Since the erection is from venous blood and the constriction band limits penile blood flow, the penis appears cyanotic and is cool to the touch and there is a fulcrum at the constriction band with a rigid penis distal to the band and flaccid penis proximal which alters functionality somewhat as well (122). Side effects are minimal and limited primarily to local bruising and anejaculation due to mechanical obstruction; but patients must be instructed to remove the constriction band as soon as possible or within 30 minutes to prevent permanent damage, including penile necrosis. Patients with bleeding diatheses or on anticoagulation therapy should use the VED with caution (121).

For patients with an excessive venous outflow but normal or slightly low arterial inflow, a condition known as a "venous leak," the use of a constriction band alone may allow for usable erections. These patients typically present with the primary complaint of early loss of erection, often during intercourse. The constriction band is available alone without having to purchase the entire VED and is far less cumbersome than the VED. The clinical diagnosis of venous leak is made after a penile Doppler ultrasound study has been performed and interpreted by a specialist, but since the constriction band is non-invasive and inexpensive, it is reasonable to try this based upon a clinical history that is consistent with venous leak.

Surgical Treatment of ED

Surgical treatments of ED should be reserved for patients who are healthy enough for sexual activity and have failed medical therapy. Penile prostheses may be inflatable or malleable. Malleable or semi-rigid prostheses are implanted into the cavernosa and have enough rigidity to facilitate penetrative intercourse. These devices can be bent downward when not in use and simply straightened when needed. This model is ideal for patients with limited manual dexterity and the implant can be placed under local anesthetic. Inflatable prostheses are, in general, the primary choice for surgeons and consist of a pump placed into the scrotum and an inflatable cylinder inserted into each cavernosal space. An erection is produced by squeezing the scrotal pump mechanism and a release valve on the pump deflates the cylinders once penile rigidity is no longer desired. Patient satisfaction rates are extremely high, in excess of 90% for patients and their partners (122). Detailed counseling prior to implantation of a penile prosthesis is critical in order to manage patient and partner expectations and minimizes subsequent dissatisfaction.

Complication rates are low but can be quite significant when they do occur. Infection rates are typically <2%, and newer prosthesis materials have been imbedded with antibiotics and other novel coatings to further decrease this risk. Another potential complication of the inflatable prosthesis is autoinflation due to increased pressure or fibrosis around the reservoir or pump valve failure, both of which may require surgical revision to correct. Patients may also complain of loss of penile length with full erection which may be due to long-standing preexisting intracorporal fibrosis, Peyronie's disease, or the fact that only the penile shaft is rigid with an inflatable penile prosthesis so glans engorgement typically does not occur resulting in the perception of lost length. These complaints can generally be addressed and mitigated preoperatively with adequate counseling from the surgeon. Overall, nearly 60% of men will still have a functional prosthesis in place 15 years after initial implantation (122).

CONCLUSION

Early palliative care and supportive oncology can provide significant benefits to patients and their families. The genitourinary system can be affected by multiple malignant and benign disease processes and their treatments. A thorough medical history and physical examination combined with an appropriate laboratory evaluation, judicious imaging, and early urology consultation can help maximize patient QOL and survival.

ACKNOWLEDGMENTS

This research was funded by the Intramural Research Program of the NIH, National Cancer Institute, Center for Cancer Research.

REFERENCES

1. Siegel R, Naishadham D, Jemal A. Cancer statistics, 2012. *CA Cancer J Clin.* 2012;62(1):10-29.
2. Dunn GP, Martensen R, Weissman D, eds. *Surgical Palliative Care: A Resident's Guide.* Chicago, IL: American College of Surgeons; 2009:278.
3. Association AU. Clinical ethics for urologists. 2008 (cited 2011 September 26). http://www.auanet.org/eforms/cme/modules.cfm?ID=407
4. EPEC. Education in palliative and end-of-life care for oncology. 2011 (cited October 17, 2011). http://epec.net/epec_oncology.php
5. Temel JS, Greer JA, Muzikansky A, et al. Early palliative care for patients with metastatic non-small-cell lung cancer. *N Engl J Med.* 2010;363(8):733-742.
6. Bakitas M, Lyons KD, Hegel MT, et al. Effects of a palliative care intervention on clinical outcomes in patients with advanced cancer: the project enable ii randomized controlled trial. *JAMA.* 2009;302(7):741-749.
7. Hofmann B, Haheim LL, Soreide JA. Ethics of palliative surgery in patients with cancer. *Br J Surg.* 2005;92(7):802-809.
8. Kwok AC, Semel ME, Lipsitz SR, et al. The intensity and variation of surgical care at the end of life: a retrospective cohort study. *Lancet.* 2011;378:1408-1413.
9. Demme RA, Singer EA, Greenlaw J, et al. Ethical issues in palliative care. *Anesthesiol Clin.* 2006;24(1):129-144.
10. O'Donoghue PM, McSweeney SE, Jhaveri K. Genitourinary imaging: current and emerging applications. *J Postgrad Med.* 2010;56(2):131-139.
11. Choyke PL, Walther MM, Wagner JR, Rayford W, Lyne JC, Linehan WM. Renal cancer: preoperative evaluation with dual-phase three-dimensional MR angiography. *Radiology.* 1997;205:767-771.
12. Chung SY, Stein RJ, Landsittel D, et al. 15-Year experience with the management of extrinsic ureteral obstruction with indwelling ureteral stents. *J Urol.* 2004;172(2):592-595.
13. Liatsikos E, Kallidonis P, Kyriazis I, et al. Ureteral obstruction: is the full metallic double-pigtail stent the way to go? *Eur Urol.* 2010;57(3):480-486.
14. Agrawal S, Brown CT, Bellamy EA, et al. The thermo-expandable metallic ureteric stent: an 11-year follow-up. *BJU Int.* 2009;103(3):372-376.
15. Ku JH, Lee SW, Jeon HG, et al. Percutaneous nephrostomy versus indwelling ureteral stents in the management of extrinsic ureteral obstruction in advanced malignancies: are there differences? *Urology.* 2004;64(5):895-899.
16. Montvilas P, Solvig J, Johansen TE. Single-centre review of radiologically guided percutaneous nephrostomy using "mixed" technique: success and complication rates. *Eur J Radiol.* 2011;80:553-538.
17. Kouba E, Wallen EM, Pruthi RS. Management of ureteral obstruction due to advanced malignancy: optimizing therapeutic and palliative outcomes. *J Urol.* 2008;180(2):444-450.
18. Boustead GB, Feneley MR. Pelvic exenterative surgery for palliation of malignant disease in the robotic era. *Clin Oncol (R Coll Radiol).* 2010;22(9):740-746.
19. McConnell J, Roehrborn CG, Bautista OM, et al. The long-term effect of doxazosin, finasteride, and combination therapy on the clinical progression of benign prostatic hyperplasia. *N Engl J Med.* 2003;349(25):2387-2398.
20. Djavan B, Margreiter M, Dianat SS. An algorithm for medical management in male lower urinary tract symptoms. *Curr Opin Urol.* 2011;21(1):5-12.
21. Sima C, Panageas KS, Schrag D. Cancer screening among patients with advanced cancer. *J Am Med Assoc.* 2010;304(14):1584-1591.
22. Lapides J, Diokno AC, Silber SJ, et al. Clean, intermittent self-catheterization in the treatment of urinary tract disease. *Trans Am Assoc Genitourin Surg.* 1971;63:92-96.
23. Trautner BW, Darouiche RO. Role of biofilm in catheter-associated urinary tract infection. *Am J Infect Control.* 2004;32(3):177-183.
24. Fitzpatrick J. Minimally invasive and endoscopic management of benign prostatic hyperplasia. In: Wein AJ, ed. *Campbell-Walsh Urology.* 10th ed. Philadelphia, PA: Saunders Elsevier; 2010:2655-2694;chap 93.
25. Marszalek M, Ponholzer A, Rauchenwald M, et al. Palliative transurethral resection of the prostate: functional outcome and impact on survival. *BJU Int.* 2007;99(1):56-59.
26. Gravas S, Bachmann A, Reich O, et al. Critical review of lasers in benign prostatic hyperplasia (bph). *BJU Int.* 2011;107(7):1030-1043.

27. Woo HH, Hossack TA. Photoselective vaporization of the prostate with the 120-w lithium triborate laser in men taking coumadin. *Urology.* 2011;78(1):142-145.

28. Grossfeld GD, Wolf JS Jr, Litwan MS, et al. Asymptomatic microscopic hematuria in adults: summary of the AUA best practice policy recommendations. *Am Fam Physician.* 2001;63(6):1145-1154.

29. Avidor Y, Nadu A, Matzkin H. Clinical significance of gross hematuria and its evaluation in patients receiving anticoagulant and aspirin treatment. *Urology.* 2000;55(1):22-24.

30. Kunkle DA, Hirshberg SJ, Greenberg RE. Urologic issues in palliative care. In: Berger AM, Shuster JL Jr, Von Roenn JH, eds. *Principles and Practice of Palliative Care and Supportive Oncology.* Baltimore, MD: Lippincott Williams & Wilkins; 2007:357-370.

31. Grossfeld GD, Litwin MS, Wolf JS Jr, et al. Evaluation of asymptomatic microscopic hematuria in adults: the American urological association best practice policy – part ii: patient evaluation, cytology, voided markers, imaging, cystoscopy, nephrology evaluation, and follow-up. *Urology.* 2001;57(4):604-610.

32. Foley SJ, Soloman LZ, Wedderburn AW, et al. A prospective study of the natural history of hematuria associated with benign prostatic hyperplasia and the effect of finasteride. *J Urol.* 2000;163(2):496-498.

33. Singh I, Laungani GB. Intravesical epsilon aminocaproic acid in management of intractable bladder hemorrhage. *Urology.* 1992;40(3):227-229.

34. Gralnick HR, Greipp P. Thrombosis with epsilon aminocaproic acid therapy. *Am J Clin Pathol.* 1971;56(2):151-154.

35. Choong SK, Walkden M, Kirby R. The management of intractable haematuria. *BJU Int.* 2000;86(9):951-959.

36. Perazella M, Brown E. Acute aluminum toxicity and alum bladder irrigation in patients with renal failure. *Am J Kidney Dis.* 1993;21(1):44-46.

37. Raghavaiah NV, Soloway MS. Anuria following silver nitrate irrigation for intractable bladder hemorrhage. *J Urol.* 1977;118(4):681-682.

38. Rastinehad AR, Ost MC, VanderBrink BA, et al. Persistent prostatic hematuria. *Nat Clin Pract Urol.* 2008;5(3):159-165.

39. Corman JM, McClure D, Pritchett R, et al. Treatment of radiation induced hemorrhagic cystitis with hyperbaric oxygen. *J Urol.* 2003;169(6):2200-2202.

40. Kaye JD, Smith EA, Kirsch AJ, et al. Preliminary experience with epsilon aminocaproic acid for treatment of intractable upper tract hematuria in children with hematological disorders. *J Urol.* 2010;184(3):1152-1157.

41. Soos G, Tsakiris I, Szanto J, et al. The prevalence of prostate carcinoma and its precursor in Hungary: an autopsy study. *Eur Urol.* 2005;48(5):739-744.

42. Stemmermann GN, Nomura AM, Chyou PH, et al. A prospective comparison of prostate cancer at autopsy and as a clinical event: the Hawaii Japanese experience. *Cancer Epidemiol Biomarkers Prev.* 1992;1(3):189-193.

43. Rullis I, Shaeffer JA, Lilien OM. Incidence of prostatic carcinoma in the elderly. *Urology.* 1975;6(3):295-297.

44. Borre M, Erichsen R, Lund L, et al. Survival of prostate cancer patients in central and northern Denmark, 1998-2009. *Clin Epidemiol.* 2011;3(suppl 1):41-46.

45. Huggins C, Hodges C. Studies on prostate cancer. I. *Cancer Res.* 1941;1:293-297.

46. Immediate versus deferred treatment for advanced prostatic cancer: initial results of the medical research council trial. The Medical Research Council Prostate Cancer Working Party Investigators Group. *Br J Urol.* 1997;79(2):235-246.

47. Byar DP. Proceedings: the Veterans Administration Cooperative Urological Research Group's studies of cancer of the prostate. *Cancer.* 1973;32(5):1126-1130.

48. Crawford ED, Eisenberger MA, McLeod DG, et al. A controlled trial of leuprolide with and without flutamide in prostatic carcinoma. *N Engl J Med.* 1989;321(7):419-424.

49. Eisenberger MA, Blumenstein BA, Crawford ED, et al. Bilateral orchiectomy with or without flutamide for metastatic prostate cancer. *N Engl J Med.* 1998;339(15):1036-1042.

50. Nyman CR, Andersen JT, Lodding P, et al. The patient's choice of androgen-deprivation therapy in locally advanced prostate cancer: bicalutamide, a gonadotrophin-releasing hormone analogue or orchidectomy. *BJU Int.* 2005;96(7):1014-1018.

51. Seidenfeld J, Samson DJ, Hasselblad V, et al. Single-therapy androgen suppression in men with advanced prostate cancer: a systematic review and meta-analysis. *Ann Intern Med.* 2000;132(7):566-577.

52. Novara G, Galfano A, Secco S, et al. Impact of surgical and medical castration on serum testosterone level in prostate cancer patients. *Urol Int.* 2009;82(3):249-255.

53. Morote J, Orsola A, Planas J, et al. Redefining clinically significant castration levels in patients with prostate cancer receiving continuous androgen deprivation therapy. *J Urol.* 2007;178 (4 pt 1):1290-1295.

54. Small EJ, Baron AD, Fippin L, et al. Ketoconazole retains activity in advanced prostate cancer patients with progression despite flutamide withdrawal. *J Urol.* 1997;157(4):1204-1207.

55. Millikan R, Baez L, Banerjee T, et al. Randomized phase 2 trial of ketoconazole and ketoconazole/doxorubicin in androgen independent prostate cancer. *Urol Oncol.* 2001;6(3): 111-115.

56. Thompson CA. FDA approves prostate cancer treatment that inhibits testosterone synthesis. *Am J Health Syst Pharm.* 2011;68(11):960.

57. Holzbeierlein JM, McLaughlin MD, Thrasher JB. Complications of androgen deprivation therapy for prostate cancer. *Curr Opin Urol.* 2004;14(3):177-183.

58. Loprinzi CL, Michalak JC, Quella SK, et al. Megestrol acetate for the prevention of hot flashes. *N Engl J Med.* 1994;331(6):347-352.

59. Dawson NA, McLeod DG. Dramatic prostate specific antigen decrease in response to discontinuation of megestrol acetate in advanced prostate cancer: expansion of the antiandrogen withdrawal syndrome. *J Urol.* 1995;153(6):1946-1947.

60. Quella SK, Loprinzi CL, Sloan J, et al. Pilot evaluation of venlafaxine for the treatment of hot flashes in men undergoing androgen ablation therapy for prostate cancer. *J Urol.* 1999;162(1):98-102.

61. Loprinzi CL, Barton DL, Carpenter LA, et al. Pilot evaluation of paroxetine for treating hot flashes in men. *Mayo Clin Proc.* 2004;79(10):1247-1251.

62. Fowler FJ Jr, McNaughton Collins M, Walker Corkery E, et al. The impact of androgen deprivation on quality of life after radical prostatectomy for prostate carcinoma. *Cancer.* 2002;95(2):287-295.

63. Potosky AL, Knopf K, Clegg LX, et al. Quality-of-life outcomes after primary androgen deprivation therapy: results from the prostate cancer outcomes study. *J Clin Oncol.* 2001;19(17):3750-3757.

64. Green HJ, Pakenham KI, Headley BC, et al. Altered cognitive function in men treated for prostate cancer with

luteinizing hormone-releasing hormone analogues and cyproterone acetate: a randomized controlled trial. *BJU Int.* 2002;90(4): 427-432.

65. Salminen EK, Portin RI, Koskinen A, et al. Associations between serum testosterone fall and cognitive function in prostate cancer patients. *Clin Cancer Res.* 2004;10(22):7575-7582.

66. Salminen E, Portin R, Korpela J, et al. Androgen deprivation and cognition in prostate cancer. *Br J Cancer.* 2003;89(6):971-976.

67. Salminen EK, Portin RI, Koskinen AI, et al. Estradiol and cognition during androgen deprivation in men with prostate carcinoma. *Cancer.* 2005;103(7):1381-1387.

68. Almeida OP, Waterreus A, Spry N, et al. One year follow-up study of the association between chemical castration, sex hormones, beta-amyloid, memory and depression in men. *Psychoneuroendocrinology.* 2004;29(8):1071-1081.

69. Nelson CJ, Lee JS, Gamboa MC, et al. Cognitive effects of hormone therapy in men with prostate cancer: a review. *Cancer.* 2008;113(5):1097-1106.

70. Hanks RA, Rapport LJ, Millis SR, et al. Measures of executive functioning as predictors of functional ability and social integration in a rehabilitation sample. *Arch Phys Med Rehabil.* 1999;80(9):1030-1037.

71. Higano CS. Bone loss and the evolving role of bisphosphonate therapy in prostate cancer. *Urol Oncol.* 2003;21(5):392-398.

72. Shahinian VB, Kuo YF, Freeman JL, et al. Risk of fracture after androgen deprivation for prostate cancer. *N Engl J Med.* 2005;352(2):154-164.

73. Fizazi K, Carducci M, Smith M, et al. Denosumab versus zoledronic acid for treatment of bone metastases in men with castration-resistant prostate cancer: a randomised, double-blind study. *Lancet.* 2011;377(9768):813-822.

74. Smith MR, Saad F, Egerdie B, et al. Effects of denosumab on bone mineral density in men receiving androgen deprivation therapy for prostate cancer. *J Urol.* 2009;182(6):2670-2675.

75. Saylor PJ, Kaufman DS, Michaelson MD, et al. Application of a fracture risk algorithm to men treated with androgen deprivation therapy for prostate cancer. *J Urol.* 2010;183(6):2200-2205.

76. Mokdad AH, Marks JS, Stroup DF, et al. Actual causes of death in the united states, 2000. *JAMA.* 2004;291(10):1238-1245.

77. Xu J, Kochanek KD, Murphy SL, et al. Deaths: final data from 2007. *Natl Vital Stat Rep.* 2010;58(19):1-135.

78. Kochanek KD, Xu JQ, Murphy SL, et al. Deaths: preliminary data for 2009. *Natl Vital Stat Rep.* 2011;59(4):1-51.

79. Peters KD, Kochanek KD, Murphy SL. Deaths: final data for 1996. *Natl Vital Stat Rep.* 1998;47(9):1-100.

80. Keating NL, O'Malley AJ, Smith MR. Diabetes and cardiovascular disease during androgen deprivation therapy for prostate cancer. *J Clin Oncol.* 2006;24(27):4448-4456.

81. Saigal CS, Gore JL, Krupski TL, et al. Androgen deprivation therapy increases cardiovascular morbidity in men with prostate cancer. *Cancer.* 2007;110(7):1493-1500.

82. Lu-Yao G, Stukel TA, Yao SL. Changing patterns in competing causes of death in men with prostate cancer: a population based study. *J Urol.* 2004;171(6 pt 1):2285-2290.

83. Newschaffer CJ, Otani K, McDonald MK, et al. Causes of death in elderly prostate cancer patients and in a comparison nonprostate cancer cohort. *J Natl Cancer Inst.* 2000;92(8): 613-621.

84. Dockery F, Bulpitt CJ, Agarwal S, et al. Testosterone suppression in men with prostate cancer leads to an increase in arterial stiffness and hyperinsulinaemia. *Clin Sci (Lond).* 2003;104(2):195-201.

85. English KM, Steeds RP, Jones TH, et al. Low-dose transdermal testosterone therapy improves angina threshold in men with chronic stable angina: a randomized, double-blind, placebo-controlled study. *Circulation.* 2000;102(16):1906-1911.

86. Webb CM, Adamson DL, de Zeigler D, et al. Effect of acute testosterone on myocardial ischemia in men with coronary artery disease. *Am J Cardiol.* 1999;83(3):437-439, A9.

87. Rosano GM, Leonardo F, Pagnotta P, et al. Acute anti-ischemic effect of testosterone in men with coronary artery disease. *Circulation.* 1999;99(13):1666-1670.

88. Azoulay L, Yin H, Benayoun S, et al. Androgen-deprivation therapy and the risk of stroke in patients with prostate cancer. *Eur Urol.* 2011;60:1244-1250.

89. Keating NL, O'Malley AJ, Freedland SJ, et al. Diabetes and cardiovascular disease during androgen deprivation therapy: observational study of veterans with prostate cancer. *J Natl Cancer Inst.* 2010;102(1):39-46.

90. Van Hemelrijck M, Garmo H, Holmberg L, et al. Absolute and relative risk of cardiovascular disease in men with prostate cancer: results from the population-based PCBaSe Sweden. *J Clin Oncol.* 2010;28(21):3448-3456.

91. Chung SD, Chen YK, Wu FJ, et al. Hormone therapy for prostate cancer and the risk of stroke: a 5-year follow-up study. *BJU Int.* 2011;109:1001-1005.

92. Alibhai SM, Duong-Hua M, Sutradhar R, et al. Impact of androgen deprivation therapy on cardiovascular disease and diabetes. *J Clin Oncol.* 2009;27(21):3452-3458.

93. Aragon-Ching JB. Cardiovascular disease with androgen deprivation: the (forgotten) role of testosterone. *J Clin Oncol.* 2009;27(35):e261; author reply e262.

94. Pitteloud N, Mootha VK, Dwyer AA, et al. Relationship between testosterone levels, insulin sensitivity, and mitochondrial function in men. *Diabetes Care.* 2005;28(7):1636-1642.

95. Braga-Basaria M, Dobs AS, Muller DC, et al. Metabolic syndrome in men with prostate cancer undergoing long-term androgen-deprivation therapy. *J Clin Oncol.* 2006;24(24):3979-3983.

96. Executive summary of the third report of the national cholesterol education program (NCEP) expert panel on detection, evaluation, and treatment of high blood cholesterol in adults (adult treatment panel III). *JAMA.* 2001;285(19):2486-2497.

97. Yannucci J, Manola J, Garnick MB, et al. The effect of androgen deprivation therapy on fasting serum lipid and glucose parameters. *J Urol.* 2006;176(2):520-525.

98. Nobes JP, Langley SE, Klopper T, et al. A prospective, randomized pilot study evaluating the effects of metformin and lifestyle intervention on patients with prostate cancer receiving androgen deprivation therapy. *BJU Int.* 2012;109:1495-1502.

99. Dacal K, Sereika SM, Greenspan SL. Quality of life in prostate cancer patients taking androgen deprivation therapy. *J Am Geriatr Soc.* 2006;54(1):85-90.

100. Herr HW, O'Sullivan M. Quality of life of asymptomatic men with nonmetastatic prostate cancer on androgen deprivation therapy. *J Urol.* 2000;163(6):1743-1746.

101. Moinpour CM, Savage MJ, Troxel A, et al. Quality of life in advanced prostate cancer: results of a randomized therapeutic trial. *J Natl Cancer Inst.* 1998;90(20):1537-1544.

102. Ayta IA, McKinlay JB, Krane RJ. The likely worldwide increase in erectile dysfunction between 1995 and 2025 and some possible policy consequences. *BJU Int.* 1999;84(1):50-56.

103. NIH Consensus Conference. Impotence. NIH Consensus Development Panel on impotence. *JAMA.* 1993;270(1):83-90.

104. Feldman HA, Goldstein I, Hatzichristou DG, et al. Impotence and its medical and psychosocial correlates: results of the Massachusetts male aging study. *J Urol.* 1994;151(1):54-61.

105. Kloner RA. Pharmacology and drug interaction effects of the phosphodiesterase 5 inhibitors: focus on alpha-blocker interactions. *Am J Cardiol.* 2005;96(12B):42M-46M.

106. Hugosson J, Stranne J, Carlsson SV. Radical retropubic prostatectomy: a review of outcomes and side-effects. *Acta Oncol.* 2011;50(suppl 1):92-97.

107. Klein T, Palisaar RJ, Holz A, et al. The impact of prostate biopsy and periprostatic nerve block on erectile and voiding function: a prospective study. *J Urol.* 2010;184(4):1447-1452.

108. Zisman A, Leibovici D, Kleinmann J, et al. The impact of prostate biopsy on patient well-being: a prospective study of pain, anxiety and erectile dysfunction. *J Urol.* 2001;165(2):445-454.

109. Bruyere F, Puichaud A, Pereira H, et al. Influence of photoselective vaporization of the prostate on sexual function: results of a prospective analysis of 149 patients with long-term follow-up. *Eur Urol.* 2010;58(2):207-211.

110. Korfage IJ, Pluijm S, Roobol M, et al. Erectile dysfunction and mental health in a general population of older men. *J Sex Med.* 2009;6(2):505-512.

111. Johannes CB, Araujo AB, Feldman HA, et al. Incidence of erectile dysfunction in men 40 to 69 years old: longitudinal results from the Massachusetts male aging study. *J Urol.* 2000;163(2):460-463.

112. Montejo-Gonzalez AL, Llorca G, Izquierdo JA, et al. Ssri-induced sexual dysfunction: fluoxetine, paroxetine, sertraline, and fluvoxamine in a prospective, multicenter, and descriptive clinical study of 344 patients. *J Sex Marital Ther.* 1997;23(3):176-194.

113. Rosen RC, Lane RM, Menza M. Effects of SSRIs on sexual function: a critical review. *J Clin Psychopharmacol.* 1999;19(1):67-85.

114. Albersen M, Shindel AW, Mwamukonda KB, et al. The future is today: emerging drugs for the treatment of erectile dysfunction. *Expert Opin Emerg Drugs.* 2010;15(3):467-480.

115. Fujisawa M, Sawada K. Clinical efficacy and safety of sildenafil in elderly patients with erectile dysfunction. *Arch Androl.* 2004;50(4):255-260.

116. Hatzimouratidis K, Hatzichristou DG. A comparative review of the options for treatment of erectile dysfunction: which treatment for which patient? *Drugs.* 2005;65(12):1621-1650.

117. Albersen M, Orabi H, Lue TF. Evaluation and treatment of erectile dysfunction in the aging male: a mini-review. *Gerontology.* 2012;58:3-14.

118. Bella AJ, Deyoung LX, Al-Numi M, et al. Daily administration of phosphodiesterase type 5 inhibitors for urological and nonurological indications. *Eur Urol.* 2007;52(4):990-1005.

119. Shindel AW. 2009 update on phosphodiesterase type 5 inhibitor therapy part 1: recent studies on routine dosing for penile rehabilitation, lower urinary tract symptoms, and other indications (CME). *J Sex Med.* 2009;6(7):1794-808; quiz 1793, 1809-1810.

120. Shabsigh R, Kaufman JM, Steidle C, et al. Randomized study of testosterone gel as adjunctive therapy to sildenafil in hypogonadal men with erectile dysfunction who do not respond to sildenafil alone. *J Urol.* 2004;172(2):658-663.

121. Hatzimouratidis K, Amar E, Eardley I, et al. Guidelines on male sexual dysfunction: erectile dysfunction and premature ejaculation. *Eur Urol.* 2010;57(5):804-814.

122. Hellstrom WJ, Montague DK, Moncada I, et al. Implants, mechanical devices, and vascular surgery for erectile dysfunction. *J Sex Med.* 2010;7(1 pt 2):501-523.

CHAPTER 34

Impact of Hepatic and Renal Dysfunction on Pharmacology of Palliative Care Drugs

Thomas Strouse

OVERVIEW

Diminished liver and kidney function are common in palliative care patients. These alterations may be transient, as in the patient with cancer who suffers reversible renal injury from nephrotoxic chemotherapy, or permanent and worsening, such as in the patient with a progressing malignancy metastatic to the liver. Although this chapter is limited to reviewing how hepatic and renal dysfunction affect the pharmacology of common palliative care drugs, it is important to note that a host of other variables are also relevant to the pharmacokinetic (how drugs are absorbed, biotransformed, and excreted) and pharmacodynamic (how drugs work at their target site and the relationship between [drug] and clinical effects) balance in the patient. The reader can consult comprehensive pharmacology textbooks for a more complete picture (1,2).

OPIOIDS

Opioids remain the cornerstone for pain management in palliative care. In the hands of a competent prescriber and responsible patient, they are also quite safe: by contrast to many of the non-opioid analgesics described below, opioids lack organotoxicity, they are broadly effective for a variety of pain states, and there are sufficient data to guide prescribing them in an informed way in end-organ failure.

For the interested reader, many comprehensive reviews of opioid metabolism and pharmacokinetics well beyond the scope of this chapter are available (3–9). For the purposes of this overview, it is useful to divide opioids into two broad metabolic categories: those that undergo little or no hepatic oxidative metabolism, requiring instead the uridine diphosphate glucuronosyltransferases (UGTs), and those that undergo primary or exclusive metabolism via CYP450/hepatic oxidative biotransformation (see also Table 34.1).

The primary UGT group is comprised of morphine, hydromorphone, and oxymorphone, while the CYP450 group includes methadone, fentanyl, oxycodone, hydrocodone, codeine, and tramadol. Not surprisingly, normal metabolism of the UGT group is more susceptible to embarrassment as a result of changes in renal function, whereas the CYP450 group is subject to pharmacokinetic variability as a result of anomalies in hepatic function. Serum levels of drugs in this latter group are also more vulnerable to the inhibitory or inductive effects on liver isoenzyme activity conferred by starting, stopping, or dose changes of other agents.

In the most general sense, the addition of potent CYP inhibitor drugs to a regimen that already includes regular dosing of an opioid that is primarily a CYP substrate (codeine, hydrocodone, oxycodone, methadone, fentanyl, and tramadol) is likely to result in higher peak plasma concentrations of the opioid parent molecule and a longer duration of action of that molecule, compared with circumstances before the addition of the inhibitor. Decrements in hepatic oxidative function will likely have similar consequences. Conversely, the addition of drugs that are potent CYP inducers may lower peak plasma concentrations of relevant opioids and shorten their duration of action, just as recovery in hepatic function from an impaired baseline will do the same.

NON-OPIOID ANALGESICS

Anticonvulsants

Nearly every commercially available anticonvulsant has been demonstrated to have at least modest analgesic efficacy (10,11). Clinician choice from among them tends to be determined by perceived ease of use: side-effect profile, dosing convenience, monitoring requirements, and increasingly whether or not the manufacturer has obtained an FDA indication for pain. Two of the most commonly prescribed anticonvulsant analgesics, gabapentin and its congener pregabalin, are mediators of the alpha-2-delta subunit of the calcium channel and show broad efficacy in neuropathic pain states. Gabapentin is FDA approved for the treatment of post-herpetic neuralgia and pregabalin for diabetic neuropathic pain, fibromyalgia, and post-herpetic neuralgia. Both drugs are biologically inert: they do not undergo oxidative metabolism and are excreted in urine unchanged, making them particularly well-suited for use in patients with complex medical illness, polypharmacy issues, and organ failure. Table 34.2 provides summary data on routes of metabolism and dosing considerations in renal and hepatic dysfunction for the commonly prescribed anticonvulsants.

TABLE 34.1	**Metabolic Pathways of Commonly Prescribed Opioids**				
Drug Category/ Name	**Uses**	**Primary Route of Metabolism**	**Renal Notes**	**Hepatic Notes**	**Comments**
Opioids					
Morphine	Analgesic	UGT2B7	M3G metabolite neuroexcitatory, antianalgesic		Avoid, and consider switching in new-onset renal insufficiency
Hydromorphone		UGT2B7	H3G in rodents neuroexcitatory, antianalgesic; human data inconclusive		In renal insufficiency, monitor patient for toxicities, otherwise no change
Oxymorphone		UGT2B7	O3G measurable but has no known pharmacologic activity		No changes unless symptoms emerge
Codeine		CYP2D6	UGT2B7 secondary		Pro-drug; 2D6-mediated biotransformation to morphine required
Hydrocodone		CYP2D6, 3A4			Lower doses in new-onset hepatic failure
Oxycodone		CYP2D6, 3A4	UGT2B7 secondary		Lower doses in new-onset hepatic failure
Methadone		CYP2C8/9/19, 2D6, 1A2			P-gp inhibitors may ↑ potency
Fentanyl		CYP3A4, 2B6, UGT secondary	UGT secondary		Lower doses in new-onset hepatic and renal failure
Tramadol		CYP2D6	CrCl < 30: max 200 mg/d immediate-release formulation only	Cirrhosis: max 100 mg/d immediate release only	
Tapentadol		CYP2C9/19, UGT secondary	PI: avoid use in "severe renal insufficiency"	PI: 50 mg q8h in "moderate" impairment; "avoid use" in severe impairment	

Adapted from Strouse TB. Pharmacokinetic drug interactions in palliative care: focus on opioids. *J Palliat Med.* 2009;12:1043–1050. Reprinted/amended with publisher's permission.

CYP, cytochrome P450 isoenzyme systems, with trailing roman numeral/letter/numeral denoting family, subfamily, etc; UGT, uridine diphosphate glucuronosyltransferase family/subfamily/etc; p-gp, p-glycoprotein cellular membrane ion pumps; CrCl, creatinine clearance; PI, package insert.

TABLE 34.2	Metabolic Pathways of Commonly Prescribed Anticonvulsants			
Drug Category/ Name	Uses	Primary Route of Metabolism	Renal Notes	Hepatic Notes	Comments
Anticonvulsants	Seizure prophylaxis Analgesia Anxiolysis				
Gabapentin		Exclusively renal; inert	CrCl 30–60: 200–700 mg BID CrCl 16–29: 200–700 mg qd CrCl 15: 100–300 mg qd CrCl < 15: dose proportionately to CrCl	None	Like lithium, may be given once orally after dialysis in patients getting renal replacement therapy at regular intervals: 125–350 mg/dose
Pregabalin		Exclusively renal; inert	CrCl 30–60: 75–300 mg/d BID or TID CrCl 15–30: 25–150 mg/d in one or two doses CrCl < 15: 25–75 mg/d	None	Like lithium, may be given once orally after dialysis in patients getting renal replacement therapy at regular intervals: 2× calculated mg/d for CrCl < 15
Topiramate		Not extensively metabolized by hepatic or renal processes	CrCl < 70: 50% of usual adult dose HD: Rapidly cleared (see comments)	Plasma levels may be increased in hepatic dysfunction; no recs in PI	May require both pre- and post-dialysis doses See PI for detail
Lamotrigine		Glucuronidation	Limited data; use with caution	No dose adjustment in mild hepatic impairment; 25% reduction in moderate/ severe; 50% in severe with ascites	Maintenance dose after dialysis in patients getting it at regular intervals
Carbamazepine		Hepatic, via CYP3A4, which it also induces	No recs in PI	No recs in PI	In view of primary hepatic route and glucuronidated metabolites, dose modification downward in hepatic and renal dysfunction is reasonable

Drug	Metabolism	Renal dysfunction	Hepatic dysfunction	Notes
Oxcarbazepine	Glucuronidation and renal clearance	CrCl < 30: start at ½ usual dose and titrate	No dose adjustment required in mild–moderate impairment	No recs in PI for patients on HD or with severe liver impairment
Phenytoin	CYP2C9 and 2C19	Little direct impact	Dose adjustment (see notes and PI)	Hypoalbuminemia (inc. free fraction of DPH) in renal and hepatic failure more important than direct impact or organ dysfunction. Dose decreases needed
Primidone	Poorly understood	No recs in PI	No recs in PI	Post-marketing studies suggest dose decrements in renal/ hepatic failure
Valproic acid	Hepatic	Valproic acid accumulates in hepatic dysfunction but PI lacks dosing recs	Per PI, no dose adjustment needed	
Felbamate	Hepatic	No recs in PI	FB clearance decreased with renal failure; no recs in PI	
Tiagabine	CYP3A3/4	No impact of mild/ moderate/severe renal dysfunction per PI	Child-Pugh class B (moderate) impairment associated with 60% decrease in clearance	
Levetiracetam	Nonenzymatic hydrolysis and renal excretion	Linear relationship to CrCl; dose decrement suggested	No impact	Dose after dialysis
Zonisamide	CYP3A4, 3A5, 3A7 acetylation to glucuronide	CrCl 50–80: caution advised; titrate slowly; CrCl < 50: contraindicated	No specific recs in PI; "caution advised, titrate slowly" in hepatic impairment	

All data referenced in this table are abstracted from the package insert for the indicated drug and is thus consistent with FDA's most current analysis of these agents. Many of the older drugs (e.g., phenytoin and primidone) were approved long before the CYP450 system had been identified. For these, there is often a paucity of what by today's standards would be considered "basic" metabolic information required for approval.

HD, hemodialysis; recs, recommendations; PI, package insert; DPH, diphenylhydantoin (dilantin); FB, felbamate.

Antidepressants

Not all drugs marketed as "antidepressants" have analgesic efficacy. Despite early optimism, investigations into the possible pain-relieving properties of the selective serotonin reuptake inhibitors were mostly disappointing (12). Two decades of clinical research supports the view that among the "modern" antidepressants, the serotonin–norepinephrine reuptake inhibitors (SNRIs) duloxetine, venlafaxine, and milnacipran reliably demonstrate analgesic efficacy. The older tricyclic antidepressants, which display some SNRI-like mechanisms of action, are also effective.

Significant differences in safety and side effects separate the older tricyclics from the modern SNRIs, however, and these differences may be magnified in the setting of polypharmacy, concomitant medical illness, end-organ dysfunction, and frank organ failure. What makes the "post-tricyclic" antidepressants so much safer than their predecessors is the absence of fast sodium channel membrane-stabilizing effects—the mechanism by which clinical doses of the tricyclics may sometimes cause benign cardiac conduction abnormalities and by which intentional or accidental overingestion can cause cardiac arrest and death. It has been repeatedly demonstrated that in renal failure, the hydroxylated metabolites of tricyclic antidepressant (TCA) parent molecules accumulate at concentrations of hundreds to thousands of times what is found in normals; these unmeasured hydroxy-metabolites may be arrhythmogenic and are present in higher than expected concentrations even after dialysis (13). Tricyclics are likely best avoided entirely in patients with renal insufficiency or dialysis dependence (14).

As a function of the FDA's more stringent requirements in recent years for testing in "special populations," the package inserts for the modern agents duloxetine, venlafaxine, and milnacipran contain recommendations for dose decrements in hepatic and renal insufficiency. It is worth pointing out that these recommendations are empirically based and do not necessarily reflect evidence of toxicity or increased side-effect burden, but rather are simply a response to measurements of elevated serum concentrations of the drugs. Specifics are outlined in Table 34.1.

NSAIDs/ASA/Acetaminophen

The potential toxicities of nonsteroidal anti-inflammatory drugs (NSAIDs)—both COX-2 specific and non-selective—are well known. There is general consensus that NSAIDs should be avoided in patients with impaired renal function since their effect on renal arteriolar tone can worsen renal insufficiency or precipitate frank renal failure. NSAIDs can be used safely and effectively in patients with static renal failure who are receiving renal replacement therapies.

End-organ toxicities of acetaminophen, particularly hepatotoxicity, are often neglected in palliative care settings. Acetaminophen is the most common co-analgesic included in short-acting compounded opioid products, and it is common for patients to inadvertently exceed the recommended maximum of 4 g of acetaminophen/24 h due to escalating opioid requirements. It is unknown whether acetaminophen exposure confers added risk to patients with established hepatic dysfunction, but common sense suggests it should be avoided. Most of the opioid molecules commonly compounded with co-analgesics are also available as single products and can be prescribed that way. Hydrocodone is the exception in North America: it is only available in compounded forms.

Salicylates are effective analgesics but, like NSAIDs, carry the risks of gastric irritation and antiplatelet properties that can cause or exacerbate bleeding. These risks may be compounded in patients with progressive hepatic dysfunction, who often have attendant coagulopathy due to synthetic impairment. Coupled with thrombocytopenia or prescribed anticoagulants, NSAID or acetylsalicylic acid–associated mild gastritis can become a life-threatening bleeding problem.

Misoprostol, H2 blockers (ranitidine and others), and proton-pump inhibitors (omeprazole and others) confer some protection.

STIMULANTS

Psychostimulants can be helpful in palliative care patients for the management of fatigue, somnolence, low mood, and other symptoms. The conventional stimulants (methylphenidate and various forms of amphetamine) are best studied and have been used for decades. They appear to work within hours of first doses. There is no evidence for toxic accumulation in renal or liver failure and they can be prescribed in immediate-release formulations at very low doses and used as needed. Modafinil and armodafinil are also used, and recently published studies support their effectiveness for fatigue and sleepiness in patients with advanced disease. In contrast to the inotropic and chronotropic effects of conventional stimulants, the newer agents have little or no impact on cardiac myocardial oxygen requirements. There is emerging evidence that modafinil and armodafinil may take weeks to exert their optimal effects, however (15,16). Since the decision to use stimulants for fatigue, lethargy, or somnolence is often taken in the last days or weeks of life, such a delayed effect may prove to limit utility. This is compounded by high per-pill costs and by the absence of an FDA indication for their use as palliative agents. Insurers therefore tend to be recalcitrant about approving payment for modafinil and armodafinil, hospice programs generally cannot afford them, and patients are understandably reluctant to pay out of pocket for agents that may take weeks to work. Modest dose decrements are recommended in organ failure (Table 34.3).

ANTIEMETICS

5-HT$_3$ Antagonists

Ondansetron revolutionized the management of chemotherapy-related nausea and vomiting. Related compounds available in North America are dolasetron, granisetron and palonosetron. Ondansetron is almost exclusively

TABLE 34.3	**Metabolic Pathways of Commonly Prescribed Stimulants / Wakefulness-promoting agents**				
Drug Category/ Name	**Uses**	**Primary Route of Metabolism**	**Renal Notes**	**Hepatic Notes**	**Comments**
Stimulants	Fatigue/ wakefulness promoting/ antidepressant augmentation				
Methylphenidate		Hepatic	Case reports: lack of accumulation in dialysis	None	
Dextroamphetamine		Hepatic	No		
Modafinil		Hepatic	Modafinil acid (inert metabolite) accumulates in CRI	↑ [SS] in cirrhotics	PI recommends dose decrement
Armodafinil		Hepatic	Same as modafinil	Same as modafinil	Same as modafinil

From Stiebel VG. Methylphenidate plasma levels in depressed patients with renal failure. *Psychosomatics*. 1994;35(5):498–500.

CRI, chronic renal insufficiency; PI, package insert; SS, steady state.

biotransformed by the liver and has biologically inactive metabolites. Not surprisingly, steady-state levels are significantly increased in liver failure, without apparent clinical consequence. There are no formal recommendations for dose alteration in organ dysfunction. Interestingly, these drugs have shown promise in managing "renal itch," an intractable symptom common to patients on chronic hemodialysis. Their off-label use in patients receiving renal replacement therapies suggests safety and effectiveness.

Phenothiazines

Prochlorperazine and related compounds are among the oldest antiemetics used in medicine. Prochlorperazine remains widely used in palliative care and home hospice; it is inexpensive and can be administered in suppositories as well as oral formulations, and recent explorations suggest a possible role for buccal administration (17). There are no FDA recommendations about usage in renal or hepatic failure.

Aprepitant

Aprepitant is a selective neurokinin/substance P receptor antagonist indicated for preventing chemotherapy-related nausea and vomiting. It is extensively metabolized by hepatic CYP450 enzymes and inhibits P450 3A3/4 in a dose-dependent manner. The package insert (18) asserts that there are no data regarding the impact of advanced liver disease on aprepitant pharmacokinetics or pharmacodynamics.

Synthetic Cannabinoids

Dronabinol was the first cannabinoid approved by the FDA to treat chemotherapy-related nausea. It is predominantly metabolized in the liver and has only recently been the subject of careful pharmacokinetic study (19). There are no recommendations regarding dose modification in organ failure, but empiric dose reduction is prudent. Nabilone is structurally similar to delta-9-tetrahydrocannabinol and also has utility in treatment-resistant nausea. Like dronabinol, it appears to be exclusively hepatically metabolized, but at the time of its approval there were no data submitted to the FDA on the impact of hepatic or renal impairment on its pharmacokinetics.

Appetite Stimulants

Megestrol acetate is the most widely used and effective agent available for appetite stimulation and the attenuation of the cachexia/anorexia syndrome in patients with cancer or HIV/AIDS. After oxidation by gut mucosa and the liver, megestrol's metabolites are excreted predominantly in urine. There is no guidance in the package insert for dosing adjustments in hepatic or renal failure.

The anti-tumor necrosis factor agents thalidomide and pentoxifylline have been studied as alternate agents to attenuate wasting. Thalidomide has shown promise in controlled trials (20) and possesses an FDA indication for use in advanced HIV. Its metabolism is complex, relying both on nonenzymatic hydrolysis and on oxidative biotransformation via CYP2C19 (21). There are no published guidelines for dose adjustment in renal or hepatic dysfunction.

The tetracyclic antidepressant mirtazapine has been noted to cause weight gain in medically well patients treated for depressive illness. A recent phase II trial supports the off-label clinical practice of using mirtazapine to stimulate appetite and promote weight gain in patients with advanced malignancies (22). Mirtazapine's label promotes use "with caution" in renal and hepatic disease, suggesting dose decrements may be indicated. There are no specific known pharmacokinetic drug interactions warranting concern, however.

Corticosteroids

Corticosteroids are used widely in the management of malignancies and other life-limiting illnesses. They are a frequent component of the palliative care pharmacopoeia for the management of pain, fatigue, nausea/appetite stimulation, itching, inflammatory processes, and other symptoms. There is essentially no evidence of toxic accumulation of corticosteroid metabolites in renal or liver failure, while at the same time the risks of adrenal insufficiency in critically ill patients continue to be elucidated (23). For the patient receiving outpatient or home-based palliative care services who has been chronically exposed to corticosteroids, it seems prudent to continue physiologic doses in order to avoid an iatrogenic crisis of acute insufficiency and to taper carefully if the eventual goal is discontinuation.

Bisphosphonates

Bisphosphonates (pamidronate, alendronate, clodronate, zoledronic acid) have revolutionized the prevention and management of skeletal complications of metastatic malignancies and the management of bone pain associated with these complications. Bisphosphonates undergo no hepatic biotransformation and are excreted unchanged in urine; occasionally, they have been implicated in acute renal injury. There are specific published drug-by-drug guidelines for dosage based on creatinine clearance (24). There are no recommendations related to hepatic dysfunction.

Stool Softeners/Laxatives

Most of the stool softeners/laxatives used in palliative care are nonabsorbed and act within the lumen of the gut to alter the water content of stool and/or to affect motility. As such, recommendations regarding use in renal or hepatic failure are moot. It is worthwhile to keep in mind that these agents are less effective in patients who are dehydrated and hypercalcemic or have other metabolic embarrassments associated with decreased bowel motility.

The osmotic laxative lactulose has long been recognized for its therapeutic effect on portosystemic encephalopathy, making it an excellent choice for the constipated patient with hepatic failure. Polyethylene glycol powder, when mixed with water, is tasteless and textureless, making it more palatable than many of the other osmotic agents.

Methylnaltrexone is the newest drug in the laxative category. This injectable peripheral opioid receptor antagonist does not reverse opioid analgesia centrally and provides rapid, reliable laxation for opioid-induced constipation. It is recommended that the dose be reduced by 50% for patients with creatinine clearance of less than 30. There are no published recommendations for patients on renal replacement therapies or who have advanced liver failure.

Octreotide

Octreotide is a somatostatin analogue used to treat neuroendocrine tumor (carcinoid). In palliative care, it is often used for symptomatic management of bowel obstruction. Its putative mechanism(s) of action involve reducing bowel contractility against a fixed obstruction, thus reducing pain and related distress; it also reduces intestinal secretions via its somatostatin-like properties. The only published guidelines pertaining to renal or hepatic insufficiency are intended to govern repeated dosing over time in patients with carcinoid or VIPoma. Octreotide's use in a palliative care setting is much more likely to be short term, for example, in the management of acute bowel obstruction near the end of life. Under such circumstances, conservative mg/kg dosing should be chosen from the nomogram in the package insert.

Antibiotics

The considerations regarding antibiotic dosing in renal or hepatic insufficiency are as varied as the numbers of antibiotics available for use. The reader is encouraged to consult the package insert or an electronic pharmacopoeia for specific information about the antibiotic being considered.

Sedative-Hypnotics

Many palliative care patients will require agents that can broadly be considered sedative-hypnotics. These can be further separated into distinct groups based on structure or mechanism of action: sedating antihistaminic anticholinergics; benzodiazepines; non-benzodiazepine sleep medicines; sedating antidepressants; sedating atypical antipsychotics; and others.

Sedating antihistaminic anticholinergics are frequently chosen because they are cheap, are available without prescription, and are perceived as safe and effective. They include diphenhydramine, chlorpheniramine, and cyproheptadine. All require some degree of hepatic oxidative metabolism and their metabolites can accumulate in patients with renal insufficiency. Because these agents have been available without prescription for decades, there has been little scientific attention paid to their pharmacokinetics. Evidence-based recommendations are scarce. General clinical caution—"start low and go slow"—is a reasonable strategy.

For the purposes of this chapter, benzodiazepines can be subdivided into two major metabolic categories: those that undergo extensive hepatic oxidative metabolism and have multiple active metabolites and/or long serum half-lives (diazepam, chlordiazepoxide, and alprazolam) and those without active metabolites (lorazepam, clonazepam, oxazepam, and temazepam) (25). It makes sense to rely on the latter group in patients with known or suspected end-organ failure. Many palliative care patients have been exposed chronically to benzodiazepines, which are prescribed routinely as part of the antiemetic regimen for most cancer chemotherapies, and may therefore have developed significant pharmacologic tolerance. Additionally, benzodiazepines confer anticonvulsant benefits, are effective anxiolytics, and are useful for insomnia with short-term use. The clinician should remain alert, however, to the potential for benzodiazepines to have new, undesirable side effects in organ failure patients: they can mimic or worsen hepatic encephalopathy in patients with liver failure (26) and can contribute to sedation, lethargy, and, in combination with opioids, to life-threatening respiratory depression. Though there is little by way of written recommendations, it is prudent in patients with organ failure to use lowest possible doses of the "no active metabolites" benzodiazepines listed above or to stop them entirely if one can rule out the possibility of withdrawal seizures or rebound anxiety.

The non-benzodiazepine sedative-hypnotics (eszopiclone, zolpidem, zaleplon in the United States) are distinct from conventional benzodiazepines by virtue of their selectivity for the GABA-A (gamma-aminobutyric acid A) subtype of the BZD receptor in the human central nervous system. It is asserted that this specificity makes them "purer" sedative-hypnotics, lacking in the anxiolytic and anticonvulsant properties of the conventional benzodiazepines and allegedly minimizing the potential for the development by users of tolerance, physiological dependence, and abuse/misuse. Clinical experience challenges some of these assertions. By virtue of their arrival to the marketplace within the last few decades, there are a bit more data about metabolism in organ failure: broadly, caution is warranted in patients who develop new-onset renal failure or hepatic failure and lowest possible doses should be sought.

REFERENCES

1. Atkinson AJ, Abnerthy DR, Daniels CE, Dedrick RL, Markey SP, eds. *Principles of Clinical Pharmacology.* New York, NY: Elsevier Academic Press; 2010.
2. Bunton L, Chabner B, Knollman B, eds. *Goodman and Gillman's the Pharmacological Basis of Therapeutics.* New York, NY: McGraw Hill; 2010.
3. Kharasch ED. Opioid analgesics. In: Levy R, Thummel KE, Trager WF, Hansten PD, Eichelbaum M, eds. *Metabolic Drug Interactions.* Philadelphia, PA: Lippincott Williams & Wilkins; 2000:297-320.
4. Holmquist G. Opioid metabolism and the effects of cytochrome P450. *Pain Med.* 2009;10:S20-S29.
5. Osborne R, Joel S, Grebenik K, Trew D, Slevin M. The pharmacokinetics of morphine and morphine glucuronides in kidney failure. *Clin Pharmacol Ther.* 1993;54:158-167.
6. Aureta K, Goucke CR, Ilett KF, Page-Sharp M, Boyd F, Ooh TE. Pharmacokinetics and pharmacodynamics of methadone enantiomers in hospice patients with cancer pain. *Ther Drug Monit.* 2006;28:359-366.
7. Shaiova L, Berger A, Blinderman CD, et al. Consensus guidelines on parenteral methadone use in pain and palliative care. *Palliat Support Care.* 2008;6:165-176.
8. Weschules DJ, Bain KT, Richeimer S. Actual and potential drug interactions associated with methadone. *Pain Med.* 2008;3:315-344.
9. Strouse TB. Pharmacokinetic drug interactions in palliative care: focus on opioids. *J Palliat Med.* 2009;12:1043-1050.
10. Martin WJ, Forouzanfar T. Efficacy of anticonvulsants in orofacial pain states: a systematic review. *Oral Surg Oral Med Oral Pathol Oral Radiol Endod.* 2011;111:627-633.
11. Brill V, England J, Franklin GM, et al. Evidence-based guidelines: treatment of painful diabetic neuropathy. Report of the American Academy of Neurology, the American Association of Neuromuscular and Electrodiagnostic Medicine, and the American Academy of Physical Medicine and Rehabilitation. *Neurology.* 2011;76(20):1758-1765.
12. Max MB, Lynch SA, Muir J, Shoaf SE, Smoller B, Dubner R. Effects of desipramine, amitryptyline, and fluoxetine on pain in diabetic neuropathy. *N Engl J Med.* 1992;326:1250-1256.
13. Cohen LM, Tessier EG, Germain MJ, Levy NB. Update on psychotropic medication use in renal disease. *Psychosomatics.* 2004;45:34-48.
14. McIntyre RS, Baghdady NT, Suman B, Swartz SA. The use of psychotropic drugs in patients with impaired renal function. *Prim Psychiatry.* 2008;15:73-88.
15. Cooper MR, Bird HM, Steinberg M. Efficacy and safety of modafinil in treatment of cancer-related fatigue. *Ann Pharmacother.* 2009;43:721-725.
16. Breitbart W, Alici Y. Psychostimulants for cancer-related fatigue. *J Natl Compr Cancer Netw.* 2010;8:933-942.
17. Finn A, Collins J, Voyksner R, Lindley C. Bioavailability and metabolism of prochlorperazine administered via the buccal and oral delivery route. *J Clin Pharmacol.* 2005;45:1383-1390.
18. Emend (Aprepitant) Package Insert.
19. Huestis MA. Pharmacokinetics and metabolism of the plant cannabinoids, Delta9-THC, cannabidiol and cannabinol. *Handb Exp Pharmacol.* 2005;168:657-690.
20. Kaplan G, Thomas S, Fierer DS, et al. Thalidomide for the Treatment of AIDS-associated Wasting. AIDS Research and Human Retroviruses. September 2000;16(14):1345-1355.
21. Gordon JN, Trebble TM, Ellis RD, Duncan HD, Johns T, Goggin PM. Thalidomide in the treatment of cancer cachexia: a randomized placebo controlled trial. *Gut.* 2005;54:540-545.
22. Lepper ER, Smith NF, Cox MC, Scipture CD, Figg WD. Thalidomide metabolism and hydrolysis: mechanisms and implications. *Curr Drug Metab.* 2006;7:677-685.
23. Riechelmann RP, Burman D, Tannock IF, Rodin G, Zimmermann C. Phase II trial of mirtazapine for cancer-related cachexia and anorexia. *Am J Hosp Palliat Med.* 2010;27:106-110.
24. Mark PE, Pastores SM, Annane D, et al. Recommendations for the diagnosis and management of corticosteroid insufficiency in critically ill adult patients: consensus statements from an international task force by the American College of Critical Care Medicine. *Crit Care Med.* 2008;36:1937-1949.
25. Hillner BE, Ingle JN, Berenson JR, et al. American Society of Clinical Oncology guidelines on the role of bisphosphonates in breast cancer. *J Clin Oncol.* 2000;18:1378-1391.
26. Butterworth RF. Complications of cirrhosis III: hepatic encephalopathy. *J Hepatol.* 2000;32:171-180.

CHAPTER **35** # Hypercalcemia

Howard Su-Hau Yeh ■ James R. Berenson

INTRODUCTION

Background and Epidemiology

Hypercalcemia of malignancy (HCM), characterized by high serum levels of calcium, is the leading malignancy-related metabolic complication in hospital practice and it is recognized as an oncologic emergency. This life-threatening incidence is reported in up to 10.9% of hospitalized patients (1–4). HCM is a condition that results from disruption of calcium homeostasis because of bone resorption secondary to skeletal invasion or indirectly through the production of endocrine factors. HCM can be divided into osteolytic hypercalcemia, where increased calcium results from the marked activity of osteoclastic bone resorption, and humoral hypercalcemia, in which increased calcium is secondary to systemic secretion of parathyroid hormone protein (PTH). Among patients with HCM, approximately 20% of cases are due to osteolytic HCM and 80% are caused by humoral HCM. Nearly 10% to 20% of patients with various solid tumors and hematologic malignancies are affected by HCM at some point during the course of their disease (5). In solid tumors, lung and breast cancers are associated with 67% of cases of HCM (2,6,7). Among hematologic malignancies, HCM occurs most commonly in patients with multiple myeloma (MM), with a prevalence of approximately 30% before the widespread use of bisphosphonates. In general, HCM usually develops either at the initial stages of cancer or late in the natural history of the disease. Patients diagnosed with HCM typically have more advanced disease and are more likely to have distant metastases and renal failure and generally have a poor prognosis (3,8).

Differential Diagnosis of Hypercalcemia

Hypercalcemia is an elevation in unbound, ionized serum calcium concentration. In the presence of hypercalcemia, it is crucial to distinguish between primary hyperparathyroidism and HCM. HCM should be suspected in patients with unexplained hypercalcemia and a low serum PTH concentration. Patients with parathyroid hormone-related protein (PTHrP)–induced hypercalcemia typically have advanced malignancy.

The diagnosis of humoral HCM can be confirmed by demonstrating a high serum concentration of PTHrP, using immunoradiometric assay (IRMA) (9). Serum PTHrP concentrations are low and undetectable in patients with primary hyperparathyroidism and in normal subjects. There is no difference in measuring serum PTHrP from assays that detect primarily amino-terminal or carboxyl-terminal epitopes of PTHrP. The main concern with the two types of assays is that patients with renal insufficiency may have high serum PTHrP values when a carboxy-terminal assay is used.

Nonetheless, some argue that the IRMA test can be time-consuming and costly for screening purposes. Therefore, one may consider using the formula described by Lind and Ljunghall (10) as a screening tool:

Values under 400 predict a malignancy, whereas values over 500 predict a parathyroid origin. This formula enables one to classify 97% of patients with cancer and 96% of patients with primary hyperparathyroidism, after excluding 5% of patients of borderline hypercalcemia that fall between the values of 400 and 500. The use of the formula is an inexpensive and easy tool to screen for a preliminary cause of HCM.

Clinical Presentation

The primary causal factor of HCM is the release of calcium into the blood from increased bone resorption that is uncoupled from bone formation, as typically occurs in patients with advanced malignancies. The excess serum calcium results in polyuria and gastrointestinal disturbances. Polyuria impairs reabsorption of sodium, potassium, and magnesium by the proximal tubules, causing hypovolemia and dehydration, which further compromise the glomerular filtration rate. The decreased glomerular filtration rate then leads to increased sodium resorption (and associated increased calcium resorption) in the proximal tubule, creating a positive feedback cycle of compromised kidney function and increasing serum calcium (5).

Normal levels of serum calcium (corrected for the concentration of serum albumin) range from 2.0 to 2.7 mmol/L (8.0 to 10.8 mg/dL) (11). Above this range, subtle symptoms of anorexia, nausea, constipation, and altered mental status begin to present. Moderate elevations of corrected serum calcium (CSC) levels at approximately 3.0 mmol/L (12 mg/dL) can lead to renal insufficiency and deposit of excess calcium in tissues. Severe HCM (CSC levels of ≥3.8 mmol/L [≥15 mg/dL]) may present with severe nausea and vomiting, dehydration, renal insufficiency, and clouding or loss of consciousness. This condition requires immediate intervention as coma and cardiac arrest may occur at these CSC levels. Although HCM can present with either subtle or dramatic symptoms, symptom development and severity in an individual patient do not always strictly correlate with serum calcium levels and may depend more on the rapidity with which HCM develops in the patient (5,12).

Prognosis of HCM

Median survival in the setting of HCM generally ranges from 1 to 3 months (6,7,13–15). Patients with high levels of calcium seem to have a shorter life span (4,15). Patients with high serum PTHrP concentrations also have shorter median survival times (16,17). When serum PTHrP concentration is above 12 pmol/L, it is often associated with both a lesser response rate to bisphosphonate therapy and a more rapid recurrence rate of hypercalcemia (16,18,19). Those who respond to intravenous (IV) bisphosphonate therapy may have a significantly better outcome, although survival duration remains short (53 vs. 19 days) (19).

Mechanisms of Disease

HCM is primarily driven by increased osteoclast-mediated bone resorption. Osteoclasts are activated by cell-to-cell contact with osteoblasts and bone marrow stromal cells. Tumor cells produce circulating soluble factors such as PTHrP, tumor necrosis factor-α, and prostaglandin E (20) These factors, along with the macrophage colony-stimulating factor, induce osteoblasts and stromal cells to express the receptor activator of nuclear factor kappa B (RANK) ligand (RANKL) (21). Membrane-bound RANKL binds to and stimulates RANK expressed by osteoclast progenitors and promotes osteoclast differentiation and activation (20). The subsequent bone-degrading osteoclast activity results in the release of calcium and several soluble growth factors, including interleukin-6 (IL-6) and transforming growth factor-β, which in turn can stimulate tumor cell growth, thereby perpetuating a cycle of bone destruction. In addition, PTHrP stimulates increased renal tubular calcium reabsorption, resulting in further increased serum calcium levels.

The potent stimulatory effects of RANKL on osteoclastogenesis are usually counteracted by secreted osteoprotegerin (OPG), which acts as a safeguard mechanism for bone destruction (20,22–24). OPG is produced by many cell types. In vitro and in vivo osteoclast differentiation from precursor cells is blocked in a dose-dependent manner by recombinant OPG. OPG also binds to tumor necrosis factor–related apoptosis-inducing ligand (TRAIL). Therefore, RANKL and OPG are important regulators produced by the marrow microenvironment, and the ratio of RANKL to OPG regulates osteoclast formation and osteoclast activity. In malignant tumors, the upregulation of the cellular machinery (osteoclasts) and molecular pathways (RANKL/RANK/OPG) results in

tumor-associated hypercalcemia, osteolysis, pathologic fractures, and severe pain.

IL-6 is also known to stimulate osteoclast formation and causes mild hypercalcemia (25). Greenfield et al. have shown that IL-6 is a downstream effector of the action of PTH on the bone. They have also suggested that IL-6, in turn, promotes PTHrP-mediated hypercalcemia and bone resorption and this cytokine can act at later stages in the osteoclast lineage (26).

Additionally, calcitriol (1,25-dihydroxyvitamin D3) may also be a cause of HCM, particularly in a variety of B-cell malignancies (27). As reported in an M.D. Anderson Cancer Center study, calcitriol is believed to be the cause of almost all cases of hypercalcemia in Hodgkin's disease and approximately one-third of cases in non-Hodgkin's lymphoma. Calcitriol-induced hypercalcemia has also been described in patients with lymphomatoid granulomatosis lymphoma (28). Calcitriol may also be associated with hypercalcemia in the setting of chronic granulomatous diseases. This aspect is of therapeutic interest because glucocorticoids and noncalcemic vitamin D analogues may be possible treatment options for counteracting this pathophysiologic mechanism.

CURRENT TREATMENT OPTIONS

Intravenous Hydration

Adequate hydration with normal saline is the key to the initial management of HCM. High serum calcium levels lead to inadequate urine concentrating ability by the nephron tubules; this results in polyuria, hypovolemia, and dehydration. Restoring normal blood volume through aggressive IV rehydration is critical and improves the glomerular filtration rate and, along with sodium, increases renal excretion of excess serum calcium (29). Patients often receive inadequate fluids initially, which does not allow either adequate rehydration or successful excretion of the excessive calcium. Use of loop diuretics following rehydration at this stage may be required (but must be carefully monitored) to counteract fluid overload, especially in those patients who are also at the risk of developing congestive heart failure (30). Careful monitoring of serum and urine electrolytes is also necessary in these patients as they often require replacement during IV hydration and diuretic therapies. However, given that HCM tends to worsen with the progression of the underlying cancer, increased calcium diuresis provides only transient relief. Effective treatment of HCM also requires pharmacologic agents to treat the underlying cause of increased calcium release from bone.

Early Inhibitors of Osteoclast-Mediated Bone Resorption

The primary pharmacologic approach for the treatment of HCM has been to decrease the rate of bone resorption. Early treatments tended to use non–bone-specific agents that researchers found lower the serum calcium. However, these treatments lacked the potency of bone-specific agents such as the bisphosphonates that were developed later. One of the first treatments for HCM was oral phosphate, which lowers serum calcium levels both by preventing dietary calcium absorption and by inhibiting osteoclast-mediated bone resorption. The major side effect of phosphate therapy is persistent diarrhea; therefore, phosphate therapy should not be used in patients with impaired renal function because calcification of soft tissues can lead to death from organ failure (11). Calcitonin was another early agent used for the treatment of HCM. Calcitonin counteracts hypercalcemia by interfering with osteoclast maturation at several points in the differentiation pathway and by simultaneously increasing renal calcium excretion (11). The onset of the action of calcitonin is rapid (within 30 minutes), although the response tends to abate within 48 hours because of downregulation of the calcitonin receptors by osteoclasts. In addition, corticosteroids are known to be a highly effective treatment for calcitriol-mediated hypercalcemia, particularly among patients with Hodgkin's disease and non-Hodgkin's lymphomas with HCM. Time to response is generally within 1 to 4 days. However, corticosteroids are not as effective in nonhematologic cancers (31). Finally, gallium nitrate and plicamycin (also known as mithramycin) were both originally used as anticancer agents and were later found to decrease serum calcium levels through cytotoxic effects on osteoclasts (11). Although these agents are effective in lowering serum calcium levels in patients with HCM, they also carry significantly higher risks of toxicity than the newer, highly effective bisphosphonate drug class (32).

Bisphosphonates

Bisphosphonates are the current standard of care in the treatment of HCM (see Table 35.1). They are nonhydrolyzable analogues of inorganic pyrophosphate that bind avidly to hydroxyapatite crystals and are subsequently released during the process of bone resorption. The released bisphosphonate is taken up by osteoclasts and inhibits the cell's activity and survival. Once internalized, bisphosphonates are cytotoxic to osteoclasts, and the more potent bisphosphonates interfere with intracellular signaling pathways required for osteoclast activity and survival. The first-generation bisphosphonates—clodronate and etidronate—were introduced clinically more than three decades ago (11). Although these agents are relatively weak inhibitors of bone resorption, they have some clinical utility for treating HCM. Several of the recently developed more potent nitrogen-containing bisphosphonates including pamidronate, zoledronic acid, and ibandronate are more effective for treating HCM. Pamidronate was approved in 1991 for the treatment of HCM. Although pamidronate is the standard of care in the United States, zoledronic acid has recently been approved by the US Food and Drug Administration (in 2001) for the treatment of HCM and shown to be more effective than pamidronate (see following text). Ibandronate has recently been approved in Europe for the treatment of HCM but is not yet approved for use in the United States.

Zoledronic acid represents the latest generation of bisphosphonates. In preclinical studies in the in vivo thyroid-parathyroidectomized rat model of vitamin D_3–induced

TABLE 35.1	Types of bisphosphonates			
	Relative Potency	Dose (mg)	Mode of Administration	Adverse Effects
Non-nitrogen				
Clodronate	1	1,600	Oral	Hypersensitivity, renal insufficiency, hypocalcemia, hyperkalemia, hyperparathyroidism, hypocalcemia, abdominal pain, arthralgia
Single nitrogen				
Pamidronate	20	90	2 h IV	Fever in 20% hypophosphatemia, hypocalcemia, hypomagnesemia, loss of appetite, nausea, vomiting
Ibandronate	857	6	1 h IV	Rash, abdominal pain, constipation, diarrhea, dyspepsia, nausea, arthralgia, back pain, dizziness, headache
		50	Oral	
Two nitrogens				
Zoledronic acid	16,700	4	15 min IV	Minor; fever, rarely hypocalcemia, hypophosphatemia, loss of appetite, nausea, vomiting

hypercalcemia and in vitro mouse calvaria cultures, zoledronic acid was shown to be more potent than both pamidronate and ibandronate (33). In fact, zoledronic acid is the most potent bisphosphonate tested to date, proving to be between 87- and 940-fold more potent than pamidronate disodium in decreasing bone resorption in in vivo models of hypercalcemia (33). Figure 35.1 represents the relative potencies of these bisphosphonates in inhibiting hypercalcemia induction in rats and reducing calcium release in bone resorption in in vitro assays (34).

In a dose-finding study, 33 patients with hypercalcemia were administered one of four escalating doses of IV zoledronic acid with a median infusion time of 30 minutes. Doses as low as 0.02 and 0.04 mg/kg of body weight (i.e., 1.2 and 2.4 mg for a 60-kg individual, respectively) effectively normalized serum calcium. After a single administration of 0.04 mg/kg zoledronic acid, 93% of patients experienced a return to normocalcemia within 2 to 3 days, and 78% of evaluable patients maintained normocalcemia throughout the 32 to 39 days of the trial. The only clinically detectable side effect was a transient fever that occurred in 30% of patients (35).

A second dose-escalation phase I trial was conducted to evaluate the effect of zoledronic acid on biochemical markers of bone resorption in patients with bone metastases. A single 1- to 16-mg infusion of zoledronic acid was administered. This trial showed a dose–response relationship of zoledronic acid with bone resorption markers. Zoledronic acid was well tolerated at all dose levels (36).

Zoledronic acid (4 or 8 mg) is superior to pamidronate disodium (90 mg) in treating patients with moderate to severe HCM. On the basis of the results of the early single-arm dose-escalation studies, two randomized, parallel, phase III trials were designed to test the efficacy of 4 or 8 mg of IV zoledronic acid compared with 90 mg pamidronate in normalizing serum calcium levels in patients with moderate to severe HCM (37). These international studies were the largest prospective, randomized, comparative clinical trials conducted comparing two different bisphosphonates in the treatment of HCM. Total enrollment was 287 patients, 275 of whom were evaluable for efficacy. Patients were randomly assigned to receive either zoledronic acid (4 or 8 mg) through a 5-minute infusion or pamidronate disodium (90 mg) through a 2-hour infusion. The primary endpoints were to define the proportion of patients with normalized serum calcium at day 10 and the duration of response. Treatment groups were well balanced for all baseline disease characteristics. Overall, 59% of patients were male, with a mean age of 59 years (range, 21 to 87 years) and a mean baseline CSC of 3.47 mmol/L (37).

Both zoledronic acid doses (4 and 8 mg) proved superior to the pamidronate disodium dose (90 mg) as shown in Table 35.2 (37). The mean patient CSC in each treatment group is represented graphically in Figure 35.2 (37). Zoledronic acid yielded a more rapid and sustained decrease in CSC than did pamidronate. By day 10, normocalcemia was achieved by 88% of patients treated with 4 mg zoledronic acid versus only 70% of patients treated with pamidronate ($P = 0.002$). Moreover, Kaplan-Meier estimation of time to relapse showed that zoledronic acid maintains normocalcemia significantly longer than pamidronate disodium

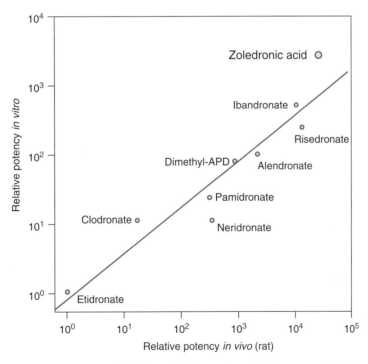

Figure 35.1. Relative potencies of bisphosphonates in inhibition of calcium release in vitro versus inhibition of hypercalcemia induction in a rat HCM model. HCM, Hypercalcemia of malignancy. Reprinted with permission from McCloskey EV, MacLennan IC, Drayson MT, et al. A randomized trial of the effect of clodronate on skeletal morbidity in multiple myeloma. MRC Working Party on Leukaemia in Adults. *Br J Haematol.* 1998;100(2):317–325.

TABLE 35.2	**Normalization of serum calcium levels by treatment with zoledronic acid or pamidronate disodium in patients with HCM**		
Agent	Patients with Normalized CSC, % Day 4 (Onset)	Patients with Normalized CSC, % Day 10	Median Days to Relapse
Pamidronate, 90 mg	33.3	69.7	17
Zoledronic acid, 4 mg	45.3*	88.4*	30*
Zoledronic acid, 8 mg	55.6*	86.7*	40*

*$P < 0.05$, as compared with pamidronate.

CSC, corrected serum calcium.

Data from Major P, Lortholary A, Hon J, et al. Zoledronic acid is superior to pamidronate in the treatment of hypercalcemia of malignancy: a pooled analysis of two randomized, controlled clinical trials. *J Clin Oncol.* 2001;19:558–567.

(Figure 35.3) (37). The median response duration was almost twice as long (30 days) for 4 mg zoledronic acid than for pamidronate (17 days; $P = 0.001$) (34). There was no significant difference in response rate between the 4 and 8 mg zoledronic acid group, implying that 4 mg of IV zoledronic acid is a sufficient dose.

The most commonly reported adverse events of zoledronic acid included fever, anemia, nausea, constipation, and diarrhea. These occurred with similar frequency between the zoledronic acid and pamidronate disodium groups. Although renal adverse events were reported more frequently in the zoledronic group than in the pamidronate disodium group,

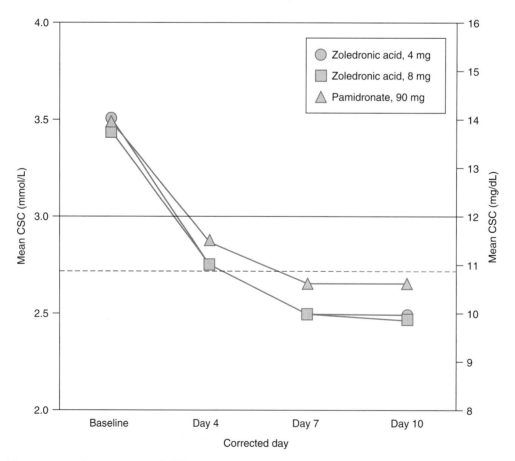

Figure 35.2. Mean corrected serum calcium (CSC) at baseline and days 4, 7, and 10 after treatment of hypercalcemia with zoledronic acid 4 mg, zoledronic acid 8 mg, or pamidronate 90 mg. Reprinted with permission from Major P, Lortholary A, Hon J, et al. Zoledronic acid is superior to pamidronate in the treatment of hypercalcemia of malignancy: a pooled analysis of two randomized, controlled clinical trials. *J Clin Oncol.* 2001;19(2):558–567.

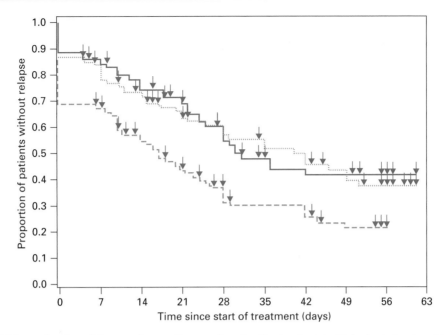

Figure 35.3. Kaplan-Meier estimation of time to relapse of hypercalcemia after treatment with (—) zoledronic acid 4 mg (median, 30 d), (----) zoledronic acid 8 mg (median, 40 d), or (—) pamidronate 90 mg (median, 17 d). Arrows denote censored time. Zoledronic acid 4 mg vs. pamidronate, *P* = 0.001; zoledronic acid 8 mg vs. pamidronate, *P* = 0.007. Reprinted with permission from Major P, Lortholary A, Hon J, et al. Zoledronic acid is superior to pamidronate in the treatment of hypercalcemia of malignancy: a pooled analysis of two randomized, controlled clinical trials. *J Clin Oncol.* 2001;19(2):558–567.

there were no differences in the National Cancer Institute's clinical toxicity criteria grade 3 or 4 for serum creatinine between treatment groups (37). Moreover, subsequent randomized clinical studies comparing these two drugs among patients with bone metastases who received long-term treatment every 3 to 4 weeks suggest that zoledronic acid (at a recommended dose of 4 mg through a 15-minute infusion) and pamidronate disodium (90 mg through 2-hour infusion) have similar renal safety profiles (37). The higher 8-mg dose showed unfavorable effects on renal function when administered on a monthly basis and is not used clinically.

Osteonecrosis of the Jaw

Osteonecrosis of the jaw is a newly reported complication that may result from long-term use of zoledronic acid or pamidronate treatment for patients with MM and other malignancies (38–41). The frequency with which this complication occurs in patients with cancer receiving bisphosphonate therapy is unknown. However, it appears that there is a higher risk of this complication among patients receiving these drugs. Most cases are associated with exposed mandibular bone with minimal symptoms, but infrequently patients may require more extensive intervention including surgical procedures to treat this problem. It is now recommended that patients receiving bisphosphonates, including most patients with myeloma, should be evaluated early on in their treatment for dental problems and encouraged to maintain excellent dental hygiene. It should be noted that there is no evidence that discontinuation of the bisphosphonate or replacement with other bisphosphonates changes the course of this complication.

Prophylactic Bisphosphonates

In studies evaluating the effects of bisphosphonates on skeletal complications among patients with breast cancer with lytic bone metastases, prevention of hypercalcemia has been demonstrated. In one study, Theriault et al. (42) assessed the efficacy of pamidronate in reducing skeletal morbidity in 372 breast cancer patients with osteolytic bone metastases, receiving hormonal therapy. Patients were randomized to receive double-blinded treatment with either 90 mg of pamidronate (through a 2-hour infusion) or placebo every 4 weeks for 24 treatment cycles. Among 371 evaluable patients, hypercalcemia was significantly lower in patients treated with pamidronate than in patients treated with placebo at 24 months. In another similar study by Hortobágyi et al. (43), 380 women with breast cancer and at least one lytic bone lesion who were receiving chemotherapy were randomly assigned to a monthly injection of pamidronate or placebo. Over the course of 1 year, the incidence of episodes of severe hypercalcemia was reduced by approximately half in the pamidronate-treated group. There were also lower incidence of pathologic fractures, bone pain, and spinal cord compression in both studies.

Bisphosphonate in the Hospice Setting

There is a paucity of studies on hospice patients using bisphosphonates. One small study was conducted using etidronate in the hospice setting. The report showed reduction in opiate use, improvement in pain control, and preservation of cognitive function (44). Control of the rate of hypercalcemia development is unknown. As bisphosphonates remain a relatively expensive therapy in patients with cancer, more studies are needed to evaluate the cost-effectiveness of this treatment in the hospice setting.

Emerging Therapeutic Approaches

In animal models, passive immunization using antisera raised against rat PTH-like peptide [PLP-(1–34) and rat PTH-(1–84)] has been studied (45). After immunization, plasma calcium in the tumor-bearing animals rapidly normalized and remained within the normal range for several days. These changes were associated with increased survival of the tumor-bearing rats. Similarly, monoclonal antibodies to PTHrP are being evaluated. The neutralizing effect of the antisera has shown specific reduction of serum calcium in the tumor-bearing animals (46). At present, however, both passive immunization and monoclonal antibodies to PTHrP are not available to patients.

A noncalcemic analogue of calcitriol in the T lymphocyte cell line was studied at the University of Tokyo (47). This study demonstrated that the analogue is capable of reducing PTHrP concentrations in vitro by approximately 50%. This compound suppresses both cell proliferation and PTHrP gene expression through binding to the vitamin D receptor that is overexpressed in T-cell lines. Whether the noncalcemic analogue of calcitriol will prove to be effective in patients remains to be determined.

Recently, OPG has been shown to inhibit osteoclast formation and activity by inhibiting RANK–RANKL signaling in a murine model of humoral HCM (45). The study showed that OPG treatment significantly returned osteoclast activity to sub-physiological range but had no effects on tumor size, tumor-induced cachexia, or PTHrP levels. These studies suggest a therapeutic potential for OPG as well as inhibitors of RANK signaling in the prevention and treatment of HCM. Ongoing early clinical trials suggest that inhibitors of RANK–RANKL may significantly reduce bone loss in patients with cancer.

It is possible that the development of antibodies to OPG may occur in patients treated with OPG, resulting in the prevention of its normal anti-bone resorptive function. To avoid potential problems with the use of OPG analogues, a recombinant form of RANKL, RANK-Fc, which is an antagonist of RANKL–RANK signaling, has recently been developed and consequently inhibits both bone disease and myeloma growth in a murine severe combined immunedeficiency human (SCID-hu) model of human myeloma (48). This recombinant protein is now being evaluated in clinical trials among patients with metastatic bone disease.

Aklilu et al. recently identified that the Ras signaling pathway is involved in PTHrP production by tumors. Treatment with Ras inhibitors in vitro produced a significant reduction in PTHrP mRNA expression and a significant decrease in cell proliferation. Treatment in mice bearing tumors with these inhibitors resulted in a significant decrease in plasma PTHrP and near-normalization of serum calcium (49). This study indicates that Ras-processing inhibitors may also be candidates for therapeutic agents to treat HCM.

CONCLUSION

HCM is a serious, often life-threatening skeletal complication. The goals of treatment for HCM are to control the underlying disorder, restore adequate hydration, increase urinary excretion of calcium, and inhibit osteoclast activity in bone. Zoledronic acid is a new, highly potent, nitrogen-containing bisphosphonate that has been recently approved for the treatment of HCM and represents a significant clinical advance in HCM treatment. The success rate is over 90%. The increased potency of zoledronic acid observed in preclinical models of HCM translated into improved clinical efficacy in the management of HCM, compared with pamidronate, the previous standard of care. Two randomized comparative trials demonstrated that zoledronic acid was superior to pamidronate disodium, safe and well tolerated. Furthermore, the recommended faster infusion time of 15 minutes of this newer agent represents a great advance over early bisphosphonate treatments for the management of HCM, which required infusion times as long as 24 hours (50,51).

As our understanding of the pathophysiology of HCM continues to increase, therapies will continue to evolve, offering new and more effective options for the management of HCM. In preclinical trials, subcutaneous injection of either OPG or antibodies against PTHrP or RANKL normalized serum calcium levels in animal models of HCM, without evidence of the nephrotoxicity that occasionally complicates the use of IV bisphosphonates (45,47,52). The antagonist of RANKL, RANK-Fc, is currently being evaluated in clinical trials among patients with metastatic bone disease (48). Moreover, inhibition of the signaling pathway, Ras-Raf MAPK-ERK, has been demonstrated to decrease PTHrP production and normalization of calcium of tumor-bearing animals (49). Ras-processing inhibitors are currently in clinical development. However, it remains to be seen whether these advances will eventually translate into more effective therapies for the management and treatment of HCM and how they will compare with the IV bisphosphonates.

REFERENCES

1. Rosol TJ, Capen CC. Mechanisms of cancer-induced hypercalcemia. *Lab Invest.* 1992;67(6):680–702.
2. O'Rourke NP, McCloskey EV, Kanis JA. Tumour induced hypercalcemia: a case for active treatment. *Clin Oncol.* 1994;6(3):172–176.
3. Vassilopoulou-Sellin R, Newman BM, Taylor SH, et al. Incidence of hypercalcemia in patients with malignancy referred to a comprehensive cancer center. *Cancer.* 1993;71:1309–1312.
4. Heath DA. Hypercalcemia in malignancy. *BMJ.* 1989;298(6686): 1468-1469.
5. Bajorunas DR. Clinical manifestations of cancer-related hypercalcemia. *Semin Oncol.* 1990;17:16–25.
6. Fisken RA, Heath DA, Bold AM. Hypercalcemia: a hospital survey. *Q J Med.* 1980;49:405–418.

7. Firkin F, Seymour JF, Watson AM, et al. Parathyroid hormone-related protein in hypercalcemia associated with hematological malignancy. *Br J Haematol.* 1996;94(3):486–492.

8. Grill V, Martin TJ. Hypercalcemia. In: Rubens RD, Mundy GR, eds. *Cancer and the Skeleton.* London: Martin Dunitz Ltd; 2000: 75–89.

9. Ratcliffe WA, Hutchesson AC, Bundred NJ, et al. Role of assays for parathyroid-hormone-related protein in investigation of hypercalcaemia. *Lancet.* 1992;339(8786):164–167.

10. Lind L, Ljunghall S. Serum chloride in the differential diagnosis of hypercalcemia. *Exp Clin Endocrinol.* 1991;98(3):179–184.

11. Mundy GR. Hypercalcemia. In: *Bone Remodeling and Its Disorders.* 2nd ed. London: Martin Dunitz Ltd; 1999: 107–122.

12. Poe CM, Radford AI. The challenge of hypercalcemia in cancer. *Oncol Nurs Forum.* 1985;12:29–34.

13. Stewart AF, Horst R, Deftos LJ, et al. Biochemical evaluation of patients with cancer-associated hypercalcemia: evidence for humoral and nonhumoral groups. *N Engl J Med.* 1980;303:1377–1383.

14. Mundy GR, Ibbotson KJ, D'Souza SM, et al. The hypercalcemia of cancer: clinical implications and pathogenic mechanisms. *N Engl J Med.* 1984;310:1718–1727.

15. Won C, Decker DA, Drelichman A, et al. Hypercalcemia in head and neck carcinoma: incidence and prognosis. *Cancer.* 1983;52(12):2261–2263.

16. Wimalawansa SJ. Significance of plasma PTH-rp in patients with hypercalcemia of malignancy treated with bisphosphonate. *Cancer.* 1994;73(8):2223–2230.

17. Pecherstorfer M, Schilling T, Blind E, et al. Parathyroid hormone-related protein and life expectancy in hypercalcemic cancer patients. *J Clin Endocrinol Metab.* 1994;78(5):1268–1270.

18. Gurney H, Grill V, Martin TJ. Parathyroid hormone-related protein and response to pamidronate in tumour-induced hypercalcaemia. *Lancet.* 1993;341(8861):1611–1613.

19. Ling PJ, A'Hern RP, Hardy JR. Analysis of survival following treatment of tumour-induced hypercalcaemia with intravenous pamidronate (APD). *Br J Cancer.* 1995;72(1):206–209.

20. Roodman GD. Biology of osteoclast activation in cancer. *J Clin Oncol.* 2001;19:3562–3571.

21. Suda T, Kobayashi K, Jimi E, et al. The molecular basis of osteoclast differentiation and activation. *Novartis Found Symp.* 2001;232:235–247; discussion 247–250.

22. Simonet WS, Lacey DL, Dunstan CR, et al. Osteoprotegerin: a novel secreted protein involved in the regulation of bone density. *Cell.* 1997;89:309–319.

23. Yasuda H, Shima N, Nakagawa N, et al. Identity of osteoclastogenesis inhibitory factor (OCIF) and osteoprotegerin (OPG): a mechanism by which OPG/OCIF inhibits osteoclastogenesis *in vitro. Endocrinology.* 1998;139:1329–1337.

24. Guise TA. Molecular mechanisms of osteolytic bone metastases. *Cancer.* 2000;88:2892–2898.

25. Greenfield EM, Shaw SM, Gornik SA, et al. Adenyl cyclase and interleukin 6 are downstream effectors of parathyroid hormone resulting in stimulation of bone resorption. *J Clin Invest.* 1995;96(3):1238–1244.

26. de la Mata J, Uy HL, Guise TA, et al. Interleukin-6 enhances hypercalcemia and bone resorption mediated by parathyroid hormone-related protein *in vivo. J Clin Invest.* 1995;95(6):2846–2852.

27. Seymour JF, Gagel RF. Calcitriol: the major humoral mediator of hypercalcemia in Hodgkin's disease and non-Hodgkin's lymphomas. *Blood.* 1993;82(5):1383–1394.

28. Scheinman SJ, Kelberman MW, Tatum AH, et al. Hypercalcemia with excess serum 1,25 dihydroxyvitamin D in lymphomatoid granulomatosis/angiocentric lymphoma. *Am J Med Sci.* 1991;301(3):178–181.

29. Davis KD, Attie MF. Management of severe hypercalcemia. *Crit Care Clin.* 1991;7:175–190.

30. Davidson TG. Conventional treatment of hypercalcemia of malignancy. *Am J Health Syst Pharm.* 2001;58(suppl 3): S8–S15.

31. Ralston SH, Gallacher SJ, Patel U, et al. Cancer-associated hypercalcemia: morbidity and mortality. *Ann Intern Med.* 1990;112(7):499–504.

32. Zojer N, Keck AV, Pecherstorfer M. Comparative tolerability of drug therapies for hypercalcaemia of malignancy. *Drug Saf.* 1999;21:389–406.

33. Green JR, Müller K, Jaeggi KA. Preclinical pharmacology of CGP 42'446, a new, potent, heterocyclic bisphosphonate compound. *J Bone Miner Res.* 1994;9:745–751.

34. Data on file. Novartis Pharma AG, Basel, Switzerland; 2000.

35. Body JJ, Borkowski A, Cleeren A, et al. Treatment of malignancy-associated hypercalcemia with intravenous aminohydroxypropylidene diphosphonate. *J Clin Oncol.* 1986;4:1177–1183.

36. Berenson JR, Vescio R, Henick K, et al. Phase I open label, dose ranging, safety trial of rapid intravenous zoledronic acid, a novel bisphosphonate, in cancer patients with osteolytic bone metastases. *Cancer.* 2001;91:144–154.

37. Major P, Lortholary A, Hon J, et al. Zoledronic acid is superior to pamidronate in the treatment of hypercalcemia of malignancy: a pooled analysis of two randomized, controlled clinical trials. *J Clin Oncol.* 2001;19:558–567.

38. Ruggiero SL, Mehrotra B, Rosenberg TJ, et al. Osteonecrosis of the jaws associated with the use of bisphosphonates: a review of 63 cases. *J Oral Maxillofac Surg.* 2004;62:527.

39. Migliorati CA. Bisphosphonates and oral cavity avascular bone necrosis. *J Clin Oncol.* 2003;21:4253.

40. Lugassy G, Shaham R, Nemets A, et al. Severe osteomyelitis of the jaw in long-term survivors of multiple myeloma: a new clinical entity. *Am J Med.* 2004;117:440.

41. Durie BG, Katz M, McCoy J, et al. Osteonecrosis of the jaws in myeloma: time dependent correlation with Aredia® and Zometa® use (abstract). *Blood.* 2004;104:216a.

42. Theriault RL, Lipton A, Hortobagyi GN, et al. Pamidronate reduces skeletal morbidity in women with advanced breast cancer and lytic bone lesions: a randomized, placebo-controlled trial. Protocol 18 Aredia Breast Cancer Study Group. *J Clin Oncol.* 1999;17:846–854.

43. Hortobágyi GN, Theriault RL, Lipton A, et al. Long-term prevention of skeletal complications of metastatic breast cancer with pamidronate. Protocol 19 Aredia Breast Cancer Study Group. *J Clin Oncol.* 1998;16:2038–2044.

44. Gloth FM III. Use of a bisphosphonate (etidronate) to improve metastatic bone pain in three hospice patients. *Clin J Pain.* 1995;11(4):333–335.

45. Henderson J, Bernier S, D'Amour P, et al. Effects of passive immunization against parathyroid hormone (PTH)-like peptide and PTH in hypercalcemic tumor-bearing rats and normocalcemic controls. *Endocrinology.* 1990;127(3): 1310–1380.

46. Kukreja SC, Shevrin DH, Wimbiscus SA, et al. Antibodies to parathyroid hormone-related protein lower serum calcium in athymic mouse models of malignancy-associated hypercalcemia due to human tumors. *J Clin Invest.* 1988;82(5):1798–1802.

47. Inoue D, Matsumoto T, Ogata E, et al. 22-Oxacalcitriol, a non-calcemic analogue of calcitriol, suppresses both cell proliferation and parathyroid hormone-related peptide gene expression in human T cell lymphotrophic virus, type I-infected T cells. *J Biol Chem.* 1993;268(22):16730–16736.

48. Sordillo EM, Pearse RN. RANK-Fc: a therapeutic antagonist for RANK-L in myeloma. *Cancer.* 2003;97(3 suppl):802–812.

49. Aklilu F, Park M, Goltzman D, et al. Induction of parathyroid hormone-related peptide by the Ras oncogene: role of Ras farnesylation inhibitors as potential therapeutic agents for hypercalcemia malignancy. *Cancer Res.* 1997;57:4517–4522.

50. Flores JF, Rude RK, Chapman RA, et al. Evaluation of a 24-hour infusion of etidronate disodium for the treatment of hypercalcemia of malignancy. *Cancer.* 1994;73:2527–2534.

51. Meunier PJ, Chapuy MC, Delmas P, et al. Intravenous disodium etidronate therapy in Paget's disease of bone and hypercalcemia of malignancy. Effects on biochemical parameters and bone histomorphometry. *Am J Med.* 1987;82:71–78.

52. Capparelli C, Kostenuik PJ, Morony S, et al. Osteoprotegerin prevents and reverses hypercalcemia in a murine model of humoral hypercalcemia of malignancy. *Cancer Res.* 2000;60(4):783–787.

CHAPTER 36

Metabolic Disorders in the Cancer Patient

Irene M. O'Shaughnessy ■ Albert L. Jochen

Endocrine disorders occur in individuals with advanced malignancy under various circumstances. Cancer may produce effects through the excess production of hormones, cytokines, and growth factors—the so-called paraneoplastic syndromes (Table 36.1). Conversely, cancer or its metastases may interfere with the normal function of endocrine organs, resulting in hormone-deficiency states. Most commonly, patients may have metabolic disorders, such as diabetes, thyroid dysfunction, and hyperparathyroidism, that predate the diagnosis of their malignancy or are diagnosed incidentally during the course of their malignancy. This chapter discusses the most common paraneoplastic syndromes and hormone-deficiency states associated with malignancy, as well as the management of diabetes and thyroid disease in the patient with cancer.

ENDOCRINE PARANEOPLASTIC SYNDROMES

Inappropriate Antidiuresis

The differential diagnosis of hyponatremia in the patient with cancer is similar to that in the general population and includes hepatic and cardiac failure, renal disease, overdiuresis, factitious hyponatremia associated with hyperglycemia, and other conditions. In the syndrome of inappropriate antidiuretic hormone (SIADH), hyponatremia results from the overproduction of arginine vasopressin (AVP) by the posterior pituitary gland in response to a stimulus by tumor cells, by the actual production of AVP or AVP-like peptides by tumor cells, or as a side effect of medications that are able to stimulate AVP production.

Epidemiology

The most common malignancies causing SIADH are small cell lung cancer and carcinoid tumors; SIADH is also seen with cancers of the esophagus, pancreas, duodenum, colon, adrenal cortex, prostate, thymomas, and lymphomas. In one series, the incidence of clinically significant SIADH was 9% among 523 patients with small cell lung cancer. A larger fraction of patients had milder abnormalities in AVP metabolism without hyponatremia. Therefore, approximately one-half of patients had abnormal renal handling of water loads that were subclinical (1, 2). Another study found that 41% of patients with all types of lung cancers and 43% of patients with colon cancer had significantly elevated levels of AVP without evidence of clinically significant SIADH (3). Hyponatremia is also a common electrolyte disorder in patients hospitalized with acquired immunodeficiency syndrome (AIDS) and AIDS-related complex. Often it is associated with gastrointestinal losses or SIADH and an increase in morbidity and mortality (4).

Clinical Features

The clinical features of hyponatremia depend on the degree of hyponatremia and the rate of its development. Most patients with chronic hyponatremia are asymptomatic. Generally, symptoms do not occur until the serum sodium falls below 115 to 120 mEq/L (5). When they occur, the signs and symptoms of SIADH are caused by water intoxication (i.e., hypo-osmolality and hyponatremia) and are manifested as confusion, lethargy, seizures, and coma. Occasionally, patients may present with focal neurologic deficits.

Diagnosis

Because most cases of SIADH are asymptomatic, the diagnosis is usually first suspected by noting a low serum sodium on routine chemistries. Other causes of hyponatremia, such as hypovolemia, hypervolemia (occurring in renal or hepatic disease or cardiac failure), hypothyroidism, and adrenal insufficiency, must be excluded before the diagnosis of SIADH can be considered. Urine chemistries show urinary osmolality that is greater than serum osmolality and a high urinary sodium concentration (Table 36.2). Medications commonly used by patients with cancer associated with SIADH include morphine sulfate, vincristine sulfate, cyclophosphamide, phenothiazines, and tricyclic antidepressants. Most drugs cause SIADH by stimulating posterior pituitary secretion of AVP.

Treatment

The treatment of SIADH is determined by the rate of development of hyponatremia and the presence of neurologic sequelae (Table 36.3). If the patient is symptomatic and has a serum sodium level below 130 mEq/L, fluid restriction to 800 to 1,000 mL per 24 hours is effective in slowly raising serum osmolality over a period of 3 to 10 days. Acute hyponatremia with neurologic symptoms has a mortality rate of 5% to 8% and warrants more aggressive treatment. For patients with more severe hyponatremia, the intravenous administration of hypertonic saline (3% saline at a rate of 0.1 mg/kg/min)

TABLE 36.1 Common paraneoplastic syndromes	
Syndrome	**Tumor Type**
Inappropriate antidiuresis (hormone vasopressin)	Lung cancer, all types
Cushing's syndrome (adrenocorticotropic hormone, corticotropic hormone)	Lung cancer, all types
Hypocalcemia	Bone metastases
Hypophosphatemia ("phosphatonin")	Mesenchymal tumors
Hyperthyroidism (human chorionic gonadotropin)	Lung cancer, all types
Gynecomastia (estrogens, follicle-stimulating hormone, luteinizing hormone)	Lung cancer, all types
Calcitoninemia (calcitonin)	Medullary carcinoma of the thyroid, lung cancer, breast cancer
Acromegaly (growth hormone, growth hormone–releasing hormone)	Carcinoids, pheochromocytoma, pancreatic cancer

and furosemide may be necessary (6). Careful monitoring of vital signs and urinary losses of sodium and potassium is indicated. Rapid correction of severe hyponatremia has been associated with central pontine myelinosis, which presents with quadriparesis and bulbar palsy 1 to 2 days after hyponatremia is corrected. A safe rate of correction in severe hyponatremia is 0.5 to 1.0 mEq/L/h until the sodium concentration reaches 125 mEq/L (7, 8).

Fluid restriction is not feasible in some patients who require long-term treatment of SIADH. In these patients, medications, including demeclocycline hydrochloride, lithium carbonate, and urea, have been tried. Demeclocycline is the drug of choice and causes partial nephrogenic diabetes insipidus by inhibiting the formation of AVP-induced cyclic adenosine monophosphate in distal tubules. It is initially administered orally in divided doses of 900 to 1,200 mg/d and then reduced to maintenance doses of 600 to 900 mg/d. Side effects are mainly gastrointestinal, although hypersensitivity and nephrotoxicity can occur. Similar to demeclocycline hydrochloride, lithium carbonate also causes a reversible, partial form of nephrogenic diabetes insipidus but is less effective. Urea acts as an osmotic diuretic and allows the patient to maintain a normal fluid intake. Urea can be

administered intravenously or orally. When given by mouth, the usual dosing is 30 g of urea dissolved in 100 mL of orange juice or water once daily (9).

CUSHING'S SYNDROME

Endogenous Cushing's syndrome is due to one of three causes: overproduction of glucocorticoid by a primary adrenal neoplasm, excessive production of adrenocorticotropic hormone (ACTH) by a pituitary adenoma, or a paraneoplastic syndrome in which either ACTH or corticotropin-releasing hormone (CRH) are produced ectopically by the tumor. A number of tumors are capable of producing ACTH, its prohormone "big ACTH," or proopiomelanocortin (POMC) (Table 36.4). The *POMC* gene is located at p23 on the short arm of chromosome 2 near N-*myc* oncogene at p24. Normally the expression of the *POMC* gene is influenced by glucocorticoids, which suppress transcription, and CRH, which stimulates transcription through cyclic adenosine monophosphate. The activation of alternative steroid-insensitive promoters may result in ectopic ACTH production that is insensitive to glucocorticoid suppression. Pituitary cells and some tumors produce the normal 1,200-base mRNA transcript; however, some nonpituitary tissues produce either a larger or smaller POMC mRNA transcript. Alternative posttranscription processing of POMC gives rise to a large number of biologically active peptides in addition to ACTH. These include pro-ACTH and a number of different peptides containing melanocyte-stimulating hormone (MSH) (α-MSH, ACTH, pro-ACTH, β-MSH, τ-lipotropin, β-lipotropin, τ-MSH, N-POMC, and pro-τ-MSH), all of which can lead to generalized hyperpigmentation (10, 11). Radioimmunoassays differ in their abilities to detect aberrant ACTH. The immunoradiometric assay for ACTH is able to distinguish between ACTH and its larger precursors, pro-ACTH, and POMC (12).

TABLE 36.2 Diagnosis of syndrome of inappropriate antidiuresis
Plasma sodium level below 135 mEq/L
Urine osmolality greater than serum osmolality
Elevated urine sodium (>20 mEq/L)
Normal extracellular fluid volume
Rule out other causes of euvolemic hyponatremia

TABLE 36.3	Usual treatment of hyponatremia	
Treatment	**Dosage**	**Uses**
Fluid restriction	800–1,000 mL limit/24 h	Serum sodium < 130 mEq/L and symptomatic
		Acute and chronic hyponatremia
Hypertonic saline (3% saline)	0.1 mg/kg/min	Rarely used
		Acute severe hyponatremia (mental status changes, coma)
Demeclocycline	Initial dose: 900–1,200 mg/d in divided doses	Chronic hyponatremia
	Maintenance: 600–900 mg/d	
Lithium carbonate (rarely used)	600–900 mg p.o. daily	Chronic hyponatremia
		Significant toxicity
Urea (rarely used)	30 g in 100 mL orange juice or water daily	Chronic hyponatremia

Epidemiology

Ectopic ACTH is most frequently secreted by lung carcinomas. A number of other tumor types are also capable of producing this syndrome (Table 36.4). In the general population, approximately 65% of patients with Cushing's syndrome have pituitary adenomas producing ACTH (Cushing's disease), 20% have primary adrenal tumors, and 14% have ectopic ACTH. Therefore, ectopic ACTH production is the least common of the three major causes in the general population.

Clinical Features of Ectopic ACTH Syndrome

Manifestations of the ectopic ACTH syndrome include hypokalemia, hyperglycemia, edema, muscle weakness (especially proximal) and atrophy, hypertension, and weight loss. Features typically seen in long-standing pituitary or adrenal Cushing's syndrome (e.g., central obesity, plethoric facies, cutaneous striae, "buffalo hump," and hyperpigmentation) are less common in highly malignant tumors such

as small cell lung carcinoma but occur more frequently in more indolent tumors such as carcinoids, thymomas, and pheochromocytomas.

Diagnosis

The biochemical diagnosis of Cushing's syndrome is suggested by an elevated 24-hour urinary-free cortisol (>100 μg per 24 hours). The other principal screening test is the overnight low-dose dexamethasone suppression test. The test is positive when 1 mg of dexamethasone given at midnight is unable to suppress the following 8:00 AM cortisol to <5 μg/dL. Failure of cortisol to suppress after high-dose dexamethasone (8 mg at midnight) suggests either ectopic ACTH or a primary adrenal tumor (13). These two are differentiated by measuring plasma ACTH. In primary adrenal tumors, ACTH levels are below 20 pg/mL, whereas in ectopic ACTH levels are generally >100 to 200 pg/mL and frequently are elevated above 1,000 pg/mL. Inferior petrosal sinus sampling of ACTH is useful in confirming the diagnosis of pituitary Cushing's syndrome (14), but it is rarely indicated in the patient with advanced malignancy secreting ectopic ACTH.

Difficulties arise in differentiating those rare tumors producing ectopic CRH from the more common ectopic ACTH production; CRH stimulates the release of pituitary ACTH. The clinical presentation and biochemical results are identical for ectopic CRH and ACTH. The prognosis and therapy are identical for the two disorders.

TABLE 36.4	**Tumors associated with ectopic adrenocorticotropic hormone/ corticotropic hormone syndrome**
Small cell lung carcinoma	
Thymoma	
Pancreatic islet cell tumor	
Carcinoid tumors (lung, gut, pancreas, ovary)	
Medullary carcinomas of the thyroid	
Pheochromocytomas	

Treatment of Ectopic ACTH Syndromes

Where possible, the treatment of ectopic ACTH syndrome should be directed primarily at the tumor. Palliative treatment of Cushing's syndrome involves inhibition of steroid synthesis. Drugs successfully used include aminoglutethimide, metyrapone, mitotane, ketoconazole, and octreotide acetate (15). Rarely, bilateral adrenalectomy is considered.

Aminoglutethimide blocks the first step in cortisol biosynthesis. At higher doses, it inhibits production of glucocorticoids, mineralocorticoids, and androgens, whereas at lower doses it primarily inhibits the conversion of androgens to estrogens, contributing to its efficacy in the treatment of postmenopausal breast cancer. At the higher doses required to treat ectopic ACTH syndrome, many patients experience sedation, ataxia, and skin rashes. Metyrapone inhibits 11-β-hydroxylase and 18-hydroxylase, resulting in adrenal atrophy and necrosis. It is a toxic drug with significant gastrointestinal side effects, including anorexia, nausea, vomiting, and diarrhea, and central nervous system (CNS) toxicity, including lethargy and somnolence. For these reasons, it is used as second-line therapy.

Ketoconazole not only acts mainly on the first step of cortisol biosynthesis but also inhibits the conversion of 11-deoxycortisol to cortisol. It can cause rare but significant reversible hepatotoxicity and is associated with nausea and vomiting.

Octreotide acetate, a long-acting analog of somatostatin, can reduce ectopic ACTH secretion. It must be injected, is expensive, and is only partially effective in most patients. The efficacy of these treatments can be monitored by 24-hour urine cortisol measurements. As levels return to normal and then fall below normal, replacement with glucocorticoids and mineralocorticoids in physiologic doses similar to patients with Addison's disease is frequently necessary. In cases of stress, these patients require stress doses of glucocorticoids (e.g., hydrocortisone 100 mg intravenously every 8 hours).

HYPERCALCEMIA

Malignancies are frequently associated with disorders of calcium metabolism, including hypercalciuria and hypercalcemia, and are the most common cause of hypercalcemia in hospitalized patients. After primary hyperparathyroidism, they are the second most common cause overall. Malignancies produce hypercalcemia by one of three mechanisms. Neoplasms may secrete parathyroid hormone–related protein (PTHrP), which, although distinct from PTH, has sufficient amino-terminal homology with PTH to mimic its effects on PTH receptors. This is the most common mechanism subserving malignancy-associated hypercalcemia, accounting for 80% of all cases (16). PTHrP is produced most commonly by squamous cell cancers (head, neck, lung, and esophagus), renal cell carcinoma, and breast cancer. Metastases with extensive localized bone destruction constitute the second most common mechanism of tumor-related hypercalcemia. Finally, hematologic neoplasms (e.g., multiple myeloma and lymphoma) cause hypercalcemia by releasing osteoclast-activating cytokines, and occasionally (in lymphomas), 1,25-dihydroxyvitamin D. Patients with malignancy may also have hypercalcemia from a cause unrelated to their cancer. In particular, hypercalcemia from primary hyperparathyroidism is a common disorder in the general population.

Most cancer-related hypercalcemia complicates an advanced malignancy that is already diagnosed and associated with a poor prognosis. Rarely, the tumor is occult and requires an extensive workup to unmask it. The features of advanced cancer typically dominate the presentation, with weight loss, anorexia, fatigue, and pain from bone metastases. Hypercalcemia is more acute and severe (often >14 mg/dL) than is typical for primary hyperparathyroidism and is more likely to cause nausea, vomiting, dehydration, and changes in mentation (hypercalcemic crisis). When possible, treatment is directed toward the primary tumor. Hypercalcemic crisis is treated medically (Table 36.5). Patients with severe hypercalcemia are typically dehydrated, with resultant diminished urine output. This further exacerbates the hypercalcemia by reducing the ability of the kidneys to eliminate calcium in the urine. Therefore, the first step in treating hypercalcemia is vigorous hydration to reestablish urine output and calciuresis. After adequate rehydration, loop diuretics such as furosemide can be used to further promote a calciuric diuresis. This therapy has the advantage of working rapidly (over hours) but is limited by incomplete calcium-lowering effects and the need for intravenous fluids. Calcitonin injections are often used concomitantly with hydration because of their rapid action, although their efficacy is somewhat limited by modest calcium-lowering effects and by tachyphylaxis. Intravenous infusion of a bisphosphonate, either pamidronate or zoledronate, is the most consistently effective treatment of cancer-related hypercalcemia, although the infusion has a delay of 1 to 2 days in the onset of action. A single infusion will normalize calcium levels in most patients with a persistent duration of action lasting a few weeks to several months. Increased bone resorption by PTHrP-activated osteoclasts is the mechanism subserving most cancer-related hypercalcemia, and intravenous bisphosphonates effectively block this pathway. Therefore, the usual therapy in hypercalcemic crisis is to begin rapid onset, partially effective therapy with hydration and calcitonin, while giving an infusion of a bisphosphonate that will have potent calcium-lowering effects in a day or two. Other therapies are used in selected cases of hypercalcemia. For example, glucocorticoids are useful calcium-lowering agents in hematologic malignancies and in hypercalcemia mediated by vitamin D intoxication. Many other therapies, commonly used in the past, have been supplanted by the safety and potency of bisphosphonates. These include intravenous and oral phosphates, gallium nitrate, plicamycin, and indomethacin.

HYPOCALCEMIA

Hypocalcemia is an uncommon paraneoplastic syndrome occurring primarily in patients with bony metastases. It occurs most commonly in association with osteoblastic metastases of the breast, prostate, and lung; its incidence is approximately 16% (17). Tetany is a rare complication of tumor-associated hypocalcemia. The etiology of the

---

TABLE 36.5   Usual treatment of hypercalcemic crisis

Treatment	Dosage	Advantages	Disadvantages
Rehydration	As needed	Rapid action	None
Saline diuresis (optional)	150–200 mL/h of normal saline with or without 40 mg/d furosemide	Rapid action	Partial response; risk of fluid overload
Calcitonin (optional)	200 units SQ q6h	Rapid action	Partial response; tachyphylaxis
Pamidronate	60 or 90 mg i.v. over 4 h	Potent; normalizes calcium in over 90% of cases. Prolonged response	1–2 d delay in action
Zoledronate	4 mg i.v. over 30 min	Potent; normalizes calcium in over 90% of cases. Prolonged response	1–2 d delay in action
Prednisone (in select cases)	60 mg daily	Suitable for oral outpatient therapy	Effective only in select patients, for example, some hematologic malignancies

hypocalcemia is not understood. Ectopic calcitonin secretion from the underlying tumor has been rarely implicated. Acute hypocalcemia is treated by i.v. calcium gluconate or calcium chloride (Table 36.6). Vitamin D and calcium supplements are the therapeutic mainstays of all forms of chronic hypocalcemia.

ONCOGENIC HYPOPHOSPHATEMIC OSTEOMALACIA

Oncogenic hypophosphatemic osteomalacia, an acquired form of adult-onset, vitamin D–resistant rickets, is associated with mesenchymal tumors, often benign, that occur in soft tissues or bones (18). These tumors are also referred to as *ossifying mesenchymal tumors, giant cell tumors of bone, sclerosing hemangioma,* or *cavernous hemangioma.* This syndrome has been rarely reported with other cancers, such as lung and prostate. The clinical syndrome can precede the discovery of the tumor by several years. Clinical and laboratory features include osteomalacia, severe phosphaturia, renal glycosuria, hypophosphatemia, normocalcemia (normal parathyroid hormone levels), and increased alkaline phosphatase. The proposed mechanisms for this syndrome include inhibition of the conversion of 25-hydroxyvitamin D to 1,25-dihydroxyvitamin D and through a substance produced by the tumor with a phosphaturic effect,

---

TABLE 36.6   Management of hypocalcemia

Acute Symptomatic Hypocalcemia (Tetany)

1. 10% calcium gluconate (90 mg of elemental calcium/10 mL ampule)

   ■ Dilute 2 × 10 mL ampules of calcium gluconate in 50–100 mL of D5 solution. Infuse 2 mg/kg body weight over 5–10 min or 10% calcium chloride (272 mg of elemental calcium/10 mL ampule)

   ■ Dilute 1 × 10 mL ampule in 50–100 mL of D5 solution. Infuse 2 mg/kg over 5–10 min.

2. Following rapid loading infusion, reduce to a slower infusion of 15 mg/kg of calcium gluconate mixed with D5 infused over 6–12 h.

Chronic Hypocalcemia

1. Oral elemental calcium 1–2 g in 2–3 divided doses

2. Vitamin D replacement (approximate doses only)

   ■ 1,25-Dihydroxyvitamin D: 0.25–2.0 µg/d

   ■ Vitamin D: 25,000–100,000 IU/d

"phosphatonin." A candidate gene for "phosphatonin" has recently been described—fibroblastic growth factor 23 (19). Treatment is directed at surgical resection of the underlying tumor. When this is not possible, treatment with high doses of vitamin D and phosphate is often required.

HYPERURICEMIA

Uric acid is a metabolite of purine catabolism. Hyperuricemia can be present in a mild form resulting from high turnover of cancer cells in large tumors, or in an acute form as a component of the tumor lysis syndrome. The tumor lysis syndrome is a complication of anticancer therapy in which abrupt necrosis of a bulky tumor releases large amounts of intracellular ions and other metabolites. The resulting metabolic abnormalities include hyperuricemia, hyperphosphatemia, hypocalcemia, and acute renal failure. The tumor lysis syndrome is not only observed most commonly in pediatric patients and young adults with lymphomas or leukemias but also occasionally recognized in older patients with solid tumors. Hyperuricemia results from rapid release and catabolism of purine-containing intracellular nucleic acids. Plasma levels of uric acid exceed secretory pathways, and uric acid crystals precipitate in the renal tubules producing acute renal failure.

Tumor lysis syndrome can usually be prevented by identifying patients at risk before initiating chemotherapy. Risk factors include large, actively growing tumors (especially lymphomas) that are expected to be sensitive to cytotoxic therapy, patients with preexisting renal insufficiency, and patients with preexisting elevations in uric acid levels. In patients with these risk factors, allopurinol and intravenous hydration can be initiated prior to cytotoxic therapy. In hyperuricemia resistant to allopurinol, the urate oxidase enzyme rasburicase can be used to rapidly normalize uric acid levels. Rasburicase infused intravenously (0.2 mg/kg/d) converts uric acid to the more soluble compound allantoin, decreasing uric acid levels by 86% within 4 hours (20). Clinical features of tumor lysis syndrome include lethargy, nausea, and vomiting from hyperuricemia; spasms, seizures, and tetany from hypocalcemia; and oliguric renal failure. Laboratory findings include hyperphosphatemia, hyperkalemia, azotemia, hyperuricemia, and hypocalcemia. Supportive care and monitoring in an intensive care unit is required. In patients with oliguric renal failure, hemodialysis is indicated for uncontrolled hyperkalemia, persistent hyperphosphatemia complicated by symptomatic hypocalcemia, or hypervolemia.

HYPERTHYROIDISM

Most commonly, human chorionic gonadotropin (hCG) is secreted by trophoblastic or germ cell tumors (21). Because of its evolutionary homology with the thyroid-stimulating hormone (TSH), hCG has intrinsic thyrotropic action. Overt hyperthyroidism usually occurs with large tumors secreting large quantities of hCG, such as gestational trophoblastic

disease (e.g., choriocarcinoma and hydatidiform mole) and testicular tumors. The hyperthyroidism resolves with surgical resection of the underlying tumor. When necessary, treatment of the hyperthyroidism is achieved by using antithyroid drugs such as propylthiouracil or methimazole.

GYNECOMASTIA

Gynecomastia is defined as *palpable breast tissue in men* (22) and may be caused by drugs that lower testosterone levels (23), including alkylating agents, vinca alkaloids, and nitrosoureas. Antiemetics, such as metoclopramide and phenothiazines, may produce gynecomastia by stimulating prolactin production. Alternatively, tumor production of gonadotropins or estrogens may result in gynecomastia; these include adrenal and testicular tumors and hepatomas. Tumors that produce hCG can stimulate estrogen production by interstitial and Sertoli cells of the testes, resulting in gynecomastia. The approach to the treatment of gynecomastia includes treatment of the underlying tumor and, if implicated, cessation of drugs known to cause gynecomastia.

Treatment of gynecomastia with antiestrogens and androgens such as tamoxifen citrate, clomiphene citrate, topical dihydrotestosterone, and danazol is generally unsuccessful. For more severe cases, long-term management with liposuction and subcutaneous mastectomy may be necessary. Low-dose radiation therapy has been used with some success for the treatment of painful gynecomastia.

CALCITONINEMIA

Calcitonin is a polypeptide hormone produced by the C cells of the thyroid. It diminishes the release of calcium from bone and increases the excretion of urine calcium, sodium, and phosphate. Interestingly, no clinical syndromes are associated with tumor production of calcitonin except for one reported case of a patient with small cell carcinoma with hypercalcitoninemia and hypocalcemia (24). Calcitonin plays an important role as a tumor marker in monitoring patients with medullary carcinoma of the thyroid and in the diagnosis of multiple endocrine neoplasia type 2, a familial disorder characterized by medullary carcinoma of the thyroid, parathyroid adenomas, and pheochromocytoma. In addition to medullary thyroid carcinoma, a number of other cancers have been associated with elevations in calcitonin, including small cell (48% to 64%) and other lung cancers, carcinoid, breast cancer, colon cancer (24%), and gastric cancer (38%). With the exception of medullary thyroid carcinoma, the clinical usefulness of serum calcitonin levels as a tumor marker remains undetermined (25).

ACROMEGALY

Most cases of acromegaly result from overproduction of growth hormone by pituitary tumors. Growth hormone elevations may also result from production of growth hormone–releasing hormone by tumors, particularly pancreatic islet cell tumors and bronchial carcinoids. Treatment of this paraneoplastic syndrome is directed at the treatment of the underlying tumor. Occasionally, growth hormone–releasing hormone secretion responds to the administration of long-acting somatostatin analogs (26).

CARCINOID SYNDROME

Carcinoid tumors are of neuroendocrine origin and are usually (74% of the time) found in the gastrointestinal tract with the most common locations being the small bowel, the appendix, and the rectum. Other gastrointestinal sites include the esophagus, bile ducts, pancreas, and liver. They are also found outside the gastrointestinal tract in the larynx, thymus, lung, breast, ovary, urethra, and testis.

The classic carcinoid syndrome is characterized by flushing, diarrhea, and bronchospasm. Less frequent signs and symptoms associated with carcinoid tumors include coronary artery spasms leading to angina pectoris, pellagra, endocardial fibrosis, arthropathy, and hypotension (Table 36.7). Cardiac symptoms can be particularly disabling in some patients, manifesting primarily as right-sided heart failure. Cardiac disease is caused by fibrous deposits on the endocardial surface of the right side of the heart, particularly on the tricuspid and pulmonary valves. This leads to valvular insufficiency or stenosis (27, 28). Because of the drainage of bronchial carcinoids into the pulmonary veins, these tumors cause fibrous deposits on the mitral valve.

Acute symptoms in the carcinoid syndrome are due primarily to the production of 5-hydroxytryptophan (serotonin), although secretion of other hormones, such as bradykinin, hydroxytryptamine, and prostaglandins, may also play a role. Useful biochemical markers include measurement of serum 5-hydroxytryptophan and 24-hour urine collections for the serotonin metabolite 5-hydroxyindoleacetic acid.

The peak incidence of carcinoid tumors is in the sixth and seventh decades. Carcinoid tumors are slow growing and tend to metastasize to regional lymph nodes and the liver. Because of their indolent nature, prognosis tends to be very good for most patients. A recent large survey of over 8,000 patients with carcinoid syndrome demonstrated a median 5-year survival of 50% (29). Patients with the most common type of carcinoid tumor, localized to the small bowel, had a 5-year survival of 80%.

Surgery is the mainstay of treatment for localized tumors. Debulkment of primary tumors remains an option for patients with metastatic involvement of regional lymph nodes or the liver. The medical treatment of the carcinoid syndrome is directed at inhibiting serotonin synthesis and at blocking its effects peripherally. Different drugs can be used to accomplish these goals (30), albeit with variable and inconsistent results. Antiserotonin agents such as cyproheptadine hydrochloride and methysergide can ameliorate the diarrhea. For long-term treatment, cyproheptadine hydrochloride is the preferred medication because of the risk of retroperitoneal, cardiac, and pulmonary fibrosis associated with methysergide. Antidiarrheal agents such as loperamide hydrochloride and diphenoxylate hydrochloride also can be quite helpful in controlling the diarrhea. Flushing appears to be due to the secretion of histamine. The administration of a combination of H_1 and H_2 histamine receptor antagonists can often control this symptom. Somatostatin analogs such as octreotide acetate are the most commonly used medications used to control symptoms of carcinoid syndrome and are effective in controlling the symptoms of flushing and diarrhea in up to 75% of patients (26). Local control of metastatic disease in the liver can also be attempted with radiofrequency ablation and arterial chemoembolization (31).

Carcinoid syndrome associated with bronchial carcinoid tumors has distinctive features. Many patients experience improvement in symptoms with glucocorticoids or phenothiazines.

ENTEROENDOCRINE TUMORS OTHER THAN CARCINOID

Recently, there has been an increased recognition and characterization of the heterogeneous group of rare gastroenteropancreatic neuroendocrine neoplasms. They vary in terms of their degree of malignancy and their biological behavior and clinical course. They may be quite small or large and bulky. Depending on their cell type, they can produce a number of different endocrine syndromes. These include hypoglycemia (insulinoma), Zollinger-Ellison syndrome (gastrinoma), watery diarrhea,

TABLE 36.7	Symptoms and complications of carcinoid tumors
Symptoms of carcinoid syndrome	Flushing, diarrhea, wheezing, hypotension, cyanosis, arthralgias
Complications of carcinoid tumors	Right-sided heart failure
	Left-sided heart failure (rare)
	Intestinal obstruction
	Biliary obstruction
	Gastrointestinal bleeding
	Pellagra

hypokalemia–achlorhydria (VIPoma), and glucagonoma syndrome (glucagonoma). The primary treatment for both cure and palliation is surgery. However, they are also treated with drugs or agents that target the tumor's specific product or its effects. Most of these tumors show some response to somatostatin analogs. Because of their slow growth, patients often survive for many years with these tumors (32).

EXTRAPANCREATIC TUMOR HYPOGLYCEMIA

Tumors most likely to cause hypoglycemia are of mesodermal origin, such as fibrosarcomas and mesotheliomas, or of epithelial origin, such as hepatomas, adrenal cortical carcinomas, and gastrointestinal adenocarcinomas. Hypoglycemia usually occurs in the late stages of malignancy. The mechanism by which hypoglycemia occurs involves a combination of impaired hepatic glucose production and increased peripheral glucose utilization. Many patients have poor nutritional status, with depleted stores of the glycogen and protein needed to sustain hepatic glycogenolysis and gluconeogenesis. Hepatic damage from metastases further limits the ability to sustain gluconeogenesis. In most patients, however, hypoglycemia results predominantly from increased peripheral glucose utilization, raising the possibility of production of hormones with insulin-like properties. Insulin levels, as well as levels of insulin-like growth factor I and growth hormone, are low, whereas insulin-like growth factor II (IGF-II) levels are usually normal. Recent work has focused on the tumor production of an abnormally processed variant of IGF-II, "big IGF-II." This variant is not measured in usual radioimmunoassays for IGF-II but possesses normal biological activity. It is likely that "big IGF-II" accounts for many or most cases of tumor hypoglycemia (33, 34).

Symptoms of hypoglycemia result from neuroglycopenia (confusion, seizures, and coma) or from activation of the adrenergic nervous system (sweating, palpitations, hunger, and tremors). The presence of tumor-associated hypoglycemia is established by demonstrating a low serum glucose level (<40 to 50 mg%) in a patient with symptoms of hypoglycemia who responds to oral or intravenous glucose. No further diagnostic workup is necessary. The primary treatment is nutritional support, either oral or intravenous. For immediate relief of symptomatic hypoglycemia, glucose is given as an intravenous bolus of 50% dextrose and then continued as a drip of 10% glucose. Refractory hypoglycemia can be treated with the counterregulatory hormones glucagon or cortisone.

SOMATOSTATIN ANALOGS

Somatostatin was first discovered as a hypothalamic hormone–inhibiting growth hormone secretion (35, 36). It is now known that it is secreted at multiple sites throughout the human body. Somatostatin has physiologic effects on multiple endocrine and exocrine secretions (37). In the pituitary, the secretion of growth hormone, prolactin, and thyrotropin is inhibited. In the gastrointestinal tract, somatostatin inhibits the secretion of cholecystokinin, gastric inhibitory

peptide, gastrin, motilin, neurotensin, and secretin. The secretion of glucagon, insulin, and pancreatic polypeptide is inhibited in the pancreas. In the CNS, somatostatin acts as a neurotransmitter in distinct pathways and as a neuromodulator, modulating the release of other neurotransmitters such as serotonin and acetylcholine. Somatostatin also inhibits a number of exocrine secretions such as amylase from the salivary glands, hydrochloric acid and pepsinogen by gastrointestinal mucosa, pancreatic enzymes and bicarbonate from the pancreatic acini, and bile by the liver. It also regulates gastrointestinal motility.

Two distinct effects of somatostatin have made it very useful in the treatment of certain cancers that express somatostatin receptors. Somatostatin has been shown to inhibit the growth of both normal and tumorous cells by inhibiting cell division and triggering cell death by apoptosis (38, 39). In patients with growth hormone–secreting pituitary tumors, somatostatin has been shown to reduce tumor size by 10% to 25% in approximately 50% of cases (40). Because a variety of endocrine tumors express somatostatin receptors, it is also used in the treatment of a number of paraneoplastic syndromes, as already mentioned. Because of its short plasma half-life, natural somatostatin has limited therapeutic potential. The first two longer acting and more potent somatostatin analogs developed were octreotide and lanreotide, but only octreotide is available in the United States. An intermediate acting form of octreotide is administered subcutaneously every 8 hours and a long-acting form is administered by intramuscular injection every 28 days (41). Radiolabeled somatostatin analogs have also been used as either tumor tracers or therapeutic agents (42).

Because of its potent antisecretory effects, somatostatin analogs are among the few oncologic agents that are continued in patients with paraneoplastic syndromes in spite of tumor progression (43). The most common side effects are a direct consequence of somatostatin's numerous actions on the endocrine and exocrine systems. Side effects are primarily gastrointestinal and include diarrhea, abdominal pain, flatulence, biliary tract abnormalities, and nausea and vomiting. More serious adverse effects include cholecystitis and ascending cholangitis (44).

ENDOCRINE DISEASES IN PATIENTS WITH CANCER

Malignancies often occur in patients with preexisting medical conditions such as diabetes mellitus and thyroid disease. Treatment of these conditions must continue during and after treatment of the malignancy and during palliative care. In each condition, goals of treatment must be reevaluated with prognosis of the underlying malignancy in mind.

DIABETES MELLITUS

Standard guidelines for the treatment of both type 1 and type 2 diabetes mellitus can generally be followed in the patient with cancer; however, the appropriateness of "tight control" needs to be addressed in these patients. On the basis of results of the Diabetes Control and Complications Trial (45), it is accepted that intensive insulin treatment of type 1 diabetes results in a decrease in microvascular complications. These results have been extrapolated to type 2 diabetes mellitus (46); however, in the patient with cancer with a limited life expectancy, intensive insulin therapy to prevent long-term complications is not a reasonable goal. The major complication of intensive insulin therapy is an increased risk of hypoglycemia. In patients with malignancies and poor nutrition, the risk of hypoglycemia is further increased. Additionally, intensive insulin treatment requires frequent blood glucose monitoring, which may place a further burden on the patient and his or her caregivers. Sulfonylurea agents are frequently included in treatment regimens for type 2 diabetes. In the cancer population with suboptimal nutrition, recent weight loss, or impaired kidney or liver function, these agents should be used with extreme caution. Severe prolonged hypoglycemia can result from the use of sulfonylurea drugs. Many patients with type 2 diabetes previously treated with these agents can have their diabetic medication discontinued because of normalization of blood glucose levels secondary to weight loss and poor calorie intake.

Diets should be tailored to meet the needs of the individual patient. Patients with poor appetite and decreased oral intake should be allowed to liberalize their diets from the traditional "diabetic diet." Patients may experience early satiety and mechanical problems with chewing and swallowing; nutritional supplementation with commercial products may be necessary. Consultation with a registered dietitian is helpful when devising an appropriate diet for the patient with cancer who has diabetes.

In summary, when choosing an appropriate treatment for diabetes mellitus in the cancer population, reasonable goals should be chosen. An attempt should be made to avoid symptomatic hyperglycemia, to decrease the risk of hypoglycemia, and to provide the patient with as many dietary choices as possible.

DIABETES AND GLUCOCORTICOID THERAPY

Glucocorticoids are used as adjunctive therapy in a number of chemotherapeutic regimens. Frequently they are given in high doses and/or intermittently. The use of steroids can increase blood glucose in patients with preexisting diabetes or can cause new hyperglycemia in patients with previously normal blood glucose. The latter is referred to as steroid-induced diabetes. In those individuals without diabetes, the risk of steroid-induced diabetes is increased with a family history of diabetes, increasing age, obesity, and increasing glucocorticoid dose (47). Glucocorticoids cause hyperglycemia by a number of different mechanisms. They increase hepatic glucose production and inhibit insulin-stimulated glucose uptake in peripheral tissues (48). They also have a direct effect on β-cell function although this is less well understood (49).

Glucocorticoids differ in their effects on carbohydrate metabolism. With hydrocortisone, produced by the adrenal glands, as a reference point, the synthetic steroids prednisone and dexamethasone are 3.5 to 4 times and 30 times more potent than hydrocortisone in decreasing carbohydrate metabolism, respectively (50).

The effect of glucocorticoids on carbohydrate metabolism is transient and reversible. This has been demonstrated in patients on alternate day steroids whose blood glucose levels were higher on the day they received steroids (51). There is a characteristic pattern of hyperglycemia caused by steroids. The fasting glucose is minimally elevated with exaggerated postprandial hyperglycemia. When steroids are dosed once a day, the blood glucose peak usually occurs 8 to 12 hours later (52). Following discontinuation of steroids, blood glucose usually returns to baseline within 2 to 3 days.

The treatment of diabetes in the face of glucocorticoid therapy can be challenging. Whereas diet therapy is important, when used alone, it is rarely effective in controlling hyperglycemia caused by high-dose steroids (53). Oral sulfonylurea agents are occasionally effective, particularly in patients with lower fasting blood glucose levels (<200 mg/dL.) However, most patients will need insulin and, in many cases, large doses of insulin. For patients receiving high doses of glucocorticoids in the hospital, a variable-rate intravenous insulin infusion should be considered (54). This is particularly useful for the patient receiving intravenous pulse steroids because insulin requirements can change rapidly throughout the day. Regular insulin is used exclusively in intravenous infusions.

For the patient receiving subcutaneous insulin, the two most common regimens consist of neutral protamine Hagedorn (NPH) insulin twice daily at breakfast and supper, and insulin glargine once daily at bedtime or in the morning. For patients whose blood glucose levels are >200 mg/dL, a reasonable starting dose of "basal" insulin is 0.3 units/kg, with the expectation that rapid increases in dosage may be necessary in the subsequent 2 to 3 days on the basis of the blood glucose response. When using NPH insulin, two-thirds of the dose is administered in the morning and one-third before supper. Regular insulin or a rapid-acting insulin analog is given pre-meal if the patient is eating or every 6 hours if the patient is nil per os (NPO) (52). Correction dose insulin therapy, also known as *supplemental insulin*, should be administered before meals and at bedtime in the patient who is eating or every 4 to 6 hours in the patient who is NPO. Blood glucose levels should be reviewed on a daily basis and the scheduled insulin doses revised if correction doses are frequently required. Alternate day steroids require alternate day insulin regimens.

EUTHYROID SICK SYNDROME

Severe illness, whether acute or chronic, can cause changes in thyroid physiology, leading to what has been referred to as the *euthyroid sick syndrome* (55). Changes can occur in levels of total thyroxine (T_4) and, to a lesser extent, free thyroxine and TSH levels. T_4 is decreased because of its decreased binding to its serum transport proteins. The decrease in tri-iodothyronine (T_3) results from inhibition of 5'-deiodinase, the enzyme that converts T_4 to T_3. Low T_4 levels are associated with a higher mortality rate; TSH levels are generally helpful in distinguishing euthyroid sick syndrome from pituitary hypothyroidism. In addition, free thyroxine levels are usually normal.

ADRENAL INSUFFICIENCY

Because of the vascular nature of the adrenal cortex, the adrenal glands are common sites of metastatic disease. Typically, adrenal metastases are found incidentally during abdominal computed tomography and magnetic resonance imaging scans and are usually of no functional significance. In a minority of cases, bilateral adrenal cortical destruction is sufficiently advanced to impair normal functioning and result in deficient production of cortisol (56). Symptoms of adrenocortical deficiency overlap with typical symptoms of advanced malignancy and include weight loss, fatigue, nausea, anorexia, and hypotension. Either hyponatremia or hyperkalemia heightens suspicion for the presence of adrenal insufficiency.

The ACTH stimulation test is the most direct diagnostic study used to exclude adrenocortical insufficiency. A normal test contains the following three elements: a morning basal cortisol of at least 7 to 9 µg/dL, an increase >7 µg/dL 30 minutes after administration of 0.25 mg intravenous ACTH, and a maximum response to intravenous ACTH of 18 to 20 µg/dL or higher.

Severely symptomatic adrenal insufficiency (*adrenal crisis*) is treated with intravenous saline and stress doses of hydrocortisone, 100 mg intravenously every 8 hours, tapered to a chronic oral maintenance dose of 20 mg every morning and 10 mg every evening. Patients with concomitant aldosterone deficiency resulting in hyperkalemia may also require the addition of the oral aldosterone analog fludrocortisone acetate (0.05 to 0.20 mg daily).

OSTEOPOROSIS IN THE PATIENT WITH CANCER

Osteoporosis has become a serious public health concern, leaving patients at risk for low trauma fractures of the hip, vertebrae, ribs, wrist, pelvis, and humerus. Patients with cancer may be at risk for osteoporosis because of preexisting factors such as age, low body weight, tobacco use, and family history of osteoporosis. Their risk may be further increased by the administration of glucocorticoids, immobilization or inactivity, and hypogonadism.

Postmenopausal women with osteoporosis should be treated according to the current National Institutes of Health consensus guidelines (57, 58). The approach to the premenopausal woman with osteoporosis is less well defined. Women with a history of malignancy are at risk for osteoporosis for a number of reasons, including premature menopause. Significant bone loss can occur within the first year after the onset of amenorrhea in patients treated with chemotherapy, including aromatase inhibitors, for breast cancer (59). Maintenance of adequate calcium and vitamin D intake is essential but may not be adequate to maintain bone density. Oral bisphosphonates, such as alendronate and risedronate, have been used with some success in the prevention of bone loss in patients with breast cancer (60). Many patients with cancer experience chemotherapy-induced nausea, vomiting, or gastrointestinal difficulties, which may preclude the use of oral bisphosphonates. Intravenous bisphosphonates such as pamidronate and zoledronate have been shown to be safe and efficacious in the prevention of bone loss in patients with premenopausal breast cancer receiving chemotherapy (61).

Though osteoporosis is considered a "woman's disease," men are also clearly at risk. Certain malignancies are associated with an increased risk of osteoporosis in both men and women, such as multiple myeloma. Recently, there has also been growing concern regarding the increased risk of osteoporosis in the patient with prostate cancer who is treated with androgen deprivation therapy (ADT). Because sex hormones are a major contributing factor for the maintenance of bone density in men, androgen deprivation has a major impact on bone loss and increased risk of fracture (62). ADT can take several forms. It may be achieved either surgically through bilateral orchiectomy or medically, usually with luteinizing hormone–releasing hormone agonist therapy. Studies indicate that men treated with ADT for prostate cancer lose bone mass to the extent of 4% to 10% and are at increased risk for fracture (63).

Given the known risk of bone loss in men treated with ADT for prostate cancer, men need a careful clinical evaluation including a comprehensive medical history and diagnostic workup, which will detect most risk factors for osteoporosis. Patients with prostate cancer who have musculoskeletal complaints should receive a prompt evaluation. If bony metastases are present, they should be treated with acute radiation therapy or surgical intervention, as needed. Currently, the indications for obtaining a bone mineral density test in men are the following: vertebral abnormalities identified on x-ray that are indicative of osteoporosis, low bone mass, or vertebral fracture; long-term glucocorticoid use; diagnosis of hyperparathyroidism; monitoring of osteoporosis treatment. However, many experts now recommend that, for patients with prostate cancer being treated with ADT, a baseline dual-energy x-ray absorptiometry (DEXA) scan be obtained before initiation of ADT. If the baseline test is normal, a DEXA should be repeated every 1 to 2 years after the patient has received at least 1 year of ADT.

Men with abnormal bone density test results should be counseled on lifestyle changes, including smoking cessation, regular weight-bearing exercise, and reduction in alcohol intake if excessive. Those individuals diagnosed with low bone density (sometimes referred to as osteopenia) or osteoporosis should begin dietary intake of calcium at 1,200 mg/d and supplemental vitamin D 400 IU/d. In addition, pharmacologic interventions may be indicated (64). Bisphosphonates are the most widely used medications for the prevention and treatment of osteoporosis in men. Alendronate is the only bisphosphonate that is FDA approved for the general treatment of osteoporosis in men, although both risedronate and alendronate are approved for the treatment of glucocorticoid-induced osteoporosis in both men and women. Bisphosphonates have two potential uses for men with advanced prostate cancer. They may help maintain bone mass and they may delay skeletal progression of the cancer. Intravenous forms of bisphosphonates such as pamidronate and zoledronic acid are indicated for the treatment of bone metastases. Other agents currently under investigation include estrogen, bicalutamide (a competitive inhibitor of androgen action with little effect on circulating testosterone levels), and raloxifene, a selective estrogen receptor modulator, currently indicated for the prevention of osteoporosis in postmenopausal women.

REFERENCES

1. Hansen M, Hammer M, Humer L. Diagnostic and therapeutic implications or ectopic hormone production in small cell lung cancer. *Thorax.* 1980;35:101.

2. Comis RL, Miller M, Ginsberg SJ. Abnormalities in water homeostasis in small cell anaplastic lung cancer. *Cancer.* 1980;45:2414.

3. Odell WD, Wolfsen AR. Humoral syndromes associated with cancer. *Annu Rev Med.* 1978;29:379–406.

4. Tang WW, Kaptein EM, Feinstein EI, et al. Hyponatremia in hospitalized patients with the acquired immunodeficiency syndrome (AIDS) and the AIDS-related complex. *Am J Med.* 1993;94:169.

5. Sorensen JB, Andersen MK, Hansen HH. Syndrome of inappropriate secretion of antidiuretic hormone (SIADH) in malignant disease. *J Intern Med.* 1995;238:97.

6. Hantman D, Rossier B, Zohlman R. Rapid correction of hyponatremia in the syndrome of inappropriate secretion of antidiuretic hormone: an alternative treatment to hypertonic saline. *Ann Intern Med.* 1973;78:870.

7. Sterns RH. Severe symptomatic hyponatraemia: treatment and outcome. *Ann Intern Med.* 1987;107:656.

8. Ayns JC, Olivero JJ, Frommer JP. Rapid correction of severe hyponatraemia with intravenous hypertonic saline solution. *Am J Med.* 1982;72:43.

9. Decaux G, Brimioulle S, Genette F. Treatment of the syndrome of inappropriate secretion of antidiuretic hormone by urea. *Am J Med.* 1980;69:99.

10. Hale AC, Besser GM, Rees LH. Characterisation of proopiomelanocortin derived peptides in pituitary and ectopic adrenocorticotrophin secreting tumors. *J Endocrinol.* 1986;108:49.

11. Tanaka K, Nicolson WE, Orth DN. The nature of immunoreactive lipotropins in human plasma and tissue extracts. *J Clin Invest.* 1978;62:94.

12. Raff H, Findling JW, Aron DC. A new immunoradiometric assay for corticotropin evaluated in normal subjects and patients with Cushing's syndrome. *Clin Chem.* 1989;35:596.

13. Tyrell JB, Findling JW, Aron DC, et al. An overnight high-dose dexamethasone suppression test for rapid differential diagnosis of Cushing's syndrome. *Ann Intern Med.* 1986;104:180.

14. Oldfield EH, Chrousos GP, Schulte HM, et al. Preoperative lateralization of ACTH-secreting pituitary microadenomas by bilateral and simultaneous inferior petrosal venous sinus sampling. *N Engl J Med.* 1985;312:100.

15. Pierce ST. Paraendocrine syndromes. *Curr Opin Oncol.* 1993;5:639.

16. Wysolmersk JJ, Broadus AE. Hypercalcemia of malignancy: the central role of parathyroid hormone-related protein. *Annu Rev Med.* 1994;45:189.

17. Raskin P, McClain CJ, Medsger TA. Hypocalcemia associated with metastatic bone disease. *Arch Intern Med.* 1973;132:539.

18. Salassa RM, Jowsey J, Arnaud C. Hypophosphatemic osteomalacia associated with "nonendocrine" tumors. *N Engl J Med.* 1970;283:65.

19. Quarles DL, Drezner MK. Pathophysiology of X-linked hypophosphatemia, tumor-induced osteomalacia, and autosomal dominant hypophosphatemia: a perPHEXing problem. *J Clin Endocrinol Metab.* 2001;86:494–496.

20. Goldman SL, Holcenberg JS, Finklestein JZ, et al. A randomized comparison between rasburicase and allopurinol in children with lymphoma or leukemia at high risk for tumor lysis. *Blood.* 2001;97:2998.

21. Caron P, Salandini AM, Plantavid M. Choriocarcinoma and endocrine paraneoplastic syndromes. *Eur J Med.* 1993;2:499.

22. Glass AR. Gynecomastia. *Endocrinol Metab Clin North Am.* 1994;23:825.

23. Thompson DF, Carter JR. Drug-induced gynecomastia. *Pharmacotherapy.* 1993;13:37.

24. Gropp C, Havemann K, Scheuer A. Ectopic hormones in lung cancer patients at diagnosis and during therapy. *Cancer.* 1980;46:347.

25. Silva OL, Broder LE, Doppman JL, et al. Calcitonin as a marker for bronchogenic cancer: a prospective study. *Cancer.* 1979;44:680.

26. Lamberts SW, van der Lely AJ, de Herder WW. Octreotide. *N Engl J Med.* 1996;334:246.

27. Pellikka PA, Tajik AJ, Khandena BK, et al. Carcinoid heart disease. Clinical and echocardiographic spectrum in 74 patients. *Circulation.* 1993;87:1188–1196.

28. Anderson AS, Karuss D, Lang R. Cardiovascular complications of malignant carcinoid disease. *Am Heart J.* 1997;134:693–702.

29. Modlin IM, Sander A. An analysis of 8305 cases of carcinoid tumors. *Cancer.* 1998;79:813–829.

30. Gregor M. Therapeutic principles in the management of metastasizing carcinoid tumors: drugs for symptomatic treatment. *Digestion.* 1994;55(suppl 3):60.

31. Diaco DS, Hajarizadeh H, Mueller CR. Treatment of metastatic carcinoid tumors using multimodality therapy of octreotide acetate, intra-arterial chemotherapy and hepatic arterial chemoembolization. *Am J Surg.* 1995;169:523.

32. Warner RRP. Enteroendocrine tumors other than carcinoid: a review of clinically significant advances. *Gastroenterology.* 2005;128:1668.

33. Phillips LS, Robertson DG. Insulin-like growth factors and non-islet cell tumor hypoglycemia. *Metabolism.* 1993;42:1093.

34. Zapf J. Role of insulin-like growth factor II and IGF binding proteins in extrapancreatic tumor hypoglycemia. *Horm Res.* 1994;42:20.

35. Reichlin S. Somatostatin. *N Engl J Med.* 1983;309:1495.

36. Reichlin S. Somatostatin. *N Engl J Med.* 1983;309:1556.

37. Krantic S, Goddard I, Saveanu A, et al. New modalities of somatostatin actions. *Eur J Endocrinol.* 2004;151:643.

38. Bevan JS. Clinical review: the antitumoral effects of somatostatin analog therapy in acromegaly. *J Clin Endocrinol Metab.* 2005;90:1856.

39. Lamberts SWJ, Reubi J-C, Krenning EP. The role of somatostatin analogues in the control of tumor growth. *Semin Oncol.* 1994;21:61.

40. Newman CB, Melmed S, George A, et al. Octreotide as primary therapy for acromegaly. *J Clin Endocrinol Metab.* 1998;83:3034.

41. Delaunoit T, Rubin J, Neczyporenko F, et al. Somatostatin analogues in the treatment of gastroenteropancreatic neuroendocrine tumors. *Mayo Clin Proc.* 2005;80:502.

42. DeJong M, Valkema R, Jamar F, et al. Somatostatin receptor-targeted radionuclide therapy of tumors: preclinical and clinical findings. *Semin Nucl Med.* 2002;32:133.

43. Oberg K, Kvols L, Caplin M, et al. Consensus report on the use of somatostatin analogs for the management of neuroendocrine tumors of the gastroenteropancreatic system. *Ann Oncol.* 2004;15:966.

44. Freda PU. Somatostatin analogs in acromegaly. *J Clin Endocrinol Metab.* 2002;87:3013.

45. DCCT Research Group. Epidemiology of severe hypoglycemia in the diabetes control and complications trial. *Am J Med.* 1991;90:450.

46. UK Prospective Study (UKPDS) Group. Intensive blood-glucose control with sulphonylureas or insulin compared with conventional treatment and risk of complication in patients with type 2 diabetes (UKPDA 33). *Lancet.* 1998;352:837–853.

47. Ruiz JO, Simmons RL, Callender CO, et al. Steroid diabetes in renal transplant recipients: pathogenic factors and prognosis. *Surgery.* 1973;73:759.

48. Boyle PJ. Cushings disease, glucocorticoid excess, glucocorticoid deficiency, and diabetes. *Diabetes Rev.* 1993;1:301.

49. Kalhan SC, Adam PAJ. Inhibitory effect of prednisone on insulin secretion in man: model for duplication of blood glucose concentration. *J Clin Endocrinol Metab.* 1975;41:600.

50. Conn JW, Fajans SS. Influence of adrenal cortical steroids on carbohydrate metabolism in man. *Metabolism.* 1956;5:114.

51. Greenstone MA, Shaw AB. Alternate day corticosteroid causes alternate day hyperglycemia. *Postgrad Med J.* 1987;63:761.

52. Clement S, Braithwaite SS, Magee MF, et al. Management of diabetes and hyperglycemia in hospitals. *Diabetes Care.* 2004;27:553.

53. Miller MB, Neilson J. Clinical features of the diabetic syndrome appearing after steroid therapy. *Postgrad Med J.* 1964;40:660.

54. Hirsch IB, Paauw DS. Diabetes management in special situations. *Endocrinol Metab Clin North Am.* 1997;26:631.

55. Docter R, Krenning EP, de Jong M. The sick euthyroid syndrome: changes in thyroid hormone serum parameters and hormone metabolism. *Clin Endocrinol.* 1993;39:499.

56. Redman BG, Pazdur R, Zingas AP. Prospective evaluation of adrenal insufficiency in patients with adrenal metastasis. *Cancer.* 1987;60:103.

57. NIH Consensus Development Panel on osteoporosis prevention, diagnosis, and therapy. *JAMA.* 2001;285:785.

58. Rosen CJ. Postmenopausal osteoporosis. *N Engl J Med.* 2005;353:595.

59. Ganz PA, Greendale GA. Menopause and breast cancer: addressing the secondary health effects of adjuvant chemotherapy. *J Clin Oncol.* 2001;19:3303.

60. Delmas PD, Balena R, Confravreux E, et al. Bisphosphonate risedronate prevents bone loss in women with artificial menopause due to chemotherapy of breast cancer: a double-blind, placebo controlled study. *J Clin Oncol.* 1997;15:955.

61. Fuleihan GE, Salamoun M, Mourad YA, et al. Pamidronate in the prevention of chemotherapy-induced bone loss in premenopausal women with breast cancer: a randomized controlled trial. *J Clin Endocrinol Metab.* 2005;90(6):3209.

62. Shahinian VB, Kuo YF, Freeman JL, et al. Risk of fracture after androgen deprivation for prostate cancer. *N Engl J Med.* 2005;352:154.

63. Preston DM, Torrens JI, Harding P, et al. Androgen deprivation in men with prostate cancer is associated with an increased rate of bone loss. *Prostate Cancer Prostatic Dis.* 2002;5:304.

64. Amin S, Felson DT. Osteoporosis in men. *Rheum Dis Clin North Am.* 2001;27:19.

CHAPTER 37

Infectious Complications/ Management

Jennifer M. Cuellar-Rodríguez ■ Juan C. Gea-Banacloche

Cancer patients have a significantly increased risk of infections (1,2). Risk factors for this increased susceptibility of infection are directly related to the underlying malignancy or to its treatment (Table 37.1) (3–5).

RISK FACTORS FOR INFECTIONS IN PATIENTS WITH CANCER

Intrinsic Host Factors

Underlying Malignancy

Some hematologic malignancies are associated with specific immune abnormalities that result in increased frequency of infections even in the absence of treatment (see Table 37.1). For instance, the rate of mycobacterial disease seems to be increased in hairy cell leukemia and Hodgkin's lymphoma. Encapsulated bacterial infections are common in patients with multiple myeloma and chronic lymphocytic leukemia, due to impaired B-cell immunity. Few studies have looked at the incidence and type of infections in non-neutropenic patients with solid tumors. Some well-recognized risk factors are related to the anatomic location of the tumor, for example, head and neck tumors predispose to serious infections by oral flora and they also increase the risk of aspiration pneumonia. Endobronchial tumors may cause postobstructive pneumonia. Neoplasias of the biliary tract significantly increase the risk of cholangitis, colon cancer increases the risk of sepsis secondary to enteric organisms and of anorectal infections, etc. (6,7). There is also a specific association of colon cancer with bacteremia caused by streptococci, in particular *Streptococcus gallolyticus* (formerly *Streptococcus bovis*) and anaerobes like *Clostridium septicum*. Tumors of the genitourinary tract may predispose to pyelonephritis. Breast tumors increase the risk of mastitis and abscess formation, usually by *Staphylococcus aureus.* Corticosteroid-producing tumors and corticotrophin hormone–secreting tumors are associated with an increased risk of bacterial and opportunistic infections. *Pneumocystis jiroveci* (formerly *Pneumocystis carinii*) and *Nocardia* infections have been reported in patients with Cushing's disease.

Other Intrinsic Host Factors

Functional asplenia is present after splenectomy and splenic irradiation and with chronic graft-versus-host disease (GVHD) (8). Functionally, asplenic patients are at risk for overwhelming sepsis by *Streptococcus pneumoniae,* but other pathogens include *Haemophilus influenzae* and *Neisseria*

meningitidis. In asplenic patients with a history of exposure to dogs, *Capnocytophaga canimorsus* should be considered. Other pathogens of concern include *Babesia* that causes babesiosis, *Plasmodium* that causes malaria, and *Salmonella* species.

In addition to the above-mentioned risk factors, other risk factors of particular importance in advanced cancer patients include immobility and poor nutritional status.

Treatment-Related Factors

Neutropenia

Most infections in cancer arise from treatment-induced neutropenia. Lack of granulocytes facilitates bacterial and fungal infections and blunts the inflammatory response allowing infections to progress much faster. The risk of infection is proportional to the degree and duration of neutropenia. There are detailed guidelines for the use of antimicrobial agents in the setting of chemotherapy-induced neutropenic fever (see below) (9).

Mucositis

Chemotherapy and radiation therapy disrupt mucosal integrity. Mucosal linings constitute the first line of host defense against a variety of pathogens, both by providing a physical barrier and by secreting a variety of antimicrobial peptides, including lactoferrin, lysozyme, proteases, phospholipases, and defensins. Chronic GVHD may also compromise mucosal immunity, including defective salivary immunoglobulin secretion. Disruption of the epithelial lining may result in local disease and bloodstream infections by local flora (i.e., aerobic and anaerobic bacteria and yeast). Palifermin, a recombinant human keratinocyte growth factor, may result in decreased infections by reduction in severity of mucositis (10–13).

Hematopoietic Stem Cell Transplantation (HSCT)

Preparative regimens, GVHD, and GVHD prophylaxis and treatment in HSCT recipients are significant drivers of infection. There are detailed guidelines for the prevention and treatment of infections in this patient population (14).

Autologous stem cell transplant may be considered a form of intensive chemotherapy. As such, it is typically associated with a few days or weeks of neutropenia and mucositis, followed by a few weeks or months of defective T-cell–mediated immunity. Allogeneic transplant is a more complex procedure, and there are many variants (i.e., conditioning regimen, degree of human leukocyte antigen

| TABLE 37.1 | Selected risk factors for infection in patients with advanced cancer |

Risk Factor	Type of Infection
Related to Underlying Malignancy	
AML	Bacterial, fungal, and viral
CLL/MM	Encapsulated bacteria
ALL	PCP
Hairy cell leukemia and Hodgkin's lymphoma	Mycobacterial and viral
ATCL	PCP, *Cryptococcus neoformans*, viral, and *Strongyloides stercoralis*
Obstructive pathology from local growth of the tumor	Bacterial
Colon cancer	Enteric bacterial sepsis, in particular *Streptococcus gallolyticus* and *Clostridium septicum*
Corticosteroid-producing tumors	PCP and *Nocardia* sp.
Related to Treatment	
Neutropenia	Bacterial (mainly gastrointestinal tract) and fungal
Mucositis	Oral flora, including gram-positive and anaerobic bacteria
Corticosteroid	PCP, bacterial, fungal, and herpes viruses
Nucleoside analogs	PCP, bacterial, fungal, and herpes viruses
Monoclonal Ab	Wide range of infections: bacterial, fungal, viral, parasitic— agent specific
GVHD prophylaxis/treatment	PCP, VZV
Miscellaneous	
Immobility	Bacterial—usually related to decubitus ulcers and atelectasis
Nutritional status	Bacterial and yeast infections
Biliary stents, ureteral ostomy tubes, and tracheostomy	Bacterial and yeast
Peripherally inserted central or central venous catheters	Bacterial and yeast

AML, acute myelogenous leukemia; CLL, chronic lymphocytic leukemia; MM, multiple myeloma; ALL, acute lymphocytic leukemia; PCP, pneumocystic jirovecii pneumonia; ATCL, adult T-cell leukemia/lymphoma; Ab, antibodies; GVHD, graft versus host disease; VZV, varicella zoster virus.

matching, source of stem cells, and GVHD prophylaxis) that result in very different infectious disease risk profiles. Early after HSCT, neutropenia and mucositis are the main host defense defects. Following engraftment, the most important risk factor for infection is the occurrence of severe GVHD and its treatment. Active GVHD is associated with immune dysregulation, may be accompanied by cytomegalovirus (CMV) reactivation or disease, and it is also an independent risk factor for mold infection (15). CMV disease delays immune reconstitution and is associated with an increased risk of bacterial and fungal infections (16).

Defects in cell-mediated immunity persist for several months even in uncomplicated allogeneic HSCT, predisposing to opportunistic infections, including candidiasis, *P. jiroveci*, CMV, and herpes zoster (HZ). Repopulation of specific T-cell subsets occurs at different rates. In addition to low T-cell number, T-cell receptor diversity is reduced (17).

In the absence of chronic GVHD, T-cell and B-cell functions are usually reconstituted by 1 to 2 years after engraftment. Chronic GVHD is associated with persistently depressed cell-mediated and humoral immunity.

Defective reconstitution of humoral immunity is a major factor contributing to increased infection susceptibility in the late transplant period. Invasive pneumococcal disease is relatively common, particularly in patients with chronic GVHD (18).

Immunomodulatory Agents and Infectious Risk

Corticosteroids

High-dose corticosteroids have profound effects on the distribution and function of neutrophils, monocytes, and lymphocytes. They blunt fever and local signs of infection. Patients treated with corticosteroids have impaired phagocytic function and cell-mediated immunity. Infections are a frequent complication of corticosteroid use, and differences in the type and frequency of infections are dependent on the dose and duration of treatment (19). Bacterial infections are most common (20); but opportunistic fungal, viral, and mycobacterial infections are also seen, particularly with high doses and long durations of systemic corticosteroids.

Fludarabine

Fludarabine is a fluorinated analog of adenine that is lymphotoxic, primarily affecting CD4+ lymphocytes. Particularly when combined with corticosteroids or cyclophosphamide, fludarabine results in a profound depression of CD4+ cells that may persist for several months after completion of therapy, resulting in opportunistic infections like *P. jiroveci* pneumonia (PCP) or listeriosis, sometimes more than a year after treatment. Mycobacterial and herpes virus infections have also been described.

Interleukin-2

High-dose interleukin-2 (IL-2), sometimes used for metastatic melanoma, is a significant risk factor for bacterial infections, possibly due to a profound but reversible defect in neutrophil chemotaxis. *S. aureus* and coagulase-negative staphylococci are common pathogens, and prophylactic oxacillin can lead to a reduction in central venous catheter–associated staphylococcal bacteremia (21).

Alemtuzumab

Alemtuzumab (Campath-1H) is a humanized monoclonal antibody that targets CD52, a glycoprotein abundantly expressed on most B and T lymphocytes, macrophages, and natural killer cells. Alemtuzumab treatment results in prolonged and severe lymphopenia, and it can also cause neutropenia in up to one-third of patients. Infections, both opportunistic and non-opportunistic, have been reported in a significant fraction of patients receiving alemtuzumab (22). Bacterial, viral, fungal, mycobacterial, and *P. jiroveci* infections are observed. CMV reactivation is seen in up to two-thirds of alemtuzumab recipients, although CMV disease seems to be uncommon.

Rituximab

Rituximab is a chimeric human/murine monoclonal antibody directed against the B-cell marker CD20. The increased risk of infection with rituximab seems to be low and related to repeated administration (23) and host co-factors (e.g., advanced HIV disease, HSCT, and specific chemotherapeutic regimen) (24). Hepatitis B virus (HBV) reactivation occurs with rituximab treatment. There have been reports of fulminant hepatitis and even death in patients that experienced hepatitis B flare. Also a "reverse seroconversion" phenomenon has been described, with loss of protective HBV surface antibodies and reactivation (25,26). Rarely, rituximab treatment for malignant and non-malignant conditions can be complicated by progressive multifocal leukoencephalopathy, a chronic encephalitis caused by the John Cunningham (JC)

virus (27). There have been several reports of PCP following rituximab, but most patients received other immunosuppressants. Other rare infections that have been described in the setting of rituximab use are enteroviral meningoencephalitis, CMV disease, disseminated varicella zoster virus, refractory babesiosis, parvovirus B19, and nocardiosis (24).

Immunosuppressive Agents for the Prevention and Treatment of GVHD

Immunosuppressive agents to prevent and treat GVHD all involve suppression of T-cell activation to inhibit donor alloreactive T-cell responses. The calcineurin inhibitors (cyclosporine A and tacrolimus), mycophenolate mofetil, sirolimus, and methotrexate are commonly used and are associated with an increased risk of common bacterial and opportunistic infections. Corticosteroids are the mainstay of therapy for GVHD. More intensive immunosuppressive therapy is used in steroid-refractory GVHD, resulting in very high risk for common and opportunistic bacterial, viral, and fungal diseases.

Lymphocyte-depleting antibodies cause severe suppression of cellular immunity. Visilizumab (a humanized anti-CD3 monoclonal antibody) is associated with a high frequency of Epstein-Barr virus reactivation and lymphoproliferative disease (28). Anti-cytokine antibodies include the IL-2 receptor antagonist, daclizumab, and tumor necrosis factor (TNF)-α inhibiting agents, infliximab, etanercept, and adalimumab. Daclizumab in steroid-refractory GVHD is associated with a significant risk of bacterial sepsis. TNF-α is a principal mediator of neutrophil and monocyte activation and inflammation. In patients with autoimmune diseases, agents that deplete TNF-α or inhibit TNF-α signaling are principally associated with an increased risk of tuberculosis and histoplasmosis. In HSCT recipients with refractory GVHD, infliximab was associated with an increased risk of invasive molds (29).

Additional Risk Factors for Infection in Advanced Cancer Patients

Although there are only scarce data on the risk factors for infection in advanced cancer patients that require palliative care (30–32), some recognized risk factors include long-term use of invasive devices such as peripherally inserted or central venous catheters, indwelling urinary catheters, ostomy tubes, biliary stents, and ureteral stents. Other risk factors include immobility, poor nutritional status, and palliative chemotherapy.

PREVENTION OF INFECTION

Preventing infections is preferable to treating them. In the case of cancer patients receiving palliative care, an acute infection may result in extreme loss of quality of life and in very difficult decisions regarding management, including the need to return to the hospital and the appropriateness of invasive diagnostic procedures. In this regard, it may be reasonable to continue prophylactic measures that are adequate to the clinical condition (e.g., antibiotics during neutropenia and opportunistic infection prophylaxis in recipients of stem cell transplantation) and administer the immunizations recommended by the American College of Physicians (ACP) to both patients and caregivers (http://www.acponline.org/clinical_information/resources/adult_immunization/).

Regarding immunizations it is important to be aware that the inactivated influenza vaccine is relatively ineffective in the elderly and that the newer, apparently more effective inhaled form is not approved for use in people older than 50 and is contraindicated in patients with a history of reactive airway disease. The zoster vaccine is a higher dose of the attenuated VZV present in the chickenpox vaccine and should be avoided in immunocompromised patients. Both the ACP and the Centers for Disease Control (CDC) (http://www.cdc.gov/vaccines/) offer up to date recommendations and answer to both common and unusual questions.

SPECIAL CONSIDERATIONS FOR ADVANCED CANCER PATIENTS

There are limited data on the incidence of infections, their management, and their effects in advanced cancer patients (30–32). Most studies have focused on current practice relating to antibiotic use in terminal cancer (32–39). There are scarce data on the impact on the quality of life of patients who receive treatment of known or suspected infections.

In general, antibiotics are not perceived as aggressive treatment such as cardiopulmonary resuscitation and artificial nutrition. Their use and possible side effects are often trivialized, and therefore there appears to be no great ethical debate on their use or non-use in terminal care patients (39–41). However, treatment of infection may indeed be considered a life-sustaining therapy that can serve to prolong life without reversing the underlying medical condition, which at times conflicts with the goals and objectives of palliative care. On the other hand, treatment of defined infections can help control symptoms and in fact be an extremely important palliative intervention. However, it is possible that at some point an acute infection may be considered by the patient and the care providers as a merciful terminal event that should not be treated. In these cases, initiating or interrupting potentially life-prolonging treatment may present a true ethical dilemma (Fig. 37.1). Ideally, before deciding to treat an episode of infection, it is necessary to reassess the goals of treatment (i.e., palliation vs. curative intent), to determine the potential benefits and burdens of treatment, and to determine the availability of alternative and adjunctive treatments that can effectively palliate infection-related symptoms, such as morphine for shortness of breath and antipyretics for fever (42). Once specific antimicrobial treatment is instituted, it is recommended to frequently reassess the effectiveness of the intervention on the control of symptoms. Additionally, new symptoms may develop that may

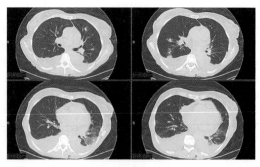

Figure 37.1. A patient with terminal multiple myeloma developed sudden respiratory insufficiency while in the hospital. A computed tomography of the chest showed worsening pleural effusions and multiple pulmonary infiltrates. A bronchoscopy with bronchoalveolar lavage was performed and was initially non-diagnostic. The patient received oxygen, morphine, and corticosteroids and her respiratory distress improved. Seventeen days later the bronchoalveolar lavage culture was positive for *Mycobacterium tuberculosis.* Treatment for tuberculosis was recommended, but the patient and her family decided against it and she remained quarantined until she passed away 1 week later.

be directly related to the use of antimicrobials and therefore affect the overall quality of life.

Currently there are no guidelines or clinical consensus on the treatment of infections in advanced cancer patients. There are no data on antimicrobial selection, efficacy, and safety profile in this susceptible population of patients, and most recommendations are based on extrapolations from other groups.

INCIDENCE AND TYPE OF INFECTIONS IN ADVANCED CANCER PATIENTS

The true incidence of infections in advanced cancer patients is difficult to discern, as many patients treated for suspected infections may not be infected. As an example, the rate of infection was as low as 29% in a study that required a positive culture for the definition of infection, but 83% in a retrospective review of infection based on a clinical diagnosis (30,32). The most common sites of infections are the urinary tract, respiratory tract, bloodstream, and skin and soft tissue. A descriptive review of published reports describing infections in 957 patients with advanced cancer in diverse settings such as palliative care unit, hospice, teaching hospital, hematology/oncology unit, and home found that 42% of terminally ill cancer patients developed infections in the final phase of their care (33). The overall frequencies of infection by organ system were as follows: urinary tract 30.5%, respiratory tract 17.9%, skin 15.7%, and blood 14.4%. The most frequent microbiologic isolates were *S. aureus, Escherichia coli,* and other Enterobacteriaceae and *Pseudomonas aeruginosa. Candida* species were the most commonly isolated fungal pathogen in the urinary tract (33).

CLINICAL EVALUATION

Typical signs and symptoms of infection may or may not be present. Fever, the cardinal sign of infection, may be nonspecific in this patient population, or suppressed by advanced age, malnutrition, comorbidities, or the use of corticosteroids. Conversely, fever may be caused by noninfectious processes, including the underlying malignancy, deep venous thrombosis, and drugs. Nonspecific signs of infection may predominate; these include decline in the functional status, confusion, and reduced oral intake. A thorough clinical examination will frequently obviate the need for extensive diagnostic workup.

DIAGNOSTIC TESTS

The use of diagnostic tests for patients with terminal cancer is controversial. A decision to pursue diagnostic workup is usually influenced by the setting in which the patients are been evaluated. Some centers will have limited diagnostic capabilities, as is the case of many palliative care units; however, advanced cancer patients are frequently hospitalized in acute care hospitals (43). A full summary of the diagnostic workup of each possible infection is beyond the scope of this chapter. However, given that the urinary tract, the respiratory tract, and blood are frequent sites of infection, the following initial workup seems reasonable, provided that the resources are available:

1. *A complete blood cell count (CBC) and differential cell counts.* The presence of an elevated white blood cell count or a left shift increases the probability of an ongoing bacterial infection. Similarly, the presence of neutropenia significantly increases the risk of bacterial or fungal infection.
2. *Urianalysis, and if abnormal a urine culture.* Urine culture should be ordered in patients with unexplained fever, altered mental status, and/or typical signs and symptoms of urinary tract infection such as pyuria, hematuria, dysuria, worsening urinary incontinence, and/or suprapubic pain (43). Asymptomatic bacteriuria does not require treatment. A dipstick urine test with a positive leukocyte esterase, nitrites, and/or pyuria should also prompt a urine culture. Appropriately collected urine culture specimens include a midstream or clean catch urine, or in patients with urethral catheters, cultures should be drawn after the removal of the catheter and insertion of a new one (44).
3. *Blood cultures.* When available blood cultures should be drawn in all advanced cancer patients in whom an infection is suspected (2). Although, in general peripherally drawn blood cultures are more reliable, if a catheter is in place, blood for culture should be drawn from the catheter. Blood from peripheral sticks should be obtained in individualized cases in which the suspicion of a catheter-related infection is very high, and positive results would impact the management of the patient.
4. *Pulse oximetry and chest x-ray.* To evaluate for pneumonia, heart failure, and pulmonary embolism.

SPECIFIC INFECTIOUS SYNDROMES

Neutropenic Fever

Fever during chemotherapy-induced neutropenia occurs in 10% to 50% of patients with solid tumors and in >80% of those with hematologic malignancies (9). Common sites of infection include the gastrointestinal tract, lung, and skin; bacteremia occurs in up to 25% of patients. Common blood isolates include coagulase-negative staphylococci, Enterobacteriaceae, and non-fermenting gram-negative rods (e.g., *P. aeruginosa*) (9). Invasive yeast (usually *Candida* spp.) infections are more commonly seen in patients with severe mucositis and neutropenia. Invasive mold infections (e.g., *Aspergillus* sp.) typically occur after prolonged neutropenia (>2 wk). The Infectious Diseases Society of America makes available detailed guidelines for the use of antimicrobial agents in the setting of chemotherapy-induced neutropenic fever (9), and these should be consulted for specific questions. The following section discusses the most important principles.

The first step in the evaluation of cancer patients with fever and neutropenia is to assess the risk of severe infection. Risk assessment may help determine the most appropriate initial management of patients with neutropenic fever (see Table 37.2). Low-risk patients are clinically defined as those with anticipated duration of neutropenia of <7 days, are clinically stable, and have no other co-morbid conditions than the underlying malignancy (9). In general terms, most consider high-risk patients as those with anticipated prolonged (>7 d) and profound neutropenia (absolute neutrophil count [ANC] ≤100 cells/mm³ following cytotoxic chemotherapy) and/or significant medical co-morbidities, including but not limited to hemodynamic instability, inability to take oral medication due to oral or gastrointestinal mucositis, nausea, vomiting, diarrhea, new pulmonary infiltrates, hypoxia or underlying chronic lung disease, new onset abdominal pain, neurologic or mental status changes, and suspected intravascular infection, especially catheter tunnel infection, or significant laboratory abnormalities such as aminotransferase levels >5 × normal or creatinine clearance of <30 ml/min. Formal risk classification may also be performed using the Multinational Association for Supportive Care in Cancer (MASCC) risk index scoring system, which uses the summation of weighted risk factors, including age, history, inpatient or outpatient status, acute clinical signs, the presence of medical conditions, and severity of the febrile neutropenic episode (45,46). An MASCC score of <21 is considered to be high risk. High-risk patients should initially receive empiric antibiotic i.v. therapy in the hospital (Table 37.2) (9).

During neutropenia, fever is the best and often the only sign of underlying infection. However, other signs or symptoms (pain and erythema) may also indicate that an infection is present. The physical examination should target commonly infected areas such as the skin (in particular around sites of existing or previous procedures or catheters), oropharynx, perineum, respiratory tract, and abdomen. Additional

| TABLE 37.2 | Initial evaluation and management in neutropenic fever |

Assessment of risk
High versus low risk[a]

⬇

Diagnostic workup
- Laboratory
  - CBC+differential
  - Serum creatinine and BUN
  - Hepatic transaminases and bilirubin
  - Electrolytes
- Blood cultures (at least two sets), and culture specimens from other sites if suspicious
- Chest radiograph is respiratory signs or symptoms

⬇

Initial Treatment High Risk
- Monotherapy with:
  - Ceftazidime or cefepime
  - Imipenem or meropenem
  - Piperacillin–tazobactam
- Consider an additional antimicrobial if resistance is suspected or hemodynamic instability:
  - Aminoglycoside
  - Fluoroquinolone
  - Vancomycin

⬇

Initial Treatment Low Risk
- Ciprofloxacin+amoxicillin/clavulanic acid (preferred)
- Ciprofloxacin or levofloxacin
- Ciprofloxacin+clindamycin

[a]High risk: anticipated prolonged (>7 d) and profound (≤100 cells/mm^3) neutropenia following cytotoxic chemotherapy and/or significant comorbidities.
CBC, complete blood count; BUN, blood urea nitrogen.

useful diagnostic tools include blood work, cultures, and radiologic studies.

In all patients being evaluated for neutropenic fever, two sets of blood cultures should be obtained. In patients with a central venous catheter (CVC), one set of blood cultures should be obtained from all the lumens, and if feasible an additional set should be obtained from a peripheral vein. If fever persists after the initial antimicrobial therapy, blood cultures should be obtained daily for the next 2 days, beyond this, blood cultures should be obtained only when there is a change in the clinical picture. Cultures from other sites should not routinely be obtained, unless there are clinical signs and symptoms to suggest their need.

Imaging studies should not be performed routinely unless clinically indicated. A chest radiograph should be obtained for patients with respiratory symptoms, bearing in mind that a negative chest radiograph does not rule out pneumonia. The computed tomography (CT) is the preferred method to evaluate all other areas (e.g., sinuses, abdomen, and pelvis).

Other laboratory analysis useful in planning supportive care and monitoring toxicity include CBC, levels of creatinine and urea nitrogen every 3 days, and weekly monitoring of serum transaminases.

Initial empiric therapy for fever and neutropenia in high-risk patients include monotherapy with an anti-pseudomonal β-lactam (Table 37.2). Other antibacterial agents may be added for the management of complications such as hypotension, pneumonia, or skin and soft tissue infection (e.g., aminoglycosides, fluoroquinolones, and/or vancomycin) or other agents as needed if antimicrobial resistance is suspected based on prior known colonization with resistant bacteria or local patterns of resistance (9).

In patients who meet stringent criteria to be considered at low risk of complications may be treated initially with oral broad-spectrum antibiotics. The regimen of choice is ciprofloxacin and amoxicillin–clavulanate (47). However, in areas where quinolone gram-negative resistance is >20%, this strategy may not be ideal (48). An outpatient course may be considered after a brief inpatient stay, during which the first dose of antibiotics is initiated, rapidly progressing infection is excluded, and prompt access to medical care can be ensured (preferably patients should be able to reach their medical facility within 1 h). Readmission to the hospital requires that patients be treated as high-risk patients (9).

Modifications to the initial regimen should be guided by clinical and microbiologic data. Patients who remain or become hemodynamically unstable after initiation of treatment should have their therapy broadened to include coverage for resistant gram-negative, gram-positive, anaerobic bacteria and fungi. Patients with persistent fever, but otherwise asymptomatic, only require a change in antimicrobials to treat identified infections, or in clinically stable patients with adequate gastrointestinal absorption, an i.v. to oral switch may be considered. Empiric gram-positive coverage (i.e., vancomycin) may be stopped in patients who after 2 days of therapy have no gram-positive bacteria identified and do not have a documented clinical infection that would require gram-positive coverage (e.g., skin and soft tissue infection). Empiric antifungal therapy with an anti-mold active agent (i.e., echinocandin, voriconazole, or amphotericin B preparation) should be considered in high-risk patients who have persistent fever after 4 to 7 days of broad-spectrum antibacterial coverage and myeloid recovery is not imminent; in these patients a CT of the chest or sinuses may reveal an occult fungal infection (9).

In high-risk patients who become afebrile after the initiation of empiric antimicrobial therapy, antimicrobial coverage should be continued for at least the duration of neutropenia; in patients with documented infections, duration of therapy should be appropriate for effective eradication of the particular infection, whichever comes last (9). In low-risk patients who have defervesced after 3 days of therapy, broad-spectrum antibiotics may be stopped before reaching an ANC > 500 cells/mm³, when there is no documented infection and there

is evidence imminent marrow recovery. The ideal duration of antimicrobial therapy in patients who remain afebrile, but in whom neutropenia recovery is not expected (e.g., refractory aplastic anemia), is unknown. A reasonable approach in patients with no identified source of infection is to give antimicrobial therapy for at least 10 to 14 days.

There are no specific recommendations for the management of neutropenic fever in palliative care patients. Risk assessment and determination goals of therapy should proceed simultaneously. Many patients with terminal cancer may not be considered "low risk" and often the automatic approach would be to admit them to an acute care facility for intravenous (i.v.) therapy. This may not always be in the best interest of quality of life. An approach that may be considered if the patient does not have an i.v. access would be to start therapy with an oral combination regimen, similar to the one recommended for low-risk neutropenic patients (i.e., ciprofloxacin or levofloxacin and amoxicillin–clavulanic acid) (Table 37.2). If i.v. access is available, then similar recommendations as in other cancer patients seem reasonable; however, the diagnostic workup should be less aggressive and limited to blood work, urinary samples, and limited imaging.

Catheter-Related Bloodstream Infections

The frequency of catheter-related bloodstream infections varies among different cancer populations (49). Definitive diagnosis usually requires that blood cultures be drawn simultaneously from the catheter and the periphery. Differential time to positivity of >2 hours from the cultures drawn from the catheter and those drawn from the periphery is a convincing evidence that the source of bacteremia is the catheter (50,51). However, peripheral blood cultures may not always be available, and deciding when the infection is secondary to an infected catheter may be problematic. Some authors have suggested that the differential time to positivity be applied to cultures drawn simultaneously from different lumens of a multi-lumen catheter. Infected nonpermanent catheters should be removed whenever feasible. Surgically implanted catheters can be salvaged when there is a rapid clearance of bacteremia after initiation of treatment and when dealing with low virulence organisms such as coagulase-negative staphylococci. In other scenarios, catheter removal should be strongly considered, although this may not always be feasible. Whenever catheter salvage is attempted in addition to i.v. antibiotics, antibiotic lock therapy has been recommended (51).

The duration of systemic antimicrobial therapy depends on several factors, including whether the catheter was removed or not, response to antimicrobial therapy within 48 to 72 hours (resolution of bacteremia and fever), and whether a complicated infection (e.g., endovascular infection or deep tissue infection) is present. In general, other than staphylococcal infections, a 14-day course of systemic antimicrobials is adequate if the catheter is removed and the patient responds to antimicrobial therapy within 72 hours. A 7-day course is adequate in patients with coagulase-negative staphylococcal infections. Cancer patients with *S. aureus* catheter–related bloodstream infections may require longer than 2 weeks of therapy. Complicated catheter-related bloodstream infection caused by any pathogen requires 4 to 6 weeks of antimicrobial therapy (9,51).

Respiratory Tract Infections

Upper Respiratory Tract Infection

Most upper respiratory tract infections in cancer patients are viral in origin (52,53). If available, a nasopharyngeal wash should be obtained for diagnosis; during influenza season, empiric anti-influenza treatment should be strongly considered. The choice of anti-viral treatment (neuraminidase inhibitors like oseltamivir or zanamivir vs. the adamantanes, amantadine, and rimantadine) should be guided by the yearly recommendations provided by the CDC, as different strains of the influenza virus exhibit different susceptibilities.

Bacterial sinusitis is common in both neutropenic and non-neutropenic cancer patients. Mold invasive infections are of particular concern in prolonged and profound neutropenia or in patients receiving high-dose steroids (54,55). Diagnosis usually requires a CT of the sinuses and an otorhinolaryngologist consultation. Suspicious lesions should be biopsied and tissue should be sent for culture and histopathology (56).

Treatment recommendations for sinusitis in non-neutropenic patients include amoxicillin/clavulanate, azithromycin, levofloxacin, moxifloxacin, cefdinir, cefprozil, or cefpodoxime. The initial treatment in neutropenic patients in whom bacterial sinusitis is suspected should include agents effective against *P. aeruginosa* and Enterobacteriaceae. *S. aureus* infection can occur and the use of an agent active against it should be considered (9). If community-acquired methicillin-resistant *S. aureus* (community-acquired MRSA) is a consideration, the antibiotic options include clindamycin, trimethoprim–sulfamethoxazole (TMP–SMX), and doxycycline. A standard approach is to start with the same agents used in fever and neutropenia (see Table 37.2), keeping in mind that MRSA is not covered by this combination and vancomycin should be added if there is a high suspicion for MRSA. When fungal sinusitis is suspected, maximal efforts should be made to establish the etiologic diagnosis because of significant differences in toxicity and convenience between amphotericin B formulations (treatment of choice for mucormycosis, but available only intravenously and quite toxic) and voriconazole (treatment of choice for almost all other invasive fungal infections, available by mouth or i.v. and much better tolerated). Pending definitive diagnosis, most experts would recommend empiric amphotericin B, in one of its lipid formulations to minimize toxicity. Once an etiologic diagnosis is established, therapy should be tailored for the specific isolate, surgical debridement may be required.

Lower Respiratory Tract Infection

There are detailed guidelines for the treatment of community-acquired and hospital-acquired pneumonia in non-neutropenic patients (57,58). Non-neutropenic patients with cancer should follow similar recommendations. When feasible, blood and sputum cultures should be carried out. Acceptable oral regimens that are also adequate for palliative care in advanced cancer patients with community-acquired pneumonia are monotherapy with a fluoroquinolone (i.e., levofloxacin, moxifloxacin, and gemifloxacin) or combination therapy with amoxicillin/clavulanate and a macrolide (azithromycin or clarithromycin) (57). First-line i.v. therapy for patients that require admission hospitalization, but do not require admission to the intensive care unit, include a third generation cephalosporin (i.e., ceftriaxone or cefotaxime) and a macrolide or monotherapy with a fluoroquinolone. In patients admitted to the intensive care unit or in neutropenic patients, a fluoroquinolone and an anti-pseudomonal β-lactam agent should be used; anti-MRSA treatment should be considered, in particular in those that are known to be colonized with MRSA (57). During influenza season, cancer patients with lower respiratory tract infection should be considered at risk for infection; rapid institution of empiric treatment should be strongly considered, and if available a respiratory viral culture should be obtained (59,60).

The 2005 guidelines for the management of health-care–associated and hospital-acquired pneumonia in adults are now being revised (58). In these guidelines, the category of health-care–associated pneumonia was introduced to include patients that had a higher likelihood than other ambulatory patients of having multidrug-resistant pathogens. In their approach, the goal of therapy is to cover broadly any patient that is at risk for multidrug-resistant pathogens (i.e., patients in whom pneumonia occurred 5 days after admission to the hospital, recent hospitalization, those with prior antibiotic exposure within the last 90 days, nursing home residents, and dialysis patients) and then de-escalate once an etiologic diagnosis is identified. Initial regimens include an anti-pseudomonal β-lactam and anti-pseudomonal fluoroquinolone or aminoglycoside and either vancomycin or linezolid. As opposed to the community-acquired pneumonia guidelines that have been widely accepted, since their publication these guidelines have been criticized (61) and concerns about its applicability, specifically as it pertains to nursing home residents or other ambulatory patients, have been raised (62). The main concerns in this triple coverage approach are not only the possibility of a treatment-related excess mortality (63) but also that the guidelines do not account for treatment restrictions in elderly or severely debilitated individuals and in particular the lack of data supporting the need of this approach in the wide classification of health-care–associated pneumonia; hence it may imply an overtreatment of many patients (61,62). Cancer patients with septic shock or severe sepsis should receive dual or triple coverage. Whether hemodynamically stable, nosocomial pneumonia patients require such wide coverage is questionable, but if instituted de-escalation should be the goal. In palliative care hospitalized advanced cancer patients, it seems reasonable to institute broad-spectrum antimicrobial coverage and to frequently reassess the goal of therapy (i.e., symptom control).

A wider range of microorganisms can cause pulmonary infiltrates in neutropenic and/or highly immunocompromised cancer patients (64–66). Bacterial pathogens are most common, but other opportunistic pathogens are also a concern and the need for etiologic diagnosis becomes more pressing. When suspicion of pneumonia arises, a chest CT can reveal infiltrates that were missed on the chest radiograph or can help to better define known lesions. Unless the etiologic diagnosis is obvious, strong consideration should be given to early broncheoalveolar lavage (BAL) and/or lung biopsy (percutaneous, transbronchial, video-assisted thoracic surgery, or even open lung biopsy) (67). When the resources are available, samples should be sent for bacterial, mycobacterial, *Nocardia*, and fungal stains and culture, as well as either viral culture or polymerase chain reaction (PCR). Adjunctive test for those at risk for fungal pneumonia are galactomannan on the BAL and serum (68,69); for those at risk for PCP (i.e., defective T-cell immunity, such as high-dose steroids or HSCT recipients) special strains for PCP on BAL fluid or tissue and/or PCR (70). Initial antimicrobial therapy should include broad antibacterial coverage, as outlined above, and depending on the pattern of infiltrates, risk factors, and severity of infections, strong consideration should be given to additional agents. In neutropenic patients that are not responding to broad antibacterial coverage or in those with nodular lung lesions, in particular in the absence of prophylaxis, the addition of voriconazole or a lipid formulation of amphotericin B is recommended (71,72). Besides mold infections, nodular and cavitated lesions in patients receiving corticosteroids should bring to mind *Nocardia*.

Intra-abdominal Infections

Intra-abdominal tumors, depending on their location, may lead to an obstructive cholangitis (e.g., pancreatic and hepatobiliary tumors) or erosion through a viscus. In some instances, tumor may replace most of the bowel wall, with perforation or bacteremia following initiation of chemotherapy.

Neutropenic enterocolitis (typhlitis—inflammation of the cecum) results from a combination of neutropenia and defects in the bowel mucosa related to cytotoxic chemotherapy and in patients with solid tumors receiving taxanes (73,74). Pathologically, typhlitis is characterized by ulceration and necrosis of the bowel wall, hemorrhage, and masses of organisms. Suggestive signs include fever, abdominal pain and tenderness, and radiologic evidence of right colonic inflammation. Nausea, vomiting, and diarrhea are the most common symptoms. Abdominal distension, tenderness, and a right lower quadrant fullness or mass reflect thickened bowel. Bacteremia with enteric flora, *P. aeruginosa* or polymicrobial may occur. Clostridial species are the most

common anaerobic pathogens. A CT scan should be performed in patients with suspected typhlitis or undiagnosed abdominal pain in the setting of neutropenia. The differential diagnosis includes *Clostridium difficile* colitis, GVHD of the bowel, CMV colitis (rarely observed during neutropenia), and bowel ischemia (75).

Treatment of typhlitis requires broad-spectrum antibiotics with activity against aerobic gram-negative bacilli and anaerobes (e.g., ceftazidime + metronidazole, imipenem, meropenem, or piperacillin/tazobactam) and supportive care, including i.v. fluids and bowel rest. The majority of patients will respond to antibiotic therapy and supportive care. Surgical indications include (1) persistent gastrointestinal bleeding after resolution of neutropenia, thrombocytopenia, and clotting abnormalities; (2) free intraperitoneal air, suggestive of perforation; (3) uncontrolled sepsis despite fluid and vasopressor support; and (4) an intra-abdominal process (such as appendicitis) that would require surgery in the absence of neutropenia (76).

Clostridium difficile Colitis

Patients with cancer are at high risk for *C. difficile* colitis due to prolonged hospitalization where environmental transmission is likely to occur and due to receiving broad-spectrum antibiotics. Both antibiotic and chemotherapy administration can result in a clinical episode of *C. difficile* colitis. The clinical spectrum ranges from asymptomatic carriage to fulminant colitis with toxic megacolon. In severe *C. difficile* disease, paralytic ileus, toxic dilatation of the colon, and bowel perforation may occur. It is important to think of it not only when patients have diarrhea but also in cases of abdominal pain or tenderness, cramping, and fever of unclear etiology. The mainstay of diagnosis is the detection of *C. difficile* toxin A, toxin B, or both in the stool with a cytotoxin test or enzyme immunoassay or PCR for the toxin gene (77,78).

Traditional options for the treatment of *C. difficile* disease include oral or i.v. metronidazole and oral vancomycin. A comparative trial suggests that oral vancomycin may be more efficacious in severe cases (79). Novel antibiotics that have been shown to be effective in *C. difficile* colitis are tigecycline, fidaxomicin, and ramoplanin (48,80,81). Nitazoxanide, which had efficacy similar to metronidazole in a randomized trial (82), may be considered for milder cases. Patients in whom oral agents cannot be administered should receive i.v. metronidazole. In cases involving toxic dilatation of the colon or perforation, subtotal colectomy, diverting ileostomy, or colostomy may be required.

The safety and efficacy of probiotic agents in immunocompromised patients and patients with cancer are unknown, but it is worth noting that bacteremia has resulted occasionally from these preparations. Management of recurrences is difficult, and many different strategies have been used (repeated courses of the same antibiotic, vancomycin "pulse" therapy, and vancomycin taper) (83). Monoclonal antibodies against *C. difficile* toxins may be an option to reduce the recurrence of *C. difficile* infection (84).

Anorectal Infections

Anorectal infections may be life threatening in patients who are receiving repeated courses of chemotherapy. Infection may follow the development of an anal fissure. Tiny abrasions may be a portal of entry or infection may originate in the anal crypts. Once anorectal infection is established, fascial extension to the external genitalia, pelvic floor, retroperitoneum, and peritoneal cavity may occur. Anorectal infections, with or without extensive regional spread, may lead to bacteremia. The most common pathogens in neutropenic patients are Enterobacteriaceae, anaerobes, enterococci, and *P. aeruginosa*. In most cases, the infection is polymicrobial (85).

Fever often precedes symptoms and signs suggestive of anorectal infection, and perirectal pain, often exacerbated by defecation, may initially occur in the absence of findings in the physical examination. Therefore, serial examinations of the perianal region are necessary, looking for point tenderness and poorly demarcated induration (86). Visual inspection should assess for the presence of perianal fissures, fistulas, cellulitis, and induration. Digital rectal examination should be avoided during neutropenia. A CT scan should be obtained to show the extent of perirectal involvement and drainable collections. Stool softeners and analgesics should be provided. Most cases of anorectal infections can be managed with appropriate broad-spectrum antibiotics and supportive measures without surgical intervention (85). Surgery is generally avoided or delayed until neutrophil recovery, unless the infection proves uncontrollable with medical management.

Urinary Tract Infection

Risk factors for bacterial urinary tract infection in cancer patients include the use of indwelling urethral or suprapubic catheters, ureteral stents, locally invasive neoplasias (i.e., prostatic cancer or colon cancer), and neurogenic bladder (44). Enteric pathogen, specifically *E. coli* is the most common cause of urinary tract infections. Other less common pathogens include *Klebsiella pneumoniae*, *Proteus mirabilis*, and *Enterococcus* sp. However, in patients with indwelling catheters infections are often polymicrobial and resistant organisms are not uncommon. If feasible, adequate urine cultures prior to initiation of therapy allow tailoring of the treatment on the basis of antimicrobial susceptibility. Acceptable empiric oral therapies are TMP–SMX if local resistance is <20% and oral fluoroquinolones (ciprofloxacin and levofloxacin) (87). In ill-appearing patients, it is reasonable to start with i.v. ceftriaxone and to rule out secondary bacteremia. If the patient is known to be colonized with resistant pathogens and urosepsis is suspected, empiric therapy should include agents that target these microorganisms. In proven catheter-associated urinary tract infection, exchange of indwelling catheter can lead to improved clinical status after 72 hours and lower rates of recurrence (44,88). In palliative care advanced cancer patients, in whom oral agents are deemed appropriate, besides TMP–SMX and quinolones, alternative agents nitrofurantoin and fosfomycin. Of note, asymptomatic bacteriuria should not be treated, except in neutropenic patients.

Candiduria is common among patients with indwelling catheters that receive broad-spectrum antibiotics; removal of the catheter or exchange of the catheter may be all that is needed to clear asymptomatic candiduria. Patients undergoing urologic manipulations are considered to be at risk for dissemination as well as neutropenic patients. In neutropenic patients, candiduria may be the only sign of disseminated candidiasis and antifungal treatment should be initiated (88,89). There is no evidence that treating candiduria in any other setting results in improved outcome.

Skin and Soft Tissue Infections

Skin and soft tissue infections are common among cancer and palliative care patients (33,64). Infections can be localized or be a manifestation of disseminated infections. Localized infections typically result from breaks in the skin or mucosa, usually related to physical trauma, maceration, pressure, or use of devices (i.e., around the sites of catheter insertion or ostomies). Most common localized infections are pressure ulcers and cellulitis. Sometimes skin lesions are manifestation of bacteremia (most notably ecthyma gangrenosum caused by *P. aeruginosa* and other gram-negative bacilli and also a variety of ulcers, nodules, hemorrhagic bullae, and violaceous or purpuric skin lesions), and patients that preset with fever or other signs of systemic toxicity should have blood cultures drawn before the initiation of antimicrobials. Common bacterial pathogens in cellulitis include streptococci and *S. aureus* (90). Emerging antibiotic resistance is problematic, and treatment should be guided by local patterns of resistance. In hospitalized patients, severely immunocompromised or in neutropenic patients, gram-negative organisms (i.e., *P. aeruginosa*, *Aeromonas* sp., *Stenotrophomonas maltophilia*, and Enterobacteriaceae) are also common culprits and therapy should target these organisms, in addition to gram-positive cocci. Pressure ulcers tend to be polymicrobial. Aerobic gram-negative bacilli and gram-positive cocci are found most commonly; however, anaerobic flora is frequently isolated when deep cultures are taken. Most pressure ulcers should be treated topically and the use of systemic antibiotics reserved for evidence of cellulitis or systemic dissemination of infection.

Necrotizing infection of the skin and deeper structures (fascia and muscle) differs from the superficial skin infections in their clinical presentation and in that their outcome can be fatal. Clinical features that suggest necrosis of deeper tissues are (1) severe constant pain, (2) bullae, (3) ecchymosis that precedes skin necrosis, (4) gas, detected by palpation or imaging, (5) edema that extends beyond the area of erythema if present, (6) anesthesia, (7) systemic toxicity, and (8) rapid spread despite antibiotic therapy. These conditions are usually secondary in that they develop from an initial break in the skin due to trauma or surgery. They can be monomicrobial (usually streptococci or *Clostridium* sp.) or polymicrobial (mixed aerobic and anaerobic flora) (90). Treatment of necrotizing infections typically requires extensive surgical debridement; antimicrobial therapy for hospitalized patients or neutropenic patients should include metronidazole and cefepime or ceftazidime or monotherapy with a meropenem, imipenem, doripenem, or piperacillin–tazobactam (91).

In prolonged neutropenia fungal infections are of particular concern, and skin and soft tissue lesions are usually a manifestation of disseminated disease, unless there is a clear history of trauma to the affected region. The incidence of disseminated candidiasis has substantially decreased, since the routine use of antifungal prophylaxis in HSCT and post-induction chemotherapy (9,71). About 10% of patients with invasive candidiasis develop single or multiple small (<1 cm) nodular non-tender erythematous skin lesions. Blood cultures are frequently positive, and skin biopsy is usually diagnostic (92).

Aspergillus spp. and *Fusarium* spp., and rarely other dematiaceous molds, can spread hematogenously to the skin and subcutaneous tissue. Lesions can begin as multiple erythematous macules or subcutaneous nodules that quickly evolve to necrotic nodules. Lesions can be painful due to angioinvasion and necrosis. Mortality from these infections is high, and a diagnostic skin biopsy should be performed. Blood cultures are positive in disseminated *Fusarium* sp. infection in up to 60% of cases (55,92,93).

Herpes simplex virus (HSV) and HZ reactivations are common infections in cancer patients. HSV infection typically present as painful vesicles or ulcerations involving the nasolabial, genital or rectal skin, or mucosa. HZ reactivations present as painful papular or vesicular lesions, usually in dermatomal distribution; however, in severely immunocompromised individuals disseminated skin lesions can appear (94). Treatment of localized HZ and HSV reactivations is with oral valacyclovir, acyclovir, or famciclovir. Treatment of disseminated disease warrants i.v. therapy. Patients with frequent reactivation could benefit from secondary prophylaxis (95,96).

CONCLUSIONS

Infections are common in neutropenic and non-neutropenic individuals with advanced cancer. Urinary tract, respiratory tract, and bloodstream infections seem to be the most common. There is only a paucity of data on how to best manage these infections in palliative care advanced cancer patients. There is an urgent need to develop home care programs, which allow the continuity of palliative care. Studies in this population need to focus on the feasibility of administering oral regimens for certain infections and to evaluate the impact on the quality of life (Table 37.3).

TABLE 37.3	Oral antimicrobial therapy for selected infectious syndromes in palliative care cancer patients
Disease	**Antimicrobial Therapy**
Neutropenic fever	*Preferred* 1. Ciprofloxacin + Amox/Clav[a] *Alternatives* 2. Levofloxacin 3. Ciprofloxacin + clindamycin 4. Levofloxacin + linezolid[b]
Bacterial sinusitis—non-neutropenic	*Preferred* 1. Amox/Clav 2. Azithromycin 3. Levofloxacin or moxifloxacin 4. Cefdinir, cefprozil, or cefpodoxime
Bacterial sinusitis—neutropenic	*Preferred* 1. Levofloxacin 2. Ciprofloxacin + Amox/clav *Alternatives* 3. Ciprofloxacin + clindamycin

(Continued)

| TABLE 37.3 | Oral antimicrobial therapy for selected infectious syndromes in palliative care cancer patients (*Continued*) |

Disease	Antimicrobial Therapy
Community-acquired pneumonia—non-neutropenic	*Preferred* 1. Levofloxacin, moxifloxacin, or gemifloxacin 2. Amox/clav and azithromycin *Alternative* 3. Amox/clav and clarithromycin
Community-acquired pneumonia—neutropenic	*Preferred* 1. Levofloxacin
Health-care–associated or hospital-acquired pneumonia	*Preferred* 1. Levofloxacin + linezolid
Suspected or known fungal pneumonia—neutropenic or high-dose steroids	*Preferred* 1. Voriconazole (preferred for all, except for mucormycosis) 2. Posaconazole
Urinary tract infection	*Preferred* 1. TMP–SMX[a] (if local resistance is <20%) 2. Ofloxacin, ciprofloxacin, or levofloxacin *Alternatives* 1. Nitrofurantoin 2. Fosfomycin
Superficial skin and soft tissue infections—community-acquired and low MRSA prevalence	*Preferred* 1. Dicloxacillin 2. Cephalexin *Alternatives* 1. Doxycycline 2. TMP–SMX 3. Clindamycin
Superficial skin and soft tissue infections—community-acquired and high MRSA prevalence	*Preferred* 1. Linezolid *Alternatives* 1. TMP–SMX 2. Doxycycline 3. Clindamycin
Skin and soft tissue infections—neutropenic	*Preferred* 1. Ciprofloxacin + linezolid
Herpes simplex virus/herpes zoster	*Preferred* 1. Valacyclovir 2. Acyclovir 3. Famciclovir

These oral regimens are reasonable alternatives to the standard of care in palliative care cancer patients in whom comfort care is the main goal of therapy.

[a]Amox/Clav: amoxicillin/clavulanate and TMP–SMX: trimethoprim–sulfamethoxazole.

[b]Linezolid should be considered when a catheter-related infection is suspected or when there are signs and symptoms of a skin and soft tissue infection or mucositis.

REFERENCES

1. Danai PA, Moss M, Mannino DM, Martin GS. The epidemiology of sepsis in patients with malignancy. *Chest.* 2006;129(6):1432-1440.

2. Thirumala R, Ramaswamy M, Chawla S. Diagnosis and management of infectious complications in critically ill patients with cancer. *Crit Care Clin.* 2010;26(1):59-91.

3. Wisplinghoff H, Seifert H, Wenzel RP, Edmond MB. Current trends in the epidemiology of nosocomial bloodstream infections in patients with hematological malignancies and solid neoplasms in hospitals in the United States. *Clin Infect Dis.* 2003;36(9):1103-1110.

4. Barker JN, Hough RE, van Burik JA, et al. Serious infections after unrelated donor transplantation in 136 children: impact of stem cell source. *Biol Blood Marrow Transplant.* 2005;11(5):362-370.

5. van Burik JA, Brunstein CG. Infectious complications following unrelated cord blood transplantation. *Vox Sang.* 2007;92(4):289-296.

6. Glenn J, Cotton D, Wesley R, Pizzo P. Anorectal infections in patients with malignant diseases. *Rev Infect Dis.* 1988;10(1):42-52.

7. Khardori N, Wong E, Carrasco CH, Wallace S, Patt Y, Bodey GP. Infections associated with biliary drainage procedures in patients with cancer. *Rev Infect Dis.* 1991;13(4):587-591.

8. Kalhs P, Kier P, Lechner K. Functional asplenia after bone marrow transplantation [letter]. *Ann Intern Med.* 1990;113(10):805-806.

9. Freifeld AG, Bow EJ, Sepkowitz KA, et al. Clinical practice guideline for the use of antimicrobial agents in neutropenic patients with cancer: 2010 update by the Infectious Diseases Society of America. *Clin Infect Dis.* 2011;52(4):e56-e93.

10. Spielberger R, Stiff P, Bensinger W, et al. Palifermin for oral mucositis after intensive therapy for hematologic cancers. *N Engl J Med.* 2004;351(25):2590-2598.

11. Rosen LS, Abdi E, Davis ID, et al. Palifermin reduces the incidence of oral mucositis in patients with metastatic colorectal cancer treated with fluorouracil-based chemotherapy. *J Clin Oncol.* 2006;24(33):5194-5200.

12. Vadhan-Raj S, Trent J, Patel S, et al. Single-dose palifermin prevents severe oral mucositis during multicycle chemotherapy in patients with cancer: a randomized trial. *Ann Intern Med.* 2010;153(6):358-367.

13. Schmidt E, Thoennissen NH, Rudat A, et al. Use of palifermin for the prevention of high-dose methotrexate-induced oral mucositis. *Ann Oncol.* 2008;19(9):1644-1649.

14. Tomblyn M, Chiller T, Einsele H, et al. Guidelines for preventing infectious complications among hematopoietic cell transplant recipients: a global perspective. Preface. *Bone Marrow Transplant.* 2009;44(8):453-455.

15. Fukuda T, Boeckh M, Carter RA, et al. Invasive fungal infections in recipients of allogeneic hematopoietic stem cell transplantation after nonmyeloablative conditioning: risks and outcomes. *Blood.* 2003;10:10.

16. Nichols WG, Corey L, Gooley T, Davis C, Boeckh M. High risk of death due to bacterial and fungal infection among cytomegalovirus (CMV)-seronegative recipients of stem cell transplants from seropositive donors: evidence for indirect effects of primary CMV infection. *J Infect Dis.* 2002;185(3):273-282.

17. Mackall CL, Gress RE. Pathways of T-cell regeneration in mice and humans: implications for bone marrow transplantation and immunotherapy. *Immunol Rev.* 1997;157:61-72.

18. Kulkarni S, Powles R, Treleaven J, et al. Chronic graft versus host disease is associated with long-term risk for pneumococcal infections in recipients of bone marrow transplants. *Blood.* 2000;95:3683-3686.

19. Lionakis MS, Kontoyiannis DP. Glucocorticoids and invasive fungal infections. *Lancet.* 2003;362(9398):1828-1838.

20. Gea-Banacloche JC, Opal SM, Jorgensen J, Carcillo JA, Sepkowitz KA, Cordonnier C. Sepsis associated with immunosuppressive medications: an evidence-based review. *Crit Care Med.* 2004;32(11 suppl):S578-S590.

21. Bock SN, Lee RE, Fisher B, et al. A prospective randomized trial evaluating prophylactic antibiotics to prevent triple-lumen catheter-related sepsis in patients treated with immunotherapy. *J Clin Oncol.* 1990;8(1):161-169.

22. Martin SI, Marty FM, Fiumara K, Treon SP, Gribben JG, Baden LR. Infectious complications associated with alemtuzumab use for lymphoproliferative disorders. *Clin Infect Dis.* 2006;43(1):16-24.

23. Vidal L, Gafter-Gvili A, Leibovici L, Shpilberg O. Rituximab as maintenance therapy for patients with follicular lymphoma. *Cochrane Database Syst Rev.* 2009;(2):CD006552.

24. Gea-Banacloche JC. Rituximab-associated infections. *Semin Hematol.* 2010;47(2):187-198.

25. Pei SN, Chen CH, Lee CM, et al. Reactivation of hepatitis B virus following rituximab-based regimens: a serious complication in both HBsAg-positive and HBsAg-negative patients. *Ann Hematol.* 2009;89(3):255-262.

26. Yeo W, Chan TC, Leung NW, et al. Hepatitis B virus reactivation in lymphoma patients with prior resolved hepatitis B undergoing anticancer therapy with or without rituximab. *J Clin Oncol.* 2009;27(4):605-611.

27. Carson KR, Evens AM, Richey EA, et al. Progressive multifocal leukoencephalopathy after rituximab therapy in HIV-negative patients: a report of 57 cases from the Research on Adverse Drug Events and Reports Project. *Blood.* 2009;113(20):4834-4840.

28. Carpenter PA, Lowder J, Johnston L, et al. A phase II multicenter study of visilizumab, humanized anti-CD3 antibody, to treat steroid-refractory acute graft-versus-host disease. *Biol Blood Marrow Transplant.* 2005;11(6):465-471.

29. Couriel D, Saliba R, Hicks K, et al. Tumor necrosis factor-alpha blockade for the treatment of acute GVHD. *Blood.* 2004;104(3):649-654.

30. Homsi J, Walsh D, Panta R, Lagman R, Nelson KA, Longworth DL. Infectious complications of advanced cancer. *Support Care Cancer.* 2000;8(6):487-492.

31. Bauduer F, Capdupuy C, Renoux M. Characteristics of deaths in a department of oncohaematology within a general hospital. A study of 81 cases. *Support Care Cancer.* 2000;8(4):302-306.

32. Ahronheim JC, Morrison RS, Baskin SA, Morris J, Meier DE. Treatment of the dying in the acute care hospital. Advanced dementia and metastatic cancer. *Arch Intern Med.* 1996;156(18):2094-2100.

33. Nagy-Agren S, Haley H. Management of infections in palliative care patients with advanced cancer. *J Pain Symptom Manage.* 2002;24(1):64-70.

34. Pereira J, Watanabe S, Wolch G. A retrospective review of the frequency of infections and patterns of antibiotic utilization on a palliative care unit. *J Pain Symptom Manage.* 1998;16(6):374-381.

35. Girmenia C, Moleti ML, Cartoni C, et al. Management of infective complications in patients with advanced hematologic malignancies in home care. *Leukemia.* 1997;11(11):1807-1812.

36. Vitetta L, Kenner D, Sali A. Bacterial infections in terminally ill hospice patients. *J Pain Symptom Manage*. 2000;20(5):326-334.

37. Lawlor PG, Gagnon B, Mancini IL, et al. Occurrence, causes, and outcome of delirium in patients with advanced cancer: a prospective study. *Arch Intern Med*. 2000;160(6):786-794.

38. Oh DY, Kim JH, Kim DW, et al. Antibiotic use during the last days of life in cancer patients. *Eur J Cancer Care (Engl)*. 2006;15(1):74-79.

39. Stiel S, Krumm N, Pestinger M, et al. Antibiotics in palliative medicine—results from a prospective epidemiological investigation from the HOPE survey. *Support Care Cancer*. 2011.

40. Enck RE. Antibiotic use in end-of-life care: a soft line? *Am J Hosp Palliat Care*. 2012;20(2):325-333.

41. Chun ED, Rodgers PE, Vitale CA, Collins CD, Malani PN. Antimicrobial use among patients receiving palliative care consultation. *Am J Hosp Palliat Care*. 2010;27(4):261-265.

42. Pizzo PA, Commers J, Cotton D, et al. Approaching the controversies in antibacterial management of cancer patients. *Am J Med*. 1984;76(3):436-449.

43. High KP, Bradley SF, Gravenstein S, et al. Clinical practice guideline for the evaluation of fever and infection in older adult residents of long-term care facilities: 2008 update by the Infectious Diseases Society of America. *Clin Infect Dis*. 2009;48(2):149-171.

44. Hooton TM, Bradley SF, Cardenas DD, et al. Diagnosis, prevention, and treatment of catheter-associated urinary tract infection in adults: 2009 International Clinical Practice Guidelines from the Infectious Diseases Society of America. *Clin Infect Dis*. 2010;50(5):625-663.

45. Klastersky J, Paesmans M, Rubenstein EB, et al. The Multinational Association for Supportive Care in Cancer risk index: a multinational scoring system for identifying low-risk febrile neutropenic cancer patients. *J Clin Oncol*. 2000;18(16):3038-3051.

46. Klastersky J, Paesmans M, Georgala A, et al. Outpatient oral antibiotics for febrile neutropenic cancer patients using a score predictive for complications. *J Clin Oncol*. 2006;24(25):4129-4134.

47. Freifeld A, Marchigiani D, Walsh T, et al. A double-blind comparison of empirical oral and intravenous antibiotic therapy for low-risk febrile patients with neutropenia during cancer chemotherapy. *N Engl J Med*. 1999;341(5):305-311.

48. Bow EJ. Fluoroquinolones, antimicrobial resistance and neutropenic cancer patients. *Curr Opin Infect Dis*. 2011;24(6):545-553.

49. Greene JN. Catheter-related complications of cancer therapy. *Infect Dis Clin North Am*. 1996;10(2):255-295.

50. Raad I, Hanna HA, Alakech B, Chatzinikolaou I, Johnson MM, Tarrand J. Differential time to positivity: a useful method for diagnosing catheter-related bloodstream infections. *Ann Intern Med*. 2004;140(1):18-25.

51. Manian FA. IDSA guidelines for the diagnosis and management of intravascular catheter-related bloodstream infection. *Clin Infect Dis*. 2009;49(11):1770-1771; author reply 1771-1772.

52. Garcia R, Raad I, Abi-Said D, et al. Nosocomial respiratory syncytial virus infections: prevention and control in bone marrow transplant patients. *Infect Control Hosp Epidemiol*. 1997;18(6):412-416.

53. Martino R, Porras RP, Rabella N, et al. Prospective study of the incidence, clinical features, and outcome of symptomatic upper and lower respiratory tract infections by respiratory viruses in adult recipients of hematopoietic stem cell transplants for hematologic malignancies. *Biol Blood Marrow Transplant*. 2005;11:781-796.

54. Walmsley S, Devi S, King S, Schneider R, Richardson S, Ford-Jones L. Invasive *Aspergillus* infections in a pediatric hospital: a ten-year review. *Pediatr Infect Dis J*. 1993;12(8):673-682.

55. Maschmeyer G, Calandra T, Singh N, Wiley J, Perfect J. Invasive mould infections: a multi-disciplinary update. *Med Mycol*. 2009;47(6):571-583.

56. De Pauw B, Walsh TJ, Donnelly JP, et al. Revised definitions of invasive fungal disease from the European Organization for Research and Treatment of Cancer/Invasive Fungal Infections Cooperative Group and the National Institute of Allergy and Infectious Diseases Mycoses Study Group (EORTC/MSG) Consensus Group. *Clin Infect Dis*. 2008;46(12):1813-1821.

57. Mandell LA, Wunderink RG, Anzueto A, et al. Infectious Diseases Society of America/American Thoracic Society consensus guidelines on the management of community-acquired pneumonia in adults. *Clin Infect Dis*. 2007;44(suppl 2):S27-S72.

58. Guidelines for the management of adults with hospital-acquired, ventilator-associated, and healthcare-associated pneumonia. *Am J Respir Crit Care Med*. 2005;171(4):388-416.

59. Casper C, Englund J, Boeckh M. How I treat influenza in patients with hematologic malignancies. *Blood*. 2010;115(7):1331-1342.

60. Chemaly RF, Ghosh S, Bodey GP, et al. Respiratory viral infections in adults with hematologic malignancies and human stem cell transplantation recipients: a retrospective study at a major cancer center. *Medicine (Baltimore)*. 2006;85(5):278-287.

61. Yu VL. Guidelines for hospital-acquired pneumonia and health-care-associated pneumonia: a vulnerability, a pitfall, and a fatal flaw. *Lancet Infect Dis*. 2011;11(3):248-252.

62. Ewig S. Nosocomial pneumonia: de-escalation is what matters. *Lancet Infect Dis*. 2011;11(3):155-157.

63. Kett DH, Cano E, Quartin AA, et al. Implementation of guidelines for management of possible multidrug-resistant pneumonia in intensive care: an observational, multicentre cohort study. *Lancet Infect Dis*. 2011;11(3):181-189.

64. Segal BH, Freifeld AG, Baden LR, et al. Prevention and treatment of cancer-related infections. *J Natl Compr Canc Netw*. 2008;6(2):122-174.

65. Commers JR, Robichaud KJ, Pizzo PA. New pulmonary infiltrates in granulocytopenic cancer patients being treated with antibiotics. *Pediatr Infect Dis*. 1984;3(5):423-428.

66. Symeonidis N, Jakubowski A, Pierre-Louis S, et al. Invasive adenoviral infections in T-cell-depleted allogeneic hematopoietic stem cell transplantation: high mortality in the era of cidofovir. *Transpl Infect Dis*. 2007;9(2):108-113.

67. Clark BD, Vezza PR, Copeland C, Wilder AM, Abati A. Diagnostic sensitivity of bronchoalveolar lavage versus lung fine needle aspirate. *Mod Pathol*. 2002;15(12):1259-1265.

68. Sherif R, Segal BH. Pulmonary aspergillosis: clinical presentation, diagnostic tests, management and complications. *Curr Opin Pulm Med*. 2010;16(3):242-250.

69. Meersseman W, Lagrou K, Maertens J, et al. Galactomannan in bronchoalveolar lavage fluid: a tool for diagnosing aspergillosis in intensive care unit patients. *Am J Respir Crit Care Med*. 2008;177(1):27-34.

70. Carmona EM, Limper AH. Update on the diagnosis and treatment of *Pneumocystis pneumonia*. *Ther Adv Respir Dis*. 2011;5(1):41-59.

71. Almyroudis NG, Segal BH. Antifungal prophylaxis and therapy in patients with hematological malignancies and hematopoietic stem cell transplant recipients. *Expert Rev Anti Infect Ther*. 2010;8(12):1451-1466.

72. Almyroudis NG, Segal BH. Prevention and treatment of invasive fungal diseases in neutropenic patients. *Curr Opin Infect Dis*. 2009;22(4):385-393.

73. Kouroussis C, Samonis G, Androulakis N, et al. Successful conservative treatment of neutropenic enterocolitis complicating taxane-based chemotherapy: a report of five cases. *Am J Clin Oncol.* 2000;23(3):309-313.

74. Ibrahim NK, Sahin AA, Dubrow RA, et al. Colitis associated with docetaxel-based chemotherapy in patients with metastatic breast cancer. *Lancet.* 2000;355(9200):281-283.

75. Kirkpatrick ID, Greenberg HM. Gastrointestinal complications in the neutropenic patient: characterization and differentiation with abdominal CT. *Radiology.* 2003;226(3):668-674.

76. Shamberger RC, Weinstein HJ, Delorey MJ, Levey RH. The medical and surgical management of typhlitis in children with acute nonlymphocytic (myelogenous) leukemia. *Cancer.* 1986;57(3):603-609.

77. McDonald LC, Killgore GE, Thompson A, et al. An epidemic, toxin gene-variant strain of *Clostridium difficile*. *N Engl J Med.* 2005;353:2433-2441.

78. Loo VG, Poirier L, Miller MA, et al. A predominantly clonal multi-institutional outbreak of *Clostridium difficile*-associated diarrhea with high morbidity and mortality. *N Engl J Med.* 2005;353:2442-2449.

79. Zar FA, Bakkanagari SR, Moorthi KM, Davis MB. A comparison of vancomycin and metronidazole for the treatment of *Clostridium difficile*-associated diarrhea, stratified by disease severity. *Clin Infect Dis.* 2007;45(3):302-307.

80. Mullane KM, Miller MA, Weiss K, et al. Efficacy of fidaxomicin versus vancomycin as therapy for *Clostridium difficile* infection in individuals taking concomitant antibiotics for other concurrent infections. *Clin Infect Dis.* 2011;53(5):440-447.

81. Herpers BL, Vlaminckx B, Burkhardt O, et al. Intravenous tigecycline as adjunctive or alternative therapy for severe refractory *Clostridium difficile* infection. *Clin Infect Dis.* 2009;48(12):1732-1735.

82. Musher DM, Logan N, Hamill RJ, et al. Nitazoxanide for the treatment of *Clostridium difficile* colitis. *Clin Infect Dis.* 2006;43:421-427.

83. Bartlett JG. Narrative review: the new epidemic of *Clostridium difficile*-associated enteric disease. *Ann Intern Med.* 2006;145(10):758-764.

84. Lowy I, Molrine DC, Leav BA, et al. Treatment with monoclonal antibodies against *Clostridium difficile* toxins. *N Engl J Med.* 2010;362(3):197-205.

85. Lehrnbecher T, Marshall D, Gao C, Chanock SJ. A second look at anorectal infections in cancer patients in a large cancer institute: the success of early intervention with antibiotics and surgery. *Infection.* 2002;30(5):272-276.

86. Barnes SG, Sattler FR, Ballard JO. Perirectal infections in acute leukemia. Improved survival after incision and debridement. *Ann Intern Med.* 1984;100(4):515-518.

87. Talan DA, Krishnadasan A, Abrahamian FM, Stamm WE, Moran GJ. Prevalence and risk factor analysis of trimethoprim–sulfamethoxazole- and fluoroquinolone-resistant *Escherichia coli* infection among emergency department patients with pyelonephritis. *Clin Infect Dis.* 2008;47(9):1150-1158.

88. Raz R, Schiller D, Nicolle LE. Chronic indwelling catheter replacement before antimicrobial therapy for symptomatic urinary tract infection. *J Urol.* 2000;164(4):1254-1258.

89. Pappas PG, Kauffman CA, Andes D, et al. Clinical practice guidelines for the management of candidiasis: 2009 update by the Infectious Diseases Society of America. *Clin Infect Dis.* 2009;48(5):503-535.

90. Stevens DL, Bisno AL, Chambers HF, et al. Practice guidelines for the diagnosis and management of skin and soft-tissue infections. *Clin Infect Dis.* 2005;41(10):1373-1406.

91. Anaya DA, Dellinger EP. Necrotizing soft-tissue infection: diagnosis and management. *Clin Infect Dis.* 2007;44(5):705-710.

92. Person AK, Kontoyiannis DP, Alexander BD. Fungal infections in transplant and oncology patients. *Infect Dis Clin North Am.* 2010;24(2):439-459.

93. Nucci M, Anaissie E. Fungal infections in hematopoietic stem cell transplantation and solid-organ transplantation—focus on aspergillosis. *Clin Chest Med.* 2009;30(2):295-306, vii.

94. Meyers JD, Reed EC, Shepp DH, et al. Acyclovir for prevention of cytomegalovirus infection and disease after allogeneic marrow transplantation. *N Engl J Med.* 1988;318(2):70-75.

95. Saral R, Ambinder RF, Burns WH, et al. Acyclovir prophylaxis against herpes simplex virus infection in patients with leukemia. A randomized, double-blind, placebo-controlled study. *Ann Intern Med.* 1983;99(6):773-776.

96. Boeckh M, Kim HW, Flowers ME, Meyers JD, Bowden RA. Long-term acyclovir for prevention of varicella zoster virus disease after allogeneic hematopoietic cell transplantation—a randomized double-blind placebo-controlled study. *Blood.* 2006;107(5):1800-1805.

CHAPTER 38

Management of Intracranial Metastases

Caroline Chung ■ Normand Laperriere

INTRODUCTION

Brain metastases are the most common brain tumors in cancer patients. The incidence is 10% to 40% in all cancer patients (1) and as high as 80% in patients with metastatic disease. Primary cancers that most commonly metastasize to the brain include lung cancer, breast cancer, renal cancer, and melanoma.

As advances in systemic therapies are improving extracranial disease control, brain metastases are having an increasing contribution to a patient's morbidity and mortality, particularly when patients present with well-controlled systemic disease. One example is the impact of trastuzumab on HER-2 positive breast cancer patients, which has prolonged the control of extracranial disease and altered the natural progression of disease with increasing brain metastatic involvement (2). Furthermore, with increasing use of more sensitive imaging modalities such as magnetic resonance imaging (MRI), patients are presenting with smaller and fewer brain metastases. Therefore, the goals of management for patients with brain metastases have now broadened to reflect the greater variation in the initial presentation, as well as expected prognosis.

Advances in surgical techniques and radiotherapy delivery have facilitated improvements in the control of brain metastases. However, a greater risk of toxicity and potentially iatrogenic morbidity are the costs of improved local tumor control with more aggressive therapies. As a result, it is now more important than ever to determine the appropriate goals of treatment for the individual patient before weighing the benefits and costs of the proposed treatment regimen. Largely, the goals of treatment will reflect the patient's expected overall prognosis, and there is a growing body of research aimed at improving our ability to estimate prognosis based on both patient and tumor factors.

CLINICAL PRESENTATION

Historically, patients have presented with signs and symptoms of increased intracranial pressure (ICP), seizures, and/or focal neurologic symptoms due to both tumor and peritumoral edema. The specific neurologic deficits are dependent on the location and size of the metastases neid the extent of peritumoral edema. These can include generalized fatigue,

headache, cognitive deficits and personality changes, motor or sensory deficits, balance disturbance, speech difficulties, or seizures. With increasing use of MRI, which has a higher sensitivity for the detection of brain metastases, a greater proportion of patients are presenting with radiologically detected asymptomatic, small brain metastases (3). Both the presence of symptoms and the number of lesions may impact management decisions and patient outcome.

In 20% of cases, a brain metastasis is the initial presentation of malignancy with or without a known primary cancer (1). A *solitary brain metastasis* is the presence of one brain metastasis with no other sites of active metastatic disease, whereas a *single brain metastasis* is the presence of one brain metastasis with other active metastatic disease. Particularly in the setting of solitary-enhancing brain lesions, the differential diagnosis should be considered and investigations should include a metastatic workup with an aim to confirm a histologic diagnosis. If a primary malignancy cannot be found, surgical resection or biopsy of the brain lesion may be required to confirm histology.

PROGNOSIS

The prognosis of patients with brain metastases is improving. This may reflect detection of earlier, lower bulk disease in patients with better performance status at the time of diagnosis, improving systemic therapy to control extracranial disease and more aggressive interventions to achieve durable control of brain metastases. Table 38.1 summarizes the range of reported overall survival rates following the different treatment for brain metastases. These differences in overall survival likely reflect the differences in treatment selection based on patients' prognostic factors such as disease extent and performance status. For instance, a patient with a single metastasis and well-controlled extracranial disease would likely receive more aggressive treatment with combined surgery and radiation than a patient with active systemic disease and multiple brain metastases.

A number of prognostic indices have been developed to help guide the appropriate goals of management and suitable care for patients with brain metastases. A key component included in most prognostic indices developed for patients with brain metastases is the Karnofsky performance status (KPS), which has been established as a reliable and valid

TABLE 38.1	Summary of outcomes following brain metastasis treatment (4,12,14,16,17)

Treatment	Overall Survival (months)
Steroids alone	1
WBRT	3–6
WBRT + surgery (single metastasis)	10–15
WBRT + radiosurgery (1–4 metastases)	6–12

WBRT, whole brain radiotherapy

measurement scale to guide appropriate treatment selection as well as measure treatment response (5).

The first prognostic index specific for patients with brain metastases was generated from a recursive partitioning analysis (RPA) of data from 1,200 patients treated with whole brain radiotherapy (WBRT) in 3 randomized controlled trials of the Radiation Therapy Oncology Group (RTOG). The RPA classification system grouped patients into three prognostic classes based on patient age, status of primary tumor control, and extent of extracranial disease (6). Several prognostic indices have been developed since the RPA, which incorporate various combinations of other factors including the extent of intracranial disease and the number of metastases (Table 38.2) (7–9). Despite the addition of more factors, these alternative prognostic indices do not appear to perform any better than the RPA classification in estimating the prognosis of cancer patients when tumor histology is not considered. More recently, the graded prognostic index was applied to patients with particular tumor histologies to develop a disease-specific graded prognostic assessment (DS-GPA). Retrospective multi-institutional analysis of 4,259 patients with brain metastasis, with incorporation of primary tumor histology, appeared to improve the accuracy of predicting patient prognosis beyond any of the prior prognostic indices (10). Emerging evidence suggests that the DS-GPA may best reflect prognosis in patients with brain metastases, although this prognostic index is not yet validated.

MANAGEMENT

Currently, the management of brain metastases may range from supportive care up to aggressive multimodal treatment with the aim of improving intracranial tumor control. The treatments that are currently used include surgery, radiosurgery, whole brain radiation, and supportive care. There are several aims for treating brain metastases and these should reflect a patient's performance status, overall disease burden and activity, and most importantly, the patient/family goals of care. In patients with limited disease burden, the aim of the treatment may be to achieve durable intracranial tumor control utilizing a combined modality approach with surgery or radiosurgery and fractionated radiotherapy. There are ongoing studies exploring the role of promising targeted agents in the management of brain metastases of particular tumor histologies.

Whole Brain Radiotherapy

WBRT, often in combination with steroids, remains the standard treatment for patients with brain metastases (11). It is an effective treatment that can provide rapid palliation and tumor response in many cases, but it yields limited survival of 3 to 6 months (12). The standard radiation treatment is usually delivered in 5 to 10 treatments to a total dose of radiation from 20 to 30 Gy. Alternate dosing schedules and

TABLE 38.2	Prognostic indices for brain metastasis (7–9)					
Prognostic Index	Age	KPS	Extracranial Disease Status	Primary Tumor Control	Volume of Largest Metastases	Number of Metastases
Golden grading system	◆	◆	◆			
Basic score for brain metastases (BS-BM)		◆	◆	◆		
Score index for radiosurgery (SIR)	◆	◆		◆	◆	◆
Graded prognostic assessment (GPA)[a]	◆	◆	◆			◆

[a]Disease-specific graded prognostic assessment, incorporating tumor histology with these prognostic factors, is currently the strongest prognostic index available.

KPS, Karnofsky performance status.

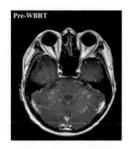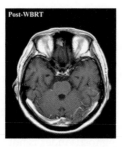

Figure 38.1. Gadolinium-enhanced axial T$_1$-weighted magnetic resonance images of a patient with leptomeningeal disease demonstrating classical enhancement within the cerebellar folia (*left*). Completed resolution of the enhancing disease was seen 2 months post-whole brain radiotherapy (post-WBRT) (*right*). Clinical improvement accompanied radiologic resolution.

higher doses of radiation have failed to show any benefit in patient outcome (13).

WBRT is associated with a number of acute toxicities, including alopecia, dermatitis, headaches, nausea, otitis externa, and otitis media, as well as short-term memory and cognitive deficits (14). Decline in neurocognitive function following WBRT has been a recent focus of research. A number of factors can contribute to neurocognitive decline in patients with cancer, including intracranial tumor progression, toxicity from systemic therapy, narcotic pain medications, and other medical causes such as infection or metabolic disturbances (15). This poses an obvious challenge in differentiating a decline due to brain radiotherapy from other causes in patients with metastatic disease. One of the current hypotheses is that irradiation of bilateral hippocampal regions may have the greatest impact on memory deficit (15). Therefore, the impact of new treatment approaches that help avoid irradiation of the hippocampal regions is currently under investigation. This includes alternative techniques to deliver WBRT while limiting the dose to the hippocampal region as well as avoidance of WBRT by treating the known metastases in selected patients with oligometastatic disease.

Despite the associated toxicities, whole brain therapy remains the most appropriate treatment in some patients, including those with diffuse multiple brain metastases and/or leptomeningeal metastases (Figs. 38.1 and 38.2). Furthermore, WBRT may be the safest and most appropriate initial treatment when lesions are not amenable to a local therapy (surgery or radiosurgery).

Surgery

Surgery has several therapeutic advantages over radiotherapy, including immediate relief of mass effect and reduced corticosteroid requirement following resection. Figure 38.3 demonstrates an example of a posterior fossa metastasis that was effectively managed with surgery. Additionally, surgical resection can provide histologic confirmation, particularly when the etiology of the detected brain lesion is unclear. However, surgical resection is an invasive treatment that is associated with a number of risks of complications, including infection, hemorrhage, thromboembolic events, and possible deterioration in neurologic function depending on the location of the tumor(s).

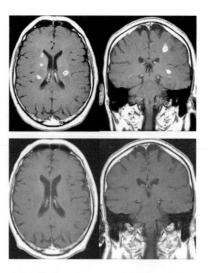

Figure 38.2. Axial (*left*) and coronal (*right*) gadolinium-enhanced T$_1$-weighted images of a patient with melanoma. The *top panel* demonstrates multiple bilateral-enhancing brain metastases. The *bottom panel* shows complete resolution of the visible-enhancing metastases 2 months after whole brain radiotherapy.

When surgery is used in combination with WBRT, local control and intracranial tumor control can be improved. In patients with good performance status and a single brain metastasis, this combination treatment can result in improved overall survival and greater functional independence compared with WBRT alone. Patchell et al. reported the seminal randomized controlled trial in 1990 comparing WBRT with surgical resection and WBRT alone for patients with single brain metastasis, which demonstrated an overall survival advantage in the combined surgery and WBRT arm with a median survival of 40 weeks compared with 15 weeks for WBRT alone. In addition, the combination treatment resulted in greater functional independence of 38 weeks versus 8 weeks for the WBRT arm (*P* < 0.005) (16). A subsequent randomized study validated the improvement in median overall survival with

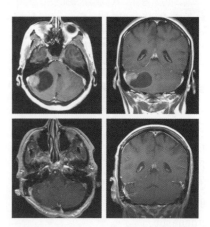

Figure 38.3. Axial (*left*) and coronal (*right*) gadolinium-enhanced T$_1$-weighted magnetic resonance images demonstrating a large cystic cerebellar brain metastases (*top panel*). The *bottom panel* shows a good surgical resection with resolution of the mass effect and no evidence of recurrence 6 months after surgery and whole brain radiotherapy.

combined surgery and WBRT compared with WBRT alone, 10 months versus 6 months (17). In an attempt to minimize the treatment-related toxicity of WBRT, there is an ongoing randomized study of surgery with radiosurgery boost versus surgery with WBRT.

Radiosurgery

Stereotactic radiosurgery (SRS) is the delivery of a single (or very few) highly accurate treatment(s) with an ablative dose of radiation focused on a radiographically distinct target (Fig. 38.4). Currently, radiosurgery treatment can be delivered using a linear accelerator, a cyberknife, or a gamma knife (11). For the treatment of brain metastases, these technologies are thought to be comparable, but no formal comparison has been reported.

For patients with a limited number of brain metastases, a recent meta-analysis has shown that the addition of radiosurgery to the visible metastases in combination with WBRT has been shown to improve local control (12). A survival benefit has not been demonstrated in patients with multiple metastases, even when limited to a maximum of four metastases. However, the addition of a radiosurgery boost to WBRT improved survival of patients with single brain metastases (median survival 6.5 mo SRS + WBRT vs. 4.9 mo WBRT, $P = 0.0393$) (12).

In addition to its benefit when utilized in combination with WBRT, radiosurgery has therapeutic advantages over surgery and WBRT. Specifically, tumors located in eloquent cortex,

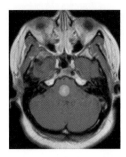
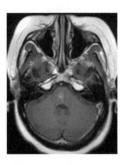

Figure 38.5. Case of brainstem metastasis from breast cancer before (*left*) and 9 months after (*right*) a single radiosurgery treatment of 15 Gy.

such as the brainstem or motor strip, that are not amenable to surgical resection can be effectively treated with radiosurgery and/or fractionated radiotherapy. For these cases, radiosurgery can be used as a boost with WBRT, for early salvage therapy following WBRT, or as the primary treatment without WBRT in selected patients. Figure 38.5 displays an example of a metastasis in the brainstem treated with radiosurgery.

Recurrent Disease

At the time of intracranial recurrence following prior therapy, the appropriate salvage therapy may depend on a number of factors, including location of the recurrence, the total number of recurrent lesions, and timing from previous treatment. Following prior WBRT, salvage therapy options may include repeat WBRT, radiosurgery, and surgery. Surgery is usually restricted to patients with one large metastasis in non-eloquent brain associated with significant mass effect with preferably minimal or stable extracranial disease. Salvage radiosurgery is usually limited to patients with a smaller number of recurrent metastases. Repeat WBRT is generally offered to those with a larger number of recurrent metastases that are not felt to be eligible for radiosurgery. Response to re-irradiation of recurrent disease following previous irradiation is variable and is not necessarily the same as the initial response to radiation. However, the timing of recurrence following whole brain radiation may impact radiation-related toxicity. Therefore, within 6 months of whole brain radiation, radiosurgery and surgery are favored options of salvage therapy for recurrence of a limited number of metastases. Recurrences in the region of previously resected metastases are often infiltrative and poor targets for radiosurgery, and when limited to the surgical region, it can be successfully managed with focal fractionated radiotherapy either via 3D conformal or intensity-modulated radiation therapy techniques.

LEPTOMENINGEAL DISEASE

Presentation

Approximately 5% to 15% of all patients with solid cancers develop leptomeningeal disease with the most common primary solid tumor histologies being breast cancer, lung cancer, and melanoma (18). Most patients presenting with leptomeningeal disease also have widely disseminated systemic cancer, and better systemic metastatic control has been

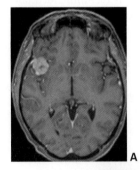
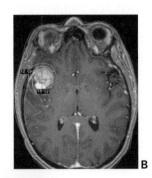
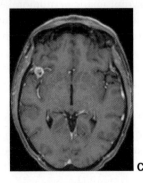

Figure 38.4. Axial T_1-weighted magnetic resonance images of a right frontal brain metastasis from primary lung cancer demonstrating (**A**) baseline tumor appearance prior to radiosurgery, (**B**) radiosurgery plan showing a very tight radiation dose targeted to the tumor with minimal dose to surrounding brain, and (**C**) magnetic resonance images at 1 year showing a durable response with significant reduction in tumor size.

associated with delayed appearance of leptomeningeal metastases (19,20). Patients can present with hydrocephalus and raised intracranial pressure or they can present with various multifocal constellations of symptoms depending on the specific areas of leptomeningeal involvement in the cerebrum, cerebellum, cranial nerves, and/or spinal cord and roots (21).

Investigation and Diagnosis

In patients with known metastatic cancer, diagnosis of leptomeningeal brain metastases is made radiologically on a gadolinium-enhanced brain MRI. Typically, there is enhancement along the meningeal lining of the brain, classically with enhancement along the cerebellar folia (21,22). In cases where neuroimaging does not show definitive evidence of leptomeningeal disease, examination of the cerebrospinal fluid (CSF) can assist in the diagnosis of leptomeningeal metastases. Although the presence of malignant cells in the CSF is diagnostic for leptomeningeal disease, a negative CSF cytology does not reliably rule out leptomeningeal disease due to the low sensitivity of CSF cytology (23). If leptomeningeal disease is found in the brain, a gadolinium-enhanced MRI of the spine is recommended to rule out leptomeningeal disease involving the spinal cord or cauda equina.

Prognosis

The prognosis of patients with leptomeningeal disease is poor and this may be compounded by their clinical presentation with both extensive systemic disease and leptomeningeal CNS disease. The median survival of patients with leptomeningeal brain metastasis is 4 to 11 weeks (20,21). Based on prior studies, which include patients with varying extent of leptomeningeal disease in the brain and/or spinal disease treated with radiotherapy and/or chemotherapy, median survival is between 4 and 6 months with cytotoxic therapy (18,21).

Treatment

Treatment of leptomeningeal metastasis can improve symptoms and in some cases prolong survival. The most common treatment for leptomeningeal brain metastasis is WBRT. Intrathecal chemotherapy or high-dose intravenous chemotherapy has been used to treat patients with leptomeningeal disease in the brain and spine (18). However, a clear survival benefit from intrathecal chemotherapy has not been demonstrated over systemic chemotherapy and/or radiotherapy (24–26). Given the uncertain benefit and the greater potential for severe complications and toxicities associated with intrathecal chemotherapy, WBRT may have the better therapeutic index for patients with radiologically visible leptomeningeal disease isolated to the brain.

SUPPORTIVE CARE

A major aim in the treatment of brain metastases is to improve symptoms and function for patients, which can include minimizing the dose and/or duration of dexamethasone required.

Surgical resection typically results in the most dramatic reduction of steroid requirements. Some patients may require higher doses of steroids following fractionated radiotherapy or radiosurgery and a slow weaning schedule can be required in this situation. In a proportion of cases, despite evidence of good tumor control radiologically, patients are unable to wean off dexamethasone completely. However, most treatments are associated with toxicities and patients with limited performance status and/or extensive disease may neither tolerate nor benefit from surgical or radiation intervention.

Steroids

Most patients who present with brain metastasis with symptomatic peritumoral edema benefit from corticosteroids. Dexamethasone is most commonly used as it has a long half-life, good absorption when taken orally, and minimal mineralocorticoid effect. The proposed mechanism of dexamethasone involves upregulation of Ang-1, a stabilizer of the blood–brain barrier and downregulation of vascular endothelial growth factor to reduce peritumoral edema (27). Evidence of reduced intracranial pressure and improvement in neurologic symptoms can be seen within hours of administration but maximal benefit is typically seen several days after starting dexamethasone.

Recommended Dosing

There is little evidence to guide the optimal dose and tapering schedule for steroids. In general, twice daily dosing at the lowest dose that alleviates symptoms is recommended and early tapering within 1 to 2 weeks is suggested, as steroid side effects have been associated with both dose and duration of steroid use. For mild to moderately symptomatic patients, an initial dose of 4 to 8 mg/d is recommended (28,29). For patients with more severe symptoms and concerns of increased intracranial pressure, a higher dose of 16 mg/d is recommended (30).

Side Effects

Although dexamethasone can provide dramatic benefits for patients with symptomatic peritumoral edema, it is also associated with many side effects that typically worsen over longer administration, including hyperglycemia, weight gain, peripheral edema, candidiasis, myopathy, Cushing's syndrome, insomnia, hypertension, psychiatric disturbances, cataracts, and susceptibility to infection (28).

Diabetic Patients and Steroids

Hyperglycemia is one of the most common medical toxicities of steroid administration, either exacerbated in known diabetic patients or unmasking previously undiagnosed Type 2 diabetes (31). Patients should be screened for symptoms such as polyuria and polydipsia and a random glucose with their other bloodwork may aid in early detection of hyperglycemia. Oral anti-diabetic agents such as metformin are typically used. However, if hyperglycemia is severe or refractory to oral agents, insulin therapy is recommended.

CONCLUSION

The treatment options for patients with brain metastases have progressed with advances in surgery and radiation techniques. The aims of treatment have also evolved to reflect the changing presentation of patients due to improving systemic therapy and increasing sensitivity of brain imaging. Although the optimal management of metastases continues to be an area of active investigation, it has been recognized that the management of individual patients should be individualized based on the patient's overall status, prognosis, tumor location, and volume, while considering the patient's goals and preferences.

REFERENCES

1. Gavrilovic IT, Posner JB. Brain metastases: epidemiology and pathophysiology. *J Neurooncol.* 2005;75(1):5-14.
2. Lin NU, Winer EP. Brain metastases: the HER2 paradigm. *Clin Cancer Res.* 2007;13(6):1648-1655.
3. Soffietti R, Ducati A, Ruda R. Brain metastases. *Handb Clin Neurol.* 2012;105:747-755.
4. Aoyama H, Shirato H, Tago M, et al. Stereotactic radiosurgery plus whole-brain radiation therapy vs stereotactic radiosurgery alone for treatment of brain metastases: a randomized controlled trial. *JAMA.* 2006;295(21):2483-2491.
5. Schag CC, Heinrich RL, Ganz PA. Karnofsky performance status revisited: reliability, validity, and guidelines. *J Clin Oncol.* 1984;2(3):187-193.
6. Gaspar L, Scott C, Rotman M, et al. Recursive partitioning analysis (RPA) of prognostic factors in three Radiation Therapy Oncology Group (RTOG) brain metastases trials. *Int J Radiat Oncol Biol Phys.* 1997;37(4):745-751.
7. Lorenzoni J, Devriendt D, Massager N, et al. Radiosurgery for treatment of brain metastases: estimation of patient eligibility using three stratification systems. *Int J Radiat Oncol Biol Phys.* 2004;60(1):218-224.
8. Viani GA, Castilho MS, Salvajoli JV, et al. Whole brain radiotherapy for brain metastases from breast cancer: estimation of survival using two stratification systems. *BMC Cancer.* 2007;7:53.
9. Golden DW, Lamborn KR, McDermott MW, et al. Prognostic factors and grading systems for overall survival in patients treated with radiosurgery for brain metastases: variation by primary site. *J Neurosurg.* 2008;109(suppl):77-86.
10. Sperduto PW, Chao ST, Sneed PK, et al. Diagnosis-specific prognostic factors, indexes, and treatment outcomes for patients with newly diagnosed brain metastases: a multi-institutional analysis of 4,259 patients. *Int J Radiat Oncol Biol Phys.* 2009;77(3):655-661.
11. Mehta MP, Tsao MN, Whelan TJ, et al. The American Society for Therapeutic Radiology and Oncology (ASTRO) evidence-based review of the role of radiosurgery for brain metastases. *Int J Radiat Oncol Biol Phys.* 2005;63(1):37-46.
12. Tsao M, Xu W, Sahgal A. A meta-analysis evaluating stereotactic radiosurgery, whole-brain radiotherapy, or both for patients presenting with a limited number of brain metastases. *Cancer.* 2012;118(9):2486-2493.
13. Tsao MN, Lloyd N, Wong R, et al. Whole brain radiotherapy for the treatment of multiple brain metastases. *Cochrane Database Syst Rev.* 2006;3:CD003869.
14. Andrews DW, Scott CB, Sperduto PW, et al. Whole brain radiation therapy with or without stereotactic radiosurgery boost for patients with one to three brain metastases: phase III results of the RTOG 9508 randomised trial. *Lancet.* 2004;363(9422):1665-1672.
15. Li J, Bentzen SM, Renschler M, Mehta MP. Regression after whole-brain radiation therapy for brain metastases correlates with survival and improved neurocognitive function. *J Clin Oncol.* 2007;25(10):1260-1266.
16. Patchell RA, Tibbs PA, Walsh JW, et al. A randomized trial of surgery in the treatment of single metastases to the brain. *N Engl J Med.* 1990;322(8):494-500.
17. Vecht CJ, Haaxma-Reiche H, Noordijk EM, et al. Treatment of single brain metastasis: radiotherapy alone or combined with neurosurgery? *Ann Neurol.* 1993;33(6):583-590.
18. Chamberlain MC. Leptomeningeal metastases: a review of evaluation and treatment. *J Neurooncol.* 1998;37(3):271-284.
19. van Oostenbrugge RJ, Twijnstra A. Presenting features and value of diagnostic procedures in leptomeningeal metastases. *Neurology.* 1999;53(2):382-385.
20. Grossman SA, Krabak MJ. Leptomeningeal carcinomatosis. *Cancer Treat Rev.* 1999;25(2):103-119.
21. Clarke JL, Perez HR, Jacks LM, et al. Leptomeningeal metastases in the MRI era. *Neurology.* 2010;74(18):1449-1454.
22. Chamberlain MC, Sandy AD, Press GA. Leptomeningeal metastasis: a comparison of gadolinium-enhanced MR and contrast-enhanced CT of the brain. *Neurology.* 1990;40(3 pt 1):435-438.
23. Wasserstrom WR, Glass JP, Posner JB. Diagnosis and treatment of leptomeningeal metastases from solid tumors: experience with 90 patients. *Cancer.* 1982;49(4):759-772.
24. Bokstein F, Lossos A, Siegal T. Leptomeningeal metastases from solid tumors: a comparison of two prospective series treated with and without intra-cerebrospinal fluid chemotherapy. *Cancer.* 1998;82(9):1756-1763.
25. Glantz MJ, Cole BF, Recht L, et al. High-dose intravenous methotrexate for patients with nonleukemic leptomeningeal cancer: is intrathecal chemotherapy necessary? *J Clin Oncol.* 1998;16(4):1561-1567.
26. Boogerd W, van den Bent MJ, Koehler PJ, et al. The relevance of intraventricular chemotherapy for leptomeningeal metastasis in breast cancer: a randomised study. *Eur J Cancer.* 2004;40(18):2726-2733.
27. Kim H, Lee JM, Park JS, et al. Dexamethasone coordinately regulates angiopoietin-1 and VEGF: a mechanism of glucocorticoid-induced stabilization of blood-brain barrier. *Biochem Biophys Res Commun.* 2008;372(1):243-248.
28. Hempen C, Weiss E, Hess CF. Dexamethasone treatment in patients with brain metastases and primary brain tumors: do the benefits outweigh the side-effects? *Support Care Cancer.* 2002;10(4):322-328.
29. Vecht CJ, Hovestadt A, Verbiest HB, van Vliet JJ, van Putten WL. Dose–effect relationship of dexamethasone on Karnofsky performance in metastatic brain tumors: a randomized study of doses of 4, 8, and 16 mg per day. *Neurology.* 1994;44(4):675-680.
30. Brainin M, Barnes M, Baron JC, et al. Guidance for the preparation of neurological management guidelines by EFNS scientific task forces—revised recommendations 2004. *Eur J Neurol.* 2004;11(9):577-581.
31. Lukins MB, Manninen PH. Hyperglycemia in patients administered dexamethasone for craniotomy. *Anesth Analg.* 2005;100(4):1129-1133.

Management of Spinal Cord and Cauda Equina Compression

Sharon M. Weinstein

EPIDEMIOLOGY

The spine is the most frequent site of bony involvement in patients with metastatic malignancy (1). The major complications of spinal neoplasm are pain and neurologic injury. Compression of neural structures may be caused directly by tumor mass and/or by displacement of bony fragments into the spinal canal. Tumor of the vertebral bodies has been demonstrated in 25% to 70% of patients with metastatic cancer (2), and spinal metastases are present in 40% of patients who die of cancer (3). Metastatic lesions from other primary malignancies are three to four times as common as primary bony tumors of the spine (4).

Each year in the United States, approximately 20,000 patients with cancer are treated for malignant epidural compression (EC) of the spinal cord and/or cauda equina. It has been estimated that EC affects 5% to 10% of adult solid tumor patients and 5% of pediatric solid tumor patients (5,6). These percentages are corroborated by autopsy series (4,7). A review of over 15,000 EC cases representing over 75,000 hospitalizations revealed that patients dying of cancer in the United States have an estimated 3.4% annual incidence of EC requiring hospitalization. Inpatient management of EC varied over time and by hospital characteristics, with inpatient radiotherapy decreasing, surgical interventions increasing, and hospitalization costs increasing during the period of 1998 to 2006 (8).

Half of all patients initially presenting with EC are not known to have cancer at the time that pain or neurologic deficits begin (9). Therefore, it is common for EC to be the presenting symptom of malignancy. The distribution of spinal tumors reflects the prevalence of the various primary malignancies as well as the physiology of metastasis. Multiple myeloma is the most common primary bone tumor, representing 10% to 15% of malignant epidural spinal disease. Osteogenic sarcoma is the second most common primary spinal tumor, usually affecting children and adolescents. Fifty percent of chordomas affect the sacrococcygeal bones and 35% affect the base of the skull. Chondrosarcoma and Ewing's sarcoma are other bone tumors that may be primary in the vertebrae, although this is rare.

Primary tumors of the breast, lung, and prostate commonly spread to the spinal column. The spine is also a frequent site of metastasis of a nonspinal primary osteogenic sarcoma. Spinal metastases are less common in renal carcinoma, melanoma, soft tissue sarcoma, Ewing's sarcoma, germ cell tumors, neuroblastoma, and carcinomas of the head and neck, thyroid, and bladder. Rarely, malignant neoplasms of the brain, pancreas, liver, or ovary affect the bony spinal column.

Ten percent of symptomatic spinal metastases originate from unknown primary tumors (3). Some malignancies spread to the intraspinal space without directly affecting the bone. Lymphoma and neuroblastoma often invade the spinal canal through the intervertebral foramina. Ewing's sarcoma, as well as osteosarcoma, may be primary in the epidural space. Primary epidural tumors are rare.

Considering distribution by location in the spinal column, thoracic metastases are estimated to occur twice as frequently as lumbar metastases and four times as frequently as cervical metastases (2). Almost two-thirds of metastatic spinal lesions present clinically in the thoracic region (10), although in some autopsy series, lesions of the lumbar spine have been most prevalent (3). The level of spinal involvement varies with the primary tumor type. Breast and lung tumor metastases are equally distributed throughout the spine. Prostate, renal, and gastrointestinal metastases are more often found in the lower thoracic, lumbar, and sacral levels. Tumors of the uterus and uterine cervix most commonly spread to the lower lumbar and sacral spine. Pancoast tumors of the apex of the lung extend directly into the cervicothoracic spine in 25% of cases (10), often by intraforaminal extension. Multiple noncontiguous levels of spinal tumor are present in 10% to 38% of cases (11); this pattern is relatively less common in patients with lung cancer (9).

EC is caused by the direct extension of the tumor from the vertebral body in 85% to 90% of cases (10). In pediatric patients, EC due to tumor of the posterior elements is more likely, and intraforaminal spread of tumor from paraspinal sites also occurs more frequently than in adults (11). It is noted, however, that tumor metastases in the epidural space seldom breach the dura (3,12).

The prevalence of EC varies according to the tumor type. In one series of 103 patients with lung cancer, 26% with squamous histology, 9% with adenocarcinoma, and 14% with small cell tumors had spinal cord compression (13). The prevalence of all neurologic complications in this series was approximately 40%.

Breast cancer accounts for almost one-fourth of EC diagnosed in cancer hospitals. Vertebral metastases are identified in 60% of patients with breast cancer, and multiple levels of involvement are common. EC is rarely the initial presentation or an early finding in breast cancer (14).

Approximately 7% of patients with prostate cancer develop EC. EC was noted in 12.2% of patients with poorly differentiated tumors and 2.9% of those with well-differentiated tumors (15). The average time from initial prostate cancer diagnosis to EC is 2 years, although it is shorter in stage D2. In approximately 30% of prostate cancer patients with EC, it is the initial manifestation of the cancer (16).

Renal cell carcinomas may also cause EC secondary to bony metastasis. Testicular cancer rarely metastasizes to bone, but it may grow into the spinal canal from the retroperitoneal space. Malignant melanoma may produce EC from vertebral disease, but intradural and leptomeningeal involvement are probably more common. Head and neck cancers rarely metastasize beyond the cervical lymph nodes; approximately 80% of distant metastases are detected within 2 years of initial diagnosis. Therefore, a patient with head and neck cancer presenting with EC after 2 years should be evaluated for a second primary malignancy. EC occurred at all levels of the spine in one small series of patients with head and neck cancers (17).

Esophageal cancers may rarely cause EC by direct invasion to the thoracic spinal column (18). Carcinoid tumors are associated with neurologic complications in <20% of cases; the most frequent is EC due to spinal metastases, generally a late complication.

In plasmacytoma and multiple myeloma, EC is usually due to bony collapse, occurring in >10% of patients. Hodgkin's disease and non–Hodgkin's lymphomas are associated with a 5% incidence of EC, usually in association with extranodal or extensive nodal disease. The thoracic spine is most often involved, in many cases by intraforaminal spread of tumor (19). Patients with EC due to lymphoma are at high risk for meningeal disease. Cerebrospinal fluid (CSF) examination should be considered along with spinal imaging, as concurrent meningeal lymphoma is common and affects the antineoplastic treatment regimen. Vertebral compression fracture with radicular pain is a rare presenting sign of acute leukemia (20).

EC is the presenting sign of cancer in up to 30% of pediatric cases. The time interval to presentation with EC may be twice as long in children without a known cancer compared with those already diagnosed with malignancy (21). Children without a cancer history presenting with EC are often initially misdiagnosed (6). EC is the most frequent neurologic complication of Ewing's sarcoma (22).

DIFFERENTIAL DIAGNOSIS

The differential diagnosis of back pain and neurologic dysfunction secondary to EC includes benign tumors; it is interesting to note that meningiomas occur frequently in patients with breast cancer (2). Given its high prevalence, coexisting nonmalignant disease of the spine may affect as many as 30% of patients with EC (23). Degenerative, inflammatory, and infectious processes commonly affect the spinal structures (24). Soft tissue injuries causing back pain are also very common. Trauma is the most common cause of back pain in children; other nonmalignant conditions such as Scheuermann's disease and scoliosis (25) are also present in this age group. Back pain in patients with cancer may be a secondary symptom caused by vertebral osteoporosis owing to radiation therapy or corticosteroids.

Spinal cord or cauda equina dysfunction may be related to direct tumor or treatment effects without EC. Leptomeningeal disease, intradural extramedullary or intramedullary spinal cord disease, paraneoplastic necrotizing myelopathy, and myelopathy induced by radiation or intrathecal chemotherapy should be considered if no compressive epidural lesion is found. Myelopathy is a late complication of radiation; epidural lipomatosis may be caused by corticosteroid therapy. Vascular events of the spinal cord may occur in association with tumor masses.

PATHOGENESIS OF NEUROLOGIC DYSFUNCTION AND PAIN

The high incidence of metastasis to the vertebrae, despite their poor blood supply, is explained by their specific physiologic features. The vertebrae have a large capillary capacity, promoting local stasis of blood. The walls of the vascular sinusoids are discontinuous and intersinusoidal cords form cul-de-sac for tumor. Tumor products and the products of bone resorption act to stimulate tumor growth (26). Monocytes produce interleukin-1, which may promote resorption of normal bone (2). Metastases may occur more commonly in previously damaged bone (27).

Batson's plexus is a valveless system of epidural veins in which blood may flow rostrally or caudally. On Valsalva's maneuver, this system drains the viscera and may be a route of metastatic spread. Tumor also reaches the bone through the arteries, lymphatics, and by direct extension.

Epidural tumor produces dysfunction of neural structures by direct compression and by secondary demyelination, ischemia, and tissue edema. Inflammation may change vascular permeability and disrupt the blood–spinal cord barrier at the tumor site. The release of excitatory amino acids by injured neurons further promotes ischemia and injury.

In the initial stage of epidural spinal cord compression, there may be white matter edema and axonal swelling with normal blood flow. These changes are due to direct compression or venous congestion. Over time, progressive compression decreases blood flow and disturbs vascular autoregulation, leading to the development of vasogenic edema. Spinal cord infarction may result from the interruption of venous outflow or occlusion of small arteries or from the interruption of the major arterial supply to the spinal cord (including the artery of Adamkiewicz) or radicular arteries in the intervertebral foramina.

A necrotic cavity, usually located in the ventral portion of the posterior columns or dorsal horn, has been visualized on magnetic resonance imaging (MRI) (11). The effects of cord compression may also be due to coup or contrecoup injury, which is not easily predicted on the basis of the tumor location in relation to the spinal cord. Demyelination as a mechanism of neural dysfunction (5) is supported by pathologic examinations, which demonstrate greater demyelination of white matter than gray matter, a pattern that does not conform to arterial supply. Animal experiments indicate that a more rapid ischemic change produces a greater degree of irreversible neurologic injury (28,29). Similar observations have been made in the human spinal cord.

Pain due to malignancy of the spine may result from activation of afferent nociceptive neurons by mechanical distortion and inflammatory mediators (nociceptive pain) or from neural dysfunction (neuropathic pain). Nociceptors innervate the periosteum of bone, soft tissues (ligaments and muscles), facet articular cartilage, dura mater, nerve root sheaths, and blood vessels. Vertebral collapse and structural instability can give rise to mechanical pain through injury to these structures, which worsens during spine loading and weight shifting. There may be secondary myofascial pain as well. Neuropathic pain results from altered peripheral and central neural activities that may be induced by injury of the nerve roots, axonal injury, or other processes such as deafferentation (loss of primary sensory input).

PATIENT EVALUATION

Although it is widely recognized that pain is often the first symptom of spinal neoplasm, accurate assessment of back and neck pain in the patient with cancer may be challenging to even the experienced clinician. Complete history and physical examination, including a thorough neurologic examination, are essential to localize the underlying pathology. Proper clinical localization is necessary to choose diagnostic and therapeutic interventions correctly (Table 39.1). The importance of obtaining a detailed understanding of the spinal lesion(s) and elucidating the relationship of pathology to symptoms (clinicopathologic correlation) cannot be overemphasized. Inadequate evaluation increases the likelihood of otherwise preventable neurologic compromise. In a retrospective survey of patients with cancer presenting with back pain, misdiagnosis was attributed to poor history, inadequate examination, and insufficient diagnostic evaluation (30). In a review of cancer pain consultations performed by a neurology-based pain service, the comprehensive evaluation of pain led to an identification of new malignant involvement in 65% of cases (31). This underscores the importance of thorough clinical evaluation.

History

Up to 95% of adult and 80% of pediatric patients with EC present with pain (10,32). The difference in pain prevalence between adults and children may reflect greater difficulty in the pain assessment of and the underreporting of pain in children. Pain may precede other symptoms and signs of EC by 1 year (11). This interval may vary by tumor type; it is generally shorter for lung cancer than breast cancer (33). Overall, patients experience pain for an average of 4 to 5 months before presentation (3).

TABLE 39.1	Patterns of spinal tumor involvement
Bone
Bone alone
Single site
Multiple contiguous sites
Multiple noncontiguous sites
Bone and paraspinal soft tissues
Bone, paraspinal tissues, and viscera
Bone and nerve roots
Bone and epidural space (without thecal compression)
Bone and epidural spinal cord compression
Bone and epidural cauda equina compression
Epidural
Intraforaminal
Isolated
Local extension
Epidural and spinal cord compression
Single site
Multiple contiguous sites
Multiple noncontiguous sites
Epidural and cauda equina compression
Single site
Multiple contiguous sites
Multiple noncontiguous sites
Diffuse

Pain may be local at the site of pathology or referred in a nonradicular or a radicular (dermatomal) distribution or have combined features. Radicular or root pain is reported in 90% of lumbosacral EC, 79% of cervical compression, and 55% of thoracic cord compression (33). Radicular pain may be bilateral in thoracic lesions and is often described as a tight band around the chest or abdomen. It is important to note that radicular pain may be experienced in only one part of a dermatome (as a partial suspended sensory level). When a nerve root lesion produces chest or abdominal pain, the complaint may be mistakenly identified as referred pain of visceral origin. Radicular lesions are usually associated with segmental findings on examination. Nonradicular referred pain may be associated with vague paresthesias and tenderness at the painful site. Pain may be continuous at rest and markedly aggravated by body movements (incident pain). Although local pain from a vertebral lesion is worsened with loading due to upright posture, pain due to EC is often greatly increased by lying supine. A lesion confined to the vertebral body may also produce nonradicular referred pain.

Disease at C7 may refer pain to the interscapular region, and pain due to disease at L1 may be referred to the iliac crests, hips, or sacroiliac region. Sacral disease often causes midline pain radiating to the buttocks, which is made worse with sitting. Radicular pain, in particular, may be paroxysmal, spontaneous, or provoked by movement or sensory stimulation. Valsalva's maneuver may produce or aggravate both local and radicular pain. Pain on neck flexion or straight leg raising implies dural traction. Lhermitte's sign (electric shock-like pain in the spine) is a symptom of spinal cord dysfunction. Compression of the cervical spinal cord rarely produces funicular pain, which is pain referred to the lower extremities, thorax, or abdomen as a band of paresthesias. "Pseudoclaudication" of legs may be an isolated lumbar root symptom (2).

The neurologic findings associated with EC also vary considerably. There can be extensive epidural tumor with no neurologic findings on examination. Upper motor neuron weakness may occur with lesions of the spinal cord (above the L1 vertebral body). This finding is present in 75% of patients with EC at diagnosis (10). Sensory changes occur in approximately half of patients at presentation, including paresthesias and sensory loss, which can be segmental or below the level of injury. Sensory complaint without pain is exceedingly rare. Bladder and bowel dysfunction are evident in more than half of patients on presentation with EC; constipation usually precedes urinary retention or incontinence (2).

Examination

The physical examination begins with the observation of posture, spinal curvature, symmetry of paraspinal muscles, extremities, and skin. The practitioner may appreciate tenderness of the spinous processes on palpation or percussion, although this may not correlate with the level of spinal disease. Gibbus deformity and vertebral misalignments are frequently palpable; actual crepitus of the spine is unusual. Tenderness or spasm of the paraspinal muscles may also be noted. Urinary retention may be demonstrated by bladder percussion. Laxity of the anal sphincter may be apparent on digital rectal examination. Specific areas of sacral or coccygeal tenderness may be identified by external palpation, rectal, or pelvic examination.

Spinal maneuvers to elicit pain should be performed carefully. Thoracic and abdominal radicular pain may be provoked on lateral flexion and rotation of the trunk. Increased pain on neck flexion and straight leg raise sign may be "pseudomeningeal" signs of dural traction due to epidural tumor. If neck rigidity is present, the examiner should use extreme caution with range-of-motion maneuvers. Muscle spasm may be triggered by bony instability of the cervical spine, and forced movements may dislodge bony fragments, causing acute spinal cord or brainstem injury.

The neurologic examination reveals positive findings in most patients with EC. The examination should include assessment of mental status, cranial nerves, motor function, reflexes, sensation, coordination, and gait. Proximal lower extremity weakness may be initially evident only as difficulty in rising from a chair. Although weakness due to upper motor neuron dysfunction is usually associated with increased tone and hyperreflexia, acute "spinal shock" can cause a flaccid areflexic paralysis. In the subacute phase of recovery from spinal shock, "mass reflexes" appear consisting of flexor spasms, hyperhidrosis, and piloerection due to autonomic dysfunction. Lower motor neuron weakness may be accompanied by flaccidity, atrophy, muscle fasciculations, and hyporeflexia. A cervical lesion can produce segmental hyporeflexia in the arm or arms and increased reflexes below. Lesions above the pyramidal decussation of the corticospinal tracts in the lower brainstem may be associated with the loss of contralateral abdominal reflexes; lesions below the decussation produce loss of ipsilateral abdominal reflexes. Segmental motor dysfunction due to thoracic nerve root disease may produce asymmetric abdominal muscle contraction and loss of abdominal reflexes. Beevor's sign (upward movement of the umbilicus on attempted flexion of the trunk) indicates a lesion at or near the T10 thoracic level. Lesions of the roots of the upper lumbar plexus produce hip flexion weakness and a dropped knee jerk reflex; lesions of the roots to the lower lumbar plexus may produce foot drop and diminished ankle jerk reflex. Loss of bulbocavernosus and anal reflexes may accompany spinal cord conus and cauda equina lesions (2).

Although the sensory examination may help in determining the level of epidural disease, EC results in a broad variation of sensory dysfunction, with incomplete lesions being the rule. The level of reduced sensation may be determined to be up to five segmental levels below, or one to two segments above, the level of cord compression. A sensory level on the trunk sparing the sacral dermatomes may occur in up to 20% of patients with thoracic or high lumbar compression (2). Suspended partial sensory levels or unilateral bands of sensory loss may be seen with spinal cord lesions up to the brainstem. Facial numbness may be due to upper cervical lesions. Lesions of the upper thoracic nerve roots may result in Horner syndrome, with autonomic dysfunction of the face and upper extremity. Compression of the conus of the spinal cord may produce sensory loss in the saddle area (buttocks and perineum) without lower extremity symptoms or signs.

Gait ataxia is an uncommon isolated sign of spinal cord compression. Other unusual features are signs of raised intracranial pressure; facial paresis, lower extremity fasciculations, or sciatica with cervical tumor; nystagmus with thoracic tumor; spinal myoclonus; an inverted knee jerk reflex; and "painful legs and moving toes" (11).

Diagnostic Evaluation

The selection of specific imaging tests is guided by the clinical presentation. Several imaging methods are available to confirm EC. Because the correct interpretation of symptomatic and asymptomatic lesions on diagnostic imaging studies requires a thorough knowledge of the patient's clinical presentation, it is strongly recommended that clinicoradiographic correlation be made by the examining physician. In each individual case, the "neurologic urgency" for further diagnostic tests must be modified according to the potential for treatment, the patient's condition, and overall prognosis (Fig. 39.1).

Plain radiographs confirm tumor and assess structural stability of the spinal elements. In the patient with cancer at risk for spinal metastases with neck, shoulder, or upper extremity pain, flexion and extension views of the cervical spine should not be forced. Although plain radiographs are >90% sensitive and 86% specific for demonstrating abnormalities in the patient with symptomatic spinal metastases, autopsy series suggest that up to 25% of spinal lesions are invisible on radiography (2). False negatives occur because of mild degree of pathology, because of poor visualization

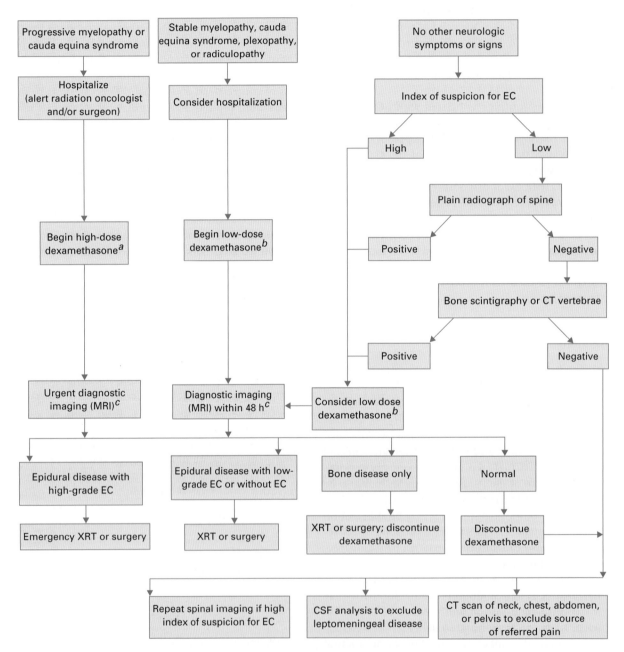

Figure 39.1. Patient with cancer and with back or neck pain—candidate for radiotherapy and/or surgery. CSF, cerebrospinal fluid; CT, computed tomography; MRI, magnetic resonance imaging; EC, epidural compression of the spinal cord and/or cauda equina; XRT, external beam radiotherapy. [a]High-dose dexamethasone, 100 mg followed by 24 mg q6h with taper over weeks. [b]Low-dose dexamethasone, 20 mg followed by 4 mg q6h with taper over weeks. [c]MRI, suggest sagittal screening of vertebral column with expanded imaging of affected areas or CT myelography (see text). (Data from Foley KM. Pain syndromes in patients with cancer. In: Portenoy RK, Kanner RM, eds. *Pain Management: Theory and Practice*. Philadelphia, PA: FA Davis Co; 1995:195; and Posner, JB. *Neurological Complications of Cancer, Contemporary Neurology Series.* Vol. 45. Philadelphia, PA: FA Davis Co; 1995:112, with permission.)

(e.g., the first thoracic vertebra), or because the abnormality is missed on interpretation. The false-positive rate for interpreting collapsed vertebrae as malignant may be as high as 20% (34).

It is estimated that a 30% to 50% change in bone mass is needed before plain films become abnormal (32). On anterior/posterior view, spinal radiographs may show pedicle erosion (the "winking owl" sign), increased interpeduncular distance, paraspinal widening, or paraspinal soft tissue shadow. On lateral view, vertebral collapse (wedging of the body), scalloped bodies, disk space destruction, a narrow spinal canal, hypertrophied facets, and disk calcification may be seen. Oblique views are needed to discriminate spondylotic osteophytic encroachment from tumor causing foraminal abnormality (5). Vertebral collapse and pedicle erosion >50% are especially predictive of EC. On plain radiography, multiple vertebral involvement is noted in up to 86% of patients with spinal tumor (5) and in >30% of patients with EC.

Computed tomography (CT) scan may be useful to better delineate pathology using restricted fields of view (2). CT is superior to other imaging techniques for demonstrating cortical bone architecture (4). Before the availability of MRI, CT scan in combination with myelography was considered the gold standard for demonstrating the level and extent of epidural disease. CT myelography may be considered if the index of suspicion for epidural disease is high and other imaging studies are normal or if MRI cannot be interpreted or performed. Lumbar puncture should precede cervical puncture in most cases. Injection of air to supplement contrast medium may better image a CSF block. If the upper and lower extent of the block cover a long spinal segment, myelography may be repeated after treatment to determine if multiple discrete lesions are present and to better define radiotherapy portals. If repeated imaging is anticipated, oil-based contrast medium may be used to allow for follow-up radiographic imaging without repeated punctures. Another advantage of myelography over other diagnostic imaging tests is the collection of CSF for analysis. However, there is a risk of worsening neurologic function after dural puncture in the patient with partial CSF block, due to the "coning" of the spinal cord as the pressure below the block is relieved. This risk may be as high as 15% (2,11). It is therefore recommended that under these conditions, corticosteroids be administered before dural puncture.

Radionuclide bone scintigrams reveal a 5% to 10% change in bone tissue (32). Bone scintigrams are more sensitive than radiographs except in multiple myeloma (11). However, they are not as specific as radiographs in identifying the level of EC. False positives may be due to nonmalignant skeletal conditions and false negatives due to lytic lesions, for example, myeloma or solid tumors such as lung and melanoma, and prior radiation therapy. If the entire skeleton is involved by tumor, no contrast in the radionuclide uptake may be appreciated. New technology of immunoscintigraphy may prove to be more sensitive (2).

MRI is now considered by many experts to be the imaging procedure of choice for EC. MRI without contrast enhancement may eliminate the need for other imaging studies. MRI sensitivity and specificity rival that of CT myelography and are better with contrast. In the patient with back pain and radicular symptoms but no bony tumor on plain radiograph, gadolinium-enhanced MRI is indicated to identify intraforaminal disease such as that which occurs in lymphoma and some solid tumors (32). Double-dose gadolinium-enhanced MRI may increase the accuracy. MRI with and without contrast excludes vertebral metastases, paravertebral lesions, EC, intramedullary tumor, and many leptomeningeal processes. Fat suppression and T_2 weighting, not supplemented by addition of contrast, may improve the detection of myeloma lesions (35). In previously irradiated bone, MRI signal intensity is increased and gadolinium contrast enhancement is decreased.

In the cancer patient with back pain and suspected EC, complete spine MRI is indicated when there is a high risk of noncontiguous or "skip" lesions. A full spine sagittal "screening" image to identify targets for more detailed imaging is suggested (5). Often, the cervical spine is not imaged because it adds significantly to sequencing time. Failure to identify multiple levels of EC may compromise radiotherapy if untreated lesions become symptomatic and are detected at a later time. The cost effectiveness of sagittal screening studies for identifying treatable lesions has not yet been determined. In patients with claustrophobia or severe pain in the supine position, conscious sedation or general anesthesia may be required to complete the MRI. The risk of sedation or anesthesia for MRI must be weighed against the risks of alternative imaging procedures, such as CT myelography, for each individual patient. Newer tumor imaging techniques may add to the diagnostic evaluation of patients with spinal malignancies in future. MRI is more efficient than bone scintigraphy in detecting metastases and is essential for treatment planning, but bone scintigraphy is more cost efficient for evaluating the entire skeleton (36). Cholewinski et al. (37) reported that fluorodeoxyglucose-Positron emission tomography/computerized tomography (FGD-PET/CT) may be needed to precisely delineate tumor pathology. Allan et al. (38) tested a telephone hotline and a rapid referral process for cancer patients to report new symptoms of neurologic urgency that resulted in more timely diagnosis and intervention.

A scale is in development to rate the severity of EC that will provide a valid reliable instrument for clinical use and that can be incorporated in a classification scheme for multicenter comparisons (39).

CSF examination is not required for the diagnosis of epidural tumor, and as noted in the preceding text, dural puncture may pose some risk to the patient with EC and should therefore be avoided. If performed, CSF analysis may show elevated protein with normal glucose and, rarely, pleocytosis in the patient with EC.

The patient presenting with EC and an unknown primary tumor generally undergoes a battery of tests to identify the primary neoplasm. At times, biopsy of a vertebral, epidural, or paraspinal lesion is needed to determine the primary tumor histology.

MANAGEMENT OF ACUTE SPINAL CORD OR CAUDA EQUINA COMPRESSION

Metastatic EC of the spinal cord and cauda equina causes significant morbidity in patients with systemic cancer. As survival in these patients is improving with improved oncologic treatment, metastatic spine involvement is encountered increasingly often. The treatment for this condition is mostly palliative. Surgical management involves early circumferential decompression of the cord with concomitant spine stabilization. Advances in surgical techniques and refining approaches according to specific patient selection criteria are leading to improved clinical outcomes. Patients with radiosensitive tumors without significant neurologic deficit will likely benefit from radiotherapy. Spinal stereotactic radiosurgery and minimally invasive techniques, such as vertebroplasty and kyphoplasty, with or without radiofrequency ablation, are being used in selected patients with spinal metastases with encouraging results.

Pharmacologic Interventions

Corticosteroids are the mainstay of pharmacologic therapy for acute EC. The administration of these agents prevents lipid peroxidation of neuronal cell membranes, ischemia, and increased intracellular calcium (40). Vasogenic edema in EC has been demonstrated to be responsive to corticosteroids. Cytotoxic edema may also play a role. Alternative steroids and other agents to treat edema, such as mannitol, may be used.

The timing of administration and dosage of corticosteroids may affect neurologic outcome, and there is some evidence for a therapeutic window (2,40). Better analgesic effect of higher dose regimens has been demonstrated in one study (41). Many authors favor a prolonged course of high-dose corticosteroids, for example, the equivalent of a bolus of 100 mg dexamethasone followed by 96 mg/d in divided doses, tapered over a few weeks for high-grade EC, and a lower dosage, for example, 20 mg dexamethasone followed by 16 mg/d in divided doses with a taper for low-grade EC (2,5,41).

High-dose corticosteroid therapy may be more analgesic, but it increases the risk of side effects. Side effects depend on the duration of drug administration, cumulative dose, and regimen. In one prospective study of patients with EC treated with high-dose corticosteroids, it was noted that depressive symptoms and neuropsychiatric disorders were more common than in similar patients not receiving such treatment (42). Suppression of the hypothalamic–pituitary–adrenal axis occurs with sustained dosing; it is suggested that dosing be readministered after withdrawal in situations of severe physiologic stress. Steroid-induced osteoporosis may be reversible in the young (43). Other withdrawal symptoms, including *Pneumocystis* infection, have been reported. Corticosteroids are metabolized by the cytochrome P-450 system, which has implications for drug interactions with anticonvulsants and other medications; this potential interaction with anticonvulsants may be the least with valproate sodium (40).

Clinicians should be aware that rapid administration of steroids causes severe burning pain in the perineum; therefore, it is preferable that doses not be given as intravenous push. Except in emergency situations, corticosteroids should be held before making the cancer diagnosis if lymphoma is suspected because of the immediate oncolytic effect, which would impede diagnosis of that condition.

Virtually all patients presenting with EC have severe pain requiring opioid analgesics. Practitioners should be prepared to rapidly titrate an opioid analgesic to effect; this may require high parenteral doses, especially in patients with neurologic involvement (44,45).

Nonpharmacologic Interventions

Radiation Therapy

Radiation therapy for EC is chosen to inhibit tumor growth, restore and preserve neurologic function, alleviate pain, and improve quality of life. The course of external beam radiotherapy (XRT) for spinal metastases and EC depends on the radiosensitivity of the tumor and its extent. Currently, XRT is considered by many clinicians to be the primary treatment for EC. The treatment course may be accelerated for patients in severe pain. The spinal section routinely treated includes two vertebral segments above and below a single site of neurologic compression. Anterior/posterior portals are set to include the vertebral body, especially in low thoracic and lumbar lesions. Fields are also designed to accommodate paravertebral tumor. A single port field can be used in very ill patients affected by cachexia. As there are no known predictive factors for epidural progression with multiple sites of spinal disease, the decision to treat asymptomatic noncontiguous sites depends on clinical judgment. In addition to the clinical condition of the patient, factors to be considered include the type of tumor, presence of vertebral collapse, and anticipated future difficulty in matching radiation portals. Special techniques are required to re-irradiate. XRT alone is >85% effective for EC in radiosensitive tumors (3). Motor improvement is seen in 49% and stabilization of function in another 31% of patients. However, <50% of patients regain their lost function (3). The possibility of progression to EC may be reduced by irradiating bony lesions. It is uncertain whether radiation treats micrometastases or prevents them. The response to XRT may be delayed in some cases; the factors accounting for this observation are not well understood (2). Brachytherapy can be used for adjacent paraspinal masses and may prevent EC (46).

American Society for Radiation Oncology (ASTRO's) Evidence-Based Guideline Task Force concluded that XRT remains the mainstay of treatment for EC (47). Stereotactic body radiotherapy (SBRT) is a promising new application. Surgical decompression with postoperative radiotherapy is recommended for certain patients. Bisphosphonates, radionuclides, vertebroplasty, and kyphoplasty also play a role.

Loblaw et al. (48) recommended 8 Gy in single fraction is as effective as multiple fractions in patients with poor prognosis, although enrollment in clinical trials is urged. Rades et al. (49)

demonstrated that long-course compared with short-course radiotherapy resulted in better progression-free survival and local disease control.

Radiosurgery of the spine was effective in a series of multiple myeloma patients, without apparent detriment to the spinal cord (50) and also in another series of patients with mixed tumor types (51). Radiosurgery following spine surgery is also being advocated to produce significantly better local disease control (52). Escalation of standard radiotherapy dose has not proven beneficial (53), but re-irradiation can be considered using high-precision techniques that are now available (54). SBRT is an emerging therapeutic option (55).

Surgery

Surgical intervention for EC may be performed for the following:

1. To establish the cancer diagnosis when it is in doubt and when tissue is required for histologic examination
2. To achieve surgical cure for a primary neoplasm
3. To treat prior irradiated radioresistant tumor with symptomatic progression of EC
4. To decompress neural structures and stabilize the spine
5. To halt a rapid clinical deterioration (2–4,23)

The specific goals of surgery are to resect pathology, restore load-bearing capacity, decompress neural structures, achieve stability, alleviate pain, and improve quality of life. Length of survival may be extended with improvement in functional status.

A long-awaited multicenter study recently concluded by Patchell et al. showed superior clinical outcomes for first-line decompressive surgery combined with postoperative radiotherapy compared with radiotherapy alone in patients with spinal cord displacement due to tumor compression. Criteria for the study entry included single-level compression, <48 hours paraplegia at the worst, prognosis of at least 3 months, and good overall condition. Patients with highly radiosensitive malignancies were excluded from participation. Study patients were treated with corticosteroids and randomized to receive 30 Gy of radiotherapy within 24 hours or surgical decompression within 24 hours followed by the same radiotherapy within 14 days of surgery. Better clinical outcomes were demonstrated for both primary end point (ability to walk) and secondary end points. The secondary end points included survival time; continence; requirement for opioid and corticosteroid medications; and function as assessed with formal functional rating scales (Frankel Functional Scale and American Spinal Injury Association Motor Score). More surgical patients retained the ability to walk ($P = 0.012$) and those able to walk at the time of enrollment retained this ability longer, having received surgery (median 153 vs. 54 d, $P = 0.024$). Continence, muscle strength, and functionality were significantly better in the surgical group ($P = 0.016$, $P = 0.001$, and $P = 0.0006$, respectively). A nonsignificant trend toward longer survival was also observed in the surgical group. Duration of hospitalization showed no difference. The results observed during the clinical trial were sufficient to meet early termination criteria, and enrollment was halted. The study supports primary surgical intervention for patients with characteristics similar to those studied (56). For patients with more complex malignant neurologic involvement and those with a higher degree of comorbidity, individualized risk/benefit analyses may favor nonsurgical treatment (57).

Many factors affect the choice of surgical technique, including tumor location, tumor extent, integrity of adjacent vertebral segments, and general debility. In vascular tumors such as renal and thyroid, operative intervention may be preceded by vascular embolization. Tumor decompression and stabilization may be achieved through either an anterior vertebrectomy or a laminectomy. Posterior decompression through wide laminectomy is generally followed by stabilization to prevent kyphosis (2,58–60). New posterolateral techniques are being developed for specific EC syndromes in patients with advanced cancer.

In one thorough retrospective study of 110 patients after aggressive surgical intervention for spinal metastases, 82% of patients showed improvement in pain relief and ambulatory status (61). The goals of the treatment were identified as gross total resection of tumor and spine reconstruction. Half of the patients had prior treatment and were deteriorating clinically. The "traditional" criteria for surgery, such as relapse after radiation therapy and the determination of histology, were expanded to include gross tumor resection for radioresistant or solitary lesions and for spinal stabilization. In this series, more complex surgical instrumentation was used than previously reported. Most patients received ongoing systemic therapy, partly confounding the analysis of long-term outcomes. The complication rate of 48% correlated with age older than 65, prior spinal treatment, and the presence of paraparesis. These factors also correlated with greater morbidity and poorer survival. However, in this series, nearly half of the patients were alive at 2 years, an improvement over prior studies that had compared the posterior surgical laminectomy and radiation therapy with radiation therapy alone. This improvement in survival was noted in patients with more advanced cancer and prior treatment. These authors concluded on the basis of prior reports (62,63) and the data from this series that the anterior surgical approach with stabilization may improve outcomes and suggested further definition of the subset of patients that might benefit from early anterior resection and spinal stabilization.

Early reviews of surgical outcomes have confirmed higher morbidity and mortality in patients with prior spine irradiation, age older than 70, and those with poor performance status at the time of surgery (64). In one reported series, the factors predictive of shorter survival were poorer preoperative neurologic status (leg strength grade 3/5 or weaker), anatomical site of the primary carcinoma (lung or colon cancer), and multiple vertebral body involvement. These authors consider that surgical intervention contraindicated if two or more of those factors are present (63). Several authors have suggested that a limited posterolateral approach to tumor resection be reserved for patients with expected survival <6 months (61,65). Few data are available with regard to surgical intervention for lateral epidural or intraforaminal disease. In a recent experience, a small group of patients, not considered candidates for major surgical procedures, benefited from limited resection of lateral epidural tumor. Surgery was preceded by careful correlation of symptoms with tumor mass, and good outcomes were recorded in all eight patients (65). This experience again supports careful consideration in each case until the criteria for primary surgical intervention are more fully delineated. Clearly, further refinement of surgical approaches depends on precise neuroanatomic localization of neoplastic involvement.

The complication rate for spinal surgery may be as high as 30% in patients who have undergone prior XRT (3). Coagulopathy and exogenous anticoagulants increase the risk of hematoma at the operative site. Difficult wound healing, infection, bony instability, nonfusion, displacement of implants, and other complications may occur.

There has been a steady evolution in the concepts and execution of surgical management for EC. In choosing primary surgical versus radiotherapeutic intervention, the prognosis for neurologic improvement and expected impact on functional status must be considered. In some series, radiation therapy has been shown to be equally effective to laminectomy and radiation, but with <50% neurologic improvement overall (9). De novo anterior–posterior resection with spine stabilization may result in better outcomes than laminectomy and radiation or radiation alone, as surgical complications are generally manageable, survival is improved (although the 2-year survival rate for lung cancer may be 10% and for colorectal cancer only 17%) and patients may remain ambulatory longer (61). The data are as yet insufficient to draw final conclusions regarding pain and quality-of-life outcomes in all patients, but as discussed in the preceding text, there is a subset of patients presenting with single-level spinal cord displacement that will benefit from primary surgical intervention. The decision to recommend initial radiation therapy versus surgical intervention must be individualized, especially in those patients with more complex presentations. To date, the cauda equina syndrome has not been well studied. It has been suggested that without bony instability, the speed of progression of neurologic deficit and radiosensitivity of the tumor are the main factors to consider in determining primary antineoplastic treatment with either surgery or radiation. Severe deficits generally hold a poor prognosis independent of treatment.

Tancioni et al. (66) advocated a mini-invasive percutaneous approach for the poor prognostic group. Chaichana et al. (67) reported that the prognostic value of the presence of vertebral fracture with EC is independently associated with decreased postoperative ambulatory status and also that preoperative nonambulatory patients required more extensive surgery and had more postoperative complications (68). Preoperative radiotherapy decreased the likelihood of regaining ambulatory status, whereas postoperative radiotherapy and symptoms of <48 hours duration predicted positively for

regaining ambulation. Putz et al. (69) found similarly and also noted individual health status to be a contributing factor to postoperative outcome. Chaichana et al. (70) also reported differences in outcomes according to primary tumor type.

Williams et al. (71) advocated aggressive surgical decompression and reconstruction for EC secondary to prostate cancer. Walcott et al. (72) and Tancioni et al. (73) reviewed their series of open spine surgeries for EC in breast cancer and concluded that aggressive therapy is warranted even in the setting of advanced and progressive systemic disease. Laufer et al. (74) suggested that reoperation in carefully selected patients can prolong ambulation and result in good functional and neurologic outcomes.

Chen et al. (75) reported good results from use of a posterolateral transpedicular approach or combined posterior anterior approaches for patients with lung cancer and also described a transpedicular partial corpectomy without anterior vertebral reconstruction in thoracic lesions (76). The posterior transpedicular approach for ventral cervical (77) and thoracic (78) spine tumors, and an extended lateral parascapular approach for thoracic spine tumors (79), have been described.

Tancioni et al. (80) also reported that combined surgery and radiotherapy yielded clinical remission of pain in 91%, neurologic improvement in 72%, and 44% overall 1-year survival that was correlated with primary tumor type.

Prolonged cancer survival has led to an increase in the incidence of spinal metastases and vertebral compression fractures with associated mechanical instability, axial pain, and progressive radiculomyelopathy. Vertebral augmentation techniques, vertebroplasty and kyphoplasty, are minimally invasive techniques of percutaneous injection of bone cement (methyl methacrylate) directly into vertebral bodies. With a low complication rate, these procedures are being used more commonly in conjunction with other treatments and even as first-line approach for management of painful malignant spine fractures. Bouza et al. (81) performed an evidence-based review of balloon kyphoplasty in malignant disease and concluded that there is level III evidence for this procedure with further investigation being warranted. Dalbayrak et al. (82) reported prospectively that there is a correlation between symptom duration and restoration of vertebral body height after kyphoplasty. Positive results were reported from a randomized controlled prospective trial of kyphoplasty (83), a retrospective review of kyphoplasty (84), and of percutaneous vertebroplasty (85,86). Zou et al. (87) suggested MRI signal localization of symptomatic myeloma lesions for targeting procedure site. Hirsch et al. (88) reported that the sequence of combined External Bean Radiation Therapy (EBRT) and Vertebral Angmentation (VA) does not affect outcomes.

Samarium 153-ethylene administered intravertebrally with kyphoplasty is a procedure to be studied further (89,90). Kyphoplasty with Intraoperative radiation therapy (IORT) (91) is also being investigated. A series of patients treated with percutaneous transpedicular coblation corpectomy followed by immediate balloon kyphoplasty and subsequent radiosurgery have been reported with good outcomes (92).

Nonsurgical stabilization of the bony spine can be accomplished with a cervical collar or body bracing. The patient with cancer, neck pain, and suspected cervical spine disease should be placed in a collar while diagnostic evaluation is being conducted. In some tumor types, chemotherapy may be the sole antineoplastic therapy against EC (94).

ONGOING CARE

Pain Management

Extended corticosteroid administration (i.e., for the duration of life in patients with EC and short prognosis) has not been well studied, but it is common in clinical practice. This practice should be discouraged unless there is an evidence of ongoing steroid-reversible neurologic deficits due to the high risk of steroid toxicities, as discussed in Section *Pharmacologic Interventions* (94).

Guidelines for the use of nonsteroidal anti-inflammatory medications, opioid analgesics, and adjuvant analgesics for neuropathic pain have been published in recent years (95–99). Chronic opioid therapy is often required for persistent pain after treatment of EC. Cases have been reported in which patients with EC required prolonged high-dose intrathecal infusion of opioid and local anesthetic to obtain adequate analgesia (100–101). Radionuclides are discussed in other chapters.

Neuroablative procedures are considered when the benefit-to-risk ratio favors analgesia over the potential for further neurologic compromise. Destruction of the nervous tissue may be accomplished by anesthetic or surgical means. Chemical epidural neurolysis may be chosen to effect single or multiple nerve root interruption. Intrathecal neurolysis would be anticipated to achieve analgesia over a wider territory and may be selected when the epidural space is compromised. Both approaches entail the risk of acute neurologic deterioration, which may be irreversible (102). Neurosurgical ablation of nerve roots (rhizotomy) involves major surgery and is less often indicated in very sick patients. Midline myelotomy may be indicated in patients with severe midline sacral pain and bladder or bowel compromise due to tumor of the sacrum. Spinothalamic tractotomy or cordotomy, although more easily performed as a percutaneous procedure, is not generally useful for pain in association with spine disease or EC. Hypophysectomy for diffuse painful metastatic bone disease may yield success rates as high as 90% in some endocrine-responsive tumors (103).

Integration of pharmacologic and nonpharmacologic analgesic therapies is needed for most patients with EC. A multidisciplinary approach to pain management and rehabilitation of patients with resected sacral chordoma has been reported (104).

Rehabilitation

Each patient's rehabilitation program must be individually tailored and continually reassessed and modified. For some patients, comprehensive care may be best accomplished in a formal inpatient rehabilitation setting (105). Specific rehabilitation goals are to improve ambulation, achieve weight bearing and transfers, restore bladder and bowel function, and protect the skin. The family is included in learning how to assist the patient with severely impaired mobility.

Spinal orthotics stabilize the spine and may decrease spinal pain by limiting motion. Physical therapy techniques for pain relief include massage, ultrasound, and transcutaneous electrical nerve stimulation.

Approximately, 50% of patients require urinary catheterization before and after XRT for EC (3). Sexual dysfunction may be treatable with physical and medical interventions.

A number of medical problems common to the cancer population may limit aggressive rehabilitation efforts. Organ failure due to the disease or its treatment, hemodynamic instability, poor nutrition, cancer cachexia, and multiple physical and psychological symptoms may complicate rehabilitation. An active exercise program may have to be modified. Weakness due to spinal cord or nerve root compression may be complicated by concurrent peripheral neuropathy or myopathy, which are common complications of antineoplastic treatment. The skin of many patients with cancer is relatively more prone to breakdown and infection. Skin care and protection are essential, especially in the bedridden patient.

Chronic musculoskeletal problems may occur in children after spine irradiation during growth, due to the development of secondary spinal deformities. The risk of fracture in osteoporotic or tumor-laden bones should be carefully evaluated before initiating a mobility program. In patients who are paraparetic or paraplegic, prophylactic fixation of upper extremity lesions may be considered to aid mobility and weight bearing. In bedridden patients with multiple impending fractures, positioning and transfers must be undertaken with great caution.

The goals of physical medicine and rehabilitation in the patient with EC range from active programs to supportive and palliative care (106). Preventive rehabilitation therapy is directed toward achieving maximal functional restoration in patients who are cured or are in stable remission from their cancer. Continued encouragement for the effort required in aggressive rehabilitation is needed for a progressive decline in function due to advancing disease. For patients with limited prognosis, usually considered as <6 months' life expectancy, family participation receives more emphasis. The needs of the patient tend toward more dependent care as the cancer progresses. Palliative rehabilitation interventions are intended to provide comfort to the patient in the terminal stages of illness, and as noted in the preceding text, include the family.

Fattal (107,108) reviewed 38 available studies, most retrospective, to conclude that with 55% overall 12-month survival, short duration (1 to 2 month) rehabilitation stays are indicated to maximize functional benefit and patients' time with family. Improvements in ambulation, pain, and bladder/bowel function were observed.

Psychological Interventions

Ongoing psychological support of the patient with metastatic spine disease is essential. Issues of loss of independence and function require careful attention. Families often benefit from emotional support for anticipatory grieving. Professional assistance may be indicated as the burden of care increases with a patient's progressing disease. The palliative care team will often assist with complex therapeutic decision analysis and provide essential psychosocial support in this setting.

CLINICAL OUTCOMES

The potential for the recovery of function in patients with tumor involvement of the spine and associated neurologic structures varies by tumor type (primary or metastatic), the number of vertebrae involved, the nature and degree of neurologic involvement, the oncologic status, and the general medical condition. In most series, approximately 50% of patients with metastatic spine tumors are ambulatory at presentation, 35% are paretic, and 15% are plegic (2). Up to 30% of patients with weakness become plegic within the first week of presentation (5). The prognosis for regaining ambulatory status in patients with EC who begin therapy while being ambulatory is 75%; prognosis declines to 30% to 50% for patients who begin therapy while being paretic and to 10% for those who begin therapy while being plegic (32). The duration of neurologic symptoms before treatment also affects the prognosis for neurologic recovery. If paraplegia has been present for days or if urinary retention is present for >30 hours, the likelihood of recovery is decreased (109). Rapidly progressing symptoms confer a worse prognosis.

Patients who remain unable to ambulate after irradiation treatment for EC have a particularly poor prognosis for survival, owing to the complications of paresis and more advanced disease. Survival rates for patients with EC are 40% at 1 year if ambulatory before and after radiation treatment, whereas patients who are nonambulatory before and ambulatory after treatment have a survival rate of 30% at 1 year and 20% at 3 years. Prognosis falls to 7% at 1 year for patients who are nonambulatory after treatment (3).

Response to treatment for EC and survival vary with the nature of the malignancy. In patients with prostate cancer, the response to the treatment of neurologic complications depends on whether the patient has received prior hormonal therapy. Better response to hormonal manipulation correlates with longer survival. The median survival of patients with prostate cancer after diagnosis with EC is 6 months; only 34% survive at least 1 year (110). Renal cancer is poorly radioresponsive and median survival time after diagnosis with EC is <4 months (111). Hemorrhagic complications of spinal surgery for metastatic renal tumor may be avoided by preoperative embolization (112). In testicular cancer, chemotherapy is effective for untreated lesions or for responsive tumors (113), but radiation and

surgery may be considered if the disease is not chemoresponsive (111). Up to 75% of patients with melanoma and EC respond to radiation therapy (114–116). Patients with carcinoid tumor and EC have a median survival of 6 months. Ambulatory status may be preserved with radiation in up to 90% of patients with carcinoid tumors (18). In myeloma, long-term survival is common. In a series of patients with multiple myeloma, the 1-year survival rate was 100% and the median survival 37 months after EC was diagnosed (117). Solitary plasmacytomas are generally irradiated and surgically removed. Patients with multiple myeloma often receive radiation therapy to maximum spinal cord tolerance before surgical intervention is considered. Most lymphomas respond to chemotherapy and radiation. In pediatric patients, surgery may be preferred for radioresistant sarcomas and small cell tumors (Ewing's sarcoma, neuroblastoma, lymphoma, and germ cell tumors) presenting with rapid neurologic deterioration. A trend toward extended survival has been shown after surgical decompression in Ewing's sarcoma. Many small cell tumors respond to chemotherapy or radiation. Younger age may confer greater risk of radiation complications (118). Complete resection of primary spinal extraosseous epidural Ewing's sarcoma may be difficult. The 18-month survival rate was <40% in a small series of patients with this unusual malignancy (119).

Chi et al. (120) estimated that the age at which surgery is no longer superior to radiotherapy is between 60 and 70 years and suggested that this may be a factor in selecting treatment.

In a recent series, median survival after first presentation with spinal cord compression was noted to be 2.9 months (120). Less than half of patients treated for EC are alive after 2 months (10). EC is an indicator of poor prognosis. Definitive intervention for EC must therefore be considered in the context of the patient's overall disease status. Systemic antineoplastic therapy may at times precede or entirely supplant intervention targeted at EC. For patients with very advanced cancer, the burden of diagnostic evaluation and intervention to reverse EC often outweighs minimal potential gains in function.

A systematic review of evidence-based treatment of EC identified in 6 trials of 544 patients concluded that ambulatory patients with stable spines may be treated with radiotherapy, while surgery may be preferred for ambulatory patients with poor prognostic factors for radiotherapy and for nonambulatory patients with a single site of compression, paraplegia for <48 hours duration, radioresistant tumors, and survival prognosis of >3 months. Serious adverse effects of high-dose corticosteroids were noted (121–122).

Although few studies of quality of life have been conducted in this population, pain control should remain a high priority regardless of prognosis. Given the emerging clinical evidence and advances in available techniques, clinicians caring for patients with spinal neoplasm must work in a coordinated interdisciplinary fashion to carefully select those interventions that will achieve therapeutic goals for each individual patient and family.

REFERENCES

1. Loeser JD. Neurosurgical approaches in palliative care. In: Doyle D, Hanks GWC, MacDonald N, eds. *Oxford Textbook of Palliative Medicine*. Oxford: Oxford University Press; 1993:221.

2. Posner JB. *Neurologic Complications of Cancer, Contemporary Neurology Series*. Vol. 45. Philadelphia, PA: FA Davis; 1995:112.

3. Perrin RG, Janjan NA, Langford LA. Spinal axis metastases. In: Levin VA, ed. *Cancer in the Nervous System*. New York, NY: Churchill Livingstone; 1996:259.

4. Byrne TN, Waxman SG. *Spinal Cord Compression: Diagnosis and Principles of Management, Contemporary Neurology Series*. Vol. 33. Philadelphia, PA: FA Davis; 1990.

5. Grant R, Papadopoulos SM, Greenberg HS. Metastatic epidural spinal cord compression. *Neurol Clin*. 1991;9(4):825.

6. Klein SL, Sanford RA, Muhlbauer MS. Pediatric spinal epidural metastases. *J Neurosurg*. 1991;74:70.

7. Barron KD, Hirano A, Araski S, et al. Experiences with metastatic neoplasms involving the spinal cord. *Neurology*. 1959;9:91.

8. Mak KS, Lee LK, Mak RH, et al. Incidence and treatment patterns in hospitalizations for malignant spinal cord compression in the United States, 1998–2006. *Int J Radiat Oncol Biol Phys*. July 2011;80(3):824-831; e-pub July 12, 2010.

9. Stark RJ, Henson RA, Evans SJW. Spinal metastases: a retrospective survey from a general hospital. *Brain*. 1982;105:189.

10. Obbens EAMT. Neurological problems in palliative medicine. In: Doyle D, Hanks GWC, MacDonald N, eds. *Oxford Textbook of Palliative Medicine*. Oxford: Oxford University Press; 1993:460.

11. Byrne TN. Spinal metastases. In: Wiley RG, ed. *Neurologic Complications of Cancer*. New York, NY: Marcel Dekker; 1995:23.

12. Harrington KD. Metastatic disease of the spine. In: Harrington KD, ed. *Orthopedic Management of Metastatic Bone Disease*. St. Louis, MO: Mosby; 1988:309.

13. Misulis KE, Wiley RG. Neurological complications of lung cancer. In: Wiley RG, ed. *Neurologic Complications of Cancer*. New York, NY: Marcel Dekker; 1995:295.

14. Anderson NE. Neurological complications of breast cancer. In: Wiley RG, ed. *Neurologic Complications of Cancer*. New York, NY: Marcel Dekker; 1995:319.

15. Kuban DA, El-Mahdi AM, Sigfred SV, et al. Characteristics of spinal cord compression in adenocarcinoma of the prostate. *Urology*. 1986;28:364.

16. Flynn DF, Shipley WU. Management of spinal cord compression secondary to metastatic prostatic carcinoma. *Urol Clin North Am*. 1991;18:145.

17. Moots PL, Wiley RG. Neurological disorders in head and neck cancers. In: Wiley RG, ed. *Neurologic Complications of Cancer*. New York, NY: Marcel Dekker; 1995:353.

18. Hagen NA. Neurological complications of gastrointestinal cancers. In: Wiley RG, ed. *Neurologic Complications of Cancer*. New York, NY: Marcel Dekker; 1995:395.

19. Friedman M, Kim TH, Panahon AM. Spinal cord compression in malignant lymphoma: treatment and results. *Cancer*. 1976;37:1485.

20. Ribeiro RC, Pui CH, Schell MJ. Vertebral compression fracture as a presenting feature of acute lymphoblastic leukemia in children. *Cancer*. 1988;61:589.

21. Jennings MT. Neurological complications of childhood cancer. In: Wiley RG, ed. *Neurologic Complications of Cancer*. New York, NY: Marcel Dekker; 1995:503.

22. Molloy PT, Phillips PC. Neurological complications of sarcomas. In: Wiley RG, ed. *Neurologic Complications of Cancer*. New York, NY: Marcel Dekker; 1995:417.

23. Galasko CSB, Sylvester BS. Back pain in patients treated for malignant tumours. *Clin Oncol*. 1978;4:273.

24. Kanner RM. Low back pain. In: Portenoy RK, Kanner RM, eds. *Pain Management: Theory and Practice, Contemporary Neurology Series*. Vol. 48. Philadelphia, PA: FA Davis; 1996:126.

25. Sty JR, Wells RG, Conway JJ. Spine pain in children. *Semin Nucl Med*. 1993;23(4):296.

26. Manishen WJ, Sivananthan K, Orr FW. Resorbing bone stimulates tumor cell growth. A role for the host microenvironment in bone metastasis. *Am J Pathol*. 1986;123:39.

27. Powell N. Metastatic carcinoma in association with Paget's disease of bone. *Br J Radiol*. 1983;56:582.

28. Tarlov IM, Klinger H. Spinal cord compression studies. II: time limits for recovery after acute compression in dogs. *Arch Neurol Psychiatry*. 1954;71:271.

29. Gledhill RF, Harrison BM, McDonald WI. Demyelination and remyelination after acute spinal cord compression. *Exp Neurol*. 1973;38:472.

30. Burger EL, Lindeque BG. Sacral and non-spinal tumors presenting as backache: a retrospective study of 17 patients. *Acta Orthop Scand*. 1994;65(3):344.

31. Gonzales GR, Elliott KJ, Portenoy RK, et al. The impact of a comprehensive evaluation in the management of cancer pain. *Pain*. 1991;47(2):141.

32. Hewitt DJ, Foley KM. Neuroimaging of pain. In: Greenberg JO, ed. *Neuroimaging*. New York, NY: McGraw-Hill; 1995:41.

33. Gilbert RW, Kim JH, Posner JB. Epidural spinal cord compression from metastatic tumor: diagnosis and treatment. *Ann Neurol*. 1978;3:40.

34. Wong DA, Fornasier VL, MacNab I. Spinal metastases: the obvious, the occult, and the imposters. *Spine*. 1990;15:1.

35. Rhamouni A, Divine M, Mathieu D, et al. Detection of multiple myeloma involving the spine: efficacy of fat-suppression and contrast-enhanced MR imaging. *AJR Am J Roentgenol*. 1993;160(5):1049.

36. Chiewvit P, Danchaivijitr N, Sirivitmaitrie K, Chiewvit S, Thephamongkhol K. Does magnetic resonance imaging give value-added than bone scintigraphy in the detection of vertebral metastasis? *J Med Assoc Thai*. June 2009;92(6):818-829.

37. Cholewinski W, Castellon I, Raphael B, Heiba SI. Value of precise localization of recurrent multiple myeloma with F-18 FDG PET/CT. *Clin Nucl Med*. January 2009;34(1):1-3.

38. Allan L, Baker L, Dewar J, et al. Suspected malignant cord compression—improving time to diagnosis via a "hotline": a prospective audit. *Br J Cancer*. June 2009;100(12):1867-1872; e-pub May 26 2009.

39. Bilsky MH, Laufer I, Fourney DR, et al. Reliability analysis of the epidural spinal cord compression scale. *J Neurosurg Spine*. September 2010;13(3):324-328.

40. Vecht CJ, Verbiest HBC. Use of glucocorticoids in neuro-oncology. In: Wiley RG, ed. *Neurologic Complications of Cancer*. New York, NY: Marcel Dekker; 1995:199.

41. Greenberg HS, Kim JH, Posner JB. Epidural spinal cord compression from metastatic tumor: results with a new treatment protocol. *Ann Neurol*. 1980;8:361.

42. Breitbart W, Stiefel F, Kornblith AB, et al. Neuropsychiatric disturbances in cancer patients with epidural spinal cord compression receiving high dose corticosteroids: a prospective comparison study. *Psychooncology*. 1993;2:233-245.

43. Pocock NA, Eisman JA, Dunstan CR, et al. Recovery from steroid induced osteoporosis. *Ann Intern Med.* 1987;107:319.

44. Yoshioka H, Tsuneto S, Kashiwagi T. Pain control with morphine for vertebral metastases and sciatica in advanced cancer patients. *J Palliat Care.* 1994;10(1):10.

45. Swarm R, Abernethy AP, Anghelescu DL, et al. NCCN Adult Cancer Pain. *J Natl Compr Canc Netw.* September 2010;8(9):1046-1086.

46. Armstrong JG, Fass DE, Bains M, et al. Paraspinal tumors: techniques and results of brachytherapy. *Int J Radiat Oncol Biol Phys.* 1991;20:787.

47. Lutz S, Berk L, Chang E, et al. Palliative radiotherapy for bone metastases: an ASTRO evidence-based guideline. *Int J Radiat Oncol Biol Phys.* March 2011;79(4):965-976; e-pub January 27, 2011.

48. Loblaw A, Mitera G. Malignant extradural spinal cord compression in men with prostate cancer. *Curr Opin Support Palliat Care.* September 2011;5(3):206-210.

49. Rades D, Lange M, Veninga T, et al. Preliminary results of spinal cord compression recurrence evaluation (score-1) study comparing short-course versus long-course radiotherapy for local control of malignant epidural spinal cord compression. *Int J Radiat Oncol Biol Phys.* January 2009;73(1):228-234; e-pub June 6, 2008.

50. Jin R, Rock J, Jin JY, et al. Single fraction spine radiosurgery for myeloma epidural spinal cord compression. *J Exp Ther Oncol.* 2009;8(1):35-41.

51. Ryu S, Rock J, Jain R, et al. Radiosurgical decompression of metastatic epidural compression. *Cancer.* May 2010;116(9):2250-2257.

52. Moulding HD, Elder JB, Lis E, et al. Local disease control after decompressive surgery and adjuvant high-dose single-fraction radiosurgery for spine metastases. *J Neurosurg Spine.* July 2010;13(1):87-93.

53. Rades D, Freundt K, Meyners T, et al. Dose escalation for metastatic spinal cord compression in patients with relatively radioresistant tumors. *Int J Radiat Oncol Biol Phys.* August 2011;80(5):1492-1497; e-pub June 25, 2010.

54. Rades D, Abrahm JL. The role of radiotherapy for metastatic epidural spinal cord compression. *Nat Rev Clin Oncol.* October 2010;7(10):590-598; e-pub August 31, 2010.

55. Sahgal A, Bilsky M, Chang EL, et al. Stereotactic body radiotherapy for spinal metastasis: current status, with a focus on its application in the postoperative patient. *J Neurosurg Spine.* February 2011;14(2):151-166; e-pub December 24, 2010.

56. Patchell RA, Tibbs PA, Regine WF, et al. Direct decompressive surgical resection in the treatment of spinal cord compression caused by metastatic cancer: a randomised trial. *Lancet.* 2005;366:643-648.

57. Gerber DE, Grossman SA. Does decompressive surgery improve outcome in patients with metastatic epidural spinal-cord compression? *Nat Clin Pract Neurol.* 2006;2:10-11.

58. Galasko CSB. Orthopaedic principles and management. In: Doyle D, Hanks GWC, MacDonald N, eds. *Oxford Textbook of Palliative Medicine.* Oxford: Oxford University Press; 1993:274.

59. Findlay GFG. Adverse effects of the management of malignant spinal cord compression. *J Neurol Neurosurg Psychiatry.* 1984;47:761.

60. McBroom R. Radiation or surgery for metastatic disease of the spine? *Soc Med Curr Med Lit—Orthop.* 1988;1:97.

61. Sundaresan N, Sachdev VP, Holland JF, et al. Surgical treatment of spinal cord compression from epidural metastasis. *J Clin Oncol.* 1995;13(9):2330.

62. Sioutos PJ, Arbit E, Meshulam BS, et al. Spinal metastases from solid tumors: analysis of factors affecting survival. *Cancer.* 1995;76(8):1453.

63. Siegal T, Siegal TZ. Surgical decompression of anterior and posterior malignant epidural tumors compressing the spinal cord: a prospective study. *Neurosurgery.* 1985;17:424-432.

64. Sundaresan N, Digiacinto GV, Hughes JEO, et al. Treatment of neoplastic spinal cord compression: results of a prospective study. *Neurosurgery.* 1991;29:645.

65. Weller SJ, Rossitch E Jr. Unilateral posterolateral decompression without stabilization for neurological palliation of symptomatic spinal metastases in debilitated patients. *J Neurosurg.* 1995;82(5):739.

66. Tancioni F, Navarria P, Pessina F, et al. Early surgical experience with minimally invasive percutaneous approach for patients with Metastatic Epidural Spinal Cord Compression (MESCC) to poor prognoses. *Ann Surg Oncol.* July 2011; e-pub ahead of print.

67. Chaichana KL, Pendleton C, Wolinsky JP, Gokaslan ZL, Sciubba DM. Vertebral compression fractures in patients presenting with metastatic epidural spinal cord compression. *Neurosurgery.* August 2009;65(2):267-274; discussion 274-275.

68. Chaichana KL, Woodworth GF, Sciubba DM, et al. Predictors of ambulatory function after decompressive surgery for metastatic epidural spinal cord compression. *Neurosurgery.* March 2008;62(3):683-692; discussion 683-692.

69. Putz C, van Middendorp JJ, Pouw MH, et al. Malignant cord compression: a critical appraisal of prognostic factors predicting functional outcome after surgical treatment. *J Craniovertebr Junction Spine.* July 2010;1(2):67-73.

70. Chaichana KL, Pendleton C, Sciubba DM, Wolinsky JP, Gokaslan ZL. Outcome following decompressive surgery for different histological types of metastatic tumors causing epidural spinal cord compression. Clinical article. *J Neurosurg Spine.* July 2009;11(1):56-63.

71. Williams BJ, Fox BD, Sciubba DM, et al. Surgical management of prostate cancer metastatic to the spine. *J Neurosurg Spine.* May 2009;10(5):414-422.

72. Walcott BP, Cvetanovich GL, Barnard ZR, Nahed BV, Kahle KT, Curry WT. Surgical treatment and outcomes of metastatic breast cancer to the spine. *J Clin Neurosci.* October 2011;18(10):1336-1339; e-pub July 22, 2011.

73. Tancioni F, Navarria P, Mancosu P, et al. Surgery followed by radiotherapy for the treatment of metastatic epidural spinal cord compression from breast cancer. *Spine (Phila Pa 1976).* September 2011;36(20):E1352-E1359.

74. Laufer I, Hanover A, Lis E, Yamada Y, Bilsky M. Repeat decompression surgery for recurrent spinal metastases. *J Neurosurg Spine.* July 2010;13(1):109-115.

75. Chen YJ, Chang GC, Chen HT, et al. Surgical results of metastatic spinal cord compression secondary to non-small cell lung cancer. *Spine (Phila Pa 1976).* July 2007;32(15):E413-E418.

76. Chen YJ, Hsu HC, Chen KH, Li TC, Lee TS. Transpedicular partial corpectomy without anterior vertebral reconstruction in thoracic spinal metastases. *Spine (Phila Pa 1976).* October 2007;32(22):E623-E626.

77. Eleraky M, Setzer M, Vrionis FD. Posterior transpedicular corpectomy for malignant cervical spine tumors. *Eur Spine J.* February 2010;19(2):257-262; e-pub October 13, 2009.

78. Cho DC, Sung JK. Palliative surgery for metastatic thoracic and lumbar tumors using posterolateral transpedicular approach with posterior instrumentation. *Surg Neurol.* April 2009;71(4):424-433; e-pub Jun 30, 2008.

79. Vecil GG, McCutcheon IE, Mendel E. Extended lateral para-scapular approach for resection of a giant multi-compartment thoracic schwannoma. *Acta Neurochir (Wien)*. December 2008;150(12):1295-1300; discussion 1300; e-pub November 18, 2008.

80. Tancioni F, Navarria P, Lorenzetti MA, et al. Multimodal approach to the management of metastatic epidural spinal cord compression (MESCC) due to solid tumors. *Int J Radiat Oncol Biol Phys*. December 2010;78(5):1467-1473; e-pub March 16, 2010.

81. Bouza C, López-Cuadrado T, Cediel P, Saz-Parkinson Z, Amate JM. Balloon kyphoplasty in malignant spinal fractures: a systematic review and meta-analysis. *BMC Palliat Care*. September 2009;8:12.

82. Dalbayrak S, Onen MR, Yilmaz M, Naderi S. Clinical and radiographic results of balloon kyphoplasty for treatment of vertebral body metastases and multiple myelomas. *J Clin Neurosci*. February 2010;17(2):219-224; e-pub December 5, 2009.

83. Berenson J, Pflugmacher R, Jarzem P, et al. Balloon kyphoplasty versus non-surgical fracture management for treatment of painful vertebral body compression fractures in patients with cancer: a multicentre, randomised controlled trial. *Lancet Oncol*. March 2011;12(3):225-235; e-pub February 16, 2011.

84. Qian Z, Sun Z, Yang H, Gu Y, Chen K, Wu G. Kyphoplasty for the treatment of malignant vertebral compression fractures caused by metastases. *J Clin Neurosci*. June 2011;18(6):763-767; e-pub April 19, 2011.

85. Saliou G, Kocheida el M, Lehmann P, et al. Percutaneous vertebroplasty for pain management in malignant fractures of the spine with epidural involvement. *Radiology*. March 2010;254(3):882-890.

86. Sun G, Jin P, Li M, et al. Percutaneous vertebroplasty for pain management in spinal metastasis with epidural involvement. *Technol Cancer Res Treat*. June 2011;10(3):267-274.

87. Zou J, Mei X, Gan M, Yang H. Kyphoplasty for spinal fractures from multiple myeloma. *J Surg Oncol*. July 2010;102(1):43-47.

88. Hirsch AE, Jha RM, Yoo AJ, et al. The use of vertebral augmentation and external beam radiation therapy in the multimodal management of malignant vertebral compression fractures. *Pain Physician*. September 2011-October;14(5):447-458.

89. Ashamalla H, Cardoso E, Macedon M, et al. Phase I trial of Vertebral Intracavitary Cement and Samarium (VICS): novel technique for treatment of painful vertebral metastasis. *Int J Radiat Oncol Biol Phys*. November 2009;75(3):836-842; e-pub April 11, 2009.

90. Gokaslan ZL, McGirt MJ. Kyphoplasty with intraspinal brachytherapy for metastatic spine tumors. *J Neurosurg Spine*. April 2009;10(4):334-335; author reply 335.

91. Wenz F, Schneider F, Neumaier C, et al. Kypho-IORT—a novel approach of intraoperative radiotherapy during kyphoplasty for vertebral metastases. *Radiat Oncol*. February 2010; 5:11.

92. Gerszten PC, Monaco EA 3rd. Complete percutaneous treatment of vertebral body tumors causing spinal canal compromise using a transpedicular cavitation, cement augmentation, and radiosurgical technique. *Neurosurg Focus*. December 2009;27(6):E9.

93. Grommes C, Bosl GJ, DeAngelis LM. Treatment of epidural spinal cord involvement from germ cell tumors with chemotherapy. *Cancer*. May 2011;117(9):1911-1916. doi:10.1002/cncr.25693; e-pub November 29, 2010.

94. Reid IR, King AR, Alexander CJ, et al. Prevention of steroid-induced osteoporosis with (3-amino-1-hydroxypropylidene)-1,1-bisphosphonate (APD). *Lancet*. 1988;1:143.

95. Portenoy RK. Pharmacologic management of chronic pain. In: Fields HL, ed. *Pain Syndromes in Neurologic Practice*. New York, NY: Butterworth–Heinemann; 1990:257.

96. Payne R, Weinstein SM, Hill CS. Management of cancer pain. In: Levin VL, ed. *Cancer in the Nervous System*. New York, NY: Churchill Livingstone; 1996:411.

97. World Health Organization. *Cancer Pain Relief and Palliative Care*. Geneva: World Health Organization; 1990.

98. Jacox A, Carr DB, Payne R, et al. *Management of Cancer Pain, Clinical Practice Guideline No 9*. Rockville, MD: Agency for Health Care Policy and Research, U.S. Department of Health and Human Services, Public Health Services; March 1994. AHCPR Publication No 94–0592.

99. American Pain Society. *Principles of Analgesic Use in the Treatment of Acute Pain and Cancer Pain*. 5th ed. Glenview, IL: American Pain Society; 2003.

100. Payne R, Cunningham M, Weinstein SM, et al. Intractable pain and suffering in a cancer patient. *Clin J Pain*. 1995;11:70.

101. Aguilar JL, Espachs P, Roca G, et al. Difficult management of pain following sacrococcygeal chordoma: thirteen months of subarachnoid infusion. *Pain*. 1994;59(2):317.

102. Morgan RJ, Steller PH. Acute paraplegias following intrathecal phenol block in the presence of occult epidural malignancy. *Anaesthesia*. 1994;49(2):142.

103. Waldman SD, Feldstein LS, Allen ML. Neuroadenolysis of the pituitary: description of a modified technique. *J Pain Symptom Manage*. 1987;2:45.

104. Watling C, Allen RR. Treatment of neuropathic pain associated with sacrectomy. In: Proceedings of the 48th Annual Scientific Meeting of the American Academy of Neurology; 1996; San Francisco, CA. Abstract 1996.

105. Schlicht LA, Smelz JK. Metastatic spinal cord compression. In: Garden FH Grabois M, eds. *Cancer Rehabilitation. Physical Medicine and Rehabilitation. State of the Art Reviews*. Vol. 8(2). Philadelphia, PA: Hanley and Belfus; 1994:345.

106. Garden FH, Gillis TA. Principles of cancer rehabilitation. In: Braddom RL, ed. *Physical Medicine and Rehabilitation*. Philadelphia, PA: WB Saunders; 1996:1199.

107. Fattal C, Fabbro M, Gelis A, Bauchet L. Metastatic paraplegia and vital prognosis: perspectives and limitations for rehabilitation care. Part 1. *Arch Phys Med Rehabil*. January 2011;92(1):125-133.

108. Fattal C, Fabbro M, Rouays-Mabit H, Verollet C, Bauchet L. Metastatic paraplegia and functional outcomes: perspectives and limitations for rehabilitation care. Part 2. *Arch Phys Med Rehabil*. 2011;92(1):134-145.

109. Bach F, Larsen BH, Rohde K, et al. Metastatic spinal cord compression: occurrence, symptoms, clinical presentation and progression in 398 patients with spinal cord compression. *Acta Neurochir (Wien)*. 1990;107(1-2):37-43.

110. Delattre JY, Krol G, Thaler HT, et al. Distribution of brain metastases. *Arch Neurol*. 1988;45:741.

111. Fadul CE. Neurological complications of genitourinary cancer. In: Wiley RG, ed. *Neurologic Complications of Cancer*. New York, NY: Marcel Dekker; 1995:388.

112. Sundaresan N, Choi IS, Hughes JEO, et al. Treatment of spinal metastases from kidney cancer by presurgical embolization and resection. *J Neurosurg*. 1990;73:548.

113. Cooper K, Bajorin D, Shapiro W, et al. Decompression of epidural metastases from germ cell tumors with chemotherapy. *J Neurooncol*. 1990;8:275.

114. Rate WR, Solin LJ, Turrisi AT. Palliative radiotherapy for metastatic malignant melanoma: brain metastases, bone metastases, and spinal cord compression. *Int J Radiat ncol Biol Phys.* 1998;15:859.

115. Herbert SH, Solin LJ, Rate WR, et al. The effect of palliative radiation therapy on epidural compression due to metastatic malignant melanoma. *Cancer.* 1991;67:2472.

116. Henson JW. Neurological complications of malignant melanoma and other cutaneous malignancies. In: Wiley RG, ed. *Neurologic Complications of Cancer.* New York, NY: Marcel Dekker; 1995:333.

117. Spiess JL, Adelstein DJ, Hines DJ. Multiple myeloma pre-senting with spinal cord compression. *Oncology.* 1988;45:88.

118. Mayfield JK, Riseborough EJ, Jaffe N, et al. Spinal deformities in children treated for neuroblastoma. *J Bone Joint Surg.* 1981;63:183.

119. Kaspars GJ, Kamphorst W, et al. Primary spinal epidural extraosseous Ewing's sarcoma. *Cancer.* 1991;68:648.

120. Chi JH, Gokaslan Z, McCormick P, Tibbs PA, Kryscio RJ, Patchell RA. Selecting treatment for patients with malignant epidural spinal cord compression—does age matter?: results from a randomized clinical trial. *Spine (Phila Pa 1976).* March 2009;34(5):431-435.

121. Loblaw DA, Laperriere NJ, Mackillop WJ. A population-based study of malignant spinal cord compression in Ontario. *Clin Oncol (R Coll Radiol).* 2003;15:211-217.

122. George R, Jeba J, Ramkumar G, Chacko AG, Leng M, Tharyan P. Interventions for the treatment of metastatic extradural spinal cord compression in adults. *Cochrane Database Syst Rev.* October 2008;(4):CD006716.

CHAPTER **40**

Recognizing and Managing Delirium

Scott A. Irwin ■ Gary T. Buckholz ■ Rosene D. Pirrello ■ Jeremy M. Hirst ■ Frank D. Ferris

INTRODUCTION

Delirium is an important medical diagnosis defined as an acute change in mental status that may fluctuate and has underlying physiologic causes (1,2). Subtypes of delirium have been defined based on the presence (hyperactive) or absence (hypoactive) of psychomotor agitation, perceptual disturbances, and/or level of consciousness (3). Often both subtypes are present (mixed) (4–12).

In the context of serious illness, delirium is highly prevalent and associated with many undesirable consequences. Most physiologic disturbances can cause delirium; however, even with serious or advanced illness, causes can often be determined and reversed. Despite this, delirium is still under-recognized and under-managed. Careful history taking, assessment of symptoms, consideration of differential diagnoses, and clear communication among the team are key to making the diagnosis. Having the diagnosis of delirium and determining prognosis, functional status, and goals of the patient/family are paramount to successful management. With this information, delirium can be conceptualized as potentially reversible or irreversible, and both workup and management strategies flow from these concepts, as well as the presence or absence of the hyperactive subtype. Both pharmacologic and non-pharmacologic interventions can be employed to improve symptoms and relieve patient/family distress.

Prevalence and Consequences

Delirium is very common in the setting of advanced illness, with reported rates of up to 56% in the hospitalized elderly (13,14), 87% in intensive care units (15–17), and 88% of patients with advanced cancer or at the end-of-life (8,9,18–22). It likely occurs in nearly 100% of patients who are actively dying. Disagreement about the most common subtype exists, but hypoactive is often reported as the most prevalent (9,10) and is the one most often under-recognized (8). One study of 228 end-stage cancer patients found the prevalence of delirium to be 47%, and of those, 68% were hypoactive (8).

Delirium leads to unnecessary medical interventions, increased hospital admissions, prolonged hospitalizations (13,14,23,24), increased healthcare utilization and costs (14,25,26), increased need for higher levels of care (24,27), functional decline (27), increased mortality

(2,8,20,21,24,27–33), and decreased life expectancy (28,34,35). It can also impair the recognition and control of other physical and psychological symptoms, such as pain (36–38). This all leads to a significant amount of distress for patients, families, and caregivers (39–42). One study of 101 cancer patients who recovered from delirium reported that 54% recalled the experience and that patients, spouses/caregivers, and nurses all reported moderate to severe distress from the experience, no matter the subtype (43).

Causes

The most common causes of delirium found in patients with serious and/or advanced illness are fluid and electrolyte imbalances, medications (benzodiazepines (44,45), opioids (21,45–47), steroids (45,46,48), and anticholinergics (49,50)), infections, hepatic or renal failure, hypoxia, and hematologic disturbances (21,51). A selected list of important causes to consider is presented in Table 40.1 (52).

Under-Recognition

Delirium is often unrecognized or misdiagnosed due to its complex and variable presentation, the inconsistent language used to describe it, preconceived notions about advanced illness and the dying process, and the difficulty of recognizing the hypoactive subtype. A retrospective study of 2,716 patients receiving hospice care found delirium was documented in only 17.8% of those in the homecare setting and 28.3% of those in an inpatient setting (53). Another study demonstrated that a palliative care team was only able to recognize delirium in 45% of all patients with an expert-confirmed delirium diagnosis, and in only 20% of those with hypoactive delirium (8).

Behaviors, Signs, and Symptoms

The diagnosis of delirium is based on a careful history that accurately captures all observed behaviors, signs, and symptoms that potentially indicate its presence, many of which are changes in mental status. To effectively communicate an evaluation, all clinicians need to know the definitions of and recognize the common behaviors, signs, and symptoms associated with delirium (Table 40.2).

| TABLE 40.1 | Selected common causes of delirium |

System	Causes
Brain	Stroke, seizure, head trauma, brain mass or metastases, normal pressure hydrocephalus, infection
Heart, lungs, circulation	Cardiac or pulmonary disease (anything that causes hypoxia), carotid disease, anemia, infection
Digestive, urinary	Hepatic or renal failure, peritonitis, bowel obstruction, fecal impaction, constipation, urinary retention, urinary tract infection
Endocrine	Thyroid, parathyroid, adrenal
Metabolic	Acid–base or electrolyte disturbances, abnormal glucose, dehydration
Toxicity and/or withdrawal	Drugs of abuse, opioids, steroids, benzodiazepines, anticholinergics, immunosuppressants, interferon, histamine-2 blockers (cimetidine and ranitidine)

ASSESSMENT

Routine screening can help identify patients at risk for delirium who can then be assessed more thoroughly. Once delirium is suspected, a careful assessment is necessary to optimally manage patients with delirium, including the following:

1. Careful description of the observed behaviors, signs, and symptoms
2. Differentiation of delirium from other related diagnoses
3. An understanding of the underlying context of the patient, that is, the primary diagnosis, associated comorbidities, functional status, and prognosis
4. The goals of care for the patient and family

| TABLE 40.2 | Behaviors/symptoms/signs often associated with delirium |

Behaviors/Symptoms/Signs	Definition
Acute onset	Rapid onset of symptoms over minutes to days, even if began or occurred in the past
Agitation	Unintentional, excessive, and purposeless cognitive and/or motor activity
Altered level of consciousness	Clinically differentiable degrees of awareness and alertness, that is, hypervigilant, alert, lethargic, cloudy, stuporous, and comatose
Confusion	Not oriented to person, place, time, or situation
Delusion	A fixed and false belief or wrong judgment that opposing evidence does not change. Can be paranoid, grandiose, somatic, and persecutory
Disinhibition	Unable to control immediate impulsive response to a situation
Disorganized thinking	Thoughts are confusing, vague, and/or do not logically flow; they are loosely or not connected
Fluctuation or waxing/waning	Intensity changes rapidly; symptoms may come and go
Hallucination	Perception of an object or event that does not exist. May be visual, auditory, olfactory, gustatory, or tactile
Inattention	Inability to focus or direct thinking
Irritable	Prone to excessive impatience, annoyance, or anger to get needs met
Labile affect	Rapidly changing and out of context mood symptoms
Psychosis	Loss of contact with reality
Restlessness	See agitation

Screening

Multiple tools have been developed to facilitate routine screening for delirium and tracking of symptom severity (52,54). The Confusion Assessment Method (CAM) is a brief, nine-item screening tool that looks at change over time (temporal profile), attention, thought processes, and levels of consciousness (55,56). It can be easily administered by non-psychiatrically trained personnel and has been validated in many populations, including patients with advanced illnesses (57). A shorter, four-question version of the CAM, which can be administered quickly, has accuracy similar to the full nine-question version (25). It has a sensitivity of 94% to 100% and specificity of 90% to 95% (55), but this can vary by setting and the administrator's clinical discipline.

Gold Standard Assessment

The gold standard for assessing delirium is a thorough history, a complete mental status and physical examination, and comparison with the DSM-IV TR criteria for delirium (2,58,59). As delirious patients are often not good historians, the gathering of collateral information is key. Caregivers, including family members and support staff, can identify and describe the behaviors, signs, and symptoms they see using simple, clear, and common language (see Table 40.2). This will help make the diagnosis of delirium and differentiate it from other diagnoses with similar presentations (see Table 40.3). Each observed behavior, sign, and symptom should be described by change over time (temporal profile), severity, and response (positive or negative) to previous therapeutic interventions (60).

A careful medication history, which documents all changes in medications and dosages over recent days, weeks, or even months, especially those leading up to the mental status changes, should be included. The types and severity of all allergic and adverse reactions need to be noted and confirmed. A careful drug and alcohol history is important; of particular interest are drugs that cause withdrawal syndromes, for example, alcohol, opioids, benzodiazepines, and muscle relaxants.

Diagnostic and Severity Rating Tools

The Delirium Rating Scale Revised-98 and the Memorial Delirium Assessment Scale are diagnostic and severity rating tools that can be used to confirm the diagnosis of delirium and to monitor changes over time (61). Both tools require that the rater have familiarity with basic psychiatric concepts.

The Delirium Rating Scale Revised-98 includes 3 specific diagnostic items and a 13-item severity rating scale (61,62). When compared with expert psychiatric diagnosis with DSM criteria, it has a sensitivity of 91% to 100% and a specificity of 85% to 100%. It has been shown to differentiate delirium from disorders with similar presentations, including depression, dementia, and schizophrenia. Its predecessor, the Delirium Rating Scale, has been used to evaluate delirium in children and adolescents (63).

The Memorial Delirium Assessment Scale is another diagnostic and severity rating scale designed for serial measurements in clinical intervention trials. It is a 10-item rating scale that can be used as frequently as every 4 hours to track the course of delirium (64). It has a sensitivity of 97% and a specificity of 95%, when compared with expert psychiatric diagnosis using DSM criteria. Other tools have been designed for use in the intensive care unit (16,65–67), with children (63,66), and by non-psychiatrically trained staff (68,69).

Several tools are often used inappropriately to screen for and assess delirium. Both the Mini-Mental State Exam and the Clock Drawing task are measures of global cognitive function, and the Mini-Mental State Exam can be used as a screen for Alzheimer's dementia. Neither of these are specific to nor should be used to assess delirium (70–72).

ALTERNATIVE DIAGNOSES TO CONSIDER

Many of the signs, symptoms, and behaviors associated with delirium can be associated with other diagnoses. As the underlying causes and management vary greatly, it is important to differentiate delirium from dementia, depression, anxiety, bipolar disorder, psychotic disorders (e.g., schizophrenia), personality disorders, developmental disorder, and adverse effects of medications (e.g., akathisia) (2), among other things. Table 40.3 lists differences in onset, changes in alertness, and frequency of fluctuation that help clinicians to make accurate diagnoses. When in doubt, assume the patient is experiencing delirium until proven otherwise, as delirium is the most common of these related diagnoses in patients with advanced illnesses. It should not be assumed that agitation is driven by pain; careful assessment of pain and consideration of other causes of agitation are important.

TABLE 40.3	**Differential diagnoses**				
	Delirium	**Dementia**	**Psychotic Disorders**	**Depression**	**Anxiety**
Onset	Hours to days	Gradual	Varies	Varies	Varies
Changes in alertness	Yes	Late	No	No	No
Frequent fluctuation	Yes	No	No	No	Varies

TABLE 40.4	Objective signs of active dying
Categories	Signs
Cardiac dysfunction	Tachycardia
	Decreased cardiac output
	Decreased intravascular volume
	Peripheral cooling
	Peripheral and central cyanosis
	Mottling of the skin (livedo reticularis)
	Venous pooling
Respiratory dysfunction	Tachypnea with progressive slowing and decreasing tidal volume
	Abnormal breathing patterns, for example, apnea, Cheyne-Stokes, agonal
Renal dysfunction	Oliguria progressing to anuria
	Darkening of urine
Neurologic dysfunction	Loss of swallow
	Loss of gag reflex
	Buildup of oral and tracheal secretions
	Loss of sphincter control
	Altered level of consciousness
	Seizures

For complex clinical situations, mental health professionals can be consulted to quickly help minimize suffering for the patient, family, and caregivers (73).

Delirium itself goes by many synonyms, including acute confusional state, ICU psychosis, encephalopathy, acute brain failure, and syndrome of cerebral insufficiency. It is important to recognize that these all refer to the same diagnosis. To ensure effective management and avoid confusion, it is best to diagnose these as "delirium."

Underlying Diagnoses and Prognosis

Delirium in patients with advanced illnesses may or may not be reversible. To establish the potential reversibility of delirium, it is important to know each patient's goals of care, principal underlying diagnosis and comorbidities, their functional status, and overall prognosis (74,75–78). If an underlying abnormal physiologic process is suspected, with appropriate investigation and therapies, the condition could be potentially reversible, even in the context of advanced illness, if consistent with patient/family goals.

Several studies have demonstrated the ability to find and reverse causes of delirium in the context of serious or advanced illness. One study of 213 hospice inpatients with cancer and delirium found a cause of the delirium in 93 (61%) of the 153 patients who chose to have a workup. The causes were found to be multifactorial in 52% of the cases, and a complete remission occurred in 20% (51). Another

study of 104 inpatients with advanced cancer who were receiving palliative care found reversible causes in 50% of the 71 who developed delirium (21). Other studies have found reversible causes in up to 68% of cases (21,34,79).

Delirium becomes irreversible (1) if workup or reversal fail, (2) in the context of a known irreversible processes (e.g., active dying or end-stage liver failure), or (3) if workup or reversal are inconsistent with patient/family goals of care. Most patients who are actively dying (exhibiting objective signs of the dying process (74,80,81), (Table 40.4) experience either a hyperactive or a hypoactive delirium (74,80). As dying is an irreversible process of multi-system organ failure, this delirium is irreversible. Management of irreversible deliria focuses on settling and supporting the patient, the family, and caregivers.

Using the terminology of reversible versus irreversible delirium (82,83) takes into account (1) that the patient has a known medical diagnosis of delirium, (2) the potential causes of the delirium, (3) the underlying diagnoses, prognosis, and functional status of the patient, and (4) the goals of care for the patient. With these, *prospective* workup and management decisions can be made that differ based on whether the delirium is potentially reversible or irreversible.

Goals of Care

Patients and families living with advance illnesses have a wide range of goals for their medical care and for their lives (75–77). Some still hope for cure, many hope for prolongation of life,

TABLE 40.5	**Potential tests for determining causes of delirium**	
Tier 1	**Subsequent Tests Guided by Clinical Picture**	
Comprehensive chemistries	PT/PTT/INR	Lumbar puncture
CBC w/differential	TSH	HIV testing
LFTs	Ammonia level	RPR testing
B$_{12}$/folate levels	ECG	EEG
X-rays	ABG	
Albumin	Cultures (blood, stool, etc.)	
UA and UC	CT or MRI	

PT, prothrombin time; PTT, partial thromboplastin time; INR, international normalized ratio; CBC, complete blood count; TSH, thyroid stimulating hormone; CT, computed tomography; MRI, magnetic resonance imaging; LFTs, liver function tests; HIV, human immunodeficiency virus; ECG, electrocardiogram; RPR, rapid plasma reagin; UA, urinalysis; UC, urine culture; ABG, arterial blood gas; EEG, electroencephalogram.

almost all hope for concurrent relief of the multiple issues that cause them suffering (as they define it) (78). At times they have what appear to be overlapping, and sometimes conflicting goals.

Goals of care frequently change over time as the patient's illness evolves and new information becomes available. Many patients nearing the end of their lives do not want to have aggressive or potentially life-prolonging medical therapies. They prefer to focus on care that gives them the best possible quality of life and a good death (as they define it).

If a delirium is potentially reversible, the patient and family goals for medical care and goals for life should guide the diagnostic workup and management of the underlying causes. A diagnosis of delirium often causes patients living with advanced illnesses, or their surrogate decision-makers, and their families to reassess their goals for medical care. Some patients and families still find simple tests, such as blood draws and urinalysis acceptable, especially if the results might indicate an easy therapeutic intervention that could potentially reverse a hyperactive delirium, reduce distress, and improve quality of life. They choose to attempt to reverse the underlying cause of the delirium and manage any associated distressing symptoms.

Others choose to forgo a diagnostic workup and/or any treatment of the underlying cause of the delirium, thus rendering it irreversible. They may choose not to attempt to reverse the underlying cause of the delirium even when the treatment is relatively easy to do (e.g., antibiotic treatment for urinary tract infection), preferring to focus on managing distressing symptoms.

Workup of Delirium

If the patient's underlying diagnoses, prognosis, functional status, and goals for medical care are consistent with a potentially reversible delirium, after a thorough history and physical examination, obtaining a comprehensive blood count, metabolic panel, vitamin levels, and limited infection workup will often reveal the most common reversible causes of delirium. Careful thought should be given before ordering tests that are potentially more invasive or burdensome to the patient. Only consider tests that will lead to definitive treatment strategies.

Delirium can be caused by any physiologic disturbance. If initial investigations do not reveal an underlying cause and the goal is a comprehensive diagnostic workup, consider any medical test consistent with confirming a suspected diagnosis using a tiered approach based on the most likely causes (Table 40.5). Always consider the benefits, risks, and burdens of every investigation.

Time-limited trials can be utilized to guide workup and/or management of underlying causes, such that clear goals and measures of success are defined over a specified period of time and unlimited workups or therapeutic trials are avoided. Should drug intoxication be suspected, reduce the dose or rotate to other medications (84,85). This is especially true for opioids (85), particularly when decreased fluid intake or urine output can lead to opioid accumulation and cause or worsen delirium.

MANAGEMENT

If consistent with the patients' diagnoses, prognosis, functional status, and goals of care, attempt to treat the underlying cause of a potentially reversible delirium. Whether attempting to reverse or not, the associated symptoms of delirium should always be managed with non-pharmacologic interventions and, when appropriate, pharmacologic interventions. Always ensure safety for the patient, caregivers, and family and address any environmental issues (2,59). Most people approaching the end of their lives want to be cared for at home in their last days to weeks, and die there

(86,87). The non-pharmacologic and pharmacologic management strategies that follow can be safely administered in any setting.

Controlling Symptoms Associated with Delirium

Non-pharmacologic Interventions

All patients can benefit from non-pharmacologic interventions, including several environmental interventions, that will minimize the risk and severity of symptoms associated with delirium (31,37,88–92). These interventions can minimize disordered thinking, disorientation, sleep disturbances, immobility, risk of falls/injury, sensory deprivation, dehydration, and address other environmental factors:

■ Engaging patients in mentally stimulating activities to help them with disordered thinking
■ Providing orienting and familiar materials to help patients know the time and date, where they are, and which staff are working with them
■ Ensuring all individuals identify themselves each time they encounter the patient, even if the encounters are minutes apart
■ Minimizing the number of people interacting with the patient and the quantity of stimulation the patient receives, for example, no television and loud music
■ Using family or volunteers as constant companions to help reassure and reorient a delirious patient. Encourage staff to sit with the patient while they do their documentation
■ Providing adequate soft lighting so patients can see without being overstimulated by bright lights
■ Managing fall risks
■ Providing warm milk, massage, warm blankets, and using relaxation tapes to optimize sleep hygiene and minimize sleep disturbances
■ Ensuring patients use their glasses, hearing aids, etc., to optimize orientation, decreased confusion, and promote better communication
■ Ensuring patients have good nutrition and an effective bowel and bladder management strategy
■ Monitoring fluid intake; rehydrate with oral fluids containing salt, for example, soups, sport drinks, red vegetable juices; when necessary, infuse fluids subcutaneously rather than intravenously (93–95)
■ Using physical restraints only as a last resort to temporarily ensure the safety of both staff and a severely agitated and not redirectable patient (31,96), and only until less restrictive interventions are possible
■ Providing education and support to help family members cope with what they are witnessing (97)

A non-pharmacologic protocol targeted at delirium was developed by Inouye and colleagues (92) to minimize the risk of delirium in geriatric patients. Using this protocol, which targets orientation, cognitive activity, mobility, sleep, hydration, and access to sensory aids, delirium developed in only 9.9% of geriatric patients admitted to a hospital medicine service versus 15% of those receiving usual care. The intervention group also had significantly fewer and shorter episodes of delirium. A follow-up study showed that this protocol reduced the risk of developing delirium in a similar population by 89% (98).

Pharmacologic Interventions

Currently, there are

■ no medications with US Food and Drug Administration (FDA)-approved indications for the management of delirium;
■ no published double-blind, randomized, placebo controlled trials to guide the pharmacologic management of delirium; and
■ no consensus among oncologists, geriatricians, psychiatrists, and palliative medicine specialists about how to pharmacologically treat delirium (99).

The following is an evidence-based and expert consensus approach to pharmacologically managing the symptoms associated with delirium. Pharmacologic management of delirium is guided by the presence or absence of hyperactive delirium and the potential reversibility of the delirium. Based on the delirium management decision tree presented in Figure 40.1, three approaches will be presented: (1) management of hyperactive (agitated), potentially reversible delirium; (2) management of hyperactive, irreversible delirium; and (3) management of hypoactive delirium, whether potentially reversible or irreversible.

Potentially Reversible, Hyperactive Delirium. The American Psychiatric Association guidelines for delirium management suggest the use of first-generation antipsychotics and the avoidance of benzodiazepines for the first-line treatment of agitation in the context of a potentially reversible delirium (NB: these guidelines do not distinguish potentially reversible from irreversible delirium, nor do they address goals of care or irreversible delirium) (2,59,100).

Antipsychotics are the medications of choice for the management of agitation associated with potentially reversible, hyperactive delirium. Some of them have sedative properties (see Tables 40.6 and 40.9) (2,58,104). They may also improve cognition and mental status (2,3,59,101,102).

No evidence exists for improved efficacy with atypical (second- or third-generation) antipsychotics (44,103–105). Also, they are more expensive and have limited routes of administration (101). With a few exceptions, benzodiazepines should not be used first line for managing potentially reversible delirium. They can worsen delirium, increase fall risk, create memory problems, and lead to withdrawal syndromes (2,44).

Likewise, opioids have no role in the treatment of agitation or delirium (Table 40.6). New or increased doses of opioids may worsen the symptoms of delirium. Care should be taken when titrating or tapering opioids: increase opioid doses carefully using a "catch-up" technique (75) that

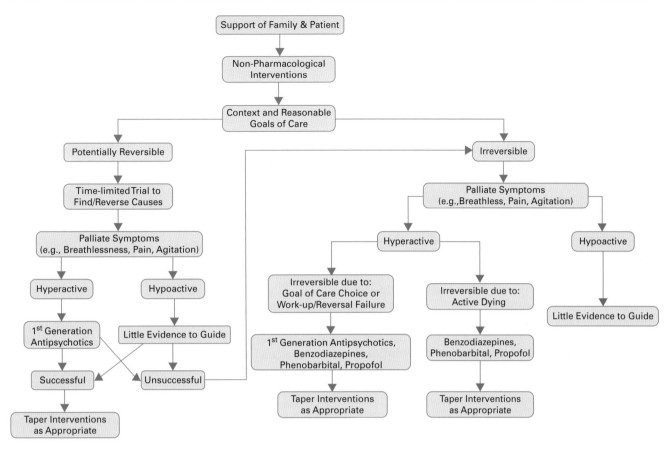

Figure 40.1. Delirium management decision tree.

minimizes the risk of adverse effects (e.g., opioid-induced delirium) and reduce opioid doses carefully to avoid withdrawal syndromes.

Irreversible, Hyperactive Delirium. When agitation occurs within the context of an irreversible delirium, a shift to management with benzodiazepines may be appropriate, especially if the patient is actively dying (i.e., there are associated objective signs of the dying process; Table 40.4) (21,52,80,84,106–114). This may also be appropriate when either (1) the patient's and family's goals for care are focused on symptom control without workup or management of the underlying causes, or (2) the initial workup or treatment of a hyperactive, potentially reversible delirium has been refractory based on predetermined time-limited trials.

When patients are dying and experiencing an irreversible hyperactive delirium, there is significant risk of muscle tension, myoclonus, seizures, and family and caregiver distress (74,80). The goal of care is to settle the patient, relieve muscle tension, and minimize the risk of seizures. Most patients would rather not "experience" the agitated delirium associated with dying or have any "memory" of the event. Likewise, witnessing this agitation causes most caregivers and families significant distress. Benzodiazepines are ideal medications to manage and prevent these symptoms (21,52,80,84,106–114). They are sedatives, anxiolytics, skeletal muscle relaxants, amnestics, and potent antiepileptics (see Table 40.6). Only the minimum benzodiazepine dose needed to achieve the desired effect should be used.

TABLE 40.6	**Antipsychotic, benzodiazepine, and opioid therapeutic properties**				
	Indication				
Drug	**Anti-agitation**	**Sedation**	**Amnesia**	**Muscle Relaxation**	**Anticonvulsant**
Antipsychotics	✔	✔/✗	✗	✗	–
Benzodiazepines	✔	✔	✔	✔	✔
Opioids	✗	✗	✗	✗	–

✔, has property; ✗, does not have property; –, has opposite property.

While some clinicians worry, evidence suggests that appropriate titration of antipsychotics and benzodiazepines for the palliation of symptoms does not hasten death, and may in fact, prolong life (113–121). Doses typically needed to control these symptoms are well below FDA maximum recommended doses and far below their median lethal dosages. If a patient has an initial paradoxical reaction with more agitation, escalating the dose rapidly can overcome this reaction. If not effective, a switch to phenobarbital (122) or propofol (123,124) to control the agitation and settle the patient may be necessary.

Hypoactive Delirium. Treatment of both potentially reversible and irreversible hypoactive delirium with medications is controversial. One approach is to avoid pharmacologic intervention, as medications are often the cause of delirium, and it is not clear if antipsychotics address anything besides agitation and psychotic symptoms (which are absent in hypoactive delirium). Another approach advocates for the use of antipsychotics, as they may improve cognition and other mental status changes (3,102). A third approach suggests that psychostimulants may improve cognitive performance in hypoactive delirium (128,129); however, the benefits must carefully be weighed against the risks of psychosis and worsening delirium. No evidence exists to guide the use of benzodiazepines to manage hypoactive delirium, though theoretically, their broad spectrum of therapeutic properties may be beneficial (Table 40.6) in the context of an irreversible delirium.

Pharmacologic Principles Improve Management

Titration of medications to control agitation or other symptoms associated with delirium should be *rapid*. All of these medications follow the same pharmacologic principles (e.g., first-order kinetics) employed when dosing medications to rapidly control other symptoms, such as pain (75).

Offer a first dose of medication. If it does not control the symptom by the time its plasma concentration is maximum (t_{CMAX}), it will not become effective with more time. To titrate rapidly and safely to control symptoms, dose the medications every t_{CMAX} until the symptom is controlled (75). Before each additional dose, ensure the patient does not have any new, undesired side effects.

Once the symptom (e.g., agitation) is controlled, provide the total dose used in the last 24 hours in divided doses administered routinely once every half-life ($t_{\frac{1}{2}}$) over a 24-hour period. To control any breakthrough agitation or other symptoms, continue to make available extra doses of the same medication once every t_{CMAX} as needed.

For example, to control agitation rapidly, antipsychotics can be safely dosed intravenously (IV) once every 15 minutes, subcutaneously (SC) once every 30 minutes, or orally (PO) once every 60 minutes until the agitation is controlled or the maximum recommended dose of the medication in a 24-hour period has been reached (75). This is similar to the protocol to rapidly control agitation in emergency situations (106,125–128). See Tables 40.7 and 40.8 for specific dosing suggestions and sample orders.

Potential Antipsychotic Side Effects

All risks of side effects must be considered alongside the potential benefits of each medication. Table 40.9 categorizes common adverse effects for five antipsychotic medications commonly used in patients with advanced illnesses (101). These side effects correlate with a drug's affinity for the neuroreceptors most implicated in the particular side effect.

The common side effects of antipsychotics include extrapyramidal symptoms (acute dystonia, akathisia, parkinsonism, and tardive dyskinesia); anticholinergic effects (delirium, urinary retention, tachycardia, blurred vision, cognitive impairment, dry mouth, constipation, sexual dysfunction, and decreased sweating); sedation; hypotension; dizziness; and orthostasis (129). Diabetes, hyperglycemia, hyperlipidemia, and weight gain may be of concern with longer term use. QTc prolongation is often cited as a concern, but the evidence to support this is lacking (101).

As lower antipsychotic doses typically control agitation in medically ill patients, their side effects are less frequent in patients with advanced illnesses (44). A Cochrane review cited one study of chlorpromazine for delirium in advanced illness that found decreased cognitive function but no increase in extrapyramidal effects (130). Another Cochrane review of the efficacy and side effects of antipsychotics in delirium cited three studies, two found no significant side effects and one found that haloperidol increased the incidence of dry mouth and extrapyramidal symptoms (131).

Black Box Warnings

The FDA has issued a black box warning about the increased risk of death (3.5% with all antipsychotics vs. 2.3% with placebos) when first- or second-generation antipsychotics are used to treat *dementia-related psychosis* in elderly patients based on a number of limited studies (132–138). Other studies have not replicated this finding (139). These data do not address the risk of short-term use of these agents to manage *delirium*. In addition, no evidence for antipsychotics being the direct cause of the increased mortality in patients with dementia or delirium has yet been produced. It is not clear how long a patient must be treated with an antipsychotic before having increased risk. While the relative risk appears large (1.7 times the risk of using a placebo), the absolute risk is small (increase of 1.2%) (137,138). Similarly, the absolute increase in the risk of cerebrovascular events related to the use of newer antipsychotics in patients with *dementia* is 1% (1.9% in treated group vs. 0.9% in the placebo group) (140).

It is important to note that none of the studies of antipsychotics in dementia were designed to evaluate the risk of mortality and cerebrovascular events, and they were not stratified by risk factors for these events. They also did not account for the multiple comorbidities and medications used by the study patients. A black box warning is a sign to use caution, but not a mandate to avoid the use of these medications. A recent survey found that 68% of geriatricians still use antipsychotics in geriatric patients with known

TABLE 40.7 **Pharmacologic parameters for medications used to manage symptoms of delirium**

Generic and Trade Name	Suggested Starting Dosage	Breakthrough Dosing based on Time C_{MAX}	Approximate Elimination t½	Recommended Scheduled Dosing Interval	Recommended Maximum Dosage
Haloperidol (non-sedating) aka **Haldol**	1–2 mg	PO: 60 min SC/IM: 30 min IV:15 min	21 h	Daily or twice daily	100 mg/d
Chlorpromazine (sedating) aka **Thorazine**	25–50 mg	PO: 60 min SC/IM: 30 min IV: 15 min	24 h	Daily or twice daily	2,000 mg/d
Risperidone (non-sedating) aka **Risperdal**	0.25–0.5 mg	PO: 60 min	3 h (metabolites: 21–30 h)	Daily or twice daily	6 mg/d
Olanzapine (sedating) aka **Zyprexa**	2.5–5 mg	PO: 6 h (onset of action 30 min) SC/IM: 30 min	30 h	Daily or twice daily	30 mg/d
Quetiapine (sedating) aka **Seroquel**	25–50 mg	PO: 90 min[a]	12 h	Up to three times daily	1200 mg/d
Lorazepam aka **Ativan**	1–2 mg	PO: 60 min SC/IM: 30 min IV: 15 min	12 h	Twice daily	40 mg/d[b]
Midazolam aka **Versed**	0.1–0.2 mg/kg loading dose, then 25% of the loading dose needed to control symptoms as a continuous infusion, for example, for a 50 kg person who required 0.2 mg/kg, = 10 mg to control, the continuous infusion would be 2.5 mg/h	SC/IM: 30 min IV: 15 min	2 h	Continuous infusion	240 mg/d[b]
Phenobarbital	10–30 mg/kg loading dose, then 20–100 mg/h continuous infusion	SC/IM: 2 h IV: 30 min	96 h	Continuous infusion	2400 mg/d
Propofol	1 mg/kg/h starting Increase by 0.5 mg/kg until effect achieved (usually <6 mg/kg/h)	IV	3–12 h[c]	Continuous infusion	12 mg/kg/h

PO, orally; PR, rectally; SC, subcutaneously; IV, intravenously; mg, milligram; kg, kilogram; h, hour.

[a]Caution increasing by more than 50–100 mg/d in ambulatory patients.

[b]Safe to use higher doses; however, management may be better with phenobarbital or propofol if symptoms are not controlled at this maximum dose.

[c]Increases with prolonged administration due to tissue distribution.

TABLE 40.8	Sample orders (routes and associated dosing schedule may differ)

Haloperidol

- 1 mg SC q30min PRN agitation
- If three doses are not effective, call MD to reassess dose, diagnosis, or medication choice
- Do not exceed 100 mg in 24 h (wide therapeutic range)
- Schedule the total dose used in the last 24 h in divided doses administered twice daily
- Continue with same PRN schedule

Chlorpromazine

- 50 mg PO q60min PRN agitation
- If three doses are not effective, call MD to reassess dose, diagnosis, or medication choice
- Do not exceed 2000 mg in 24 h
- Schedule the total dose used in the last 24 h in divided doses administered twice daily
- Continue with same PRN schedule

Risperidone

- 0.5 mg PO q60min PRN agitation
- If three doses are not effective, call MD to reassess dose, diagnosis, or medication choice
- Do not exceed 6 mg in 24 h (wide therapeutic range)
- Schedule the total dose used in the last 24 h in divided doses administered twice daily
- Continue with same PRN schedule

Olanzapine

- 2.5 mg SC q30min PRN agitation
- If three doses are not effective, call MD to reassess dose, diagnosis, or medication choice
- Do not exceed 30 mg in 24 h (wide therapeutic range)
- Schedule the total dose used in the last 24 h in divided doses administered twice daily
- Continue with same PRN schedule

Lorazepam

- 1 mg PO q60min PRN agitation
- If three doses are not effective, call MD to reassess dose, diagnosis, or medication choice
- Do not exceed 40 mg in 24 h (wide therapeutic range)
- Schedule the total dose used in the last 24 h in three divided doses administered every 12 h
- Continue with same PRN schedule

Midazolam

- 0.2 mg/kg loading dose SC
- If needed give 0.1 mg/kg q30min × 2 PRN
- Continuously infuse 25% of total dose needed for symptom control per hour
- Consider alternative if need >10 mg/h

vascular risk due to lack of alternatives, lack of solid evidence, and lack of clear guidelines (141). The bottom line is (1) take account of patient/family goals for care and (2) weigh the risks, benefits, burdens, and alternatives of treatment. Often, families are willing to accept these risks, if necessary, to control the severe distress everyone experiences when a patient has a delirium.

CONCLUSIONS

In patients with serious and advanced illnesses, delirium is a common diagnosis. It is associated with many negative consequences, including significant distress for patients, families, and caregivers. With a careful history, physical examination, and investigation as appropriate, the causes of delirium are often discoverable and reversible, even in this patient population.

Delirium can be conceptualized as potentially reversible or irreversible. By knowing patients underlying diagnoses,

prognosis, functional status, and goals of care, clinicians can treat or manage the underlying cause and use non-pharmacologic and pharmacologic therapies to minimize the symptoms and reduce the distress caused by delirium. In all cases, through careful attention to the pharmacokinetics of medications, clinicians can rapidly control agitation and other symptoms associated with delirium, even in actively dying and seemingly refractory patients.

ACKNOWLEDGMENTS

We wish to acknowledge the support from the staff and patients of San Diego Hospice and The Institute for Palliative Medicine. This work was supported, in part, by the John A Hartford Center of Excellence in Geriatric Psychiatry at the University of California, San Diego (Scott A. Irwin), The National Institute of Mental Health K23MH091176 (Scott A. Irwin), a National Palliative Care Research Center Career Development Grant (Scott A. Irwin), and by donations from

TABLE 40.9	Side effects associated with antipsychotic medications				
	Adverse Event (receptor)				
Drug	**Anticholinergic (M$_1$)**	**Sedation (H$_1$)**	**Orthostasis (α_1)**	**QTc Prolongation**	**EPS (D$_2$)**
Haloperidol	✗	✔	✗	✗ (PO) ✔ (IV)	✔✔✔
Chlorpromazine	✔✔	✔✔✔	✔	✔	✔
Risperidone	✗	✔	✗	✗	✔✔
Olanzapine	✔✔	✔✔	✗	✗	✔
Quetiapine	✗	✔✔✔	✔	✗	✗

✔, relative strength of effect; ✗, does not have effect; EPS, extrapyramidal side effects.

the generous benefactors of the education and research programs at San Diego Hospice and the Institute for Palliative Medicine.

REFERENCES

1. American Psychiatric Association. *Diagnostic and Statistical Manual of Mental Disorders.* Washington, DC: American Psychiatric Association; 2000:943.
2. American Psychiatric Association. Practice guideline for the treatment of patients with delirium. *Am J Psychiatry.* 1999;156:1-20.
3. Boettger S, Breitbart W. Phenomenology of the subtypes of delirium: phenomenological differences between hyperactive and hypoactive delirium. *Palliat Support Care.* 2011;9: 129-135.
4. Stagno D, Gibson C, Breitbart W. The delirium subtypes: a review of prevalence, phenomenology, pathophysiology, and treatment response. *Palliat Support Care.* 2004;2:171-179.
5. O'Keeffe ST. Clinical subtypes of delirium in the elderly. *Dement Geriatr Cogn Disord.* 1999;10:380-385.
6. Lipowski ZJ. Delirium in the elderly patient. *N Engl J Med.* 1989;320:578-582.
7. Meagher D, Moran M, Raju B, et al. A new data-based motor subtype schema for delirium. *J Neuropsychiatry Clin Neurosci.* 2008;20:185-193.
8. Fang CK, Chen HW, Liu SI, Lin CJ, Tsai LY, Lai YL. Prevalence, detection and treatment of delirium in terminal cancer inpatients: a prospective survey. *Jpn J Clin Oncol.* 2008;38: 56-63.
9. Spiller JA, Keen JC. Hypoactive delirium: assessing the extent of the problem for inpatient specialist palliative care. *Palliat Med.* 2006;20:17-23.
10. Ross CA, Peyser CE, Shapiro I, Folstein MF. Delirium: phenomenologic and etiologic subtypes. *Int Psychogeriatr.* 1991;3:135-147.
11. Meagher DJ, Moran M, Raju B, et al. Motor symptoms in 100 patients with delirium versus control subjects: comparison of subtyping methods. *Psychosomatics.* 2008;49:300-308.
12. Peterson JF, Pun BT, Dittus RS, et al. Delirium and its motoric subtypes: a study of 614 critically ill patients. *J Am Geriatr Soc.* 2006;54:479-484.
13. Pompei P, Foreman M, Rudberg MA, Inouye SK, Braund V, Cassel CK. Delirium in hospitalized older persons: outcomes and predictors. *J Am Geriatr Soc.* 1994;42:809-815.
14. Inouye SK. Delirium in hospitalized older patients. *Clin Geriatr Med.* 1998;14:745-764.
15. McNicoll L, Pisani MA, Zhang Y, Ely EW, Siegel MD, Inouye SK. Delirium in the intensive care unit: occurrence and clinical course in older patients. *J Am Geriatr Soc.* 2003;51: 591-598.
16. Ely EW, Margolin R, Francis J, et al. Evaluation of delirium in critically ill patients: validation of the Confusion Assessment Method for the Intensive Care Unit (CAM-ICU). *Crit Care Med.* 2001;29:1370-1379.
17. Hart RP, Levenson JL, Sessler CN, Best AM, Schwartz SM, Rutherford LE. Validation of a cognitive test for delirium in medical ICU patients. *Psychosomatics.* 1996;37:533-546.
18. Massie MJ, Holland J, Glass E. Delirium in terminally ill cancer patients. *Am J Psychiatry.* 1983;140:1048-1050.
19. Breitbart W, Strout D. Delirium in the terminally ill. *Clin Geriatr Med.* 2000;16:357-372.
20. Bruera E, Miller L, McCallion J, Macmillan K, Krefting L, Hanson J. Cognitive failure in patients with terminal cancer: a prospective study. *J Pain Symptom Manage.* 1992;7:192-195.
21. Lawlor PG, Gagnon B, Mancini IL, et al. Occurrence, causes, and outcome of delirium in patients with advanced cancer: a prospective study. *Arch Intern Med.* 2000;160:786-794.
22. Gagnon P, Allard P, Masse B, DeSerres M. Delirium in terminal cancer: a prospective study using daily screening, early diagnosis, and continuous monitoring. *J Pain Symptom Manage.* 2000;19:412-426.
23. Thomas RI, Cameron DJ, Fahs MC. A prospective study of delirium and prolonged hospital stay. Exploratory study. *Arch Gen Psychiatry.* 1988;45:937-940.
24. Cole MG, Primeau FJ. Prognosis of delirium in elderly hospital patients. *CMAJ.* 1993;149:41-46.
25. Inouye SK. Delirium in hospitalized older patients: recognition and risk factors. *J Geriatr Psychiatry Neurol.* 1998;11:118-125; discussion 157-118.
26. Inouye SK. Delirium in hospitalized older patients. *Clinics in Geriatric Medicine.* 1998;14:745.
27. Inouye SK, Rushing JT, Foreman MD, Palmer RM, Pompei P. Does delirium contribute to poor hospital outcomes? A three-site epidemiologic study. *J Gen Intern Med.* 1998;13:234-242.

28. Trzepacz PT, Teague GB, Lipowski ZJ. Delirium and other organic mental disorders in a general hospital. *Gen Hosp Psychiatry.* 1985;7:101-106.

29. Inouye SK. The dilemma of delirium: clinical and research controversies regarding diagnosis and evaluation of delirium in hospitalized elderly medical patients. *Am J Med.* 1994;97: 278-288.

30. Maltoni M, Amadori D. Prognosis in advanced cancer. *Hematol Oncol Clin North Am.* 2002;16:715-729.

31. Casarett DJ, Inouye SK. Diagnosis and management of delirium near the end of life. *Ann Intern Med.* 2001;135:32-40.

32. Cole MG, Ciampi A, Belzile E, Zhong L. Persistent delirium in older hospital patients: a systematic review of frequency and prognosis. *Age Ageing.* 2009;38:19-26.

33. Kiely DK, Marcantonio ER, Inouye SK, et al. Persistent delirium predicts greater mortality. *J Am Geriatr Soc.* 2009;57:55-61.

34. Fainsinger R, Bruera E. Treatment of delirium in a terminally ill patient. *J Pain Symptom Manage.* 1992;7:54-56.

35. Morita T, Tsunoda J, Inoue S, Chihara S. Survival prediction of terminally ill cancer patients by clinical symptoms: development of a simple indicator. *Jpn J Clin Oncol.* 1999;29: 156-159.

36. Bruera E, Fainsinger RL, Miller MJ, Kuehn N. The assessment of pain intensity in patients with cognitive failure: a preliminary report. *J Pain Symptom Manage.* 1992;7:267-270.

37. Fainsinger R, Miller MJ, Bruera E, Hanson J, Maceachern T. Symptom control during the last week of life on a palliative care unit. *J Palliat Care.* 1991;7:5-11.

38. Coyle N, Breitbart W, Weaver S, Portenoy R. Delirium as a contributing factor to "crescendo" pain: three case reports. *J Pain Symptom Manage.* 1994;9:44-47.

39. Namba M, Morita T, Imura C, Kiyohara E, Ishikawa S, Hirai K. Terminal delirium: families' experience. *Palliat Med.* 2007;21:587-594.

40. Morita T, Akechi T, Ikenaga M, et al. Terminal delirium: recommendations from bereaved families' experiences. *J Pain Symptom Manage.* 2007;34:579-589.

41. Bruera E, Bush SH, Willey J, et al. Impact of delirium and recall on the level of distress in patients with advanced cancer and their family caregivers. *Cancer.* 2009;115:2004-2012.

42. Cohen MZ, Pace EA, Kaur G, Bruera E. Delirium in advanced cancer leading to distress in patients and family caregivers. *J Palliat Care.* 2009;25:164-171.

43. Breitbart W, Gibson C, Tremblay A. The delirium experience: delirium recall and delirium-related distress in hospitalized patients with cancer, their spouses/caregivers, and their nurses. *Psychosomatics.* 2002;43:183-194.

44. Breitbart W, Marotta R, Platt MM, et al. A double-blind trial of haloperidol, chlorpromazine, and lorazepam in the treatment of delirium in hospitalized AIDS patients. *Am J Psychiatry.* 1996;153:231-237.

45. Gaudreau JD, Gagnon P, Harel F, Roy MA, Tremblay A. Psychoactive medications and risk of delirium in hospitalized cancer patients. *J Clin Oncol.* 2005;23:6712-6718.

46. Gaudreau JD, Gagnon P, Roy MA, Harel F, Tremblay A. Opioid medications and longitudinal risk of delirium in hospitalized cancer patients. *Cancer.* 2007;109:2365-2373.

47. Bruera E, Macmillan K, Hanson J, MacDonald RN. The cognitive effects of the administration of narcotic analgesics in patients with cancer pain. *Pain.* 1989;39:13-16.

48. Stiefel FC, Breitbart WS, Holland JC. Corticosteroids in cancer: neuropsychiatric complications. *Cancer Invest.* 1989;7:479-491.

49. Han L, McCusker J, Cole M, Abrahamowicz M, Primeau F, Elie M. Use of medications with anticholinergic effect predicts clinical severity of delirium symptoms in older medical inpatients. *Arch Intern Med.* 2001;161:1099-1105.

50. Ancelin ML, Artero S, Portet F, Dupuy AM, Touchon J, Ritchie K. Non-degenerative mild cognitive impairment in elderly people and use of anticholinergic drugs: longitudinal cohort study. *BMJ.* 2006;332:455-459.

51. Morita T, Tei Y, Tsunoda J, Inoue S, Chihara S. Underlying pathologies and their associations with clinical features in terminal delirium of cancer patients. *J Pain Symptom Manage.* 2001;22:997-1006.

52. Levenson JL. *Textbook of Psychosomatic Medicine.* Washington, DC: American Psychiatric Publishing; 2005:xxi, 1092 p.

53. Irwin SA, Rao S, Bower KA, et al. Psychiatric issues in palliative care: recognition of *delirium* in patients enrolled in hospice care. *Palliat Support Care.* 2008;6:159-164.

54. Schuurmans MJ, Deschamps PI, Markham SW, Shortridge-Baggett LM, Duursma SA. The measurement of delirium: review of scales. *Res Theory Nurs Pract.* 2003;17:207-224.

55. Inouye SK, van Dyck CH, Alessi CA, Balkin S, Siegal AP, Horwitz RI. Clarifying confusion: the confusion assessment method. A new method for detection of delirium. *Ann Intern Med.* 1990;113:941-948.

56. Inouye SK. *The Confusion Assessment Method (CAM): Training Manual and Coding Guide.* Yale University School of Medicine, New Haven Connecticut 2003.

57. Ryan K, Leonard M, Guerin S, Donnelly S, Conroy M, Meagher D. Validation of the confusion assessment method in the palliative care setting. *Palliat Med.* 2009;23:40-45.

58. *Diagnostic and Statistical Manual of Mental Disorders: DSM-IV.* Washington, DC: American Psychiatric Association; 1994: 886.

59. Cook IA. Guideline watch: practice guideline for the treatment of patients with delirium. Updated 2004. http://psychiatryonline.org/content.aspx?bookid=28&sectionid=1681952

60. Bickley LS, Szilagyi PG, Bates B. *Bates' Guide to Physical Examination and History Taking.* Philadelphia, PA: Lippincott Williams & Wilkins; 2007.

61. Trzepacz PT, Mittal D, Torres R, Kanary K, Norton J, Jimerson N. Validation of the delirium rating scale-revised-98: comparison with the delirium rating scale and the cognitive test for delirium. *J Neuropsychiatry Clin Neurosci.* 2001;13:229-242.

62. Trzepacz PT. The Delirium Rating Scale. Its use in consultation-liaison research. *Psychosomatics.* 1999;40:193-204.

63. Turkel SB, Braslow K, Tavare CJ, Trzepacz PT. The delirium rating scale in children and adolescents. *Psychosomatics.* 2003;44:126-129.

64. Breitbart W, Rosenfeld B, Roth A, Smith MJ, Cohen K, Passik S. The memorial delirium assessment scale. *J Pain Symptom Manage.* 1997;13:128-137.

65. Ely EW, Inouye SK, Bernard GR, et al. Delirium in mechanically ventilated patients: validity and reliability of the confusion assessment method for the intensive care unit (CAM-ICU). *JAMA.* 2001;286:2703-2710.

66. Smith HA, Fuchs DC, Pandharipande PP, Barr FE, Ely EW. Delirium: an emerging frontier in the management of critically ill children. *Crit Care Clin.* 2009;25:593-614, x.

67. Truman B, Ely EW. Monitoring delirium in critically ill patients. Using the confusion assessment method for the intensive care unit. *Crit Care Nurse.* 2003;23:25-36; quiz 37-28.

68. Neelon VJ, Champagne MT, Carlson JR, Funk SG. The NEECHAM confusion scale: construction, validation, and clinical testing. Nursing Research: November/December 1996;45(6):324-330.

69. Gaudreau JD, Gagnon P, Harel F, Tremblay A, Roy MA. Fast, systematic, and continuous delirium assessment in hospitalized patients: the nursing delirium screening scale. *J Pain Symptom Manage.* 2005;29:368-375.

70. Folstein MF, Folstein SE, McHugh PR. "Mini-mental state". A practical method for grading the cognitive state of patients for the clinician. *J Psychiatr Res.* 1975;12:189-198.

71. Folstein MF, Folstein SE, McHugh PR, Fanjiang G. *Mini-Mental State Examination User's Guide.* Odessa, FL: Psychological Assessment Resources; 2001.

72. Task Force for the Handbook of Psychiatric Measures. *Handbook of Psychiatric Measures.* Washington, DC: American Psychiatric Association; 2000:820.

73. Irwin SA, Ferris FD. The opportunity for psychiatry in palliative care. *Can J Psychiatry.* 2008;53:713-724.

74. Ferris FD, Danilychev M, Siegel A. Last hours of living. In: Emanuel LL, Librach SL, eds. *Palliative Care: Core Skills and Clinical Competencies.* Philadelphia, PA: Saunders Elsevier; 2007:267-293.

75. Emanuel EJ, Ferris FD, von Gunten CF, von Roenn J. *Education in Palliative and End-of-Life Care for Oncology.* The EPEC project. Chicago; 2005.

76. von Gunten CF, Sloan PA, Portenoy RK, Schonwetter RS. Physician board certification in hospice and palliative medicine. *J Palliat Med.* 2000;3:441-447.

77. Emanuel LL, Librach SL. *Palliative Care: Core Skills and Clinical Competencies.* Philadelphia, PA: Saunders/Elsevier; 2007.

78. Ferris FD, Balfour HM, Bowen K, et al. A model to guide patient and family care: based on nationally accepted principles and norms of practice. *J Pain Symptom Manage.* 2002;24:106-123.

79. Leonard M, Raju B, Conroy M, et al. Reversibility of delirium in terminally ill patients and predictors of mortality. *Palliat Med.* 2008;22:848-854.

80. Ferris FD. Last hours of living. *Clin Geriatr Med.* 2004;20:641-667.

81. Rao S, Ferris FD, Irwin SA. Ease of screening for depression and delirium in patients enrolled in inpatient hospice care. *J Palliat Med.* 2011;14:275-279.

82. Breibart WS, Gibson C, Chochinov H. Palliative care. In: Levenson JL, ed. *Textbook of Psychosomatic Medicine.* Washington, DC: American Psychiatric Publishing; 2005:979-1007.

83. Lawlor PG, Bruera ED. Delirium in patients with advanced cancer. *Hematol Oncol Clin North Am.* 2002;16:701-714.

84. Breitbart W, Cohen K. Delirium in the terminally ill. In: Chochinov HM, Breitbart W, eds. *Handbook of Psychiatry in Palliative Medicine.* New York, NY: Oxford University Press; 2000:435.

85. de Stoutz ND, Bruera E, Suarez-Almazor M. Opioid rotation for toxicity reduction in terminal cancer patients. *J Pain Symptom Manage.* 1995;10:378-384.

86. Plonk WM Jr, Arnold RM. Terminal care: the last weeks of life. *J Palliat Med.* 2005;8:1042-1054.

87. Tang ST. Supporting cancer patients dying at home or at a hospital for Taiwanese family caregivers. *Cancer Nurs.* 2009;32:151-157.

88. Cole MG, Primeau FJ, Bailey RF, et al. Systematic intervention for elderly inpatients with delirium: a randomized trial. *CMAJ.* 1994;151:965-970.

89. Cole MG, McCusker J, Bellavance F, et al. Systematic detection and multidisciplinary care of delirium in older medical inpatients: a randomized trial. *CMAJ.* 2002;167:753-759.

90. Pitkala KH, Laurila JV, Strandberg TE, Tilvis RS. Multicomponent geriatric intervention for elderly inpatients with delirium: a randomized, controlled trial. *J Gerontol A Biol Sci Med Sci.* 2006;61:176-181.

91. Pitkala KH, Laurila JV, Strandberg TE, Kautiainen H, Sintonen H, Tilvis RS. Multicomponent geriatric intervention for elderly inpatients with delirium: effects on costs and health-related quality of life. *J Gerontol A Biol Sci Med Sci.* 2008;63:56-61.

92. Inouye SK, Bogardus ST Jr, Charpentier PA, et al. A multicomponent intervention to prevent delirium in hospitalized older patients. *N Engl J Med.* 1999;340:669-676.

93. Bruera E, Belzile M, Watanabe S, Fainsinger RL. Volume of hydration in terminal cancer patients. *Support Care Cancer.* 1996;4:147-150.

94. Dalal S, Bruera E. Dehydration in cancer patients: to treat or not to treat. *J Support Oncol.* 2004;2:467-479, 483.

95. Steiner N, Bruera E. Methods of hydration in palliative care patients. *J Palliat Care.* 1998;14:6-13.

96. Inouye SK, Zhang Y, Jones RN, Kiely DK, Yang F, Marcantonio ER. Risk factors for delirium at discharge: development and validation of a predictive model. *Arch Intern Med.* 2007;167:1406-1413.

97. Gagnon P, Charbonneau C, Allard P, Soulard C, Dumont S, Fillion L. Delirium in advanced cancer: a psychoeducational intervention for family caregivers. *J Palliat Care.* 2002;18:253-261.

98. Inouye SK, Bogardus ST Jr, Williams CS, Leo-Summers L, Agostini JV. The role of adherence on the effectiveness of nonpharmacologic interventions: evidence from the delirium prevention trial. *Arch Intern Med.* 2003;163:958-964.

99. Agar M, Currow D, Plummer J, Chye R, Draper B. Differing management of people with advanced cancer and delirium by four sub-specialties. *Palliat Med.* 2008;22:633-640.

100. Rundell JR, Wise MG, Press AP. *Essentials of Consultation-Liaison Psychiatry: Based on the American Psychiatric Press Textbook of Consultation-Liaison Psychiatry.* Washington, DC: American Psychiatric Press; 1999:xxi, 671 p.

101. Stahl SM. *Stahl's Essential Psychopharmacology: Neuroscientific Basis and Practical Applications.* Cambridge; New York, NY: Cambridge University Press; 2008:1117.

102. Boettger S, Breitbart W. An open trial of aripiprazole for the treatment of delirium in hospitalized cancer patients. *Palliat Support Care.* 2011;9:351-357.

103. Skrobik YK, Bergeron N, Dumont M, Gottfried SB. Olanzapine vs haloperidol: treating delirium in a critical care setting. *Intensive Care Med.* 2004;30:444-449.

104. Sipahimalani A, Masand PS. Olanzapine in the treatment of delirium. *Psychosomatics.* 1998;39:422-430.

105. Han CS, Kim YK. A double-blind trial of risperidone and haloperidol for the treatment of delirium. *Psychosomatics.* 2004;45:297-301.

106. Bottomley DM, Hanks GW. Subcutaneous midazolam infusion in palliative care. *J Pain Symptom Manage.* 1990;5:259-261.

107. Rousseau P. Palliative sedation in the management of refractory symptoms. *J Support Oncol.* 2004;2:181-186.

108. Rousseau P. Palliative sedation in the control of refractory symptoms. *J Palliat Med.* 2005;8:10-12.

109. Morita T, Tei Y, Inoue S. Agitated terminal delirium and association with partial opioid substitution and hydration. *J Palliat Med*. 2003;6:557-563.

110. Stiefel F, Fainsinger R, Bruera E. Acute confusional states in patients with advanced cancer. *J Pain Symptom Manage*. 1992;7:94-98.

111. Ventafridda V, Ripamonti C, De Conno F, Tamburini M, Cassileth BR. Symptom prevalence and control during cancer patients' last days of life. *J Palliat Care*. 1990;6:7-11.

112. Fainsinger RL, Waller A, Bercovici M, et al. A multicentre international study of sedation for uncontrolled symptoms in terminally ill patients. *Palliat Med*. 2000;14:257-265.

113. Rietjens JA, van Zuylen L, van Veluw H, van der Wijk L, van der Heide A, van der Rijt CC. Palliative sedation in a specialized unit for acute palliative care in a cancer hospital: comparing patients dying with and without palliative sedation. *J Pain Symptom Manage*. 2008;36:228-234.

114. Connor SR, Pyenson B, Fitch K, Spence C, Iwasaki K. Comparing hospice and nonhospice patient survival among patients who die within a three-year window. *J Pain Symptom Manage*. 2007;33:238-246.

115. Sykes N, Thorns A. Sedative use in the last week of life and the implications for end-of-life decision making. *Arch Intern Med*. 2003;163:341-344.

116. Vitetta L, Kenner D, Sali A. Sedation and analgesia-prescribing patterns in terminally ill patients at the end of life. *Am J Hosp Palliat Care*. 2005;22:465-473.

117. Morita T, Chinone Y, Ikenaga M, et al. Efficacy and safety of palliative sedation therapy: a multicenter, prospective, observational study conducted on specialized palliative care units in Japan. *J Pain Symptom Manage*. 2005;30:320-328.

118. Good PD, Ravenscroft PJ, Cavenagh J. Effects of opioids and sedatives on survival in an Australian inpatient palliative care population. *Intern Med J*. 2005;35:512-517.

119. Bercovitch M, Adunsky A. Patterns of high-dose morphine use in a home-care hospice service: should we be afraid of it? *Cancer*. 2004;101:1473-1477.

120. Bercovitch M, Waller A, Adunsky A. High dose morphine use in the hospice setting. A database survey of patient characteristics and effect on life expectancy. *Cancer*. 1999;86:871-877.

121. Portenoy RK, Sibirceva U, Smout R, et al. Opioid use and survival at the end of life: a survey of a hospice population. *J Pain Symptom Manage*. 2006;32:532-540.

122. Stirling LC, Kurowska A, Tookman A. The use of phenobarbitone in the management of agitation and seizures at the end of life. *J Pain Symptom Manage*. 1999;17:363-368.

123. Lundstrom S, Zachrisson U, Furst CJ. When nothing helps: propofol as sedative and antiemetic in palliative cancer care. *J Pain Symptom Manage*. 2005;30:570-577.

124. Lundstrom S, Twycross R, Mihalyo M, Wilcock A. Propofol. *J Pain Symptom Manage*. 2010;40:466-470.

125. Schatzberg AF, Cole JO, DeBattista C. *Manual of Clinical Psychopharmacology*. Washington, DC: American Psychiatric Publishing; 2007:xxv, 697 p.

126. Clinical Pharmacology Online. Updated 2008. http://www.clinicalpharmacology-ipcom/defaultaspx

127. Allen MH, Currier GW, Hughes DH, Reyes-Harde M, Docherty JP. The expert consensus guideline series. Treatment of behavioral emergencies. *Postgrad Med*. 2001;1-88; quiz 89-90.

128. Wise MG, Rundell JR. *Clinical Manual of Psychosomatic Medicine: A Guide to Consultation-Liaison Psychiatry*. Arlington, VA: American Psychiatric Publishing; 2005:xi, 338 p.

129. Richelson E. Preclinical pharmacology of neuroleptics: focus on new generation compounds. *J Clin Psychiatry*. 1996;57(suppl 11):4-11.

130. Jackson KC, Lipman AG. Drug therapy for delirium in terminally ill patients. *Cochrane Database Syst Rev*. 2004:(2); CD004770.

131. Lonergan E, Britton Annette M, Luxenberg J. *Antipsychotics for Delirium*. Cochrane Database of Systematic Reviews. Chichester, UK: Wiley; 2007.

132. Wang PS, Schneeweiss S, Avorn J, et al. Risk of death in elderly users of conventional vs. atypical antipsychotic medications. *N Engl J Med*. 2005;353:2335-2341.

133. Ballard C, Hanney ML, Theodoulou M, et al. The dementia antipsychotic withdrawal trial (DART-AD): long-term follow-up of a randomised placebo-controlled trial. *Lancet Neurol*. 2009;8:151-157.

134. Ray WA, Chung CP, Murray KT, Hall K, Stein CM. Atypical antipsychotic drugs and the risk of sudden cardiac death. *N Engl J Med*. 2009;360:225-235.

135. Gill SS, Bronskill SE, Normand S-LT, et al. Antipsychotic drug use and mortality in older adults with dementia. *Ann Intern Med*. 2007;146:775-786.

136. Schneeweiss S, Setoguchi S, Brookhart A, Dormuth C, Wang PS. Risk of death associated with the use of conventional versus atypical antipsychotic drugs among elderly patients. *CMAJ*. 2007;176:627-632.

137. Schneider LS, Dagerman KS, Insel P. Risk of death with atypical antipsychotic drug treatment for dementia: meta-analysis of randomized placebo-controlled trials. *JAMA*. 2005;294:1934-1943.

138. Jeste DV, Blazer D, Casey D, et al. ACNP White paper: update on use of antipsychotic drugs in elderly persons with dementia. *Neuropsychopharmacology*. 2008;33:957-970.

139. Elie D, Poirier M, Chianetta J, Durand M, Gregoire C, Grignon S. Cognitive effects of antipsychotic dosage and polypharmacy: a study with the BACS in patients with schizophrenia and schizoaffective disorder. *J Psychopharmacol*. 2010;24:1037-1044.

140. Schneider LS, Tariot PN, Dagerman KS, et al. Effectiveness of atypical antipsychotic drugs in patients with Alzheimer's disease. *N Engl J Med*. 2006;355:1525-1538.

141. Saad M, Cassagnol M, Ahmed E. The impact of FDA's warning on the use of antipsychotics in clinical practice: a survey. *Consultant Pharm*. 2010;25:739-744.

CHAPTER 41

Treating Depression at the End of Life

Donna B. Greenberg

DEPRESSION

Sadness is a natural emotion in the setting of illness and particularly grave illness. Sickness stands in the way of a person's pursuit of life dreams and starkly defines mortality and vulnerability. It is not surprising to find a sick person uncomfortable, frustrated, irritable, and blue. The healer's challenge is to find the right techniques in the armamentarium to relieve suffering and to allow the patient's life force to go forward with the patient's unique style and individual values.

Since patients come for help when they are overwhelmed or worried about being overwhelmed, we facilitate the patient's ability to cope with the challenge of illness and augment the ability to make choices about the life that remains. We do this ideally by treating each patient with respect and attention. That respect and furthermore, the appreciation of who the patient is, supports the patient's morale and self-esteem and sustains the ability to hope (1).

In that process, we are supporting the patient's ability to sustain a desirable self-image. We allow each patient to find a path to more control or more influence over the world. This goal or sense of purpose contributes to the value of life whether it is framed by a day or a week or a year.

In the process of normal coping, particularly at times of transitions, patients variably acknowledge the facts of the illness, the implications, and mortality. Choices must be made in the presence of an illness and life continues. Acknowledgment may be private, connected to intimates, or perhaps public; but acknowledgment of mortality clearly has a social dimension with implications for the patient and those connected to the patient.

The healer must learn with the patient the facts of the illness, implications for the patient, and how these relate to survival or death. If we understand the medical predicament, we can help by clarification of what is known. Reliable and pertinent information can be organized and sought from the appropriate medical specialists. Often a great deal of unknown remains and in that we find possibility.

It helps the physician to have a sense of the time course of the illness, its treatment, plateaus, and setbacks. In emergencies, patients cope with what is most immediate. Complex implications are put to the back. Sometimes emotions and fuller understanding of the personal dimension of illness are put aside until the long marathon of initial anti-cancer surgery, radiation treatment, and chemotherapy has been completed. Changes in status with new losses set new

emergencies and then more subtle, subsequent complex coping. The interpersonal crisis, the challenge of getting medical care, and the effects on family or work occur over this longitudinal trajectory.

Depressive symptoms are common. In 365 patients with advanced gastrointestinal and lung cancers, depressive symptoms were assessed longitudinally every 2 months (2). Mild depressive symptoms were seen in 35% of patients with 16% having moderate to severe symptoms. At first, about 5% had persistent moderate to severe depressive symptoms. Compared with the setting of patients more than 1 year before death, the prevalence of moderate to severe symptoms tripled in the final 3 months of life. Those who were more apt to have depressive symptoms were younger, had a greater physical burden of disease, and had greater proximity to death. They were the patients more apt to have been treated with antidepressants before the study with lower self-esteem and less sense of spiritual well-being, greater anguish about rejection and abandonment, and greater hopelessness.

The convergence of physical and mental symptoms was ultimately associated with the highest risk of depression (2), suggesting that the growing physical symptom burden over time has psychological consequences manifest in cognitive and affective symptoms. Here, depressive symptoms are seen as a final common pathway of distress, particularly in those who have psychosocial vulnerability and greater physical symptoms before death.

Against this backdrop of normal coping with illness, we discuss the nature of depression, the different syndromes that overlap, and the value of diagnosis and treatment.

Major Depressive Disorder

Major depressive disorder is a defined neuropsychiatric syndrome that has been extensively studied separate from major medical illness and cancer. As wheezing is the symptom of asthma, an element of the serious, relapsing condition of asthmatic illness, depressive symptoms are elements of the serious relapsing condition of major depressive disorder. On its own without medical illness, depressive disorder is a painful, anguishing state with serious morbidity and mortality. We have no laboratory test for the condition, and its presence is all the more difficult to diagnose in the setting of other causes of the mental and physical symptoms. However, because it is serious and treatable, it should not be missed.

The official diagnosis refers to a condition of key symptoms, which included depressed mood or loss of interest or pleasure in what is usually pleasurable, that persists 2 weeks or more, accompanied by 5 or more secondary signs or symptoms:

(a) thoughts of death, suicidal ideation, or action
(b) reduced concentration or indecisiveness
(c) worthlessness or inordinate guilt
(d) fatigue
(e) psychomotor agitation or retardation
(f) insomnia or hypersomnia
(g) weight loss or gain

Because the vegetative or physical symptoms have multiple causes, different approaches to the list of symptoms in diagnosis have been suggested (3). A combination of the exclusive, substitutive, etiologic, or inclusive approaches is more apt to be used in clinical practice. The inclusive approach uses all symptoms of depression regardless of whether they are secondary to a physical illness. The etiologic approach counts as symptoms of depression only those symptoms that are clearly not the result of the physical illness. The substitutive approach replaces symptoms that may relate to physical illness with added cognitive symptoms like indecisiveness, hopelessness, and pessimism. Endicott proposed that appetite, sleep disturbance, fatigue, or poor concentration be substituted by other criteria: a tearful or depressed appearance, social withdrawal, brooding self-pity, or inability to be cheered up (4). The exclusive approach eliminates two common symptoms of depression, fatigue, and appetite or weight change and uses only the other symptoms. The etiologic and substitutive approaches together obtained a lower prevalence rate and more reliable diagnosis than any one approach used alone (3). Each approach has its own merit (5).

The lifetime prevalence of major depressive disorder is 16.2% and the 12-month prevalence is 6.6% in adults (6). It is more common in women than in men, with a risk ratio of 1.7 to 1.0 over a lifetime and 1.4 to 1.0 for 12 months. Risk factors include personal or family history of depressive disorder, prior suicide attempts, lack of social supports, stressful life events, and current substance abuse. More than 50% of those who have one episode have another (7). The second episode is often within 2 years, but the majority (75%) of recurrences occur within 10 years (8).

The prevalence of depression in cancer patients has a wide range (9). It makes sense that lifetime history and past personal history of major depressive disorder would raise the threshold of suspicion for depression in a patient with advanced medical illness. For instance, Pirl et al. found that past history of major depressive disorder was a predictor of clinical depression in men with prostate cancer on antiandrogen treatment (10).

Depression adds to the gravity of medical illness. In patients with medical illness, major depressive disorder and even sub-threshold depression have higher mortality rates (11). Medical illness, past depression, and present depression predict in-hospital mortality (12). Over the course of a chronic illness like cancer, depression is associated with more functional impairment and poorer quality of life (13,14).

Major depressive disorder puts a veil of negativity on perception; patients say that they are under a cloud. The hopelessness and persistent suicidal thoughts of depressed terminally ill patients may affect choices in care (15). Untreated depression can lead to earlier admission to hospice or inpatient care (16). Oncology outpatients are more apt to hoard drugs to prepare for a possible suicide attempt due to major depressive disorder even more than pain (17). Even when depressed, patients with cancer can express a convincing benefit analysis of the burdens of continued life despite hopelessness, poor self-esteem, and pessimism (18). Because of the ambiguity of the presentation of major depressive disorder, even physicians who know what clinical depression looks like, the majority of Oregon psychiatrists, did not think that they could in a single evaluation adequately assess whether a psychiatric disorder was impairing the judgment of a patient desiring assisted suicide (19). We do know, however, that antidepressant treatment of hospitalized depressed patients can alter the patient's outlook and, therefore, the desire for death (20).

The nature of depressive illness itself, thoughts of hopelessness and worthlessness, inhibits active pursuit of care for the depressive syndrome, impairs adherence to a treatment, and affects the ability of the patient to recognize what is emotional distortion rather than cancer itself. Oncology staff deal with many patients who are unhappy about their predicament, and the staff do not always have the conviction that treating those with major depressive disorder will make a difference. Often cancer physicians do not ask, and patients with cancer do not tell. They do not want their physicians to give up on them or to see them as crazy or weak (21,22). The patients themselves may never have had cancer before and attribute dysphoria to the knowledge of the diagnosis and difficulty of treatment rather than to clinical depression itself.

Suicidal Thoughts

The desire for hastened death, death sooner than natural disease progression, and passive or active suicidal wishes in the setting of advanced disease are associated with depressive disorder and its feature of hopelessness. Chochinov et al. found that 8.5% of those admitted to the hospital for terminal illness in Canada wished to die sooner and most were depressed (15).

Some ambulatory cancer patients do have thoughts that they would be better off dead or the thoughts of hurting themselves. One study of almost 3,000 patients in Scotland found that 8% reported such thoughts in the previous 2 weeks (23). Those patients with suicidal thoughts were more apt to have clinically significant emotional distress, substantial pain, and to a lesser extent older age.

In the setting of a cancer diagnosis, the likelihood of suicide is greatest when the diagnosis is new and when it seems to the patient more likely to be advanced and progressive. The most common cancers associated with suicide are lung, stomach, oral cavity and pharynx, larynx, and pancreatic cancers. Even with pancreatic cancer, which had the highest rate, however, suicide is extremely rare (24,25). The presence of suicidal thoughts should directly lead to further assessment of the diagnosis of depressive disorder.

The narrowed thinking that comes with depression makes it harder to see any window of light or any sense that an individual's life matters. Often intoxicants like alcohol or the medications for a medical illness like narcotics contribute to impulsivity and distortions of thinking.

Questions about the wish to die should be part of a basic evaluation of depression. The seriousness and persistence of the thoughts and the seriousness of a plan convey the gravity of the danger for a patient. Safety is a priority. Sometimes, the idea of suicide offers patients a sense of ultimate control over a worse fate, untreated pain or helplessness, and loss of respect in illness. The caretakers' attention to relief of pain, to hearing the patient out, to amplifying the patient's control as much as possible has value. Evaluation and treatment for clinical depression, a syndrome that comes with suicidal thoughts even when patients are not physically ill, is critical. If there has been a suicide attempt, understanding what made the patient think that suicide was the best choice can open a dialogue. In the setting of depression, thinking is pessimistic and distorted. Self-esteem is small. Patients may acutely underestimate their ability to cope and underestimate what can be done, room for hope, and the caring of loved ones. Medical intervention to increase comfort, to treat depression, and to change the psychosocial reality becomes paramount.

Delirium

Patients with clinical depression have a hard time concentrating and persisting in concentration. They may not read the newspaper or follow their favorite team as usual. However, usually when pressed to do basic cognitive functions, they are able to. In the setting of systemic illness, multiple medications, including especially narcotics and benzodiazepines, the likelihood of syndromes of cognitive impairment increases. The lack of function that comes with cognitive impairment may be misunderstood as depression. Once confusion is documented, medical interventions or reduction in medication to improve cognition becomes the first priority.

Malaise

Sickness, that is, anything that causes injury and inflammation, triggers cytokines and sickness behavior that can mimic the vegetative somatic symptoms of major depressive disorder (26). Malaise is the syndrome associated with fever or flu syndromes like the syndrome caused by interferon treatment. It is listlessness, inability to concentrate, hypersomnia, social withdrawal, anorexia, loss of interest, and poor grooming. Interleukin (IL)-1 and tumor necrosis factor foster slow wave sleep. Proinflammatory cytokines, IL-α and IL-β, tumor necrosis factor-α, and IL-6, generally, can trigger a constellation of behavioral changes that include fatigue, sleep disturbance, and depressive-like symptoms in animal models. There is a fatigue syndrome that follows procedures like surgery and radiation treatment. Bower et al. found that among breast cancer patients after the complex initial multi-modal treatment of the first year, 25% had depressive symptoms

and 60% were fatigued. Fatigue was associated with soluble tumor necrosis factor receptor II levels and with recent treatment with chemotherapy. Depressive symptoms were associated with fatigue but not with inflammatory markers. These data support the idea that systemic chemotherapy is followed by a somatic fatigue syndrome characterized by inflammation that is distinct from the fatigue of major depressive disorder (27).

The fatigue of depression is typically associated with a sense of effort, a dread of the day, and insomnia, rather than the sleepiness and lack of stamina that come with the fatigue of sickness behavior.

Demoralization

Demoralization is a condition seen in medically ill patients, experienced as existential despair, hopelessness, helplessness, and loss of meaning and purpose in life. According to Clark and Kissane, who wrote about this syndrome and its history in the setting of those with advanced illness, this condition is distinguished from depression by the emphasis on a feeling of subjective incompetence rather than anhedonia. Its hallmark is hopelessness and the wish to die. The demoralized "feel inhibited in action by not knowing what to do, feeling helpless and incompetent, in the face of uncertainty, a failure of knowing how to cope" (28). Kissane et al. have developed a scale with distinct dimensions of loss of meaning, dysphoria, disheartenment, helplessness, and sense of failure (29). Demoralization has been seen as a normal response to adversity analogous to grief. These authors called upon Frank's description of demoralization in combat soldiers (30) and Schmale and Engel's giving up–given up complex (31). Griffith and Gaby (32) suggested that a pragmatic explanation of demoralization in medically ill patients is a set of different existential postures that position a patient to retreat from the challenges of illness. Helplessness, despair, or meaninglessness may to different degrees combine in contributing to the sense of subjective incompetence. Shader (33) noted that it is difficult to distinguish the presence or absence of depressive disorder in the demoralized patient since such a patient would feel more helpless in the presence of a persistent negative mood. He argued that the recognition of demoralization implies, beyond somatic treatments, that the clinician must work with patients to promote a sense of mastery and return of hope.

Melancholia

Melancholia is a distinct syndrome within the diagnosis of major depressive disorder that has a long history. It is a particularly severe form of depressive disorder. Its importance in the setting of cancer and progressive illness is its distinct features, which may be misdiagnosed as progressive medical illness. Whether melancholia should be separated from major depressive disorder within the newest lexicon of diagnosis has been discussed (34). The key features are disturbances in affect disproportionate to stressors, marked by unremitting apprehension and morbid statements, blunted emotional response, nonreactive mood, and pervasive anhedonia, regardless of improved circumstances. The risk of recurrence and suicide is high. Psychomotor findings, retardation (slowed thought, movement, and speech and anergia) or spontaneous agitation (motor restlessness and stereotypic movements and speech) are common. Cognitive impairment with reduced concentration and working memory are noted. Psychotic features are often present with nihilistic conviction of hopelessness, guilt, sin, and ruin. While the usual vegetative problems in sleep, appetite, and libido are prominent, symptoms are especially worse in the morning and get better as the day goes on. Melancholia is thought to be more responsive to electroconvulsive treatment and to broad action antidepressants rather than pure serotonin reuptake inhibitors (SSRIs). Antipsychotics and electroconvulsive treatment may have a role.

Specific Anti-cancer Drugs Inducing Depression

The majority of cancer treatments do not directly cause a destabilization of mood. The exceptions are two treatments that destabilize mood, namely corticosteroids and interferon. Drugs that lead to estrogen withdrawal can also be associated with mood disorder.

Corticosteroids. Corticosteroids, particularly dexamethasone and prednisone, are used in anti-cancer treatments. These include protocols, for instance, anti-lymphoma protocols, prednisone 100 mg each day for 5 days in CHOP (cyclophosphamide, adriamycin, vincristine, and prednisone); dexamethasone to treat central nervous system edema, dexamethasone as an anti-emetic for acute chemotherapy-related nausea and delayed nausea associated with cisplatin, and prevention of hypersensitivity to taxanes. In general, psychiatric side effects are common with a dose above prednisone 60 mg or the parallel potency dexamethasone 9 mg. Depression can occur with addition of steroids or as they are tapered. Lability of mood is often seen.

Interferon. The depressive syndrome associated with alpha-interferon develops insidiously over weeks or months. It responds to serotonergic antidepressants, like paroxetine, and can be prevented (35). Manic state has been observed, usually during interferon dose reductions or pauses in therapy or as interferon-induced depression is treated with antidepressants. Nearly all patients develop adverse effects on memory after six doses of therapy in the doses used for advanced melanoma. Generally, mild to moderate neuropsychiatric symptoms resolve in 2 to 3 weeks of interferon discontinuation (36,37).

Tamoxifen and Other Contributors to Menopause. The late transition in menopause is associated with a greater risk of depression (38). Some women are more sensitive to withdrawal or fluctuations of female hormones. Tamoxifen by inducing an anti-estrogenic state in the brain with hot flashes, insomnia, and dysphoria has the clearest record of association with depression. However, dysphoria can also result from aromatase inhibitors in a similar minority of patients (39).

Since tamoxifen has a complex metabolism, there has been some concern that drugs like paroxetine, fluoxetine, and bupropion, which cause 2D6 inhibition should not be used during tamoxifen treatment. This matter is in debate, but it is prudent to use an alternate agent like venlafaxine or citalopram and to minimize the use of bupropion unless the risk benefit ratio is considered.

Recognition and Treatment

Treatment of major depressive disorder in the setting of cancer or other systemic illness means persistent assessment of treatment approaches, medications and psychosocial interventions, and continuous monitoring of the effectiveness of treatment, so that treatments can be adjusted, combined, or diagnosis reconsidered.

Screening tests for depression have been used to advantage. A distress thermometer has been used widely to begin a conversation about the needs of the patient (40). The Zung Depression Scale was used in an Indiana oncology setting to trigger brief diagnostic interviews for assessment of the need for antidepressants (41,42). Strong et al. used the Physician's Health Questionnaire (PHQ) to follow severity of depression (43,44). The screening led to effective models to improve the outcome of depression care in oncology settings.

The Beck Depression Inventory (BDI) was used as a laboratory test in Australia (45) to call the attention of oncology staff to the diagnosis of depression. The BDI score reported immediately to an oncologist via a computer-generated patient report signaled them that a patient had moderate to severe depressive symptoms. Physicians who received these reports were more likely to offer the patient counseling. Six months later, the level of depression was significantly reduced in such patients compared with patients whose BDI scores of moderate/severe depression were not made known to their physicians. In the intervention group, 68% were offered counseling and 47% accepted.

Collaborative care for depression has been effective in the cancer setting. In a regional cancer centre in Scotland, United Kingdom, patients with cancer and major depressive disorder identified by screening were randomized to usual care or to an intervention delivered by a cancer nurse at the centre over an average of seven sessions. The intervention proved better than usual care, and the treatment effect was sustained at 6 and 12 months (44). In the United Kingdom, usual care includes both specialist cancer care and primary care. The primary care doctors of patients in the usual care group were told that their patients had major depressive disorder; so prescription of antidepressants was higher in both groups than commonly seen. Very few patients in either groups were referred to specialist mental health services (44).

The intervention used specially trained cancer nurses as care managers, supervised by psychiatrists. The goal was to maximize acceptability to patients and integration with existing medical care. Patients were excluded who had cancers with poor prognoses and who had treatment needs more appropriately met by readily available specialist psychiatric services, such as chronic depression that antedated the diagnosis of cancer. About 40% of eligible patients declined to take part. Patients in the intervention group were offered a maximum of 10 one-to-one sessions over 3 months, preferably in person at the cancer centre but occasionally by telephone or at patients' homes if they were unable to attend the centre. The content of the intervention comprised education about depression and its treatment, including antidepressant medication, problem-solving treatment to teach the patients coping strategies designed to overcome feelings of helplessness, and communication about management of major depressive disorder with each patient's oncologist and primary care doctor. For 3 months after treatment, session progress was monitored by monthly telephone calls. The Patient Health Questionnaire was used to assess the severity of depression. Each 45 minutes session was delivered by one of three cancer nurses who followed a detailed manual. All sessions were video recorded and 10% of sessions were randomly selected to be independently assessed for adherence to the manual. A psychiatrist reviewed patients' progress with the nurses every week. Nurses presented each patient's scores on the PHQ, their antidepressant dose, and their progress with problem-solving treatment. Primary care doctors prescribed the antidepressant medication. If the patient decided during discussion with the nurse to start or change antidepressant medication, they were encouraged to contact their primary care physician for this purpose. The patient's doctor was then contacted by the nurse by fax or telephone before their appointment to provide information about the patient and offer advice from a study psychiatrist. This study outlines the principles of a pragmatic method to insure quality of depression care in the oncology setting. The medical team must have the conviction that major depressive disorder is worth treating, must engage the patient in adherence to the drug regimen, and must continue to adjust the doses and types of antidepressants to maximize outcome and minimize side effects. The outcome is often best when medications are augmented with a psychosocial intervention that is integrated into their care.

Treatment

Antidepressants. Antidepressant medications succeed in treating major depressive disorder better than placebo even in cancer patients. This is the conclusion of evidence-based *Cochrane Reviews*, for cancer patients and for the medically ill (46). Most patients tolerated these medications. Only 1 of 10 patients dropped out of antidepressant treatment because of treatment with drug rather than placebo. The response rate was not affected by the severity of comorbid conditions (47).

For patients with major depressive disorder, antidepressant medications lead to a response, 50% reduction in symptoms, in two-thirds of patients compared with a third who may respond to placebo. The benefit occurs over 8 weeks in two-thirds, but some symptoms persist in half. Those who respond and continue medication are less likely to relapse compared with patients on placebo. When the standard is higher, a remission of all symptoms, one-third remit on the first antidepressant and two-thirds remit after a year of treatment with a sequence of four different antidepressants. Only 10% to 20% stay well if the

patient continues with placebo. The relapse rate is related to the completeness of response; the more complete the remission, the less likely the patient is to relapse. Younger patients (25–65) have the best chance at response. Therefore, antidepressants are more effective than placebo, 2 to 3 times better for acute treatment and 3 to 4 times better for continuation and maintenance. The same response rate generally applies for all drugs in the class of antidepressants (48).

Since any antidepressant has a fair chance of being effective, they should be chosen with their side-effect profile in mind. Initial side effects may be minimized by slow increase of dose. It takes perhaps 4 to 8 weeks to see a full benefit from these medications, so a commitment from the patient to persist beyond the negotiation of initial side effects becomes important.

SSRIs are common first-line agents. These include fluoxetine, sertraline, paroxetine, fluvoxamine, citalopram, and escitalopram. They are well tolerated. The most common initial side effects are nausea, headache, and appetite suppression. Occasionally, the drug causes diarrhea. There can be a brief period of anxiety. Many of these side effects remit with time. Slow initiation of dose can be helpful.

Fluoxetine and paroxetine are inhibitors of the P450 system and may interact with medications metabolized by those cytochromes. SSRIs have a well-established record in treating anxiety disorders as well.

Later side effects can include weight gain, but this is inconsistent. Delay in orgasm as well as decrease in sexual interest can be a feature. Since depression itself affects appetite and sexual interest, the benefits of treatment may outweigh the side effects of treatment. There are various methods of reducing side effects later. Sudden discontinuation of a drug of this class, particularly in those with a short half-life like paroxetine or venlafaxine is associated with a flu-like syndrome associated with paresthesias. The remedy is to restart the antidepressant or to use a pure SSRI like fluoxetine, which has a long half-life. These antidepressants can be slowly tapered if discontinuation is the goal.

Bupropion is a very effective dopaminergic antidepressant with a different side-effect profile. It is also used for smoking cessation. It can cause headache, jitteriness, or constipation, but not weight gain or sexual dysfunction. It has a risk of causing seizures in the setting of metabolic abnormalities or structural brain pathology.

Mirtazapine is a sedating antidepressant associated with weight gain. This may be the proper side-effect profile in a patient who is losing weight and not sleeping.

Serotonin–norepinephrine reuptake inhibitors like venlafaxine or duloxetine are also effective. These drugs have had benefit for neuropathic pain.

Tricyclic antidepressants are equally effective but used more infrequently in recent years. They have benefit for neuropathic pain and fibromyalgia so are more often added by neurologists or rheumatologists in low dose. They may be contributing antidepressant benefit and prevention of depressive episode recurrence. When discontinued, the patient may be more at risk of depression. Amitriptyline, nortriptyline, and desipramine are quinidine-like antiarrhythmics that can widen the QRS complex and prolong the QT interval and should not be used in patients with bundle branch blocks. They are anticholinergic and can cause postural hypotension. They are dangerous in overdose.

Any antidepressant may induce hypomania in a patient who is vulnerable. The tendency to become grandiose, irritable, talkative, preoccupied and hyperfocused on a specific goal, imprudently traveling, spending, not sleeping, and talking with hyperactivity should be recognized, particularly in those who have had this response in the past.

Psychostimulants, methylphenidate and dextroamphetamine, have been used in the medically ill to improve concentration and attention, mood, and energy. They have the advantage of a quick effect. Recent meta-analyses have shown marginal improvement for depression or cancer-related fatigue with more benefit in those more fatigued (49). Modafinil has also been useful to help improve alertness in cancer patients.

Atypical antipsychotics have been used to alleviate the antipsychotic symptoms of psychotic depression, to reduce fear, and to augment antidepressant response, particularly aripiprazole, quetiapine, and olanzapine.

Lithium is a distinct drug used to stabilize a patient with bipolar disorder. In the setting of medical illness, the first consideration is whether the serum level is stable for that person. Toxicity is associated with confusion, nausea, trouble speaking, and tremor. Since it is associated with baseline diabetes insipidus, a setting in which the patient is sedated and cannot drink water may be hazardous. The patient should be monitored for hypothyroidism and sudden changes in renal function that would contribute to higher serum levels. Therapeutic levels are usually 0.4 to 1.0 mmol/L, lower in older patients with vulnerable brains.

OTHER PSYCHOSOCIAL INTERVENTIONS

The best treatment for major depressive disorder combines psychotherapeutic interventions and antidepressant medication. Hopelessness and humiliation may be eased by psychotherapeutic interventions that sustain dignity and meaning (50,51). Group therapy for patients with metastatic cancer, a supportive–expressive approach, has reduced distress and facilitated the patient's confrontation with what had to be confronted (52). Most interventions to prevent distress in cancer patients, however, have not focused on the most depressed (53).

One recent phase II trial combined a biobehavioral intervention useful to reduce stress in cancer patients and cognitive behavioral treatment for depression for cancer patients with depressive disorder on antidepressant medication. Significant improvements in 19/21 study completers were noted with syndromal criteria for remission. Fatigue and quality of life improved. Concurrent anxiety disorders and high levels of cancer stress were each associated with more depressive symptoms at the beginning and ending of treatment. The program included progressive muscle relaxation

training, emphasis on coping with the cancer crisis, behavioral activation, communication with healthcare providers, social support, cognitive reappraisal, communicating needs, problem solving, core beliefs, rhythmic walking, review of therapy components, and strategies for successful maintenance; 21 of 36 were on psychotropic medication. Only two increased dose during treatment (54).

In order to treat demoralization, Griffith and Gaby (32) focus questions at the bedside to find the dominant existential theme, the patient's experience of illness, and then nudge forward with a series of questions oriented to attributes of resilience: coherence, communion, hope, agency, purpose, courage, and gratitude rather than confusion, isolation, despair, helplessness, meaninglessness, cowardice, and resentment. Among the questions that they pose to patients are those listed in Table 41.1.

Chochinov et al. (55) evaluated the effect of dignity therapy on distress and end-of-life experience in terminally ill patients in a randomized controlled trial. This brief psychotherapy was developed to relieve distress.

The therapeutic process begins with a framework of questions. These conversations, guided by a trained therapist, are flexible to accommodate the patients' needs and choices about what they specifically wish to address. The conversation is audio recorded and transcribed with an edited version of the transcript given to patients to share or bequeath to individuals of their choice. The protocol for questions about dignity therapy is listed in Table 41.2.

This treatment was compared with client-centered care, a supportive psychotherapeutic approach focusing on the here-and-now and to standard palliative care, which involved a range of disciplines, including psychologists, psychiatrists, social workers, and chaplains.

Patients were shown the framework of questions and asked to consider what they might wish to speak about during their sessions. Within a few days, the therapist used the framework to elicit patients' recollections. The document was returned in four working days. No specific treatment led to different distress levels in the three groups or differences in desire for death or depression. Patients did report that this therapy was more likely than the other two interventions to increase sense of dignity, quality of life, change how their family saw and appreciated them, and be helpful to their family. It lessened sadness or depression more than the standard palliative care approach. However, the patients who participated were not severely depressed, and the treatment was feasible only for patients mentally capable of providing personally meaningful responses.

In conclusion, sadness is a natural emotion in the setting of serious illness, but persistent severe anhedonia and hopelessness, the syndrome of major depressive disorder, is a serious and treatable condition that can occur at the same time as medical illness. The best treatment includes both antidepressant medications and psychosocial interventions. Suicidal thoughts are a signal calling attention to the suffering of the patient and to the possibility of clinical depression. An experienced clinician will distinguish delirium,

TABLE 41.1	Questions concerning different existential themes posed to patients with demoralization in order to challenge their withdrawal from the challenges of illness as suggested by Griffith and Gaby (32)

Coherence vs. Confusion

How do you make sense of what you are going through?

When you are uncertain how to make sense of it, how do you deal with feeling confused?

To whom do you turn for help when you feel confused?

(For a religious patient) Do you have a sense that God has a way of making sense of it? Do you sense that God sees meaning in your suffering?

Communion vs. Isolation

Who really understands your situation?

When you have difficult days, with whom do you talk?

In whose presence do you feel a bodily sense of peace?

(For religious patients) Do you feel the presence of God? How? What does God know about your experience that other people may not understand?

Hope vs. Despair

From what sources do you draw hope?

On difficult days, what keeps you from giving up?

Who have you known in your life who would not be surprised to see you stay hopeful amid adversity? What did this person know about you that other people may not have known?

Purpose vs. Meaninglessness

What keeps you going on difficult days?

For whom, or for what, does it matter that you continue to live?

(For terminally ill patients) What do you hope to contribute in the time you have remaining?

(For religious patients) What does God hope you will do with your life in days to come?

Agency vs. Helplessness

What is your prioritized list of concerns/what concerns you most? What next most?

What most helps you to stand strong against the challenges of this illness?

What should I know about you as a person that lies beyond your illness?

How have you kept this illness from taking charge of your entire life?

Courage vs. Cowardice

Have there been moments when you felt tempted to give up but didn't?

How did you make a decision to persevere?

If you were to see someone else taking such a step even though feeling afraid, would you consider that an act of courage? If so, can you imagine viewing yourself as a courageous person? Is that a description of yourself that you would desire?

Can you imagine that others who witness how you cope with this illness might describe you as a courageous person?

Gratitude vs. Resentment

For what are you most deeply grateful?

Are there moments when you can still feel joy despite the sorrow you have been through?

If you could look back on this illness from some future time, what would you say that you took from the experience that added to your life?

TABLE 41.2	**Protocol for questions about dignity therapy**

- Tell me a little about your life history, particularly the parts that you either remember most or think are the most important? When did you feel most alive?

- Are there specific things that you would want your family to know about you, and are there particular things you would want them to remember?

- What are the most important roles you have had in life (e.g., family roles, vocational roles, and community service roles)? Why were they so important to you and what do you think you accomplished in those roles?

- What are your most important accomplishments and what do you feel most proud of?

- Are there particular things that you feel still need to be said to your loved ones or things that you would want to take the time to say once again?

- What are your hopes and dreams for your loved ones?

- What have you learned about life that you would want to pass along to others? What advice or words of guidance would you wish to pass along to your son, daughter, husband, wife, parents, or others?

- Are there words or perhaps even instructions that you would like to offer your family to help prepare them for the future?

- In creating this permanent record, are there other things that you would like included?

Adapted from Panel 1 in Chochinov HM, Kristjanson LJ, Breitbart W, et al. Effect of dignity therapy on distress and end-of-life experience in terminally ill patients: a randomized controlled trial. *Lancet Oncol.* 2011:12:753–762, 754.

malaise, drug side effects, and melancholia with psychotic features from the symptoms of physical illness. Report of a depression score to physicians as laboratory data and collaborative care models for depression in cancer centers improve patient outcomes. The clinician can engage the patient in active coping through an interview that pays attention to demoralization and to what has meaning for the patient at the end of life.

REFERENCES

1. Weisman AD. *Coping with Cancer.* New York, NY: McGraw-Hill; 1979.
2. Lo C, Zimmermann C, Rydall A, et al. Longitudinal study of depressive symptoms in patients with metastatic gastrointestinal and lung cancer. *J Clin Oncol.* 2010;28:3084-3089.
3. Trask PC. Assessment of depression in cancer patients. *J Natl Cancer Inst Monogr.* 2004;32:80-92.
4. Endicott J. Measurement of depression in patients with cancer. *Cancer.* 1984;53:2243-2249.
5. Kathol R, Mutgi A, Williams J, et al. Diagnosis of major depression according to 4 sets of criteria. *Am J Psychiatry.* 1990;147:1021.
6. Kessler RC, Berglund P, Bemler O, et al. The epidemiology of major depressive disorder. *J Am Med Assoc.* 2003;289:3095-3105.
7. Depression Guideline Panel. *Depression in Primary Care: Detection and Diagnosis.* Vol 1. Rockville, MD: US Dept Health and Human Services; 1993. Clinical Practice Guideline #5. Public Health Service, Agency for Health Care Policy and Research.
8. Glick ID, Suppes T, DeBattista C, et al. Psychopharmacologic treatment strategies for depression, bipolar disorder, and schizophrenia. *Ann Intern Med.* 2001;134:47-60.
9. Massie MJ. Prevalence of depression in patients with cancer. *J Natl Cancer Inst Monogr.* 2004;32:57.
10. Pirl WF, Siegel GI, Goode MJ, Smith MR. Depression in men receiving androgen deprivation therapy for prostate cancer: a pilot study. *Psycho-Oncology.* 2002;11:518-523.
11. Roach MJ, Connors AF, Dawson NV, et al. Depressed mood and survival in seriously ill hospitalized adults. *Arch Intern Med.* 1998;158:397-404.
12. Cavanaugh SA, Furlanetto LM, Creech SD, Powell LH. Medical illness, past depression, and present depression: a predictive triad for in-hospital mortality. *Am J Psychiatry.* 2001;158:43-48.
13. Katon W, Sullivan M. Depression and chronic medical illness. *J Clin Psychiatry.* 1990;11:3-11.
14. Weitzner MA, Meyers CA, Steuebing KK, Saleeba AK. Relationship between quality of life and mood in long-term survivors of breast cancer treated with mastectomy. *Support Care Cancer.* 1997;5:241-248.
15. Chochinov HM, Wilson KG, Enns M, Lander S. Depression, hopelessness, and suicidal ideation in the terminally ill. *Psychosomatics.* 1998;39:366-370.
16. Christakis NA. Timing of referral of terminally ill patients to an outpatient hospice. *J Gen Intern Med.* 1994;9:314-320.
17. Emmanuel EJ, Fairclough DL, Daniels ER, Claridge BR. Euthanasia and physician-assisted suicide: attitudes and experience of oncology patients, oncologists, and the public. *Lancet.* 1996;347:1805-1810.
18. Ganzini L, Lee MA. Psychiatry and assisted suicide in the United States. *N Engl J Med.* 1997;336:1824-1826.
19. Ganzini L, Fenn DS, Lee MA, Heintz RT, Bloom JD. Attitudes of Oregon psychiatrists toward physician-assisted suicide. *Am J Psychiatry.* 1996;153:1469-1475.
20. Ganzini L, Lee MA, Heintz RT, Bloom JD, Fenn DS. The effect of depression treatment on elderly patients' preferences for life-sustaining medical therapy [comment]. *Am J Psychiatry.* 1994;151:1631-1636.

21. Valente SM, Saunders JM, Cohen MZ. Evaluating depression among patients with cancer. *Cancer Pract.* 1994;2:65-71.

22. Maguire P. Improving the detection of psychiatric problems in cancer patients. *Soc Sci Med.* 1985;20:819-823.

23. Walker J, Waters RA, Murray G, et al. Better off dead: suicidal thoughts in cancer patients. *J Clin Oncol.* 2008;26:4725-4730.

24. Turaga KK, Malafa MP, Jacobsen PB, Schell MJ, Sarr MG. Suicide in patients with pancreatic cancer. *Cancer.* 2011;117:642-647.

25. Greenberg DB. The signal of suicide rates seen from a distance in patients with pancreatic cancer. *Cancer.* 2011;117:446-448.

26. Dantzer R, O'Connor JC, Freund GG, Johnson RW, Kelley KW. From inflammation to sickness and depression: when the immune system subjugates the brain. *Nat Rev/Neurosci.* 2008;9:46-57.

27. Bower JE, Ganz Pa, Irwin MR, et al. Inflammation and behavioral symptoms after breast cancer treatment: do fatigue, depression, and sleep disturbance share a common underlying mechanism? *J Clin Oncol.* 2011;29:3517-3522.

28. Clarke DM, Kissane DW. Demoralization: its phenomenology and importance. *Aust N Z J Psychiatry.* 2002;36:733-742.

29. Kissane DW, Wein S, Love A, et al. The demoralization scale: a report of its development and preliminary validation. *J Palliat Care.* 2004;20:269-276.

30. Frank JD. *Persuasion and Healing.* 2nd ed. Baltimore, MD: The Johns Hopkins University Press. 1998.

31. Schmale AH. Giving up as a final common pathway to changes in health. *Adv Psychosom Med.* 1972;8:20-40.

32. Griffith JL, Gaby L. Brief psychotherapy at the bedside: countering demoralization from medical illness. *Psychosomatics.* 2005;46:109-116.

33. Shader RI. Demoralization revisited. *J Clin Psychopharm.* 2005;25:291-292.

34. Parker G, Fink M, Shorter E, et al. Issues for DSM-5: whither melancholia? The case for its classification as a distinct mood disorder. *Am J Psychiatry.* 2010;167:745-746.

35. Musselman DL, Lawson DH, Gumnick JF, et al. Paroxetine for the prevention of depression induced by high-dose interferon alfa. *N Engl J Med.* 2001;344.

36. Kirkwood JM, Bender C, Agarawala S, et al. Mechanisms and management of toxicities associated with high-dose interferon alfa-2b therapy. *J Clin Oncol.* 2002;17:3703-3718.

37. Hauschild A, Goagas H, Tarhini A, et al. Practical guidelines for the management of interferon-alpha-2b side effects in patients receiving adjuvant treatment for melanoma: expert opinion. *Cancer.* 2008;112:982-984.

38. Schmidt PJ, Rubinow DR. Sex hormones and mood in the perimenopause. *Ann N Y Acad Sci.* 2009;1179:70-85.

39. Cella D, Fallowfield L, Barker P, et al. Quality of life in postmenopausal women in ATAC after 5 years. *Breast Cancer Res Treat.* 2006; 100:273-284.

40. Holland JC, Andersen B, Breitbart WS, et al.; NCCN Distress Management Panel. Distress management. *J Natl Compr Canc Netw.* 2010;8:448-485.

41. Passik SD, Donaghy KB, Theobald DE, et al. Oncology staff recognition of depressive symptoms on videotaped interviews of depressed cancer patients: implications for designing a training program. *J Pain Symptom Manage.* 2000;19:329-338.

42. Passik SD, Kirsh KL, Donaghy KB, et al. An attempt to employ the Zung self-rating depression scale as a "lab test" to trigger follow-up in ambulatory oncology clinics: criterion validity and detection. *J Pain Symptom Manage.* 2001;21:273-281.

43. Kroenke K, Spitzer R, Williams JB. The PHQ-9 validity of a brief depression severity measure. *J Gen Intern Med.* 2001;16:606-613.

44. Strong V, Waters R, Hibberd C, et al. Management of depression for people with cancer (SMaRT oncology 1): a randomized trial. *Lancet.* 2008;372:40-48.

45. McLachan S, Allenby A, Matthews J, et al. Randomized trial of coordinated psychosocial interventions based on patients self-assessments versus standard care to improve the psychosocial functioning of patients with cancer. *J Clin Oncol.* 2001;19:4117-4125.

46. Gill D, Hartcher S. Antidepressants for depression in medical illness. *Cochrane Database Syst Rev.* 2000;4:CD001312.

47. Steffens DC, McQuoid Dr, Krishnan KRR. The Duke somatic treatment algorithm for geriatric depression (STAGED) approach. *Psychopharmacol Bull.* 2002;36:58-68.

48. Stahl SM. Antidepressants. In *Stahl's Essential Psychopharmacology.* 3rd ed. New York, NY: Cambridge University Press; 2008: 511-666.

49. Minton O, Richardson A, Sharpe M, Hotopf M, Stone PC. Psychostimulants for the management of cancer-related fatigue: a systematic review and meta-analysis. *J Pain Symptom Manage.* 2011;41:761-767.

50. Chochinov HM. Dignity-conserving care—a new model for palliative care helping the patient feel valued. *JAMA.* 2002;287:2253-2260.

51. McClain CS, Rosenfeld B, Breitbart W. Effect of spiritual well-being on end of life despair in terminally ill cancer patients. *Lancet.* 2003;361:1603-1607.

52. Spiegel D, Butler LD, Giese-Davis J, et al. Effects of supportive-expressive group therapy on survival of patients with metastatic breast cancer. A randomized prospective trial. *Cancer.* 2007;110:1130-1137.

53. Sheard T, Maguire P. The effect of psychological interventions on anxiety and depression in cancer patients: results of 2 meta-analyses. *Br J Cancer.* 1999;80:1770-1780.

54. Brothers BM, Yang HC, Strunk DR, Andersen BL. Cancer patients with major depressive disorder: testing a biobehavioral/cognitive behavior intervention. *J Consult Clin Psychol.* 2011;79:253-260.

55. Chochinov HM, Kristjanson LJ, Breitbart W, et al. Effect of dignity therapy on distress and end-of-life experience in terminally ill patients: a randomized controlled trial. *Lancet Oncol.* 2011:12:753-762.

Anxiety is an experience of worry, apprehension, unease, tension, or nervousness that is unpleasant and distressing. Almost any person facing a serious illness will experience some feelings of anxiety from time to time. When these emotions are brief and of low intensity, they may not be a source of significant distress. In fact, as an indicator signal of threat and a stimulus to seek safety or find solutions to life's problems or challenges, anxiety can serve an important adaptive function. However, once anxiety becomes severe, frequent, or pervasive enough to cause distress, disability, or functional impairment in important roles, anxiety has crossed the threshold to become the legitimate focus of attention and treatment, as described in the Diagnostic and Statistical Manual of Mental Disorders, Fourth Edition (DSM-IV) (1).

Though anxiety is commonly comorbid with depression and other mental disorders, anxiety is the most common category of mental disorder, with 31.2% of the general population meeting criteria for a formal anxiety diagnosis at some point in their lifetime (36.4% in women and 25.4% in men) (2). A meta-analysis of studies examining the prevalence of anxiety, depression, and adjustment disorders among patients with cancer found the prevalence of anxiety disorders among patients with cancer to be 10.3% compared with 9.8% among those in palliative care settings (3). Reported rates of adjustment disorder and mixed anxiety/depressive states were 19.4% and 38.2%, respectively, among patients with cancer and 15.4% and 29% among those receiving palliative care. There were substantial data heterogeneity reported for the studies used in this meta-analysis.

Wilson et al. found that 24.4% of 381 patients receiving palliative care for cancer met diagnostic criteria for at least one anxiety or depressive disorder (4). In this sample, 13.9% met diagnostic criteria for any anxiety-related diagnosis. Generalized anxiety disorder (GAD) was diagnosed in 5.8% of the sample, panic disorder was diagnosed in 5.5%, and anxiety disorder due to a general medical condition in 1.8%. In 4.7% of the sample, sub-syndromic but clinically significant anxiety (anxiety disorder not otherwise specified) was diagnosed. Kolva et al. looked at anxiety-related symptoms and distress, as measured by the Hospital Anxiety and Depression Scale (HADS), among 194 terminally ill cancer patients receiving care in inpatient and outpatient settings (5). Scores indicative of clinically significant anxiety were detected in 12.4% of the sample and 18.6% had at least moderately elevated levels of anxiety.

There are a variety of anxiety disorders, as described below, but it would be a mistake to focus only on formal anxiety disorders for intervention. There are a number of problems or situations that can cause non-specific anxiety symptoms or mimic anxiety disorders, as listed in Table 42.1. It is important for the clinician to be willing to address and treat anxiety-related distress, whether or not it reaches the threshold of a formal diagnosis. The National Comprehensive Cancer Network has published a guideline for the approach to distress in patients with cancer, including distress related to or manifest as anxiety symptoms (6). The overall goals of management are reduction of anxiety-related distress, restoration of peace, morale, and quality of life, and resolution of underlying fears, worries, or conflicts that drive anxiety symptoms.

APPROACH TO THE PATIENT WITH ANXIETY

Chronic versus Acute

When evaluating a patient with anxiety-related distress, it is important to determine the temporal course of the symptoms. Patients whose anxiety problems are chronic, predating the onset of their cancer diagnosis, are likely to have a formal anxiety disorder. Whether or not an anxiety disorder has been previously diagnosed, it is useful to determine if the quality and pattern of anxiety symptoms are familiar to the patient. The stress of a cancer diagnosis, its treatment, or other life stresses coincident with cancer can exacerbate a long-standing anxiety problem. For example, patients with a history of panic disorder are likely to have more frequent or intense panic attacks. Similarly, patients with GAD are likely to have an increase in troublesome worry and so on. In patients with chronic anxiety states, previously effective management strategies are likely to give relief from recurrent symptoms.

If the anxiety complaints are new or qualitatively different from a pattern characteristic for the patient, the distress is more likely to be related to a specific event. Open-ended questioning about sources and causes of anxiety, focusing on temporal associations, will often give important clues about the source.

Anxiety versus Fear versus Loss of Control

Fear differs from anxiety in that the source of the distressed feeling is obvious to the patient. Often, patients may have distress related to specific fears (e.g., dying, uncontrolled symptoms, loss of function, dependence on others, and family conflicts). For example, patients may paradoxically feel more

TABLE 42.1	Causes and mimics of anxiety

Anger

Anxiety disorders

Coping style—pattern of poor coping with stresses

Delirium

Fear

Financial concerns

Grief and bereavement

Interpersonal stresses

Legitimate worries and concerns

Loss of control and acute emotional disruption (feeling "in a tailspin")

Pain

Physical symptoms (e.g., nausea and dyspnea)

Side effects of medications (including akathisia from antipsychotic or antiemetic medications)

Spiritual and existential crises

Withdrawal states

worried and distressed as the end of a prolonged course of treatment, such as a course of radiation therapy, approaches. While one might expect the end of a taxing course of therapy to be greeted with relief as the goal of completion is reached, patients often become accustomed to and comforted by close monitoring, supportive contact from treating staff, and the routine of care. Feelings of worry and apprehension about losing these positive aspects of the therapy can be distressing, all the more so because they are unexpected. It is important to determine early on whether there are specific worries and fears, as opposed to a more non-specific feeling of anxiety or tension. While anxiolytic medications may be of some help, specific fears and worries should be addressed with exploration of the problem and therapeutic approaches, including supportive or problem-solving therapy.

Often, patients with cancer are distressed by an acute sense of being out of control. Combined with worries about mortality, the disruption in life and routines caused by cancer, cancer-related symptoms, and cancer treatments can provoke a great deal of distress. Often described as being overwhelmed or "in a tailspin," this experience can easily be misdiagnosed as clinical anxiety. Again, though anxiolytic medications may provide some degree of relief, they are not typically sufficient. Acute feelings of dyscontrol are often related to important milestones in illness (e.g., initial diagnosis, completing courses of radiation or chemotherapy treatment, and receiving bad prognostic news) or major changes in life roles and routines (e.g., job loss and separation from family). Much like specific fears, acute dyscontrol should be addressed with exploration of the problem and therapeutic approaches including supportive or problem-solving therapy.

Search for Precipitants

The patient's perspectives about causes and precipitants of anxiety are important to explore. Special attention should be paid to temporal associations between events and onset or worsening of anxiety symptoms. Are there specific worries, fears, or concerns? Have there been conflicts with family, friends, or care providers? Are there financial or transportation problems? Are there spiritual or existential concerns? Any of these items, alone or in combination, can lead to anxiety-related distress.

Are there other symptoms that cause or exacerbate the anxiety? Depression and anxiety are commonly comorbid, and addressing depression can reduce the burden of anxiety. Pain, dyspnea, and nausea are all symptoms that are commonly associated with anxiety. All these symptoms have an adaptive function making them a priority for the attention of the nervous system. Pain is a signal that attention needs to be paid to a source of tissue injury. Dyspnea is a signal that attention needs to be paid to a cause of poor oxygenation. Nausea is a signal that toxic contents of the gastrointestinal tract need to be expelled. These symptoms are hard-wired to be priority stimuli and, even when their presence is not an adaptively meaningful signal, persistence of these symptoms leaves the nervous system on "red alert" status, manifest as anxiety. Understandably, control of these and other distressing symptoms is anxiolytic.

Are there medications that are temporally related to the onset of anxiety symptoms? It is important to explore whether the onset of anxiety was associated with starting a new medication. It is also important to determine whether the onset of anxiety was associated with medication discontinuation, with particular attention paid to alcohol and sedative-hypnotic medications with potential for withdrawal states. Table 42.2 lists medications associated with anxiety.

Older antiemetic medications, and especially metoclopramide, can cause an adverse effect known as akathisia. Akathisia is a sensation of motor restlessness that is commonly seen with medications related to first-generation antipsychotic drugs. An elegant description of akathisia once provided by a patient is that the feeling is like "an itch in my muscles that can only be scratched by moving around." While akathisia is primarily a feeling of motor restlessness, when unrelieved it can be quite distressing and the fidgeting and emotional upset it causes can easily be mistaken for anxiety. In extreme cases, patients are frankly agitated and restless and can complain of feeling like "jumping out of my skin." Treatment centers on discontinuation of the offending drug.

History of Effective Treatments

Particularly in patients with a history of chronic anxiety or a formal anxiety disorder, inquiry should be made into what treatments were effective in the past. Were there anxiolytic medications that provided reliable relief? Were there non-pharmacologic approaches that were effective? How has the patient best managed these symptoms in the past? If the current anxiety-related distress is consistent with past episodes of anxiety, past treatment response is a good predictor of treatment response in the present.

TABLE	42.2	**Medications associated with anxiety**

Alcohol

Analgesics

Anticholinergics

Anticonvulsants

Antiemetics

Antihistamines and decongestants

Antihypertensives

Antiparkinsonian drugs

Antipsychotics

Bronchodilators and sympathomimetics

Caffeine

Corticosteroids and anabolic steroids

Hallucinogens

Psychostimulants (amphetamines and methylphenidate) and cocaine

Thyroid hormones

Sources of Relief

Patients should be asked about actions or activities that worsen or relieve anxiety symptoms. Can the patient distract herself/himself from distressed feelings by engaging in pleasurable activities, hobbies, or conversation with families and friends? Are relaxation techniques, exercise, meditation, or prayer reliably effective? What are the sources of inner strength and social support available to the patient and how can he/she access them?

Is a Trial of Anxiolytic Medication Indicated?

Though not all sources of anxiety-related distress are best treated with medication alone, prompt relief from a significant burden of anxiety usually requires a treatment plan that includes medication, if acceptable to the patient. Formal anxiety disorders are usually best managed with anxiolytics and/or antidepressants. Benzodiazepines and antipsychotic medications can reduce anxiety rapidly, while antidepressant medications may take longer to work. Explicit fears and worries should be addressed directly with supportive therapeutic intervention, though anxiolytic medication can be useful as an adjunct.

ANXIETY DISORDERS

Although not all presentations of anxiety represent formal anxiety disorders, attention should be paid to diagnosis of a specific disorder or disorders, if present, since there are

variations in treatment approach and prognosis for different anxiety disorders and for anxiety symptoms not related to a formal disorder. Anxiety disorders tend to be chronic, even lifelong, problems and may require long-term maintenance of effective therapy. Detailed descriptions of the diagnostic criteria for anxiety disorders, as well as information about associated features and comorbidities, demographics, and the typical course of illness, are contained in the DSM-IV (1).

Panic Disorder

A panic attack, while not sufficient for a diagnosis in and of itself, is the essential feature of panic disorder. Panic attacks are discrete, brief, intense episodes of intense anxiety associated with symptoms such as

> palpitations, pounding heartbeat, or tachycardia;
> diaphoresis;
> tremor;
> dyspnea or a sensation of smothering;
> a sensation of choking;
> chest pain or discomfort;
> nausea or gastrointestinal distress;
> dizziness or lightheadedness;
> derealization or depersonalization;
> fear of losing control as a result of the panic attack;
> fear of dying as a result of the panic attack;
> paresthesias; and/or
> chills or hot flashes.

The typical panic attack has rapid onset and crescendo to full intensity in a matter of minutes. Though the patient's perception may be that a panic attack lasts much longer, the attack usually dissipates over the course of 15 to 20 minutes, though the experience may leave the sufferer tense, fearful, and apprehensive for some longer period of time. Panic attacks may occur as a response to a perception of overwhelming threat, a reaction to anxiogenic medications, or as a result of spontaneous misfire of the brain's "fight or flight" response. Those who describe a persistent level of baseline anxiety as "panic" are not describing panic attacks.

Presence of panic attacks is necessary but not sufficient for a diagnosis for panic disorder, which is characterized by the presence of recurrent panic attacks that are frequently or typically unexpected and unprovoked. During a panic attack, the sufferer often attributes the attack to some unseen threat and has an urge to escape the environment, so those with recurrent panic may move suddenly and seemingly irrationally to another setting, avoid situations from which escape would be difficult or embarrassing, or (in extreme cases) avoid placing themselves in such settings altogether. Patients with recurrent panic attacks often live with fear and dread of recurrent attacks. The burden of recurrent panic, the impairment caused by ongoing dread of recurrence, and the disruption caused by maladaptive lifestyle adaptations are the hallmarks of panic disorder.

In one study of panic disorder among hospitalized cancer patients, approximately one-fifth of the patients referred for psychiatric consultation suffered from panic anxiety (7). Reported complications of panic anxiety in this population included the urge to elope from hospital, requests for discharge against medical advice, disruptions in adherence to cancer therapy protocols, and a request for discontinuation of cancer therapy in order to hasten death (7).

Therapeutic approaches for panic disorder center on pharmacologic therapy to reduce the frequency and intensity of panic attacks, restore functioning, and improve quality of life (8). However, a thorough assessment to rule out medical causes of panic anxiety (e.g., secondary panic related to medical problems producing episodic hypoxia) is an indispensible first step. Another important aspect of care is patient education about the nature and causes of panic attacks to maximize a sense of control and minimize misattribution of symptoms (e.g., misinterpretation of panic symptoms as a manifestation of disease progression or a heart attack). Cognitive-behavioral therapy (CBT) is among the non-pharmacologic therapies recommended for the treatment of panic disorder (8).

Recommended pharmacologic therapies generally include anxiolytic antidepressants and benzodiazepines (8,9). Most antidepressant medications are reliably effective for anxiety disorders, including panic disorder, but may take weeks of daily administration to have optimal effect. Benzodiazepines have the advantage of rapid onset of relief, but they have liabilities including the potential for misuse and addiction. For this reason, benzodiazepines are often co-prescribed with anxiolytic antidepressants at the onset of treatment for panic disorder and then tapered to discontinuation as the antidepressant medication has time to take effect. This approach can also help reduce the risk of anxiety exacerbation sometimes seen in the first few days of initiation of an antidepressant for a primary anxiety diagnosis (9). Some patients with panic disorder may need chronic co-administration of anxiolytic antidepressants and benzodiazepines or a small amount of benzodiazepines for PRN use to abort panic attacks.

Generalized Anxiety Disorder

GAD is characterized by a pattern of excessive worry that the patient has difficulty controlling. Typically, others in the patient's social network would readily identify him or her as an excessive worrier. The worrying itself becomes a distressing or even disabling problem and is associated with other symptoms, such as

- restlessness, feeling keyed-up, or feeling on edge;
- fatigue;
- problems with concentration;
- irritability;
- muscle tension; and
- disturbance in sleeping.

The worrying is a long-standing pattern of behavior, is pervasive, and involves worry about a broad range of things (not just having a medical illness such as cancer). That said,

a diagnosis with cancer, especially an illness with poor prognosis or high symptom burden, can exacerbate the level of worry-related distress in a patient with GAD to new heights.

Patients with GAD are managed primarily with anxiolytic antidepressants. A meta-analysis of randomized controlled trials of pharmacotherapy for GAD found that while a broad range of antidepressant medications are effective for GAD, fluoxetine ranked first among those drugs studied, in terms of response and remission rates (10). Sertraline was the best-tolerated drug studied in this meta-analysis (10). Nutt recommends venlafaxine as the initial pharmacologic approach to GAD (9). The non-antidepressant, non-benzodiazepine serotonergic agent buspirone is also effective for GAD (9). CBT and other non-pharmacologic therapies aimed at reducing the burden of worry and worry-related distress are also helpful.

Posttraumatic Stress Disorder

Posttraumatic stress disorder (PTSD) is one of the few mental disorders in DSM-IV with a known etiology, though this etiology is determined by definition. PTSD is a pervasive pattern of distress developing as a consequence of an overwhelmingly traumatic experience. The characteristics of the kinds of experience that cause PTSD include a sudden and unexpected nature of the traumatic event, a traumatic threat that is outside one's control, a realistic threat of death or severe injury to oneself or others, and a response to this event that involves fear, helplessness, or horror. Symptoms of PTSD are manifest as re-experiencing phenomena, avoidance of reminders of the trauma, increased startle response and hyperarousal, and emotional numbness or detachment. The re-experiencing phenomena (e.g., nightmares, flashbacks, intrusive daydreams, and ruminations) usually feel more like a virtual recurrence of the traumatic event than an intense memory. A variety of factors appear to increase the chance that a given person will develop PTSD in response to trauma, including having recurrent traumas, the intensity of the fear produced (related to the patient's interpretation of the severity of the threat), and innate coping capacities.

Severe or advanced illness in and of itself can produce PTSD, especially if there is an acute, overwhelming, and life-threatening event associated with an illness. Often, patients with this degree of illness are delirious (and therefore amnestic) for much of this experience, which can be protective in terms of developing PTSD related to acute medical illness. More typical precipitants of PTSD include experiences of abuse in childhood, sexual assault, severe accidents with physical trauma, surviving natural disasters, and combat. PTSD is common and if unrecognized and untreated impairs quality of life and adds substantially to the burden of suffering in patients with advanced or terminal illnesses (11).

Acute stress disorder (ASD) is a response to traumatic stress that does not become chronic. If the pattern of symptoms described above develops within days of the trauma and resolves within 4 weeks, ASD is the proper diagnosis. More chronic symptoms as the result of trauma are best diagnosed as PTSD.

Treatment for PTSD and ASD is aimed at soothing an overstimulated and hyperaroused central nervous system. An obvious first step is to take measures to prevent re-exposure of the patient to ongoing or repetitive traumas. Psychotherapeutic interventions, generally in combination with medication therapies, are of primary importance, and patients with chronic PTSD should be directed to clinicians with expertise in providing these therapies. Supportive therapy, debriefing, rallying the patient's support networks, and anxiolytic medications in the immediate posttrauma period may facilitate recovery and reduce the risk of progression to PTSD (12). CBT, eye movement desensitization and reprocessing (EMDR) therapy, relaxation-based therapies, and exposure/desensitization therapies can be of benefit (12).

There is good evidence that antidepressants, particularly the selective serotonin reuptake inhibitors (SSRIs), are effective in reducing the symptom burden of PTSD. SSRIs are recommended as first-line therapy, though other anxiolytic antidepressants are often useful if SSRIs are ineffective, not well tolerated, or contraindicated (12,13). Nutt's review recommends mirtazapine and tricyclic antidepressants (TCAs) as second-line treatments for PTSD (9). Benzodiazepines, atypical antipsychotics, anticonvulsants, and a variety of other agents, including α- and β-adrenergic blockers, have demonstrated some efficacy in reducing symptoms in PTSD (12). Benzodiazepines are not recommended in the long-term management of PTSD, and especially not as monotherapy over the long term (12). The α-adrenergic agent prazosin has been shown to reduce the frequency and intensity of trauma-related nightmares and to improve the quality of sleep (14).

In the next revision of the DSM, PTSD and ASD are likely to be removed from the category of anxiety disorders and become a separate category, trauma- and stressor-related disorders (15).

Obsessive–Compulsive Disorder

Obsessive–compulsive disorder (OCD) is a long-standing pattern of recurrent, intrusive thoughts, impulses, or images that prompt repetitive, often purposeless behaviors. Common themes of these obsessions and compulsions include contamination (often manifest as compulsive hand washing), safety (repetitive checking of items like door locks or stove knobs), counting rituals, or intolerance of items out of a particular order. These are not simply people who are meticulously organized—the obsessions and compulsions are distressing to the patient and often consume a significant amount of time (more than an hour a day by definition). Patients have insight into the purposelessness of the obsessions (differentiating these thoughts from delusions), and typically try to resist them, but attempts to suppress or ignore the repetitive, obsessive thoughts often lead to significant distress. The most effective means to gain relief from the obsessive thoughts, at least in the short term, is to give in and perform the compulsive behavior. This often produces embarrassment, self-consciousness, and despair.

Treatment for OCD involves behavioral psychotherapy in combination with serotonergic antidepressants, typically SSRIs (9). The TCA clomipramine is a second-line treatment for OCD (9). Often, antidepressant doses must be raised to the upper limits of the recommended dose range to gain significant benefit for OCD.

Compulsive hair-pulling (trichotillomania), nail biting, and skin picking are likely OCD-spectrum illnesses, and initial therapeutic approaches are similar to those recommended for OCD.

Specific Phobia

Phobias are consistent patterns of anxiety consistently and reliably provoked by an identified stimulus. Specific phobias are marked and persistent fear of a specific object or situation and are the most common of the anxiety disorders (2). Common specific phobias involve enclosed spaces (claustrophobia), heights, blood, needles, crossing bridges, or flying in airplanes. These reactive fears are recognized as excessive or unreasonable and are often managed effectively by simply avoiding the phobic stimulus.

When a patient's phobic stimulus cannot be avoided (e.g., the patient with a needle phobia who requires chemotherapy), anxiolytic medications can be of help, usually benzodiazepines or antipsychotics for acute and severe anxiety and antidepressants for symptom control in the longer term. The primary long-term approach for specific phobias, however, is psychotherapeutic, using CBT, relaxation approaches, or desensitization approaches.

Social Phobia

Social phobia is a pattern of marked and persistent fear of one or more social or performance situations, such as public speaking or being in crowds or public places. The underlying fears and worries often center around being embarrassed or humiliated. Like specific phobias, these fears are recognized as excessive or unreasonable and are often managed effectively by simply avoiding anxiety-provoking situations. Treatment approaches are similar to those recommended for specific phobias.

Akechi et al. reported on two cases of social phobia in cancer patients (16). In addition to the burden of anxiety experienced by the patient, this disorder can interfere with cancer care when patients avoid hospitalization, miss ambulatory medical visits, or request discharge against medical advice due to phobic anxiety.

Substance-Induced Anxiety Disorder

The diagnosis of substance-induced anxiety disorder should be used when symptoms of anxiety are the direct consequence of a drug or medication, either substances of abuse or prescribed therapeutic drugs. A number of substances of abuse can produce anxiety during periods of intoxication (e.g., alcohol, cocaine, and amphetamines) or withdrawal (e.g., alcohol and sedative hypnotics). An example of an anxiety state related to a prescription medication is the distress related to akathisia sometimes seen as an adverse effect of antipsychotics, antiemetics, and metoclopramide, as described above. Table 42.2 lists medications associated with anxiety.

In addition to dose reduction or discontinuation of the offending medication, if possible, and management of a withdrawal state, if present, treatment generally follows the predominant anxiety symptom (e.g., panic).

Anxiety Disorder Due to a General Medical Condition

This diagnosis is made when the anxiety state is judged to be the consequence of an underlying general medical condition, such as cancer. The DSM-IV criteria state that the anxiety symptoms must be a *direct physiological consequence* of the medical illness, but this is often very difficult to judge. Many clinicians use this diagnosis when there is a clear temporal association between the detection or progression of the medical diagnosis and the onset or exacerbation of the anxiety symptom and the anxiety symptoms are not better explained by another anxiety disorder. Treatment generally follows the predominant anxiety symptom (e.g., panic).

Anxiety Disorder Not Otherwise Specialized

This diagnosis is used when an anxiety state clearly surpasses the threshold of severity, distress, and/or impairment that renders it a mental disorder, but does not fit the diagnostic pattern of any of the other anxiety disorders.

Adjustment Disorder

Adjustment disorders are states of emotional disturbance that occur in reaction to identified stressors, such as illness, that are not better explained by another mental disorder. The diagnosis of an adjustment disorder requires a fair amount of clinical judgment, since the emotional or behavioral symptoms must be deemed to both be in excess of what would be expected in response to the identified stressor and to be an independent source of significant distress or impairment. By definition, the symptoms must have their onset within 3 months of the stressor and cannot persist beyond 6 months past the termination or resolution of the stressor.

As with non-specific anxiety states, it is important for the clinician to be willing to address and treat anxiety-related distress. Many of the patients with distressing specific fears and feelings of being out of control or "in a tailspin," as described above, could be properly diagnosed as having an adjustment disorder with anxiety. Unfortunately, the name of this diagnosis implies that the syndrome it describes is trivial—as if one simply needed to be advised to adjust. The distress related to an adjustment disorder is not trivial, since the diagnosis requires symptoms that clearly surpass the threshold of severity, distress, and/or impairment that indicates a formal mental disorder.

Treatment involves identification and management of the stressor, to the extent possible, augmented by supportive or problem-solving therapy and anxiolytic medications for symptom relief. Pharmacologic treatment generally follows the predominant anxiety symptom.

MEASUREMENT OF ANXIETY IN PATIENTS WITH CANCER

Given the impact of anxiety-related distress, including sub-syndromic and non-specific anxiety states, it is important to consider a general approach to screening for anxiety. Detection of anxiety and anxiety disorders provides the opportunity to intervene to reduce the burden of anxiety on the patient. Less obviously, detection and treatment of anxiety has the potential to improve the relief of comorbid physical and psychological symptoms. Anxiety has been associated with poorer physical performance status among patients with advanced cancer (17). Anxiety and depression are also associated with a greater frequency and intensity of symptoms, including pain, nausea, dyspnea, and fatigue among patients with cancer receiving palliative care (18). Patients with substantial symptom burden, especially those not responding satisfactorily to first-line therapies, should be screened for anxiety and depression. Clinicians can use the diagnostic criteria from the DSM-IV to screen for anxiety disorders, but this can be time consuming and complicated for the clinician unfamiliar with the subtleties of anxiety disorder diagnosis.

The HADS is probably the most commonly used screening tool for anxiety in cancer patients (19). The HADS has the advantage of being a rapidly administered, patient-completed measure that screens for both anxiety and depression. While it has been used in numerous studies and clinical care settings and has been widely recommended (20), recent analyses have questioned the accuracy and utility of the HADS as a clinical screening measure for anxiety in cancer patients (21,22).

Spitzer et al. (23) developed a seven-item, patient-completed anxiety screening measure called the GAD-7, since it was initially developed to screen for GAD. In subsequent study, the GAD-7 was found to have good sensitivity and specificity as a screening measure for panic disorder, PTSD, and social phobia, as well as for GAD (24). The GAD-7 contains seven items scored from 0 to 3, yielding a score range from 0 to 21. Score cutpoints of 5, 10, and 15 are recommended for mild, moderate, and severe anxiety, respectively. When using the GAD-7 as a stand-alone screen for anxiety, a cutoff score of 10 is the recommended cutpoint to trigger a more detailed evaluation. The GAD-7 form, along with instruction and scoring materials, is available online (25).

MANAGEMENT STRATEGIES

The first step in the management of anxiety states in patients with cancer is to address the underlying fears, concerns, and comorbid physical symptoms (e.g., pain, dyspnea, and nausea) that can drive or complicate anxiety. A search for medications that may cause anxiety and appropriate streamlining of the patient's pharmacologic regimen is also a primary consideration. If a formal anxiety disorder is diagnosed, management generally includes anxiolytic medications.

While a recent systematic review of drug therapies for anxiety in palliative care concluded that there were insufficient data in the published medical literature to make recommendations for evidence-based therapies (26), a more recent review of evidence-based treatments for anxiety in patients with cancer summarizes a substantial number of studies of treatments that appear to be effective in this setting (27). Table 42.3 summarizes doses and properties of medications commonly used for the management of anxiety.

TABLE 42.3	Common anxiolytic medications used for patients with cancer	
Generic Name	**Approximate Daily Dosage Range (mg)**	**Comment**
Benzodiazepines		
Alprazolam	0.25–2 tid–qid	Short acting
Clonazepam	0.5–2 bid–qid	Long acting
Diazepam	5–10 bid–qid	Long acting; rapid onset with single PO dose
Lorazepam	0.5–2 tid–qid	Short acting; multiple routes (PO, SL, IV, and IM); no active metabolites
Azapirones		
Buspirone	5–20 tid	Lag time to effect similar to antidepressants
Antidepressants		
Serotonin Reuptake Inhibitors		
Citalopram	20–40 daily	New FDA warning about doses above 40 mg
Fluoxetine	10–80 daily	Longest half-life among serotonin reuptake inhibitors
Paroxetine	10–60 daily	
Sertraline	50–200 daily	
Tricyclics		
Desipramine	12.5–150 daily	Least sedating tricyclic antidepressant
Imipramine	12.5–150 daily	
Nortriptyline	10–125 daily	Least likely tricyclic antidepressant to cause orthostasis; most reliable blood level
Other Antidepressants		
Duloxetine	40–60 daily	
Venlafaxine	75–375 daily	
Mirtazapine	15–60 daily	Promotes sleep and appetite at low doses; orally disintegrating tab available
Antipsychotics		
Olanzapine	5–15 daily[a]	Orally disintegrating tab available
Quetiapine	25–200 daily[a]	Preferred for patients with Parkinson's disease
Risperidone	1–3 daily[a]	
Haloperidol	0.5–5 q2-12h	Inexpensive and multiple routes of administration (IV, PO, and IM)
Antihistamines		
Hydroxyzine	25–50 q4-6h	Risk of anticholinergic side effects and delirium

PO, per oral; IM, intramuscular; PR, per rectum; IV, intravenous; SC, subcutaneous; SL, sublingual; bid, two times a day; tid, three times a day; qid, four times a day. Parenteral doses are generally twice as potent as oral doses; intravenous bolus injections should be administered slowly.

[a]In divided doses.

Antidepressants

Most antidepressant medications are also effective for anxiety, though not all have formal FDA indications for anxiety disorders (28). A notable exception is bupropion, which offers little benefit for anxiety. Antidepressants are especially important to consider as a primary long-term treatment for anxiety since mixed anxiety/depression states are so common. Antidepressants are not habit forming, can often be effective when taken once daily, and maintain effectiveness in the long term. Like their efficacy for depression, however, the onset of full benefit for anxiety may take several weeks of regular administration. Doses in the lower end of the dose range are often better tolerated and can be effective when antidepressant medications are used for anxiety.

SSRIs are the first-line medications for many anxiety disorders (9), since they are reliably effective and relatively simple to prescribe. Various SSRIs have formal FDA indications for a variety of anxiety disorders, including panic disorder, GAD, PTSD, and OCD. They are not constipating and have a low liability for precipitating delirium, but have little benefit as adjunctive treatments for pain. Common side effects are gastrointestinal upset, dizziness, headaches, and jitteriness, which may appear to be a manifestation of anxiety. These problems are generally manageable by slow dose titration.

Serotonin–norepinephrine reuptake inhibitors (SNRIs) include venlafaxine, desvenlafaxine, duloxetine, and milnacipran. Venlafaxine is FDA-approved for GAD, panic disorder, and social phobia. Duloxetine is FDA-approved for GAD. SNRIs have the advantage of being effective for a variety of painful conditions. Milnacipran is FDA-approved for treating fibromyalgia, but not depression or anxiety.

Mirtazapine is a tetracyclic antidepressant with common side effects of appetite stimulation and sedation, particularly at the lower end of its dose range. These side effects are often therapeutically advantageous in cancer patients (29). Mirtazapine also demonstrates 5HT3 antagonism and may therefore be helpful in reducing nausea.

TCAs are reliably effective for anxiety, relatively inexpensive, and effective as adjunctive treatments for neuropathic pain. TCAs can also help promote sleep and appetite. Their side-effect burden, however, is higher than most other antidepressant drugs. Anticholinergic effects, sedation, resting tachycardia, constipation, orthostasis, and the risk of ventricular arrhythmias due to slowing down of cardiac conduction are the main reasons that newer antidepressant agents have come into more common use compared with TCAs. This class of drugs still deserves consideration, however, for management of anxiety resistant to other agents such as SSRIs.

Benzodiazepines

Benzodiazepines have long been the mainstay for the relief of acute anxiety and are also commonly used for nausea in cancer patients. Their chief advantage over other medication classes is the rapid onset of anxiolysis. Benzodiazepines are toxic in overdose, can suppress respiratory drive in patients with lung disease, and can cause or exacerbate cognitive impairment (28). These problems and the liability for abuse and addiction make other drug classes preferable as first-line treatments for long-term use, but there is evidence that benzodiazepines are effective in the long term, without loss of efficacy due to tolerance or need for dose escalation (28). Some patients with panic disorder may need chronic co-administration of anxiolytic antidepressants and benzodiazepines or a small amount of benzodiazepines for PRN use to abort panic attacks.

Long-acting agents (e.g., clonazepam) can prevent loss of efficacy between doses sometimes seen with short-acting agents. Lorazepam is metabolized by conjugation, does not have active metabolites, and is reliably absorbed by a variety of administration routes, making it the preferred agent in acutely ill patients (28).

Antipsychotics

Antipsychotic drugs are reliably anxiolytic, but their risks with long-term use (including the risk of developing movement disorders) make them second-line maintenance treatments for chronic anxiety, at best. However, when rapid anxiolysis is needed in patients with mixed anxiety and delirium, patients who do not tolerate benzodiazepines (e.g., elderly or cognitively impaired patients who exhibit paradoxical disinhibition to benzodiazepine administration), or patients with tenuous respiratory drive due to severe lung disease, antipsychotics are a valuable option. Additionally, a variety of antipsychotic medications have been studied as augmentation strategies for PTSD and OCD (28).

Anticonvulsants

Pregabalin has been studied as a treatment for GAD and social phobia, with the most substantial evidence base as a treatment for GAD (28). Lamotrigine and topiramate have shown benefit for PTSD (28). Anticonvulsants are not first-line therapy for anxiety symptoms or disorders.

Other Agents

Buspirone is an azapirone anxiolytic and a good alternative to consider as a primary therapy for GAD or as an augmentation strategy for other anxiety disorders. Buspirone has a significant lag time to effect, analogos to antidepressants, and requires divided dosing, usually three times daily (28). The antihistamine hydroxyzine has anxiolytic properties and is a useful second or third-line option. A recent case report describes rapid resolution of anxiety and depression in two hospice patients treated with ketamine (30).

There is significant potential for drug interactions with use of anxiolytic medications (31). For benzodiazepines, the primary concern is additive sedation with other sedating medications. Antidepressants, particularly SSRIs and SNRIs, have substantial potential for metabolic drug interactions mediated by their effects on the cytochrome P450 system. For example, fluoxetine and paroxetine are likely to impair the efficacy of tamoxifen through their inhibition of CYP2D6, which converts tamoxifen to its active metabolite, endoxifen (31). Prescribers should familiarize themselves with common drug interactions with anxiolytic drugs.

Psychotherapies

A recent review has complied the evidence for effectiveness of psychosocial interventions in cancer patients (27,32). CBT is effective for anxiety in patients with cancer, and CBT approaches have been modified and abbreviated to fit the needs of patients with advanced cancer and patients receiving hospice care, demonstrating feasibility of delivering CBT interventions to these patient populations (33–35). Relaxation therapies, psychoeducation, and supportive and supportive–expressive therapies have also been shown to be effective for anxiety in patients with cancer (32).

Other Approaches

A variety of complementary and alternative therapies have been reported to be effective for anxiety in patients with cancer. Anti-anxiety effects have been reported for hospice and palliative care patients treated with aromatherapy (36,37), massage therapy (38), hypnotherapy (39), and music therapy and progressive muscle relaxation (alone or in combination) (40).

REFERENCES

1. American Psychiatric Association. *Diagnostic and Statistical Manual of Mental Disorders.* 4th ed. Washington, DC: American Psychiatric Association; 2000.
2. National Comorbidity Survey. http://www.hcp.med.harvard.edu/ncs/ftpdir/NCS-R_Lifetime_Prevalence_Estimates.pdf. Accessed March 28, 2012.
3. Mitchell AJ, Chan M, Bhatti H, et al. Prevalence of depression, anxiety, and adjustment disorder in oncological, haematological, and palliative-care settings: a meta-analysis of 94 interview-based studies. *Lancet Oncol.* 2011;12:160-174.
4. Wilson KG, Chochinov HM, Skirko MG, et al. Depression and anxiety disorders in palliative cancer care. *J Pain Symptom Manage.* 2007;33:118-129.
5. Kolva E, Rosenfeld B, Pessin H, Breitbart W, Brescia R. Anxiety in terminally ill cancer patients. *J Pain Symptom Manage.* 2011;42:691-701.
6. National Comprehensive Cancer Network Guidelines for Supportive Care. http://www.nccn.org/professionals/physician_gls/f_guidelines.asp#supportive. Accessed March 28, 2012.
7. Slaughter JR, Jain A, Holmes S, et al. Panic disorder in hospitalized cancer patients. *Psychooncology.* 2000;9:253-258.
8. American Psychiatric Association. Practice guideline for the treatment of patients with panic disorder. Work Group on Panic Disorder. *Am J Psychiatry.* 1998;155(5 suppl):1-34.
9. Nutt DJ. Overview of diagnosis and drug treatments of anxiety disorders. *CNS Spectr.* 2005;10:49-56.
10. Baldwin D, Woods R, Lawson R, Taylor D. Efficacy of drug treatments for generalised anxiety disorder: systematic review and meta-analysis. *BMJ.* 2011;342:d1199. doi:10.1136/bmj.d1199.
11. Feldman DB. Posttraumatic stress disorder at the end of life: extant research and proposed psychosocial treatment approach. *Palliat Support Care.* 2011;9:407-418.
12. Ursano RJ, Bell C, Eth S, et al. Practice guideline for the treatment of patients with acute stress disorder and posttraumatic stress disorder. *Am J Psychiatry.* 2004;161(11 suppl):3-31.
13. Stein DJ, Ipser J, McAnda N. Pharmacotherapy of posttraumatic stress disorder: a review of meta-analyses and treatment guidelines. *CNS Spectr.* 2009;14(1 suppl 1):25-31.
14. Miller LJ. Prazosin for the treatment of posttraumatic stress disorder sleep disturbances. *Pharmacotherapy.* 2008;28:656-666.
15. American Psychiatric Association, DSM-5 Development. http://www.dsm5.org/proposedrevision/Pages/TraumaandStressorRelatedDisorders.aspx. Accessed March 28, 2012.
16. Akechi T, Okuyama T, Sagawa R, et al. Social anxiety disorder as a hidden psychiatric comorbidity among cancer patients. *Palliat Support Care.* 2011;9:103-105.
17. Spencer R, Nilsson M, Wright A, Pirl W, Prigerson H. Anxiety disorders in advanced cancer patients: correlates and predictors of end-of-life outcomes. *Cancer.* 2010;116:1810-1819.
18. Delgado-Guay M, Parsons HA, Li Z, Palmer JL, Bruera E. Symptom distress in advanced cancer patients with anxiety and depression in the palliative care setting. *Support Care Cancer.* 2009;17:573-579.
19. Zigmond AS, Snaith RP. The Hospital Anxiety and Depression Scale. *Acta Psychiatr Scand.* 1983;67:361-370.
20. Luckett T, Butow PN, King MT, et al. A review and recommendations for optimal outcome measures of anxiety, depression and general distress in studies evaluating psychosocial interventions for English-speaking adults with heterogeneous cancer diagnoses. *Support Care Cancer.* 2010;18:1241-1262.
21. Vodermaier A, Millman RD. Accuracy of the Hospital Anxiety and Depression Scale as a screening tool in cancer patients: a systematic review and meta-analysis. *Support Care Cancer.* 2011;19:1899-1908.
22. Carey M, Noble N, Sanson-Fisher R, Mackenzie L. Identifying psychological morbidity among people with cancer using the Hospital Anxiety and Depression Scale: time to revisit first principles? *Psychooncology.* 2012;21:229-238.
23. Spitzer RL, Kroenke K, Williams JB, Löwe B. A brief measure for assessing generalized anxiety disorder: the GAD-7. *Arch Intern Med.* 2006;166:1092-1097.
24. Kroenke K, Spitzer RL, Williams JB, Monahan PO, Löwe B. Anxiety disorders in primary care: prevalence, impairment, comorbidity, and detection. *Ann Intern Med.* 2007;146:317-325.
25. Patient Health Questionnaire (PHQ) Screeners. http://www.phqscreeners.com. Accessed March 28, 2012.
26. Jackson KC, Lipman AG. Drug therapy for anxiety in palliative care. *Cochrane Database Syst Rev.* 2004;(1):CD004596.
27. Traeger L, Greer JA, Fernandez-Robles C, Temel JS, Pirl WF. Evidence-based treatment of anxiety in patients with cancer. *J Clin Oncol.* 2012;30:1197-1205.
28. Ravindran LN, Stein MB. The pharmacologic treatment of anxiety disorders: a review of progress. *J Clin Psychiatry.* 2010;71:839-854.
29. Cankurtaran ES, Ozalp E, Soygur H, et al. Mirtazapine improves sleep and lowers anxiety and depression in cancer patients: superiority over imipramine. *Support Care Cancer.* 2008;16:1291-1298.
30. Irwin SA, Iglewicz A. Oral ketamine for the rapid treatment of depression and anxiety in patients receiving hospice care. *J Palliat Med.* 2010;13:903-908.

31. Muscatello MR, Spina E, Bandelow B, Baldwin DS. Clinically relevant drug interactions in anxiety disorders. *Hum Psychopharmacol*. February 2012. doi:10.1002/hup.2217. e-pub ahead of print.

32. Jacobsen PB, Jim HS. Psychosocial interventions for anxiety and depression in adult cancer patients: achievements and challenges. *CA Cancer J Clin*. 2008;58:214-230.

33. Greer JA, Park ER, Prigerson HG, Safren SA. Tailoring cognitive-behavioral therapy to treat anxiety comorbid with advanced cancer. *J Cogn Psychother*. 2010;24:294-313.

34. Anderson T, Watson M, Davidson R. The use of cognitive behavioural therapy techniques for anxiety and depression in hospice patients: a feasibility study. *Palliat Med*. 2008;22:814-821.

35. Pitceathly C, Maguire P, Fletcher I, et al. Can a brief psychological intervention prevent anxiety or depressive disorders in cancer patients? A randomised controlled trial. *Ann Oncol*. 2009;20:928-934.

36. Louis M, Kowalski SD. Use of aromatherapy with hospice patients to decrease pain, anxiety, and depression and to promote an increased sense of well-being. *Am J Hosp Palliat Care*. 2002;19:381-386.

37. Kyle G. Evaluating the effectiveness of aromatherapy in reducing levels of anxiety in palliative care patients: results of a pilot study. *Complement Ther Clin Pract*. 2006;12:148-155.

38. Falkensteiner M, Mantovan F, Müller I, Them C. The use of massage therapy for reducing pain, anxiety, and depression in oncological palliative care patients: a narrative review of the literature. *ISRN Nurs*. 2011:929868. e-pub ahead of print August 23 2011.

39. Plaskota M, Lucas C, Evans R, et al. A hypnotherapy intervention for the treatment of anxiety in patients with cancer receiving palliative care. *Int J Palliat Nurs*. 2012;18:69-75.

40. Choi YK. The effect of music and progressive muscle relaxation on anxiety, fatigue, and quality of life in family caregivers of hospice patients. *J Music Ther*. 2010;47:53-69.

43 Cognitive Decline Following Cancer Treatment

James C. Root ■ Elizabeth Ryan ■ Timothy Ahles

INTRODUCTION

Cognitive decline following cancer diagnosis and treatment is an important clinical problem for cancer survivors that may have far-reaching consequences in home-life, educational attainment, and vocational success. Increasingly, cognitive decline has been identified in individuals treated for non-CNS cancers, in which no primary neurological etiology can be identified. Reports from patients and their physicians of cognitive decline in breast and other cancers following treatment has led to a focus on various treatment modalities and their potential effect on cognition in these groups. While earlier reports generally focused on the effects of chemotherapy exposure ("chemobrain"), other factors and treatment modalities are increasingly recognized as potential contributors to ultimate cognitive dysfunction. In addition to chemotherapy exposure, hormone treatment, pain medications, genetic susceptibilities, immune system dysfunction, and the psychological and physical stress of diagnosis and treatment may all potentially affect self-report and objective findings of cognitive dysfunction. For this reason, we focus on post-treatment difficulties in cognition with a focus on chemotherapy exposure, mainly derived from studies in women with breast cancer, but with the caveat that several other factors may also contribute to reported and observed dysfunction. Studies utilizing neuropsychological measures have defined the objective cognitive effects following treatment and have been extended through the use of structural and functional neuroimaging to better understand potential pathology underlying cognitive dysfunction. In addition, while still in the early stages of investigation, mechanisms by which cancer treatments might influence cognitive abilities and brain function have been proposed that might help to explain resulting cognitive dysfunction.

In this chapter, we will first describe a typical case of cognitive dysfunction putatively associated with cancer treatment to provide the reader a better understanding of how this syndrome presents in a routine clinical setting. We will then review research literature documenting the self-report of individuals' post-treatment in regard to their most prominent cognitive symptoms and how these affect day-to-day functioning. Research documenting formal, objective measurement of cognitive abilities in this group is then reviewed and contrasted. Contributions of structural and functional imaging, which may help to clarify the underlying changes in brain structure and function following treatment, are then discussed, followed by potential mechanisms by which

treatment may exert an effect on the brain and cognition. We then close with a review of the emerging literature on cognitive rehabilitation and pharmacologic interventions that have been developed for the treatment of cognitive changes following treatment.

CASE SUMMARY

Ms. C., a 25-year-old woman diagnosed with non-Hodgkins lymphoma approximately 2 years before, was referred to our service with reports of forgetfulness, poor concentration, and difficulties in understanding instructions and learning new tasks. Ms. C. had undergone chemotherapy treatment consisting of four rounds: rituximab, cyclophosphamide, doxorubicin hydrochloride, vincristine sulfate, and prednisone (R-CHOP), and two rounds: ifosfamide, carboplatin, and etoposide (ICE) after her diagnosis, with no evidence of disease since then. While she had had no difficulties performing her work in office administration before treatment, she found herself making increasing errors on routine assignments, felt more easily distracted, and experienced difficulties when new tasks were assigned to her. These difficulties only increased when she took a new position with similar responsibilities in a different, faster-paced environment with new co-workers. She found herself making significant errors on a daily basis and increasingly relying on her co-workers around her for additional help, both of which led to reprimands from her supervisors. Ms. C. expressed considerable anxiety about her situation, fearing that her many mistakes were putting her job in jeopardy.

Ms. C. was administered a standard neuropsychological test battery, which included measures of processing speed, attention, language functioning, verbal and visuospatial reasoning, learning and memory, as well as executive functioning; psychological and emotional factors that may have been contributing to the reported issues were also assessed by self-report. Our assessment found mildly impaired cognitive and motor slowing across all timed tasks in which speed and efficiency are prerequisites, as well as difficulties in recollection of previously learned information. Complicating the clinical picture, Ms. C.'s profile was also notable for considerable anxiety, manifested by rumination, tension, and constant worry. These difficulties were discussed with Ms. C., who found the objective results broadly overlapping with the issues she had identified at work and at home; specifically, she identified feelings of being forgetful, "slower," "less efficient," difficulties in real-time, pressured situations, and constant anxiety that appeared in reaction to mistakes as well as distracted her from tasks at hand. Cognitive rehabilitation, tailored to her specific tasks and difficulties at work, was recommended, as well as regular psychotherapy for treatment of the attendant anxiety in relation to her diagnosis and current difficulties.

SELF-REPORTED COGNITIVE DECLINE FOLLOWING TREATMENT

The kinds of difficulties described above are widely cited in literature studying self-reported cognitive issues following treatment. Slowing, inattention, distraction, forgetfulness, difficulties in multi-tasking, and language function are all implicated in patients' self-report to varying degrees. Early research on self-reported cognitive difficulties in mixed etiology cancer patients found that roughly half of patients reported difficulties in memory or concentration at some point in their treatment (1). Follow-up by this group in a sample of 91 lymphoma patients six or more months post-treatment found 30% of patients reported difficulties in concentration, with significant forgetfulness being reported by 52% of patients (2). That these self-reported cognitive difficulties persisted for longer interims post-treatment was confirmed by Schagen et al. (3), who found persistent reported cognitive difficulties, including poor concentration (31%) and forgetfulness (21%) in breast cancer survivors treated with cyclophosphamide, methotrexate, and fluorouracil 5FU (CMF) compared with surgery and radiation treatment alone. Similarly, Ahles et al. (4) found persistent reports of difficulties in concentration and complex attention up to 10 years post-treatment in individuals who received systemic chemotherapy for breast cancer and lymphoma. Several other studies, including patients with different cancers at various time points during and after completion of treatment, have found similar increased incidence of reported cognitive difficulties putatively associated with chemotherapy and hormone exposure (5–13).

OBJECTIVE MEASUREMENT OF COGNITION FOLLOWING TREATMENT

The first studies that investigated objective differences in cognition of individuals post-treatment were cross-sectional, contrasting individuals post-treatment with healthy controls or cancer diagnosed controls undergoing a different treatment. Initial cross-sectional studies of breast cancer survivors found that 17% to 75% of patients experienced cognitive difficulties anywhere between 6 months and 10 years post-treatment. A meta-analysis that included mainly cross-sectional studies (5–6, 14) found small to moderate effect sizes across motor function, executive function, learning and memory, spatial reasoning, and language function; these results square with reports of cancer survivors and their clinicians, which document difficulties including forgetfulness, difficulties in attention and multi-tasking, cognitive slowing, and difficulties in word finding (15,16). Ahles et al. (4) documented that

a subset of cognitive difficulties appear even at longer intervals post-treatment, with chemotherapy-exposed individuals exhibiting significantly worse performance overall and lower performance specifically in verbal ability and psychomotor speed 10 years post-treatment.

The cross-sectional design of these studies, which do not include pre-treatment baseline assessments, qualifies the interpretation of their results. Cancer patients may present with pre-treatment, baseline cognitive dysfunction, with these difficulties persisting through treatment and post-treatment testing (17,18). Wefel et al. (18) found that 35% of women pre-chemotherapy treatment exhibited cognitive impairment. Ahles et al. (2008) investigated pre-treatment cognitive ability in healthy controls and patients diagnosed with invasive (stages I to III) and non-invasive (stage 0) breast cancer and found significantly slowed reaction time in the invasive group compared with healthy controls, and lower overall performance in the invasive group compared with the healthy and non-invasive patient groups. While pre-treatment/baseline differences remain poorly understood in regard to mechanism or etiology, the fact that differences are present between groups prior to treatment requires that longitudinal assessments be conducted.

More recent longitudinal studies that can control for these pre-treatment differences have contrasted cancer diagnosed individuals undergoing different treatment regimens with each other and with healthy, non-cancer diagnosed individuals. Results of these longitudinal studies suggest more specific and more subtle cognitive decline associated with chemotherapy treatment than previous cross-sectional studies would indicate. A subset of these studies find no observable cognitive effect of chemotherapy exposure (19), observable decline in only a subset of patients treated with a specific regimen of chemotherapy (CTC vs. FEC) (20), or declines in only a subset of cognitive abilities with no overall decline in neuropsychological performance (21). Positive studies generally suggest that declines in performance following chemotherapy exposure will be in specific cognitive abilities and that these declines will only be exhibited in a subset of individuals. Quesnel et al. (22) compared chemotherapy-exposed and radiotherapy-treated patients pre-treatment and at 3 months post-treatment and found that verbal memory was affected in both groups regardless of treatment, but with a specific effect on verbal fluency in the chemotherapy-exposed group.

Recent work complicates the interpretation that chemotherapy, in isolation, is responsible for cognitive decline post-treatment and reinforces the argument that effects post-treatment are likely multi-factorial. In addition to chemotherapy treatment, longitudinal studies that included patients not exposed to chemotherapy and healthy controls revealed that the no chemotherapy group frequently performed as poorly as the chemotherapy group or at an intermediate level between the chemotherapy-exposed group and the healthy controls. This pattern of results raised the question of whether endocrine therapy could impact cognitive functioning. Initial examination of this issue produced mixed results; however, most studies were not powered to adequately examine the independent effects of endocrine therapy. A recent longitudinal study examining patients not treated with chemotherapy who were randomized to tamoxifen or exemestane revealed that patients treated with tamoxifen, but not with exemestane, experienced cognitive problems compared with healthy controls (23). Even though investigators assumed that they were studying the effects of chemotherapy, in reality, most breast cancer patients receive multi-modality treatment including surgery with exposure to general anesthesia, radiation therapy, and endocrine therapy in addition to chemotherapy. This, in combination with the evidence for pre-treatment cognitive issues, lead Hurria and colleagues to propose the phrase "cancer and cancer treatment–associated cognitive change" as a more accurate descriptor of the phenomenon (24).

The research cited above confirms the presence of objective cognitive difficulties in a subset of cancer patients post-treatment, and these difficulties have been linked specifically to chemotherapy treatment as well as to several other variables, including endocrine therapies. Significantly, while both subjective reports and objective assessment have found significant changes post-treatment, outcomes appear to differ depending on whether cognition is assessed by self-report or neuropsychological testing.

SUBJECTIVE VERSUS OBJECTIVE MEASUREMENT OF COGNITION FOLLOWING TREATMENT

Similar to findings in other disorders, subjective cognitive reports exhibit poor agreement with results of objective testing at the level of the individual. Depending on the study, this discrepancy appears to be due either to a tendency to overestimate cognitive difficulties by self-report where objective measures find no significant issue or a failure to report cognitive dysfunction where objective measures would suggest significant difficulties. Importantly, most studies do find increased objective cognitive difficulties in individuals post-treatment but report little overlap with subjective reports.

As an example, following on their observation of patient reports of cognitive difficulties described above, Cull et al. (2) found no significant difference in performance on objective memory or concentration tasks between those reporting cognitive difficulties and those reporting no issues. Similarly, Schagen et al. (3) found no relationship between the cognitive reports and objective cognitive performance of breast cancer survivors treated with CMF, despite a higher rate of objective cognitive difficulties in the CMF-exposed group. This same inconsistency between self-report and objective measures is found across several later studies and in those described above, with studies either finding no relationship between subjective and objective measures or that subjective reports were better accounted for by other variables.

The source of this discrepancy has received increasing attention as these inconsistencies have come to light (for review, see Ref. 25) and is important to understand when assessing the reports of patients' post-treatment. While objective findings of cognitive dysfunction have been documented in previous studies, it is important to note that use of these objective measures either clinically or in research applications may tend to underestimate cognitive dysfunction. To what extent these measures are actually predictive of day-to-day functioning, that is, their ecological validity is not clear; to what extent neuropsychological measures are adequately sensitive to what are likely subtle deficits is also in question. Additionally, formal assessments typically take place in a somewhat rarefied environment that includes no distractions and no competing demands in a quiet, generally predictable setting, all important factors for individuals who complain of attentional difficulties and distractibility. In the research context, in addition to being subject to all of the caveats described in the clinical setting, prior research has excluded individuals who may be at most risk for cognitive dysfunction because of a history of neurological, medical, or psychological difficulties that may in fact act as risk factors to treatment-related effects. As Pullens et al. (25) note, several factors may be in play: 1) The sensitivity of objective measures may be questioned in their ability to identify what may be subtle cognitive deficits; 2) objective measures may fail to measure the kinds of difficulties that most affect patients post-treatment; 3) patients may be describing their worst functioning over a period of months versus a one-time, cross-sectional objective measurement; 4) increasing patient exposure and knowledge of "chemobrain" may lead to increased reporting; 5) subjective reports may reflect poor-self evaluation as a result of depression, anxiety, or stress. Emotional factors, in particular, have been found to be associated with increased reporting of cognitive decline post-treatment in the absence of objective decline. Van Dam et al. (13) found a higher incidence of objective cognitive difficulties in high versus low dose and healthy control patients as well as a higher incidence of reported cognitive difficulties between chemotherapy-treated patients and healthy control participants. Significantly, while objective performance and subjective reports were not associated, subjective reports were associated with elevated scores on the anxiety and depression subscales of the Hopkins Symptom Checklist, with similar findings in a subset of other studies (3,7,12,26,27). Subjective expectation of cognitive difficulties may also affect increased self-reporting as a result of increasing awareness of treatment-related effects. This is suggested by Schagen et al. (28), who found that, similar to other schema induction research (29,30), individuals who had pre-existing knowledge of potential treatment effects reported more cognitive difficulties.

Despite this disagreement between subjective and objective measures, findings of objective cognitive decline post-treatment are replete in the literature. Objective measures provide what may be considered the most conservative estimate of cognitive decline. The limitations of objective measures, including potentially poor sensitivity, poor ecological validity, and differences between the testing environment and real-world settings, however, may tend to underestimate actual cognitive dysfunction in cancer patients post-treatment.

RISK FACTORS AND MODERATORS OF COGNITIVE CHANGE FOLLOWING TREATMENT

In light of previous research finding pre-treatment differences in a subset of cancer-diagnosed individuals together with the more recent research that suggests only a subset of individuals experience cognitive decline following treatment, a next logical step is to examine risk factors that increase vulnerability to cognitive change and factors that may compensate for, or confer resilience to, these changes. Cognitive changes may be understood as the product of intrinsic factors—age appropriate and pathological changes in structural and functional integrity in the brain—together with what may be broadly characterized as environmental exposures, either currently or by history, that may be either protective or represent a risk factor to cognitive functioning. Work on the concept of brain reserve, that is, the theory that structural integrity or burden in the brain can influence the course of cognitive function in the face of new onset insults, has realized increasing attention in studies of dementing conditions and traumatic brain insult (31). This work has mainly focused on resilience to cognitive deterioration in conditions in which progressive decline is a natural course (Alzheimer's disease, frontotemporal dementia, Lewy body disease) (32) (for review, see Ref. 33). The concept of cognitive reserve, that is, innate and developed cognitive capacity which is influenced by various factors including genetics, education, occupational attainment, and life style, is related to brain reserve but is defined as a more active, compensatory process (34). Age, premorbid cognitive ability, and genetic inheritance have all been identified as significant factors that may moderate or mediate cognitive difficulties following treatment. Age is a well-established risk factor for cognitive decline in other disorders; researchers have speculated that older adults may be more vulnerable to a variety of insults partly as a result of decreased brain reserve

mediated by brain pathology and the accumulated effects of age-appropriate changes in brain structure (35). Individuals with lesser cognitive abilities pre-treatment, which may be indicative of lesser cognitive reserve, may also be at greater risk for post-treatment cognitive changes. Research has demonstrated that people with low cognitive reserve are more vulnerable to the development of neurocognitive disorders (Alzheimer's disease) and to cognitive decline following a variety of insults to the brain. Further, research has demonstrated poorer cognitive outcomes secondary to neurotoxic exposures (e.g., lead) in people with low cognitive reserve (36). Based on the concepts of brain and cognitive reserve, one would predict that older patients with lower than expected cognitive performance at pre-treatment would demonstrate poorer cognitive performance post-treatment. Ahles and colleagues found support for an interaction of age, cognitive reserve, and exposure to chemotherapy as risk factors for cognitive decline. In the context of a longitudinal study, they demonstrated that older patients who had lower levels of estimated premorbid function demonstrated significantly reduced performance on post-treatment measures of processing speed (see Figure 43.1) (37).

Genetic factors have also been examined as potential risk factors for cognitive decline. Apolipoprotein E (ApoE) is a complex glycolipoprotein that facilitates the uptake, transport, and distribution of lipids. It appears to play an important role in neuronal repair and plasticity after injury. A four exon gene codes for ApoE on chromosome 19 in humans. There are three major alleles: E2, E3, and E4. These alleles differ in amino acids at positions 112 and 158: E2 (cysteine/cysteine), E3 (cysteine/arginine), and E4 (arginine/arginine). Animal models suggest a link between the E4 allele and increased mortality, extent of damage, and poor repair following trauma (38). The human E4 allele has been associated with a variety of disorders with prominent cognitive dysfunction including healthy individuals with memory difficulties,

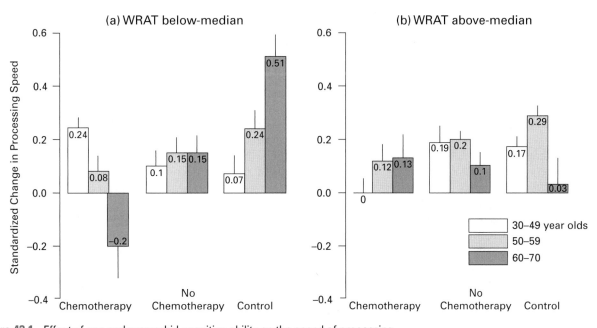

Figure 43.1. Effect of age and premorbid cognitive ability on the speed of processing.

Alzheimer's disease, and poor outcomes in stroke and traumatic brain injury. Ahles et al. (39) evaluated the relationship between the ApoE genotype and neuropsychological performance in long-term cancer survivors treated with standard dose chemotherapy. The results demonstrated that survivors with at least one E4 allele scored significantly lower in the visual memory and spatial ability domains, with a trend to score lower in the psychomotor domain, compared with survivors who did not carry an E4 allele.

Small et al. (40) studied catechol-o-methyltransferase (COMT), which influences the metabolic breakdown of catecholamines through the methylation of dopamine (DA). The valine version (val allele) is almost four times as active as the methionine version of the gene (met allele). Thus individuals homozygous for the val allele presumably metabolize DA much more rapidly than those with the met allele. COMT becomes a major modulator of dopaminergic tone in the frontal cortex, accounting for ~60% of the metabolic degradation of DA. These researchers found that breast cancer patients who had the COMT-Val allele and were treated with chemotherapy performed more poorly on tests of attention, verbal fluency, and motor speed compared with COMT-Met homozygotes.

Other genetic factors that have been suggested as potential candidates for increasing risk for chemotherapy-induced cognitive change include genes that regulate DNA repair (e.g., X-ray repair cross complementing protein 1, XRCC1; Meiotic recombination 11 homolog A, MRE11A), cytokine regulation (e.g., Interleukin 1, IL1; IL6; tumor necrosis factor alpha, TNF-alpha), neurotransmitter activity (e.g., BDNF), and blood–brain barrier efficiency (e.g., multidrug resistance 1, MDR1; organic anion transporting polypeptide, OATP). However, no studies have directly examined the relationship between these genes and chemotherapy-induced cognitive function (41).

STRUCTURAL AND FUNCTIONAL MRI FINDINGS

A crucial, intermediate step in understanding potential mechanisms of chemotherapy-induced cognitive decline will utilize structural brain imaging techniques that enable measurement of changes in regional cerebral volume and cortical thickness. A handful of relatively recent investigations utilizing various methodologies have studied this issue, with a focus on changes in gray matter volumes in individuals post-chemotherapy. These studies utilize voxel-based morphometry (VBM), which estimates gray matter volume after segmentation of MRI-derived structural images. In a cross-sectional study, which incorporated data collection points at 1- and 3-years post chemotherapy treatment in a cohort of breast cancer survivors, brain structure and neuropsychological performance was compared between a chemotherapy and healthy control group (42). Results suggested significantly decreased gray matter volume in prefrontal cortex, precuneus, cingulate cortex, and parahippocampal gyri relative to healthy controls initially, with no difference observed at a 3-year follow-up. A more recent cross-sectional study utilized

diffusion tensor imaging (DTI) to examine white matter tract integrity in breast cancer survivors treated with chemotherapy and unaffected controls (43). While complimentary to VBM analysis, DTI relies on measures of regional diffusion to estimate white matter tract integrity and efficiency. Significantly, results suggest decreased white matter tract integrity indicated by increased fractional anisotropy and mean diffusion measures in chemotherapy-treated individuals relative to controls. Focal deficits were exhibited in frontal and temporal white matter tracts, consistent with VBM gray matter findings described above, and correlated with neuropsychological measures of processing speed and attention.

While suggestive, interpretation of the results from the above studies is qualified given the relatively small patient groups, the absence of control groups of cancer survivors with no chemotherapy treatment, and the use of cross-sectional designs that prevent interpretation of interval changes from pre-treatment baseline. As noted above, pre-treatment baseline structural measurement is an important element in any investigation because of pre-treatment differences in cognition in individuals prior to adjuvant chemotherapy treatment (17). Results from Ahles et al.'s study also underscore the importance of the inclusion of cancer-diagnosed individuals who are not treated with chemotherapy to delineate the effects of chemotherapy treatment versus cancer diagnosis alone on cognition. Recently, the first longitudinal study of structural changes associated with chemotherapy treatment, including pre-treatment baseline and a cancer diagnosed, non-chemotherapy cohort, was reported (44). Pre-treatment baseline scans were collected in breast cancer survivors treated with (CTx+) and without (CTx−) chemotherapy and healthy controls and compared with structural scans at 1-month and 1-year post-treatment in the same individuals. VBM analysis found decreases in frontotemporal cortex and cerebellum at 1 month relative to baseline in the chemotherapy-treated group, with partial recovery of volume at 1 year. While the CTx-group exhibited gray matter reduction in cerebellum at 1 month, the CTx+ group exhibited more widely distributed gray matter reductions across frontal and temporal cortical regions as well as cerebellum and thalamus. Partial recovery of volume in these same regions was exhibited in the CTx+ group at 1 year post-treatment but reduced volume remained relative to pre-treatment baseline. The course of recovery of gray matter volume described in this study is in agreement with the report of individuals reporting cognitive changes following chemotherapy treatment, in that neuropsychological deficits are most pronounced immediately following treatment, with subsequent, partial recovery of function over time (26,45).

Studies utilizing functional imaging methods such as functional magnetic resonance imaging (fMRI), positron emission tomography (PET), or single proton emission computed tomography are relatively sparse in the literature at this point. An early study investigated putative effects of chemotherapy on cognitive function as well as fMRI-derived estimates of brain structure and function in a pair of monozygotic twins discordant for breast cancer diagnosis and chemotherapy treatment (46). Results suggested significantly increased self-reported cognitive difficulties in the affected twin, together with higher incidence of white matter hyperintensities and differential activity in frontal cortices in a functional activation task. Significantly, standard neuropsychological measures revealed only slight decreases in performance in the affected twin, which may suggest that clinical neuropsychological measures may lack some level of sensitivity to the kinds of cognitive difficulties typically reported by individuals treated with chemotherapy. This lack of sensitivity may be due in part to compensatory strategies that help to obscure behavioral differences, evidence of which may be found in wider and more diffuse regional brain recruitment. In a cross-sectional study comparing verbal memory performance between 14 women post-chemotherapy treatment and 14 healthy controls (47), patients exhibited increased prefrontal cortex recruitment during the recall task. The areas of increased recruitment were described as atypical for the declarative memory task based on previous findings associated with this task, and interpreted, again, as compensatory for more typical cortical sites recruited in this paradigm; behavioral performance and accuracy did not significantly differ between groups. Two studies investigated functional activation in chemotherapy-exposed individuals at longer intervals post-treatment. In a PET study, Silverman et al. (48) investigated differences in regional recruitment between women who had been treated with chemotherapy 5 to 10 years earlier and control subjects who had not been exposed to chemotherapy while performing a memory task. While task performance was equivalent between groups, increased inferior frontal gyrus recruitment was exhibited in the chemotherapy-exposed group during task completion, suggesting that increased prefrontal activity may be compensatory. The suggestion that the chemotherapy group employed compensatory strategies for task completion is further supported by the fact that this inferior frontal gyrus recruitment was not found in the control group, in whom parietal and occipital cortex recruitment was more typical. De Ruiter et al. (49) studied 19 women approximately 10 years post-chemotherapy treatment compared with 15 women previously diagnosed with breast cancer but not treated with chemotherapy on a task of executive functioning and planning (Tower of London) and on a paired associate memory task. In contrast to the previously described studies, the chemotherapy-exposed group exhibited decreased recruitment in dorsolateral prefrontal cortex on the executive functioning task, as well as decreased recruitment in parahippocampal gyri on the paired associates task, with corresponding poorer performance on each task in the chemotherapy group. Similar to previous research in objective neurocognitive assessment of cancer-diagnosed patients, a recent fMRI study (50) compared 10 cancer-diagnosed women prior to chemotherapy with nine healthy controls on a working memory task. Consistent with findings of pretreatment cognitive issues in cancer-diagnosed individuals, the patient group was less accurate on the working memory task in the context of wider and more diffuse recruitment of prefrontal cortex, and specifically inferior frontal gyrus. This study, similar to studies using objective neuropsychological testing that found pre-treatment differences in cognition in cancer diagnosed individuals, underscores the need for longitudinal design in fMRI studies that would account for pretreatment differences.

Collectively, functional imaging studies suggest that in tasks in which performance is essentially equivalent between groups, the affected group generally employs compensatory prefrontal mechanisms for task completion; there is also evidence that in the subset of studies in which performance was decreased in the affected group, typical brain regions that would otherwise be recruited exhibit reduced recruitment. Still unclear are the precise mechanisms by which treatment may influence brain structure and function.

MECHANISMS

As treatment-related cognitive changes have been increasingly supported in previous studies, central to understanding the etiology of these changes will be the investigation of how prescribed treatments affect underlying brain structure and function. While a number of mechanisms have been proposed to explain cognitive dysfunction associated with cancer treatments, still little is known regarding biological risk factors or mechanisms of damage (41).

The most intuitive explanation for the effects of treatment, and specifically chemotherapy, on brain structure and function is the direct effect of chemotherapy agents on the brain (e.g., neurotoxic or inflammatory mechanisms). Chemotherapy agents exhibit different profiles in their ability to cross the blood–brain barrier, although in rare cases, most agents can cause CNS disorders, suggesting that some permeability of the blood–brain barrier is common to these drugs under certain conditions. Research utilizing positron emission tomography (PET), a neuroimaging technique that is capable of radiolabeling chemotherapy agents including cisplatin, BCNU, and paclitaxel, has found evidence of these agents in the CNS post-administration (51–53). It is clear, however, that the absolute levels of chemotherapy reaching the CNS are much lower than outside the CNS, as evidenced by the poor efficacy of systemic chemotherapy treatment on CNS tumors. This may suggest that, while chemotherapy permeability of the blood–brain barrier is relatively low, little drug is necessary to have an effect on the brain. Evidence of this is found in non-human animal studies that find cell death and decreased cell division in hippocampal, parahippocampal, and corpus callosum regions following systemic chemotherapy treatment in mice (54). Differences in blood–brain barrier permeability between individuals may also be an important factor in the extent of chemotherapy exposure in the CNS. The gene multi-drug resistance 1 (MDR1) has been found to play a role in blood–brain barrier functioning through its role in encoding the protein P-glycoprotein (P-gp) which is implicated in transporting toxic substances out of the cell. Select MDR1 polymorphisms may be associated with P-gp function, which may in turn alter the efficiency with which toxic agents, including chemotherapy, are transported from the blood–brain barrier (55).

DNA damage as a result of oxidative stress has also been proposed as a potential intermediate mechanism to CNS damage. One mechanism through which chemotherapy agents affect tumor cell growth is through DNA damage to tumor cells. Importantly, chemotherapy treatment also leads to DNA damage in non-tumor cells and is associated with increased levels of non-protein bound iron, free radicals, and reduced anti-oxidant capacity, leading to increased oxidative stress more generally. Evidence of an association between increased oxidative DNA damage and cognitive dysfunction has been found in previous studies of neurocognitive disorders, including Alzheimer's disease, and mild cognitive impairment (56). At this point, it is not clear how DNA damage might affect the CNS. The production of defective proteins leading to neuronal apoptosis, deficient DNA repair mechanisms, as well as the loss of essential gene products as a result of DNA damage have all been considered (57,58). Finally, chemotherapy treatment may have a direct effect on telomere length (59–61). With each DNA replication, telomeres become shorter, and past a given threshold, this shortening leads to cell death or cell senescence. Chemotherapy treatment therefore may essentially accelerate the aging process either through direct effect on telomere length in the CNS or the more general effect on genomic stability and biological systems.

Cytokines, cell-signaling proteins that play an important role in immune system functioning as well as in the nervous system, have also been identified as one potential mechanism in CNS damage related to treatment. Cytokines have been found to modulate neuronal and glial cell functioning, neural repair, as well as the action of the neurotransmitters dopamine and serotonin, and cytokine dysregulation has been associated with neural cell death and degenerative neurological disorders associated with aging. In cancer patients, the role of cytokines in cognitive functioning is most clear in patients undergoing IL2 or IFN-α treatment, which are associated with increased fatigue, depression, and cognitive difficulties (62). Importantly, chemotherapy treatment has been associated with increased cytokine levels in the acute phase of treatment (63–65). While the association of chemotherapy-associated cytokine increases with cognitive dysfunction has not been studied, chemotherapy-exposed individuals with significant and chronic fatigue at longer intervals post-treatment exhibit elevated levels of cytokines (66,67).

Research has been initiated and continues in our lab and others that seek to better understand and locate mechanistic explanations for treatment-related cognitive dysfunction. Regardless of how such changes come about, an important clinical issue is how best to measure and define these difficulties such that treatment recommendations can be made with an aim toward ameliorating difficulties in cognition.

CLINICAL NEUROPSYCHOLOGICAL TESTING OF POST-TREATMENT COGNITIVE DYSFUNCTION

Neuropsychology is a subspeciality of psychology with a primary interest in understanding brain–behavior relationships, with a particular focus on higher level cognitive processes

and their dysfunction in clinical syndromes. Given the disagreement between subjective reports and objective cognitive measures, neuropsychological testing remains the most direct and accurate way in which to measure cognitive effects post-cancer treatment. Even given this disagreement, the most typical reason for referral is generally subjective complaint of difficulties or caregiver/family observation of cognitive difficulties in the patient.

Depending on the setting, referrals may be made by the primary oncologist involved in the patient's care, rehabilitation medicine, psychiatry, by a general practitioner, or, most often in older patients, by the primary geriatrician. There are many questions to consider when contemplating referral for assessment of post-cancer treatment, and more generally, in any medically ill population: Is the patient at their "new" baseline? Are they currently on an active treatment regimen that may have acute effects not predictive of longer term adjustment (current chemotherapy treatment, intracranial irradiation, etc.)? Will their medical care change dramatically in the near future and would this alteration be expected to affect cognition (initiation of chemotherapy regimen, initiation of intracranial irradiation)? Is there a significant psychiatric issue that may affect cognition (uncontrolled depression, anxiety, adjustment reaction)? Is there significant fatigue, pain, or physical discomfort that may influence cognitive testing? These considerations are meant to ensure that the results of the assessment will be indicative and predictive of long-term, future cognitive function and will not be overwhelmed by state-like transient factors or subject to change because of a change in treatment, physical condition, or emotional/psychological status.

Once a referral is made, a typical neuropsychological consultation begins with a full diagnostic interview, which gathers information on the chief cognitive difficulties, cancer, medical, neurological, psychiatric, psychosocial, substance use, and educational/vocational history, all of which will help to contextualize the results of the neuropsychological assessment. If a neuropsychological assessment is considered appropriate, formal testing is recommended, which will vary in terms of time and measures administered depending on patient characteristics and referral question; time for an assessment may range from as little as 30 minutes to an hour, to several hours. Older patients, patients with significant fatigue, or patients with significant pain who cannot tolerate a full evaluation may be given briefer screening measures or stand-alone batteries.

A flexible approach to test selection will allow tailoring of the assessment to the specific referral question; while most practitioners will employ a somewhat standard, "core" battery of measures, additional measures may be administered for specific issues or difficulties (multi-tasking, attention/concentration issues over longer periods of time). Neuropsychological and psychological measures are generally in a paper and pencil as well as interview and computer administered formats, and should have acceptable validity and reliability. Most assessments will attempt to sample cognitive ability in multiple domains, including attention and concentration, psychomotor speed, verbal functioning, visuospatial reasoning, praxis and construction, verbal and visual learning and recall, and executive functioning (abstraction, reasoning, cognitive flexibility, problem solving, planning and organization) (see Table 43.1 for a list of typical measures used in our Neuropsychological Evaluation Service). Depending on the patient's presentation, stand-alone measures of personality, emotional, and psychological functioning may also be administered either by course or when there is suspicion that a significant psychiatric issue may be affecting cognition.

TABLE 43.1	List of commonly used neuropsychological measures in assessment of post-treatment cognitive dysfunction

Measure	Function
Premorbid Intelligence	
Wide Range Achievement Test-Reading subtest (WRAT 4)	A measure estimating premorbid cognitive abilities, highly correlated with general intellectual abilities
Verbal Ability	
FAS-Controlled Oral Word Association Test	A timed measure of phonemic fluency
Animal Naming Test	A timed measure of semantic fluency
Boston Naming Test	A measure of confrontation naming (word finding)
Learning and Memory	
California Verbal Learning Test II (CVLT-II)	A measure of verbal list learning and recall
Logical Memory I and II (WMS-IV)	A measure of verbal story learning and recall
Rey-Osterreith Complex Figure	A measure of visual figure learning and memory
Attention	
Digit Span (WAIS-IV)	A measure of brief span of attention
Arithmetic (WAIS-IV)	A measure of brief span of attention and working memory
Continuous Performance Test (CPT)	A measure of sustained attention
Processing Speed	
The Trail Making Test (Part A)	A measure of visual scanning and graphomotor speed
The Trail Making Test (Part B)	A measure of visual scanning, graphomotor speed and set-shifting
Digit Symbol—Coding (WAIS-IV)	A speeded graphomotor measure
Symbol Search (WAIS-IV)	A speeded measure of visual scanning and attention
Visual Reasoning/Construction	
Rey-Osterreith Complex Figure	A measure of visual construction
Judgment of Line Orientation	A measure of visuospatial judgment and reasoning
Block Design (WAIS-IV)	A timed measure of visual construction and reasoning
Executive Functioning	
Wisconsin Card Sorting Task (WCST)	A measure of abstract reasoning and problem solving
Stroop	A measure of speeded word reading, color naming, and inhibition
Psychological/Emotional	
Personality Assessment Inventory (PAI)	A self-report measure of psychological functioning
Beck Depression Inventory (BDI)	A self-report measure of depressive symptomatology
State Trait Anxiety Inventory (STAI)	A self-report measure of anxiety symptomatology

Once testing is complete, patient performance on individual measures is compared with normative groups defined by age, or, increasingly, age, education, gender, and ethnicity to ensure the most exact matching of patients to their respective cohorts. In contrast to a "deficit testing" model of assessment, in which performance is categorized as either normal or aberrant, comparison of patients' performance with that of normative groups, and with their own premorbid functioning, allows for finer gradations of interpretation; test results can indicate how well, or how poorly, an individual patient performs on a given task and also allows for detection not only of absolute deficits but also of deficits that are relative to the patient's normative cohort or to their own premorbid functioning.

Results are then integrated and contextualized with the patient's report of difficulty as well as with their medical and other history. Differential diagnosis is a particularly important aspect of neuropsychological assessment in cancer survivors. Because the incidence of a subset of cancers increases with age, referrals for neuropsychological assessment in a cancer center typically skew to older patients. Since older patients may present with several possible etiologies or, at the very least, contributors to cognitive dysfunction, a detailed assessment and analysis of the pattern of strengths and weaknesses is especially necessary. While some etiologies or syndromes may express a typical pattern of neuropsychological performance, few exhibit pathognomonic signs, and it is more likely that a combination of a given pattern of performance together with an association of history of treatment and onset of difficulties will guide interpretation. Once the pattern of neuropsychological performance is analyzed and interpreted, recommendations for further treatment, evaluations, and rehabilitation can be made. These can include referrals for neurological evaluation and neuroimaging studies, psychiatric evaluation, and cognitive rehabilitation.

TREATMENT OPTIONS

Treatment options following cancer therapy will depend on the nature of the cognitive impairment, the presence of additional potential etiologies, and patient preference. The two discussed here are cognitive rehabilitation and pharmacologic intervention. Follow-up treatment by psychiatry, neurology, and physical therapy are also potential directions in the event that the patient has a significant psychological or emotional component, there is suspicion of a primary neurological disorder that better explains results of neuropsychological testing, or there is a significant impact of physical limitations.

Cognitive Rehabilitation

In traditional rehabilitation settings, cognitive rehabilitation has been employed to assist individuals in learning, or in most cases relearning, ways to concentrate, remember, and solve problems after an illness or injury affecting the brain. Cognitive rehabilitation involves a structured set of therapeutic activities designed to retrain an individual's ability to think, use judgment, and make decisions. The focus is on improving deficits in memory, attention, perception, learning, planning, and judgment through both restoration and compensatory strategies (68). The desired outcome of cognitive rehabilitation is an improved quality of life or an improved ability to function in home and community life. Cognitive rehabilitation has been generally characterized as either restorative, which focuses on retraining basic cognitive skills, or compensatory, which focuses on developing skills and strategies that work around the presenting cognitive issue. Often, interventions may consist of a mixture of both strategies in treating cognitive issues.

Research on the efficacy of cognitive rehabilitation has been mixed in other neurological disorders (minimal cognitive impairment, traumatic brain injury), as well as in post-treatment issues. Ferguson and colleagues (69) conducted a single-arm pilot study utilizing a cognitive behavioral treatment approach to aid breast cancer survivors in managing deficits with attention and memory following treatment with adjuvant chemotherapy. In brief, 29 adult women who received adjuvant chemotherapy for stage I or II breast cancer underwent Memory and Attention Adaptation Training (MAAT) at least 3 years post-treatment (mean years post-chemotherapy was 8.20 (sd = 4.40). Inclusion criteria included complaint of memory and attention problems post-chemotherapy but not a deficit on neuropsychological testing. The program consisted of seven contact sessions: four individual, in-person monthly sessions and three phone contacts. Participants were given a workbook that reviewed knowledge of chemotherapy-associated memory deficits, introduced self-awareness training, gave instruction on self-regulation including relaxation training and activity scheduling, and supplied compensatory strategies and tailored recommendations. Participants demonstrated significant improvements in verbal memory and executive functions and reported improvement in overall cognitive functioning and quality of life. While MAAT demonstrated efficacy, there was no control group and treatment was participant specific, thus limiting generalization. Given these limitations, Ferguson and colleagues (70) recently conducted a randomized clinical trial to further evaluate the efficacy of MAAT. Forty adult women who received adjuvant chemotherapy for stage I or II breast cancer were enrolled in the study; 19 were randomized to the treatment condition (MAAT) and 21 were randomized to the waitlist control condition. Inclusion criteria were a memory or attention complaint but an actual cognitive deficit was not a pre-requisite. Participants in the treatment condition underwent MAAT training as described above. Results indicated that MAAT participants demonstrated a significant improvement in verbal memory and spiritual well-being compared with controls. This randomized clinical trial did not replicate the previous finding of improved executive functioning or improvement in self-reported cognitive functioning or quality of life.

In contrast to the positive findings of cognitive interventions in this population, Poppelreuter and colleagues (71) failed to find a specific cognitive intervention effect in their recent study. They investigated two forms of cognitive rehabilitation training: a Neuropsychological Training Group (NTG), which consisted of functional training groups in which participants practiced compensatory strategies and techniques to improve attention and memory as they relate to everyday activities, and an individualized, computer-based training software package (PC) under direct supervision also targeted at improving attention and memory. These intervention groups were compared with a control group of participants that received no training. Participants had received high-dose chemotherapy and hematopoietic stem cell transplantation for systemic cancer; median time since therapy conclusion was 3 months. At the time of the study, they were undergoing inpatient rehabilitation following their oncological therapy, which is standard care for individuals in Germany. Participants had to have demonstrated a cognitive deficit in order to be in the study. Subtests from the Test Battery for Attentional Performance were used and participants had to score in the lowest quartile of the normative sample in at least two of the five parameters (61.1% of participants screened had a cognitive deficit). Eligible participants were randomly assigned to either one of the two treatment groups (NTG: $n = 21$; PC: $n = 26$) or a control group ($n = 28$). Training was implemented four times per week for 1 hour a day over the course of their inpatient stay. They found significant improvements across all cognitive domains among the three study groups concluding no specific intervention effect. Poppelreuter and colleagues (72) replicated this study with stage I or II breast cancer patients. Participants had to have demonstrated a cognitive deficit in order to be in the study. Subtests from the Test Battery for Attentional Performance were used and participants had to score in the lowest quartile of the normative sample in at least two of the five parameters (47.1% of participants screened had a cognitive deficit). They found similar results as with the hematopoietic stem cell transplantation study in that there were no specific intervention effects.

As can be seen from the above studies, current research on the efficacy of cognitive rehabilitation for post-treatment cognitive difficulties is mixed and this may reflect research findings on cognitive rehabilitation more generally. One complicating issue is whether restorative or compensatory therapy is prescribed and the manner in which post-rehabilitation abilities are measured. A restorative model would predict that objective performance should improve since training is focused on the underlying ability and this should generalize to other tasks in which that ability is a prerequisite. In contrast, compensatory rehabilitation, with its focus on developing strategies and managing the environment in which cognitive tasks are performed, would likely not lead to changes in objective measures since at least a subset of alternate strategies most likely cannot be used (e.g., patients could not keep a list of memory items). At this point, given the paucity of literature in this area, more research needs to be conducted to measure the efficacy of various treatment approaches.

Pharmacologic Interventions

Pharmacologic interventions have generally taken the form of stimulant treatment with more recent research in the efficacy of Modafinil. Dexymethylphenidate (Focalin) has been approved for the treatment of attentional symptoms in attention deficit disorder through its action as a psychostimulant. To test for more generalized effects of dexymethylphenidate on attention in other etiologies, its effect on cognition and fatigue was studied in women undergoing adjuvant chemotherapy (73). During chemotherapy for breast cancer women were randomized to D-methylphenidate ($N = 29$) or placebo ($N = 28$) to see if it improved cognitive functioning, QOL, or fatigue. In the D-MPH group, the percentage of patients classified as having moderate to severe cognitive dysfunction by the High Sensitivity Cognitive Screen, a test of six major neuropsychological domains, decreased from 3.6% at baseline to 0% at the end of chemotherapy. Rate of impairment was stable at 11% in the placebo group. However, a correction factor applied for practice effects at the follow-up assessments led to 11% with moderate to severe impairment in the D-MPH group and 22% in the placebo group with no statistically significant difference in cognitive outcomes between groups. In another study, Lower et al. (2005) conducted a randomized placebo control trial of D-methylphenidate as a treatment for cognitive dysfunction and fatigue in 250 non-anemic breast and ovarian cancer patients. Patients (76% breast cancer and 13.6% ovarian cancer) were randomized to placebo ($N = 75$) or D-methylphenidate ($N = 77$). Significant improvement in memory and fatigue was observed in the D-methylphenidate group.

Modafinil (Provigil) has been approved for the treatment of narcolepsy and shift-work disorder and, as such, has been considered in the treatment of attentional and fatigue symptoms in several other disorders. Kohli and colleagues (74) examined the effects of modafinil on cognitive functioning in patients with breast cancer. Sixty-eight participants with breast cancer who had completed treatment with chemotherapy and/or radiation more than 1 month prior to commencement of the study completed both the open-label phase of the study (phase 1) and the randomization phase to continued treatment with modafinil or placebo (phase 2). Results indicated that 200 mg/day of modafinil during phase 1 significantly increased participants' ability to store, retain, and retrieve verbal and non-verbal information and that they were more accurate in doing so. These results were also found at the end of phase 2 for individuals receiving continued treatment with modafinil. Further, increased attention was also found at the end of phase 2 for individuals receiving modafinil. Lundorff and colleagues (75) also examined the effects of modafinil on cancer-related cognitive dysfunction. They conducted a double-blind, randomized, cross-over, single-dose trial of modafinil in an advanced cancer patient population. Twenty-eight patients with advanced cancer (breast, genitourinary, gastrointestinal, head/neck, hematologic, lung, other) were randomly assigned to receive a single dose of 200 mg modafinil or placebo on day one and were crossed over to the alternative treatment on day four. Attention and psychomotor speed were assessed with the Finger Tapping Test (FTT) and Trail Making Test B (TMT-B), which were administered before tablet intake on each day and again four and a half hours after tablet intake. Statistically significant improvements were found in both FTT with the dominant hand and TMT-B after treatment with modafinil compared with placebo. Taken together, these studies demonstrate that modafinil is effective in improving cancer-related cognitive dysfunction.

CONCLUSIONS

Since the early studies documenting patients' report of cognitive difficulties putatively associated with treatment, significant progress has been made in better defining these issues objectively and understanding potential mechanisms. We have discussed the nature of subjective reports and objective cognitive performance post-treatment, as well as potential reasons for their disagreement. Changes in cortical thickness and subcortical volumes from pre- to post-treatment were also discussed together with their association with changes in brain function following treatment. Potential risk factors and mediators of cognitive dysfunction were identified that may explain individual outcome differences post-treatment. The role of neuropsychological assessment was discussed in clarifying cognitive dysfunction post-treatment, together with identification of specific cognitive issues that may be a focus of treatment through rehabilitation or pharmacologic intervention. Some qualifications and caveats are suggested given what we now know in regard to cancer therapies and cognitive issues. Cognitive decline is most likely associated with broader treatment variables and chemotherapy treatment alone does not fully explain cognitive dysfunction. Cognitive changes following treatment are far from uniform; subsets of individuals, as a result of age, premorbid cognitive reserve, brain reserve, or genetic variants, may be more likely or more severely affected by treatment. Cognitive differences are also exhibited in cancer-diagnosed individuals pre-treatment, underscoring the necessity of longitudinal studies; this observation also suggests that cancer diagnosis and pre-treatment cognitive differences may be related by an as yet undetermined factor. The exact mechanism of treatment variables' effect on brain structure and function is not clear; research studying oxidative stress, DNA repair mechanisms, and cytokine deregulation in response to treatment is ongoing.

REFERENCES

1. Cull A, Stewart M, Altman DG. Assessment of and intervention for psychosocial problems in routine oncology practice. *Br J Cancer*. 1995;72(1):229-235.
2. Cull A, et al. What do cancer patients mean when they complain of concentration and memory problems? *Br J Cancer*. 1996;74(10):1674-1679.
3. Schagen SB, et al. Cognitive deficits after postoperative adjuvant chemotherapy for breast carcinoma. *Cancer*. 1999;85(3):640-650.
4. Ahles TA, et al. Neuropsychologic impact of standard-dose systemic chemotherapy in long-term survivors of breast cancer and lymphoma. *J Clin Oncol*. 2002;20(2):485-493.
5. Castellon SA, et al. Neurocognitive performance in breast cancer survivors exposed to adjuvant chemotherapy and tamoxifen. *J Clin Exp Neuropsychol*. 2004;26(7):955-969.
6. Downie FP, et al. Cognitive function, fatigue, and menopausal symptoms in breast cancer patients receiving adjuvant chemotherapy: evaluation with patient interview after formal assessment. *Psychooncology*. 2006;15(10):921-930.
7. Hermelink K, et al. Cognitive function during neoadjuvant chemotherapy for breast cancer: results of a prospective, multicenter, longitudinal study. *Cancer*. 2007;109(9):1905-1913.
8. Jansen CE, et al. Preliminary results of a longitudinal study of changes in cognitive function in breast cancer patients undergoing chemotherapy with doxorubicin and cyclophosphamide. *Psychooncology*. 2008;17(12):1189-1195.
9. Mehnert A, et al. The association between neuropsychological impairment, self-perceived cognitive deficits, fatigue and health related quality of life in breast cancer survivors following standard adjuvant versus high-dose chemotherapy. *Patient Educ Couns*. 2007;66(1):108-118.
10. Poppelreuter M, et al. Cognitive dysfunction and subjective complaints of cancer patients. a cross-sectional study in a cancer rehabilitation centre. *Eur J Cancer*. 2004;40(1):43-49.
11. Schagen SB, et al. Cognitive complaints and cognitive impairment following BEP chemotherapy in patients with testicular cancer. *Acta Oncol*. 2008;47(1):63-70.
12. Shilling V, Jenkins V. Self-reported cognitive problems in women receiving adjuvant therapy for breast cancer. *Eur J Oncol Nurs*. 2007;11(1):6-15.
13. van Dam FS, et al. Impairment of cognitive function in women receiving adjuvant treatment for high-risk breast cancer: high-dose versus standard-dose chemotherapy. *J Natl Cancer Inst*. 1998;90(3):210-218.
14. Falleti MG, et al. The nature and severity of cognitive impairment associated with adjuvant chemotherapy in women with breast cancer: a meta-analysis of the current literature. *Brain Cogn*. 2005;59(1):60-70.
15. Berglund G, et al. Late effects of adjuvant chemotherapy and postoperative radiotherapy on quality of life among breast cancer patients. *Eur J Cancer*. 1991;27(9):1075-1081.
16. Phillips KA, Bernhard J. Adjuvant breast cancer treatment and cognitive function: current knowledge and research directions. *J Natl Cancer Inst*. 2003;95(3):190-197.
17. Ahles TA, et al. Cognitive function in breast cancer patients prior to adjuvant treatment. *Breast Cancer Res Treat*. 2008;110(1):143-152.
18. Wefel JS, et al. "Chemobrain" in breast carcinoma? A prologue. *Cancer*. 2004;101(3):466-475.
19. Jenkins V, et al. A 3-year prospective study of the effects of adjuvant treatments on cognition in women with early stage breast cancer. *Br J Cancer*. 2006;94(6):828-834.
20. Schagen SB, et al. Change in cognitive function after chemotherapy: a prospective longitudinal study in breast cancer patients. *J Natl Cancer Inst*. 2006;98(23):1742-1745.
21. Wefel JS, et al. The cognitive sequelae of standard-dose adjuvant chemotherapy in women with breast carcinoma: results of a prospective, randomized, longitudinal trial. *Cancer*. 2004;100(11):2292-2299.
22. Quesnel C, Savard J, Ivers H. Cognitive impairments associated with breast cancer treatments: results from a longitudinal study. *Breast Cancer Res Treat*. 2009;116(1):113-123.

23. Schilder CM, et al. Effects of tamoxifen and exemestane on cognitive functioning of postmenopausal patients with breast cancer: results from the neuropsychological side study of the tamoxifen and exemestane adjuvant multinational trial. *J Clin Oncol*. 2010;28(8):1294-1300.

24. Hurria A, Somlo G, Ahles T. Renaming "chemobrain." *Cancer Invest*. 2007;25(6):373-377.

25. Pullens MJ, De Vries J, Roukema JA. Subjective cognitive dysfunction in breast cancer patients: a systematic review. *Psychooncology*. 2010;19(11):1127-1138.

26. Weis J, Poppelreuter M, Bartsch HH. Cognitive deficits as long-term side-effects of adjuvant therapy in breast cancer patients: "subjective" complaints and "objective" neuropsychological test results. *Psychooncology*. 2009;18(7):775-782.

27. Tannock IF, et al. Cognitive impairment associated with chemotherapy for cancer: report of a workshop. *J Clin Oncol*. 2004;22(11):2233-2239.

28. Schagen SB, Das E, van Dam FS. The influence of priming and pre-existing knowledge of chemotherapy-associated cognitive complaints on the reporting of such complaints in breast cancer patients. *Psychooncology*. 2009;18(6):674-678.

29. Steele CM. A threat in the air. How stereotypes shape intellectual identity and performance. *Am Psychol*. 1997;52(6):613-629.

30. van Wijk CM, Kolk AM. Sex differences in physical symptoms: the contribution of symptom perception theory. *Soc Sci Med*. 1997;45(2):231-246.

31. Sole-Padulles C, et al. Brain structure and function related to cognitive reserve variables in normal aging, mild cognitive impairment and Alzheimer's disease. *Neurobiol Aging*. 2009;30(7):1114-1124.

32. Mortimer JA, et al. Very early detection of Alzheimer neuropathology and the role of brain reserve in modifying its clinical expression. *J Geriatr Psychiatry Neurol*. 2005;18(4):218-223.

33. Fratiglioni L, Wang HX. Brain reserve hypothesis in dementia. *J Alzheimers Dis*. 2007;12(1):11-22.

34. Stern Y. What is cognitive reserve? Theory and research application of the reserve concept. *J Int Neuropsychol Soc*. 2002;8(3):448-460.

35. Bartres-Faz D, Arenaza-Urquijo EM. Structural and functional imaging correlates of cognitive and brain reserve hypotheses in healthy and pathological aging. *Brain Topogr*. 2011;24(3-4):340-357.

36. Bleecker ML, et al. Impact of cognitive reserve on the relationship of lead exposure and neurobehavioral performance. *Neurology*. 2007;69(5):470-476.

37. Ahles TA, et al. Longitudinal assessment of cognitive changes associated with adjuvant treatment for breast cancer: impact of age and cognitive reserve. *J Clin Oncol*. 2010;28(29):4434-4440.

38. Bookheimer S, Burggren A. APOE-4 genotype and neurophysiological vulnerability to Alzheimer's and cognitive aging. *Annu Rev Clin Psychol*. 2009;5:343-362.

39. Ahles TA, et al. The relationship of APOE genotype to neuropsychological performance in long-term cancer survivors treated with standard dose chemotherapy. *Psychooncology*. 2003;12(6):612-619.

40. Small BJ, et al. Catechol-O-methyltransferase genotype modulates cancer treatment-related cognitive deficits in breast cancer survivors. *Cancer*. 2011;117(7):1369-1376.

41. Ahles TA, Saykin AJ. Candidate mechanisms for chemotherapy-induced cognitive changes. *Nat Rev Cancer*. 2007;7(3):192-201.

42. Inagaki M, et al. Smaller regional volumes of brain gray and white matter demonstrated in breast cancer survivors exposed to adjuvant chemotherapy. *Cancer*. 2007;109(1):146-156.

43. Deprez S, et al. Chemotherapy-induced structural changes in cerebral white matter and its correlation with impaired cognitive functioning in breast cancer patients. *Hum Brain Mapp*. 2011;32(3):480-493.

44. McDonald BC, et al. Gray matter reduction associated with systemic chemotherapy for breast cancer: a prospective MRI study. *Breast Cancer Res Treat*. 2010;123(3):819-828.

45. Yamada TH, et al. Neuropsychological outcomes of older breast cancer survivors: cognitive features ten or more years after chemotherapy. *J Neuropsychiatry Clin Neurosci*. 2010;22(1):48-54.

46. Ferguson RJ, et al. Brain structure and function differences in monozygotic twins: possible effects of breast cancer chemotherapy. *J Clin Oncol*. 2007;25(25):3866-3870.

47. Kesler SR, et al. Regional brain activation during verbal declarative memory in metastatic breast cancer. *Clin Cancer Res*. 2009;15(21):6665-6673.

48. Silverman DH, et al. Altered frontocortical, cerebellar, and basal ganglia activity in adjuvant-treated breast cancer survivors 5-10 years after chemotherapy. *Breast Cancer Res Treat*. 2007;103(3):303-311.

49. de Ruiter MB, et al. Cerebral hyporesponsiveness and cognitive impairment 10 years after chemotherapy for breast cancer. *Hum Brain Mapp*. 2011;32(8):1206-1219.

50. Cimprich B, et al. Prechemotherapy alterations in brain function in women with breast cancer. *J Clin Exp Neuropsychol*. 2010;32(3):324-331.

51. Gangloff A, et al. Estimation of paclitaxel biodistribution and uptake in human-derived xenografts in vivo with (18) F-fluoropaclitaxel. *J Nucl Med*. 2005;46(11):1866-1871.

52. Ginos JZ, et al. (13N)cisplatin PET to assess pharmacokinetics of intra-arterial versus intravenous chemotherapy for malignant brain tumors. *J Nucl Med*. 1987;28(12):1844-1852.

53. Mitsuki S, et al. Pharmacokinetics of 11C-labelled BCNU and SarCNU in gliomas studied by PET. *J Neurooncol*. 1991;10(1):47-55.

54. Dietrich J, et al. CNS progenitor cells and oligodendrocytes are targets of chemotherapeutic agents in vitro and in vivo. *J Biol*. 2006;5(7):22.

55. Muramatsu T, et al. Age-related differences in vincristine toxicity and biodistribution in wild-type and transporter-deficient mice. *Oncol Res*. 2004;14(7-8):331-343.

56. Mariani E, et al. Oxidative stress in brain aging, neurodegenerative and vascular diseases: an overview. *J Chromatogr B Analyt Technol Biomed Life Sci*. 2005;827(1):65-75.

57. Caldecott KW. DNA single-strand breaks and neurodegeneration. *DNA Repair (Amst)*. 2004;3(8-9):875-882.

58. Harrison JF, et al. Oxidative stress-induced apoptosis in neurons correlates with mitochondrial DNA base excision repair pathway imbalance. *Nucleic Acids Res*. 2005;33(14):4660-4671.

59. Schroder CP, et al. Telomere length in breast cancer patients before and after chemotherapy with or without stem cell transplantation. *Br J Cancer*. 2001;84(10):1348-1353.

60. Lahav M, et al. Nonmyeloablative conditioning does not prevent telomere shortening after allogeneic stem cell transplantation. *Transplantation*. 2005;80(7):969-976.

61. Maccormick RE. Possible acceleration of aging by adjuvant chemotherapy: a cause of early onset frailty? *Med Hypotheses*. 2006;67(2):212-215.

62. Trask PC, et al. Psychiatric side effects of interferon therapy: prevalence, proposed mechanisms, and future directions. *J Clin Oncol*. 2000;18(11):2316-2326.

63. Penson RT, et al. Cytokines IL-1beta, IL-2, IL-6, IL-8, MCP-1, GM-CSF and TNFalpha in patients with epithelial ovarian cancer and their relationship to treatment with paclitaxel. *Int J Gynecol Cancer*. 2000;10(1):33-41.

64. Pusztai L, et al. Changes in plasma levels of inflammatory cytokines in response to paclitaxel chemotherapy. *Cytokine*. 2004;25(3):94-102.

65. Tsavaris N, et al. Immune changes in patients with advanced breast cancer undergoing chemotherapy with taxanes. *Br J Cancer*. 2002;87(1):21-27.

66. Bower JE, et al. Fatigue and proinflammatory cytokine activity in breast cancer survivors. *Psychosom Med*. 2002;64(4):604-611.

67. Collado-Hidalgo A, et al. Inflammatory biomarkers for persistent fatigue in breast cancer survivors. *Clin Cancer Res*. 2006;12(9):2759-2766.

68. Lustig C, et al. Aging, training, and the brain: a review and future directions. *Neuropsychol Rev*. 2009;19(4):504-522.

69. Ferguson RJ, et al. Cognitive-behavioral management of chemotherapy-related cognitive change. *Psychooncology*. 2007;16(8):772-777.

70. Ferguson RJ, et al. Development of CBT for chemotherapy-related cognitive change: results of a waitlist control trial. *Psychooncology*. 2012;21(2):176-186.

71. Poppelreuter M, et al. Rehabilitation of therapy-related cognitive deficits in patients after hematopoietic stem cell transplantation. *Bone Marrow Transplant*. 2008;41(1):79-90.

72. Poppelreuter M, Weis J, Bartsch HH. Effects of specific neuropsychological training programs for breast cancer patients after adjuvant chemotherapy. *J Psychosoc Oncol*. 2009;27(2):274-296.

73. Mar Fan HG, et al. A randomised, placebo-controlled, double-blind trial of the effects of d-methylphenidate on fatigue and cognitive dysfunction in women undergoing adjuvant chemotherapy for breast cancer. *Support Care Cancer*. 2008;16(6):577-583.

74. Kohli S, et al. The effect of modafinil on cognitive function in breast cancer survivors. *Cancer*. 2009;115(12):2605-2616.

75. Lundorff LE, Jonsson BH, Sjogren P. Modafinil for attentional and psychomotor dysfunction in advanced cancer: a double-blind, randomised, cross-over trial. *Palliat Med*. 2009;23(8):731-738.

CHAPTER 44

Substance-Abuse Issues in Palliative Care

Julie R. Hamrick ■ Steven D. Passik ■ Kenneth L. Kirsh

INTRODUCTION

Chemical dependency in patients with advanced illness poses complex clinical challenges. Particularly alarming is the sharp increase in controlled prescription drug abuse in the United States in the past decade (1). Physicians and other medical staff need to be continually mindful of the potential for substance abuse and diversion in the palliative care setting. The severity of substance-related problems varies significantly: some patients exhibit minor difficult behaviors, such as escalating drug dosages without informing their physicians or using analgesics to treat symptoms other than those intended. At the other end of the continuum, some patients present to the palliative care team with a known history of, or current substance dependence on, illicit drugs or prescription medications that requires aggressive drug control on the part of the treatment team. Proper identification, assessment, and clinical management of the entire spectrum of substance-related problems are critically important for optimal treatment of patients in palliative care settings.

Clinicians must balance the obligation to be thorough in assessing potential opioid abuse or diversion with the duty to ensure that patients' pain is not undertreated. Regulatory pressures only add to this burden, leading some physicians to believe that they must avoid being duped by those abusing prescription pain medications at all costs. Although it is tempting to reduce the clinical implications of patient behavior to dichotomous labels of "addiction" or "not addiction," this oversimplification is not in the patient's best interests. In fact, pain management can be adapted to address the multiple possibilities that might be behind the problematic behaviors noted in an assessment. Physicians can assert control over prescriptions without necessarily ceasing to prescribe controlled substances entirely. Although these situations invariably defy simple solutions, knowledgeable clinicians can implement strategies to simultaneously address the need for compassionate care and management of problematic drug use.

PREVALENCE

Approximately half the individuals aged 15 to 54 in the United States have used illegal drugs at some point in their lives and an estimated 6% to 15% have a current or past substance use disorder of some type (2–7). In less than a decade, sharp increases in the rate of controlled prescription drug abuse have been noted, with rates climbing by nearly 94%, from 7.8 million in 1992 to 15.1 million in 2003 (1). As a result of the high prevalence of substance abuse in the US population and the association between drug abuse and life-threatening diseases such as acquired immunodeficiency syndrome (AIDS), cirrhosis, and some types of cancer (8–12), patients with substance-abuse–related issues are encountered commonly in palliative care settings. In diverse patient populations with progressive life-threatening diseases, the presence of a current or past drug problem complicates the management of the underlying disease and can undermine palliative treatment. The balance between the therapeutic use of potentially abusable drugs and the abuse of these drugs must be understood to optimize care.

The rapid rise in controlled prescription drug abuse is of particular concern for the palliative care team. When misused, prescription opioids and central nervous system depressants and stimulants can be deadly. In 2002, controlled prescription drugs were implicated in 30% of drug-related emergency room deaths and in at least 23% of emergency department admissions (1). Contrary to past data suggesting that most controlled prescription drug abusers were regular or experienced users, approximately one-third of abusers in 2000 were new users of controlled prescriptions according to the data from the National Center of Addiction and Substance Abuse (1). Between the years 1992 and 2003, there has been a 225% increase in new opioid abusers, a 150% increase in new tranquilizer abusers, a 127% increase in new sedative abusers, and a 171% increase in new stimulant abusers (1). Particular regions of the country, most notably the south and west, have been hardest hit.

The growing rates of abuse of controlled prescription drugs raise questions about the prevalence of substance abuse in patient populations with cancer and how palliative care physicians can best address the needs of their patients. Despite its prevalence in the general population, substance abuse appears to be very uncommon within the tertiary care population with cancer. In a 6-month period in 2005, fewer than 1% of inpatient and outpatient consultations performed by the psychiatry service at Memorial Sloan-Kettering Cancer Center (MSKCC) were requested for substance-abuse–related issues and only 3% of patients who were referred to the psychiatry department were subsequently diagnosed with a substance-abuse disorder of any type (13). This prevalence is much lower than the frequency of substance-abuse disorders in society at large, in general medical populations, and in emergency medical departments (2,6,14–16). A 1983 study of the Psychiatric Collaborative Oncology Group, which

TABLE 44.1	DSM-IV diagnostic criteria for substance abuse and substance dependence

Criteria for Substance Abuse

A maladaptive pattern of substance use leading to clinically significant impairment or distress, as manifested by one (or more) of the following, occurring within a 12-month period:

  Recurrent substance use resulting in a failure to fulfill major role obligations at work, school, or home (e.g., repeated absences or poor work performance related to substance use; substance-related absences, suspensions, or expulsions from school; neglect of children or household)

  Recurrent substance use in situations in which it is physically hazardous (e.g., driving an automobile or operating a machine when impaired by substance use)

  Recurrent substance-related legal problems (e.g., arrests for substance-related disorderly conduct)

  Continued substance use despite having persistent or recurrent social or interpersonal problems caused or exacerbated by the effects of the substance (e.g., arguments with spouse about consequences of intoxication and physical fights)

The symptoms have never met the criteria for substance dependence for this class of disorder

Criteria for Substance Dependence

A maladaptive pattern of substance use, leading to clinically significant impairment or distress, as manifested by three (or more) of the following, occurring at any time in the same 12-month period:

  Tolerance, as defined by either a need for markedly increased amounts of the substance to achieve intoxication or desired effect or markedly diminished effect with continued use of the same amount of the substance

  Withdrawal, as manifested by either the characteristic withdrawal syndrome for the substance or the same (or a closely related) substance taken to relieve or avoid withdrawal symptoms

  The substance is often taken in larger amounts over a longer period than was intended

  There is persistent desire or unsuccessful effort to cut down or control substance use

  A great deal of time is spent in activities necessary to obtain the substance (e.g., visiting multiple physicians or driving long distances), use the substance (e.g., chain smoking), or recover from its effects

  Important social, occupational, or recreational activities are given up or reduced because of substance use

  The substance use is continued despite knowledge of having a persistent or recurrent physical or psychological problem that is likely to have been caused or exacerbated by the substance (e.g., current cocaine use despite recognition of cocaine-induced depression or continued drinking despite recognition that an ulcer was made worse by alcohol consumption)

From American Psychiatric Association. *Diagnostic and Statistical Manual for Mental Disorders—IV.* Washington, DC: American Psychiatric Association; 1983.

assessed psychiatric diagnoses in ambulatory patients with cancer from several tertiary care hospitals (15), also found a low prevalence of substance-related disorders. Following structured clinical interviews, fewer than 5% of 215 patients with cancer met the Diagnostic and Statistical Manual for Mental Disorders (DSM) III Edition criteria for a substance-use disorder (17) (Table 44.1).

The relatively low prevalence of substance abuse among patients with cancer treated in tertiary care hospitals may reflect institutional biases or a tendency for patients to underreport in these settings. Many drug abusers are poor, feel alienated from the health care system, may not seek care in tertiary centers, and may be reluctant to acknowledge the stigmatizing history of drug abuse. For these reasons, the low prevalence of drug abuse in cancer centers may not be representative of the true prevalence in the cancer population overall. In support of this conclusion, the findings of a 1995

survey of patients admitted to a palliative care unit indicate alcohol abuse in more than 25% of patients (18). Additional studies are needed to clarify the current epidemiology of substance abuse and dependence in patients with cancer and others with progressive medical diseases. These patients can be adequately and successfully treated only when their substance problems are noted by staff and their needs addressed.

DEFINITIONS OF SUBSTANCE ABUSE AND DEPENDENCE

Both epidemiologic studies and clinical management depend on an accepted, valid nomenclature for substance abuse and dependence. Unfortunately, this terminology is highly problematic. The pharmacologic phenomena of tolerance and physical dependence are commonly confused with abuse and true substance dependence as defined by

TABLE 44.2	Substance-abuse definitions in the medically ill
Tolerance	The need for increasing doses to maintain analgesic effects
Addiction	Continuing and compulsive use despite physical, psychological, or social harm
Physical dependence	Presence of withdrawal following abrupt dose reduction

the DSM-IV (Table 44.1), and the definitions applied to medical patients have been developed from experience with substance-abusing populations. The clarification of this terminology is an essential step in improving the diagnosis and management of substance abuse in the palliative care setting (Table 44.2).

Tolerance

Tolerance is a pharmacologic property defined by the need for increasing doses to maintain effects (19,20). An extensive clinical experience with opioid drugs in the medical context has not confirmed that tolerance causes substantial problems (21,22). Although tolerance to a variety of opioid effects, including analgesia, can be reliably observed in animal models (23), and tolerance to nonanalgesic effects, such as respiratory depression and cognitive impairment (24), occurs routinely in the clinical setting, analgesic tolerance seldom interferes with the clinical efficacy of opioid drugs. Indeed, most patients attain stable doses associated with a favorable balance between analgesia and side effects for prolonged periods; dose escalation, when it is required, usually heralds the appearance of a progressive painful lesion (25–31). Unlike tolerance to the side effects of opioids, clinically meaningful analgesic tolerance, which would yield the need for dose escalation to maintain analgesia in the absence of progressive disease, appears to be a rare phenomenon. Clinical observation also fails to support the conclusion that analgesic tolerance is a substantial contributor to the development of substance dependence.

Physical Dependence

Physical dependence is defined solely by the occurrence of an abstinence syndrome (withdrawal) following abrupt dose reduction or administration of an antagonist (19,20,32). There is great confusion among clinicians about the differences between physical dependence and true substance dependence. Physical dependence, like tolerance, has been suggested to be a component of substance dependence (33,34), and the avoidance of withdrawal has been postulated to create behavioral contingencies that reinforce drug-seeking behavior (35). These speculations, however, are not

supported by experience acquired during opioid therapy for chronic pain. Physical dependence does not preclude the uncomplicated discontinuation of opioids during multidisciplinary pain management of nonmalignant pain (36), and opioid therapy is routinely stopped without difficulty in the patients with cancer whose pain disappears following effective antineoplastic therapy. Indirect evidence for a fundamental distinction between physical dependence and substance dependence is even provided by animal models of opioid self-administration, which have demonstrated that persistent drug-taking behavior can be maintained in the absence of physical dependence (37).

Addiction

The terms addiction and addict are particularly troublesome. These labels are often inappropriately applied to describe both aberrant drug use (reminiscent of the behaviors that characterize active abusers of illicit drugs) and phenomena related to tolerance or physical dependence. The labels "addict" and "addiction" should never be used to describe patients who are only perceived to have the capacity for an abstinence syndrome. These patients must be labeled "physically dependent." Use of the word "dependent" alone also should be discouraged, because it fosters confusion between physical dependence and psychological dependence, a component of substance dependence. For the same reason, the term habituation should not be used. It is recommended that the DSM-IV (17) terms substance abuse and substance dependence be applied as appropriate.

Definitions of "substance abuse" and "substance dependence" must be based on the identification of drug-related behaviors that are outside of cultural or societal norms. The ability to categorize questionable behaviors (e.g., consuming a few extra doses of a prescribed opioid, particularly if this behavior was not specifically prescribed by the clinician, or using an opioid drug prescribed for pain as a nighttime hypnotic) as nonnormative presupposes that there is certainty about the parameters of normative behavior. In fact, even experienced pain clinicians disagree on the interpretation of varied drug-taking patterns. In a recent survey, pain clinicians expressed significant individual differences in the perception of which behaviors were the most problematic when asked to rank order a list of aberrant drug-taking behaviors (38). In general, physicians rated illegal behaviors as the most aberrant, followed by alteration of the route of delivery and self-escalation of dose.

Unfortunately, there are few empirical data in medically ill populations that define the meaning of specific drug-related behaviors in relation to substance-use disorders or future drug abuse; as a result, the boundaries of normative behavior remain ill defined. The confusing nature of normative drug taking was highlighted in a pilot survey performed in 2000 at MSKCC, which revealed that inpatients with cancer harbor attitudes supporting misuse of drugs in the face of symptom management problems and that women with human immunodeficiency virus (at MSKCC for palliative care) engage in such behaviors commonly (39). The prevalence of such behaviors and attitudes among the medically ill raises concern about their predictive validity as a marker of any diagnosis related to substance abuse. Clearly, there is a need for empirical data that illuminate the prevalence of drug-taking attitudes and behaviors in different populations of medically ill patients.

The core concepts used to define substance dependence also may be problematic as a result of changes induced by a progressive disease. Deterioration in physical or psychosocial functioning caused by the disease and its treatment may be difficult to separate from the morbidity associated with drug abuse. This may particularly complicate efforts to evaluate the concept of "use despite harm," which is critical to the diagnosis of substance abuse or dependence. For example, the nature of questionable drug-related behaviors can be difficult to discern in the patient who develops social withdrawal or cognitive changes following brain irradiation for metastases. Even if impaired cognition is clearly related to the drugs used to treat symptoms, this outcome might only reflect a narrow therapeutic window, rather than a desire on the patient's part for these psychic effects.

Definitions of Substance Dependence in the Medically Ill

Previous definitions that include phenomena related to physical dependence or tolerance cannot be the model terminology for medically ill populations who receive potentially abusable drugs for legitimate medical purposes. A more appropriate definition of substance dependence notes that it is a chronic disorder characterized by "the compulsive use of a substance resulting in physical, psychological, or social harm to the user and continued use despite that harm" (40). Although this definition was developed from experience in substance-abusing populations without medical illness, it appropriately emphasizes that substance dependence is, fundamentally, a psychological and behavioral syndrome. Any appropriate definition of substance abuse or dependence must include the concepts of loss of control over drug use, compulsive drug use, and continued use despite harm.

Even appropriate definitions of substance dependence will have limited utility, however, unless operationalized for a clinical setting. The concept of "aberrant drug-related behavior" is a useful first step in operationalizing the definitions of substance abuse and dependence and recognizes the broad range of behaviors that may be considered problematic by prescribers. Although the assessment and interpretation of these behaviors can be challenging, as discussed previously, the occurrence of aberrant behaviors signals the need to reevaluate and manage drug taking, even in the context of an appropriate medical indication for a drug.

If drug-taking behavior in a medical patient can be characterized as aberrant, a "differential diagnosis" for this behavior can be explored. That a patient has a true substance-dependent disorder is only one of several possible explanations. The challenging diagnosis of pseudoaddiction must be considered if the patient is reporting distress associated

with unrelieved symptoms. In the case of pseudoaddiction, behaviors such as aggressively complaining about the need for higher doses and occasional unilateral drug escalations indicate desperation caused by pain and disappear if pain management improves.

Alternatively, impulsive drug use may indicate the existence of another psychiatric disorder, the diagnosis of which may have therapeutic implications. Patients with borderline personality disorder can express fear and rage through aberrant drug taking and behave impulsively and self-destructively during pain therapy. Passik and Hay (41) reported a case in which one of the more worrisome aberrant drug-related behaviors, forging of a prescription for a controlled substance, was an impulsive expression of fears of abandonment, having little to do with true substance abuse in a borderline patient. Such patients are challenging and often require firm limit-setting and careful monitoring to avoid impulsive drug taking.

Similarly, patients who self-medicate for anxiety, panic, depression, or even periodic dysphoria and loneliness can present as aberrant drug takers. In such instances, careful diagnosis and treatment of these problems can at times obviate the need for such self-medication. Occasionally, aberrant drug-related behavior appears to be causally related to a mild encephalopathy, with confusion about the appropriate therapeutic regimen. This may be a concern in the treatment of the elderly patient. Low doses of neuroleptic medications, simplified drug regimens, and help with organizing medications can address such problems. Rarely, problematic behaviors indicate criminal intent, such as when patients report pain but intend to sell or divert medications.

These diagnoses are not mutually exclusive. A thorough psychiatric assessment is critically important, both in the population without a prior history of substance abuse and the population of known abusers, who have a high prevalence of psychiatric comorbidity (42,43).

In assessing the differential diagnosis for drug-related behavior, it is useful to consider the degree of aberrancy (Table 44.3). The less aberrant behaviors (such as aggressively complaining about the need for medications) are more likely to reflect untreated distress of some type, rather than substance dependence–related concerns. Conversely, the more aberrant behaviors (such as injection of an oral formulation) are more likely to reflect true substance dependence. Although empirical studies are needed to validate this conceptualization, it may be a useful model when evaluating aberrant behaviors.

EMPIRICAL STUDIES USING THE ABERRANT DRUG-TAKING CONCEPT

Several studies have investigated the usefulness of considering aberrant drug taking as occurring on a continuum. Although the studies performed to date all involve small samples, they have shown that conceptualizing aberrant drug taking in this way has important implications for clinicians. The first study examined the relationship between aberrant drug-taking behaviors and compliance-related outcomes in patients with a history of substance abuse receiving

TABLE 44.3	Degrees of aberrance in drug-taking behavior
Mildly aberrant	Requests for specific pain medication
	Aggressive complaints about the need for medication
	Using drugs prescribed for a friend or family member
	Frequent prescription losses
	Hoarding drugs
More highly aberrant	Forging prescriptions
	Obtaining drugs from nonmedical source
	Sale of prescription drugs
	Crushing sustained-release tablets for snorting or injecting

From Passik SD, Kirsh KL, Whitcomb L, et al. Pain clinicians' rankings of aberrant drug-taking behaviors. *J Pain Palliat Care Pharmacother.* 2002;16:39–49.

chronic opioid therapy for nonmalignant pain. Dunbar and Katz (44) examined outcomes and drug taking in 20 patients with diverse histories of drug abuse who underwent a year of chronic opioid therapy. During the year of therapy, 11 patients were adherent with the drug regimen and 9 were not. The authors examined patient characteristics and aberrant drug-taking behaviors that differentiated the two groups. The patients who did not abuse the therapy were abusers of solely alcohol (or had remote histories of polysubstance abuse), were participating in 12-step programs, and had good social support. The patients who abused the therapy were polysubstance abusers, were not participating in 12-step programs, and had poor social support. The specific behaviors that were recorded more frequently by those who abused the therapy were unscheduled visits and multiple phone calls to the clinic, unsanctioned dose escalations, and acquisition of opioids from more than one source.

A second study examined the relationship between aberrant drug taking and the presence or absence of a psychiatric diagnosis of substance-use disorder in pain patients. Compton et al. (45) studied 56 patients seeking pain treatment in a multidisciplinary pain program who were referred for "problematic drug taking." The patients all underwent structured psychiatric interviews, and the sample was divided between those qualifying and those not qualifying for psychiatric diagnoses of substance-use disorders. The authors then examined the subjects' reports of aberrant drug-taking behaviors on a structured interview assessment. The patients who qualified for a substance-use disorder diagnosis were more likely to have engaged in unsanctioned dose escalations, received opioids from multiple sources, and reported a subjective impression of loss of control of their prescribed medications.

Passik and researchers at a major cancer center (39) examined the self-reports of aberrant drug-taking attitudes and behaviors in samples of patients with cancer ($N = 52$) and patients with AIDS ($N = 111$) on a questionnaire designed for the purposes of the study. Reports of past drug use and abuse were more frequent than the present reports in both groups. Current aberrant drug-related behaviors were seldom reported, but attitude items revealed that patients would consider engaging in aberrant behaviors or would possibly excuse them in others, if pain or symptom management were inadequate. It was found that aberrant behaviors and attitudes were endorsed more frequently by the women with AIDS than by male and female patients with cancer. Overall, patients greatly overestimated the risk of substance dependence during pain treatment. Experience with this questionnaire suggests that patients both with cancer and AIDS respond in a forthcoming fashion to drug-taking behavior questions and describe attitudes and behaviors which may be highly relevant to the diagnosis and management of substance-use disorders.

These studies help clarify the meanings ascribed by clinicians to the various behaviors that occur during long-term administration of a potentially abusable drug. Ultimately, such studies may define the true "red flags" in a given population.

Far too often, anecdotal accounts shape the way clinicians view drug-related behaviors. Some behaviors are regarded almost universally as aberrant despite limited systematic data to suggest that this is the case. Consider, for example, the patient who requests a specific pain medication or a specific route or dose. Although this behavior may reflect a patient who is knowledgeable and assertive—favorable characteristics in other contexts—it is often greeted with suspicion on the part of practitioners. Other behaviors may be common in medically ill non–substance-abusing populations, and although aberrant, they may have little predictive value for true substance dependence. For example, the finding that many non–substance-abusing patients with cancer use anxiolytic medications prescribed for a friend or others (39) more than likely reflects the undertreatment and underreporting of anxiety in patients with cancer than true substance abuse.

RISK OF SUBSTANCE ABUSE AND DEPENDENCE IN THE MEDICALLY ILL

Opioid administration in patients with cancer having no prior history of substance abuse is only rarely associated with the development of significant substance abuse or dependence (46–58). Indeed, concerns about abuse in this population are now characterized by an interesting paradox: although the lay public and inexperienced clinicians still fear the development of substance abuse or dependence when opioids are used to treat cancer pain, specialists in cancer pain and palliative care widely believe that the major problem related to potential abuse is not the phenomenon itself, but rather the persistent undertreatment of pain driven by inappropriate fear that it will occur.

The very sanguine experience in the cancer population has contributed to a desire for a reappraisal of the risks and benefits associated with the long-term opioid treatment of chronic nonmalignant pain (31,59). The traditional view of this therapy is negative, and early surveys of substance abusers, which noted that a relatively large proportion began their abuse as patients on medication administered opioid drugs for pain (60–62), provided some indirect support for this perspective. The most influential of these surveys recorded a history of medical opioid use for pain in 27% of white male addicts and 1.2% of black male abusers (62).

Surveys of substance-abusing populations, however, do not provide a valid measure of the liability associated with chronic opioid therapy in medically ill populations without known drug abuse. Prospective patient surveys are needed to define this risk accurately. Studies of relatively short-term opioid exposure have been reassuring. The Boston Collaborative Drug Surveillance Project evaluated 11,882 inpatients who had no prior history of substance abuse and were administered an opioid while hospitalized; only 4 cases of substance abuse or dependence could be identified subsequently (63). A national survey of burn centers could find no cases of abuse in a sample of more than 10,000 patients without prior drug-abuse history who were administered opioids for pain (64), and a survey of a large headache clinic identified opioid abuse in only 3 of 2,369 patients admitted for treatment, most of whom had access to opioids (65). These surveys do not, however, define the risk of substance abuse or dependence during long-term, open-ended opioid therapy. Other supporting data derive from surveys of patients with cancer and postoperative patients, which indicate that euphoria, a phenomenon believed to be common during the abuse of opioids, is extremely uncommon following administration of an opioid for pain; dysphoria is observed more typically, especially in those who receive meperidine (66).

The inaccurate perception that opioid therapy inherently yields a relatively high likelihood of substance abuse or dependence has encouraged assumptions that are not supportable given the current understanding of substance abuse. Perhaps most important, the relevance of a genetically determined predisposition to substance abuse (67) tends to be minimized or dismissed by such a view. A more critical evaluation of the extant literature (28–31,67–69) actually yields little substantive support for the view that large numbers of individuals with no personal or family history of substance abuse or dependence, no affiliation with a substance-abusing subculture, and no significant premorbid psychopathology will develop abuse or dependence de novo when administered potentially abusable drugs for appropriate medical indications.

RISK IN PATIENT WITH CURRENT OR REMOTE DRUG ABUSE

There is very little information about the risk of substance abuse or dependence during, or after, the therapeutic administration of a potentially abusable drug to patients with a current or remote history of substance abuse or dependence. Anecdotal reports have suggested that successful long-term opioid therapy in patients with cancer pain or chronic

nonmalignant pain is possible, particularly if the history of substance abuse or dependence is remote (44,70,71). Indeed, a 1992 study showed that patients with AIDS-related pain could be successfully treated with morphine whether or not they were substance users or nonusers. The major group difference found in this survey was that substance users required considerably more morphine to reach stable pain control (72).

These data are reassuring but do not obviate the need for caution. For example, although there is no empirical evidence that the use of short-acting drugs or the parenteral route is more likely to lead to problematic drug-related behaviors than other therapeutic approaches, it may be prudent to avoid such therapies in patients with histories of substance abuse.

CLINICAL MANAGEMENT

Aberrant drug taking among patients with advanced illnesses (with or without a prior history of substance abuse) represents a serious and complex clinical occurrence. Perhaps, the more difficult situations involve the patient who is actively abusing illicit or prescription drugs or alcohol concomitantly with medical therapies. Whether the patient is an active drug abuser, has a history of substance abuse, or is not complying with the therapeutic regimen, the clinician should establish structure, control, and monitoring so that they can prescribe freely and without prejudice.

Multidisciplinary Approach

A multidisciplinary team approach is usually optimal for the management of substance abusers in the palliative care setting. If available, mental health professionals with specialization in substance abuse can be instrumental in helping palliative care team members develop strategies for management and patient treatment compliance. Providing care to these patients can lead to feelings of anger and frustration among staff. Such feelings can unintentionally compromise pain management and contribute to feelings of isolation and alienation by the patient. A structured multidisciplinary approach can be effective in helping the staff better understand the patient's needs and develop effective strategies for controlling pain and aberrant drug use simultaneously. Staff meetings can be helpful in establishing treatment goals, facilitating compliance, and coordinating the multidisciplinary team.

Assessment

The first member of the medical team (frequently a nurse) to suspect problematic drug taking or a history of drug abuse should alert the patient's palliative care team, thereby beginning the multidisciplinary assessment and management process (73). A physician should assess the potential of withdrawal or other pressing concerns and begin involving other staff (i.e., social work, psychology, and/or psychiatry) to initiate the planning of management strategies (Table 44.4). Obtaining as detailed as possible a history of the duration, frequency, and desired effect of drug use is crucial. Frequently,

TABLE 44.4	Screening for substance abuse and treatment recommendations

Assessment Guidelines

Use graduated interview approach beginning with broad questions about substances such as nicotine or caffeine and becoming more specific

Assess for comorbid psychiatric disorders, such as anxiety, personality disorders, and mood disorders

Consider diagnostic instruments, such as Screener and Opioid Assessment for Patients with Pain (74)

Treatment Recommendations	
General	Listen and accept patient's report of distress
	Use behavioral and nonopioid interventions for pain when possible
	Consider drugs with slower onset and longer duration (e.g., transdermal fentanyl and modified-release opioids). Note that higher doses may be needed for adequate pain control in patients with a history of abuse or dependence
	Frequently assess adequacy of symptom and pain control
Outpatients	Limit amount of drug dispensed per prescription
	Make refills contingent on clinic attendance
	Consider urine toxicology screenings to assess usage
	Involve family members and friends in the treatment plan
Inpatients	Consider placing the patient in a private room near the nurses' station
	Consider daily urine collection

clinicians avoid asking patients about substance abuse because of fear that they will anger the patient or that they are incorrect in their suspicion of abuse. This stance can contribute to continued problems. Empathic and truthful communication is always the best approach.

The use of a careful, graduated interview can be instrumental to assess drug use. This approach entails starting the assessment interview with broad questions about the role of drugs (e.g., nicotine and caffeine) in the patient's life and gradually becoming more specific in focus to include illicit drugs. Such an approach is helpful in reducing denial and resistance.

This interviewing style may also assist in the detection of coexisting psychiatric disorders. Comorbid psychiatric disorders can significantly contribute to aberrant drug-taking behavior. Studies suggest that 37% to 62% of alcoholics have one or more coexisting psychiatric disorders, and the patient's drug history may be a clue to comorbid psychiatric disorders (e.g., drinking to quell panic symptoms). Anxiety, personality disorders, and mood disorders are those most commonly encountered (7,43,75). The assessment and treatment of comorbid psychiatric disorders can greatly enhance management strategies and reduce the risk of relapse.

Prescreening Patients

Most of the recent research has focused on screening tools that can be used to prescreen patients to determine the level of risk when considering opioids as part of the treatment regimen. While mislabeling patients as either a good or bad risk can have negative consequence, safe opioid prescribing relies on proper risk stratification and the accommodation of that risk into a treatment plan. In addition, we must always keep in mind that a spectrum of nonadherence exists and that this spectrum is distinct for pain patients versus those who use these medications for nonmedical purposes (76) (Fig. 44.1). Nonmedical users can be seen as self-treating personal issues, purely as recreational users, or as having a more severe and consistent substance use disorder or addiction. On the other hand, pain patients are more complex and their behaviors might range from strict adherence to chemically coping to a frank addiction. Thus, scores indicating increased risk on the following tools do not necessarily indicate addiction, but might be uncovering some of the gray areas of noncompliance.

Assessment tools have been developed for chronic pain populations for the purpose of evaluating the likelihood of problematic drug use during therapy. In the most recent effort, Butler et al. (74) tested a screening measure for patients suffering from chronic pain. An initial 24-item self-administered Screener and Opioid Assessment for Patients with Pain (SOAPP) was validated in a sample of 175 chronic nonmalignant pain patients, 95 of whom were available for a 6-month follow-up. From these results, a 14-item short form was derived that has good psychometrics and shows promise as a way to screen chronic pain patients who might be at risk for substance abuse and dependence, although the data available to date are correlational and not causal in nature. In 2005, Webster and Webster (77) developed the Opioid Risk Tool (ORT), a 5-question self-report measure which addresses such issues as personal and family history of substance abuse, age, history of preadolescent sexual abuse, and certain psychological diseases.

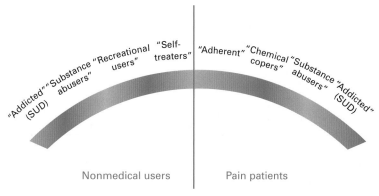

Figure 44.1. The spectrum of adherence for pain patients versus the spectrum of illicit use by nonmedical users. From Kirsh KL, Passik SD. The interface between pain and drug abuse and the evolution of strategies to optimize pain management while minimizing drug abuse. *Exp Clin Psychopharmacol.* 2008;16(5):400–404.

SUD, substance use disorder.

The ORT was tested on 185 consecutive patients and displayed excellent discriminatory ability in both men and women for identifying patients who will go on to abuse their medications or develop an addiction. The ORT is useful due to its brevity and ease of scoring, but the face-valid nature of the ORT brings up the issue of susceptibility to deception. For many, this will be an acceptable risk tool, but it may not be sufficient for all.

Moore et al. (78) completed a comparison of common screening methods for predicting aberrant drug-related behavior among patients receiving opioids for chronic pain management. Patients referred for opioid medication for pain management participated in a semi-structured clinical interview with the staff psychologist and completed the SOAPP; the Diagnosis, Intractability, Risk, and Efficacy inventory (DIRE); and/or the ORT. Results showed the highest sensitivity for the clinical interview (0.77) and the SOAPP (0.72), followed by the ORT (0.45) and the DIRE (0.17). Combining the clinical interview with the SOAPP increased sensitivity to 0.90. Among patients who were discontinued from opioids for aberrant drug-related behaviors, the clinical interview and the SOAPP were most effective at predicting risk at baseline. The applicability of these instruments, or others developed for this purpose, in populations with medical illness remains to be determined in future studies.

The Four A's for Ongoing Monitoring

On the basis of extensive clinical experience, four domains have been proposed as most relevant for ongoing monitoring of patients with chronic pain on opioids. These domains have been summarized as the "Four A's" (analgesia, activities of daily living, adverse side effects, and aberrant drug-taking behaviors) (79). The monitoring of these outcomes over time should inform therapeutic decision-making and provide a framework for documentation. A checklist tool has been developed to aid in monitoring of the four A's (80) (Table 44.5).

Development of a Treatment Plan—General Consideration

Clear treatment goals are essential in managing aberrant drug-related behaviors. Depending on the history, a complete remission of the patient's substance use problems may

not be a reasonable goal. The distress of coping with a life-threatening illness and the availability of prescription drugs for symptom control can undermine efforts to maintain control over comorbid substance abuse or dependence (81). For some patients, "harm reduction" may be a better model. It aims to enhance social support, maximize treatment compliance, and contain harm done through episodic relapse.

Several elements are key in this approach. First, clinicians must establish a relationship based on empathic listening and accept the patient's report of distress. Second, it is important to use nonopioid and behavioral interventions for pain when possible, but not as substitutes for appropriate pharmacologic management. Third, specific aspects of drug selection and dosing should be informed by a history of problematic drug use. For example, a history of active opioid abuse usually means that higher doses may be needed more rapidly than commonly observed in patients who are opioid-naive. Underdosing may lead to a degree of persistent pain that drives the patient's attempts to self-medicate. The use of medications with slow onset and longer duration (e.g., transdermal fentanyl and modified-release opioids) should be considered in those with substance-use disorders. Patients who are perceived to be at high risk should not be given short-acting opioids for breakthrough pain. Finally, the team should make plans to frequently reassess the adequacy of pain and symptom control.

Urine Toxicology Screening

Clinicians must control and monitor drug use in all patients, a daunting task in some active abusers. In some cases, a major issue is compliance with treatments for the underlying disease, which may be so poor that the substance abuse actually shortens life expectancy by preventing the effective administration of primary therapy. Prognosis may also be worsened by the use of drugs in a manner that negatively interacts with therapy or predisposes to other serious morbidity. The goals of care can be very difficult to define when poor compliance and risky behavior appear to contradict a reported desire for disease-modifying therapies.

Urine toxicology screening has the potential to be a useful tool to the practicing clinician for both diagnosing potential abuse problems and monitoring patients with an established

TABLE 44.5	Four A's for ongoing monitoring
Analgesia	Document and monitor patient's pain, using scales such as a 0–10 pain rating scale. Although listed as the first "A," analgesia is not necessarily to be considered the most important outcome of pain management. An alternate view is how much relief it takes for a patient to feel that their life is meaningfully changed so they can work toward the attainment of their own goals.
Activities of daily living	Monitor patient's typical level of daily activities and psychosocial functioning to observe increases over time. The second "A" concerning activities of daily living refers to quality of life issues and functionality. It is necessary that patients understand that they must comply with all of their recommended treatment options so that they are better able to return to work, avocation, and social activities.
Adverse effects	Strive for highest analgesia with most benign side-effect profile. Patients must also be made aware of the adverse side effects inherent in the treatment of their pain condition with opioids and other medications. Side effects must be aggressively managed so that sedation and other side effects do not overshadow the potential benefits of drug therapy. The most common side effects of opioid analgesics include constipation, sedation, nausea and vomiting, dry mouth, respiratory depression, confusion, urinary retention, and itching.
Aberrant behaviors	Be aware of aberrant behaviors suggestive of drug use, such as multiple "lost" prescriptions or unauthorized dose escalations. Patients must be educated through agreements, or other means, about the parameters of acceptable drug taking. Even an overall good outcome in every other domain might not constitute satisfactory treatment if the patient is not compliant with the contract in worrisome ways. Dispensing pain medicine in a highly structured fashion may become necessary for some patients who are in violation or constantly on the fringes of appropriate drug taking.

history of abuse. However, a 2000 chart review of the ordering and documentation of urine toxicology screens suggests that urine toxicology screens are employed infrequently in tertiary care centers (82). In addition, when urine tests are ordered, documentation tends to be inconsistent regarding the reasons for ordering as well as any follow-up recommendations based on the results. Indeed, the chart review found that nearly 40% of the charts surveyed listed no reason for obtaining the urine toxicology screen and the ordering physician could not be identified nearly 30% of the time. Staff education efforts can help to address this problem.

One might wonder how good clinicians are at detecting adherence and misuse in their patients. Bronstein et al (83) addressed this question by asking clinicians to identify patients who they thought were at risk for medication misuse and those who were not based on risk assessment methods used in their practice. Urine drug testing results were then compared with these assessments. A total of 755 samples were received from 62 clinicians in 50 practices. Patients who were thought to potentially be misusing their medications ($N = 226$) had urine drug tests (UDTs) showing illicits, missing prescribed medication, unprescribed medication present, and/or results above or below the range using Rx Guardian methodology 79% of the time. In patients who clinicians thought were not at risk for misuse of medications ($N = 297$), 72% had UDTs showing illicits, missing prescribed medication, unprescribed medication present, and/or results above or below the range using Rx Guardian methodology. The third group (random with no risk assessment

identified, $N = 232$) showed 71% of samples had illicits, missing prescribed medication, unprescribed medication present, and/or results above or below the range using Rx Guardian methodology. Bronstein et al. (83) went on to relax the criteria for labeling a test abnormal to see if that lead to improved clinician's accuracy. For this data cut, tests were considered abnormal only if illicits were present and/or prescribed drug was not found. This resulted in a data set of 549 samples. In group A ($N = 204$, those patients not suspected of medication misuse), 60% still had abnormal results; group B ($N = 173$, those suspected of medication misuse), 72% had abnormal results; and the random group C ($N = 172$) had 61% abnormal tests.

As demonstrated by Bronstein et al. (83) it is difficult to predict which patients are likely to be misusing opioids or taking an illicit drug. Clinicians were better able to predict medication misuse in patients where they thought there might be an issue based on whatever risk assessments they used in the clinic. Thus, if clinicians only test patients suspected of likely misusing medications, they are missing a significant group of patients, up to 72% in the large data set and 60% in the narrower data set that were likely misusing their medications without any identifiable risk behaviors.

Patients with Advanced Disease

Managing substance abuse in patients with advanced medical illness may be particularly challenging. Although clinicians may be tempted to overlook a patient's use of illicit substances or alcohol, viewing these behaviors as a last source of pleasure for the patient, drug use that is out of control may have a highly deleterious impact on palliative care efforts. Aberrant drug-related behaviors may be associated with poor symptom control, distress, increased stress for family members, family concern over the misuse of medication, poor compliance with the treatment regimen, and diminished quality of life. Complete abstinence from drugs of abuse may not be a realistic outcome, but reduction in use can certainly have positive effects for the patient (84).

Management of risk is a "package deal." It comprises a suite of assessment, monitoring, and treatment tools that need to be considered for each patient and individualized as clinically indicated (76) (Table 44.6). Screening tools are available to help in the assessment of known risk factors for opioid abuse, including smoking, psychiatric disorders, and personal or family history of substance abuse. When available, prescription monitoring programs, which exist in 35 states and monitor when and where prescriptions are filled, can provide physicians with valuable information about prescription compliance (85). Patients determined to be at minimal risk can receive minimal structure, whereas those determined to be at greater risk can receive more structure, such as more frequent visits, fewer pills per prescription, specialist-level care (e.g., an addiction specialist or psychotherapist), and UDTs. Patients must be made aware of the responsibility of safeguarding these medications against diversion by friends, family, or visitors who may have access to medications left out or in unlocked locations. Multiple studies have shown that 50% or more of prescription opioids diverted for nonmedical use are obtained from friends and family (85). Finally, opioid formulations that incorporate barriers to common forms of manipulation are an emerging component of risk management. Novel subclasses of opioid formulations, incorporating pharmacological strategies and physical barriers, are designed to deter or resist misuse and abuse by making it difficult to obtain euphoric effects from opioid use.

Outpatient Management

There are a number of additional strategies for promoting treatment adherence in an outpatient setting. A written contract between the team and patient helps provide structure to the treatment plan, establishes clear expectations of the roles played by both parties, and outlines the consequences of aberrant drug taking. The inclusion of spot urine toxicology screens in the contract can be useful in maximizing treatment compliance. Expectations regarding follow-up visits and management of drug supply also should be stated. For example, clinicians may wish to limit the amount of drug dispensed per prescription and make refills contingent upon clinic attendance. The clinician may consider the requirement for joint management by a specialist in substance abuse or required attendance at a 12-step program. With the patient's consent, the clinician may wish to contact the patient's sponsor and make him or her aware that the patient is being treated for a chronic illness that requires medications (e.g., opioids). This action will reduce the potential for stigmatization of the patient as being noncompliant with the ideals of the 12-step program. Finally, clinicians should involve family members and friends in the treatment to help bolster social support and functioning. Becoming familiar with the family may help the team to identify family members who are themselves drug abusers and who may potentially divert the patient's medications. Mental health professionals can help family members with referrals to drug treatment and codependency groups as a way to help the patient receive optimal medical care.

Inpatient Management

The management of patients with active substance-abuse problems who have been admitted to the hospital for treatment of a life-threatening illness is based on the guidelines discussed in the preceding text for outpatient settings. These guidelines aim to promote the safety of patients and staff, contain manipulative behaviors by patients, enhance the appropriate use of medication for pain and symptom management, and communicate an understanding of pain and substance-abuse management. First, the patient's drug use needs to be discussed in an open manner. It may be necessary to reassure the patient that steps will be taken to avoid adverse events such as drug or alcohol withdrawal. In some challenging cases, it would be best to admit a patient several days in advance of a planned procedure for stabilization of the drug regimen.

If the patient is actively abusing drugs, it is often best to place the patient on the unit in a private room, if possible, near the nurses' station. This aids in monitoring the patient and may discourage attempts to leave the hospital for the purchase of illicit drugs. Further, the team should require

TABLE 44.6	Risk management package for patients undergoing opioid therapy

Screening and risk stratification
Use of prescription monitoring program data
Compliance monitoring
Urine drug testing
Pill or patch counts
Education about drug storage and sharing
Psychotherapy and highly structured approaches
Abuse-deterrent or abuse-resistant strategies in opioid formulation

From Kirsh KL, Passik SD. The interface between pain and drug abuse and the evolution of strategies to optimize pain management while minimizing drug abuse. *Exp Clin Psychopharmacol.* 2008;16(5):400–404.

visitors to check in with nursing staff prior to visitation. In some cases, it may be necessary to search the packages of visitors in order to stem a patient's access to drugs. Depending on the severity of the problem, the clinician should consider ordering daily urine collection, which may or may not be sent for random toxicology analysis. In all cases, pain and symptoms should be frequently assessed.

Management approaches should be tailored to reflect the clinician's assessment of the severity of drug abuse. Open and honest communication between the clinician and the patient throughout the admission reassures the patient that these guidelines were established in their best interest.

In some cases, these guidelines fail to curtail aberrant drug use despite repeated interventions by staff. At that point, the patient should be considered for discharge. This appears to be necessary only in the most recalcitrant of cases. The clinician should involve members of the staff and administration for discussion about the ethical and legal implications of such a decision.

Methadone

Oral methadone can be used safely and effectively as an analgesic (84–89). Once-daily methadone is rarely useful as an analgesic, and patients receiving maintenance methadone for opioid dependence cannot obtain pain relief merely by increasing their dose. Indeed, practitioners sometimes assume that patients receiving methadone from a maintenance program do not need further pain medication, but this is simply not true (90,91). Methadone can be used for pain management by increasing the dose and dividing it during the day. Alternately, an entirely separate pharmacologic therapy can be chosen and incorporated into the patient's treatment plan.

Alcohol

Patients with life-threatening illness who are dependent on alcohol require careful assessment and management. When these patients are not identified and are admitted to the hospital, alcohol withdrawal can be an unexpected complication. Patients at the end of life can also inadvertently experience withdrawal symptoms if they decrease their alcohol intake as their physical condition declines. Withdrawal symptoms may be mistaken for simple anxiety when the full extent of the patient's use of alcohol is not known (92). The first symptoms of withdrawal usually manifest a few hours following the cessation of alcohol intake and often consist of tremors, agitation, and insomnia. In mild to moderate cases, these symptoms lessen within 2 days. Patients with advanced illness are more likely than the physically healthy to progress from these milder symptoms to a state of delirium characterized by autonomic hyperactivity, hallucinations, incoherence, and disorientation (73). Delirium tremens (DTs) occur in approximately 5% to 15% of patients in alcohol withdrawal (93), typically within the first 72 to 96 hours of withdrawal. Severe DTs is a medical emergency and requires prompt treatment.

In surgical settings, alcohol withdrawal can cause up to a threefold increase in postoperative mortality when unrecognized and not addressed (94,95). Because patients with cancer who abuse alcohol are already at high risk for delirium postoperatively due to poor nutrition, prior head trauma, and other causes of brain injury, the impact of severe alcohol withdrawal may be life-threatening (73).

The extreme vulnerability of patients who are terminally ill necessitates that potential withdrawal symptoms be managed aggressively and prevented whenever possible (94). To date, no research exists to determine the best approach to treat acute alcohol withdrawal in the palliative care setting; in its absence, basic management steps, such as the use of hydration, benzodiazepines, and in some cases, neuroleptics, should be taken to manage alcohol withdrawal syndrome (73,92). The administration of a vitamin–mineral solution is indicated, including parenteral thiamine 100 g for 3 days before switching to oral administration to prevent the development of Korsakoff's syndrome. A daily dose of folate 1 mg should also be given throughout treatment (73).

Patients in Recovery

Pain management with patients in recovery presents a unique challenge. Depending on the structure of the recovery program (e.g., alcoholics anonymous and methadone maintenance programs), a patient may fear ostracism from the program's members or have intense fear regarding susceptibility to relapsing into substance-abuse behaviors. Nonopioid therapies should be optimized, which may require referral to a pain center or other specialists (90). If opioids are required, therapy should be structured based on a thorough assessment, the goals of care, and the life expectancy of the patient. In some cases, it is necessary to use opioid management contracts, random urine toxicology screens, and occasional pill counts. If possible, attempts should be made to include the patient's recovery program sponsor in order to garner their cooperation in monitoring of the patient.

CONCLUSION

The effective management of patients who engage in aberrant drug-related behavior necessitates a comprehensive approach that recognizes the biological, chemical, social, and psychiatric aspects of substance abuse and provides practical means to manage risk, treat pain effectively, and assure patient safety. An accepted nomenclature for substance abuse and dependence and an operational approach to the assessment of patients with medical illness are prerequisites to an accurate definition of risk in populations with and without histories of substance abuse. Unfortunately, there are very limited data relevant to risk assessment in the medically ill. Also, there is almost no information about the risk of less serious aberrant drug-related behaviors, the risk of these outcomes in populations that do have a history of abuse, or the risk associated with the use of potentially abusable drugs other than opioids.

REFERENCES

1. National Center on Addiction and Substance Abuse of Columbia University. Paper presented at: Under the Counter: the Diversion and Abuse of Controlled Prescription Drugs in the U.S.; July 2005; New York, NY.

2. Colliver JD, Kopstein AN. Trends in cocaine abuse reflected in emergency room episodes reported to DAWN. *Public Health Rep.* 1991;106:59-68.

3. Warner LA, Kessler RC, Hughes M, et al. Prevalence and correlates of drug use and dependence in the United States. Results from the National Comorbidity Survey. *Arch Gen Psychiatry.* 1995;52:219-229.

4. Kessler RC, Chui WT, Demler O, et al. Prevalence, severity, and comorbidity of 12-month DSM-IV disorders in the National comorbidity survey replication. *Arch Gen Psychiatry.* 2005;62:617-627.

5. Kessler RC, Berglund P, Demler O, et al. Lifetime prevalence and age-of-onset distributions of DSM-IV disorders in the National comorbidity survey replication. *Arch Gen Psychiatry.* 2005;62:593-602.

6. Groerer J, Brodsky M. The incidence of illicit drug use in the United States, 1962-1989. *Br J Addict.* 1992;87:1345.

7. Regier DA, Farmer ME, Rae DS, et al. Comorbidity of mental disorders with alcohol and other drug abuse. *J Am Med Assoc.* 1990;264:2511-2518.

8. Wells KB, Golding JM, Burnam MA. Chronic medical conditions in a sample of the general population with anxiety, affective, and substance use disorders. *Am J Psychiatry.* 1989;146:1440.

9. Smith-Warner SA, Spiegelman D, Yaun S, et al. Alcohol and breast cancer in women: a pooled analysis of cohort studies. *J Am Med Assoc.* 1998;279:535-540.

10. Blot WJ. Alcohol and cancer. *Cancer Res.* 1992;52:S2119-S2123.

11. Thun MJ, Peto R, Lopez AD, et al. Alcohol consumption and mortality among middle-aged and elderly U.S. adults. *N Engl J Med.* 1997;337:1705-1714.

12. Room R, Babor T, Rehm J. Alcohol and public health. *Lancet.* 2005;365:519-530.

13. Yu, DK. Review of Memorial Sloan-Kettering Counselling Center Database (Unpublished) 2005.

14. Burton RW, Lyons JS, Devens M, et al. Psychiatric consults for psychoactive substance disorders in the general hospital. *Gen Hosp Psychiatry.* 1991;13:83.

15. Derogatis LR, Morrow GR, Fetting J, et al. The prevalence of psychiatric disorders among cancer patients. *J Am Med Assoc.* 1983;249:751.

16. Regier DA, Meyers JK, Dramer M, et al. The NIMH epidemiologic catchment area program. *Arch Gen Psychiatry.* 1984;41:934.

17. American Psychiatric Association. *Diagnostic and Statistical Manual for Mental Disorders—III.* Washington, DC: American Psychiatric Association; 1983.

18. Bruera E, Moyano J, Seifert L, et al. The frequency of alcoholism among patients with pain due to terminal cancer. *J Pain Symptom Manage.* 1995;10(8):599.

19. Dole VP. Narcotic addiction, physical dependence and relapse. *N Engl J Med.* 1972;286:988.

20. Martin WR, Jasinski DR. Physiological parameters of morphine dependence in man-tolerance, early abstinence, protracted abstinence. *J Psychiatr Res.* 1969;7:9.

21. Portenoy RK. Opioid tolerance and efficacy: basic research and clinical observations. In: Gebhardt G, Hammond D, Jensen T, eds. *Proceedings of the VII World Congress on Pain, Progress in Pain Research and Management.* Vol 2. Seattle, WA: IASP Press; 1994:595.

22. Foley KM. Clinical tolerance to opioids. In: Basbaum AI, Besson J-M, eds. *Towards a New Pharmacotherapy of Pain.* Chichester: Wiley; 1991:181.

23. Ling GSF, Paul D, Simantov R, et al. Differential development of acute tolerance to analgesia, respiratory depression, gastrointestinal transit and hormone release in a morphine infusion model. *Life Sci.* 1989;45:1627.

24. Bruera E, Macmillan K, Hanson JA, et al. The cognitive effects of the administration of narcotic analgesics in patients with cancer pain. *Pain.* 1989;39:13.

25. Twycross RG. Clinical experience with diamorphine in advanced malignant disease. *Int J Clin Pharmacol Ther Toxicol.* 1974;9:184.

26. Kanner RM, Foley KM. Patterns of narcotic drug use in a cancer pain clinic. *Ann N Y Acad Sci.* 1981;362:161.

27. Chapman CR, Hill HF. Prolonged morphine self-administration and addiction liability: evaluation of two theories in a bone marrow transplant unit. *Cancer.* 1989;63:1636.

28. Meuser T, Pietruck C, Radruch L, et al. Symptoms during cancer pain treatment following WHO guidelines: a longitudinal follow-up study of symptom prevalence, severity, and etiology. *Pain.* 2001;93:247-257.

29. McCarberg BH, Barkin RC. Long-acting opioids for chronic pain: pharmacotherapeutic opportunities to enhance compliance, quality of life, and analgesia. *Am J Ther.* 2001;8:181-186.

30. Aronoff GM. Opioids in chronic pain management: is there a significant risk of addiction? *Curr Rev Pain.* 2000;4:112-121.

31. Zenz M, Strumpf M, Tryba M. Long-term opioid therapy in patients with chronic nonmalignant pain. *J Pain Symptom Manage.* 1992;7:69.

32. Redmond DE, Krystal JH. Multiple mechanisms of withdrawal from opioid drugs. *Annu Rev Neurosci.* 1984;7:443-478.

33. World Health Organization. *Technical Report No. 516, Youth and Drugs.* Geneva: World Health Organization; 1973.

34. American Psychiatric Association. *Diagnostic and Statistical Manual for Mental Disorders—IV.* Washington, DC: American Psychiatric Association; 1994.

35. Wikler A. *Opioid Dependence: Mechanisms and Treatment.* New York, NY: Plenum Press; 1980.

36. Halpern LM, Robinson J. Prescribing practices for pain in drug dependence: a lesson in ignorance. *Adv Alcohol Subst Abuse.* 1985;5:184.

37. Dai S, Corrigal WA, Coen KM, et al. Heroin self—administration by rats: influence of dose and physical dependence. *Pharmacol Biochem Behav.* 1989;32:1009.

38. Passik SD, Kirsh KL, Whitcomb L, et al. Pain clinicians' rankings of aberrant drug- behaviors. *J Pain Palliat Care Pharmacother.* 2002;16:39-49.

39. Passik S, Kirsh KL, McDonald M, et al. A pilot survey of aberrant drug-taking attitudes and behaviors in samples of cancer and AIDS patients. *J Pain Symptom Manage.* 2000;19:274-286.

40. Rinaldi RC, Steindler EM, Wilford BB, et al. Clarification and standardization of substance abuse terminology. *J Am Med Assoc.* 1988;259:555.

41. Hay J, Passik SD. The cancer patient with borderline personality disorder: suggestions for symptom-focused management in the medical setting. *Psychooncology.* 2000;9:91-100.

42. Khantzian EJ, Treece C. DSM-III psychiatric diagnosis of narcotic addicts. *Arch Gen Psychiatry.* 1985;42:1067.

43. Grant BF, Stinson FS, Dawson DA, et al. Prevalence and co-occurrence of substance use disorders and independent mood and anxiety disorders. *Arch Gen Psychiatry.* 2004;61:807-816.

44. Dunbar SA, Katz NP. Chronic opioid therapy for nonmalignant pain in patients with a history of substance abuse: report of 20 cases. *J Pain Symptom Manage.* 1996;11:163.

45. Compton P, Darakjian J, Miotto K. Screening for addiction in patients with chronic pain with "problematic" substance use: evaluation of a pilot assessment tool. *J Pain Symptom Manage.* 1998;16:355-363.

46. Jorgensen L, Mortensen M-J, Jensen N-H, et al. Treatment of cancer pain patients in a multidisciplinary pain clinic. *Pain Clinic.* 1990;3:83.

47. Moulin DE, Foley KM. Review of a hospital-based pain service. In: Foley KM, Bonica JJ, Ventafridda V, eds. *Advances in Pain Research and Therapy, Second International Congress on Cancer Pain.* Vol 16. New York, NY: Raven Press; 1990:413.

48. Schug SA, Zech D, Dorr U. Cancer pain management according to who analgesic guidelines. *J Pain Symptom Manage.* 1990;5:27.

49. Schug SA, Zech D, Grond S, et al. A long-term survey of morphine in cancer pain patients. *J Pain Symptom Manage.* 1992;7:259.

50. Ventafridda V, Tamburini M, DeConno F. Comprehensive treatment in cancer pain. In: Fields HL, Dubner R, Cervero F, eds. *Advances in Pain Research and Therapy, Proceedings of the Fourth World Congress on Pain.* Vol 9. New York, NY: Raven Press; 1985:617.

51. Ventafridda V, Tamburini M, Caraceni A, et al. A validation study of the WHO method for cancer pain relief. *Cancer.* 1990;59:850.

52. Walker VA, Hoskin PJ, Hanks GW, et al. Evaluation of WHO analgesic guidelines for cancer pain in a hospital-based palliative care unit. *J Pain Symptom Manage.* 1988;3:145.

53. World Health Organization. *Cancer Pain Relief and Palliative Care.* Geneva: World Health Organization; 1990.

54. Health and Public Policy Committee. American College of Physicians. Drug therapy for severe chronic pain in terminal illness. *Ann Intern Med.* 1983;99:870.

55. Agency for Health Care Policy and Research, U.S. Department of Health and Human Services. *Clinical Practice Guideline Number 9: Management of Cancer Pain.* Washington, DC: U.S. Department of Health and Human Services; 1994.

56. Ad Hoc Committee on Cancer Pain, American Society of Clinical Oncology. Cancer pain assessment and treatment curriculum guidelines. *J Clin Oncol.* 1992;10:1976.

57. American Pain Society. *Principles of Analgesic Use in the Treatment of Acute Pain and Cancer Pain.* Skokie, IL: American Pain Society; 1992.

58. Zech DFJ, Grond S, Lynch J, et al. Validation of the World Health Organization Guidelines for cancer pain relief: a 10 year prospective study. *Pain.* 1995;63:65.

59. Portenoy RK. Opioid therapy for chronic nonmalignant pain: current status. In: Fields HL, Liebeskind JC, eds. *Progress in Pain Research and Management, Pharmacological Approaches to the Treatment of Chronic Pain: New Concepts and Critical Issues.* Vol 1. Seattle, WA: IASP Publications; 1994:247.

60. Kolb L. Types and characteristics of drug addicts. *Ment Hyg.* 1925;9:300.

61. Pescor MJ. The Kolb classification of drug addicts. *Public Health Rep Suppl.* 1939:155.

62. Rayport M. Experience in the management of patients medically addicted to narcotics. *J Am Med Assoc.* 1954;156:684.

63. Porter J, Jick H. Addiction rare in patients treated with narcotics. *N Engl J Med.* 1980;302:123.

64. Perry S, Heidrich G. Management of pain during debridement: a survey of U.S. burn units. *Pain.* 1982;13:267.

65. Medina JL, Diamond S. Drug dependency in patients with chronic headache. *Headache.* 1977;17:12.

66. Kaiko RF, Foley KM, Grabinski PY, et al. Central nervous system excitatory effects of meperidine in cancer patients. *Ann Neurol.* 1983;13:180.

67. Grove WM, Eckert ED, Heston L, et al. Heritability of substance abuse and antisocial behavior: a study of monozygotic twins reared apart. *Biol Psychiatry.* 1990;27:1293.

68. Gardner-Nix JS. Oral methadone for managing chronic nonmalignant pain. *J Pain Symptom Manage.* 1996;11:321.

69. Potter JS, Hennessy G, Borrow JA, et al. Substance use histories in patients seeking treatment for controlled-release oxycodone dependence. *Drug Alcohol Depend.* 2004;76:213-215.

70. Macaluso C, Weinberg D, Foley KM. Opioid abuse and misuse in a cancer pain population [abstract]. *J Pain Symptom.* 1988;3:S24.

71. Gonzales GR, Coyle N. Treatment of cancer pain in a former opioid abuser: fears of the patient and staff and their influence on care. *J Pain Symptom Manage.* 1992;7:246.

72. Kaplan R, Slywka J, Slagle S, et al. A titrated analgesic regimen comparing substance users and non-users with AIDS-related pain. *J Pain Symptom Manage.* 2000;19:265-271.

73. Lundberg JC, Passik SD. Alcohol and cancer: a review for psycho-oncologists. *Psychooncology.* 1997;6:253-266.

74. Butler SF, Budman SH, Fernandez K, et al. Validation of a screener and opioid assessment measure for patients with chronic pain. *Pain.* 2004;112:65-75.

75. Penick E, Powell B, Nickel E, et al. Comorbidity of lifetime psychiatric disorders among male alcoholics. *Alcohol Clin Exp Res.* 1994;18:1289-1293.

76. Kirsh KL, Passik SD. The interface between pain and drug abuse the evolution of strategies to optimize pain management while minimizing drug abuse. *Exp Clin Psychopharmacol.* 2008;16(5):400-404.

77. Webster LR, Webster RM. Predicting aberrant behaviors in opioid-treated patients: preliminary validation of the opioid risk tool. *Pain Med.* 2005;6:432-442.

78. Moore TM, Jones T, Browder JH, et al. A comparison of common screening methods for predicting aberrant drug-related behavior among patients receiving opioids for chronic pain management. *Pain Med.* 2009;10(8):1426-1433.

79. Passik SD, Weinreb HJ. Managing chronic nonmalignant pain: overcoming obstacles to the use of opioids. *Adv Ther.* 2000;17:70-80.

80. Passik SD, Kirsh KL, Whitcomb LA, et al. A new tool to assess and document pain outcomes in chronic pain patients receiving opioid therapy. *Clin Ther.* 2004;26:552-561.

81. Passik SD, Portenoy RK, Ricketts PL. Substance abuse issues in cancer patients: part 2: evaluation and treatment. *Oncology (Huntingt).* 1998;12:729-734.

82. Passik S, Schreiber J, Kirsh KL, et al. A chart review of the ordering and documentation of urine toxicology screens in a cancer center: do they influence patient management? *J Pain Symptom Manage.* 2000;19:40-44.

83. Bronstein K, Passik S, Munitz L, et al. Can clinicians accurately predict which patients are misusing their medications? Poster presentation at: The 30th Annual Scientific Meeting of the American Pain Society; May 2011; Austin, TX.

84. Passik S, Theobald D. Managing addiction in advanced cancer patients: why bother? *J Pain Symptom Manage.* 2000;19:229-234.

85. Passik SD. Issues in long-term opioid therapy: unmet needs, risks, and solutions. *Mayo Clin Proc.* 2009;84(7):593-601.

86. Ripamonti C, Groff L, Brunelli D, et al. Switching from morphine to oral methadone in treating cancer pain: what is the equianalgesic dose ratio? *J Clin Oncol.* 1998;16:3216-3221.

87. Mercadante S, Sapio R, Serretta M, et al. Patient-controlled analgesia with oral methadone in cancer pain: preliminary report. *Ann Oncol.* 1996;7:613-617.

88. Carrol E, Fine E, Ruff R, et al. A four-drug pain regimen for head and neck cancers. *Laryngoscope.* 1994;104:694-700.

89. Lawlor P, Turner K, Hanson J, et al. Dose ratio between morphine and methadone in patients with cancer pain: a retrospective study. *Cancer.* 1998;82:1167-1173.

90. Parrino M. *State Methadone Treatment Guidelines, Treatment Improvement Protocol (TIP)—Series 1.*. Rockville, MD: Center for Substance Abuse Treatment; 1993. DHHS publication no. (SMA) 93-1991.

91. Zweben JE, Payte JT. Methadone maintenance in the treatment of opioid dependence: a current perspective. *West J Med.* 1990;152:588-599.

92. Myrick H, Anton RF. Treatment of alcohol withdrawal. *Alcohol Health Res World.* 1998;22:38-43.

93. Sonne NM, Tonnesen H. The influence of alcoholism on outcome after evacuation of subdural haematoma. *Br J Neurosurg.* 1992;6:125-130.

94. Maxmen JS, Ward NG. Substance-related disorders. In: Julie Hamrick, ed. *Essential Psychopathology and Its Treatment.* New York, NY: WW. Norton and Company; 1995:132-172.

95. Spies CD, Nordmann A, Brummer G, et al. Intensive care unit stay is prolonged in chronic alcoholic men following tumor resection of the upper digestive tract. *Acta Anaesthesiol Scand.* 1996;40:649-656.

ISSUES IN PALLIATIVE CARE

CHAPTER 45

Epidemiology and Prognostication in Advanced Cancer

Paul A. Glare

"I want to die at home, Paul Newman tells his family as he's given 'weeks to live.'" So read the headline in the London Daily Mail newspaper in August 2008. Mr. Newman died 6 weeks later. Patients and families both dread and crave this kind of precise, accurate prognostic information as they make their plans for care at the end of life. Unfortunately, however, most clinicians have trouble estimating and talking about patient's prognoses. Because one-third of the population now dies from cancer and close to 90% die from chronic life-limiting illnesses in which death can be anticipated, contemporary physicians need to develop their prognostic abilities.

Prognostication, along with diagnosis and therapeutics, has always been a cardinal clinical skill of physicians. In fact, in 400 BC, Hippocrates wrote a *Book of Prognostics* and began with the following invocation:"It appears to me a most excellent thing for physicians to cultivate Prognosis; for by foreseeing and foretelling, in the presence of the sick, the present, the past and the future and explaining the omissions which patients have been guilty of, he will be the more readily believed to be acquainted with the circumstances of the sick; so that men will have the confidence to entrust themselves to such a physician" (http://classics.mit.edu/Hippocrates/prognost.html, translated by Francis Adams. Accessed October 7, 2011).

Until 150 years ago, prognosis was closely linked to diagnosis—because there were very few effective options for treating diseases (at least morphine was available to make the death less distressing). This all began to change in the Civil War era with the development of anesthetics and safe surgical techniques. The discovery in the early 20th century of antibiotics and other pharmacotherapy led to an uncoupling of this historic nexus between diagnosis and prognosis, with prognosis being displaced by therapeutics. Nicholas Christakis has referred to this as the "ellipsis of prognosis in modern medical thought" (1).

It is now 40 years since President Richard Nixon signed the National Cancer Act. Although the death rates for cancer in the United States have dropped by 22% for men and 14% for women and there are more than 10 million survivors (AACR Progress Report for 2011. http://www.aacr.org/Uploads/DocumentRepository/2011CPR/2011_AACR_CPR_Text_web.pdf. Accessed September 23, 2011), the reality is that more than 570,000 people died of cancer in 2011 and it will soon become the number 1 killer of Americans. As we move into the second decade of the 21st century, predicting the survival of patients who will die from their cancer continues to be an abiding clinical competency.

The reasons why prognostication needs to be revived as a core clinical skill that is a competency of palliative and supportive care physicians are shown in Table 45.1. Patients and families need prognostic information to make their plans, but there are many other reasons why predicting survival of patients with advanced cancer is an important clinical skill. Time-to-death is also important as a technical prerequisite for high-quality clinical decision making such as whether to perform a surgery, place an intrathecal pump, or refer a patient to hospice. Prognostication is gaining greater legal and regulatory importance, beyond the qualification for hospice benefits. In New York State, the Palliative Care Information and Counseling Act of 2010 mandates that physicians and nurse practitioners will discuss palliative care options with all patients who have a prognosis of 6 months or less. Prognosis is also important for the design (inclusion/exclusion criteria) and analysis (stratification according to survival) of clinical trials. Lastly, and perhaps most importantly, prognostic categories could also form the basis for a common language in palliative care. Oncologists have the TNM classification that allows them to distinguish between different stages of cancer independent of other factors, but palliative care physicians lack such taxonomy.

Because of the ellipsis of prognosis in modern medical thought, most physicians still do not receive any formal training in how to go about this ancient clinical skill. Therefore, it is not surprising that modern physicians avoid prognosticating and do not like doing it when they cannot avoid it. A decade ago, a random sample of internists revealed that although the typical internist not infrequently addressed the question "How long do I have to live?" withdrew or withheld life support, and referred patients to hospice, they generally disdained prognostication (2). Some 60% found it stressful or difficult; almost half wait to be asked by a patient before offering predictions; more than three-quarters believed patients expect too much certainty; exactly half believed that if they were to make an error, patients might lose confidence; 90% believed they should avoid being too specific; and more than half reported inadequate training in prognostication. These attitudes clearly have significant consequences for patient care.

TABLE 45.1	Why is prognosis an important clinical skill in palliative and supportive care?

- Patients and families need prognostic information to make their plans
- It is a technical pre-requisite for clinical decision making
- Legal and regulatory issues
- The design and analysis of clinical trials
- To provide a common language in palliative and supportive care

There are several other forces operating against physicians' prognostications, in addition to not being well educated on how to do it. First, given that prognosis is concerned with what is arguably the most inherently uncertain, and often the most troubling, domain of clinical knowledge, it seems likely that physicians will continue to adopt variable, meaningful, and consequential responses to it in an effort to cope. Second, until recently survival predictions have been in the realm of subjective judgment and there has been no rational basis on which approach to it. Subjective judgments are known to be inaccurate and physicians only want to base their treatment decisions on accurate information. Third, for some physicians prognosis is not only unscientific but should not be attempted, "Only the Father knows the hour" (Mark13:32). Stories like that of Oscar the Cat, the resident feline in a Providence, RI nursing home with almost absolutely accurate prognostic skills, superior to any human being do not help in this regard, either (3). Finally, physicians in general and oncologists in particular do not like to take away a patient's hope (4).

As a result of these negative attitudes toward predicting survival, several "norms" of prognostication had developed. Do not do it unless asked. Be vague. Put an optimistic spin on it. Do not discuss it with colleagues (5). In reviving prognostication as a core clinical skill in palliative care, all of these barriers need to be removed, and a new set of attitudes developed. Fortunately, a new science of prognosis has begun to emerge in the last 10 years. Some of the important concepts are as follows.

Prognostication has two components: formulation of the prediction or "foreseeing" and communicating the prediction or "foretelling." There is a growing body of evidence supporting both of these skills. Both are equally important because there is no point being a good communicator if the content of the message is erroneous. And there is no point formulating an accurate prognosis if the way it is delivered has an undesired effect on the patient.

Two types of judgment may be used when formulating a prognosis: subjective or actuarial. With subjective judgment, the clinician formulates the prognosis in his or her head. With actuarial judgment, the human judge is replaced by a decision based on a prognosis factor, or combination of factors, whose importance and weighting has been predetermined from data (6). In general, actuarial judgment is preferred in medicine to subjective judgment. However, in the case of prognostication, the actuarial models we have as yet are only as good as subjective judgment. There are various advantages and disadvantages to using these two kinds of judgment for prognosis, to be discussed later.

This chapter mainly focuses on predicting survival in patients with advanced cancer. But it is important to understand that there is more to prognosis than answering the question "How long do I have?" The definition of prognosis found in clinical epidemiology textbooks is more generic. It is "the relative probabilities of the various outcomes of the natural history of a disease." In the case of patients with advanced cancer, palliative and supportive care clinicians may be called on to predict many outcomes other than death. These could include further progression of disease; occurrence or recurrence of complications such as bowel obstruction, spinal cord compression, or hypercalcemia; structural or functional limitations due to the disease or its treatment and their impact on the activities of daily living; pain, other physical symptoms, and psychosocial distress; adverse effects of therapies; and the cost of care (see Table 45.2). These different domains of prognostication have been labeled the "five D's" of prognosis: Death, Disease progression, Disability, Drug toxicity, and Dollars (cost) (7). A sixth D—"Derivative health"—could perhaps be added, representing the externalities of a disease on others. For example, morbidity and mortality are known to increase in the bereaved spouses of patients who have passed, and this effect has been shown to be ameliorated by hospice (8).

Little information is available on the kind of rules or principles which clinicians follow or the kind of observations and interpretations they utilize when making a clinical estimate of survival in a patient with advanced cancer. Subjective judgments are widely used in general life and many important decisions depend on them. Subjective judgments should not be mistaken as necessarily haphazard guesswork if they may follow a well-defined process. For example, specified criteria can be set down for the judge of a singing contest to evaluate. These include singing ability, originality, stage presence, and

TABLE 45.2	The six "D's" of prognosis

- Death
- Disease progression or recurrence
- Disability/discomfort
- Drug toxicity
- Dollar cost
- Derivative health

TABLE 45.3	**Some principles to consider when making a subjective judgment of the prognosis**

- What is the death trajectory for this disease and where is the patient on it?
- Is this patient's disease progressing rapidly or slowly?
- Is the volume of disease large or small?
- Do they have a complication of cancer usually associated with a poor survival (e.g., brain metastases, bowel obstruction, spinal cord compression, and hypercalcemia)?
- Has they been responding to treatment?
- Is the patient's performance status good, intermediate, or bad?
- Are they very symptomatic or not?

overall performance. The judgment will have more credibility if there is a scoring sheet and a panel of judges.

The factors that influence clinicians when they are formulating a prognosis have not been studied, but a prospective list is shown in Table 45.3. Even a junior medical student can recognize a patient who is actively dying: the patient is pale, malnourished, bedridden, has poor oral intake, the vital signs are unstable, and the biochemistry is abnormal. The prognosis is then measured in hours to days. But how prognoses of so many weeks, months, or years are formulated is unclear. Recent developments in the science of prognosis can provide a framework for developing, improving, and teaching better clinical predictions of survival (CPS).

First, guidance for subjective judgment of survival comes from the so-called death trajectories of life-limiting illnesses (Figs. 45.1 and 45.2) (9,10). Figure 45.1 shows the typical death trajectory of the solid tumor patient once they have limited treatment options. There has been a long period of good function on treatment (with the assistance of a supportive or palliative care program). This is followed by a relatively short period once the cancer becomes overwhelming, of a monophasic decline with losses in function and well-being which are obvious each week. The individual's death is relatively predictable, and referral to hospice should occur earlier than it currently does.

The death trajectory of hematology/oncology patients is less clear cut. It may be more like that of the organ failure patient (Fig. 45.2), with a more gradual decline punctuated by acute, life-threatening episodes that are potentially treatable (e.g., sepsis, respiratory failure, and bleeding). Each acute episode is met by rescue treatment and followed by nearly the prior function status. Eventually, though, one of the complications will be lethal. Since it is not possible in advance to know which one, the current hospice program

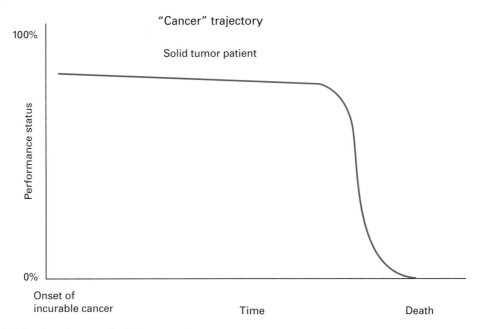

Figure 45.1. Typical death trajectory of solid tumor patients.

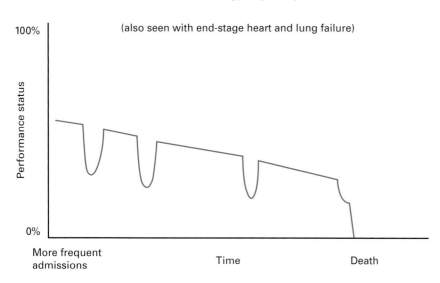

Figure 45.2. Typical death trajectory of liquid tumor patients.

is mostly unavailable. Death in this course is usually experienced as sudden and unexpected for each patient, even though the median survival time of these diseases is well known.

Second, a conceptual framework has been proposed by Mackillop (11) and begins with the diagnosis, which is associated with a general prognosis (e.g., 6 months for the typical Stage IV lung cancer patient). This general prognosis then needs to be individualized by adjusting for other clinical findings such as the patient's performance status, symptoms, complications of the cancer and comorbid conditions, and psychosocial factors such as mood and social support. The relative importance of different prognostic factors varies across the course of the disease. In early-stage cancer, the prognosis is most influenced by attributes of the cancer (primary, metastases, tumor grade, and volume) and the effects of treatment. In patients with advanced disease, clinical factors' performance status, symptoms and laboratory measures, and psychological factors (mood and social support)—referred to as "interactions between the host, tumor and treatment"— have most impact on the prognosis (12).

Third, unlike the diagnosis and treatment, the prognosis is dynamic, especially if there is an effective treatment. Therefore, it should be reviewed and revised at clinically relevant intervals. If the lung cancer responds to therapy and shrinks, then the prognosis would need to be revised upward. If there is no response or the patient develops high-grade toxicities, then it may need to be downgraded.

Fourth, prognosis can be formulated as two different types of predictions. One is a prediction of the time-to-death (or other event), referred to as a "temporal" prediction. The other type is a prediction of the absolute risk of the death occurring, for example, percentage chance of surviving 1 month, referred to as a probabilistic prediction. The accuracy of temporal predictions is poor; the accuracy of probabilistic predictions can be quite high, and they are generally well calibrated if imprecise (13).

SUBJECTIVE JUDGMENT OF PROGNOSIS

In modern medicine, it is preferable to use data to determine diagnosis, therapy, toxicity, or prognosis, rather than relying on the clinician's subjective judgment. To be accurate with subjective judgment requires a lot of experience with the condition; the experience to have been broadly representative and unbiased; the possession of a good memory; the ability to be discriminate (dying or not) and well calibrated (patients with a worse prognosis die sooner); a dispassionate temperament. Valid, reliable tools for actuarial judgment of survival in advanced cancer are becoming increasingly available, reducing the need for clinical predictions, but subjective judgment still has a place. Some of the actuarial tools are hybrids that incorporate a score for the clinician's prediction of survival; the appropriate tool is less accurate than subjective judgment; inputs for the tool are not available (e.g., recent blood work); the patient may not have a disease in which the tool was validated or the tool may need recalibration for this patient population; and the output may not be easily calculable or does not provide the type of prognostic information that is required in this clinical situation. Principles of subjection judgment of prognosis are listed in Table 45.3.

Numerous studies over the last 40 years have shown that clinicians are not very good at subjective judgment of survival, especially when the predictions are temporal. One of the earliest studies evaluating the performance of physicians' temporal predictions in terminally ill cancer patients was performed at St. Christopher's Hospice, London, in 1969 to 1970 (14). Referring physicians and the admitting physician at the hospice were asked to estimate individual patients' prognoses in terms of weeks. These CPSs were then compared with the actual survival (AS). The median CPS was 2 months but the median AS was only 3.5 weeks. Less than 10% of CPSs were accurate. More than half were out by factor of 2 and approximately 40% were out by even more. Two-thirds of inaccurate predictions overestimated the AS. It was noteworthy that there was no difference in accuracy between the referring physicians' CPS and the hospice physicians' CPS.

In a systematic review of studies, the accuracy of CPS subsequently confirmed this tendency to be overoptimistic when predicting survival in terminal cancer patients (15). The CPS generally overestimated the survival (median CPS of 42 d vs. median AS of 29 d). CPS was correct to within 1 week in only 25% of cases, and overestimated AS l by at least 4 weeks in 27%. The longer the CPS, the greater the variability in the AS. Although agreement between CPS and AS was poor, the two were highly correlated out to 6 months. These data suggested that clinicians can discriminate but are poorly calibrated when it comes to predicting survival in terminal cancer.

Some studies included in the review also provided data on prognostic factors such as performance status, symptoms, and use of steroids. Combining these factors with the CPS improved the accuracy of the prediction, although the additional value was small. The explained variance in AS increased from 0.51 to 0.54 when these actuarial data were added.

One of the studies included in the review evaluated the reasons why CPS tends to overestimate survival (16). Almost 350 physicians provided CPS in more than 450 patients at the time of referral to five outpatient hospice programs in Chicago. The average time on hospice was 24 days. Only 20% of the CPSs were accurate (defined here as being within 33% of the AS); two-thirds were overoptimistic. Overall, physicians overestimated survival by a factor of 5.3.

Because this study involved a large number of referring physicians, the authors were able to look at the patient and physician-related factors influencing the accuracy of CPS. The results were surprising; few patient or physician-related characteristics were associated with prognostic accuracy. In particular, patient characteristics such as age, race, diagnosis, functional status, and illness duration were not associated with prognostic error (with the exception that male patients were less likely to have overly pessimistic predictions). Several physician attributes were also generally not associated with error, including age, sex, race, specialty, and dispositional optimism, although non-oncology medical specialists were more than three times more likely to make overly pessimistic predictions than general internists. Experience did matter, with physicians in the upper quartile of practice experience being the most accurate. The length and the intensity of doctor–patient relationship were also associated with prognostic error, but the results were counterintuitive: As the duration of physician–patient relationship increased and the time since last contact decreased, prognostic accuracy decreased. The better the physician knew the patient, the more likely the error was to be overoptimistic. It could be argued based on these data that if an accurate CPS is required, an experienced specialist who does not know the patient should be called in for a "second opinion."

ACTUARIAL JUDGMENT OF PROGNOSIS

Given the deficiencies of clinical judgment of prognosis, a method that eliminates the need for the human judge would be desirable. Actuarial judgment refers to combining or interpreting information in which clinical judgment is eliminated in reaching conclusions. Actuarial decision making is defined by two necessary characteristics: (a) the same data are always used and always lead to the same conclusion and (b) the conclusion rests exclusively on the empirically established relationships in the data. An example of actuarial judgment in clinical medicine is when a statistically defined cutoff score is strictly followed in determining whether an individual has a certain condition or not, and this diagnosis is not modified by clinical judgment. For example, one elevated troponin level above the established cutoff makes a diagnosis of acute myocardial infarction (MI), according to the American College of Cardiology's guidelines for non-ST elevation MI (17).

Progress in the actuarial judgment of survival at the end of life has burgeoned in the past decade. The kinds of data that have been tested for statistical associations with an increased risk of dying or in patients with advanced cancer are mostly those due to interactions between the host, tumor, and treatment, rather than characteristics of the tumor itself. The main factors that have been evaluated include performance status, symptoms, quality of life (QoL) scores, and laboratory measures (see Table 45.4). With modern statistical computing, the hazard ratios for each can be determined and these can then be combined into mathematical models which can be used for making survival predictions.

While it is relatively easy to collect clinical data, measure survival, and generate a prognostic model, design of the study is just as important as in any clinical trial to ensure the results of the model are valid (18). A key point is that the cohort of patients who is followed until death is a "defined representative sample of patients assembled at a similar point in the course of the disease" (19). This is challenging for prognostic studies in patients referred to palliative care or supportive care programs, because referral is the prerogative of the referring physician. Patients failing first-line or standard chemotherapy would comprise a well-defined cohort, but very few studies have used this definition for their sample (20).

Performance Status

The Karnofsky Performance Status (KPS) scale was developed in the 1940s to assess the effects of chemotherapy on functional level. Ever since then, performance status has been recognized as a predictor of oncologic outcomes, including survival. Perhaps the first study of actuarial judgment of survival in advanced cancer was a 1980 study to establish the reliability and validity of the KPS scale (21). An association was observed between poor performance status (KPS score < 50%) and shortened survival, indicating construct validity of the scale. In this study, KPS scores began to decline about 3 months before death and the score continued to fall as death approached. In the National Hospice Study (22), each increase in the KPS level (e.g., from 10 to 20) accounted for approximately 2 weeks of the remaining time-to-death, and the KPS scores were used to group patients into survival risk classes (KPS score 10% to 20%: median survival 2 wk; KPS score 30% to 40%: 7 wk; KPS score ≥ 50% 12 wk).

Factors associated with survival in patients with advanced cancer

TABLE 45.4

Tumor Related
- Primary site
- Number and sites of metastases
- Time since diagnosis
- Failure of standard treatment options

Performance Status
- Performance status scale scores (e.g., Palliative Performance Scale)
- Activities of daily living scores

Symptoms
- Anorexia and weight loss
- Dysphagia
- Dyspnea
- Fatigue
- Poor sense of well-being
- Pain
- Depression (data less consistent)

Physical Examination Findings
- Vital signs (tachycardia)
- Pleural effusion
- Edema
- Altered mental status/delirium

Quality of Life Scores
- Symptom assessment schedules
- Multidimensional scales
- Self-rated health

Lab Values
- Hemoglobin
- White cell count and lymphocyte percentage
- Bilirubin, alanine transaminase, alkaline phosphatase, lactate dehydrogenase, alpha-1-acid glycoprotein
- Blood urea nitrogen
- Acute phase reactants (e.g., C-reactive protein)
- Pro-inflammatory cytokines (e.g., interleukin-6)

The association between KPS score and survival is highly statistically significant, and performance status is retained in all the main models for predicting survival (see below). However, it accounts for only a small amount of the variance in observed survival. Because of this, the KPS alone is not very useful for actuarial judgment, and mixed results have been obtained when compared with CPS (23,24). The fact that KPS score and the CPS were closely correlated suggests that experienced clinicians have learnt to base their CPS on performance status score when formulating the prognosis. Patients can also self-report their performance status. Patient-rated KPS scores have been shown to provide prognostic information that is independent of physician-rated KPS scores (25).

The Palliative Performance Scale (PPS) was developed in Canada in the 1990s to address the limitations of the KPS, including the outdated definitions and lack of objectivity for the lower scores (<50%) (26), and to add categories for oral intake and conscious levels. The KPS and PPS definitions are compared in Table 45.5. Initial testing of PPS showed that performance status in terminal cancer could be used for predicting various outcomes, including short-term survival. For example, patients admitted to a hospice unit with a PPS of 10% all died in the unit, with an average survival of 1.9 days, while 56% of those with a PPS of 40% on admission died in the unit, with an average survival of 10 days.

Similar results have been obtained in various settings internationally, including inpatients admitted to an Australian palliative care unit (27), and a Japanese palliative care unit where the PPS scores were highly correlated with KPS scores (Spearman's $\rho = 0.94$). The PPS scores stratified patients into three homogeneous survival groups (PPS 10% to 20%, median survival 6 d; PPS 30% to 50%, median survival 41 d; and PPS 60% to 70%, median survival 108 d) (28). This grouping was also seen in a community-based hospice (29).

Another study of 733 Canadian patients showed admission PPS score as a strong predictor of survival in patients already identified as palliative, along with gender and age, but diagnosis was not significantly related to survival (30). Further, PPS scores from PPS 10% to PPS 50% demonstrated distinct survival curves, rather than three PPS bands. Such differences are likely to be attributed to the size and characteristics of the patient populations involved. PPS performs well as a predictor of prognosis in a heterogeneous hospice population and performs particularly well for nursing home residents and for patients with non-cancer diagnoses (31). A study of 396 patients admitted to a community-based hospice program confirmed its predictive ability for PPS scores and length of survival with negative-change scores predictive of patient decline toward death, while stable PPS ratings over time resulted in discharge consideration (29). Similar associations have been demonstrated in an acute tertiary hospital consultation program (32). When these four studies are combined in a meta-analysis, each PPS level is distinct and without grouping (see Table 45.5) (33).

By the summer of 2011, more than 20 studies of the PPS have now been published for various diseases and in different care locations. The PPS is well calibrated; the lower the level, the shorter the survival (34). Because referral to palliative care services does not represent a true inception cohort, local calibration of the PPS (median survival and survival rates for each level) is recommended. PPSv2, a minor wording clarification, is emerging as a strong predictor of survival

TABLE 45.5 Comparison of Karnofsky Performance Status scale score and Palliative Performance Scale score

Score (%)	Karnofsky Performance Scale	Palliative Performance Scale					
		Ambulation	Activity Level	Evidence of Disease	Self-Care	Intake	Conscious Level
100	Normal; no complaints; no evidence of disease	Full	Normal activity	No evidence of disease	Full	Normal	Full
90	Able to carry on normal activity; minor signs or symptoms of disease	Full	Normal activity	Some evidence of disease	Full	Normal	Full
80	Normal activity with effort; some signs or symptoms of disease	Full	Normal activity with effort	Some evidence of disease	Full	Normal or reduced	Full
70	Cares for self; unable to carry on normal activity or do active work	Reduced	Unable to do normal job/work	Some evidence of disease	Full	Normal or reduced	Full
60	Requires occasional assistance but is able to care for most of his needs	Reduced	Unable to do hobby/house work	Significant disease	Occasional assistance necessary	Normal or reduced	Full or confusion
50	Requires considerable assistance and frequent medical care	Mainly sit/lie	Unable to do any work	Extensive disease	Considerable assistance necessary	Normal or reduced	Full or drowsy or confusion
40	Disabled; requires special care and assistance	Mainly in bed	Unable to do any work	Extensive disease	Mainly assistance	Normal or reduced	Full or drowsy or confusion
30	Severely disabled; hospitalization is indicated although death not imminent	Totally bed bound	Unable to do any work	Extensive disease	Total care	Reduced	Full or drowsy or confusion
20	Very sick; hospitalization necessary; active supportive treatment necessary	Totally bed bound	Unable to do any work	Extensive disease	Total care	Minimal sips	Full or drowsy or confusion
10	Moribund; fatal process progressing rapidly	Totally bed bound	Unable to do any work	Extensive disease	Total care	Mouth care only	Drowsy or coma
0	Dead	Dead					

in palliative patients. An inter- and intra-rater reliability study of 53 physicians and nurses showed a high intra-class correlation coefficient of 0.96 (CI 0.864, 0.886) for PPSv2, and it was again shown to be useful for prognostication, transitional-point disease monitoring, care planning, communication, resource allocation, administrative planning, and research (35).

The other performance status scales, such as Eastern Cooperative Oncology Group—Performance Status (ECOG-PS) scale, have not been investigated as extensively as KPS or PPS. The ECOG score has been shown to be predictive of survival in advanced cancer (25,36,37). Activity of Daily Living scores have also been associated with the survival of cancer patients (38).

Symptoms

Various symptoms have been associated with poor survival in patients with advanced cancer. Classic work on this topic was first published by Feinstein in the 1960s. He posited that symptoms such as weight loss were a more robust indicator of cancer progression and prognosis than alternative pathology-based systems (39).

Anorexia and weight loss are the symptoms most commonly associated with a poor survival. Cachexia has been referred to as the "final common pathway" in patients dying from cancer (25,40–42). Dyspnea and cognitive failure are other symptoms that have been repeatedly found to be present in patients close to death. Somewhat surprisingly, pain is not usually found to be predictive of a poor survival, even though cancer pain is progressive, and severe uncontrollable pain episodes are more common in the last few weeks of life (43,44). There may be two explanations for this counterintuitive finding. First, it may reflect lead time bias because pain is often a trigger for referral to the services from whom the cohorts to study survival are taken. Second, effective treatment is available to relieve pain, masking its prognostic properties, and treatment with morphine was associated with a shorter survival in the one study in which it has been evaluated (45).

There is growing interest in changes in symptoms as predictors of approaching death from cancer. Edmonton Symptom Assessment Scale (ESAS) scores have been used to track changes. In a large study of ambulatory cancer patients, pain, nausea, anxiety, and depression remained relatively stable over the 6 months prior to death, while shortness of breath, drowsiness, lack of well-being, lack of appetite, and tiredness increased in severity, particularly in the month before death (10). Again, it is unclear if the symptoms that did not increase were truly non-progressive or whether they were well palliated pharmacologically. More than one-third of the cohort of patients followed in this study reported moderate-to-severe scores for most symptoms in the last month of life.

In a smaller study of ambulatory patients having palliative radiotherapy, all nine ESAS significantly deteriorated in the month before death when compared with those scores in the preceding months. At 1 week prior to death, the worst

ESAS experienced by patients were fatigue, appetite, and well-being. It was concluded that sudden deterioration of the global ESAS may predict impending death and that future studies of prognostic models should incorporate both ESAS severity and trends (46).

Cancer patients and health care providers often believe that psychological variables influence the course of cancer. Marital status and socioeconomic status have also been shown to influence survival. Depression is associated with an increased mortality risk in the general population, especially in men (47). Numerous studies have examined the association between depression and cancer survival. Two recent meta-analyses assessing the extent to which depressive symptoms and major depressive disorder predict cancer mortality both concluded that there is an associated risk which is statistically significant but relatively small (48,49). Mortality rates are typically 25% higher in patients with depressive symptoms and 40% higher in patients diagnosed with depression. Adjusting for known clinical prognostic factors did not diminish the effect of depression on mortality in cancer patients.

As with physical symptoms, changes in severity of depression over time could also be predictive of an early death. A retrospective chart review of cancer patients admitted to an acute PCU found that worsened depression was associated with a 30% increased risk of death, but this association was not independently significant. In another study, depression scores remained relatively stable over the final 6 months (10). In a clinical trial of psychotherapy in women with metastatic breast cancer, decreasing depression symptoms over the first year were associated with longer subsequent survival (53 mo vs. 25 mo) (50).

Quality of Life

Comprehensive QoL scores should provide prognostic information beyond tumor burden by integrating all other aspects of disease severity. QoL has also been shown to be prognostic in early-stage cancer, but it is currently unclear why that should be. One hypothesis is that patient reporting poor QoL might be producing cytokines and other tumor factors that affect general health. This could also affect patients with micrometastatic disease before it is clinically or radiologically apparent (51). However, the data on the prognostic role of QoL in cancer are conflicting and inconsistent. Some studies found no association between QoL and survival (52). One problem is that there is no "gold standard" cancer QoL questionnaire available and the choice of selecting a QoL questionnaire for a particular study is governed for the most part by the research goals of that study. The problem may also be methodological, such as ill-defined patient population, inappropriate study measures, or deficient statistical analysis. Improvement in the study design could overcome these problems. Another explanation could be that by integrating all clinical aspects of disease severity, QoL scores are not independent of the individual parameters.

TABLE 45.6 Median survival in months, according to the Glasgow Prognostic Score and B$_{12}$/CRP index				
Tool	**Population**	**Low Score**	**Intermediate Score**	**High Score**
Glasgow Prognostic Score (64)	Lung cancer on chemotherapy	17	12	7
Glasgow Prognostic Score (65)	Colorectal cancer	12	6	2
Glasgow Prognostic Score (65)	Gastric cancer	6	3	2
B$_{12}$/CRP index (63)	Hospice	3	1.5	<1

CRP, C-reactive protein.

Other studies have shown that baseline global QoL provides useful prognostic information. In one study of lung cancer patients, every 10-point increase in global QoL measured with the European Organization of Research and Treatment of Cancer (EORTC) QLQ C30 was associated with a 10% increase in survival (53). These data are consistent with other studies using the QLQ C30, the Functional Assessment of Cancer Therapy-Generic (FACT-G) score (54) and the Functional Living Index-Cancer (55). QoL scores have also predicted survival in advanced breast cancer (56), prostate cancer (53), and metastatic melanoma (57).

Studies of QoL scores in terminally ill cancer patients will be the most methodologically challenging to conduct. A validated Italian QoL questionnaire designed for use in hospice patients, called the Therapeutic Impact Questionnaire (TIQ), uses four-point Likert scales to rate four major components of QOL—physical symptoms, function, psychological state, and family and social relationships to determine global QoL (58). When TIQ was evaluated as a prognostic tool, only the patient-rated perception of cognitive function and the global well-being scores were independently associated with survival. Patients had median survivals of 137, 50, and 17 days for impairment of neither, one, or both scores, respectively.

Comorbid Conditions

Many patients with cancer have comorbid conditions that are in themselves life threatening, or else severe enough to prohibit the use of the preferred anticancer therapy, thereby impacting adversely on survival. Comorbidity is particularly important in cancers that are not rapidly fatal and people older than 65 years. In some cancers, prognostic impact of comorbidity has to be independent of clinical aggressiveness, including lung, head and neck, bladder, and prostate cancer (59). It has been suggested that comorbidity information should be included in cancer staging systems because it will improve accuracy in determining prognosis and in assessing treatment effectiveness (60).

Comorbidities and comorbidity scores have not been evaluated very much in the survival of heterogeneous patient populations with advanced cancer. None of the prognostic models listed below include comorbidity scores. The interplay between age, symptoms, performance status, and QoL in sick patients with advanced disease is complex. Even if comorbidity scores were significant in a univariate analysis they may not remain independently significant on multivariate analysis.

Laboratory Parameters

Interest in simple biological parameters as prognostic markers in advanced cancer has gradually increased in the past two decades. The first large study in Italian hospice patients (with median survival of 32 d) found that high total white blood cell (WBC) count, high neutrophil percentage, low lymphocyte percentage, low serum albumin, low serum pseudocholinesterase; and proteinuria were all associated with reduced survival, but on multivariate analysis, only high WBC and low lymphocyte percentage retained independent prognostic significance.

Other laboratory parameters that have been shown to be prognostic in advanced cancer, mostly indicators of liver function, include alpha-1-acid glycoprotein, bilirubin, alanine transferase, alkaline phosphatase, lactate dehydrogenase, and pre-albumin. More recently, inflammatory markers have been evaluated for their prognostic impact because of their implication in the genesis of the cancer cachexia syndrome (61). Acute phase reactants, such as C-reactive protein (CRP) and vitamin B$_{12}$, and cytokines, such as tumor necrosis factor, interleukin-6, and vascular endothelial growth factor, have been associated with a shortened survival. While a blood test for predicting survival which performs as well as the troponin level does in diagnosing an MI is yet to be identified, objective prognostic scores relying solely on lab results are available. These include the Glasgow Prognostic Score (elevated CRP and hypoalbuminemia), which has been evaluated in lung cancer and gastrointestinal malignancies (62), and the B$_{12}$/CRP index (both elevated), which has been evaluated in hospice patients (63). Survival data from several studies of these two indices are shown in Table 45.6.

MATHEMATICAL MODELS PREDICTING SURVIVAL IN ADVANCED CANCER

Modern statistical computing allows multiple prognostic factors to be combined into a model which can then provide output in the form of a score, nomogram, or other decision aid. As a precursor to more sophisticated models, data collected during the National Hospice Study were re-analyzed to develop a prognostic model based on performance status and symptom prevalence (44). Five out of 14 symptoms which were evaluated were found to be predictive of survival. These were anorexia, weight loss, xerostomia, dysphagia, and dyspnea. The beauty of this model is that it is easy to calculate, the prognostic information is available in a business card-sized contingency table for easy reference, and temporal and probabilistic predictions are provided. Patients with a KPS score > 50% and none of the five key symptoms typically live for 6 months and have a 10% chance of living for 1.5 years; conversely patients with a KPS score < 50% and all five symptoms have a temporal prognosis of 2 months and a 10% chance of living for only 9 months. Symptoms have less of an impact in patients with a poor performance status: in patients with a KPS score of 10% to 20%, the prognosis is 8 weeks when none of the key symptoms are present, versus 2 weeks when all are present.

The Palliative Performance Index also combines performance status with three symptoms (dyspnea at rest, delirium, and edema) to predict survival in hospice patients (66). Patients' survival for <3, 3 to 6, or >6 weeks is predicted, with moderately high levels (75% to 85%) of sensitivity and specificity, although the accuracy (area under receiver operating characteristic curve) was not calculated.

The Study to Understand Prognoses and Preferences for Outcomes and Risks of Treatments (SUPPORT) Prognostic Model

This model estimates 6-month survival in seriously ill hospitalized adults (67). Independent variables include diagnosis, age, number of days in the hospital before entry to the SUPPORT study, presence of cancer, neurologic function, and 11 physiologic measures recorded on day 3 after study entry. The predictions were accurate 78% to 79% of the time. The model had equal discrimination and slightly improved calibration compared with physician's estimates. Combining the SUPPORT model with physician's estimates improved predictive accuracy slightly to 82%. The physiological measures were similar to those used in APACHE and the formula for the model is complex. It needed a computer to calculate, hence, it was not feasible to use at the bedside. The SUPPORT model did show for the first time that actuarial judgment had the potential to provide survival estimates that are as accurate as physicians' estimates.

The Palliative Prognostic (PaP) Score

The PaP score was developed in Italian hospice-home care patients, so it predicts shorter term survival than the SUPPORT model (68). The advantages of the PaP score over SUPPORT are its use of simple clinical–biological variables that are readily available to any clinician, and it can be easily calculated with pen and paper at the bedside. A drawback of the PaP score is that it is a hybrid of subjective and actuarial

judgment, as the final model contains the CPS. The actuarial variables in the model include two symptoms (anorexia and dyspnea), a very poor performance status (KPS < 30), and two lab results (an elevated total white cell count and a reduced lymphocyte percentage).

The statistical parameters of the model were used to devise a score from 0 to 17.5, and the CPS is the most heavily weighted factor for predictions of less than 2 months. Cut points were determined to separate patients who are likely (>70% chance), intermediate (30% to 70% chance), or unlikely (<30% chance) to be alive in 1 month. The presence of delirium was later shown to impact the PaP score (69). The model has been externally validated and shown to be predictive in other populations (70–72). The Japan Palliative Oncology Study-Prognostic Index (JPOS-PI) is similar to the PaP score, also consisting of the CPS plus four clinical variables: conscious level, pleural effusion, WBC count, and lymphocyte percentage (73). JPOS-PI also divides patients into low (group A), intermediate (group B), and high (group C) populations for the likelihood of surviving 1 month. When tested, these subgroups were well calibrated with the proportion alive at 30 days being 81%, 48%, and 11% for groups A, B, and C, respectively.

Prognosis in Palliative Care Study (PiPS)

This new model is also for the hospice population but has several improvements over the PaP and JPOS-PI models (74). First, it does not depend on the CPS so is truly actuarial. Second, its primary outputs (alive or not at 2 wk and 2 mo) are closer to clinical reality ("days," "weeks," and "months"), than a high, intermediate, or low chance of surviving 1 month. Third, separate prognostic models were created for patients without PiPS-A or with PiPS-B blood results.

In detail, 2-week and 2-month survival were both independently predicted by seven core clinical variables (presence of any site of metastatic disease, presence of liver metastases, performance status, pulse rate, general health status, mental test score, and presence of anorexia) and four core lab results (white blood count, platelet count, urea, and CRP). Four variables had prognostic significance only for 2-week survival (dyspnea, dysphagia, bone metastases, and alanine transaminase) and eight variables had prognostic significance only for 2-month survival (primary breast cancer, male genital cancer, tiredness, loss of weight, lymphocyte count, neutrophil count, alkaline phosphatase, and albumin). The accuracy of all models was high, 79% to 86%. Absolute agreement between AS and PiPS predictions was 57%, after correcting for overoptimism. The median survival across the PiPS-A categories was 5, 33, and 92 days and across PiPS-B categories was 7, 32, and 100.5 days. All PiPS models performed as well or better than CPS. Like the SUPPORT model, PiPS has shown that actuarial judgment of survival in terminally ill cancer patients can perform as well as physician judgment. Also, like SUPPORT, the actuarial model is arcane and a computer is needed to calculate it; an electronic application is being developed so it can be calculated on a smart phone.

Of the many other less well-established models that are available, two are worth mentioning. These include a model that combines QoL scores with performance status and symptom distress (75), and another that specifically predicts intra-hospital mortality risk of cancer patients (76). The variables in this model include performance status, short duration of illness, emergency admission, hemoglobin, and lactate dehydrogenase.

MATHEMATICAL MODELS FOR PALLIATIVE CARE/SUPPORTIVE CARE PATIENTS

The regular oncology literature is full of models for predicting response to treatment and/or survival for specific cancer types at an early stage. There has been much less research done on predicting survival in ambulatory patients with heterogeneous types of metastatic cancer who would be encountered in a palliative care or supportive care clinic before they reach the hospice stage. A simple model has been derived for this purpose and validated in patients with metastatic cancer attending a palliative radiotherapy clinic. In the first version of this model, six prognostic factors were included: primary cancer site, site of metastases, KPS score, and three symptoms (fatigue, appetite, and shortness of breath) (77). Subsequently, the model was evaluated when only three factors were included: primary cancer site other than breast, metastases other than osseous, and KPS score < 70% (78). The ability of the three- and six-variable models to separate patients into three prognostic groups and to predict their survival was found to be similar, whether the factors were weighted or just counted. In the validation study of the three-factor model, patients had a median survival of approximately 12, 6, or 3 months if they had 0 to 1, 2, or 3 affirmative factors.

Foretelling: Communicating Prognosis

Most doctors in Western countries now tell patients about their diagnosis of cancer, but information about prognosis is less commonly presented. A decade ago, only a quarter of cancer patients could recall a discussion of prognosis around the time of their initial diagnosis, although an audiotape audit of visits with the oncologist revealed about half were given some information about life expectancy (79). Only one-third were given a quantified estimate. In a recent survey, physicians were asked to divulge what they would discuss at the first consultation with an asymptomatic cancer with an expected survival of 6 months. Some two-thirds of respondents affirmed that they would talk now about the prognosis, while less than half would discuss the code status and only a quarter would discuss hospice (80).

Although physicians may not offer information about prognosis, patients generally want it. In developing and testing a question prompt list designed to improve communication when cancer patients see an oncologist for the first time, it was found in three separate randomized trials of this intervention that prognosis was the only topic about which patients who received the prompt list asked more questions. This was despite the fact that only 2 of the 17 suggested questions on the list were related to the prognosis (81).

At present, there is limited evidence for the best method of communicating prognosis (82). In the absence of evidence to the contrary, foretelling in advanced disease should be approached like other "breaking bad news." While the discussion can be pre-planned, the request for prognostic information may pop up unexpectedly on rounds or after breaking other bad news. So the physician needs to have a framework for approaching foretelling when put in a tough spot. Finding out what patient and family know and want to know is considered to be a very important first step in this process (83,84). Patients get divergent prognostic information from multiple sources, including other physicians as well as the Internet, televisions, family, and friends. Patients both dread and crave this information, wanting realism with compassion, maintaining hope but lessening uncertainty. Their information needs are affected by various factors, including age, culture, education, mood, and proximity to death. Individuals may also be inconsistent and ambivalent about being told their prognosis. Once it is established what they already know and want to know now, the medical situation can be reviewed and the prognostic information shared. After the news is broken, the foreteller should respond empathically, identify and resolve conflicts, and then move on to goal setting and future planning.

Survival curves of patients with advanced cancer tend to have a declining exponential shape, even if it does not provide an exact fit (steeper at the beginning and flatter at the end). Foreseeing and foretelling come together when the clinician keeps the exponential shape in mind when thinking and talking about predictions of life expectancy. In an exponential distribution, the time taken for a group to be halved (half still alive and half already dead) is constant along the whole curve, analogous to the half-life of radioactive decay. So, in an exponential distribution the proportion remaining after two half-lives is 25%, after three half-lives is 12.5%, and after four half-lives is 6.25%.

Therefore, if the median is known or can be estimated, then these other predications can be made as simple multiples of the median. If the median survival of a group of patients is known to be 6 months and they follow an exponential survival curve, then 25% will still be alive in twice the median and approximately 10% (actually 12.5%) in quadruple the median. When presenting this information to patients, some other principles need to be considered (13). CPS is typically imprecise, so it is probably better to think and talk about ranges than single point estimates. It is helpful to think of median survivals as half-lives and to use simple multiples of the predicted median survival (e.g., half to double) to construct ranges. Survival times are skewed to the right, toward longer times, so ranges around any point estimate such as the predicted median survival should be asymmetrical with wider intervals above than below. Rough predictions of the best- and worst-case scenarios might be estimated as about three to four times, and 1/6 of the predicted median, respectively.

It is recommended deliberately to leave estimates rough and to accurately convey their inherent imprecision.

The question "Doc, how long do I have?" begs a simple, single-number answer. Unfortunately, a response like "6 months" is inappropriate, although it is a reasonable starting point if it is the median. Taking the caveats listed above into account, a longer but more helpful response would be "In group patients similar to you I would expect half to still be alive/to have died in around 6 months. About a quarter will still be alive in 12 months, and perhaps a 10% chance of still being alive in 2 years. But the 10% who do worst may have already died in 1 or 2 months." Tables, graphs, or figures can be employed to supplement this kind of verbal information.

CONCLUSION: PROGNOSTICATION AS A CLINICAL COMPETENCY FOR PALLIATIVE AND SUPPORTIVE CARE IN THE 21ST CENTURY

Competency in the contemporary physician is defined by the above average levels of medical knowledge, patient care, interpersonal and communication skills, professionalism, practice-based learning and improvement, and systems-based practice (85). Because prognostication is a core clinical skill required to care for patients with advanced cancer and other life-limiting diseases, the goals and objectives for each of the competencies with respect to prognosis need to be laid down. Medical knowledge for competent prognosis would include the ability to define prognosis in modern epidemiological terms, beyond predicting death; explain key terms such as subjective judgment, actuarial judgment, death trajectories, and general and individual prognoses; and list the prognostic factors that are important in advanced cancer. Goals and objectives for prognosis-based patient care would include the use of prognostic tools or CPS where indicated to provide care that is compassionate, appropriate, and effective for the patient which is based on their predicted survival. Competency in practice-based learning related to prognosis would include incorporating into daily practice the systematic analysis of the accuracy of one's predictions, whether subjective or actuarial; identifying the strengths and weaknesses of one's predictions in different clinical settings; and locating and appraising scientific studies of prognosis for patient's various situations. Competency in interpersonal and communication skills would require expertise in using the approaches described above to effectively exchange prognostic information with patients, family, and other health professionals. The old norm of avoiding prognostication, being vague, and always being optimistic is obsolete. Professionalism is closely linked to this competency. Professionalism in the formulation and communication of prognosis means practicing them with compassion, honesty, and empathy; being patient centered when prognosticating; and sharing the prognosis in a way that is sensitive to patient's diversity of age, gender, and culture. Finally, systems-based practice of prognosis would require the physician to use prognosis to co-ordinate patient care within the health care system with the aim of enhancing patient care.

REFERENCES

1. Christakis NA. The ellipsis of prognosis in modern medical thought. *Soc Sci Med*. February 1997;44(3):301-315.
2. Christakis NA, Iwashyna TJ. Attitude and self-reported practice regarding prognostication in a national sample of internists. *Arch Intern Med*. November 1998;158(21):2389-2395.
3. Dosa DM. A day in the life of Oscar the cat. *N Engl J Med*. July 2007;357(4):328-329.
4. Delvecchio Good MJ, Good BJ, Schaffer C, Lind SE. American oncology and the discourse on hope. *Cult Med Psychiatry*. March 1990;14(1):59-79.
5. Christakis N. *Death Foretold*. Chicago: Chicago University Press; 2000.
6. Dawes RM, Faust D, Meehl PE. Clinical versus actuarial judgment. *Science*. March 1989;243(4899):1668-1674.
7. Fries JF, Ehrlich GE. *Prognosis: Contemporary Outcomes of Disease*. Baltimore, MD: Charles Press; 1981.
8. Christakis NA, Iwashyna TJ. The health impact of health care on families: a matched cohort study of hospice use by decedents and mortality outcomes in surviving, widowed spouses. *Soc Sci Med*. August 2003;57(3):465-475.
9. Lunney JR, Lynn J, Foley DJ, Lipson S, Guralnik JM. Patterns of functional decline at the end of life. *JAMA*. May 2003;289(18):2387-2392.
10. Seow H, Barbera L, Sutradhar R, et al. Trajectory of performance status and symptom scores for patients with cancer during the last six months of life. *J Clin Oncol*. March 2011;29(9):1151-1158.
11. Mackillop WJ. The importance of prognosis in cancer medicine. In: Gospodarowicz MK, O'Sullivan B, Sobin LH, eds. *Prognostic Factors in Cancer*. 3rd ed. Hoboken, NJ: Wiley-Liss; 2006:3-22.
12. Hauser CA, Stockler MR, Tattersall MH. Prognostic factors in patients with recently diagnosed incurable cancer: a systematic review. *Support Care Cancer*. October 2006;14(10):999-1011.
13. Stockler MR, Tattersall MH, Boyer MJ, Clarke SJ, Beale PJ, Simes RJ. Disarming the guarded prognosis: predicting survival in newly referred patients with incurable cancer. *Br J Cancer*. January 2006;94(2):208-212.
14. Parkes CM. Accuracy of predictions of survival in later stages of cancer. *Br Med J*. April 1972;2(5804):29-31.
15. Glare P, Virik K, Jones M, et al. A systematic review of physicians' survival predictions in terminally ill cancer patients. *BMJ*. July 2003;327(7408):195-198.
16. Christakis NA, Lamont EB. Extent and determinants of error in doctors' prognoses in terminally ill patients: prospective cohort study. *BMJ*. February 2000;320(7233):469-472.
17. Anderson JL, Adams CD, Antman EM, et al. ACC/AHA 2007 guidelines for the management of patients with unstable angina/non-ST-elevation myocardial infarction: a report of the American College of Cardiology/American Heart Association Task Force on practice guidelines (writing committee to revise the 2002 guidelines for the management of patients with unstable angina/non-ST-elevation myocardial infarction) developed in collaboration with the American College of Emergency Physicians, the Society for Cardiovascular Angiography and Interventions, and the Society of Thoracic Surgeons endorsed by the American Association of Cardiovascular and Pulmonary Rehabilitation and the Society for Academic Emergency Medicine. *J Am Coll Cardiol*. August 2007;50(7):e1-e157.
18. Glare P. Predicting and communicating prognosis in palliative care. *BMJ*. 2011;343:d5171.

19. Laupacis A, Wells G, Richardson WS, Tugwell P. Users' guides to the medical literature. V. How to use an article about prognosis. Evidence-Based Medicine Working Group. *JAMA.* July 1994;272(3):234-237.

20. Llobera J, Esteva M, Rifa J, et al. Terminal cancer. duration and prediction of survival time. *Eur J Cancer.* October 2000;36(16):2036-2043.

21. Yates J, Chalmer B, McKegney FP. Evaluation of patients with advanced cancer using the Karnofsky performance status. *Cancer.* 1980;45(8):2220-2224.

22. Mor V, Laliberte L, Morris JN, Wiemann M. The Karnofsky Performance Status Scale. An examination of its reliability and validity in a research setting. *Cancer.* May 1984;53(9): 2002-2007.

23. Evans C, McCarthy M. Prognostic uncertainty in terminal care: can the Karnofsky index help? *Lancet.* May 1985;1(8439):1204-1206.

24. Maltoni M, Nanni O, Derni S, et al. Clinical prediction of survival is more accurate than the Karnofsky performance status in estimating life span of terminally ill cancer patients. *Eur J Cancer.* 1994;30A(6):764-766.

25. Loprinzi CL, Laurie JA, Wieand HS, et al. Prospective evaluation of prognostic variables from patient-completed questionnaires. North Central Cancer Treatment Group. *J Clin Oncol.* 1994;12(3):601-607.

26. Anderson F, Downing GM, Hill J, Casorso L, Lerch N. Palliative performance scale (PPS): a new tool. *J Palliat Care.* 1996;12(1):5-11.

27. Virik K, Glare P. Validation of the palliative performance scale for inpatients admitted to a palliative care unit in Sydney, Australia. *J Pain Symptom Manage.* 2002;23(6):455-457.

28. Morita T, Tsunoda J, Inoue S, Chihara S. Validity of the palliative performance scale from a survival perspective. *J Pain Symptom Manage.* 1999;18:2-3.

29. Head B, Ritchie CS, Smoot TM. Prognostication in hospice care: can the palliative performance scale help? *J Palliat Med.* 2005;8(3):492-502.

30. Lau F, Downing GM, Lesperance M, Shaw J, Kuziemsky C. Use of Palliative Performance Scale in end-of-life prognostication. *J Palliat Med.* October 2006;9(5):1066-1075.

31. Harrold J, Rickerson E, Carroll JT, et al. Is the palliative performance scale a useful predictor of mortality in a heterogeneous hospice population? *J Palliat Med.* 2005;8(3):503-509.

32. Olajide O, Hanson L, Usher BM, Qaqish BF, Schwartz R, Bernard S. Validation of the palliative performance scale in the acute tertiary care hospital setting. *J Palliat Med.* 2007;10(1):111-117.

33. Downing GM, Lau F, Lesperance M, et al. Meta-analysis of survival prediction with the Palliative Performance Scale. *J Palliat Med.* 2007;23(4):245-252. In press.

34. Lau F, Downing M, Lesperance M, Karlson N, Kuziemsky C, Yang J. Using the Palliative Performance Scale to provide meaningful survival estimates. *J Pain Symptom Manage.* July 2009;38(1): 134-144.

35. Ho F, Lau F, Downing MG, Lesperance M. A reliability and validity study of the Palliative Performance Scale. *BMC Palliat Care.* 2008;7:10. http://www.biomedcentral.com/1472-684X/7/10

36. Dewys WD, Begg C, Lavin PT, et al. Prognostic effect of weight loss prior to chemotherapy in cancer patients. Eastern Cooperative Oncology Group. *Am J Med.* October 1980;69(4): 491-497.

37. Rosenthal M, Gebski V, Kefford R, Stuart-Harris R. Prediction of life-expectancy in hospice patients: identification of novel prognostic factors. *Palliat Med.* 1993;7:199-204.

38. Bennett M, Ryall N. Using the modified Barthel index to estimate survival in cancer patients in hospice: observational study. *BMJ.* 2000;321(7273):1381-1382.

39. Feinstein A. Symptoms as an index of biological behaviour and prognosis in human cancer. *Nature.* 1966;209:241-245.

40. Wachtel T, Masterson S, Reuben D, Goldberg R, Mor V. The end stage cancer patient: terminal common pathway. *Hosp J.* 1989;4(4):43-80.

41. Ma G, Alexander H. Prevalence and pathophysiology of cancer cachexia. In: Bruera E, Portenoy R, eds. *Topics in Palliative Care.* Vol 2. New York, NY: Oxford University Press; 1998:91-129.

42. Vigano A, Dorgan M, Bruera E, Suarez-Almazor M. Terminal cancer syndrome: myth or reality. *J Palliat Care.* 1999;15(4):32-39.

43. Bruera E, Miller MJ, Kuehn N, MacEachern T, Hanson J. Estimate of survival of patients admitted to a palliative care unit: a prospective study. *J Pain Symptom Manage.* 1992;7(2):82-86.

44. Reuben DB, Mor V, Hiris J. Clinical symptoms and length of survival in patients with terminal cancer. *Arch Intern Med.* July 1988;148(7):1586-1591.

45. Gripp S, Moeller S, Bolke E, et al. Survival prediction in terminally ill cancer patients by clinical estimates, laboratory tests, and self-rated anxiety and depression. *J Clin Oncol.* August 2007;25(22):3313-3320.

46. Zeng L, Zhang L, Culleton S, et al. Edmonton symptom assessment scale as a prognosticative indicator in patients with advanced cancer. *J Palliat Med.* March 2011;14(3):337-342.

47. Murphy JM, Gilman SE, Lesage A, et al. Time trends in mortality associated with depression: findings from the Stirling County study. *Can J Psychiatry.* December 2010;55(12):776-783.

48. Satin JR, Linden W, Phillips MJ. Depression as a predictor of disease progression and mortality in cancer patients: a meta-analysis. *Cancer.* November 2009;115(22):5349-5361.

49. Pinquart M, Duberstein PR. Depression and cancer mortality: a meta-analysis. *Psychol Med.* November 2010;40(11):1797-1810.

50. Giese-Davis J, Collie K, Rancourt KM, Neri E, Kraemer HC, Spiegel D. Decrease in depression symptoms is associated with longer survival in patients with metastatic breast cancer: a secondary analysis. *J Clin Oncol.* February 2011;29(4):413-420.

51. Halyard MY, Ferrans CE. Quality-of-Life assessment for routine oncology clinical practice. *J Support Oncol.* May-June 2008;6(5):221-229, 233.

52. Herndon JE 2nd, Fleishman S, Kornblith AB, Kosty M, Green MR, Holland J. Is quality of life predictive of the survival of patients with advanced nonsmall cell lung carcinoma? *Cancer.* January 1999;85(2):333-340.

53. Braun DP, Gupta D, Staren ED. Predicting survival in prostate cancer: the role of quality of life assessment. *Support Care Cancer.* June 2012;20(6):1267-1274.

54. Dharma-Wardene M, Au HJ, Hanson J, Dupere D, Hewitt J, Feeny D. Baseline FACT-G score is a predictor of survival for advanced lung cancer. *Qual Life Res.* September 2004;13(7):1209-1216.

55. Ganz P, Lee JJ, Siau J. Quality of life assessment: an independent prognostic variable for survival in lung cancer. *Cancer.* 1991;67(12):3131-3135.

56. Coates A, Gebski V, Signorini D, et al. Prognostic value of quality-of-life scores during chemotherapy for advanced breast cancer. Australian New Zealand Breast Cancer Trials Group. *J Clin Oncol.* 1992;10(12):1833-1838.

57. Coates A, Thomson D, McLeod GRM, et al. Prognostic value of quality of life scores in a trail of chemotherapy with or without interferon in patients with metastatic malignant melanoma. *Eur J Cancer*. 1993;29A(12):1731-1734.

58. Tamburini M, Brunelli C, Rosso S, Ventafridda V. Prognostic value of quality of life scores in terminal cancer patients. *J Pain Symptom Manage*. 1996;11:32-41.

59. Megwalu, II, Vlahiotis A, Radwan M, Piccirillo JF, Kibel AS. Prognostic impact of comorbidity in patients with bladder cancer. *Eur Urol*. March 2008;53(3):581-589.

60. Piccirillo JF, Feinstein AR. Clinical symptoms and comorbidity: significance for the prognostic classification of cancer. *Cancer*. March 1996;77(5):834-842.

61. Lee BN, Dantzer R, Langley KE, et al. A cytokine-based neuroimmunologic mechanism of cancer-related symptoms. *Neuroimmunomodulation*. 2004;11(5):279-292.

62. Forrest LM, McMillan DC, McArdle CS, Angerson WJ, Dunlop DJ. Evaluation of cumulative prognostic scores based on the systemic inflammatory response in patients with inoperable non-small-cell lung cancer. *Br J Cancer*. September 2003;89(6):1028-1030.

63. Geissbuhler P, Mermillod B, Rapin CH. Elevated serum vitamin B12 levels associated with CRP as a predictive factor of mortality in palliative care cancer patients: a prospective study over five years. *J Pain Symptom Manage*. August 2000;20(2):93-103.

64. Forrest LM, McMillan DC, McArdle CS, Angerson WJ, Dunlop DJ. Comparison of an inflammation-based prognostic score (GPS) with performance status (ECOG) in patients receiving platinum-based chemotherapy for inoperable non-small-cell lung cancer. *Br J Cancer*. May 2004;90(9):1704-1706.

65. Elahi MM, McMillan DC, McArdle CS, Angerson WJ, Sattar N. Score based on hypoalbuminemia and elevated C-reactive protein predicts survival in patients with advanced gastrointestinal cancer. *Nutr Cancer*. 2004;48(2):171-173.

66. Morita T, Tsunoda J, Inoue S, Chihara S. The Palliative Prognostic Index: a scoring system for survival prediction of terminally ill cancer patients. *Support Care Cancer*. May 1999;7(3):128-133.

67. Knaus WA, Harrell FE Jr, Lynn J, et al. The SUPPORT prognostic model. Objective estimates of survival for seriously ill hospitalized adults. Study to understand prognoses and preferences for outcomes and risks of treatments. *Ann Intern Med*. February 1995;122(3):191-203.

68. Pirovano M, Maltoni M, Nanni O, et al. A new palliative prognostic score: a first step for the staging of terminally ill cancer patients. Italian Multicenter and Study Group on Palliative Care. *J Pain Symptom Manage*. April 1999;17(4):231-239.

69. Caraceni A, Nanni O, Maltoni M, et al. Impact of delirium on the short term prognosis of advanced cancer patients. Italian Multicenter Study Group on Palliative Care. *Cancer*. September 2000;89(5):1145-1149.

70. Glare PA, Eychmueller S, McMahon P. Diagnostic accuracy of the palliative prognostic score in hospitalized patients with advanced cancer. *J Clin Oncol*. December 2004;22(23):4823-4828.

71. Glare P, Virik K. Independent prospective validation of the PaP score in terminally ill patients referred to a hospital-based palliative medicine consultation service. *J Pain Symptom Manage*. November 2001;22(5):891-898.

72. Glare P, Eychmueller S, Virik K. The use of the palliative prognostic score in patients with diagnoses other than cancer. *J Pain Symptom Manage*. October 2003;26(4):883-885.

73. Hyodo I, Morita T, Adachi I, Shima Y, Yoshizawa A, Hiraga K. Development of a predicting tool for survival of terminally ill cancer patients. *Jpn J Clinl Oncol*. May 2010;40(5):442-448.

74. Gwilliam B, Keeley V, Todd C, et al. Development of prognosis in palliative care study (PiPS) predictor models to improve prognostication in advanced cancer: prospective cohort study. *BMJ*. 2011;343:d4920.

75. Hwang SS, Scott CB, Chang VT, Cogswell J, Srinivas S, Kasimis B. Prediction of survival for advanced cancer patients by recursive partitioning analysis: role of Karnofsky performance status, quality of life, and symptom distress. *Cancer Invest*. 2004;22(5):678-687.

76. Bozcuk H, Koyuncu E, Yildiz M, et al. A simple and accurate prediction model to estimate the intrahospital mortality risk of hospitalised cancer patients. *Int J Clin Pract*. November2004;58(11):1014-1019.

77. Chow E, Fung K, Panzarella T, Bezjak A, Danjoux C, Tannock I. A predictive model for survival in metastatic cancer patients attending an outpatient palliative radiotherapy clinic. *Int J Radiat Oncol Biol Phys*. August 2002;53(5):1291-1302.

78. Chow E, Abdolell M, Panzarella T, et al. Predictive model for survival in patients with advanced cancer. *J Clin Oncol*. December 2008;26(36):5863-5869.

79. Gattellari M, Voigt KJ, Butow PN, Tattersall MH. When the treatment goal is not cure: are cancer patients equipped to make informed decisions? *J Clin Oncol*. January 2002;20(2):503-513.

80. Keating NL, Landrum MB, Rogers SO Jr, et al. Physician factors associated with discussions about end-of-life care. *Cancer*. February 2010;116(4):998-1006.

81. Brown R, Butow PN, Boyer MJ, Tattersall MH. Promoting patient participation in the cancer consultation: evaluation of a prompt sheet and coaching in question-asking. *Br J Cancer*. April 1999;80(1-2):242-248.

82. Hagerty RG, Butow PN, Ellis PM, Dimitry S, Tattersall MH. Communicating prognosis in cancer care: a systematic review of the literature. *Ann Oncol*. July 2005;16(7):1005-1053.

83. Back AL, Arnold RM. Discussing prognosis: "how much do you want to know?" talking to patients who are prepared for explicit information. *J Clin Oncol*. September 2006;24(25):4209-4213.

84. Back AL, Arnold RM. Discussing prognosis: "how much do you want to know?" talking to patients who do not want information or who are ambivalent. *J Clin Oncol*. September 2006;24(25):4214-4217.

85. *Program Director Guide to the Common Program Requirements*. Chicago: American College of Graduate Medical Education; 2009.

46 Hospice

Martha L. Twaddle ■ Sally A. Kelley

END-OF-LIFE CARE

> For each of us, the sounds of our time passing are amplified in our feelings and emotions, in our fears and anxieties, in our loves and our guilts, in our thoughts, beliefs, and hopes. It is to these that we must listen if we are to hear the sounds of time passing and if we are to capture the meaning of those sounds. However, we can neither listen for and to, nor can we really hear, the sounds of our time and others' time passing if we are fragmented, scattered, and drawn here and there under the force of untold stresses, through one distraction after another. David Roy (1)

National data reports tell us that over 80% of those who die in the United States do so after a lengthy, progressively debilitating illness (2). In essence, over 80% of the time, the outcome of the disease is predictable, but it is likely that the timing of the outcome is not. In the oncology model, the trajectory of the illness has changed over the recent decades to increasingly be one of a chronic progressively debilitating illness, punctuated by acute exacerbations with temporary recoveries. Like nonmalignant illness, oncology patients may likely experience more frequent exacerbations in their final months and years, these crises coming closer and closer together with less and less time or capacity for an interval sustained recovery. These frequent exacerbations may be related directly to the malignant illness or are oft times caused by associated morbidities or infections. This pattern of closely occurring crises focuses the healthcare teams on "rescue" behaviors and may obscure their perspective as to the overall pattern of decline. Unlike nonmalignant illnesses, more has been clarified as to the pattern of far-advanced malignant diseases, characteristically punctuated by a precipitous decline in functional status, with the trajectory toward death more typically predictable, or at the least, recognizable (3,4).

PATIENT AND FAMILY GOALS MAY LACK SYNERGY WITH MODERN HEALTH CARE

The data also tell us that when faced with approaching death, modern Americans prefer to maximize the time with those activities that are meaningful to them and speak to the integrity of their individual well-being (5–9). Unfortunately, with encroaching illness, the time spent in organizing resources, navigating the complexity of healthcare systems, and receiving institutional-based "care" through procedures, tests, and products tends to overwhelm the energies of individuals and families. When given the choice, most patients likely would not elect to focus their last days and energies on interactions with healthcare systems. But the operative phrase within that statement is "when given the choice." Informed consent regarding procedures is the standard of care in health care; however, advance care planning discussions that might provide opportunity for patients and families to modify or decline further disease-focused interventions without the risk of abandonment, real or perceived, are not yet routine practice in all settings of care (10–13).

In the disease management model, resources are focused on the eradication of the disease and prolongation of life. The goals and resources of care are focused on disease intervention. The physician, nurse, and others work in the warrior roles of fighting disease and within this context, see death as failure, and the lack of disease-interventional treatments as "doing nothing." It is normative for a physician who has exhausted all protocols in fighting a malignancy to say "I have nothing left to offer you" when in fact, an armamentarium of supportive care modalities may be available and of benefit. The warriors of health care do not typically have the perspective to ask the questions that would thereby generate the choices. This may not be for any lack of empathy on their part but rather attests to the emphasis of their training and practice, the finely honed intervention skills that are prioritized within the highly technologic, science-based environment of healthcare centers.

PALLIATIVE CARE COMPLEMENTS TREATMENTS

Palliative care by definition and practice is not an alternative, *per se*, to this approach, but rather represents the foundation of good medical care (14). This approach views the patient as a whole person in the context of his or her family and his or her community and seeks to understand the cultural, social, spiritual, and psychological aspects that will influence the provision or acceptance of professional medical care. The emphasis of palliative care is to clarify the goals of care in the light of how the individual defines the quality and meaning of his or her life. With the goals defined and documented, care ideally moves from crisis intervention to crisis avoidance, resources for support and advocacy are defined earlier in the illness, and discussions of the burden and benefit of interventions are recurrently pursued. Palliative care is thereby a continuum of supportive care

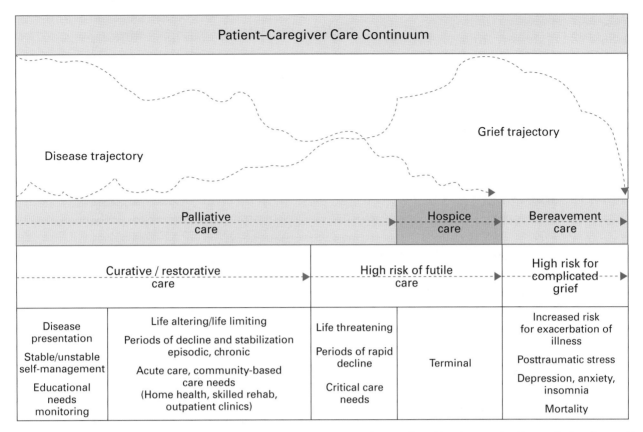

Figure 46.1. Diagram of the continuum of palliative care through hospice (AsceraCare Hospice, used with permission. Created by Bob Parker, RN, MSN/ED; Angie Hollis-Sells, RN CHPN; Martha L. Twaddle, MD, FACP, FAAHPM; and David B. Friend, MD, MBA).

that ideally begins at the time of a potentially life-limiting diagnosis and actively supports the patient and family throughout the course of illness, however long that journey may be (Fig. 46.1) (15–17).

HOSPICE CULMINATES THE CONTINUUM

Within this continuum of palliative care, and most often at its end, is hospice, which is best defined as the most intensive, refined form of palliative care. Hospice is a philosophy of care that recognizes that the disease is not curable, that time is limited to months at best, and that symptom control and quality of life are preeminent goals. In this paradigm, *all* interventions and therapies must have immediate, tangible benefit to the patient and family, consistent with their personally defined goals. Hospice views death as an expected outcome within a discrete time frame. It offers a support system to patients, families, and professionals that affirms the outcome of death not as failure, but its heralded approach as opportunity to maximize quality so that the patient might live well until death. Recognizing the time limitations of life allows patients and families to prioritize the activities and interactions that have meaning, to seek closure personally and practically, and to have an opportunity to "leave a legacy," if so desired, or to have some focused intent as to how or even in what manner one will be remembered after death.

ROOTS OF HOSPICE CARE

Hospice is a term with deep history. Originally, places of safety for travelers on pilgrimage throughout the ancient Middle East (c. AD 400), these centers of "hospitality" evolved into the earlier hospitals of Europe, oft times operated and staffed by religious orders. Dame Cicely Saunders of Great Britain is credited with launching the modern concept of hospice care (Fig. 46.2) (18). Dame Saunders initially practiced as a nurse during World War II, but a back injury forced her to redirect her career to medical social work. In this context, she cared for and befriended a young man, David Tasma, a 40-year-old dying of inoperable cancer. Visiting him frequently in hospital, she witnessed how his symptoms were controlled by the administration of morphine and noted particularly how, when free of pain, he "had time to sort out who he was, dying at the age of 40, and coming from the Warsaw ghetto. Of course, leaving nobody behind and feeling he had made no impression on the world for ever having lived in it. But as we were talking, he said he would leave me something in his will, he had insurance, and he said, 'I'll be a window in your home.' And the idea of openness to everybody who might come, openness to every future challenge, really stems from that gift, which was, I think, the founding gift of the whole hospice movement, made by David Tasma, who thought his name would never mean anything to anybody" (19).

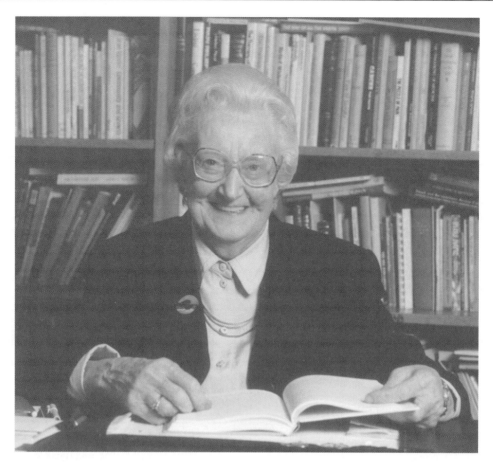

Figure 46.2. Dame Cicely Saunders of Great Britain is credited as launching the modern concept of hospice care.

THE EXPANSION OF THE BRITISH MODEL OF HOSPICE

The original concept of hospice in England, sparked into being by Dame Saunders and David Tasma's gift, was care for those with advanced cancer provided in an institutional setting, in essence, a specialty hospital. St. Christopher's hospice opened in 1967 and in this setting, Dame Saunders pioneered the application of the scientific approach to the care of the dying, establishing many of the current best practices of palliative medicine, in particular, the around-the-clock administration of analgesic therapy to control pain symptoms. Dame Saunder's trainees further developed hospice in the world.

■ Dr. Robert Twycross established the World Health Organization's Collaborating Center for Hospice/Palliative Care at the Sir Michael Sobell House in Oxford. A prolific writer and erudite teacher, he has written and published extensively on pharmacologic interventions in pain and symptom management.
■ Dr. Balfour Mount (Fig. 46.3), a urologic surgeon at McGill University, is credited with having coined the term "palliative medicine" to describe the medical discipline of hospice care. His work at the Royal Victoria Hospital in Montreal helped moved forward the integration of this care model throughout North American and, along with

Dr. Josephina Magno, contributed substantially to the formation in 1988 of the Academy of Hospice Physicians which later evolved to the American Academy of Hospice and Palliative Medicine (AAHPM) (20).
■ Florence Wald, PhD, Dean of the Graduate School of Nursing at Yale University, opened the New Haven Connecticut Hospice in 1974. This was a sentinel event for hospice, the introduction of the hospice care model into the United States; and the form of hospice care being delivered in the home setting, a model that is most common within the United States to this day. Early models of inpatient hospice care were established at Calvary Hospital and St. Luke's-Roosevelt Hospital in New York City; however, the model that has grown prolifically in the United States has been home care (21).

GROWTH WITHIN THE UNITED STATES

The growth of hospice in the United States found fertile soil in the work of Dr. Elizabeth Kubler-Ross, who raised the awareness of death and the recognition of the patient's coping mechanisms through her observational studies published in *Death and Dying* in 1969 (22). In keeping with the grassroots psychology of the American, hospice programs were established at the community level, often by professional

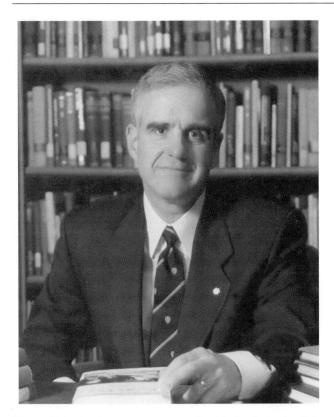

Figure 46.3. Dr. Balfour Mount is credited for having coined the term "palliative medicine" to describe the medical discipline of hospice care.

volunteers, to provide an alternative to institutional-based dying. The early pioneers of hospice in the United States were vocal in their condemnation of "modern" health care's inattention to the needs of dying patients and their families and sought to establish healthcare systems that existed outside of the mainstream in reaction to this deficit. Within the United States, terminally ill patients with diagnoses other than cancer were increasingly served by hospice programs: by 2009, nearly 60% of patients were admitted with noncancer diagnoses, with the most common being end-stage heart disease (23). The New Haven program brought together hospice leaders and advocates in the late 1970s to establish guidelines for the operations of hospice programs in the United States. This led to the development of the National Hospice Organization, now the National Hospice and Palliative Care Organization (NHPCO). The mission of this membership organization that represents the nation's hospice programs is "to lead and mobilize social change for improved care at the end of life" (24).

Through the involvement and advocacy of such leaders, the United States Congress authorized the Medicare Hospice Benefit (MHB) in 1982. This entitlement benefit addresses the types of services provided within hospice care, the persons eligible to elect the benefit, and the payment system that supports the care. Hospice programs throughout the United States moved to become Medicare certified by adhering to these federal regulations. Medicaid and commercial insurance developed similar guidelines, and hospice programs thereby could bill and receive insurance dollars to support care. The Hospice Medicare benefit is divided into periods, the initial being two 90-day periods with an unlimited number of 60-day increments to follow. Each benefit period requires physician recertification around prognosis and goals of care (25,26).

The regulations for Medicare certified hospice providers were published in the Federal Register as the *Hospice Conditions of Participation* in 1983 and updated further in 2008. The 2008 update reflects the Centers for Medicare and Medicaid Services' (CMS) increased emphasis on both patient-centered care and the development of quality and performance measures to monitor hospice care and its outcomes. The stated goal of CMS is to ensure access to high-quality end-of-life care for Medicare beneficiaries electing the benefit and the agency has thus contracted for the development of quality measurement tools. Currently, the *Assessment Intervention and Measurement* (AIM) toolkit, an outgrowth of the Carolinas Center for Medical Excellence's *Prepare, Embrace, Attend, Communicate, Empower* (PEACE) Project is being developed and tested (27–29). Communications from CMS suggest that hospices will be required to submit data on quality measures beginning in 2014 with possible payment reductions as a penalty for noncompliance.

In addition, CMS' requirements for the determination of *continued* hospice eligibility have become more accountable with the enactment of the face-to-face visit requirement (Federal Register May 9, 2010). As of January 2011, the hospice physician or hospice nurse practitioner is required to have a face-to-face encounter with the Medicare beneficiary within 30 days of the start of the third and each subsequent benefit period. The goal of this increased clinician involvement is to improve the documentation of the patient's medical condition and clinical justification that supports the prognosis of a life expectancy of 6 months or less. As such, it is part of the overall effort to administer healthcare resources to guarantee affordable, quality health care for all Americans, as outlined in the Patient Protection and Affordable Care Act in March 2010.

THE BUSINESS OF HOSPICE CARE

As is typical with any philosophical approach that moves to a business model, hospice care in America has been challenged by the tension between its philosophy and what is economically feasible to support. In truth, the MHB was one of the first capitated insurance programs and also one of the most successful. With a flat per diem rate of roughly a hundred and fifty dollars, the hospice program is responsible to provide the professional care of nurses, social workers, chaplains, and therapists in an interdisciplinary team structure. The per diem also covers all the medications, therapies, and procedures related to the hospice diagnosis and any durable medical equipment necessary to care for the patient. The MHB also specifically calls for the involvement of volunteers to provide support to the patient and family. The benefit requires the participation of a hospice medical director to oversee the medical management and, along with the primary attending physician, to certify the patient has a life expectancy of 6 months or less if the disease follows its normal course. Clinical care provided by a physician in the domain of either primary care or palliative medicine is not part of the per diem and is reimbursed through established billing protocols that cover physician services. The benefit also requires a minimum of 12 months of bereavement support for the survivors of the deceased; the per diem payment does not continue through that time period (Table 46.1) (26).

The MHB also requires and covers three other levels of care. The general inpatient (GIP) level of care was established to address the short-term needs of hospice patients when an acute condition precluded the safe delivery of care in any other setting. Under this portion of the benefit, the hospice patient could be hospitalized for acute symptom exacerbations or physical, psychological, or existential issues around dying that could not be safely or effectively managed in an another setting. The goal of GIP is to stabilize or resolve the issue(s) that led to inpatient care and return the patient to a less acute setting. No more than 20% of the hospice's overall patient days can be at the GIP level of care. Continuous care is available to address high-acuity situations in the home setting that require additional care in a low-tech environment for a finite period of time. By definition, the hospice team is providing continuous care to the patient; the majority must be nursing care. The MHB also provides respite care, a 5-day provision that is allowed within each benefit period to ease caregiving strain. Under this provision, the patient

TABLE 46.1	Comparison of home health and hospice requirements and services	
	Home Health	**Hospice**
Eligibility	Any diagnosis	Any diagnosis
	Need to have a skilled need (this can be nursing or therapy)	No such requirement
	Need to be homebound	No such requirement
Site of care delivery	Can only be provided in the home or assisted living (not skilled, LTCF or hospital)	Many sites of care: home, LTCF, ALF, hospital, adult day care, etc.
Certification	Only one medical director certifies	Need two physicians to certify
	Certification periods are 60 d	Certification periods are two 90 d and then 60 d
	Face-to-face encounter and attestation by eligible healthcare provider required 90 d prior or 30 d after initiation of benefit	Face-to-face encounter and attestation by eligible healthcare provider within 30 days of the third and all subsequent benefit periods. Certification for continued eligibility within 15 days of the benefit periods.
Care management	Physician directed; prescriptive	Interdisciplinary team directed
Services covered	Payment does not include meds or DME	Does include meds and DME
	Includes supplies related to admitting diagnosis	Includes supplies related to admitting diagnosis plus general care (diapers, skin care, etc.)
	Can only be provided in the home or assisted living (not skilled, LTCF, or hospital)	Many sites of care: home, LTCF, ALF, hospital, adult day care, etc.
Levels of care	N/A	Four different levels of care: routine home care, inpatient respite, continuous care, and general inpatient
Hours of coverage	Varies from agency to agency. Most will direct patient to ER after hours	24 h on call support
Physician reimbursement	*Attending Physician* may bill for accumulation of 30-min increments of "oversight" care. *Medical director* is salaried if has no medical practice	*Attending Physician* bills insurance with a GW or GV modifier if not employed by hospice. *Consulting physicians* bill hospice program. *Hospice medical director* receives administrative salary or stipend

LTCF, long-term care facility; ALF, assisted living facility; DME, durable medical equipment; N/A, not applicable; ER, emergency room.

is typically transferred from a home to a nursing home or other inpatient facility for a finite period of time, and a small per diem rate goes for room and board as well as to cover all medications and equipment related to the hospice diagnosis supplied within the facility. Most commercial insurance programs mimic the MHB, but with variations that require hospice programs to negotiate and clarify the scope of coverage.

The MHB is a capitated reimbursement program. The CMS determines the adjusted cap amount and works through Medicare Administrative Contractors (MACs) to distribute the funds for hospice services. The MAC is responsible for calculating each hospice's cap amount by multiplying the adjusted cap by the number of Medicare beneficiaries who elected to receive hospice care from each hospice during a 12-month period ending with September 30 of each year. If in excess of the cap, each hospice must refund Medicare payments in excess of this aggregated cap amount (25).

CHALLENGES AND LIMITATIONS TO ACCESS

The challenges of fully utilizing hospice care exist more in its business model than philosophy. Given the regulatory issues and cost constraints, many hospice programs accept patients who have made the decision to forego further disease-related treatments and disease-modifying therapies, consistent with the Medicare regulations. Late referrals to hospice programs may frequently result from physicians and/or families waiting until death is imminent, resulting in short lengths of stay within the benefit. Some hospice programs still require for the patient to have caregivers in place to support them safely in the home setting until death. Despite the steady growth in the utilization of hospice services in the United States, increasing from 340,000 in 1994 to 885,000 in 2002 to an estimated 1.56 million in 2009, the median length of stay in hospice programs in 2009 was only 21 days, down from 22 days in 2003, with 34% of hospice patients dying within 7 days or less of accessing hospice support. In a study of referral patterns, those patients referred by oncologists typically have the shortest length of stay in hospice care, as opposed to patients referred from primary care practitioners (30).

INCREASING ACCESS—THE NATIONAL AGENDA

Despite the financial and regulatory limitations of hospice care, larger hospice programs in the United States have sought ways to increase access and provide the fullness of support to patients who are grappling with the decisions of foregoing further disease-modifying treatment. The NHPCO and the National Association of Home Care and Hospice (NAHC) have focused many resources on improving access to care, particularly for underserved patients. More common now are hospice programs that accept patients who are still receiving disease-modifying treatments with palliative intent, who have not yet established a "Do Not Attempt Resuscitation Order" or who do not have a caregiver living with them. Hospice programs will more typically underwrite

such therapies as palliative radiation or palliative chemotherapy if the goals of care are clearly for enhanced quality of life and symptom management, and if the treatments have little, if any, associated morbidity. The developments within the field of oncology of improved supportive therapies that may slow the progression of the disease with little, if any, dose-limiting side effects have fueled the discussions further regarding continuing such therapies in the setting of hospice. Although great variations exist in the field of hospice as to eligibility around admissions, the overarching theme is to enhance access and stretch the model of care beyond confines that limit its utilization (31).

PEDIATRIC HOSPICE CARE

The pediatric population benefits significantly from this enhanced access model. Pediatric palliative and/or hospice care (PP/HC) is a philosophical and organized method to provide competent, compassionate, and consistent care to children with chronic, complex, and/or life-threatening conditions and their families. PP/HC differs significantly from the models of hospice care provided to adults because of the wide age and developmental ranges of the patients, the inherent differences in the pediatric trajectories of illness, clinical models of care delivery, funding support for care, communication strategies with patients and their families, staffing models and ratios, symptom management interventions, and the ethical concerns that can arise during care (32).

In the United States, cancer is the second most common cause of death for children aged 1 to 14. More than 16 out of 100,000 children are diagnosed with cancer; 3 out of 100,000 die. Over the past 25 years, the 5-year survival rate for all major childhood cancers has improved significantly and a large percentage of children may survive childhood cancer. Pediatric palliative care and hospice service programs may serve patients and their families with chronic complex illness over a much longer period of time. While most chronic conditions do not lead to death in childhood, the death rate is more than twice that of an age-matched unaffected populations, and death can occur suddenly for the affected children (32).

In October 2001, the Children's International Project on Palliative/Hospice Services issued a white paper of specific recommendations for change and improvement in the care of children living with life-threatening conditions. Of the 53,000 children who died that year, only 5,000 received hospice services and most for only a brief period of time (33). The Institute of Medicine's *When Children Die; Improving Palliative and End-of-Life Care for Children and their Families* reinforced that the best model to approach the care for these children is palliative care (34). The cessation of supportive modalities such as fluids and many medications is typically not feasible for a child; palliative care allows continued active physical support with intensive psychosocial spiritual care for the child and their parents. Bereavement care for parents following the death of a child is critically important. Morbidity and mortality increase in this circumstance, particularly for the mother who has experience the death of her child (35).

DOES HOSPICE MEAN GIVING UP?

The philosophical barriers regarding access to hospice care are matters of ongoing debate. Physicians and patients will argue that accepting hospice support is "giving up." There is, however, a substantive difference in acceptance of a terminal diagnosis and resignation to the illness. Acceptance confers that the reality is acknowledged, and plans, attitudes, and priorities are adjusted given this reality. Patients live within this new reality—with new limitations. Resignation confers passivity, an inactive waiting. Although some individuals may live their lives and their last days in this manner, it is not the imposed paradigm for those receiving a terminal diagnosis or choosing the support of hospice care. Many in hospice care speak of hope and would likely define that as trust and reliance in the people and process of support as opposed to hope as an expectation of fulfillment (cure) (36). In hospice, these individuals and families are *hopeful* in living well despite advanced disease, seeking active supportive care to enhance their living in the time they have left. There are, in addition, a percentage of patients who survive hospice care, discharged after a period in hospice with stabilization of their disease process, if not improvement in their condition. These patients are most often those with noncancer diagnoses and a higher functional status (37).

HOSPICE OUTCOMES ARE POSITIVE

The reported satisfaction ratings of hospice care are extremely high, and the testimonials of individuals who access hospice support further fuel the passion of its advocates (7,38,39). The data also suggest that the well-being and survival of the survivors themselves is directly impacted by hospice support. A 2003 retrospective cohort study by Dr. Nicholas Christakis matched over 30,000 couples who used hospice care with an equal number who did not. The results suggested strongly that hospice care might attenuate the ordinarily increased mortality following the death of a spouse, particularly so for women (40).

Along with high satisfaction ratings of hospice care are significant cost savings. The cost of provisioning care to patients choosing palliative care or hospice support services is significantly less compared with those expenditures for patients who pursue a disease-intervention model until death (41,42). This is particularly significant because Medicare recipients tend to consume the highest percentage of their healthcare dollars in the weeks and months just prior to death, in large part due to the utilization of intensive care services (43). Of concern is the trend toward the increasingly aggressive treatment of cancer patients in the weeks just before death, which is reflected in higher utilization of emergency rooms and intensive care units (44). In a study of over 8,700 Medicare patients, mean and median costs were lower for patients enrolled in hospice care. The data also show that the maximum reduction in Medicare expenditures per user occurred when a decedent with a primary diagnosis of cancer used hospice care for their last 58 to 103 days of life (45).

Lower costs, however, were not associated with a shorter time frame until death; in fact, the patients in hospice care tended to live longer than matched controls that did not elect hospice care (46).

THE GROWTH OF MEDICAL PROFESSIONALISM IN HOSPICE CARE

A significant shift in hospice care has occurred gradually throughout the 1990s and is ongoing. This is best defined as the reintegration of hospice into the mainstream of health care. The integration has occurred through many routes. President Clinton's healthcare reform proposals of 1993 recognized hospice care as an accepted part of the healthcare continuum. Hospital systems have increasingly recognized the benefits in terms of clinical outcomes, patient satisfaction, and cost savings achieved through the integration of hospice services (47). The MHB GIP level of care allows patients to activate their hospice benefit while still hospitalized: in essence, discharging them from the acute care admission and readmitting them to hospice care with a series of medical orders, as opposed to any physical changes in setting. Hospices and hospitals often have partnered in these arrangements to facilitate hospice patients receiving inpatient hospice care and also accessing a revenue stream that can help support the care (48,49). These integrative models have been further developed on the national level through the encouragement and mentoring of NHPCO, NAHC, and the Center for Advancement of Palliative Care (CAPC) (50). CAPC has taught and mentored several different models for the integration of palliative care and hospice into the hospital/institution settings through its national meetings and training sites. Leaders from NHPCO, CAPC, AAHPM, and the Hospice and Palliative Nursing Association along with the now defunct Last Acts Project collaborated to create the *National Consensus Project in Quality Palliative Care*, which was published in April 2004 and revised in 2009, providing institutions and agencies with best practice guidelines in palliative care (14). Intrinsic to these guidelines is the idea of the continuum of palliative and hospice care and the defining presence of the interdisciplinary team. In addition, the compilation of over 1,400 references was a sizable advancement toward establishing the evidence base of palliative care in the United States.

CONCLUSION

Hospice, as a vital support system for the end-of-life care for patients and families, has steadily integrated into traditional health care. As the medical community and the public become increasingly aware of the benefits of hospice, the phrase "There's nothing more I can offer you" will become a relic of the past. The utilization of the palliative care continuum, the emphasis on access to care, and the expansion of insurance and regulatory guidelines allow more patients and families who face life-limiting illnesses to experience the fullness of hospice support. Hospice care clearly promotes the concept of "live until you die" by actively supporting patients and families with attention to the physical, psychological, social, cultural, and spiritual aspects of care. Patients who elect hospice care may live longer than those who forego this support, and yet their healthcare costs are significantly less. Ongoing support for families in bereavement promotes wellness and opportunities for healing and positively protects against the raised mortality risk of the bereaved.

ACKNOWLEDGMENTS

The authors owe special thanks to Donald Schumacher PsyD and Judi Lund Person MPH at NHPCO for their contributions and review.

WEB-BASED RESOURCES

American Academy of Hospice and Palliative Medicine (AAHPM)
    http://www.aahpm.org
Center for Advancement of Palliative Care (CAPC)
    http://www.capc.org
End-of-Life Palliative Educational Resource Center (EPERC)
    http://www.eperc.mcw.edu
National Association of Homecare (NAHC)
    http://www.nahc.org
National Consensus Project (NCP)
    http://www.nationalconsensusproject.org
National Hospice and Palliative Care Organization
    http://www.nhpco.org
Pediatric Palliative Care
    http://www.nhpco.org/files/public/ChIPPSCallforChange.pdf
    http://www.nhpco.org/files/public/quality/Pediatric_Facts-Figures.pdf

REFERENCES

1. Roy D. Palliative care in a technological age. *J Palliat Care.* 2004;20:267-268.
2. Pickle L, Mungiole M, Jones GK, et al. *Atlas of United States Mortality.* US Department of Health and Human Services; 1996. Publication (PHS) 97-1015.
3. Teno JM, Weitzen S, Fennell ML, et al. Dying trajectory in the last year of life: does cancer trajectory fit other diseases? *J Palliat Med.* 2001;4:457-464.
4. Constantini M, Beccaro M, Higginson IJ. Cancer trajectories at the end of life: is there an effect of age and gender? *BMC Cancer.* 2008;8:127-131.
5. McSkimming S, London M, Lieberman C, et al. Improving response to life-threatening illness. *Health Prog.* 2004;1:26-56.
6. Steinhauser KD, Clipp EC, McNeilly M, et al. In search of a good death: observations of patients, families, and providers. *Ann Intern Med.* 2000;132:825-832.
7. Teno JM, Clarridge BR, Casey V, et al. Family perspectives on end-of-life care at the last place of care. *JAMA.* 2004;291:88-93.
8. Steinhauser KE, Christakis NA, Clipp EC, et al. Preparing for the end of life: preferences of patients, families, physicians, and other care providers. *J Pain Symptom Manage.* 2001;22:727-737.
9. Steinhauser KE, Christakis NA, Clipp EC, et al. Factors considered important at the end of life by patients, family, physicians and other care providers. *JAMA.* 2000;284:2476-2482.
10. Lamont EB, Christakis NA. Prognostic disclosure to patients with cancer near the end of life. *Ann Intern Med.* 2001;134:1096-1105.
11. Casarett D, Crowley R, Stevenson C, et al. Making difficult decisions about hospice enrollment: what do patients and families want to know? *J Am Geriatr Soc.* 2005;53:249-254.
12. The SUPPORT principle investigators. A controlled trial to improve care for seriously ill hospitalized patients. The study to understand prognoses and preferences for outcomes and risks of treatments (SUPPORT). *JAMA.* 1995;274:1591-1598.
13. Baker R, Wu AW, Teno JM, et al. Family satisfaction with end-of-life care in seriously ill hospitalized adults. *J Am Geriatr Soc.* 2000;48(5 suppl):S61-S69.
14. National Consensus Project for Quality Palliative Care. *Clinical Practice Guidelines for Quality Palliative Care.* 2nd ed. Brooklyn, NY: National Consensus Project; 2009. http://www.nationalconsensusproject.org/guideline.pdf. Accessed October 7, 2011.
15. Von Gunten CF. Secondary and tertiary palliative care in US hospitals. *JAMA.* 2002;287:875-881.
16. Selwyn PA, Forstein M. Overcoming the false dichotomy of curative vs palliative care for late-stage HIV/AIDS: "let me live the way I want to live, until I can't". *JAMA.* 2003;290:806-814.
17. Meyers FJ, Linder J. Simultaneous care: disease treatment and palliative care throughout illness. *J Clin Oncol.* 2003;21:1412-1415.
18. Clark D. *Cicely Saunders—Founder of the Hospice Movement.* Oxford: Oxford University Press; 2002.
19. Curriculum Emanuel LL, von Gunten CF, Ferris FD, eds. *The Education in Palliative and End-of-Life Care (EPEC) Curriculum: © The EPEC Project.* Chicago, IL: Northwestern University, Feinberg School of Medicine; 1999, 2003.
20. Holman GH, Forman WB. On the 10th anniversary of the organization of the American Academy of Hospice and Palliative Medicine (AAHPM): the first 10 years. *Am J Hosp Palliat Care.* 2001;18:275-278.
21. Buck J. Home hospice versus home health. *Nurs Hist Rev.* 2004;12:25-46.
22. Kubler-Ross E. *On Death and Dying.* New York, NY: Macmillan; 1969.
23. Hospice Facts and Figures. NHPCO. http://www.nhpco.org/files/public/Statistics_Research/Hospice_Facts_Figures_Oct-2010.pdf. Accessed October 7, 2011.
24. Mission and Vision. NHPCO. http://my.nhpco.org/about-ourcommunity/aboutnhpco/nhpcomissionvision/. Accessed October 7, 2011.
25. Conditions for Coverage (CfC) & Conditions of Participation (COPs); Hospice. 42 CFR 418.3, 418.52-116. https://www.cms.gov/CFCsAndCoPs/05_Hospice.asp. Accessed October 7, 2011.
26. Hospice Facts and Statistics. National Association for Home Care & Hospice, 2010. http://www.nahc.org/facts/HospiceStats10.pdf. Accessed October 7, 2011.
27. Hanson LC, Scheunemann LP, Zimmerman S, Rokoske FS, Schenck AP. The PEACE project review of clinical instruments for hospice and palliative care. *J Palliat Med.* October 2010;13(10):1253-1260.
28. Ross C. QAPI, how do you measure up? Preparing for public reporting in hospice: an overview for success. *Home Healthcare Nurse.* 2011;29:45-51.
29. Hospice AIM Toolkit. http://www.ipro.org/index/hospice-aim. Accessed October 7, 2011.
30. Lamont EB, Christakis NA. Physician factors in the timing of cancer patient referral to hospice palliative care. *Cancer.* 2002;94:2733-2737.
31. Jennings B, Ryndes T, D'Onofrio C, et al. Access to hospice care: expanding boundaries, overcoming barriers. *Hastings Cent Rep Spec Suppl.* 2003;2:S3-S9, S9-S13, S15-S21.

32. Friebert S. NHPCO facts and figures: pediatric palliative and hospice care in America, 2009. http://www.nhpco.org/files/public/quality/Pediatric_Facts-Figures.pdf. Accessed October 7, 2011.

33. Children's International Project on Palliative/Hospice Services. A Call for Change: recommendations to improve the care of children living with life-threatening conditions, 2001. http://www.nhpco.org/files/public/ChIPPSCallforChange.pdf. Accessed October 7, 2011.

34. Institute of Medicine Board on Health Science Policy. When children die: improving palliative and end-of-life care for children and their families, 2003. http://www.nap.edu/catalog.php?record_id=10390. Accessed October 7, 2011.

35. Li J, Precht DH, Mortensen PB, et al. Mortality in parents after death of a child in Denmark: a nationwide follow-up study. *Lancet.* 2003;361(9355):363-367.

36. Tulsky J. Hope and hubris. *J Palliat Med.* 2002;5:339-341.

37. Kutner JS, Blake M, Meyer SA. Predictors of live hospice discharge: data from the National Home and Hospice Care Survey (NHHCS). *Am J Hosp Palliat Care.* 2002;19:331-337.

38. Casarett DJ, Hirschman KB, Crowley R, et al. Caregivers' satisfaction with hospice care in the last 24 hours of life. *Am J Hosp Palliat Care.* 2003;20:205-210.

39. Miceli PJ, Mylod DE. Satisfaction of families using end-of-life care: current successes and challenges in the hospice industry. *Am J Hosp Palliat Care.* 2003;20:360-370.

40. Christakis NA, Iwashyna TJ. The health impact of health care on families: a matched cohort study of hospice use by decedents and mortality outcomes in surviving, widowed spouses. *Soc Sci Med.* 2003;57:465-475.

41. Elsayem A, Swint K, Fisch M, et al. Palliative care inpatient service in a comprehensive cancer center: clinical and financial outcomes. *Clin Oncol.* 2004;22:2008-2014.

42. Campbell ML, Frank RR. Experience with an end-of-life practice at a university hospital. *Crit Care Med.* 1997; 25:197-202.

43. Harrison JP, Ford D, Wilson K. The impact of hospice programs on US hospitals. *Nurs Econ.* 2005;23:78-84.

44. Earle CC, Neville BA, Landrum MB, et al. Trends in the aggressiveness of cancer care near the end of life. *J Clin Oncol.* 2004;22:315-321.

45. Taylor DH, Osterman J, Van Houtven CH, Tulsky J, Steinhauser K. What length of hospice use maximizes reduction in medical expenditures near death in the US Medicare program? *Soc Sci Med.* 2007;65:1466-1478.

46. Pyenson B, Connor S, Fitch K, et al. Medicare cost in matched hospice and non-hospice cohorts. *J Pain Symptom Manage.* 2004;28:200-210.

47. Higginson IJ, Finlay IG, Goodwin DM, et al. Do hospital-based palliative teams improve care for patients or families at the end of life? *J Pain Symptom Manage.* 2002;23:96-106.

48. Dunlop RJ, Hockey JM. *Hospital-Based Palliative Care Teams: The Hospital-Hospice Interface.* New York, NY: Oxford University Press; 1998.

49. Meier DE. When pain and suffering do not require a prognosis: working toward meaningful hospital-hospice partnership. *J Palliat Med.* 2003;6:109-115.

50. Center for Advancement of Palliative Care. http://www.capc.org/. Accessed October 7, 2011.

James Hallenbeck

People experience health and illness in cultural contexts. A better understanding of culture helps the clinician avoid certain common pitfalls, thereby improving the chances of good outcomes. Very sick and dying patients in our society are often dependent upon care from people of very different cultural backgrounds, making cross-cultural misunderstandings and conflict common. Following an introductory discussion of culture and ethnicity and their relation to palliative care, this chapter will explore cultural issues in palliative care from a framework of three interrelated concepts—cultural sensitivity, competence, and effectiveness (1). Cultural sensitivity refers to an awareness of cultural influences on beliefs, practices, communication styles, and system issues as they affect the patient, the family, and the clinician. Cultural competence refers to skills and behaviors that serve to decrease cross-cultural conflict and improve care outcomes (2). Finally, the chapter will conclude with a discussion of the effectiveness of various interventions that might be used to improve care across cultures.

WHAT IS CULTURE?

Various definitions of culture exist in the literature. Helman (3) defines culture as "a set of guidelines (both explicit and implicit) which individuals inherit as members of a particular society and which tells them how to view the world, how to experience it emotionally, and how to *behave* in it in relation to other people, to supernatural forces or gods, and to the natural environment." This definition suggests culture, as a *noun*, exists as a pervasive set of guidelines shaping the individual. Culture, as a *verb*, is in fact more than an inheritance; it is a dynamic *process* wherein people interact with each other and thereby actively create an ever-changing world experience (4). Culture can also be viewed as a complex and overlapping set of descriptors, adjectives, and adverbs, giving meaning, shading, and even texture to various patterns of human organization and behavior.

IMPORTANCE OF CULTURE TO PALLIATIVE CARE

Recent American national consensus guidelines identified cultural aspects of care as a major domain of palliative care, highlighting its importance (5). Criteria under this domain

are outlined in Table 47.1. Although the criterion list is short, it suggests a broad array of concerns to be addressed: knowledge of and sensitivity to cultural backgrounds, awareness regarding cultural influences on bioethics and communication skills, and system issues. At both the individual clinician and the program level the challenge is taking such a list and translating it into discrete skills and actions that will result in more culturally effective care. Before considering specific interventions, let us consider why culture is so important in palliative care.

We live in an increasingly pluralistic society, although the extent of diversity varies dramatically by geographic region. Pluralism exists in terms of not only ethnicity but also other cultural attributes. National and geographic origin, current home (geographic location and urban/rural), gender, sexual orientation, marital status, family, professional and community roles, religion, and economic and educational status—these cultural attributes and others contribute to our cultural personae (4). Social factors associated with these attributes can create barriers to care, limiting the availability and effectiveness of palliative care for certain populations. Pluralism also exists among healthcare workers (6). When people become chronically ill, they are more likely to come under the care of clinicians and others from very different backgrounds than their own (7,8). Relationships in such situations are often imposed. That is, healthcare workers, whether physicians working in an intensive care unit or nurse's aides in a nursing home, and patients have limited choices as to who will care for whom. Because hands-on care, such as that provided by nurse's aides, is devalued in our society, immigrant and underclass workers make up a substantial portion of this workforce. These workers have little choice but to accept positions at the bottom of the social ladder, which in our society includes the provision of the most intimate care for chronically ill and dying patients. Conversely, patients and families are increasingly dependent upon care provided by such workers. Imposed relationships at such a fragile stage in the life cycle can create a problematic environment. Efforts to understand each other are not only desirable but also essential.

Although culture lurks in the background of all human experience, it comes alive and overt during transition periods in the human life cycle. Death and dying are obviously major transitions and as such are heavily invested with culture.

TABLE 47.1 Cultural aspects of care
National Consensus Project Criteria
The cultural background, concerns, and needs of the patient and their family are elicited and documented
Cultural needs identified by team and family are addressed in the interdisciplinary team care plan
Communication, in all forms, with patient and family is respectful of their cultural preferences regarding disclosure, truth telling, and decision making
The program aims to respect and accommodate the range of language, dietary, and ritual practices of patients and their families
Communication should occur in a language and manner that the patient and family understand. For the patient and family who do not speak or understand English, the palliative care program should make all reasonable efforts to use appropriate interpreter services. Interpreters can be accessed both by person and phone. When professional interpreters are unavailable, other healthcare providers may be used to provide translation. In the absence of all other alternatives, family members may be used in an emergency situation and if the patient is in agreement
Recruitment and hiring practices strive to reflect the cultural diversity of the community

From National Consensus Project for Quality Palliative Care. *Clinical Practice Guidelines for Quality Palliative Care.* 2nd ed. Pittsburgh, PA: National Consensus Project for Quality Palliative Care; 2009.

Cultural transitions are often marked by rituals and rites wherein meaning is expressed and created through particular behaviors. Beyond this, ritual is used to change reality or at least to create a particular human expression of reality. Rites and rituals related to palliative care are most obvious in considering death and dying practices (9). More subtle may be myriad behaviors, some of a very personal nature, that are used to cope with transitions in chronic illness. For example, ritual is involved in the process of making a person a patient in a hospital. Wristbands and hospital gowns serve ritual purposes beyond mere technical efficiency. The ritual use of wigs or caps after hair loss through chemotherapy is another example that may serve the purpose of maintaining a certain image of self (in addition to keeping one's head warm). Conversely, "going bald" after hair loss may serve a ritual purpose of declaring acceptance as a new member of a class of cancer patients. Clinicians also engage in ritual behavior. For example, death pronouncement is more a ritual than a diagnosis of death (10). The importance of ritual as a cultural activity related to dying (and birth) is highlighted by Grimes in his book, *Deeply into the Bone—Reinventing Rites of Passage*:

> If we do not birth and die ritually, we will do so technologically, inscribing technocratic values in our very bones. Technology without ritual (or worse, technology *as* ritual) easily degenerates into knowledge without respect (9, p13).

Culture shapes how we relate to and communicate about major aspects of life, including serious and chronic illness. As discussed further in the subsequent text, if clinicians, patients, and families approach illness from differing cultural perspectives, miscommunication is almost inevitable, barring serious efforts to compensate for such differences. Finally, culture is inexorably intertwined with society and the healthcare system. It would be a mistake to view "culture" as

a disembodied set of beliefs and practices, somehow separate from the social and organizational forces that shape our lives. As will be discussed at the end of the chapter, understanding this relationship and effecting systemic change may be one of the most useful ways to improve cross-cultural outcomes.

ETHNICITY

Most clinician training regarding culture has focused on ethnicity, as have many palliative care texts and articles (11–21). The tendency in many such texts is to describe beliefs and practices of particular ethnic groups relative to health care. Lipson et al. (22), for example, provides overviews of how 24 ethnic groups construct illness, relate to symptoms such as pain, decision making, relations with clinicians, preparations for dying, grief practices, and death rites. Although this and similar texts may be helpful to clinicians struggling to care for patients from very foreign ethnic groups, some caution is in order. Excessive reliance on such texts risks stereotyping by underestimating the extent of cultural diversity within ethnic groups (23). Culture tends to be portrayed more as a determinant *thing*, much like a genetic code, rather than an active *process* of social engagement. An exclusive focus on ethnicity and associated beliefs and practices also tends to narrowly define culture and limits the ability to appreciate other important aspects of culture (4,24). Problematic, cross-cultural encounters between individuals and healthcare systems may too easily be ascribed to differences in belief systems, with inadequate attention to social forces associated with ethnicity such as those arising from poverty or racism. As a case in point, a follow-up analysis of the SUPPORT study population demonstrated that African Americans (among other nonwhite groups) were more likely than Caucasians to die in acute care hospitals (odds ratio 1.88) (25). Other studies have suggested that as a group, African Americans are more likely to desire aggressive, life-prolonging care and less likely to complete written advance directives (26). While all this may be true, it would be a mistake to *assume* a connection between the probability of dying in the hospital and ascribed cultural beliefs of African Americans. Other demographic variables correlated with African American ethnicity, such as higher population densities in urban areas, proximity to certain hospitals, or socioeconomic factors such as poverty, might play as great or a greater role than beliefs (27). As a practical matter, it is far easier to classify people by ethnicity than to sort out the influences of related and overlapping factors such as these.

Still, ethnicity is a useful starting point for considering the forces that affect care, as long as one understands that considerably more than "beliefs and practices" are at work. Correlated with ethnicity are important factors such as immigrant status, educational background, socioeconomic status, geographic and demographic distribution relative to healthcare resources, communication styles, and other social roles (28,29). Space does not allow for a detailed discussion of all these factors, although they undeniably affect clinician interactions with patients and families in profound ways. If seeking to learn more about a particular ethnic group, the clinician will likely be disappointed by a traditional Medline search. Although some good books are available, few journal articles are specific to cultural aspects of particular ethnic groups. In contrast, the Internet is a particularly rich source for material with a number of web sites specializing in this area. A selected list of Internet references is listed in Table 47.2.

Cultural sensitivity requires an awareness of and respect for differences. This is far easier said than done. As one anthropologist puts it, "culture hides much more than it reveals, and strangely enough what it hides, it hides most effectively from its own participants" (30). This statement suggests that examination of one's own culture, a form of cultural self-reflection, is a natural starting point for increasing cultural sensitivity. Such reflection is furthered by contrasting one's understanding and assumptions with those of other cultural groups. Of particular importance is contrasting differing understandings of illness, medical systems, and styles of communication. To a degree, such reflection can be stimulated by formal medical education. Unfortunately, medical curricula have rarely included cultural aspects of care, despite calls for such inclusion. A study in 1992 queried 126 medical schools regarding possible courses in "cultural sensitivity." Of 98 respondents only 13 schools reported offering such courses and all but one were elective. Fifty-nine schools indicated that they had incorporated cultural sensitivity in other courses such as courses on medical ethics (31). A systematic review of the literature from 1963 to 1998 published in 1999 found 17 reports of curricula meeting search criteria (32). Thirteen of these programs were in North America and 11 were exclusively for students in years 1 and 2 of medical school. The focus of most of the content was on ethnicity, attitudes, health beliefs, and language barriers. Only one program is reported to have considered anthropologic and sociologic theories (33). The lack of breadth and the apparent lack of depth of training suggested in this review are discouraging. However, there are some encouraging signs of change. Carrillo et al. (34) published a description of a course for medical students and residents consisting of four 2-hour modules covering *basic concepts, core cultural issues, understanding the meaning of the illness, determining the patient's social context, and negotiating across cultures*, which seems to be more in keeping with recent anthropologic and sociologic trends. In an intervention designed to assist internal medicine programs in the United States in improving palliative care education, Dr. David Weissman found that teaching regarding cross-cultural issues was high on the list of unmet needs of residency training programs

TABLE 47.2	Internet references

Internet Links for Cross-Cultural Issues in Health

The Cross-Cultural Health Care Program. Specializes in issues related to medical interpreters and other cultural competency issues: http:/www.xculture.org

Stanford Geriatric Education Center. Specializing in ethnogeriatrics. Includes online training modules on cross-cultural communication: http:/sgec.stanford.edu/

Ethnomed. Ethnic Medicine Information from Harborview Medical Center. Contains healthcare information pertinent to health care of recent immigrants: http:/www.ethnomed.org

CultureMed. From SUNY, this web site promotes culturally competent health care for immigrants and refugees. Superb bibliographies: http://culturedmed.binghamton.edu/

International Association for Hospice and Palliative Care. Leading international hospice and palliative care organization for a more global perspective: http://www.hospicecare.com/

Multi-Cultural Resources for Health Information, U.S. Dept. of Health & Human Services. Links to multiple health care–related sites with a particular emphasis on government and regulatory agencies: http://sis.nlm.nih.gov/outreach/multicultural.html

(Weissman, D., personal communication, 1998). In response to this, a module on addressing cross-cultural concerns was developed (35). This suggests that physicians are generally interested in improving their training in cultural issues, which bodes well for future educational efforts.

CULTURE OF BIOMEDICINE AND PALLIATIVE CARE

In keeping with the notion of cultural self-reflection, let us consider biomedicine as a culture, particularly as it has evolved in the United States and the relation between biomedicine and palliative care. Originating in western Europe, the evolution of biomedicine has been guided by complex historical, religious, philosophical, and economic forces (36). Biomedicine has now become, arguably, the dominant medical system throughout the world, being integrated, or at least coexisting, with numerous other medical systems. Insight into cultural aspects of biomedicine is critical for the practitioner trying to work with individuals across cultures.

Although sharing with other medical systems a fundamental charge to heal the sick, biomedicine's emphasis in recent decades has been increasingly to fix broken bodies (36,37). Pursuing a western rationalist belief that the *good* is best approached through scientific inquiry, biomedicine has developed a mechanistic approach to care. Through a progressively refined and reductionist understanding of the origins of illness, labeled *disease*, the hope (and the myth) of biomedicine is to eliminate physical disease entirely. Although suffering is not entirely ignored in biomedicine, it does take second place to biology as an issue of concern in that it is often presumed that suffering will disappear once disease has been eliminated. This belief that suffering is derivative to biological malfunctioning is naïve on two fronts. First, it simply takes no account of aspects of suffering not arising from the body (38,39). Second, almost too obviously, biomedicine to date has failed to eliminate disease. Given our continuing mortality, inevitably the elimination of one illness must, by default, increase the probability of becoming ill and eventually dying from something else. Therefore, suffering continues. Indeed, biomedicine "creates" new forms of illness and associated suffering, as the field of supportive oncology, dealing in large part with the sequelae of oncologic treatment, is ample testimony. The evolution of palliative and supportive care, pain clinics, and hospices as social phenomena on the margin of biomedicine can be understood in part as reactions to the failure of this dominant myth of biomedicine.

Biomedicine is unusual as a medical system in its inattention to any concept of a "life force" (40,41). Most other medical systems include some notion of a life force and commonly frame the understanding of health and illness in terms of balance and imbalance between aspects of energy (often positive and negative) that give rise to a life force (24). Examples include Chinese (yin-yang) and Hispanic (hot-cold) systems. A medicine that identifies healing as a process of *balancing* seems philosophically closer to the spirit of palliative care than a medicine based on *cure* and is arguably more

relevant when cure is no longer possible. Balance need not be approached solely in terms of energy. For example, palliative approaches to congestive heart failure and skin disorders often emphasize a balance between wetness and dryness.

Biomedical culture influences our behavior as clinicians at more intimate levels as well. Our cultural personae as clinicians are shaped to a large degree by innumerable small interactions with teachers and peers. For example, in learning to *take* a history, clinicians come to understand that the Social History should primarily focus on behavioral risk factors for disease, such as alcohol intake and sexual activity, not the social network of the patient (42). Nor is there usually a section for a Personal History of the patient as a *person*. Such a bias is a reflection of the biomedical emphasis on disease and relative neglect of more social aspects of illness. With chronic or terminal illness, preventive health care, emphasized in the traditional H&P, becomes less relevant and the social network upon which the patient increasingly relies becomes more relevant. Insensitive application of a biomedically oriented approach to care risks neglect of social and cultural aspects of the patient's illness, which tend to grow in importance with progressive severity and chronicity of illness.

Palliative care, working at the margin of biomedicine, constitutes a radical challenge to many of biomedicine's tenets. The emphasis in palliative care is on the person and family as the unit of care. Attention to suffering and quality of life assumes primacy in care provision. It should come as little surprise that resistance to such an approach has been engendered by many in biomedicine. Resistance is less a conscious opposition to palliative goals of care (nobody is *against* relief of suffering) than a reflection of a cross-cultural conflict between the traditional biomedical culture and the evolving subculture of palliative care.

BIOETHICS, BIOMEDICINE, AND CROSS-CULTURAL ENCOUNTERS IN PALLIATIVE CARE

The relevance of bioethical concerns to palliative care should be obvious. It is more difficult to appreciate that bioethics is the product of western biomedicine and as such is prone to cultural biases. The national consensus guidelines list three topics more commonly discussed as bioethical issues as "cultural preferences": disclosure, truth telling, and decision making. Other topics such as hydration and nutrition could be added to this list. Such topics do indeed raise ethical concerns. However, to address the ethics of such concerns separate from the diverse belief and value systems shaping "cultural preferences" is to risk cultural insensitivity. Therefore, the practice of bioethics must be informed by a consideration of intrinsic cultural biases as the first step in the development of a culturally sensitive bioethics.

Anthropologic critiques of bioethics are limited but raise important issues of concern (43). Often noted as "ethnocentric" positions of bioethics are the following:

■ The dominance of abstract ethical "principles" as prime movers for decision making, based on tenets of western philosophy.

Classically, four such principles are identified—autonomy, beneficence, nonmaleficence, and justice. The process of using abstract principles as prime movers betrays a cultural bias. So too does the choice of specific principles. For example, *interdependence*, valued by so many non-western cultures as a principle for decision making, might be posited as the counterweight to autonomy, rather than justice (44,45):

■ A tendency to make such abstractions "practical" through the practice of consultations on ethics, especially in the United Sates.
■ Codification of such abstractions in a plethora of laws, regulations, and policies, reflecting bureaucratic and litigious tendencies, especially in American society.
■ The dominance of autonomy as a guiding principle (46,47).
■ Suffering as a derivative, not a primary concern of ethics.

An almost unassailable insistence on surrogate decision making as the only proper vehicle for deciding a course of action for patients lacking capacity derives from the dominance of autonomy as a principle of bioethics. The anthropologic basis for the primacy of surrogate decision making and substituted judgment, in which the proxy is supposed to decide *as if* he or she were the patient, is highly questionable (48). Even a cursory examination of decision making for incapacitated patients across world cultures would find very few examples of groups espousing surrogate decision making as a guiding value. One could argue that the primacy given to surrogate decision making reflects the limited view of a very small subculture of western bioethicists (and the courts and many policy makers who seem to share this view) (7).

CULTURAL COMPETENCE

The prior section on cultural sensitivity stressed the importance of an appreciation and respect for differences among cultural groups. Such awareness is an important step in moving toward cultural competence and effectiveness but is inadequate in and of itself. Cultural competence requires the acquisition of new skills and behaviors to address differences identified through greater sensitivity and awareness. The term cultural competence, which has become broadly accepted in the literature, is somewhat unfortunate in that it implies that clinicians are either *competent* or *incompetent* in their practices, when in fact cultural competence should be understood as existing along a broad spectrum of abilities; one does not *become* culturally competent, the best one can do is to *improve* one's competency. In this section, the issue of nondisclosure will be discussed as an example of a skill used to address a bioethical issue in a culturally sensitive manner and then the broader issue of cross-cultural communication will be addressed.

EXAMPLE OF NONDISCLOSURE

The scene is well known to most clinicians (49). A relative requests that the clinician not inform a patient of some bad news such as a diagnosis of cancer or a terminal prognosis (50,51). Such a request appears to conflict with autonomy as a guiding principle and multiple healthcare policies that stress the importance of informed consent. The dilemma is doubly difficult because the request is that clinicians either not talk to or blatantly lie to the patient, inhibiting open communication that might resolve the issue.

A narrowly applied bioethics could do serious harm in such a case. Rigidly insisting that the patient has "the right to know" could both alienate family members and damage the patient by forcing undesired information. Anecdotal case reports suggest that some patients, if bluntly told of their prognosis, will in fact lose the will to live, as families sometimes warn. Orona et al. (46) suggest a possible resolution to the problem based on a twist of logic, which recognizes that autonomy can be reframed as a choice *not* to act independently but to defer to others. The trick is how to identify such a choice on the part of the patient without giving undesired information. Skill must be used in exploring the understandings of the patient and the family and then negotiating a resolution.

At the simplest level, the clinician should state and demonstrate *respect* in the face of such a request (35,52). Recalling that family-based decision making and nondisclosure are common worldwide, and recognizing that courage is often needed to make such a request in the face of a powerful healthcare system that generally disapproves of nondisclosure, may help the clinician engender respect.

Exploration of the context may begin with the person(s) making the request for nondisclosure. Why are they making this request? How do they understand the roles of participants, both in the family and among clinicians, relative to care? What do they fear might happen if the person knew? What are their hopes?

Just as cultures are not monoliths, neither are families. It is quite possible for a family to believe the patient does not want to know, when in fact he or she does. The clinician might then inquire how the family and specifically the patient have dealt with similar situations in the past. The clinician might ask questions such as, *"Do you think or know that she would agree with this? Have you discussed this approach with her? How has she dealt with similar situations in the past?"*

Exploration is not a one-way street; it is not the same as *taking* a history. Clinicians are advised to share their (often equally foreign) biomedical viewpoints as well. The clinician might explain that he or she values truth telling and could not lie if asked a question directly. Hopefully, finding the presumed common ground of wishing the best for the patient will foster some mutual understanding.

The clinician will probably want to explore the patient's understanding and concerns. The intent and desire to explore the patient's wishes regarding disclosure without coercion may be explained to family members. At a simple level, one may simply need to confirm that the patient wishes to "defer" decision making to the family, although a richer exploration is encouraged. What to do if the patient states that she wants to know the truth or to be in charge should be worked out before such an encounter. Most clinicians will want to be clear on certain ground rules such as not lying. If the patient requests to be informed, rather than simply telling the patient, the clinician may change roles and facilitate improved communication between the patient and family.

Dealing with difficult dilemmas in real life cannot be done as prescriptively as the preceding text might imply. The preceding text is presented to offer the clinician some guidance on how to explore and negotiate such a situation and to illustrate an approach to conflict resolution.

INTERCULTURAL COMMUNICATION

As the prior discussion highlights, good communication is critical to the practice of medicine in general and palliative care in particular (53,54). Generic communication skills in palliative care, such as the ability to listen or give bad news, will not be discussed here. A number of recent texts explore intercultural communication in health care (55,56). Cultural aspects of communication specific to palliative care are beginning to be addressed in the literature and will be discussed further here (52,54,57).

The most obvious cultural communication barrier is language. Communication will be largely ineffective and prone to serious misunderstanding without competent translation/interpretation. Relying on family members as translators, although sometimes unavoidable, is problematic, as messages between the clinician and patient may be filtered (58). Using family members as translators also puts both patients and family members in awkward positions. They may be forced to discuss sensitive topics inappropriate for their family roles. *Role conflict*, in which new social roles conflict with established roles, may result. For example, in using a bilingual child as a translator, as is common, there may be a role reversal between the patient/parent and the child in which the parent becomes dependent upon the child. Professional medical interpreters, where available, are generally recommended, although their use does not eliminate communication challenges (59). Skilled interpreters can do more than translate words. They may act as "cultural guides," facilitating broader understanding (60).

In considering language as a cultural barrier, the tendency is to view the other's language as the problem, something that needs only to be *translated*. More difficult is recognition of the barriers intrinsic to the language of biomedicine. The language of biomedicine emphasizes scientific, technologic, and cognitive concerns and tends to neglect more human concerns such as emotion. Patients and families often attempt to express their concerns through this biomedical language, trying to speak to us in our peculiar, foreign tongue. Consider, for example, the use of pain scores. Clinicians use pain scores (0 to 10) as a means of quantifying the severity of pain at any point in time. Scoring systems such as this work well across cultures and languages for this purpose. However, people do not innately experience pain in terms of numbers. Natural communication about pain is more likely to stress the desired urgency of response from other people. Patients become acculturated by clinicians to the use of pain

scores as a means of communicating about pain and often "co-opt" this language for their own purposes, which may differ from the clinician's original intent. A patient may, for example, report "15/10" pain as a means of stressing the perceived urgency of response, even though such a statement is absurd in terms of the formal purpose of the scale (61). Clinicians are prone to hear and respond more to the technical and medically sanctioned aspects of the communication and ignore relational and affective subtexts, such as a call of distress (62). Therefore, the specialized language of biomedicine can pose particular communication challenges for those attempting to address more human concerns, as palliative care leaders have rightfully advocated is necessary. A specific communication skill of particular value in palliative care is to learn to recognize and address subtexts of a message in terms of both affect and underlying cultural values (62).

Cross-cultural communication in palliative care is particularly difficult because key content issues, such as serious illness, difficult decisions, and dying, are very sensitive for many people. Discussion of certain topics may frankly be taboo. In many cultures and for many people, words have power. To speak of illness or dying is to increase the chance of illness or death occurring. Carrese, discussing Navajo difficulties with western bioethics, quotes a Navajo medicine man:

> In my practice, when I'm working with the patient, I am very careful of what I say, because any negative words could hurt the patient. So, with Western medicine, a doctor could be treating a patient, and he can mention death, and that is sharper than any needle (63).

Communication is far more than simple transmission of data from one source to another. Without some understanding of the context within which communication occurs, mutual understanding is impossible. A branch of anthropology has focused on intercultural communication, based largely upon the pioneering work of anthropologist Edward Hall (30,64,65). Hall recognized that cultural contexts are not inert boxes within which communication exists, but important aspects of communication itself. Hall and others have identified some cultures as being relatively high and others as relatively low in the degree to which communication is shaped by context (66). High-context cultures tend to depend more on the context of the situation than on explicit verbal expression for communication. Context refers to things such as *who* is speaking to *whom*, the setting for the discussion, relationships among participants, and the physical use of space and shared meanings. Nonverbal communication is closely linked to context (67). Context may be imbedded in verbal communication as well. The very different meanings in two expressions for dying, "kick the bucket" and "passing on," derive from shared contextual meanings (68). High-context cultures tend to stress the importance of relationships in their communication, verbal and nonverbal. In contrast, low-context cultures tend to stress direct verbal communication that focuses on non-relational, technical tasks. High- and low-context communication styles have different advantages and disadvantages; one style is not better than the other. The greater problem is the serious risk of miscommunication and misunderstanding when differing communication styles collide. From a high-context perspective, direct, task-oriented low-context communication may appear cold, uncaring, and disrespectful. From a low-context perspective, high-context communication may seem unfocused, and wasteful of time.

Biomedicine, arising from a western, predominantly northern European scientific tradition, is very low in context. Although such a low-context approach may serve well where efficiency is needed and accurate transmission of data is required across cultures and languages, it becomes problematic when dealing with the more human issues, which commonly arise in palliative care.

Just as cultures may be higher or lower in context, so too can different human activities. Very personal, taboo, or dangerous situations or activities, which rely on intimate human interaction, tend to involve high-context communication styles. Serious illness and dying are very personal and involve a complex web of relationships. Illness and the provision of care for illness entail both great risks and potential benefits. Therefore, they are intrinsically high in context. Major communication problems arise when clinicians practicing within the world of biomedicine use low-context communication strategies in dealing with patients and families experiencing illness as a high-context event. Very direct, scientifically oriented communication, emphasizing reason over emotion, as typical of western biomedicine, can easily clash with more indirect, contextual styles typical of many cultural groups. Clinicians engaging with others in encounters suggestive of a high-context framing may benefit from first cultivating awareness of this framing. Hints to a high-context encounter include strong emotional undertones to the encounter, references to relationships among individuals, and vagueness of speech in association with strong body language or ritual behavior. Requests for nondisclosure, previously discussed, typically occur in high-context encounters. Although the low-context tendency is to "get down to business" and resolve an issue quickly, perhaps by too directly emphasizing the patient's right to know, this approach often backfires when inadequate attention has been paid to relationship building, which is usually critical to the resolution of high-context problems. The low-context clinician may need to slow down and build new relationships before negotiating a specific course of action. Adjusting one's speed of communication, using spatial positioning and surroundings to convey intended meanings, and building relationships are examples of explicit high-context communication skills (62).

MODELS AND ILLNESS NARRATIVES

Serious and life-limiting illnesses pose threats to personhood (37,69,70). People tend to live optimistically, creating life stories that end with everyone living "happily ever after." Serious illnesses are radical interruptions in these stories. Sick individuals and those involved with them struggle to make some sense of this negation, to fill in the blank by reinterpreting illnesses

and eventually incorporating them into revised life stories. In revising their stories people tend to fall back on traditional patterns and understandings. These understandings of illness often differ significantly from biomedical understandings.

Kleinman introduced the term *explanatory model* as a means of exploring different understandings of illness (71,72). "Explanatory models are the notions that patients, families, *and practitioners* have about a specific illness episode" (71, p. 121) (italics mine). As this quotation points out, clinicians also have their own explanatory models for illness, most typically revolving around the concept of *disease*. Kleinman has suggested that eliciting a patient's explanatory model (and reciprocally reflecting and sharing one's one model) can further mutual understanding and help form a basis for collaborative decision-making (71, pp. 227–251). He writes that in the face of illness two questions seem to dominate—*why* did this happen and *what* should be done about it. Specific questions useful in eliciting an explanatory model are included in Table 47.3:

> I meant the explanatory models technique to be a device that would privilege meanings, especially the voices of patients and families, and that would design respect for difference. I intended it to be a *modus operandi* to get at what is at stake in suffering. I saw explanatory models as a methodology for clinical self-reflexivity, for pressing against biomedical crystallizations, for laying hold of the sources of clinical miscommunication. I wanted to encourage the use of open-ended questions, negotiation, and listening, not the usual mode of clinical interrogation (40, pp. 8–9).

The preceding passage suggests that Kleinman understood the explanatory model technique as a means to enhance both cultural sensitivity and competence in clinical encounters.

Exploring explanatory models is critical for effective communication. This is a process not only of listening to the patient but also of sharing and interpreting the clinician's explanatory model of the patient's illness. Such exploration serves as a basis for collaboration and negotiation as to goals and choices. Exploration itself is often therapeutic in its own right, as it enhances relationship building and mutual understanding.

TABLE 47.3	**Explanatory model questions**

What—do you call the problem, do you think the illness does, do you think the natural course of the illness is, do you fear?

Why—do you think this illness or problem has occurred?

How—do you think the sickness should be treated, do you want us to help you?

Who—should you turn to for help and who should be involved in decision making? What are their roles in your illness?

TABLE 47.4 Patient and physician explanatory models of pain		
Question	Patient's Model	Clinician's Model
Why do you think you are in pain?	The cancer (superficial level)	The cancer (superficial level)
	I deserve to suffer for mistakes I have made in the past (deeper level)	A combination of nociceptive and neuropathic pain, due to nerve compression (deeper, biomedical level)
What do you think the natural course of your illness and pain will be?	There is not much that can be done about it. The pain and my illness will worsen until I die. The situation is hopeless	While this is a terminal illness, this particular pain syndrome seems eminently treatable. The patient could feel much better
What do you think would happen if you took morphine?	I would just get addicted, which would make matters worse	The pain would improve. The patient would not become addicted, although certain side effects such as constipation would need to be managed
Who should be involved in dealing with your pain?	It is really up to God. Perhaps, this is also a test for me to see how I handle all this. I wonder if I am up to it	Whereas there is a physical cause for the pain, it is also clear that the patient is struggling with other issues. Perhaps others on our team could be of help

EXAMPLE OF THE USE OF THE EXPLANATORY MODEL IN PALLIATIVE CARE

Consider the following common dilemma: a patient with cancer does not want to take an opioid a clinician believes would be helpful in managing the patient's pain. Although it might be tempting to simply explain common misperceptions regarding opioid management, exploration of explanatory models might be more productive in the long run, as outlined in Table 47.4.

As this hypothetical example shows, there are areas of overlap and difference in the two explanatory models. In the process of exploring the model the clinician comes to understand that far more is involved than clearing up misunderstandings of addiction. The patient is struggling with whether or not the pain can or *should* be relieved. Statements made reflect spiritual and psychologic distress, which might best be addressed by others.

Kleinman points out that explanatory models are not complete accounts of illness in and of themselves. They are part of broader *illness narratives*, which in turn are actively created out of rich life experiences in response to a disruption in life stories—a process of *integration* in the face of the disintegrating forces of illness (69,70). This process of healing work in the face of certain unalterable realities of illness seems to get to the heart of what palliative care is all about.

CULTURAL EFFECTIVENESS

Cultural effectiveness refers to outcomes resulting from individual provider or healthcare system actions arising from efforts toward cultural sensitivity and competence. The question, quite simply, is what interventions, processes, or behaviors result in *effective* change for the better?

One systematic review of 34 educational initiatives found that most studies of courses on cultural sensitivity and competence demonstrated measurable changes in attitudes and skills over short to intermediate time ranges (73). However, this review found only three studies demonstrating improved patient satisfaction and no article addressing patient health outcomes such as access to or provision of care. None of the reviewed studies was specific to palliative care. Obviously, more research is needed.

Interventions that might be effective could work at either interpersonal or system levels. As the referenced review demonstrates, courses addressing knowledge, attitudes, and skills related to cultural competence can clearly affect the clinician. Despite a lack of studies, it seems highly probable that such courses also improve patient and family satisfaction, to the extent they result in more sensitive and effective communication. Where particular tensions exist between clinicians and particular patient populations, as where most providers

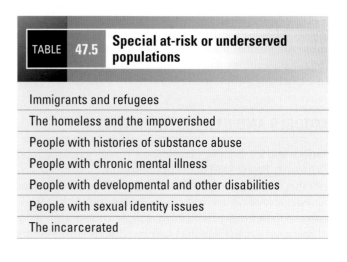

TABLE 47.5 Special at-risk or underserved populations
Immigrants and refugees
The homeless and the impoverished
People with histories of substance abuse
People with chronic mental illness
People with developmental and other disabilities
People with sexual identity issues
The incarcerated

TABLE 47.6	Suggestions for programmatic changes to improve cultural effectiveness

Inclusion of cultural sensitivity and competency training as a staff requirement

Staff recruitment, reflecting community diversity

Community needs assessment

Identify and make accessible resources useful in meeting the needs of target populations including

    Internet resources

    Local community agencies and support groups

    Library of relevant books, journals, educational material

    Establishment of policies and procedures addressing translation needs

    Inclusion of a cultural assessment as part of routine patient and family assessment

Outreach efforts to disadvantaged groups with palliative care needs

    Partnerships and educational efforts with community organizations

    Brochures and educational material linguistically and culturally appropriate for target populations

are from a different ethnic or religious group than are most patients, targeted educational interventions addressing such tensions would seem particularly important.

The bigger challenge seems to be to identify interventions that would likely improve access to care and clinical outcomes for underserved groups. This is a major challenge for palliative, supportive, and hospice care programs, as a number of studies have demonstrated underutilization and barriers to care for minority groups and special populations (28,74–78). A partial list of at-risk populations that would likely benefit from special attention is presented in Table 47.5. It is not hard to imagine that these groups, among others, might have very special palliative needs that currently are poorly addressed within existing systems of care. Hospice and palliative care organizations are rightly concerned that the care they provide too often is for those in privileged classes.

Although a variety of macroscopic social forces, related to patient demographics and healthcare system factors, undoubtedly serve as barriers to good palliative and supportive care, these should not prohibit system changes at a local level. Table 47.6 provides a partial list of interventions that local programs might consider. Of note, formal training becomes a system change, when it is required and monitored. A community needs assessment might start with a review of patients historically served by the program and then a study of cultural groups in the program's catchment area to identify underserved populations. Outreach to and collaborative problem solving with leaders of underserved populations might then improve access and hopefully outcomes for patients.

SUMMARY

Culture is all around us and yet for the most part, we are blind to it. We may recognize culture in others, very different from ourselves; it is far more difficult to be aware of how our own culture invisibly influences our own thoughts, actions, and organizations. It is the very ubiquitous nature of culture that makes it so difficult to move from good intentions to action. The temptation is to rest on our intentions or to narrowly circumscribe "cultural competence" with isolated educational courses. As has been demonstrated admirably elsewhere in the palliative care movement, the most effective changes are likely to result from systemic changes that institute new patterns of care.

ACKNOWLEDGMENTS

This work was supported by the Department of Veterans Affairs, VA Palo Alto Health Care System.

REFERENCES

1. Crawley LM, Marshall PA, Lo B, et al. Strategies for culturally effective end-of-life care. *Ann Intern Med.* 2002;136(9):673-679.
2. Betancourt JR, Green AR, Carrillo JE, et al. Defining cultural competence: a practical framework for addressing racial/ethnic disparities in health and health care. *Public Health Rep.* 2003;118(4):293-302.
3. Helman C. *Culture Health and Illness.* 3rd ed. London: Butterworth-Heineman; 1994.
4. Chan LS, Macdonald ME, Cohen SR. Moving culture beyond ethnicity: examining dying in hospital through a cultural lens. *J Palliat Care.* 2009;25(2):117-124.
5. National Consensus Project for Quality Palliative Care. *Clinical Practice Guidelines for Quality Palliative Care.* 2nd ed. Pittsburgh, PA: National Consensus Project for Quality Palliative Care; 2009.
6. Koenig BA. Cultural diversity in decision making about care at the end of life. In: Field M, Cassel C, eds. *Approaching Death: Improving Care at the End of Life* (Institute of Medicine). Washington, DC: National Academy Press; 1997:363-382.
7. Hallenbeck J, Goldstein MK. Decisions at the end of life: cultural considerations beyond medical ethics. *Generations.* 1999;23(1):24-29.

8. Barker JC. Cultural diversity—changing the context of medical practice. *West J Med.* 1992;157(3):248-254.

9. Grimes R. *Deeply into the Bone—Reinventing Rites of Passage.* Berkeley, CA: University of California Press; 2000.

10. Hallenbeck J. Palliative care in the final days of life—"they were expecting it at any time." *JAMA.* 2005;293(18):2265-2271.

11. Braun K, Pietsch J, Blanchette P. *Cultural Issues in End-of-Life Decision Making.* Thousand Oaks, CA: Sage; 2000.

12. Connor SR, Elwert F, Spence C, Christakis NA. Racial disparity in hospice use in the United States in 2002. *Palliat Med.* 2008;22(3):205-213.

13. Koffman J, Morgan M, Edmonds P, et al. Cultural meanings of pain: a qualitative study of Black Caribbean and White British patients with advanced cancer. *Palliat Med.* 2008;22(4):350-359.

14. Barnato AE, Chang CC, Saynina O, Garber AM. Influence of race on inpatient treatment intensity at the end of life. *J Gen Intern Med.* 2007;22(3):338-345.

15. Rabow MW, Dibble SL. Ethnic differences in pain among outpatients with terminal and end-stage chronic illness. *Pain Med.* 2005;6(3):235-241.

16. Crawley LM. Racial, cultural, and ethnic factors influencing end-of-life care. *J Palliat Med.* 2005;8(suppl 1):S58-S69.

17. Barnato AE, Enguídanos S, Siciliano M, Coulourides-Kogan A. Racial and ethnic differences in preferences for end-of-life treatment. *J Gen Intern Med.* 2009;24(6):695-701.

18. Mancuso L. Providing culturally sensitive palliative care. *Nursing.* 2009;39(5):50-53.

19. Field A, Maher P, Webb D. Cross cultural research in palliative care. *Soc Work Health Care.* 2002;35(1-2):523-543.

20. Gatrad AR, Brown E, Notta H, Sheikh A. Palliative care needs of minorities. *BMJ.* 2003;327(7408):176-177.

21. Periyakoil VS, Noda AM, Kraemer HC. Assessment of factors influencing preservation of dignity at life's end: creation and the cross-cultural validation of the preservation of dignity card-sort tool. *J Palliat Med.* 13(5):495-500.

22. Lipson J, Minarik P, Dibble S. *Culture and Nursing Care: A Pocket Guide.* San Francisco, CA: UCSF Nursing Press; 1996.

23. Gunaratnam Y. Culture is not enough: a critique of multiculturalism in palliative care. In: Small N, ed. *Death, Gender and Ethnicity.* London: Routledge; 1997:166-186.

24. Good B. *Medicine, Rationality, and Experience: An Anthropological Perspective.* New York, NY: Cambridge University Press; 1994.

25. Pritchard R, Fisher ES, Teno J, et al. Influence of patient preferences and local health system characteristics on the place of death. *J Am Geriatr Soc.* 1998;46(10):1242-1250.

26. Eleazer G, Horunung C, Egbert C, et al. The relationship between ethnicity and advance directives in a frail older population. *J Am Geriatr Soc.* 1996;44(8):938-943.

27. Barnato AE, Berhane Z, Weissfeld LA, et al. Racial variation in end-of-life intensive care use: a race or hospital effect? *Health Serv Res.* 2006;41(6):2219-2237.

28. Oliviere D, Monroe B. *Death, Dying, and Social Differences.* New York, NY: Oxford University Press; 2004.

29. Field D, Hockey J, Small N, eds. *Death, Gender and Ethnicity.* New York, NY: Routledge; 1997.

30. Hall E. *The Silent Language.* New York, NY: Anchor; 1990.

31. Lum C, Korenman S. Cultural-sensitivity training in U.S. medical schools. *Acad Med.* 1994;69:239-241.

32. Loudon RF, Anderson PM, Gills PS, Greenfield SM. Educating medical students for work in culturally diverse societies. *JAMA.* 1999;282(9):875-880.

33. Wells KB, Benson MC, Hoff P. Teaching cultural aspects of medicine. *J Med Educ.* 1985;60(6):493-495.

34. Carrillo JE, Green AR, Betancourt JR. Cross-cultural primary care: a patient-based approach. *Ann Intern Med.* 1999;130(10):829-834.

35. Hallenbeck J. Cross-cultural issues in end-of-life care. In: Weissman D, Ambuel B, Hallenbeck J, eds. *Improving End-of-Life Care: A Resource Guide for Physician Education.* Madison, WI: Medical College of Wisconsin; 2000:142-147.

36. Fabrega H. *Evolution of Sickness and Healing.* Berkeley, CA: University of California Press; 1997.

37. Hahn R. *Sickness and Healing—An Anthropological Perspective.* New London: Yale University Press; 1995.

38. Cassell E. *The Nature of Suffering and the Goals of Medicine.* New York, NY: Oxford University Press; 1991:xvi, 254.

39. Byock IR. The nature of suffering and the nature of opportunity at the end of life. *Clin Geriatr Med.* 1996;12(2):237-252.

40. Kleinman A. *Writing in the Margin: Discourse Between Anthropology and Medicine.* Berkeley, CA: University of California Press; 1995.

41. Brady E, ed. *Healing Logics—Culture and Medicine in Modern Health Belief Systems.* Logan: Utah State University Press; 2001.

42. Green AR, Betancourt JR, Carrillo JE. Integrating social factors into cross-cultural medical education. *Acad Med.* 2002;77(3):193-197.

43. Marshall PA, Koenig B. Bioethics in anthropology: perspectives on culture, medicine and morality. In: Sargent C, Johnson T, eds. *Handbook of Medical Anthropology—Contemporary Theory and Method.* Westport, CT: Greenwood; 1996:349-373.

44. Bowman K. Communication, negotiation, and mediation: dealing with conflict in end-of-life decisions. *J Palliat Care.* 2000;16(suppl):S17-S23.

45. Chan HM. Sharing death and dying: advance directives, autonomy and the family. *Bioethics.* 2004;18(2):87-103.

46. Orona C, Koenig B, Davis A. Cultural aspects of nondisclosure. *Camb Q Healthc Ethics.* 1994;3:338-346.

47. Frank G, Blackhall LJ, Michel V, et al. A discourse of relationships in bioethics: patient autonomy and end-of-life decision making among elderly Korean Americans. *Med Anthropol Q.* 1998;12(4):403-423.

48. High D. Families' roles in advance directives. *Hastings Cent Rep.* 1994;24(suppl):S16-S18.

49. Hallenbeck J, Arnold R. A request for nondisclosure: don't tell mother. *J Clin Oncol.* 2007;25(31):5030-5034.

50. Charlton R. The dilemma of truth disclosure: Stoke-on-Trent, England. *Am J Hosp Palliat Care.* 1997;14(4):166-168.

51. Muller J. Ethical dilemmas in cross-cultural context. *West J Med.* 1992;1992(157):323-327.

52. Hallenbeck JL. Intercultural differences and communication at the end of life. *Prim Care.* 2001;28(2):401-413.

53. von Gunten CF, Ferris F, Emanuel L. Ensuring competency in end-of-life care. *JAMA.* 2000;284(23):3051-3057.

54. Kissane D, Bultz BD, Butow PN, et al., eds. *Handbook of Communication in Oncology and Palliative Care.* Oxford: Oxford University Press; 2010.

55. Krept G, Kunimoto E. *Effective Communication in Multicultural Health Care Settings.* Thousand Oaks, CA: Sage; 1994.

56. Luckman J. *Transcultural Communication in Health Care.* Albany, NY: Delmar; 2000.

57. Kogan S, Blanchette P, Masaki K. Talking to patients and death and dying: improving communication across cultures. In: Braun K, Pietsch J, Blanchette P, eds. *Cultural Issues in End-of-Life Decision Making.* Thousand Oaks, CA: Sage; 2000:305-325.

58. Chan A, Woodruff RK. Comparison of palliative care needs of English- and non-English-speaking patients. *J Palliat Care.* 1999;15(1):26-30.

59. Rivadeneyra R, Elderkin-Thompson V, Silver RC, et al. Patient centeredness in medical encounters requiring an interpreter. *Am J Med.* 2000;108(6):470-474.

60. Yeo G. Ethical considerations in Asian and Pacific island elders. *Clin Geriatr Med.* 1995;11:139-152.

61. Hallenbeck J. Pain and intercultural communication. In: Moore RJ, ed. *Handbook of Pain and Palliative Care.* New York, NY: Springer; 2011.

62. Hallenbeck J, Periyakoil VS. Intercultural communication in palliative care. In: Kissane D, Bulz B, Butow P, et al., eds. *Handbook of Communication in Oncology and Palliative Care.* Oxford: Oxford University Press; 2010:301-309.

63. Carrese J, Rhodes L. Western bioethics on the Navajo reservation. *JAMA.* 1995;274:826-829.

64. Hall E. *Beyond Culture.* Garden City, NY: Anchor Press; 1976.

65. Hall E. *The Dance of Life.* New York, NY: Anchor Press; 1983.

66. Porter R, Samovar L. An introduction to intercultural communication. In: Porter R, Samovar L, eds. *Intercultural Communication.* Wadsworth: Belmont; 1997:5-26.

67. Martin J, Nakyama T. *Experiencing Intercultural Communication.* Mountain View, CA: Mayfield Publishing; 2001.

68. Lee W. That's Greek to me: between a rock and a hard place in intercultural encounters. In: Samovar L, Porter R, eds. *Intercultural Communication.* Belmont, CA: Wadsworth; 1997:213-216.

69. Frank A. *The Wounded Storyteller—Body, Illness, and Ethics.* Chicago: University of Chicago Press; 1995.

70. Becker G. *Disrupted Lives—How People Create Meaning in a Chaotic World.* Berkeley, CA: University of California Press; 1999.

71. Kleinman A. *The Illness Narratives—Suffering Healing and the Human Condition.* New York, NY: Basic Books; 1988.

72. Hallenbeck J. The explanatory model #26. *J Palliat Med.* 2003;6(6):931.

73. Beach MC, Price EG, Gary TL, et al. Cultural competence: a systematic review of health care provider educational interventions. *Med Care.* 2005;43(4):356-373.

74. Jennings B, Ryndes T, D'Onofrio C, Baily MA. Access to hospice care. Expanding boundaries, overcoming barriers. *Hastings Cent Rep.* 2003;2:(suppl):S3-7, S9-13, S15-21 passim.

75. Reese DJ, Melton E, Ciaravino K. Programmatic barriers to providing culturally competent end-of-life care. *Am J Hosp Palliat Care.* 2004;21(5):357-364.

76. Kessler D, Peters TJ, Lee L, et al. Social class and access to specialist palliative care services. *Palliat Med.* 2005; 19(2): 105-110.

77. Greiner KA, Perera S, Ahluwalia JS. Hospice usage by minorities in the last year of life: results from the National Mortality Followback Survey. *J Am Geriatr Soc.* 2003;51(7): 970-978.

78. Moller D. *Dancing with Broken Bones-Portraits of Death and Dying Among Inner-City Poor.* New York, NY: Oxford University Press; 2004.

CHAPTER 48

Communication during Transitions of Care

James A. Tulsky ■ Robert M. Arnold

Palliative care aims to improve quality of life for patients and families living with serious illness. Good communication is indispensable to uncovering patient and family needs and individually negotiating the goals of care. Everyone defines a good death differently (1), and whether a patient's suffering is caused by pain, nausea, unwanted medical intervention, or spiritual crisis, the common pathway to treatment is through a provider who is able to elicit these concerns and is equipped to help the patient and family address them.

Good communication brings real and tangible benefits. In patients with cancer, the number and severity of unresolved concerns has been shown to predict high levels of emotional distress and future anxiety and depression (2,3). Conversely, considerable evidence suggests that improved physician–patient communication correlates with improved health outcomes, patient satisfaction, and emotional wellbeing (4–6). For example, primary care patients exhibit decreased anxiety and are more satisfied with their physicians if they discuss advance care planning (7). And, trust in physicians may be increased when physicians respond empathically to patient distress (8). Communication itself appears to be therapeutic, as simply telling one's story may improve objective health outcomes (9). Finally, families who are better prepared for their loved one's deaths may experience less difficult bereavement.

This chapter is designed to:

1. Review recent literature concerning health-care provider communication;
2. Survey basic communication issues relevant to palliative care, particularly the role of affect in communication; and
3. Give the reader practical advice regarding some of the common topics that arise when caring for patients with life-limiting illness—giving bad news, discussing advance care planning, introducing palliative care, and talking about prognostic issues.

HEALTH-CARE PROVIDERS DO NOT COMMUNICATE WELL

Unfortunately, the general quality of communication between health care providers and patients with life-limiting disease is suboptimal. Studies show that the discussion of bad news frequently does not meet patient needs or falls short of expert recommendations (10–12). Both physicians and nurses tend to underestimate and not elicit cancer patients' concerns (13) and commonly do not attend to patients'

affect or even recognize their emotional cues (14,15). When patients express negative emotion, physicians respond with empathic language only about 25% of the time (15,16). Rather than using facilitative communication techniques, such as open-ended questions or empathic responses when inquiring about psychosocial issues, they often block discussion of these issues by changing the subject or not attending to patients' emotional states (17). Even in a hospice setting, one study revealed that only 40% of patient concerns were elicited (18). As a result, patients with cancer tend to disclose fewer than 50% of their concerns (17,18), which leads further to physicians' inaccurate assessments of patient distress (19). Two large studies of audio-recorded oncology visits with terminally ill patients found that physicians dedicated only a small percentage of their time to health-related, quality-of-life issues, including psychosocial concerns, frequently missed opportunities to address issues that seemed to be most important to patients, and did not often check for patient's understanding (20,21). Finally, physicians rarely talk with seriously ill patients about their goals, values, or even treatment decisions (22–24). A significant gap exists between the idealized model of provider–patient communication at the end of life and the reality of practice.

WHAT CAUSES POOR COMMUNICATION?

Why is the "state-of-the-art" so poor? First, health-care providers are not selected for their communication skills. Expertise in cognitive areas is not always positively correlated with empathy or an interest in understanding another person's experience. Medical education emphasizes cognitive teaching techniques and cognitive material rather than the psychosocial and spiritual aspects of care. Second, until recently there has been little training regarding communication skills in general, not to mention communication about these difficult topics. For example, in a survey of over 3,200 oncologists, few had any formal training in end-of-life care or communication skills. Oncology programs are not alone in devoting little attention to this subject. At both the medical school and residency level, inadequate attention is given to care of the dying (25). Among graduating students at two medical schools, only 48% said they had adequate role models for how to discuss end-of-life issues. At another school, 41% of medical students on a medicine rotation and 73% on a surgery rotation had never observed a staff physician talk with a dying patient. Happily, educational interventions have improved this situation; over 60% of medical students now report "adequate" training on end-of-life care. Unfortunately, these interventions continue to focus on cognitive aspects of care. Students report that death is still viewed as a loss not to be discussed and that they are discouraged from showing their emotions (26,27). Finally, physicians have difficulty inquiring directly about the emotional status of dying patients because of their feelings about the patient or their own mortality. We will particularly focus on this issue.

Considerable evidence suggests that physicians' personal feelings toward their patients are important to the doctor–patient relationship (28), and many have suggested that physicians' emotional responses to their dying patients may interfere with their care (29). Physicians dealing with dying patients are not objective observers. They are active participants whose beliefs and feelings influence the interaction. For example, a study of surrogate decision making found that physicians' predictions of their patients' wishes regarding life-sustaining treatment were closer to their own choices than to the choices expressed by their patients (30).

Caring for the dying may elicit significant stress in physicians and a variety of reactions, including guilt ("If only I'd convinced him to get that screening colonoscopy."), impotence ("There's nothing I can do for her."), failure ("I messed up. I'm a bad doctor."), loss ("I'm really going to miss this person."), resentment ("This patient is going to keep me in the hospital all night."), and fear ("I know they're going to sue me.") (31). According to Spikes and Holland (29), many physicians have unconscious feelings of omnipotence and troublesome responses stem from a physician's need to preserve his or her image as a "powerful healer" who can master any situation. Feeling that he or she has failed the dying patient, a physician may respond by acting defensively, wishing that the patient would die (to avoid dealing with the patient), or by treating too aggressively (to ensure that "everything has been done to save the patient").

Empathizing with a dying patient often evokes anxiety about a physician's own mortality. Physicians respond by withdrawing from terminally ill patients, avoiding threatening topics (17,32), employing blocking behaviors that distance them from addressing affective concerns of patients (33), or falsely reassuring them that "everything is OK" (29).

Empirical data support these claims about physicians' anxieties regarding death. Physicians score higher on death anxiety scales than other professional groups (34). They also find caring for terminally ill patients stressful. For example, in a survey of 598 oncologists, 56% reported being burned out and 53% attributed these feelings to continuous exposure to fatal illness (35). When caring for dying patients, physicians often report sadness, helplessness, failure, disappointment, and loneliness (36). These feelings, particularly if unrecognized, may affect patient care. Residents who are more burned out endorse more negative attitudes and behaviors related to patient care (37). Conversely, residents who report better personal well-being score higher on empathy scales (38). A study of 25 pediatric residents explored the relationship between their orientation toward death and their response to a clinical vignette. Residents with a high death threat and anxiety scores were more likely to adopt avoidance and denial strategies for dealing with the vignette (39).

Although these issues are profound, awareness of their own emotional responses to caring for dying patients can help physicians begin to focus more objectively on the effect of their behavior on the patient.

BASIC COMMUNICATION SKILLS

Talking to dying patients is just like, and completely unlike, all other communication with patients (40). Whether one is explaining the implications of hypertension, or talking about impending death, basic principles of good communication are useful. The primary difference between these communication tasks is the meaning of the conversation to the patient and the provider, and the attendant level of emotional significance. When the situation is more likely to make the patient (or physician) feel vulnerable, sad, or inadequate, one should focus extra attention on the task. In this section, we will address basic communication skills that are universal to all encounters.

A little effort spent on advance preparation can have a tremendous impact on the quality of the encounter. Whenever possible, important medical information, particularly bad or sad news, should be delivered during a scheduled meeting. This allows patients to prepare themselves for the type of information they will hear and to make sure that appropriate family members or friends are present. It also allows the physician to allocate the necessary time to the encounter and to come prepared with basic medical information and anticipating the most likely questions regarding treatment options, prognosis, and resources for support and guidance.

Communication best occurs face to face. Telephones accentuate physical communication difficulties and there is no opportunity to employ the benefits of nonverbal communication. Given that over 50% of communication is nonverbal, both parties operate at a disadvantage if they cannot see each other. The physician should sit at eye level and within reach of the patient. If possible, one's pager or cellular phone should be turned off, or at least put on a quiet mode, and one should avoid interruptions. Finally, as many physicians are now compelled to interact with electronic medical record systems during the office visit, they must be careful that accessing and inputting data do not compromise direct human interaction.

Increasingly, we encounter non-English-speaking patients. One must absolutely employ the assistance of an interpreter in such settings. However, it is equally important to avoid using family members as interpreters. Not only does this run the risk of faulty translation or reinterpretation of the physician's statements, it also places family members into the uncomfortable position of being the physician's and patient's spokesperson (41). The common practice of using bilingual young children as translators is particularly problematic. Most hospitals and health-care facilities in regions with high numbers of immigrants employ professional translators or maintain lists of language skills among facility staff members.

Regarding the dialogue itself, considerable data exist from the medical and psychological literature to support certain general techniques that allow more accurate assessment of anxiety and depression and increased disclosure of concerns (14,42). One should maintain good eye contact, ask open-ended rather than closed-ended questions, focus on the patient's concerns as well as the agenda for the visit, respond to the patient's affect, ask about the patient's life outside of medicine, attend to psychosocial concerns, and ensure that nonverbal behavior signifies attentiveness (Table 48.1). In contrast, disclosure of concerns is inhibited by closed-ended or leading questions, focusing on physical aspects of illness, and offering of advice and premature reassurance (14).

One core precept is not to assume that one knows what is on the patient's agenda. For example, while many patients will want to discuss end-of-life issues, approximately 25% will not. This may have to do with cultural particularities or with how individuals cope with illness. Physicians are not very good at predicting which patients want more and which patients want less information. Instead of assuming one should ask. For example, on a first visit one could say, "I want to touch base with you about how you want me to handle information we get about your illness. Some patients want to know everything that is going on with their illness, the good and the bad. Other people do not want as much information and want me to speak more generally. And some would really prefer I do not discuss bad news with them but want me to discuss these issues with their family. Which kind of person do you think you are?"

Another important precept of communication is to "ask before telling." Patients often carry misperceptions or incomplete information obtained from the popular media, folklore, or friends and family. It is easier to deal with this information if it is discussed directly. Thus, it is usually helpful to ask patients about their understanding of their illness

before educating them. Furthermore, one study of intensive care unit (ICU) family conferences observed that allowing families more opportunity to speak may improve family satisfaction (43).

WHAT IS EFFECTIVE COMMUNICATION AT THE END OF LIFE?

According to seriously ill patients, family members, and health-care providers, goals for communication at the end of life include talking with patients in an honest and straightforward way, being willing to talk about dying, giving bad news in a sensitive way, listening to patients, encouraging questions from patients, and being responsive to patients' readiness to talk about death (44). Patients want physicians to achieve a balance between being honest and straightforward and not being discouraging. For some this requires leaving open the possibility that unexpected "miracles" might happen, discussing outcomes other than a cure that can offer patients hope and meaning, and helping patients prepare for the losses they may experience. Patients cope better when physicians emphasize what can be done, explore realistic goals, and discuss day-to-day living (45). Although patients must receive adequate information to make informed choices, they wish to receive that information in an emotionally supportive way (46). Patients want to discuss emotional concerns but are frequently unwilling to bring them up spontaneously and may need to be prompted (47).

This may sound impossible. How can one be honest and be hopeful? How can one ensure informed consent and let patients decide they do not want to hear all the information? While many models have been proposed (48–52) they have in common several principles:

1. Given that patients vary greatly in their desire for information and participation in decision making, one should assess patients' preferences for communication as part of the medical encounter (53,54). One cannot presume to "intuit" patient's wants and needs, therefore one should ask.
2. One should give information non-technically and in brief, understandable chunks. This allows the physician to constantly reassess the patient's verbal or nonverbal reaction to the information, as well as their desire for more information.
3. Patients and their family members may have different goals and needs for information; thus, one needs to assess each person in a group conversation.
4. While doctors focus on medical treatments and dying, patients focus on function and relationships. Therefore, treatments should be discussed within the framework of the patient's goals rather than in abstraction.
5. Attention to the affective component of the conversation is as important as the cognitive aspects. Thus, all models stress the critical role of empathy in communication. In the rest of this chapter, we will focus on the role of emotions in such discussions.

TABLE 48.1	**General communication skills to enhance disclosure of concerns**

Maintain good eye contact

Ask open-ended rather than closed-ended questions

Focus on the patient's concerns as well as the agenda for the visit

Observe and respond to the patient's affect

Attend to psychosocial concerns

Ask about the patient's life outside of medicine

Ensure that nonverbal behavior signifies attentiveness

THE ROLE OF AFFECT

Most difficulties in communication at the end of life are the result of inattention to affect. *Affect* refers to the feelings and emotions associated with the content of the conversation. Feelings such as anger, guilt, frustration, sadness, and fear modify our ability to hear, to communicate, and to make decisions. For example, after hearing bad news, most patients are so overwhelmed emotionally that they are unable to comprehend very much about the details of the illness or a treatment plan. Some studies have shown that emotion affects processing; people who are in negative moods may pay more attention to how messages are given than to the content of the messages (55). Thus, when patients are experiencing high levels of negative affect and caregivers do not ameliorate this affect, patients may be less likely to receive the health-care providers' messages. Unfortunately, conversations between doctors and patients often transpire only in the cognitive realm; emotion is frequently not acknowledged or handled directly and physicians miss opportunities to do so (56).

Dealing with Physician's Emotions

Physicians, as well as patients, experience many emotions as they care for people approaching the end of life. In addition to its effect on their own communication, physician affect plays an important role in patients' reactions to medical information. In one study, women were randomly assigned to view of video of an oncologist presenting mammogram results, and who was portrayed as either worried or not worried. Those watching the "worried" physician received less information, experienced higher anxiety levels, and perceived the situation as more severe compared with those watching the "nonworried" physician (57).

For physicians, the first step toward managing feelings of loss, helplessness, or anxiety is to acknowledge that they exist and to recognize that they are normal. When experiencing a strong emotion while interacting with a patient, one should ask oneself, "Where is this coming from?" Although it may be a result of what the physician brings to the encounter (e.g., one's own sense of mortality or how it makes one think of one's grandmother who died), it may also be a clue into what the patient is feeling. Thus, many doctors report feeling anxious when talking with a patient who has an anxiety disorder, or feeling overly sad when talking with a depressed patient. If the physician gets a sense that he or she is reflecting the patient's emotion, it may help to ask the patient about this (e.g., "I wonder if you're feeling sad?").

If the emotion is a result of the physician's reaction to the encounter, the next step is to discuss this with colleagues or confidants. In most cases, however, patients do not benefit from hearing such thoughts. When considering sharing such feelings with a patient, a good rule of thumb is to ask oneself, "Am I doing this for me or for the patient?" If the answer is truly the latter, then it may be appropriate to share.

Dealing with Patient's Emotions

One barrier to engaging patient affect is the fear of being unable to manage the emotional response. This section will describe an approach to handling emotions that is also likely to further elicit the sorts of patient concerns described earlier.

The primary goal when responding to emotions is to convey a sense of empathy. Empathy is the sense that "I could be you" and is what patients are usually feeling when they comment about a physician who really cared for them (58). Empathy can be expressed either verbally or nonverbally. The acronym SOLER is used to identify the following non-verbal behaviors that have been shown to reflect empathy:

1. Facing the patient **S**quarely indicates involvement and interest in the patient's story.
2. Adopting an **O**pen body position is a sign that you are open to the patient.
3. **L**eaning toward the patient reflects intimacy and flexibility to the patient's position.
4. **E**ye contact reflects attention in North American cultures, although it is impolite in other cultures.
5. One should maintain a **R**elaxed and natural body posture (59).

Robert Smith has created a useful mnemonic to recall four basic techniques to use when confronted by patient emotions, NURS (*N*ame, *U*nderstand, *R*espect, and *S*upport) (60). This discussion adds a final "E" for *E*xplore (Table 48.2). Naming the emotion serves to acknowledge the feeling and to demonstrate that it is a legitimate area for discussion. Statements such as, "That seems sad for you," can serve this purpose well, although one needs to be careful not to inappropriately label the patient. Therefore, naming is often best done in a quizzical fashion that does not presuppose the emotion (e.g., "Many people would feel angry if that happened to them. I wonder if you ever feel that way?").

Expressing a sense of understanding normalizes the patient's emotion and conveys empathy. However, expressing understanding must be done cautiously to prevent a response such as, "How can you possibly understand what I'm going through? Have you ever had a stroke?" A typical statement might be, "Although I've never shared your

TABLE 48.2	*Nurse*ing an emotion
Name the emotion	
Understand the emotion	
Respect or praise the patient	
Support the patient	
Explore what underlies the emotion	

Fischer GS, Tulsky JA, Arnold RM. Communicating a poor prognosis. In: Portenoy RK, Bruera E, eds. *Topics in Palliative Care*. Vol 4. New York, NY: Oxford University Press; 2000.

experience, I do understand that this has been a really hard time for you."

Respect reminds us to praise patients and families for what they are doing and how they are managing with a difficult situation. Offering respect defuses defensiveness and makes people feel good about themselves and more capable of handling the future. A useful statement might be, "I am so impressed with how you've continued to provide excellent care for your mother as her dementia has progressed" (61).

Support is essential to helping people in distress not to feel alone. Simple statements such as, "I will be there with you throughout this illness," can be tremendously comforting. Health-care providers ought not to feel the entire support burden on their shoulders—support offered can include other members of a team. For example, "We will send a nurse to your home to check in on you in a couple of days and if you'd like, I could ask the chaplain to visit you."

Finally, patients will frequently make statements that deserve further exploration. For example, a patient may say, "After you gave me the results of the test, I thought that this is going to be it." A simple response such as, "Tell me more," may help reveal the patient's fears and concerns about cancer that will be helpful in planning future treatment.

Hope in the Context of Palliative Care

Physicians struggle to promote hope in the patient with advanced disease and to support a positive outlook, fearing that discussing death may decrease the patient's hopefulness (44,62,63). As a result, they frequently convey prognosis with an optimistic bias or do not give this information at all. This is relevant to treatment choices; patients with more optimistic assessments of their own prognosis are more likely to choose aggressive therapies at the end of life (64). In turn, fearing the loss of hope, patients frequently cope by expressing denial and may be unwilling to hear what is said.

It is not clear if health-care providers can either steal or instill hope. However, they can provide an empathic, reflective presence that will help patients draw strength from their existing resources. Physicians should recognize that it is not their job to "correct" the patient's hope for a miracle. The key question is whether the hope is interfering with appropriate planning and behavior. A patient who has completed his will and said his good-byes but is still hoping for a miracle is different from a patient who is making long-term investments and does not plan for custody of a minor child despite a 3-month prognosis.

Physicians can respond in several ways (in addition to demonstrations of empathy discussed earlier). Acknowledging the hope may allow the physician and the patient to "hope for the best but prepare for the worst." They can also recognize that people hope for many different things and leave space for patients to hope for outcomes and futures that are more likely to occur. One might say, "I know you are hoping that your disease will be cured. Are there other things that you want to focus on?" Or, "If we cannot make that happen, what other shorter term goals might we focus

on?" Finally, one can ask about what tasks are left undone as a way to get patients to begin to think in a shorter time course.

Managing Conflict

Conflict occurs frequently in discussions about the end-of-life care. In one study of 102 consecutive cases of decisions to limit life-sustaining care in ICUs at an academic medical center, conflict of some type was described in 78% of cases and clinician–family conflict occurred nearly half the time (65). Although often avoided by clinicians and patients, conflict managed well can be productive (66). However, when clinicians engage in behaviors such as denying the conflict, assuming they know the whole story or the other party's intentions, repeatedly trying to convince the other party and ignoring their own strong emotions, they are likely to exacerbate the problem. Useful tools to address conflict include many of the communication techniques already described: active listening, empathizing, reframing, explaining, and self-disclosure. Back and Arnold (66) have described a stepwise approach to addressing conflicts that recognizes the emotional content of these situations and focuses on interests, rather than positions. They encourage clinicians to:

1. Notice the conflict.
2. Prepare themselves by getting into a ready state of mind, examine what has happened and their feelings and decide on the purpose of working through the conflict.
3. Find a nonjudgmental starting point.
4. Reframe emotionally charged issues.
5. Respond empathically.
6. Look for options that meet the needs of both parties.
7. Get help if no satisfactory agreement can be reached.

Such an approach will likely achieve a resolution in most cases and improve relationships with patients, family members, and other clinicians.

PRACTICAL SUGGESTIONS FOR SPECIFIC SITUATIONS

Communicating Bad News

Communicating bad news draws upon the skills discussed previously (see the Section What is Effective Communication at the End of Life?). Many protocols exist for the delivery of bad news; however, the behaviors tend to be grouped into several key domains: preparation, content of message, dealing with patient responses, and ending the encounter (Table 48.3) (12). The primary elements of preparation have been addressed above (see the Section Basic Communication Skills).

Content of Message

Knowledge of what the patient already knows or believes is extremely valuable to have, before revealing bad news to a patient. This allows the physician to begin the explanation

| TABLE 48.3 | Key elements of delivering bad news |

Preparation

Find out what patient knows and believes

Find out what patient wants to know

Suggest a supportive person accompany the patient

Learn about the patient's condition

Arrange the encounter in a private place with enough time

Content

Get to the point quickly

Fire "warning shot" (e.g., "I have bad news.")

State the news clearly, simply, and sensitively

Avoid false reassurance

Make truthful, hopeful statements

Provide information in small chunks

Handle patient's reactions

Inquire about meaning of the condition for the patient

NURSE expressed emotions

Assure continued support

Wrap-up

Set up a meeting within next few days

Offer to talk to relatives/friends

Suggest that patients write down questions

Provide a way to be reached in emergencies

Assess tendency to commit suicide

Fischer GS, Tulsky JA, Arnold RM. Communicating a poor prognosis. In: Portenoy RK, Bruera E, eds. *Topics in Palliative Care.* Vol 4. New York, NY: Oxford University Press; 2000.

from the patient's perspective, aligning oneself with the patient and making communication more efficient and effective. The time that a test is ordered is a good time to assess this. One might ask, "Is there anything that you are particularly concerned about?" If the patient mentions a serious illness that might be present, the physician can follow up by asking about the patient's specific fears and concerns.

When prepared to deliver the content of the message, the physician should begin by firing a brief "warning shot," and then stating the news in clear and direct terms. One should avoid spending any time "beating around the bush" before sharing the news, as this only serves to heighten anxiety. Patients also prefer that physicians merely deliver the news objectively rather than pre-judging it as "bad" (67). After this brief exchange, the physician should remain silent and allow the patient an opportunity for the news to sink in. One

can strike an empathic posture, maintain comfortable eye contact, and perhaps use a nonverbal gesture such as reaching out and touching the patient's hand. However, silence is imperative to allow the patient an opportunity to process the information, formulate a response, and to experience his or her emotions. Physicians who feel uncomfortable during this silent phase need to appreciate that the discomfort is rarely shared by the patient, who is engrossed in thought about the meaning of the news and thoughts about the future. Furthermore, very little that is said by the physician at this time will be remembered by the patient, so it is best not to say it at all. If the patient makes no verbal response after, perhaps, 2 minutes, it can be useful to check in: "I just told you some pretty serious news, do you feel comfortable sharing your thoughts about this?"

Dealing with the Response

The remainder of the conversation should be spent primarily dealing with the patient's response. This includes using the SOLER and NURSE skills to legitimize and empathize with the patient's experience. It is also important to explore the meaning the news has for the patient and to achieve a shared understanding of the disease and its implications. For example:

MD: What is most troubling to you about having cancer?

PT : It's a death sentence—my mother died from cancer, my brother died from cancer. I guess it's my turn now.

MD: Given your experience, I can see how this is really scary for you. And cancer can be very serious. However, in your case, there are a lot of treatment options, and you have a good chance of surviving with this disease.

PT : So this won't kill me?

MD: I certainly hope not. And, I'll be there with you every step of the way fighting this illness.

Hopeful messages need to be tailored to patients' specific concerns, particularly addressing patient's misconceptions and fears. Once patients' concerns have been explored, patients can be reassured more effectively. When effective treatment is available, this fact should be explained. When the treatment options are poor, hope may be found by alleviating the patients' worst fears. Doctors may reassure patients that they will not be abandoned during their illness, that the doctor will remain available if things get worse, that everything will be done to maintain patients' comfort, and that they will continue to watch for new treatment developments. Often people find hope and strength from their religious or spiritual beliefs, from having their individuality respected, from meaningful relationships with others, and from finding meaning in their lives. Exploring these with the patient over time may help to foster realistic hope. Although physicians may have a desire to make an overly reassuring statement to the patient right after revealing the diagnosis, hopeful statements that are truthful and that are made after taking the time to first explore the patient's concerns are more likely to be accepted by the patient. One can offer a realistic sense of hope, whether biomedical ("We'll keep our eyes open for new treatments and discuss them as they become available") or psychosocial ("I look forward to talking with you more about how we can help you live everyday as fully as possible, despite this illness").

Patients may have specific questions about further tests, treatment options, and prognosis. It is important to respond to these seriously. However, many patients will suffer difficulties in comprehension in such emotionally challenging situations. Information, particularly a plan, is helpful, as it allows the patient to reconceptualize the future as a safer, more predictable place. The exact details matter less than the clarity of the plan and the reassurance that the physician will be available. Giving simple, focused bits of information, using nonvague language that patients can understand, carefully observing the patient's verbal and nonverbal reactions to what is said, and most importantly, avoiding information-packed speeches helps.

Ending the Encounter

The clinician must end the encounter in a way that leaves the patient feeling supported and with some sense of hope. Support can be provided through meeting patients' immediate health needs and risks. One must treat pain and palliate other symptoms. Patients should be asked how they plan to cope with the news, and if their response raises any concerns about suicide this should be asked about directly and addressed. One should try to minimize aloneness through statements of nonabandonment and referral to other resources, such as support groups, counselors, or pastoral care.

Lastly, one should provide a specific follow-up plan: "I'd like you to keep a list of questions so I can answer them for you on our next visit this Tuesday. We'll talk about all your options again at that time... Okay? And please feel free to call me." The physician needs to remember that the goal of this conversation is not to leave a happy patient. That is rarely possible (or even desirable) after delivering bad news. Instead, one hopes to leave a patient who feels supported and cared for, and can look forward to a specific plan of action.

Advance Care Planning

Discussions about advance care planning encompass many goals. These include preparing for death and dying, exercising control, relieving burdens placed on loved ones, helping patients make decisions consistent with their values, and leaving patients feeling supported and understood (68). The first step in preparing to discuss advance care plans is deciding upon the appropriate goals for the discussion. What one hopes to accomplish will vary depending on the clinical situation (69). Advance care planning includes many different tasks: informing the patient, eliciting preferences, identifying a surrogate decision maker, and providing emotional support. Frequently, one cannot accomplish all of this in one conversation and

focusing on the goals of the discussion allows the physician to tailor the encounter. Advance care planning is completed as a process over time that allows patients an opportunity for thoughtful reflection and interaction with others.

For a healthy, older patient, physicians might establish whom the patient would like to appoint as a health-care surrogate. They might ask whether the patient already has a written advance directive and explore the patient's thoughts about dying and the general views about life-sustaining treatments. For a patient with a life-limiting chronic illness, the doctor might also discuss the patient's attitudes about specific interventions that are likely to occur (e.g., mechanical ventilation in severe chronic obstructive pulmonary disease). Finally, for a patient who will soon die, the doctor will shift the focus from future treatment in hypothetical scenarios to establishing what the goals should be for care provided in the present. In all cases, advance care planning can help patients prepare for death, discuss their values with their loved ones, and achieve a sense of control (68). It can help build trust between doctors and their patients, so that when difficult treatment decisions arise, doctors, patients, and their loved ones can communicate openly and achieve resolution.

Initiating the Conversation

There are a number of ways to begin the discussion. Often physicians can relate the topic to a recent serious event such as a hospitalization. Another way to begin is to ask about experiences with relatives or friends who have died. Many patients are likely to have observed serious illness closely and perhaps have had loved ones in some of the situations that the physician is describing. They are likely to have much information and misinformation about the end-of-life care and are likely to have thought about their own deaths. Opening a discussion in this manner can naturally lead to a discussion about how decisions were made and what the patient thought of that particular death. This will provide valuable insights into the patient's own values.

Providing Information

Patients must have adequate information to make informed decisions. It helps to start by asking patients what they understand about their medical illness. If the patient's condition is more serious than what he or she realizes, then the physician will need to shift focus. The physician will want to put off discussing advance care planning, focusing the discussion instead on explaining to the patient the seriousness of his or her condition.

Studies indicate that patients are more interested in what the expected health outcome will be than in details about the interventions themselves (70,71). The primary reason for patients to consider withholding treatments is to avoid an outcome judged by them to be worse than death (72). The other reason is that the burden of the treatment, on themselves or their loved ones, outweighs the potential benefit. Therefore, patients should achieve an understanding of the impact of common, life-sustaining interventions on one's quality of life. In contrast, vivid descriptions of the nature of the treatments themselves (e.g., intubation, cardioversion, and ICU care) may alarm patients and be less helpful.

Eliciting Preferences

Patients state preferences after learning about potential options and evaluating these in light of their personal values. Values refer to deeply held beliefs such as a desire for personal independence or the importance of a religious practice. By exploring patients' values and goals, clinicians can help them clarify their specific preferences. Sometimes one can ask explicitly about such values (e.g., "What makes life worth living for you?"). Alternatively, values may be elicited in the process of asking about specific treatment preferences. For example, after a patient makes a statement about the end-of-life care (e.g., "I'd never want to be on one of those machines"), the clinician may respond by simply asking, "Why?" The answer to this question (e.g., "Because I never want to be a burden on my family or society") may uncover a patient's core values that will impact greatly on treatment decisions.

Identifying what conditions the patient would find unacceptable can also help clarify a patient's preferences. A useful question is, "Can you imagine any situations in which life would not be worth living (73)?" This question can be followed by asking what the patient would be willing to forgo in order to avoid such states.

For many patients, dealing with uncertainty is the most difficult aspect of decision making. When doctors ask patients if they would want a particular treatment, like a ventilator, patients will often state that the treatment should be provided "if it will help me, but if it won't help me, don't do it." Statements like this ignore the reality that physicians are often uncertain about the outcome. Everyone responds to uncertainty differently, and the patient's approach to this issue should be discussed explicitly as well. For example, one may ask, "What if we are not sure whether we will be able to get you off the breathing machine?" Depending on the patient's answer to this question, the doctor can explore what the chance of success needs to be in order to pursue aggressive treatment. Some patients will state that any possibility of recovery is worth pursuing while others will refuse curative treatment when the likelihood of recovery drops below a particular threshold (64). Some patients are comfortable using numbers talking about probabilities, others are less quantitatively facile (74,75). The patient's preferences should dictate the extent to which numbers are used in this discussion. Many patients will be satisfied, leaving it to the judgment of the physician and family members, with only general instructions. The option of a treatment trial is also a useful way to provide clarity in the face of uncertainty.

It is impossible to elicit meaningful preferences for every intervention in every possible situation. By focusing on a patient's values and goals, the physician can then help the patient make decisions about current or future treatments that are consistent with those goals. Discussions should move back and forth from preferences to reasons and values to information and back again, ensuring that the patient understands the implications of his or her stated preferences and that the doctor understands the patient's values. In this way, when the physician is faced with an unanticipated clinical situation, he or she can use the patient's stated values and goals to help determine the appropriate course of action. In such discussions, it is frequently worthwhile to inquire specifically about some controversial treatments such as artificial nutrition and hydration. This is particularly true in states that require the patients' specific directive to withhold these treatments.

Patients and physicians often use vague terms that ought to be avoided. For example, a statement that a treatment should be continued as long as "quality of life is good" begs further clarification. How does the patient (or his or her surrogate, or the physician) define a good quality of life? In fact, it is always important to ensure that the patient and physician have a shared understanding of the conversation and its implications. Similarly, medical jargon should be avoided, one should always define technical terms, and patients must be encouraged to ask questions.

Choosing Surrogate Decision Makers

Identifying who is to act as the patient's health-care proxy may be the most important outcome of a conversation about advance care planning. Does the patient wish this to be a single individual or an entire family? Given the literature demonstrating poor concordance between patient preferences and surrogate perceptions of those preferences, the clinician would be wise to stress the need for the patient to communicate with the selected proxy decision maker (76). Patients should also be asked how much leeway their proxies should have in decision making (77). Should proxies adhere strictly to patients' stated preferences or ought they to have more flexibility when making actual decisions?

These discussions can be emotionally difficult, even when they are welcome. It is important to draw upon the emotion-handling skills described earlier (see the Section "The Role of Affect") and to acknowledge patient's feelings of sadness, fear, or anger, when they come up, and to validate those feelings by stating your understanding of their reaction. The physician can admit that the discussion can be difficult and support the patient by stating how helpful he or she has been in helping to understand his or her preferences. Another way doctors can provide support to patients is to assure them that they will do whatever they can to meet their goals (such as comfort) and to articulate what some of those things might be. In this way, doctors can assure patients that they will continue to care for them, even if they are in a condition in which they would not want life-sustaining treatment.

Communicating Over the Transition

It is possible that the greatest communication challenges face physicians and patients as they discuss progression of disease, the transition from curative therapy to palliation only, and the referral to hospice care. Such times of transition involve the recognition of loss, redefinition of self-concept and social role, and great emotional stress. Patients are likely to feel sadness, anger, and denial. Physicians frequently have difficulty with such discussions because they feel a sense of failure, are worried that patients will feel abandoned, or that they will be overcome in the conversation by anxiety or despair. Furthermore, they may have their own unresolved issues about mortality or fear the patient's anticipated emotional response.

Again, it is useful to identify the goals of these conversations. They include eliciting emotional, psychologic, and spiritual concerns and providing empathic and practical support. Of course, it is also important to help patients acknowledge their illness and to make appropriate health-care decisions, such as enrolling in hospice. However, conversations should not be dominated by the physician's agenda, and patients must be given ample space to make decisions according to their own timetables. Physicians should employ behaviors that promote the sharing of concerns by patients and avoid behaviors such as reassurance that inhibit such sharing. See Table 48.4 for useful, open-ended questions with which one can initiate such conversations.

As patients respond to these questions, the physician should continue to focus on the psychosocial and spiritual aspects of their illness and not allow the biomedical issues to dominate. It is important to avoid false reassurance. A particular form of response that can be extremely effective at these times is the "wish statement" (78). This is particularly effective in response to statements that appear to demonstrate significant denial of the severity of illness. For example:

PT: I'm going to get better. I know that this new chemotherapy they're offering at the university will make the difference.

MD: I wish that there was a treatment that would make this cancer go away.

TABLE 48.4	**Open-ended questions to initiate conversations about dying**

"What concerns you most about your illness?"

"How is treatment going for you (your family)?"

"As you think about your illness, what is the best and the worst that might happen?"

"What has been most difficult about this illness for you?"

"What are your hopes (your expectations and your fears) for the future?"

"As you think about the future, what is most important to you (what matters the most to you)?"

Lo B, Quill T, Tulsky J. Discussing palliative care with patients. *Ann Intern Med.* 1999;130:744–749.

PT : You mean that you don't think it will work.

MD: It's hard to come to terms with this, but, unfortunately, I don't believe it would help you overcome your cancer.

PT : I was afraid you might say that. What do we do now?

MD: There's a lot that we can do. Let's talk about what is most important for you right now.

The wish statement allows the doctor to demonstrate empathy toward the patient and to align the doctor with the patient's hopes. Yet, at the same time it implicitly conveys the message that certain goals are unrealistic. In this way, the physician can address the patient's denial without losing the therapeutic alliance.

Dreaded Questions

Finally, it is useful to consider several of the questions that many physicians find most difficult to answer (e.g., "Why me?" "How long do I have to live?"). Responding to such questions draws upon the many skills described in this chapter and it is useful to keep several additional points in mind. The most important thing a physician can do is to remain curious. One should not assume that one knows what the question is "really" about. A patient who is asking, "How long do I have?" may be wondering if she is going to live until Christmas, whether reports she has heard that the disease is fatal are accurate or whether she is going to get out of the hospital. Acknowledge the question, but make sure you understand it before trying to answer (e.g., "That is a really tough question. What are you concerned about?"). It is also important to recognize that it is not necessarily the physician's job to solve the problem. Physicians do not have the answers to questions such as "Why me?" and may not be able to diminish the feelings of sadness and loss. What one can do is to acknowledge and normalize the feelings. In allowing the patient to be heard, the physician may decrease the patient's sense of being alone in their disease and thus decrease their suffering. (An illustrative example is to imagine you have had a very bad day at work. When you come home and start to share this with your family, how would you feel if they began to brainstorm different solutions to the problem? Most individuals would prefer their loved ones to acknowledge their feelings—"sounds like it was a really tough day"—rather than to try to solve their problem.)

Having anticipated replies can be useful and several examples follow (50):

PT : How long do I have to live?

MD: I wonder if it is frightening not knowing what will happen next, or when.

This response acknowledges that underlying such a question is tremendous emotion, most likely fear. It will be important for the physician to give a factual response to this question. However, the patient will not be prepared to hear this response until the doctor has addressed his or her emotional concerns. The suggested answer above allows patients to speak about their fears and worries. When the physician needs to use a more factual response, the following is a way of being honest while maintaining hope: "On average, a person in your situation lives up to 3 to 4 months, but some people have much less time, and others may live over a year. I would now take care of any practical or family matters that you wish to have completed before you die, but continue to hope that you are one of the lucky people who gets a bit more time."

FM: Does this mean you're giving up on him?
MD: Absolutely not. But tell me, what do you mean by giving up?

Suggesting that a patient receives palliative care risks conveying a sense of abandonment. Physicians must be emphatic that palliative care and hospice are active forms of care that meet patients' varying goals at the end of life. However, further exploration of patients' or family's concerns about abandonment are important to understanding their perceptions and attitudes toward care at the end of life:

Patient: "Are you telling me that I am going to die?"
Physician: "I wish that were not the case. I am also asking, how do you want to spend your remaining time, recognizing that it's limited?"

This wish statement helps the physician identify with the patient's loss. The following sentence is an attempt by the physician to reframe the patient's understanding of the situation. He has acknowledged that the patient is dying, but now he seeks to understand what the patient's goals might be in light of this new information. Creating new goals in this way provides an outlet for the patient's hope.

Bereavement

Palliative care does not end when a patient dies. An awareness of bereavement can help one communicate with family and loved ones after the loss. Bereaved people ought to be encouraged to tell their stories of loss, including describing details of the days and weeks around the death of their loved ones. Similarly, family members and friends benefit by recalling earlier positive memories of the person. Physicians can explore how the bereaved person has responded to the grief ("How have things been different for you because your husband died?") and identify their social support and coping resources. One should not overlook the frequently enormous practical ramifications of loss such as financial difficulties, the need to leave a home, and transportation. Finally, physicians need to be aware that a significant minority of bereaved family members and friends, 10% to 20%, have difficulty regaining their normal functioning after the loss. This syndrome—complicated grief—seems distinct from depression and is characterized by excessive rumination and preoccupation with the dead individual (79).

Good communication skills are central to the provision of palliative care. The fundamentals of such communication are listening, recognizing one's own affective responses, attending to patients' emotional needs, and achieving a shared understanding of the concerns at hand. Specific tasks, such as delivering bad news, discussing advance care planning, helping patients through the transition to hospice care, and responding to difficult questions, require using these skills to ensure that patients' concerns are elicited and addressed, and they are informed and feel supported.

REFERENCES

1. Steinhauser KE, Christakis NA, Clipp EC, et al. Factors considered important at the end of life by patients, family, physicians, and other care providers. *JAMA.* 2000;284:2476-2482.
2. Heaven CM, Maguire P. The relationship between patients' concerns and psychological distress in a hospice setting. *Psychooncology.* 1998;7(6):502-507.
3. Parle M, Jones B, Maguire P. Maladaptive coping and affective disorders among cancer patients. *Psychol Med.* 1996;26(4):735-744.
4. Bertakis KD, Roter D, Putnam SM. The relationship of physician medical interview style to patient satisfaction. *J Fam Pract.* 1991;32(2):175-181.
5. Kaplan SH, Greenfield S, Ware JE Jr. Assessing the effects of physician-patient interaction on the outcomes of chronic disease. *Med Care.* 1989;27:S110-S127.
6. Roter DL, Hall JA, Kern DE, et al. Improving physicians' interviewing skills and reducing patients' emotional distress. A randomized clinical trial. *Arch Intern Med.* 1995;155(17):1877-1884.
7. Tierney WM, Dexter PR, Gramelspacher GP, et al. The effect of discussions about advance directives on patients satisfaction with primary care. *J Gen Intern Med.* 2001;16:32-40.
8. Tulsky JA, Arnold RM, Alexander SC, et al. Enhancing communication between oncologists and patients with a computer-based training program: a randomized trial. *Ann Intern Med.* 2011;155(9):593-602.
9. Smyth JM, Stone AA, Hurewitz A, et al. Effects of writing about stressful experiences on symptom reduction in patients with asthma or rheumatoid arthritis: a randomized trial. *JAMA.* 1999;281(14):1304-1309.
10. Butow PN, Kazemi JN, Beeney LJ, et al. When the diagnosis is cancer: patient communication experiences and preferences. *Cancer.* 1996;77(12):2630-2637.
11. Friedrichsen MJ, Strang PM, Carlsson ME. Breaking bad news in the transition from curative to palliative cancer care-patient's view of the doctor giving the information. *Support Care Cancer.* 2000;8(6):472-478.
12. Ptacek JT, Eberhardt TL. Breaking bad news. A review of the literature. *JAMA.* 1996;276(6):496-502.
13. Goldberg R, Guadagnoli E, Silliman RA, et al. Cancer patients' concerns: congruence between patients and primary care physicians. *J Cancer Educ.* 1990;5(3):193-199.
14. Maguire P, Faulkner A, Booth K, et al. Helping cancer patients disclose their concerns. *Eur J Cancer.* 1996;32A(1):78-81.
15. Butow PN, Brown RF, Cogar S, et al. Oncologists' reactions to cancer patients' verbal cues. *Psychooncology.* 2002;11(1):47-58.
16. Pollak KI, Arnold RM, Jeffreys A, et al. Oncologist communication about emotion during visits with advanced cancer patients. *J Clin Oncol.* 2007;25(36):5748-5752.
17. Maguire P. Improving communication with cancer patients. *Eur J Cancer.* 1999;35(10):1415-1422.

18. Heaven CM, Maguire P. Disclosure of concerns by hospice patients and their identification by nurses. *Palliat Med.* 1997;11(4):283-290.

19. Ford S, Fallowfield L, Lewis S. Doctor-patient interactions in oncology. *Soc Sci Med.* 1996;42(11):1511.

20. Detmar SB, Muller MJ, Wever LD, et al. The patient-physician relationship. Patient-physician communication during outpatient palliative treatment visits: an observational study. *JAMA.* 2001;285(10):1351-1357.

21. Gattellari M, Voigt KJ, Butow PN, et al. When the treatment goal is not cure: are cancer patients equipped to make informed decisions? *J Clin Oncol.* 2002;20(2):503-513.

22. Emanuel LL, Barry MJ, Stoeckle JD, et al. Advance directives for medical care—a case for greater use. *N Engl J Med.* 1991;324(13):889-895.

23. Tulsky JA, Chesney MA, Lo B. How do medical residents discuss resuscitation with patients? *J Gen Intern Med.* 1995;10(8):436-442.

24. Tulsky JA, Fischer GS, Rose MR, et al. Opening the black box: how do physicians communicate about advance directives? *Ann Intern Med.* 1998;129(6):441-449.

25. Billings JA, Block S. Palliative care in undergraduate medical education. Status report and future directions. *JAMA.* 1997;278(9):733-738.

26. Rhodes-Kropf J, Carmody SS, Seltzer D, et al. This is just too awful; I just can't believe I experienced that. Medical students' reactions to their "most memorable" patient death. *Acad Med.* 2005;80(7):634-640.

27. Sung AD, Collins ME, Smith A, Sanders A, Block S, Arnold RM. Crying, stress and sadness: the experience and attitudes of 3rd year medical students and interns. *Teach Learn Med.* 2009;21(3):180-187.

28. Smith RC, Zimny GH. Physicians' emotional reactions to patients. *Psychosomatics.* 1988;29(4):392-397.

29. Spikes J, Holland J. The physician's response to the dying patient. In: Strain JJ, Grossman S, eds. *Psychological Care of the Medically Ill: A Primer in Liaison Psychiatry.* New York, NY: Appleton-Century-Crofts; 1975:138-148.

30. Schneiderman LJ, Kaplan RM, Pearlman RA. Do physicians own preferences for life-sustaining treatment influence their perceptions of patients' preferences? *J Clin Ethics.* 1993;4:28-33.

31. Quill TE, Townsend P. Bad news: delivery, dialogue, and dilemmas. *Arch Intern Med.* 1991;151(3):463-468.

32. The AM, Hak T, Koeter G, et al. Collusion in doctor-patient communication about imminent death: an ethnographic study. *BMJ.* 2000;321(7273):1376-1381.

33. Maguire P. Barriers to psychological care of the dying. *BMJ.* 1985;291:1711-1713.

34. Benoliel JQ. Health care delivery: not conducive to teaching palliative care. *J Palliat Care.* 1988;4(1&2):41-42.

35. Whippen DA, Canellos GP. Burnout syndrome in the practice of oncology: results of a random survey of 1,000 oncologists. *J Clin Oncol.* 1991;9:1916-1920.

36. Schaerer R. Suffering of the doctor linked with death of patients. *Palliat Med.* 1993;7:27-37.

37. Shanafelt TD, Bradley KA, Wipf JE, et al. Burnout and self-reported patient care in an internal medicine residency program. *Ann Intern Med.* 2002;136(5):358-367.

38. Shanafelt TD, West C, Zhao X, et al. Relationship between increased personal well-being and enhanced empathy among internal medicine residents. *J Gen Intern Med.* 2005;20(7):612-617.

39. Neimeyer GJ, Behnke M, Reiss J. Constructs and coping: physicians' response to patient death. *Death Educ.* 1983;7:245-264.

40. Back AL, Arnold RM, Tulsky JA. *Mastering Communication with Seriously Ill Patients: Balancing Honesty with Empathy and Hope.* New York, NY: Cambridge University Press; 2009.

41. Schenker Y, Lo B, Ettinger KM, Fernandez A. Navigating language barriers under difficult circumstances. *Ann Intern Med.* 2008;149(4):264-269.

42. Fogarty LA, Curbow BA, Wingard JR, et al. Can 40 seconds of compassion reduce patient anxiety? *J Clin Oncol.* 1999;17(1):371-379.

43. McDonagh JR, Elliott TB, Engelberg RA, et al. Family satisfaction with family conferences about end-of-life care in the intensive care unit: increased proportion of family speech is associated with increased satisfaction. *Crit Care Med.* 2004;32(7):1484-1488.

44. Wenrich MD, Curtis JR, Shannon SE, et al. Communicating with dying patients within the spectrum of medical care from terminal diagnosis to death. *Arch Intern Med.* 2001;161(6):868-874.

45. Clayton JM, Butow PN, Arnold RM, et al. Fostering coping and nurturing hope when discussing the future with terminally ill cancer patients and their caregivers. *Cancer.* 2005;103(9):1965-1975.

46. Parker PA, Baile WF, de Moor C, et al. Breaking bad news about cancer: patients' preferences for communication. *J Clin Oncol.* 2001;19(7):2049-2056.

47. Detmar SB, Aaronson NK, Wever LD, et al. How are you feeling? Who wants to know? Patients' and oncologists' preferences for discussing health-related quality-of-life issues. *J Clin Oncol.* 2000;18(18):3295-3301.

48. Baile WF, Glober GA, Lenzi R, et al. Discussing disease progression and end-of-life decisions. *Oncology.* 1999;13(7):1021-1031.

49. Larson DG, Tobin DR. End-of-life conversations: evolving practice and theory. *JAMA.* 2000;284(12):1573-1578.

50. Lo B, Quill T, Tulsky J. Discussing palliative care with patients. *Ann Intern Med.* 1999;130(9):744-749.

51. Parle M, Maguire P, Heaven C. The development of a training model to improve health professionals' skills, self-efficacy and outcome expectancies when communicating with cancer patients. *Soc Sci Med.* 1997;44(2):231-240.

52. von Gunten CF, Ferris FD, Emanuel LL. The patient-physician relationship. Ensuring competency in end-of-life care: communication and relational skills. *JAMA.* 2000;284(23):3051-3057.

53. Hagerty RG, Butow PN, Ellis PA, et al. Cancer patient preferences for communication of prognosis in the metastatic setting. *J Clin Oncol.* 2004;22(9):1721-1730.

54. Pfeifer MP, Mitchell CK, Chamberlain L. The value of disease severity in predicting patient readiness to address end-of-life issues. *Arch Intern Med.* 2003;163(5):609-612.

55. Bohner G, Chaiken S, Hunyadi P. The role of mood and message ambiguity in the interplay of heuristic and systematic processing. *Eur J Soc Psychol.* 1994;24(1):207-221.

56. Levinson W, Gorawara-Bhat R, Lamb J. A study of patient clues and physician responses in primary care and surgical settings. *JAMA.* 2000;284(8):1021-1027.

57. Shapiro DE, Boggs SR, Melamed BG, et al. The effect of varied physician affect on recall, anxiety, and perceptions in women at risk for breast cancer: an analogue study. *Health Psychol.* 1992;11(1):61-66.

58. Spiro HM. What is empathy and can it be taught? In: Spiro HM, ed. *Empathy and Practice of Medicine: Beyond Pills and the Scalpel.* New Haven, CT: Yale University Press; 1993:7-14.

59. Egan G. *The Skilled Helper: A Problem-Management and Opportunity-Development Approach to Helping.* 7th ed. California, CA: Brooks/Cole; 2002.

60. Smith RC, Hoppe RB. The patient's story: integrating the patient- and physician-centered approaches to interviewing. *Ann Intern Med.* 1991;115(6):470-477.

61. Back A, Arnold RM, Baile WF, Fryer-Edwards K, Tulsky JA. The clinical use of praise. *Lancet.* 2010:376(9744):866-867.

62. Christakis NA. *Death Foretold: Prophecy and Prognosis in Medical Care.* Chicago, IL: University of Chicago Press; 2000.

63. Delvecchio MJ, Good BJ, Schaffer C, et al. American oncology and the discourse on hope. *Cult Med Psychiatry.* 1990;14(1):59-79.

64. Weeks JC, Cook EF, O'Day SJ, et al. Relationship between cancer patients' predictions of prognosis and their treatment preferences. *JAMA.* 1998;279(21):1709-1714.

65. Breen CM, Abernethy AP, Abbott KH, et al. Conflict associated with decisions to limit life-sustaining treatment in intensive care units. *J Gen Intern Med.* 2001;16(5):283-289.

66. Back AL, Arnold RM. Dealing with conflict in caring for the seriously ill: "it was just out of the question." *JAMA.* 2005;293(11):1374-1381.

67. Back AL, Trinidad SB, Hopeley EK, Arnold RM, Baile WF, Edwards KA. What patients value when physicians give news of cancer recurrence: commentary from 'at-risk' patients on physician audiorecording. *Oncologist.* 2011;16(3):342-350.

68. Singer PA, Martin DK, Lavery JV, et al. Reconceptualizing advance care planning from the patient's perspective. *Arch Intern Med.* 1998;158:879-884.

69. Teno JM, Lynn J. Putting advance-care planning into action. *J Clin Ethics.* 1996;7:205-213.

70. Frankl D, Oye RK, Bellamy PE. Attitudes of hospitalized patient toward life support: a survey of 200 medical inpatients. *Am J Med.* 1989;86:645-648.

71. Pfeifer MP, Sidorov JE, Smith AC, et al. The discussion of end-of-life medical care by primary care patients and physicians: a multicenter study using structured qualitative interviews. *J Gen Intern Med.* 1994;9:82-88.

72. Patrick DL, Starks HE, Cain KC, et al. Measuring preferences for health states worse than death. *Med Decis Mak.* 1994;14(1):9-18.

73. Pearlman RA, Cain KC, Patrick DL, et al. Insights pertaining to patient assessments of states worse than death. *J Clin Ethics.* 1993;4(1):33-41.

74. Mazur DJ, Hickam DH. Patients' interpretations of probability terms. *J Gen Intern Med.* 1991;6(3):237-240.

75. Woloshin KK, Ruffin MT, Gorenflo DW. Patients' interpretation of qualitative probability statements. *Arch Fam Med.* 1994;3:961-966.

76. Seckler AB, Meier DE, Mulvihill M, et al. Substituted judgment: how accurate are proxy predictions? *Ann Intern Med.* 1991;115(2):92-98.

77. Sehgal A, Galbraith A, Chesney M, et al. How strictly do dialysis patients want their advance directives followed? *JAMA.* 1992;267(1):59-63.

78. Quill TE, Arnold RM, Platt F. "I wish things were different": expressing wishes in response to loss, futility, and unrealistic hopes. *Ann Intern Med.* 2001;135(7):551-555.

79. Lichtenthal WG, Cruess DG, Prigerson HG. A case for establishing complicated grief as a distinct mental disorder in DSM-V. *Clin Psychol Rev.* 2004;24(6):637-662.

CHAPTER 49

The Family Meetings

Lori L. Olson ■ Sumi K. Misra ■ Mohana B. Karlekar ■ Sara F. Martin

INTRODUCTION

The goal of excellent palliative care is to collaboratively meet the needs of the patients, families, and treatment teams during times of transition in the context of life-limiting and serious illness. Good communication between medical clinicians and families of seriously ill patients is recognized as a key factor in successful shared decision-making and family perception of quality care (1–3).

Formal family meetings have increasingly been seen as an effective tool to facilitate this dialogue (4,5). Not only do families improve their understanding of the patient's diagnosis, therapeutic options, and prognosis, clinicians better recognize the emotional weight and the personal meaning of the patient's illness. Through family meetings, clinicians and families build honest relationships based on each other's desire to provide the best care for the patient (6). Family meetings should allow for families to identify patient's goals and patient's views of quality of life which allows clinicians to provide medical recommendations based on those identified goals. This process results in a shared decision plan (7).

This chapter is designed to:

1. Review recent literature relevant to optimal communication during family meetings.
2. Outline the anatomy of a family meeting, including setting, population targeted, planning, execution, pitfalls, and documentation of the event.
3. Highlight the family meeting as a tool for enhanced shared decision-making.

THE ROLE OF THE FAMILY MEETING

Communication occurs best, face to face. Given that over 50% of communication is non-verbal, it is a disadvantage to lose an opportunity for clarity and connection at a time of confusion, potential conflict, and impactful decision-making (8). While most patients and family members want to receive support and hope from clinicians, they also request honest information about the patient's medical condition and prognosis (9,10). Yet, studies reveal that up to a third of families of critically ill patients are dissatisfied with the lack of communication or conflicting information from different clinicians (11,12).

Even when clinicians spend time communicating the patient's medical diagnosis, treatment, and prognosis with the family, only half of families actually comprehend what was said despite both clinicians' and families' perception of understanding (13). This disconnect is alarming since clinical decisions are made based upon these misunderstandings.

Physicians rarely effectively communicate with their seriously ill patients about their goals, values, or basic treatment decisions. When physicians communicate effectively they are more apt to understand and address the issues that are important for the patient or the patient–family unit. Consequently, patients are better able to understand their medical situation in the context of their psychosocial situation. This could affect their understanding of their medical issues and treatment options more concretely (14). In addition, effective communication improves patient satisfaction and reduces anxiety and distress (15,16). Even brief expressions of empathy may reduce patient anxiety (17).

Optimal communication has been identified by patients and their families as one of the more important aspects of medical care at a time of serious illness and at the end of life (18–20). The family meeting is a useful format for clarification ensuring that everyone involved is on the same page regarding the patient's condition.

WHEN SHOULD A FAMILY MEETING BE CONSIDERED?

A family meeting should be considered when multiple teams are involved in a patient with complicated care and decisions need to be made about further treatment. Family meetings provide an opportunity to clarify treatment goals, advocate for the patient, and ensure that all parties involved in care (both medical and nonmedical) understand treatment decisions and prognosis (21). Family meetings are an invaluable part of all levels of hospital-based care and are an important step in providing best care to patients and their loved ones. Meetings are recommended during transitions in care and critical decision-making points in a patient's disease trajectory. For the cancer patient, a proactive meeting soon after the initial diagnosis may help the patient and family ask questions and begin to think about quality-of-life issues as they make treatment decisions. Consider follow-up family meetings when there is progression of cancer despite current therapy, complications from therapy, and when patient would be eligible for hospice (see Table 49.1).

Currently, the majority of family meetings happen in the hospital in situations where the patient is not able to make decisions for himself such as the intensive care unit

TABLE 49.1	Patient- and family-centered reasons to conduct a family meeting

To provide a sense of autonomy and control

To understand their illness, disease trajectory, and treatment options

To present and understand their illness in their unique psychosocial context

To have a preference and value-based discussion for goals of care

To gain realistic expectations aligned with their goals

To actively participate in the care plan

To provide a coping mechanism and plan and prioritize for the future

To provide a platform to reframe "hope"

TABLE 49.2	The pre-meeting

Identify and gather key stakeholders

Review medical issues and advance directives

Identify and address areas of potential conflict

Discuss and reach consensus

Designate the "leader"

Identify key additional "presenters"

Emphasize role of empathetic active listening

(ICU). Meetings should take place upon admission to the ICU, if a patient's condition changes, if there is conflict within the family, or if there is conflict between family and clinicians (8,22).

Lilly et al. (1) instituted early family meetings for critically ill patients which identified patient's goals sooner and paved the road for follow-up family meetings when the clinical course became incompatible with either the patient's goals or restoring life which subsequently permitted earlier withdrawal of life-sustaining therapy (1). Family members were more satisfied about the quality of a patient's death in the ICU if a family meeting was held to discuss patient's goals (23).

The data on the pediatric population mirror the adult side. The majority of parents believed they shared the same beliefs on prognosis of their children's illness; however, 70% of parents were more optimistic than their physicians regarding prognosis again highlighting this chasm between clinicians and families (24). In the pediatric ICU, a single formal meeting results in increased shared decision-making (25).

THE FAMILY MEETING SETUP (THE PRE-MEETING)

Planning is an essential component to the success of any conference, and family meetings are no different. It is important that a "pre-meeting" occurs prior to the actual designated meeting with family to prevent common pitfalls (26) (Table 49.2). It is an important step to help identify the stakeholders from the medical staff who are going to be involved in the meeting. Physicians, nurses, social workers, and chaplains should be included in this step if they plan to participate in the meeting. This allows time for the medical

team to discuss potential family dynamics (e.g., siblings that do not get along or distrust of medical staff) (27).

The medical staff should jointly discuss the patient's current medical condition and hospital course to date and come to a consensus regarding prognosis and treatment course. This is an opportunity to discuss with any other consultants their medical opinions and ensure that a cohesive plan is being presented to the family. Proposed treatments should be reviewed and consensus reached about what will be recommended to the family.

During the pre-meeting, the person that will lead the meeting should be designated. Each member involved should be informed of any information they will be asked to give in the meeting (update on medical condition, discuss current "brain function," etc.). By telling each participant what they will be expected to present, they can begin to prepare what they wish to communicate to the family prior to the actual meeting (21,26). Attempts should be made to minimize "surprise revelations and opinions" during the actual family meeting.

The medical participants should review any pertinent advance directives and ensure that they understand them and are proposing a treatment plan in alignment with those directives. Careful attention should be paid to review if the patient has identified a surrogate decision maker or made any explicit statements about treatment options (e.g., feeding tubes).

By attempting to do the above prior to a family meeting, all the providers can enter the meeting adequately prepared and, more importantly, with an understanding of their role in the meeting. Each step in this pre-meeting is a potential pitfall, where things can go wrong in the family meeting. If a leader is not designated, medical provider roles are not clear, or communication regarding prognosis is not consistent, then it will be challenging to establish trust with the family and reach any conclusive shared patient-centered decisions (28–30).

THE ANATOMY OF THE FAMILY MEETING

The majority of evidence discussing the family meeting originates from the ICU and medical oncology literature. Though there are many different well-established methods on how to conduct a family meeting, the fundamental

TABLE 49.3	The 12-step process for an effective family meeting

Step 1: The pre-meeting

Step 2: Meeting logistics and physical setup

Step 3: Introductions, setting expectations, and a framework

Step 4: Eliciting patient and family position, perspectives, and concerns

Step 5: Establishing boundaries (if any) on information sharing

Step 6: Communication of relevant medical fact

Step 7: Responding to emotions and managing conflict

Step 8: Eliciting patient-centered goals of care

Step 9: Establishing and summarizing mutually acceptable plans of care

Step 10: Outlining the "next steps"

Step 11: Expressing appreciation for involvement and attendance

Step 12: Communicating, debriefing, and documenting, in written form, a summary of the interaction

principles remain constant. As discussed above, much of the work for the family meeting is done before the actual meeting. Von Gunten et al. (27) divided the actual family meeting into a seven-step process (27). We recommend a 12-step process (Table 49.3).

Step 1: The pre-meeting (Tables 49.1 and 49.2). Here the clinician must ascertain the following: What is the purpose of the meeting? Which individuals in the family need to attend? Who are the relevant medical team members from both the primary team and consulting team? The clinicians chosen to participate in the family meeting should meet prior to the meeting and determine who will lead the discussion. Each participant should know what the other will communicate.

Step 2: A mutually acceptable time needs to be agreed upon with sufficient prior notice to all, in order to maximize attendance (31). In an effort to better prepare the family prior to the meeting, Nelson et al. (32) discussed giving family members a written checklist of what they should consider prior to the meeting. A decisional patient can be asked who he or she wants to participate from his or her family and community, including faith leaders. In general, it is wise not to set any arbitrary limits on the number of attendees. The medical care team should likewise decide who they want to participate. It is wise to not overwhelm a family with too many health professionals. On the other hand, a physician from the primary team as well as a nurse and social worker

should attend when possible; these individuals can help ensure the consistency of information as well as help deal with complicated dynamics. If the patient has a long-time treating physician whom he or she trusts, this person should ideally be present (22,26,28,33,34).

The ideal setting is private and quiet, with chairs arranged in a circle or around a table. Everyone should be able to sit down if they wish. All pagers and cellular telephones should be turned off.

Step 3: At the start of the meeting, the clinician leading the meeting should initiate introductions and have each individual present to explain their role in the patient's care. Family should be asked to introduce themselves. Ground rules should be established, emphasizing that everyone interested in speaking will have an opportunity to do so.

Phrases that may be helpful: "We are here to discuss the next steps in the care of Mrs. X."

If you do not know the patient or family well, take a moment to build relationship. Ask a nonmedical question such as, "I am just getting to know you. I had a chance to look at your chart and learn about your medical condition but it does not say much about your life before you got sick. Can you tell us about the things you liked to do before you got sick?" Similarly, if the patient is not able to participate in the meeting, ask family to describe the patient prior to his becoming ill: "As we get started, can you describe what Mrs. X was like before she became ill?" (35).

Step 4: Determine what the family understands. Prior to imparting information, it is recommended that the team actively listen to the patient and family and elicit their full list of concerns (14). Physicians cannot assume that patients will volunteer all their concerns spontaneously. It is important to ask the family what they know about the patient's condition, treatment options, and prognosis using open-ended questions. The extent to which the patient's concerns have been disclosed and resolved directly correlate with lower levels of depression and anxiety. When a holistic and thoughtful approach is taken to establish a safe space for the patient and family to discuss the issues, they feel more satisfied and may comply better with the offered advice (36–38).

Phrases that may be helpful: "What is your understanding of what is going on with Mrs. X?" "What has been most difficult about this illness for you?"

"As you think about your illness, what is the best and worst that can happen?"

Step 5: Multiple factors determine how much information is to be shared (Table 49.4). This will be a function of both the family's ability to process information and how much they would like to know. The majority of English-speaking people in North America who have a serious illness prefer to be fully informed about a variety of topics related to their health, including diagnosis, prognosis, and treatment options (39–41). However, not all patients want very extensive information about their illness and prognosis (42). It is noted that patients' information needs may be strongly influenced by their unique culture, country of

TABLE 49.4	**Factors that could influence information disclosure to patients**

Culture

Country of origin

Disease progression and life expectancy

Age

Sex

Socioeconomic background

Level of education

Relationship with healthcare team

origin, or by subculture within a country. Some patients may want minimal information or nondisclosure when their life expectancy is very short (43). The evidence is inconclusive in non-western countries, but the overall trend has been more disclosure based on insightful understanding of where the patient and family are in their journey of experiencing the serious illness. Patients from some cultural backgrounds may prefer disclosure negotiated through the family when the prognosis is poor (43). Higher levels of information are often sought by younger patients (40,44,45), females (40), individuals in a middle socioeconomic class (46), and those who have a higher level of education (44).

Phrases that may be helpful: "Is there anything you are particularly concerned about, that would help us understand your/your loved ones illness better?" "How have you adapted to difficult circumstances in the past?" "Would it help to have someone with you as we discuss this further?"

Step 6: Communicate the relevant medical facts. The information delivered should be done so with clarity without the use of medical jargon or excessive and complex physiology. Some patients and surrogates are comfortable using numbers when talking about probabilities, whereas others could be quantitatively challenged (47,48). Information should be presented based on elicited patient preferences, and many patients will leave decisions to the judgment of the medical team, based on the team's best interpretation of wide-ranging medical data.

Phrases that may be helpful:

"I would like to update everyone here about Mrs. X's condition."

"Mrs. X has been in the ICU for 27 days. She has had many people involved in her medical care and has had many test and procedures. I would like to summarize these for you."

Step 7: Acknowledge, validate, and respond to emotions. It is important to tolerate and allow silence. Although conflict is often avoided by clinicians and patients, conflict managed well can be productive. Denial of conflict and non-revelation

of "hidden agendas" and unexplored strong negative emotions can derail honest communication and exacerbate indecision in goal setting. Back and Arnold (49) have described a seven-step approach to conflict management and resolution that takes into account active listening, empathizing, reframing, explaining, self-disclosure, and trying to reach a "middle ground."

Phrases that may be helpful: "Although I have never shared your experience, I do understand that this is a really difficult time for you."

"Many people would feel angry/sad/overwhelmed if this happened to them. I wonder if you ever feel that way."

Step 8: Elicit patient-centered goals of care and establish treatment plans based on the patient's wishes, values, goals, and treatment priorities. Discussions based on vague terms such as "quality of life" should be avoided; instead, it is more important to identify how a patient or their surrogates identify a good quality of life. Identifying what conditions the patient would find unacceptable can also help clarify a patient's preferences. A useful question is, "Can you imagine any situations in which life would not be worth living?" (50). This question can be followed by asking what the patient would want in the current context of illness and treatment plans. Emphasize to family members that they should be communicating the wishes of their loved one, not their own. The literature clearly demonstrates poor concordance between patient preferences and surrogate perceptions of those preferences. It is recommended that it be stressed that the patient communicates his preference with the proxy decision maker as well as communicates how much leeway the proxy should have in the decision-making (51,52).

Phrases that may be helpful:

"What makes life worth living for you?"

"What do you think Mrs. X would say if she were at this table and listening to this question/discussion?"

"We realize it is sometimes very difficult to take our own emotions and feelings out of a decision regarding a loved one, knowing that, we could face a life without them."

Step 9: Establish the plan of care and summarize this to the group at the conclusion of the meeting.

Phrases that may be helpful: "I appreciate everybody's input into Mrs. X's plan to help us jointly make some decisions. We can now agree to move forward with…."

"I believe, after this very helpful discussion, that you would prefer…."

Step 10: Outline the next steps. Patients may have specific questions about further tests, treatment options, and interventions. A succinct short-term plan as well as a general clear overview of the next immediate few hours to days can go a long way in allowing the patient and family to reframe and re-conceptualize their future. It could provide a "safe haven" during the current period of turmoil and transition.

Phrases that may be helpful:

"We have covered a lot of ground today, let's go over some of the things we have discussed and see what we will be doing over the next few hours/days."

"I will keep you updated about his breathing over the next few hours, as well as his x-ray results while you think about your decision regarding the breathing machine."

"There is a lot that we can do. Let's talk about what goals are most important for your loved one."

Step 11: Express appreciation for involvement and attendance: One cannot always achieve a happy ending or make the participants happy in a family meeting, given the circumstance under which most meetings are held. Instead, a closing statement that focuses on appreciation of the attendees' support of and dedication to the patient's best interests is recommended. Emphasize that the meeting is an important step in a series of communications that may occur in the care and caring of the patient.

Phrases that may be helpful:

"Thank you for being here today. Your presence and involvement was very helpful in coming to these important decisions."

"Mrs. X is so very fortunate to have you keeping her best interests in mind at a time like this. Thanks you for being there for her and us."

Step 12: Communication, debriefing, and documentation of the meeting. It is critically important to communicate all relevant information to the healthcare team both verbally and in the medical record immediately following the family meeting. Family meetings are often billed using time as the factor in determining the appropriate E/M code (53).

SKILL SETS AND COMMUNICATION TOOLS TO CONDUCT THE FAMILY MEETING

All clinicians should strive to improve their communication strategies in the family meeting setting. A good physician–patient relationship is the cornerstone of effective communication in the scenario of advancing chronic as well as sudden illnesses (54,55). Unfortunately, most physicians have received little to no training regarding effective communication. For many, this skill set has been learned by trial and error. Clinicians are often very uncomfortable when they must discuss prognosis and treatment options with the patient if the information is unfavorable. Based on our own observations and those of others (56–62), we believe that the discomfort is based on a number of concerns that physicians experience. These include uncertainty about the patient's expectations, fear of destroying the patient's hope, fear of their own inadequacy in the face of uncontrollable disease, not feeling prepared to manage the patient's anticipated emotional reactions, and sometimes embarrassment at having previously painted too optimistic a picture for the patient.

Communication Skills

In general, it is recommended that the healthcare team create a holistic patient-centered climate where the patient is treated as a "whole person" and it clearly communicates that the physician is interested, is attuned and is sensitive to their

TABLE 49.5	The SPIKES protocol for breaking bad news
Setting up	
Perception	
Invitation	
Knowledge	
Emotions/empathy	
Strategy and summary	

medical needs as well as their psychosocial needs and emotions of the patient (14). Over the last decade, communication tools have been developed to help clinicians become more adept at family meetings. The SPIKES protocol is a commonly used practical protocol for disclosing unfavorable information—"breaking bad news"—to cancer patients about their illness. The protocol (SPIKES) consists of six steps (63) (Table 49.5).

The goal is to enable the clinician fulfill the four most important objectives of the interview disclosing bad news: gathering information from the patient, transmitting the medical information, providing support to the patient, and eliciting the patient's collaboration in developing a strategy or treatment plan for the future. Oncologists, oncology trainees, and medical students who have been taught the protocol have reported increased confidence in their ability to disclose unfavorable medical information to patients. Another such tool is an acronym VALUE that incorporates the following techniques (64):

- Value and appreciate what families communicate
- Acknowledge emotions with reflective summary statements
- Listen carefully
- Understand who the patient is as a person by asking open-ended questions
- Eliciting questions from families

Leadership Skills

A cornerstone skill in palliative medicine is leadership of family meetings to establish goals of care, typically completed at a time of patient change in status, where the value of current treatments needs to be reevaluated. Leading a family meeting requires considerable flexibility to ensure that all relevant participants have the opportunity to have their points of view expressed. Although it is useful to have one person designated as the main orchestrator and coordinator of the meeting, the essential skills for making a family meeting successful can come from more than one participant. These skills include group facilitation skills, counseling skills, knowledge of medical and prognostic information, and a willingness to provide leadership and guidance in decision-making (26).

Conflict Management and Resolution Skills

Conflicts about medical care occur frequently at the end of life. These conflicts threaten therapeutic relationships and lead to patient, healthcare provider, and family dissatisfaction. Conflict between the patient/family and physician may arise from simple factual misunderstandings about medical care. Frequently, however, conflict is driven by a patient's or family's emotions such as feeling unheard or ignored, as well as having goals that conflict with those of the medical team. In these instances, attempting to convince a patient or family with additional medical information will not work (Table 49.6).

Information gaps can arise when there is an inaccurate understanding of the patient's medical condition. Inconsistent information that varies between providers or confusing information that is embedded in medical jargon and presented in an illogical and non-sequential manner can create informational gaps, leading to conflict. Additionally, information in excess of what needs to be communicated at a certain time or information that is presented at times of genuine uncertainty such as immediate post cerebrovascular accident and brain injury in children as well as in adults can cause information disconnects. All the above can be exacerbated if additional issues of language and cultural barriers exist.

Treatment goal confusion arises from a disparity between the perception of the treating team and the patient–family dynamics. This includes lack of clarity about short-term and long-term goals when multiple issues need to be addressed and inconsistent and illogical treatment plans that are driven on emotion rather than logic. This can also arise when phrases and terms such as "comfort care" and "do everything" are used, which can mean different things to different people unless clarified explicitly (65).

Humans are intensely emotional beings and the combination of uncertainty in the context of serious, life-limiting, and sometimes sudden illness can give rise to situations fraught with conflict. Emotions such as grief, fear, anxiety, guilt, anger, hope, and despair can all cause conflict situations and should be recognized in context and addressed directly and with empathy if possible.

Family dynamics can often cause conflict between family members and between the family and healthcare team or between the family and patient. Issues pertinent are families and surrogates confusing patients' best interests and wishes with their own needs, poor coping and decision-making capacity of surrogate decision makers, and unrecognized history/presence of psychiatric illness in family that impedes rational decision-making.

Healthcare team dynamics, such as disagreement with regard to prognosis, approach to treatment plan, and level of disclosure, when not recognized and addressed appropriately in a timely fashion can unfairly and unfortunately jeopardize the family meeting, putting the patient/family in the middle of the dispute.

The relationship between the clinician and the patient/surrogate has a potential to play a significant role in conflict development, management, and resolution during times of crisis. Lack of trust in the healthcare team/healthcare system, past experiences where the patient has had a better outcome than predicted by the healthcare team, and genuine value differences in the arena of cultural/religious values concerning life, dying, and death can all play an important role in how issues could be addressed and resolved (34,49,66–68).

Addressing the underlying roots of conflict will have considerable impact. The following method emphasizes resolving conflict through mutual trust and shared goals between physicians, patients, and families. Weissman's approach to conflict resolution is based on understanding a patient's or a family's story, attending to their emotions, and establishing shared decision-making (30).

Principled negotiation is an approach to resolving conflict that avoids power struggles and unwanted compromises (Table 49.7) (29,67). The process recommends that one identify the fundamental problem, separating this from

TABLE 49.6	Potential causes for conflict during a family meeting

Information gaps

Treatment goal confusion

Emotions

Family/team dynamics

Relationship between the clinician and the patient/surrogate

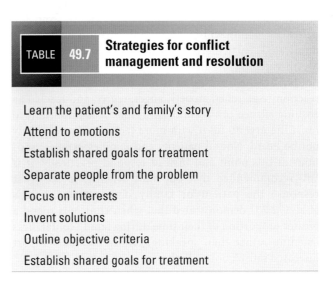

TABLE 49.7	Strategies for conflict management and resolution

Learn the patient's and family's story

Attend to emotions

Establish shared goals for treatment

Separate people from the problem

Focus on interests

Invent solutions

Outline objective criteria

Establish shared goals for treatment

the individual's judgment on both sides. It next involves listening to requests and demands but making an attempt to look into underlying interests, for all parties concerned. This would include a clear expression of the intentions and goals of the medical team. It is recommended that one avoid contrasting different philosophies of medical care. Instead, it would be prudent to propose a plan of care that meets a family's expectations without detracting from good medical care. Provision of objective information to substantiate medical recommendations rather than anecdotes is also recommended in this approach.

Empathetic Truth-Telling Skills

Healthcare providers are often afraid that by telling someone the truth about his/her diagnosis, they would be responsible for taking away hope. The conflict, between truth telling and fear of destroying hope, is commonly noted by patients and families who feel that "the doctor is not really telling me everything," a feeling that is highly corrosive to the doctor–patient relationship (69).

Brody (70) writes, "Hope means different things to different people, and different things to the same person as he/she moves through stages of illness." The physician can play a valuable role in helping the individual patient define his/her hopes and fears. When close to death, hope often becomes refocused away from long-term goals and toward short-term or spiritual goals. Hope may mean a pain-free day, a sense of security, love and non-abandonment, or a wedding to attend in the near future. Factors that often increase hope in the terminally ill include feeling valued, maintaining meaningful relationships, reminiscence, humor, realistic goals, and optimal symptom relief. Factors that often decrease hope include feeling devalued, abandoned or, lack of direction and goals, and unrelieved pain and discomfort (71).

Strategic Use of a Therapeutic Silence

When communicating distressing information it is important to allow for silence. In the authors' experience, no matter what one might imagine the response from the patient or family will be to any information being communicated, particularly information in the setting of a life-threatening or life-limiting illness, one really cannot predict their expressed as well as repressed emotional reaction (e.g., relief, anxiety, anger, regret, and fear). The ensuing silence can be uncomfortable. It is important to resist the urge to fill it with more facts as they will likely not be heard. Not all patients and families express emotions at this point and instead respond practically. It is still recommended that one wait, silently, to see what response the patient or family demonstrates. Curtis et al. (72,73) demonstrated that when clinicians spend a greater proportion of their time during family conferences listening rather than speaking, family members report increased satisfaction with the communication.

POPULATIONS, SITUATIONS, AND CIRCUMSTANCES THAT REQUIRE A SPECIAL MENTION

Pediatrics

Caring for the seriously ill and dying children is a stressful job. Insufficient training and competence in communication skills may exacerbate staff members' stress and affect the quality of care (74). This stress affects not only the physicians and nurses who work closely with children and families in the palliative phases of treatment but also a host of other hospital staff members. The staff members and family members often experience anguish at watching children suffer and a sense of helplessness with respect to alleviating the pain (74–76). Staff members also conveyed concerns about their lack of preparation and their feelings of inadequacy in pain management. In addition, they described instances of disagreements among attending physicians and refusal to consult with the pain management team (74,76). The expanding literature and experiences of families and staff members emphasize the continuing need for improvements in communication (77) and caring at the end of life for the pediatric population. An abundance of adequate and timely support is necessary for staff members as well as families (74,78). Although children are typically allowed to assent, rather than consent to plans regarding their care, parents and healthcare providers must recognize the subjective personal nature of suffering and respect the child's autonomy and capacity to make decisions, particularly for emancipated and mature minors.

Trauma

There are several unique characteristics of trauma patients that make family meetings imperative. First, there is a 10% to 20% mortality incidence in trauma ICUs. A significant minority of these patients are young, healthy patients who become critically ill in a matter of seconds. Second, the illness course is usually either brief (patient succumbing to devastating neurologic injury in the first 72 h) or long and drawn out (patient who initially survives trauma injury but has complications from multiple organ failure and sepsis) (79). The prognostication tools for these patients are of limited value at the individual patient level (80). Often, communication about the end-of-life decisions are not done until the last hours of a patient's life. Measures to hold a family meeting early on to address prognosis or prognostic uncertainty and goals of care have improved communication in the trauma setting (81).

Withdrawal of Life-Sustaining Measures

It is important not to directly ask the family to make a decision about withdrawal of life support but to rather make a shared decision based on your medical knowledge and the family's input about patient's goals or wishes. Do not use language that causes fear of abandonment such as "There's nothing more we can do" or "I've done all I can." Instead, empathetic phrases such as "I wish your dad's liver could be fixed. Unfortunately, it can't be fixed. Based on what you've told me about your dad's wishes, I recommend focusing on your dad's comfort." Discussing what the patient would want rather than what the family desires also relieves family guilt (82). Giving concrete information about what withdrawal of life support looks like, including anticipated time of death, reassurance that the patient will be continued to be cared for, and common terminal symptoms, decreases caregivers' depression and anxiety (83).

Language Barrier

During times of emotional stress and during conversations that are ripe with emotion, vulnerability, and those that touch the very sense and core of the inner soul, it is most comforting and safe for patients and families to describe feelings and thoughts in their primary language. Although using family members as interpreters may seem convenient, and tempting, it is fraught with problems. There is no assurance they will have the necessary language skills to convey medical information, and the patient may not feel comfortable expressing their feelings through family members. Family members may misinterpret medical phrases, censor sensitive/taboo topics, or summarize discussions rather than translating them completely (84). Family members may have strong emotions that affect their objectivity and impartiality. In addition, being the bearer of bad news or discussing contentious information may have negative implications for a family member following the encounter.

When communicating to patients and families with limited English proficiency, one should utilize a medical interpreter who has acquired the specific training and meet the national standards/ethics of practice (National Council on Interpreting in Healthcare) (85). The need to use an interpreter implies that significant cultural differences exist between the practitioner and the patient/family. Professional interpreters can help one to provide effective and efficient communication that is culturally sensitive and factually accurate upon translation. Accomplished and qualified uses of translators prevent the "lost in translation" phenomenon, which can cause conflict and misunderstandings in communications (86).

Cultural Beliefs

The cultural backgrounds of not only patients and families but also of healthcare teams profoundly influence their preferences and needs regarding discussing bad news, decision-making, and the dying experience (Table 49.8).

It is important to identify the patient's preferences regarding how and with whom medical information is shared. For those who request that the physician discuss their condition with family members, identify the main contacts to give information to, about the patient's condition. Use respectful,

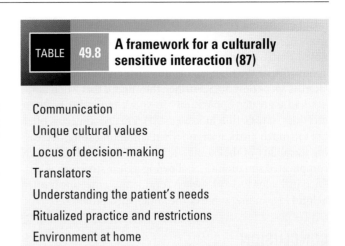

TABLE 49.8	A framework for a culturally sensitive interaction (87)

Communication

Unique cultural values

Locus of decision-making

Translators

Understanding the patient's needs

Ritualized practice and restrictions

Environment at home

curious, and open-ended questions about a patient's cultural heritage to identify their values (87).

For some patients, medical decision-making is communally driven rather than individualistic. Multiple family members or a community elder or leader may need to be involved, often without prior official documentation because it is assumed or understood from the patient's perspective. As discussed in a previous section, language barriers are extremely challenging, especially during times of severe illness. Utilize medical interpreters frequently and effectively.

Reassess what is being heard, understood, and agreed upon frequently, from both the patient's and clinician's standpoint. Specifically confirm that the patient understands (88). This is particularly important if a medical translator is involved, as miscommunication is common even when using trained medical interpreters. Determine if there are specific customs the patient desires to be followed. These must be communicated to other healthcare providers, especially in the hospital setting. It may be necessary to advocate for the patient and negotiate with healthcare facility administrators to find an agreeable way to honor a patient's wishes. Given that a majority of hospice care happens in the patient's home environment, respectfully explore whether there are any needs that can be met by the healthcare system, and how open the patient, family, or community is to receiving care at home. Even if a trusting, collaborative relationship has developed between a patient/family and clinicians in the hospital, this may not immediately translate into the home setting. With the patient's permission, expectations about cultural-specific aspects of a patient's care should be explicitly communicated to care providers outside the hospital (89–92).

WHAT CAN GO WRONG?

The family meeting can be the most effective tool for clinicians when handled well. However, when conducted poorly, it can be catastrophic. What can go wrong? Often there is insufficient preparation that is done prior to the meeting. Clinicians may not agree on treatment decisions. This gets reflected in the meetings causing confusion among the family members, ultimately making it difficult to delineate a cohesive plan (22). Physicians often talk too much. McDonagh et al. noted that typically in the ICU settings, physicians spent about 70% of the time talking during family meetings while families spent only 30%. Further, they found that when families had a greater opportunity to speak more during these meetings, satisfaction increased (73). Finally, clinicians often use too much medical jargon when communicating, decreasing the ability of the families to truly understand an already complicated situation (5). Following a clear structure as outlined in Tables 49.1–49.3 when conducting a meeting is often helpful in avoiding some of the anticipated pitfalls.

CONCLUSION

Good communication and organizational skills are critical to delivering effective and timely care to all patients, particularly those with serious illnesses. Using a stepwise approach to family meetings provides a framework to optimize shared decision-making. A family meeting and other patient–physician interactions when executed well have correlated with improved health outcomes, patient satisfactions, and emotional well-being and should be considered (7,93–95).

REFERENCES

1. Lilly CM, De Meo DL, Sonna LA, et al. An intensive communication intervention for the critically ill. *Am J Med.* October 2000;109(6):469-475.

2. Lautrette A, Darmaon M, Megarbane B, et al. A communication strategy and brochure for relatives of patients dying in the ICU. *N Engl J Med.* February 2007;356(5):469-478.

3. Stapleton RD, Engelberg RA, Wenrich MD, Goss CH, Curtis JR. Clinician statements and family satisfaction with family conferences in the intensive care unit. *Crit Care Med.* June 2006;34(6):1679-1685.

4. Mularski RA, Curtis JR, Billings JA, et al. Proposed quality measures for palliative care in the critically ill: a consensus from the Robert Wood Johnson Foundation Critical Care Workgroup. *Crit Care Med.* November 2006;34(11):S404-S411.

5. Curtis JR, Patrick DL, Shannon SE, Treece PD, Engelberg RA, Rubenfeld GD. The family conference as a focus to improve communication about end-of-life care in the intensive care unit: opportunities for improvement. *Crit Care Med.* February 2001;29(2):N26-N33.

6. Billings JA. The end-of-life family meeting in intensive care part I: indications, outcomes, and family needs. *J Palliat Med.* September 2011;14(9):1042-1050.

7. Billings JA. The end-of-life family meeting in intensive care part II: family-centered decision making. *J Palliat Med.* September 2011;14(9):1051-1057.

8. Breen CM, Abernethy AP, Abbott KH, Tulsky JA. Conflict associated with decisions to limit life-sustaining treatment in intensive care units. *J Gen Intern Med.* May 2001;16(5):283-289.

9. Hofmann JC, Wenger NS, Davis RB. et al. Patient preferences for communication with physicians about end-of-life decisions. SUPPORT Investigators. Study to Understand Prognoses and Preference for Outcomes and Risks of Treatment. *Ann Intern Med.* July 1997;127(1):1-12.

10. Clarke EB, Curtis JR, Lucw JM, et al. Quality indicators for end-of-life care in the intensive care unit. *Crit Care Med.* September 2003;31(9):2255-2262.

11. Abbott KH, Sago JG, Breen CM, Abernethy AP, Tulsky JA. Families looking back: one year after discussion of withdrawal or withholding of life-sustaining support. *Crit Care Med.* January 2001;29(1):197-201.

12. Baker R, Wu AW, Teno JM, et al. Family satisfaction with end-of-life care in seriously ill hospitalized adults. *J Am Geriatr Soc.* May 2000;48(5):S61-S69.

13. Azoulay E, Chevret S, Leleu G, et al. Half the families of intensive care unit patients experience inadequate communication with physicians. *Crit Care Med.* August 2000;28(8):3044-3049.

14. Maguire P, Pitceathly C. Key communication skills and how to acquire them. *BMJ (Clin Res Ed.).* September 2002;325(7366):697-700.

15. Roberts CS, Cox CE, Reintgen DS, Baile WF, Gibertini M. Influence of physician communication on newly diagnosed breast patients' psychologic adjustment and decision-making. *Cancer.* July 1994;74(1):336-341.

16. Kaplan SH, Ware JE. The patients role in healthcare and quality assessment. In: Goldfield N, Nash DB, eds. *Providing Quality Care: Future Challenges.* Chicago, IL: Health Administration Press; 1995:26-27.

17. Fogarty LA, Curbow BA, Wingard JR, McDonnell K, Somerfield MR. Can 40 seconds of compassion reduce patient anxiety? *J Clin Oncol Off J Am Soc Clin Oncol.* January 1999;17(1):371-379.

18. Curtis JR, Wenrich MD, Carline JD, Shannon SE, Ambrozy DM, Ramsey PG. Understanding physicians' skills at providing end-of-life care perspectives of patients, families, and health care workers. *J Gen Intern Med.* January 2001;16(1):41-49.

19. Steinhauser KE, Clipp EC, McNeilly M, Christakis NA, McIntyre LM, Tulsky JA. In search of a good death: observations of patients, families, and providers. *Ann Intern Med.* May 2000;132(10):825-832.

20. Wenrich MD, Curtis JR, Shannon SE, Carline JD, Ambrozy DM, Ramsey PG. Communicating with dying patients within the spectrum of medical care from terminal diagnosis to death. *Arch Intern Med.* March 2001;161(6):868-874.

21. Weissman DE, Quill TE, Arnold RM. The family meeting: end-of-life goal setting and future planning #227. *J Palliat Med.* April 2010;13(4):462-463.

22. Lautrette A, Ciroldi M, Ksibi H, Azoulay E. End-of-life family conferences: rooted in the evidence. *Crit Care Med.* November 2006;34(11):S364-S372.

23. Lilly CM, Sonna LA, Haley KJ, Massaro AF. Intensive communication: four-year follow-up from a clinical practice study. *Crit Care Med.* May 2003;31(5):S394-S399.

24. Mack JW, Cook EF, Wolfe J, Grier HE, Cleary PD, Weeks JC. Understanding of prognosis among parents of children with cancer: parental optimism and the parent-physician interaction. *J Clin Oncol Off J Am Soc Clin Oncol.* April 2007;25(11):1357-1362.

25. Garros D, Rosychuk RJ, Cox PN. Circumstances surrounding end of life in a pediatric intensive care unit. *Pediatrics.* November 2003;112(5):e371.

26. Weissman DE, Quill TE, Arnold RM. Preparing for the family meeting #222. *J Palliat Med.* February 2010;13(2):203-204.

27. von Gunten CF, Ferris FD, Emanuel LL. The patient-physician relationship. Ensuring competency in end-of-life care: communication and relational skills. *JAMA.* December 2000;284(23):3051-3057.

28. Curtis JR, Engelberg RA, Wenrich MD, Shannon SE, Treece PD, Rubenfeld GD. Missed opportunities during family conferences about end-of-life care in the intensive care unit. *Am J Respir Crit Care Med.* April 2005;171(8):844-849.

29. King DA, Quill T. Working with families in palliative care: one size does not fit all. *J Palliat Med.* June 2006;9(3):704-715.

30. Weissman DE, Quill TE, Arnold RM. The family meeting: causes of conflict #225. *J Palliat Med.* March 2010;13(3):328-329.

31. Hudson P, Quinn K, O'Hanlon B, Aranda S. Family meetings in palliative care: multidisciplinary clinical practice guidelines. *BMC Palliat Care.* 2008;7:12.

32. Nelson JE, Walker AS, Luhrs CA, Cortez TB, Pronovost PJ. Family meetings made simpler: a toolkit for the intensive care unit. *J Crit Care.* December 2009;24(4):626.e7-e14.

33. Tobin B, Lobb E, Roper E, Ingham J. Is the patient's voice under-heard in family conferences in palliative care? A question from Sydney, Australia. *J Pain Symptom Manage.* February 2011;41(2):e3-e6.

34. Back A. *Mastering Communication with Seriously Ill Patients: Balancing Honesty with Empathy and Hope.* Cambridge and New York, NY: Cambridge University Press; 2009.

35. Weissman DE, Quill TE, Arnold RM. The family meeting: starting the conversation #223. *J Palliat Med.* February 2010;13(2):204-205.

36. Radwany S, Albanese T, Clough L, Sims L, Mason H, Jahangiri S. End-of-life decision making and emotional burden: placing family meetings in context. *Am J Hosp Palliat Care.* November 2009;26(5):376-383.

37. Parle M, Jones B, Maguire P. Maladaptive coping and affective disorders among cancer patients. *Psychol Med.* July 1996;26(4):735-744.

38. Maguire P. Improving communication with cancer patients. *Eur J Cancer.* December 1999;35(14):2058-2065.

39. Butow PN, Maclean M, Dunn SM, Tattersall MH, Boyer MJ. The dynamics of change: cancer patients' preferences for information, involvement and support. *Ann Oncol Off J Eur Soc Med Oncol ESMO.* September 1997;8(9):857-863.

40. Jenkins V, Fallowfield L, Saul J. Information needs of patients with cancer: results from a large study in UK cancer centres. *Br J Cancer.* January 2001;84(1):48-51.

41. Kutner JS, Steiner JF, Corbett KK, Jahnigen DW, Barton PL. Information needs in terminal illness. *Soc Sci Med (1982).* May 1999;48(10):1341-1352.

42. Leydon GM, Boulton M, Moynihan C, et al. Cancer patients' information needs and information seeking behaviour: in depth interview study. *BMJ (Clin Res Ed.).* April 2000;320(7239):909-913.

43. Goldstein D, Thewes B, Butow P. Communicating in a multicultural society. II: Greek community attitudes towards cancer in Australia. *Intern Med J.* July 2002;32(7):289-296.

44. Cassileth BR, Zupkis RV, Sutton-Smith K, March V. Information and participation preferences among cancer patients. *Ann Intern Med.* June 1980;92(6):832-836.

45. Blanchard CG, Labrecque MS, Ruckdeschel JC, Blanchard EB. Information and decision-making preferences of hospitalized adult cancer patients. *Soc Sci Med 1982.* 1988;27(11):1139-1145.

46. Jones R, Pearson J, McGregor S, et al. Cross sectional survey of patients' satisfaction with information about cancer. *BMJ (Clin Res Ed.).* November 1999;319(7219):1247-1248.

47. Mazur DJ, Hickam DH. Patients' interpretations of probability terms. *J Gen Intern Med.* June 1991;6(3):237-240.

48. Woloshin KK, Ruffin MT 4th, Gorenflo DW. Patients' interpretation of qualitative probability statements. *Arch Fam Med.* November 1994;3(11):961-966.

49. Back AL, Arnold RM. Dealing with conflict in caring for the seriously ill: 'it was just out of the question'. *JAMA.* March 2005;293(11):1374-1381.

50. Pearlman RA, Cain KC, Patrick DL, et al. Insights pertaining to patient assessments of states worse than death. *J Clin Ethics.* 1993;4(1):33-41.

51. Seckler AB, Meier DE, Mulvihill M, Paris BE. Substituted judgment: how accurate are proxy predictions? *Ann Intern Med.* July 1991;115(2):92-98.

52. Sehgal A, Galbraith A, Chesney M, Schoenfeld P, Charles G, Lo B. How strictly do dialysis patients want their advance directives followed? *JAMA.* January 1992;267(1):59-63.

53. von Gunten CF, Ferris FD, Kirschner C, Emanuel LL. Coding and reimbursement mechanisms for physician services in hospice and palliative care. *J Palliat Med.* 2000;3(2):157-164.

54. Wenrich MD, Curtis JR, Ambrozy DA, Carline JD, Shannon SE, Ramsey PG. Dying patients' need for emotional support and personalized care from physicians: perspectives of patients with terminal illness, families, and health care providers. *J Pain Symptom Manage.* March 2003;25(3):236-246.

55. Steinhauser KE, Christakis NA, Clipp EC, McNeilly M, McIntyre L, Tulsky JA. Factors considered important at the end of life by patients, family, physicians, and other care providers. *JAMA.* November 2000;284(19):2476-2482.

56. OKEN D. What to tell cancer patients. A study of medical attitudes. *JAMA.* April 1961;175:1120-1128.

57. Taylor KM. 'Telling bad news': physicians and the disclosure of undesirable information. *Soc Health Illn.* June 1988;10(2):109-132.

58. Miyaji NT. The power of compassion: truth-telling among American doctors in the care of dying patients. *Soc Sci Med 1982.* February 1993;36(3):249-264.

59. Siminoff LA, Fetting JH, Abeloff MD. Doctor-patient communication about breast cancer adjuvant therapy. *J Clin Oncol Off J Am Soc Clin Oncol.* September 1989;7(9):1192-1200.

60. Maguire P. Barriers to psychological care of the dying. *BMJ (Clin Res Ed.).* December 1985;291(6510):1711-1713.

61. Buckman R. Breaking bad news: why is it still so difficult? *BMJ (Clin Res Ed.).* May 1984;288(6430):1597-1599.

62. Delvecchio MJ Good, Good BJ, Schaffer C, Lind SE. American oncology and the discourse on hope. *Cult Med Psychiatry.* March 1990;14(1):59-79.

63. Baile WF, Buckman R, Lenzi R, Glober G, Beale EA, Kudelka AP. SPIKES-A six-step protocol for delivering bad news: application to the patient with cancer. *Oncologist.* 2000;5(4):302-311.

64. Curtis JR, White DB. Practical guidance for evidence-based ICU family conferences. *Chest.* October 2008;134(4):835-843.

65. Quill TE, Arnold R, Back AL. Discussing treatment preferences with patients who want 'everything'. *Ann Intern Med.* September 2009;151(5):345-349.

66. Lazare A, Eisenthal S, Frank A. Clinician/patient relations II: conflict and negotiation. In: *Outpatient Psychiatry.* Baltimore, MD: Williams and Wilkins; 1989:137-157.

67. Fisher R. *Getting to Yes: Negotiating Agreement Without Giving In.* 2nd ed. Boston, MA: Houghton Mifflin; 1991.

68. Quill TE. Recognizing and adjusting to barriers in doctor-patient communication. *Ann Intern Med.* July 1989;111(1):51-57.

69. Tywcross R, Lichter I. The terminal phase. In: Doyle D, Hanks, G, and MacDonald N. eds. *Oxford Textbook of Palliative Medicine.* 2nd ed. New York, NY: Oxford University Press; 1998: 977-978.

70. Brody H. Hope. *JAMA.* September 1981;246(13):1411-1412.

71. Ambuel B, Weissman DE. Discussing spiritual issues and maintaining hope. In: Weissman DE, Ambuel B, eds. *Improving End-of-Life Care: A Resource Guide for Physician Education,* 2nd Edition. Milwaukee, WI: Medical College of Wisconsin; 1999:113-121.

72. Curtis JR, Engelberg RA, Wenrich MD, et al. Studying communication about end-of-life care during the ICU family conference: development of a framework. *J Crit Care.* September 2002;17(3):147-160.

73. McDonagh JR, Elliott TB, Engelberg RA, et al. Family satisfaction with family conferences about end-of-life care in the intensive care unit: increased proportion of family speech is associated with increased satisfaction. *Crit Care Med.* July 2004;32(7):1484-1488.

74. Hilden JM, Emanuel EJ, Fairclough DL, et al. Attitudes and practices among pediatric oncologists regarding end-of-life care: results of the 1998 American Society of Clinical Oncology survey. *J Clin Oncol Off J Am Soc Clin Oncol.* January 2001;19(1):205-212.

75. Contro NA, Larson J, Scofield S, Sourkes B, Cohen HJ. Hospital staff and family perspectives regarding quality of pediatric palliative care. *Pediatrics.* November 2004;114(5):1248-1252.

76. Contro N, Larson J, Scofield S, Sourkes B, Cohen H. Family perspectives on the quality of pediatric palliative care. *Arch Pediatr Adolesc Med.* January 2002;156(1):14-19.

77. Khaneja S, Milrod B. Educational needs among pediatricians regarding caring for terminally ill children. *Arch Pediatr Adolesc Med.* September 1998;152(9):909-914.

78. Vachon ML. Staff stress in hospice/palliative care: a review. *Palliat Med.* April 1995;9(2):91-122.

79. Mosenthal AC, Murphy PA, Barker LK, Lavery R, Retano A, Livingston DH. Changing the culture around end-of-life care in the trauma intensive care unit. *J Trauma.* June 2008;64(6):1587-1593.

80. Sinuff T, Adhikari NK, Cook DJ, et al. Mortality predictions in the intensive care unit: comparing physicians with scoring systems. *Crit Care Med.* March 2006;34(3):878-885.

81. Mosenthal AC, Murphy PA. Interdisciplinary model for palliative care in the trauma and surgical intensive care unit: Robert Wood Johnson Foundation Demonstration Project for Improving Palliative Care in the Intensive Care Unit. *Crit Care Med.* November 2006;34(11):S399-S403.

82. Way J, Back AL, Curtis JR. Withdrawing life support and resolution of conflict with families. *BMJ (Clin Res Ed.).* December 2002;325(7376):1342-1345.

83. Kirchhoff KT, Palzkill J, Kowalkowski J, Mork A, Gretarsdottir E. Preparing families of intensive care patients for withdrawal of life support: a pilot study. *Am J Crit Care.* March 2008;17(2):113-121; quiz 122.

84. Haffner L. Translation is not enough. Interpreting in a medical setting. *West J Med.* September 1992;157(3):255-259.

85. Howard S. Use of interpreters in palliative care. Fast facts and concepts #154. April 2006.

86. Haffner L. Guide to interpreter positioning in health care settings. *The National Council on Interpreting in Health Care Working Paper Series,* 2003. [Online]. http://www.ncihc.org/mc/page.do?sitePageId=57022&orgId=ncihc

87. Lum H, Arnold R. Asking about cultural beliefs in palliative care. Fast facts and concepts #216." June 2009.

88. Maugans TA. The SPIRITual history. *Arch Fam Med.* January 1996;5(1):11-16.

89. Pham K, Thornton JD, Engelberg RA, Jackson JC, Curtis JR. Alterations during medical interpretation of ICU family conferences that interfere with or enhance communication. *Chest.* July 2008;134(1):109-116.

90. Searight HR, Gafford J. Cultural diversity at the end of life: issues and guidelines for family physicians. *Am Fam Physician.* February 2005;71(3):515-522.

91. Crawley LM, Marshall PA, Lo B, Koenig BA. Strategies for culturally effective end-of-life care. *Ann Intern Med.* May 2002;136(9):673-679.

92. Arnold R. Palliative care case of the month: the family says not to tell. *University of Pittsburgh Institute to Enhance Palliative Care,* May 2006. [Online]. http://www.dom.pitt.edu/dgim/IEPC/case-of-the-month.html

93. Hallenbeck J, Arnold R. A request for nondisclosure: don't tell mother. *J Clin Oncol Off J Am Soc Clin Oncol.* November 2007;25(31):5030-5034.

94. Bertakis KD, Roter D, Putnam SM. The relationship of physician medical interview style to patient satisfaction. *J Fam Pract.* February 1991;32(2):175-181.

95. Roter DL, Hall JA, Kern DE, Barker LR, Cole KA, Roca RP. Improving physicians' interviewing skills and reducing patients' emotional distress. A randomized clinical trial. *Arch Intern Med.* September 1995;155(17):1877-1884.

CHAPTER 50

Psychosocial Consequences of Advanced Cancer

James R. Zabora ■ Matthew J. Loscalzo

All psychosocial care is palliative in nature. Attention must be directed to the realities of one's life within their unique social context in order to maximize internal resources, activate external support systems, and focus on the dignity and quality of life (QOL). Psychosocial care within palliative care programs seeks ongoing evidence of effectiveness and clear benefit to patients, caregivers, and the healthcare system. Palliative care is provided by interdisciplinary teams of compassionate experts, but if there is no team in place, true whole-patient-centered care is not possible (1). The creation of palliative care in hospitals has dramatically increased over the past 5 years (2); however, institutional support and integration into standard clinical care is still far less than is desirable.

Psychosocial concerns, to varying degrees, based on context and predisposition, are always at the core of the cancer experience. Life-limiting illness and related demands are always stressful. However, there are also opportunities for the repairing and deepening of relationships and to live a meaningful life. In the absence of moderate to severe distress caused by physical symptoms, such as pain, nausea, and difficulty in breathing, the psychosocial and spiritual aspects of a person's identity and life become paramount. The psychosocial aspects of a person's life are what give them a sense of being vital human beings within a social context for living with a life-threatening illness with the possibility for emotional growth and transcendence.

Despite significant progress in research and treatments, the diagnosis of cancer creates fear and turmoil in the lives of every patient and family. In many respects, cancer generates a greater sense of dread than other life-threatening illnesses with similar prognoses (3). Some studies have found that patients with cancer are sicker and have more symptoms than patients without cancer in the year before death, and most often, it is easier to predict the course of the illness (4). Yabroff and Youngmee (5) documented that many noxious physical and psychological symptoms are prevalent in the year after diagnosis, after disease-directed treatments have ceased, regardless of prognosis.

Frequently, the greatest concern of patients with cancer is not death, pain, or physical symptoms, but rather the impact of the disease on their families (6). People see themselves as imbedded in a larger social construct that gives them a sense of place and meaning. For most cancer patients, it is the family that is at the most basic core of that identity. According to the World Health Organization (7), family refers to those individuals who are either relatives or other significant people as defined by the patient. Healthcare professionals must acknowledge the role of the family to maximize treatment outcomes. If the family is actively incorporated into patient care, the healthcare team gains valuable allies and resources. Families are the primary source of support and also fill in the caregiving roles for persons with cancer. Of note, men are taking a greater responsibility for the care of seriously ill spouses, but women still comprise most of the individuals who serve in these caregiving roles (8,9).

Although access to ongoing palliative care could potentially provide needed support for both patient and family, resources for palliative care remain consistently limited. In the United States most palliative care is still invested in hospice programs, but only the median length of service for hospice patients continues at 3 weeks or less (10,11). Furthermore, a discussion concerning a referral to hospice can seem quite sudden, and the patient and family can experience this transition as rejection. Despite the sobering survival statistics for many cancers, relatively few hospitals have truly developed a continuum of cancer care, which informs patients and families that most antineoplastic therapy in advanced disease is palliative and not curative. In particular, this is true for patients with cancer who enroll in phase I and II clinical trials (12). This is significant given that most patients with cancer overestimate the probability of long-term survival (13). At present, patients and family members enter hospice care, which is the primary resource for comprehensive palliative care services, and attempt to accept that prolongation of life is no longer the goal of care. In addition to the shift in the focus from cure to care, the patient and family experience the loss of the healthcare team with whom trust has been imbued over months and sometimes many years. The loss occurs simultaneously at multiple levels. Although palliative care at the end of life should be a time of refocusing and resolution, the hospice referral process may cause an iatrogenic crisis rather than comfort. But even when patients are not transferred to an external setting trauma is common. This is especially true of patients who are admitted to ICUs where the caregivers of deceased patients all too frequently report symptoms (up to 20%) of posttraumatic distress disorder from the experience many years after the death (14). Consequently, the focus of care for patients with advanced disease needs to be the early identification of vulnerability, such as significantly elevated distress, that is followed by evidence-based psychosocial interventions.

PSYCHOLOGICAL RESPONSES TO ADVANCED CANCER

The psychological impact of advanced cancer and its management is directly influenced by the interactions among the degree of physical disability, the severity of symptoms, the internal resources of the patient, the level of social support, the intensity of the treatment, side effects and other adverse reactions, and the relationship with the healthcare team. The degree of physical distress placed on any individual and the inevitable drive to give meaning to the experience is the core from which the psychosocial concerns arise. At present, active support for aspects of palliative care is sporadic at best, especially in non-academic medical settings (15).

Adaptation to advancing disease begins with an appraisal of the extent of perceived harm, loss, threat, and challenge that this experience generates. In many respects, this appraisal is linked to the intensity and quality of the patient's emotional response. Emotional regulation is at the core of coping and has significant implications for maintaining a sense of direction and control. Overall, this primary appraisal, efficiency of emotional regulation, and definition of the meaning of advanced cancer result in an assessment of the extent of the potential harm and threat, which then requires a secondary appraisal to be made. In this secondary level, patients must assess their personal (internal) and social (external) resources necessary to begin to address the demands and problems associated with advanced cancer. This process can be significantly influenced by the patient's ability to maintain emotional regulation (16).

In addition, two salient continuums related to patient and family adaptation must be considered. The level of psychological distress forms the first continuum and the second consists of the predictable and transitional phases of the disease process. Patients with a preexisting high level of psychological distress can experience significant difficulty with any attempt to adapt to the stressors associated with a cancer diagnosis. Although most patients experience significant distress at the time of their diagnosis, most patients gradually adjust during the following 6 months (17). Evidence indicates that the best predictor of positive adaptation is the psychological state of the patient with cancer before the initiation of any therapeutic regimens (18). Although clinical experience would clearly indicate that the health system can influence the ability of patients and their families to adapt, literature to support this premise empirically is not available. Clinically, it is quite evident that hospitals do a very poor job at key (very common and entirely predictable) transition points in the care of seriously ill patients. But, there are now strong data that indicate palliative care for specific groups of cancer patients with advancing disease can extend both QOL and length of life (19).

Figure 50.1 details potential interventions along the disease and distress continuums. The level of psychological vulnerability also falls along a continuum from low to high distress and should guide this selection of interventions (20). In addition, problem-solving interventions have been demonstrated to reduce distress among patients with cancer as well as among family members (21,22). Prevalence studies demonstrate that one of every three newly diagnosed patients (regardless of prognosis) needs psychosocial or psychiatric intervention (23–26). As disease advances, a positive relationship exists between the increase in the occurrence and severity of physiologic symptoms and the patient's level of emotional distress and overall QOL. For example, a study of 268 patients with cancer having recurrent disease observed that patients with higher symptomatology, greater financial concerns, and a pessimistic outlook experience higher levels of psychological distress and lower levels of general wellbeing (27).

In an effort to establish early identification of patients at high risk for poor adaptation, the National Comprehensive Cancer Network (NCCN) developed guidelines for the

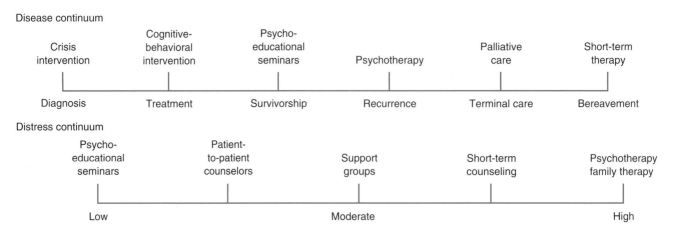

Figure 50.1. Continuum of care for patients with cancer and their families.

management of psychological distress among cancer patients across the disease continuum. The NCCN described distress in a manner consistent with the focus and goals of palliative care, as an experience that can be psychological, social, or spiritual which interferes with one's ability to manage or problem-solve in relation to the diagnosis, treatment, side effects, and symptoms associated with cancer (28). These guidelines provide a framework for the development and implementation of psychosocial interventions based on the perspectives of psychiatry, social work, psychology, nursing, and pastoral care. Psychosocial screening serves as the mechanism to identify patients at higher levels of risk in order to provide interventions at a much earlier point in time. These guidelines can be accessed at www.nccs.org.

If distress levels can be identified through techniques such as psychosocial screening, patients can then be introduced into supportive care systems earlier in the treatment or palliative care process. In fact, nationally and internationally, a number of investigators have successfully implemented robust biopsychosocial screening initiatives as part of the standard of clinical care in cancer setting (e.g., J. Zabora, M. Loscalzo, B. Bultz, and A. Mitchell). All of these screening programs use instruments that include psychological and physical symptoms, as well as social, spiritual, and practical concerns (28). Some of these programs use automated referrals or triages, provide educational information, and send clinical summary alerts to the physician and team during the clinical encounter (29). Of significant importance, the influential Institute of Medicine report in 2007, Cancer Care for the Whole Patient: Meeting Psychosocial Health Needs, has endorsed biopsychosocial screening as the minimum standard of quality cancer care (30). Subsequently, the American College of Surgeons (ACoS) has established a new standard that requires screening for distress in ACoS accredited programs. In Canada, distress has been endorsed as the sixth vital sign (31).

Accordingly, any attempt to identify vulnerable patients and families in a prospective manner is worthwhile. Screening techniques are available through the use of standardized instruments that are able to prospectively identify patients and families that may be more vulnerable to the cancer experience (32,33). Preexisting psychosocial resources are critical in any predictive or screening process. In one approach, Weisman et al. (34) delineated key psychosocial variables in the format of a structured interview accompanied by a self-report measure (Table 50.1). However, in hospitals, clinics, or community agencies, which provide care to a high volume of patients and family members, a structured interview by a psychosocial provider is seldom feasible or even warranted. Consequently, brief and rapid methods of screening are necessary. Brief screening techniques that examine components of distress, such as anxiety or depression, can be incorporated into the routine clinical care of the patient. But only screening for psychiatric symptoms is not adequate. Just as cancer patients should not have to be dying to receive the full suite of palliative care services, patients and their families should not have to manifest psychiatric symptoms to receive psychosocial support. Early psychosocial interventions may be less stigmatizing to the patient, and more readily accepted by patients, families, and staff if screening identifies the management of distress as one component of comprehensive care (35). Screening is also a cost-effective technique for case identification in comparison to an assessment of all new patients (36). Although screening for distress and disease-related problems have received much attention recently, there are relatively few screening programs in place, even in comprehensive cancer centers (37). The City of Hope National Medical Center and NCI-designated Comprehensive Cancer Center in Duarte, California, is one of the few cancer programs that is screening patients with cancer for common problems and related distress. A fully automated touchscreen system (*SupportScreen*) has been in place since 2009 and has been licensed to a number of hospitals (29). *SupportScreen* provides an opportunity for the patients (and in some clinics family caregivers) to input their own information (in English and Spanish) relating to

TABLE 50.1	Variables associated with psychosocial adaptation		
Social Support	**History**	**Current Concerns**	**Other Variables**
Marital status	Substance abuse	Health	Education
Living arrangements	Depression	Religion	Employment
Number of family members and relatives in vicinity	Mental health	Work-finance	Physical symptoms
Church attendance	Major illness	Family	Anatomic staging
	Past regrets	Friends	
	Optimism vs. pessimism	Existential	
		Self-appraisal	

From Weisman AD, Worden JW, Sobel HJ. *Psychosocial Screening and Interventions with Patients with Cancer: A Research Report.* Boston, MA: Harvard Medical School and Massachusetts Hospital; 1980, with permission.

immediate psychological and physical symptoms as well as social, spiritual, and practical concerns. Patients are able to indicate the degree of distress they are experiencing as well as the kind of assistance they are seeking from the healthcare team. Personalized educational sheets and resources are also provided, all in real time during the actual clinical encounter. The physician and healthcare team also automatically receive paper and electronic clinical alerts right before they meet with the patient. This technology has been very well received by physicians and staff, patients (of all adult ages), and family members. The experience at the City of Hope and other hospitals has demonstrated that patients prefer touchscreen technology to either paper and pencil and to a personal interviews and provide more personal information in this medium (38). The items on the screening instrument have also been tailored for individual clinics by medical specialty. The implications for the integration of palliative care into the standard of clinical care are of major importance. Many of the domains that relate to serious illness are emotionally laden and many physicians and healthcare providers lack the time, training, or inclination to open conversations that are essential to the psychological well-being of patients and their concerned family members. In this instance, it is quite evident that this technology and biopsychosocial content have the potential to transform the clinical encounter and the relationship between patients and their healthcare providers.

For each of the problems listed, a triage plan is in place and can be accessed during the clinical visit by the physician, nurse, or social worker. The social worker assesses the potential need for referrals to psychology and psychiatry. Not surprisingly, the 10 most common problems in rank order manifested by the first 300 patients with cancer at the City of Hope were fatigue (feeling tired), fear and worry about the future, finances, pain, feeling down, depressed or blue, being dependent on others, understanding my treatment options, sleeping, managing my emotions, and solving problems due to my illness. Of particular note, although pain was not the most frequently endorsed problem, it was the most emotionally distressing.

Standardized measures of psychological distress can differentiate patients into low, moderate, or high degrees of vulnerability. Patients with a low or moderate level of distress may benefit from a psychoeducational program, which can enhance adaptive capabilities and problem-solving skills; high distress patients possess more complex psychosocial needs that require brief therapy or family therapy along with psychotropic drug therapy for the patient. For some patients ongoing mental health services are essential, whereas other patients may require assistance only at critical transition points. Clinical practice suggests that virtually all patients could benefit from some type of psychosocial intervention at some point along the disease continuum, especially at the end of life. Psychosocial interventions include educational programs, support groups, cognitive-behavioral techniques, problem-solving therapy or education, and psychotherapy (39). To further

facilitate the process of screening, the brief standardized instruments have been developed to create greater ease of administration and scoring and to develop gender-based norms (40,41).

The second continuum relates to the predictable phases of the disease process. This disease continuum extends from the point of diagnosis to cancer therapies and beyond. Across this continuum, patients acquire experiences, knowledge, and skills that enable them to respond to the demands of their disease. The needs of a newly diagnosed patient with intractable symptoms differ significantly from a patient who has advanced disease and no further options for curative treatments.

The patient and family may be supported throughout the illness process and the family requires continuing support following the death of the patient. At times families are overwhelmed by the illness and as a result are unable to effectively respond. For some families, a death may represent a major loss of the family's identity and may paralyze the family's coping and problem-solving responses. Failure to respond and solve problems leads to a lack of control and may generate a significant potential for a chronic grief reaction (42). Although the disease continuum consists of specific points, Table 50.2 identifies a series of predictable and relevant crisis events and psychosocial challenges that occur as patients and families confront advanced disease.

FAMILY ADAPTABILITY AND COHESION

The circumplex model of family functioning, as developed by Olson et al. (43), categorizes families in a manner that explains the variation in their behavior. Although not specifically developed for cancer, this model conceptualizes families' responses to stressful events based on two constructs: adaptability and cohesion. The end-of-life care simultaneously generates significant stressors for both patients and families, especially in issues related to power, structure, and role assignments. Adaptability reflects the capability of a family to reorganize internal roles, rules, and power structure in response to a significant stressor. Given the impact of advancing cancer on the total family unit, families must frequently reassign roles, alter rules for daily living, and revise long-held methods for problem solving. Dysfunction in the family can relate to either low adaptability (rigidity) or excessively high adaptability (chaotic). A family characterized as rigid in its adaptability persists in the use of coping behaviors, such as frequent manifestations of anger, even when they are ineffective. Those that exhibit high adaptability create a chaotic response within the power structure, roles, and rules of the family; such families lack structure in their responses and attempt different coping strategies with every new stress. Although most families are in the more functional category of "structured adaptability," 30% are rigid or chaotic. These latter families are likely to exhibit problematic behaviors such as excessive demands of staff time or interference with the delivery of medical care that the healthcare team may find difficult to manage (44).

TABLE 50.2	**Advancing disease and psychosocial treatment**				
Crisis Event	**Personal Meaning**	**Manifestation**	**Coping Tasks**	**Survivor Goals**	**Professional Interventions**
Recurrence/ new primary	What did I do wrong?	Anger	Reestablish hope	Integrate reality with family functioning, maintain self-worth	Information
	Was it my negative attitude?	Fear	Accept the uncertainty about the future		Support
		Depression			Education
	Was I foolish to hope this was over forever?	Anxiety	Understand information about new situation		Cognitive/behavioral skills training
		Shock			
	God has failed me	Loss of hope	Regain a life focus and time perspective appropriate to the changed prognosis		Physical availability
	I beat this last time, I will beat it again	Denial			Supportive psychotherapy
		Guilt			Resource provision/referral
	Nothing ever works out good for me	Loss of trust	Communicate new status to others		
		Feelings of alienation			
	They said I was okay but I am not	Increased vulnerability	Make decisions about the new treatment course		
		Loss of control			
	Do I have to start all over again?	Confronting mortality	Integrate reality of ongoing nature of disease to probable death from cancer		
		Search for meaning			
			Tolerate changes in routine and roles again		
			Adjust to increased dependency again		
			Reinvest in treatment		
Advanced disease	I am out of control	Depression	Maintain hope and direction	Dignity	Support
	Will they offer new treatment?	Anxiety	Tolerate medical care	Direction	Cognitive/behavioral skills training
		Demoralization	Enhance coping skills	Role in work, family, and community	Supportive psychotherapy
	What am I doing wrong?	Fear	Maintain open communication with family, friends, and healthcare professionals		Physical availability
	Will it be as bad as the last time?	Denial			Resource provision/referral
		Anger	Assess treatment and care options		Information
	Will I go broke?	Fear of intimacy	Maintain relationships with medical team		Education

(Continued)

TABLE 50.2   Advancing disease and psychosocial treatment (*Continued*)

Crisis Event	Personal Meaning	Manifestation	Coping Tasks	Survivor Goals	Professional Interventions
Terminal	When am I going to die?	Depression	Maintain a meaningful quality of life	Dignity	Physical availability
	Does dying hurt?	Fear	Adjust to physical deterioration	Family support and bereavement	Support
	What happens after you die?	Anxiety	Plan for surviving family members		Cognitive/behavioral skills training
		Denial	Accept reality of prognosis		Therapeutic rituals
	Why me? Why now?	Demoralization	Mourn actual losses		Coordination of services
	What did I do to deserve this?	Self-destructive behavior	Mourn the death of dreams		Advocacy
	What will happen to my family?	Loss of control	Get things in order		Information
	Will I be remembered by my family and friends?	Guilt	Maintain and end significant relationships		
		Anger			
	What if I start to die and I am all alone?	Fear of abandonment	Say good-bye to family and friends		
		Fear of isolation			
	Can't the doctors do something else, are they holding back on me, have they given up on me?	Increased dependency	Accept impending death		
		Acceptance	Confront the relevant existential and spiritual issues		
		Withdrawal			
		Search for meaning in past as well as present	Talk about feelings		
		Pain/suffering	Review one's life		
		Need to discuss afterlife			

From Mitchell SL, Teno JM, Miller SC, Mor V. A national study of the location of death for older persons with dementia. *J Am Geriatr Soc.* 2005;53(2):299–305.

The second construct of Olson et al.—cohesion—is indicative of the family's ability to provide adequate support (43). Cohesion is the level of emotional bonding that exists among family members and is also conceptualized on a continuum from low to high. Low cohesion (disengagement) suggests little or no connectedness among family members. A commitment to care for other family members is not evident, and, as a result, these families are frequently unavailable to the medical staff for support of the patient or for participation in the decision-making process. At the other extreme, high cohesion (enmeshment) blurs the boundaries among family members. This results in the perception by healthcare providers that some family members seem to be just as affected by the diagnosis or treatment or by each symptom, as the patient. Enmeshed families may demand excessive amounts of time from the healthcare team and be incapable of following simple medical directives. These families are not able to objectively receive and comprehend information that may be in the best interest of the patient. Also these families may assume a highly overprotective position in relation to the patient and may speak for the patient even when the patient's self-expression could be encouraged.

When engaging families, it is necessary to gain an appreciation for the rules and regulations within each particular family. Each family has its own rules, regulations, and communication styles. In gaining an understanding of the role of the patient in the family, it is helpful to ask the patient to describe the specific responsibilities he or she performs in the family, especially during a crisis. Generalities are less informative than descriptions of the specific experiences and duties of each family member during a crisis. These queries enable the patient to openly communicate and objectively evaluate his or her role and importance in the family system and provide a clinical opportunity to assess ongoing progress or deterioration. Patients and families can usually tolerate even the worst news or the most dire prognosis as long as it is framed within a context in which the patient and family know how they are expected to respond and that the healthcare team will not abandon them.

IMPACT OF PHYSICAL AND PSYCHOLOGICAL SYMPTOMS

Patients with advanced illness experience pain, delirium, dyspnea, fatigue, nausea, anxiety, depression, sleeplessness, and many other symptoms that impair QOL. These noxious symptoms also compromise cognition, concentration, and memory (45) and may override the underlying mental schema of patients. For the person in pain or acute physical distress, perception is confined to only the most immediate and essential elements of his or her sensory experience, and there is only a distant remnant of a past or future. The immediate need and goal is to stop or minimize the noxious experience. In some sense, pain and other symptoms absorb the limited psychic energy of the patient, and valuable energy can only be made available if physical distress is effectively managed. The psychic life is subservient and dependent to the bodily experience. This is an important point for healthcare providers. Therefore, psychosocial interventions must simultaneously focus on physical symptoms in order to be effective. Furthermore, interventions that do not address the physical concerns of the patient may be unethical. The essence of psychosocial care is to raise the "bar" of what humanistic medical care means so that all of the concerns and needs of patients are effectively addressed and resolved. Unless physical and psychosocial distress are managed simultaneously, psychosocial interventions are less likely to be effective.

Moderate to severe pain is reported by 30% to 45% of patients undergoing (34) cancer treatments and 75% to 90% of patients with advanced disease (46). Pain seems to stand alone in its ability to gain the active attention of others although dramatically demonstrating a sense of being alone and vulnerable. This is especially true of patients with advanced disease and their families. Although a patient is experiencing pain, another person only inches away is incapable of truly understanding what is so central and undeniable to the patient. This invisible and almost palpable boundary between the person in pain and his or her caregivers has significant implications for the quality and effectiveness of the therapeutic relationship (47,48).

Given that cancer pain can be adequately managed in almost all circumstances, its deleterious and at times life-threatening impact on the physical, psychological, and spiritual resources of both the patient and family are not only unnecessary but also evil. There is no known benefit to ongoing unrelieved pain. There are many known negative consequences. For example, O'Mahony et al. (49) found that the desire for death was correlated with ratings of pain and low family support but most significantly with depression. Given the relationship between pain and depression, the importance of adequate pain management can hardly be overstated. Recently Cobb et al. (50), in their comprehensive review of the delirium literature, found that poor pain control was identified as the number one cause or contributor for delirium. Given the obvious importance and prevalence of delirium as an indicator of QOL at the end of life, this is very important information.

Serlin et al. (51) were able to demonstrate that there is a positive correlation between pain intensity and function. As expected, low levels of pain intensity cause low levels of interference with life, whereas moderate to high levels of pain make it virtually impossible to have meaningful interactions with others and to feel part of a larger whole. Clinical experience consistently demonstrates that people with physical illness accompanied by high levels of pain intensity experience acute isolation, are unable to advocate for themselves, and are at very high risk to be badly cared for even in the best medical centers. Family and healthcare providers can be sensitive, caring, supportive, and concerned, but if pain is not adequately managed, the person confronting death has little possibility to think clearly, express his or her concerns, make a contribution, and have anything resembling a peaceful death.

It is generally accepted that pain is poorly managed despite the availability of effective therapies (52–54). Of particular note, effective pain management may also be influenced by the race and ethnicity of the patient, but socioeconomic disadvantage is the more important predictor of disabling pain (55). Patients, families, and professional staff may share a reluctance to use opioid analgesics even when life expectancy is quite limited. Dysfunctional processes continue to exist which enable patients to accept suffering and to allow the healthcare team to permit unnecessary pain. This type of response represents an adaptive, but "dark side" of professional care. Although most patients with cancer are psychologically healthy (23,56), inadequately managed cancer pain and other symptoms can produce a variety of "pseudopsychiatric" syndromes, which are anxiety-provoking and confusing to patients, families, and clinicians. Patients with cancer and pain are also more likely to develop psychiatric disorders than patients with cancer without significant pain (54). In the short term, pain provokes anxiety; over the long term, it generates depression and demoralization. Misguided priorities in the heathcare system frequently result in needless pain and suffering in patients, and long-term guilt in family members and permanent mistrust of the intentions of healthcare providers.

The differences between depression and demoralization as clinical constructs have yet to be empirically explored. Depression is significantly related to higher levels of cancer pain and pain is likely to play a causal role related to depression. Overall depression rates for cancer patients are 20% to 25% (57) and estimates as high as 50% to 70% have been applied to populations with advanced disease (58). Patients who are demoralized are disheartened or discouraged by their circumstances but not in a pathologic sense. There is a significant correlation between affective disorders and pain and among the negative emotional states associated with pain (dysphoria, hopelessness, guilt, suicidal ideation, etc.). Anecdotal clinical experience consistently demonstrates that once pain and related distressing physical symptoms are relieved, and suffering, anxiety, depression, demoralization, and suicidal ideation are ameliorated, the impact on the family is equally significant (59).

Patients who are depressed distort reality and grossly minimize their perceived abilities in managing the demands of the illness and its treatment. Furthermore, patients with cancer who are depressed and have inadequately controlled pain are at increased risk for suicide (49,60). For the patient who is depressed, acute sensitivity to physical sensations may lead to or exaggerate preexisting morbid or catastrophizing thoughts. The complex and interactive associations among physical sensations (neutral or noxious sensations), mentation (personal meaning given to the sensations), and behaviors (attempts to minimize threat and regain control) are all negatively influenced by depression. The destructive synergy of unrelieved pain and depression may lead to overwhelming suffering in patients and families and to a shared sense of helplessness and hopelessness (61). Consequently, a patient or family may develop the faulty perception that suicide is

their only remaining vestige of control. From this perspective, the value of a multimodality approach that combines pharmacology, supportive psychotherapy, and cognitive-behavioral skills training is clear (62). From a psychological perspective, promotion of compliance with medical regimens; correction of distorted cognitive perceptions; acquisition of coping skills to manage physical tension, stress, and pain; and the effective use of valuable physical energy to maximize engagement of life become the focus of care.

SOCIOCULTURAL INFLUENCES ON PATIENT AND FAMILY ADAPTATION

Perceptions of illness and death can be conceptualized as experiences with both conscious and unconscious associations. These perceptions include concerns and fears that are beyond the limits of objective knowledge. Sociocultural beliefs may soothe anxiety or fear by providing comfort when a vacuum exists due to a lack of experience in the management of a chronic illness. Sociocultural attitudes also exert considerable influence as patients approach the end of their lives (63,64). These beliefs and attitudes are evident in direct observations of how the family cares for the patient, views of an afterlife, and rituals related to how the corpse is to be managed.

Koenig and Gates-Williams (65) offer a framework to assess cultural responses relevant to palliative care. This framework, which is consistent with a comprehensive psychosocial assessment, posits that "culture is only meaningful when interpreted in the context of a patient's unique history, family constellation, and socioeconomic status. Dangers exist in creating negative stereotypes—in simply supplying clinicians with an atlas or map of "cultural traits common among particular ethnic groups."

Patients and their families can simply not be adequately understood without knowledge of their sociocultural backgrounds (66). Patients and families vary according to interests, beliefs, values, and attitudes. Individuals learn attitudes or values through family interactions and these patterns influence how patients respond to the healthcare team. Although the healthcare team represents expertise, safety, and authority, it is also an external and foreign force, which only through necessity has gained influence and power within the family system. In stressful situations, the patient and family may project their own perceptions about themselves onto the healthcare team.

Although cultural characteristics are important, these influences often diminish over time as families are assimilated into the predominant culture. Second-generation families are more similar to the host country than the country of origin. First-generation immigrants may possess old-world attitudes and values about authority and illness, whereas the perspectives of their offspring will be more consistent with the healthcare team.

Given the many and complex demands already made on healthcare professionals and the rapidly increasing diversity of institutions, is it reasonable to expect that staff be informed about the myriad cultures represented in such a pluralistic environment? For example, it is estimated that there are over 150 different languages spoken among the Native Americans, with each tribe having its own rituals around the end of life (67). One can only imagine trying to provide bereavement services to a group that demands that the name of the deceased never be mentioned again. Or that believes that even mentioning the word death will cause the event to happen. These barriers to effective and open communication, so respected by healthcare professionals in the United States, are not unique to Native Americans (68). Furthermore, evidence exists that African Americans are far less likely to discuss the end-of-life issues due to a belief that these discussions may result in less care being delivered (69).

Although there is no formula to making a connection with another person when he or she is ill, there are some areas that can be explored together that can be mutually enriching. The healthcare provider needs to specifically ask the patient and family about them as a system, patient, family, tribe, group, and so on. Some examples are as follows:

- Because everyone is different, can you teach me how to help you get the information you need about your illness?
- How would you like me to share information with you about your illness?
- How much information, if any, would you like me to share with your family and others?
- Is there a particular person you would like me to include when you and I talk about serious matters?
- Would you like me to give you an overview of what is happening to you each time we meet, or would you like me to simply answer your specific questions?
- What is your understanding of your health right now?
- What kinds of information would you like me to tell you?
- You have a very serious illness. Some people want to know what they have to prepare for in the near future. Is there anything that you would like to know now?
- Is there anything you think we need to share with your family and others that may be helpful to them and you?
- Is there anything we can do together to make this time meaningful for you and your family?
- Would you feel comfortable contacting me if you have any questions?

Ultimately, a relationship is always between two people at a time. Opening up one's self to be taught by the patient and family about who they are and how they want to manage the illness is the perfect counterpoint to the awesome power held by healthcare professionals.

PRINCIPLES OF EFFECTIVE PATIENT AND FAMILY MANAGEMENT

The family, as defined by the patient, is virtually always the primary supportive structure for the patient. The family serves as a supportive environment, which provides instrumental assistance, psychological support, and consistent encouragement, so that the patient seeks the best available medical care. Early in the diagnostic and treatment planning phases, a family's

primary functions are to instill hope and facilitate communication. For the patient whose disease is beyond life-prolonging therapy, caregiving becomes the primary focus for the family. In the latter situation, families must prepare psychologically and financially for the experience of life without the patient (anticipatory grief). Cancer and its treatments is always a crisis and an assault on the family system. As an uninvited intruder, cancer challenges the viability of the family structure to tolerate and integrate a harsh and threatening reality, which cannot be overcome by force, denial, or even joint action. Joint action can be successful in terms of adaptation, and if the goals are clearly defined, there is an ongoing plan that promotes the optimal opportunity for successful goal attainment.

The healthcare team can guide the family in developing a problem-solving approach to the demands of the illness. Problem-solving therapy conceived by D'Zurilla, Nezu, and others defines problem solving as a series of tasks rather than a single skill. According to the theoretical model, successful problem solving requires five component processes, each of which contributes directly to effective problem resolution (70,71). The five components are as follows:

1. Problem orientation, definition, and formulation
2. Generation of alternatives
3. Decision making
4. Solution implementation
5. Verification

Problem orientation involves a motivational process; the other components consist of specific skills and abilities that enable a person to effectively solve a particular problem. Because problem solving is a set of skills, this approach has also been provided as an educational format.

The basic notion underlying the relevance of problem solving for cancer patients lies in the moderating role of coping through problem-solving serves in the general stress–distress relationship (72). The more effective people are in resolving or coping with stressful problems, the more probable it is that they will experience a higher QOL as compared with those persons facing similar problems who have difficulty in coping. Families also require guidance and support in managing the multiple problems associated with cancer, related treatments, adverse reactions, and rehabilitation. Following the diagnosis of cancer, families need to have honest, intelligible, and timely information whereas being reassured that competent healthcare professionals are genuinely caring for their family member.

Previous research indicates that problem-solving education for family caregivers improves their ability to manage care better and cope more effectively with the stressors generated by caregiving. D'Zurilla, Nezu, and others (73,74) have developed conceptual frameworks for problem-solving therapy and have conducted research that demonstrates that counseling caregivers, who are under stress, reduces their distress while increasing their problem-solving competence. This conceptual model has been applied successfully with a number of diverse health-related problems, including cancer (75). Toseland et al. (76) have shown that problem-solving counseling of family caregivers lessened caregiver distress and reduced long-term depression in the patients.

Therapeutic treatment plans must always be clearly communicated because it delineates each individual's responsibility so that the potential for goal attainment is maximized. For many families with histories of effective functioning, the cancer experience represents the first time that their joint action may not overcome an external threat. Consequently, the cancer experience must be reframed into more realistic terms so that the threat can be perceived as manageable rather than destructive. If this is not achieved, the family can manifest anger, avoidance, displacement, or other forms of regressive behavior. For the family with a history of multiple defeats and failures, the cancer experience may be perceived as more evidence that they are incapable of managing the demands of an overwhelming world. The cancer experience temporarily alters the family structure, but it also has the potential to inflict permanent change. The healthcare team can significantly influence how these changes are interpreted and integrated into family life.

Patients often identify the effect on the family as the most upsetting repercussion of the cancer (5). Therefore, any effective intervention must include the patient, family, and other social support networks. When patients consider their families, they may experience guilt, shame, anger, frustration, and fear of abandonment. Family members may experience anger, fear, powerlessness, survivor guilt, and confusion as they attempt to care for the patient. Family members may demonstrate the defense mechanism of displacement, transferring emotion from one person or situation to another and potentially confusing healthcare professionals. This confusion can create tension for family members and providers at a time when clarity and effective interactions are essential.

With little exception, assessment of the primary players in the family system is a rather straightforward process. The patient can be asked the following directly:

- Who do you rely on most to assist you in relation to the practical needs of your illness (e.g., transportation and insurance company negotiations)?
- With whom do you share your emotional concerns? (e.g., the kind of thoughts you have if you wake up in the middle of the night and fears about dying)?
- When you get scared or confused, with whom in your family are you most able to talk?
- Who in your family most concerns you?
- Is anyone in your family overwhelmed with your ongoing medical and practical needs?
- Who in your family is coping least well with your illness?
- Is anyone in your family openly angry with you because of your illness?
- Are you particularly worried about how a specific person in your family is coping?
- Who is most dependent on you in your family?
- For what are they dependent on you?
- What would happen to your family if you were unable to maintain your present level of functioning?
- Are you ever concerned that the demands of your illness will be too much for your family?

The answers to these questions communicate to the patient and family that it is appropriate and necessary to gauge the impact of the cancer and its treatment on their lives and also provide the groundwork for the coordination of patient and family functions. In addition, role modeling of open communication provides an environment of emotional support, flexibility in roles, trust, and the implied and spoken promise never to abandon each other. This cannot be achieved unless the patient and family accept that some treatment effects and life events are beyond their control and there are limits to what is possible. The medical team has the responsibility to manage the physical aspects of the disease, whereas the patient and family actively strive to integrate change, maintain normalcy, and accept the reality of the illness. The course of the illness—including death—must be identified as one of the potentially uncontrollable issues so the patient and family can focus on areas that are amenable to their influence.

Financial resources are virtually always a major concern of patients and families. When discussions of money and resources occur within the family system, shame and guilt are common. These emotions are frequently alluded to but not openly discussed. This can be a barrier to open communication and can lead to patient's fears and fantasies of abandonment. This is especially true for patients with advancing disease. Simultaneously, the family may have concerns about life goals after the patient's acute need is past or death occurs. The expected range of emotional reactions within the family includes anger, fear, guilt, anxiety, frustration, powerlessness, and confusion. Cancer confronts people with the reality of limitations.

In addition to the increasing costs of health insurance and home care, there is a wide variety of nonreimbursable, illness-related costs that can be financially devastating to patients and families. Transportation, nutritional supplements, temporary housing, child care, and lost work days are but a few examples of costs borne almost totally by patients and families for which there is seldom any form of reimbursement (77). Schulz et al. (27) found that respondents spent more than $200 per month on health-related expenses and reported significant negative effects on the amount of time worked. Other studies have confirmed the negative financial impact of advanced cancer (78,79).

Money is almost always a metaphor for value, control, and power (80). How patients and family members communicate about money can be an indication of their perceptions of whether treatment is progressing or not. Therefore, interchanges about financial matters can actively represent latent communications about the perceived but unexpressed value of care and its potential outcome. For example, the patient and family may at the beginning of treatment state that money is no object and all resources must be expended so that the patient survives. When treatment becomes prolonged, however, a much more sober and realistic view concerning valuable and vanishing resources may become evident, and a greater discussion of investment and return may ensue. At this point in time, both patient and family may be actually talking about their ability to persevere. Concerns about money may then be an expression of exhaustion, diminishing hope, or anger. It is important that this metaphorical communication be seen as inadequate for open and direct communication. A metaphor is a signal and cue that indicate the need for open discussion. Openness is essential for the patient and family to discuss both their common and increasingly diverging needs. Patients and families must discuss their physical and spiritual fatigue, as well as specific financial concerns related to diminishing resources as a result of their struggle with cancer. The following clinical example illustrates a number of these points.

A 54-year-old married woman with three adolescent daughters expressed concern to the medical team about the ongoing cost of care for her terminally ill husband. The team felt that she was selfish and that it was unethical for them to consider the financial impact on the family in caring for the patient. Sensing their resistance to her plight, she felt rejected and became irate. A meeting with the patient, family, and relevant staff was organized by the social worker to openly address her financial concerns. The family had existing financial debts due to past medical treatments and consequently had ample reason for its concern related to the additional costs of care. Once this meeting resolved concerns over additional unneeded expenditures, the focus shifted to the much more emotionally laden issues related to the slow deterioration of the patient and the family's intense grief over the impending loss. It became evident that money for the family represented the loss of "everything."

In some cases, the family may begin to perceive the dying patient as already being deceased. Anticipatory grief and premature emotional withdrawal from the dying patient creates confusion and a sense of terror in the patient. As a result, the family experiences guilt and shame because they are prepared for the loss but the patient is still alive.

SPECIFIC PROBLEMATIC PATIENT AND FAMILY BEHAVIORS

Physicians almost always identify "difficult families" as one of the most challenging tasks as a medical provider. Within the context of the family milieu, conflicts with staff may be unavoidable. It is the management of these conflicts that will determine the quality of the relationship between the patient, family, and professional staff. Conflicts may result if a family cannot follow simple guidelines or is intolerant of any physical discomfort that the patient may experience. Families that frequently criticize staff may be held to more rigid standards of behavior. Unit guidelines become laws, and the struggle for control results in fear and mistrust. Conversely, patients and families who endear themselves to staff through verbal praise of the quality of care often receive warmth and flexibility, and, as a result, unit guidelines, such as visiting hours or number of visitors, may be relaxed.

The professional staff must be flexible in their communication styles or they may be perceived as violating family boundaries. This type of interaction can devolve into a

battle for power and control. Conflicts that remain at the level of power and control make it virtually impossible to work with the patient and family to develop action-oriented, problem-solving strategies, which unite all in a common set of values and goals. Effective symptom management is essential to engage the patient, family, and the staff toward a common goal. Poor management can lead to estrangement and abandonment (81). Open communication can establish goals within the context of the family and significantly reduce the strain. However, healthcare providers must accept that at times any approach may be ineffective because the family structure cannot tolerate the influence of external forces. When this occurs continued attempts at open communication is the only alternative that can achieve some sense of mutual understanding and trust.

Families can exhibit a range of behaviors that the healthcare team defines as problematic and can potentially interfere with the delivery of medical care. Families can delay or prevent the completion of a procedure, verbally abuse the staff, or divide the team. Families may demand excessive amounts of staff time, repeatedly demanding sessions to review the same information. Confusion may reflect intense anxiety and the overwhelming nature of this experience for caregivers. Some families have unrealistic expectations and compare the responses of staff members searching for inconsistencies. Others fail to follow unit guidelines, consistently arriving well before visiting hours or delaying their departure from the hospital at the end of the day. Families may encourage patients to refuse medical recommendations or directives. Family members at times may speak for the patient and encourage the patient to withdraw and regress. Families may also possess unrealistic expectations of staff. Family members may perceive the staff as their own medical providers and seek personal care from the team (44).

Family functions include facilitation of medical decision making, reduction of stress, initiation of effective problem solving, and provision of comfort to the patient. If the family cannot provide these functions or is unavailable to the patient and staff, the staff may need to assume and fulfill these roles. At times, the staff may be resentful when families are unavailable or withdraw from participation. The burden on staff to care for these patients can be dramatically increased.

SPECIAL PATIENT AND FAMILY ISSUES

Children in the Home

Children of adult patients with cancer may be an unseen and forgotten population. In acute care settings, children are not observed due to the patients' daytime appointments or policies that prohibit visits to inpatient units. Within the palliative setting, however, children and grandchildren are often present and may play an active role in the caregiving process.

Although salient developmental differences exist among children of different ages, those 3 years or older are able to verbally communicate their concerns so that an ongoing dialogue can occur. Highly sensitive to emotional and physical changes, children benefit most from an environment where they are continually given information in a manner that they can understand and are then encouraged to ask questions. Adults should be prepared for questions to be rather concrete and egocentric, centered around the immediate needs of the child and any potential change in the immediate family. Children are specifically concerned about the continued presence of parents and their own safety. Questions from children usually come one or two at a time. Children often need time to interpret and integrate the adult responses before returning for additional information, which may occur days or weeks later.

Methods to deliver medical information or relieve distress must vary according to each child's developmental stage. Children have fantasies about the etiology, meaning, and duration of a parent's illness. Young children need consistent information about the chronic nature of the disease so that they can anticipate changes and incorporate an understanding of these medical events into their world. Young children cannot fully appreciate the concept of permanence. The permanence of death or abstract terms, such as "forever," are beyond their ability to integrate on a cognitive level. Children need consistent support, measured doses of information, and an environment that can respond to their questions.

Developmentally, adolescence is the time for resolution of conflicts with parents as well as a quickened pace to individuation from the family. These processes can be delayed or significantly complicated by the family's focus on a loved one who is slowly deteriorating and dying. Competitiveness, sexuality, aggression, and peer relationships may compound and confuse attempts to cope with a loss and the end of a specific relationship.

Familial roles can be disrupted or confused during a parent's illness, and, as a result, adolescents may be required to assume adult responsibilities. There is a danger in treating an adolescent as an adult. The demands of adolescence under normal circumstances generate numerous stressors for the family, and a chronic illness at this point in the life cycle can significantly exacerbate the family's level of distress. Of particular concern, adolescents may be "parentified." Physical maturity should not be equated with emotional, intellectual, or spiritual development. Adolescents can easily be overwhelmed with guilt and shame when their normal sense of power and grandiosity cannot control symptoms or death. This may have a long-term negative effect on the ability to tolerate emotional relationships. If the death of a parent or grandparent is to occur in the home, children must be carefully assessed, and appropriate interventions and support should be offered.

Psychiatric Illness

Histories of psychiatric disorders present further challenges in the effective management of patients and families. Psychiatric symptoms must be assessed and appropriately managed if the patient is to truly benefit from supportive care interventions. For example, symptoms, such as severe depression, may dramatically influence a patient's perception of pain and the ability of the healthcare team to control it. Furthermore, psychiatric symptoms of a family member can also cause a significant concern given the healthcare team's expectations concerning caregiving in the home by family members. Frequently, expectations of family members as caregivers are relatively uniform despite the significant variation that exists in each family's level of functioning. Families must be assessed not only for their availability but also for their ability to provide adequate supportive care.

Patients or family members with a history of physical or sexual abuse may exhibit significant difficulty in the ability to develop a trusting relationship with the healthcare team and may require psychiatric management. Families with a history of abuse may try to withhold information related to the abuse and any attempt to assess the patient or family as an intrusion. Trust can only be developed over time as the healthcare team consistently verbalizes their concern for patient and family as well as their availability for support and intervention. Families with severe dysfunction isolate and protect themselves from the outside world with rigid outer boundaries. Healthcare providers may define such a family as problematic when initial offers of assistance are refused. The team may experience frustration and rejection, which is inevitably communicated directly to the patient and family. Consequently, the family is lost as an ally and resource and, as a result, their isolation is increased. Although few in number, timely psychiatric referrals for these patients and family members are essential.

Addictions

A current or past history of substance abuse or an active addiction within the patient or the family creates a sense of alarm within the healthcare team. For example, the patient with a history of substance abuse may simply not be trusted by healthcare providers. The patient's behavior may be viewed as manipulative and if pain is a problem, there may be reticence to prescribe higher opioid doses if the patient is in pain or even when dying.

Patients should not needlessly suffer as a result of a prior history of substance abuse or their current treatment in a methadone clinic. Patients with a history of substance addiction that is remote or has been effectively managed in a drug treatment program are at much greater risk for the undertreatment of cancer pain. Consultation with a drug treatment facility may be necessary to plan effective management strategies.

Family members of a substance abuser can negatively influence or reinforce the patient's drug-seeking behavior. These families frequently possess an extremely high level of cohesion, which can be characterized as enmeshed. Within this type of family, boundaries between family members are nebulous, and, as a result, family members may appear to be equally affected by the status of the patient. The care provided to the patient may be sporadic or inconsistent because the family may be overwhelmed by the severity of the illness.

Careful medical and psychosocial coordination between patient, family, staff, and, when appropriate, a drug treatment center is necessary to maximize cooperation and maintain quality care. Despite the level of frustration associated with this group of patients, dignified care is possible and attainable.

Intimacy and Sexuality

Advanced disease always affects sexuality and sexual functioning. Notwithstanding, the lack of libido and impaired sexual functioning are frequently overlooked or ignored as a concern of the patient. Open discussion of intimacy and sexuality with the team can actually result in enhancement of emotional vitality. In fact, an increase in intimacy can evolve as closeness is redefined and openly discussed. Patients' needs for intimacy and sexual activity must be examined and supported. A couple's expression of intimacy, even during terminal care, can create a sense of normalcy and relief in the midst of a highly traumatic course of medical events. As patients enter the terminal phase, these discussions require a high level of sensitivity. Most patients long to be touched and held, and it is not uncommon for spouses or children to lie in bed with a dying patient to provide comfort and experience closeness or intimacy. Models for assessment of these issues with effective interventions are available (82).

Dying at Home

Although many patients and families describe a preference for death to occur in the comfort of their homes, this goal is not always attainable. While the majority of patient deaths continue to occur in medical institutions, the return to home, nursing homes, or hospices as the chosen places of death continues to increase, primarily as a result of the Medicare Hospice Benefit (83,84) and physician availability for home visits (85,86). A number of key psychosocial variables (Table 50.2) may inhibit or prevent the occurrence of death in the home even with the highest level of supportive care or hospice services. Families must be carefully assessed and prepared for the death event. Key family members can be specifically questioned concerning their level of comfort or toleration for stressful events within the home. Preparations, including advance directives, wills, and do-not-resuscitate orders, should begin as early as possible to resolve all questions and informational needs that the family may have. Typically, hospice services are only available in the home for a fraction of each day. Consequently, the patient's death will probably occur when the family is alone (87).

A family that wants to maintain a dying member at home despite complex needs may suddenly request that the patient die in the hospital. Reasons for rapid changes may be obvious and practical or may be irrational and unconscious. Either way, the resources and limitations of the family must be assessed and supported. Many patients who are terminally ill possess acute care needs (e.g., pain control and mental status changes), and admission may be warranted to provide brief respite for the family or to actually manage the death event.

When the Patient Dies

The final hours of the patient's life have significant meaning for the family and offer an opportunity for closure (88,89). The ritualistic need to be present at the exact moment of death can be very powerful for family members. The desire to be present for the death event is common, and for family members who are absent, significant regrets may result (90,91). Unexpected deaths occur in approximately 30% of patients; attempts to notify the family of the impending event is possible in 70% of cases (92).

Family members may require objective information concerning the cause of death, especially if the death was unexpected. Despite the terminal prognosis, many families need to understand why the patient died when he or she did. This information can mitigate a high level of mistrust and resulting distress and address any irrational concerns and fears associated with the death as it is happening.

Interactions with staff that occur immediately following the death can have a long-term effect. Emotional reactions of family members are expected, and crying, sobbing, and wailing are common. The therapeutic demands associated with the provision of terminal care challenges the healthcare professional to communicate with empathy while facilitating the initiation of essential tasks such as removal of the body and funeral arrangements. Families vary in their ability to receive information and emotional support during this time. The relationship between the family and the healthcare team influences how much of these preparations can be made prior to the death event and how much clinical intervention the family requires and can tolerate. Generally, families elect a spokesperson to provide and receive information but care must be taken to assess other members of the family. A follow-up meeting with the family by a social worker or nurse in the home can be very helpful to identify any family member who may be at risk for an abnormal grief response (42,91).

CONCLUSIONS

All patients and families possess a personal meaning of disease, prolonged illness, and death. These meanings are influenced over time by numerous factors. A clear understanding of these meanings, associated emotions, and their antecedents enhances the healthcare team's ability to provide care and anticipate potential problems. Information and education must be consistently available as the patient and family move across the disease continuum toward and post the death event (90).

Variables, such as family cohesion, describe the quality and intensity of relationships within the family. High cohesion or enmeshed families lose more than a family member when the patient dies. For these families, part of their identity is also lost. Given their extreme level of dependence on one another, these families may experience the death as catastrophic, which prevents the effective resolution of the loss. Chronic grief can exacerbate current psychological symptoms and influence healthcare practices. Bereavement follow-up among high-risk families is essential as a means to develop psychosocial prevention programs. The psychosocial obligation to the family does not end with the patient's death, and some families may require follow-up beyond the customary 1-year period as the bereaved experience salient dates such as a birthday or anniversary for the first time without the loved one who has died. Most often, bereaved family members must experience the "four seasons of the year" as they attempt to celebrate holidays or experience a vacation following the death of their loved one (27). Given the intensity of the loss and the family's level of risk, grief must be monitored and resolved.

As with palliative care, despite data supporting effectiveness and benefits to patients, their caregivers, and to the system, psychosocial services have been actively supported and increasingly demanded by consumers of these services. In addition, professional organizations are now creating clinical standards that support the importance of whole-patient-centered care. To its detriment, the health system has for too long resisted a wider view of the patient experience. Paradoxically, just as professional groups and the public are demanding a more comprehensive model of cancer care that minimally includes a full biopsychosocial (and sometimes spiritual) approach to care and caring, the recent worldwide financial crisis and American politicization of end-of-life care by demagogues are in stark conflict. This leads to great uncertainty in the near, but not distant future. Given international demographics relating to aging, population growth, the obesity epidemic, and increasingly sedentary lifestyles palliative care is being recognized as an essential element to healthcare systems. Recent empirical support for the value of palliative care will only accelerate this process.

Palliative care has actively promoted the importance of psychosocial services and has created an opportunity to give a strong voice to the humanistic agenda, where respect, dignity, and identifying personal and social strengths are synergized into a healthcaring system where the needs of people are more wisely and appropriately balanced with the inquisitiveness and natural desire to defy the limits of what humans can presently accomplish while still maintaining our humanity.

Ultimately, the role of the healthcare team and the compassionate expertise they provide is to create an environment with exquisite symptom management and honest and open communication (92). If these components are present, the opportunity exists to provide meaning to the death event. If this occurs, a sense of growth is possible for patients who are dying, their surviving family members, their healthcare providers, and society at large.

ACKNOWLEDGMENTS

The authors thank Sheri and Les Biller for their generous and ongoing support of the Sheri & Les Biller Patient and Family Resource Center and for City of Hope administrative leadership who had the audacity and vision to create the integrated interdisciplinary Department of Supportive Care Medicine.

REFERENCES

1. Loscalzo MJ. Palliative care: an historical perspective. *Hematology Am Soc Hematol Educ Program.* 2008;2008:465.
2. National Hospice and Palliative Care Organization. *Facts and Figures: Hospice Care in America.* Alexandria, VA: NHPCO; September 2010.
3. Mishel MH. Reconceptualization of the uncertainty in illness theory. *Image J Nurs Sch.* 1990;22:256.
4. Seale C, Cartwright A. *The Year before Death.* Brookfield, WI: Ashgate Publishing Company; 1994.
5. Yabroff CR, Youngmee K. Time costs associated with informal caregiving for cancer survivors. *Cancer.* Supplement: Cancer Survivorship Research: Mapping the New Challenges Atlanta, Georgia, Supplement to Cancer. September 2009;115(suppl 18):4362–4373.
6. Levin DN, Cleeland CS, Dar R. Public attitudes toward cancer pain. *Cancer.* 1985;56:2337.
7. World Health Organization. *Cancer Pain and Palliative Care,* Technical Report 804. Geneva: World Health Organization; 1990.
8. Zarit SH, Todd PA, Zarit JM. Subjective burdens of husbands and wives as caregivers: a longitudinal study. *Gerontologist.* 1986;26:260.
9. Brody EM. Women in the middle and family help to older people. *Gerontologist.* 1981;21:471.
10. Iwashyna TJ, Christakis NA. Attitude and self-reported practice regarding hospice referral in a national sample. *J Palliat Med.* 1998;1(3):241.
11. Bomba PA. Enabling the transition to hospice through effective palliative care. *Case Manager.* 2005;16(1):48.
12. Zwerding T, Hamann K, Meyers F. Extending palliative care: is there a role for preventive medicine? *J Palliat Med.* 2005;8(3):486.
13. Weeks JC, Cook EF, O'Day SJ, et al. Relationship between cancer patients' predictions of prognosis and their treatment preferences. *JAMA.* 1998;279:1709.
14. Azoulay E, Pochard F, Kentish-Barnes N, et al. Risk of post-traumatic stress symptoms in family members of intensive care unit patients. *Am J Respir Crit Care Med.* 2005;171:987–994.
15. Gott M, Ingleton C, Bennett MI, Gardiner C. Transitions to palliative care in acute hospitals in England: qualitative study. *BMJ.* March 2011;342:d1773.
16. Lazarus RS. *Emotion and Adaptation.* New York, NY: Oxford University Press; 1991.
17. Weisman AD, Worden JW. The existential plight in cancer: significance of the first 100 days. *Int J Psychiatry Med.* 1976–1977;7:1.
18. Carlsson M, Mamrin E. Psychological and psychosocial aspects of breast cancer treatments. *Cancer Nurs.* 1994;17:418.
19. Ternel JS, Greer JA, Muzinkansky A, et al. Early palliative care for patients with metastatic non-small-cell lung cancer. *N Engl J Med.* August 2010;363(8):733–742.
20. Zabora JR, Loscalzo MJ, Weber J. Managing complications in cancer: identifying and responding to the patient's perspective. *Semin Oncol Nurs.* 2003;19(4 suppl 2):1.
21. Houts PS, Nezu AM, Nezu CM, et al. A problem-solving model of family care giving for cancer patients. *Patient Educ Couns.* 1996;27:63.
22. Bucher J, Loscalzo MJ, Zabora JR, et al. Problem-solving cancer care education for patients and caregivers. *Cancer Pract.* 2001;9(2):66.

23. Derogatis LR, Morrow GR, Fetting J. The prevalence of psychiatric disorders among cancer patients. *JAMA*. 1983;249(6):751.

24. Farber JM, Weinerman BH, Kuypers JA. Psychosocial distress in oncology outpatients. *J Psychosoc Oncol*. 1984;2:109.

25. Stefanek M, Derogatis L, Shaw A. Psychological distress among oncology outpatients. *Psychosomatics*. 1987;28:530.

26. Zabora J, BrintzenhofeSzoc K, Curbow B, et al. The prevalence of psychological distress by cancer site. *Psychooncology*. 2001;10:19.

27. Schulz R, Williamson GM, Knapp JE, et al. The psychological, social, and economic impact of illness among patients with recurrent cancer. *J Psychosoc Oncol*. 1995;13(3):21.

28. National Comprehensive Cancer Network. *The NCCN Distress Practice Guidelines in Oncology*. Vol 1.2011. Fort Washington, PA: NCCN; 2011:2.

29. Clark K, Bardwell WA, Arsenault, T, DeTeresa, D, Loscalzo, M. Implementing touch-screen technology to enhance recognition of distress. *Psycho-Oncology*. August 2009;18(8):822–830.

30. Institute of Medicine. *Cancer Care for the Whole Patient: Meeting Psychosocial Health Needs*. Washington, DC: Institute of Medicine; October 2007.

31. Bultz BD, Johansen C. Screening for distress, the 6th vital sign: where are we, and where are we going? *Psycho-Oncology*. June 2011;Special Issue: Screening for Distress, the 6th Vital Sign. 20(6):569–571.

32. Zabora JR. Pragmatic approaches in the psychosocial screening of cancer patients. In: Holland J, Breitbart P, Loscalzo M, eds. *Handbook of Psychooncology*. 2nd ed. London: Oxford Press; 1998.

33. Jacobsen PB, Donovan KA, Trask PC, et al. Screening for distress in ambulatory cancer patients. *Cancer*. 2005;103(7):1494.

34. Weisman AD, Worden JW, Sobel HJ. *Psychosocial Screening and Interventions with Cancer Patients: A Research Report*. Boston, MA: Harvard Medical School and Massachusetts Hospital; 1980.

35. Fawzy FI, Fawzy NW, Arndt LA, et al. Critical review of psychosocial interventions in cancer care. *Arch Gen Psychiatry*. 1995;52:100.

36. Zabora JR, Smith-Wilson R, Fetting JH, et al. An efficient method for the psychosocial screening of cancer patients. *Psychosomatics*. 1990;31(2):192.

37. Jacobsen PB, Ransom S. Implementation of NCCN Distress Management Guidelines by Member Institutions. *J Natl Compr Canc Netw*. January 2007;5(1):99–103.

38. Velikova G, Booth L, Smith AB, et al. Measuring quality of life in routine oncology practice improves communication and patient well-being: a randomized controlled trial. *J Clin Oncol*. February 2004;22(4):714–724.

39. Zabora JR, Loscalzo MJ, Smith ED. Psychosocial rehabilitation. In: Abeloff MD, Armitage JO, Lichter AS, et al., eds. *Clinical Oncology*. New York, NY: Churchill Livingstone; 2002.

40. Derogatis LR. *BSI-18: Administration, Scoring and Procedures Manual*. Minneapolis, MN: National Computer Systems; 2000.

41. Zabora J, BrintzenhofeSzoc K, Jacobsen P, et al. Development of a new psychosocial screening instrument for use with cancer patients. *Psychosomatics*. 2001;42(3):19.

42. BrintzenhofeSzoc K, Smith E, Zabora J. Development of a screening approach to predict complicated grief in surviving spouses of cancer patients. *Cancer Pract*. 1999;7(5):233.

43. Olson DH, McCubbin HI, Barnes HL, et al. Predicting conflict with staff among families of cancer patients during prolonged hospitalizations. *J Psychosoc Oncol*. 1989;7(3):103.

44. Zabora JR, Fetting JH, Shaley VB, et al. Predicting conflict with staff among families of cancer patients during prolonged hospitalization. *J Psychosoc Oncol*. 1989;7(3):103.

45. Jamison RN, Sbrocco T, Parris W. The influence of problems in concentration and memory on emotional distress and daily activities in chronic pain patients. *Int J Psychiatry Med*. 1988;18:183.

46. Daut RL, Cleeland CS. The prevalence and severity of pain in cancer. *Cancer*. 1982;50(9):1913.

47. Bond MR, Pearson IB. Psychological aspects of pain in women with advanced cancer of the cervix. *J Psychosom Res*. 1969;13:13.

48. Cleeland CS. The impact of pain on the patient with cancer. *Cancer*. 1984;54:2635.

49. O'Mahony S, Goulet J, Kornblith A, et al. Desire for hastened death, cancer pain and depression: report of a longitudinal observational study. *J Pain Symptom Manage*. 2005;29(5):446.

50. Cobb JL, Glantz MJ, Martin EW, et al. Delirium in patients with cancer at the end of life. *Cancer Pract*. 2000;8(4):172.

51. Serlin RC, Mendoza TR, Nakamura Y, et al. When is cancer pain mild, moderate or severe? *Pain*. 1995;61(2):277.

52. Von Roemn JH, Cleeland CS, Gonin R, et al. Physician attitudes and practice in cancer pain management. *Ann Intern Med*. 1993;119:121.

53. Cleeland CS, Gonin R, Hatfield AK, et al. Pain and its treatment in outpatients with metastatic cancer. *N Engl J Med*. 1994;330(9):592.

54. Grossman SA, Sheidler VR, Sweeden K, et al. Correlation of patient and caregiver ratings of cancer pain. *J Pain Symptom Manage*. 1991;692:53.

55. Portenoy RK, Ugarte C, Fuller I, et al. Population-based survey of pain in the United States: differences among white, African American, and Hispanic subjects. *J Pain*. 2004;5(6):317.

56. Spiegel D, Sands SS, Koopman C. Pain and depression in patients with cancer. *Cancer*. 1994;74:2579.

57. Razavi D, Delvaux N, Farvacques C, et al. Screening for adjustment disorders and major depressive disorders in cancer inpatients. *Br J Psychiatry*. 1990;156:79.

58. Shacham S, Reinhart LC, Raubertas RF, et al. Emotional states and pain: intraindividual and interindividual measures of association. *J Behav Med*. 1983;6:405.

59. Bucher JA, Trostle GB, Moore M. Family reports of cancer pain, pain relief, and prescription access. *Cancer Pract*. 1999;792:71.

60. Bolund C. Suicide and cancer II: medical and care factors in suicide by cancer patients in Sweden, 1973–1976. *J Psychosoc Oncol*. 1985;3:17.

61. Breitbart W, Rosenfeld B, Pessin H, et al. Depression, hopelessness, and desire for hastened death in terminally ill patients with cancer. *JAMA*. 2000;284(22):2907.

62. Massie MJ, Holland JC. Depression and the cancer patient. *J Clin Psychiatry*. 1990;51(suppl 7):12.

63. Kagawa-Singer M. Diverse cultural beliefs and practices about death and dying in the elderly. In: Wieland D, ed. Cultural diversity and geriatric care: challenges to the health professions. New York, NY: Haworth Press; 1994.

64. Hellman C. *Culture, Health and Illness*. 3rd ed. Newton, MA: Butterworth–Heinemann; 1995.

65. Koenig BA, Gates-Williams J. Understanding cultural difference in caring for dying patients. Caring for patients at the end of life. *West J Med*. 1995;163(3):244.

66. Power PW, Dell Orto AE. Understanding the family. In: Power PW, Dell Orto AE, eds. *Role of the Family in the Rehabilitation of the Physically Disabled*. Baltimore, MD: University Park Press; 1980.

67. Van Winkle NM. End of life decision making in American Indian and Alaska Native cultures. In: *Cultural Issues in End-of-Life Decision Making.* Thousand Oaks, CA: Sage Publications Inc; 2000.

68. Parker SG. The challenge of bringing hospice to the Zuni Tribe. *Last Acts* 2001;10.

69. Hopp F, Duffy SA. Racial variations in end-of-life care. *J Am Geriatr Soc.* 2000;48(6):658.

70. Nezu AM, Nezu CM, Friedman SH, et al. *Helping Cancer Patients Cope.* Washington, DC: American Psychological Associates; 1998.

71. Meyers FJ, Carducci M, Loscalzo MJ, et al. Effects of a problem-solving intervention (COPE) on quality of life for patients with advanced cancer on clinical trials and their caregivers: simultaneous care educational intervention (SCEI): linking palliation and clinical trials. *J Palliat Med.* April 2011;14(4):465–473.

72. Nezu AM, Nezu CM, Perri MG. *Problem-Solving Therapy for Depression: Theory, Research, and Clinical Guidelines.* New York, NY: Wiley; 1989.

73. D'Zurilla TJ, Nezu AM. Social problem-solving in adults. In: Kendall P, ed. *Cognitive-Behavioral Research and Therapy.* New York, NY: Academic Press; 1982.

74. Nezu AM, Nezu CM, Houts PS, et al. Relevance of problem-solving therapy to psychosocial oncology. *J Psychosoc Oncol.* 1999;16(3–4):5–26.

75. Nezu AM, D'Zurilla TJ, Social problem-solving and negative affective states. In: Kendall P, Watson D, eds. *Anxiety and Depression: Distinctive and Overlapping Features.* New York, NY: Academic Press; 1989.

76. Toseland RW, Blanchard CG, McCallion P. A problem solving intervention for caregivers of cancer patients. *Soc Sci Med.* 1995;40(4):517.

77. Lansky SB, Cairns N, Lowman J, et al. Childhood cancer: nonmedical costs of the illness. *Cancer.* 1979;43(1):403.

78. Houts PS, Lipton A, Harvey HA, et al. Nonmedical costs to patients and their families associated with outpatient chemotherapy. *Cancer.* 1984;53:2388.

79. Mor V, Guadagnoli E, Wool M. An examination of the concrete service needs of advanced cancer patients. *J Psychosoc Oncol.* 1987;5(1):1.

80. Farkas C, Loscalzo M. Death without indignity. In: Kutscher AH, Carr AC, Kutscher LG, eds. *Principles of Thanatology.* New York, NY: Columbia University Press; 1987:133.

81. Loscalzo M, Amendola J. Psychosocial and behavioral management of cancer pain: the social work contribution. In: Foley KM, Bonica JJ, Ventafridda V, eds. *Advances in Pain Research and Therapy.* Vol 16. New York, NY: Raven Press; 1990:429.

82. Cagle JG, Bolte S. Sexuality and life-threatening illness: implications for social work and palliative care. *Health Soc Work.* 34(3):223–233.

83. Jordhoy MS, Saltvedt I, Fayers P, et al. Which cancer patients die in nursing homes? Quality of life, medical and sociodemographic characteristics. *Palliat Med.* 2003;17(5):433.

84. Bruera E, Sweeney C, Russell N, et al. Place of death of Houston area residents with cancer over a two-year period. *J Pain Symptom Manage.* 2003;26(1):637.

85. Sager M, Easterling D, Kindig D, et al. Changes in the location of death after passage of Medicare's prospective payment system. A national study. *N Engl J Med.* 1989;320:433.

86. McMullan A, Mentnech R, Lubitz J, et al. Trends and patterns in place of death for medicare enrollees. *Health Care Financ Rev.* 1990;12:1.

87. Leff B, Kaffenbarger KP, Remsburg RN. Prevalence, effectiveness, and predictors of planning the place of death among older persons followed in community-based long term care. *J Am Geriatr Soc.* 2000;48(8):943.

88. Tolle SW, Bascom PB, Hickam DA, et al. Communication between physicians and surviving spouses following patient death. *J Gen Intern Med.* 1986;1:309.

89. Tolle SW, Girard DW. The physician's role in the events surrounding patient death. *Arch Intern Med.* 1982;143:1447.

90. Abbott KH, Sago JG, Breen CM, et al. Families looking back: one year after discussion of withdrawal or withholding of life-sustaining support. *Crit Care Med.* 2001;25(1):197.

91. Worden JW. *Grief Counseling and Grief Therapy: A Handbook for the Mental Health Practitioner.* 2nd ed. New York, NY: Springer Publishing Company; 1991.

92. Steinhauser KE, Christakis NA, Clipp EC, et al. Factors considered important at the end of life by patients, families, physicians, and other care providers. *JAMA.* 2000;284(19):2476.

CHAPTER 51

Disorders of Sexuality and Reproduction

Mary K. Hughes

INTRODUCTION

Palliative care applies to the entire course of cancer, from diagnosis to death, and enhances quality of life (1). Bruner and Boyd (2) assert that the promotion of sexual health is vital for preserving quality of life and is an integral part of total or holistic cancer management. Often, the innate desire to express and experience sexual and emotional closeness is abruptly and irreversibly changed by the cancer diagnosis and/or its treatments (3). Schover et al. (4) report sexuality to be one of the first elements of daily living disrupted by a cancer diagnosis. Treatments and/or the disease itself can cause changes in sexuality, but healthcare providers rarely ask about sexuality issues because of concepts about the importance of sexuality in the context of the disease (5). According to Leiblum et al. (6), all patients regardless of age, sexual orientation, marital status, or life circumstances should have the opportunity to discuss sexual matters with their healthcare professional. But it is not easy to talk about despite living in a culture that is saturated with overtly sexual images, graphic lyrics, and explicit advertising (7).

According to Tomlinson (8), the main difference between taking a history about a sexual problem and an ordinary medical history is the level of embarrassment and discomfort of the patient and the healthcare provider. A discussion of sexual changes can begin by acknowledging the sexual changes brought about by the cancer or the treatment of the cancer (9). Sexual changes after treatment is not routinely addressed or only barely touched on despite patients having significant needs for education, support, and practical help with managing them. Maslow (10) described sexual activity to be a basic need on his hierarchy of needs while love and connection to others were at a higher level. Everyone has a lifelong need for touch and emotional connection to others regardless of current relationship status (11). But touching changes with cancer. Often the partner becomes the caregiver, changing dressings, and managing drains and wounds, and intimate touching decreases and becomes treatment related. Sexual intercourse is not the defining characteristic of a person's sexuality; a sexual relationship includes the need to be touched and held along with closeness and tenderness (12,13). Malcarne et al. (14) report that because of the emotional and physical changes in the person with cancer, the quality of a couple's relationship can be altered even by successful treatment.

SEXUALITY

In order for providers to begin assessing sexuality in people with cancer, they must first understand what sexuality encompasses. It is a broad term including social, emotional, and physical components (15). It is not just genitals or gender but includes body image, love of self and others, relating to others, and pleasure (15). It is genetically endowed, phenotypically embodied, hormonally nurtured, is not age related, but is matured by experience and cannot be destroyed despite what is done to a person (16,17). Sexuality includes affection, sexual orientation, sexual activity, eroticism, reproduction, intimacy, and gender roles and encompasses feelings of trust (18,19).

Masters and Johnson (20) described the human sexual response cycle that begins with libido or the desire for sexual activity. Gregoire (21) reports that men are more attracted to visual sexual stimuli, whereas women are more attracted to auditory and written material, particularly stimuli associated within the context of a loving and positive relationship. Women are not linear in their sexual response, but more circular (22) and may experience sexual excitement before they have a desire for sexual activity. Sexual excitement is the phase where the penis becomes rigid enough to use and in the female, the vagina lubricates and enlarges in depth and width, and the clitoris enlarges (23–25). Erection is the male counterpart to vaginal lubrication from the sexual physiology perspective (26). Orgasm is the height of sexual pleasure and the release of sexual tension. The penis emits semen through muscular spasms and there are rhythmic contractions of the vagina and the cervix lifts up out of the vaginal vault. The last phase of the cycle is the resolution phase where the genitals return to their normal, non-excited state. During this phase, there is an evaluation of the sexual experience as well as relaxation and contentment (27,28). The refractory period, where the genitals are resistant to sexual stimulation, happens during this stage. In males, this period can be a matter of minutes in youth, but take days in older men or with certain medications or medical conditions like cancer.

Sexual expression is influenced by cultural norms, past experiences, and the developmental stage of the individual (19,24,29). Expressions of sexuality include style of dress, values and attitudes, as well as hugging, touching, kissing, acting out scenarios/fantasies, sex toys, masturbation, sexual intercourse, oral genital stimulation, either alone or with others (11,19,30). Sexual behaviors may involve oral, vaginal, and/or anal penetration (30). Sexual behavior is influenced by religious beliefs, age, education, level of comfort with one's body and physical functioning, experiences of sexual abuse and trauma, their partner's wishes, and comfort level with one's own sexual orientation and gender identity (31,32).

SEXUAL DYSFUNCTION

Sexual dysfunction is failure of any aspect of the sexual response cycle to function properly (33). Goldstein et al. (34) report that 90% of sexual dysfunction cases have a psychological component and 75% have clear physiologic sources, so there is a significant overlap. But when a person with cancer has sexual dysfunction, it is mostly physiological. Causes of sexual dysfunction include psychosocial/interpersonal stressors, medical illness, depressive illness, medication, and sexual disorders (DSM-IV) (35). According to Gregoire (21), a sexual problem includes physiological dysfunction, altered experiences, one's own perceptions and beliefs, partner's perceptions and expectations, altered circumstances, and past experiences. Causes of sexual dysfunction in a person with cancer are often treatment related due to the changes in physiological, psychological, and social dimensions of sexuality and disruption in one or more phases of the sexual response cycle (11,36). Radiation and surgery can have long-lasting effects on sexuality due to chronic pain, scarring, and body image issues. Besides chemotherapy, biologic agents, and hormones, there are numerous medications that can have sexual side effects that range from decreased desire to difficulty reaching orgasm. Many of these medications are used in palliative care (21,37–41) and include the following:

- Neurotransmitters
- Stimulants
- Hallucinogens
- Sedatives
- Narcotics
- Anxiolytics
- Anticholinergics
- Antipsychotics
- Lipid-lowering drugs
- H_2 antagonists
- Many antidepressants
- Phenothiazines
- Antihypertensives
- Recreational drugs
- Alcohol
- Herbals and vitamins
- Serotonin reuptake inhibitors
- Anticonvulsants

Table 51.1 provides a list of menopausal symptoms and sexual side effects.

Menopausal symptoms can be very distressing to women and interfere with sexuality because of the changes on her body (53). These changes happen gradually in women without cancer and they have time to adjust and enjoy sexual activity 5 to 10 years longer with fewer sexual problems than women with cancer who rapidly experience menopause

(54,55). One should note that while dyspareunia assumes pain with penile–vaginal intercourse, it may be a source of distress as well for women with same-sexed partners, where touch and/or finger or object penetration is uncomfortable (56). Katz (57) found that physical appearance was important in gay culture and having a partner show acceptance of treatment- or disease-related physical changes was comforting. Table 51.2 describes types of sexual dysfunction (35,58–61) as defined by the DSM-IV (35).

It should be remembered that sexual dysfunctions are not all or nothing phenomena, but occur on a continuum in terms of frequency and severity. Comorbidity of sexual dysfunctions is common. Gregoire (21) reports that almost half the men with low libido also have another sexual dysfunction, and 20% of men with erectile dysfunction have low libido. The patient's partner and their relationship probably have a more profound effect on sexual health than on any other aspect of health. Sexual dysfunction in men is not as complicated as in women and is usually associated with age and illness. Ideally male testosterone levels should be tested before beginning cancer treatment as a baseline indicator of a man's normal level (62). Table 51.3 describes sexual dysfunctions and possible causes (21,35,38,63–72).

Men with colorectal cancer report more problems with sexual function related to their surgeries than women with similar treatment for similar diagnoses (73,74). Some studies show that partners of patients with cancer experience more psychological distress than their cancer-affected mate (75–79). Neese et al. (80) note that less than half of men with sexual dysfunction believed that their partners supported them in their efforts to find help.

Body image is a key aspect of sexuality and includes one's feelings and attitudes about one's body (18,81). Body image changes can profoundly alter feelings of attractiveness, an important aspect of sexuality (9). External changes that are visible to others as well as internal changes affect body image (18,82). Temporary body changes include the following:

- Alopecia
- Change in facial hair growth
- Skin changes (color and texture)
- Ostomies and stomas
- Placement of drains and venous access lines
- Weight changes
- Incontinence of bowel and/or bladder
- Gynecomastia
- Penile/testicular atrophy
- Change in shape of breasts
- Rashes, acne, peeling of palms, and soles of feet
- Fertility
- Neuropathies

Permanent body changes may have been temporary, but became permanent and affect body image and include the following:

- Alopecia from radiation
- Change in facial hair growth
- Scarring

TABLE 51.1 Menopausal symptoms (42–52)	
Menopausal Symptoms	**Sexual Affects**
Vaginal dryness and atrophy	Painful intercourse
Decreased vaginal ridges	Decreased friction on the vagina
Labia minora and vulvar atrophy	Painful intercourse
Hot flashes	Decreased libido and arousal and difficulty having an orgasm, hard to remain physically close
Change in body aroma	Decreased libido and arousal
Decreased clitoral sensation	Decreased arousal and longer time to achieve orgasm
Insomnia	Fatigue
Joint pain and decreased muscle mass	Harder to engage in sexual activities due to pain
Irritability; mood swings	Lower libido and arousal; partner doesn't know what to expect
Decreased bone density	Fear of fractures with sexual activity
Skin and hair changes	Poor body image, decreased libido, altered sense of sexual self
Migraine headaches	Decreased libido
Stature loss	Poor body image
Decreased sexual hair	Poor body image, less cushioning during sex, altered sense of sexual self
Increased urinary tract infections	Painful intercourse
Vaginal itching	Painful intercourse
Loss of tissue elasticity	Painful intercourse
Infertility	Change in body image
Urogenital atrophy	Dyspareunia, vaginal dryness, decreased libido

- Ostomies and stomas
- Pain control pumps
- Skin changes
- Amputations
- Incontinence of bowel and/or bladder
- Thinning hair
- Penile/testicular atrophy
- Change in shape of breasts
- Pelvic exenteration
- Hemipelvectomy
- Vaginal stenosis
- Fertility
- Neuropathies

Mitchell et al. (83) assert that mood can affect sexual functioning in a negative or positive way. Psychological issues that can alter sexual functioning include the following:

- Frustration
- Stigma
- Embarrassment
- Anxiety

- Anger
- Irritability
- Depression
- Loneliness
- Despair
- Grief
- Interference of age-appropriate goals (education, marriage, child bearing, and retirement)
- Performance anxiety
- Changes in personality
- Mood swings
- Misinformation
- Guilt and shame
- Disappointment
- Fear of
  - Death
  - Rejection
  - Never feeling better
  - Abandonment
  - How cancer will affect others
  - Social role change

TABLE 51.2	Sexual dysfunction according to DSM IV (35,58–61)

Type of Sexual Dysfunction	Description
Persistent or recurrent disorders of interest/desire (hypoactive sexual desire disorder)	An absence of sexual fantasies or thoughts, desire, or receptivity to sexual activity at anytime during the sexual experience designates disorder
Disorders of subjective and genital arousal	If subjective, no response to any type of sexual stimulation but may have genital arousal
	If genital arousal disorder, subjective arousal to nongenital stimulation (usually postmenopausal women), but impaired or absent genital sexual arousal. Inability to attain or maintain adequate lubrication or swelling response during sexual activity
	Combined: Absence or very diminished feelings of sexual arousal from any type of sexual stimulation as well as absent genital sexual arousal
Persistent sexual arousal disorder	In the absence of sexual interest and desire, spontaneous, intrusive, unwanted genital throbbing unrelieved by orgasm
Male erectile disorder	Episodic or continuous inability to obtain and/or maintain an erection during sexual activity
Orgasmic disorder (female orgasmic disorder)	Lack of, markedly diminished, or delay of orgasms despite sexual arousal regardless of stimulation. Body image, relationship satisfaction, and self-esteem may affect the ability of women to orgasm
Vaginismus	Reflexive tightening around the vagina when vaginal entry is attempted despite woman's desire for penetration. No physical abnormalities present. Often associated with fear, anticipation, or pain
Dyspareunia	Recurrent genital pain with attempted vaginal penetration or penile thrusting
Orgasmic disorder	Episodic, continuous, or complete absence of orgasm following excitement phase
Sexual aversion disorder involving dysfunctions of sexual desire (female sexual arousal disorder)	Extreme anxiety and/or disgust at the anticipation of or attempt to have any sexual activity. Avoidance of sexual contact with a partner
Sexual dysfunction secondary to a general medical condition or substance induced	Medications, chronic or acute illnesses, fatigue, pain

- How attractiveness changes
- Never finishing treatment
- Pain—major obstacle to enjoying sex
- Recurrence with sexual activity
- Cancer spread with sexual activity
- Loss of control
- Dependency (43,53,81,84–90)

FERTILITY

Treatment decisions made at the time of diagnosis impact interpersonal relationships, sexuality, and reproductive capacity of all survivors (9). One of the greatest concerns of cancer survivors of childbearing age is the effect of treatment on fertility (91). Reproductive concerns that emerge within

the cancer experience are negatively associated with quality of life (92). Studies show that most young survivors are interested in having children, especially if they were childless at the time of their cancer diagnosis (91,93). Difficulties with fertility increase with age and are much more common for women greater than 40 years (94,95). Pregnancy does not appear to increase the risk of cancer recurrence (96). The ability to preserve fertility depends on these variables: age, type of cancer, and types of treatment (97–100).

The American Society of Clinical Oncologists recommends that

- Oncologists address the possibility of infertility with patients in their reproductive years
- Fertility preservation should be considered as early as possible during treatment

TABLE 51.3	Causes of sexual dysfunction (21,35,38,63–72)
Sexual Dysfunction	**Causes**
Low libido	Chemotherapy, androgen deprivation therapy, fatigue, pain, dementia, delirium, depression, boredom, benzodiazepines, antipsychotics, neuroleptics, sedatives, opioids, diuretics, brain tumors, low testosterone, histamine-2 antagonists
Erectile dysfunction/female arousal	Antihypertensives, chemotherapy, androgen deprivation therapy, surgery, loss of a willing partner, opportunity, privacy, decreased frequency of activity, decreased tactile sensation, increased refractory period after orgasm, peripheral vascular disease, diabetic neuropathy, nicotine, diuretics, alcohol, opioids, neuroleptics, brain and spine tumors, anxiety, antihistamines, histamine-2 antagonists, high body mass, St. John's wort, cocaine, marijuana, lipid-lowering agents
Ejaculation problems: retrograde, dry, premature, delayed	SSRIs, surgery, radiation, opioids, antipsychotics, neuroleptics
Orgasmic disorder	Antidepressants, antihypertensives, diuretics, neuroleptics, antipsychotics, anxiety, neuropathy, radiation

SSRIs, serotonin reuptake inhibitors.

- Standard fertility preservation practice is:
  - Sperm cryopreservation for men
  - Embryo cryopreservation for women
  - Other methods considered investigational (101,102)

Fertility preservation takes time, is expensive and can delay treatment and many cancers need to be treated promptly (86). One study showed significant depression, grief, and sexual difficulties in women whose cancer treatment caused infertility (103). Psychological responses to infertility include a variety of emotions such as grief, anger, depression, sadness, loss of femininity/masculinity, and/or changes in self-image (9). Traditional reproductive options are seen in Table 51.4 (93).

Psychosocial issues surrounding infertility are complicated. There are emotional aspects of losing one's fertility which can include the whole spectrum of grieving. The patient may have fear of undergoing additional treatment as well as fear of abandonment by the partner. There are numerous financial issues related to pursuing treatment for infertility. How does one tell the family, friends, and significant others? Often it makes the patient feel like a failure. The couple has to address issues of child-free living.

SEXUAL ASSESSMENT AND TREATMENT

According to Ritchie (104), the most important factor in improving care of sexual problems in cancer is to ask about them. In most published studies, patients have stated that they would like more information about sex than they received from their physician. The patient usually does not voluntarily ask sex-related questions, so it is up to the healthcare provider to integrate sexuality into the routine care of all oncology patients (86). Regardless of our role in providing care to the patient, most of us do not have experience talking about sexuality and intimacy in a frank, direct, and authentic manner (7). Annon's (105) PLISSIT model can provide a framework for doing a sexual assessment. It has four components: P, permission; LI, limited information; SS, specific suggestions; and IT, intensive therapy. The practitioner gives the patient permission (P) to think about cancer and sexuality at the same time by asking, "What sexuality changes have you noticed since your cancer?" which lets them know that they are not the only ones to experience sexuality changes. By asking open-ended questions, the healthcare provider is better able to get a thoughtful response from the patient (87). Giving them the time to

TABLE 51.4	Reproductive options (93)	
Option	**Challenge**	
Adoption	Limited availability of infants	
	Emotional and financial constraints	
	Discrimination	
Third-party reproduction	Society often considers this a less favorable option	
	Some major religions forbid this	
	Expensive	

answer is important. Try to remain relaxed with good eye contact to let them know that you are interested in this area of their lives. Addressing sexuality issues early on in the assessment and treatment of the patient allows the practitioner to open up a line of communication with the patient so that these issues can be addressed as they come up in the future (87). Giving them limited information (LI) about side effects from treatments by saying, "Sometimes people notice sexuality changes when they get this treatment," lets them know that you are comfortable talking about sexuality issues. One of the first steps toward sexual rehabilitation is sex education (106). Ways to incorporate assessment of sexuality concerns into clinical practice include addressing sexuality through patients' perceptions of their body image, family roles and functions, relationships, and sexual function (107). Describing specific suggestions (SS) such as books to read, or positions to use, can offer them help with the problem.

Some patients are in difficult relationships, which only get worse with cancer treatment and need intensive therapy (IT) from a marital or a sex therapist. Having a list of those resources in the community can be helpful to the patient. But Schover (108) reports that patients often prefer to receive information from a member of the healthcare team instead of being sent to a sex specialist. Giving referrals depends on what specialized assistance would benefit the patient.

The culture in which the person grew up as well as the culture in which the person currently lives will affect not only how one copes with cancer but influences one's sexuality (53). Katz's study found that homophobia does not affect current cancer care experiences of gay and lesbian patients, and healthcare providers accepted the support of the patient's same-sexed partners (57). Often the healthcare practitioner does not know the sexual orientation or gender identity of their patients. Dibble et al. (30) state that because of heterosexism, those who do not share a heterosexual orientation may have difficult lives especially when they are ill. Heterosexism is the belief that heterosexuality is the only "normal" option for relationships (30). Most of the research on the effects of cancer and its treatment on sexuality has been limited to heterosexual women or women assumed to be heterosexual (109).

People in isolated, rural areas may feel a lack of support and resources to address sexuality changes. Someone with cancer may mistakenly feel they are contagious. Partners of women with cancer often are fearful of inflicting pain, causing fractures, or infecting them because of lack of information or misinformation from the practitioner about resuming sexual activity (44,110). Cancer is expensive to treat and often financial and insurance concerns interfere with sexuality because of the patient being distracted. The stress of cancer and its treatments can exacerbate underlying marital tension and likewise affect the sexual relationship (54). There are many socioeconomic factors that can affect sexuality and include marital status, race, education, attitude toward cancer/treatment, gender preference, family traditions, religion, lack of partner, significance of body part, role change, job loss/pressures, end of life issues, and relationship inequalities (4,43,44,86,111–113).

Sexual morbidities after breast cancer diagnosis include an immediate reduction in sexual activity and responsiveness (114–116). Andersen (117) found that women diagnosed with breast cancer recurrence initially were less sexually active but increased their activity to pre-recurrence rates unless they had distance metastases. Even when patients are dealing with end-of-life issues, it is important to be aware of their sexuality concerns and address these (87). Interventions for sexual dysfunction resulting from cancer treatment can be limited because of the hormone status of the tumor. Women with estrogen-receptive positive breast cancer are often unable to use any estrogen products, while some oncologists give them the go-ahead to use an estrogen vaginal ring, vaginal creams, or tablets. A study reported that the use of vaginal estradiol tablet was associated with a rise in systemic estradiol levels which reverses estrogen suppression achieved by aromatase inhibitors and should be avoided (46). Greenwald and McCorkle (118) reported that women with cervical cancer had their sexual desire and enjoyment rebound 6 years after treatment, but they struggled with sexuality issues until then. Most of the symptoms of sexual dysfunction in patients with breast cancer are related to estrogen deprivation due to premature menopause caused by chemotherapy and antiestrogen hormonal therapy. There are some oncologists that will approve the use of off-label androgen gel for those women to improve libido. Studies have shown that testosterone has positive effects on women's sexuality and higher doses show greater effects (119, 120). It is controversial and should be left to the discretion of the medical oncologist. Women with other types of cancer can use oral estrogen replacement if they are comfortable with this and their oncologist gives them the approval. Maintenance of vaginal health through hormonal and nonhormonal methods is important not only for the overall well-being in the postmenopausal female but also for the elimination of sexual dysfunctions that occur because of urogenital atrophy (50,120).

Levine (121) reports that sexual activity serves as a re-bonding mechanism by serving as an eraser for ordinary annoyances; preventing hostility between partners; decreasing extramarital temptations; and providing psychological intimacy. Treatment options for female and male sexual dysfunction are shown in Table 51.5 (4,24,44,53,112,122–128).

Men with prostate cancer do not have the option to take testosterone replacements for low libido for fear of stimulating the tumor. However, men with other types of cancer can take testosterone replacements without fear of increasing their risk of prostate cancer (129). Asking about desire includes inquiring about sexual fantasies and dreams which are dependent on testosterone levels.

Many people have adopted a pattern of sexual behavior before their diagnosis and attempt to return to it after treatment. If they experience discomfort or failure to function as before, they will stop trying and feel they cannot enjoy sexual activity (117). Some couples who are cancer

TABLE 51.5	Treatment of sexual dysfunction (4,24,44,53,112,122–128)
Treatment	**Example**
Vaginal dilator (use with lubricant)	Different sizes to find comfortable fit with partner or to be able to tolerate gynecological examination. Silicone ones can be heated or cooled
Erotica	Videos, magazines, books, music, web sites
Water-soluble or silicone vaginal lubricants and moisturizers	K-Y, Astroglide or other lubricants for sexual activity, Replens, or other vaginal moisturizers for vaginal health and comfort
Videos	Better Sex Videos, an inexpensive, tastefully done option
Contraceptive options	Oral contraceptives may not be option, use barrier protection (female or male condoms and diaphragm)
Planning for sexual activity	Take medications to control symptoms 30 min before encounter. Schedule encounters when energy is highest
Communicating more openly about sexual needs	Tell partner what feels good, when sexual desire is highest
Exploring one's own body	Finding out new erogenous zones, pleasuring self
Safer sexual practices	If not in committed relationship, use barrier protection (condoms)
Different means of sexual expression	Oral–genital activity, manual stimulation, different sexual positions
Better symptom control	Take medications for pain, nausea, fatigue, diarrhea as needed
Using erotic devices	Vibrators can enhance sexual activity and improve blood flow in the vagina
Sensate focus	Focuses on receiver's pleasure, no genital activity, uses all of the senses
PDE-5 inhibitors	Tadafil, vardenafil, sildenafil. Best if taken on an empty stomach 30 min prior to sexual activity. Needs sexual stimulation to be effective
Penile implants	Genitourinary specialist referral
Penile injections	Alprostadil, Caverject. Needs prescription
Penile bands	Over the counter; improve sustainability of erection
Vacuum erection device	Need prescription
Fertility specialists	Both male and female
EROS-CT for women	Vacuum device for female (need prescription)
Physical therapist for pelvic floor exercises	P.T. must have specialized training
Reconstructive surgery	Plastic surgeon, dentists, wound ostomy nurses
Breast implants	Plastic surgeon
Acupuncture	Improve erectile dysfunction
Yohimbine	Improve erectile dysfunction
L-Arginine	Reportedly improves genital blood flow to improve arousal. Does not stimulate estrogen
Hormone therapy	Endocrinology; improves libido and erections
Psychosexual therapy	Sexual therapist
Lymphedema	P.T. who specializes in treating this

PDE-5, phosphodiesterase 5.

survivors and are in a stressful relationship with an unsupportive partner tend to have more distress which can lead to avoidant coping behaviors (130). They avoid talking about difficult issues, including sexuality. Conversely, during the time of treatment, the cancer experience encourages a more intimate and intense interpersonal relationship (9). There are few studies that have attempted any type of psychosocial intervention to assist survivors in integrating the cancer experience into their personal life (9). If one is not partnered, there is the question of when to reveal one's cancer history: at the beginning of a relationship or wait until the relationship develops.

CONCLUSION

The Institute of Medicine report, *From Cancer Patient to Survivor: Lost in Transition*, recommends intervention for consequences of cancer and its treatment including sexual side effects (131). Palliative care can address these side effects as they treat other side effects the patient experiences. By legitimizing the topic of sexuality from the onset of patient assessment, healthcare providers support patients who then find it easier to raise issues of sexuality as they evolve. According to Taylor and Davis (132), sexual well-being includes participation in sexual activity, satisfaction with sexual experiences, and sexual function. Recognizing the importance of sexual well-being for the patient can prompt the healthcare provider to include a sexual assessment on all patients. The patient will realize that the practitioner is interested in all aspects of his/her quality of life, not just pain.

REFERENCES

1. World Health Organization. Palliative care, 2011. http://www.who.int/cancer/palliative/definition/en/. Accessed September 17, 2011.
2. Bruner DW, Boyd CP. Assessing women's sexuality after cancer therapy: checking assumptions with the focus group technique. *Cancer Nurs.* 1999;22:438-447.
3. Lee JJ. Sexual dysfunction after hematopoietic stem cell transplantation. *Oncol Nurs Forum.* 2011;38(4):online article: www.ons.org accessed September 23, 2011.
4. Schover L, Montague D, Lakin M. Sexual problems. In: Devita VT, Hellman S, Rosenberg SA, eds. *Cancer: Principles and Practices of Oncology.* 5th ed. Philadelphia, PA: Lippincott-Raven; 1997:2857-2871.
5. Bitzer J, Platano G, Tschudin S, Alder J. Sexual counseling for women in the context of physical diseases: a teaching model for physicians. *J Sex Med.* 2007;4:29-37.
6. Leiblum SR, Baume RM, Croog SH. The sexual functioning of elderly hypertensive women. *J Sex Marital Ther.* 1994;20:259-270.
7. Bober SL. From the guest editor: out in the open: addressing sexual health after cancer. *Cancer J.* 2009;15:13-14.
8. Tomlinson JM. Talking a sexual history. In: Tomlinson JM, ed. *ABC of Sexual Health.* Malden, MA: Blackwell Publishing, Inc; 2005:13-16.
9. Thaler-DeMers D. Intimacy issues: sexuality, fertility, and relationships. *Semin Oncol Nurs.* 2001;17:255-262.
10. Maslow A. A theory of human motivation. *Psychol Rev.* 1943;50:370-396.
11. Tierney DK. Sexuality: a quality-of-life issue for cancer survivors. *Semin Oncol Nurs.* 2008;24:71-79.
12. Shell JA. Sexuality. In: Carroll-Johnson R, Gorman L, Bush N, eds. *Oncology Nursing.* St. Louis, MO: Mosby; 2007:546-564.
13. Stausmire JM. Sexuality at the end of life. *Am J Hosp Palliat Care.* 2004;21:33-39.
14. Malcarne VL, Banthia R, Varni JW, Sadler GR, Greenbergs HL, Ko CM. Problem-solving skills and emotional distress in spouses of men with prostate cancer. *J Cancer Educ.* 2002;17:150-154.
15. Southard NZ, Keller J. The importance of assessing sexuality: a patient perspective. *Clin J Oncol Nurs.* 2009;13:213-217.
16. Smith DB. Sexuality and the patient with cancer: what nurses need to know. *Oncol Patient Care Pract Guidel Special Nurse.* 1994;4:1-3.
17. Winze JP, Carey MP. *Sexual Dysfunction: A Guide for Assessment and Treatment.* New York, NY: Guilford Press; 1991.
18. Krebs L. What should I say? Talking with patients about sexuality issues. *Clin J Oncol Nurs.* 2006;10:313-315.
19. Wilmoth MC. Life after cancer: what does sexuality have to do with it? 2006 Mara Mogensen Flaherty Memorial Lectureship. *Oncol Nurs Forum.* 2006;33:905-910.
20. Masters WH, Johnson VE. *Human Sexual Response.* 1st ed. Boston, MA: Little Brown; 1966.
21. Gregoire A. Male sexual problems. In: Tomlinson JM, ed. *ABC of Sexual Health.* 2nd ed. Malden, MA: Blackwell Publishing, Inc; 2005:37-39.
22. Basson R. Human sex-response cycles. *J Sex Marital Ther.* 2001;27:33-43.
23. Kandeel FR, Koussa VK, Swerdloff RS. Male sexual function and its disorders: physiology, pathophysiology, clinical investigation, and treatment. *Endocr Rev.* 2001;22:342-388.
24. Katz A. *Breaking the Silence on Cancer and Sexuality.* Pittsburgh, PA: Oncology Nursing Society; 2007.
25. Schiavi RC, Segraves RT. The biology of sexual function. *Psychiatr Clin North Am.* 1995;18:7-23.
26. Sarrel P. Genital blood flow and ovarian secretions. *J Clin Pract Sex,* 1990;14-15.
27. Zilbergeld B, Ellison C. Desire discrepancies and arousal problems in sex therapy. In: Leiblum S Pervin L, eds. *Principles and Practice of Sex Therapy.* New York, NY: Guilford Press; 1980:65-104.
28. Gallo-Silver L. The sexual rehabilitation of persons with cancer. *Cancer Pract.* 2000;8,10-15.
29. Pelusi J. Sexuality and body image. Research on breast cancer survivors documents altered body image and sexuality. *Am J Nurs.* 2006;106:32-38.
30. Dibble S, Eliason MJ, Dejoseph JF, Chinn P. Sexual issues in special populations: lesbian and gay individuals. *Semin Oncol Nurs.* 2008;24:127-130.
31. Dibble SL, Eliason MJ, Christiansen MA. Chronic illness care for lesbian, gay, bisexual individuals. *Nurs Clin North Am.* 2007;42:655-674; viii.
32. Bruner DW. Quality of life: sexuality issues for cancer patients. Presented at NCCN Conference, Hollywood, FL. February 2005.
33. Maurice WL. *Sexual Medicine in Primary Care.* St. Louis, MO: Mosby; 1999.

34. Goldstein I, Meston CM, Traish AM, et al. Future directions. In: *Women's Sexual Function and Dysfunction: Study, Diagnosis, and Treatment.* London: Taylor & Francis; 2007:745-748.

35. American Psychiatric Association. *Diagnostic and Statistical Manual of Mental Disorders: DSM-IV-TR.* Washington, DC: Author; 2000.

36. Schover L. Reproductive complications and sexual dysfunction in cancer survivors. In: Ganz PA, ed. *Cancer Survivorship; Today and Tomorrow.* New York, NY: Springer; 2007:251-271.

37. Galbraith ME, Crighton F. Alterations of sexual function in men with cancer. *Semin Oncol Nurs.* 2008;24:102-114.

38. Crenshaw TL, Goldberg JP, eds. *Sexual Pharmacology: Drugs that Effect Sexual Functioning.* New York, NY: WW Norton; 1996.

39. Sadock V. Psychotropic drugs and sexual dysfunction. *Prim Psychiatry.* 1995;4:16-17.

40. Ofman US. Psychosocial aspects of sexuality in the patient with cancer. *Oncol Patient Care Pract Guidel Special Nurse.* 1994;4:14-15.

41. Montejo-Gonzalez AL, Llorca G, Izquierdo JA, et al. SSRI-induced sexual dysfunction: fluoxetine, paroxetine, sertraline, and fluvoxamine in a prospective, multicenter, and descriptive clinical study of 344 patients. *J Sex Marital Ther.* 1997;23:176-194.

42. Derogatis LR, Kourlesis SM. An approach to evaluation of sexual problems in the cancer patient. *CA Cancer J Clin.* 1981;31:46-50.

43. Auchincloss SS, Holland J, Hughes M. Gynecological. In: Holland J, Greenberg D, Hughes M, eds. *Quick Reference for Oncology Clinicians: The Psychiatric and Psychological Dimensions of Cancer Symptom Management.* Charlottesville, VA: IPOS Press; 2006:128-134.

44. Hughes M. Sexual dysfunction. In: Holland J, Greenberg D, Hughes M, eds. *Quick Reference for Oncology Clinicians: The Psychiatric and Psychological Dimensions of Cancer Symptom Management.* Charlottesville, VA: IPOS Press; 2006.

45. Stein KD, Jacobsen PB, Hann DM, Greenberg H, Lyman G. Impact of hot flashes on quality of life among postmenopausal women being treated for breast cancer. *J Pain Symptom Manage.* 2000;19:436-445.

46. Kendall A, Dowsett M, Folkerd E, Smith I. Caution: vaginal estradiol appears to be contraindicated in postmenopausal women on adjuvant aromatase inhibitors. *Ann Oncol.* 2006;17:584-587.

47. Gupta P, Sturdee DW, Palin SL, et al. Menopausal symptoms in women treated for breast cancer: the prevalence and severity of symptoms and their perceived effects on quality of life. *Climacteric.* 2006;9(1):49-58.

48. Santoro N. The menopause transition. *Am J Med.* 2005;118(12B):85-135.

49. Ganz PA, Desmond KA, Belin TR, Meyerowitz BE, Rowland JH. Predictors of sexual health in women after a breast cancer diagnosis. *J Clin Oncol.* 1999;17(8):2371-2380.

50. Lester JL, Bernhard LA. Urogenital atrophy in breast cancer survivors. *Oncol Nurs Forum.* 2009;36(6):693-698.

51. Barton D, Wilwerding M, Carpenter L, Loprinzi C. Libido as part of sexuality in female cancer survivors, *Oncol Nurs Forum.* 2004;31(3):599-609.

52. Wilmoth MC. The aftermath of breast cancer: an altered sexual self. *Cancer Nurs.* 2001;24:278-286.

53. Hughes MK. Alterations of sexual function in women with cancer. *Semin Oncol Nurs.* 2008;24:91-101.

54. Conde DM, Pinto-Neto AM, Cabello C, Sa DS, Costa-Paiva L, Martinez EZ. Menopause symptoms and quality of life in women aged 45 to 65 years with and without breast cancer. *Menopause.* 2005;12:436-443.

55. Fobair P, Stewart SL, Chang S, D'Onofrio C, Banks PJ, Bloom JR. Body image and sexual problems in young women with breast cancer. *Psycho-Oncology.* 2006;15:579-594.

56. Rosenbaum TY. Managing postmenopausal dyspareunia: beyond hormone therapy. *Fem Patient.* 2006;31:1-5.

57. Katz A. Gay and lesbian patients with cancer. *Oncol Nurs Forum.* 2009;36:203-207.

58. Basson R, Leiblum S, Brotto L, et al. Revised definitions of women's sexual dysfunction. *J Sex Med.* 2004;1:40-48.

59. Basson R. Women's sexual dysfunction: revised and expanded definitions. *CMAJ.* 2005;172:1327-1333.

60. Clayton AH. Sexual function and dysfunction in women. *Psychiatr Clin North Am.* 2003;26:673-682.

61. Basson R, Althof S, Davis S, et al. Summary of the recommendations on sexual dysfunctions in women. *J Sex Med.* 2004;1:24-34.

62. Yi JC, Syrjala KL. Sexuality after hematopoietic stem cell transplantation. *Cancer J.* 2009;15:57-64.

63. Feldman HA, Goldstein I, Hatzichristou DG, Krane RJ, McKinlay JB. Impotence and its medical and psychosocial correlates: results of the Massachusetts Male Aging Study. *J Urol.* 1994;151:54-61.

64. Kupelian V, Shabsigh R, Araujo AB, O'Donnell AB, McKinlay JB. Erectile dysfunction as a predictor of the metabolic syndrome in aging men: results from the Massachusetts Male Aging Study. *J Urol.* 2006;176:222-226.

65. Krychman ML, Carter J, Aghajanian CA, Dizon DS, Castiel M. Chemotherapy induced dyspareunia: A case study of vaginal mucositis and pegylated liposomal doxorubicin injection in advanced stage ovarian carcinoma, *Gynecol Oncol.* 2004;93:561-563.

66. Taylor MJ, Rudkin L, Hawton K. Strategies for managing antidepressant-induced sexual dysfunction: Systematic review of randomized controlled trials. *J Affect Disord.* 2005;88:241-254.

67. Zemishlany Z, Weizman A. The impact of mental illness on sexual dysfunction. *Adv Psychosom Med.* 2008;29:89-106.

68. Basson R, Schultz WW. Sexual sequelae of general medical disorders. *Lancet* 2007;369:409-424.

69. Hitiris N, Barrett JA, Brodie JJ. Erectile dysfunction associated with pregablin Add-on treatment in patients with partial seizures: Five case reports. *Epilepsy Behav.* 2006;8: 418-421.

70. Hypericum Depression Trial Study Group. Effect of *Hypericum perforatum* (St. John's wort) in major depressive disorder. A randomized controlled trial. *JAMA.* 2002;287:1807-1814.

71. Lue T. Physiology of penile erection and pathophysiology of erectile dysfunction and priaprism. In: Walsh C, ed. *Campbell's Urology.* 8th ed. Philadelphia, PA: W.B. Saunders; 2002:1591-618.

72. Do C, Huyghe E, Lapeyre-Mestre M, Montastruc JI, Bagheri H. Statins and erectile dysfunction: results of a case/noncase study using the French Pharmacovigilance System Database. *Drug Saf.* 2009;32:591-597.

73. Maurer CA, Z'Graggen K, Renzulli P, Schilling MK, Netzer P, Buchler MW. Total mesorectal excision preserves male genital function compared with conventional rectal cancer surgery. *Br J Surg.* 2001;88:1501-1505.

74. Schmidt CE, Bestmann B, Kuchler T, Kremer B. Factors influencing sexual function in patients with rectal cancer. *Int J Impot Res.* 2005;17:231-238.

75. Harden J. Developmental life stage and couples' experiences with prostate cancer: a review of the literature. *Cancer Nurs.* 2005;28:85-98.

76. Carlson LE, Bultz BD, Speca M, St. Pierre M. Partners of cancer patients. part 1: impact, adjustment, and coping across the illness trajectory. *J Psychosoc Oncol.* 2000;18:39-63.

77. Kiss A, Meryn S. Effect of sex and gender on psychosocial aspects of prostate and breast cancer. *Br Med J.* 2001;323:1055-1058.

78. Perez MA, Skinner EC, Meyerowitz BE. Sexuality and intimacy following radical prostatectomy: patient and partner perspectives. *Health Psychol.* 2002;21:288-293.

79. Sestini AJ, Pakenham KI. Cancer of the prostate – a biopsychosocial review. *J Psychosoc Oncol.* 2000;18:17-38.

80. Neese LE, Schover LR, Klein EA, Zippe C, Kupelian PA. Finding help for sexual problems after prostate cancer treatment: a phone survey of men's and women's perspectives. *Psychooncology.* 2003;12:463-473.

81. DeFrank JT, Mehta CC, Stein KD, Baker F. Body image dissatisfaction in cancer survivors. *Oncol Nurs Forum.* 2007;34:E36-E41.

82. Butler L, Banfield V, Sveinson T, Allen K. Conceptualizing sexual health in cancer care. *West J Nurs Res.* 1998;20:683-699; discussion 700-705.

83. Mitchell WB, DiBartolo PM, Brown TA, Barlow DH. Effects of positive and negative mood on sexual arousal in sexually functional males. *Arch Sex Behav.* 1998;27:197-207.

84. Massie M. Breast. In: Holland J, Greenberg D, Hughes M, eds. *Quick Reference for Oncology Clinicians: The Psychiatric and Psychological Dimensions of Cancer Symptom Management.* Charlottesville, VA: IPOS Press; 2006:113-118.

85. Fisher SG. The psychosexual effects of cancer and cancer treatment. *Oncol Nurs Forum.* 1983;10:63-68.

86. Hughes MK. Sexuality and the cancer survivor: a silent coexistence. *Cancer Nurs.* 2000;23:477-482.

87. Shell JA, Carolan M, Zhang Y, Meneses KD. The longitudinal effects of cancer treatment on sexuality in individuals with lung cancer. *Oncol Nurs Forum.* 2008;35:73-79.

88. Cull A, Cowie VJ, Farquharson DI, Livingstone JR, Smart GE, Elton RA. Early stage cervical cancer: psychosocial and sexual outcomes of treatment. *Br J Cancer.* 1993;68:1216-1220.

89. Kritcharoen S, Suwan K, Jirojwong S. Perceptions of gender roles, gender power relationships, and sexuality in Thai women following diagnosis and treatment for cervical cancer. *Oncol Nurs Forum.* 2005;32:682-688.

90. Gevirtz C. How chronic pain affects sexuality. *Nursing.* January 2008;38:17.

91. Schover LR. Sexuality and fertility after cancer. *Hematol Am Soc Hematol Educ Program.* 2005;523:7.

92. Wenzel L, Dogan-Ates A, Habbal R, et al. Defining and measuring reproductive concerns of female cancer survivors. *J Natl Cancer Inst Monogr.* 2005;94:8.

93. Schover LR. Psychosocial aspects of infertility and decisions about reproduction in young cancer survivors: a review. *Med Pediatr Oncol.* 1999;33:53-59.

94. Simon B, Lee SJ, Partridge AH, Runowicz CD. Preserving fertility after cancer. *CA Cancer J Clin.* 2005;55:211-228; quiz 63-64.

95. Partridge AH, Burstein HJ, Winer EP. Side effects of chemotherapy and combined chemohormonal therapy in women with early-stage breast cancer. *J Natl Cancer Inst Monogr.* 2001; 135-142.

96. Fossa SD, Dahl AA. Fertility and sexuality in young cancer survivors who have adult-onset malignancies. *Hematol Oncol Clin North Am.* 2008;22:291-303, vii.

97. Dow KH, Kuhn D. Fertility options in young breast cancer survivors: a review of the literature. *Oncol Nurs Forum.* 2004;31:E46-E53.

98. Leonard M, Hammelef K, Smith GD. Fertility considerations, counseling, and semen cryopreservation for males prior to the initiation of cancer therapy. *Clin J Oncol Nurs.* 2004;8(127-131):45.

99. Wallace WH, Anderson RA, Irvine DS. Fertility preservation for young patients with cancer: who is at risk and what can be offered? *Lancet Oncol.* 2005;6:209-218.

100. Lamb MA. Effects of cancer on the sexuality and fertility of women. *Semin Oncol Nurs.* 1995;11:120-127.

101. American Society of Clinical Oncology. ASCO recommendations on fertility preservation in cancer patients: guideline summary. *J Oncol Pract.* 2006;2:143-146.

102. Oktay K, Sonmezer M. Ovarian tissue banking for cancer patients: fertility preservation, not just ovarian cryopreservation. *Hum Reprod.* 2004;19:477-480.

103. Carter J. Cancer-related infertility. *Gynecol Oncol.* 2005;99:S122-S123.

104. Ritchie K. Sexual issues in gynecologic cancer. *Clin Consult Obstet Gynecol.* 1997;3:118-121.

105. Annon JS. The PLISSIT model: a proposed conceptual scheme for the behavioral treatment of sexual problems. *J Sex Educ Ther.* 1976;2:1-15.

106. Smith DB, Babaian RJ. The effects of treatment for cancer on male fertility and sexuality. *Cancer Nurs.* 1992;15: 271-275.

107. Mick JM. Sexuality assessment: 10 strategies for improvement. *Clin J Oncol Nurs.* 2007;11:671-675.

108. Schover LR. Sexual rehabilitation after treatment for prostate cancer. *Cancer.* 1993;71:1024-1030.

109. Boehmer U, Potter J, Bowen DJ. Sexual functioning after cancer in sexual minority women. *Cancer J.* 2009;15: 65-69.

110. Kwan KSH, Roberts LJ, Swalm DM. Sexual dysfunction and chronic pain: the role of psychological variables and impact on quality of life. *Eur J Pain.* 2005;9:643-652.

111. Hughes MK. Sexuality changes in the cancer patient: M.D. Anderson case reports and review. *Nurs Interv Oncol.* 1996;8:15-18.

112. Ferrell BR, Dow KH, Leigh S, Ly J, Gulasekaram P. Quality of life in long-term cancer survivors. *Oncol Nurs Forum.* 1995;22:915-922.

113. Dobkin PL, Bradley I. Assessment of sexual dysfunction in oncology patients: review, critique, and suggestions. *J Psychosoc Oncol.* 1991;9:43-75.

114. Yurek D, Farrar W, Andersen BL. Breast cancer surgery: comparing surgical groups and determining individual differences in postoperative sexuality and body change stress. *J Consult Clin Psychol.* 2000;68:697-709.

115. Ganz PA, Rowland JH, Desmond K, Meyerowitz BE, Wyatt GE. Life after breast cancer: understanding women's health-related quality of life and sexual functioning. *J Clin Oncol.* 1998;16:501-514.

116. Henson HK. Breast cancer and sexuality. *Sex Disabil.* 2002;20:261-275.

117. Andersen BL. In sickness and in health: maintaining intimacy after breast cancer recurrence. *Cancer J.* 2009;15:70-73.

118. Greenwald HP, McCorkle R. Sexuality and sexual function in long-term survivors of cervical cancer. *J Womens Health*. 2008;17:955-963.

119. Heiman JR. Treating low sexual desire – new findings for testosterone in women. *N Engl J Med*. 2008;359:2047-2949.

120. Bachmann GA. Sexual issues at menopause. *Ann N Y Acad Sci*. 1990;592:87-94; discussion 123-133.

121. Levine SB. What patients mean by love, intimacy, and sexual desire. In: Levine SB, Risen CB, Althof SE, eds. *Handbook of Clinical Sexuality for Mental Health Professionals*. 2nd ed. Routledge, New York, NY. 2010:19-34.

122. Masters WH, Johnson VE, Kolodny RC. *Human Sexuality*. New York, NY: HarperCollins; 1992.

123. Notelovitz M. Management of the changing vagina. *J Clin Pract Sex*. 1990;16-21.

124. Guirguis WR. Oral treatment of erectile dysfunction: from herbal remedies to designer drugs. *J Sex Marital Ther*. 1998;24:69-73.

125. Albaugh JA. Intracavernosal injection algorithm. *Urol Nurs*. 2006;26:449-453.

126. Aung HH, Dey I, Rand V, Yuan CS. Alternative therapies for male and female sexual dysfunction. *Am J Chin Med*. 2004;32:161-173.

127. Bruner DW, Calvano T. The sexual impact of cancer and cancer treatments in men. *Nurs Clin North Am*. 2007;42: 555-580.

128. White A, Hayhoe S, Hart A, Ernst E, and Volunteers from BMAS and AACP. Adverse events following acupuncture (SAFA): a prospective survey of 32,000 consultations. *Acupunct Med*. 2001;19:84-92.

129. Slater S, Oliver RT. Testosterone: its role in development of prostate cancer and potential risk from use as hormone replacement therapy. *Drugs Aging*. 2000;17:431-439.

130. Manne SL, Ostroff J, Winkel G, Grana G, Fox K. Partner unsupportive responses, avoidant coping, and distress among women with early stage breast cancer: patient and partner perspectives. *Health Psychol*. 2005;24,635-641.

131. Institute of Medicine. *From Cancer Patient to Cancer Survivor: Lost in Transition*. Washington, DC: National Academies Press; 2005.

132. Taylor B, Davis S. The extended PLISIT model for addressing the sexual wellbeing of individuals with an acquired disability or chronic illness. *Sex Disabil*. 2007;25:135-139.

CHAPTER 52

Caregiving in the Home

Betty Ferrell ■ Jo Hanson

CAREGIVING

Background

In the United States, caring for the patient in the home setting has undergone marked shifts over the last 30 years. Prior to the 1980s, most home care was provided by informal (family/unpaid) caregivers (1). Home care consisted mainly of non-complex interventions, such as administering oral medications or changing simple dressings. Patients requiring more complicated care remained as inpatients in the hospital.

In the mid-1980s, with large increases in access to and use of Medicare, home care shifted toward the formal (unlicensed or licensed paid) caregiver, that is, home health, to provide patient care and to support the family. The formal and informal caregivers worked as a team managing the patient's needs. It was common for a home health nurse to visit the patient's home prior to discharge. The visit provided an opportunity for the nurse to meet the family, to introduce the treatment plan, and to assess the home for any potential care issues. Meeting the nurse and reviewing the treatment plan greatly alleviated the family's anxiety concerning their loved ones' special home care needs. When the patient came home, the supplies and/or medications were already in place and the nurse–family caregiver team was prepared to start the treatment plan.

The Balanced Budget Act of 1997 enactment initiated a shift away from the formal caregivers (2). Although home health benefits were not eliminated, for many they were greatly reduced. Eligibility parameters were narrowed and frequent and complicated documentation was required. The newly enacted Budget Act, along with the combination of the increasing trend toward managed care and growing reimbursement restrictions on hospital and home care services, accelerated the shift toward the family caregivers shouldering the home care responsibilities (3,4). Patients were discharged earlier, sicker, and with fewer support resources; suddenly family caregivers were overwhelmed and ill prepared to meet the demands of the complex and multiple responsibilities thrust upon them (5–8). With minimal support or training, family caregivers struggled to manage pain and other symptoms, dispense medications, support emotional needs, pay bills, run errands, administer complex and highly technical treatments, coordinate care, communicate with multiple providers, provide meals, change dressings, and transport as needed (4,9–11).

In the 21st century, new technologies, innovative surgical techniques, and advances in medication modalities are changing how and where cancer care is delivered. In contrast to just 10 years ago, the majority of care is now provided in freestanding or outpatient hospital clinics, offices, ambulatory care centers, or outpatient surgical units. For example, a newly diagnosed non-surgical lung cancer patient, scheduled for several months of chemotherapy followed by weeks of daily radiation, may receive all tests, procedures, and treatments in the outpatient clinic or in an ambulatory cancer care center. While keeping people out of the inpatient hospital setting is a positive trend, it creates an even greater need for more support from the healthcare system for the patients and the families providing care in the home setting (12).

Complex Care in the Home Setting

In the past, most studies of symptom management have been largely concentrated on major symptoms, such as cancer pain, and acute care settings. More recent studies have focused on the broader needs of patients in the home settings (13). Several factors influence home care, especially the delivery of palliative care. Heavy reliance on the family caregivers, access to diagnostic facilities, and often the limited pharmacy services influence the effectiveness of pain and symptom management at home (12).

It is often assumed that comfort is enhanced in home setting, as it has been considered preferable to institutional settings. In fact, patients, families, and healthcare professionals frequently elect care at home assuming patients will be more comfortable (14,15). As researchers have extended studies into the home care setting, barriers that impede pain management have been revealed. Issues of patient and family fears of addiction, failure to report pain, and limited access to needed services have limited the effectiveness of pain management (11). When planning cancer home care, consideration must be given to the accessibility of services and to family caregivers' knowledge, values, and abilities. If potential home care issues have not been identified, not only can patient comfort level be compromised but also it can evoke a sense of inadequacy and despair in family caregivers.

Symptom management at home is different from that in the hospital and other institutional settings. Hospitals provide technical equipment and services for acutely ill patients. For patients with complex problems, inpatient care includes a variety of aggressive or invasive strategies for diagnosis and definitive treatment of the underlying conditions. With immediate access to specialists and high-tech equipment, an appropriate plan can be determined and immediately initiated. In contrast, care provided in the home is slow to change and relies mostly on low-tech strategies that concentrate on symptom management. The dynamic nature of cancer and its treatment side effects make effective symptom management especially challenging for home care patients and family caregivers. A change in symptoms may indicate disease progression or treatment-related side effects. Determining the best overall strategies for symptom management in the home setting is difficult. Further research is needed to better understand and support the inherent challenges of providing cancer care in the home (16,17).

Cancer as a Family Experience

A cancer diagnosis is recognized as a disease that affects the whole family (7,11,17–19). As cancer care shifts toward the outpatient setting, there is a heightened awareness of the importance of families and their understanding of and involvement in the total care needs of the patient (11,20). It is remarkable that care which only a decade ago was reserved for intensive care units (ICUs), to be delivered by specially trained healthcare providers, is now delegated to families in the home who have had little or no preparation for the physical and emotional demands of caregiving (21,22). Family caregiving has advanced from caring for patients with mostly low-tech needs to providing high-tech active treatments, such as chemotherapy regimens, intravenous fluid administration, complex wound care, and many other technical procedures (17). Recent literature has acknowledged the intense demands of family caregiving at home, especially in the areas of technical care, acquisition of skills, and provision of intense 24-hour physical caregiving (11,23). Less emphasis has been placed on the family caregiver's emotional burdens of assuming responsibilities for the patient's well-being or peaceful death in the home (16,19,24–26). Studies have found that family caregivers report feelings of unpreparedness, uncertainty, and extreme anxiety in providing care and a home death. Further research is needed to understand the family caregivers' feelings and to develop interventions that will provide the needed support (27).

Care in the home setting can be a delicate balance for families. At one end of the spectrum are the many patient needs; if out of balance, it can result in intense burdens for family caregivers and compromised care for patients (8). At the other end of the spectrum are the many benefits of providing the care at home (28,29). Home care may offer the patient improved physical comfort and the psychological well-being of familiar surroundings. Together patients and families may find opportunities to heal relationships, to benefit from the compassion of giving and receiving comfort care, and to share in the transition from life to death (13,25).

Families have been greatly impacted by their limited ability to choose the primary healthcare setting. In the late 1970s and early 1980s, patient and family preferences and abilities were major considerations when healthcare professionals determined whether to discharge a patient to the home

setting or extend the inpatient stay. In the 1990s, care began to shift to the home as the primary setting for active treatment as well as palliative care. Insurance and managed care benefits became the driving force in the care setting decision, leaving patient and family choices as secondary considerations. Although many patients and families may volitionally have chosen home as the primary care setting, others had no choice; the healthcare system or hospital relegated care to the home.

The outcomes of home caregiving may best be evaluated by the effects on families following the death of the patient and during bereavement. Hospice providers have long recognized that positive experiences with caregiving in the home result in positive bereavement and adaptation by family members after the patient's death. However, feelings of inadequacy in providing care in the home, patient complications, and deaths that are less optimal than anticipated can result not only in the patient's diminished quality of life (QOL) or quality of death but also in long-term consequences for the family (13,27,30).

Case Study

To further illustrate cancer as a family experience and the long-term consequences, a case study is included.

Six-year-old Trevor was diagnosed with acute lymphoblastic leukemia 3 months ago. He has two older sisters, 8 and 10 years old. His parents, Amy and Sam, both teach in an inner city high school 45 minutes from their home. For the first 6 weeks, Sam took time off to be with Trevor while he was an inpatient receiving high-dose chemotherapy. He has no more paid time off. Trevor's mother is worried about taking time off now, in case he gets "really sick from the chemo" and has to go back into the hospital. He has two more years of outpatient chemotherapy.

On discharge, his parents were given the 35 medications and a 2-page list of instructions on diet, activity, infection prevention, and signs of infection, such as redness, tenderness, or pus at his Port-a-Cath site or if the temperature was ≥38.3°C they were to rush him to the hospital immediately. He started his outpatient chemotherapy a month ago. Since then he has been to the emergency room twice and admitted to the hospital once for 4 days.

Fortunately, they live in a closely knit neighborhood that has reached out to support the family. Transportation for the sisters' school and activities has been organized by their neighbors who have also insured that the food is well supplied and have cared for the dog. Amy's parents live nearby and spend the day with Trevor while the rest of the family is away at work and school.

Amy no longer allows the girls to have friends over to their house, fearing they may bring germs into the house. She disinfects the whole house twice a day and has established "Trevor only" items such as keyboards, toys, and furniture. Upon their return from work and school, everyone has to shower before they are allowed in the same room with Trevor. Other than work and school, the family has stopped outside activities, including church. Even the dog, which has always slept in the girls' room, is no longer allowed in the house.

Sam is anxious to keep Trevor "normal" during his 2-year treatment period. He feels like Amy is overreacting and is making the girls feel as if they don't matter. When Sam tries to discuss this with Amy, she gets defensive telling him he doesn't care about his son. She says it's just for 2 years and that he and girls will just have to adjust.

THE FAMILY CAREGIVER

"In 2009, about 42.1 million family caregivers in the United States provided care to an adult with limitations in daily activities at any given period in time; and about 61.6 million provided care at some time during this year. The estimated economic value of their unpaid contributions was approximately $450 billion" (1).

Definition

Family caregivers have been defined as follows:

- A relative, friend, or partner who has a significant relationship and provides assistance (physical, social, and/or psychological) to a person with a life-threatening, incurable illness (31).
- An unpaid family member, friend, or neighbor who provides care to an individual who has an acute or chronic condition and needs assistance to manage a variety of tasks, from bathing, dressing, and taking medications to tube feeding and ventilator care (11).
- Any relative, partner, friend, or neighbor who has a significant personal relationship with, and provides a broad range of assistance for, an older person or an adult with a chronic or disabling condition. These individuals may be primary or secondary caregivers and live with, or separately from, the person receiving care (6).

Commonalities in each definition include (1) significant relationship; (2) unpaid; and (3) breadth of caregiving responsibilities. Throughout this chapter, family caregivers refers to those who provide uncompensated care in the home and who have a pre-existing relationship (either through friendship or kinship) with the person for whom care is being provided. This care can be in any of the QOL domains, including physical, social, psychological, and spiritual care.

Demographics

Today, in the United States, 65 million people are family caregivers. A typical family caregiver is a 49-year-old woman caring for her widowed 69-year-old mother who does not live with her. She is married and employed. Approximately, 66% are women and more than 37% have children or grandchildren <18 years old living with them. They average 20 hours per week caring for loved ones; however, 13% provide care for 40 or more hours per week. More than 3 in 10 households (31.2%) report that at least 1 person has been a caregiver of the last 12 months. They have been in the family caregiver role for an average of 4.6 years, with 3 in 10 having given care to their loved ones for 5 or more years (31%). The majority care for a relative (86%) and 36% are taking care of a parent (9).

Elderly

The changing demographics are of special significance for the cancer family caregiver. Cancer is associated with aging; over half of all cancers occur in those 65 years and older (32). Between the years 2005 and 2030, the number of older adults in the United States will almost double, making up 20% of the population. The 2008 Institute of Medicine (IOM) report warned that the nation is not prepared to meet the elderly healthcare needs (33). The Seer Cancer Statistics Review reported approximately 60% of cancer diagnosis and 70% of cancer mortality occur in patients 65 years of age or older (34). The average adult care recipient's age is 69.2 years old. Eighty percent of their care is provided by family caregivers and of these caregiver 80% are their spouses (9).

Care for the cancer patient at home becomes far more difficult when the patient and the family caregiver are elderly and also have concomitant illnesses themselves, such as cardiac disease, hypertension, and diabetes, with their associated medications and treatments. The current trend toward earlier discharge from acute care hospitals and the increase in home care leads to more adult children becoming involved in caring for a physically dependent parent. Advances in cancer treatment have led to increased survivorship, which in turn has led to caregiving demands that may exist for several months to years (18). Importantly, the majority of the family caregivers are women, many over the age of 65. They suffer from multiple role responsibilities and co-morbidities, making them especially vulnerable to the significant physical, emotional, social, and spiritual toll of caregiving (35). There is limited attention focused on the special care needs of the geriatric population at home and that of their caregiver. Expanded efforts in attending to complex needs of the aging need to be adopted, especially given the growing percentage of population over the age of 65 (33).

Children

Although there are over 10,000 new childhood cancer diagnoses each year and even though cancer is the leading cause of childhood death due to disease (36), most of the literature regarding family caregivers has focused on the care of adults. The care of children is often perceived to be less demanding or even normal as family caregivers usually provide pediatric home care. However, studies reveal that when a child is diagnosed with cancer, the family equilibrium is disrupted, often with the adverse affects of the family caregivers experiencing post-traumatic stress disorder, anxiety, depression, financial distress, marital discord, social and behavioral problems, and/or prolonged/complicated mourning (37). Expectations of pediatric cancer family caregivers include managing frequent medical appointments and hospital stays; learning rigorous treatment protocols; providing high-tech medical care in the home; responding to severe side effects; partnering with the medical team for invasive procedures; and getting the child to cooperate/comply with treatments and procedures. The parent–caregiver role/parent–healthcare provider role presents a parental dilemma. Parents view their role as one that nurtures, protects, and avoids suffering; however, in the healthcare provider role, the parent is often providing or assisting in painful care. Parents struggle with the desire to reflect child's preferences, to receive positive feedback from the staff concerning the wisdom of decision-making, and to still feel like they are still being a "good parent" (38).

Recent studies have explored the experience of parents in caring for a child with cancer. These studies have added a dimension to the previous research related to family caregivers and described the decisions and conflicts of caring for children with cancer. Jones identified the needs of family caregivers who are providing pediatric palliative and end-of-life care. They are as follows: (1) adequate pain control and symptom management; (2) companionship, counseling, and support; and (3) information, control, and advocacy for the medical decisions they must make (37).

Parents of pediatric patients with cancer in pain have reported that healthcare providers did not take their child's pain seriously and did not provide adequate analgesia to relieve the pain (39,40). This is consistent with literature describing the inadequate assessment and management of pediatric pain and the overall deficiencies in pediatric palliative care. However, when specialized pain teams were involved, they were better able to relieve not only the child's pain but also the parent's emotional suffering as well (41). The parents' role in decision-making varied from allowing the child to have control whenever possible regarding his or her treatment to personally administering nondrug methods of pain relief that temporarily alleviated both the child's pain and the parents' feelings of helplessness.

Distance

The number of distance caregivers is rapidly growing. It is estimated that more than 7 million Americans are distant caregivers (8,34). Mazanec defines distant caregiving as the experience of providing instrumental and emotional support to an ill loved one who lives far away (28). In distance caregiving, generally the focus is more on gathering information and available resources, coordinating services, and putting together a team (i.e., friends or paid help) that can provide the care for the family's loved one rather than providing hands-on care. Caregiver burden increases for many distant caregivers as they struggle to gain information and for some to participate in the care of their loved ones. For instance, an adult daughter caregiver, living 500 miles away from her 89-year-old mother with breast cancer, is unable to participate in her mother's day-to-day caregiving and is challenged by complicated communication issues. Feelings of guilt and anxiety heighten her already heavy caregiver burden. In a study of caregivers living at least 100 miles from their loved ones, issues concerning lack of control and information were identified as major caregiver challenges (42). More research is needed to change the way information is delivered to distance caregivers and to identify their unique needs in supporting their loved ones.

Roles/Responsibilities

Family caregiver roles and responsibilities are varied and multidimensional, reaching across the QOL domains: physical; psychological; social; and spiritual (43,44) (Table 52.1). Family members' roles change as they learn and adapt to the nuances of family caregiving responsibilities, such as providing care and support, dealing with stress and grief, and managing finances. One of the most important responsibilities of the cancer family caregiving is that of pain management. In the early stages of cancer 30% to 45% of patients experience pain; by the advanced stages this increases to 75% (7). Although each family navigates the cancer journey differently, all families go through a learning process in determining the best plan in caring for their loved ones.

A primary task of family caregivers is management of medications. It is enlightening to realize that healthcare professionals assume similar responsibilities in inpatient and other settings only after formal courses in pharmacology and with support available from professional colleagues, such as pharmacists, reached by direct access. For family caregivers in the home setting, this is particularly challenging when symptom management is often either accomplished on an as-needed basis for symptoms such as nausea or anxiety or with necessary titration of around-the-clock dosing of medication such as analgesics.

TABLE 52.1	**Family caregiver responsibilities**
Activity	**QOL Domain**[a]
Symptom management	P, Ps, S, Sp
Medication acquisition/ dispensing	P, Ps
Emotional support	P, Ps, S, Sp
Communication with providers	Ps, S, Sp
Coordinating care	P, Ps
Transportation	P, S
Errands/bill paying	P, Ps
Supervision, adherence	P, Ps
Monitoring using electronic devices	P, Ps
Meals and nutritional assistance	P, Ps, S, Sp

[a]P, physical; Ps, psychological; S, social; Sp, spiritual.
QOL, quality of life.

Management of medications is important not only to preserve the patient's comfort but also to diminish the burden on the family caregiver and to avoid costly complications such as repeat hospitalizations when medications are not effectively used. Often patients and family caregivers do not have the necessary knowledge to judge indications for administration of medications or the delicate issues involved with titration or the side effects of medications. Healthcare providers can make a valuable contribution to the care of patients at home by insuring that medication schedules are made as simple as possible using single agents rather than multiple drugs and maintaining the simplest possible routes of administration and dosage schedules. Patients and family caregivers require assistance with important decisions regarding the use and titration of medications and practical techniques such as written dosage schedules, use of logs, and provision of guidelines to help in medication choices.

Another factor of caregiver burden is the costs assumed by cancer patients and their caregivers related to symptom management and home care (45). Family caregivers incur significant expenses related to caregiving responsibilities, much of which is not reimbursed (46). Costs may include direct expenses, such as medications, increases in insurance coverage, and higher co-pays, as well as extensive indirect costs such as loss of wages, missed work, missed promotions, and loss in pension/social security/wages (1,45,47). Most of the cost savings to third-party payers have resulted in increased costs assumed by patients and families, which have only added to the financial burden.

In addition to the extensive responsibilities related to the pharmacologic management of pain and other symptoms, patients and family caregivers use many nondrug strategies at home such as hot/cold compresses, lotion/ointments, positioning, or fans for air circulation. The home care setting offers the benefit of access to nondrug symptom management methods. Patients and family caregivers often feel more comfortable with these complementary methods. Typically, patients and family caregivers receive minimal formal information or guidance regarding nondrug strategies; instead they rely on advice from friends to find methods that may add to the patient's comfort. It is important for healthcare providers to explore the nondrug interventions with the family caregiver in order to assess for possible interactions with ongoing treatments.

Patients and families are eager to add nondrug interventions to their overall symptom management arsenal. These activities have the potential to greatly benefit patients by not only enhancing physical relief but also alleviating their anxiety and providing a better sense of control. Additionally, family caregivers find nondrug comfort measures to be extremely valuable in reducing their sense of helplessness. Studies found family caregivers trained to provide safe massage therapy felt empowered by their ability to add to the patient's comfort. They described feelings of making a positive difference, connecting with their loved ones, and finding deep satisfaction in caring for their loved ones (48–50). This type of intervention is often recalled by family caregivers during bereavement as positive memories of their ability to provide greater comfort during terminal illness.

Case Study

To further illustrate the impact cancer has on the caregiver's roles and responsibilities this case study is included.

Chen, a 45-year-old Chinese-American woman, works 7 days a week with her husband, Hui, in their small grocery store. In addition to shop keeping, she is responsible for their household, which includes a teenage son and Hui's non–English speaking aging parents. The son does not drive and is involved in many after school activities. Hui is the leader of the family.

Several months ago Hui began experiencing nausea, vomiting, and gastric pain. After many doctor visits, tests, and treatment regimens, he was diagnosed with stage III gastric cancer. He is scheduled for surgery, which will be followed by chemotherapy. Although the surgery will be inpatient, the 6 months of chemotherapy will be outpatient at the same site, 15 miles away. The chemotherapy will require a minimum of three visits per week.

Neither Hui's parents nor the son has been told of his cancer diagnosis. His obvious illness has been explained as a passing virus. Chen is a reluctant driver but has been able to transport Hui to his medical appointments and take their son to his frequent after school activities. She is feeling overwhelmed as she struggles to keep the grocery store (their only income) open, to transport/support their son at school, to protect her in-laws and son from any knowledge of the diagnosis, and to take care of all of Hui's needs. Hui's only brother, who lives in China, has been told about the cancer diagnosis; he is unable to leave his job to come for help. He agrees that his parents should not be told about the cancer diagnosis. At this point, the surgery is only 1 week away. Chen is bravely trying to embrace her new role as the quasi-family leader while shouldering all her new responsibilities.

FAMILY CAREGIVER NEEDS

Family caregivers, like cancer patients themselves, have diverse needs and health concerns (51). The impact of the disease on the family is multifocal. Caring for a loved one with cancer at home entails inherent physical, psychological, and financial burdens (7,37,52). Complex symptom management represents a challenge for the patients and their family caregivers. Whether or not they feel competent to do so, and despite the stress of incorporating caregiving into their daily lives, family members become active caregivers (16). Family caregivers report feelings of anxiety, depression, fear, helplessness, anger, guilt, and uncertainty (13,25). Studies reveal that more family caregivers are stressed and depressed and have lower levels of subjective well-being, physical health, and self-efficacy than their non–caregiver peers (53). Although these feelings have been recognized, there are few model programs to address these needs (24). Family caregiver needs have a broad scope reaching across the informational, personal, household, and patient care spheres. It is essential for healthcare providers to acknowledge these needs to avoid potential consequent impact upon adherence and delays in medical decision-making (16,51,54).

Caregiver needs and access to resources vary; consideration must be given to demographic characteristics, including gender, age, culture, education, economics, and geographic setting (rural vs. urban) (55). They also vary according to the nature and closeness of the relationship to the patient. Those caring for an especially vulnerable loved one with cognitive impairments or one who is physically or emotionally dependent (52,56) and who requires substitutive decision-making are at even greater risk for increased guilt and complicated bereavement (57). Family caregivers vary regarding their abilities to deal with the challenges and burdens of care and require additional time and attention from professional providers (27,51). Patients and their family caregivers may vary regarding preferred coping styles, which can further stress a relationship challenged by illness (18,58). Perhaps most importantly, caregiver needs vary in the trajectory of illness from diagnosis through treatment, survivorship, and end-of-life care (18).

Cancer caregivers are distinguished from other family caregivers as a result of the unique nature of the disease and its treatment (25). Attention to the impact on family caregivers' QOL has been a focus of concern for more than a decade (16). There is growing attention to the impact of home deaths upon family caregivers' coping and bereavement needs (18,24). Developing and standardizing appropriate bereavement support services for differing caregiver groups remains problematic (18,25).

At the time of diagnosis family caregivers, like patients themselves, may be overwhelmed by the need to adapt to the myriad of new information, decision-making, and adjustments to the impact of the illness upon their lives (22,59). Due to new advances in care, many with cancer find themselves facing their illness as a chronic disease requiring months or even years of active treatment resulting in long-term impact upon family caregiver (18). Although the survivorship phase may now last for decades, patients are often left with an illness or treatment legacy that continues to require ongoing attention from family caregivers. For those facing end of life, caregiving needs typically escalate as family caregivers cope with the increasing burden of illness upon their loved ones (18,25).

Despite these differing needs, family caregivers have many concerns in common. Family caregivers consistently express a desire for increased communication with their healthcare team (60). Communication patterns are particularly distressing surrounding the concept of the delivery of "bad news" to patients and family caregivers. Issues surrounding advance care planning, not just with patients but with family caregivers, benefit from skilled communication by healthcare providers regarding their understanding and readiness for transitions in prognosis (61).

Family caregivers request education and support to better prepare themselves for their caregiving responsibilities (20).

They are especially challenged with communication needs when the patient is in a critical care unit (60). Because family caregivers may assume their caregiving role under unexpected and emotionally difficult circumstances, anticipatory guidance and education regarding effective coping strategies are often desperately needed (7,25). Sophisticated assessment and intervention skills are needed by the entire oncology team to maximize health outcomes (19). Failure to address these complex needs impacts adherence to healthcare treatment and satisfaction with care and is a factor increasing risk for complicated bereavement (60).

Self-Care

Much of the health-related research in family caregivers has focused on health-related problems as a result of caregiving duties. In a study with 60 patients with incurable cancer and their caregivers, Gibbins et al. found that poor sleep was a frequent complaint, sleep fragmentation was high in both groups, and poor sleep was significantly related to higher anxiety in caregivers (62). Other studies have found that caregiving is associated with negative physical health consequences of fatigue, pain, sleep problems, loss of physical strength, loss of appetite, and loss of weight (17,63). However, there is increasing recognition that the ability of family members to care for patients is dependent on caring for themselves (18). Examples of health-promoting self-care include getting enough rest, eating nutritiously, exercising, seeking psychological counseling or spiritual support, maintaining routine health checks, and attention to the caregivers' own chronic illnesses and health conditions (64,65).

Given the benefits of health maintenance, engaging in self-care behaviors should reduce caregiver burden. The emerging literature in this research area supports this hypothesis. Acton explored the effect of health-promoting self-care behavior on caregiver stress and well-being. The findings suggest that caregivers who practiced more self-care behaviors were better protected from stress, and the effects of stress on well-being were reduced (64). Many of the self-care strategies recommended for nurses and other healthcare professionals (66), such as meditation, relaxation, and exercise, are applicable to family caregivers. Adopting these self-care strategies to support family caregivers will improve their QOL as well as the lives of their loved ones.

Quality of Life

The cancer experience profoundly affects the patients' and family caregivers' QOL, including their physical, psychological, social, and spiritual well-being (46). The patient and family caregiver make up a unit of care as they go through the cancer experience in constellation with each other (67). Mellon et al.'s study findings revealed that one of the most robust predictors of cancer survivors' and family caregivers' QOL is social support. QOL for survivor and family caregiver independently contributed to the other's QOL (68) (Fig. 52.1).

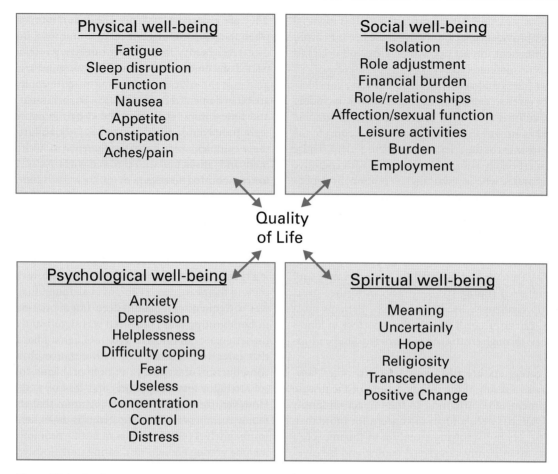

Figure 52.1. Quality of life model applied to family caregivers (69).

Physical Well-Being. Physical demands of caregiving are generally related to the patient's medical situation (1,7,10,11). Adverse physical outcomes associated with cancer family caregivers are far reaching, affecting the overall state of physical well-being (21,70,71) (Table 52.2) (72). Research indicates that as the patient's disease progresses, the physical well-being of the family caregivers decreases (3,14). In the

TABLE 52.2	Caregiver's most common worsened health effects as a result of caregiving (72)
Energy and sleep	87%
Stress and/or panic attacks	70%
Pain and aching	60%
Depression	52%
Headaches	41%
Weight gain/loss	38%

Evercare® study, family caregivers reported that their health worsened as a result of caregiving and rated their overall health as fair to poor (72). The degree of deterioration was directly proportional to the intensity of care provided and the amount of time spent caregiving. Bishop et al. found that while health status is initially similar to that of the normal population, over time, family caregivers report more problems with fatigue, sleep disturbances, and impaired cognitive function (3,73,74). Other studies have found that stressful caregiving experiences of elderly spouses have a 63% higher mortality rate for 5 years following their caregiver experience when compared with their non–caregiver peers (11). Serious physical repercussions can result when family caregivers neglect their own health needs in order to provide care to their loved ones (35,75). With the dynamic nature of cancer triggering changes in caregiver responsibilities, family caregivers' physical well-being must be assessed and reassessed throughout the caregiving period.

Psychological Well-Being. Distress is a critical factor in psychological well-being and QOL for patients and their caregivers. Family caregivers, often referred to as the backbone of health care, report as much distress as their ill loved ones (76,77). This distress is fueled from the demands of the caregiver role along with the stress from watching their loved ones suffer (46). Increased anxiety, depression, marital and family conflicts, embarrassment, guilt, resentment, low morale, and severe emotional exhaustion are commonly reported by distressed family caregivers. Distress puts family caregivers at risk for mental and physical problems of their own (16). At points in the cancer trajectory (diagnosis, treatment, post-treatment/survivorship, recurrence, and end of life), the distress level can change in relation to the disease phase. In the diagnosis phase, shock, uncertainty, and a sense of helplessness/hopelessness can lead to significant distress. It has been described as a feeling of "nailed by cancer" (59). During the treatment phase, levels of depressive symptoms are often higher for the family caregiver than for the patient (78). Recognized as a transition stage either to survivorship or to palliative care, in the post-treatment phase family caregivers report experiencing more fear of recurrence than does the patient (79). The recurrence phase has been called the most stressful event in the course of the illness (18) and creates serious impairment in family caregivers' emotional well-being. In the end-of-life phase, depression is three times higher compared with their non–caregiver peers (80). Consideration of the cancer trajectory is an essential component when assessing the family caregivers' psychological well-being (46).

Social Well-Being. The social demands of family caregiving are primarily related to relationships and financial factors. While assessing family caregivers' social well-being, factors to consider include (1) patient/family caregiver communication and relationships, for example, marital quality, marital tension, emotional and physical intimacy, and role adaptation; (2) family members' way of interrelating, for example, family cohesion, conflict, communication, interpersonal support, and relationship quality with patient; and (3) parenting behavior and parenting quality. Social well-being studies have examined the interpersonal effect of cancer on patients and their family caregivers mostly with a focus on couples. A study exploring the concerns of couples living with early-stage breast cancer found that 66% of the couples wanted to work on ways to better deal with tension in the marriage or be together as a couple with cancer (81). Marital relationships can be strained; research has found that depression in both patient and spouse negatively affected marital relationships. Family communication patterns, roles, and coping methods are crucial components of family functioning. Difficulties in these components can be exacerbated by cancer and increased family caregiver burden. In a qualitative study with 12 lung cancer caregivers, Badr and Taylor found that couples coping with lung cancer experience a wide variety of social constraints, such as denial, avoidance, and conflict, that may compromise open communication and spousal support (82).

The complexities of family communication are especially profound during the cancer experience, challenging

caregivers' social well-being. The Clinical Practice Guidelines for Quality Palliative Care established by the National Consensus Project (NCP) recommend that routine patient and family meetings be conducted with the interdisciplinary care team to facilitate communication and develop an individualized plan of care (83). The family meeting has become increasingly more common. It is an ideal forum for eliciting family caregivers' concerns and identifying their unmet needs.

Spiritual Well-Being. Spirituality has been increasingly recognized as an important factor in cancer patients and their family caregivers (84). "Spirituality is the way we experience our connectedness to the moment, to self, to others, to nature, and to the significant or sacred" (85). Spiritual well-being refers to the way people make sense of and find meaning in their daily lives. Research suggests that the cancer patients and their family caregivers derive meaning in their cancer experience (3,7,86). For instance, in a cancer caregiver QOL study, results indicate that many cancer family caregivers experience personal growth from providing care to their loved ones (86). In another study of bone marrow transplant family caregivers, Fife found that those with a sense of spiritual connectedness experienced lower emotional distress (87). Tang et al. found that the QOL of family caregivers has been closely correlated with the QOL of patients with terminal illness (88). This would suggest that the suffering of terminally ill patients and their caregivers is interrelated; the suffering of one amplifies the distress of the other (14,89). It is crucial that healthcare professionals routinely assess (and reassess) spiritual well-being and help family caregivers find meaning and benefit in their caregiving experience.

Case Study

The case of Renee, a distance caregiver for her mother, illustrates how communication issues fostered feelings of distress and impacted Renee's overall QOL.

Renee is an African-American woman born in Washington D.C. where she was raised by her single parent mother, Dorothy. Dorothy was the sole provider for their household and worked as an appointment clerk in a downtown hospital. Her priority was to provide good education for Renee so "she can do whatever she wants to do." Although the rent has doubled, Dorothy still lives in the same rented row house. After graduating from law school a year ago, Renee moved 100 miles away to Richmond, VA, where she works for the state of Virginia. Although the job requires her to work 80 hour weeks, she loves it.

At the age of 53, Dorothy was diagnosed with breast cancer and retired from her hospital job. Renee begged her mother to come to Richmond for her surgery and treatment, but Dorothy wanted to be close to her Baptist Church and go to "her" hospital.

Dorothy's surgery was on a Friday in "her" hospital, which enabled Renee to be with her for the overnight inpatient stay and at her home through the weekend. Dorothy's church friends promised to care for her and assured Renee they would call her if her mother needed anything. Nevertheless, when Renee left on Sunday to return to Richmond, she was overcome with feelings of guilt. "My mother gave up her life for me, now I can't even be with her when she needs me the most."

Since the surgery, there have been issues with lymphedema and pain. Renee's long-distance attempts to talk to the oncologist or surgeon have been unsuccessful. Even though she travels to be with her mother every weekend, Renee has been unable to meet with her mother's healthcare providers or to establish a communication plan. Her mother is scheduled to start her chemotherapy within the next 2 weeks. Renee has become depressed and is unable to concentrate at work.

SUPPORTING THE FAMILY CAREGIVER

Family Caregiver Bill of Rights

Caregivers often struggle to find a balance between the needs of their loved ones and the need to take care of themselves. The Caregiver's Bill of Rights (90) is helpful in providing a guideline for caregivers to appreciate their responsibilities and their limitations as they partner with their loved ones in the cancer experience (Fig. 52.2).

CAREGIVER'S BILL OF RIGHTS

Adapted from: Home, J. (1985). *CareGiving: Helping an Aging Loved One.* Washington, D.C.: American Association of Retired Persons. pp 300.

I HAVE THE RIGHT TO:

- To take care of myself. It will enable me to take better care of my loved one.

- To seek help from others even though my loved one may object. I recognize the limits of my own endurance and strength.

- To maintain facets of my own life that do not include the person I care for, just as I would if he or she was healthy.

- To get angry, be depressed, and to express other difficult emotions occasionally.

- To reject any attempt by my loved one (either conscious or unconscious) to manipulate me through guilt, anger or depression.

- To receive consideration, affection, forgiveness and acceptance from my loved one for as long as I offer these qualities in return.

- To take pride in what I am accomplishing and to applaud the courage it sometimes takes to meet the needs of my loved one.

- To protect my individuality and to make a life for myself.

- To expect as new strides are made in finding resources to aid physically and mentally impaired persons, similar strides will be made toward supporting their caregivers.

Figure 52.2. Caregiver's Bill of Rights.

Intervention Supporting Family Caregivers: Lung Cancer Family Caregivers Intervention (FCPCI)

An ongoing 5-year interventional study, *Family Caregivers of Patients with Lung Cancer*, provides support to family caregivers using a psycho-educational program. The FCPCI program is offered to caregivers of lung cancer patients who were currently enrolled in the patient lung cancer program. Family caregivers are taught how to best care for their loved ones and manage their symptoms and how to care for themselves as well. The program framework is guided by the QOL model, which includes the four domains: (1) physical; (2) psychological; (3) social; and (4) spiritual. In the interventional phase, a nurse meets with the family caregiver for four teaching sessions to discuss the physical, psychological, social, and spiritual issues of caregiving. Included in each of these sessions is the development of a personalized self-care plan with strategies addressing the four QOL domains. In three follow-up phone calls, at 16, 20, and 24 weeks post-sessions, the nurse reviews any questions regarding care; assesses symptom management, community resources, and supports; and reviews the caregiver's self-care plan. Family caregivers receive a notebook containing educational information, and the nurse helps each family caregiver come up with a self-care plan to take care of themselves. Positive outcomes will reflect a decrease in family caregiver burden, an increase in skills preparedness, an improvement in family caregiver QOL, and a decrease in psychological distress (Table 52.3).

Case Study

In this case, Ellen and Joe, long married and dependent on each other, illustrate the need for early intervention to support patients and families throughout the cancer experience.

Ellen and Joe have been married for 65 years. Joe retired from his bus driver job 20 years ago; now he spends most of his time watching sports on television. He is diabetic and arthritic and has congestive heart failure. Ellen was a homemaker and stay-at-home mother and had many close friends. She says most of them have died, "I miss them; I don't have anyone to talk to anymore." She has been healthy, "just a little arthritis," but recently she has lost weight and has fallen several times. They have lived in their two-bedroom two-level condo in a run-down area of Los Angles for the past 10 years. Most of their neighbors are new and they do not know them. They have two children (one married and one divorced) who live within 45 miles, but with LA traffic taking at least 2 hours, they get to their house only every few months. Ellen and Joe's three adult grandchildren rarely visit as they are busy taking care of their own grandchildren.

When Ellen started having difficulty breathing she attributed it to age. The problem progressively worsened and she was too fatigued to leave the house. Ellen was ultimately diagnosed with stage IV lung cancer and referred to her local oncologist. Joe was devastated by the diagnosis. He insisted she have every treatment available. The children and grandchildren agreed to help Joe with the caregiving

TABLE 52.3	Family caregiver palliative care intervention

Time	Lung Cancer Family Caregivers Intervention Content
Week 1	Administer baseline assessment: caregiver demographics, preparedness scale, caregiver burden, family QOL, distress thermometer, self-care practices form, and resources use.
Week 7	Administer pre-intervention assessment: preparedness scale, caregiver burden, family QOL, distress thermometer, self-care practices form, and resources use.
Week 7, visit #1	Focus on caregiver burden, describing family caregiving (1) post-surgery for early-stage lung cancer or (2) caregiving during chemotherapy or radiation for late-stage lung cancer QOL of the FC and the patient; FC role in caregiving, the burdens and benefits of caregiving, and introduce role of palliative care in early disease.
	Assess self-care and begin wellness plan (e.g., physical: exercise and nutrition).
Week 8, visit #2	Review previous session.
	Focus on skill preparedness for management of symptoms in (1) early-stage lung cancer patients (post-operative pain, resuming nutrition, importance of hydration, post-operative activities, and report of new symptoms) or (2) late-stage lung cancer patients (e.g., pain, dyspnea, and cough, anorexia/cachexia, dysphagia, fatigue, sleep, nausea, vomiting, constipation, and diarrhea; physical care of the lung cancer patient [bathing and ambulation]).
	Review and revise wellness plan.
Week 10, visit #3	Review previous session.
	Focus on management of psychological symptoms in (1) early-stage lung cancer patients post-operatively (anxiety, distress, depression, and guilt) or (2) late-stage lung cancer patients (anxiety, distress, depression, guilt, and fear of death), management of FC distress, social issues (communication, financial concerns, sexuality, and support groups), and spiritual needs of the lung cancer patient.
	Review wellness plan.
Week 12, visit #4	Review previous session.
	Focus on the continuing role of FC in caring for the patient with (1) early-stage lung cancer after surgery and moving to survivorship or (2) late-stage lung cancer continuation of care. Monitoring chronic and palliative care grief support for FC in (1) living with serious illness with possible recurrence or (2) grief and bereavement support for FC.
	Review wellness plan.
Week 12—data collection, post-intervention	Administer post-intervention assessment: preparedness scale, caregiver burden, family QOL, distress thermometer, self-care practices form, and resources use.
Weeks 16, 20, and 24— phone calls monthly × 3	Review any questions regarding post-operative care.
	Assessment of symptom management, community resources, and supports.
	Review wellness plan.
Week 24—data collection	Final assessment: preparedness scale, caregiver burden, family QOL, distress thermometer, self-care practices form, and resources use.

QOL, quality of life; FC, family caregiver.

responsibilities. Even though Ellen wanted to talk about advance directives, her family refused, saying that was giving up. She started her chemotherapy 3 days after her diagnosis. The first day Joe and Ellen arrived at the clinic at 7:00 a.m. for blood tests, x-rays, doctors' visits, and then 4 hours of chemotherapy. They did not eat breakfast, as Ellen was too nervous to cook or eat. By mid-day, Joe was in a wheelchair needing medical assistance for his low blood sugar. By the end of the 12-hour day they had to call their son to pick them up; Joe could not drive home.

As the chemotherapy treatment continued, Ellen became weaker and weaker. She was constantly nauseated, had diarrhea, and could not eat. Joe's health deteriorated faster than Ellen's. She no longer could administer his insulin or make his meals. They did not want to burden their children/grandchildren with their caregiving needs. Joe discouraged the children's and grandchildren's offers of help.

CONCLUSION

The home care setting can best be described as the ICU of the future. Home care is complex as a result of changing patient and family caregiver characteristics, changing healthcare delivery systems, and changing payer benefits. Although the home setting is rich with benefits to enhance patient comfort, it also provides challenges in providing optimum physical, psychological, social, and spiritual care. The literature has addressed many interventions that are helpful in assisting family caregivers in home care. These interventions include a range of suggestions about physical care, including the transferring of information about physical caregiving to family caregivers, offering validation and support to family caregivers for their caregiving efforts, and offering interventions to improve communication.

There is a tremendous need for continuity of care as patients are increasingly cared for across many settings. It is essential that issues of care in the home are communicated to those involved, including the healthcare professionals, patients, and family caregivers. Quality care for patients at home, similar to all aspects of palliative care, begins with a thorough assessment of the patients' and the family caregivers' needs. Organized care based on a comprehensive perspective, which recognizes the needs for physical, psychological, social, and spiritual well-being during the cancer experience, is best accomplished by empowering family caregivers to provide excellent care for their loved ones and to care for themselves.

APPENDIX

Family Caregiver Resources

Cancer Caregiving

■ American Cancer Society (ACS). Caring for the Patient with Cancer at Home: A Guide for Patients and Families (http://www.cancer.org/acs/groups/cid/documents/webcontent/002818-pdf.pdf)
■ Cancer Care: Caregivers (http://www.cancercare.org/get_help/loved_one.php)
■ Cancer Hope Network: Cancer: You Can Talk to Someone Who's Been There (http://www.cancerhopenetwork.org/index.php?page=brochures)
■ Families Facing Cancer (http://familiesfacingcancer.org/)

■ Journey Forward (http://journeyforward.org/)
■ National Cancer Institute (http://www.cancer.gov/cancertopics/pdq/supportivecare/caregivers/patient/page1)
■ National Comprehensive Cancer Network (NCCN): About: Caregiver Concerns Column (http://www.nccn.org/about/news/ebulletin/2011-02-07/jai_pausch.asp)
■ Navigating Cancer (https://www.navigatingcancer.com/caregivers-intro)
■ Osher Center for Integrative Medicine: Caregivers: Support for Family Caregivers of Loved Ones with Serious Illness (http://www.osher.ucsf.edu/patient-care/self-care-resources/caregivers/)
■ Strength for Caring: A Place for Caregivers (http://www.strengthforcaring.com/manual/about-you-you-are-not-alone/cancer-caregivers/)

Caregiving:

■ Aging Parents and Elder Care (http://www.aging-parents-and-elder-care.com)
■ AARP: Caregiving Resource Center (http://www.aarp.org/relationships/caregiving-resource-center/)
■ American College of Physicians Ethics, Professionalism and Human Rights Committee Information Resources for Physicians Supporting Family Caregivers (http://www.acponline.org/running_practice/ethics/issues/policy/caregivers_appendix.pdf)
■ Caring.com (http://www.caring.com/cancer)
■ Family Caregiver Alliance (http://www.caregiver.org/caregiver/jsp/home.jsp)
■ Family Caregiving 101 (http://www.familycaregiving101.org/)
■ National Alliance for Caregiving (http://www.caregiving.org/)
■ National Family Caregivers Association (http://www.nfcacares.org)
■ Rosalynn Carter Institute for Caregiving (http://www.rosalynncarter.org/)

REFERENCES

1. Feinberg L, Reinhard S, Houser A. Choula R. *Valuing the Invaluable: 2011 Update—The Growing Contributions and Costs of Family Caregiving.* Washington, DC: AARP Public Policy Institute; 2011.
2. Schneider A. *Overview of Medicaid Provisions in the Balanced Budget Act of 1997, P.L. 105-33.* Washington, DC: Center on Budget and Policy Priorities; 1997.
3. Northouse LL. Helping families of patients with cancer. *Oncol Nurs Forum.* 2005;32(4):743-750.
4. Ferrell BR, Grant M, Borneman T, Juarez G, ter Veer A. Family caregiving in cancer pain management. *J Palliat Med.* Summer 1999;2(2):185-195.

5. Family Caregiver Alliance. *Caregiver Assessment: Principles, Guidelines and Strategies for Change.* Report from a National Consensus Development Conference. San Francisco, CA: National Center on Caregiving, Family Caregiver Alliance; 2006.

6. Family Caregiver Alliance. *Caregiver Assessment: Voices and Views from the Field.* Report from a National Consensus Development Conference. San Francisco, CA Family Caregiver Alliance; 2006.

7. Glajchen M. The emerging role and needs of family caregivers in cancer care. *J Support Oncol.* March–April 2004;2(2):145-155.

8. Ferrell B, Mazanec, P. Family caregivers. In: Hurria A, Balducci, L, eds. *Geriatric Oncology: Treatment Assessment & Management.* New York, NY: Springer; 2009:135-155.

9. National Alliance for Caregiving. Caregiving in the U.S. 2009. http://www.caregiving.org/pdf/research/CaregivingUS AllAgesExecSum.pdf. Accessed July 18, 2012.

10. National Cancer Institute (NCI). Family Caregivers in Cancer: Roles and Challenges (PDQ®). Resources regarding interventions for caregivers. http://www.cancer.gov/cancertopics/pdq/supportivecare/caregivers/HealthProfessional/. Accessed July 10, 2011.

11. Reinhard S, Given B, Huhtala Petlick N, Bemis A. Supporting family caregivers in providing care. In: Hughes RG, ed. *Patient Safety and Quality an Evidence-Based Handbook for Nurses.* Rockville, MD: Agency for Healthcare Research and Quality (US); 2008:1400.

12. Meeker MA, Finnell D, Othman AK. Family caregivers and cancer pain management: a review. *J Fam Nurs.* 2011;17(1):29-60.

13. Hudson PL, Thomas K, Trauer T, Remedios C, Clarke D. Psychological and social profile of family caregivers on commencement of palliative care. *J Pain Symptom Manage.* 2011;41(3):522-534.

14. Stajduhar KI, Martin WL, Barwich D, Fyles G. Factors influencing family caregivers' ability to cope with providing end-of-life cancer care at home. *Cancer Nurs.* 2008;31(1):77-85.

15. Wright AA, Keating NL, Balboni TA, Matulonis UA, Block SD, Prigerson HG. Place of death: correlations with quality of life of patients with cancer and predictors of bereaved caregivers' mental health. *J Clin Oncol.* October 2010;28(29):4457-4464.

16. Northouse LL, Katapodi MC, Song L, Zhang L, Mood DW. Interventions with family caregivers of cancer patients: meta-analysis of randomized trials. *CA Cancer J Clin.* September–October 2010;60(5):317-339.

17. Stenberg U, Ruland CM, Miaskowski C. Review of the literature on the effects of caring for a patient with cancer. *Psycho-Oncology.* 2010;19(10):1013-1025.

18. Kim Y, Given BA. Quality of life of family caregivers of cancer survivors. *Cancer.* 2008;112(S11):2556-2568.

19. Houldin A. A qualitative study of caregivers' experiences with newly diagnosed advanced colorectal cancer. *Oncol Nurs Forum.* 2007;34(2):323-330.

20. Tamayo G, Broxson A, Munsell M, Cohen M. Caring for the caregiver. *Oncol Nurs Forum.* 2010;37(1):E50-E57.

21. Teschendorf BS, Ferrans C, O'Mara A, Novotny P, Sloan J. Caregiver role stress: when families become providers. *ACS Cancer Control.* 2007;14(5):183-189.

22. Bart H, Osse, BH, Vernooij-Dassen MJ, Schade E, Grol RP. Problems experienced by the informal caregivers of cancer patients and their needs for support. *Cancer Nurs.* September–October 2006;29(5):378-388; quiz 389-390.

23. van Ryn M, Sanders S, Kahn K, et al. Objective burden, resources, and other stressors among informal cancer caregivers: a hidden quality issue? *Psycho-Oncology.* 2011;20(1):44-52.

24. Jones C, Drake, R, Leurent B, King M. Interventions for supporting informal caregivers of patients in the terminal phase of a disease. *Cochrane Database Syst Rev.* 2011;Issue 6. Art. No.:CD007617. http://onlinelibrary.wiley.com/store/10.1002/14651858.CD007617.pub2/asset/CD007617.pdf?v=1&t=gsmcpgco&s=68cfaa06c1f1b05aca574c816ee19590699a794e. Accessed July 10, 2011.

25. Williams AL, McCorkle R. Cancer family caregivers during the palliative, hospice, and bereavement phases: a review of the descriptive psychosocial literature. *Palliat Support Care.* September 2011;9(3):315-325.

26. Sherwood PR, Given BA, Donovan H, et al. Guiding research in family care: a new approach to oncology caregiving. *Psycho-Oncology.* 2008;17(10):986-996.

27. Funk L, Stajduhar K, Toye C, Aoun S, Grande G, Todd C. Part 2: home-based family caregiving at the end of life: a comprehensive review of published qualitative research (1998–2008). *Palliat Med.* September 2010;24(6):594-607.

28. Mazanec P. Distant Caregiving of a Parent with Advanced Cancer [Doctoral dissertation], Case Western Reserve University; 2008.

29. Wong WKT, Ussher J, Perz J. Strength through adversity: bereaved cancer carers' accounts of rewards and personal growth from caring. *Palliat Support Care.* 2009;7(2):187-196.

30. National Consensus Project for Quality Palliative Care. *Clinical Practice Guidelines for Quality Palliative Care.* 2nd ed. Pittsburgh, PA: National Consensus Project for Quality Palliative Care; 2009.

31. Hudson P, Payne, S. The future of family caregiving: research, social policy and clinical practice. In: Hudson P, Payne S, eds. *Family Carers in Palliative Care: A Guide for Health and Social Care Professionals.* New York, NY: Oxford University Press; 2009:277-303.

32. Deimling GT, Bowman KF, Sterns S, Wagner LJ, Kahana B. Cancer-related health worries and psychological distress among older adult, long-term cancer survivors. *Psycho-Oncology.* 2006;15(4):306-320.

33. Institute of Medicine (IOM). *Retooling for an Aging America: Building the Health Care Workforce.* Washington, DC: The National Academies Press; 2008.

34. Ries LAG HD, Krapcho M, Mariotto A, Miller BA, Feuer EJ, Clegg L, Eisner MP, Horner MJ, Howlader N, Hayat M, Hankey BF, Edwards BK (eds)., National Cancer Institute. Bethesda, MD, based on November 2005 SEER data submission. *SEER Cancer Statistics Review, 1975-2003.* Bethesda, MD: National Cancer Institute; 2006.

35. Given B, Sherwood PR. Family care for the older person with cancer. *Semin Oncol Nurs.* 2006;22(1):43-50.

36. American Cancer Society. *Cancer Facts & Figures 2012.* Atlanta: American Cancer Society; 2012.

37. Jones BL. Companionship, control, and compassion: a social work perspective on the needs of children with cancer and their families at the end of life. *J Palliat Med.* June 2006;9(3):774-788.

38. Hinds PS, Oakes LL, Hicks J, et al. "Trying to be a good parent" as defined by interviews with parents who made phase I, terminal care, and resuscitation decisions for their children. *J Clin Oncol.* December 2009;27(35):5979-5985.

39. Ferrell B, Rhiner M, Shapiro B, Dierkes M. The experience of pediatric cancer pain, part I: impact of pain on the family. *J Pediatr Nurs.* 1994;9(6):368-379.

40. Hooke C, Hellsten MB, Stutzer C, Forte K. Pain management for the child with cancer in end-of-life care: APON position paper. *J Pediatr Oncol Nurs.* March 2002;19(2):43-47.

41. Hinds PS. Progress in quality of life in children and adolescents with cancer. *Semin Oncol Nurs.* February 2010;26(1):18-25.

42. Mazanec P, Daly B, Ferrell B, Prince-Paul M. Lack of communication and control: experiences of distance caregivers of parents with advanced cancer. *Oncol Nurs Forum.* 2011;38(3):307-313.

43. Glajchen M. Role of family caregivers in cancer pain management. In: Bruera ED, Portenoy RK, eds. *Cancer Pain: Assessment and Management.* 2nd ed. New York, NY: Cambridge University Press; 2009:597-607.

44. Honea NJ, Brintnall R, Given B, et al. Putting evidence into practice: nursing assessment and interventions to reduce family caregiver strain and burden. *Clin J Oncol Nurs.* June 2008;12(3):507-516.

45. Caregiving E-NAf. *Family Caregivers—What They Spend, What They Sacrifice: The Personal Financial Toll of Caring for a Loved One.* Minnetonka, MN; Bethesda, MD: Evercare and NAC; 2007.

46. Juarez G, Ferrell B, Uman G, Podnos Y, Wagman L. Distress and quality of life concerns of family caregivers of patients undergoing palliative surgery. *Cancer Nurs.* 2008;31(1):2-10.

47. van Houtven CH, Ramsey SD, Hornbrook MC, Atienza AA, van Ryn M. Economic burden for informal caregivers of lung and colorectal cancer patients. *Oncologist.* 2010;15(8):883-893.

48. Myers CD, Walton T, Small BJ. The value of massage therapy in cancer care. *Hematol Oncol Clin North Am.* 2008;22(4):649-660.

49. Collinge W. *Touch, Caring & Cancer: Guide for Professionals.* 1st ed. Kittery Point, ME: Collinge and Associates; 2009.

50. Walton T. *Medical Conditions in Massage Therapy: A Decision Tree Approach.* London: Lippincott Williams and Wilkins; 2010.

51. King D, Quill, T. Working with families in palliative care: one size does not fit all. *J Palliat Med.* 2006;9(3):704-715.

52. Hudson P. How well do family caregivers cope after caring for a relative with advanced disease and how can health professionals enhance their support? *J Palliat Med.* 2006;9(3):694-703.

53. del-Pino-Casado R, Frías-Osuna A, Palomino-Moral PA. Subjective burden and cultural motives for caregiving in informal caregivers of older people. *J Nurs Sch.* 2011;43(3):282-291.

54. Given B, Given CW, Sikorskii A, Jeon S, Sherwood P, Rahbar M. The impact of providing symptom management assistance on caregiver reaction: results of a randomized trial. *J Pain Symptom Manage.* 2006;32(5):433-443.

55. Sherwood PR, Given BA, Given CW, et al. The influence of caregiver mastery on depressive symptoms. *J Nurs Sch.* 2007;39(3):249-255.

56. Schumacher KL, Stewart BJ, Archbold PG, Caparro M, Mutale F, Agrawal S. Effects of caregiving demand, mutuality, and preparedness on family caregiver outcomes during cancer treatment. *Oncol Nurs Forum.* January 2008;35(1):49-56.

57. Wilson D. Quality care at the end of life: the lived experience of surrogate decision makers. *J Hosp Palliat Nurs.* 2011;13(4):249-256.

58. Oh S, Meyerowitz BE, Perez MA, Thornton A. Need for cognition and psychosocial adjustment in prostate cancer patients and partners. *J Psychosoc Oncol.* 2007;25(1):1-19.

59. Zahlis EH, Lewis FM. Coming to grips with breast cancer: the spouse's experience with his wife's first six months. *J Psychosoc Oncol.* January 2010;28(1):79-97.

60. Dobrof J, Ebenstein H, Dodd S-J, Epstein I. Caregivers and professionals partnership caregiver resource center: assessing a hospital support program for family caregivers. *J Palliat Med.* February 2006;9(1):196-205.

61. Mitnick S, Leffler C, Hood V. For the American College of Physicians Ethics, Professionalism and Human Rights Committee. Family caregivers, patients and physicians: ethical guidance to optimize relationships *J Gen Intern Med.* 2010;25(3):255-260.

62. Gibbins J, McCoubrie R, Kendrick AH, Senior-Smith G, Davies AN, Hanks GW. Sleep–wake disturbances in patients with advanced cancer and their family carers. *J Pain Symptom Manage.* 2009;38(6):860-870.

63. Fletcher BS, Paul SM, Dodd MJ, et al. Prevalence, severity, and impact of symptoms on female family caregivers of patients at the initiation of radiation therapy for prostate cancer. *J Clin Oncol.* February 2008;26(4):599-605.

64. Acton GJ. Health-promoting self-care in family caregivers. *West J Nurs Res.* February 2002;24(1):73-86.

65. Bowman KF, Rose JH, Deimling GT. Families of long-term cancer survivors: health maintenance advocacy and practice. *Psycho-Oncology.* 2005;14(12):1008-1017.

66. Kravits K, McAllister-Black R, Grant M, Kirk C. Self-care strategies for nurses: a psycho-educational intervention for stress reduction and the prevention of burnout. *Appl Nurs Res.* 2010;23(3):130-138.

67. Wittenberg-Lyles E, Goldsmith J, Ragan S, Sanchez-Reilly S, ed. *Dying with Comfort: Family Illness Narrative and Early Palliative Care.* Cresskill, NJ: Hampton Press; 2010.

68. Mellon S, Northouse LL, Weiss LK. A population-based study of the quality of life of cancer survivors and their family caregivers. *Cancer Nurs.* 2006;29(2):120-131.

69. Ferrell BR, Ferrell FB, Rhiner M, Grant M. Family factors influencing cancer pain management. *PostGrad Med J.* 1991;67(S64-S69):S64-S69.

70. Johansson L, Guo X, Waern M, et al. Midlife psychological stress and risk of dementia: a 35-year longitudinal population study. *Brain.* August 2010;133(pt 8):2217-2224.

71. Willette-Murphy K, Lee KA, Dodd M, et al. Relationship between sleep and physical activity in female family caregivers at the initiation of patients' radiation therapy. *J Obstetr Gynecol Neonatal Nurs.* 2009;38(3):367-374.

72. National Alliance for Caregiving & Evercare. *Evercare® Study of Caregivers in Decline: A Close-Up Look at the Health Risks of Caring for a Loved One.* Bethesda, MD; Minnetonka, MN: National Alliance for Caregiving and Evercare; 2006.

73. Hearson B, McClement S, McMillan D, Harlos M. Sleeping with one eye open: the sleep experience of family members providing palliative care at home. *J Palliat Care.* 2011;27(2):69.

74. Bishop MM, Beaumont JL, Hahn EA, et al. Late effects of cancer and hematopoietic stem-cell transplantation on spouses or partners compared with survivors and survivor-matched controls. *J Clin Oncol.* 2007;25(11):1403-1411.

75. Blum K, Sherman DW. Understanding the experience of caregivers: a focus on transitions. *Semin Oncol Nurs.* 2010;26(4):243-258.

76. Hodges LJ, Humphris GM, Macfarlane G. A meta-analytic investigation of the relationship between the psychological distress of cancer patients and their carers. *Soc Sci Med.* January 2005;60(1):1-12.

77. Hagedoorn M, Sanderman R, Bolks HN, Tuinstra J, Coyne JC. Distress in couples coping with cancer: a meta-analysis and critical review of role and gender effects. *Psychol Bullet.* January 2008;134(1):1-30.

78. Lewis FM, Fletcher KA, Cochrane BB, Fann JR. Predictors of depressed mood in spouses of women with breast cancer. *J Clin Oncol.* March 2008;26(8):1289-1295.

79. Mellon S, Kershaw TS, Northouse LL, Freeman-Gibb L. A family-based model to predict fear of recurrence for cancer survivors and their caregivers. *Psycho-Oncology.* March 2007;16(3):214-223.

80. Given B, Wyatt G, Given C, et al. Burden and depression among caregivers of patients with cancer at the end of life. *Oncol Nurs Forum.* November 2004;31(6):1105-1117.

81. Shand M, Lewis F, Sinsheimer J, Cochrane B. Core concerns of couples living with early stage breast cancer. *Psycho-Oncology.* 2006;15:1055-1064.

82. Badr H, Taylor CLC. Social constraints and spousal communication in lung cancer. *Psycho-Oncology.* 2006;15(8): 673-683.

83. National Consensus Project for Quality Palliative Care. *Clinical Practice Guidelines for Quality Palliative Care.* 2nd ed. Pittsburgh, PA:National Consensus Project for Quality Palliative Care; 2009.

84. Colgrove LA, Kim Y, Thompson N. The effect of spirituality and gender on the quality of life of spousal caregivers of cancer survivors. *Ann Behav Med.* February 2007;33(1):90-98.

85. Puchalski C, Ferrell, B. *Making Health Care Whole.* West Conshohocken, PA: Templeton Press; 2010.

86. Kim Y, Schulz R, Carver CS. Benefit-finding in the cancer caregiving experience. *Psychosom Med.* April 2007;69(3):283-291.

87. Fife BL, Monahan PO, Abonour R, Wood LL, Stump TE. Adaptation of family caregivers during the acute phase of adult BMT. *Bone Marrow Transplant.* 2008;43(12):959-966.

88. Tang WR. Hospice family caregivers' quality of life. *J Clin Nurs.* September 2009;18(18):2563-2572.

89. Lim J, Zebrack B. Caring for family members with chronic physical illness: a critical review of caregiver literature. *Health Qual Life Outcomes.* 2004;2:50.

90. Horne J. *Caregiving: Helping an Aging Loved One.* Washington, DC: American Association of Retired Persons Books; 1985.

CHAPTER 53

Management of Symptoms in the Actively Dying Patient

Paul Rousseau ■ Leigh Vaughan

The obligation of physicians to relieve suffering is universal, particularly when death is imminent and the indignities of illness consume patients' final days and hours of life. This honored encumbrance transcends all other duties accorded by physicians and is fundamental to a death free of interminable symptoms and a satisfactory bereavement for surviving family members (1). Lamentably, the dying process can be a time of untold loss and suffering, and although spiritual and psychosocial concerns are basic domains in the inherent makeup of an individual, unrelieved physical suffering can detract the attention from important spiritual and psychosocial issues at the end of life. Accordingly, physicians must be competent in relieving physical distress and, in so doing, maintaining patient dignity and familial equanimity (2).

During the last days of life, there are characteristic symptoms that commonly occur, including dyspnea and noisy, gurgling respirations frequently referred to as the "death rattle," anxiety, restlessness, delirium, nausea and vomiting (NV), and pain (2–9). Although such symptoms are often multifactorial in etiology, treatment is usually empiric and palliative. Diagnostic evaluation is limited in recognition of the short life expectancy and impending death. Nevertheless, empiric treatment strategies do not suggest or encourage clinical indifference but rather mandate ongoing clinical assessment of therapeutic interventions in a continual effort to allay suffering. From time to time, terminal symptoms are refractory and unresponsive to aggressive and exhaustive interventions. In such cases, palliative sedation (PS) is an ethically and morally appropriate option that may be utilized to afford a more peaceful and tranquil death for the patient and a satisfactory grieving.

DYSPNEA AND THE DEATH RATTLE

Dyspnea

Dyspnea occurs in 29% to 90% of terminally ill patients and is the most common severe symptom as death approaches (9–13). Although it is more common in patients with pulmonary disorders, 23.9% of dyspneic patients in the National Hospice Study did not exhibit cardiac or pulmonary disease (11). Dyspnea is also reportedly more common in children dying of cancer, occurring in 80% of such patients (14,15). Dyspnea in terminally ill patients derives from five primary causes, namely:

1. Existing disease (i.e., chronic obstructive pulmonary disease [COPD] and congestive heart failure)
2. Acute superimposed illness (i.e., pneumonia and pulmonary embolus)
3. Cancer-related complications (i.e., pleural effusion, lymphangitic carcinomatosis, tumor-induced bronchial obstruction, and ascites)
4. Effects of cancer therapy (i.e., radiation and chemotherapy–induced pulmonary fibrosis), and
5. Miscellaneous causes (i.e., anemia, uremia, and anxiety) (9,13,16).

As with any symptom, the treatment of dyspnea should address any easily correctable underlying cause, all the while recognizing and considering the limited life expectancy of the imminently dying patient and the invasiveness and discomfort of the proposed therapeutic interventions. Consequently, for most patients near death, opioids, benzodiazepines, phenothiazines, and corticosteroids are the mainstays of therapy (2,7–9,12,13,16,17).

Opioids purportedly relieve dyspnea by altering the perception of breathlessness (10,18), decreasing ventilatory response to hypoxia and hypercapnia (10,19), and reducing oxygen consumption at rest and with exercise (10,20). Controlled trials and anecdotal case reports on the use of systemic opioids in the treatment of malignant and COPD-associated dyspnea have generally demonstrated a reduction in dyspnea (10,17,21–25), including a *Cochrane Review* that further confirmed the benefit of oral and parenteral opioids in improving dyspnea in patients with life-limiting disease (26–28). In 2008, opioids were endorsed as the preferred drug to control dyspnea by the American Thoracic Society and the American College of Physicians (29,30) followed by The American College of Chest Physicians in 2010 (31). Although morphine preparations are generally utilized, any opioid should potentially alleviate dyspnea (Table 53.1). Opioids can be administered orally, rectally, sublingually, subcutaneously, intravenously, and by inhalation, but during the final hours of life when the ability to swallow declines and consciousness wanes, rectal, subcutaneous, and intravenous routes are more commonly used.

Inhalation of opioids is a unique and innovative approach to drug delivery. Controlled trials have revealed conflicting results (17,21,25,32–40), including a *Cochrane Review* that showed no benefit of nebulized morphine over nebulized saline (26–28,41), but anecdotal reports have generally been favorable (13,42–44). In addition, a recent study by Bruera

TABLE 53.1	**Pharmacologic treatment of terminal dyspnea**

Drug	Dose[a]
Opioids	
Morphine	5–10 mg p.o., s.l., i.m., i.v., s.q., p.r. q1-4h; i.v. or s.q. doses should be adjusted accordingly using a 3:1 oral to parenteral ratio; titrate dose 30–50% daily or more frequently until symptoms improve or sedation becomes problematic; patients already on morphine may need to increase their regular dose by 25–50%; when dyspnea is severe and acute, 2–5 mg i.v. q15min or 5 mg s.q. q20min until dyspnea is relieved
Oxycodone	5–10 mg p.o., s.l., p.r. q1-4h
Hydromorphone	1–2 mg p.o., s.l., i.m., i.v., s.q., p.r. q1-4h; i.v.or s.q. doses should be adjusted accordingly using a 5:1 oral to parenteral ratio; titrate dose as per morphine recommendation
Nebulized morphine[b]	5 mg in 2 mL of normal saline q1-4h through nebulizer, may titrate to 20 mg q2-4h; hydromorphone may be substituted for morphine and started at 2 mg q1-4h
Corticosteroids	
Dexamethasone	4–8 mg p.o., s.l., i.m., i.v., s.q., p.r. daily
Prednisone	20–40 mg p.o., s.l. daily
Benzodiazepines	
Lorazepam	0.5–2 mg p.o., s.l., i.m., i.v., s.q., p.r. q1-4h
Diazepam	5–10 mg p.o., s.l., i.m., i.v., p.r. q1-4h
Midazolam	0.5 mg i.v. q15min until settled; 2.5–5 mg s.q., then 10–30 mg CSI q24h
Phenothiazine	
Chlorpromazine	12.5–25 mg i.v. q2-4h; 25 mg p.o., p.r. q2-4h

CSI, continuous subcutaneous infusion; I.M, intramuscular; I.V, intravenous; P.O, oral; P.R, rectal; S.L, sublingual; S.Q, subcutaneous.

[a]Suggested starting doses may need to be clinically titrated; older frail patients may need doses adjusted appropriately.

[b]Nebulized morphine may cause histamine-mediated bronchospasm, particularly in opioid-naive patients or during the first nebulization; may be difficult for actively dying patients to take oral medications.

et al. noted that nebulized morphine was as good as subcutaneous morphine in relieving dyspnea in patients with cancer; however, only 11 patients were included in the study, limiting its value (45). It is postulated that inhaled opioids exert their effect by means of opioid receptors that have been identified in the bronchial mucosa, as pharmacokinetic studies suggest that systemic bioavailability of nebulized morphine is extremely poor, varying from 4% to 8% (21,35,46). However, opioids may also stimulate histamine release from pulmonary mast cells and precipitate bronchospasm, worsening terminal dyspnea. Because this complication is usually a first-dose effect, careful observation is required during initial administration and may warrant the prophylactic use of an antihistamine such as diphenhydramine. Although studies are generally nonsupportive and further research with randomized controlled trials is unquestionably warranted, in the dyspneic patient near death, nebulized opioids may be efficacious and worth a trial in an attempt to reduce breathlessness and assuage the horrific fear of suffocation when all other palliative measures have failed.

Benzodiazepines have been frequently utilized in dyspnea primarily when a component of anxiety is involved. However, studies and anecdotal reports are contradictory (17), with most well-designed randomized controlled trials failing to find significant benefit (47–50). Nevertheless, benzodiazepines are frequently beneficial in reducing dyspnea, particularly during the final days of life (51), and are increasingly used in hospice and palliative care programs. Midazolam when used as an adjuvant to opioids showed significant benefit in the relief of dyspnea when compared with opioids as a single agent (52) without further risk of respiratory depression (53). Buspirone, a popular nonbenzodiazepine anxiolytic and serotonin agonist, has been shown to relieve dyspnea in patients with anxiety and COPD at a dose of 15 to 45 mg daily (54). Because of its delayed onset of action, it may be of limited use in actively dying patients. Although not a benzodiazepine, the neuroleptic chlorpromazine has been used in dyspnea refractory to other medications. It appears to reduce air hunger and anxiety with minimal side effects (primarily sedation and hypotension) and has been efficacious in patients near death (9,55,56).

Although corticosteroids are useful when bronchospasm is associated with inflammation, most studies suggest that only 20% to 30% of patients with COPD show improvement with corticosteroid therapy. In the final days of life, corticosteroids are most useful when prescribed for dyspnea associated with airway obstruction, lymphangitic carcinomatosis, radiation pneumonitis, and superior vena cava syndrome (9,16). Corticosteroids can be administered orally, rectally, subcutaneously, intravenously, and by inhalation. Although side effects are of concern during chronic use, such concerns are negated by short-term use in dying patients.

Other medications are also available to attenuate dyspnea in the dying patient. These include diuretics, bronchodilators, and inhaled anesthetics. Oral and intravenous diuretics are useful when pulmonary edema and ascites contribute to dyspnea. The diuretic furosemide can also be administered through inhalation in a dose of 20 mg every 2 to 4 hours as needed and appears to reduce dyspnea, irrespective of the underlying etiology (57–60). Although bronchodilators are best utilized in patients with a bronchospastic component to dyspnea (i.e., asthma and COPD with reactive airways), these drugs are frequently used when there is little-to-no evidence of bronchospasm and appear to provide subjective reduction of dyspnea in many patients. The use of adrenergic agonist bronchodilators, such as albuterol and metaproterenol, should be tempered by the possibility of resultant agitation, tremor, and heightened anxiety, potentially aggravating terminal dyspnea (9).

Nebulized anesthetics have been used infrequently for dyspnea in dying patients. In a study comparing nebulized saline and lidocaine, saline exerted a greater effect on the reduction of breathlessness (35,61). However, nebulized anesthetics have been useful for cough and may be considered when persistent coughing contributes to or aggravates dyspnea (35).

Nonpharmacologic interventions that are useful for terminal dyspnea include oxygen, a bedside fan, thoracentesis for pleural effusion, and paracentesis for ascites. The role of oxygen therapy in reducing dyspnea in patients near the end of life is somewhat controversial. In hypoxemic patients with disorders such as COPD, congestive heart failure, or pulmonary fibrosis, most studies suggest that there is a significant symptomatic improvement (21,32,62). In patients without hypoxemia, however, its use is not advantageous (35,63,64). Even so, the medical symbolism inherent in oxygen therapy may alleviate dyspnea by way of a placebo effect and should be considered in actively dying patients (a nasal cannula is better tolerated than a mask in most patients) (9,49). Moreover, oxygen therapy may provide many family members with the symbolic solace that "something is being done" to help their loved one, in spite of the fact that oxygen may actually provide only little therapeutic benefit.

A bedside fan may also be useful in alleviating dyspnea by reportedly stimulating thermal and mechanical receptors of the trigeminal nerve (V2 branch) in the cheek and nasopharynx, altering the central perception of breathlessness (9,55,65,66). The fan should be placed at the bedside, set on a low speed, and directed at the patient's face (9).

Thoracentesis and paracentesis may be useful when pleural effusion and ascites contribute to dyspnea (particularly if previous drainage has reduced dyspnea). In the final days

of life, however, generally other strategies should be utilized unless noninterventional approaches have failed and breathlessness aggravates suffering. An indwelling thoracentesis or paracentesis catheter may obviate the need for repeated and painful intermittent thoracenteses and paracenteses and should be considered in recurrent and disabling pleural effusions and ascites depending on estimated life expectancy.

Death Rattle

In the last 24 to 48 hours of life, most patients retain secretions in the back of the throat that produces a gurgling type of respiration frequently referred to as the death rattle (9,67). The presence of these enhanced secretions is felt to predict death within 48 hours in over 75% of patients (68). Fortunately, the patient is usually unaware of the noise. It can, however, be very disturbing to family members. Oropharyngeal suctioning is usually provided, but gagging and coughing may generate patient discomfort and further distress for relatives and caregivers. Instead, treatment with anticholinergic drugs is recommended to desiccate bronchial secretions and abolish the need for suctioning. Suggested medications include atropine, glycopyrrolate, scopolamine, and hyoscyamine (Table 53.2) (9,16,69). In one study, subcutaneous scopolamine was more immediately efficacious when compared with subcutaneous glycopyrrolate; however, glycopyrrolate has a longer duration of action (26,36). Nevertheless, most anticholinergic medications work relatively well and are widely used in clinical practice, although the overall efficacy has been challenged by a recent *Cochrane Review* (70). These antisialagogues do not dry up secretions that are already present, and they should therefore be used at the first sign of noisy respirations (7). In addition, placing patients in a lateral recumbent position with the head slightly elevated may help reduce the pooling of secretions and diminish noisy respirations (2), as may discontinuing parenteral and enteral infusions whenever possible (14).

ANXIETY, RESTLESSNESS, AND DELIRIUM

Anxiety

Anxiety is one of the most common psychological problems in terminally ill patients and like most symptoms can have numerous etiologies (67,71–75). Anxiety can be a component of a preexisting anxiety disorder or, more commonly in actively dying patients, accompany medical disorders and complications of illness and medications (72,74). Medical disorders that can cause anxiety include hyperthyroidism, pheochromocytoma, and primary and metastatic brain tumors. Medical complications and medications that can precipitate anxiety include hypoxia, sepsis, unrelieved pain, dyspnea, and medications such as corticosteroids, bronchodilators, and antiemetics that cause akathisia (71–74). In addition, withdrawal states from benzodiazepines and opioids can result in anxiety and may occur inadvertently when medications are suddenly discontinued after admission to a hospital or a long-term care facility (73).

| TABLE 53.2 | **Pharmacologic treatment of the death rattle** |

Drug	Dose
Scopolamine	0.4–0.6 mg s.q. q2-4h; 0.8–2.0 mg CSI q24h; 1–3 transdermal patches q3d
Hyoscyamine	0.125–0.250 mg s.l. q2-4h; 0.25–0.5 mg s.q. q2-4h; 1–2 mg CSI q24h
Glycopyrrolate	0.2 mg s.l., s.q. q2-4h
Atropine	0.4 mg s.q. q2-4h; may give 2 mg of atropine, 2.5–5.0 mg of morphine, and 2 mg of dexamethasone q2-4h through nebulizer

CSI, continuous subcutaneous infusion; S.L, sublingual; S.Q, subcutaneous.

The treatment of anxiety in the terminally ill often depends on etiology, but it generally involves nondrug maneuvers, specific interventions, and pharmacotherapy. Nondrug measures include meditation, biofeedback, progressive relaxation, and psychotherapy (73). In actively dying patients, these nondrug methods are of little value. In some cases, specific interventions can be of benefit and include such measures as oxygen and opioids for dyspnea, opioids and other analgesics for pain, and discontinuing medications that cause akathisia, a movement disorder precipitated by neuroleptic medications (i.e., haloperidol, chlorpromazine, and prochlorperazine) and characterized by motor restlessness, compulsive moving, and anxiety.

The principal therapy for anxiety includes the judicious use of benzodiazepines, neuroleptics, and antihistamines (71–74). Benzodiazepines are the mainstay of treatment in the terminally ill patient, with the shorter-acting agents, such as lorazepam and oxazepam, preferred in the patient with advanced disease (Table 53.3). These drugs are metabolized by conjugation in the liver and are the safest when hepatic disease is present (71–74). This is in contrast to alprazolam and other benzodiazepines, which are metabolized through oxidative pathways and may accumulate in debilitated patients (76). Midazolam, a water-soluble benzodiazepine, may be infused intravenously or subcutaneously and is very useful in controlling anxiety in the terminal phase of illness. The cost of midazolam may limit its use (71–74,77), particularly in managed care and capitated health systems, although a generic version is now available. Diazepam, an older but efficacious benzodiazepine, may be used rectally when no other route is available and the cost is of concern, with recommended dosages equivalent to oral regimens. Clonazepam, a long-acting benzodiazepine used for seizure disorders and myoclonus, is useful in patients who experience end-of-dose recurrence of anxiety on shorter-acting benzodiazepine medications (71–74).

Other nonbenzodiazepine medications that are useful for anxiety include the neuroleptics chlorpromazine, thioridazine, and haloperidol and the antihistamine hydroxyzine (Table 53.3). Neuroleptics may be used when benzodiazepines fail to relieve anxiety, when psychotic symptoms accompany anxiety, or when there is concern regarding the respiratory depressant effects of benzodiazepines (78). Hydroxyzine,

an effective antihistaminic anxiolytic, may have coanalgesic effects (79) and may be a particularly useful alternative to benzodiazepines when pain accompanies or exacerbates anxiety or when benzodiazepines and neuroleptics are contraindicated (i.e., allergy, respiratory depression, and akathisia).

Restlessness

Restlessness is commonly observed during the last hours of life. Although it has multiple causes (and may overlap with delirium), specific treatment may not be possible (7). Restless

| TABLE 53.3 | **Pharmacologic treatment of anxiety** |

Drug	Dose[a]
Benzodiazepines	
Lorazepam	0.5–2.0 mg p.o., s.l., i.m., i.v., s.q. q1-4h
Midazolam	0.5–5.0 mg i.v., s.q. q1-4h; 10–30 mg CSI q24h
Diazepam	2.5–10.0 mg p.o., i.m., i.v., p.r. q1-4h
Clonazepam	0.5–2.0 mg p.o. b.i.d.–q.i.d.
Oxazepam	15 mg p.o. t.i.d.–q.i.d.
Neuroleptics	
Haloperidol	0.5–1.0 mg p.o., i.m., i.v., s.q. q1-6h
Chlorpromazine	10–25 mg p.o., i.m., i.v., p.r. q4-6h
Thioridazine	10–75 mg p.o. t.i.d.–q.i.d.
Antihistamines	
Hydroxyzine	10–50 mg p.o., i.m., i.v., s.q. q2-4h

CSI, continuous subcutaneous infusion; I.M, intramuscular; I.V, intravenous; P.O, oral; P.R, rectal; S.L, sublingual; S.Q, subcutaneous.

[a]Suggested starting doses, may need to be clinically titrated; older frail patients may need doses adjusted appropriately, may be difficult for actively dying patients to take oral medications.

patients may have diverse symptoms, including impaired consciousness, intermittent sleepiness, tossing and turning, moaning, grunting, crying out, and agitation, and muscle spasms or twitching (2). Restlessness may be caused by spiritual conflicts; by physical discomfort, such as a distended urinary bladder or bladder spasms, fecal impaction, unrelieved pain, and pressure ulcers; or by nausea, dyspnea, pruritus, hypoxia, extreme weakness, corticosteroids, and sudden withdrawal from benzodiazepines. Treatment involves identifying and managing the underlying cause or, if that is not possible, providing spiritual support, verbal and tactile reassurance, and utilizing a benzodiazepine such as midazolam or a neuroleptic such as chlorpromazine (Table 53.3) (2,7).

Delirium

Delirium is a nonspecific global disorder of cognition and attention that occurs in 8% to 75% of hospitalized patients with cancer (73,74,80,81) and in 62% to 83% of patients just before death (82–85). It is a significant sign of physiologic disturbance and, analogous to anxiety, may be secondary to multiple etiologies, including primary or metastatic brain tumors, infection, organ failure, metabolic disturbances, vascular complications, nutritional deficiencies, medication side effects, radiotherapy, and paraneoplastic syndromes (82). In contrast to dementia, delirium is considered a reversible disorder with rapid onset; in the last 24 to 48 hours of life, however, it may be irreversible. According to the *Diagnostic and Statistical Manual of the American Psychiatric Association* (86), delirium is characterized by

- Disturbance of consciousness (reduced awareness of the environment), with reduced ability to focus, sustain, or shift attention
- Change in cognition (memory deficit, disorientation, and perceptual disturbances such as hallucinations, illusions, and delusions) that is not related to a preexisting dementia

- Development over a short period of time, with usual fluctuation throughout the day
- Evidence from the history, physical examination, or laboratory tests of a general medical condition judged to be etiologically related to the causation of delirium

The assessment of delirium must take into consideration the life expectancy of the patient and the patient's goals for care. Most palliative care clinicians would undertake a diagnostic workup only when a clinically suspected cause can be easily identified and treated effectively with simple interventions that carry a minimal burden or risk of causing further distress (i.e., hypodermoclysis for dehydration). Most often, the cause of delirium in the actively dying patient is multifactorial and irreversible and treatment is usually empiric (82). Similar to anxiety, nondrug supportive measures are of limited value (other than the presence of family members, a well-lit room, and familiar sounds and music). Consequently, pharmacologic interventions are the primary methods for treating delirium in patients near death.

Neuroleptic medications are the preferred pharmacologic agents and are particularly safe and efficacious in reducing disturbing cognitive symptoms in dying patients (Table 53.4) (16,71,73,74,80,82). Haloperidol is the usual drug of choice and may be given orally, intravenously, and subcutaneously, with its use supported by three recent studies (87–90). However, clinicians should be aware that parenteral doses are approximately twice as potent as oral doses (80,82). It is the drug of choice because of its short half-life, lack of active metabolites, and minimal anticholingeric and cardiovascular side effects. It is also less likely to cause sedation or paradoxical delirium (91). The atypical antipsychotics such as olanzapine, risperidone, and quetiapine can also be considered in the management of delirium.

A short-acting benzodiazepine can be added if the patient is overly agitated, although (26) benzodiazepines alone are

| TABLE 53.4 | **Pharmacologic treatment of delirium** |

Drug	Dose[a]
Neuroleptics	
Haloperidol	0.5–1.0 mg p.o., i.m., i.v., s.q. q1-6h; 5–15 mg CSI q24h; in acute situations, 0.5–1.0 mg i.v., s.q. q45-60min until symptoms controlled
Chlorpromazine	10–25 mg p.o., i.m., i.v., p.r. q4-6h
Risperidone	0.5–1.0 mg p.o. b.i.d.
Olanzapine	2.5–5 mg p.o. q.d.
Benzodiazepines	
Lorazepam	0.5–2.0 mg p.o., s.l., i.m., i.v., s.q. q1-4h
Midazolam	0.5–5.0 mg i.v., s.q. q1-4h; 10–30 mg CSI q24h

CSI, continuous subcutaneous infusion; I.M, intramuscular; I.V, intravenous; P.O, oral; P.R, rectal; S.L, sublingual; S.Q, subcutaneous.
[a]Suggested starting doses, may need to be clinically titrated.

not indicated in the treatment of delirium. In fact, benzodiazepines may actually exacerbate the delirious state and should be used cautiously and discontinued if delirium worsens. When delirium is difficult to control in the last days of life, PS to the point of unconsciousness may be needed (6,92). In such situations a benzodiazepine, such as lorazepam or midazolam, is the drug of choice, either alone or in conjunction with a neuroleptic.

NAUSEA AND VOMITING

NV occurs in 62% of patients with terminal cancer. Although the prevalence is 40% to 46% during the last 6 weeks of life (93), it rarely develops as a new symptom during the last days of life (8). NV is observed more frequently in women, individuals younger than 65, and patients with stomach and breast cancer (93).

The etiology of NV in terminal illness varies and is frequently multifactorial (9), particularly as death approaches. Although diagnostic evaluation can be done in the actively dying patient, treatment usually involves the empiric use of nonpharmacologic measures and antiemetics. However, if the clinician, patient, or family insists on an evaluation, simple tests, such as measurement of electrolytes, blood urea nitrogen, creatinine, calcium, albumin, glucose, and digoxin or anticonvulsant drug levels, are recommended and may readily disclose a reversible cause.

Nonpharmacologic measures used to treat NV include dietary manipulations (Table 53.5), elimination of emetogenic medications (i.e., nonsteroidal anti-inflammatories, digoxin, and iron (94)), and the limited use of nasogastric suctioning, particularly for high gastrointestinal bowel obstruction. Nasogastric tubes can be uncomfortable and difficult to place, especially in the home environment, but intermittent use may be considered for severe and intractable vomiting refractory to antiemetic therapy. A percutaneous

TABLE 53.5	Dietary manipulations for nausea and vomiting

Minimize unpleasant odors

Sounds and smells of food preparation should be excluded

Avoid foods known to precipitate nausea and vomiting

Clear liquid diet may be best tolerated

Cold foods may be preferred

Sour foods, such as lemons, and rinsing of the mouth with weak lemon juice may reduce nausea

Utilize frequent small feedings if the patient wants to eat

Adapted from Lichter I. Nausea and vomiting in patients with cancer. *Hematol Oncol Clin North Am.* 1996;10:207–220, with permission.

venting gastrostomy is useful if placed prior to the active dying process. However, its placement in the patient near death is usually not practical.

Nine types of antiemetics are utilized in the treatment of terminal NV: dopamine antagonists, metoclopramide, anticholinergics, antihistamines, corticosteroids, serotonin antagonists, octreotide, cannabinoids, and benzodiazepines (Table 53.6) (9,94–96).

Dopamine antagonists include haloperidol and prochlorperazine and are the usual first-line antiemetics chosen by most clinicians. Haloperidol is an excellent antiemetic and is particularly useful in delirious patients with NV because the symptoms may be improved with a single medication, although a recent *Cochrane Review* cited insufficient evidence to support its usefulness (97). As mentioned earlier (see Section "Delirium"), parenteral doses are twice as potent as oral doses, and there is a reported ceiling effect at approximately 30 mg a day. Prochlorperazine is also efficacious and a favorite of many clinicians, and while promethazine and chlorpromazine are also prescribed, there is probably little advantage in using them over prochlorperazine (94), except in the treatment of NV as an effect of increased intercranial pressure for which promethazine is preferred (98). Although combination therapy for NV is common in the terminally ill, two or more dopamine antagonists should not be prescribed concurrently as the potential for adverse extrapyramidal reactions is increased without additional antiemetic benefit.

Metoclopramide is both a dopamine antagonist and a serotonin (5-HT4) agonist, but at doses >120 mg a day it becomes a serotonin (5-HT3) antagonist (99). It is very useful as an antiemetic and a prokinetic agent for gastroparesis-induced vomiting but caution must be exercised with older patients as it may cause extrapyramidal reactions that may not be dose dependent (94).

Anticholinergic medications are most efficacious in NV related to colic and mechanical bowel obstruction (94,100). They include scopolamine, hyoscyamine, and glycopyrrolate. Antihistamines are effective in motion sickness, mechanical bowel obstruction, and increased intracranial pressure. These drugs comprise buclizine, meclizine, and diphenhydramine.

Corticosteroids have a synergistic effect with metoclopramide and the serotonin antagonists (94), but they are rarely useful as single agents (however, they may reduce peritumor edema of gastrointestinal malignancies and brain metastases and, in so doing, lessen emetic episodes). Dexamethasone is the favored agent due to the small pill size, minimal mineralocorticoid activity, and availability of intravenous and subcutaneous administration. Serotonin antagonists are relatively new and expensive agents. Although quite useful in chemotherapy-induced and radiation-induced emesis, their value in terminal NV is unknown. Nevertheless, they are frequently utilized in dying patients and are reportedly quite effective in reducing emesis, particularly NV associated with radiation, bowel obstruction, and renal failure (94,101).

Octreotide is a somatostatin analog that is useful in reducing NV associated with intestinal obstruction. This drug

TABLE 53.6	Pharmacologic treatment of nausea and vomiting

Drug	Dose[a]
Dopamine antagonists	
Haloperidol	0.5–2.0 mg p.o., i.m., i.v., s.q. q4-6h; 5–15 mg CSI q24h
Prochlorperazine	5–20 mg p.o., i.m., i.v. q4-6h; 25 mg p.r. q4h
Droperidol	2.5–5.0 mg i.v. q4-6h
Promethazine	25 mg p.o., p.r. q4-6h; 12.5–25.0 mg i.v. q4-6h
Substituted benzamide	
Metoclopramide[b]	5–20 mg p.o., i.m., i.v., s.q. q6h; 20–80 mg CSI q24h
Anticholinergics	
Scopolamine	0.3–0.8 mg p.o., s.q. q4-6h; 1–3 transdermal patches q3d; 0.8–2.0 mg CSI q24h
Hyoscyamine	0.125–0.250 mg p.o., s.l. q4h; 0.25–0.50 mg s.q. q4-6h; 1–2 mg CSI q24h
Antihistamines	
Buclizine	50 mg p.o. q4-6h
Meclizine	25–50 mg p.o. q4-6h
Diphenhydramine	25–50 mg p.o., i.m., i.v. q4-6h
Corticosteroids	
Dexamethasone	1–4 mg p.o., i.v., s.q. q6h; 2–12 mg CSI q24h
Serotonin antagonists	
Ondansetron	8 mg p.o., i.v., s.q. q8h; 8–24 mg CSI q24h
Granisetron	0.5–1.0 mg p.o., i.v., s.q. q12h
Somatostatin analog	
Octreotide	150 μg s.q. t.i.d.; 0.2–0.9 μg CSI q24h
Cannabinoid	
Dronabinol	2.5–7.5 mg p.o. b.i.d.–t.i.d.
Benzodiazepines	
Lorazepam	0.5–2.0 mg p.o., s.l., i.m., i.v., s.q. q4h
Compounded medication[c]	
ABHR, ABHRD, ABHRDC[d]	1 p.r. q4-6h

CSI, continuous subcutaneous infusion; I.M, intramuscular; I.V, intravenous; P.O, oral; P.R, rectal; S.L, sublingual; S.Q, subcutaneous.

[a]Suggested starting doses, may need to be clinically titrated; older frail patients may need doses adjusted appropriately.

[b]Metoclopramide is a serotonin antagonist at high doses.

[c]Needs to be prepared by a compounding pharmacist.

[d]ABHR compounded medications have not been tested in a research setting and their use is not supported by well-designed trials.

decreases gastrointestinal secretions, stimulates absorption of water and electrolytes, and inhibits intestinal peristalsis (102,103).

Dronabinol is the only commercially available cannabinoid available in the United States. It is rarely used in terminal NV. It exhibits antikinetic properties in the stomach and small bowel (94) and may be most useful in emesis related to small bowel obstruction. It may, however, potentially worsen gastroparetic conditions.

The benzodiazepines have little role as singular antiemetics in the actively dying patient unless anxiety is a dominant component. They are best utilized as adjuncts to other antiemetics through their amnesic, anxiolytic, and sedative properties (104).

Many hospice programs utilize compounding pharmacists to prepare diverse and innovative medications and delivery systems for symptom control in dying patients. A compounding pharmacist can prepare a topical gel and/or suppository variously known as *ABHR*, *ABHRD*, or *ABHRDC* that contain commercially available antiemetics, including Ativan (lorazepam), Benadryl or Dramamine (diphenhydramine), Haldol (haloperidol), Reglan (metoclopramide), Decadron (dexamethasone), or Cogentin (benztropine). These drugs are combined in various dosages (i.e., Ativan, 1.0 mg; Benadryl, 12.5 to 25.0 mg or Dramamine, 25 to 50 mg; Haldol, 0.5 to 1.0 mg; Reglan, 5 to 10 mg; Decadron, 10 mg; and Cogentin, 1 mg). The suppositories have been quite useful in refractory NV and may be very effective in patients near death. Although there have been no studies that support the use of varied combinations, they appear to benefit some patients because of both antiemetic and sedative effects.

PAIN

As death approaches, pain may become less problematic because the patient becomes bedbound and experiences less movement–related pain. Nevertheless, opioids must not be stopped abruptly, and clinicians should be cognizant that patients may be disturbed by pain, even when comatose (7). Assessment of pain may become difficult and, in the final hours of life, patients may appear to show signs of pain when turned or repositioned, even when unconscious. Such pain may be due to an underlying medical disorder or due to joint stiffness secondary to bed rest and minimal body movement (105). Conversely, moaning and groaning is not uncommon in actively dying patients and may be interpreted as pain by family members. However, it is rare for uncontrolled pain to develop during the last hours of life, and in such patients, it is helpful to look for tension across the forehead, furrowing of the eyebrows, or facial grimacing, all evidence that the moaning and groaning may be secondary to pain (106,107).

Assessing pain in confused or demented patients may be problematic. Such patients frequently exhibit pain by facial grimacing, resistance to turning or repositioning, agitation, and a reduction in functional abilities. Conversely, signs of apparent discomfort may be noted when a patient who is hearing or visually impaired or confused is touched without forewarning. Such response may not in fact be pain but rather the result of a startled response from tactile stimulation without prior warning.

In the final hours of life, patients may be unable to swallow and sublingual/buccal, transdermal, rectal, intravenous, or subcutaneous administration of analgesics may be necessary (Tables 53.7 and 53.8). Although rectal administration of sustained-release opioids is not approved by the U.S. Food and Drug Administration (FDA), studies suggest that rectal absorption is similar to oral administration. In addition, suppositories are available for nonsteroidal anti-inflammatory drugs, the tricyclic antidepressant doxepin, and the corticosteroid dexamethasone. The antiepileptics carbamazepine and valproic acid are frequently administered rectally by placing them in gelatin capsules.

Unfortunately, many patients and family members are reluctant to utilize the rectal route for administration of medications, especially if pain is not controlled and frequent supplementary doses of analgesics are required. In such cases, subcutaneous infusions are appropriate and well tolerated. Opioids; the nonsteroidal anti-inflammatory ketorolac (108); the anticholinergics scopolamine, atropine, hyoscyamine, and glycopyrrolate; and the corticosteroid dexamethasone can all be given by means of the subcutaneous route in an effort to maintain or improve pain control. Epidural and other invasive analgesic interventions are rarely utilized when the patient is near death and should ideally be considered for use earlier in the disease process.

PALLIATIVE SEDATION

PS, also referred to as terminal sedation or controlled sedation, is the intentional use of pharmacologic agents to induce and maintain a deep sleep, but not deliberately cause death, in specific clinical circumstances complicated by refractory symptoms (109–112). The incidence of PS varies from 5% to 52% (113). This variation is attributable to diverse definitions of PS, the retrospective nature of studies, and cultural and ethnic diversities. A refractory symptom is at times subjective and nonspecific and includes physical as well as psychological symptoms (114). Cherny and Portenoy clarify the boundaries of a refractory symptom by offering three criteria that suggest a symptom is refractory:

1. It cannot be controlled adequately despite aggressive efforts to identify a tolerable therapy that does not compromise consciousness.
2. Additional invasive and noninvasive interventions are incapable of providing adequate relief.
3. The therapy directed at the symptom is associated with excessive and intolerable acute or chronic morbidity and is unlikely to provide relief within a tolerable time frame (109).

The ethical validity of PS derives from the doctrine of double effect, a doctrine that is applied to situations in which it is impossible for a person to avoid all harmful actions, and the precept of informed consent. The traditional formulations of the doctrine of double effect involve four basic conditions:

1. The nature of the act must be good or morally neutral and not in a category that is absolutely prohibited and intrinsically wrong.
2. The intent of the clinician must be good, and the good effect, not the bad effect, must be intended.
3. The demarcation between the means and effects must be acceptable, in other words, the bad effect must not be the means to the good effect.
4. Proportionality, whereby the good effect must exceed or balance the bad effect (115).

Contentious issues regarding PS revolve around the use of tube feedings and eventual dehydration and the relationship of PS to physician-assisted suicide and euthanasia. Opponents of PS claim that the sedated patient dies of malnutrition and/ or dehydration, not the underlying disease, although most

TABLE 53.7	Alternative routes of delivery for pharmacologic treatment of pain

Opioids That Can Be Delivered Subcutaneously	
Morphine	
Hydromorphone	
Methadone	
Fentanyl	
Opioids That Can Be Delivered Topically	
Fentanyl[a]	
Morphine[b]	
Oral Opioids That Can Be Delivered Rectally	
Morphine[c]	
Oxycodone	
Anesthetics That Can Be Delivered Subcutaneously	
Lidocaine[d]	
Adjuvant Medications and Alternative Routes of Delivery	
Dexamethasone	s.q., i.m., i.v., p.r.
Indomethacin	p.r.
Diclofenac	p.r.
Ketorolac[e]	s.q.
Carbamazepine[f]	p.r.
Valproic acid	p.r.
Doxepin	p.r.

I.M, intramuscular; I.V, intravenous; P.R, rectal; S.Q, subcutaneous.

[a]Available as a topical patch; to convert from an oral opioid, convert the opioid to a morphine equivalent dose, then divide the morphine dose by 2 to get the approximate strength of the fentanyl patch. From Storey P, Knight CF. *UNIPAC Three: Assessment and Treatment of Pain in the Terminally Ill.* Gainesville, FL: American Academy of Hospice and Palliative Medicine; 1996, with permission.

[b]Also available as a suppository; hydromorphone also available as a suppository.

[c]Morphine can be compounded into a gel for topical use, bioavailability is unknown.

[d]1–3 mg/kg (often 100 mg) i.v. over 20–30 min or s.q. over 30–60 min—if pain relieved, start an infusion either i.v.or s.q. at 0.5–2 mg/kg/h; serum levels may be monitored. See: Ferrini R. Parenteral lidocaine for severe intractable pain in six hospice patients continued at home. *J Palliat Med.* 2000;3:193–200.

[e]Can be administered by a continuous subcutaneous infusion, 60 mg q24h.

[f]Crush the tablets, put in a gelatin capsule, and place rectally.

patients have stopped eating and drinking before the initiation of PS, negating the argument of clinician-induced food and fluid deprivation. Nevertheless, if patients or surrogate family members wish to continue tube feedings, most clinicians discuss the futility of nutritional support but acquiesce to such requests, or more favorably suggest a time-limited use of enteral nutrition, and initiate PS.

Opponents of PS also contend that PS is nothing more than slow euthanasia. As proffered by the doctrine of double effect, however, the intent of the clinician must be considered. In the case of refractory symptoms, the intent is to alleviate suffering, not assist in suicide or euthanasia, although PS may undeniably hasten death. Auspiciously, the US Supreme Court fundamentally sanctioned PS in its decision opposing the constitutional right to physician-assisted suicide in 1997 (116,117) and, in so doing, helped establish its value in the palliative armamentarium.

If PS is employed in a dying patient, guidelines should be followed (Table 53.9), including obtaining informed consent, as it is intimately integrated with autonomy and self-determination, and allowing a reasonable person or surrogate to make independent and noncoerced treatment decisions (118). The reason for PS should be documented, as should the people present during the discussion, and if required by institutional or corporate policy, a completed consent form placed in the patient's chart. The choice of medications for PS is practitioner dependent; clinicians should choose the drugs they are most familiar with, considering efficacy,

TABLE 53.8	Alternative routes of medication administration[a]

Route	Medication
Rectal	Valproic acid
	Carbamazepine
	Diazepam
	Indomethacin
	Doxepin
	Pentobarbital
	Phenobarbital
	Chlorpromazine
	Opioids
Inhalation	Furosemide
	Vasopressin
Sublingual	Liquid opioids[b]
	Hyoscyamine
	Atropine
	Lorazepam
Subcutaneous	Morphine
	Hydromorphone
	Midazolam
	Lorazepam
	Haloperidol
	Hyoscyamine
	Glycopyrrolate
	Metoclopramide
	Dexamethasone
	Lidocaine
	Ketorolac
Transdermal	Fentanyl
	Scopolamine

[a]List is not all inclusive.

[b]Methadone is lipophilic and therefore better absorbed across the buccal membrane than the other opioids.

TABLE 53.9	Guidelines for palliative sedation

Presence of a terminal illness with refractory symptom(s)
A do-not-resuscitate order
Exhaustion of all palliative treatments, including treatment for depression, delirium, anxiety, and familial discord
Consideration of ethical and psychiatric consultations
Consideration of assessment for spiritual issues by a skilled clinician or clergy member
Discussion regarding the discontinuation of parenteral or enteral nutrition or hydration
Obtaining informed consent
Consideration of respite sedation, particularly in patients with refractory existential distress

Adapted from Rousseau P. Palliative sedation in the management of refractory symptoms. *J Support Oncol.* 2004;2:181–186.

cost, and clinical circumstance. Drugs frequently used for PS include benzodiazepines, barbiturates, neuroleptics, and propofol (Table 53.10).

FAMILY VIGIL

As death nears, family members tend to gather for comfort, solace, and support of themselves and their dying loved one. Emotions may become capricious and volatile, and aggressive treatments may be requested in an attempt to delay or preclude death. A "long-lost" family member may also suddenly appear and precipitate dissension among family members. Such disruption can distract healthcare providers as well as family members from providing the care and sustenance the dying patient needs. The clinician must keep in mind that such actions are often a manifestation of grief and fear, a desire to control an uncontrollable situation, or apprehension regarding one's own predestined death. It is important to maintain open communication with family members and reaffirm the goal of comfort care. Social work, nursing, and chaplain involvement can help direct family members in accepting the inevitable death of their loved one and provide reassurance that they will be there during this final journey.

Involving family members in the plan of care for the patient will enhance cooperation and a sense of contribution, as will frequent interaction with and discussion of their loved ones decline. They should be encouraged to assist in care by swabbing the oral mucosa, applying cool compresses to the eyes, performing gentle range of motion, and holding the hand of their loved one. The signs and events of the dying process should be reinforced, and personal, cultural, and religious beliefs and rituals honored (119,120). Family members may also be encouraged to convey the five affirmations recommended by Ira Byock: I forgive you, forgive me, I love you, thank you, and good-bye (121). Facilitating and supporting the opportunity for resolution and closure, personal and spiritual growth, and emotional healing is cardinal to a constructive death and bereavement and should be provided for and encouraged.

To preclude confusion and turmoil during a home death, family members should be advised not to call "911."

TABLE 53.10	**Medications for palliative sedation**

Drug	Dose
Benzodiazepines	
Midazolam	5 mg s.q. bolus, then 1 mg/h s.q., titrate as needed
Lorazepam	2–5 mg s.q. bolus, then 0.5–1.0 mg/h s.q., titrate as needed; 1–4 mg q1-4h s.l., p.r.
Barbiturates	
Thiopental	5–7 mg/kg/h i.v. bolus, then 20–80 mg/h i.v., titrate as needed
Pentobarbital[a]	2–3 mg/kg i.v. bolus, then 1 mg/h i.v., titrate as needed; 60–120 mg p.r. q4h
Phenobarbital	200 mg i.v., s.q. bolus, then 25 mg/h i.v., s.q., titrate as needed
Neuroleptics	
Haloperidol	2–10 mg i.v., s.q. bolus, then 5–15 mg/d, titrate as needed
Chlorpromazine[a]	25–100 mg p.r. q4h
Anesthetic	
Propofol	10 mg/h i.v., titrate as needed; boluses of 20–50 mg may be administered for urgent sedation

I.V, intravenous; P.R, rectal; S.L, sublingual; S.Q, subcutaneous.

[a]Available as a suppository.

Specific instructions should be given about whom to call (i.e., hospice nurse, social worker, chaplain, or physician). Family members should also be instructed about the physiologic events that occur as the patient dies (e.g., the heart stops beating, breathing stops, pupils may dilate, eyes may remain open, urine and stool may be released, and jaw may drop open (119)) and offered sufficient time to ask questions. Once death occurs, there is no immediacy to deliver the body to the morgue or funeral home, and family members should be allowed private time with their deceased loved one. Intravenous lines and catheters should be removed and, if desired by the spouse or children, the deceased bathed by family members; the latter can facilitate closure and allow expressions of immediate grief in a supportive setting (120). Finally, if the clinician is present to pronounce the patient, forthright and candid respect should be shown to the patient and family. Words such as "I'm sorry, he/she has died" and "My deepest condolences" are appropriate. However, silence, touch, and mere presence can be the greatest forms of communication and compassion at the time of death.

TIME OF DEATH

No matter how well family members and healthcare professionals are prepared, the time of death can be challenging and difficult (106). If the patient is at home, family members should have been instructed to call the hospice program or their family physician if hospice was not involved. Rarely is it necessary to involve the coroner, unless the death was unexpected or surrounded by suspicious circumstances. If the death occurs in an institution, a medical student or resident may be called to certify or pronounce death; in nonteaching

institutions, the responsibility may fall on the nurse (107). However, one issue that may arise before and after death is what are the signs of death, especially if the patient is dying at home away from professional caregivers. Family members should be counseled on the signs of death, particularly in homebound patients (106,107). Basic signs of death include absence of heart sounds, pulses, and respiration, fixed pupils, pale and waxen color as blood settles, and release of urine and stool with relaxation of sphincter tone (106).

Once death has occurred, the focus of care should immediately shift from the patient to the family and caregivers; although death had been expected, no one understands the emotions and depth of loss until it actually occurs. Families should be allowed to spend time with their deceased loved one before the body is moved; time spent with the body immediately after death reportedly helps family members assimilate and deal with acute grief (106,107). Moreover, moving the body is a direct confrontation with the reality of death, so providing ample time with the body and asking whether family members wish to witness the removal is suggested (106). Finally, professional caregivers should offer to assist the family in notifying other family members and friends and provide a telephone number where they can be reached should unforeseen issues or questions arise.

REFERENCES

1. Rousseau PC. The losses and suffering of terminal illness. *Mayo Clin Proc.* 2000;75:197-198.
2. Abrahm JL. *A Physician's Guide to Pain and Symptom Management in Cancer Patients.* Baltimore, MD: The Johns Hopkins University Press; 2000.

3. Nelson KA, Walsh D, Behrens C, et al. The dying cancer patient. *Semin Oncol.* 2000;27:84-89.

4. Conill C, Verger E, Henriquez I, et al. Symptom prevalence in the last week of life. *J Pain Symptom Manage.* 1997;14:328-331.

5. Fainsinger R, Miller M, Bruera E, et al. Symptom control during the last week of life on a palliative care unit. *J Palliat Care.* 1991;7:5-11.

6. Ventafridda V, Ripamonti C, DeConno F, et al. Symptom prevalence and control during cancer patients' last days of life. *J Palliat Care.* 1990;6:7-11.

7. Twycross R, Lichter I. The terminal phase. In: Doyle D, Hanks GWC, MacDonald N, eds. *Oxford Textbook of Palliative Medicine.* 2nd ed. Oxford: Oxford University Press; 1998:977-992.

8. Adam J. ABC of palliative care. The last 48 hours. *BMJ.* 1997;315:1600-1603.

9. Rousseau PC. Nonpain symptom management in terminal care. *Clin Geriatr Med.* 1996;12:313-327.

10. Bruera E, MacMillan K, Pither J, et al. The effects of morphine on the dyspnea of terminal cancer patients. *J Pain Symptom Manage.* 1990;5:341-344.

11. Reuben DB, Mor V. Dyspnea in terminally ill cancer patients. *Chest.* 1986;89:234-236.

12. Sykes NP. Advances in symptom control for dysphagia and dyspnea. *J Cancer Care.* 1992;1:47-52.

13. Hsu DHS. Dyspnea in dying patients. *Can Fam Physician.* 1993;39:1635-1638.

14. Von Roenn JH, Paice JA. Control of common, non-pain cancer symptoms. *J Support Oncol.* 2005;32:200-210.

15. Wolfe J, Grier HE, Klar N, et al. Symptoms and suffering at the end of life in children with cancer. *N Engl J Med.* 2000;342: 326-333.

16. Rousseau PC. Hospice and palliative care. *Dis Mon.* 1995;41: 769-844.

17. Manning HL. Dyspnea treatment. *Respir Care.* 2000;45: 1342-1351.

18. Light RW, Muro JR, Sato RI, et al. Effects of oral morphine on breathlessness and exercise tolerance in patients with chronic obstructive pulmonary disease. *Am Rev Respir Dis.* 1989;139: 126-133.

19. Weil JV, McCullough RE, Kline JS, et al. Diminished ventilatory response to hypoxia and hypercapnia after morphine in normal man. *N Engl J Med.* 1975;292:1103-1106.

20. Woodcock AA, Gross ER, Gellert A, et al. Effects of dihydrocodeine, alcohol, and caffeine on breathlessness and exercise tolerance in patients with chronic obstructive lung disease and normal blood gases. *N Engl J Med.* 1981;305:1611-1616.

21. Ripamonti C. Management of dyspnea in advanced cancer patients. *Support Care Cancer.* 1999;7:233-243.

22. Allard P, Lamontagne C, Bernard P, et al. How effective are supplementary doses of opioids for dyspnea in terminally ill cancer patients? A randomized continuous sequential clinical trial. *J Pain Symptom Manage.* 1999;17:256-265.

23. Boyd KJ, Kelly M. Oral morphine as symptomatic treatment of dyspnea in patients with advanced cancer. *Palliat Med.* 1997;11:277-281.

24. Bruera E, MacEachern T, Ripamonti C, et al. Subcutaneous morphine for dyspnea in cancer patients. *Ann Intern Med.* 1993;119:906-907.

25. LeGrand SB, Walsh D. Palliative management of dyspnea in advanced cancer. *Curr Opin Oncol.* 1999;11:250-254.

26. Plonk WM, Arnold RM. Terminal care: the last weeks of life. *J Palliat Med.* 2005;8:1042-1054.

27. Jennings AL, Davies AN, Higgins JP, et al. Opioids for the palliation of breathlessness in terminal illness. *Cochrane Database Syst Rev.* 2001;(4):CD002066; www.cochrane.org.

28. Abernethy AP, Currow DC, Frith P, et al. Randomized double blind placebo controlled trial of sustained release morphine in the management of refractory dyspnea. *BMJ.* 2003;327:523-528.

29. Lanken PN, Terry PB, DeLisser HM, et al. An official American Thoracic Society clinical policy statement: palliative care for patients with respiratory diseases and critical illnesses. *Am J Respir Crit Care Med.* 2008;177:912-927.

30. Qaseem A, Snow V, Shekelle P, et al. Evidence-based interventions to improve the palliative care of pain, dyspnea, and depression at the end of life: a clinical practice guideline from the American College of Physicians. *Ann Intern Med.* 2008;148(2):141-146.

31. Mahler DA, Selecky PA, Harrod CG, et al. American College of Chest Physicians Consensus statement on the management of dyspnea in patients with advanced lung cancer or heart disease. *Chest.* 2010;137:674-691.

32. Ripamonti C, Fulfaro F, Bruera E. Dyspnoea in patients with advanced cancer: incidence, causes, and treatments. *Cancer Treat Rev.* 1998;24:69-80.

33. Chrubasik J, Wust H, Friedrich G, et al. Absorption and bioavailability of nebulized morphine. *Br J Anaesth.* 1988;61:228-230.

34. Ripamonti C, Bruera E. Transdermal and inhalatory routes of opioid administration: the potential application in cancer pain. *Palliat Med.* 1992;6:98.

35. Davis C. The role of nebulised drugs in palliating respiratory symptoms of malignant disease. *Eur J Palliat Care.* 1995;2:9-15.

36. Zeppetella G. Nebulized morphine in the palliation of dyspnea. *Palliat Med.* 1997;11:267.

37. Coyne P, Viswanathan R, Smith TJ. Fentanyl by nebulizer reduces dyspnea (Abstract). *Proc Am Soc Clin Oncol.* 2001; 20:402A.

38. Leung R, Hill P, Burdon J. Effect of inhaled morphine on the development of breathlessness during exercise in patients with chronic lung disease. *Thorax.* 1996;51:596-600.

39. Masood AR, Reed JW, Thomas SH. Lack of effect of inhaled morphine on exercise induced breathlessness in chronic obstructive pulmonary disease. *Thorax.* 1995;50:629-634.

40. Viola R, Kiteley C, Lloyd NS, et al. The management of dyspnea in cancer patients: a systematic review. *Support Care Cancer.* 2008;16(4):329-337.

41. Jennings AL, Davies AN, Higgins JP. A systematic review of the use of opioids in the management of dyspnea. *Thorax.* 2002;57:939-944.

42. Farncombe M, Chater S. Case studies outlining use of nebulized morphine for patients with end-stage chronic lung and cardiac disease. *J Pain Symptom Manage.* 1993;8:221-225.

43. Quelch PC, Faulkner DE, Yun JWS. Nebulized opioids in the treatment of dyspnea. *J Palliat Care.* 1997;13:48-52.

44. Farncombe M, Chater S. Clinical application of nebulized opioids for treatment of dyspnea in patients with malignant disease. *Support Care Cancer.* 1994;2:184-187.

45. Bruera E, Sala R, Spruyt O, et al. Nebulized versus subcutaneous morphine for patients with cancer dyspnea: a preliminary study. *J Pain Symptom Manage.* 2005;29:613-618.

46. Masood AR, Thomas SHL. Systemic absorption of nebulized morphine compared with oral morphine in healthy subjects. *Br J Clin Pharmacol.* 1996;41:250-252.

47. Zeppetella G. The palliation of dyspnea in terminal disease. *Am J Hosp Palliat Care.* 1998;15:322-330.

48. Booth S, Wade R, Johnson M, et al. For the Expert Working Group of the Scientific Community of the Association of Palliative Medicine. The use of oxygen in the palliation of breathlessness. *Respir Med.* 2004;98:66-77.

49. Bruera E. Symptom control in the terminally ill cancer patient. UpToDate®. www.uptodateonline.com. Accessed April 19, 2005.

50. Simon ST, Higginson IJ, Booth S, et al. Benzodiazepines for the relief of breathlessness in advanced disease in adults. *Cochrane Review System Rev.* 2010;(1):CD007354; www.cochrane.org. Accessed January 20, 2010.

51. Storey P. Symptom control in advanced cancer. *Semin Oncol.* 1994;21:748-753.

52. Navigante AH, Cerchietti LC, Castro MA, et al. Midazolam as adjunct therapy to morphine in the alleviation of severe dyspnea perception in patients with advanced cancer. *J Pain Symptom Manage.* 2006;31(1):38-47.

53. Ben-Aharon I, Gafter-Gvili A, Paul M, et al. Interventions for alleviating cancer-related dyspnea: a systematic review. *J Clin Oncol.* 2008;26(14):2396-2404.

54. Craven J, Sutherland A. Buspirone for anxiety disorders in patients with severe lung disease. *Lancet.* 1991;338:249.

55. McIver B, Walsh D, Nelson K. The use of chlorpromazine for symptom control in dying cancer patients. *J Pain Symptom Manage.* 1994;9:341-345.

56. Walsh D. Dyspnoea in advanced cancer. *Lancet.* 1993;324:450-451.

57. Ong KC, Kor AC, Chong WF, et al. Effects of inhaled furosemide on exertional dyspnea in chronic obstructive lung disease. *Am J Respir Crit Care Med.* 2004;169:1029-1033.

58. Stone P, Kurowska A, Tookman A. Nebulized furosemide for dyspnea. *Palliat Med.* 1994;8:256.

59. Shimoyama N, Shimoyama M. Nebulized furosemide as a novel treatment for dyspnea in terminal cancer patients. *J Pain Symptom Manage.* 2002;23:73-76.

60. Kohara H, Ueoka H, Aoe K, et al. Effect of nebulized furosemide in terminally ill cancer patients with dyspnea. *J Pain Symptom Manage.* 2003;26:962-967.

61. Wilcock A, Corcoran R, Tattersfield AE. Safety and efficacy of nebulised lignocaine in patients with cancer and breathlessness. *Palliat Med.* 1994;8:35-38.

62. Bruera E, de Stoutz ND, Velasco-Leiva A, et al. Effects of oxygen on dyspnoea in hypoxaemic terminal cancer patients. *Lancet.* 1993;342:13-14.

63. Clemens KE, Quednau I, Klaschik E. Use of oxygen and opioids in the palliation of dyspnea in hypoxic and non-hypoxic palliative care patients: a prospective study. *Support Care Cancer.* 2008;17(4):367-377.

64. Phillip J, Gold M, Miner A, et al. A randomized, double-blind, crossover trial of the effects of oxygen on dyspnea in patients with advanced cancer. *J Pain Symptom Manage.* 2006;32(6):541-550.

65. Enck RE. *The Medical Care of Terminally Ill Patients.* Baltimore, MD: The Johns Hopkins University Press; 1994.

66. Dudgeon DJ, Rosenthal S. Management of dyspnea and cough in patients with cancer. *Hematol Oncol Clin North Am.* 1996;10:157-171.

67. Sorenson HM. Managing secretions in dying persons. *Respir Care.* 2000;45:1355-1362.

68. Kompanje EJ. "The death rattle" in the intensive care unit after withdrawal of mechanical ventilation in neurological patients. *Neurocrit Care.* 2005;3(2):107-110.

69. Wildiers H, Dhaenekit C, Demeulenaere P, et al. Atropine, hyoscine butylbromide, or scopolamine are equally effective for the treatment of death rattle in terminal care. *J Pain Symptom Manage.* 2009;38(1):124-133.

70. Wee B, Hillier R. Interventions for noisy breathing in patients near to death. *Cochrane Database System Rev.* 2008;(1):CD005177; www.cochrane.org. Accessed February 17, 2010.

71. Breitbart W, Chochinov HM, Passik S. Psychiatric aspects of palliative care. In: Doyle D, Hanks GWC, MacDonald N, eds. *Oxford Textbook of Palliative Medicine.* 2nd ed. Oxford: Oxford University Press; 1998:933-954.

72. Breitbart W, Jacobsen PB. Psychiatric symptom management in terminal care. *Clin Geriatr Med.* 1996;12:329-347.

73. Roth AJ, Breitbart W. Psychiatric emergencies in terminally ill cancer patients. *Hematol Oncol Clin North Am.* 1996;10:235-259.

74. Breitbart W. Psycho-oncology: depression, anxiety, delirium. *Semin Oncol.* 1994;21:754-769.

75. Holland JC. Anxiety and cancer: the patient and family. *J Clin Psychiatry.* 1989;50:20-25.

76. Hollister LE. Pharmacotherapeutic considerations in anxiety disorders. *J Clin Psychiatry.* 1986;47:33-36.

77. Bottomley DM, Hanks GW. Subcutaneous midazolam infusion in palliative care. *J Pain Symptom Manage.* 1990;5:259-261.

78. Massie MJ, Holland JC. Depression and the cancer patient. *J Clin Psychiatry.* 1990;51:12-17.

79. Beaver WT, Feise G. Comparison of the analgesic effects of morphine, hydroxyzine and their combination in patients with post-operative pain. In: Bonica JJ, Albe-Fessard D, eds. *Advances in Pain Research and Therapy.* New York, NY: Raven Press; 1976:553-557.

80. Ingham J, Breitbart W. Epidemiology and clinical features of delirium. In: Portenoy RK, Bruera E, eds. *Topics in Palliative Care.* Vol 1. New York, NY: Oxford University Press; 1997:7-19.

81. Massie MJ, Holland JC, Glass E. Delirium in terminally ill cancer patients. *Am J Psychiatry.* 1983;140:1048-1050.

82. Breitbart W, Strout D. Delirium in the terminally ill. *Clin Geriatr Med.* 2000;16:357-372.

83. Pereira J, Hanson J, Bruera E. The frequency and clinical course of cognitive impairment in patients with terminal cancer. *Cancer.* 1997;79:835-842.

84. Back IN, Jenkins K, Blower A, et al. A study comparing hyoscine hydrobromide and glycopyrrolate in the treatment of death rattle. *Palliat Med.* 2001;15:329-336.

85. Casarett DJ, Inouye SK. Diagnosis and management of delirium near the end of life. *Ann Intern Med.* 2001;135:32-40.

86. American Psychiatric Association. *Diagnostic and Statistical Manual of Mental Disorders.* 4th ed. Washington, DC: American Psychiatric Association; 1994.

87. Jackson KC, Lipman AG. Drug therapy for delirium in terminally ill patients. *Cochrane Database System Rev.* 2004;(2):CD004770; www.cochrane.org. Accessed October 7, 2009.

88. Kehl KA. Treatment of terminal restlessness: a review of evidence. *J Pain Palliat Care Pharmacother.* 2004;18:5-30.

89. Breitbart W, Marotta R, Platt NM, et al. A double blind trial of haloperidol, chlorpromazine, and lorazepam in the treatment of delirium in hospitalized AIDS patients. *Am J Psychiatry.* 1996;153:231-237.

90. Finucane TE. Delirium at the end of life. *Ann Intern Med.* 2002;137:295.

91. Stiefel F, Fainsinger R, Bruera E. Acute confusional states in patients with advanced cancer. *J Pain Symptom Manage.* 1992;7:94-98.

92. Fainsinger R, Bruera E. Treatment of delirium in a terminally ill patient. *J Pain Symptom Manage.* 1992;7:54-56.

93. Reuben DB, Mor V. Nausea and vomiting in terminal cancer patients. *Arch Intern Med.* 1986;146:2021-2023.

94. Davis MP, Walsh D. Treatment of nausea and vomiting in advanced cancer. *Support Care Cancer.* 2000;8:444-452.

95. Lichter I. Nausea and vomiting in patients with cancer. *Hematol Oncol Clin North Am.* 1996;10:207-220.

96. Baines M. Nausea and vomiting in the patient with advanced cancer. *J Pain Symptom Manage.* 1988;3:81-85.

97. Perkins P, Dorman S. Haloperidol for the treatment of nausea and vomiting in palliative care patients. *Cochrane Database System Rev.* 2009;(2):CD006271; www.cochrane.org. Accessed January 20, 2010.

98. Glare PA, Dunwoodie D, Clark K, et al. Treatment of nausea and vomiting in terminally ill cancer patients. *Drugs.* 2008;68(18):2575-2590.

99. Axelrod R. Antiemetic therapy. *Compr Ther.* 1997;23:539-545.

100. Rousseau PC. Management of malignant bowel obstruction in advanced cancer: a brief review. *J Palliat Med.* 1998;1:65-72.

101. Currow D, Coughlan M, Fardell B, et al. Use of ondansetron in palliative medicine. *J Pain Symptom Manage.* 1997;13:302-307.

102. Riley J, Fallon MT. Octreotide in terminal malignant obstruction of the gastrointestinal tract. *Eur J Palliat Care.* 1994;1:23-25.

103. Hisanaga T, Shinjo T, Morita T, et al. Multicenter prospective study of efficacy and safety of octreotide for inoperable malignant bowel obstruction. *Jpn J Clin Oncol.* 2010;40(8):739-745.

104. Rousseau P. Antiemetic therapy in adults with terminal disease: a brief review. *Am J Hosp Palliat Care.* 1995;12:13-18.

105. Saunders C. Pain and impending death. In: Wall PD, Melzack E, eds. *Textbook of Pain.* London: Churchill Livingstone; 1989:624-631.

106. Ferris FD. Last hours of living. *Clin Geriatr Med.* 2004;20:641-667.

107. Ferris FD, von Gunten CF, Emanuel LL. Competency in end-of-life care: last hours of life. *J Palliat Med.* 2003;4:605-613.

108. Trotman IF, Myers KG. Use of ketorolac by continuous subcutaneous infusion for control of cancer-related pain. *Postgrad Med J.* 1994;70:359-362.

109. Cherny NI, Portenoy RK. Sedation in the management of refractory symptoms: guidelines for evaluation and treatment. *J Palliat Care.* 1994;10:31-38.

110. Maltoni M, Scarpi E, Rosati M, et al. Palliative sedation in end-of-life care and survival: asystematic review. *J Clin Oncol.* 2012;30(12):1378-1383.

111. Mercadante S, Porzio G, Valle A, et al. Palliative sedation in patients with advanced cancer followed at home: a systematic review. *J Pain Symptom Manage.* 2011;41(4):754-760.

112. Cherny NI, Radbruch L, Board of the European Association for Palliative Care. European Association for Palliative Care recommended framework for the use of sedation in palliative care. *Palliat Med.* 2009;23(7):581-593.

113. Rousseau PC. Terminal sedation in the care of dying patients. *Arch Intern Med.* 1996;156:1785-1786.

114. Rousseau PC. The ethical validity and clinical experience with palliative sedation. *Mayo Clin Proc.* 2000;75:1064-1069.

115. Quill TE, Dresser R, Brock DW. The role of double effect—a critique of its role in end-of-life decision making. *N Engl J Med.* 1997;337:1768-1771.

116. *Vacco v Quill,* 117 SCt 2293 (1997).

117. *Washington v Glucksberg,* 117 SCt 2258 (1997).

118. Rousseau P. Palliative sedation in the management of refractory symptoms. *J Support Oncol.* 2004;2:181-186.

119. American Medical Association. *Education for Physicians on End-of-Life Care, Module 12.* Chicago, IL: American Medical Association; 1999:M12-1-M12-37.

120. Twaddle M. The process of dying and managing the death event. *Prim Care.* 2001;28(2):329-338.

121. Byock I. *Dying Well: Peace and Possibilities at the End of Life.* New York, NY: Riverhead Books; 1997.

CHAPTER 54

Spirituality

Christina M. Puchalski

Palliative care is a specialty based in the whole person care model. Thus, care of the patient and family includes addressing psychosocial and spiritual needs as well as the physical needs. In a whole person–centered model, preservation of human dignity is considered an important part of quality of life. Spiritual care is based in honoring the dignity of each person. In doing so, spiritual care supports the whole person and recognizes that a goal of care is helping each patient find a sense of wholeness and integrity in the midst of suffering and illness. This is especially important in caring for seriously ill and dying patients.

Illness can strip away one's meaning and purpose, one's important relationships in life; illness can call into question patients' beliefs and values thus triggering profound questions of deep meaning purpose and what is most important to a person. It can be an opportunity for deep reflection and growth. Healthcare professionals can hinder that opportunity by not providing attention and space for patients to address these deeper questions in their lives. Illness can also cause deep suffering. Addressing only the physical pain does not address the spiritual and existential suffering seriously ill and dying patients experience. How the healthcare professionals interact with patients in the midst of their illness can have profound effects on how that person will understand their illness, cope with it, find a will to live and persevere, or the strength to let go and die peacefully when it is time. This process, that is, the patients' confronting their illness and the healthcare system working with the patients to treat that illness, is a spiritual one. Spiritual care is the act of partnering with patients to help them find meaning, wholeness, and healing. Spirituality and spiritual care are the fabrics that underlie the process of honoring the dignity of each person.

THE BIOPSYCHOSOCIAL–SPIRITUAL MODEL

The basic tenets of whole person, patient-centered care are rooted in the biopsychosocial–spiritual model: attention to all the dimensions of a patient—physical, emotional, social, and spiritual (Table 54.1) (1).

The biopsychosocial care model developed by Engel (2) and White et al. (3) forms another theoretical framework for spiritual care by recognizing that each person is a "being-in-relationship." In support of extending the biopsychosocial care model to encompass the spiritual, Jonas said, "Life is essentially a relationship; and relation as such implies 'transcendence,' a going-beyond-itself on the part of that which entertains the relation" (4). Sulmasy took the association a step farther by describing disease as a disturbance in the right relationships that constitute the unity and integrity of what we know to be a human being (see Fig. 54.1) (5,6).

Spiritual care recognizes that a person's relationships—from those inside the physical body that define health to external relationships that give a person's life meaning—are disrupted by illness and, thus, all relationships must be attended to in the treatment or care plan to enhance quality of life.

According to the biopsychosocial–spiritual model, everyone has a spiritual history. For many people, this spiritual history unfolds within the context of an explicit religious tradition; for others it unfolds as a set of philosophical principles or significant experiences. Regardless, this spiritual history helps shape who each patient is as a whole person. An illness experience is unique to each individual in his or her totality (7). This totality includes not only simply the biologic, psychological, and social aspects of the person (8) but also the spiritual aspects as well (9,10). The biologic, psychological, social, and spiritual are distinct dimensions of each person. No one aspect can be disaggregated from the whole. Each aspect can be affected differently by a person's history and illness and each aspect can interact and affect other aspects of the person (6).

Based on this model, one can reframe the standard assessment and plan to include all dimensions of the person, not just the physical. This radically changes how we approach the patient as person. By attending to the whole person, spiritual care embraces the definition of health as not just absence of disease, but as a state of well-being that includes a sense that life has purpose and meaning (11) as stated in the Pew-Fetzer definition of health: "We are coming to understand health not as the absence of disease, but rather as the process by which individuals maintain their sense of coherence (i.e. sense that life is comprehensible, manageable and meaningful) and ability to function in the face of changes in themselves and their relationship with the environment."

MEANING AND PURPOSE

Illness and the prospect of dying can call into question the very meaning and purpose of a person's life. Illness can also cause people to suffer deeply. Victor Frankl wrote that man is not destroyed by suffering; he is destroyed by suffering without meaning (12). Writing about concentration camp victims, he noted that survival itself might depend on seeking and finding meaning. Harold Kushner also noted that pain may be the reason, and out of pain and suffering may come

TABLE 54.1	Dimensions of the dying experience
Physical	Pain and other symptom management
Psychological	Anxiety and depression
Social	Social isolation and economic issues
Spiritual	Purpose and meaning, relationships with the transcendent, search for ultimate meaning, hope, reconciliation, and despair

the answer (13). In my own clinical experience, I have found that people may cope with their suffering by finding meaning in it. Illness can present people with the opportunity to find new meaning in their lives. Many patients say that out of their despair they were able to realize an entirely new and more fulfilling meaning in their lives. Rabbi Cohen wrote,

> When my mother died, I inherited her needlepoint tapestries. When I was a little boy, I used to sit at her feet as she worked on them. Have you ever seen needlepoint from underneath? All I could see was chaos; strands of thread all over with no seeming purpose. As I grew, I was able to see her work from above. I came to appreciate the patterns, the need for the dark threads as well as the light and gaily colored ones. Life is like that. From our human perspective, we cannot see the whole picture, but we should not despair or feel that there is no purpose. There is meaning and purpose even for the dark threads, but we cannot see that right away (14).

Spirituality helps people find hope in the midst of despair. As caregivers, we need to engage our patients on that spiritual level. This is where spirituality plays such a critical

role—the relationship with a transcendent being or concept can give meaning and purpose to people's lives, to their joys, and to their sufferings. Spirituality is concerned with a transcendental or existential way to live one's life at a deeper level, "with the person as human being" (15). All people seek meaning and purpose in life; this search may be intensified when someone is facing death.

There are many different ways people can derive meaning from their lives:

- Work
- Relationships
- Hobbies
- Art, music, and dance
- Reflective writing
- Sports
- Relationship with God/sacred/Divine
- Religious, spiritual, philosophical, or existential beliefs
- Religious, spiritual, or cultural rituals

Some of these activities or practices provide an important but perhaps transient meaning (meaning with a small m); others provide a more transcendent and spiritual meaning (meaning with a large M). For example, work may provide an immense amount of meaning to a person. But when that person is ill or dying and unable to work, what then will provide meaning? Therefore, there are activities, relationships, and values that are meaningful but do not define the ultimate purpose of one's life. Illness, aging, and dying strip away all those things that were meaningful but that do not ultimately sustain us. When we confront ourselves in the nakedness of our dying, it is then that we have the opportunity to find deep and transcendent meaning, that is, values, beliefs, practices, relationships, expressions that lead one to the awareness of transcendence/God/Divine and to a sense of ultimate value and purpose in life. Everyone's sense of meaning evolves over their life in response to experiences and life in general. People can fluctuate between "meaning" and "Meaning."

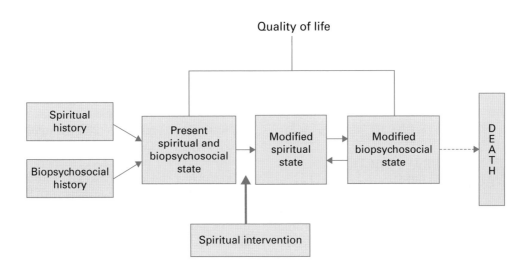

Figure 54.1. The biopsychosocial–spiritual model of care. (From Sulmasy DP. A biopsychosocial–spiritual model for the care of patients at the end of life. *Gerontologist*. 2002;42(spec 3):24–33. Used with permission.)

Downey defined spirituality as "an awareness that there are levels of reality not immediately apparent and that there is a quest for personal integration in the face of forces of fragmentation and depersonalization" (16). Spirituality is that aspect of human beings that seeks to heal or be whole. Foglio and Brody wrote,

> For many people religion [spirituality] forms a basis of meaning and purpose in life. The profoundly disturbing effects of illness can call into question a person's purpose in life and work; responsibilities to spouse, children, and parents … Healing, the restoration of wholeness (as opposed to merely technical healing) requires answers to these questions (17).

Healing, then, is not synonymous with recovery. Indeed, healing may occur at any time, independent of recovery from illness. In dying, for example, restoration of wholeness may be manifested by a transcendent set of meaningful experiences while very ill. It may be reflected by a peaceful death. In chronic illness, healing may be experienced as the acceptance of limitations (15). A person may look to medical care to alleviate his or her suffering, and when the medical system fails to do so, begin to look toward spirituality for meaning, purpose, and understanding. As people are faced with serious illness or the prospect of dying, questions often arise:

- Why did this happen to me?
- What will happen to me after I die?
- Why would God allow me to suffer this way?
- Will I be remembered?
- Will I be missed?

These questions can cause people to undergo a life review whereby they analyze their lives, accomplishments, relationships, and perceived failings (18). This questioning can result in fears, anxieties, and unresolved feelings, which in turn can result in despair and suffering as people face themselves and their eventual mortality. Cassell wrote, "Since in suffering, disruption of the whole person is the dominant theme, we know of the losses and their meaning by what we know of others out of compassion for their suffering" (19). Compassion is essential in the care of all patients, particularly those who are dealing with chronic and serious illnesses and are dying. Two Latin words form the root of the word compassion: "cum," meaning "with," and "passio," meaning "suffering with" (20). What compassionate care asks us to do is to suffer with our patients, that is, to be present to them fully as they suffer and to partner with them in the midst of their pain.

SPIRITUALITY IN CLINICAL PRACTICE PROFESSIONAL GUIDELINES

Guidelines from several organizations, including the American College of Physicians (ACP) and The Joint Commission on Healthcare Accreditation, American Association of Nursing, and National Association of Social Workers, recognize the need for spiritual care. In a recent ACP consensus conference on end of life, it was concluded that physicians have the obligation to address all dimensions of suffering, including spiritual, religious, and existential suffering (21). It also developed guidelines for communicating with patients about spiritual and religious matters (22). JCAHO (Joint Commission on Accreditation of Healthcare Organizations) requires that spiritual care be available to patients in hospital settings (23). In 1978, the first nursing diagnosis related to spirituality, spiritual distress, was established in the North American Nursing Diagnosis Association (NANDA). Spiritual distress is the "impaired ability to experience and integrate meaning and purpose in life through a person's connectedness with self, others, art, music, literature, nature, or a power greater than oneself" (24). The Code of Ethics for professional nurses in the United States recognizes the importance of spirituality and health, illustrated by Provision 1 of the code, which states, "The nurse, in all professional relationships, practices with compassion and respect for the inherent dignity, worth, and uniqueness of each individual, unrestricted by considerations of social and economic status, personal attributes, or the nature of health problems" (25). The National Association of Social Workers' Code of Ethics declares that a social worker must include spirituality when completing an assessment (26).

The National Quality Forum identified spiritual care as one of eight domains of the Clinical Practice Guidelines developed by the National Consensus Project for Quality Palliative Care (NCP) (27). The NCP is a coalition of the leading palliative care organizations in the United States. The NCP recommendations for spiritual care emphasize regular and ongoing assessment and response to patients' spiritual and existential issues and concerns. They emphasize the use of a spiritual assessment to identify religious or spiritual/existential preferences, beliefs, rituals, and practices of the patient and family. These guidelines also recognize the need for inclusion of pastoral care in the interdisciplinary care team.

DATA DEMONSTRATING PATIENT NEED

Studies, as well as theoretical and philosophical literature, demonstrate the impact of religious and spiritual beliefs on people's moral decision-making, way of life, ability to transcend suffering, dealing with life's challenges, interactions with others, and life choices. Spiritual and religious beliefs have been shown to have an impact on how people cope with serious illness, aging, and life stresses. Spiritual practices can foster coping resources (28,29), promote health-related behavior (30), enhance a sense of well-being and improve quality of life (31), provide social support (32), and generate feelings of love and forgiveness (33). Spiritual beliefs can also impact healthcare decision-making (34). Spiritual/religious beliefs, however, can also be harmful (35). Thus, spirituality may be a critical dynamic of how patients understand their illness and cope with it either positively or negatively.

Research also indicates that patients would like their spiritual beliefs addressed by physicians and other healthcare professionals in a variety of healthcare circumstances (36).

One study shows that patients feel increased trust in their clinicians if a spiritual history is obtained. They also note that they experience an increased sense of being listened to (36). Interestingly, a study by Balboni et al. showed that 75% of dying cancer patients did not have their spiritual needs met even when 95% of them said spirituality was important to them (37). These data indicate the importance of developing guidelines and resources for patients and clinicians.

RELATIONSHIP BETWEEN SPIRITUALITY AND COPING

The beneficial effects of spirituality in helping people cope with serious illness and dying are well documented (38). Furthermore, researchers have noted that most patients with cancer in a palliative care setting experience spiritual pain, which is expressed as an internal conflict, a loss or interpersonal conflict, or in relation to God/Divine. Fitchett et al. have shown that spiritual struggles are associated with poor physical outcome and higher rates of morbidity (39). Spiritual pain is also related to psychological distress so that patients presenting with depression or anxiety may actually be suffering from spiritual conflict (40).

Quality of life instruments used in end-of-life care try to measure an existential domain, which addresses purpose, meaning in life, and capacity for self-transcendence. In studies of one such instrument, three items have been found to correlate with good quality of life for patients with advanced disease: if the patient's personal existence is meaningful; if the patient finds fulfillment in achieving life goals; and if life to this point has been meaningful (41). This supports the importance of addressing meaning and purpose in a dying person's life. Spirituality and nonorganized religion have also been associated positively with the will to live in patients with acquired immunodeficiency syndrome (HIV) (42).

The observations noted in patient stories (15) and in the writings of Foglio and Brody (17)—that illness can cause people to question their lives, their identities, and what gives their life meaning—are supported by research. For example, in a study of 108 women undergoing treatment for gynecologic cancer, 49% noted becoming more spiritual after their diagnosis (29). In a study of parents with a child who had died of cancer, 40% of those parents reported a strengthening of their own spiritual commitment over the course of the year before their child's death (43). Illness, facing one's mortality, is an opportunity for new experience, self-awareness, and meaning in life.

Religion and religious beliefs can play an important role in how patients understand their illness. In a study asking older adults about God's role in health and illness, many respondents saw health and illness as being partly attributable to God and, to some extent, God's interventions (44). Pargament et al. have studied both positive and negative coping and have found that religious experiences and practices, such as seeking God's help or having a vision of God, extend the individual's coping resources and are associated with improvement in healthcare outcomes (45). Patients showed less psychological distress if they sought control through a partnership with God or a higher power in a problem-solving way, if they asked God's forgiveness or were able to forgive others, if they reported finding strength and comfort from their spiritual beliefs, and if they found support in a spiritual community. Patients had more depression, poorer quality of life, and callousness toward others if they saw the crisis as a punishment from God, if they had excessive guilt, or if they had an absolute belief in prayer and cure and an inability to resolve their anger if cure did not occur. Pargament et al. have also noted that sometimes patients refuse medical treatment based on religious beliefs (35).

There are a number of studies on meditation as well as other spiritual and religious practices that demonstrate a positive physical response, especially in relation to levels of stress hormones and modulation of the stress response (46). Although more solid evidence is needed, there appears to be an association between meditation and some spiritual or religious practices and certain physiologic processes, including cardiovascular, neuroendocrine, and immune function.

SPIRITUAL COPING

How does spirituality work to help people cope with their dying (Table 54.2)? One mechanism might be through hope. Hope is a powerful inner strength that helps one transcend the present situation and helps foster a positive belief or outlook. Spirituality and religion offer people hope and help people find hope in the midst of the despair that often occurs in the course of serious illness and dying. Hope can change during a course of an illness. Early on, the person may hope for a cure; later, when a cure becomes unlikely, the person may hope for time to finish important projects or goals, travel, make peace with loved ones or with God, and have a peaceful death. This can result in a healing, which can be manifested as a restoration of one's relationships or sense of self. Often our society thinks in terms of cures. Whereas cures may not always be possible, healing—the restoration of wholeness—may be possible to the very end of life. Hope has also been shown to be an effective coping mechanism. Patients who are more hopeful tend to be less depressed.

Religious beliefs offer a sense of hope. For example, in Catholicism, hope in Jesus' promise of victory over death through resurrection and salvation gives Catholics hope in a

TABLE 54.2	Spiritual coping
Hope: for a cure, for healing, for finishing important goals, and for a peaceful death
Sense of control
Acceptance of the situation
Strength to deal with the situation
Meaning and purpose: in life and in midst of suffering

life beyond death. In the funeral rites, it is stated, "I believe in the resurrection of the dead and the life of the world to come" (47). In the Protestant view, the concept of salvation in death gives hope. Jesus' dying and rising from the dead means that those who participate in His death no longer participate in the sinful human nature (48). In Eastern traditions such as Buddhism and Hinduism, the hope of rebirth and a belief in karma offer people hope in the face of mortality (49). In Judaism, there are many diverse ways of viewing death. For some, hope is found in living on through one's children. In the orthodox and conservative views, there is a belief in a resurrection in which the body arises to be united with the soul (50). For patients with and without specific religious beliefs, there is a need to transcend death, which may also be manifested through living on through one's relationships or one's accomplishments and deeds (51). Irion suggests that humans may create abstractions by portraying a life after death (52). For the religious, this may take the form of concepts found in their religious traditions. For others, life after death might be in terms of one's descendants. For some, it might be being immortalized in the memory of others or in the contributions one makes in life. Cultural beliefs and traditions can also contribute to how people find meaning and hope in the midst of despair (53).

Finding meaning in the midst of suffering and uncertainty is critical to effective coping. Spiritual beliefs in general and religious, in particular, can help people find this meaning and purpose. Religion provides a system of beliefs, ritual, and community that can help people find meaning in the context of their illness and dying (54). One very powerful intervention that addresses meaning with patients with advanced cancer has had positive outcomes in these patients. It involved a brief meaning-centered group psychotherapy intervention that is centered on helping patients find meaning in the midst of their suffering (55).

Spirituality can offer people a sense of control. Illness can disrupt life completely. Some people find a sense of control by turning worries or a situation over to a higher power or to God (56). Similarly, people can use their beliefs to help them accept their illness and find strength to deal with their situation (57). Reconciliation may be an important aspect of a dying person's spiritual journey. Often people seek to forgive others or themselves as they review their lives and their relationships.

SPIRITUAL ISSUES: DIAGNOSIS AND RESOURCES OF STRENGTH

The diagnosis of chronic or life-threatening illness or other adverse life events can lead to spiritual struggles for patients. The turmoil may be short for some patients and protracted for others as individuals attempt to integrate the reality of their diagnosis with their spiritual beliefs. The journey may result in growth and transformation for some people and to distress and despair for others (58).

Studies have found that patients with spiritual or religious struggles had poorer physical health, worse quality of life, and greater depression (59); those with chronic spiritual

or religious struggles also had increased disability (58) and higher indices of pain and fatigue and more difficulties with daily physical functioning (60). Religious struggle has also been found to be a significant predictor of increased mortality, even when controlling for demographic, physical health, and mental health factors (61). Poorer quality of life and greater emotional distress were found among patients with diabetes and congestive heart failure who experience religious struggle (40).

Spirituality may also present as a source of strength for patients. The act of seeking forgiveness or the willingness to forgive may be a spiritual strength. The Joint Commission notes that adult and older adult strengths may include, "cultural/spiritual/religious and community involvement" (62). Another example of spiritual strength may be a patient's connection to God or the sacred. Spiritual strengths may help patients cope, find hope in the midst of suffering, find joy in life, and/or find the ability to be grateful (63).

Some of the spiritual issues, which might present as distress, are as follows:

- Lack of meaning and purpose
- Hopelessness
- Despair
- Not being remembered
- Guilt/shame
- Anger at God/others
- Abandonment by God/others
- Feeling out of control
- Existential suffering
- Trust
- Reconciliation
- Grief/loss
- Loneliness
- Lack of love or connection to others or to God
- Fear

Personal and professional caregivers also have similar spiritual issues, as well as spiritual issues that relate to the caregiving role:

- Loss of meaning (no time for activities and relationships)
- Guilt/shame (not being able to be present 100% to patient)
- Questions of faith/God
- Anger at God
- Sense of abandonment
- Powerlessness
- Loneliness
- Fear

In addition to identifying and addressing the spiritual issues discussed in the preceding section, it is important to assess the spiritual resources of strength for patients—hope, sense of meaning and purpose, ability to transcend suffering, as well as support from spiritual or religious community, family, or friends.

Communities, such as churches, temples, mosques, spiritual, or other support groups or a group of like-minded friends, can serve as strong support systems for some patients. The absence of these resources could impact in an adverse way on how patients cope with illness and/or dying.

SPIRITUAL CARE: FRAMEWORK OF CARE

An approach to the care of a patient is to recognize that spirituality is an essential part of being human. It is the part of a person that seeks transcendent meaning and purpose in life. It is that part of each individual from which each person can heal by becoming whole again in the midst of suffering, loss, and stress. Therefore, in caring for patients, healthcare professionals must not only attend to the physical, emotional, and social domains of a patient's life as is supported by the biopsychosocial model of care but also the spiritual domain, therefore a biopsychosocial–spiritual model of care. In a recent Ethics Conference with the George Washington Institute of Spirituality and Health, as well as the AAMC, spiritual care was described as an essential element of health care and not an amenity (64).

During the time a person experiences illness, suffering, loss, or stress, he/she will engage actively in the healthcare system. Healthcare professionals will often meet people during profoundly difficult times in their patients' lives. During these times, patients are vulnerable and often afraid, lonely, and confused. Spiritual care offers a framework for healthcare professionals to connect with their patients, listen to their fears, dreams, and pain, collaborate with their patients as partners in their care, and provide through the therapeutic relationship an opportunity for healing. Healing is distinguished from cure in this context. It refers to the ability of a person to find solace, comfort, connection, meaning, and purpose in the midst of suffering, disarray, and pain. The care the clinician provides is rooted in spirituality through compassion, hopefulness, and the recognition that although a person's life may be limited or no longer socially productive, it remains full of possibility (65).

There are studies that document the importance of the doctor–patient relationship (66). Dr. Francis Peabody wrote in his 1927 medical classic, *The Care of the Patient,* "One of the essential qualities of the clinician is interest in humanity, for the secret care of the patient is in caring for the patient" (67). This relationship can have potential positive impact on healthcare outcomes, compliance, and patient satisfaction (66). Because healing springs from the therapeutic relationship, spiritual care is grounded in relationship-centered care. Spiritual care begins from the moment the healthcare professional enters the patient's room.

SPIRITUAL CARE: PRACTICE WITH INTENTION

The healthcare practitioner intentionally opens himself/herself to the possibility of openness, connection, and mystery. Intention to openness refers to the willingness to listen to the patient without a preconceived agenda, with full respect of the patient as an individual with a unique story (cultural, personal, and spiritual), and a commitment to be fully present in the encounter with the patient. Intention to connection refers to the willingness and ability to actively and appropriately form a connection with the patient on a spiritual and emotional level thereby affording the patient the opportunity to experience a sense of belonging, care, and love. By relating from our humanness, we can help to form deeper and more meaningful connections with our patients. Intention to mystery refers to the acceptance that none of us controls another, life, outcome, or ourselves. Life is full of mysteries—being open to mystery allows the healthcare practitioner to let go of a need to be in control and fully responsible for outcome. It implies a humbleness as one accepts that both the healthcare practitioner and the patient are walking a journey together, which may have many unplanned and unexpected turns. This reframes the commitment from fixing or solving to a commitment of presence, persistence, partnership, and a willingness to walk with the unknown and handle situations as they arise together. It removes the illusion of expert and client and offers the reality of spiritually equal partners.

In order to be able to engage in spiritual care, healthcare professionals need training on how to be intentionally open, willing, and accepting of mystery. This means that the clinician brings his or her whole being to the encounter and places full attention on the patient, not allowing distractions to interfere with that attention. Integral to this is the ability to listen and to be attentive to all dimensions of patients' and their family's lives. Some clinicians suggest that current medical practices do not allow enough time for this. However, being wholly present to the patient is not time dependent. It simply requires the intention on the part of the physician to be fully present for their patients. One becomes fully present when one approaches the patient with deep respect, respect stemming from a commitment to honoring of the whole person. Mohamad Reaz Abdullah of the Asian Institute for Development Communication (AidCom) said, "When we say 'I respect you,' what exactly are we saying? We are really respecting a quality that has been expressed by the person, and we are forming a symbiotic relationship with a quality that we admire. However, when the divinity in the individual that is common to all beings is respected, then the meaning of respect is taken on golden wings to a new height." This is the essence of a spiritually based relationship with others.

Relationship-centered care is intense and personal as it opens up to the possibility of emotional and spiritual reaction on the part of both patient and healthcare professional. Both patients and healthcare professionals can be transformed as a result of their interaction in clinical environments. This requires an awareness of the clinician's own values, beliefs, and attitudes, particularly toward their own mortality. By confronting one's own mortality, one can better understand what the patient is facing. Many clinicians speak of their own spiritual practices and how those practices help them in their ability to deliver good spiritual care and, in fact, good medical care (15,68). Therefore, in order to practice spiritual care effectively, the healthcare professional needs to be aware of and supported in their spiritual needs and journey. It is also critical to train and support the healthcare professional on how to practice relationship-centered care in a way that respects the power differential of the contextual relationship—doctor–patient, nurse–patient, and so on.

INTRINSIC AND EXTRINSIC SPIRITUAL CARE

All medical care has intrinsic (the behavior, attitudes, and values the healthcare professionals bring to the encounter) and extrinsic aspects (the knowledge and skills applied in the encounter). The relationship-centered aspect of medical care is the intrinsic essential aspect of all care from which extrinsic care emanates, including physical, emotional, and social care. That is, spiritual intrinsic care refers to the intention of presence; physical extrinsic care refers to taking vital signs, for example, and spiritual extrinsic care refers to the ability to reorganize spiritual issues and problems as they present in relationship to the presenting healthcare problem or situation. It also refers to recognizing patients' inner resources of strength or a lack of those resources. Once these are recognized, clinicians then incorporate patients' spirituality into the care plan if appropriate to the clinical situation. Everyone on the interdisciplinary healthcare team practices spiritual care, but the specifics of how the spiritual care is delivered is dependent on the context, which it is given. A chaplain provides spiritual care in the context of his/her training as a spiritual counselor in healthcare setting, a clergy provides spiritual care in the context of a religious setting, and a nurse and physician practice spiritual care in the context of caring for patients in a spiritual healthcare situation (hospital, clinic, patient visits, and education). Although the relationship-centered caring aspects are similar in how each profession deals with the patient, how patient's spiritual issues and problems are dealt with depend on the healthcare professional's level of training and context. Chaplains and clergy work primarily with spiritual issues and spiritual problems in-depth and not necessarily in relation to health and illness. They may be secondarily aware of and interface with social, emotional, and physical issues but deal with them more in a supportive way. Nurses and doctors are trained primarily to address the physical issues with which patients present. However, emotional, social, and spiritual issues may affect or be related to the physical issue. Therefore, nurses and doctors recognize, support, and/ or triage those spiritual issues appropriately to the spiritual care professionals (Table 54.3).

A CONSENSUS-BASED INTERPROFESSIONAL MODEL OF SPIRITUAL CARE

In 2009, 40 interdisciplinary experts in palliative care participated in the 2009 National Consensus Conference for Spiritual Care in Palliative Care (NCC) to develop recommendations for improving spiritual care in palliative care settings, with palliative care broadly defined as care for patients with chronic or life-threatening illness (6). Conference participants produced a consensus-based definition of spirituality for clinical settings that recognizes that each person's

TABLE 54.3	Spiritual care
Compassionate Presence	
Intention to openness	
Intention to connection	
Intention to mystery	
Relationship-Centered Care	
Partnership	
Not agenda driven	
Listening to patients' fears, hopes, dreams, and meaning	
Spirituality of Healthcare Professional	
Awareness of one's own spirituality	
Awareness of one's own mortality	
Having a spiritual practice	
Extrinsic Spiritual Care	
Taking a spiritual history	
Recognizing patients' spiritual issues	
Recognizing patients' spiritual problems or spiritual pain	
Recognizing patients' resources of inner strength or lack of resources	
Incorporating patients' spirituality into treatment or care plans (presence, referral, rituals, meditation, etc.)	

spirituality is unique and may or may not include religious beliefs and/or cultural practices:

> Spirituality is the aspect of humanity that refers to the way individuals seek and express meaning and purpose, and the way they experience their connectedness to the moment, to self, to others, to nature, and to the significant or sacred.

Spiritual care defined by this group is a broad term that refers to many different aspects of care ranging from the intrinsic (presence to patients' suffering, honoring dignity of patients, recognition of the concept of healing, and the role of spirituality in the healing process) to extrinsic (doing a spiritual history, integration of spirituality into the treatment plan, and follow-up on spiritual issues as appropriate). The consensus process also described the obligation that all clinicians have: First, to attend to all dimensions of the suffering of the patient and the patient's family; second, to elicit the patient's spiritual needs; and third, to respect those beliefs and struggles. The participants also highlighted the interprofessional model as a spiritual generalist–specialist model, where board-certified chaplains are the spiritual specialist with all other clinicians on the team being the spiritual generalists. Nonchaplain clinicians need to recognize the limits of their expertise (63) and should not engage in significant spiritual counseling. The separation of responsibilities between clinicians and chaplains and/or the patient's personal clergy recognizes both specific expertise and ethical concerns—patients may tell physicians things they would not tell clergy and vice versa.

Thus the physician, nurse, and social worker should engage in the spiritual aspects of illness by being present to all patients, honoring their dignity, and taking a spiritual history or a screening to identify patients' spiritual issues. For simple issues, as discussed below, medical clinicians may work with patients to address those needs. For more complex issues or if the simple issues are not resolved, then patients should be referred to board-certified or board-eligible chaplains. All issues, whether simple or complex, should be documented in the patient's chart appropriately and shared with the healthcare team.

The NCC also described the concept of spiritual distress as a diagnosis, which should be treated with the same intensity as physical pain. An algorithm was developed whereby clinicians would evaluate patient distress in the biopsychosocial–spiritual framework. This framework recognized that pain not only may be physical but also may have psychosocial or spiritual aspects as well, that is, suffering. Spiritual screening would identify if a patient is in spiritual distress and should therefore need an urgent chaplain referral. Spiritual history, a more complete assessment done by clinicians doing a treatment or care plan, would further identify more about types of spiritual issues that cause the distress as well as identify spiritual resources of strength. Clinicians would then refer to chaplains for a more complete spiritual assessment as well as treatment of spiritual distress. Ideally, the treatment or care plan is developed by the interdisciplinary team, which should also include a chaplain.

The NCC produced guidelines, for taking a spiritual history and for the formulation of spiritual treatment or care plans, include

- All healthcare professionals should be trained in doing a spiritual screening or history as part of their routine history and evaluation
- Spiritual screenings, histories, and assessments should be communicated and documented in patient records (e.g., charts and computerized databases shared with the interprofessional healthcare team)
- Follow-up spiritual histories or assessments should be conducted for all patients whose medical, psychosocial, or spiritual condition changes and as part of routine follow-up in a medical history
- A spiritual issue becomes a diagnosis if the following criteria are met, (1) the spiritual issue leads to distress or suffering (e.g., lack of meaning, conflicted religious beliefs, and inability to forgive); (2) the spiritual issue is the cause of a psychological or physical diagnosis such as depression, anxiety, or acute or chronic pain (e.g., severe meaninglessness that leads to depression or suicidality and guilt that leads to chronic physical pain); and (3) the spiritual issue is a secondary cause or affects the presenting psychological or physical diagnosis (e.g., hypertension is difficult to control because the patient refuses to take medications because of his or her religious beliefs)
- Treatment or care plans should include but not be limited to referral to chaplains, spiritual directors, pastoral counselors, and other spiritual care providers, including clergy or faith-community healers for spiritual counseling; development of spiritual goals; meaning-oriented therapy; mind–body interventions; rituals, spiritual practices; and contemplative interventions
- Spiritual diagnosis, resources of strength, as well as the spiritual treatment plan should be documented in the chart

Obtaining a spiritual history is one way of listening to what is deeply important to the patient (69). When one gets involved in a discussion with a patient about his or her spirituality, one enters the domain of what gives the person meaning and purpose in life and how that person copes with stress, illness, and dying. The spiritual history affords the patient the space and opportunity to address his or her suffering and hopes. A spiritual history validates the importance of a patient's spirituality and gives the patient permission to discuss their spirituality, if they desire to. Having the physician or other clinician inquire about the patient's spiritual beliefs gives the patient an opening and an invitation to discuss spiritual beliefs, if that is what the patient would like to do. It also enables the physician to connect with the patient on a deep, caring level. In fact, many physicians who obtain spiritual histories remark that the nature of the doctor–patient relationship changes. As soon as they bring up these questions, they feel that it establishes a level of intimacy and an understanding of who the person is at a much deeper level than is typical. The relationship feels less superficial (69). Patients note that they feel more trusting of a physician who addresses and respects their spiritual beliefs. In one survey, 65% of patients in a pulmonary outpatient clinic noted that a physician's inquiry about spiritual beliefs would strengthen their trust in the physician (70).

TREATMENT OF CARE PLAN

Once the clinician identifies the spiritual distress or spiritual resources of strength or resources for coping, the clinician should then integrate that into the patient treatment or care plan and document this in the chart. Spiritual distress needs to be attended with the same urgency as any other distress. Thus patients with moderate or severe spiritual distress or with religious-specific needs should be referred to the board-certified chaplain. Some types of spiritual distress, which one might classify as minimal or mild, might be able to be attended to by other clinicians on the team. In the NCC, these would be classified as simple spiritual issues. An example might be patient not clear about meaning and purpose but is not particularly distressed by this. Talking about this to the clinician might be helpful as just telling of one's story can sometimes be enough for the patient to find an answer for themselves. Or other providers, such as art therapists, might be a helpful resource. The patient might also share spiritual practices that are important to the patient. These might be prayer, meditation, listening to certain music, enjoying solitude, writing poetry, or journeying. The clinician can then incorporate these practices as appropriate. However, if the patient is in significant spiritual distress this would be a complex spiritual issue and therefore a referral to the chaplain would be recommended. If the clinician initially thought the spiritual issue was simple but the initial interventions did not work, then a referral should be made to the board-certified chaplain.

Possible options for a spiritual care plan, then, are as follows:

- Referrals to:
  - Appropriate spiritual care professionals, such as chaplains, pastoral counselors, and spiritual directors especially with complex spiritual issues
  - A meaning-centered psychotherapy group
  - Music thanatologists
  - Art therapy
  - Meditation
  - Yoga and tai chi
  - Specific spiritual support groups
  - Religious or sacred spiritual reading or rituals (based on what the patient has identified as appropriate for them)
- Incorporating spiritual practices or rituals as appropriate
- Presence to patient as he/she works on spiritual issues with the healthcare Professional

SPIRITUAL HISTORY

The main elements of a spiritual history, which have been developed for physicians and other healthcare providers, can be recalled by using the acronym "FICA" (Table 54.4)

(69). This acronym helps clinicians to structure questions that help elicit patients' spiritual beliefs and values. This tool was developed with a focus group of primary care physicians. The goal was to identify the basic information clinicians need to know in order to determine how a patient's spirituality might impact their care. The tool is primarily used as a way to invite the patient to share their spiritual beliefs and values with their clinician, if they would like to. Anecdotal evidence suggests that patients experienced increased trust in their clinician once these conversations are initiated. Patients also express feeling respected and that the clinician is interested in who they are as people. Clinicians also find that the information obtained from the spiritual history allows the clinician to come up with a more comprehensive treatment plan.

The initial question of FICA affords the patient the opportunity to talk about spiritual matters. These spiritual issues can be religious, spiritual, or other sources of deep meaning and purpose in life. In this first question, it is important to assess what the patient's belief system is and also if that belief system or something else gives meaning to the person's life. The second question allows the clinician to determine if these belief systems are important to the patient. For some people, identified spiritual beliefs may not be important to them but there may be other philosophies or activities that give deeper meaning or purpose. This is also the place where patients might reveal if they have any spiritual issues that need attending to. For example, patients might reveal spiritual distress, such as meaninglessness or guilt. It is also important to know if there is anything else about the belief system that might impact healthcare decision-making. This is particularly important with advanced directives: wishes for how a patient would like to be treated and who should be involved in the decision-making process. Many patients would like their

TABLE 54.4	**FICA**

F—Faith and Belief

"Do you consider yourself spiritual or religious?" or "Do you have spiritual beliefs that help you cope with stress or difficult times?" If the patient asks what is meant by the word spiritual, reflect back to the patient to define that for themselves. If a patient relates to the question as only religious, suggest that spiritual can be broader than religion and often refers to what gives a deep meaning to a person's life. Also ask what gives deep meaning to the patients' life.

I—Importance

"What importance does your belief system or faith have in your life? Have your beliefs influenced how you take care of yourself in this illness? What role do your beliefs play in coping with your illness or in healing?" Do your beliefs affect your health care decision-making?

C—Community

"Are you a part of a spiritual or religious community? Is this of support to you and how? Is there a group of people you really love or who are important to you?"

A—Address/Action in Care

The physician and other healthcare providers can think about what needs to be done with the information the patient shared—referral to chaplain, other spiritual care provider, or other resource. This is the part of the history that is used for formulating a treatment plan.

clergy or culturally based healers involved. The fourth question has to do with the extrinsic aspect of the patient's belief system—is there a community that the patient identifies as their spiritual or main support community. This could be church, temple, or mosque or could be like-minded friends, family, or other spiritual support group (e.g., a cancer support group could be thought of by some as a spiritual support group). Finally, the "A" (assessment or action) section is not a specific question one has to ask, but rather it is one to be considered in terms of what specific aspects of the treatment plan might be affected. So, if the patient is in spiritual distress, a referral to a chaplain might be appropriate. Or if a patient would like to learn to meditate, then a referral to a teacher or class might be beneficial.

FICA is not meant to be used as a checklist, but rather as a guide as to how to start the spiritual history and what to listen for as the patient talks about his or her beliefs. Mostly, FICA is a tool to help physicians and other healthcare providers know how to open a conversation to spiritual issues and issues of meaning and value. In the context of the spiritual history, patients may relate those fears, dreams, and hopes to their care provider. The spiritual history can be done in the context of a routine history or at any time in the patient interview, usually as a part of the social history. In addition to religious or spiritual beliefs and values and other aspects of the spiritual history, the social history should address lifestyle, home situation, and primary relationships; other important relationships and social environment; work situation and employment; social interests/avocation; life stresses; and lifestyle risk factors (e.g., tobacco, alcohol, or illicit drugs).

The spiritual history is patient centered. One should always respect patients' wishes and understand appropriate boundaries. Physicians and other healthcare providers must respect patients' privacy regarding matters of spirituality and religion and should avoid imposing their own beliefs on the patient (71).

The following case illustrates how FICA can be used. A patient who died of metastatic malignant melanoma was an Episcopalian. Her religious beliefs were central to her life and, in fact, were the means through which she came to be at peace with dying. During her last hospitalization, the house officers caring for her were apprehensive about discussing advance directives and dying. However, during the spiritual history, the patient told them how her religious beliefs helped her come to terms with dying and how she was ready to die naturally. She handed them her living will. She also asked that her church members be allowed to visit her often. She later told me that being asked about her beliefs helped her feel respected and valued by the physicians and that she felt that she could trust them more. The physicians stated that once they asked a spiritual history, the nature of the interaction between themselves and this patient changed. It felt "more natural, more comfortable, warmer, and more honest."

Another case illustrates the variability encountered in practice. When asked "if you have any spiritual beliefs that help you with stress," a patient undergoing a routine examination answered that she found meaning and purpose while sitting in the woods near her house—that nature brought her peace. This was very important to her, as she noted that on days when she did not meditate there in the morning, she would become scattered and tense. Her community consisted of a group of like-minded friends who shared her beliefs. She asked that her medical record indicate that when she became seriously ill or dying, she wanted a room in her hospice overlooking the trees. She also asked to learn basic meditation techniques. In a subsequent visit many months later, she reported that she had stopped meditating, with negative results; resuming meditation helped her cope better with her stress.

ETHICAL ISSUES: ROLE OF SPIRITUALITY IN THE CLINICAL SETTING

It is critical for physicians and other healthcare providers to address spiritual issues with their patients because spirituality affects patients' clinical care in a direct manner. Spiritual issues can impact clinical care in various ways, which are illustrated by the following cases.

Case 1

Spiritual beliefs may be a dynamic in patients' understanding of their illness. Julie was a 28-year-old woman whose husband left her recently. She learned through the family grapevine that he has HIV. She came into a clinic and saw a physician for the first time to get tested for HIV. When she returned to the clinic for her test results, she found out that she was HIV positive. The physician attempted to present an optimistic picture by relaying all the newest information on treatment for HIV. The patient, however, continued to cry out about "God doing this to me." The physician persisted in discussion of the medical and technical aspects of the diagnosis while the patient continued to make references to God. After some time, the physician asked the patient why she thought her illness was coming from God. She told the physician that she was raped as a teenager, got pregnant, and had an abortion. She said, "I have been waiting for the punishment for 15 years, and this is it." The patient refused all medications and treatment.

Patients come to understand their health, illness, and dying through their beliefs, cultural backgrounds, past experience, and values. In this case, Julie had been carrying guilt for an event that happened many years before. The temptation for the physician was to alleviate this guilt by talking about how understandable the abortion was in the context of the rape. However, this is not what the patient felt, and by trying to erase her guilt, it actually precluded the patient from talking about her feelings. The physician instead listened to the patient and did not force the issue of medications and preventive care. The physician continued to see the patient regularly, listening to her issues around the diagnosis. She also referred Julie to a chaplain who worked further with Julie on these issues. It took approximately a year before Julie was able to see God as forgiving and was able to forgive herself. It was then that she could focus on the treatment of her HIV disease. Issues like these can be complicated. What part of Julie's beliefs came from strongly held religious dogma and what part from low self-esteem or depression? Chaplains are trained to understand the difference in the roots of these beliefs, and they are trained to help patients resolve these types of conflicts. In addition, physicians can be helpful by listening to patients, giving patients the time to resolve conflicts, and respecting patients' rights to their own beliefs.

Case 2

Religious convictions/beliefs may affect healthcare decision-making. Frank was an 88-year-old man dying of pancreatic cancer in the intensive care unit. He was on pressors and a ventilator. The team approached the family about withdrawing support. The family was very religious and believed that their father's life was in God's hands; they believed there would be a miracle and that their father would survive.

These types of cases are very common and are often handled poorly. Physicians and intensive care unit teams get frustrated that patients' families cannot see that their loved one is dying, and the family feels hurt and angry that the medical teams do not understand their beliefs. The discussion often gets polarized and difficult to resolve. It is critical that the medical teams, even if they do not agree with the family, respect family beliefs. Often, simply listening to the family about what they mean by a "miracle" can open up the conversation to many feelings that the family is experiencing. For example, the physician could simply say, "I can understand that a miracle would be wonderful," and then wait to see what the family says. Or the physician could ask, "What does a miracle mean to you?" If families feel respected, they are not as likely to feel threatened and that the medical team opposes them. The medical team, in turn, can get to know the values and beliefs of the family. Referral to a chaplain would be critical in this case. The chaplain, someone who is not perceived as being a part of the medical team per se, can explore the issues of miracles in a very nonthreatening way.

In Frank's case, the chaplain worked with the family. Over time, they began to see the possibility of a miracle independent of whether their father was on a ventilator. The family was then at peace with withdrawing ventilator support. The family was invited to bring their minister in during the whole process, and there were prayers and rituals at the bedside. Their father lived for several days and then died at peace.

Case 3

Spirituality may be a patient need. Rebecca was a 60-year-old woman who had a stroke and had had diabetes and hypertension for many years. She was very debilitated, being wheelchair bound with a speech impediment. Her major coping strategy was prayer. She was Catholic. Her church group and family were her major social supports. It was very important for her to discuss her spiritual beliefs with her physician.

Rebecca's faith was central to her life and was the basis of all her decisions. It was the way she coped with the effects of her chronic illnesses and with her dying. It was important for her to talk about her faith at every visit. She had an inner strength that was rooted in her religious beliefs and enabled her to withstand numerous physical and emotional challenges. In the end, it was her faith that probably gave her the will to live beyond what medical statistics would have predicted for someone as ill as she was. Daily prayer was so important to her that it also became an indicator for her well-being. At one point in her illness, she became very depressed. Although she denied symptoms of depression, she related that she was too tired to pray. She was then able to recognize symptoms of depression. Her church group was also a strong support. In fact, they were so present to her that they were clearly part of her extended family.

Case 4

Spirituality may be important in patient coping. Ronda was a 54-year-old woman with advanced ovarian cancer. Her husband, who was her major support, died unexpectedly. Ronda, who was Jewish, dealt with her suffering and depression through her faith in God. She also joined Jewish Healing Services for support and guidance.

Ronda was raised Jewish but was not observant throughout her adult life. She described herself as an optimist and saw that attitude as an inner strength. Her will to live was strong, and her fight to survive her cancer in the face of dismal odds gave her meaning in life. She spoke of her cancer as a gift in that it gave her a new perspective of life. She came to understand her life in a different, deeper way. She expressed a sense of gratitude for being alive each moment of the day and did not take anything, or anyone, for granted. During times of stress and loss, she relied on her inner strength as a resource. She reached out to support networks, such as the Jewish Healing Services. When her cancer metastasized, she looked at her religious roots for an understanding of death and of suffering. It was important for her to talk with her physicians about these issues and for her to be respected. For a physician to dismiss her will to live and try new therapies simply because of a statistical understanding of her disease would be to dismiss who she is as a person, a "statistic of one," as she said. It was important for her to be able to talk with her physician about her will to live and also about her search for meaning in the midst of suffering. She made a "dream list" as to what was important for her to accomplish before her death. Therapy was adjusted around her ability to complete her dream list.

Case 5

Spirituality may be integral to whole patient care. Joe was a 42-year-old man with irritable bowel syndrome. He had major stressors in his life, including a failed marriage and dissatisfaction at work. He had signs of depression, including insomnia, excessive worrying, decreased appetite, and anhedonia. Overall, he felt that he had no meaning and purpose in life.

Joe did not respond to medication and diet changes alone. However, with the addition of meditation and counseling, Joe improved. In this case, the physical, emotional, social, and spiritual issues all interplayed and affected how he coped with illness.

ETHICAL ISSUES: PROFESSIONAL AND PERSONAL BOUNDARIES

Performing a spiritual history has been included in coursework on spirituality and medicine (49). The spiritual history emphasizes the practice of compassion with one's patients and helps the clinician learn to integrate patients' spiritual concerns into the therapeutic plans. Given the data suggesting that spirituality may be beneficial for patients who are coping with illness, healthcare institutions should have written policies stating that the patient has a right to express his or her spirituality and religiosity in a respectful and supportive clinical environment.

Physicians should strive to discuss patients' spiritual concerns in a respectful manner and as directed by the patient. The spiritual history is patient centered, not physician centered (Table 54.5). A physician should always respect patients' privacy regarding matters of spirituality and religion and must be vigilant in avoiding imposing his or her beliefs on the patients. The relationship between physician and patient is not an equal one. There is an intimacy in the relationship, but it is intimacy with formality. The patient comes to the physician in a vulnerable time of his or her life, often looking to the physician as a person of authority. The physician should not abuse that authority by imposing his or her own beliefs, or lack of beliefs, onto patients. A vulnerable patient may adopt a physician's belief simply because the patient is fearful and assumes the physician knows more. In

terms of spiritual intervention, physicians can recommend a variety of interventions, such as chaplain referral, meditation, yoga, prayer, or other spiritual practice. But the decision to recommend these comes from the patient. For example, physicians could recommend religious and spiritual practices to a patient if these practices are already part of that patient's belief system. However, an agnostic patient should not be told to engage in worship any more than a highly religious patient should be criticized for frequent church attendance. Therefore, if a patient states that prayer helps with stress, the physician could suggest that prayer might help in dealing with a serious diagnosis. Or, if a patient finds meaning and purpose in nature, a physician might suggest meditation techniques focused on nature.

Patients sometimes ask their physician about the physician's beliefs. Given the unequal relationship between patient and physician, it is important that the question be handled carefully and with the same guidelines that are used when addressing other sensitive issues such as sexual history or domestic violence. Patients sometimes ask personal questions of their physicians to take the attention off themselves. Sometimes, it is to see if they can connect with the physician by reassuring themselves that the physician has the same beliefs as they. In general, if asked about his or her own beliefs, the physician could ask the patient why it is important for him or her to know that information. The physician can reassure the patient that the focus of the encounter is on the patient's needs and issues, not the doctor's. In some cases, patients still feel the need to know. A patient of a certain religious belief may want to work only with a doctor of that same religion. In some cases, it may not be possible to accommodate the patient, but at least the physician can explore with the patient the reasons for the request. Some patients want to know that their beliefs will not be ridiculed. A response from the physician that he or she respects and supports a patient's beliefs might serve to reassure the patient. In general, it is best to avoid sharing one's personal beliefs unless one already knows the patient and is comfortable that this sharing would not coerce the patient into adopting the physician's beliefs or intimidate the patient from sharing more about his or her own beliefs. A physician should not do anything that violates his or her own comfort level as well. Many physicians prefer to keep their private lives private in the professional context of the doctor–patient relationship.

Patients often ask physicians to pray with them. A physician need not worry that it is somehow inappropriate to allow a moment of silence or a prayer if the patient requests this. In fact, walking away and not showing respect for the request may leave the patient with a sense of abandonment by the physician. If the physician feels conflicted about praying with patients, he or she needs to only stand by quietly as the patient prays in his or her own tradition. Alternatively, the physician could suggest calling in the chaplain or the patient's clergyperson to lead a prayer. Physician-led prayer is generally not recommended, as that is usually the role of the clergy or chaplain. In addition, having the physician lead a prayer opens the possibility of having the prayer be of the

TABLE 54.5	Ethical and professional boundaries

Spiritual history: patient centered

Recognition of pastoral care professionals as experts

Proselytizing is not acceptable in professional settings

More in-depth spiritual counseling should be under the direction of chaplains and other spiritual leaders

Praying with patients:

    Not initiated by physicians unless there is no pastoral care available and the patient requests it

    Physician can stand in silence as patient prays in his/her tradition

    Referral to pastoral care for chaplain-led prayer

physician's belief, not of the patient's. Furthermore, clergy and chaplains are trained specifically in techniques of leading prayer in ecumenical and healthcare contexts.

Appropriate referrals to chaplains are important to good healthcare practice and are as appropriate as referrals to other specialists. Chaplains are clergy or laypersons certified in a pastoral training program designed to train them as chaplains. Chaplains work in hospital settings, outpatient clinics, businesses, schools, and prisons. They are trained to be spiritual care providers working with people to explore meaning in life, cope with suffering, and use their beliefs to help them cope with illness or stress. Chaplains work with people of all faiths, as well as with nonreligious people. Clergy are trained to provide religious care usually only to people of their specific denomination.

Where are the boundaries between what chaplains do and what physicians do? Some would argue that discussions with patients about spiritual matters should be initiated solely by chaplains (72). Physicians can use spiritual histories as a screening tool. By inquiring about a patient's beliefs, the physician can evaluate whether the beliefs are helpful or harmful to the patient's health and medical care. If a patient has beliefs that support him or her and give meaning and peace of mind, the physician can encourage those beliefs. In cases in which spiritual beliefs interfere with a patient's getting needed therapy, for example, a patient who thinks an illness is a punishment caused by God and therefore refuses medicine or treatment because of a feeling that the punishment is deserved, a referral to a chaplain would be very helpful. Patients have the right to refuse medical treatment. However, it is important that the choice be made with full informed consent. Therefore, if a patient refuses treatment based on a religious or spiritual belief, it may be appropriate to refer the patient to a chaplain so that the chaplain can explore these beliefs with the patient.

Sometimes, refusal of treatment is based on accepted religious tenets. Other times, the patient may attribute the reasons for refusal to religious beliefs when it actually stems from other concerns, such as lack of self-esteem or depression. The chaplain is trained to explore the beliefs with the patient further and help the patient differentiate between the two. The physician should be respectful of the patient's beliefs, but still explain the consequences of refusal of treatment without being coercive. This way the patient can have enough medical and spiritual information to make a fully informed decision. Physicians in general are not trained to explore the theological aspects of belief, although they can listen and learn about belief from patients. However, physicians can listen to and support patients as they make decisions for themselves. Sometimes, simply listening to a patient in a nonjudgmental fashion and asking a few open-ended questions, such as "tell me more about your belief," can help patients resolve issues of belief and treatment for themselves.

Although many studies suggest that spirituality can be helpful, there are also circumstances in which spirituality can have a negative effect on health. It is important for healthcare providers to recognize this dynamic. For example, a person who interprets his or her illness as a punishment from God might attempt to refuse treatment. In such a scenario, a chaplain or other religious advisor could perhaps work with the patient's beliefs to help him or her work through the guilt issues. The patient might accept treatment or refuse it, but at least the decision would not be motivated solely by guilt and would be more of an informed decision. Some people who feel guilt in their relationships with God might also relate to others in their lives in a similar way. Counseling may also be helpful. Some religious beliefs forbid certain medical practices, such as Jehovah's Witnesses' refusal to accept blood transfusions. It is important to recognize the difference between refusing treatment based on an established religious principle versus refusal of treatment stemming from depression, unwarranted guilt, or a misperceived sense of punishment from God. Some patients may have complicated ethical and spiritual issues. Physicians need not feel that they must solve these dilemmas on their own. Chaplains, members of ethics committees, and counselors often work with physicians in the care of patients.

It is important to recognize that spirituality in the healthcare setting is not in any one person's domain. Physicians, nurses, social workers, and chaplains all can deal with patient's spirituality. It also is true, however, that most physicians are not trained to deal with complex spiritual crises and conflicts. Chaplains and other spiritual caregivers are. Therefore, it is important that physicians obtain a spiritual history as a way of inquiry about spiritual issues that might impact a patient but that physicians also recognize when to make a referral to these specialists.

CARING FOR OUR PATIENTS

Beyond the data, writings, and courses are personal stories from physicians and their patients. In the experience of many physicians who care for patients with chronic and terminal illnesses, there is a feeling of being privileged and honored to care for people who are facing death. Their strength and courage in the midst of suffering is inspiring. Our patients are greater teachers to us and to our students on the meaning of life than any philosophical text. The stories they share are ones of personal transcendence, courage, and dignity. Our patients continually live with dying and, in the midst of that, are often able to face their losses, their fears, and their pain, and transcend to a place where they see their lives as rich and fulfilling. They reprioritize and thereby are able to find a place of deep meaning and purpose in their lives. It is often humbling for us to recognize that what we now place importance on in life may have little or no importance in the end when facing our own mortality. Annoyance at rush hour traffic when late or our emphasis on academic success pale in comparison to our patients' descriptions of a glowing sunrise or the deep love they feel for another. We would encourage all students reading this text to look on your patients as teachers and to approach dying patients not with trepidation and fear but with openness to all the joy and wisdom you can experience with them.

We should have systems of care that allow for people to die in peace, to die the way they want to, and to be able to engage in those activities that bring peace to them: prayer, meditation, listening to music, art, journaling, sacred ritual, and relationships with others. Our systems of care should be interdisciplinary, with physicians, nurses, social workers, chaplains, and other spiritual care providers all working together to provide spiritual and holistic care for our patients. It is then that healthcare systems will become caring communities rather than impersonal, technologically driven ones.

Our culture and our profession as a whole must look at dying very differently from the way it currently does. We need to see dying not as a medical problem but as a natural part of life that can be meaningful and peaceful. We can broaden and perhaps even enhance our lives now by knowing that one day we will die. By thinking about our mortality early in life, we will not be caught off guard and pressured by the dilemmas of choices at the end of life. We will have had a chance to think about some of those choices sooner and to come to peace with our mortality. This is where religious organizations can be particularly helpful. They can facilitate our discussions of dying and what that means to us. They can educate their members about the importance of preparing themselves for the choices, both spiritual and medical that need to be made near the end of life. We, the interdisciplinary care team, can jointly assist the dying person come to peace in life's last moments.

All of us, whether actively dying or helping care for the dying, have one thing in common: we all will die. The personal transformation that is often seen in patients as they face death can occur in all of our lives. By facing our inevitable dying, we can ask ourselves the same questions that dying patients face—what gives meaning and purpose to our lives, who are we at our deepest core, and what are the important things we want to do in our lives. By attending to the spiritual dimensions of our personal and professional lives, however, we express that, we can better provide care to our patients (73).

Wayne Muller has written

There are times in all of our lives when we are forced to reach deep into ourselves to feel the truth of our real nature. For each of us there comes a moment when we can no longer live our lives by accident. Life throws us into questions that some of us refuse to ask until we are confronted by death or some tragedy in our lives. What do I know to be most deeply true? What do I love, and have I loved well? Who do I believe myself to be and what have I placed on the center of the altar of my life? Where do I belong? What will people find in the ashes of my incarnation when it is over? How shall I live my life knowing that I will die? And what is my gift to the family of earth? (74)

Of all life's difficult yet important experiences, dying may be the most difficult one we will ever have. The moment of death, and the dying that precedes it, brings to a close the journey that each one of us has been on. We are the privileged persons who attend people while they are dying, be they our patients or our loved ones and friends. We are the persons who can bring hope and comfort to dying patients as they complete their lives. We need to ensure that our society and our systems of care preserve and enhance the dignity of all people, especially when they are made vulnerable by illness and suffering. We need to listen to the dying and to all our patients, and be with them, for them. The process of dying can be a meaningful one, one that we can all embrace and celebrate rather than fear and dread.

How might the assessment and plan look for an 87-year-old female with history of dementia and hypertension now hospitalized for pneumonia?

Physical:

- Pneumonia, oxygen saturation 98%, on Zithromax, blood and urine culture pending
- Dementia: stable, continue Aricept
- Hypertension: stable continue Vasotec

Psychological: No evidence of depression; some anxiety about being in the hospital.

- Reassurance, private room, family to stay with her, consider massage and music

Social: strong family support

- Plan to discharge home with home Physical Therapy (PT)
- Offer additional resource education to family

Spiritual: faith important to patient and family. Patient appears peaceful and accepting of her situation

- Faith important to patient, gets comfort from prayer and the Eucharist. Will contact chaplain as well as patients' family priest.
- Staff to offer continued presence and compassion to patient and family.
- Encourage husband to sing to patient in hospital to bring her comfort and connection.

COMMUNICATING WITH PATIENTS ABOUT SPIRITUAL ISSUES

A key component of spiritual care is the spiritual assessment. Every person on the interdisciplinary team has a role in assessing patients' spiritual issues, as well as the physical, emotional, and social issues. Every person on the team also has a different area of expertise. Thus, physical issues may be dealt with in depth by the nurse or physician; social issues by the social worker; emotional issues by the psychologist; and spiritual by the chaplain. The chaplain will identify and discuss physical pain, for example, with the patient. The chaplain will then refer to the physician for more specialized handling of the pain issues. The physician will identify and discuss spiritual issues with patient but will also refer to the chaplain for more in-depth counseling on these issues. All healthcare professionals ideally should communicate with each other and develop a treatment plan together so that the practice of the biopsychosocial–spiritual model of care is seamless and fully integrated.

The spiritual assessment that non-chaplain healthcare professionals do is, therefore, more of a history and a screening than the full assessment chaplains do. The spiritual history can be done as part of the social history in an intake or initial visit and then be brought up at follow-up visits as appropriate. The goal of the spiritual history is to offer the patient and their family the opportunity to discuss issues that relate to meaning, purpose, hope, suffering, transcendence, as well as values and beliefs that may affect healthcare decision-making. The spiritual history invites people to share their experiences of the sacred in their lives or of hope, joy, or sadness. It is listening to their inmost stories. There are several spiritual history tools that have been developed. These include SPIRIT (75), FICA (69), and HOPE (76). FICA is given in Table 54.4.

Anecdotal evidence from healthcare professionals who use the FICA tool suggests that the act of taking the spiritual history is transformative to the clinical encounter. One medical student noted, "The whole feeling of the interview changed. My patient became more open, more comfortable. There was less tension and more trust, it seemed, in me. I also felt more human. It felt like we moved from the purely technical visit to a human encounter." The patient said, "I really felt she (the medical student) cared deeply for me, was interested in me, … in who I really am and what I really feel." Spirituality is an essential element of what makes a person human. Talking about spirituality reaches the human being, not just the patient. The spiritual history gives the healthcare professional the opportunity to be compassionate and to know of their patient's suffering through the act of being present to that suffering, being open to caring, and being committed to honoring the dignity of that patient.

CONCLUSION

Two weeks before my mother died, she was in the hospital. The nurse was tender and caring, making sure my mother and I were comfortable and that my mother's needs were attended to. She bathed her with the utmost tenderness, respecting her privacy and dignity. This time, her physician was open, warm, and honored her for who she was. He asked her how she felt and responded to her nonverbal answer in her facial expression. He asked her about her family. He knew her faith was important to her and asked us if she would like to see the chaplain. He reassured her with his touch. He told her that he saw in her a strong yet tender woman, a loving mother and wife. My mother was so happy with her visit with him that even with the difficulty she had with speech, she was able to tell him "you are so nice" and then offer him part of the banana she was eating. When the chaplain came, she offered my mother and me communion. In her prayer, she honored my mother's life, her strength, and her holiness in her suffering with dementia. The healthcare team created an atmosphere of trust and peace in which my mother was happy and I was able to come to a deep sense of acceptance that my mother would die soon. Most importantly, she was honored for who she was as a person. Her illness was obscured by the enormity of her life, her passions, and her love. Spirituality is the expression of all that is meaningful in one's life, it is the foundation of the dignity and worth of a person, and it is essential to healing and wholeness.

REFERENCES

1. Sulmasy DP. A biopsychosocial–spiritual model for the care of patients at the end of life. *Gerontologist.* 2002;42:24-33.
2. Engel GL. The need for a new medical model: a challenge for biomedicine. *Science.* 1977;196:129-136.
3. White KL, Williams TF, Greenberg BG. The ecology of medical care. *Acad Med.* 1996;73:187-205.
4. Jonas H. *The Phenomenon of Life: Towards a Philosophical Biology.* Evanston, IL: Northwestern University Press; 2001.
5. Sulmasy DP. *The Rebirth of the Clinic: An Introduction to Spirituality in Health Care.* Washington, DC: Georgetown University Press; 2006.
6. Puchalski CM, Ferrell B, Virani R, et al. Improving the quality of spiritual care as a dimension of palliative care: the report of the Consensus Conference. *J Palliat Med.* 2009;12(10):885-904.
7. Ramsey P. *The Patient as Person.* New Haven, CT: Yale University Press; 1970.
8. Engel GL. How much longer must medicine's science be bound by a seventeenth century world view? *Psychother Psychosom.* 1992;57(1-2):3-16.
9. King DE. *Faith, Spirituality and Medicine: Toward the Making of a Healing Practitioner.* Binghamton, NY: Haworth Pastoral Press; 2000.
10. McKee DD, Chappel JN. Spirituality and medical practice. *J Fam Pract.* 1992;5:201, 205-208.
11. Medical School Objectives Project (MSOP). *Report III: Contemporary Issues in Medicine: Communication in Medicine.* Washington, DC: AAMC; October 1999:21.
12. Frankl V. *Man's Search for Meaning.* New York, NY: Simon & Schuster; 1984.
13. Kushner HS. *When Bad Things Happen to Good People.* New York, NY: Schocken Books; 1981.
14. Cohen KL. In: Lynn J, Harrold J, eds. *Handbook for Mortals.* New York, NY: Oxford University Press; 1999:31.
15. Doka KJ, Morgan JD, eds. *Death and Spirituality.* Amityville, NY: Baywood Publishing; 1993.
16. Downey M. *Understanding Christian Spirituality.* New York, NY: Paulist Press; 1997.
17. Foglio JP, Brody H. Religion, faith and family medicine. *J Fam Pract.* 1988;27:473-474.
18. Kubler-Ross E. *On Death and Dying.* New York, NY: Collier Books/Macmillan; 1997.
19. Cassell EJ. *The Nature of Suffering and Goals of Medicine.* New York, NY: Oxford University Press; 1991.
20. *Webster's 7th New Collegiate Dictionary.* Springfield, MA: Merriam-Webster; 1965.
21. Lo B, Quill T, Tulsky J. Discussing palliative care with patients. ACP-ASIM End-of-Life Care Consensus Panel. *Ann Intern Med.* 1999;130:744-749.
22. Karlawish J, Quill T, Meier D. A consensus-based approach to providing palliative care to patients who lack decision-making capacity. ACP-ASIM End-of-Life Care Consensus Panel. *Ann Intern Med.* 1999;130:835-840.
23. Joint Commission for Accreditation of Healthcare Organizations (JCAHO). Spiritual assessment, 2004. http://www.jointcommission.org/AccreditationPrograms/ HomeCare/Standards/FAQs/Provision+of+Care/Assessment/ Spiritual_Assessment.htm. Accessed November 15, 2007.

24. Burkhart, L. Documenting spiritual care. *J Christian Nurses.* 2005;22(1):6-12.

25. American Nursing Association. *Nursings Social Policy Statement.* 2nd ed. Washington, DC: ANA; 2003.

26. National Association of Social Workers. Code of ethics, 1996 (revised 1999). http://www.socialworkers.org/pubs/code/code.asp. Accessed August 2007.

27. National Consensus Guidelines for Quality Palliative Care. American Academy of Palliative Care, 2004. www.nationalconsensusproject.org/guideline.pdf. Accessed June 29, 2008.

28. Keonig HG, McCullough ME, Larson DB. *Handbook of Religion and Health.* New York, NY: Oxford University Press; 2001.

29. Roberts JA, Brown D, Elkins T, Larson DB. Factors influencing views of patients with gynecologic cancer about end-of-life decisions. *AM J Obstet Gynecol.* 1997;176(1):166-172.

30. Powell LH, Shabbi L, Thoreson CE. Religion and spirituality linkages to physical health. *Am Psychol.* 2003;58:36-52.

31. Cohen SR, Mount BM, Tomas JJ, Mount LF. Existential well-being is an important determinant of quality of life. Evidence from the McGill Quality of Life Questionnaire. *Cancer.* 1996;77:576-586.

32. Burgener SC. Predicting quality of life in caregivers of Alzheimer's patients: the role of support from and involvement with the religious community. *J Pastoral Care.* 1999;53:443-446.

33. Worthington E. *Five Steps to Forgiveness: The Art and Science of Forgiveness.* New York, NY: Crown Publishers; 2001.

34. Silvestri GA, Knittig S, Zoller JS, Nietert PJ. Importance of faith on medical decisions regarding cancer care. *J Clin Oncol.* 2003;21:1379-1382.

35. Pargament KI, Smith BW, Koenig HG, Perez L. Patterns of positive and negative religious coping with major life stresses. *J Sci Study Relig.* 1998;37(4):710-724.

36. McCord G, Gilchrist V, Grossman S, et al. Discussing spirituality with patients: a rational and ethical approach. *Ann Fam Med.* 2004;2(4):356-361.

37. Balboni TA, Vanderwerker LC, Block SD, et al. Religiousness and spiritual support among advanced cancer patients and associations with end-of-life treatment preferences and quality of life. *J Clin Oncol.* 2007;25(5):555-560.

38. Cohen SR, Boston P, Mount BM, et al. Changes in quality of life following admission to palliative care units. *Palliat Med.* 2001;15(5):363-371.

39. Fitchett G, Rybarczyk BD, DeMarco GA, et al. The role of religion in medical rehabilitation outcomes: a longitudinal study. *Rehabil Psychol.* 1999;44(4):333-353.

40. Fitchett G, Murphy PE, Kim J, Gibbons JL, Cameron JR, Davis JA. Religious struggle: prevalence, correlates and mental health risks in diabetic, congestive heart failure, and oncology patients. *Int J Psychiatry Med.* 2004;34(2):179-196.

41. Cohen SR, Mount BM, Strobel MG, et al. The McGill Quality of Life Questionnaire: a measure of quality of life appropriate for people with advanced disease. A preliminary study of validity and acceptability. *Palliat Med.* 1995;9:207-219.

42. Cotton S, Puchalski, CM, Sherman SN, et al. Spirituality and religion in patients with HIV/AIDS. *J Gen Intern Med.* 2006;21:S5-S13.

43. Cook JA, Wimberly DW. If I should die before I wake: religious commitment and adjustment to death of a child. *J Sci Study Relig.* 1983;22:222-238.

44. Bearon LB, Koenig RG. Religious cognitions and use of prayer in health and illness. *Gerontologist.* 1990;30:249-253.

45. Pargament KI, David SE, Kathryn F, et al. God help me: I, religious coping efforts as predictors of the outcomes to significant negative life events. *Am J Community Psychol.* 1990;18:793-824.

46. Seeman TE, Aubin LF, Seema M. Religiosity/spirituality and health: a critical review of the evidence for biological pathways. *Am Psychol.* 2003;58(1):53-63.

47. Rutherford R. *The Death of a Christian: The Rite of Funerals.* New York, NY: Pueblo; 1980.

48. Klass D. Spirituality, Protestantism and death. In: Doka KJ, Morgan JD, eds. *Death and Spirituality.* Amityville, NY: Baywood Publishing; 1993:61.

49. Ryan D. Death: eastern perspectives. In: Doka KJ, Morgan JD, eds. *Death and Spirituality.* Amityville, NY: Baywood Publishing; 1993:81.

50. Grollman EA. Death in Jewish thought. In: Doka KJ, Morgan JD, eds. *Death and Spirituality.* Amityville, NY: Baywood Publishing; 1993:25-27.

51. VandeCreek L, Nye C. Trying to live forever: correlates to the belief in life after death. *J Pastoral Care.* 1994;48(3):273-280.

52. Irion PE. Spiritual issues in death and dying for those who do not have conventional religious beliefs. In: Doka KJ, Morgan JD, eds. *Death and Spirituality.* Amityville, NY: Baywood Publishing; 1993.

53. Meagher D, Bell CP. Perspectives on death in the African American community. In: Doka KJ, Morgan JD, eds. *Death and Spirituality.* Amityville, NY: Baywood Publishing; 1993:113-130.

54. Puchalski CM, O'Donnell E. Religious and spiritual beliefs in end-of-life care: how major religions view death and dying. *Techniques Reg Anesth Pain Manage.* 2005;9(3):114-121.

55. Breithart W. Spirituality and meaning in supportive care. Spirituality and meaning-centered group psychotherapy interventions in advanced cancer. *Support Care Center.* 2002;10:272-280.

56. *44 Questions: Questions and Answers About Alcoholics Anonymous.* General Service Office of Great Britian: AA World Services; 1952.

57. Strachan JG. *Alcoholism, Treatable Illness: An Honorable Approach to Man's Alcoholism Problem.* Center City, MN: Hazelden; 1982.

58. Pargament KI, Koenig HG, Tarakeshwar N, Hahn J. Religious coping methods as predictors of psychological, physical and spiritual outcomes among medically ill elderly patients: a two-year longitudinal study. *J Health Psychol.* 2004; 9(6):713-730.

59. Koenig HG, Pargament KI, Nelson J. Religious coping and health status in medically ill hospitalized older adults. *J Nerv Ment Dis.* 1998;186(9):513-521.

60. Sherman AC, Simonton S, Latif U, Spohn R, Tricot G. Religious struggle and religious comfort in response to illness: health outcomes among stem cell transplant patients. *J Behav Med.* 2005;28(4):359-367.

61. Pargament KI, Koenig HG, Tarakeshwar N, Hahn J. Religious struggle as a predictor of mortality among medically ill elderly patients: a two-year longitudinal study. *Archiv Intern Med.* 2001;161(15):1881-1885.

62. Joint Commission. Specifications Manual for Joint Commission National Quality Core Measures, 2010. http://manual.jointcommission.org/releases/TJC2010A2/rsrc/Manual/TableOfContentsTJC/HBIPS_2010A2.pdf

63. Puchalski CM, Ferrell B. *Making Health Care Whole: Integrating Spirituality into Patient Care.* West Conshohocken, PA: Templeton Press; 2010.

64. Puchalski CM, Anderson BM, Lo B, et al. *Ethical Guidelines for Spiritual Care.* 2006. Washington D.C.:AAMC Report. In press.

65. O'Connor P. The role of spiritual care in hospice. Are we meeting patients' needs? *Am J Hosp Care.* 1988;5:31-37.

66. DiBlasi Z, Harkness E, Ernst E, et al. Influence of context effects on health outcomes: a systematic review. *Lancet.* 2001;357(9258):757-762.

67. Peabody FW. *The Care of the Patient.* Cambridge, MA: Harvard University Press; 1927.

68. Sulmasy DP. *The Healer's Calling: A Spirituality for Physicians and Other Health Care Professionals.* New York, NY: Paulist Press; 1997.

69. Puchalski CM, Romer AL. Taking a spiritual history allows clinicians to understand patients more fully. *J Palliat Med.* 2000;3(1):129-137.

70. Ehman JW, Ott BB, Short TH, et al. Do patients want physicians to inquire about their spiritual or religious beliefs if they become gravely ill? *Arch Intern Med.* 1999;159:1803-1806.

71. Post SG, Puchalski CM, Larson DB. Physicians and patient spirituality: professional boundaries, competency, and ethics. *Ann Intern Med.* 2000;132(7):578-583.

72. Sloan RP, Bagiella E, VandeCreek L, et al. Should physicians prescribe religious activities? *N Engl J Med.* 2000;342(25):1913-1916.

73. Newman LF, Epstein L. Doctor–patient relationships: know thy patient, know thyself. *Med Health R I.* 1996;79(8):308-310.

74. Muller W. *Touching the Divine: Teachings, Meditations and Contemplations to Awaken Your True Nature* [Audiocassettes]. Louisville, CO: Sounds True; 1994.

75. Maugans, TA, The SPIRITual history. *Arch Fam Med.* 1996;5(1):11-16.

76. Anandarajah G, Hight E. Spirituality and medical practice: using HOPE questions as a practical tool for spiritual assessment. *Am Fam Physician.* 2001;63(1):81-89.

Justin Banerdt ■ Paul R. Duberstein ■ Holly G. Prigerson

BEREAVEMENT

Bereavement refers to the situation of being deprived of someone or something, typically referring to the loss through death of an individual to whom one is attached. Grief refers to the emotional and psychological response to that loss and has been characterized as a yearning for what one cannot have (1). Bereavement and grief are universal experiences that almost all individuals must confront at some point in their lifetime. Approximately, 2.4 million US citizens die annually each leaving behind many to grieve their loss (2). Approximately, 9.7% of women and 2.5% of men in the United States are widows and widowers, respectively (3). Most of those experiencing widowhood are older than 64, when their health is likely to be already compromised, and bereavement may compound their health difficulties. Although it is often considered in the post-loss context, grief can also be anticipatory as loved ones confront the loss of health and normal functioning in the patient, the looming threat of an impending death, and the changes in social roles, responsibilities, and relationships that follow (4).

Bereavement is considered one of life's most stressful experiences (5,6). Hospitalizations are more common following bereavement and mortality risk is increased (7–11). Associated with an increased risk of cardiac events, hypertension, cancer, and suicidal ideation (12–17), bereavement also compromises quality of life and can lead to disability, functional impairments (social, family, and occupational), and health-damaging behaviors. Bereavement is a well-established risk factor for elevated depressive symptomatology and an increased likelihood of major depressive episodes (18–22) and anxiety-related symptoms and disorders (23–25). Bereaved individuals who experience an abnormally lengthy and extreme response to their loss may be suffering from "prolonged grief disorder" (PGD), the phenomenology of which differs from other mood or anxiety disorders. The severe psychological, functional, and emotional impairment associated with PGD places these individuals at substantial risk for morbidity (7–17).

Given the health risks associated with bereavement, it would be useful to develop preventive interventions. In many circumstances, this is not feasible. Deaths due to cardiac events or violence occur with little or no forewarning. In contrast, palliative and cancer care providers are well positioned to minimize the potential negative health consequences of bereavement as many deaths in these treatment settings follow a relatively predictable course. In particular, health-care providers working in these settings are uniquely placed during the dying process to facilitate preparedness and a degree of acceptance among the patient's family of the approaching loss, which helps alleviate future distress and suffering (4,26,27). Additionally, bereavement care could be the final phase of any comprehensive palliative care plan. One must look at the family as the unit of care when providing palliative services and hence bereavement care becomes an essential aspect to complete and facilitate the family's healing process.

NORMAL GRIEF: ANTICIPATORY AND POST-LOSS

Normal grief reactions are those that, though painful, move the survivor toward an acceptance of the loss and an ability to carry on with his or her life. Approximately, 80% to 90% of bereaved individuals experience normal grief (28), but personal, familial, and cultural factors may influence its progression and manifestation (29). It is important to recognize that most people adjust to the loss over time in a fairly satisfactory way.

Anticipatory grief encompasses grief-like symptoms experienced by patients and families leading up to the time of death (30). For many individuals, anticipatory grief is a natural response to a terminal prognosis and the prospect of inevitable loss (4). Families may react negatively in scenarios of anticipatory grief as escalating levels of hostility, anger, and poor communication lead to or exacerbate relationship dysfunction and conflict. Such families are at risk for psychosocial morbidity and may benefit from intervention. Supportive families, however, are notable for their cohesion and effective communication as they respond to their grief (31). Predictors of anticipatory grief include female gender, adult children, high-perceived stress, and difficulty coping (32,33). Anticipatory grief in surviving spouses and adult children has been documented as more intense than post-loss grief and predicts adjustment to the patient's death (34,35). We recognize that many clinicians may feel uneasy about assessing risk for poor bereavement outcomes. To facilitate these assessments, clinicians may wish to administer the PG-12, a scale we have developed to assess symptoms of pre-loss grief, both to start a conversation about bereavement and to identify people at risk, using the well-established cut-scores (35).

There has been much debate about whether grief follows a direct stage-by-stage pathway from denial to anger, separation distress, depression, and finally recovery (36). Results of a recent empirical test of the stage theory of grief (36) provide mixed support for the theory. The data reveal a gradual reduction in distress over time from loss. Contrary to the stage theory of the course of grief, disbelief was not found to be the most frequently endorsed initial reaction to loss. The predominant symptom throughout the first 6 months post-loss was yearning. Depressed mood did not peak after disbelief, yearning, and anger had subsided; rather, disbelief, yearning, and depressed mood all declined significantly from 2 to 20 months post-loss. Levels of anger remained stably low and did not peak after disbelief had faded (36). Additionally, acceptance of death increased significantly over time and revealed a pattern inverse to disbelief and yearning (36). The data suggest a parallel shift downward in all the grief indicators over time from loss (36).

When these five grief indicators (so-called stages or what we prefer to call "states") are all placed on the same scale (i.e., response format), they can be compared directly. This analysis revealed that the five indicators of grief peak in the exact sequence proposed by Kübler-Ross. The likelihood that this would happen by chance was miniscule ($P < 0.008$). Therefore, there does appear to be some empirical support for the notion that a first reaction involves disbelief, followed by yearning, anger, depression, and ultimately acceptance. In these ways, our results offer evidence that supports and also refutes the stage theory of grief.

How to make sense of it all? It appears that some generalizations can be made. First, the initial response is one that involves disbelief. Second, acceptance, recovery, or some form of adaptation to the new "normal" gradually increases over time. Third, depressive symptoms, anger, and yearning serve to bridge the initial shock and ultimate acceptance. Fourth, as yearning, anger, and depression decrease, acceptance increases. The human psyche appears preprogrammed to disbelieve when confronted with significant life changes; adjustment and reorganization is a gradual process that occurs over time. Not all people will adjust adaptively (e.g., those with PGD), but the vast majority will.

Although uncomplicated grief can be an extremely painful and sad experience, by 6 months following a death in later life from natural causes, bereaved individuals develop some sense of acceptance and may rediscover or find meaning or purpose in their lives with renewed zeal. They see the future holding potential enjoyment for them and are capable of engaging in productive activities and functioning without substantial impairment (28). They are also able to maintain connections with others and their sense of competence and self-esteem are not markedly changed by their loss. Survivors may initially exhibit many symptoms of PGD, but by 6 months post-loss there is usually improvement in their ability to focus on other things and move beyond the loss. Those who have elevated levels of a specific set of symptoms (Table 55.1) (36) after more than 6 months after the death may require clinical intervention.

TABLE 55.1	Criteria for prolonged grief disorder

Category	Definition
A.	*Event*: Bereavement (loss of a significant other)
B.	*Separation distress*: The bereaved person experiences yearning (e.g. craving, pining, or longing for the deceased: physical or emotional suffering as a result of the desired, but unfulfilled, reunion with the deceased) daily or to a disabling degree
C.	*Cognitive, emotional, and behavioral symptoms*: The bereaved person must have five (or more) of the following symptoms experienced daily or to a disabling degree.
	1. Confusion about one's rose in life or diminished sense of self (i.e., feeling that a part of oneself has died)
	2. Difficulty accepting the loss
	3. Avoidance of reminders of the reality of the loss
	4. Inability to trust others since the loss
	5. Bitterness or anger related to the loss
	6. Difficulty moving on with life (e.g., making new friends, pursuing interests)
	7. Numbness (absence of emotion) since the loss
	8. Feeling that life is unfulfilling, empty, or meaningless since the loss
	9. Feeling stunned, dazed, or shocked by the loss
D.	*Timing*: Diagnosis should not be made until at least 6 months have elapsed since the death
E.	*Impairment*: The disturbance causes clinically significant impairment in social, occupational, or other important areas of functioning (e.g., domestic responsibilities)
F.	*Relation to other mental disorders*: The disturbance is not better accounted for by major depressive disorder, generalized anxiety disorder, or posttraumatic stress disorder

From Prigerson HG, Horowitz MJ, Jacobs SC, et al. Prolonged grief disorder: psychometric validation of criteria proposed for DSM-V and ICD-11. *PLoS Med.* 2009;6:e100–e121.

PGD: DIAGNOSTIC CRITERIA, COURSE, AND OUTCOMES

Following a death from natural causes, approximately 10% to 20% of bereaved survivors find themselves unable to recover and suffer from a debilitating grief response (9,37,38). A recent study found that the sudden death of a parent results in about a 10% rate of PGD in children and adolescent survivors (39). Rates following parental death from war, however, are much higher (34.6%) (40). Deaths of children reveal higher rates of PGD in parents than other kinship relationships (41). Studies are underway to compare the prevalence rates and performance of the diagnostic criteria for PGD in countries throughout the world, across various circumstances of the death (e.g., from war to tsunami and earthquakes and fires), and kinship relationships to the deceased (e.g., parents vs. offspring).

Bereaved individuals with PGD experience disruptive and distressing yearning, pining, and longing for the deceased that remain elevated for 6 months or longer after the death. They also report extreme difficulty "moving on" with their life (feeling "stuck" in their grief), as well as feelings of numbness and detachment, bitterness, and a lack of meaning in life without the deceased. They have trouble accepting the death and see no potential for future happiness. Bereaved individuals experiencing PGD report having these symptoms several times a day and find these symptoms impair their ability to function normally (9,14,30,42–52). Table 55.1 presents recently validated criteria for diagnosing PGD in bereaved individuals (36).

It is important to note that this conceptualization of PGD specifies that these particular distress symptoms are elevated for at least 6 months. Hence, delayed and chronic subtypes of grief may both come under the PGD diagnosis as long as, whatever the delay in onset, symptoms are severe at 6 months post-loss. Typically, however, the overwhelming feelings of those who are diagnosed with PGD are not delayed; it is much more often the case that their grief has been intense and unrelenting since the death (28,38).

Recent research demonstrates that bereaved individuals with high levels of PGD symptoms have substantially greater dysfunction than those with lower levels of these symptoms. PGD symptoms may endure for several years and predict substantial morbidity and adverse health behaviors beyond depressive symptoms (7–17,38). PGD has been shown to be a substantial risk for suicidal thoughts and behaviors, with incidence of cardiac events, high blood pressure, and even cancer, in studies that took into account the effect of major depression and generalized anxiety disorder (7–12,28). It is a risk factor for quality of life impairments such as poor social interactions and role functioning, loss of energy, and self perception of illness, disability and functional impairments, loss of work days, and adverse health behaviors such as changes in patterns of consumption of alcohol, food, and tobacco (7–12,28). It has also been shown that PGD increases the risk for ulcerative colitis (11). Table 55.2 provides a summary of the several negative health consequences associated with PGD.

TABLE 55.2	Outcomes of prolonged grief disorder
Increased risk of suicidal thoughts and behaviors
Increased risk of major depressive disorder
Increased risk of anxiety disorders (generalized anxiety disorder, posttraumatic stress disorder, and panic disorder)
Increased incidence of cardiac events
Increased incidence of high blood pressure
Significant changes in consumption of food, alcohol, and tobacco
Increased risk of impairment in social and occupational functioning
Impaired quality of life

Research has shown that PGD at 6 months predicts impairment and complications at 13 to 23 months post-loss (8–10,12,38). Hence, health-care professionals can identify survivors who may experience further adjustment difficulties in the future by recognizing the signs and symptoms of PGD (Table 55.1) at 6 months. Since palliative care and oncology providers who were present during the loss may no longer be in regular contact with survivors at 6 months post-loss, it is particularly important that primary care providers are aware of the PGD diagnostic criteria outlined in Table 55.1 (36). Primary care physicians are well positioned to monitor bereaved patients and connect them with appropriate interventions if a PGD diagnosis is made.

WHY DO CLINICIANS NEED TO CARE FOR BEREAVED PERSONS?

When looking at the outcomes of PGD, one is able to see why clinicians should play a role in all aspects of bereavement care. There remains little doubt about the excess morbidity associated with bereavement, and with PGD, specifically. Bereavement tends to occur most often in later life, when health and adaptive capacities may already be compromised and hence physicians and other health-care professionals need to play an integral role in caring for bereaved patients and in preventing the unchecked progression of PGD. Additionally, severe grief reactions are not limited to the context of losing a loved one later in life. There are a number of particularly vulnerable groups at risk for substantial bereavement-associated morbidities. Grief response in parents who lose a child to cancer has been shown to be more severe and lengthy than from the passing of a spouse or parent (53,54). Rates of sick leave and health-care utilization increased in bereaved parents compared with non-bereaved parents (55). Adolescents and young adults (individuals 15 to 39 years old) who lose a loved one during the psychosocially formative years of their life may experience challenges to the formation of their adult identity (56). Children who experience the death of a parent may fear for their own safety and well-being (57). All three groups are at risk for prolonged depression and chronic anxiety (58–62).

There are several compelling reasons for physicians, and most especially palliative and cancer care providers, to actively engage themselves in bereavement care. First, they are already involved in caring for bereaved patients and will become increasingly so as the population ages. Empathic "aftercare" for bereaved patients demonstrates the physicians' respect for the deceased and concern for the surviving family members. It may reduce the family's sense of abandonment by the health-care system and soften the psychological blow of losing a loved one. Enhanced discussion between bereaved family members and physicians may help both in attaining a sense of closure. Finally, engaging in the active care of bereaved individuals may reduce the negative health consequences and complications associated with the bereavement process in the surviving family members.

WHAT SHOULD CLINICIANS DO TO ASSIST BEREAVED PATIENTS?

Health-care professionals can use the algorithm in Table 55.1 to diagnose PGD. Although many of these signs and symptoms are similar to the manifestation of normal grief during the first 6 months following the loss, it is the persistence of these symptoms and their overall effects on the functioning of the bereaved individuals that are the hallmarks of PGD (Fig. 55.1). Figure 55.1 shows the mean grief resolution scores (a summation of the nine symptoms presented in Table 55.1) over time from loss for those with and without PGD (diagnosed at 6 months post-loss). In contrast to the significant average decline in grief and associated distress over time found

in bereaved individuals with normal grief (36), Figure 55.1 illustrates how the mean grief score remains stably high from 2 to 20 months post-loss for the group diagnosed with PGD. These results indicate that bereaved persons diagnosed with PGD at 6 months post-loss are unlikely to resolve their grief naturally and may benefit from interventions (see Section *Treatment of PGD*).

DISTINCTIONS BETWEEN PGD AND OTHER PSYCHIATRIC DISORDERS SECONDARY TO BEREAVEMENT

PGD is distinct from other psychiatric disorders. Research has found the symptoms of PGD to be distinct from symptoms of major depressive disorder, generalized anxiety disorder, and posttraumatic stress disorder (PTSD) (7,8,10–15). Data have shown that symptoms of PGD form a cluster that hold together cohesively and that they are distinct from depression and anxiety symptoms (8,10–12,16,42).

Considering the substantial associated morbidity and evidence for unique symptomatology, PGD has been proposed for and approved for inclusion in the upcoming *Diagnostic and Statistical Manual of Mental Disorders 5* (38) as a subtype of an Axis I, Adjustment Disorder. While PGD has been variously termed "complicated" and "traumatic" grief in the literature, Prigerson et al. have made the case for "prolonged" as the best descriptor of an abnormally lengthy and severe grief reaction (38). Objections to this proposal have raised concern that pathologizing grief will place bereaved patients at risk for stigma and needless medical treatment in what should be a natural healing process. In response, proponents of PGD recognition emphasize that agreed upon diagnostic criteria will allow health practitioners to accurately and reliably identify and address cases of severe grief that are associated with

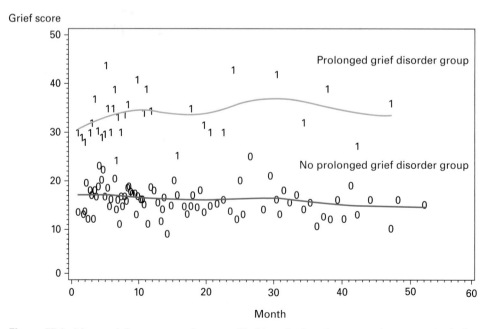

Figure 55.1. Mean grief score over time, stratified by whether the respondent met criteria for prolonged grief disorder or not.

excess suffering and disability, the principal treatment goal for any currently recognized disorder (37,38,63). A recent study of widowers diagnosed by PGD criteria found that 100% would be receptive to treatment for mental illness (64).

DISTINGUISHING PGD FROM PTSD

Traumatized individuals are typically anxious about the threat related to the traumatic event, whereas for persons bereaved from nontraumatic deaths separation anxiety is more prominent (63). In general, fears of violent harm to self or significant others play a less significant role for the bereaved than it does among trauma victims. Additionally, grieving individuals uniquely experience yearning and pining. Efforts to cope with PGD involve reorienting oneself in a world without the deceased rather than processing the events of the death, as might occur following a traumatic event (63). Furthermore, one's personal sense of safety is frequently challenged after a trauma and often but not necessarily following bereavement.

Despite the similarities in the phenomenology of PTSD and PGD such as reexperiencing (intrusive thoughts), and agitation, the core meaning behind the symptoms of these two disorders is quite dissimilar (63). In PTSD, intrusive thoughts and reexperiencing involve memories of the traumatic event that are negative and distressing. Intrusions experienced by individuals with PGD, in contrast, are often positive and comforting (63). In fact, PTSD and PGD are further distinguished by the tendency of some grieving individuals to treasure and retain positive memories in their consciousness, often to the extent that they become maladaptive because they prohibit forward movement and personal development (63). When looking at avoidance, traumatized individuals more frequently avoid reminders of the event, whereas the bereaved might seek reminders of the deceased (63). Individuals with PGD do not appear to avoid reminders of threat as individuals with PTSD often do, but rather avoid reminders of the absence of the deceased through denial (63). In fact, they tend to seek out reminders of the deceased's presence. They are more likely to speak with others about the loss including the deceased, whereas individuals with PTSD try to avoid discussions that will entail a painful return to the traumatic experience (63).

DISTINGUISHING PGD FROM BEREAVEMENT-RELATED DEPRESSION

Distinguishing PGD from the major depressive disorder is clinically difficult because the disorders may coexist following bereavement (10,12). Yet, their symptom profiles are distinct (10,12). Symptoms of yearning, intrusive thoughts, preoccupation with thoughts of the deceased, disbelief regarding the death, and feeling that a part of oneself died with the deceased are all specific to PGD and are distinct from depressive symptoms (10,12). Symptoms of sad mood, psychomotor retardation, and damaged

self-esteem are indicators of depression (10,12). The recognition of the differences between these disorders is essential in guiding decisions for effective intervention. Later in this chapter, we will discuss the treatments of PGD and bereavement-related psychiatric complications such as depression.

RISK FACTORS FOR PGD

Understanding the risk factors that predispose certain individuals to experiencing PGD will help health-care providers identify individuals at risk and provide the necessary support to help survivors through their grieving process. PGD is associated with attachment disturbance and a high degree of insecurity and unstable sense of self and one's relationship with others (45,65,66). Other personal psychiatric vulnerabilities for PGD include a history of psychiatric illnesses such as depression or childhood separation anxiety (67). Survivors who were in a dependent, relationship with the deceased are more likely to experience PGD (45,65,68,69). Individuals who have experienced childhood abuse and serious neglect have also been shown to have a higher risk of PGD (70). Individuals who are generally averse to lifestyle changes are also more likely to experience complications (71). PGD is less likely to be seen in survivors with a good social support network and with some advance preparation for the death (27,72).

Table 55.3 shows a list of risk factors that health-care professionals can keep an eye on when dealing with bereaved individuals. Monitoring these risk factors can be a clue to identify bereaved individuals who may be at risk. Those at risk should be connected early on to psychosocial resources that can prevent unchecked progression of PGD. For example, individuals lacking a good social support structure should be encouraged to participate in support groups and in bereavement organizations such as the American association of retired persons (AARP) Widowed Persons Service to reduce isolation, normalize the challenges that they face, and obtain useful practical advice and empathy, as well as companionship.

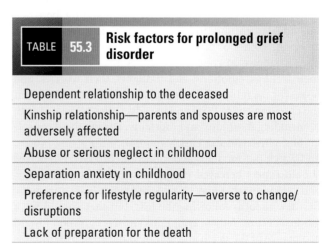

TABLE 55.3	Risk factors for prolonged grief disorder
Dependent relationship to the deceased
Kinship relationship—parents and spouses are most adversely affected
Abuse or serious neglect in childhood
Separation anxiety in childhood
Preference for lifestyle regularity—averse to change/disruptions
Lack of preparation for the death

GENERAL MANAGEMENT OF BEREAVED INDIVIDUALS

Health-care professionals can make the grieving process a more tolerable experience for the survivors. If health-care professionals consider care for the bereaved as part of their duty and as an integral part of end-of-life care, some incidents of PGD might be prevented, detected early, and/or brought under control before causing significant damage to health and quality of life.

As noted earlier, preparedness for the death tends to decrease the risks of developing PGD and hence the first task for health-care professionals who may have a chance to make family members more prepared for their loss is to encourage them to say goodbye to their loved ones and to deal with any guilt or regrets they might have. Health-care providers can also facilitate a peaceful and dignified death by engaging patients and family members in discussions of end-of-life care preferences. Observational findings suggest that physician–patient/caregiver communication about care and care preferences can decrease the technological intensity of end-of-life treatments (73,74) and have positive effects on patient quality of life and caregiver mental and physical health prior to death (75). Further, when patients receive less technologically intensive medical care (e.g., being placed on a ventilator and resuscitated), caregiver bereavement outcomes are often better (76).

Following the death, health-care professionals should provide an opportunity for survivors to spend some time with the body of the deceased, when possible. This will facilitate acceptance of the death and help in overcoming the denial and shock due to the loss. Additionally, staff may develop a close relationship with the patient's family over the course of treatment. Recognizing and sustaining that relationship through small actions of sympathy (a card, home visit, or attendance at the funeral, for example) are appreciated a great deal and provide a much needed, yet often absent, source of compassionate support (4).

In the first couple of months post-loss, the physician or other clinic staff members might make telephone calls to offer condolences and also to recommend a visit to evaluate and then monitor the survivors' health-care needs. The content of office visits between the physician and the bereaved individual might shift from ordinary practice to a discussion about the course of grief, the ways the bereaved individual have attempted to cope with the loss, their daily practices, their feelings, emotions, and thoughts, their worries, and hopes for the future. This type of intervention could prevent the development of PGD and the adversities associated with it, including morbidity and mortality. During these consultations, physicians can closely monitor the grieving process and watch out for signs and indicators of PGD. Physicians should expect bereaved individuals to exhibit some signs and symptoms that may be associated with PGD during the first few months following the loss, but they should see a gradual decline in these symptoms and a progression toward acceptance of the death and ability to move on by 6 months post-loss.

Physicians sometimes feel reluctant to approach the deceased patient's surviving family out of fear that the family is angry with them and perhaps due to a sense of guilt and/or helplessness about being unable to prevent the death. In a study of reactions to terminal care, 30% of surviving family members reported dissatisfaction with the information provided about the cause of death (13). Physicians who contact bereaved patients and express sorrow and concern may minimize the anger directed toward them.

The physician's discomfort or uncertainty about what to say or do when taking care of bereaved patients must be overcome in favor of taking active steps to help them. Some important practices to implement include setting up a system of death notification, outreach, having a list of resources available, and follow-up (13). Physicians should acknowledge the loss and let the bereaved person know that they feel for him/her. Furthermore, they should acknowledge their inability to fully comprehend the magnitude of their loss and the feelings that the bereaved individuals may be experiencing. Physicians should encourage conversations about the deceased, remembering him/her and allowing the bereaved individual to talk freely about their thoughts of the deceased. Additionally, physicians should provide an opportunity for the bereaved individuals to ask any of their unanswered questions and to address their concerns about the final moments in the deceased's life. Physicians should always express concern for the bereaved individuals and provide them with an opportunity to talk about their loss and its effect on their lives (13).

In managing bereaved individuals, health-care professionals can facilitate healing and minimize the risk of PGD by encouraging certain behaviors and providing some helpful advice for bereaved individuals. Physicians can encourage bereaved individuals to socialize, develop new routines and skills, and maintain an active lifestyle. Furthermore, health-care professionals can serve as advocates for good health behaviors such as discouraging bereaved persons from excessive drinking, smoking, or eating and maintaining good sleep hygiene (e.g., regular sleep–wake hours and not eating or watching TV in bed).

Bereaved people with PGD are less likely to seek medical care than those without prolonged grief, perhaps because they think prolonged grief is normal and not worthy of professional attention (35,77). Consequently, health-care professionals must make an extra effort to identify appropriate services and encourage those with PGD to use them. Many of the bereaved with PGD are suicidal, heightening the need for detection and intervention with this gravely at-risk group.

INTERVENTIONS AND TREATMENTS FOR BEREAVED INDIVIDUALS

Although a variety of interventions and treatments for grief have been described, results have only recently demonstrated significant efficacy/effectiveness. Meta-analyses of the expansive research on psychotherapeutic interventions have attempted to explain inconsistencies across these studies and why many authors find weak or nonsignificant treatment effect (78–80). Patients with severe grief reactions who may be at risk for PGD, however, are more likely to respond to treatments (32,78).

Psychodynamic and interpersonal treatments focus on the unresolved social, attachment, and relational issues that may underlie the patient's grief symptoms (81). Psychodynamic therapy may be particularly helpful for patients with long-standing patterns of anxious attachment, dependency, and problems stemming from problematic childhood relationships (4). In interpersonal psychotherapy (IPT), a therapist works with a patient to create an inventory of relationships from which problem areas (grief, disputes, transitions, and deficits) can be identified. Treatment then focuses on addressing these relational problem areas through communication and problem-solving techniques (78). IPT effectiveness has been inconclusive, with some studies (4,78) demonstrating a stronger treatment effect than others (82).

Cognitive-behavioral therapy (CBT) provides a framework through which to understand dysfunctional thoughts, beliefs, and associated maladaptive behaviors. Within this framework, a patient's grief may be connected to an inability to fully integrate the loss into a coherent self-narrative (83). CBT may be most effective when the individual suffers from debilitating feelings of anger and guilt that may be connected to catastrophic beliefs surrounding the death (4). CBT may also be used to address avoidant behaviors in bereaved individuals who may be unable to perform daily activities and live peaceably within their life once shared with a loved one (83).

Group-oriented therapeutic approaches provide an opportunity for participants to support each other through a network of shared experiences. Participants can also share coping strategies with each other, creating a pool of knowledge about personal grief management. Group therapy has been shown to be the most effective among patients diagnosed with PGD who are able to contribute in an open and conscientious way and who have a history of social support and healthy relationships (84–86).

In caring for the deceased, health-care professionals often become aware of the difficulties that surviving family members may experience together in coping with their grief and as a result may recommend family therapy. Family-focused grief therapy aims to prevent the morbidity associated with a family's maladaptive response to bereavement by addressing problems with communication, cohesion, and conflict resolution (31). Families are screened for these relational problems and, if selected, enter therapy that continues after loss. Family therapy has been demonstrated to have a moderate effect size, but it had the most impact with sullen families that demonstrated intermediate functioning (31). Early identification and enrollment of vulnerable families may prevent excess morbidity after death of the patient.

Internet-based therapy has been found to reduce distress associated with avoidance and depression (87). Patients may prefer Internet-based interventions for a number of reasons: low cost, convenience, anonymity, and avoidance of clinical settings that may bring forth distressing memories of the deceased's passing (4). Several studies have demonstrated the effectiveness of Internet-based therapies in reducing symptoms associated with PGD, depression, and PTSD (88,89).

TREATMENT OF PGD

While managing bereaved individuals, being able to recognize risk factors and symptoms of PGD will help health-care professionals in identifying individuals who are having an exceptionally difficult time coping with the loss and in recommending further counseling and support. Treatment and counseling that get at the meaning of the loss to the survivor's sense of self and attitudes toward their surrounding environment and interventions that enhance the survivor's sense of their prospects for future fulfillment would target the core attachment issues that lay at the root of PGD (13). Treatments that foster a sense of competence and independence in the survivor, that promote development of new, meaningful relationships, and that encourage new routines and skills would be beneficial (90,91). When dealing with patients suffering from PGD, health-care providers should recommend maintaining an active daily routine, monitoring caloric intake, getting adequate sleep (6.5 to 9 h/night), and exercising several times each week just as they would with any bereaved individual. Bereaved individuals experiencing difficulties, adjusting to the loss as predicted, should also be encouraged to participate in support groups that will help them find empathic support, feel less isolated or abnormal, and potentially learn ways to enhance their sense of independence and "survival" skills and generally assist them in coping with their loss (13,90–96).

William Piper's interpretative and supportive therapies (84,98) and Mardi Horowitz's eclectic integrated cognitive-dynamic approach to case formulation and treatment (95) are all promising psychotherapeutic techniques for PGD, although conclusive results await publication of randomized controlled trials. Katherine Shear's complicated grief therapy (CGT) (99) is the first randomized controlled trial for PGD with proven efficacy for the reduction of PGD symptomatology. Because PGD includes depressive symptoms such as sadness, guilt, and social withdrawal, Shear used a framework for the treatment based on previous research with IPT for grief-related depression (99). Because of the presence of PTSD-like symptoms of disbelief, as well as unique symptoms related to the death, Shear modified IPT techniques to include CBT-based techniques for addressing death trauma (99). The cognitive strategies were used when working with loss-specific distress. Shear reports that her new integrated approach, her targeted CGT, is an improved treatment over IPT that shows higher response rates and faster time to response for symptoms of PGD, specifically (99).

Preliminary results from our Healthy Experiences After Loss (HEAL, NIMH R34: Litz, PI) online self-management intervention are showing large effects for the reduction of PGD symptoms specifically. Work is underway to conduct a multi-center randomized, controlled trial of HEAL to demonstrate more conclusively and generalizably the effectiveness of this secondary, Internet-based prevention for PGD onset.

It is important for health-care professionals to be able to distinguish between PGD and bereavement-related psychiatric complications such as bereavement-related depression because they might call for different treatment protocols and different therapies.

TREATMENT OF BEREAVEMENT-RELATED PSYCHIATRIC COMPLICATIONS

The results of research on bereavement interventions suggest that treatment selection should be based on the patient's specific psychiatric diagnosis or diagnoses (13). For patients diagnosed with bereavement-related depression, the treatment should follow the guidelines for treating a major depressive disorder including the prescription of selective serotonin reuptake inhibitors (SSRIs) or tricyclic antidepressants (TCAs) (13). Similarly, if the bereaved individuals show distinct signs and symptoms of any other major psychiatric disorder, treatment should follow the guidelines for treating that specific disorder independent of the PGD treatment.

Several studies have shown that SSRIs and TCAs are able to reduce depressive symptoms in bereaved individuals (79,100,101). Research has also indicated that a combination of antidepressants and psychotherapy may be particularly effective in treating depression during bereavement (82). However, neither the TCA nortriptyline nor IPT was found to have a significant effect on symptoms of PGD (82). Initial studies indicated that IPT and TCAs have not proven to be effective in ameliorating symptoms of PGD compared with placebo (82,102).

Here, once again, one can see the importance of an accurate understanding of the distinct differences between the clinical presentation of PGD and other psychiatric disorders in the bereavement setting. The success of treating the patient's symptoms will depend on the ability to diagnose their symptoms and monitor their illness course.

IMPLICATIONS FOR PALLIATIVE CARE

Barry et al. evaluated the association between the bereaved persons' perceptions of death (e.g., extent of suffering and violent vs. peaceful death) and preparedness for the death and psychiatric disorders (27). Barry et al. showed that the perception of death as more violent was associated with major depressive disorder at 4 months post-loss. More importantly, this work indicated that the perception of lack of preparedness for the death was associated with PGD at 4 and 9 months post-loss.

Recent work (103) suggests that earlier hospice enrollment may reduce the risk for major depressive disorder during the first 6 to 8 months of bereavement. This is consistent with Barry's work because earlier hospice enrollment might indicate more preparedness for the death. Additionally, another study in the Netherlands indicated that the bereaved family and friends of cancer patients who died by euthanasia coped better with respect to grief symptoms and posttraumatic stress reactions than the bereaved of comparable cancer patients who died a natural death (104). Research has demonstrated that hospice use may reduce the increased risk of mortality among widowed spouses and thus could positively influence health outcomes for the deceased's love ones (105). Deaths that occurred within hospice were associated with lower risk of PGD in surviving family members compared with those that occurred with a hospital setting (76).

These data strongly suggest that preparation in advance for the loss may help reduce the risk of developing PGD and make the grieving process less painful for the survivors.

This information can have important implications for palliative care services and hospices by allowing them to play a key role in reducing the risks of developing complications in bereaved individuals during their grieving process. Palliative care services as well as hospices can help families orient to their loss and provide them with a chance to accept and deal with that loss. Furthermore, this information should also be used by health-care professionals when dealing with patients suffering from terminal illnesses. Health-care professionals should be encouraged to recommend hospice and palliative care services to their patients when it is appropriate to do so to prevent prolongation of suffering in them, allow them a peaceful ending, and also help their families prepare for their loss, which may lower their risk of developing PGD.

CONCLUSION

Bereavement is a natural and nearly universal experience that causes a great deal of distress and sorrow. However, an individual's experience with grief and bereavement may vary depending on many factors including the circumstances of the death and social elements, relationship (e.g., parents and spouses) and closeness to the deceased, and, particularly, emotional dependency on the deceased. Past experiences with loss, intrapersonal factors, and interpersonal factors are all influential in determining bereavement adjustment.

Because of the many negative health care consequences associated with bereavement and PGD, bereavement care should be a responsibility assumed by health-care providers and an integral part of any comprehensive palliative care plan that focuses on providing good quality end-of-life care for the dying patient as well as support for the survivors. Health-care professionals need to recognize the symptoms associated with PGD and identify the persons having difficulties in coping with their loss. Additionally, having a solid understanding of the various risk factors that predispose certain individuals to PGD will help health-care providers in closely monitoring individuals at risk and also in recommending proper treatment and support options.

Bereavement care currently does not get the proper attention in the education and the development of tomorrow's physicians. This cannot be understood apart from a broader understanding of health economics. Preventive medicine in general is poorly reimbursed, and this is particularly true of the prevention of bereavement-associated morbidity, which is not specifically reimbursed, although services that reduce maladjustment in bereavement (e.g., hospice) may be. Medical and psychiatric training often devotes little time to the recognition of PGD. Without the proper education, physicians might not be able to recognize the signs and symptoms of PGD, comprehend their duty to take care of the family and survivors who are left behind, and provide adequate help and encouragement for bereaved individuals attempting to cope with their loss. Furthermore, all health-care professionals will probably be exposed to grieving individuals, and survivors will probably be greatly helped by having a doctor who is comfortable in addressing their grief, capable of helping them cope with their loss, and supporting their efforts to bring closure to the loss and to move on with their lives. Hence, it is essential that bereavement care becomes an integral part of current educational programs directed at developing better physicians who are capable of managing all aspects of their patient's struggles, including their grieving process.

In this chapter, we have also tried to outline the importance of preparing families for their loss, for experiencing a peaceful resolution and a nonviolent death when possible, and for the advantages of early hospice enrollment in lowering the risk of developing PGD. This provides yet another reason for health-care professionals to reassess their priorities and their efforts when providing quality end-of-life care for their patients and their families. Aggressive therapies and prolongation of life above all else might not be the best strategy to implement when taking care of patients and their families. Instead, preparing the families for the loss and accepting death as part of the natural life cycle rather than a failure in the medical care provided may prove extremely helpful for the bereaved individuals and their grieving process. Finally, we hope that the research findings outlined in this chapter will help in shaping palliative care programs and hospices' roles in the bereavement process as well as in physicians' attitudes, perceptions, and actions when providing end-of-life and bereavement care for their patients and for those who are left behind.

REFERENCES

1. Prigerson HG, Maciejewski PK. Grief and acceptance as opposite sides of the same coin: setting a research agenda to study peaceful acceptance of loss. *Br J Psychiatry.* 2008;193:435-437.
2. Summary of Current Surveys and Data Collection Systems. National Center for Health Statistics, Center for Disease Control, June 2012;18. http://www.cdc.gov/nchs/data/factsheets/factsheet_summary1.pdf. Accessed July 18, 2012.
3. America's Families and Living. Arrangement 2003 March. Current Population Survey Report, U.S. Census Bureau, March 2003. http://www.census.gov/prod/2004pubs/p20-553.pdf. Accessed July 18, 2012.
4. Licthenthal WG, Prigerson HG, Kissane DW. Bereavement: A special issue in Oncology" in: Holland JC, Breitbart WS, Jacobsen PB, Lederberg MS, Loscalzo Mj, McCorkle R (eds). Psycho-Oncology (2nd edition). New York; NY, New York, USA: Oxford University Press, 2010: 537-543.
5. Holmes TH, Rahe RH. The social readjustment rating scale. *J Psychosom Res.* 1967;11:213-218.
6. Osterweis M, Solomon F, Green M, eds. *Bereavement: Reactions, Consequences and Care.* Washington, DC: National Academy Press; 1984:86-88.
7. Prigerson HG, Jacobs Sc. Perspectives on care at the close of life. Caring for bereaved patients: "all the doctors just suddenly go." *JAMA.* 2001;286:1369-1376.
8. Silverman GK, Jacobs SC, Kasl SV, et al. Quality of life impairments associated with diagnostic criteria for traumatic grief. *Psychol Med.* 2000;30:857-862.
9. Prigerson HG, Shear MK, Jacobs SC, et al. Consensus criteria for traumatic grief. A preliminary empirical test. *Br J Psychiatry.* 1999;174:67-73.

10. Boelen PA, van den Bout J, de Keijser J. Traumatic grief as a disorder distinct from bereavement-related depression and anxiety: a replication study with bereaved mental health care patients. *Am J Psychiatry.* 2003;160:1229-1241.
11. Ott CH. The impact of complicated grief on mental and physical health at various points in the bereavement process. *Death Stud.* 2003;27:249-272.
12. Prigerson HG, Bridge J, Maciejewski PK, et al. Influence of traumatic grief on suicidal ideation among young adults. *Am J Psychiatry.* 1999;156:1994-1995.
13. Chen JH, Bierhals AJ, Prigerson HG, et al. Gender differences in the effects of bereavement-related psychological distress in health outcomes. *Psychol Med.* 1999;29:367-380.
14. Prigerson HG, Bierhals AJ, Kasl SV, et al. Traumatic grief as a risk factor for mental and physical morbidity. *Am J Psychiatry.* 1997;154:616-623.
15. Prigerson HG, Bierhals AJ, Kasl SV, et al. Complicated grief as a disorder distinct from bereavement-related depression and anxiety: a replication study. *Am J Psychiatry.* 1996;153:1484-1486.
16. Prigerson HG, Maciejewski PK, Reynolds CF III, et al. Inventory of complicated grief: a scale to measure maladaptive symptoms of loss. *Psychiatry Res.* 1995;59:65-79.
17. Prigerson HG, Frank E, Kasl SV, et al. Complicated GRIEF and bereavement-related depression as distinct disorders: preliminary empirical validation in elderly bereaved spouses. *Am J Psychiatry.* 1995;152:22-30.
18. Brown GW, Harris TO. Depression. In: Brown GW, Harris TO, eds. *Life Events and Illness.* New York, NY: Guilford Press; 1989:49-94.
19. Bruce ML, Kim K, Leaf PJ, et al. Depressive episodes and dysphoria resulting from conjugal bereavement in a prospective community sample. *Am J Psychiatry.* 1990;147:608-611.
20. Clayton PJ. Bereavement and depression. *J Clin Psychiatry.* 1990;51:34-38.
21. Lund D, Dimond M, Caserta MS. Identifying elderly with coping difficulties two years after bereavement. *Omega.* 1985;16:213-224.
22. Zisook S, Shuchter S. Uncomplicated bereavement. *J Clin Psychiatry.* 1993;54:365-372.
23. Bornstein PE, Clayton PJ, Halikas JA, et al. The depression of widowhood after 13 months. *Br J Psychiatry.* 1973;122:561-566.
24. Parkes CM, Wiss RS. *Recovery of Bereavement.* New York, NY: Basic Books; 1983.
25. Jacobs S, Hansen F, Kasl S, et al. Anxiety disorders during acute bereavement: risk and risk factors. *J Clin Psychiatry.* 1990;51:269-274.
26. Metzger PL, Gray MJ. End-of-life communication and adjustment: pre-loss communication as a predictor of bereavement-related outcomes. *Death Stud.* 2008;32:301-325.
27. Barry LC, Kasl SV, Prigerson HG. Psychiatric disorders among bereaved persons: the role of perceived circumstances of death and preparedness for death. *Am J Geriatr Psychiatry.* 2001;10:447-457.
28. Prigerson HG. Complicated grief: when the path of adjustment leads to a dead-end. *Bereavement Care.* 2004;23:38-40.
29. Parkes CM, Prigerson HG. *Bereavement: Studies of Grief in Adult Life.* 4th ed. London: Penguin Books; 2010.
30. Lindemann E. Symptomatology and management of acute grief. *Am J Psychiatry.* 1944;151:155-160.
31. Kissane DW, McKenzie M, Bloch S, Moskowitz C, McKenzie DP, O'Neill I. Family focused grief therapy: a randomized,

controlled trial in palliative care and bereavement. *Am J Psychiatry*. 2006;163:1208-1218.

32. Gilliland G, Fleming S. A comparison of spousal anticipatory grief and conventional grief. *Death Stud*. 1998;22:541-569.

33. Chapman KJ, Pepler C. Coping, hope, and anticipatory grief in family members in palliative home care. *Cancer Nurs*. 1998;21:226-234.

34. Smith SH. Anticipatory grief and psychological adjustment to grieving in middle-aged children. *Am J Hosp Palliat Care*. 2005;22:283-286.

35. Lichtenthal W, Breitbart W, Jones E, Kissane D, Prigerson HG. Underutilization of mental health services among bereaved caregivers with prolonged grief disorder. *Psychiatr Serv*. October 2011;62(10):1225-1229.

36. Maciejewski PK, Zhang B, Block SD, Prigerson HG. An empirical examination of the stage theory of grief. *JAMA*. February 2007;297(7):716-723.

37. Prigerson HG, Horowitz MJ, Jacobs SC, et al. Prolonged grief disorder: psychometric validation of criteria proposed for DSM-V and ICD-11. *PLoS Med*. 2009;6:e100-e121.

38. Prigerson HG, Vanderwerker LC, Maciejewski PK. A case for inclusion of prolonged grief disorder in DSM-V. In: Stroebe MS, Hansson RO, Schut H, Stroebe W, eds. *Handbook of Bereavement Research and Practice: Advances in Theory and Intervention*. Washington, DC: American Psychological Association; 2008:165-186.

39. Melhem NM, Porta G, Shamseddeen W, Walker Payne M, Brent DA. Grief in children and adolescents bereaved by sudden parental death. *Arch Gen Psychiatry*. September 2011;68(9):911-919.

40. Morina N, von Lersner U, Prigerson HG. *PLoS One*. 2011;6(7):e22140. e-pub July 12, 2011.

41. Cleiren M, Diekstra RF, Kerkhof AJ, van der Wal J. Mode of death and kinship in bereavement: focusing on "who" rather than "how." *Crisis*. 1994;15(1):22-36.

42. Prigerson HG, Bridge J, Maciejewski PK, et al. Traumatic grief as a risk factor for suicidal ideation among young adults. *Am J Psychiatry*. 1997;156:1994-1995.

43. Bowlby J. *Loss: Sadness and Depression*. New York, NY: Basic Books; 1980.

44. Prigerson HG, Shear MK, Frank E, et al. Traumatic grief: a case of loss-induced distress. *Am J Psychiatry*. 1997;154:1003-1009.

45. Schut HA, De Keijser J, Van den Bout J, et al. Post-traumatic stress symptoms in the first years of conjugal bereavement. *Anxiety Res*. 1991;4:225-234.

46. Zisook S, Chentsova-Dutton Y, Shuchter SR. PTSD following bereavement. *Ann Clin Psychiatry*. 1998;10:157-163.

47. Lewis CS. *A Grief Observed*. New York, NY: Bantam Seabury Press; 1963.

48. Middleton W, Burnett P, Paphael B, et al. The bereavement response: a cluster analysis. *Br J Psychiatry*. 1996;169:167-171.

49. Horowitz MJ, Siegel B, Holen A, et al. Criteria for complicated grief disorder. *Am J Psychiatry*. 1997;154:905-910.

50. Jacobs S, Kasl S, Schaefer C, et al. Conscious and unconscious coping with loss. *Psychosom Med*. 1994;56:557-563.

51. Bonanno GA, Keltner D, Holen A, et al. When avoiding unpleasant emotions might not be such a bad thing: verbal-autonomic response dissociation and midlife conjugal bereavement. *J Pers Soc Psychol*. 1995;69:975-989.

52. Stroebe MS, Stroebe W. Does "grief work" work? *J Consult Clin Psychol*. 1991;59:479-482.

53. Sanders CM. A comparison of adult bereavement in the death of a spouse, child, and parent. *Omega*. 1980;10:303-322.

54. Rando TA. *Parental Loss of a Child*. Champaign, IL: Research Press; 1986.

55. Lannen PK, Wolfe J, Prigerson HG, Onelov E, Kreicbergs UC. Unresolved grief in a national sample of bereaved parents: impaired mental and physical health 4 to 9 years later. *J Clin Oncol*. 2008;26:5870-5876.

56. Meshot CM, Leitner LM. Adolescent mourning and parental death. *Omega*. 1993;26:287-299.

57. Geis HK, Whittlesey SW, McDonald NB, Smith KL, Pfefferbaum B. Bereavement and loss in childhood. *Child Adolesc Psychiatr Clin N Am*. 1998;7:73-85, viii.

58. Kreicbergs U, Valdimarsdottir U, Onelov E, Henter J, Steineck G. Anxiety and depression in parents 4-9 years after the loss of a child owing to a malignancy: a population-based follow-up. *Psychol Med*. 2004;34:1431-1441.

59. Mireault GC, Bond LA. Parental death in childhood: perceived vulnerability, and adult depression and anxiety. *Am J Orthopsychiatry*. 1992;62:517-524.

60. Tyrka AR, Wier L, Price LH, Ross NS, Carpenter LL. Childhood parental loss and adult psychopathology: effects of loss characteristics and contextual factors. *Int J Psychiatry Med*. 2008;38:329-344.

61. Saler L, Skolnick N. Childhood parental death and depression in adulthood: roles of surviving parent and family environment. *Am J Orthopsychiatry*. 1992;62:504-516.

62. Harris ES. Adolescent bereavement following the death of a parent: an exploratory study. *Child Psychiatry Hum Dev*. 1991;21:267-281.

63. Lichtenthal WG, Cruess DG, Prigerson HG. A case for establishing complicated grief as a distinct mental disorder in DSM-V. *Clin Psychol Rev*. 2004;24:637-662.

64. Johnson JG, First MB, Block S, et al. Stigmatization and receptivity to mental health services among recently bereaved adults. *Death Stud*. 2009; 33(8):691-711.

65. Carr D, House JS, Wortman C, et al. Psychological adjustments to sudden and anticipated spousal loss among older widowed persons. *J Gerontol Psychol Soc Sci*. 2001;56:S237-S248.

66. van Doorn C, Kasl SV, Beery LC, et al. The influence of marital quality and attachment styles on traumatic grief and depressive symptoms. *J Nerv Ment Dis*. 1998;186:566-573.

67. Vanderwerker LC, Jacobs SC, Parkes CM, Prigerson HG. An exploration of associations between separation anxiety in childhood and complicated grief in later life. *J Nerv Ment Dis*. 2006;194:121-123.

68. Prigerson HG, Maciejewski PK, Rosenheck R. The interactive effects of marital harmony and widowhood on health, health service utilization and costs. *Gerontologist*. 2000;40:349-357.

69. Johnson JG, Vanderwerker LC, Bornstein RF, et al. Development and validation of an instrument for the assessment of dependency among bereaved persons. *J Psychopathol Behav*. 28:263-272.

70. Silverman GK, Johnson JG, Prigerson HG. Preliminary explorations of the effects of prior trauma and loss on risk of psychiatric disorders in recently widowed people. *Isr J Psychiatry Relat Sci*. 2001;38:202-215.

71. Beery LC, Prigerson HG. Lifestyle regularity as a unique risk factor for complicated grief. In press.

72. Vanderwerker LC, Prigerson HG. Social support, technological connectedness and periodical readings as protective factors in bereavement. *J Loss Trauma*. 2004;9:45-57.

73. Wright AA, Mack JW, Kritek PA, et al. Influence of patients' preferences and treatment site on cancer patients' end-of-life care. *Cancer*. 2010;116(19):4656-4663.

74. Mack JW, Paulk ME, Viswanath K, et al. Racial disparities in the outcomes of communication on medical care received near death. *Arch Intern Med*. 2010;170(17):1533-1540.

75. Wright AA, Zhang B, Ray A, et al. Associations between end-of-life discussions, patient mental health, medical care near death, and caregiver bereavement adjustment. *JAMA*. 2008;300(14):1665-1673.

76. Wright AA, Keating NL, Balboni TA, et al. Place of death: correlations with quality of life of patients with cancer and predictors of bereaved caregivers' mental health. *J Clin Oncol*. 2010;28(29):4457-4464.

77. Prigerson HG, Silverman GK, Jacobs SC, et al. Disability, traumatic grief, and the underutilization of health services. *Prim Psychiatry*. 2001;8:61-69.

78. Kato PM, Mann T. A synthesis of psychological interventions for the bereaved. *Clin Psychol Rev*. 1999;19:275-296.

79. Currier JM, Neimeyer RA, Berman JS. The effectiveness of the psychotherapeutic interventions for bereaved persons: a comprehensive quantitative review. *Psychol Bull*. 2008;134:648-661.

80. Jordan JR, Neimeyer RA. Does grief counseling work? *Death Stud*. 2003;27:765-786.

81. Luty SE, Carter JD, McKenzie JM, et al. Randomized controlled trial of interpersonal psychotherapy and cognitive-behavioral therapy for depression. *Br J Psychiatry*. 2007;190:96-502.

82. Reynolds CF III, Miller MD, Pasternak RE, et al. Treatment of bereavement-related major depressive episodes in later life: a controlled study of acute and continuation treatment with nortriptyline and interpersonal psychotherapy. *Am J Psychiatry*. 1999;156:202-208.

83. Boelen PA, van den Hout MA, van den Bout J. A cognitive-behavioral conceptualization of complicated grief. *Clin Psychol*. 2006;13:109-128.

84. Piper WE, Ogrodniczuk JS, Joyce AS, Weideman R, Rosie JS. Group composition and group therapy for complicated grief. *J Consult Clin Psychol*. 2007;75:116-125.

85. Ogrodniczuk JS, Piper WE, Joyce AS, McCallum M, Rosie JS. Social support as a predictor of response to group therapy for complicated grief. *Psychiatry*. 2002;65:346-357.

86. Ogrodniczuk JS, Piper WE, Joyce AS, McCallum M, Rosie JS. NEO-five factor personality traits as predictors of response to two forms of group psychotherapy. *Int J Group Psychother*. 2003;53:417-442.

87. Lange A, van de Ven JP, Schrieken B. Interapy: treatment of posttraumatic stress via the Internet. *Cogn Behav Ther*. 2003;32:110-124.

88. Litz BT, Engel CC, Bryant RA, Papa A. A randomized, controlled proof-of-concept trial of an Internet-based, therapist-assisted self-management treatment for posttraumatic stress disorder. *Am J Psychiatry*. 2007;164:1676-1683.

89. Wagner B, Maercker A. An Internet-based cognitive-behavioral preventive intervention for complicated grief: a pilot study. *G Ital Med Lav Ergon*. 2008;30:B47-B53.

90. Brown LF, Reynolds CF, Monk TH, et al. Social rhythm stability following late-life spousal bereavement: associations with depression and sleep impairment. *Psychiatry Res*. 1996;62:161-169.

91. Prigerson HG, Reynolds CF III, Frank E, et al. Stressful life events, social rhythms, and depressive symptoms among the elderly: an examination of hypothesized causal linkages. *Psychiatry Res*. 1991;51:33-49.

92. Main J. Improving management of bereavement in general practice based on a survey of recently bereaved subjects in a single general practice. *Br J Gen Pract*. 2000;50:863-866.

93. Morgan DL. Adjusting to widowhood: do social networks really make it easier? *Gerontologist*. 1989;29:101-107.

94. Schneider DS, Sledge PA, Shuchter SR, et al. Dating and remarriage over the first two years of widowhood. *Ann Clin Psychiatry*. 1996;8:51-57.

95. Marmar CR, Horowitz MJ, Weiss DS, et al. A controlled trial of brief psychotherapy and mutual-help group treatment of conjugal bereavement. *Am J Psychiatry*. 1988;145:203-309.

96. Pennebaker JW, Zech E, Rime B. Disclosing and sharing emotion: psychological, social and health consequences. In: Stroebe MS, Hansson RO, Stroebe W, et al., eds. *Handbook of Bereavement Research: Consequences, Coping and Care*. Washington, DC: American Psychological Association; 2001:517-544.

97. Esterling BA, Antoni MH, Fletcher MA, et al. Emotional disclosure through writing or speaking modulates latent Epstein-Barr virus antibody titers. *J Consult Clin Psychol*. 1994;62:130-140.

98. Piper WE, McCallum M, Joyce AS, et al. Patients personality and time-limited group psychotherapy for complicated grief. *Int J Group Psychother*. 2001;51:525-555.

99. Shear MK, Frank E, Houck P, et al. Treatment of complicated grief: a randomized controlled trial. *JAMA*. 2005;293:2601-2659.

100. Jacobs SC, Nelson JC, Zisook S. Treating depressions of bereavement with antidepressants. A pilot study. *Psychiatr Clin North Am*. 1987;10:501-510.

101. Pasternak RE, Reynolds CF 3rd, Schlernitzauer M, et al. Acute open-trial nortriptyline therapy of bereavement-related depression in late life. *J Clin Psychiatry*. 1991;52:307-310.

102. Rosenzweig AS, Pasternak RE, Prigerson HG, et al. Bereavement-related depression in the elderly. Is drug treatment justified? *Drugs Aging*. 1996;8:323-328.

103. Bradley EH, Prigerson HG, Carlson MD. Depression among surviving caregivers: does length of hospice enrollment matter? *Am J Psychiatry*. 2004;161:2257-2262.

104. Swarte NB, Van der Lee ML, Van der Born JG, et al. Effects of euthanasia on the bereaved family and friends: a cross sectional study. *Br Med J*. 2003;327:189-194.

105. Christakis NA, Iwashyna TJ. The health impact of health care on families: a matched cohort study of hospice use by decedents and mortality outcomes in surviving, widowed spouses. *Soc Sci Med*. 2003;57:465-475.

Alvin L. Reaves III ■ Hunter Groninger

INTRODUCTION

In this ever-changing world of health-care reform, limited resources, and reduced reimbursement, as well as increased demands for quality performance measures, clinicians are experiencing less autonomy in their scope of practice due to these growing restrictions (1–9). Health-care providers, particularly physicians, are reporting more job-related stressors, including employee dissatisfaction and mental exhaustion (10,11), over the last several decades, as the availability of their human resources (time and emotion/empathy) to invest in their clientele/patients is diminishing; however, consumer demand, partly due to increased complexity and severity of illness, is not (12).

This is particularly true in the disciplines of oncology and palliative care, examples of subspecialties in which clinicians care for individuals with chronic, progressive, often life-limiting diseases, with whom they develop deep, meaningful doctor–patient relationships. The well-being and job satisfaction of individuals practicing in these fields should be tantamount to the wellness that they expect from the delivery of their services to their patients (1). It has been noted that the wellness of a care provider has direct negative effects on important outcomes, including quality of patient care, efficiency, and productivity, as well as increased resource utilization. These stressors often lead to problems with substance abuse and psychiatric or medical illnesses. They can affect interpersonal relationships, subsequently causing compassion fatigue before culminating later in burnout or even early retirement (1,6,9,10,13–20). This rippling effect has the potential to decrease clinical workforce substantially, creating gaps in the ability to provide expert care (1).

Research over the last several decades, however, consistently elucidates that no significant advances have been made to improve upon these factors, reducing stress, burnout, and compassion fatigue (21–24). Therefore, it is imperative that workers in the human service industry incorporate measures into their daily routine to effectuate professional sustainability and find tenable ways to ensure adequate and frequent maintenance of their mind, body, and soul so that delivery of quality care may persist.

The aim of this chapter is to describe job-related stressors in the field of oncology and palliative care and to delineate its impact on provider performance as it relates to burnout and compassion fatigue. It has been noted that higher levels of burnout exist in oncologists (82). Although, there has been a paucity of major advances in mitigating burnout and compassion fatigue over the last decades, we will provide a recent selective review of the literature to further understand and attempt to improve upon this potentially career destructive syndrome. Finally, we provide an overview of strategies for sustained self-care.

DEFINING COMPASSION FATIGUE VERSUS BURNOUT

One is often bewildered as to the differences between burnout and compassion fatigue. These terms are frequently used interchangeably in our profession. Commonalities between the two experiences do exist; however, there are striking distinguishing features. These are perhaps two distinct entities on a spectrum of job satisfaction.

Much attention has been given to the concept of *burnout* or *burnout syndrome* over the last 40 years, more so from an organizational business model, but of late from a health-care perspective (21–24). Less is known, however, about the entity of *compassion fatigue*. Historically, most of the existing literature on burnout and compassion fatigue has stemmed from studies conducted in the nursing population. In recent years, however, increasing attention has focused on physician experiences of burnout and compassion fatigue. The literature that does exist on physicians deals primarily with physician job satisfaction (13,25–29). It is possible, though, to see how this topic might be extrapolated further to theorize about physician burnout and compassion fatigue.

Burnout is a term first described in the 1970s by psychologist and psychoanalyst Herbert Freudenberger, Ph.D. (6,30–32), endowed with quantifiable measures two decades later by Christina Maslach, Ph.D., at the University of California, Berkley, CA, United States. Burnout is felt to be a "stress-induced occupational disease" affecting many health-care professionals (33–35). The Maslach Burnout Inventory-Human Services Survey (MBI-HSS) is now considered the gold standard in measuring the burnout syndrome, in which the domain metrics are emotional exhaustion, depersonalization, and personal accomplishment (6,33,35). The MBI consists of a 22-item questionnaire assessing the frequency with which clinicians experience certain feelings related to their jobs in the three aforementioned subscales where scores are rated low, moderate, and high (Table 56.1) (35). One is said to have burnout when emotional exhaustion or depersonalization scores are high (52).

Emotional exhaustion encompasses the feelings of being overextended with loss of emotional and physical resources

TABLE 56.1	**Maslach Burnout Inventory scale**
Depersonalization	I feel I treat some patients as if they were impersonal objects.
	I do not really care what happens to some patients.
Emotional exhaustion	I still feel tired when I wake up on the workday mornings.
Personal accomplishment	I deal effectively with my patient's problems.
	I can easily create a relaxed atmosphere for my patients.
	I feel exhilarated after working closely with my patients.

Adapted from Maslach C, Schaufeli WB, Leiter MP. Job burnout. *Ann Rev Psychol.* 2001;52:397–422/Excerpts from modified Maslach Burnout Inventory (MBI). MBI consists of a 22-item questionnaire consisting of three domains: depersonalization, emotional exhaustion, and personal accomplishment. The frequency with which one experiences these feelings is scored on a seven-point Likert scale and rated low, moderate, and high. The hallmark of burnout is high emotional exhaustion (32,35,71).

and reserve. *Depersonalization* refers to "negative, callous, or excessively detached responses" to various aspects of the job. Both of these entities, which are deemed high in burnout syndrome, are mechanisms by which one distances himself/herself from the job. Sense of *personal accomplishment*, which is low in burnout, refers to the feelings of incompetence and underachievement at work (36–38). In a 1991 study of oncologists by Whippen et al., 56% of members surveyed from the American Society of Clinical Oncology met the criteria for burnout syndrome. These individuals displayed increased emotional exhaustion, increased levels of depersonalization, and low levels of personal accomplishment. Researching burnout in oncology and palliative care has yielded mixed, but striking, statistics. According to two studies using the MBI scale, 53.3% and 69% of oncologists, respectively, documented high rates of emotional exhaustion compared with only 37.1% of allied health professionals caring for their patients (23,36,39). Additional studies illustrate rates of depersonalization ranging from 10% to 25%, both in the United States and internationally, where oncology physicians scored higher in this domain, suggesting they may be more vulnerable to burnout than their oncology nurse colleagues. Compared with Canadian and Japanese oncologists and palliative care physicians (33% to 50%) and allied health professionals, American oncologists were less likely (9%) to exhibit feelings of low personal accomplishment (23,36,40,41).

Burnout has been described as "an individual experience that is specific to the work context" (6). It might be best for one to conceptualize burnout in terms of individual job fit. In other words, one may be more prone to experiencing feelings of "being burned out," if one's work conditions are not congruent with one's work goals. Maslach et al. noted that burnout occurs when there is a mismatch of the person and the job, as it relates to workload, control, reward, community, fairness, and values (32,42,43). This is not to say that one will find perfection in each of the aforementioned domains—rather that there will be acceptable or substantial levels of satisfaction in them such that one remains satisfied and committed to his/her job. This commitment or job engagement may help mitigate job burnout.

For all intents and purposes, these domains reflect organizational, often modifiable elements, more so than personal, perhaps less modifiable traits. Therefore, burnout, in its deconstruction, seems to stem from external influences that are beyond the care provider's own locus of control. Potter cites Gentry and Baranowsky who describe burnout as "the chronic psychological syndrome of perceived demands from work outweighing perceived resources in the work environment" (10). Thus, this imbalance produces a stress reaction in the individual; if such stress persists unaddressed, it manifests fertile conditions for burnout.

By contrast, where burnout relates to extrinsic issues of the workplace environment, the basis of compassion fatigue seems due to internal qualities of the care provider: giving high levels of energy and compassion over a prolonged period to those who are suffering, often without experiencing the positive outcomes of seeing patients improve (44,45). Joinson initially described the phenomenon of compassion fatigue in 1992, a concept derived from research on burnout in emergency department nurses (10). She suggested that compassion fatigue was "a unique form of burnout that affects people in care giving profession" (10,44,46). She noted particular behaviors characteristic of compassion fatigue in "cancer-care providers," which included the following: chronic fatigue, irritability, dread going to work, aggravation of physical ailments, and a lack of joy in life (44).

Some investigators purport that the "cost of caring" (47) for patients with cancer and other chronic life-limiting diseases in which deep emotional, empathic investment is made undergirds the concept of compassion fatigue. They suggest that repeated exposure to highly emotional care, often with frequent losses, is akin to post-traumatic stress disorder (PTSD). Compassion fatigue has also been described as *secondary trauma* or *vicarious trauma*—a consequence of trauma of another rather than trauma to oneself (36,47,48). It is characterized by classic symptomatology of PTSD, including recurring and intrusive thoughts, avoidance, and emotional hyper-arousal. Compassion fatigue can lead to burnout (36,48).

Orlovsky (44,49) helped to differentiate compassion fatigue from job dissatisfaction or frustration with the organizational mechanics of the workplace. Compassion fatigue may be considered a loss of the continued "ability to nurture" (46) as it relates to loss of empathic restoration due to repeated encounters with those dying from their chronic diseases. Although one may be unable to nurture anymore and is suffering from compassion fatigue or perhaps is even burned out, there can still exist a degree of compassion satisfaction. *Compassion satisfaction*, as noted by Stamm in 2002 (50), is defined as "the positive benefits that helping professionals derive from working with traumatized or suffering persons and the degree to which they feel successful in their jobs." Therefore, it is appears possible to experience compassion fatigue concomitantly with compassion satisfaction. Furthermore, research conducted by Costa (51) postulates that compassion satisfaction subdues compassion fatigue and burnout.

Reviewing the limited, but growing, body of literature on the phenomenon of compassion fatigue has yielded many descriptions of the caregiver's experience. Emotions include discontentment, depression, and loss of self-worth, in addition to feelings of mental and physical exhaustion (10,33,36,79). Although none of these emotions is wholly unique to compassion fatigue per se, it is in a context of simultaneous expression of such characteristics that compassion fatigue manifests itself. It is normal for a health-care provider to feel exhausted, both physically and emotionally, at times during one's career. However, it is the loss of the caregiver's ability to be an empathic witness for one's patients and their families that constitutes compassion fatigue. Colloquially, compassion fatigue has been characterized as when "the well runs dry" or when one's "cup is empty" and is unable to be replenished (44). For our purposes, we consider compassion fatigue to be a unique form of burnout that occurs earlier on the "trajectory" of job burnout where there is the loss of "ability to nurture" (46). It is a phenomenon where timely and upstream intervention can ameliorate its vastly devastating effects. Interventions are listed in Table 56.2.

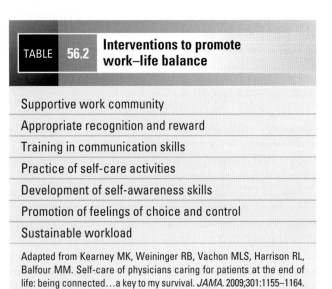

TABLE 56.2	Interventions to promote work–life balance
Supportive work community	
Appropriate recognition and reward	
Training in communication skills	
Practice of self-care activities	
Development of self-awareness skills	
Promotion of feelings of choice and control	
Sustainable workload	

Adapted from Kearney MK, Weininger RB, Vachon MLS, Harrison RL, Balfour MM. Self-care of physicians caring for patients at the end of life: being connected…a key to my survival. *JAMA.* 2009;301:1155–1164.

ETIOLOGIES/MANIFESTATIONS OF COMPASSION FATIGUE

In a study examining the prevalence of burnout in oncologists in the United States, 61% of the more than 1,700 physicians that were surveyed possessed symptoms suggestive of burnout as defined by Maslach's assessment tool (36,39). Research has demonstrated that young physicians are more prone to burnout than their older counterparts, the sentiments of which are speculated to start as early as residency (1,52). Nearly, one-quarter of medical residents who were surveyed in a study by Cohen and Patten would likely pursue a career other than medicine if they were able likely due to long work hours, heavy workload, little autonomy, and control (1,53). Additional risk factors for burnout found in this demographic included unmarried individuals—particularly those who had never married; poor self-esteem; external locus of control situations in which individuals allow themselves to be governed by circumstances over which they feel a lack of control—the "victim mentality" (6); personality traits of perfectionism, workaholism, and/or type A personality (1,54).

One might ask, why is compassion fatigue, or burnout, significant, particularly in the medical world? These phenomena are associated with negative clinical adverse events such as increased medical errors and less optimal patient care and some studies purport that patient adherence and compliance to prescribed medical regimens, both in the outpatient setting and post acute care discharge, are also diminished. In a study examining the effects of workload on physicians' quality of care, Firth-Cozens and Greenhalgh found that 57% of those studied purported that exhaustion, fatigue, or sleep deprivation resulted in suboptimal patient care (1,55). Additional studies further highlight the dangers of fatigue, tiredness, and sleep deprivation in health-care professionals as sleep deprivation was noted to be more incapacitating than a high blood alcohol concentration (1,56). Again, these symptoms are not unique to physicians, nurses, and other health-care professionals, but are noteworthy due to the work demands, particularly longer work hours, experienced by these professionals (1,69) and the negative consequences to patient care.

Professionally, burned out health-care providers have experienced increased absenteeism, decreased productivity, and increased job turnover (6,16,19,34,57–59). Such loss of physician power is costly to organizations as it has to recruit additional work force and is also counter-productive to those team members that remain, as their workload often increases in response to the loss. The expense of replacing a physician who is lost to burnout, which includes the advertising, interviewing, and use of a locums tenens to fill the void, was estimated at $150,000 to 300,000 according to one study (1,60). Although one does not often consider medicine from a consumer service perspective, it is ultimately the consumer (patient and family member) who suffers the greatest from physicians' and other caregivers' compassion fatigue and burnout, as continuity of care is sacrificed. Patients who trust and have confidence in their physicians because of the physician's job satisfaction are more likely to comply with the prescribed regimen of care (13,61).

Physicians are noted to have greater job stress and emotional distress than the general population with burnout rates ranging from 24% to 75% in some studies (1,52,62–66). It is not surprising that clinicians in oncology are more vulnerable to burnout due to the intensity and frequency of losses in the field (10,67). With respect to oncology nursing burnout, the following stress factors have been identified: the nature of the cancer, complex treatments, death, a personal sense of failure and futility, intense involvement with patients and families, ethical issues in treatment, surrogate decision-making, and palliative care issues (44,68). The issues, although identified in nursing literature, are likely applicable to the entire interdisciplinary team caring for the individual patient.

Physicians were also found to work longer hours per week (50 to 60 h/wk) even when not on call (1,69). Over the last decade, the Accreditation Council of Graduate Medical Education (ACGME)—the organization responsible for resident and fellow physicians' training in the United States—has become interested in the amount of duty hours spent in the hospital and on call by these physicians. There are now stringent guidelines in place to ensure that house staff are able to sleep and have time for self-care. Research efforts have shown that more serious medical mistakes are made by those physicians working shifts longer than 24 hours compared with those working less hours (1,70). Therefore, it is easily demonstrable how fatigue, lack of restorative sleep, and an increased workload might have negative consequences on the health-care provider's overall well-being.

More interestingly, researchers investigating the negative impact of stress upon one's physical being found abnormal biological markers, including ketonuria (indicative of starvation), cardiac arrhythmias, and heart rate abnormalities on examination of subjects (71). In a study of the association between workload and burnout in intensive care unit physicians, these findings correlated with more intense workloads and were factors suggestive of future burnout (72). With this objective evidence, one might be better able to conceptualize that burnout is not merely a subjective phenomenon, but it gives merit to stress serving as the forerunner to disease.

Occupational injuries such as percutaneous needle sticks (1,73) increase with fatigue and lack of attentiveness. For individuals working 16 consecutive hours or more, a rise in medical errors occurred due to lack of attentiveness (1,74). In addition, these factors are also likely culprits in the increased motor vehicle accidents noted within the profession.

Physician personal lives are also impacted by such rigorous work hours and demanding workloads. Researchers have found that substance abuse and increased alcohol use are often evident in the lives of those providers who have a difficult time with the person–job fit due to factors, both intrinsic and extrinsic (2–5,9,14,15,36). These negative coping mechanisms of avoidance and denial underscore how this type of self-medication can be a slippery slope, as often there are real underlying psychiatric disorders (depression, anxiety, and suicide) that should be professionally addressed (1,75,76). Interpersonal relations, those that are considered beneficial in protecting one from burnout, often suffer as a result of unrecognized and untreated compassion fatigue and burnout (2–5).

SELF-CARE

Characterizing compassion fatigue and burnout helps delineate where things can go wrong. For more sustainable professional development—including within the fields of oncology and palliative medicine—one must routinely incorporate principles of self-care. These deliberate practices help to ensure self-preservation and daily restoration of the care provider; they function to keep work–life balance at greater equilibrium, lessening the effects of compassion fatigue that can lead to burnout (44,49). It should be noted, however, that one may likely never find a true, static steady state/balance, as the stressors and factors, both internal and external, that influence work–life balance are dynamic, lifelong, and in a state of continuous flux (77). Therefore, it is important for one to recognize and understand multiple variables that impact an individual's perception of the world around them, both personally and professionally, and how one reacts to the stressful situations it evokes.

It might be helpful for one to conceptualize stress as a multidimensional entity that has repercussions that are expressed in as many ways. In the palliative care world, Dame Cicely Saunders, who put extensive efforts in the development of modern hospice care, theorized a model for total pain. She postulated that pain, in its finer analysis, is a constellation of physical, social, psychological, and spiritual pain elements, coexisting in one individual, with dynamic interplay on the other. Using this paradigm of total pain as an example, one might consider an analogous model of *total stress*. Total stress is then influenced by physical, social, psychological, and spiritual factors (Fig. 56.1). The interplay of these components can either ameliorate or exacerbate one's stress response.

Implementation of self-care practices into one's routine can be challenging. As busy health-care professionals with seemingly limited time resources and other constraints, taking care of one's main tool, oneself, is often neglected. However, although discrete data are lacking, daily participation in self-care practices that address all domains of "total stress" is likely beneficial in preventing or combating compassion fatigue and burnout (Table 56.3). Clinical literature reinforces anecdotal findings that physicians often work when sick, self-medicate their ailments, and are less likely to be open about physical or mental illness as sharing these situations with colleagues, or even to have patients witness them, is thought to be perceived as a care provider's weakness and (medical) incompetence (1,78). This underscores the importance of obtaining preventative medical care, appropriate screening tests, and routine dental care as integral parts of self-care practices (77). However, as we have already discussed, not disclosing or recognizing one's limitations has profound negative influences on the care provider, the patient/families, and the organization (inadequate sleep and poor eating habits).

Wallace et al. (1) postulate a "conspiracy of silence" as it relates to poor coping abilities noted in some physicians. As stated above, traditionally, there is a culture in medicine that stigmatizes the one which appears weak and vulnerable. Realizing that stoicism can create untenable situations, care

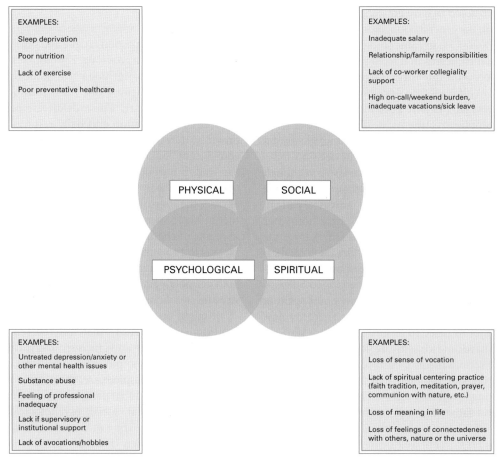

Figure 56.1. Conceptual model of total stress and examples.

providers must communicate to others what their needs are so that personal and professional productivity and efficiency are maintained. Care providers must come to expect the same of themselves, as it relates to personal self-care, as they hope for their patients.

Self-care research findings consistently show important trends. Physical activity, particularly exercise, is a key component to self-care and is consistently noted in the literature (77,79). Intuitively, exercise likely promotes overall general cardiovascular health in this population. As it has been suggested that the cardiovascular mortality in physicians is "higher than average," one might speculate that this is one intervention in the practitioner's control to help reduce stress and promote vigor and vitality (1). However, more studies are needed to determine the exact mechanisms of benefit of exercise in physicians versus the general public.

TABLE 56.3	**Table of self-care interventions**
Do	**Don't**
Honor yourself	Blame others
Recharge, renew daily: regular exercise program, mediation, a walk	Ignore the problem
Have a meaningful conversation each day; value time with family, friends	Complain to coworkers or look for a new job (make rash decisions)
Get enough sleep and rest	Self-medicate
Identify your own personal goals	Neglect your own needs, interests, and desires
Take some time off	Work harder and longer

Adapted from Showalter SE. Compassion fatigue: what is it? Why does it matter? Recognizing the symptoms, acknowledging the impact, developing the tools to prevent compassion fatigue, and strengthen the professional already suffering from the effects. *Am J Hosp Palliat Care*. 2010;27:239–242.

In order to be an effective care provider, one has to be not only physically but also emotionally well to function at a high and sustainable level of service. Thus, fostering interpersonal relationships (professionally with colleagues and personally with family members) is one protective mechanism against burnout (44,80–82). One mitigation strategy employed by Scandinavian researchers in burned out clinicians (physicians, nurses, therapists, and social workers) included the use of peer support groups (6,83). The culture of medicine suggests that physicians are reluctant to talk about their own health issues or distress or even those problems affecting their colleagues. This "conspiracy of silence" often fosters feelings of isolation without access to supportive resources (1,84).

Though the Interdisciplinary Care Team in hospice was created by Dame Saunders to facilitate the best care for the dying patient experiencing total pain, the interconnectedness of the various members of the team—doctor, nurse, chaplain, social worker, etc.—seemingly helps to balance the care-giving investment of any one provider. Saunders expressed that

> The care of the dying patient should not be an individual work but one that is shared. Shared with the relative with all the various members of the staff, spiritual, medical, and lay; and, as far as we can, with the patient himself. Where this is so we are left with the sense of completion and fulfillment which makes this such a rewarding branch of medical and nursing care (85).

In the late 1950s, Dr. Michael Balint, a psychoanalyst in the United Kingdom understood the dynamics of the doctor–patient relationship realizing that it can evoke considerable stress in the physician (44,80). Thus, he provided regular forums for physicians to meet and discuss challenging patients, as it was felt that such cathartic venues helped to stave off internal turmoil, stresses generated by such patients. In later years, continued emphasis has been placed on the importance of this type of group intervention for health-care providers in an effort to further combat compassion fatigue and burnout (44,81,82). It is the "presence" of other colleagues that lends support as empathic/sympathetic witnesses when one has encountered a difficult family member or a dying child; had to deliver bad news; or make a difficult decision to withdraw or forgo care in someone who has experienced an unexpected trauma. Challenges even occur when discussing any of the above clinical scenarios with nursing and other supportive staff caring for the patient/family who themselves are experiencing a difficult time with the clinical situation, from executing orders to grappling with their own morals and beliefs regarding difficult decisions, particularly at the end-of-life care.

Recent research examining burnout in intensive care unit physicians demonstrated that the quality of collegial relationships and the support derived from them are protective against compassion fatigue (71). In hospice care, this is known as the Interdisciplinary Team. Some postulate that because of this unique mandatory feature in hospice care—also common in oncology and palliative care— less burnout is experienced in palliative care practice than in oncology (36,86,87). This again underscores the importance

of communication and sharing the caregiver burden as it helps to increase compassion satisfaction, lessen compassion fatigue and hopefully, to prevent later burnout.

Communication, however, can be the source of great conflict, particularly in oncology and palliative care. Ramirez et al. noted that oncologists and other clinicians working with cancer patients were more susceptible to burning out if they felt poorly equipped to handle the emotional needs of this patient population (86). This ineffective doctor–patient communication dyad causes conflict in the workplace and can likely be a precipitant of burnout. Continued efforts must be invested into implementation of communication and interpersonal skills early on in medical education as research has proven it beneficial in building therapeutic alliance with patients, particularly those with cancer (44,86,88,89).

Spirituality remains an important, often overlooked area in holistic support of the patient and caregiver. Spirituality is often used interchangeably with religiosity and faith. However, spirituality also pertains to what gives meaning to one's life or experiences. As caregivers in oncology and palliative care repeatedly, often daily, encounter death and dying, they are witness to meaning-making experiences of their patients. Naturally, these interactions can and do bring pause to the health professional allowing for introspection and reflection regarding one's own significance and mortality. Several researchers have postulated that a clinician's spirituality or spiritual well-being is protective against burnout and is inversely related to burnout (90–92).

Personal accomplishment, one of the three domains of burnout that was discussed earlier, also seems to be a protective factor in preventing burnout. In those physician and nursing populations where the risk of burnout was deemed to be the highest, personal accomplishment was found to be "a buffering element" (6–8,93–95). Literature has demonstrated in populations where the other two domains of burnout were high (emotional exhaustion and depersonalization), if the sense of personal accomplishment was high, then burnout could be avoided. This is perhaps due to the influence of spirituality; how a caregiver's work gives meaning to another's life including their own (91).

From an institutional perspective, it may behoove the global medical profession to borrow from organizational management strategies researched and developed by Kaiser Permanante Medical Group over the last several years in their thrust to enhance physicians' professional satisfaction and job retention (96). They have recognized that in order to quell the severity of the experience of compassion fatigue, subsequent burnout, and eventual loss of their physician work pool, they must be more attentive to the needs of their physicians. Anticipating their needs prior to their official start times with the company, during the early affiliation/working for the organization, and throughout the tenure of their employment with the company is one of the ways that the organization has tried to achieve this. Striving to find and maintain a work-life balance is dynamic force changing from day to day, so are the needs of physicians/employees. King and Speckhart concluded that there exist 10 evidence-based practices that are needed for successful physician retention (96) (Table 56.4).

TABLE 56.4	Practice strategies for physician retention
Realistic job preview and behavioral interviewing
Essential startup resources and administrative processes planned and in place
Practical, timely, comprehensive orientation programs delivered in multiple ways
Physician enculturation, socialization, and fostering feelings of belonging
Mentoring program
Perceived control over the practice environment
Accurate, effective, and timely feedback
Recognition, rewards, and opportunities for advancement/career development
Open and trustworthy communication; belief that management listens and acts on suggestions
Reduction of stress in the workplace

Adapted from King H, Speckart C. Ten evidence-based practices for successful physician retention. *Perm J.* 2002;6:52–54.

Therefore, organizations, such as hospitals, health maintenance organizations, or physician practices, should reasonably attend to those institutional factors that will enhance physician job satisfaction and promote job engagement as much as possible. This is facilitated by prioritizing physicians' and health providers' needs in the organizational hierarchy such that there is a greater sense of control and autonomy in shaping the work environment with the aim of maintaining as ideal a person–job fit as possible (Table 56.4). In addition, Wallace et al. (1) suggest routinely measuring physician wellness as a quality of care indicator. These experts underscore how clinicians with high compassion fatigue provide substandard clinical care.

SUMMARY

As an empathic witness to a patient's stress and distress, caregivers must be able to respond to the emotional needs of the patient. This is best enhanced through effective communication skills (44,86). The corollary of this is that health-care providers in oncology and palliative care must practice recognizing their own limitations, when they feel "stressed out" or unable to find the appropriate words to effectively mediate difficult patient/family situations. There must be an impetus to move from tacit isolation to finding a voice to let others know that one needs help. Relationship building, rapport, and teamwork, where effective communication is timely and frequent, along with daily, multidimensional self-care interventions, are perhaps the most effective tools against compassion fatigue and subsequent burnout.

Traditionally, the medical education curriculum, however, has not met the needs of young clinicians in this regard. With more research and clarity on burnout and compassion fatigue, perhaps this awareness will trickle down to young trainees in the profession. Future research endeavors might focus on the field of palliative care, as it is a relatively new and growing discipline, to assess how self-care interventions affect rates of attrition and retention of its workforce.

Work–life balance is crucial to self-preservation and diminishing, if not preventing, compassion fatigue. One must set appropriate boundaries and expectations and recognize limitations so that the empathic presence required to help others is not emotionally depleted. If depleted, the caregiver may certainly become less productive or efficacious. Attention must be given to foster a sense of well-being and wholeness in the physicians and other health-care professionals to thwart the infectious and destructive pattern of burnout that permeates and threatens to undermine the future of medicine. If physicians, nurses, social workers, and chaplains are enduring more stress and feeling less supported and more overworked, they then are less likely to encourage subsequent generations to pursue careers in the profession, thus jeopardizing the quality of our health-care system (13).

REFERENCES

1. Wallace JE, Lemaire JB, Ghali WA. Physician wellness: a missing quality indicator. *Lancet.* 2009;374:1714-1721.
2. Sargent MC, Sotile W, Sotile MO, Rubash H, Barrack RL. Stress and coping among orthopaedic surgery residents and faculty. *J Bone Joint Surg Am.* 2004;86:1579-1586.
3. Firth-Cozens J. Individual and organizational predictors of depression in general practitioners. *Br J Gen Pract.* 1998;48:1647-1651.
4. Frank E, Dingle AD. Self-reported depression and suicide attempts among U.S. women physicians. *Am J Psychiatry.* 1999;156:1887-1894.
5. Graham J, Albery IP, Ramirez AJ, Richards MA. How hospital consultants cope with stress at work: implications for their mental health. *Stress Health.* 2001;17:85-89.
6. Hyman SA, Michaels DR, Berry JM, Schildcrout JS, Mercaldo ND, Weinger MB. Risk of burnout in perioperative clinicians: a survey study and literature review. *Anesthesiology.* 2011; 114:194-204.
7. Gabbe SG, Melville J, Mandel L, Walker E. Burnout in chairs of obstetrics and gynecology: diagnosis, treatment and prevention. *Am J Obstet Gynecol.* 2002;186:601-612.

8. Ramirez AJ, Graham J, Richards MA, Cull A, Gregory WM. Mental health of hospital consultants: the effects of stress and satisfaction at work. *Lancet*. 1996;347:724-728.

9. Spickard A Jr, Gabbe SG, Christensen JF. Mid-career burnout in generalist and specialist physicians. *JAMA*. 2002;288:1447-1450.

10. Potter P, Deshields T, Divanbeigi J, et al. Compassion Fatigue and Burnout: Prevalence Among Oncology Nurses. *Clin J Oncol Nurs*. 2010;14:e56-e62.

11. Ferrans C. Quality of life: conceptual issues. *Semin Oncol Nurs*. 1990;6:248-254.

12. Saint S, Zemencuk JK, Hayward RA, et al. What effect does increasing inpatient time have on outpatient-oriented internist satisfaction? *J Gen Intern Med*. 2003;18:725-729.

13. Scheurer D, McKean S, Miller J, Wetterneck T. U.S. physician satisfaction: a systematic review. *J Hosp Med*. 2009;4:560-568.

14. Brooke D, Edwards G, Taylor C. Addiction as an occupational hazard: 144 doctors with drug and alcohol problems. *Br J Addict*. 1991;86:1011-1016.

15. Juntunen J, Asp S, Olkinuora M, Aarimaa M, Strid L, Kauttu K. Doctors' drinking habits and consumption of alcohol. *BMJ*. 1988;297:951-954.

16. Ahola K, Kivimaki M, Honkonen T, et al. Occupational burnout and medically certified sickness absence: a population-based study of Finnish employees. *J Psychosom Res*. 2008;64:185-193.

17. Gardulf A, Soderstrom IL, Orton ML, Ericksson LE, Arnetz B, Nordstrom G. Why do nurses at a university hospital want to quit their jobs? *J Nurs Manage*. 2005;13:329-337.

18. Sharma A, Sharp DM, Walker LG, Monson JR. Stress and burnout among colorectal surgeons and colorectal nurse specialists working in the National Health Service. *Colorectal Dis*. 2008;10:397-406.

19. Borritz M, Rugulies R, Christensen KB, Villadsen E, Kristensen TS. Burnout as a predictor of self-reported sickness absence among human service workers: prospective findings from three year follow up of the PUMA study. *Occup Environ Med*. 2006;63:98-106.

20. Garelick AI, Gross SR, Richardson I, von der Tann M, Bland J, Hale R. Which doctors and with what problems contact a specialist service for doctors? *BMC Med*. 2007;5:26.

21. Rochester SR, Vachon MLS, Lyall WAL. Immediacy in language: a channel to care of the dying patient. *J Comp Psychol*. 1974;2:75-76.

22. Lyall WAL, Vachon MLS, Rogers J. A study of the degree of stress experienced by professionals caring for dying patients. In: Ajemian I, Mount BM, eds. *The RVH Manual on Hospice/ Palliative Care*. New York, NY: ARNO Press; 1980:498-508.

23. Grunfeld, E, Whelan TJ, Zitzelsberger L, et al. Cancer care workers in Ontario: prevalence of burnout, job stress and job satisfaction. *Can Med Assoc J*. 2000;163:166-169.

24. Grunfeld E, Zitzelsberger L, Coristine M, et al. Job stress and job satisfaction of cancer care workers. *Psychooncology*. 2005;14:61-69.

25. Keeton, K, Fenner DE, Johnson TRB, Hayward RA. Predictors of physician career satisfaction, work–life balance, and burnout. *Obstet Gynecol*. 2007;109:949-955.

26. Doan-Wiggins L, Zun L, Cooper MA, Meyers DL, Chen EH. Practice satisfaction, occupational stress, and attrition of emergency physicians. Wellness Task Force, Illinois College of Emergency Physicians. *Acad Emerg Med*. 1995;2:556-563.

27. Freeobrn DK. Satisfaction, commitment, and psychological well-being among HMO physicians. *West J Med*. 2001;174:13-18.

28. Gallery ME, Whitley TW, Klonic LK, Anzinger RK, Revicki, DA. A study of occupational stress and depression among emergency physicians. *Ann Emerg Med*. 1992;21:58-64.

29. Linzer M, Visser MR, Oort FJ, et al. Predicting and preventing physician burnout: results from the United States and Netherlands. *Am J Med*. 2001;111:170-175.

30. Freudenberger HJ. The staff burn-out syndrome in alternative institutions. *Psychother Theory, Res Pract*. 1971;12:73-82.

31. Freudenberger HJ. Burn-out: occupational hazard of the child care worker. *Child Care Q*. 1977;6:90-99.

32. Maslach C, Schaufeli WB, Leiter MP. Job burnout. *Ann Rev Psychol*. 2001;52:397-422.

33. Trufelli DC, Bensi CG, Garcia JB, et al. Burnout in cancer professionals: a systematic review and meta-analysis. *Eur J Cancer Care*. 2008;17:524-531.

34. Felton JS. Burnout as a clinical entity—its importance in health care workers. *Occup Med*. 1998;48:237-250.

35. Maslach C, Jackson S, Leiter MP. *Maslach Burnout Inventory Manual*. Palo Alto, CA: Consulting Psychologists Press; 1996.

36. Kearney MK, Weininger RB, Vachon MLS, Harrison RL, Balfour MM. Self-care of physicians caring for patients at the end of life: being connected … a key to my survival. *JAMA*. 2009;301:1155-1164.

37. Maslach C, Leiter MP. Early predictors of job burnout and engagement. *J Appl Psychol*. 2008;93:498-512.

38. Maslach C. Job burnout: new directions in research and intervention. *Curr Dir Psychol Sci*. 2003;12:189-192.

39. Allegra CJ, Hall R, Yothers G. Prevalence of burnout in the US oncology community. *J Oncol Pract*. 2005;1:140-147.

40. Kuerer HM, Eberlein TJ, Pollock RE, et al. Career satisfaction, practice patterns and burnout among surgical oncologists: report on the quality of life of members of the Society of Surgical Oncology. *Ann Surg Oncol*. 2007;14:3043-3053.

41. Elit L, Trim K, Mand-Bains IH, Sussman J, Grunfeld E; Society of Gynecologic Oncology Canada. Job satisfaction, stress, burnout among Canadian gynecologic oncologists. *Gynecol Oncol*. 2004;94:134-139.

42. Vachon MLS, Sherwood C. Staff stress and burnout. In: Berger AM, Shuster DL Jr, Von Roenn JH, eds. *Principles and Practice of Palliative Oncology and Supportive Oncology*. Philadelphia, PA: Lippincott, Williams and Wilkins; 2007:667-683.

43. French JRP, Rodgers W, Cobb S. Adjustment as person–environment fit. In: Coelho GV, Hamburg DA, Adams E, eds. *Coping and Adaptation*. New York, NY: Basic Books; 1974; 316-333.

44. Najjar N, Davis LW, Beck-Coon K, Doebbeling CC. Compassion fatigue: a review of the research to date and relevance to cancer-care providers. *J Health Psychol*. 2009;14:267-277.

45. McHolm F. Rx for compassion fatigue. *J Christ Nurs*. 2006; 23:12-19;quiz 20-11.

46. Joinson C. Coping with compassion fatigue. *Nursing*. 1992; 22:116-121.

47. Figley CR, ed. *Compassion Fatigue: Coping with Secondary Traumatic Stress Disorder in Those Who Treat the Traumatized*. New York, NY: Brunner/Mazel; 1995:7-12.

48. Figley CR, ed. *Treating Compassion Fatigue*. New York, NY: Brunner-Routledge; 2002.

49. Orlovsky C. Compassion fatigue. *Prairie Rose*. 2006;75:13.

50. Stamm B. Measuring compassion fatigue as well as fatigue: developmental history of the compassion satisfaction and fatigue testing. In: Figley C, ed. *Treating Compassion Fatigue*. New York, NY: Brunner-Routledge; 2002.

51. Costa D. Compassion fatigue: self-care skills for practitioners. *OT Pract*. 2005;10:13-18.

52. Shanafelt TD, Bradley KA, Wipf JW, Back AL. Burnout and self-reported patient care in an internal medicine residency program. *Ann Intern Med*. 2002;136:358-367.

53. Cohen JS, Patten S. Well being in residency training: a survey examining resident physician satisfaction both within and outside of residency training and mental health in Alberta. *BMC Med Educ*. 2005;5:21.

54. Firth-Cozens J, King J. Are psychological factors linked to performance? In: Firth-Cozens J, King J, Hutchinson A, McAvoy P, eds. *Understanding Doctors' Performance.* Oxford: Radcliffe Publishing; 2006.

55. Firth-Cozens J, Greenhalgh J. Doctors' perceptions of the links between stress and lowered clinical care. *Soc Sci Med.* 1997;44:1017-1022.

56. Williamson AM, Feyer AM. Moderate sleep deprivation produces impairments in cognitive and motor performance equivalent to legally prescribed levels of alcohol intoxication. *Occup Environ Med.* 2000;57:649-655.

57. Middaugh DJ. Presenteeism: sick and tired at work. *Dermatol Nurs.* 2007;19:172-173,185.

58. Pilette PC. Presenteeism in nursing: a clear and present danger to productivity. *J Nurs Adm.* 2005;35:300-303.

59. Toppinen-Tanner S, Ojajarvi A, Vaananen A, Kalimo R, Japinen P. Burnout as a predictor of medically certified sick-leave absences and their diagnosed causes. *Behav Med.* 2005;31:18-27.

60. Shi L. *Managing Human Resources in Health Care Organizations.* 1st ed. Sudbury, MA: Jones and Bartlett; 2006.

61. DiMatteo MR, Sherbourne CD, Hays RD, et al. Physicians' characteristics influence patients' adherence to medical treatment: results from the Medical Outcomes Study. *Health Psychol.* 1993;12: 93-102.

62. Fahrenkopf AM, Sectish TC, Barger LK, et al. Rates of medication errors among depressed and burnt out residents: prospective cohort study. *BMJ.* 2008;336:488-491.

63. Goehring C, Bouvier Gallacchi M, Kunzi B, Bovier P. Psychological and professional characteristics of burnout in Swiss primary care practitioners: a cross-sectional survey. *Swiss Med Wkly.* 2005;135:101-108.

64. Panagopoulou EA, Montgomery A, Benos A. Burnout in internal medicine physician: differences between residents and specialists. *Eur J Intern Med.* 2006;17:195-200.

65. Renzi C, Tabolli S, Ianni A, Di Petro C, Puddo P. Burnout and job satisfaction comparing healthcare staff of a dermatological hospital and a general hospital. *J Eur Acad Dermatol Venerol.* 2005;19:153-157.

66. Goitein L, Shanafelt TD, Wipf JE, Slatore CG, Back AL. The effects of work-hour limitations on resident well being, patient care, and education in an internal medicine residency program. *Arch Intern Med.* 2005;165(22):2601-2606.

67. Lewis AE. Reducing burnout: development of an oncology staff bereavement program. *Oncol Nurs Forum.* 1999;26:1065-1069.

68. Kash K, Breitbart W. The stress of caring for cancer patients. In: Breitbart W, Holland JC, eds. *Psychiatric Aspects of Symptom Management in Cancer Patients.* Washington, DC: American Psychiatric Press; 1993:243-260.

69. Williams ES, Rondeau KV, Xiao Q, Francescutti LH. Heavy physician workloads: impact on physician attitudes and outcomes. *Health Serv Manage Res.* 2007;20:261-269.

70. O'Connor C, Adhikari NK, DeCaire K, Friedrich JO. Medical admission order sets to improve deep vein thrombosis prophylaxis rates and other outcomes. *J Hosp Med.* 2009;4:81-89.

71. Embriaco N, Papazian L, Kentish-Barnes N, Pochard F, Azoulay E. Burnout syndrome among critical care healthcare workers. *Curr Opin Crit Care.* 2007;13:482-488.

72. Parshuram C, Dhanni S, Kirsch J, Cox P. Fellowship training, workload, fatigue and physical stress: a prospective observational study. *CMAJ.* 2004;170:965-970.

73. Ayas NT, Barger LK, Cade BE, et al. Extended work duration and the risk of self-reported percutaneous injuries in interns. *JAMA.* 2006;296:1055-1062.

74. Lockley SW, Cronin JW, Evans EE, et al. for the Harvard Work Hours, Health and Safety Group. Effect of reducing interns' weekly work hours on sleep and attentional failures. *N Engl J Med.* 2004;351:1829-1837.

75. Baldisseri MR. Impaired healthcare professional. *Crit Care Med.* 2007;35(suppl):S106-S116.

76. Firth-Cozens J. Interventions to improve physicians' well being and patient care. *Soc Sci Med.* 2001;52:215-222.

77. Chittenden EH, Ritchie CS. Work–life balancing: challenges and strategies. *J Palliat Med.* 2011;14:870-874.

78. Thompson WT, Cupples ME, Sibbett CH, Skan DI, Bradley T. Challenges of Culture, Conscience, and Contract to General Practitioners' 2008; 63 care of their own health: qualitative study. *BMJ.* 2001;323:728-731.

79. Showalter SE. Compassion fatigue: what is it? Why does it matter? Recognizing the symptoms, acknowledging the impact, developing the tools to prevent compassion fatigue, and strengthen the professional already suffering from the effects. *Am J Hosp Palliat Care.* 2010;27:239-242.

80. Balint M. *The Doctor, His Patient and the Illness.* New York, NY: International University Press; 1957.

81. Benson J, Magraith K. Compassion fatigue and burnout. *Aust Fam Physician.* 2005;34:497-498.

82. Lyckholm, L. Dealing with stress, burnout, and grief in the practice of oncology. *Lancet Oncol.* 2001;2:750-755.

83. Peterson U, Bergstrom G, Samuelsson M, Asberg M, Nygren A. Reflecting peer-support groups in the prevention of stress and burnout: randomized controlled trail. *J Adv Nurs.* 2008;63: 506-516.

84. Arnetz BB. Psychological challenges facing physicians of today. *Soc Sci Med.* 2001;52:203-213.

85. Saunders C. The last achievement. *Nurs Times.* 1976;72: 1247-1249.

86. Ramirez A, Graham J, Richards M, et al. Burnout and psychiatric disorder among cancer clinicians. *Br J Cancer.* 1995;71:1263-1269.

87. Vachon MLS. Staff stress in hospice/palliative care: a review. *Palliat Med.* 1995;9:91-122.

88. Gysels M, Richardson A, Higginson IJ. Communication training for health professionals who care for patients with cancer: a systematic review of effectiveness. *Support Care Cancer.* 2004;12:692-700.

89. Fellowes D, Wikinson S, Moore P. Communication skills training for health care professionals working with cancer patients, their families and/or carers. *Cochrane Database System Rev.* 2004:(2) CD003751.

90. Harrison RL, Westwood MJ. Preventing vicarious traumatization of mental health therapists: identifying protective practices. *Psychother Theory Res Pract Train.* In Press. 2009;46(2): 203-219.

91. Boston PH, Mount BM. The caregiver's perspective on existential and spiritual distress in palliative care. *J Pain Symptom Manage.* 2006;32:13-26.

92. Huggard PK. *Managing Compassion Fatigue: Implications for Medical Education* [dissertation]. Aukland, New Zealand: University of Aukland; 2008.

93. Johns MM 3rd, Ossoff RH. Burnout in academic chairs of otolaryngology: head and neck surgery. *Laryngoscope.* 2005;115:2056-2061.

94. Bertges YW, Eshelman A, Raoufi M, Aboujoud MS. A national study of burnout among American transplant surgeons. *Transplant Proc.* 2005;37:1399-1401.

95. Guntupalli KK, Fromm RE Jr. Burnout in the internist–intensivist. *Intensive Care Med.* 1996;22625-22630.

96. King H, Speckart C. Ten evidence-based practices for successful physician retention. *Perm J.* 2002;6:52-54.

Ethical Considerations in Palliative Care

CHAPTER 57

Advance Directives, Decision Making, and Withholding and Withdrawing Treatment

Christine Grady

Advance directives and advance care planning evolved as a response to the wishes of most people to have some control over their medical care now and into the future. Advance directives were conceived of as a way to give individuals some control over future treatment and care decisions by providing an opportunity to specify choices and preferences in advance for use at a time when they might be too sick or incapacitated to participate in making decisions themselves. Progress in our ability to prolong life through the use of available technologies especially over the last several decades has increased awareness of the challenges of deciding when and how to employ such technologies. Public attention about the complexities of making decisions about end-of-life care and treatment, especially in the face of uncertainty about individuals' previously expressed wishes, was stirred up by publicly debated cases such as Nancy Cruzan and Terry Schiavo (1,2). Most Americans die in the hospital, although an estimated 80% say they want to die at home. More than half a million Americans die of cancer annually, often supported by technology in the impersonal and isolated environment of an intensive care unit. Only an estimated 10% of people dying in intensive care can make decisions for themselves (3). Alzheimer's dementia is increasingly common in the United States and a leading cause of death in people over 65 years of age (4). A study of elderly Americans who had died showed that approximately 30% required decision making at the end of life but lacked decision-making capacity (5). Facilitating treatment decisions, including those about treatment at the end of life, is essential for patients who cannot make decisions for themselves and for the patients' loved ones.

The US Patient Self-Determination Act of 1990 requires all Medicare participating healthcare facilities to provide patients with information about their rights to make healthcare decisions, to ask patients at admission about advance directives, and to provide further information if desired (6). In the United States, all 50 states and the District of Columbia have statutes that support advance directives and make it permissible for physicians to follow them without fear of liability. Although there are some differences among state statutes, most allow the use of instructional directives and/or the designation of a proxy decision maker for healthcare decisions, and many states honor documents completed in accordance with another state's laws. Meisel et al. pointed out that even if the legal formalities are not all met, written advance directives, as well as oral statements previously made

by patients, can help to guide decisions about treatment (7). Available online resources allow anyone to download the specific forms and instructions for advance directives from each of the 50 states (8). State-specific forms are also available from state or municipal Departments of Health, hospitals, and some physicians' offices. Forms and instructions are often available in languages besides English and sometimes can be found online, for example, Spanish and Chinese language California forms are available at http://coalitionccc.org/advance-health-planning.php. Recent initiatives in certain states provide the opportunity for individuals to complete their advance directive online and store it in a registry (9). Advance Directive/Living Will Registries are public or proprietary databases that electronically store advance directives and make them available to patients and providers when they are needed.

TYPES OF ADVANCE DIRECTIVES

Traditionally, there are two distinct general types of advance directives: the instructional directive and designation of a proxy. Most available forms—developed at the state level or by specialty organizations—allow one or the other or both. An instructional directive is a tool that allows an individual to express preferences or give instructions about future medical treatment and care for such a time when the individual is no longer able to make his or her own decisions. One of the earliest instructional directives, the living will, gives individuals the opportunity to state in writing their desire to accept or refuse a limited set of life-prolonging treatments, such as cardiopulmonary resuscitation (CPR) or artificial ventilation, under certain conditions.

Unfortunately, early living will statements of preference were often written so nonspecifically that they were not very effective in guiding treatment decisions. Over time, there were efforts to make instructional directives more treatment specific, to develop directives that better articulated patients' general values and beliefs, and to use validated predrafted instructional directives (10–13).

Designating a proxy to make decisions at such a time a person cannot make them for himself or herself is the other traditional advance directive option. The designated proxy is referred to by several names, including Durable Power of Attorney for Health Care (DPA), Health Care Agent, Health Care Proxy, or medical power of attorney, often depending on the state laws. Importantly, a DPA or medical power of attorney is distinct from a traditional power of attorney, which is a legal document that grants a proxy jurisdiction over financial and personal matters, an issue that sometimes causes confusion.

Most people who have completed advance directives have assigned a DPA. Instructional directives and assignment of a DPA are complementary and patients may be well served by both designating a DPA and providing instructions. Assigning a DPA or proxy is helpful because it is difficult to anticipate many possible future healthcare situations and decisions, and specific instructions related to held preferences are helpful, since these can provide welcome guidance for the assigned DPA and medical team when making decisions.

Unfortunately, despite considerable efforts, evidence accumulated that advance directives were not as successful in facilitating patient-centered decisions at the end of life as originally anticipated (14). Large studies found that a relatively small percentage (20% to 30%) of patients—even seriously ill patients—had advance directives and that even when an advance directive existed it often had limited influence on treatment decisions at the end of life (15). Hickman et al. described several reasons that might explain the limitations on the usefulness of advance directives including (1) disproportionate focus on the legal right to refuse treatment rather than understanding patients' underlying goals and values; (2) vague or unclear instructions or expressions of patients' wishes (such as "Don't keep me alive if I am a vegetable"); (3) inadequate attention to ongoing discussion and re-evaluation of previously expressed preferences; (4) little attention to integrating planning into clinical care; (5) narrowly privileging individual autonomy rather than recognizing the importance of social networks and relationships; (6) difficulty and significant stress for the designated proxy when asked to make decisions because of inadequate discussion about values and goals; and (7) uncertainty about whether the patient would want decisions to be made using a substituted judgment standard or want their proxies to take other considerations into account (16). Others pointed out that practical details such as where an advanced directive is kept and who knows about it often make it difficult or impossible to honor. A Pew Research Center's 2006 survey found that over the years since the Patient Self-Determination Act, more people are thinking about and planning for their own medical treatment in the event of a terminal illness or incapacitating medical condition. About 42% of their survey cohort had experienced a friend or relative's terminal illness or coma in the previous 5 years, and the issue of withholding life-sustaining treatment came up for the majority. In addition, most Americans are aware of living wills and in 2005, 29% said they had one compared with 12% in 1990 (17). Two studies that evaluated advance directives among elderly Americans who had recently died found that about two-thirds of the total (18), or of those who needed surrogate decision making, had an advance directive (19). Studies have shown that people who are older, have serious diseases and certain types of disease such as cancer, are Caucasian, of a relatively high socioeconomic status, know about advance directives, have a positive attitude toward end-of-life discussions, and have a long-standing relationship with their primary care physician are more likely to have an advance directive (6).

Focus on advance care planning as well as expansion of the types of advance directive processes and forms and complementary initiatives have attempted to preserve the goal of advancing patient autonomy and respect for surviving interests. Initiatives such as Five Wishes, Let Me Decide, Respecting Choices, Physicians Orders for Life-Sustaining Treatment (POLST) paradigm, and others have aimed to find ways to provide patients with the opportunity to direct some future treatment decisions, while trying to overcome some of the previously documented challenges. "Five Wishes" includes appointment of a proxy and documentation of a range of issues that people might care about but are not usually included in a traditional advance directive, including emotional, spiritual, and personal needs (20). "Let Me Decide" was developed in Canada based on empirical research and the booklet and forms have been translated into multiple languages. The program offers patients and families an opportunity to document choices about level of care, nutrition, CPR, and treatment of life-threatening illness (21). "Respecting Choices" began in Lacrosse Wisconsin through the Gundersen Lutheran Hospital system as a community-wide planning system (22). It uses a staged approach to advance care planning, emphasizes training of physicians and healthcare providers and advance care planning facilitators, and encourages the use of hospice and palliative care services. Besides the fact that most Lacrosse residents have advance directives, the hospital system has experienced a reduced number of hospital days at the end of life and lowered Medicare spending compared with other centers. Ironically, this successful program urged coverage for end-of-life conversations between physicians and patients that was labeled "death panels" and pulled from consideration as part of the 2010 health care reform proposals (23). POLST is a system of advance care planning and documentation that offers patients an opportunity to indicate the types of life-sustaining treatment that they want and converts their preferences into written medical orders (on a brightly colored form) that transfer with patients across treatment settings (24). POLST is an actionable medical order that can be based on a previously completed advance directive or on expressed wishes for patients who do not have advance directives. Patients are informed about available treatment options for their current conditions and their preferences for CPR, feeding tubes, and other medical treatments are discussed. These wishes are then documented on a standardized medical order form. Healthcare providers in hospitals or nursing homes agree to honor these orders in an effort to improve the quality of end-of-life care. POLST enables patients to make choices about care options that range from aggressive treatment to limited interventions to comfort care.

ADVANCE CARE PLANNING

The process of advance care planning encompasses a number of important and related activities, including discussion of clinical circumstances, prognosis, and goals in context, deliberation and communication about values and goals, and the development of plans and preferences for future care to approximate those goals (25). Advance care planning is a more iterative and interactive process than simply filling out an advance directive and precedes and surrounds the completion of a written advance directive (Chapter 57). As part of an advance care planning process, healthcare providers give patients and families information about the patient's current clinical circumstances, likely trajectory and possibilities, and available treatment options. Discussion of the patient's values and goals can help guide clinicians and proxy decision makers when called upon later to make decisions. Any plans and decisions made and documented should be revisited if possible whenever the patient's clinical or social situation changes or when a patient wishes to re-examine the goals or directives. A written advance directive serves as documentation of decisions made through the process of advance care planning and connects the process of deliberation with specification about who and how decisions will be made for the patient in the future.

HELPING PATIENTS CHOOSE AND ASSIGN A HEALTHCARE PROXY OR DPA

Physicians and other healthcare providers can do several things to help patients and the selected DPA understand important aspects of selecting a healthcare proxy or DPA. The patient should be reassured that his or her DPA will only be invoked and asked to make decisions, when the patient is unable to make decisions for himself/herself, after a determination of decision-making capacity. (Assessment of decision-making capacity is addressed below.) Both patient and DPA should be informed that, when invoked, the DPA will have the authority to make all treatment and care decisions that the patient would be asked to make if he or she were able. These might include decisions about treatment options, choosing a doctor, a caregiver, and a place of care, accepting or refusing medical treatments including life-sustaining treatments, making discharge and transfer decisions, and authorizing the release of medical information, among others.

Most commonly, a DPA is asked to make decisions based on the patient's previously expressed wishes. However, in situations where previously expressed wishes do not provide sufficient or any guidance, the DPA might be asked to use their knowledge of the patient to imagine what the patient would have wanted and make a decision using "substituted judgment." Substituted judgment is a complex concept and can be very hard to implement, especially when the patient is in a situation that neither he/she nor the DPA had previously considered or discussed. When substituted judgment is not feasible, the DPA may be asked to make decisions based on the patient's best interests. Some individuals may want to specifically authorize their DPA to have more discretion or instruct them to consult with other family members or loved ones when making health-related decisions. Data suggest that surrogates often do rely on other factors, including their own best interests or mutual interests that they share with the patient (26).

Physicians and other healthcare providers should inform patients and their designated DPAs about growing evidence that shows that proxies, even or especially those who are close to the patient, are not very good at accurately guessing what patients would have wanted and often choose more aggressive care than the patient would have chosen (27). Although there is limited evidence, more specific and frequent discussion during the advance care planning process about medical aspects of end-of-life care, especially circumstances or types of treatments that the patient cares strongly about, could be helpful. Making decisions for a loved one can be emotionally difficult for the DPA and other family and close friends. Surrogates are sometimes left with feelings of stress, guilt, and doubt, but knowing that the treatment selected was consistent with the patient's preferences appears to reduce the negative effect on surrogates (28). Sometimes the emotional burden of making end-of-life decisions and letting go of a loved one can also present conflicts for the DPA about what decisions to make.

In light of these considerations, patients may need some assistance in deliberating and deciding when choosing a DPA or healthcare agent and the opportunity to discuss it with a healthcare provider. For legal and practical reasons, the person designated as DPA should be an adult (usually 18 years or older to be legally able to serve as a proxy) and someone who will be available when needed and willing to speak on the patient's behalf. In addition, the DPA should be someone the patient trusts, who knows the patient well, understands the patient's values and beliefs, will be comfortable asking questions to the healthcare team and advocating for the patient even at emotionally difficult times, and who is willing to make decisions that represent the patient's wishes and values. Sometimes, for well-considered reasons, a patient will choose a DPA who is not the most obvious choice, for example, selecting a sister as DPA instead of a spouse or a friend instead of a parent. Although there may be very good reasons for these choices, the patient may need support in making and communicating this decision to their loved ones.

Once an agent is chosen and agrees to be the DPA, it should be documented (with DPA's name and contact information) on an advance directive form and copies given to the patient, the DPA, the primary physician, and when appropriate placed in the medical record. Many advance directive forms also ask patients to designate an alternate, which is very useful in the event that the primary DPA is unavailable or no longer willing or able to serve in this role. The patient should be encouraged to talk with the designated DPA about treatment preferences and values that are important to him/her and that will help the DPA make health-related decisions on the patient's behalf. Healthcare providers can provide information about the kinds of choices people might need to make and can guide patients and their DPAs to be as specific as possible in these discussions and to repeat the discussions periodically, and especially whenever there are important health or life changes.

HELPING PATIENTS COMPLETE INSTRUCTIONAL DIRECTIVES

Most instructions that are available to guide patients in completing living wills and other instructional directives recommend discussion about certain interventions used in serious illnesses, including mechanical ventilation, CPR, dialysis, chemotherapy or radiation, blood transfusions, and pain control. Patients often need information about what these interventions are, how they might be utilized, and the advantages or disadvantages of choosing them under certain circumstances. Healthcare providers can offer patients realistic and accessible information about these and other interventions and provide an opportunity for discussion and questions. Certain individuals may already have strong preferences for or against certain interventions based on previous experience with a friend or a relative or exposure to the issue through a news story, a movie, or other experience. Strong preferences should be explored to ensure that they are based on a realistic understanding of the interventions involved. Patients who want to make and document specific decisions regarding certain interventions might want to write out their preferences clearly or might find the use of certain validated and predrafted instruments helpful. For example, the medical directive describes a number of situations and then presents choices for the patient to make (29). One scenario, for example, asks the patient to consider the following situation and choose one of the options below it.

> If I am in a coma or a persistent vegetative state and, in the opinion of my physician and two consultants, have no known hope of regaining awareness and higher mental functions no matter what is done, then my goals and specific wishes—if medically reasonable—for this and any additional illness would be

- Prolong life; Treat everything
- Attempt to cure, but re-evaluate often
- Limit to less invasive and less burdensome interventions
- Provide comfort care only
- Other (please specify)

For some patients it may be more useful to discuss general parameters and use these as guides to their wishes rather than to make a series of specific treatment decisions. With either choice of writing instructions, it is helpful to inform patients that it is very difficult to imagine all the possible interventions that may need to be decided upon.

Whether using a predrafted or open-ended format, patient preferences should be documented in writing whenever possible. Most states require one or more witnesses who

are asked to sign the instructional advance directive form. The designated DPA/proxy or the physician should not serve as witnesses. Some states require advance directives to be notarized. Written instructions can be very useful, but are usually more useful in guiding decision making when complemented by discussions with proxies, family members, physicians, and others who might be involved in later decisions. As described above with documentation of a DPA, copies of instructional directives should be available to the patient, the DPA, the primary physician, and when appropriate put in the medical record.

Advance directives do not automatically expire, although it is wise for patients to periodically revisit their choices and any specific parameter that they set. A capacitated patient can change or revoke an advance directive at any time. Once the patient loses capacity, the advance directive will be activated.

ASSESSING DECISION-MAKING CAPACITY

When possible, patients should be allowed to make health-related decisions for themselves. When a patient lacks or loses the capacity to make decisions, the DPA or surrogate will become the legal decision maker for health-related decisions. Deciding when a DPA should be called upon to make decisions or when a patient is unable to make decisions for himself/herself is rarely straightforward. Sometimes, the capacity of a patient waxes and wanes and often a patient will have the capacity for some decisions but not for others. In most cases, the patient's physician will make the determination that the patient does not have the capacity to make the decision at hand. Often, the physician makes this determination with the help of other members of the healthcare team and sometimes with the help of a consultant psychiatrist or neurologist. A patient with decisional capacity is able to receive information, evaluate and deliberate about the information, and communicate a preference or choice. Capacity to make a treatment or care decision further requires (1) a basic understanding of the medical situation, (2) an understanding of the nature of the decision, including the risks and benefits of any treatment being considered and the alternatives, and (3) the ability to communicate a decision that is logical and consistent with the patient's values. Several instruments are available to assist the physician in determining capacity for decision making. A recent review evaluating 19 instruments identified 3 as easy to use and useful: the Aid to Capacity Evaluation, The Hopkins Competency Assessment Test, and the Understanding Treatment Disclosure (30). The authors note that the Aid to Capacity Evaluation was validated in the largest cohort and is available for free online (31). When the treating physician is uncertain about the assessment of capacity, consultation from a psychiatrist, an ethics consultant or committee, or social services can be helpful. Some states require additional safeguards specifically related to decisions about discontinuing life-sustaining treatments, for example, the law may require confirmation by a second physician of a patient's incapacity to make decisions before allowing a DPA to discontinue life-sustaining treatment.

When assessing understanding, physicians and other healthcare providers should minimize the influence of any possible barriers to understanding, such as language, timing, and sedating medications. They should also assure that the patient has received the information he/she would need to make an informed decision. When the patient communicates a decision, his/her decisions should make sense within the context of his/her values and history and be reasonably consistent and reasonably free of influence from other people. Decision-making capacity is not the same as competence, which is a legal determination. Decision-making capacity is also understood to be task specific. Some decisions are more complex than the others and the treatment choice is likely to expose the patient to higher risk. For example, the information is more complex and there is more at stake when deciding about a bone marrow transplantation for a serious illness than about antibiotics for an infection. The capacity to make the former decision requires a higher threshold of understanding and ability to deliberate and make a choice.

When a patient is determined to have compromised capacity or is unable to make a decision or set of decisions about his/her own medical care and treatment then that determination should be documented in the medical record and the DPA or legally authorized representative asked to make decisions on the patient's behalf. Because decision-making capacity is usually in degrees, and people may have the capacity for some decisions but not for others, the patient should be kept involved in the treatment decisions to the extent possible. When someone else is making treatment and care decisions, the patient should be informed about decisions made if he/she is capable of receiving the information. Depending on the circumstances, it may be appropriate to repeat assessment of a patient's capacity to make decisions on a regular basis, as some patients regain the ability to make decisions.

In certain cases, the healthcare team may have doubt or even be certain that a patient does not have the capacity to make the necessary medical care decisions but there is no previous advance directive with instructions or designation of a proxy. Recent research has shown that some patients may retain the capacity to assign a surrogate even if they have lost the capacity to make medical decisions (32). Importantly, however, an advance directive cannot be completed for a patient who does not himself/herself have the capacity to assign a surrogate or provide instructions. In these cases, in lieu of a DPA, a relative can be asked to make medical decisions according to the next-of-kin hierarchy as specified by state law. Although the hierarchy varies by state, usually the list includes spouses, adult children, parents, siblings, and others in that or a similar order.

HONORING ADVANCE DIRECTIVES

State laws, professional ethics, and respect for persons underlie an obligation to honor a patient's expressed wishes in a valid advance directive. Unfortunately, the completion of an advance directive does not always ensure that expressed wishes will be followed. One critical barrier to effectively using advance directives is the difficulty in ensuring that they are available when needed. In order to follow an advance directive, the treating physician and healthcare team need to have a copy of it and need to be able to understand what it expresses and apply it to the situation at hand. In a summary of studies supported by the US Agency for Healthcare Research and Quality, fewer than 50% of the severely or terminally ill patients studied had an advance directive available in their medical record and almost three-fourths of physicians whose patient had an advance directive were not aware that it existed (19).

Findings from the early SUPPORT study (Study to Understand Prognoses and Preferences for Outcomes and Risks of Treatment) showed that many patients had aggressive, invasive treatments even against their previously stated wishes (15). More recent studies have shown, however, that advance directives seem to substantially improve the correlation between what patients want and the care they receive at the end of life. Studies have shown, for example, that patients with advance directives were less likely to die in the hospital (5,19,33,34) and less likely to have certain procedures such as feeding tubes or respirators (33). Silveira et al. found a strong agreement between stated preferences on a living will and care received and said their data indicated that "living wills have an important effect on care received and that a durable power of attorney for health care is necessary to account for unforeseen factors" at least in elderly patients (5, p. 1217). Nicholas et al. found that fewer hospital deaths, more use of hospice, and lower spending were associated with advance directives but only in regions characterized by high levels of Medicare spending (34).

WITHHOLDING AND WITHDRAWING TREATMENT

Recommendations for treatment of disease or clinical symptoms are based on evidence of what is effective and the clinician's experience as well as judgment about what is appropriate in the particular case (Table 57.1). Adult patients who retain decision-making capacity when provided with a recommendation for treatment can consent or refuse based on their understanding of how it comports with their interests. At a certain point in the trajectory of many serious illnesses, continued aggressive treatment of disease is inappropriate and a decision is made to reorder the goals so that comfort and palliation of symptoms are primary. Sometimes this reordering raises questions about withholding or withdrawing treatment, including life-sustaining treatment. When the burdens of a treatment outweigh the benefits of the treatment as determined by the overall goals for the patient, withholding, changing, or withdrawing the treatment may be the most appropriate course of action, even when that course anticipates the patient's death. Even when aggressive treatment is withheld or withdrawn, treatment of symptoms is an integral goal of all health care. In that regard, symptom management and

TABLE 57.1	**Common misperceptions**	
Question	**Misperceptions**	**Realities**
Does an advance directive have to be on a particular form or in a particular format to be valid?	Healthcare providers will only follow an advance directive if it is on the approved state form	Written advance directives on state forms or commonly available forms are useful in guiding decision making by proxies and healthcare providers, even if all the legal formalities are not met. Oral expressions of a patient's wishes can also be useful and valid guides to decision makers
When the DPA is asked to make a decision for a patient, will he or she make all future health-related decisions?	Once the DPA is activated, the patient cannot make any more decisions	Capacity can wax and wane in some people and capacity is task specific. Even if a patient was determined not to have capacity, his/her decision-making capacity should be re-assessed in some cases and the patient should be involved in decisions to the extent possible
If a patient or surrogate decides to withhold a life-sustaining intervention, will other care provided to the patient change?	Patients, families, and some healthcare providers fear that a decision to limit a life-sustaining intervention means limited care	Patients and proxies and the healthcare team should agree on the goals of care. Treatment will be provided consistent with those goals and an analysis of the benefits and burdens. Symptoms will be treated regardless of other treatment choices throughout a person's life
Is it illegal to prescribe large doses of opiates to relieve pain, dyspnea, or other symptoms?	If a physician administers drugs to treat pain and the patient dies, the physician could be criminally liable	Large doses of opiates are permitted and appropriate if titrated to the patient's need for pain or symptom relief. It is common practice for a physician to choose medications and doses appropriate for symptom relief and not with the primary intent of causing death
Is it ethically or legally better to withhold treatment than to withdraw it?	Once a treatment is begun, it is ethically more problematic to stop it	Patients or their legally authorized representatives consent to or refuse treatment. Treatment is withdrawn most often because the patient or proxy no longer consents to receiving it. Although withdrawing treatment is ethically and legally similar to withholding treatment, healthcare providers and families usually find withdrawal more difficult
Can a physician withdraw life-sustaining treatment?	When withdrawing a treatment leads to a patient's death, it could be seen as murder or euthanasia	Termination of life support at the request of the patient or family is seen as honoring their right to make treatment decisions. Death is understood as a result of the patient's underlying disease. Current law supports the termination of life support that is consistent with the patient's wishes or his/her best interests

DPA, Durable Power of Attorney for Health Care.

Adapted from Meisel A, Snyder L, Quill T. Seven legal barriers to end-of-life care: myths, realities and grains of truth. *J Am Med Assoc.* 2000;284(19):2495–2501 and from Ackermann, Chapter 32, Table 63.2.

palliation are management goals at every stage of illness, including during aggressive treatment of the disease and at such a time that treatment may be limited to palliation and pain control. Some patients and their families worry that if they opt for palliative or comfort care, they will not receive good care and they will die sooner. Yet, a recent study showed that patients with metastatic non–small cell lung cancer who received early palliative care had improvements in their quality of life and mood and lived on average a few months longer than those who continued to receive standard aggressive care (35). Nonetheless, cancer patients in some places are receiving more aggressive care at the end of life in 2008 than in 2002 despite the availability of palliative care (36).

There are several reasons a physician might agree to withhold or withdraw life-sustaining treatment from a patient: (1) to comply with an adult patient's competent wishes or wishes expressed through an authorized proxy; (2) because the treatment cannot achieve the goal; and (3) because the therapy has failed and is simply prolonging the dying process (37).

In the first case, a decision to withhold or withdraw treatment is a demonstration of respect for the patient's autonomy or the right of a competent adult to accept or refuse treatments and interventions. When the request of the patient is informed, clear, consistent, and well-considered treatment can be withheld or stopped in accord with the patient's wishes, even if it results in the patient's death. Gerstel et al. noted that "the majority of deaths in the intensive care setting involve withholding or withdrawing multiple life-sustaining therapies" (38).

If a patient lacks the capacity to make decisions about starting a treatment or stopping it, the previously appointed DPA or other legally authorized surrogate can act to make such decisions. A decision to withhold or withdraw treatment for a seriously or terminally ill patient is stressful for all involved, including the DPA and family members, and also for healthcare providers, especially those who have been caring for a patient over an extended period of time. As described above, a decision to withhold treatment may be made at the request of the patient or family and is usually made when the expected burdens of the treatment outweigh its likely benefits. Withdrawing treatment, including life-sustaining treatments (e.g., ventilator and respiratory support, nutrition, and hydration) once they have been started can also be ethically appropriate when the burdens of treatment outweigh its benefits. Withdrawing treatment often creates more controversy and psychological distress for the family and healthcare team than not starting a treatment to begin with. It has been long recognized that withholding and withdrawing treatment in certain circumstances are both legally and morally acceptable and that circumstances that would morally justify not starting life-sustaining treatment could also justify stopping it (39-41). Respecting the considered choice of the patient or his/her legally authorized representative to refuse treatment or to have a treatment withdrawn is consistent with respect for patient autonomy. Although it is often emotionally more difficult to stop a treatment once it has been provided, in certain cases it may be preferable to start a treatment with the later option of stopping it rather than not starting the treatment at all, especially if there is uncertainty about the burdens and benefits or about the patient's wishes. Despite some consensus that both withholding and withdrawing treatment are morally and legally comparable and acceptable, healthcare providers do not always agree and practices vary (42). Healthcare teams may find assistance and helpful advice in making determinations about withholding or withdrawing care from hospital ethics committees, legal counsel, and professional society guidelines.

Because such decisions can be stressful and difficult, the more communication between the patient, DPA or family, and the treating team, the better. Members of the healthcare team can facilitate decision making about withholding or withdrawing treatment by offering the patient, DPA, and/or family opportunities to discuss the medical situation as well as the patient's cultural, spiritual, and other values and preferences. Multidisciplinary patient care conferences as well as family conferences provide useful opportunities to review goals for care, decipher complex medical and prognostic information, update everyone about the patient's clinical course, and discuss options (Chapter 49). The Medical College of Wisconsin's End of Life/Palliative Education Resource Center publishes a useful set of *Fast Facts and Concepts for Clinicians*, including one entitled *Moderating an End-of-Life Family Conference* (43). The DPA and the family may need assistance in deciphering complex medical and prognostic information about the patient and in understanding the various intervention options. The Society for Critical Care Medicine has developed online reader-friendly descriptions of many interventions that might be used in the intensive care unit (44). Patients and their families may have different preferences in terms of how decisions are made; some will prefer recommendations from the physician while others may prefer a more shared decision-making process. Effective communication between the patient or legally designated decision maker and healthcare professionals helps to ensure that decisions are sound and based on an understanding of the medical condition, prognosis, the benefits and burdens of the life-sustaining treatment, and the goals of care.

Despite a considerable amount of effort and attention, most agree that much more can be done to improve the quality of patient-centered care at the end of life (45,46). Advance care planning and advance directives, although underutilized and imperfect in realizing the original goals, can be helpful tools by facilitating deliberation and discussion and helping us to understand patients' preferences and values. Thoughtful and respectful consideration of patients' wishes—expressed presently or previously—and of the difficult and emotional challenges facing surrogate decision makers and loved ones can help guide our actions as healthcare providers in providing quality care for all patients.

CONFLICTS OF INTERESTS

The views expressed are those of the author and do not represent any policies or positions of the Department of Bioethics, the Clinical Center, National Institutes of Health, or Department of Health and Human Services.

REFERENCES

1. Annas G. Culture of life: politics at the bedside—the case of Terri Schiavo. *N Engl J Med.* 2005;352:1710-1715.
2. Quill T, Terri Schiavo A. Tragedy compounded. *N Engl J Med.* 2005;352:1630-1633.
3. Ackermann RJ. *Chapter 63, 3e: Withholding and Withdrawing Potentially Life-Sustaining Treatment.*
4. Alzheimers Association Facts and Figures. http://www.alz.org/alzheimers_disease_facts_and_figures.asp. Accessed October, 2011.
5. Silveira M, Kim S, Langa K. Advance directives and outcomes of surrogate decision making before death. *N Engl J Med.* 2010;362:1211-1218.
6. Patient Self-Determination Act. 42 C.F.R. § 489.102.

7. Meisel A, Snyder L, Quill T. Seven legal barriers to end-of-life care: myths, realities and grains of truth. *J Am Med Assoc.* 2000;284(19):2495-2501.

8. See for example, National Hospice and Palliative Care Organization, Caring Connections. http://www.caringinfo.org/i4a/pages/index.cfm?pageid=1. Accessed October, 2011.

9. See for example, Texas Living Will Online Completion. http://texaslivingwill.org/.

10. Berry SR, Singer PA. The cancer-specific advance directive. *Cancer.* 1998;82(8):1570-1577.

11. Doukas DJ, McCullough LB. The values history: the evaluation of the patient's values and advance directives. *J Fam Pract.* 1991;32:145-153.

12. Emanuel LL, Emanuel EJ. The medical directive: a new comprehensive advance care document. *J Am Med Assoc.* 1989;261:3288-3293.

13. Relman AS. Michigan's sensible living will. *N Engl J Med.* 1979;300:1270-1272.

14. Fagerlin A, Schneider C. Enough. The failure of the living will. *Hastings Cent Rep.* 2004;34(2)30-42.

15. The SUPPORT Investigators. A controlled trial to improve decision-making for seriously ill hospitalized patients: the struggle to understand prognoses and preferences for outcomes and risks of treatments (SUPPORT). *J Am Med Assoc.* 1995;274(20):1591-1598.

16. Hickman S, Hammes B, Moss A, Tolle S. Hope for the future: achieving the original intent of advance directives. *Hastings Cent Spec Rep.* Improving End of Life Care: Why Has it Been So Difficult? 2005;Special Report35(6):S26-S30.

17. Pew Research Center for the People and the Press. More Americans discussing—and planning—end-of-life treatment. http://people-press.org/http://people-press.org/files/legacy-pdf/266.pdf.

18. Teno J, Grunier A, Schwartz Z, Nanda A, Wetle T. Association between advance directives and quality of end-of-life care: a national study. *J Am Geriatr Assoc.* 2007;55:189-194.

19. Kass-Bartelmes BL, Hughes R, Rutherford MK. *Advance Care Planning: Preferences for Care at the End of Life.* Rockville, MD: Agency for Healthcare Research and Quality; 2003. Research in Action Issue #12. AHRQ Pub No. 03-0018. http://www.scribd.com/fullscreen/47966710.

20. Aging with Dignity. Five Wishes Online. www.agingwithdignity.org.

21. Geriatric Research Group. Advance Directives. Let Me Decide. http://fhs.mcmaster.ca/grg/advanced.htm.

22. Gunderson Lutheran Medical Foundation. Respecting choices. www.gundersenlutheran.com/eolprograms. Accessed December, 2011.

23. MacGillis A. Debate over end-of-life care began in small town. Washington Post, Friday, Sept. 4 2009. http://www.washingtonpost.com/wp-dyn/content/article/2009/09/03/AR2009090303833.html.

24. Physicians Orders for Life-Sustaining Treatment Paradigm, POLST. www.polst.org.

25. Emanuel LL, Danis M, Pearlman RA, et al. Advance care planning as a process. *J Am Geriatr Soc.* 1995;43:440-446

26. Vig E, Taylor J, Starks H, Hopley E, Fryer-Edwards K. Beyond substituted judgment: how surrogates navigate end-of-life decision-making. *J Am Geriatr Soc.* 2006;54:1688-1693.

27. Shalowitz DI, Garrett-Mayer E, Wendler D. The accuracy of surrogate decision makers: a systematic review. *Ann Intern Med.* 2006;166(5):493-497

28. Wendler D, Rid A. Systematic review: the effect on surrogates of making treatment decisions for others. *Ann Intern Med.* 2011;154(5):336-346.

29. The Medical Directive. http://www.medicaldirective.net/#.

30. Sessums L, Zembrzuska H, Jackson J. Does this patient have medical decision-making capacity? *J Am Med Assoc.* 2011;306(4):420-427.

31. Aid to Capacity Evaluation. http://www.rgpc.ca/best/GiiC%20Resources/GiiC/pdfs/3%20An%20Aid%20To%20Capacity%20Evaluation.pdf.

32. Kim S, Karlawish J, Kim M, Wall I, Bozoki A, Appelbaum P. Preservation of the capacity to appoint a proxy decision maker. *Arch Gen Psychiatry.* 2011;68(2):214-220.

33. Degenholtz H, Rhee Y, Arnold R. The relationship between having a living will and dying in place. *Ann Intern Med.* 2004;141:113-117

34. Nicholas L, Langa K, Iwashyna T, Weir D. Regional variation in the association between advance directives and end-of-life Medicare expenditures. *J Am Med Assoc.* 2011;306(13):1447-1453.

35. Temel J, Greer J, Muzikansky A, et al. Early palliative care for patients with metastatic non–small-cell lung cancer. *N Engl J Med.* 2010;363:733-742.

36. Gonsalves W, Tashi T, Davies T, et al. Aggressiveness of end-of-life care before and after the utilization of a palliative care service. *J Clin Oncol.* 2011;29(suppl):abstr 9135.

37. Prendergast TJ, Puntillo KA. Withdrawal of life support. Intensive caring at the end of life. *J Am Med Assoc.* 2002;288:2732-2740.

38. Gerstel E, Engelberg RA, Koepsell T, Curtis J. Duration of withdrawal of life support in the intensive care unit and association with family satisfaction. *Am J Respir Crit Care Med.* 2008;178:798-804.

39. President's Commission for the Study of Ethical Problems in Medicine and Biomedical Research. *Deciding to Forego Life-Sustaining Treatment: A Report on the Ethical, Medical, and Legal Issues in Treatment Decisions.* Washington, DC: Government Printing Office; 1983.

40. Hastings Center Task Force. *Guidelines on the Termination of Life-Sustaining Treatment and the Care of the Dying: A Report of the Hastings Center.* New York, NY: Briarcliff Manor; 1987.

41. Dickensen D. Are medical ethicists out of touch? Practitioner attitudes in the US and UK towards decisions at the end of life. *J Med Ethics.* 2000;26:254-260.

42. Glick S. Withholding versus withdrawal of life support: is there an ethical difference? *BMJ.* 2011;342:d728.

43. Ambuel B, Weissman D. Fast fact and concept #016: moderating an end-of-life family conference. www.eperc.mcw.edu.

44. Society of Critical Care Medicine. What are my choices regarding life support? A guide to understanding types of life support and end-of-life care offered in the intensive care unit. http://www.myicucare.org/Support_Brochures/Pages/Life_Support.aspx.

45. Assistant Secretary for Planning and Evaluation, Department of Health and Human Services. Advance Directives and Advance Care Planning: Report to Congress, August 2008. http://aspe.hhs.gov/daltcp/reports/2008/ADCongRpt.pdf.

46. Lorenz K, Lynn J, Morton SC, et al. *End-of-Life Care and Outcomes.* Rockville, MD: Agency for Healthcare Research and Quality (AHRQ); December 2004; Evidence Report/Technology Assessment #110, Publication #05-E004-1, Contract No. 290-02-0003.

CHAPTER 58

Palliative Care: Ethics and the Law

Ryan R. Nash

INTRODUCTION TO ETHICS

Ethics is the study of right and wrong, good and evil. Ethics assumes that such categories exist, although these categories are not always dichotomous. Ethics does not always deal with absolutes; instead, it entails trying to find the better option on the moral gradient. The ultimate determination of right and wrong, or the meta-ethical claim, is based on how one knows truth and how one values or orders life. Therefore, the ultimate ethical determination is based on epistemology. Epistemologies are diverse. Various philosophical theories and religions have made claim to define the good, the evil, virtue, and vice. However, they often do not agree. One may place the highest value on self-determination and freedom, another on equal opportunity for all, and yet another on self-sacrifice and love of another. When there is no agreement on where humankind comes from, where it is going, and what in life is most valuable and good, then agreement on what is ethical is all but impossible. Even if two persons from competing epistemologies find that they agree on an ethical claim they may do so for very different reasons. Thus, making a claim that something is ethical or unethical begs the question, "according to whose ethics? and why?" In a pluralistic society such as that of the United States, it is expected that two may meet as moral strangers (1), not having an agreed upon epistemology or understanding of right and wrong. In such as anticipated scenario, how are we to "do ethics" and determine the best path forward? We strive to come to an agreement of mutual consent, a modus vivendi (way of life). This is not a claim that we are agreeing on the ultimate ethic, nor is it saying that all of ethics is personal and relative. It is claiming that we come to an agreed upon operation that allows for variation on points of disagreement. Mistakenly many in health care use the phrase ethical or unethical as an ultimate truth claim and pretend, perhaps unknowingly, that all ethics is agreed upon. Much in ethics is not agreed upon. Thus, how we "do ethics" in health care is more procedural, based on agreements and precedence over time. Though consensus statements exist (2, 3), we fail to give ethics and ultimate truth claims their due if we think our laws, procedures, or professional statements are the ultimate source of right and wrong, good and evil. This chapter will not focus on the ultimate meta-ethical claims or differing epistemological approaches to finding the good but deals with the practical approach of doing bedside clinical medical ethics, describing the usual modus vivendi and shared wisdom of those that have wrestled with what to do in the past. It will not attempt to solve the legion of disagreements that do and will exist.

DIVERSE FOUNDATIONS

Many ethical systems or approaches have been promoted. Some of these are summarized in Table 58.1. However, these ethical systems are often an attempt to identify or at least define the ultimate ethical nature of an action. As previously mentioned, all attempts to reach the ultimate ethical judgment depends on presuppositions of how life is valued or ordered. These systems do give focus for reflection and are helpful in ethical discourse by giving a shared vocabulary. However, at the bedside they too often fail to give sufficient clarity and direction. For instance, how does one decide if differing ethical principles conflict? Should autonomy or beneficence receive greater ethical weight?

PALLIATIVE CARE TERMS

To establish a common ground of meaning, palliative care terms are defined in Table 58.2. These terms reflect hospice and palliative medicine's emphasis on improving quality of life for patients with serious disease through management of pain and other distressing symptoms. Misunderstanding of these terms often leads to needless ethical conflicts or false dilemmas.

RESPONSIBILITY AND OBLIGATIONS OF PALLIATIVE CARE

Related to the definition of palliative care is its responsibilities. It has been proclaimed that the role of medicine is to restore health or to fight disease and death. More realistic views have emphasized the sentiment attributed to a number of famous physicians including Sir William Osler and Edward Trudeau, "to cure sometimes, to relieve often, to comfort (or to care) always" (4,5). Palliative care professionals have understood this later call and have championed it. However, some have taken the call for comfort and relief of all suffering as responsibilities and obligations. Although relief of suffering is a worthy goal and should be attempted with great effort and skill, the hospice and palliative medicine specialist's responsibility is not to perfectly relieve

---

This material is also covered with modification and greater depth in Nash RR, Nelson LJ. *UNIPAC 6: Ethical and Legal Dimensions of Care.* 4th ed. AAHPM; 2012.

TABLE 58.1	Selected ethical frameworks and foundations

Principle based

Focuses on the following ethical principles:

- Beneficence—promote patient well-being
- Autonomy—respect patient self-determination
- Nonmaleficence—do no harm
- Justice—protect vulnerable populations and provide fair allocation of resources

Professionalism

Professionalism involves the qualities that make a good professional or a good physician. The ways in which a practitioner is true to a standard when honoring established principles, oaths, or examples determines his or her level of professionalism.

Virtue based

Virtues defining the character of a good physician include the following:

- Fidelity to trust and promise—honoring the ineradicable trust of the patient–physician relationship
- Effacement of self-interest—protecting the patient from exploitation and refraining from using the patient as a means to advance power, prestige, profit, or pleasure
- Compassion and caring—exhibiting concern, empathy, and consideration for the patient's plight
- Intellectual honesty—knowing when to say "I do not know"
- Prudence—deliberating and discerning alternatives in situations of uncertainty and stress

Caring based

The ethics of caring assumes that connections to others are central to what it means to be human. Caring requires empathy and compassion for patients, assuming responsibility for patients by performing actions that meet their needs and creating an educational environment that fosters caring

Respect for personhood

Respect for personhood proposes the following:

- Treatment of patients must reflect the inherent dignity of every person regardless of age, debility, dependence, race, color, or creed.
- Actions must reflect the patient's current needs.
- Decisions must value the person and accept human mortality and medical finitude.

Humanities

Uses literature, history, the arts, and narrative to arrive at principles or sentiment of the right and wrong

Religious and cultural

Application of deep and rich contextual understandings of the good or ways of life. Such considerations may or may not be able to be reduced into philosophical categories or language. The truth claims are at times exclusive to the group.

all suffering but to use the best of one's knowledge, skill, and abilities to provide the best possible care (6). Palliative care teams also must appreciate the finitude of medicine. Not only is medicine not the source of eternal life but it often fails at being the source of perfect relief of suffering or "a good death." Attempts to "totalize" the dying experience with medicine can lead to actions held by many to be wrong or evil in the name of compassion (7). Ironically, palliative care providers must be reminded of the original hospice

movement goals of not medicinalizing, institutionalizing, or trying to hide death.

Ethics, Law, and Practice

In giving clinical ethics advice, it is common for a clinical ethicist to address three perspectives: the legal, the professional, and the consultant's judgment or opinion on the case. This chapter provides a suggested framework to practically

TABLE 58.2	**Definitions associated with hospice and palliative care**

Palliative care is patient- and family-centered care that anticipates, prevents, and treats burdens of disease. Palliative care throughout the continuum of illness involves addressing physical, intellectual, emotional, social, and spiritual needs and facilitating patient access to information and choice. Palliative care is ideally delivered by an interprofessional team including a physician, nurse, social worker, chaplain, counselor, and others. (Modified from 73 FR 32204, June 5, 2008, Medicare—Final Rule.) **Palliative care deals with the burden of disease regardless of the stage of disease and attempts to encourage effective and desired interventions delivered in the right place and at the right time.**

Palliative treatments are treatments and interventions that enhance comfort and improve the quality of a patient's life. No specific therapy is excluded from consideration. The decision to intervene with a palliative treatment is based on the treatment's ability to meet the stated goals rather than on its effect on the underlying disease. The treatments are explored and evaluated within the context of the patient's values, symptoms, and clinical circumstances.

What palliative care is not

Palliative care is **not only end-of-life care**. Palliative care deals with the burden of disease regardless of the stage of disease. It includes treating patients with serious, but not necessarily life-limiting, illnesses as well as those who likely are dying.

Palliative care is **not** an attempt to **contain medical costs or ration care**. Palliative care attempts to encourage effective and desired interventions in the right place and at the right time. Palliative care has been shown to be a good steward of medical resources and sometimes is associated with cost savings, but controlling costs is not its primary aim.

Palliative care does **not hasten death**. In fact, many patients receiving palliative care may live longer and have opportunity to pursue additional "aggressive" or curative interventions due to enhanced symptom management, communication, and coordination of care. Appropriate pain and symptom management and addressing other burdens of disease have not been shown to hasten death.

Palliative care is **not** a dichotomy of care between **"do everything" vs. "do nothing"** or aggressive care vs. comfort care only. Palliative care helps involved parties navigate the complex range of medical choices and make the best possible medical decisions under difficult circumstances.

Palliative care is **not** always a **choice**. Most patients receiving palliative care will have a goal to live longer and have a better quality life. Many would choose life-prolonging, curative therapies if they were available and could be effective for them, but often they are not. For those with incurable disease, palliative care is an essential part of their treatment plan alongside the disease-directed therapies they continue to try.

Palliative care is **not** an attempt to force one definition of **"the good death"** upon all patients.

---

address clinical ethical decision making and describes key legal considerations and give an overview of issues important in palliative care. Hospice and palliative medicine, unlike many other specialities, has less univocity regarding many ethical issues. Thus, the chapter will not emphasize professional standards. The American Academy of Hospice and Palliative Medicine (AAHPM) has ethical statements readily available, which are frequently updated and sometimes changed (www.aahpm.org).

The Law

The law and ethics are not synonyms. We hope that our laws are ethical but history has shown that such is not guaranteed. At least theoretically, if a law were ethically wrong then one may willfully disobey the law. Further, some may suggest that we may have duty to try to change unethical laws. However, the laws we currently have throughout the United States are an attempt for a modus vivendi (mentioned in the Introduction). Laws vary from state to state and a description

of each is beyond the scope of this chapter. Needless to say, it behooves all health-care professionals to know the laws of their land (8,9), as many myths and misconceptions exist (10–12). Failure to correct these misconceptions may result in physicians stepping outside of accepted standards of medical practice (13). Most state laws are a reaction to landmark court cases around the country that became precedence. These cases, at times, had misinformation or needless court involvement, but they have defined the current legal terrain. Upon review of state laws and landmark cases, one may be surprised how often the well-intended laws are impractical and often not followed in clinical settings.

RIGHT TO REFUSE AND RIGHT TO DIE

Two distinct but related movements occurred in end-of-life law during the recent technological age of medicine and in part a reaction against the perception of a paternalistic medicine. The *right to refuse* is the belief that medical care is optional for adults with decisional capacity (or determined by their appropriate proxy decision maker). This negative or material right has become accepted in clinical care and ethical discourse and is legal precedence. Further, it is constitutive of palliative care.[1]

The *right to die* movement agrees that medical care is optional and can be refused, but adds a claim or positive right for a person to choose the method, manner, and timing of death. Some advocates argue for the right to demand help in causing death from health-care professionals and systems. The right to die movement advocates assisted suicide and some types of euthanasia. The right to die has not been broadly accepted legally, ethically, or clinically. The right to die is not constitutive of palliative care.

Finally, another positive or claim right, the *right to demand medical care*, movement has come to the fore, as seen in several court cases (14). This right to demand is similar to the right to die (which is a type of demand) in that they are both positive or claim rights. Currently, the right to demand is mainly being considered in the context of reproductive technologies and chronic treatments such as hemodialysis. Currently, a right to demand a particular treatment is not broadly accepted in law or medical ethics.

LANDMARK CASES ON THE RIGHT TO REFUSE

The Quinlan Case[1]

In April 1975, at age 21 years, Karen Ann suffered severe anoxic brain injury. Karen Ann was eventually diagnosed to be in a persistent vegetative state. She had been on a mechanical ventilator. Her father requested guardianship and requested the mechanical ventilator be removed. Mr. Quinlan's requests were opposed by the treating physicians, the hospital, the local prosecutor, the State of New Jersey, and Karen's guardian ad litem. The Supreme Court of New Jersey authorized the withdrawal of life support and the appointment of Mr. Quinlan as guardian for that purpose if it was concluded, after appropriate consultation with a hospital ethics committee, that there was no reasonable possibility of Karen ever emerging from a persistent vegetative state. The court also noted that this decision was consistent with Karen Ann's and Mr. Quinlan's Roman Catholic faith (the decision had been endorsed by their bishop).

The Supreme Court of New Jersey found that the right of Karen Ann Quinlan to refuse medical treatment, even if exercised by her surrogate or proxy, was protected by a right of privacy. The court noted that the claimed interests of the state were to preserve life and protect the right of physicians to administer treatment in accordance with their best judgment, but these interests were outweighed by the poor prognosis of the patient and great bodily invasion involved in sustaining her life. The court endorsed the use of a substituted judgment standard (i.e., allowing her guardian and family "to render their best judgment" regarding whether she would refuse the continuation of

treatment if she could wake up for a few minutes and tell her family what she would want them to do before returning to her vegetative state). The court also endorsed the use of hospital ethics committees in reviewing decisions to withdraw life-sustaining treatment as preferable to court proceedings. After this decision, mechanical ventilation was removed, but Karen Ann Quinlan was able to breathe on her own (as predicted by only one expert witness). She lived for several years being fed by artificial nutrition and hydration (ANH) and died from an "overwhelming infection in 1985 without regaining consciousness" (15). Despite the expanded role for ethics committees envisioned in the *Quinlan* decision, few hospitals created such committees (16). The failure of hospitals to adopt ethics committees was attributed to a "reluctance to disturb the status quo, together with a sense of confusion over what an ethics committee could accomplish" (16).

The Cruzan Case[2]

In January 1983, Nancy Cruzan, a 25 year-old Missourian, was seriously injured in an automobile accident. When she was found lying face down, there was no detectable heartbeat or respiration, but these functions were restored at the scene by paramedics. She was taken to a hospital where she remained unconscious. Physicians implanted a gastrostomy tube with permission. Her condition subsequently was diagnosed as a persistent vegetative state. Eventually, Cruzan's parents asked hospital employees to stop ANH administration, but hospital employees refused to accede without a court order. The trial court recognized a constitutional right to refuse life-sustaining treatment and authorized withdrawal of ANH based upon its finding that before her injury Cruzan had told a friend that if she were seriously injured she would not want to live unless she could live "halfway normally." The Missouri Supreme Court reversed the decision of the trial court. Although the court recognized a right to refuse treatment under the common law doctrine of informed consent, it refused to recognize a constitutional right. It found strong state interest in preservation of life as expressed in the Missouri Living Will Statute. On that basis, the court found that treatment could not be terminated in the absence of a valid living will unless it could be shown by "clear and convincing evidence" that the patient would have wanted it terminated. It found that the statements relied on by the trial court were unreliable and did not meet the clear and convincing evidence standard. The US Supreme Court affirmed the decision of the Supreme Court of Missouri, holding that the state could require clear and convincing evidence of a person's expressed wishes made while competent. While the majority opinion upheld the constitutionality of the State of Missouri's requirement of clear and convincing evidence, it also acknowledged that "a constitutionally protected liberty interest in refusing unwanted medical treatment may be inferred from our prior decisions." The court stated, however, that because incompetent patients need certain

---

[1]*In re Quinlan*, 355 A2d 647 (NJ 1976).

[2]*Cruzan v Director, Missouri Department of Health*, 497 US 261 (1990).

protection given they cannot exercise this right of refusal, it was appropriate for the State of Missouri to impose additional safeguards in the form of the clear and convincing evidence standard in light of its interest in preserving life. After the Supreme Court's decision, the Cruzans petitioned the trial court in Missouri, again requesting discontinuation of tube feedings. Her coworkers testified that Cruzan stated she would not like to live "like a vegetable." Cruzan's treating physician and court-appointed guardian also supported discontinuation of ANH. As a result, the Missouri court authorized the discontinuation of feeding, and Cruzan died shortly thereafter. The publicity surrounding this case fostered interest in advance directives and health-care proxy appointments. It also generated support for the federal Patient Self-Determination Act passed in 1991 (17), which requires some health facilities to present patients with information on advance health-care directives.

The Schiavo Case

On February 25, 1990, Theresa Schiavo suffered anoxic brain injury following a cardiac arrest as the result of a potassium imbalance. She never regained consciousness and eventually her condition was diagnosed as a persistent vegetative state. A feeding tube was inserted and ANH started, but in 1998 her husband asked a Florida state trial court for permission to remove the feeding tube. The court granted permission after determining this was what she would have wanted. At the time feeding tube removal was sought, it was clear that with ANH Terri Schiavo could continue to live for many years, but, if withdrawn, she would die in a few days. The Florida trial court authorized the withdrawal of ANH. The trial court decision was affirmed by the Florida District Court of Appeals, holding that the trial judge had properly found under the clear and convincing evidence standard that Theresa would have wanted the feeding discontinued.[3] The Florida courts—applying a substituted judgment standard—authorized the withdrawal of ANH based on the assumption that she, if competent to make the decision, would have wanted it withdrawn. Schiavo and her family were Roman Catholic, so Catholic teaching was an issue in the case, bearing on the question of what she would have wanted. In the original proceedings before the trial court, a Catholic priest from the Diocese of St. Petersburg, FL, testified regarding Church teaching on the withdrawal of ANH from patients in a persistent vegetative state. Schiavo's husband's attorney asked the priest whether removal of ANH would be consistent with the teaching of the Catholic Church. He further asked the priest to assume, for purposes of this question, that Theresa Schiavo had told her husband she would not want to live "if she was dependent on the care of others" and further that she "mentioned to her husband and to her brother and sister-in-law that she would not want to be kept alive artificially." The priest answered: "After all that has transpired, I believe, yes, it would be consistent with the teaching of the

Catholic Church." On cross-examination, Fr. Murphy was asked if he was familiar with Directive 58 in the 1994 Ethical and Religious Directives for Catholic Health Care Services, which states there should be a presumption in favor of providing ANH. He stated that he was familiar with Directive 58, but characterized it as providing an ideal standard; further, "You have to go back and evaluate the proportion" (18). The appellate court sided with the husband, permitting the husband to order the withdrawal of treatment. After this decision came several years of additional legal wrangling in both state and federal courts between her parents, who opposed removal of the feeding tube, and her husband, who sought its removal. The parents continued to contend that Theresa was in a minimally conscious state rather than in a persistent vegetative state and that in light of her Catholic faith she would want the feeding continued. On October 15, 2003, Theresa's feeding tube was removed. Six days later, the Florida legislature passed a law allowing Governor Jeb Bush to order that the feeding be resumed. The feeding tube was reinserted, but this law subsequently was declared unconstitutional by the Florida Supreme Court.[4]

Theresa Schiavo died on March 31, 2005, approximately 2 weeks after the removal of her feeding tube pursuant to a court order (19).

The Schiavo case focused attention on Catholic teaching on withdrawal of ANH from patients in a persistent vegetative state and eventually resulted in a revision of Directive 58 of the Ethical and Religious Directives for Catholic Health Care Services (see box below).

Catholic Health Care Directives

The 2009 version of Ethical and Religious Directives for Health Care Services, 5th edition (20) (the norms adopted by Catholic bishops in the United States that apply to Catholic hospitals) states

56. A person has a moral obligation to use ordinary or proportionate means of preserving his or her life. Proportionate means are those that in the judgment of the patient offer a reasonable hope of benefit and do not entail an excessive burden or impose excessive expense on the family or the community.

57. A person may forgo extraordinary or disproportionate means of preserving life. Disproportionate means are those that in the patient's judgment do not offer a reasonable hope of benefit or entail an excessive burden, or impose excessive expense on the family or the community.

58. In principle, there is an obligation to provide patients with food and water, including medically assisted nutrition and hydration for those who cannot take food orally. This obligation extends to patients in chronic and presumably irreversible

---

[3] *In re Guardianship of Schiavo*, 780 So2d 176, 180 (FL App. Ct. 2001).

[4] *Bush v Schiavo*, 885 So2d 321 (FL 2004).

conditions (e.g., the "persistent vegetative state") who can reasonably be expected to live indefinitely if given such care. Medically assisted nutrition and hydration become morally optional when they cannot reasonably be expected to prolong life or when they would be "excessively burdensome for the patient or [would] cause significant physical discomfort, for example resulting from complications in the use of the means employed." For instance, as a patient draws close to inevitable death from an underlying progressive and fatal condition, certain measures to provide nutrition and hydration may become excessively burdensome and therefore not obligatory in light of their very limited ability to prolong life or provide comfort.

59. The free and informed judgment made by a competent adult patient concerning the use or withdrawal of life-sustaining procedures should always be respected and normally complied with, unless it is contrary to Catholic moral teaching.

Other noteworthy cases include the following.

The Barber Case[5]

Two physicians were found not guilty of murder and conspiracy to commit murder when they withdrew ANH from a patient in a persistent vegetative state at the request of the patient's family and the patient died. The ruling held that ANH should be viewed as medical treatment, that it was permissible to withdraw ANH without appointment of a legal guardian, and that the patient's wife and children could act as surrogate decision makers. The panel noted that surrogate decision makers should apply a substituted judgment standard (what the patient would want), but, even in the absence of evidence of the patient's wishes, ANH could be withdrawn under a best interests standard (what seems to be the best for the patient) when its burdens exceeded its benefits.

Vacco v Quill[6]

In this case, the US Supreme Court upheld state laws prohibiting physician-assisted death, the court rejected an argument that the ban irrationally distinguished between physician-assisted suicide or euthanasia and palliative sedation (21). The US Supreme Court also has recognized that the withdrawal of life-sustaining treatment is not equivalent to physician-assisted death. The right to die was not recognized though the right to refuse was again affirmed.

[5]*Barber v Superior Court*, 147 CA Rptr 484 (Ct App 1983).
[6]*Vacco v Quill*, 521 US 793, 807 (1997).

Ethical Decision Making

The decisions made by terminally ill patients and their physicians can profoundly affect the life of the patient and his or her family. When physicians and patients face ethical decisions about emotionally charged issues, such as withholding or withdrawing life-sustaining treatment, the palliative medicine model of care recognizes the importance of shared communication and respect for the multiple and sometimes conflicting needs of physicians, patients and family members, and interdisciplinary team members. Palliative medicine also acknowledges the intellectual, emotional, and spiritual challenges accompanying ethical decision making for everyone involved in the process—patients, family members, physicians, and other health-care professionals. To arrive at the best decision for a patient and to minimize unnecessary decision-making burden while honoring patient self-determination, an informed consent process using shared decision making should be used. Patients should be given the opportunity to accept or refuse potentially effective treatments; however, physicians are not ethically obligated to provide any and all treatments a patient or family may demand. Shared decision also helps align patient goals and values with available treatments.

The shared decision-making process is a response to past medical paternalism, when physicians decided for patients and often acted without adequate communication or opportunity for refusal. Medical paternalism assumed that the physician knew what was best for the patient. Shared decision-making models reflect the fact that physicians and patients have differing spheres of expertise: the physician has knowledge of diseases and their treatments, while the patient has a lifetime of personal experiences and knowledge about their own values and priorities. The goal of a shared decision-making or informed consent process is to give an opportunity for *informed refusal* (protect the patient from unwanted treatments or advice from health-care professionals) and to have the best plan for a patient.

THE PHYSICIAN IN DECISION MAKING

The physician plays a key role as facilitator of the decision-making process. In an understandable reaction against paternalism, many physicians may be reluctant to share their recommendations with patients for fear of overly influencing them and diminishing patient autonomy; however, this reluctance may deprive patients and families of the physician's expertise and guidance. Physicians should make recommendations based on their medical knowledge and what they have learned about the patient's values and priorities.

In hospice and palliative care settings, the physician is responsible for decisions about medical care and recommending courses of action with input from members of the interdisciplinary team. Non-physician team members must advise the patient's physician about changes in the patient's condition and include the physician in treatment-related decisions. The hospice and palliative care physician also is an integral member of the interdisciplinary team.

When difficult decisions must be made, other team members can and should help with the decision and help communicate with and educate patients and families. However, it is not ethically appropriate for professionals to work outside of their scope of practice and competency. It is vital that physicians take a leadership role in assisting patients in making these decisions.

It is the responsibility of the care provider to gather all relevant information about the decision to be made. The potentially important questions are included in the 4-Box Model (22) (Table 58.3). Practical procedural approaches such as the 4-Box Model may not address the ultimate ethical nature of an action, but they provide a practical construct or approach to attempting to reach the best decision. An approach such as the 4-Box Model can help with the vast majority of ethical dilemmas in clinical practice.

The 4-Box Model is organized with a hierarchy in mind; clinical and biographical facts that focus on what makes sense medically and respects patient wishes are given more weight than quality of life or cultural facts. This hierarchy does not suggest that the questions in the bottom two boxes are insignificant but rather is more attuned to the avoidance of unnecessary conflicts or dilemmas. If a plan of care makes practical medical sense, the patient agrees, and the physician and team agree, there is a reduced likelihood of conflict.

THE PATIENT IN DECISION MAKING

Hospice and palliative medicine recognizes the patient and family as the unit of care. When possible the patient is the key decision maker, with authority to give consent or refuse treatment.

Decision-Making Capacity

It is important to confirm decision-making capacity to ensure the patient has the ability to execute an informed refusal or give informed consent (23). In medical settings, it is the physician's responsibility to determine decisional capacity. Capacity may change depending on the patient's condition and the complexity of the decision in question. Decision-making capacity is decision specific. The same patient may be able to express a simple value judgment (e.g., "I want my son to make decisions for me because I trust him") but not be able to understand the risks, benefits, and alternatives of a complex treatment (e.g., aortic valve replacement with

TABLE 58.3 **The 4-Box Model**	
I. Medical information	**II. Patient and professional preferences**
What is the patient's diagnosis and prognosis?	What is known about the patient's wishes and values?
How has the patient's condition changed?	What is known about the wishes of surrogates, family members, and other involved parties?
Are symptoms adequately treated?	Does the patient have the capacity to make decisions about medical treatments?
What is the proposed intervention?	Who is involved in making the decision and what is his or her involvement?
How effective is the intervention likely to be for this patient?	What is the recommendation of the physician and interdisciplinary team?
What is the intention of the proposed intervention?	
What are possible alternatives?	
III. Benefits and burdens	**IV. Contextual features**
What are the potential benefits and burdens/risks of the treatment in question?	Who is this patient?
How does the patient describe his or her quality of life or burden of life?	What are the patient's life story and primary values?
What brings meaning or sustains the patient?	What is the patient's relationship with family members and significant others?
How has the patient made treatment decisions in the past?	What are the patient's cultural, religious, and spiritual beliefs and values?
What types of treatments would provide a satisfactory outcome for this patient's life?	What are the potential benefits and burdens of each alternative for the patient and family, including financial and emotional costs?
What is achievable with regard to the patient's preferences?	What are the legal considerations?
	How will the decision affect the patient and family physically, emotionally, spiritually, socially, and economically?

Adapted with modification from Jonsen AR, Siegler M, Winslade WJ. *Clinical Ethics: A Practical Approach to Ethical Decisions in Clinical Medicine.* 7th ed. New York, NY: McGraw-Hill; 2010:8. © 2010 by McGraw-Hill.

lifelong warfarin therapy). To have capacity to make a specific decision, a patient needs to be able to (22)

- *express insight* (express sufficient understanding of relevant information and the implications of various treatment choices)
- make an *internally rational* choice (a decision that is in accordance with personal values and goals); external rationality standards usually equate to whether a person agrees with a decision
- demonstrate that he or she is *not delusional* as a consequence of delirium or other psychiatric diseases (capacity evaluation in the latter may necessitate a psychiatrist)
- express a *static preference* (not change their mind rapidly based on cognitive difficulties)

SURROGATE DECISION MAKERS

If a patient becomes incapacitated, treatment decisions may be made by a proxy or surrogate decision maker (i.e., a third person who has the authority to make medical decisions). Most states have adopted laws permitting a legally competent individual to execute a document authorizing a proxy to make health-care decisions on behalf of a patient after that patient loses decision-making capacity. Sometimes, these documents are referred to as *durable powers of attorney for health care*. It is becoming more common to combine a proxy appointment with an instructive advance directive (e.g., Five Wishes document) or advance physician orders (e.g., POLST). While some states by statute specifically authorize proxies to make decisions to withhold or withdraw life-sustaining treatment, other states by statute limit the authority of a proxy, setting standards of evidence required for certain decisions in that regard (24). Even if there is an advance directive, its instructions often will not be sufficient to cover the current situation. Designation of a surrogate should always be recommended. A proxy appointment is important particularly in certain circumstances, such as a patient naming someone other than a legal spouse to act as their surrogate. A proxy also is important when disagreements among family members cannot be resolved or when family members are unavailable or nonexistent.

When the patient is incapacitated and there is no proxy or guardian with authority to make a medical decision, many states have statutes designating the patient's spouse, then adult children, then parents or siblings to act as the patient's surrogate decision maker. Even in the absence of such a statute, it may be appropriate to presume that close family members who know the patient well have decision-making authority (24).

In the case of an incapacitated patient with no proxy, no guardian with authority to make medical decisions, and no family, court designation of a surrogate may be necessary. Sometimes a patient may have indicated that a friend should act as a surrogate when he or she becomes incapacitated. It may be appropriate in some cases for the physician to accept this designation. Neither the patient's physician nor members of an interdisciplinary care team should serve as a patient's surrogate decision maker.

Decisions by Surrogates

The basic role of the surrogate is to make decisions in accordance with the "substituted judgment" standard that attempts to mirror the decisions the patient would make under the same circumstances. If unknown or uncertain, it is appropriate for a surrogate to apply the best interests standard. Although ethicists and clinicians expect surrogates to use substituted judgment or patients' best interests when making decisions, data indicate that many surrogates rely on other factors such as their own best interests or mutual interests of themselves and the patient (25).

The term *substituted interests*, coined in a 2010 *Journal of the American Medical Association* article, describes the practical approach employed by many experienced physicians. This definition includes physician leadership in listening to the values and wishes of patients, contextualizing medical recommendations appropriately for patients, and offering guidance to surrogates in decision making, but not in such a way that reverts to paternalism (Table 58.4) (26).

SELECTED ETHICAL ISSUES

Proportionate Pain and Symptom Management

Some physicians fail to prescribe adequate amounts of pain medication because they fear the required dosages may inadvertently shorten a patient's life. They tend to grossly overestimate the toxicity of carefully titrated dosages of opioids.

Although advocates of effective pain management may invoke the principle of double effect (see box below) to encourage adequate pain control, in most cases the principle is irrelevant. Carefully titrated opioid dosages are not likely to shorten a patient's life (27). The principle of double effect may be more applicable in treating severe terminal dyspnea; however, this is an unproven speculation. In fact, many hospice and palliative care physicians have observed that prescribing dosages of an opioid sufficient to relieve pain and dyspnea can improve activity levels, quality of life (28), and perhaps even survival (29). Formal informed consent processes and drug agreements can be used to enhance understanding and shared expectations for symptom treatment (these should not be viewed as "drug contracts" (30)).

Principle of Double Effect

Although it has been criticized in recent years, the principle of double effect has had a significant role in secular and religious bioethics and also has influenced criminal law (31).

It validates the use of treatments that are honestly intended to relieve suffering or restore health even if the

(Continued)

TABLE 58.4 The substituted interests model of surrogate decision making	
Step	**Sample Conversation Starters and Points**
Empathy and connection: acknowledge stresses of the situation and difficulty of the task and attend to needs of the surrogate	"It must be very difficult to see your loved one so sick."
Authentic values: understand the patient as a person *Values*: interpersonal, moral, religious, familial, psychological *Directives*: substantive treatment preferences and process considerations, such as who should decide and how	"Tell us about your loved one." "Has anyone else in the family ever experienced a situation like this?"
Clinical data: share understanding of the patient's clinical circumstances and prognosis	"All of that is important for us to know as we face the current situation." "Here is what is wrong ..." "This is what is likely to happen ..."
Substituted interests: determine what the patient's real interests are, given the patient's values and these circumstances	"Knowing your loved one, what do you think would be the most important for him/her right now? Avoiding pain? Having family members here?"
Clinical judgment: share understanding of the options and offer recommendation based on clinical experience, tailored to the particular patient's real interests	"Here's what could be done." "This is what we would recommend, based on what we know and what you've told us about your loved one."
Best judgment for the patient: best path to promote the good of this patient as a unique person, in the context of his or her relationships, authentic values, known wishes, and real interests, given the circumstances and options	"Knowing your loved one, does our recommendation seem right for him or her? Do you think another plan would be better, given his or her values, preferences, relationships?"

Adapted from Sulmasy DP, Snyder L. Substituted interests and best judgments: an integrated model of surrogate decision making. *JAMA*. 2010;304(17): 1946–1947. © 2010 by the American Medical Association.

intervention has potential untoward effects. The four elements of the doctrine are as follows:

1. The good effect has to be intended (e.g., relieving pain or dyspnea).
2. The bad effect can be foreseen but not intended (could possibly shorten life, but not the intent).
3. The bad effect cannot be the means to the good effect (cannot end the patient's life to relieve the pain).
4. The symptom must be severe enough to warrant taking risks; this is known as proportionality.

Medical Futility

The concept of futility has been controversial, and attempts to implement it to limit treatment despite the wishes of the patient's family have led to serious disagreements (32). Texas, alone, has enacted legislation giving physicians the authority, upon approval of a hospital ethics committee, to remove life-sustaining medical treatment without consent of the patient or family under circumstances deemed medically futile (33, 34). The Texas law remains very controversial.

Difficulties regarding medical futility are partly attributable to varying definitions. Medical futility can be defined on quantitative and qualitative grounds (35). If an intervention has a theoretical chance of providing benefit but has failed to do so in the last 100 cases, it is *quantitatively medically futile*. A treatment is *qualitatively futile* when it is perceived that the burdens outweigh the benefits of the treatment in the context of a certain patient. Qualitative futility often is considered if a technology is perceived as merely maintaining a patient in a state of permanent unconsciousness or in a state that continues to require management in an ICU with no hope of benefit other than maintenance. Consent from the patient or family to forgo (withhold or withdraw) quantitatively futile treatments may not be required, but qualitatively futile treatments generally require at least assent prior to forgoing treatment. The Texas law does not distinguish between the two types.

When physicians use the term *futile* to describe a treatment, they often are reacting to a profound sense that it would be "wrong" to provide the treatment for a particular patient in a specific situation (36). The challenge is to honor the physician's sense of wrongdoing by exploring relevant issues with the patient instead of implying the existence of objective and dispassionate standards of medical futility that do not exist. When a patient or family demands treatment the physician believes is medically futile, full disclosure and compassionate communication usually result in medically appropriate decisions without resorting to the legal system. When treatment issues cannot be resolved, the case should be referred to an ethics consultant. Throughout this process, it is important for the treatment team to remember that in most cases family members are struggling with how to love their loved one.

Organ Donation

Although organ procurement and transplantation generally are not the domain of palliative care, it is important to realize that it is a potential source for concern, comfort, or both for patients and their families (37). If a patient or their family is interested in organ donation, it is the responsibility of the health-care team to contact the appropriate organ procurement organization (OPO). Early contact with the OPO staff gives the patient and family time to discuss their concerns about organ donation such as logistics, cost, and time. The OPO staff is trained at effectively discussing these issues with families and providing appropriate psychosocial support (38–40). Increasingly, palliative care teams may be asked to participate in certain types of organ procurement called donation after circulatory death. Palliative care teams should become familiar with the protocols used at their institution, as they vary. Controversially, the determination of death after circulatory death no longer has a verification time requirement. Participation in organ procurement without verification of death over several minutes may violate the ethical standards of some health-care workers and patients (41).

Health-Care Provider Conscientious Refusal

Federal laws known as the Church Amendments support the rights of health-care providers to conscientiously refuse to participate in any "program or activity that would be contrary to his religious beliefs or moral convictions."[7] Violations of these laws are to be reported to the Office of Civil Rights Enforcement (42). Those invoking conscience protection may not be doing so only to protect themselves from being involved in an action they believe to be morally wrong. They may be attempting to protect the patient from an action they believe may be harmful.

Withdrawing ANH

ANH is a medical procedure that involves placing a tube or needle into the alimentary tract, in a vein, or under the skin to deliver fluids and nutrients. It does not refer to assisted oral feeding. Physicians must consider the withdrawal of ANH within an ethical framework, using all of the medical data available. As with other medical interventions, ANH should have a clearly defined therapeutic goal. The treatment can be discontinued when the patient's condition or appropriate time-limited trials

indicate that the therapeutic goal is not achievable, when the intervention has become more burdensome than beneficial, or when it no longer serves the patient's goals (43).

The decision to withdraw ANH is complicated by many issues. There is debate and uncertainty among the general public and some care providers whether this is a basic need or a medical intervention. The fear of death by starvation and dehydration remains an emotionally charged subject.

A judicial and increasingly an ethical consensus has emerged that ANH is a medical treatment and may be refused under the same standards as other medical treatment and there is now no question that adult patients with decision-making capacity can refuse ANH (24). In the aftermath of the Cruzan case, discussed in this chapter, many states revised their advance directive and proxy appointment statutes to permit refusal of ANH. But sometimes the instructions in an advance directive may not adequately cover the situation (44). And some states by statute limit the right of proxies to refuse ANH.

Palliative Sedation

Palliative sedation at the end of life refers to the use of high-dose sedatives to relieve extreme suffering as a last resort (45,46). Some physicians believe sedation at the end of life offers a humane alternative to suicide and assisted suicide. Others fear a "slippery slope" to euthanasia. *The intent of sedation is to provide relief and not to hasten death* (47).

The nomenclature for palliative sedation has changed and remains of poor consistency. Some will refer to palliative sedation as a situation in which a person dies sleepy from disease or drug. This is inaccurate. Some will include in the term *palliative sedation* the following: ordinary sedation (sedation as a side effect of regular symptom management), intermittent sedation (intentional sedation for a limited time period), and sedation to decreased awareness but not to unconsciousness, but these are not particularly ethically controversial issues. *Palliative sedation to unconsciousness* and continued until death is the controversial form, and this usually is referred to as palliative sedation. Before instituting palliative sedation to unconsciousness, the following conditions should be met (48):

- The patient is diagnosed with a terminal illness with a very short prognosis.
- All palliative treatment has been exhausted and profound symptoms persist.
- A psychological assessment has been made.
- A spiritual assessment has been made.
- There is a DNAR order (Do Not Attempt Resuscitation).
- There is informed consent.
- ANH was discussed before sedation.
- A policy and procedure should be in place and followed.
- Appropriate documentation is assured.
- Complicated bereavement follow-up for family is available.

In the past, sedation at the end of life was referred to as "terminal sedation." However, use of this phrase often is

---

[7]Sterilization or Abortion Act, 42 USC, §300a-7 (1973).

discouraged because it may be misinterpreted to imply an intent to "terminate" a patient's life (49). It may be prudent to further modify our nomenclature to refer only to sedation to unconsciousness until death as palliative sedation. If we did so, "ordinary sedation" and palliative sedation that is not to unconsciousness or intermittent sedation would not potentially fall under the same heading. In the meantime, this nomenclature has yet to be agreed upon.

The debate regarding palliative sedation is that for the wrong patient or if inappropriately applied it can be a form of "slow euthanasia" (50); however, this is possibly not true if reserved for the rare case described here. The other issue of debate is that some centers seem to use palliative sedation to unconsciousness quite frequently, while other top centers use it rarely, if at all. Such variation is difficult to explain based on patient characteristics and values. Further, many world religions and cultures value awareness at the end of life and are opposed to intentional sedation at that time, even if symptoms are not optimally managed. Most experienced palliative care clinicians believe that palliative sedation to unconsciousness should be needed quite rarely, and only after other rigorous attempts have been made to relieve the patient's suffering.

Physician-Assisted Death

AAHPM defines *physician-assisted death* "as a physician providing, at the patient's request, a lethal medication that the patient can take by his own hand to end otherwise intolerable suffering" (51). *Euthanasia* is when a physician personally ends a patient's life (52). The US Supreme Court has rejected arguments that there is a constitutional right to physician-assisted death, and it is illegal in most states.[8,9] Oregon[10] and Washington state[11] now have laws permitting physician-assisted death that were adopted by the vote of the people. The Montana Supreme Court has ruled that patients with terminal illness have a right to physician-assisted death.[12] The protection offered by this court ruling is questionable. Other states are free to legalize physician-assisted death. No state at this time has legalized euthanasia.

The Oregon and Washington laws contain exemption clauses for health-care providers who conscientiously object to participation in physician-assisted death. Under the Affordable Care Act, federal and state governments and health-care providers receiving federal financial assistance may not discriminate against individuals and institutions for refusing to offer physician-assisted death, euthanasia, or mercy killing.[13]

---

[8] *Vacco v Quill*, 521 US 793, 807 (1997).

[9] *Washington v Glucksberg*, 521 US 702 (1997).

[10] Oregon Death with Dignity Act, Or Rev Stat, §127.805, 2.01 (2003).

[11] Washington Death with Dignity Act, Wash Rev Code, §70.245 (2008).

[12] *Baxter v State*, 224 P3d 1211 (2009).

[13] Patient Protection and Affordable Care Act, Pub L No. 111–48, 124 Stat 119, §1553 (2010).

The Debate

Thoughtful and compassionate people have compelling arguments for both prohibiting physician-assisted death and allowing it under carefully defined circumstances (53). Proponents of physician-assisted death base their arguments on autonomy and compassion (54). Proponents view physician-assisted death—in compelling cases and with adequate safeguards—as a humane way to end a life characterized by intense suffering resulting from uncontrollable physical, psychosocial, or spiritual pain. They also point out that such practices have historical and cultural precedence. When a patient's life has become intolerable, some proponents view a refusal to participate in assisted death as contrary to the principle of patient autonomy, which, they argue, includes the patient's right to determine when and how life ends. Some believe assisted death is compatible with a physician's professional integrity, but only when it is used as a last resort to relieve intractable physical suffering (55). Those supporting physician-assisted death tend to believe society is systematically diverging from what is right by forcing dying patients to endure unwanted days of meaningless suffering (56).

Opponents of physician-assisted death and euthanasia often base their arguments on moral codes or religious traditions that assert the wrongness or evil of intentionally killing innocents even at their request. Physicians, opponents believe, have a professional obligation to avoid harming a patient. They will point to a history of medical professionalism opposed to such practices. They will point out that most physicians, hospice groups, and physician societies oppose physician-assisted dying. Opponents also voice concerns about the dangers of social policies that condone killing; the initiation of a "slippery slope" that could be used to justify the elimination of disabled or expensive patients; and subtle family, societal, or financial pressures on patients to choose assisted death. Many believe in the likelihood that pain and suffering can be alleviated with skillful palliative interventions that will help patients view life as worth living until death occurs, and that the nature of requests for assisted death, which generally are withdrawn when pain and depression effectively are treated, are temporary. Further, people may believe that suicide may be harmful to bereaved families, or even harmful transcendentally to the patient after death. Opponents often express fears that societal trust toward medicine (and particularly hospice and palliative care) will wane if medicine becomes an instrument of death. They often want to respect autonomy, but they embrace the long-held view that suicide presents a limit to respecting self-determination (57). Finally, they often lament the societal denigration of all that is not youth, beauty, sexuality, independence, and productivity (52,58,59).

Common Ground

Proponents and opponents of physician-assisted death should share an ethic of compassion and must agree that abandonment is not a viable alternative to assisted death.

Further, universal agreement should exist that suffering among dying patients remains all too prevalent, and lack of access to expert hospice and palliative care contributes to the suffering. Although this chapter *about* ethics cannot offer an universally accepted answer (though the author believes one exists) for physicians grappling with the issue of physician-assisted death, it does offer unequivocal recognition of the need to support improved access to expert palliative care.

REFERENCES

1. Engelhardt HT. *Foundations of Bioethics.* 2nd ed. London: Oxford University Press; 1996.
2. Meisel A. The legal consensus about foregoing lifesustaining treatment: its status and its prospects. *Kennedy Inst Ethics J.* 1992;2(4):309-345.
3. Snyder L. *Ethics Manual.* 6th ed. Philadelphia, PA: American College of Physicians; 2012.
4. Stoneberg JN, von Gunten CF. Assessment of palliative care needs. *Anesthesiol Clin.* 2006;24(1):1-17.
5. Cayley WE Jr. Our most important role as a physician is being a comforter to the sick. *Fam Pract Manag.* October 2006;13(9):74.
6. Daneault S, Lussier V, Mongeau S, et al. The nature of suffering and its relief in the terminally ill: a qualitative study. *J Palliat Care.* 2004;20(1):7-11.
7. Bishop, J. *The Anticipatory Corpse: Medicine, Power, and the Care of the Dying.* Notre Dame, IN: Notre Dame Press; 2011 (theme of the book). www.aahpm.org
8. Koppel A, Sullivan SM. Legal considerations in end-of-life decision making in Louisiana. *Ochsner J.* 2011;11(4):330-333.
9. Schuklenk U, van Delden JJ, Downie J, McLean SA, Upshur R, Weinstock D. End-of-life decision making in Canada: the report by the Royal Society of Canada expert panel on end-of-life decision making. *Bioethics.* 2011;25(suppl 1):1-73.
10. Sato K, Miyashita M, Morita T, Suzuki M. The long-term effect of a population-based educational intervention focusing on end-of-life home care, life-prolongation treatment, and knowledge about palliative care. *J Palliat Care.* 2009;25(3):206-212.
11. Feltman DM, Du H, Leuthner SR. Survey of neonatologists' attitudes toward limiting life-sustaining treatments in the neonatal intensive care unit. *J Perinatol.* 2011.
12. Solomon MZ, O'Donnell L, Jennings B, et al. Decisions near the end of life: professional views on life-sustaining treatments. *Am J Public Health.* 1993;83(1):14-23.
13. Meisel A, Snyder L, Quill T. Seven legal barriers to end-of-life care: myths, realities, and grains of truth. *JAMA.* 2000;284(19):2495-2501.
14. Bradley A. Positive rights, negative rights and health care. *J Med Ethics.* 2010;36(12):838-841.
15. Kinney HC, Korein J, Panigrahy A, Dikkes P, Goode R. Neuropathological findings in the brain of Karen Ann Quinlan. The role of the thalamus in the persistent vegetative state. *N Engl J Med.* 1994;330(21):1469-1475.
16. Cranford RE, Doudera AE. The emergence of institutional ethics committees. *Law Med Health Care.* 1984;12(1):13-20.
17. Lewin T. Nancy Cruzan dies, outlived by a debate over the right to die. *New York Times.* December 27, 1990.
18. University of Miami Ethics Programs, Shepard Broad Law Center at Nova Southeastern University. Key events in the case of Theresa Marie Schiavo. http://www6.miami.edu/ethics/schiavo/timeline.htm. Accessed January 12, 2012.
19. Goodnough A. The Schiavo case: the overview. *New York Times.* April 1, 2005: A1.
20. United States Conference of Catholic Bishops. *Ethical and Religious Directives for Catholic Health Care Services.* 5th ed. http://www.ncbcenter.org/document.doc?id=147. Accessed January 11, 2012.
21. Burt RA. The Supreme Court speaks—not assisted suicide but a constitutional right to palliative care. *N Engl J Med.* 1997;337(17):1234-1236.
22. Jonsen AR, Siegler M, Winslade WJ. *Clinical Ethics: A Practical Approach to Ethical Decisions in Clinical Medicine.* 7th ed. New York, NY: McGraw-Hill; 2010.
23. Miller SS, Marin DB. Assessing capacity. *Emerg Med Clin North Am.* 2000;18(2):233-242.
24. Meisel A, Cerminara KL. *Right to Die: The Law of End-of-Life Decision Making.* 3rd ed. Riverwoods, IL: Aspen Publishers; 2011.
25. Vig EK, Taylor JS, Starks H, Hopley EK, Fryer-Edwards K. Beyond substituted judgment: how surrogates navigate end-of-life decision-making. *J Am Geriatr Soc.* 2006;54(11):1688-1693.
26. Sulmasy DP, Snyder L. Substituted interests and best judgments: an integrated model of surrogate decision making. *JAMA.* 2010;304(17):1946-1947. © 2010 by the American Medical Association.
27. Brown DJ. Palliation of breathlessness. *Clin Med.* 2006;6(2):133-136.
28. El-Jawahri A, Greer JA, Temel JS. Does palliative care improve outcomes for patients with incurable illness? A review of the evidence. *J Support Oncol.* 2011;9(3):87-94.
29. Temel JS, Greer JA, Muzikansky A, et al. Early palliative care for patients with metastatic non-small-cell lung cancer. *N Engl J Med.* 2010;363(8):733-742.
30. Payne R, Anderson E, Arnold R, et al. A rose by any other name: pain contracts/agreements. *Am J Bioeth.* 2010;10(11):5-12.
31. Quill TE, Dresser R, Brock DW. The rule of double effect—a critique of its role in end-of-life decision making. *N Engl J Med.* 1997;337(24):1768-1771.
32. Bernat JL. Medical futility: definition, determination, and disputes in critical care. *Neurocrit Care.* 2005;2(2):198-205.
33. Procedure if Not Effectuating a Directive or Treatment Decision, Texas Health & Safety Code, §166.046 (2003).
34. Burge CR. Texas Advance Directives Act versus "state-created danger" theory: a prima facie analysis. *Am J Trial Advoc.* 2009; 32:552.
35. Schneiderman LJ, Jecker NS, Jonsen AR. Medical futility: its meaning and ethical implications. *Ann Intern Med.* 1990;112(12):949-954.
36. Alpers A, Lo B. When is CPR futile? *JAMA.* 1995;273(2):156-158.
37. Nelson JL. Internal organs, integral selves, and good communities: opt-out organ procurement policies and the 'separateness of persons'. *Theor Med Bioeth.* 2011;32(5):289-300.
38. Arnold RM. Fast facts and concepts #79: discussing organ donation with families. 2006. www.aahpm.org/cgi-bin/wkcgi/view?status=A%20&search=155&id=390&offset=0&limit=258. Accessed August 3, 2007.
39. Arnold RM, Siminoff LA, Frader JE. Ethical issues in organ procurement: a review for intensivists. *Crit Care Clin.* 1996;12(1):29-48.
40. Siminoff LA, Arnold RM, Caplan AL, Virnig BA, Seltzer DL. Public policy governing organ and tissue procurement in the United States. Results from the National Organ and Tissue Procurement Study. *Ann Intern Med.* 1995;123(1):10-17.

41. Stein R. Changes in controversial organ donation method stir fears. *Washington Post.* September 19, 2011.

42. Public Welfare: Definitions. To be codified at 45 CFR §88.2. *Fed Regist.* 2008;73:414-415.

43. Fuhrman MP, Herrmann VM. Bridging the continuum: nutrition support in palliative and hospice care. *Nutr Clin Pract.* 2006;21(2):134-141.

44. Gillick MR. The use of advance care planning to guide decisions about artificial nutrition and hydration. *Nutr Clin Pract.* 2006;21(2):126-133.

45. Quill TE, Lo B, Brock DW, Meisel A. Last-resort options for palliative sedation. *Ann Intern Med.* 2009;151(6): 421-424.

46. Quill TE, Byock IR. Responding to intractable terminal suffering. *Ann Intern Med.* 2000;133(7):561-562.

47. Lo B, Rubenfeld G. Palliative sedation in dying patients: "we turn to it when everything else hasn't worked." *JAMA.* October 2005;294(14):1810-1816.

48. Rousseau P. Palliative sedation in the management of refractory symptoms. *J Support Oncol.* 2004;2(2):181-186.

49. Krakauer EL, Penson RT, Truog RD, King LA, Chabner BA, Lynch TJ Jr. Sedation for intractable distress of a dying patient: acute palliative care and the principle of double effect. *Oncologist.* 2000;5(1):53-62.

50. Billings JA, Block SD. Slow euthanasia. *J Palliat Care.* 1996;12(4):21-30.

51. American Academy of Hospice and Palliative Medicine. AAHPM Statement on Physician-Assisted Suicide. www.aahpm.org/positions/default/suicide.html. Accessed December 15, 2011.

52. Moulin DE, Latimer EJ, Macdonald N, et al. Statement on euthanasia and physician-assisted suicide. *J Palliat Care.* 1994;10(2):80-81.

53. Foley KM. Competent care for the dying instead of physician-assisted suicide. *N Engl J Med.* 1997;336(1):54-58.

54. Battin MP. *Ethical Issues in Suicide.* 2nd ed. Englewood Cliffs, NJ: Prentice-Hall; 1995.

55. Emanuel EJ, Fairclough D, Clarridge BC, et al. Attitudes and practices of U.S. oncologists regarding euthanasia and physician-assisted suicide. *Ann Intern Med.* 2000;133(7):527-532.

56. Warnock M. *Easeful Death: Is There a Case for Assisted Dying?* New York, NY: Oxford University Press; 2009.

57. Foley KM, Hendin H, eds. *The Case Against Assisted Suicide: For the Right to End-of-Life Care.* Baltimore, MD: Johns Hopkins University Press; 2004.

58. Hendin H. Selling death and dignity. *Hastings Cent Rep.* 1995;25(3):19-23.

59. Cherny NI, Coyle N, Foley KM. The treatment of suffering when patients request elective death. *J Palliat Care.* 1994;10(2):71-79.

Special Interventions in Supportive and Palliative Care

CHAPTER 59

Hematologic Support of the Cancer Patient

Lee S. Schwartzberg

INTRODUCTION

The bone marrow, site of origin for blood cells, is the organ most at risk for collateral damage from the modalities of modern cancer therapy. Each of the constituent components of blood—granulocytes, erythrocytes, and platelets—is at risk for compromise. Reduction in quantity and/or function in any component can lead to profound consequences for the patient. Moreover, the bone marrow itself is a frequent site of metastases for many solid tumors and the primary site of many hematologic malignancies, rendering it particularly vulnerable to insult. Indeed, neutropenia, anemia, and thrombocytopenia are the most common complications of cancer and its treatment. Physicians caring for cancer patients must be fully versed in the consequences of cytopenias.

In the early decades of oncology, the armamentarium for hematologic support was limited to transfusions, antibiotics, and the passage of time. The development of growth factors was a technologic tour de force, which profoundly transformed hematologic supportive care. However, growth factors are expensive and are associated with real and theoretical complications. Clinicians should recognize the reasons to consider hematologic support for patients and carefully evaluate the risk–benefit ratio of growth factors and other available measures to maximize patient outcome. By utilizing appropriate supportive care, cancer patients can undergo more effective therapy with reduced morbidity and mortality.

ANEMIA

Anemia is defined as a reduction in the number of circulating red blood cells (RBCs) or by the hemoglobin (Hb) level and the hematocrit (Hct), all reported on a complete blood count. It is the most common hematologic abnormality in patients with cancer. Depending on the tumor type, between 32% and 49% of patients are anemic at the time of cancer diagnosis (1) and approximately 50% of all patients will develop anemia at some time during their treatment. Anemia is graded as mild, moderate, severe, or life threatening (Table 59.1).

When oxygen delivery to tissue is impaired by anemia, subtle or profound organ dysfunction occurs depending on the rapidity of the fall of RBCs, availability of compensatory mechanisms, absolute RBC levels, baseline functional state, and comorbid conditions. Signs of anemia include pallor in mucous membranes, conjunctiva, and nail beds,

tachycardia, and increased respiratory rate and may progress to hypoxemia and orthostatic hypotension in patients with acute blood loss and hypovolemia. A widened pulse pressure, hyperdynamic precordium, and systolic flow murmur can be ascertained along with, in decompensated states, signs of high output cardiac failure, peripheral edema, S_3 and S_4 gallops, and pulmonary rales.

Symptoms of anemia can be insidious and include early decrease in exercise tolerance, shortness of breath on exertion, and fatigue that does not resolve with rest. Some patients describe muscle cramps, irritability, and other signs of neuropsychiatric dysfunction, including depression and confusion. Strain on the cardiovascular system is manifest by breathlessness and rapid heartbeat and can precipitate angina. While cancer-related fatigue itself has many etiologic causes, anemia is a common and contributing factor (2–4).

Anemia can have a direct impact on cancer responsiveness to radiation therapy and may impact the ability to deliver full doses of curative chemotherapy on schedule (5). Cancer-associated anemia is an independent risk factor for survival regardless of tumor type (6).

Etiologies of Anemia in Cancer Patients

There are a myriad of possible etiologies for anemia in cancer patients. The particular type of cancer, patient comorbidities, and the treatment itself may all act independently or together to result in anemia (7). Non-cancer-related causes include pre-existing nutritional deficiencies, renal dysfunction, bleeding, hemolysis, hemoglobinopathies, and infection (8). Malignancy itself can promote the development of anemia (anemia of cancer [AOC]) and anemia frequently develops as a consequence of cancer treatment (chemotherapy-induced anemia [CIA]).

Due to the numerous potential etiologies of anemia in patients with cancer, the evaluation may be complex. Thus, knowledge of the pathophysiology behind cancer and chemotherapy resulting in anemia is an important step in gaining a more thorough understanding of cancer-related anemia. The most common anemias in the world are nutritional, particularly those resulting from iron deficiency as well as deficiencies of folate and vitamin B_{12} (9). These are more often seen in non–cancer populations but should always be considered in patients with cancer. In a study of anemic cancer patients receiving chemotherapy, 17% had ferritin levels <100 mg/L, 6% had low vitamin B_{12} levels, and 2% had high creatinine levels (10).

TABLE 59.1 Anemia grade

Grade	Scale (Hb g/dL)
1 (mild)	10 to lower limit of normal
2 (moderate)	8 to <10
3 (severe)	6.5 to <8
4 (life threatening)	<6.5
5 (death)	Death

Adapted from the Common Terminology Criteria for Adverse Events. http://evs.nci.nih.gov/ftp1/CTCAE/About.html.

It is critical for clinicians to recognize nutritional deficiency as a cause or component of multifactorial etiologies for anemia since it is easily and effectively treated. Patients with cancer may develop nutritional anemia secondary to decreased caloric intake in general or due to decreased ability of the gastrointestinal (GI) tract to absorb nutrients. Iron deficiency anemia due to blood loss or due to the inability to absorb iron often occurs in patients with malignancies of the GI tract, including gastric and colorectal cancers. Iron deficiency may also frequently occur in premenopausal women with heavy menses.

A useful framework for the assessment of anemia arises from evaluating three factors: the degree of RBC proliferation, the size of the RBCs, and the quality of hemoglobinization. Proliferation is estimated by the reticulocyte production index (RPI), which is calculated by multiplying the reticulocyte count by the actual Hct divided by the normal expected Hct and corrected for the longer life span of prematurely released reticulocytes (11). The RBC size is determined by the mean corpuscular volume and can be normal (normocytic), small (microcytic), or large (macrocytic). The degree of hemoglobinization is derived from the mean corpuscular hemoglobin concentration (MCHC). RBCs may have normal levels of Hb (normochromic), low amounts of Hb (hypochromic), or high amounts of Hb (hyperchromic). These simple tests, along with serum iron, total iron-binding capacity, ferritin, vitamin B_{12}, folate, and creatinine levels, and a visual examination of the peripheral blood smear can help diagnose the majority of anemias quickly.

Iron deficiency leads to a microcytic, hypochromic anemia. Conversely, vitamin B_{12} or folate deficiencies typically lead to macrocytic and normochromic anemias. In the absence of therapy, anemia associated with myelodysplastic syndrome (MDS) will be normocytic to macrocytic and is often associated with other cytopenias. The RPI will be low in nutritional anemias, but it will be high in the setting of acute or chronic hemolysis and may also be high in occult or acute blood loss. A careful history is always a cost-effective tool in determining if there is a hereditary component to anemia such as a hemoglobinopathy or a prior GI surgical procedure that could lead to nutritional deficiency. Endocrine and metabolic deficiencies should be ruled out as well, as they frequently have anemia as a consequence.

Anemia of Cancer

RBCs developed from primitive bone marrow progenitor cells that are functionally defined as burst forming units-erythroid. These red cell precursors are simulated to proliferate and differentiate largely as a result of the actions of erythropoietin, a growth factor hormone synthesized and secreted by the kidney in response to sensing tissue hypoxemia. There is an inverse relationship between the Hb and Hct and erythropoietin levels, which begin to rise above normal when the Hb is <10 g/dL and/or the Hct is <30% (12). Erythropoietin production can be impaired in multiple ways and is frequently compromised in individuals with reduced renal function from any cause, including nephrotoxic chemotherapy, diabetes, and aging.

Many cancer patients experience activation of the immune system. At its most extreme, autoantibodies can destroy RBCs leading to autoimmune hemolytic anemia or even profound suppression of RBC production (RBC aplasia). More commonly, there appears to be a less-specific activation of the immune system in the bone marrow leading to increased cytokine production, reduction in erythropoietin production, and increased apoptosis of RBC precursors. Inflammatory cytokines are generated either by cancer cells directly or through tumor–stromal interactions leading to production of interferon gamma, interleukin-1 (IL-1), interleukin-6 (IL-6), and tumor necrosis factor, each of which can suppress erythropoietin production (13,14). These cytokines may also interact synergistically and perpetuate each other's production leading to a chronically elevated cytokine state and reduction in erythropoietin (Fig. 59.1) (15,16).

Iron metabolism is intrinsically linked to RBC production as iron is incorporated into the functioning Hb molecule through a complex physiology. There is abundant evidence that abnormalities of iron metabolism play a significant role in etiology of AOC. Hepcidin, a small peptide, serves a critical regulatory role in the transfer of iron to RBC precursors. Hepcidin is upregulated by IL-6, acts principally to decrease both iron absorption in the GI tract and macrophage iron release, and decreases erythropoietin levels (17) with a net effect of decreased iron available for erythropoiesis (18).

RBC life span, typically around 90 days in normal individuals, is reduced by cytokines and shortened survival cannot be overcome by compensatory increase in production. Finally, AOC can occur due to myelophthisis, which is replacement of the marrow-forming elements by cancer, a situation frequently seen in prostate cancer, breast cancer, and small cell lung cancer.

The clinical manifestations of AOC are a hypoproliferative state with normocytic to microcytic RBCs, normal to mildly reduced MCHC, and a low reticulocyte count. Serum ferritin levels are typically normal to increased while both serum iron and serum transferrin may be low. These studies

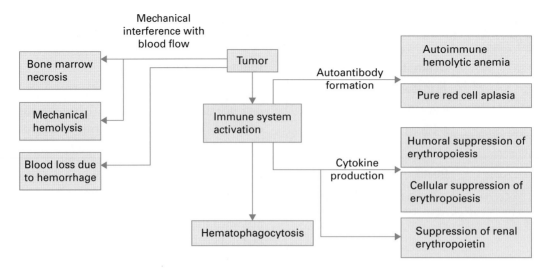

Figure 59.1. Causes of anemia of cancer. Solid tumors can cause anemia by a range of mechanisms. Immune system activation with direct and indirect inhibition of red blood cell (RBC) production is most common, but other factors as described are also operant. Hematopoietic tumors involve similar mechanisms with the addition of intrinsic genetic abnormalities in the erythroid progenitor cells as the most common cause of reduced RBCs.

help to differentiate AOC from iron deficiency anemia. Severe AOC with an Hb <8 g/dL is rare. Other etiologies should be entertained in this circumstance.

Chemotherapy-Induced Anemia

The use of chemotherapy significantly increases the proportion of cancer patients with anemia. Myelosuppressive effects of cytotoxic chemotherapy on erythropoiesis are generally cumulative in nature and up to 50% of patients with cancer may develop CIA over the course of treatment (19). A steady increase in the rate of anemia occurs with additional cycles of chemotherapy as demonstrated by the European Cancer Anemia Survey (ECAS), which followed 15,367 patients in 24 countries (20). This study showed that the rate of anemia, defined as an Hb <12 g/dL, increased from 19.5% in cycle 1 to 46.7% by cycle 5. The percentage of patients with more severe, grade 2/3 anemia also increased with greater number of chemotherapy cycles.

Patients frequently become anemic within the first two cycles of chemotherapy as evidenced from a separate analysis of ECAS data in patients who were not anemic (Hb > 12 g/ dL) prior to initiating chemotherapy (21). In this analysis, 62% of patients experienced an Hb decline of 1.5 g/dL within a median time of 6.1 to 7.2 weeks and 51% experienced an Hb reduction of ≥2 g/dL within a median time of 7.3 to 8.9 weeks. Over a 6-month period of observation, 67% of surveyed patients became anemic.

A more recent, retrospective study of US community-based oncology practices shed additional light on the variations and prevalence of anemia by cancer type (22). In this observational cohort study of adult patients with cancer conducted between 2001 and 2007, anemia was defined by an Hb <11 g/dL at any time during chemotherapy. At baseline,

20.9% of the 42,923 patients evaluated were anemic. Fifty-six percent of ovarian cancer patients were anemic during chemotherapy representing the most common group. The next highest prevalences were breast cancer at 53.3% and non–small cell lung cancer at 50.9%.

Type of chemotherapy and the length and intensity of treatment can affect the prevalence of anemia. The commonly used platinum-based agents can cause anemia through a variety of mechanisms, including direct effect on renal function as well as occasionally causing hemolytic anemia (23). Patients who received gemcitabine-based regimens (59%), platinum-based regimens (50.7%), and anthracycline-based regimens (50.8%) were the most likely to develop anemia (22).

Additionally as we move into the era of biologic agents, there may be a greater risk for the development of anemia with the newer drugs. For example, imatinib therapy for GI stromal tumors resulted in almost 90% of patients developing anemia, with 10% developing grade 3 or 4 anemia (24). Patients with metastatic renal cell carcinoma receiving temsirolimus as monotherapy experienced an increased rate of clinically significant anemia compared with patients receiving sunitinib or sorafenib (25–27).

Erythropoiesis-stimulating agents to Treat Anemia

The use of blood transfusions to ameliorate anemia dates back to the early 20th century and this method was the only treatment available to increase circulating RBCs until the 1980s. The discovery of erythropoietin as the hormone responsible for RBC production led to the purification, cloning, and manufacture of recombinant human erythropoietin (rHuEPO) in quantities useful as a therapeutic agent. First approved to treat anemia associated with chronic renal disease, in 1993 rHuEPO was approved to treat CIA. Several varieties of rHuEPO are available commercially including epoetin alfa (Procrit, Ortho Biotech) and darbepoetin alfa (Aranesp, Amgen) in North America and epoetin beta (NeoRecormon, Roche) in Europe. Together, they are termed *erythropoiesis*-stimulating agents (ESAs).

The use of ESAs rapidly increased through the 1990s and early 2000s, based on randomized trials that demonstrated improvement in Hb levels, reduction in the need for blood transfusions, and improvement in quality of life (28–30). In the mid-2000s, safety concerns were raised with ESA use, leading to a series of US Food and Drug Administration (FDA) advisory boards examining the issue and ultimately to several FDA label changes and a black box warning. As a result, ESA usage dropped very substantially in patients with CIA. It is now likely that once again anemia remains an undertreated problem in the clinical oncology setting.

Large community-based prospective trials of rHuEPO were completed and reported in the late 1990s. The first trial enrolled 2,370 patients with a variety of nonmyeloid malignancies with Hb levels <11 g/dL (31). Patients received 10,000 units (U) of epoetin alfa subcutaneously (SQ) every 3 weeks. Sixty-three percent of patients had a >1 g/dL rise in Hb after 4 weeks and after 16 weeks, 61% had a 2 g/dL rise or Hb >12 g/dL and a mean rise of Hb of 2 g/dL. A weekly fixed dosing schedule of 40,000 U fixed (32) demonstrated an Hb response of 68%, mean Hb rise of 1.8 g/dL, and reduction in transfusion requirement. Given the convenience of weekly compared with thrice a week dosing, 40,000 U weekly of epoetin alfa quickly became the community standard dosage.

Darbepoetin alfa is a modified recombinant form of erythropoietin with a slightly different amino acid structure that adds additional glycosylation to the native glycoprotein (33). Due to these changes, darbepoetin alfa has a prolonged half-life and altered receptor affinity. Darbepoetin alfa was FDA approved for treatment of CIA in 2002. Randomized clinical trials (RCTs) showed a reduction in transfusion requirements, an increase in Hb levels, and an improvement in quality of life in patients with solid tumors and nonmyeloid hematologic malignancies (27,34,35).

A 2005 meta-analysis of 27 randomized trials examining treatment with epoetin alfa or beta demonstrated a reduction in transfusion rate by 33% over untreated patients (relative risk [RR] 0.67 [0.62 to 0.73]) (36). A sub-analysis of 14 trials demonstrated that 48% of patients receiving epoetin alfa had an Hb response, defined as a 2 g/dL rise or achievement of Hb >12 g/dL. Subsequent RCTs and systemic reviews have reinforced the value of ESAs in reducing transfusion requirements (37).

Several clinical trials have compared weekly epoetin alpha with darbepoetin alfa given less frequently (every 2 to 3 wk) and have demonstrated similar efficacy end points (38,39). Therefore, the decision of the agent to be used should be based on scheduling and economic considerations. Darbepoetin alfa was initially FDA approved on a weight-based weekly dosage. More recent trials have demonstrated that a fixed dosage given as infrequently as every 3 weeks

retains efficacy with far greater patient convenience (40–42). The American Society of Clinical Oncology (ASCO) and the American Society of Hematology (ASH) 2010 guidelines state that epoetin alfa and darbepoetin alfa are therapeutically equivalent with regard to both efficacy and safety (37).

Risks of ESAs

Initial studies with ESAs suggested a potential survival advantage for patients treated for CIA. There was rationale for this signal; anemic patients in many different settings including cancer have an inferior survival over non-anemic-matched controls, and hypoxia can potentially reduce the effectiveness of radiotherapy and even chemotherapy. This hypothesis led to the conduct of several trials in non–anemic patients designed either to prevent significant anemia from occurring or to increase Hb levels to supranormal values. However, a trial in non–anemic head and neck cancer patients receiving radiation therapy and a study in metastatic breast cancer receiving first-line chemotherapy showed higher mortality rates with this strategy (43,44).

Overall, inferior outcomes were demonstrated in 8 of 59 controlled phase III trials of ESAs in a variety of cancers. Only four of these eight trials included patients with CIA, the FDA label indication for ESAs, and all four targeted higher than normal Hb levels as the end point for stopping the ESA. A cervical cancer trial was terminated early in 2003 before the primary end point could be assessed (45). In another breast cancer trial with intent of ESA to increase Hb in non–anemic patients, the event-free survival and overall survival were unplanned analyses (46). No difference in survival was detected in a more mature analysis (47).

An individual patient-level data meta-analysis was published in 2009 (48). This involved 53 studies with 13,933 cancer patients receiving ESAs and included both concurrently chemotherapy-treated patients and those not receiving chemotherapy while on study with the ESA. A significantly increased RR for mortality on study Hazard Ratio (HR 1.17, $P = 0.003$) and for overall survival duration (HR 1.06, $P = 0.005$) was noted. When analysis was restricted to 10,441 patients receiving chemotherapy, there was a nonsignificant increase in on-study mortality (HR 1.10, $P = 0.12$) and shortened survival (HR 1.04, $P = 0.26$). Other meta-analyses published subsequently have reached conflicting conclusions (49).

Based on these results, the consensus of expert opinion concurs that ESAs should not be administered to patients with AOC not receiving chemotherapy. However, it is important to keep in mind that there are no trials published to date that suggest that ESAs given in accordance with guidelines and as per FDA label for CIA result in inferior survival. A number of clinical trials involving ESAs in CIA with survival at the end point are currently in progress.

In contrast to the still unclear signal of survival in CIA patients treated with ESAs, there is substantial evidence that ESAs are associated with an increased risk of thrombovascular events in cancer patients. Venous thromboembolism (VTE) is a frequent complication of cancer in the absence of

ESA therapy. Multiple risk factors for VTE in cancer patients include cancer type, stage, chemotherapy regimen, comorbidities, and immobilization (50).

Several recent meta-analyses have evaluated the risk of VTE in patients receiving ESAs with chemotherapy, radiotherapy, or without additional treatment, and each showed a significant increase in the RR for VTE events. The Agency for Healthcare Research and Quality (AHRQ) comparative effectiveness review of 30 RCTs published in 2006 revealed an RR of 1.69 (95% CI 1.36 to 2.10, $P < 0.001$) (51). The event rate for VTE was 7% (range 0% to 30%) in patients treated with epoetin alfa versus 4% in controls (range 1% to 23%) and 5% in patients treated with darbepoetin alfa versus 3% in controls. A pooled analysis of individual patient-level data from RCTs comparing darbepoetin with placebo showed an increased risk for VTE (HR 1.5, 95% CI 1.10 to 2.26) (52). No increase was observed in mortality in progression-free survival (HR 0.93, 95% CI 0.84 to 1.04) or disease progression. A meta-analysis of long-term follow-up in 18 RCTs utilizing ESAs in CIA demonstrated an odds ratio of 1.47 and 95% CI of 1.24 to 1.74 for VTE (49).

The relative rate for VTE appears to be dependent on target Hb, increasing as Hb rises to ≥13 g/dL. The actual dose or schedule of ESAs utilized does not seem to play a role in the RR of VTEs. None of the trials evaluated specific factors that might impact VTE risk. It is reasonable to weigh the risks and benefits of ESAs carefully in patients judged to be at increased risk for VTE based on history or clinical findings.

ESAs Dosing

Table 59.2 summarizes dosing of ESAs. Epoetin alfa can be initiated at doses of 150 U/kg SQ three times per week (t.i.w) or 40,000 U weekly in patients with CIA as per the FDA label. The dose should be increased to 300 U/kg t.i.w or 60,000 U weekly, respectively, if no response in Hb or no reduction in transfusion requirement is noted after 4 to 6 weeks of therapy. Doses can be reduced or held once target Hb levels are obtained

---

TABLE 59.2	Common dosing options for epoetin alfa and darbepoetin alfa	
	Starting Dose	**Escalation**
Epoetin alfa (Procrit, Ortho Biotech)		
FDA label doses	Epoetin alfa 150 U/kg t.i.w.	Increase to 300 U/kg 3 t.i.w.
	OR	
	Epoetin alfa 40,000 U qwk	Increase to 60,000 U qwk
Darbepoetin alfa (Aranesp, Amgen)		
FDA label doses	Darbepoetin alfa 2.25 μg/kg qwk	Increase Darbepoetin alfa to up to 4.5 μg/kg qwk
	OR	
	Darbepoetin alfa 500 μg q3wk	NONE
Alternative regimens		
Evaluated in RCTs	Darbepoetin alfa 100 μg fixed dose qwk	Increase darbepoetin alfa to up to 150–200 μg fixed dose qwk
	OR	
	Darbepoetin alfa 200 μg fixed dose q2wk	Increase darbepoetin alfa to up to 300 μg fixed dose q2wk
	OR	
	Darbepoetin alfa 300 μg fixed dose q3wk	Increase darbepoetin alfa to up to 500 μg fixed dose q3wk
	OR	
	Epoetin alfa 80,000 U q2wk	NONE
	OR	
	Epoetin alfa 120,000 U q3wk	NONE

All doses developed subcutaneously. Escalation at weeks 6–9 if <1 g/dL rise in Hb from baseline. FDA, Food and Drug Administration; RCT, randomized clinical trial.

with careful monitoring, reinitiating when Hb levels begin to drop toward a level where transfusion might be contemplated. Extended dosing with epoetin alfa at 80,000 U every 2 weeks or 120,000 U every 3 weeks has also been evaluated (53,54).

Darbepoetin alfa can be initiated at 2.25 µg/kg SQ weekly or 500 µg every 3 weeks as per the FDA-approved dose. In addition, randomized trials support starting doses of darbepoetin at 200 µg every 2 weeks or 300 µg every 3 weeks (39,55). The weekly dose of darbepoetin should be doubled to 4.5 µg/kg, the biweekly dose increased to 300 µg, and a starting dose of 300 µg every 3 weeks can be escalated to 500 µg if inadequate response by week 6. There is no evidence to support doses of darbepoetin >500 µg every 3 weeks.

ESAs should be discontinued following completion of chemotherapy or if there is no response after 8 to 9 weeks of therapy as measured by Hb levels or continued need for transfusions. Overall, approximately 50% to 70% of patients will achieve an Hb response, and unfortunately no pretreatment factors predictive of response or nonresponsiveness have yet been identified (56).

Attempts to improve the response to ESAs have focused on providing additional iron, given the functional iron deficiency that occurs in both AOC and CIA. Nine prospective RCTs of intravenous (IV) iron supplementation to oral iron or no iron in CIA patients receiving ESAs have been conducted (57). Eight of these trials showed benefit from the addition of IV iron as measured by Hb response, decrease in blood transfusions, or less ESA requirement (58–61). Patients had ferritin levels from 160 to 460 mg/L and transferrin saturations from 19% to 36%.

Only one trial, the largest so far conducted, detected no benefit of oral or IV iron (62). A possible explanation for the discordant results in this study is that the rate of IV iron delivery was far lower in this trial than in other studies of IV iron. Given the weight of the data, all patients initiating ESA therapy should be screened for iron deficiency and functional iron deficiency. Concurrent IV iron should be strongly considered for those with evidence of functional iron deficiency.

The FDA labels for epoetin alfa and darbepoetin state that ESA should be initiated when the Hb level falls below 10 g/dL. Additionally, the labels recommend using the lowest dose necessary to avoid transfusion. In contrast, clinical trials in CIA establishing the worth of ESAs generally initiated therapy at a starting Hb of <11 g/dL and discontinued when the Hb rose to the 11 to 12 g/dL range. In the RCTs, significant improvement in quality of life and transfusion reduction were established based on those parameters. It is not clear that utilizing <10 g/dL as an arbitrary starting point and discontinuing when Hb is >10 g/dL as mandated by the Centers for Medicare and Medicaid Services National Coverage Determination will lead to the benefits documented by the RCTs in CIA.

Current FDA labels for ESAs include a black box warning against usage in patients with curative malignancies given the potential risk from harm from ESAs. A risk evaluation and mitigation strategy (REMS) program is mandated for all practitioners prescribing an ESA. The patient receives a medication guide and must sign a consent form attesting to receiving explanation of the risks and benefits of the drug. The REMS program for ESA usage is periodically audited.

Transfusion to Treat Cancer-Associated Anemia

Modern day blood banks typically fractionate whole blood collections into packed red blood cells (PRBCs), fresh frozen plasma, and platelet concentrates. In general, use of blood products is more appropriate than administering whole blood except in the rare instance of severe hypovolemia from large volume acute blood loss. In cancer patients, anemia is generally treated with PRBC units. One 300-mL unit typically raises the recipient's Hb by approximately 1 g/dL and the Hct by 3% to 4%.

Indications for a transfusion in anemia associated with cancer are not clearly defined. The US Department of Health and Human Services suggests that transfusion should be used for "treatment of symptomatic deficit oxygen-carrying capacity" and should not be used "to treat anemias that could be corrected with specific medications should as iron, vitamin B_{12}, folic acid or erythropoietin" (57).

Many clinicians utilize an Hb of ≤8 g/dL or Hct of ≤25 to initiate transfusions in relatively asymptomatic patients, but there is little evidence base around this recommendation in ambulatory patients. Symptomatic patients and in those where anemia develops rapidly may require PRBCs at a higher Hb level. The availability of PRBCs varies by season, blood type, and other local and regional factors. Considerable resource utilization occurs with blood transfusions, requiring several hours to perform and crossmatch followed by several hours to deliver the transfusion, typically in an outpatient setting, but occasionally as an inpatient at significantly higher costs.

Transfusion Risks

Blood transfusions are generally safe but not without a consequence. Transfusion-related mortality remains a reality (Fig. 59.2). The annual number of transfusion-related deaths increased from 16 in 1976 to 105 in 2005 with an estimated rate of 2.3 deaths per million transfused components (63). Hemolytic transfusion reactions occur infrequently but may be responsible for 1.0 to 1.2 deaths per 100,000 patients transfused. Transfusion-related circulatory overload is also associated with morbidity and possible mortality.

Alloimmunization is the most frequent complication of transfusions with estimates of rates ranging from 7% to 31%. A retrospective analysis of patients with myeloproliferative or lymphoproliferative disorders found an overall immunization rate in 9% of patients receiving long-term transfusion support with the risk of immunization approximately 0.5% for each unit of PRBC transfused (64). Acute reactions to blood transfusions range from an allergic skin reaction with urticaria to life-threatening hemolysis and multi-organ dysfunction. Modern molecular techniques of crossmatching have reduced acute hemolytic reactions to rare events, <1/200 U transfused (65).

As a biologic product, blood transfusions carry the risk of transmitting infection. Remarkable progress has been made over the years in reducing the chance of infection

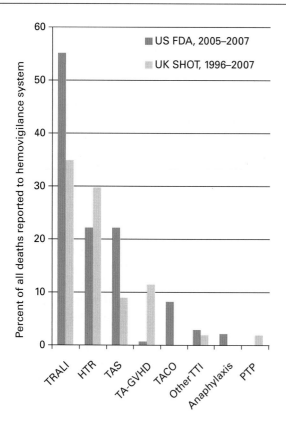

Figure 59.2. Causes of allogeneic blood transfusion deaths in United Kingdom and United States. The figure shows the causes of death that accounted for at least 1% of all deaths. Transfusion-associated circulatory overload (TACO) was not specifically captured, and anaphylaxis not specifically reported, by the UK Serious Hazards of Transfusion (SHOT) surveillance system in 1996 to 2007. There were no deaths due to posttransfusion purpura (PTP) reported to the US Food and Drug Administration (FDA) from 2005 to 2007. TRALI, transfusion-related acute lung injury; TA-GVHD, transfusion-associated graft-versus-host disease; HTR, hemolytic transfusion reactions; TAS, transfusion-associated sepsis; and TTI, transfusion-transmitted infections.

from hepatitis C to <1:100,000 and <1:500,000 for HIV (66). However, there remains the possibility of infection from other transmissible agents, including bacteria, parasites, and other viruses. Cases of blood transfusion–related infection from West Nile Virus have been reported (67), and there are other viruses and infectious agents such as prions capable of causing hepatitis, which are not currently screenable. Bacterial infection is rare, but it can occur as an outgrowth of contaminated blood products (68).

The most common cause of treatment-related deaths from transfusion occurs from transfusion-related acute lung injury (TRALI). TRALI develops during or within 6 hours of a transfusion and is characterized by rapid onset of dyspnea, tachypnea, cyanosis, fever, and hypoxemia. Radiographic studies reveal diffuse fluffy infiltrates consistent with non-cardiogenic pulmonary edema. Treatment consists of supplemental oxygen and mechanical ventilation. Milder forms of the disease have also been reported (69). The reported incidence of TRALI is between 1:300 and 1:5,000 transfusions in

North America. TRALI is thought to originate from granulocyte-mediated lung tissue injury. Mortality from TRALI may be as high as 6% to 10%. At the moment, there is no method of predicting which donors and transfusions may increase the risk of TRALI and no screening method is available.

Cytomegalovirus (CMV) is worthy of mention because of the high seroprevalence in the United States (35% to 80% by region). There is a risk of acute infection in immunosuppressed hosts, particularly bone marrow/stem cell transplant patients. CMV is a leukocyte-associated virus. Therefore, any blood product containing white blood cells is capable of transmitting infection. With the widespread use of leukodepleted blood products, the risk of CMV infection is lessened. However, in the absence of prospective trials comparing leukocyte depleted with seronegative CMV products, CMV-negative donors are still the standard of care for severely immunocompromised CMV-seronegative recipients (70).

Irradiated blood products should be given to cancer patients at increased risk for graft-versus-host disease. Such groups would include allogeneic and autologous bone marrow/stem cell transplant patients and patients who are severely immunocompromised including Hodgkin's disease and other lymphomas (71).

NEUTROPENIA

Neutrophils are the immune system's first line of defense against bacterial and fungal infection. As the neutrophil count drops to <1,000 cells/μL, the risk of infection begins to rise. This level of neutropenia is termed severe neutropenia (SN). Patients with absolute neutrophil counts (ANCs) <500 cells/μL for several days or <100 cells/μL for even 1 day are at substantial risk for blood-borne infection. Fever associated with neutropenia, or febrile neutropenia (FN), is defined as a temperature of 38.3°C orally with an ANC of <1,000 cells/μL. A broad range of symptomatology is associated with FN, from none to severe sepsis syndrome. Because in the early stages of FN the outcome cannot be predicted, all patients with FN should be carefully evaluated and presumed to be infected (72). It should be kept in mind that the absence of neutrophils markedly reduces the inflammatory response characteristically seen with infections, for example, pulmonary infiltrates in the setting of pneumonia. Signs and symptoms of infection may therefore be lacking. As a result, broad-spectrum antibiotics should be initiated immediately after a careful search for localizing sources of infection and pan culturing.

There is significant morbidity and mortality risk for FN. In-hospital mortality determined from a large US survey of hospitalized patients between 1995 and 2000 was 9.5% and rose with increasing number of patient comorbidities. Hospitalization for FN is associated with substantial resource utilization, including a mean length of stay of 11.5 days and a mean cost of $19,100 for an episode of FN (73). More recent surveys suggest that the cost of hospitalization and/or emergency department visits for FN continue to rise (74). A scoring system can help predict the risk of complications in patients with FN (75,76).

Patients presenting with FN can be characterized into low-risk groups who could be treated as outpatients with oral antibiotics and higher risk groups requiring IV antibiotics and prolonged hospitalizations (77,78). Low-risk patients tend to have solid tumors under control, are without serious comorbidities, and expect relatively shorter duration of SN/FN. At least two prediction models are validated and are useful to make decisions or hospitalization for patients who present with FN (79,80). Given the expense of hospitalization for FN and the ability to reliably identify low-risk patients (81), utilizing risk stratification in FN is a cost-effective strategy.

The use of antibiotic prophylaxis to prevent FN is not well established for solid tumors, although often utilized along with colony-stimulating factor (CSF) support in hematologic malignancies when long periods of neutropenia are expected. Two meta-analysis and a systematic review suggest that evidence is too limited to recommend prophylactic antibiotics in patients receiving myelosuppressive chemotherapy (82–84).

Determination of Risk of Neutropenia

The likelihood of SN/FN with chemotherapy is dependent mainly on the intrinsic myelosuppression of the regimen utilized, but patient and disease factors should also be considered. Many clinical trials, which determined the efficacy of a particular chemotherapy regimen, did not formally establish the risk of FN as a component of the trial. Therefore, there is still a knowledge gap for many established combination chemotherapy programs. However, the National Comprehensive Cancer Network (NCCN) guidelines has grouped regimens into a moderate risk of FN, defined as 10% to 20%, or high risk, >20% chance of FN.

Patient factors should also be taken into consideration when determining the risk of SN/FN (Table 59.3) (90). The most important patient risk factor is age, with patients >65 years old at highest risk for any given chemotherapy regimen (85,86). Other important factors include previous exposure to chemotherapy or radiation therapy, prior chemotherapy-induced neutropenia, bone marrow involvement with tumor, poor performance status, poor renal function, liver dysfunction, and pre-existing conditions including neutropenia, infection, or recent surgery (87,88).

Several risk models have been developed to integrate patient-related factors into a useful tool to predict SN/FN, particularly when regimens with intermediate intrinsic risk are utilized (89). Lyman et al. developed a predictive model that was retrospectively validated with a data set of over 3,760 patients (90). Cycle 1 neutropenic events were predicted in 34% of high-risk and 4% of low-risk patients with a sensitivity of 90% and specificity of 59%. Another model utilizes a validated web-based tool for predicting the severity of hematologic toxicity in lymphoma patients receiving cyclophosphamide, doxorubicin, vincristine, and prednisone (CHOP)-like regimens (91) and another for non–Hodgkin's lymphoma (NHL) showed high sensitivity of 81% and specificity of 80% for predicting cycle 1 FN with 28% positive and

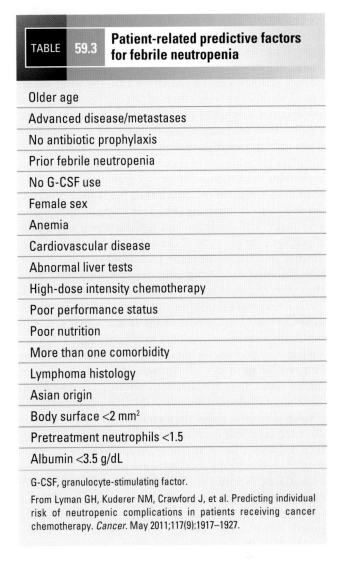

TABLE 59.3	Patient-related predictive factors for febrile neutropenia
Older age	
Advanced disease/metastases	
No antibiotic prophylaxis	
Prior febrile neutropenia	
No G-CSF use	
Female sex	
Anemia	
Cardiovascular disease	
Abnormal liver tests	
High-dose intensity chemotherapy	
Poor performance status	
Poor nutrition	
More than one comorbidity	
Lymphoma histology	
Asian origin	
Body surface <2 mm^2	
Pretreatment neutrophils <1.5	
Albumin <3.5 g/dL	

G-CSF, granulocyte-stimulating factor.

From Lyman GH, Kuderer NM, Crawford J, et al. Predicting individual risk of neutropenic complications in patients receiving cancer chemotherapy. *Cancer.* May 2011;117(9):1917–1927.

98% negative predictive value (92). All of the models to date suffer from a lack of prospective validation, but they can still serve as useful adjuncts to decision making for primary prophylaxis with growth factors.

Growth Factor Use for Prevention of FN

Granulocyte colony-stimulating factor (G-CSF) is a lineage-specific myeloid growth factor that hastens maturation and release of the committed progenitor pool, prolongs circulation of released granulocytes, and stimulates demargination of neutrophils in the vascular pool. It also enhances neutrophil function through increases in chemotaxis, phagocytosis, and primes granulocytes for respiratory burst. The normal proliferation and maturation of neutrophils from progenitors in the bone marrow is markedly enhanced by the addition of pharmacologic doses of recombinant human G-CSF (Filgrastim [Neupogen], Amgen), such that the normal 5-day maturation process may occur within a single day. Normal volunteers receiving filgrastim experience a dose-dependent increase in ANC (93).

Pegfilgrastim (Neulasta, Amgen) is a modified version of recombinant G-CSF with a 20-kDa polyethylene glycol molecule attached to the N-terminus of the standard molecule. Due to this modification, pegfilgrastim is not cleared by the kidneys and has a prolonged serum half-life, while maintaining all other biologic effects of G-CSF. The clearance of pegfilgrastim is by ligand–receptor binding at the neutrophil, which is then internalized and metabolized intracellularly. When patients receive myelosuppressive chemotherapy, pegfilgrastim given afterward remains at high circulating concentrations until stimulation of accelerated recovery of the neutrophil compartment, which then binds the pegfilgrastim and clears it internally (94). This mode of metabolism is termed as self-regulation and explains why a single dose of pegfilgrastim per cycle of chemotherapy can be clinically effective in reducing duration and depth of neutropenia. Both filgrastim and pegfilgrastim are FDA approved for the prevention of chemotherapy-induced neutropenia.

Granulocyte–macrophage colony-stimulating factor (GM-CSF) is a lineage-nonspecific factor, which acts synergistically with other cytokines to enhance myeloid, macrophage, and erythrocyte lineage expansion and maturation with resulting broader hematologic effects. Recombinant human GM-CSF is available commercially (sargramostim [Leukine], Genzyme). Clinically, GM-CSF can increase the neutrophil count as well as the monocyte count and modestly affect the erythroid compartment; immunologic enhancement is also seen. GM-CSF is not FDA approved for the treatment of chemotherapy-induced neutropenia.

Initial RCTs testing G-CSF as primary prophylaxis after myelotoxic chemotherapy with an expected risk of FN of >40% demonstrated a 50% reduction in FN rate with daily growth factor administration until neutrophil recovery (95,96). Subsequent trials examined less myelosuppressive regimens and showed reduction in FN rate with G-CSF prophylaxis. Pegfilgrastim compared with daily filgrastim showed equal or better efficacy with the benefit of administration of only one dose per cycle compared with an average of 10 daily doses of filgrastim for equivalent effects (97,98).

A trial examining the use of primary prophylaxis with pegfilgrastim versus placebo in patients receiving myelosuppressive doses of docetaxel in breast cancer demonstrated a dramatic reduction in the rate of FN from 17% to 1% (99). Additionally, use of anti-infective agents declined from 10% to 2% and hospitalizations were reduced from 14% to 1%. Notably, the first cycle rate of FN was 11% in the placebo arm versus 1% in patients receiving pegfilgrastim.

A systematic analysis of RCTs including 3,493 patients utilizing G-CSF as primary prophylaxis against FN showed a risk reduction of 46% (RR 0.54, 95% CI 0.43 to 0.67, $P < 0.001$) for the incidence of FN (100). Moreover, the relative dose intensity (RDI) of chemotherapy delivered was improved by 8.4%, $P = 0.001$. Notably, this meta-analysis demonstrated a reduction in infection-related mortality (RR 0.55, 95% CI 0.33 to 0.90, $P = 0.018$) and also for early

mortality during chemotherapy (RR 0.60, 95% CI 0.43 to 0.83, $P = 0.002$). A more recent systematic review of 25 randomized trials involving 12,000 patients showed an RR of 0.897 for all-cause mortality with the use of prophylactic growth factor, translating into a 3.4% absolute reduction in mortality (101).

Growth Factor Indications and Dosing

Given the documented marked reduction in FN with the use of myeloid growth factors, G-CSF prophylaxis is recommended for patients receiving myelotoxic chemotherapy with an expected FN rate of around 20% or higher (Table 59.4). NCCN (1), ASCO (102), and European Organization for Research and Treatment of Cancer (EORTC) guidelines (103) are concordant on this recommendation. The NCCN usefully subdivides recommendations for growth factor usage by intent of therapy. For patients receiving curative intent therapy, where delivered dose intensity may be extremely important, growth factor support is considered for regimens with a 10% to 20% risk of FN (Table 59.5). Prophylaxis is also suggested to treat patients with full-dose chemotherapy in the setting of life-prolonging treatment when the risk is 10% to 20%.

Alternatively, for patients receiving purely palliative chemotherapy it may be more appropriate to reduce doses of chemotherapy when the risk of FN is high or after a prior episode of FN to a particular treatment regimen. Prophylactic G-CSF is recommended for any patient considered to be at high risk for FN regardless of the intent of therapy. Moreover, patients receiving a lower risk regimen should be considered for growth factor support when there is a high chance for serious morbidity or mortality.

Growth factor support allows for the delivery of full dose of chemotherapy on schedule. Reduction in RDI of even modest amounts has been associated with inferior outcomes in curative disease settings such as NHL treated with CHOP and adjuvant chemotherapy in early-stage breast cancer (104,105). First-cycle FN is associated with lower subsequent RDI. Neutropenia remains the major dose-limiting toxicity of adjuvant chemotherapy for early-stage breast cancer (106). A meta-analysis of 10 studies that reported RDI and compared prophylaxis with growth factors versus none showed an increase in RDI to 95.1% of anticipated in patients who received G-CSF compared with 86.7% in those without growth factor support (100).

Filgrastim and pegfilgrastim should be administered 1 to 3 days after completion of chemotherapy to achieve optimal effects and reduce potential complications. Filgrastim is dosed at 5 µg/kg SQ daily, adjusted to the closest vial size available, until recovery of the neutrophil count. Pegfilgrastim is given at a single fixed dose of 6 mg SQ to adults, with chemotherapy occurring every 2 weeks or greater. Studies examining alternative or shorter programs of growth factor support have generally demonstrated inferior results (107,108). Trials examining giving growth factors on

TABLE 59.4 Disease settings and chemotherapy regimens with a high risk of febrile neutropenia (>20%)

Bladder Cancer

- MVAC (methotrexate, vinblastine, doxorubicin, cisplatin)

Breast Cancer

- Docetaxel + trastuzumab
- Dose dense AC → T (doxorubicin and cyclophosphamide, paclitaxel)
- AT (doxorubicin, paclitaxel)
- AT (doxorubicin, docetaxel)
- TAC (docetaxel, doxorubicin, cyclophosphamide)

Esophageal and Gastric Cancer

- Docetaxel/cisplatin/fluorouracil

Hodgkin's Lymphoma

- BEACOPP (bleomycin, etoposide, doxorubicin, cyclophosphamide, vincristine, procarbazine, prednisone)

Kidney Cancer

- Doxorubicin/gemcitabine

Non–Hodgkin's Lymphoma

- CFAR (cyclophosphamide, fludarabine, alemtuzumab, rituximab)
- ICE (ifosfamide, carboplatin, etoposide)
- RICE (rituximab, ifosfamide, carboplatin, etoposide)
- CHOP-14 (cyclophosphamide, doxorubicin, vincristine, prednisone)
- MINE (mesna, ifosfamide, novantrone, etoposide)
- DHAP (dexamethasone, cisplatin, cytarabine)
- ESHAP (etoposide, methylprednisolone, cisplatin, cytarabine)
- HyperCVAD + rituximab (cyclophosphamide, vincristine, doxorubicin, dexamethasone + rituximab)

Melanoma

- Dacarbazine-based combination (dacarbazine, cisplatin, vinblastine)
- Dacarbazine-based combination with IL-2, interferon alfa (dacarbazine, cisplatin, vinblastine, IL-2, interferon alfa)

Multiple Myeloma

- Modified HyperCVAD

Myelodysplastic Syndrome

- Antithymocyte globulin, rabbit/cyclosporine
- Decitabine

Ovarian Cancer

- Topotecan
- Paclitaxel
- Docetaxel

Sarcoma

- MAID (mesna, doxorubicin, ifosfamide, dacarbazine)
- Doxorubicin

Small Cell Lung Cancer

- Topotecan

Testicular Cancer

- VeIP (vinblastine, ifosfamide, cisplatin)
- VIP (etoposide, ifosfamide, cisplatin)
- BEP (bleomycin, etoposide, cisplatin)
- TIP (paclitaxel, ifosfamide, cisplatin)

From The NCCN Clinical Practice Guidelines in Oncology. Cancer- and chemotherapy-induced anemia. http://www.nccn.org/professionals/physician_gls/f_guidelines.asp.

the same day as chemotherapy have also shown to be less effective than beginning at least 1 day after chemotherapy, and same day administration is not recommended (109,110).

The first cycle of a myelosuppressive regimen is associated with the highest risk of FN (111). Indeed, in many prospective and retrospective analyses the first cycle constitutes up to 50% of the risk of FN for the entire chemotherapy program (Vogel C., etc. need others). Therefore, primary prophylaxis beginning with the first cycle of therapy and continuing with each cycle represents the most effective way to reduce the chance of FN with appropriately myelotoxic chemotherapy. A patient who develops FN after chemotherapy not supported by prophylactic growth factors should be strongly considered for subsequent cycle prevention with CSF.

Patients who develop FN without growth factors can be treated with filgrastim at the time of neutropenia until the ANC recovers. Studies examining this secondary prevention have not demonstrated a robust effect for

| TABLE 59.5 | Disease settings and chemotherapy regimens with an intermediate risk of febrile neutropenia (10% to 20%) |

Occult Primary Adenocarcinoma

Gemcitabine, docetaxel

Breast Cancer

Docetaxel every 21 d

Epirubicin

Epirubicin + sequential cyclophosphamide + methotrexate + 5-fluorouracil

CMF classic (cyclophosphamide, methotrexate, fluorouracil)

AC (doxorubicin, cyclophosphamide)+ sequential docetaxel

AC + sequential docetaxel + trastuzumab

FEC (fluorouracil, epirubicin, cyclophosphamide) + sequential docetaxel

Paclitaxel every 21 d

Vinblastine

Cervical Cancer

Cisplatin + topotecan

Topotecan

Irinotecan

Colorectal Cancer

FOLFOX (fluorouracil, leucovorin, oxaliplatin)

Esophageal and Gastric Cancer

Irinotecan/cisplatin

Epirubicin/cisplatin/5-fluorouracil

Epirubicin/cisplatin/capecitabine

Hodgkin's Lymphoma

ABVD (doxorubicin, bleomycin, vinblastine, dacarbazine)

Stanford V (mechlorethamine, doxorubicin, vinblastine, bleomycin)

Non–Hodgkin's Lymophomas

EPOCH (etoposide, prednisone, vincristine, cyclophosphamide, doxorubicin)

EPOCH (etoposide, prednisone, vincristine, cyclophosphamide, doxorubicin + IT chemotherapy)

Non–Hodgkin's Lymophomas

ACOD (modified CHOP–doxorubicin, cyclophosphamide, vincristine, prednisone)

GDP (gemcitabine, dexamethasone, cisplatin)

GDP (gemcitabine, dexamethasone, cisplatin) + rituximab

FM (fludarabine, mitoxantrone)

CHOP + rituximab (cyclophosphamide, doxorubicin, vincristine, prednisone, rituximab)

Non–Small Cell Lung Cancer

Cisplatin/paclitaxel

Cisplatin/vinorelbine

Cisplatin/docetaxel

Cisplatin/irinotecan

Cisplatin/etoposide

Carboplatin/paclitaxel

Docetaxel

Cyclophosphamide, doxorubicin + IT chemotherapy

Ovarian Cancer

Carboplatin/docetaxel

Prostate

Cabazitaxel

Small Cell Lung Cancer

Etoposide/carboplatin

Testicular Cancer

Etoposide/cisplatin

Uterine Cancer

Docetaxel

Uterine Cancer

Docetaxel

treatment of established FN, although neutrophil recovery may be hastened by 1 to 2 days. Nonetheless, older patients, those with comorbidities or complications like pneumonia or sepsis, should be strongly considered for treatment with growth factors during FN. A patient who receives pegfilgrastim following myelosuppressive chemotherapy and still develops SN or FN should not receive further filgrastim as circulating levels of G-CSF will be high and there is no benefit of additional growth factor in this situation.

Toxicity of Growth Factors

Filgrastim and pegfilgrastim are generally considered safe. Occasional skin and other allergic reactions have been reported. The most common adverse reaction is mild to moderate bone pain and myalgias, probably secondary to the marrow stimulation. Typical onset is 2 to 5 days after the growth factor administration. Pretreatment patient education and early intervention with nonsteroidal anti-inflammatory drugs or other non-opioid analgesics work well to alleviate the symptoms. Anecdotally, long-acting H_1-blockers have been reported to reduce bone pain, but no formal prospective evaluations of this strategy have been conducted. Evaluation of RCTs has demonstrated no evidence that pegfilgrastim is more likely to cause bone pain compared with daily filgrastim (113). GM-CSF has a broader range of toxicities, including fever, nausea, headache, diarrhea, and thrombosis in addition to bone pain. Myeloid growth factors should be used with caution if at all in patients with sickle cell disease due to the chance of precipitating a crisis.

There is a small increased risk of secondary malignancies, notably acute myeloid leukemia and MDS, in patients receiving growth factors with chemotherapy (101). Some of the increase may well be due to dose escalation of chemotherapy, which was a strategy attempted to improve the efficacy of the regimen, usually without benefit. It is difficult to distinguish the growth factor effect from the high-dose chemotherapy effect. The benefits of growth factor in preventing FN, hospitalization, and potential early mortality outweigh the small risk.

THROMBOCYTOPENIA

Reduction in platelet counts is common in patients with cancer. Causes of thrombocytopenia include chemotherapy, radiation therapy, bone marrow infiltration by tumor, nutritional deficiencies, and tumor-associated immune effects, including autoimmune thrombocytopenic purpura. Thrombocytopenia is particularly prevalent in patients with hematologic malignancies, including MDS and acute and chronic leukemia. Patients with solid tumors increasingly experience thrombocytopenia with the chronicity of sequential multi-agent chemotherapy as well as newer biologic agents, which exacerbate hematologic toxicity and may also independently increase bleeding. Complications from thrombocytopenia vary from asymptomatic to mild bleeding characterized by ecchymosis and petechiae through disruptive epistaxis and gingival bleeding to life-threatening GI or intracranial hemorrhage.

The treatment of thrombocytopenia largely remains prophylactic platelet transfusions for asymptomatic patients with severe thrombocytopenia and therapeutic platelet transfusions in the setting of active bleeding. Platelets for transfusion are either collected as a fraction of whole blood which is then pooled with 4 to 6 donors or collected from a single donor by apheresis to constitute an adequate transfusion dose. The quality of apheresis platelets is similar to that of pooled random donor platelet concentrates (114,115) and

therefore these two products can be used interchangeably based on availability and cost considerations (116).

Prophylactic platelet transfusions should be initiated when a platelet count declines to 10,000/μL as per most recent ASCO guidelines (117). Several randomized studies have demonstrated no difference in bleeding events when a trigger of 10,000/μL is utilized versus a higher trigger of 20,000/μL (118,119). Additional trials are ongoing to compare 10,000/μL with no prophylaxis in thrombocytopenic patients with hematologic malignancies (120).

Therapeutic platelet transfusions are generally initiated when there is an evidence of active bleeding due to platelet dysfunction or thrombocytopenia. For chronic thrombocytopenia, evidence of gross bleeding with or without the need for PRBC transfusions usually triggers platelet transfusions. Some other factors like anatomical abnormalities, quantitative platelet dysfunction, coagulation factor deficiencies, and others contribute to bleeding. It is not surprising that therapeutic platelet transfusions are only modestly effective in controlling bleeding in clinical trials (121). For major surgical procedures, a platelet count of at least 50,000/μL should be established. Because the count itself is not the only indication of hemostatic function, patients undergoing neurosurgical procedures should have platelet counts closer to 100,000/μL.

Platelet Refractoriness

Cancer patients who require frequent platelet transfusions often show inadequate rise in platelet count afterward, termed refractoriness to transfusions. Both immune and non-immune mechanisms play a role in this inadequate response. However, alloimmunization against major histocompatability antigens is the major determinant of refractoriness. Providing ABO compatible platelets achieves the highest posttransfusion platelet count and reduces the incidence of alloimmunization.

A large trial in leukemia patients demonstrated the value of leukoreduced platelets (and PRBC) compared with standard blood products to prevent the development of human leukocyte antigen (HLA) antibodies (122). Leukodepleted transfusions are also less likely to cause transfusion reaction, which is thought to be mediated by cytokines from leukocytes. Many institutes have instituted universal leukoreduction of the blood supply (123).

Strategies for dealing with alloimmunized recipients include selecting HLA-matched donors from an HLA-typed registry of apheresis donors, identifying HLA–antibody specificities, and selecting antigen-compatible apheresis donors or perform platelet crossmatch tests to select compatible donors (124). Even with these techniques, up to one-third of the patients will remain refractory likely due to non-alloimmunization factors like splenomegaly, concurrent heparin use, disseminated intravascular coagulation, sepsis, and idiopathic thrombocytopenic purpura (ITP). Persistently, refractory patients with ongoing bleeding may derive some benefit from immunoglobulin G (IgG) infusions, fibrinolytic inhibitors, or recombinant Factor VIIa (124).

Thrombopoietic Agents

Platelet transfusions are costly, at times ineffective and place the recipient at risk for transfusion reactions and infectious exposure. Given the proven benefit of utilizing pharmacologic doses of erythroid and myeloid growth factors, there has been considerable interest in developing a biologic treatment for thrombocytopenia. Analogous to G-CSF and erythropoietin, thrombopoietin (TPO) is the endogenous ligand for the TPO receptor expressed on the surface of megakaryocytes, platelet precursors, and platelets. First-generation recombinant human TPO and its derivatives were ineffective and led to prolonged thrombocytopenia and autoantibodies in some patients (125). Clinical development of these agents was therefore abandoned.

rHIL-11, also known as oprelvekin (Neumega, Wyeth), has been approved as a thrombopoietic agent based on a 30% reduction in platelet transfusions in patients with breast cancer (126). IL-11 has multiple effects on both hematopoietic cells and other organ systems. In vivo, it promotes megakaryocytopoeisis and increases platelet production. However, side effects of IL-11 are substantial and include edema, fatigue, myalgias, and cardiovascular events. The modest activity and significant toxicity of this drug have markedly limited use in general clinical practice and fueled the drive to find other agents to stimulate platelet production.

Second-generation thrombopoiesis-stimulating agents, including romiplostim (Nplate, Amgen) an IV peptide–antibody construct and eltrombopag (Promacta, GlaxoSmithKline) an oral small molecule, are now commercially available. Both of these drugs carry an FDA label for treating chronic ITP, a condition occasionally encountered in cancer patients, particularly those with lymphoma. Phase II and III trials evaluating these agents in MDS-related thrombocytopenia and chemotherapy-induced thrombocytopenia are ongoing.

CONCLUSION

Cancer patients remain highly susceptible to hematologic complications, which impact every aspect of oncologic care. The clinical complications of neutropenia, anemia, and thrombocytopenia are now well characterized and range from minimal to life threatening. The discovery of hematopoietic growth factors and their introduction into clinical practice dramatically changed our treatment approach to hematologic support of cancer patients. Over the last decade, better understanding of the risks and benefits of hematopoietic growth factors has been defined.

Many questions still remain unanswered regarding the optimal use of growth factors from clinical and cost perspectives. Advances in blood product transfusions have improved safe delivery of blood components but better pharmacologic approaches to hematologic support remains the preferred approach. In this dynamic supportive care environment, readers are encouraged to follow the results of ongoing RCTs as well as frequent updates of evidence-based clinical practice guidelines to best incorporate use of hematopoietic growth factors, transfusion support, and antibiotics in the clinical care of their patients.

REFERENCES

1. The NCCN Clinical Practice Guidelines in Oncology. Cancer-and chemotherapy-induced anemia. http://www.nccn.org/professionals/physician_gls/f_guidelines.asp. Accessed August 14, 2012.
2. Berger AM, Abernethy AP, Atkinson A, et al. Cancer-related fatigue. *J Natl Compr Canc Netw*. August 2010;8(8):904-931.
3. Balducci L. Anemia, fatigue and aging. *Transfus Clin Biol*. December 2010;17(5-6):375-381.
4. Wagner LI, Cella D. Fatigue and cancer: causes, prevalence and treatment approaches. *Br J Cancer*. August 2004;91(5):822-828.
5. Glaser CM, Millesi W, Kornek GV, et al. Impact of hemoglobin level and use of recombinant erythropoietin on efficacy of pre-operative chemoradiation therapy for squamous cell carcinoma of the oral cavity and oropharynx. *Int J Radiat Oncol Biol Phys*. July 2001;50(3):705-715.
6. Caro JJ, Salas M, Ward A, Goss G. Anemia as an independent prognostic factor for survival in patients with cancer: a systemic, quantitative review. *Cancer*. June 2001;91(12):2214-2221.
7. Birgegard G, Aapro MS, Bokemeyer C, et al. Cancer-related anemia: pathogenesis, prevalence and treatment. *Oncology*. 2005;68(suppl 1):3-11.
8. Marks P. *Hematologic Manifestations of Systemic Disease: Infection, Chronic Inflammation, and Cancer*. 5th ed. Philadelphia, PA: Churchill Livingstone Elsevier; 2009.
9. Kaushansky K, Kipps TJ. *Hematopoietic Agents: Growth Factors, Minerals, and Vitamins*. 11th ed. New York, NY: McGraw Hill; 2005.
10. Henry D. Iron or vitamin B_{12} deficiency in anemic cancer patients prior to erythropoiesis-stimulating agent therapy. *Community Oncol*. February 2007;4(2):95-101.
11. Hillman RS, Finch CA. Erythropoiesis: normal and abnormal. *Semin Hematol*. October 1967;4(4):327-336.
12. Spivak JL. The anaemia of cancer: death by a thousand cuts. *Nat Rev Cancer*. July 2005;5(7):543-555.
13. Maccio A, Madeddu C, Massa D, et al. Hemoglobin levels correlate with interleukin-6 levels in patients with advanced untreated epithelial ovarian cancer: role of inflammation in cancer-related anemia. *Blood*. July 2005;106(1):362-367.
14. Faquin WC, Schneider TJ, Goldberg MA. Effect of inflammatory cytokines on hypoxia-induced erythropoietin production. *Blood*. April 1992;79(8):1987-1994.
15. Hellwig-Burgel T, Rutkowski K, Metzen E, Fandrey J, Jelkmann W. Interleukin-1beta and tumor necrosis factor-alpha stimulate DNA binding of hypoxia-inducible factor-1. *Blood*. September 1999;94(5):1561-1567.
16. Herrmann F, Gebauer G, Lindemann A, Brach M, Mertelsmann R. Interleukin-2 and interferon-gamma recruit different subsets of human peripheral blood monocytes to secrete interleukin-1 beta and tumour necrosis factor-alpha. *Clin Exp Immunol*. July 1989;77(1):97-100.
17. Nicolas G, Chauvet C, Viatte L, et al. The gene encoding the iron regulatory peptide hepcidin is regulated by anemia, hypoxia, and inflammation. *J Clin Invest*. October 2002;110(7):1037-1044.
18. Weiss G, Goodnough LT. Anemia of chronic disease. *N Engl J Med*. March 2005;352(10):1011-1023.
19. Groopman JE, Itri LM. Chemotherapy-induced anemia in adults: incidence and treatment. *J Natl Cancer Inst*. October 1999;91(19):1616-1634.
20. Ludwig H, Van Belle S, Barrett-Lee P, et al. The European Cancer Anaemia Survey (ECAS): a large, multinational, prospective survey defining the prevalence, incidence, and

treatment of anaemia in cancer patients. *Eur J Cancer*. October 2004;40(15):2293-2306.

21. Barrett-Lee PJ, Ludwig H, Birgegard G, et al. Independent risk factors for anemia in cancer patients receiving chemotherapy: results from the European Cancer Anaemia Survey. *Oncology*. 2006;70(1):34-48.

22. Wu Y, Aravind S, Ranganathan G, Martin A, Nalysnyk L. Anemia and thrombocytopenia in patients undergoing chemotherapy for solid tumors: a descriptive study of a large outpatient oncology practice database, 2000-2007. *Clin Ther*. 2009;31(pt 2):2416-2432.

23. Wood PA, Hrushesky WJ. Cisplatin-associated anemia: an erythropoietin deficiency syndrome. *J Clin Invest*. April 1995;95(4):1650-1659.

24. Duffaud F, Lecesne A, Ray-Coquard I. Erythropoietin for anemia treatment of patients with GIST receiving imatinib. *J Clin Oncol*. 2004;22(14):9046.

25. Hutson TE, Figlin RA, Kuhn JG, Motzer RJ. Targeted therapies for metastatic renal cell carcinoma: an overview of toxicity and dosing strategies. *Oncologist*. October 2008;13(10):1084-1096.

26. Sher A, Wu S. Anti-vascular endothelial growth factor antibody bevacizumab reduced the risk of anemia associated with chemotherapy—a meta-analysis. *Acta Oncol*. October 2011;50(7):997-1005.

27. Glaspy JA, Jadeja JS, Justice G, et al. Darbepoetin alfa given every 1 or 2 weeks alleviates anaemia associated with cancer chemotherapy. *Br J Cancer*. July 2002;87(3):268-276.

28. Littlewood TJ, Bajetta E, Nortier JW, Vercammen E, Rapoport B. Effects of epoetin alfa on hematologic parameters and quality of life in cancer patients receiving nonplatinum chemotherapy: results of a randomized, double-blind, placebo-controlled trial. *J Clin Oncol*. June 2001;19(11):2865-2874.

29. Lyman GH, Glaspy J. Are there clinical benefits with early erythropoietic intervention for chemotherapy-induced anemia? A systematic review. *Cancer*. January 2006;106(1):223-233.

30. Crawford J, Cella D, Cleeland CS, et al. Relationship between changes in hemoglobin level and quality of life during chemotherapy in anemic cancer patients receiving epoetin alfa therapy. *Cancer*. August 2002;95(4):888-895.

31. Demetri GD, Kris M, Wade J, Degos L, Cella D. Quality-of-life benefit in chemotherapy patients treated with epoetin alfa is independent of disease response or tumor type: results from a prospective community oncology study. Procrit Study Group. *J Clin Oncol*. October 1998;16(10):3412-3425.

32. Gabrilove JL, Cleeland CS, Livingston RB, Sarokhan B, Winer E, Einhorn LH. Clinical evaluation of once-weekly dosing of epoetin alfa in chemotherapy patients: improvements in hemoglobin and quality of life are similar to three-times-weekly dosing. *J Clin Oncol*. June 2001;19(11):2875-2882.

33. Macdougall IC, Gray SJ, Elston O, et al. Pharmacokinetics of novel erythropoiesis stimulating protein compared with epoetin alfa in dialysis patients. *J Am Soc Nephrol*. November 1999;10(11):2392-2395.

34. Vansteenkiste J, Pirker R, Massuti B, et al. Double-blind, placebo-controlled, randomized phase III trial of darbepoetin alfa in lung cancer patients receiving chemotherapy. *J Natl Cancer Inst*. August 2002;94(16):1211-1220.

35. Glaspy JA, Jadeja JS, Justice G, Fleishman A, Rossi G, Colowick AB. A randomized, active-control, pilot trial of front-loaded dosing regimens of darbepoetin-alfa for the treatment of patients with anemia during chemotherapy for malignant disease. *Cancer*. March 2003;97(5):1312-1320.

36. Bohlius J, Langensiepen S, Schwarzer G, et al. Recombinant human erythropoietin and overall survival in cancer patients: results of a comprehensive meta-analysis. *J Natl Cancer Inst*. April 2005;97(7):489-498.

37. Rizzo JD, Brouwers M, Hurley P, et al. American Society of Clinical Oncology/American Society of Hematology clinical practice guideline update on the use of epoetin and darbepoetin in adult patients with cancer. *J Clin Oncol*. November 2010;28(33):4996-5010.

38. Schwartzberg LS, Yee LK, Senecal FM, et al. A randomized comparison of every-2-week darbepoetin alfa and weekly epoetin alfa for the treatment of chemotherapy-induced anemia in patients with breast, lung, or gynecologic cancer. *Oncologist*. 2004;9(6):696-707.

39. Glaspy J, Vadhan-Raj S, Patel R, et al. Randomized comparison of every-2-week darbepoetin alfa and weekly epoetin alfa for the treatment of chemotherapy-induced anemia: the 20030125 Study Group Trial. *J Clin Oncol*. May 2006;24(15):2290-2297.

40. Schwartzberg L, Burkes R, Mirtsching B, et al. Comparison of darbepoetin alfa dosed weekly (QW) vs. extended dosing schedule (EDS) in the treatment of anemia in patients receiving multicycle chemotherapy in a randomized, phase 2, open-label trial. *BMC Cancer*. 2010;10:581.

41. Muller RJ, Baribeault D. Extended-dosage-interval regimens of erythropoietic agents in chemotherapy-induced anemia. *Am J Health Syst Pharm*. December 2007;64(24):2547-2556.

42. Canon JL, Vansteenkiste J, Bodoky G, et al. Randomized, double-blind, active-controlled trial of every-3-week darbepoetin alfa for the treatment of chemotherapy-induced anemia. *J Natl Cancer Inst*. February 2006;98(4):273-284.

43. Henke M, Laszig R, Rube C, et al. Erythropoietin to treat head and neck cancer patients with anaemia undergoing radiotherapy: randomised, double-blind, placebo-controlled trial. *Lancet*. October 2003;362(9392):1255-1260.

44. Leyland-Jones B, Semiglazov V, Pawlicki M, et al. Maintaining normal hemoglobin levels with epoetin alfa in mainly nonanemic patients with metastatic breast cancer receiving first-line chemotherapy: a survival study. *J Clin Oncol*. September 2005;23(25):5960-5972.

45. Thomas G, Ali S, Hoebers FJ, et al. Phase III trial to evaluate the efficacy of maintaining hemoglobin levels above 12.0 g/dL with erythropoietin vs above 10.0 g/dL without erythropoietin in anemic patients receiving concurrent radiation and cisplatin for cervical cancer. *Gynecol Oncol*. February 2008;108(2):317-325.

46. Untch M, Fasching P, Bauerfeind I, et al. PREPARE trial: a randomized phase III trial comparing preoperative, dose-dense, dose-intensified chemotherapy with epirubicin, paclitaxel and CMF with a standard dosed epirubicin/cyclophosphamide followed by paclitaxel (+/−) darbepoetin alfa in primary breast cancer: a preplanned interim analysis of efficacy at surgery. *J Clin Oncol*. 2008;26(15):517.

47. Untch M, von Minckwitz G, Konecny GE, et al. PREPARE trial: a randomized phase III trial comparing preoperative, dose-dense, dose-intensified chemotherapy with epirubicin, paclitaxel, and CMF versus a standard-dosed epirubicin–cyclophosphamide followed by paclitaxel with or without darbepoetin alfa in primary breast cancer—outcome on prognosis. *Ann Oncol*. September 2011;22(9):1999-2006.

48. Bohlius J, Schmidlin K, Brillant C, et al. Erythropoietin or darbepoetin for patients with cancer—meta-analysis based on individual patient data. *Cochrane Database Syst Rev*. 2009;(3):CD007303.

49. Glaspy J, Crawford J, Vansteenkiste J, et al. Erythropoiesis-stimulating agents in oncology: a study-level meta-analysis of survival and other safety outcomes. *Br J Cancer.* January 2010;102(2):301-315.

50. Khorana AA, Connolly GC. Assessing risk of venous thromboembolism in the patient with cancer. *J Clin Oncol.* October 2009;27(29):4839-4847.

51. Seidenfeld J, Piper M, Bohlius J, et al. Agency for Healthcare Research and Quality (US). *Comparative Effectiveness of Epoetin and Darbepoetin for Managing Anemia in Patients Undergoing Cancer Treatment.* Rockville, MD; 2006.

52. Ludwig H, Crawford J, Osterborg A, et al. Pooled analysis of individual patient-level data from all randomized, double-blind, placebo-controlled trials of darbepoetin alfa in the treatment of patients with chemotherapy-induced anemia. *J Clin Oncol.* June 2009;27(17):2838-2847.

53. Glaspy JA, Charu V, Luo D, Moyo V, Kamin M, Wilhelm FE. Initiation of epoetin-alpha therapy at a starting dose of 120,000 units once every 3 weeks in patients with cancer receiving chemotherapy: an open-label, multicenter study with randomized and nonrandomized treatment arms. *Cancer.* March 2009; 115(5):1121-1131.

54. Henry DH, Gordan LN, Charu V, et al. Randomized, open-label comparison of epoetin alfa extended dosing (80 000 U Q2W) vs weekly dosing (40 000 U QW) in patients with chemotherapy-induced anemia. *Curr Med Res Opin.* July 2006;22(7):1403-1413.

55. Boccia R, Malik IA, Raja V, et al. Darbepoetin alfa administered every three weeks is effective for the treatment of chemotherapy-induced anemia. *Oncologist.* April 2006;11(4):409-417.

56. Littlewood TJ, Zagari M, Pallister C, Perkins A. Baseline and early treatment factors are not clinically useful for predicting individual response to erythropoietin in anemic cancer patients. *Oncologist.* 2003;8(1):99-107.

57. Henry DH. Parenteral iron therapy in cancer-associated anemia. *Hematology (Am soc Hematol Educ Program)* 2010;351-356.

58. Auerbach M, Ballard H, Trout JR, et al. Intravenous iron optimizes the response to recombinant human erythropoietin in cancer patients with chemotherapy-related anemia: a multicenter, open-label, randomized trial. *J Clin Oncol.* April 2004; 22(7):1301-1307.

59. Hedenus M, Birgegard G, Nasman P, et al. Addition of intravenous iron to epoetin beta increases hemoglobin response and decreases epoetin dose requirement in anemic patients with lymphoproliferative malignancies: a randomized multicenter study. *Leukemia.* April 2007;21(4):627-632.

60. Bastit L, Vandebroek A, Altintas S, et al. Randomized, multicenter, controlled trial comparing the efficacy and safety of darbepoetin alpha administered every 3 weeks with or without intravenous iron in patients with chemotherapy-induced anemia. *J Clin Oncol.* April 2008;26(10):1611-1618.

61. Pedrazzoli P, Farris A, Del Prete S, et al. Randomized trial of intravenous iron supplementation in patients with chemotherapy-related anemia without iron deficiency treated with darbepoetin alpha. *J Clin Oncol.* April 2008;26(10):1619-1625.

62. Steensma DP, Sloan JA, Dakhil SR, et al. Phase III, randomized study of the effects of parenteral iron, oral iron, or no iron supplementation on the erythropoietic response to darbepoetin alfa for patients with chemotherapy-associated anemia. *J Clin Oncol.* January 2011;29(1):97-105.

63. Vamvakas EC, Blajchman MA. Transfusion-related mortality: the ongoing risks of allogeneic blood transfusion and the available strategies for their prevention. *Blood.* April 2009;113(15):3406-3417.

64. Schonewille H, Haak HL, van Zijl AM. Alloimmunization after blood transfusion in patients with hematologic and oncologic diseases. *Transfusion.* July 1999;39(7):763-771.

65. Goodnough LT, Brecher ME, Kanter MH, AuBuchon JP. Transfusion medicine. First of two parts—blood transfusion. *N Engl J Med.* February 1999;340(6):438-447.

66. Dodd RY, Notari EPt, Stramer SL. Current prevalence and incidence of infectious disease markers and estimated window-period risk in the American Red Cross blood donor population. *Transfusion.* August 2002;42(8):975-979.

67. Pealer LN, Marfin AA, Petersen LR, et al. Transmission of West Nile virus through blood transfusion in the United States in 2002. *N Engl J Med.* September 2003;349(13):1236-1245.

68. Brecher ME, Hay SN. Bacterial contamination of blood components. *Clin Microbiol Rev.* January 2005;18(1):195-204.

69. Cherry T, Steciuk M, Reddy VV, Marques MB. Transfusion-related acute lung injury: past, present, and future. *Am J Clin Pathol.* February 2008;129(2):287-297.

70. Vamvakas EC. Is white blood cell reduction equivalent to antibody screening in preventing transmission of cytomegalovirus by transfusion? A review of the literature and meta-analysis. *Transfus Med Rev.* July 2005;19(3):181-199.

71. Ruhl H, Bein G, Sachs UJ. Transfusion-associated graft-versus-host disease. *Transfus Med Rev.* January 2009;23(1):62-71.

72. Freifeld AG, Bow EJ, Sepkowitz KA, et al. Clinical practice guideline for the use of antimicrobial agents in neutropenic patients with cancer: 2010 update by the Infectious Diseases Society of America. *Clin Infect Dis.* February 2011;52(4):e56-e93.

73. Kuderer NM, Dale DC, Crawford J, Cosler LE, Lyman GH. Mortality, morbidity, and cost associated with febrile neutropenia in adult cancer patients. *Cancer.* May 2006;106(10): 2258-2266.

74. Courtney DM, Aldeen AZ, Gorman SM, et al. Cancer-associated neutropenic fever: clinical outcome and economic costs of emergency department care. *Oncologist.* August 2007;12(8): 1019-1026.

75. Klastersky J, Paesmans M, Rubenstein EB, et al. The Multinational Association for Supportive Care in Cancer risk index: a multinational scoring system for identifying low-risk febrile neutropenic cancer patients. *J Clin Oncol.* August 2000; 18(16):3038-3051.

76. de Souza Viana L, Serufo JC, da Costa Rocha MO, Costa RN, Duarte RC. Performance of a modified MASCC index score for identifying low-risk febrile neutropenic cancer patients. *Support Care Cancer.* July 2008;16(7):841-846.

77. Talcott JA, Whalen A, Clark J, Rieker PP, Finberg R. Home antibiotic therapy for low-risk cancer patients with fever and neutropenia: a pilot study of 30 patients based on a validated prediction rule. *J Clin Oncol.* January 1994;12(1):107-114.

78. Raber-Durlacher JE, Epstein JB, Raber J, et al. Periodontal infection in cancer patients treated with high-dose chemotherapy. *Support Care Cancer.* September 2002;10(6):466-473.

79. Talcott JA, Yeap BY, Clark JA, et al. Safety of early discharge for low-risk patients with febrile neutropenia: a multicenter randomized controlled trial. *J Clin Oncol.* October 2011; 29(30):3977-3983.

80. Klastersky J, Paesmans M, Georgala A, et al. Outpatient oral antibiotics for febrile neutropenic cancer patients using a score predictive for complications. *J Clin Oncol.* September 2006; 24(25):4129-4134.

81. Carstensen M, Sorensen JB. Outpatient management of febrile neutropenia: time to revise the present treatment strategy. *J Support Oncol.* May–June 2008;6(5):199-208.

82. Gafter-Gvili A, Fraser A, Paul M, Leibovici L. Meta-analysis: antibiotic prophylaxis reduces mortality in neutropenic patients. *Ann Intern Med.* June 2005;142(12 pt 1):979-995.

83. Herbst C, Naumann F, Kruse EB, et al. Prophylactic antibiotics or G-CSF for the prevention of infections and improvement of survival in cancer patients undergoing chemotherapy. *Cochrane Database Syst Rev.* 2009;(1):CD007107.

84. van de Wetering MD, de Witte MA, Kremer LC, Offringa M, Scholten RJ, Caron HN. Efficacy of oral prophylactic antibiotics in neutropenic afebrile oncology patients: a systematic review of randomised controlled trials. *Eur J Cancer.* July 2005;41(10):1372-1382.

85. Dees EC, O'Reilly S, Goodman SN, et al. A prospective pharmacologic evaluation of age-related toxicity of adjuvant chemotherapy in women with breast cancer. *Cancer Invest.* 2000;18(6):521-529.

86. Lyman GH, Morrison VA, Dale DC, Crawford J, Delgado DJ, Fridman M. Risk of febrile neutropenia among patients with intermediate-grade non-Hodgkin's lymphoma receiving CHOP chemotherapy. *Leuk Lymphoma.* December 2003;44(12):2069-2076.

87. Jenkins P, Freeman S. Pretreatment haematological laboratory values predict for excessive myelosuppression in patients receiving adjuvant FEC chemotherapy for breast cancer. *Ann Oncol.* January 2009;20(1):34-40.

88. Matter-Walstra KW, Dedes KJ, Schwenkglenks M, Brauchli P, Szucs TD, Pestalozzi BC. Trastuzumab beyond progression: a cost–utility analysis. *Ann Oncol.* November 2010;21(11):2161-2168.

89. Aapro M, Crawford J, Kamioner D. Prophylaxis of chemotherapy-induced febrile neutropenia with granulocyte colony-stimulating factors: where are we now? *Support Care Cancer.* May 2010;18(5):529-541.

90. Lyman GH, Kuderer NM, Crawford J, et al. Predicting individual risk of neutropenic complications in patients receiving cancer chemotherapy. *Cancer.* May 2011;117(9):1917-1927.

91. Ziepert M, Schmits R, Trumper L, Pfreundschuh M, Loeffler M. Prognostic factors for hematotoxicity of chemotherapy in aggressive non-Hodgkin's lymphoma. *Ann Oncol.* April 2008;19(4):752-762.

92. Pettengell R, Bosly A, Szucs TD, et al. Multivariate analysis of febrile neutropenia occurrence in patients with non-Hodgkin lymphoma: data from the INC-EU Prospective Observational European Neutropenia Study. *Br J Haematol.* March 2009;144(5):677-685.

93. Bensinger WI, Price TH, Dale DC, et al. The effects of daily recombinant human granulocyte colony-stimulating factor administration on normal granulocyte donors undergoing leukapheresis. *Blood.* April 1993;81(7):1883-1888.

94. Holmes FA, Jones SE, O'Shaughnessy J, et al. Comparable efficacy and safety profiles of once-per-cycle pegfilgrastim and daily injection filgrastim in chemotherapy-induced neutropenia: a multicenter dose-finding study in women with breast cancer. *Ann Oncol.* June 2002;13(6):903-909.

95. Crawford J, Ozer H, Stoller R, et al. Reduction by granulocyte colony-stimulating factor of fever and neutropenia induced by chemotherapy in patients with small-cell lung cancer. *N Engl J Med.* July 1991;325(3):164-170.

96. Trillet-Lenoir V, Arpin D, Brune J. Optimal delivery of dose in cancer chemotherapy with the support of haematopoietic growth factors. *Eur J Cancer.* 1993;29A(suppl 5):S14-S16.

97. Holmes FA, O'Shaughnessy JA, Vukelja S, et al. Blinded, randomized, multicenter study to evaluate single administration pegfilgrastim once per cycle versus daily filgrastim as an adjunct to chemotherapy in patients with high-risk stage II or stage III/IV breast cancer. *J Clin Oncol.* February 2002;20(3):727-731.

98. Green MD, Koelbl H, Baselga J, et al. A randomized double-blind multicenter phase III study of fixed-dose single-administration pegfilgrastim versus daily filgrastim in patients receiving myelosuppressive chemotherapy. *Ann Oncol.* January 2003;14(1):29-35.

99. Vogel CL, Wojtukiewicz MZ, Carroll RR, et al. First and subsequent cycle use of pegfilgrastim prevents febrile neutropenia in patients with breast cancer: a multicenter, double-blind, placebo-controlled phase III study. *J Clin Oncol.* February 2005;23(6):1178-1184.

100. Kuderer NM, Dale DC, Crawford J, Lyman GH. Impact of primary prophylaxis with granulocyte colony-stimulating factor on febrile neutropenia and mortality in adult cancer patients receiving chemotherapy: a systematic review. *J Clin Oncol.* July 2007;25(21):3158-3167.

101. Lyman GH, Dale DC, Wolff DA, et al. Acute myeloid leukemia or myelodysplastic syndrome in randomized controlled clinical trials of cancer chemotherapy with granulocyte colony-stimulating factor: a systematic review. *J Clin Oncol.* June 2010;28(17):2914-2924.

102. Smith TJ, Khatcheressian J, Lyman GH, et al. 2006 update of recommendations for the use of white blood cell growth factors: an evidence-based clinical practice guideline. *J Clin Oncol.* July 2006;24(19):3187-3205.

103. Aapro MS, Bohlius J, Cameron DA, et al. 2010 update of EORTC guidelines for the use of granulocyte-colony stimulating factor to reduce the incidence of chemotherapy-induced febrile neutropenia in adult patients with lymphoproliferative disorders and solid tumours. *Eur J Cancer.* January 2011;47(1):8-32.

104. Kwak LW, Halpern J, Olshen RA, Horning SJ. Prognostic significance of actual dose intensity in diffuse large-cell lymphoma: results of a tree-structured survival analysis. *J Clin Oncol.* June 1990;8(6):963-977.

105. Budman DR, Berry DA, Cirrincione CT, et al. Dose and dose intensity as determinants of outcome in the adjuvant treatment of breast cancer. The Cancer and Leukemia Group B. *J Natl Cancer Inst.* August 1998;90(16):1205-1211.

106. Link BK, Budd GT, Scott S, et al. Delivering adjuvant chemotherapy to women with early-stage breast carcinoma: current patterns of care. *Cancer.* September 2001;92(6):1354-1367.

107. Papaldo P, Lopez M, Marolla P, et al. Impact of five prophylactic filgrastim schedules on hematologic toxicity in early breast cancer patients treated with epirubicin and cyclophosphamide. *J Clin Oncol.* October 2005;23(28):6908-6918.

108. Nabholtz JM, Cantin J, Chang J, et al. Phase III trial comparing granulocyte colony-stimulating factor to leridistim in the prevention of neutropenic complications in breast cancer patients treated with docetaxel/doxorubicin/cyclophosphamide: results of the BCIRG 004 trial. *Clin Breast Cancer.* October 2002;3(4):268-275.

109. Burris HA, Belani CP, Kaufman PA, et al. Pegfilgrastim on the same day versus next day of chemotherapy in patients with breast cancer, non-small-cell lung cancer, ovarian cancer, and non-Hodgkin's lymphoma: results of four multicenter, double-blind, randomized phase II studies. *J Oncol Pract/Am Soc Clin Oncol.* May 2010;6(3):133-140.

110. Skarlos DV, Timotheadou E, Galani E, et al. Pegfilgrastim administered on the same day with dose-dense adjuvant chemotherapy for breast cancer is associated with a higher incidence of febrile neutropenia as compared to conventional growth

factor support: matched case–control study of the Hellenic Cooperative Oncology Group. *Oncology.* 2009;77(2):107-112.

111. Dale, DC Advances in the treatment of neutropenia. Curr Opin Support Palliat Care 2009;3(3):207-212.

112. Crawford J, Dale DC, Kuderer NM, et al. Risk and timing of neutropenic events in adult cancer patients receiving chemotherapy: the results of a prospective nationwide study of oncology practice. *J Natl Compr Canc Netw.* February 2008;6(2):109-118.

113. Pinto L, Liu Z, Doan Q, Bernal M, Dubois R, Lyman G. Comparison of pegfilgrastim with filgrastim on febrile neutropenia, grade IV neutropenia and bone pain: a meta-analysis of randomized controlled trials. *Curr Med Res Opin.* September 2007;23(9):2283-2295.

114. Keegan T, Heaton A, Holme S, Owens M, Nelson E, Carmen R. Paired comparison of platelet concentrates prepared from platelet-rich plasma and buffy coats using a new technique with ^{111}In and ^{51}Cr. *Transfusion.* February 1992;32(2):113-120.

115. Cardigan R, Williamson LM. The quality of platelets after storage for 7 days. *Transfus Med.* August 2003;13(4):173-187.

116. Chambers LA, Herman JH. Considerations in the selection of a platelet component: apheresis versus whole blood-derived. *Transfus Med Rev.* October 1999;13(4):311-322.

117. Schiffer CA, Anderson KC, Bennett CL, et al. Platelet transfusion for patients with cancer: clinical practice guidelines of the American Society of Clinical Oncology. *J Clin Oncol.* March 2001;19(5):1519-1538.

118. Wandt H, Frank M, Ehninger G, et al. Safety and cost effectiveness of a 10 × 10(9)/L trigger for prophylactic platelet transfusions compared with the traditional 20 × 10(9)/L trigger: a prospective comparative trial in 105 patients with acute myeloid leukemia. *Blood.* May 1998;91(10):3601-3606.

119. Rebulla P, Finazzi G, Marangoni F, et al. The threshold for prophylactic platelet transfusions in adults with acute myeloid leukemia. Gruppo Italiano Malattie Ematologiche Maligne dell'Adulto. *N Engl J Med.* December 1997;337(26):1870-1875.

120. Stanworth SJ, Dyer C, Choo L, et al. Do all patients with hematologic malignancies and severe thrombocytopenia need prophylactic platelet transfusions? Background, rationale, and design of a clinical trial (trial of platelet prophylaxis) to assess the effectiveness of prophylactic platelet transfusions. *Transfus Med Rev.* July 2010;24(3):163-171.

121. Heddle NM, Cook RJ, Sigouin C, Slichter SJ, Murphy M, Rebulla P. A descriptive analysis of international transfusion practice and bleeding outcomes in patients with acute leukemia. *Transfusion.* June 2006;46(6):903-911.

122. Leukocyte reduction and ultraviolet B irradiation of platelets to prevent alloimmunization and refractoriness to platelet transfusions. The Trial to Reduce Alloimmunization to Platelets Study Group. *N Engl J Med.* December 1997;337(26):1861-1869.

123. Slichter SJ. Evidence-based platelet transfusion guidelines. *Hematology (Am Soc Hematol Educ Program).* 2007:172-178.

124. Delaflor-Weiss E, Mintz PD. The evaluation and management of platelet refractoriness and alloimmunization. *Transfus Med Rev.* April 2000;14(2):180-196.

125. Vadhan-Raj S. Management of chemotherapy-induced thrombocytopenia: current status of thrombopoietic agents. *Semin Hematol.* January 2009;46(1 suppl 2):S26-S32.

126. Tepler I, Elias L, Smith JW 2nd, et al. A randomized placebo-controlled trial of recombinant human interleukin-11 in cancer patients with severe thrombocytopenia due to chemotherapy. *Blood.* May 1996;87(9):3607-3614.

CHAPTER 60

Issues in Nutrition and Hydration

Elizabeth Kvale ■ Christine S. Ritchie

The issues surrounding artificial nutrition and hydration (ANH) pose challenges for clinicians, patients, families, and society. Legal precedent and ethical principles guide medical practice; yet with regard to critical questions in this area our scientific base for establishing benefit or harm is inadequate to provide guidance that is fully evidence based. Two recent *Cochrane Reviews* evaluated the use of ANH in palliative populations, including the terminal and dying phases of illness. It concluded that the evidence base is insufficient to make any recommendation for practice with regard to the use of ANH in patients receiving palliative care (1,2). Decisions regarding the use of hydration and nutrition in palliative care often boil down to an honest if imperfect discussion of the potential harm and benefit of nutrition and hydration in a particular setting, filtered through the values of each patient and their family. This chapter reviews some of the elements to consider in such a discussion, including the historic context of artificial hydration and nutrition, the legal and ethical framework for decision making, and a review of the evidence base related to the benefits and potential harms of ANH.

WHAT IS NUTRITION AND HYDRATION?

Definitions

Artificial hydration is the provision of water or electrolyte solutions through any nonoral route. *Artificial nutrition* includes total parenteral nutrition (TPN) and enteral nutrition (EN) by nasogastric tube (NGT), percutaneous endoscopic gastrostomy (PEG) tube, percutaneous endoscopic gastrostomy jejunostomy (PEG-J) tube, gastrostomy tube, or gastrojejunostomy tube.

History

In the 1920s, continuous infusion of i.v. glucose was introduced in humans. It was not until the 1960s that parenteral nutrition was used, first in seriously ill adult surgical patients and then in children and adults with short bowel syndrome (3). These children, who before these therapies died of starvation, were able to live for years, sustained with artificial nutrition. Parenteral nutrition use then expanded to many other patient populations, often without clear or well-established indications. Only in the last decade has some light been shed in critical care settings as to when TPN is beneficial and when it may be more harmful (4,5).

In the late 1970s, gastrostomies began to be performed and were often used for swallowing problems in children (6). Their use became widely generalized to adults such that EN is now commonly used among patients with stroke, neurologic disease, and cancer (7). Between 1988 and 1995, the number of tubes placed in the United States doubled; in 2000, more than 216,000 tubes were placed. Recent data from Veterans Administration (VA) and Medicare database reviews suggest a stabilization of this trend in some settings (Fig. 60.1).

Whereas i.v. hydration is a well-established part of medical practice, its role in end-of-life care remains less clear. Intravenous hydration is often used for the treatment of terminal delirium and agitation. Whether it is beneficial, and if so, for what outcomes and at what rate of infusion, remains an area of controversy.

ETHICAL AND LEGAL FRAMEWORK

Nutrition and hydration decisions may be more difficult for some families than ventilator support or cardiac resuscitation. Families may equate foregoing of artificial nutrition with starvation. The potential harms associated with artificial nutrition (such as restraint use, immobility, and decreased social contact) are often not considered. Because of the dearth of good scientific data to assist clinicians in addressing whether or not artificial nutrition has meaningful benefit, it is often difficult to provide guidance to patients' families.

In medicine, ethical principles guide how a patient should be treated or how a treatment dilemma should be handled. The ethical principle of *autonomy* states that a person should have the ability to govern oneself. This principle was applied in the court decisions of Barber in 1983, Bouvia in 1986, and Cruzan in 1990, all of which stated that competent adults should be the final arbiters of decisions regarding their own health care. If nutritional support is unwanted, then providing artificial nutrition does not adhere to the principle of *autonomy* and lessens patient dignity. *Beneficence* is the ethical principle that states that physicians should always provide care that benefits the patient. In the case of artificial nutrition, the physician needs to ask if the artificial nutrition is actually "doing good" for their patient. The principle of *nonmaleficence* addresses the complimentary principle that one should "do no harm"—primum non nocere. In the case of ANH, physicians must weigh the potential for this medical treatment to harm their patient in any way. If ANH were contributing to more harm than benefit, then the principle of *nonmaleficence* would support its discontinuation (Fig. 60.2).

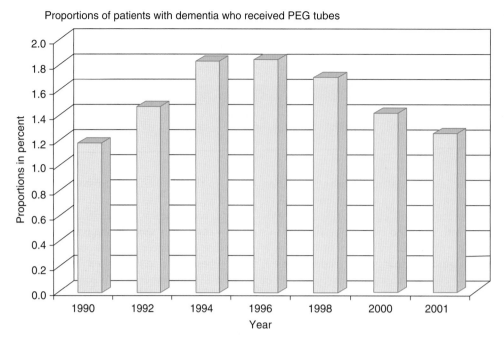

Figure 60.1. Time trends in the use of percutaneous endoscopic gastrostomy (PEG) tube feeding: proportion of demented patients in the administrative database of the Veterans Health Administration shown as percentage of total number of demented patients. A decreasing trend since 1996 is identified.

The argument for the discontinuation of nutritional support states that ANH are indistinguishable from other medical treatments. In the 1990 Cruzan decision, the US Supreme Court stated that "the law does not distinguish artificial feeding from other forms of medical treatment" (8). The right of patients to refuse this treatment is supported, and within this framework artificial nutrition is considered medical intervention and not basic care. Withdrawing artificial nutritional support and allowing a patient to die is *not* considered equivalent to euthanasia. In the former instance, the goal of discontinuing therapy is to remove burdensome interventions; in the latter, the intended result is the death

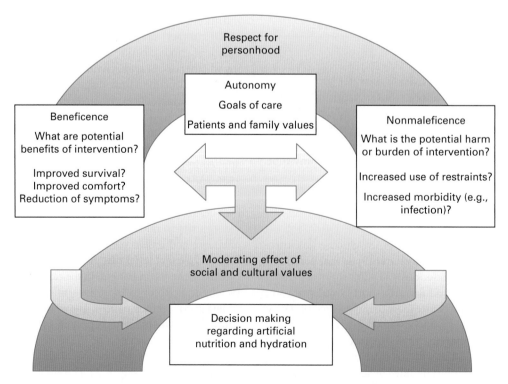

Figure 60.2. Integration of ethical principles into decision making regarding artificial nutrition and hydration.

of the patient. Nevertheless, as demonstrated by the Schiavo case, public acceptance of these distinguishing features in nutritional support varies greatly. Furthermore, some faith communities take issue with the distinction between artificial and basic nutrition (proposition 52).

In addition, much legal confusion persists because advance directive statutes may make it more difficult for a person capable of making decisions to prospectively forego ANH and many state statutes are poorly written and confusing (9).

INDICATIONS

No clear palliative indications exist for artificial nutrition. The American Gastroenterological Association (AGA) endorses PEG tube placement for prolonged tube feeding (specifically more than 30 d) and nasogastric feeding when enteral feeding is required for shorter periods (Table 60.1). In practice, PEG tubes are placed for a variety of different clinical conditions, including dysphagia, prolonged illness, anorexia, neurologic/psychiatric disorders, oropharyngeal or esophageal disorders or cancers, or increased nutritional needs that the patient is unable to meet with oral intake. Studies show that neurologic illnesses (e.g., dysphagia following stroke and dementia), cancer (obstruction secondary to tumor, postradiation, postchemotherapy, or postresection), and the prevention of aspiration account for most placements (10–12).

Indications for artificial hydration are relatively straightforward in critical care settings or when an otherwise healthy patient presents with volume depletion. Indications for hydration at the end of life have not been established. In the acute care setting, parenteral hydration is routinely given. In the hospice setting, parenteral hydration is not routine, but may be considered in instances where the patient is experiencing neuropsychiatric symptoms such as delirium, myoclonus, and agitation.

With regards to ANH, the scientific literature lacks high-quality randomized trials that might yield clear indications to guide practice. Benefits and harms are often gleaned from imperfect evidence from heterogeneous populations.

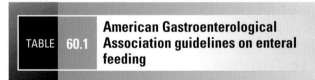

| TABLE 60.1 | **American Gastroenterological Association guidelines on enteral feeding** |

- The patient cannot or will not eat
- The gut is functional
- The patient can tolerate the placement of the device[a]

[a]American Gastroenterological Association. American Gastroenterological Association medical position statement: guidelines for the use of enteral nutrition. *Gastroenterology.* 1995;108:1280–1301.

POTENTIAL BENEFIT OF ARTIFICIAL NUTRITION

Common rationale for use of artificial nutrition includes improved survival, comfort, reduction or healing in pressure ulcers, and reduction in aspiration. Although most of the studies performed to date are compromised by substantial methodological problems, none have consistently demonstrated improved outcomes in these arenas with the exceptions of improved survival for short bowel syndrome, decreased hepatic encephalopathy in alcoholic cirrhosis, decreased length of hospital stay in hip fracture patients, and decreased postoperative complications of patients with gastric cancer given artificial nutrition preoperatively (13,14). Although no controlled trials exist, follow-up studies suggest increased survival of patients in persistent vegetative state who are likely to die within weeks without artificial nutrition, but they may live for many years with artificial nutrition (15). There is also moderately strong evidence that artificial nutrition can prolong life when it is used in short-term critical care (16). A summary of the levels of evidence for benefit from artificial nutrition is given in Tables 60.2 and 60.3.

Survival

A number of retrospective studies and a few prospective studies have been performed in patients to ascertain survival benefit in patients receiving artificial nutrition. The largest study to date was a retrospective review by Grant et al. of 81,105 Medicare beneficiaries who received gastrostomies in 1991. No comparison group was identified for this study. Cerebrovascular disease, neoplasms, fluid and electrolyte disorders, and aspiration pneumonia were the most common primary diagnoses. The mortality rate at 1 and 3 years was 63.0% to 81.3%. The median survival was 28.9 weeks for women and 17.6 weeks for men. At 30 days, primary diagnoses of malnutrition and fluid and electrolyte disorders and secondary diagnoses of swallowing disorders, dementia, or cerebrovascular disease were characterized by the *lowest* mortality rates. Thirty-day mortality rates were *highest* among those with primary diagnoses of nonaspiration pneumonia or influenza and secondary diagnoses of congestive heart failure or any neoplasm (12). Rabeneck et al. studied 7,369 patients receiving PEG tubes at VA facilities between 1990 and 1992. In this retrospective cohort study, 23.5% died during their index hospitalization. The median survival of the full cohort was 7.5 months from the time of tube placement. The overall mortality rates at 1, 2, and 3 years were 59%, 71%, and 77%, respectively. The highest mortality rates were observed for patients with lung or pleural cancer (46.4%), followed by esophageal cancer (20.8%) and head and neck cancer (18.8%) (17). Survival decreased with increasing age. The median survival across clinical diagnostic categories was 13.9 months for cerebrovascular disease, 13.4 months for other organic neurologic diseases, 9.6 months for nutritional deficiency, 8.0 months for head and neck cancer, and 4 or fewer months for all other cancers. Among 674 older

TABLE 60.2	Levels of evidence for artificial nutrition		
Population/Type of Artificial Nutrition	**Outcome**	**Classification**	**Level of Evidence**
Stroke			
PEG vs. NG tube	Improved albumin/weight	IIa	B1
PEG vs. NG tube/oral feeding	Survival	IIb	B1
Acquired Immunodeficiency Syndrome			
TPN in advanced disease	Increased weight	IIa	B1
TPN in advanced disease	Survival	IIb	B1
Cancer			
TPN	During chemotherapy	III	B1
Prophylactic enteral nutrition[a] before treatment in head and neck cancer	Weight stabilization	IIa	B2
Enteral nutrition before surgery	Gastrointestinal cancer	IIa	A
Dementia			
Enteral nutrition	Survival	III	B2
Enteral nutrition	Aspiration	III	B2
Enteral nutrition	Pressure sores	IIb	C

PEG, percutaneous endoscopic gastrostomy; NG, nasogastric; TPN, total parenteral nutrition.

[a]Enteral nutrition includes NG, gastrostomy, and PEG tube feeding.

(age >50 yr) adults referred to a community gastroenterology group for PEG insertion over a 10-year period, mortality rates at 1, 2, and 3 years were 54.3%, 73.2%, and 84.5%, respectively. Like Rabeneck's study, the overall median survival was between 6 months and 1 year; however, those receiving tube feeding in this cohort were much more likely to be patients with stroke or other neurologic conditions. Very few of the PEGs were placed in patients with cancer. Risk factors for mortality in this cohort were being male, having feeding difficulty, having diabetes, being referred from a hospital, and being 80 years of age or greater (18). Similar to Grant's cohort, dementia was *not* an independent risk factor for decreased survival. Because these studies used large databases, identification of truly comparable control groups would have been challenging. Nevertheless, because there was no comparable control group, the impact of gastrostomies on survival could not be ascertained.

Comfort

The small body of literature evaluating the patient symptoms at the end of life suggests a relatively low prevalence of hunger (19). In McCann's study of 32 patients in a comfort care unit, 63% denied hunger entirely, while 34% reported

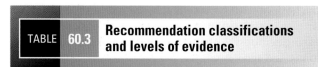

TABLE 60.3	Recommendation classifications and levels of evidence

Classification

Class I: Intervention is useful and effective

Class IIa: Weight of evidence/opinion is in favor of usefulness/efficacy

Class IIb: Usefulness/efficacy less well established by evidence/opinion

Class III: Intervention is not useful/effective and may be harmful

Level of Evidence

A: Sufficient evidence from multiple randomized trials

B: Limited evidence from

   1. Single, randomized trial or

   2. Other nonrandomized studies

C: Based on expert opinion, case studies, or standard of care hunger during the first quarter of their course in the unit. In all patients reporting either hunger or thirst, these symptoms were consistently and completely relieved by oral care or the ingestion of small amounts of food and fluid. In a case study of a patient refusing nutrition and hydration, the patient experienced no discomfort and died peacefully (19). A survey of Oregon hospice nurses found that among those who had cared for patients who declined nutrition and hydration, the majority reported the ensuing death to be peaceful (20).

Studies of healthy volunteers engaged in fasting report resolution of hunger in <24 hours. The resulting ketosis is associated with the relief of hunger and a mild euphoria. Animal studies suggest that ketosis may also have a mild analgesic effect. When ketosis is minimized by small feedings, hunger may persist (21).

Reduction in Pressure Ulcers

There is some evidence that malnutrition is positively correlated with pressure ulcer incidence and severity (22,23). However, only two nutrition intervention studies for pressure ulcer prevention or treatment included artificial nutrition. Hartgrink et al. performed a randomized controlled trial (RCT) of 140 patients with fracture of the hip and an increased pressure ulcer risk. The intervention group was treated with a standard hospital diet and an additional NGT feeding administered overnight. The comparison group received the standard hospital diet alone (24). No significant difference was found between the groups. Ohura et al. utilized artificial nutrition in a trial that enrolled 60 tube-fed patients. The treatment comparison, however, was protein and micronutrient intake, not tube feeding (25). Thus, while it is not possible to draw any firm conclusions on the effect of enteral and parenteral nutrition on the prevention and treatment of pressure ulcers, there is growing evidence that disease-specific nutrition support may offer benefit with regard to pressure ulcer incidence and healing (26).

Reduction in Aspiration Rates

In prospective studies of EN, aspiration pneumonia is not demonstrably decreased. Progression of aspiration to pneumonia is difficult to predict and is influenced by a number of factors, including decreased level of alertness, prolonged supine position, and colonization of the oropharynx (27). Tube feeding is a risk factor for the development of aspiration pneumonia among nursing home residents (odds ratio 3.0) (28). A recent meta-analysis suggests that small bowel feeding reduces the frequency of aspiration pneumonia compared with intragastric feeding in critical care settings (29).

POTENTIAL HARM

Complications

Complications from nasal intubation can include pharyngeal or esophageal perforation and accidental bronchial insertion. Approximately 25% of NGTs "fall out" or are pulled out by patients soon after insertion; fine bore tubes can be displaced by coughing or vomiting. Immediate complications of percutaneous gastrostomy and jejunostomy tubes include abdominal wall or intraperitoneal bleeding and bowel perforation (30). Significant surgical intervention is needed in fewer than 5% of cases. Postinsertion tube–related complications from percutaneous gastrostomy and jejunostomy tubes include infection at the insertion site, peristomal leaks, accidental tube removal, peritonitis, sepsis, and necrotizing fasciitis.

Restraints

Families are often unaware that patients with PEG tubes may require restraints (31). In Peck's study of nursing home residents with dementia, those receiving EN were more likely to be restrained (71%) than those who were not (56%) (32). When a select cohort of nursing home residents were asked, a third stated that they would prefer tube feeds if they were unable to eat. But 25% then declined when they were informed that restraints are sometimes applied during the feeding process.

Social Isolation

Patients fed enterally may be given fewer opportunities to taste food or experience the social interaction that can occur at mealtimes. They may experience sensory deprivation and social isolation if feeding comprises simply hanging a bag of nutrients on a pole for delivery through a tube. Hand-feeding, though more labor intensive than EN, enhances the dietary impact of feeding through touch, social engagement, and nurturing interactions.

CONDITIONS FOR WHICH ARTIFICIAL NUTRITION IS OFTEN CONSIDERED

Stroke

Two randomized studies of stroke patients with dysphagia who received PEG tube feeds showed improvement in albumin and weight gain at 6 weeks follow-up (33,34). Norton et al. performed a prospective randomized comparison of PEG versus NGT feeding after acute dysphagic stroke (33). Thirty patients with persisting dysphagia 14 days after acute stroke were randomly assigned to PEG (16 patients) versus NGT feeding (14 patients). Mortality at 6 weeks was significantly lower in the PEG group, with two deaths compared with eight deaths in the NGT group. Patients with PEG were more likely to have received the total amount of prescribed feeding and showed statistically greater improvement in nutritional state as well as discharge rate at 6 weeks. The comparison groups for both of these studies were patients receiving NGT feeding, not oral feeding. A meta-analysis of the three completed trials comparing PEG and NGTs estimated that the odds ratio for death is 0.88 (95% confidence interval [CI], 0.59–1.33) in favor of PEG. This value is not significant; CIs were wide and included the possibility of a large advantage or disadvantage with respect to survival for PEG over nasogastric feeding.

More recently, Iizuka and Reding performed a case-matched control of PEG versus no-PEG for 193 PEG patients. Controls were matched to the greatest extent possible on (from highest to lowest priority):

1. Sex
2. Duration from onset to stroke unit admission (interval poststroke)
3. Functional status on admission
4. Age
5. Diagnosis (ischemic vs. hemorrhagic)
6. Year of admission

No significant differences were found between the two groups except for functional status, which was significantly lower for the PEG group. There was a 4.7-fold greater frequency of death in the PEG group. Medical complications (pneumonia, cardiac events, and stroke progression) were also greater in this group. Both groups, however, showed a similar frequency of home discharge for survivors (35).

The largest controlled trials in stroke patients are the Feed or Ordinary Diet (FOOD) trials, which consisted of two trials for dysphagic stroke patients. In one trial, patients enrolled within 7 days of admission were randomly allocated to early enteral tube feeding or no tube feeding for more than 7 days (early vs. avoid). In the other, patients were assigned to PEG or nasogastric feeding. In the early versus avoid trial, early tube feeding was associated with a nonsignificant reduction in absolute risk of death of 5.8% (95% CI, 0.8–12.5; $P = 0.09$). There was no increase in pneumonia associated with early tube feeding; however, the improved survival was offset by a 4.7% excess of survivors with a poor outcome, with a worse quality of life. Thus, early feeding might have kept patients alive in a severely disabled state when they would otherwise have died. This finding is reinforced by a study utilizing data from the Centers for Medicare and Medicaid Services that evaluated outcomes related to PEG tube placement among 31,301 patients discharged with acute ischemic stroke. This study identified no association between PEG placement and mortality at 30 days; however, at 1 year PEG patients had a 2.59-fold greater mortality hazard (95% CI, 2.38–2.82) (36). In the PEG versus nasogastric trial, PEG feeding was associated with a nonsignificant increase in the absolute risk of death of 1.0% (37).

End-Stage Acquired Immunodeficiency Syndrome

Retrospective and prospective observational studies have reported conflicting results regarding the impact of TPN or EN on body weight and body composition in patients with human immunodeficiency virus infections. In a 2-month RCT of 31 malnourished and severely immunodepressed acquired immunodeficiency syndrome patients, subjects were assigned to receive either dietary counseling ($n = 15$) or home TPN ($n = 16$). Bodyweight increased by 8 kg in the TPN group and decreased by 3 kg in the control group ($P < 0.0006$). Lean body mass increased in the TPN group and decreased in the control group ($P < 0.004$). However, no difference in survival rate was noted. Quality of life in this trial was measured with a self-assessed "subjective health feeling" that demonstrated improvement in 83% of participants in the intervention arm, while 91% of participants in the control group reported feeling worse. Karnofsky scores stabilized in the intervention group and decreased in the control group (−12%), though this change was only statistically significant at one-time point (38). Other studies of TPN have also demonstrated increases in lean body mass and body weight, but only in patients who do not have a systemic infection (39).

Cancer

TPN and EN cancer–randomized studies in patients with a variety of tumors and therapies have generated inconsistent results. In a meta-analysis of 28 prospective RCTs evaluating the use of TPN in patients with cancer, TPN was found to be possibly useful when used preoperatively in patients with gastrointestinal tract cancer. It appeared to be beneficial in reducing major surgical complications and operative mortality, but it increased risk of infection. No statistically significant benefit from TPN could be demonstrated in survival, treatment tolerance, treatment toxicity, or tumor response in patients receiving chemotherapy or radiotherapy (40). A meta-analysis of patients receiving TPN during chemotherapy failed to demonstrate any clinical benefit (41). The poor outcomes observed in these trials culminated in a consensus statement from the American College of Physicians. This statement advised that the routine use of parenteral nutrition should be discouraged in patients undergoing chemotherapy and that when it is used in patients with cancer with malnutrition, physicians should consider the possibility of increased risk (42). This statement and the clinical trials that led to its issuance have curbed the use of TPN in the United States in patients with metastatic, incurable disease. However, subsequent studies evaluating TPN and EN remain mixed. In other countries, TPN continues to be used regularly for patients with advanced cancer.

Like TPN, EN in patients with cancer has not been shown to improve survival, improve tumor response, decrease toxicity, or decrease surgical complications. The only exception is in patients with cancer in head and neck and esophagus (43). In a retrospective case–control study of 88 patients treated for locally advanced head and neck cancer with accelerated radiation or concurrent chemoradiotherapy, prophylactic gastrostomy tubes (PGTs) were associated with half of the weight loss compared with the control group. There were significantly fewer hospitalizations for nutritional or dehydration issues in those with PGTs than in the control group; the use of PGTs had no influence on overall survival or local control. Although in animal studies nutritional support has been shown to increase rates of tumor growth, this has not been demonstrated consistently in humans (44).

Both TPN and EN have been able to improve some nutritional indices, such as body weight, fat mass, nitrogen balance, and whole body potassium. Thyroxine-binding prealbumin and retinol-binding protein levels increase only with TPN, whereas some immune response indices (complement factors and lymphocyte number) improve only with EN. EN appears to be more available for use in protein synthesis than TPN (45). The results of randomized studies comparing TPN and EN have been conflicting, but demonstrated a potential marginal advantage to TPN with regard to weight gain and nitrogen balance (46,47). Taken as a whole, TPN and EN both appear able to prevent further deterioration of the nutritional state and sometimes improve some metabolic indices in patients with cancer. However, no real demonstrable benefit has been shown on quality of life, and no large randomized trials have been performed in patients with advanced cancer.

Dementia

Dementia is a progressive disease that worsens in recognizable stages. In the Functional Assessment Staging System (FAST), one system used to follow the course of Alzheimer's disease; it is at the final stage seven when Alzheimer's disease patients may stop eating spontaneously. At stage seven, patients usually die within a year. They lose the ability to speak, ambulate, eat, control their muscles, and smile. When patients reach this stage, it is very difficult to maintain nutrition because encouragement to eat becomes less successful. In this instance, difficulty eating is a marker for the terminal phase of Alzheimer's dementia.

The same is not true in other forms of dementia. For example, patients with Parkinson's disease often lose the ability to maintain adequate caloric intake at an earlier stage of their disease; in this setting, a feeding tube may be required. Weight loss is characteristic of Parkinson's disease even in the early phases of the illness, thus some authors speculate that the role of dysphagia as a mediator of weight loss is limited (48). PEG tube placement does not prevent aspiration; aspiration rates may continue to range between 25% and 40% (49). PEG tubes in patients with advanced dementia do not prevent aspiration pneumonia, reduce the risk of infection or pressure sores, or improve function. Based on Rimon's findings and those of others not showing dementia to be a risk factor for increased mortality, the impact of EN on survival remains unclear (18).

Amyotrophic Lateral Sclerosis

Some studies suggest that the benefits of a PEG in amyotrophic lateral sclerosis are adequate nutritional intake and weight stabilization (50–52). Studies indicate lower survival in malnourished patients. Whether PEG increases survival time remains unclear (53). One study indicates that PEG tube placement is associated with greater survival than NGT placement. This study was retrospective, however, and the indications for treatment and nutritional indices differed between groups (54). PEG placement may be associated with increased pulmonary risks and shorter survival time when done in patients with reduced vital capacity, defined as forced vital capacity <50% of predicted. Recent studies, however, call this into question (55,56).

POTENTIAL BENEFIT FROM ARTIFICIAL HYDRATION

Comfort

A common argument for providing artificial hydration in palliative care is to alleviate thirst. Healthy volunteers who undergo experimentally induced dehydration often report thirst, yet this sensation is relieved by ad lib sips of fluid in cumulative volumes insufficient to restore physiologic fluid balance. The few studies evaluating patient symptoms at the end of life suggest a high prevalence of dry mouth and thirst that is not correlated with hydration status, but it can be alleviated with ice chips and sips of water (19). In several studies of palliative care patients, no statistically significant association was found between thirst and fluid intake, serum sodium, urea, or osmolality (57,58).

Reduction of Delirium or Opioid Toxicity

Retrospective studies have suggested that hydration might be able to reduce neuropsychiatric symptoms such as sedation, hallucinations, myoclonus, and agitation. In the first RCT of hydration versus placebo in patients with cancer, Bruera et al. compared the effects of hydration with either 1,000 or 100 mL of normal saline on target symptoms of sedation, fatigue, hallucinations, and myoclonus (59). Although the study did not meet its accrual goals, 53 (73%) of 73 target symptoms experienced by the treatment group improved compared with 33 (49%) of 67 target symptoms in the placebo group ($P = 0.006$), suggesting a potential benefit of hydration in this population. This study was underpowered and characterized by many subjective measures and was not performed in hospice patients. Nevertheless, it highlights the importance of further study in this controversial area.

POTENTIAL HARM FROM ARTIFICIAL HYDRATION

Commonly cited side effects of artificial hydration in palliative care include fluid overload and increased respiratory secretions. Because no controlled trials exist, the association between these adverse effects and artificial hydration is hard to measure.

Fluid Overload

Concerns regarding hydration often center on the potential impact such hydration might have on edema, ascites, and respiratory distress. A comparison of two different healthcare settings (a palliative care unit and an acute care unit) demonstrated marked differences in volume of hydration ordered. The acute care group ordered higher volumes of hydration, but it also prescribed a higher number of diuretics, suggesting that increased hydration could be associated with greater likelihood for fluid overload (60). Morita's study of terminally ill patients also noted an association between hydration and symptom scores for edema, ascites, and pleural effusion (61).

Increased Respiratory Secretions

Many palliative care providers believe that hydration may worsen retained respiratory secretions at the very end of life. However, the effect of hydration on respiratory secretions at the end of life is unclear. Neither Ellershaw nor Morita found a correlation between hydration status and bronchial secretions.

METHODOLOGICAL ISSUES IN EVALUATING EFFECTIVENESS OF NUTRITION INTERVENTIONS

In reviewing the current ANH literature, one is struck by the dearth of methodologically rigorous studies available to inform practice. With the exception of several large retrospective cohort studies, most studies had small sample sizes and heterogeneous patient populations. These cohort studies did not include meaningful comparison groups, so evaluating the true impact of ANH is problematic.

Very little attention has been given to the nature of the nutritional intervention being provided through artificial nutrition. PEG placement or tube feeding might or might not lead to adequate caloric intake. Evaluating differences in outcome between those receiving adequate nutrients and those that did not would elucidate whether or not outcomes varied by actual caloric intake. In most studies, the composition of the nutrition or fluid formulations in these studies was rarely addressed or identified.

In almost all instances, RCTs either do not exist or are underpowered to evaluate the main outcomes. Most studies had difficulty with recruitment and high dropout rates. Furthermore, the follow-up time was often very short (days to weeks). Hence, these trials are not likely to detect true effects of the intervention.

For the preponderance of observational studies influencing this field, confounding is not adequately addressed. For example, in observational studies of patients with dementia receiving EN, it is possible that tubes are placed primarily in a subgroup of patients whose oral intake has become insufficient to sustain life, thus prolonging their survival from 0 to 1 month to 6 to 7 months (confounding by indication). On the other hand, it is likely that tubes were not placed in the subgroup of patients who retained some capacity to eat; those patients also survived a median of roughly 6 to 7 months. The ability to eat could then be a confounding factor that explains the similar survival between groups receiving and not receiving artificial nutrition. Measuring the ability to eat and controlling for this risk factor in the analysis could help to ascertain the true association between tube placement and survival. Because many patients have multiple conditions, the nature and severity of these conditions (especially in Medicare databases) may be difficult to capture and therefore adequately control for in analyses.

Many of the outcomes chosen in these studies provide inadequate information for clinicians to guide patients. Most studies have evaluated survival and nutritional or medical indicators. Most have not addressed quality-of-life outcomes or quality-adjusted life years.

WHAT ARE CULTURAL AND RELIGIOUS DIMENSIONS TO THESE FORMS OF TREATMENT?

Ethnicity

Among nursing home residents with severe cognitive impairment, African Americans were almost four times more likely than Whites to have a feeding tube (62). Despite a recent trend toward decreased PEG tube placement in dementia patients, racial discrepancies persist. In a review of the Veterans Health Administration database, Braun et al. found that although only 18.4% of dementia patients were African Americans, they accounted for 28.8% of all PEG tube recipients with dementia (63). Reasons cited for this discrepancy include mistrust of the healthcare system, a greater desire for more aggressive medical treatment near the end of life, and differences in underlying religious beliefs and values. The possibility remains that African Americans are receiving a different standard of care with regard to ANH at end of life.

Religious Background

Jewish, Islamic, and Catholic traditions place a priority on "sanctity of life," often preferring greater life-sustaining treatments over "quality of life." Jewish and Islamic traditions do not distinguish tube feeding from other forms of basic nutrition (64). According to most Jewish religious authorities, "nutrition in any form is a basic human need and should be provided to all patients" (65). How cognitively impaired the patient is, is not relevant, because human life of any quality is of supreme value. Jewish tradition, however, does not argue for *any* treatment that is not of benefit to the patient and relies on scientific evidence in making an ethical judgment on a particular treatment modality.

GUIDELINES FOR ENTERAL/PARENTERAL NUTRITION IN PALLIATIVE CARE

Improve the Scientific Literature Base

Because all the current data regarding ANH have significant methodological weaknesses, providers should be circumspect about the true benefits and harm of nutrition support, especially in the enteral form. Improvements in the overall quality could be made by:

1. Collaboration with epidemiologists/biostatisticians from the beginning stages of the study
2. Agreement on appropriate outcome measures
3. Use of the highest quality design for the clinical question at hand

More rigorous studies are needed to increase the confidence that current clinical practice is based on the higher levels of evidence.

Improve the Assessment Process

Before initiating artificial nutrition, it is worth asking the following questions:

1. Is the patient able to swallow properly? If so, oral nutrition is preferable and safer than tube feeding.
2. If the patient can swallow properly, is the patient maintaining adequate nutritional intake to meet nutritional needs? If not, dietary supplementation is preferable and safer than tube feeding.
3. If the patient can swallow but cannot maintain adequate nutritional intake, is it due to a specific modifiable cause? If so, addressing the underlying cause is preferable and safer than tube feeding. For example,

   ■ Does the patient have a psychological condition such as depression that affects nutritional intake?
   ■ Does the patient have mouth pain, poorly fitted dentures, or loss of teeth?
   ■ Is the food or the eating environment unappealing?
   ■ Does the patient have the physical dexterity needed to eat without assistance?
   ■ Does the patient need to be reminded how to chew and swallow?
   ■ Is the patient receiving the help he or she needs to eat?
   ■ Are language barriers, ethnic or cultural dietary restrictions, or religious beliefs keeping the patient from taking an adequate amount of nutrition?

4. If the patient is unable to eat or does not have adequate nutritional intake, address the following questions before considering tube feeding:

   ■ Does the clinical decision to employ tube feeding respect the autonomy of the patient and family to decline the intervention?
   ■ Is conservative treatment a better option? Has it been tried? If not, why?
   ■ Is there scientific evidence that supports tube feeding as a better option than oral intake in this situation?
   ■ Are there any contraindications to artificial feeding in this patient?
   ■ When and how will the effectiveness of and continued need for tube feeding be reassessed (i.e., reaching a specific therapeutic goal or a prespecified time period)?

Improve the Informed Consent Process

The current quality of informed consent for EN and, in particular, placement of gastrostomy tubes is poor. In a review of 154 consecutive hospitalized adults undergoing placement of gastrostomy tubes, only 1 medical record documented a procedure-specific discussion of benefits and burdens of and alternatives to tube feeding (66).

Specific Information that Should Be Provided

The informed consent process should include discussion of median, 1-year, and 3-year survival rates. It should also identify both physical (restraints) and potential psychosocial (social isolation and sensory deprivation) adverse effects associated with artificial nutrition. In patients who are not imminently dying, alternatives such as carefully monitored hand-feeding should be discussed, including the observation that there is no difference in survival for PEG tubes versus hand-feeding for demented and nondemented patients (67). In patients who are in the terminal phase of their illness, findings regarding the common lack of hunger experienced by patients should be communicated to patients' families to allay concerns regarding potential patient distress associated with minimal oral intake.

Poor prognostic factors consistently noted in the literature should be described, including increased age (>80 yr), chewing and swallowing disorders, and the presence of underlying malignancies (68).

GUIDELINES FOR HYDRATION IN PALLIATIVE CARE

Hydration may be of benefit in patients with potential opioid toxicity, confusion, or nausea. Patients and families should be informed regarding the lack of correlation between hydration and thirst and the finding that sips of water, ice chips, lip moisteners, salivary substitutes, mouth swabs, hard candy, and routine mouth care are more effective at addressing the sense of dry mouth and thirst than is artificial hydration.

CONCLUSION

Evidence regarding the potential benefit or harm associated with ANH in palliative care continues to be limited by underpowered or poorly designed studies. Decisions regarding ANH should be informed by treatment goals and patient preference (autonomy) and the application of the principles of nonmaleficence and beneficence where potential harm or benefits can be determined. While case law regards artificial nutrition as medical treatment, in the absence of a developed literature to provide a scientific basis for decision making, social values may continue to guide decisions in some instances. Many religious traditions do not distinguish artificial nutrition from basic food and water, a point that renders moot discussion of harm and benefits for some decision makers. Physicians should inform the patient or their family as fully as possible regarding the potential benefit and harm associated with ANH and assist them to make the best decision possible based on the patient's values and available information about risks and benefits.

REFERENCES

1. Good P, Cavenagh J, Mather M, Ravenscroft P. Medically assisted nutrition for palliative care in adult patients. *Cochrane Database Syst Rev.* 2008(4):CD006274.
2. Good P, Cavenagh J, Mather M, Ravenscroft P. Medically assisted hydration for palliative care patients. *Cochrane Database Syst Rev.* 2008(2):CD006273.
3. Dudrick SJ. Rhoads Lecture: a 45-year obsession and passionate pursuit of optimal nutrition support: puppies, pediatrics, surgery, geriatrics, home TPN, A.S.P.E.N., et cetera. *JPEN J Parenter Enteral Nutr.* 2005;29(4):272-287.

4. Heyland DK, Montalvo M, MacDonald S, Keefe L, Su XY, Drover JW. Total parenteral nutrition in the surgical patient: a meta-analysis. *Can J Surg.* 2001;44(2):102-111.

5. Heyland DK, MacDonald S, Keefe L, Drover JW. Total parenteral nutrition in the critically ill patient: a meta-analysis. *JAMA.* 1998;280(23):2013-2019.

6. Gauderer MW. Percutaneous endoscopic gastrostomy-20 years later: a historical perspective. *J Pediatr Surg.* 2001;36(1):217-219.

7. Callahan CM, Haag KM, Buchanan NN, Nisi R. Decision-making for percutaneous endoscopic gastrostomy among older adults in a community setting. *J Am Geriatr Soc.* 1999;47(9):1105-1109.

8. Cruzan v Director, Missouri Department of Public Health. In: 110 S. Court; 1990; 2841.

9. Kapp MB. Regulating the foregoing of artificial nutrition and hydration: first, do some harm. *J Am Geriatr Soc.* 2002;50(3):586-588.

10. Taylor CA, Larson DE, Ballard DJ, et al. Predictors of outcome after percutaneous endoscopic gastrostomy: a community-based study. *Mayo Clin Proc.* 1992;67(11):1042-1049.

11. Light VL, Slezak FA, Porter JA, Gerson LW, McCord G. Predictive factors for early mortality after percutaneous endoscopic gastrostomy. *Gastrointest Endosc.* 1995;42(4):330-335.

12. Grant MD, Rudberg MA, Brody JA. Gastrostomy placement and mortality among hospitalized Medicare beneficiaries. *JAMA.* 1998;279(24):1973-1976.

13. Wasa M, Takagi Y, Sando K, Harada T, Okada A. Long-term outcome of short bowel syndrome in adult and pediatric patients. *JPEN J Parenter Enteral Nutr.* 1999;23(5 suppl):S110-S112.

14. Klein S, Kinney J, Jeejeebhoy K, et al. Nutrition support in clinical practice: review of published data and recommendations for future research directions. *Clin Nutr.* 1997;16(4):193-218.

15. Tresch DD, Sims FH, Duthie EH, Goldstein MD, Lane PS. Clinical characteristics of patients in the persistent vegetative state. *Arch Intern Med.* 1991;151(5):930-932.

16. Heyland DK, Dhaliwal R, Drover JW, Gramlich L, Dodek P. Canadian clinical practice guidelines for nutrition support in mechanically ventilated, critically ill adult patients. *JPEN J Parenter Enteral Nutr.* 2003;27(5):355-373.

17. Rabeneck L, Wray NP, Petersen NJ. Long-term outcomes of patients receiving percutaneous endoscopic gastrostomy tubes. *J Gen Intern Med.* 1996;11(5):287-293.

18. Rimon E, Kagansky N, Levy S. Percutaneous endoscopic gastrostomy: evidence of different prognosis in various patient subgroups. *Age Ageing.* 2005;34(4):353-357.

19. McCann RM, Hall WJ, Groth-Juncker A. Comfort care for terminally ill patients. The appropriate use of nutrition and hydration. *JAMA.* 1994;272(16):1263-1266.

20. Ganzini L, Goy ER, Miller LL, Harvath TA, Jackson A, Delorit MA. Nurses' experiences with hospice patients who refuse food and fluids to hasten death. *N Engl J Med.* 2003;349(4):359-365.

21. Byock I. Patient refusal of nutrition and hydration: walking the ever-finer line. *Am J Hosp Palliat Care.* 1995;12(2):8, 9-13.

22. Berlowitz DR, Wilking SV. Risk factors for pressure sores. A comparison of cross-sectional and cohort-derived data. *J Am Geriatr Soc.* 1989;37(11):1043-1050.

23. Bergstrom N, Braden B. A prospective study of pressure sore risk among institutionalized elderly. *J Am Geriatr Soc.* 1992;40(8):747-758.

24. Hartgrink HH, Wille J, Konig P, Hermans J, Breslau PJ. Pressure sores and tube feeding in patients with a fracture of the hip: a randomized clinical trial. *Clin Nutr.* 1998;17(6):287-292.

25. Ohura T, Nakajo T, Okada S, Omura K, Adachi K. Evaluation of effects of nutrition intervention on healing of pressure ulcers and nutritional states (randomized controlled trial). *Wound Repair Regen.* 2011;19(3):330-336.

26. Stratton RJ, Ek AC, Engfer M, et al. Enteral nutritional support in prevention and treatment of pressure ulcers: a systematic review and meta-analysis. *Ageing Res Rev.* 2005;4(3):422-450.

27. McClave SA, DeMeo MT, DeLegge MH, et al. North American Summit on Aspiration in the critically ill patient: consensus statement. *JPEN J Parenter Enteral Nutr.* 2002;26 (6 suppl):S80-S85.

28. Langmore SE, Terpenning MS, Schork A, et al. Predictors of aspiration pneumonia: how important is dysphagia? *Dysphagia.* 1998;13(2):69-81.

29. Heyland DK, Drover JW, MacDonald S, Novak F, Lam M. Effect of postpyloric feeding on gastroesophageal regurgitation and pulmonary microaspiration: results of a randomized controlled trial. *Crit Care Med.* 2001;29(8):1495-1501.

30. Stroud M, Duncan H, Nightingale J. Guidelines for enteral feeding in adult hospital patients. *Gut.* 2003;52(suppl 7):vii1-vii12.

31. Sullivan-Marx EM, Strumpf NE, Evans LK, Baumgarten M, Maislin G. Predictors of continued physical restraint use in nursing home residents following restraint reduction efforts. *J Am Geriatr Soc.* 1999;47(3):342-348.

32. Peck A, Cohen CE, Mulvihill MN. Long-term enteral feeding of aged demented nursing home patients. *J Am Geriatr Soc.* 1990;38(11):1195-1198.

33. Norton B, Homer-Ward M, Donnelly MT, Long RG, Holmes GK. A randomised prospective comparison of percutaneous endoscopic gastrostomy and nasogastric tube feeding after acute dysphagic stroke. *BMJ.* 1996;312(7022):13-16.

34. Park RH, Allison MC, Lang J, et al. Randomised comparison of percutaneous endoscopic gastrostomy and nasogastric tube feeding in patients with persisting neurological dysphagia. *BMJ.* 1992;304(6839):1406-1409.

35. Iizuka M, Reding M. Use of percutaneous endoscopic gastrostomy feeding tubes and functional recovery in stroke rehabilitation: a case-matched controlled study. *Arch Phys Med Rehabil.* 2005;86(5):1049-1052.

36. Golestanian E, Liou JI, Smith MA. Long-term survival in older critically ill patients with acute ischemic stroke. *Crit Care Med.* 2009;37(12):3107-3113.

37. Dennis MS, Lewis SC, Warlow C. Effect of timing and method of enteral tube feeding for dysphagic stroke patients (FOOD): a multicentre randomised controlled trial. *Lancet.* 2005;365(9461):764-772.

38. Melchior JC, Chastang C, Gelas P, et al. Efficacy of 2-month total parenteral nutrition in AIDS patients: a controlled randomized prospective trial. The French Multicenter Total Parenteral Nutrition Cooperative Group Study. *AIDS.* 1996;10(4):379-384.

39. Klein S, Kinney J, Jeejeebhoy K, et al. Nutrition support in clinical practice: review of published data and recommendations for future research directions. Summary of a conference sponsored by the National Institutes of Health, American Society for Parenteral and Enteral Nutrition, and American Society for Clinical Nutrition. *Am J Clin Nutr.* 1997;66(3):683-706.

40. Klein S, Simes J, Blackburn GL. Total parenteral nutrition and cancer clinical trials. *Cancer.* 1986;58(6):1378-1386.

41. McGeer AJ, Detsky AS, O'Rourke K. Parenteral nutrition in cancer patients undergoing chemotherapy: a meta-analysis. *Nutrition.* 1990;6(3):233-240.

42. Parenteral nutrition in patients receiving cancer chemotherapy. American College of Physicians. *Ann Intern Med.* 1989;110(9):734-736.

43. Lee JH, Machtay M, Unger LD, et al. Prophylactic gastrostomy tubes in patients undergoing intensive irradiation for cancer of the head and neck. *Arch Otolaryngol Head Neck Surg.* 1998;124(8):871-875.

44. Bozzetti F, Gavazzi C, Mariani L, Crippa F. Artificial nutrition in cancer patients: which route, what composition? *World J Surg.* 1999;23(6):577-583.

45. Dresler CM, Jeevanandam M, Brennan MF. Metabolic efficacy of enteral feeding in malnourished cancer and noncancer patients. *Metabolism.* 1987;36(1):82-88.

46. Burt ME, Gorschboth CM, Brennan MF. A controlled, prospective, randomized trial evaluating the metabolic effects of enteral and parenteral nutrition in the cancer patient. *Cancer.* 1982;49(6):1092-1105.

47. Lim ST, Choa RG, Lam KH, Wong J, Ong GB. Total parenteral nutrition versus gastrostomy in the preoperative preparation of patients with carcinoma of the oesophagus. *Br J Surg.* 1981;68(2):69-72.

48. Barichella M, Cereda E, Pezzoli G. Major nutritional issues in the management of Parkinson's disease. *Mov Disord.* 2009;24(13):1881-1892.

49. McClave SA, Chang WK. Complications of enteral access. *Gastrointest Endosc.* 2003;58(5):739-751.

50. Klor BM, Milianti FJ. Rehabilitation of neurogenic dysphagia with percutaneous endoscopic gastrostomy. *Dysphagia.* 1999;14(3):162-164.

51. Mazzini L, Corra T, Zaccala M, Mora G, Del Piano M, Galante M. Percutaneous endoscopic gastrostomy and enteral nutrition in amyotrophic lateral sclerosis. *J Neurol.* 1995;242(10):695-698.

52. Kasarskis EJ, Scarlata D, Hill R, Fuller C, Stambler N, Cedarbaum JM. A retrospective study of percutaneous endoscopic gastrostomy in ALS patients during the BDNF and CNTF trials. *J Neurol Sci.* 1999;169(1-2):118-125.

53. Desport JC, Preux PM, Truong CT, Courat L, Vallat JM, Couratier P. Nutritional assessment and survival in ALS patients. *Amyotroph Lateral Scler Other Motor Neuron Disord.* 2000;1(2):91-96.

54. Rio A, Ellis C, Shaw C, et al. Nutritional factors associated with survival following enteral tube feeding in patients with motor neurone disease. *J Hum Nutr Diet.* 2010;23(4):408-415.

55. Gregory S, Siderowf A, Golaszewski AL, McCluskey L. Gastrostomy insertion in ALS patients with low vital capacity: respiratory support and survival. *Neurology.* 2002;58(3):485-487.

56. Boitano LJ, Jordan T, Benditt JO. Noninvasive ventilation allows gastrostomy tube placement in patients with advanced ALS. *Neurology.* 2001;56(3):413-414.

57. Ellershaw JE, Sutcliffe JM, Saunders CM. Dehydration and the dying patient. *J Pain Symptom Manage.* 1995;10(3):192-197.

58. Burge FI. Dehydration symptoms of palliative care cancer patients. *J Pain Symptom Manage.* 1993;8(7):454-464.

59. Bruera E, Franco JJ, Maltoni M, Watanabe S, Suarez-Almazor M. Changing pattern of agitated impaired mental status in patients with advanced cancer: association with cognitive monitoring, hydration, and opioid rotation. *J Pain Symptom Manage.* 1995;10(4):287-291.

60. Lanuke K, Fainsinger RL, DeMoissac D. Hydration management at the end of life. *J Palliat Med.* 2004;7(2):257-263.

61. Morita T, Hyodo I, Yoshimi T, et al. Association between hydration volume and symptoms in terminally ill cancer patients with abdominal malignancies. *Ann Oncol.* 2005;16(4):640-647.

62. Gessert CE, Curry NM, Robinson A. Ethnicity and end-of-life care: the use of feeding tubes. *Ethn Dis.* 2001;11(1):97-106.

63. Braun UK, Rabeneck L, McCullough LB, et al. Decreasing use of percutaneous endoscopic gastrostomy tube feeding for veterans with dementia-racial differences remain. *J Am Geriatr Soc.* 2005;53(2):242-248.

64. Gordon M, Alibhai SH. Ethics of PEG tubes—Jewish and Islamic perspectives. *Am J Gastroenterol.* 2004;99(6):1194.

65. Jotkowitz AB, Clarfield AM, Glick S. The care of patients with dementia: a modern Jewish ethical perspective. *J Am Geriatr Soc.* 2005;53(5):881-884.

66. Brett AS, Rosenberg JC. The adequacy of informed consent for placement of gastrostomy tubes. *Arch Intern Med.* 2001;161(5):745-748.

67. Franzoni S, Frisoni GB, Boffelli S, Rozzini R, Trabucchi M. Good nutritional oral intake is associated with equal survival in demented and nondemented very old patients. *J Am Geriatr Soc.* 1996;44(11):1366-1370.

68. Mitchell SL, Buchanan JL, Littlehale S, Hamel MB. Tube-feeding versus hand-feeding nursing home residents with advanced dementia: a cost comparison. *J Am Med Dir Assoc.* 2003;4(1):27-33.

CHAPTER 61

Complementary, Alternative, and Integrative Therapies in Oncology

M. Jennifer Cheng ■ Daniel L. Handel

omplementary and alternative medicine (CAM) includes a group of diverse medical and health care systems, practices, and products that are distinct from conventional medical modalities and used in conjunction with (complementary) or in lieu of (alternative) standard biomedical management (1,2). The use of CAM in the United States has substantially increased since the 1990s. The National Center for Health Statistics reported in 2008 that 38% of Americans use some form of CAM, reflecting CAM's continued popularity through the past decade (3).

The use of CAM among people with cancer is particularly common, with up to 54% of patients initiating CAM after cancer diagnosis (4) and up to 80% of all cancer patients using some form of CAM during the course of their disease (5,6). A recent analysis by Mao et al. of the 2007 National Health Interview Survey shows that cancer survivors are more likely to use CAM than the general population. The researchers find that 65% of cancer survivors have used CAM in their lifetime; in contrast, only 53% of the non-cancer respondents used CAM in their lifetime (7).

While used in the same acronym, a distinction must be made between complementary and alternative therapies. Alternative therapies are used *instead* of mainstream treatments. There has not been convincing evidence to date of the effectiveness of alternative cancer treatments. On the other hand, complementary therapies *complement* mainstream oncologic treatments, and there is growing research supporting their safety and efficacy.

Patients are increasingly seeking holistic cancer care that is tailored to the unique needs of the individual. This trend has fueled the establishment of the field of Integrative Oncology in 2000, which interweaves conventional and evidence-based complementary therapies in oncology (5). Complementary therapies usually serve as adjuncts to mainstream cancer treatments to enhance well-being and self-empowerment (4,8), manage cancer and cancer treatment symptoms, and provide survivor care (9,10). There is limited evidence that CAM therapies might improve immune system function (11); however, there is not yet strong evidence for improved survival from this effect (12).

This chapter will review various modalities of complementary therapies in integrative oncology: mind–body interventions (hypnosis, relaxation therapies, meditation/mindfulness-based stress reduction (MBSR), biofeedback, yoga, and creative therapy), energy therapies (Reiki, healing/therapeutic touch), manipulative and body-based methods (chiropractic, massage therapy, exercise, Qigong, and Tai Chi Chuan), acupuncture, and biologically based therapies (herbs and vitamins). The biologically based therapies section also examines specific phytochemicals and vitamins that are under investigation for cancer prevention, cancer treatment, and symptom management.

MIND–BODY INTERVENTIONS

Mind–body interventions utilize the interactions among the brain, mind, body, and behavior and are defined by the National Institutes of Health Center for Complementary and Alternative Medicine as "a variety of techniques designed to enhance the mind's capacity to affect bodily function and symptoms" (13,14). For the purposes of this chapter we will limit our discussions to select the better studied mind–body interventions, reviewing their characteristics and recommendations for use.

Hypnosis

In 1985, Kihlstrom (15) defined hypnosis as "a social interaction in which one person, designated the subject, responds to suggestions offered by another person, designated the hypnotist, for experiences involving alterations in perception, memory, and voluntary action". Hypnosis allows for a highly relaxed state in which the patient's conscious and unconscious mind is open to therapeutic suggestions (13).

Hypnosis has been well researched in randomized clinical studies as treatment interventions for outcomes in controlling chronic pain including alleviating cancer-related pain (16–18); improving acute and procedural pain in adults and children including procedures such as bone marrow aspiration, lumpectomy/breast cancer surgery, and vascular access procedures (19,20); alleviating stress, anxiety, and depression in breast cancer surgery patients and terminally ill cancer patients (21,22); improving anticipatory nausea and vomiting in children and adults receiving chemotherapy use (23–25); and reducing frequency and intensity of hot flashes among breast cancer survivors (26). Some studies support the use of self-hypnosis in the medical setting, where brief training sessions that build self-hypnosis skills result in improved clinical outcomes, coupled with increased sense of mastery and self-control (27,28).

Self-hypnosis has also been utilized in conjunction with other complementary therapies. In a 1989 prospective study by Spiegel et al. published in *The Lancet*, women with metastatic breast cancer are randomly assigned to the intervention or control groups. Intervention includes 1 year of group therapy led by a psychiatrist or social worker with a therapist, and self-hypnosis training for pain control. At 10-year follow-up, there was significantly improved survival in the intervention group, with a mean survival of 36.6 months compared with 18.9 months in the control group, (29). However, subsequent multicenter randomized clinical trials (RCTs) did not replicate the survival benefit found by Spiegel et al. This may be due to the innovations in breast cancer treatment subsequent to Spiegel's publication, including selective estrogen receptor modulators and earlier detection of breast cancer through routine cancer screening. However, all of these studies demonstrate improvements in quality of life and reductions in distress and pain among women utilizing self-hypnosis and group support strategies (30).

Relaxation Therapies

Beginning in the early 1900s with Jacobson's progressive muscle relaxation technique (31), many relaxation techniques have evolved, such as jaw relaxation, focused breathing, and abdominal breathing, that aim to engender a state free of mental and/or physical tension (13).

A literature review by Kwekkeboom et al. found six studies where relaxation was implemented as the key intervention in treating two or more symptoms in the pain–fatigue–sleep disturbance cancer symptom cluster. Pain benefit was demonstrated in three of the four studies in which it was the key outcome. Other cancer-related symptoms mitigated by relaxation intervention include physical tension and sleep (32). Populations studied include hospitalized patients with cancer pain, outpatients with chronic cancer pain, and women with early-stage breast cancer. While symptoms generally improved compared with no treatment group, results have not been consistent (33).

Guided Imagery

Guided imagery engages the imagination in creating a sensory experience to achieve a specific clinical outcome (34). Imagery is often utilized with other mind–body techniques such as relaxation techniques and music therapy.

Guided imagery is one of the mind–body modalities recommended by the National Comprehensive Cancer Network for treatment of anticipatory nausea and vomiting. In one study, guided imagery with music therapy was found to improve the quality of life and mood disturbance in cancer survivors (35). Mood and quality of life improved significantly in the guided imagery group as well as the progressive muscle relaxation group compared with usual care in an RCT of 56 participants with advanced cancer receiving palliative care at home (36). While studies evaluating the use of guided imagery in participants receiving chemotherapy did not find significant improvements in nausea and vomiting prior to and hours to days after chemotherapy, there have generally been significant improvements in emotional response and

anxiety during chemotherapy treatment associated with the use of guided imagery (37,38).

Only six RCTs compared imagery alone with a no treatment or another active intervention group. In general, imagery alone is more effective than no treatment in improving symptoms of depression, anxiety, pain, and quality of life. Its effects are generally comparable to other mind–body techniques such as hypnosis or relaxation (34,35). However, more stringently designed clinical trials are needed, as current studies lack explicit descriptions of the intervention procedures, duration, and outcome measures.

Meditation/Mindfulness-Based Stress Reduction

Meditation is a family of techniques with the goal of training the mind to focus on a single target perception to realize an ultimate benefit. While purported to have its origin from Eastern traditions, many religious and spiritual traditions have developed their own meditative practices. The most well-studied meditation technique is the MBSR, a secular meditation technique developed by Jon Kabat-Zinn and colleagues with its roots in Buddhist Vipassana and Zen practices (39). The primary goal of mindfulness meditation to complete engagement in the present moment experience with a nonjudgmental attitude of acceptance and patience—without ruminations about prior or future experience. Through this training, one develops a nonreactive awareness even during stressful situations (40).

MBSR is a well-defined patient-focused intervention typically offered in 7 to 10 weekly group sessions, each lasting for 1 to 1.5 hours. Breast and prostate cancer patients are the oncology populations most studied in MBSR intervention. Most interventions are one-group pretest–posttest design and generally demonstrate improvements in mood and stress (41), quality of life (42), cytokine production (42), sleep quality (43), coping styles, decreases in helplessness–hopelessness (44), and pain. Speca's prospective, randomized, treatment controlled trial demonstrated significant decreases in overall symptoms of stress, depression, anxiety, anger, and confusion following a mindfulness meditation-based stress reduction program in cancer outpatients with various stages of disease. A study by Carlson et al. demonstrated improvements at 1 year following MBSR interventions in quality of life and stress symptoms. This study also found clinical and lab evidence consistent with reductions in the stress response, including hormonal, immunological, and vascular parameters (42,45).

Mindfulness-based cognitive therapy, a refinement of MBSR, focuses on the ruminative processes in major depression and recently has been evaluated in effectiveness for individuals with variety of cancer diagnoses. Preliminary evidence suggests improvement in depression and anxiety.

Overall, meta-analysis demonstrates that MBSR is effective in oncology populations for psychological stressors, with more modest effect sizes for physiological measurements and physical health measures. Larger RCTs are needed to fully determine the efficacy of mindfulness in oncology.

Yoga

The practice of yoga originates from Eastern traditions. The word *yoga* is derived from the Sanskrit root *yuj*, meaning to bind, join, and yoke. The goal of yoga is to strengthen the union between mind, body, and spirit through ethical disciplines, physical postures, and spiritual practices (13,46). Listed in Table 61.1 are various styles of yoga and corresponding clinical studies assessing its effectiveness in symptom management among cancer patients (13,46,56).

Overall, there has been preliminary positive evidence supporting the use of yoga through single-arm pilot trials and small-scale RCTs. Data suggest improved overall quality of life, emotional well-being, mood, hot flashes, spiritual well-being, and sleep (Table 61.1). Larger clinical trials are underway or have recently been completed. For example, the first nationwide, multisite, phase II/III RCT led by Mustain et al. has recently been completed with promising results. The National Cancer Institute is sponsoring a large phase III, three-arm clinical study comparing yoga, meditation, and simple stretching in radiation therapy patients with stage zero to III breast cancer.

Biofeedback

Biofeedback enables an individual to learn how to change physiologic functions by measuring these activities and providing real-time "feedback" to patients in order to facilitate changes in behavior, emotions, and cognition. Physiologic measures can include brainwaves, heart function, breathing, muscle activity, and skin temperature. The goal is for the physiologic changes to persist without the need for an instrument (57).

A small randomized control study in advanced cancer patients demonstrates reduction in cancer-related pain using electromyography biofeedback-assisted relaxation over a 4-week period. The mechanism of action is thought to be associated with attenuation of physiologic arousal (58).

The study of audio-visual feedback in respiratory-gated radiotherapy for lung cancer patients by George et al. assesses the effect of 5 weekly breath-training sessions with a goal of improved compliance during radiotherapy. Within each session the patients initially breathed without any instruction (free breathing), then with audio instructions, and finally with audio-visual biofeedback. Audio-visual biofeedback significantly reduces residual motion compared with free breathing and audio instruction (59). However, results in biofeedback have not been consistent. Bladder ultrasound biofeedback training did not produce a reproducible increase in bladder filling in prostate cancer patients during pelvic tumor irradiation (60).

Biofeedback is often used in conjunction with other integrative techniques. For example, a model for social work teaches cancer patients and their relatives ways of coping through a combination of cognitive behavioral intervention, relaxation methods with guided imagery, and biofeedback (61).

Creative Therapies

Creative therapies are a group of creative processes that aim to enhance individuals' physical, mental, and emotional well-being. This category includes visual arts, music therapy, creative writing, and mixed-modality programs. Music therapy is one of the best studied creative therapies in the literature.

Music therapy in its strictest definition is provided by professional musicians trained at the university level whose training includes music theory, psychology, supervision, and personal psychotherapy (62). In recent years, the definition has broadened to include listening to pre-recorded music offered by medical staff.

In a descriptive review written by Gallagher from the Cleveland Clinic Arts and Medicine Institute, music therapy can be used throughout the spectrum of the cancer care process, including palliation, hospice, the active dying process, and bereavement. Common interventions include instrument playing, lyric analysis, musical entrainment, music-assisted relaxation, musical life review, music listening (live or recorded), participation (i.e., clapping, humming, and tapping foot), planning funeral music, singing, song-writing, and verbal processing (63).

A Cochrane review by Bradt et al. in 2011 examines the effects of music intervention on physical and psychological outcomes in cancer patients. The review includes all randomized controlled trials and quasi-randomized trials—30 trials with a total of 1,891 participants are included. The results suggest that music interventions may have beneficial effects in people with cancer, including quality of life and symptoms such as mood, anxiety, and pain. No strong evidence is found for improvements in fatigue, physical status, or depression. Authors conclude that the systematic review suggests beneficial effects of music therapy in aforementioned outcome, but caution that these trials are at high risk for bias (64).

Art therapy is another creative therapy modality commonly utilized by cancer patients; however, there is currently a dearth of controlled empirical studies evaluating this intervention. A literature review by Geue et al. in 2010 identifies 17 papers evaluating the effectiveness of using painting/drawing intervention for adult cancer patients. Nine out of the 17 papers are quantitative papers with two studies using randomization, the rest are qualitative studies. The sample sizes range from 7 and 70 participants with considerable variation in the structure and content of interventions. Results are generally positive, revealing decreases in anxiety and depression, increases in quality of life, and positive effects on personal growth, coping, and social interactions (65). More systematic evaluations are needed in this fertile field.

Acupuncture

Acupuncture is considered to be a part of mind–body medicine, but it is also considered a component of energy medicine, manipulative and body-based practices, and traditional Chinese medicine (66). Acupuncture involves the insertion

TABLE 61.1   **Various styles of yoga with corresponding clinical studies in symptom management among cancer patients**

		Selected Studies	Design	Result
Hatha yoga	Focuses on postures (asanas) and breathing exercises (pranayama).	Moadel et al. (47)	RCT 128 patients (stages I–III) breast cancer. ECOG performance status of < 3 recruited from urban cancer center to a 12-wk yoga intervention or a 12-wk waitlist control group	Improved overall QOL ($P < 0.008$), emotional well-being ($P < 0.015$), social well-being ($P < 0.004$), spiritual well-being ($P < 0.009$), and distressed mood ($P < 0.031$)
Iyengar yoga	Focuses on body alignment, precision, and sequencing of poses; uses props such as blankets and blocks.	Blank et al. (48)	RCT Pilot study of 18 women diagnosed with stage I–III breast cancer and receiving antiestrogen or aromatase inhibitor hormonal therapy. Yoga classes were conducted two times per week for 8 wk	More than 60% experienced less anxiety and improved mood
		Duncan et al. (49)	Single-arm pilot trial 24 postmenopausal women with stage I–III breast cancer who reported aromatase inhibitor–associated arthralgia were enrolled in a single-arm pilot trial. A yoga program was provided twice a week for 8 wk	Improvement in patient-reported QOL, spiritual well-being, and mood
		Speed-Andrews et al. (50)	Single-arm pilot trial 24 breast cancer survivors participated in 12-wk classes in Iyengar yoga and completed a questionnaire measuring generic and disease-specific QOL and psychosocial function before and after the intervention	Improvement in mental health (mean change, $+4.2$; $P = 0.045$), vitality (mean change, $+4.9$; $P = 0.033$), role-emotional (mean change, $+6.4$; $P = 0.010$), and bodily pain (mean change, $+4.4$; $P = 0.024$).
Restorative Yoga	"Gentle type" of yoga. Traditional poses performed with props (e.g., an exercise ball) to support the body	Danhauer et al. (51)	Single-arm pilot trial 51 women with ovarian ($n = 37$) or breast cancer ($n = 14$). The majority (61%) were actively undergoing cancer treatment. All study participants participated in 10 weekly classes	Significant improvements in depression, negative affect, state anxiety, mental health, and quality of life

(Continued)

TABLE **61.1** **Various styles of yoga with corresponding clinical studies in symptom management among cancer patients** (*Continued*)

	Selected Studies	Design	Result
	Danhauer et al. (52)	RCT 44 women with breast cancer enrolled, 34% were actively undergoing cancer treatment. Study participants were randomized to the intervention (10 weekly 75-min classes) or a waitlist control group	Improved mental health, depression, fatigue, positive affect, and spirituality
	Cohen et al. (53)	Single-arm pilot trial A pilot trial in 14 postmenopausal women experiencing ≥4 moderate to severe hot flushes per day or ≥30 moderate to severe hot flashes per week. Eight restorative yoga poses taught in a 3-h introductory session and 8 weekly 90-min sessions	Mean number of hot flushes per week decreased by 30.8% (95% CI 15.6–45.9%) and mean hot-flash score decreased 34.2% (95% CI 16.0–52.5%) from baseline to week 8
Yoga of awareness program	Carson et al. (54)	RCT 37 breast cancer disease-free women experiencing hot flashes were randomized to the 8-wk yoga of awareness program (gentle yoga poses, meditation, and breathing exercises) or to waitlist control	Improvements in hot-flash frequency, severity, and total scores and in levels of joint pain, fatigue, sleep disturbance, symptom-related bother, and vigor
UR yoga for cancer survivors (YOCAS)	Mustain et al. (55)	RCT; nationwide, multisite, phase II/III study 410 early-stage cancer survivors randomized to usual care or 75-min yoga class twice a week for 4 wk	Treatment group reported 22% improvement in sleep quality compared with a 12% improvement in control group. Treatment group reduced the use of sleep medication by 12% compared with 5% increase in sleep medication in the control. Treatment group with 42% reduction in fatigue compared with the 12% in control group

8-wk protocol involving gentle yoga postures, breathing exercises, meditation, didactic, and group exchanges

Mindfulness exercises that covered breathing, meditation, visualization, and 18 poses

RCT, randomized clinical trial; QOL, quality of life; ECOG, Eastern Cooperative Oncology Group.

of fine needles into predefined meridian acupuncture points to relieve symptoms and improve disease processes. The World Health Organization reports 28 diseases, symptoms, and conditions for which evidence from controlled trials suggests benefit from acupuncture (67).

Capodice's (68) review of the evidence supports the use of acupuncture in oncologic settings for pain, xerostomia, and fatigue (Table 61.2). Stone and Johnstone (80) further discuss the evidence behind acupuncture use in peripheral neuropathy, post-surgical pain and dysfunction, joint pain from aromatase inhibitors, cancer-related fatigue, and hyperemesis associated with chemotherapy.

The strength of the evidence supporting acupuncture use varies, with randomized controlled trials available for postoperative pain in head and neck cancer patients (81), fatigue (82,83), hyperemesis (84), xerostomia (85), and aromatase inhibitor–induced arthralgias (86).

Lu and Rosenthal (87) discuss safety considerations in acupuncture use and recommend against acupuncture use in the following conditions: absolute neutrophil count <500/μL; platelet count <25,000/μL; altered mental state; clinically significant cardiac arrhythmias; and other unstable medical conditions evaluated on a case-by-case basis.

ENERGY HEALING

Energy healing techniques include a group of therapies where the healer transfers and/or channels energy from an external source through their hands to the patient. Among the more commonly used energy healing are Reiki, therapeutic touch, and healing touch.

Reiki was developed in Japan by Mikao Usui in 1922 and brought to the West in 1938. It is widely practiced in the United States. Reiki is a Japanese word for "spirit-guided life energy" (88) and is administered through gentle touch with hands placed on or near the recipient's body. Energy is thought to be channeled to the patient. The benefits from Reiki and other healing touch therapies are proposed to derive from improved flow of life energy (chi) that is associated with achieving and maintaining good health. According to a 2007 National Health Interview Survey, 1.2 million adults and 161,000 children in the United States received one or more sessions of energy healing such as Reiki during the year 2006 (89).

The 2010 scientific review of Reiki by Baldwin et al. reveals 26 peer-reviewed Reiki articles, including 7 qualitative and 19 quantitative trials. In total, 11 (42%) of the 26 studies are categorized as "weak" and 8 (30%) as "very good" to "excellent." The eight studies classified as "very good" to "excellent" published between 2001 and 2009 suggest improved quality of research in Reiki with time. Most weaknesses relate to experimental design such as lack of blinding, small sample size, lack of controls, lack of standardization of Reiki treatments within study, and lack of information about participants (such as gender, age, and race). The articles classified as "very good" or "excellent" provide mixed results for using Reiki as a healing modality. Additional studies with

robust study designs are encouraged to further elucidate the role and benefit of Reiki specifically for cancer patients (88).

A systematic review by Agdal et al. (90) of the use of energy healing in cancer patients in 2011 identifies a total of six quantitative and two qualitative studies in which practitioners explicitly intend to direct energy to the cancer patient for therapeutic purpose without the use of other technical devices, remedies, or massage. Studies utilizing prayer or ritual healing interventions are not included in this review, although there is acknowledged similarity between these modalities and energy healing.

Positive marginal to moderate effects of energy healing are found on pain, fatigue, well-being, and quality of life. There are mixed results concerning anxiety, physical indicators, and medication use for symptom management.

Methodological weaknesses such as lack of or inadequately described blinding process, modest sample size, self-selection, and sparse descriptions on the interaction between practitioner and patient limit the interpretation of many studies in energy healing. Lack of documented working mechanisms makes it a challenge to design sham treatments that do not activate the same working mechanism as the intervention. Thus far, the differences between intervention and sham treatments are small and patient expectation may be a large factor influencing outcome (91,92). It cannot be excluded that the so-called placebo effects may be an integral part of energy healing and other therapies. Psychosocial processes should be taken into account and explored, rather than dismissed. Additional validated spiritual healing outcome tools will hopefully improve the reliable measurement of efficacy in energy healing techniques (93).

MANIPULATIVE AND BODY-BASED THERAPIES

Exercise Therapy

The benefit of regular exercise has been well recognized in chronic illnesses such as coronary artery disease and chronic obstructive pulmonary disease. More recently, the American Cancer Society (ACS) recommends regular exercise to reduce the risk of colon, breast, renal, and other cancers (94). The field of exercise oncology began with the first studies exploring the effect of exercise training on fatigue and nausea associated with chemotherapy and radiation and loss of fitness found in breast cancer patients (95–97). Since then, the number of studies in this field has increased steadily, covering the spectrum of cancer survivorship—from cancer diagnosis through palliation (98).

The beneficial effects of regular exercise on cancer-specific and all-cause mortality in breast cancer was first demonstrated in a study by Holmes et al. in 2005 (99). Jones et al. demonstrate that peak oxygen consumption ($Vo_{2\,peak}$) is a strong independent predictor of long-term overall survival in non–small cell lung cancer (NSCLC) (100). In a single-arm intervention study, NSCLC patients undergoing lung resection engaged in pre-surgical daily exercise training at intensities varying from

	Source	Intervention	Design	No. of Participants	Setting	Outcomes	Results
Aromatase Inhibitor–Induced Arthralgia	Crew et al. (86)	Full body/auricular acupuncture and joint-specific point prescriptions vs. sham acupuncture of superficial needle insertion at nonacupoint locations	RCT[a]; blinded study	51	Women with breast cancer treated with aromatase inhibitors with joint symptoms	Difference in mean Brief Pain Inventory-Short Form worst pain scores at 6 wk	Lower pain score for intervention group compared with sham acupuncture (3.0 vs. 5.5; $P < 0.001$).
	Mao et al. (69)	Based on Chinese medicine diagnosis of "Bi" syndrome with electrostimulation of needles around the painful joint(s)	Single-arm feasibility trial	12	Postmenopausal women with stage I–III breast cancer who reported aromatase inhibitor-related arthralgia	Pain severity of the modified Brief Pain Inventory was used as the primary outcome	Patients reported reduction in pain severity (from 5.3 to 1.9), stiffness (from 6.9 to 2.4), and joint symptom interference (from 4.7 to 0.8), all $P < 0.001$
Metastatic and Advanced Cancer Pain	Dean-Clower et al. (70)	Manual acupuncture with a standardized acupuncture point protocol	Single-armed prospective pilot	40	Women with advanced ovarian or breast cancer at an outpatient academic oncology center (Karnofsky performance scale >60)	Symptom severity and quality of life questionnaires over 8 wk of treatment	There was improvement in anxiety ($P = 0.001$), fatigue ($P = 0.0002$), pain ($P = 0.0002$), and depression ($P = 0.003$) as well as general quality of life relief

TABLE 61.2 Clinical trials of acupuncture use in cancer-related symptoms

Pfister et al. (81)	Manual acupuncture once a week. Acupuncture needles were placed at both standard and customized anatomic points	RCT; acupuncture once a week for 4 wk vs. usual care	58	Patients at a tertiary cancer center with chronic pain or dysfunction attributed to neck dissection	The Constant-Murley score, a composite measure of pain, function, and activities of daily living, was the primary outcome measure. Xerostomia, a secondary end point, was assessed using the Xerostomia Inventory	Constant-Murley scores improved more in the acupuncture group (adjusted difference between groups = 11.2; 95% CI, 3.0 to 19.3; $P = 0.008$). No significant difference in medication use. Acupuncture produced greater improvement in reported xerostomia (adjusted difference in Xerostomia Inventory = −5.8; 95% CI, −0.9 to −10.7; $P = 0.02$)
Deng et al. (71)	Preoperative implantation of small intradermal needles that were retained for 4 wk	RCT; acupuncture vs. preoperative placement of sham needles at the same schedule	162	Patients with cancer undergoing thoracotomy	Comparison of Brief Pain Inventory pain intensity scores at the 30-d follow-up	A special acupuncture technique did not reduce pain or use of pain medication after thoracotomy more than a sham technique
Deng et al. (85)	Unilateral manual acupuncture stimulation at LI-2, a point commonly used in clinical practice to treat xerostomia	RCT; sham acupuncture controlled	20	Healthy volunteers	Cortical regions that were activated or deactivated during the interventions were evaluated by functional magnetic resonance imaging. Saliva production was also measured	Acupuncture at LI-2 was associated with neuronal activations absent during sham acupuncture stimulation. True acupuncture induced more saliva production than sham acupuncture

Post-surgical Cancer Pain

Xerostomia

(Continued)

TABLE 61.2 **Clinical trials of acupuncture use in cancer-related symptoms** (*Continued*)

Source	Intervention	Design	No. of Participants	Setting	Outcomes	Results
Wong et al. (72)	ALTENS[b] daily with radiotherapy for radiation-induced xerostomia	RCT	56	Head and neck cancer patients	Stimulated and basal unstimulated WSP[c] plus RIXVAS[d] were assessed at specific time points	There was no significant difference in mean WSP and RIXVAS between the two groups, so ALTENS is not recommended as a prophylactic intervention
Simock et al. (73)	Each received eight weekly sessions of acupuncture using four bilateral acupuncture points (Salivary Gland 2; Modified Point Zero; Shen Men and one point in the distal radial aspect of each index finger [LI1])	Single-armed study	12	Men with established radiation induced xerostomia	Sialometry and quality of life assessments were performed at baseline and at the end of treatment	There were objective increases in the amounts of saliva produced for 6/12 patients post intervention and the majority also reported subjective improvements. Mean quality of life scores for domains related to salivation and xerostomia also showed improvement
Mao et al. (74)	Manual acupuncture. Patients received up to 12 treatments of acupuncture over the entire course of their RT[e]	Cross-sectional survey study and a single-arm acupuncture clinical trial	16	Patients undergoing radiation therapy	The LFS[f] was administered at baseline, in the middle of RT, and at the end of RT, along with the PGIC[g]	Among the 16 trial participants, average fatigue and energy domains of the LFS remained stable during and after RT, without any expected statistical decline owing to RT. Based on the PGIC at the end of RT, 2 subjects (13%) reported their fatigue as worse, 8 (50%) as stable, and 6 (37%) as better

Cancer Cancer fatigue

Balk et al. (83)	Manual acupuncture once to twice per week during the 6-wk course of radiation therapy	RCT; Modified double blind	27	Cancer patients receiving external radiation therapy	Fatigue, fatigue distress, quality of life, and depression	Both true and sham acupuncture groups had improved fatigue, fatigue distress, quality of life, and depression from baseline to 10 wk, but the differences between the groups were not statistically significant
Molassiotis et al. (75)	Manual acupuncture vs. acupressure vs. sham acupressure group	RCT	47	Patients with cancer who experienced moderate to severe fatigue after chemotherapy	Patients completed the Multidimensional Fatigue Inventory before randomization, at the end of the 2-wk intervention and again about 2 wk after the end of the intervention	Significant improvements were found with regards to General fatigue ($P < 0.001$), Physical fatigue ($P = 0.016$), Activity ($P = 0.004$) and Motivation ($P = 0.024$). At the end of the intervention, there was a 36% improvement in fatigue levels in the acupuncture group, while the acupressure group improved by 19% and the sham acupressure by 0.6%
Chemotherapy-Induced Neuropathy	Wong et al. (76)	Manual acupuncture	Prospective case series	5	Patients with advanced gynecological cancers requiring chemotherapy with carboplatin and paclitaxel and developed severe paresthesia	Patient self-reported pain score (0–10), analgesic dosage	Average pain score was reduced to 3 out of 10 (range 1 to 5). All patients had a reduction in analgesic dosage

(Continued)

TABLE 61.2 **Clinical trials of acupuncture use in cancer-related symptoms** (*Continued*)

Source	Intervention	Design	No. of Participants	Setting	Outcomes	Results
Walker et al. (77)	12 wk of manual acupuncture or venlafaxine treatment (37.5 mg orally at night for 1 wk, then 75 mg at night for the remaining 11 wk)	RCT	50	Women with stage 0–III pre- or postmenopausal breast cancer patients on hormone therapy with tamoxifen or arimidex with ≥14 hot flashes per week; must be within 5 yr after treatment; Karnofsky performance status >70	The primary end point was hot-flash frequency via the Hot Flash diary; the MenQOL[h] Questionnaire; the SF-12[i] Survey; the BDI-PC[j]; and the National Cancer Institute Common Toxicity Criteria scale. Patients were observed for 1-yr posttreatment	Both groups exhibited significant decreases in hot flashes, depressive symptoms, and other quality of life symptoms, indicating that acupuncture was as effective as venlafaxine. The acupuncture group experienced no negative adverse effects
Ashamalla et al. (78)	Electroacupuncture twice a week for 4 wk	Single-arm prospective study	14	Men with hot flashes and history of androgen ablation therapy for prostate cancer	An HFS[k] was used to measure daily hot flashes. The composite daily score was calculated as the product of frequency × severity	The mean initial HFS was 28.3; it dropped to 10.3 (*P* = 0.0001) at 2 wk posttreatment, 7.5 (*P* = 0.0001) at 6 wk, and 7.0 (*P* = 0.001) at 8 mo
Beer et al. (79)	Acupuncture with electrostimulation biweekly for 4 wk, then weekly for 6 wk	Single-arm prospective study	22	Men who had a hot-flash score >4 who were receiving androgen deprivation therapy for prostate cancer	The primary end point was a 50% reduction in the hot-flash score after 4 wk of therapy, calculated from the patients' daily hot-flash diaries	Of the 22 patients, 41% had responded by week 4 and 55% had a >50% reduction in the hot-flash score at any point during the therapy course

Vasomotor Symptoms in Breast and Prostate Cancers

[a]RCT, randomized clinical trial.
[b]Acupuncture-like transcutaneous electrical nerve stimulation.
[c]Whole saliva production.
[d]RIX symptoms visual analogue score.
[e]Radiation treatment.
[f]Lee Fatigue Scale.
[g]Patient Global Impression of Change.
[h]Menopause Specific Quality of Life.
[i]Short Form 12-Item.
[j]Beck Depression Inventory-Primary Care.
[k]Hot-flash score.

60% to 100% of baseline peak oxygen consumption $Vo_{2\,peak}$. This training was associated with significant Vo_{2peak} increases of 2.4 mL/kg/min that did not decrease below baseline values following surgery (101). However, exercise training did not improve the quality of life from baseline (102).

Current studies provide promising evidence that structured exercise training during and after adjuvant cancer therapy is a well-tolerated adjunct therapy for mitigating common treatment-related side effects. Improvements in cancer-related fatigue, anxiety, cardiopulmonary fitness, and enhanced activities of daily living have been demonstrated with exercise training programs. The majority of studies utilize aerobic training alone, resistance training alone, or the combination of both in accordance with the traditional exercise prescription guidelines (3 to 5 d/wk at 50% to 75% of baseline Vo_{2peak} for 12 to 15 weeks) (103). Further studies clarifying the optimal frequency, intensity, type, and duration of exercise intervention, tailored for different types and/or stages of cancer, are needed (103–107).

Finally, a systematic review by Lowe et al. identifies six studies that evaluated the effect of exercise on quality of life, (108) fatigue, or physical function in patients with advanced cancer. While findings are generally positive, more rigorously designed studies are needed before exercise therapies should be routinely recommended as effective for this population.

The aforementioned exercise intervention mainly consists of aerobic, resistance training, or a combination of both. In recent years, alternative forms of exercise, such as Tai Chi Chuan and Qigong, had gained increasing popularity in the Western Hemisphere. Both forms of exercise originated from China, and while practiced extensively in their native country for hundreds of years, currently rigorous clinical trials are lacking for their effectiveness in cancer care (109).

Massage Therapy

Massage therapy focuses on manual manipulation of soft tissue of whole body areas using pressure and traction (110). It is one of the oldest forms of therapeutic interventions, and various cultures have developed their unique styles of massage. A US survey done in 2008 concluded that 11.2% of 4,139 cancer survivors used massage therapy for symptoms relief and/or relaxation (111).

Classical massage, described as manual treatment, using effleurage (long, light strokes), friction (small circular strokes), percussion (chopping motion), and petrissage (kneading action) has been demonstrated in several RCTs to alleviate pain, nausea, depression, anxiety, stress, and fatigue. However, the effect sizes in most trials are small to moderate, with a paucity of high-quality studies (110). Similarly, reflexology is another popular form of massage in which manual pressure is applied to the feet or hands, under the premise that internal organs can be stimulated by pressing particular areas of the extremity. Currently, there is no convincing evidence of efficacy for reflexology in cancer care, but studies are ongoing (112,113).

Chiropractic

Chiropractic comes from the Greek words *cheir* (hands) and *praktikos* (efficient) and is defined by the ACS as "a health care system that focuses on the relationship between the body's skeletal and muscular structure and its functions. Treatment often involves manipulating (moving) the bones of the spine to correct medical problems." In addition to chiropractic adjustments, techniques such as massage, stretching, electrical stimulation of the muscles, traction, heat, and ice can be employed (114). While studies suggest chiropractic is effective in some forms of acute lower back pain (115), there is no strong evidence for efficacy in chronic lower back pain. Currently, the nature of the chiropractic clinical encounter and its reported benefits remain to be fully investigated for cancer-related symptoms. A systematic review in 2011 found 60 case reports, 2 case series, 21 commentaries, 2 survey studies, and 2 literature reviews thus far for chiropractic care of patients with cancer (116). More research is encouraged in this field as chiropractic services remain well utilized among cancer patients (117).

BIOLOGICALLY BASED THERAPIES

Biologically based therapies, such as phytochemicals and vitamins, are consistently polled to be the most frequently utilized complementary and alternative therapy by cancer patients (4). For some cancer patients, using botanicals and vitamins may provide an increased sense of control and participation in their health care. For others, these supplements may be viewed as natural complementary therapies that help with cancer and therapy-related side effects. For still others, herbs and vitamins may represent an alternative to cancer treatment, especially if conventional therapies have failed (118). Despite the frequent use of phytochemicals and vitamins, many healthcare providers are not aware of the use of supplements by their patients (119). There is the common assumption that "natural" means safe, when many biologically based therapies may interact with cancer treatments (120). Furthermore, patients are commonly unaware that dietary supplements are not regulated by the Food and Drug Administration, and preparations of herbs and supplements may vary from manufacturer to manufacturer (121). It is therefore important for clinicians to encourage open discussions of complementary and alternative therapies that patients may be using.

Phytochemicals

Phytochemicals consist of bioactive compounds found in plants. It is estimated that approximately 50% of drugs used in the last few decades are either derived directly from plants or chemically similar to naturally occurring compounds (122). In the field of cancer treatment, there is currently an abundance of cancer research invested in finding other phytochemicals that may have anti-cancer properties like paclitaxel (derived from the Pacific yew). Table 61.3 lists some of

TABLE 61.3   Phytochemicals and their properties, in cancer-related studies, and safety considerations

Phytochemicals	Properties	Study findings	Safety Considerations	General Comment/Other
Ginger (*Zingiber officinale*)	The rhizome (underground stem) can be used fresh, dried, and powdered, or as a juice or oil	Mixed results for use of ginger for chemotherapy-induced nausea when compared with standard antiemetics though overall more effective than placebo (123)	May inhibit platelet function with increased risk of bleeding, gastrointestinal upset, bloating May have estrogenic modulating effect based on in vitro evidence (124)	Special consideration should be taken in estrogen receptor-positive patients and those at increased risk for bleeding
Gingko biloba	Extract from the leaves of the Gingko tree	Mostly in vitro and animal studies on the effects of gingko extract on ovarian and colon cancer cells	May inhibit platelet function Common side effects include headache and gastrointestinal discomfort	Insufficient data to recommend its use for cancer-related symptoms Avoid use with NSAID and anticoagulants.
Ginseng (*Panax* spp. and American)	The root is used to make medicine. It is a common ingredient in traditional Chinese medicine	Trials using American ginseng to treat cancer-related fatigue showed nonsignificant trends toward benefit (125)	Headache, insomnia, gastrointestinal toxicities, increased risk of bleeding American ginseng preparations that contain chemicals called ginsenosides might act like estrogen	Further clinical trials are needed for the use of ginseng in cancer patients and its effect on cancer treatment Caution when used with medications metabolized by cytochrome P450 2D6 and in estrogen receptor–positive patients
Green tea (*Camellia sinesis*)	A product made from the *Camellia sinensis* plant. Can be prepared as a beverage or an extract from the leaves	Decreased occurrence of prostate cancer treated with green tea extract vs. placebo with high-grade prostate intraepithelial neoplasia (126) Green tea ingestion associated with improved prognosis in stage I and II breast cancer among Japanese women (127)	Interfere with the action of boronic acid–based proteasome inhibitors	Additional human research is needed in the use of green tea in prevention and treatment of cancer Avoid use in combination with boronic acid–based chemotherapy agents

Milk thistle (*Silybum marianum*)	The above-ground parts and seeds of this plant are used	In vitro and animal model studies show that silibinin, the flavonoid found in the milk thistle, may have anti-tumorigenesis properties. For example, silibinin has been shown to inhibit mouse lung tumorigenesis (128), induce a loss of cell viability and apoptotic cell death in MCF-7 human breast cancer cells (129), and inhibit the growth of colorectal cancer (130)	Oral milk thistle has generally been well tolerated for up to 6 yr (131). Some side effects include mild gastrointestinal symptoms, urticaria, eczema, and headache. Case reports of anaphylactic reactions Inhibition of cytochrome P450 3A4 and 2C9	Preliminary studies are promising for silibinin's potential anti-cancer effects, but more studies are needed before it can be recommended as an anti-cancer treatment Extracts from milk thistle plant might have estrogen-like properties. Milk thistle seed extracts do not seem to act like estrogen
Mistletoe (*Viscum album*)	Mistletoe is a semiparasitic plant that grows on several species of trees native to Great Britain, Europe, and western Asia. The plant's leaves and twigs are used in herbal remedies; the berries are not used (132). Mistletoe injections are one of the most widely used unconventional cancer treatment in Europe (121)	While numerous studies have evaluated the effect of mistletoe in survival and quality of life and suggest positive effects among cancer patients, most were of poor methodological quality with publication bias. Further well-designed randomized controlled trials are needed (121,133).	Contraindicated in patients with protein hypersensitivity or chronic progressive infections Most common reactions are erythema and hyperemia (134)	The mistletoe plant should not be eaten because all parts of it are poisonous Patients generally tolerate the intervention well and may have quality of life benefit when used as an adjunct therapy in cancer treatment (135,136). Until more high-quality studies are available, cannot recommend its use as alternative cancer treatment
Turmeric (*Curcuma longa*)	Used as the main spice in curry. The root of the turmeric plant is used to make medicine Curcumin is the hydrophobic polyphenol derived from turmeric and is the active ingredient studied in cancer research	Multiple clinical trials are underway to evaluate the use of turmeric in treatment of cancer In vitro and in vivo research has shown various activities, such as anti-inflammatory, cytokines release, antioxidant, immunomodulatory, enhancing of the apoptotic process, and anti-angiogenic properties (137)	The most common side effect is epigastric burning, dyspepsia, nausea, and diarrhea (121) Phase I trial found limited toxicity with doses as high as 8 g daily (121). Can induce liver transaminase abnormalities (in rats) Increased bleeding risk with high doses of curcumin	Use in caution with hepatotoxic agents and those at increased risk of bleeding

NSAIDs, non-steroidal anti-inflammatory drugs.

the botanically based therapies currently under investigation for cancer treatment or as adjunctive therapy for symptom alleviation as described by Ulbricht and Chao (121).

Vitamins

Vitamins are organic compounds that organisms are required to ingest as nutrients as it cannot be synthesized in sufficient quantities by the organism and must be taken in through diet or the environment. Vitamins have a variety of functions, including hormone-like properties (vitamin D), regulation of cell and tissue growth and differentiation (vitamin A), and act as antioxidants (vitamins E and C) and enzyme co-factors (vitamin B complex) (138). The majority of data in the cancer literature regarding vitamins focuses on cancer prevention and investigates potential anti-cancer properties of vitamin supplements.

β-Carotene is a group of carotenoids that can be found in fruits, vegetables, and whole grains and provide vitamin A. Two large RCTs demonstrate no efficacy from β-carotene supplementation in the prevention of lung cancer (Alpha-Tocopherol and Beta-Carotene Cancer Prevention Trial [ATBC] and Beta-Carotene and Retinol Efficacy Trial); in fact, ATBC study demonstrates an increase in the incidence of lung cancer for those who received β-carotene. In people who smoke, β-carotene supplements might increase the risk of lung and prostate cancer (139). β-Carotene intake is currently recommended through food sources rather than nutritional supplements.

Vitamin B complex includes thiamine (B1), riboflavin (B2), niacin (B3), pantothenic acid (B5), pyridoxine (B6), biotin (B7), folic acid (B9), and cobalamin (B12). Folic acid is one of the more well-studied B vitamins. Through the years, there have been conflicting results on how folic acid may affect cancer risk. The Nurses' Health Study which followed nurses from 1980 to 1994 reports that the women receiving more than 400 μg of folic acid per day are much less likely to develop colon cancer than those with less than 200 μg intake (140). However, the large European Prospective Investigation into Cancer and Nutrition (EPIC) study in Europe published in 2010 reports no significant link between folic acid levels in the blood and colon or rectal cancer risk (141). A similarly mixed result is seen in breast cancer risk and folic acid intake (142). Until more is known, the ACS recommends eating a variety of healthful foods—with most of them coming from plant sources—rather than relying on supplements. As high doses of folic acid may interfere with the actions of methotrexate and other similar class of agents, the use of over-the-counter supplements and vitamins should routinely be investigated in the cancer patient.

Vitamin C is a water-soluble vitamin found in abundance in citrus fruits and in green leafy vegetables. Many studies demonstrate a connection between eating foods rich in vitamin C and a reduced risk of cancer. However, clinical trials of high doses of vitamin C as a treatment for cancer show no benefit (143,144). This suggests that the beneficial effects may be the combination of vitamin C and other phytochemicals found in food products, rather than vitamin C alone. Most oncologists recommend that people with cancer avoid large doses of vitamin C during treatment due to its potential antioxidant effects (145).

Observational epidemiologic studies suggest that higher levels of vitamin D in the body might be linked to lower cancer risk. In a study of more than 3,000 adults who had colonoscopies between 1994 and 1997, those with the highest vitamin D intake are less likely to have advanced cancer than those with low intake. In randomized control trials, the Women's Health Initiative study published in 2006 randomly divides 36,000 menopausal women into the intervention group of vitamin D with calcium and placebo (sham pill) group. After 7 years, the cancer risk is not significantly different between the two groups. Criticisms of this study cite the low dose of vitamin D given (400 IU/d) and the allowance of supplemental vitamin D and calcium possibly diluting the effect of intervention (146,147).

Lappe's randomized control trial (148), including calcium, calcium plus vitamin D3, and placebo arms, demonstrates a reduction in cancer risk conferred to women receiving supplemental calcium and vitamin D. However, it is difficult to tease out the effect of calcium from vitamin D in many of these studies, and more studies are needed to confirm this finding.

There are several pilot studies evaluating the use of vitamin D in prostate cancer treatment and its use in combination with chemotherapy agents (Taxotere). More studies are likely to follow, and further investigations are needed before conclusions can be made (149,150).

Vitamin E represents a group of fat-soluble substances that function as antioxidants in the body. The Woman Health Study published in 2005 showed that vitamin E has no effect on lung, breast, and colorectal cancers (151). The Selenium and Vitamin E Cancer Prevention Trial (SELECT) looks at the effect of vitamin E alone or in combination with selenium on prostate cancer risk, and the preliminary analysis in 2008 does not show a significant difference between the intervention groups and placebo. In fact, slight increase in the risk of prostate cancer and diabetes in the vitamin E and selenium groups is seen, respectively (152). It is unclear how the antioxidant effect of vitamin E interacts with radiation therapy and some chemotherapy agents—whether reducing or potentiating the treatments' effectiveness (153).

Finally, small clinical studies on the effect of menatetrenone, a vitamin K2 analog, on liver cancer development and recurrence show promising results. More research is needed to demonstrate the strength of this effect (154,155).

FUTURE DIRECTIONS

In this chapter, we reviewed the indications and evidence for mind–body interventions, energy therapies, manipulative and body-based methods, and biologically based therapies in integrative oncologic care. While integrative oncology is a relatively young field, preliminary results from some clinical trials and bench research are promising, and certain complementary interventions have shown to significantly affect a person's well-being during conventional cancer treatment and cancer survivorship.

The trend in oncologic care over the past decades has been toward a multidisciplinary as well as a multidimensional approach to patient care. There is a growing recognition of cancer patients' needs beyond conventional cancer treatment, and the importance of an interdisciplinary team that includes nurse, social worker, chaplain, physical therapist, occupational therapist, recreational therapist, and physician to address problems and concerns that arise through cancer diagnosis, management, remission, and end-of-life care. Similarly, the goal of integrative oncology is to assess the needs of the whole person and to utilize safe, effective, and well-tolerated complementary interventions to manage symptoms, be they physical, psychological, or spiritual.

Future research should focus on standardizing definition of various complementary therapies and performing studies with larger sample sizes and more stringent study designs. Ongoing research is also underway in the field of phytochemicals and vitamins, exploring their roles in cancer risk and cancer treatment. Finally, increasing awareness of complementary therapies throughout the professional and public communities will promote evidence-based recommendations, encourage open dialogue between patients and physicians regarding CAM use, and encourage critical appraisal of inadequately studied and regulated products and therapies. It is likely that the field of integrative oncology will continue to evolve and increasingly inform and influence the care of cancer patients.

USEFUL WEB SITES

Cancer Consultants: www.cancerconsultants.com

National Center for Complementary and Alternative Medicine: http://nccam.nih.gov/

NCI's Office of Cancer and Complementary and Alternative Medicine: http://www.cancer.gov/cam/cam_at_nci.html

University of Maryland Medical Center Medical Alternative Medicine Index: http://www.umm.edu/altmed/

Natural Standard Research Collaboration: www.naturalstandard.com

Dietary Supplements Labels Database: http://dietarysupplements.nlm.nih.gov/dietary/

Medline Plus: herbs and supplements: http://www.nlm.nih.gov/medlineplus/druginfo/herb_All.html

American Cancer Society: http://www.cancer.org/index

REFERENCES

1. National Center for Complementary and Alternative Medicine. [Online]. http://www.nccam.nih.gov/health/whatiscam/. Accessed September 20, 2011.
2. Verhoef MJ, Mulkins A, Carlson LE, Hilsden RJ, Kania A. Assessing the role of evidence in patients' evaluation of complementary therapies: a quality study. *Integr Cancer Ther.* 2007;6(4):345-353.
3. Barnes PM, Powell-Griner E, McFann K, Nahin RL. Complementary and alternative medicine use among adults: United States 2002. *Adv Data.* May 2004;27(343):1-19.
4. Vapiwala N, Mick R, Hampshire MK, Metz JM, DeNittis AS. Patient initiation of complementary and alternative medical therapies (CAM) following cancer diagnosis. *Cancer J.* 2006;12(6):467-474.
5. Geffen JR. Integrative oncology for the whole person: a multidimensional approach to cancer care. *Integr Cancer Ther.* 2010;9(1):105-121.
6. Yates JS, Mustian KM, Morrow GR, et al. Prevalence of CAM use in cancer patients during treatment. *Support Care Cancer.* 2005;13:806-811.
7. Mao JJ, Palmer CS, Healy KE, et al. Complementary and alternative medicine use among cancer survivors: a population-based study. *J Cancer Surviv Res Pract.* 2011;5(1):8-17.
8. Paltiel O, Avitzour M, Peretz T, et al. Determinants of the use of complementary therapies by patients with cancer. *J Clin Oncol.* 2001;19:2439-2448.
9. White MA, Verhoef MJ. Decision-making control: why men decline treatment for prostate cancer. *Integr Cancer Ther.* 2003;2:217-224.
10. Wesa KM, Cassileth BR. Introduction to section on integrative oncology. *Curr Treat Options Oncol.* 2010;11(3-4):70-72.
11. Humpel N, Jones SC. Gaining insight into the what, why, and where of CAM use by cancer pts and survivors. *Eur J Cancer Care.* 2006;15:362-268.
12. Singh H, Maskarinec G, Shumay DM. Understanding the motivation for conventional and complementary/alternative medicine use among men with prostate cancer. *Integr Cancer Ther.* 2005;4:187-194.
13. Elkins G, Fisher W, Johnson A. Mind-body therapies in integrative oncology. *Curr Treat Options Oncol.* 2010;11(3-4):128-140.
14. What is CAM?. [Online]. http://nccam.nih.gov/health/whatiscam/. Accessed September 15, 2011.
15. Kihlstrom JF. Hypnosis. *Annu Rev Psychol.* 1985;36:385-418.
16. Elkins G, Jensen MP, Patterson DR. Hypnotherapy for the management of chronic pain. *Int J Clin Exp Hypn.* 2007;(3):275-287.
17. NIH Technology Assessment Panel on Integration of Behavioral and Relaxation Approaches into the Treatment of Chronic Pain and Insomnia. Integration of behavioral and relaxation approaches into the treatment of chronic pain and insomnia. *JAMA.* 1996;276:313.
18. Patterson DR, Jensen MP. Hypnosis and clinical pain. *Psychol Bull.* 2003;129(4):495-521.
19. Liossi C, White P, Hatira P. Randomized clinical trial of local anesthetic versus a combination of local anesthetic with self-hypnosis in the management of pediatric procedure-related pain. *Health Psychol.* 2006;25(3):307-315.
20. Stoelb BL, Molton IR, Jensen MP, Patterson DR. The efficacy of hypnotic analgesia in adults: a review of the literature. *Contemp Hypn.* March 2009;26(1):24-39.
21. Neron S, Stephenson R. Effectiveness of hypnotherapy with cancer patients' trajectory: emesis, acute pain, and analgesia and anxiolysis in procedures. *Int J Clin Exp Hypn.* 2007;55(3):336-354.
22. Peynovska R, Fisher J, Oliver D, Mathew VM. Efficacy of hypnotherapy as a supplement therapy in cancer intervention. *Eur J Clin Hypn.* 2005;6(1):2-7.
23. Zeltzer LK, Dolgin MJ, LeBaron S, LeBaron C. A randomized controlled-study of behavioral intervention for chemotherapy distress in children with cancer. *Pediatrics.* 1991;88:34-42.
24. Jacknow DS, Tschann JM, Link MP, Boyce WT. Hypnosis in the prevention of chemotherapy-related nausea and

vomiting in children: a prospective study. *J Dev Behav Pediatr.* 1994;15:258-264.

25. Syrjala KL, Cummings C, Donaldson GW. Hypnosis or cognitive behavioral training for the reduction of pain and nausea during cancer treatment: a controlled clinical trial. *Pain.* 1992;48:137-146.

26. Elkins G, Marcus J, Stearns V, et al. Randomized trial of a hypnosis intervention for treatment of hot flashes among breast cancer survivors. *J Clin Oncol.* 2008;26:5022-5026.

27. Liossi C, Hatira P. Clinical hypnosis in the alleviation of procedure-related pain in pediatric oncology patients. *Int J Clin Exp Hypn.* 2003;51:4-28.

28. Lang EV, Benotsch EG, Fick LJ, et al. Adjunctive non-pharmacological analgesia for invasive medical procedures: a randomized trial. *Lancet.* April 2000;355(9214):1486-1490.

29. Spiegel D, Bloom JR, Kraemer HC, Gottheil E. Effect of psychosocial treatment on survival of patients with metastatic breast cancer. *The Lancet.* October 1989;2(8668):888-891.

30. Spiegel, D. Mind matters – Group therapy and survival in breast cancer. *N Engl J Med.* December 2001;345(24):1767-1768.

31. Jacobson E. *Progressive Relaxation.* Chicago, IL: University of Chicago Press; 1929.

32. Cannici J, Malcolm R, Peek LA. Treatment of insomnia in cancer patients using muscle relaxation training. *J Behav Ther Exp Psychiatry.* 1983;14:251-256.

33. Kwekkeboom KL, Cherwin CH, Lee JW, Wanta B. Mind-body treatments for the pain-fatigue-sleep disturbance symptom cluster in persons with cancer. *J Pain Symptom Manage.* 2010;39(1):126-138.

34. Carlson LE, Bultz BD. Mind-body interventions in oncology. *Curr Treat Options Oncol.* 2008;9(2-3):127-134.

35. Roffe L, Schmidt K, Ernst E. A systematic review of guided imagery as an adjuvant cancer therapy. *Psychooncology.* 2005;14(8):607-617.

36. Sloman R. Relaxation and imagery for anxiety and depression control in community patients with advanced cancer. *Cancer Nurs.* 2002;25:432-435.

37. Feldman CS, Salzberg HC. The role of imagery in the hypnotic treatment of adverse reactions to cancer therapy. *J S C Med Assoc.* 1990;86:303-306.

38. Troesch LM, Rodehaver CB, Delaney EA, Yanes B. The influence of guided imagery on chemotherapy-related nausea and vomiting. *Oncol Nurs Forum.* 1993;20:1179-1185.

39. Jon Kabat-Zinn. *Full catastrophe living: using the wisdom of your body and mind to face stress, pain, and illness.* Delta Trade Paperbacks, 1991. ISBN 0-385-3012-2.

40. Ott MJ, Norris RL, Bauer-Wu SM. Mindfulness meditation for oncology patients: a discussion and critical review. *Integr Cancer Ther.* June 2006;5(2):98-108.

41. Brown KW, Ryan RM. The benefits of being present: mindfulness and its role in psychological well-being. *J Pers Soc Psychol.* April 2003;84(4):822-848.

42. Carlson LE, Speca M, Patel KD, Goodey E. Mindfulness-based stress reduction in relation to quality of life, mood, symptoms of stress, and immune parameters in breast and prostate cancer outpatients. *Psychosom Med.* 2003;65(4):571-581.

43. Shapiro SL, Bootzin RR, Figueredo AJ, Lopez AM, Schwartz GE. The efficacy of mindfulness-based stress reduction in the treatment of sleep disturbance in women with breast cancer: an exploratory study. *J Psychosom Res.* January 2003;54(1):85-91.

44. Tacón AM, Caldera YM, Ronaghan C. Mindfulness-based stress reduction in women with breast cancer. *Fam Syst Health.* 2004;22(2):193-203.

45. Carlson LE, Speca M, Patel KD, Goodey E. Mindfulness-based stress reduction in relation to quality of life, mood, symptoms of stress and levels of cortisol, dehydroepiandrosterone-sulfate (DHEAS) and melatonin in breast and prostate cancer outpatients. *Psychoneuroendocrinology.* 2004;29:448-474.

46. DiStasio SA. Integrating yoga into cancer care. *Clin J Oncol Nurs.* 2008;12(1):125-130.

47. Moadel AB, Shah C, Wylie-Rosett J, et al. Randomized controlled trial of yoga among multiethical sample of breast cancer patients: effects on quality of life. *J Clin Oncol.* 2007;25:4387-4395.

48. Blank S, Kittel J, Haberman MR. Active practice of Iyengar Yoga as an intervention for breast cancer survivors. *Int J Yoga Ther.* 2005;15:51-59.

49. Duncan MD, Leis A, Taylor-Brown JW. Impact and outcomes of an Iyengar Yoga program in a cancer centre. *Curr Oncol.* 2008;15:51-59.

50. Speed-Andrews AE, Stevinson C, Belanger LJ, Mirus JJ, Courneya KS. Pilot evaluation of an Iyengar Yoga program for breast cancer survivors. *Cancer Nurs.* 2010;33:369-381.

51. Danhauer SC, Tooze JA, Farmer DF, et al. Restorative yoga for women with ovarian or breast cancer: findings from a pilot study. *J Soc Integr Oncol.* 2008;6:47-58.

52. Danhauer SC, Mihalko SL, Russell GB, et al. Restorative yoga for women with breast cancer: findings from a randomized pilot study. *Psycho-Oncology.* 2009;18:360-368.

53. Cohen B, Kanaya AM, Macer JL, Shen H, Chang AA, Grady D. Feasibility and acceptability of restorative yoga for treatment of hot flushes: a pilot trial. *Maturitas.* 2007;56:198-204.

54. Carson JW, Carson KM, Porter LS, Keefe FJ, Seewaldt VL. Yoga of awareness program for menopausal symptoms in breast cancer survivors: results from a randomized trial. *Support Care Cancer.* October 2009;17(10):1301-1309.

55. Mustain KM, Palesh O, Sprod L, et al. Effect of YOCAS yoga on sleep, fatigue, and quality of life: a URCC CCOP randomized, controlled clinical trial among 410 cancer survivors. *J Clin Oncol.* 2010;28:15s.

56. Hede K. Supportive care: large studies ease yoga, exercise into mainstream oncology. *J Natl Cancer Inst.* 2011;103(1):11-12.

57. Applied psychophysiology and biofeedback. [Online]. http://www.aapb.org/. Accessed September 17, 2011.

58. Tsai PS, Chen PL, Lai YL, Lee MB, Lin CC. Effects of electromyography biofeedback-assisted relaxation on pain in patients with advanced cancer in palliative care unit. *Cancer Nurs.* September-October 2007;30(5):347-353.

59. George R, Chung TD, Vedamm SS, et al. Audio-visual biofeedback for respiratory-gated radiotherapy: impact of audio instruction and audio-visual biofeedback on respiratory-gated radiotherapy. *Int J Radiat Oncol Biol Phys.* July 2006;65(3):924-933.

60. Stam MR, van Lin EN, van der Vight LP, Kaanders JH, Visser AG. Bladder filling variation during radiation treatment of prostate cancer: can the use of a bladder ultrasound scanner and biofeedback optimize bladder filling? *Int J Radiat Oncol Biol Phys.* June 2006;65(2):371-377.

61. Cohen M. A model of group cognitive behavioral intervention combined with bio-feedback in oncology settings. *Soc Work Health Care.* 2010;49(2):149-164.

62. Olofsson A, Fossum B. Perspectives on music therapy in adult cancer care: a hermeneutic study. *Oncol Nurs Forum.* July 2009; 36(4):E223-E231.

63. Gallagher LM. The role of music therapy in palliative medicine and supportive care. *Semin Oncol.* June 2011;38(3):403-406.

64. Bradt J, Dileo C, Grocke D, Magill L. Music interventions for improving psychological and physical outcomes in cancer patients. *Cochrane Database Syst Rev.* August 2011;1(8):CD006911.

65. Geue K, Goetze H, Buttstaedt M, Kleinert E, Richter D, Singer S. An overview of art therapy interventions for cancer patients and the results of research. *Complement Ther Med.* June–August 2010;18(3-4):160-170.

66. National Center for Complementary and Alternative Medicine. What is complementary and alternative medicine? [Online] July 2011. http://www.nccam.nih.gov/health/whatiscam/#mindbody. Accessed September 17, 2011

67. World Health Organization. Acupuncture: Review and Analysis of Reports on Controlled Clinical Trials. [Online] http://apps.who.int/medicinedocs/en/d/Js4926e/5.html. Accessed July 18, 2012.

68. Capodice JL. Acupuncture in the oncology setting: clinical trial update. *Curr Treat Options Oncol.* December 2010;11(3-4):87-94.

69. Mao JJ, Bruner DW, Stricker C, et al. Feasibility trial of electroacupuncture for aromatase inhibitor-related arthralgia in breast cancer survivors. *Integr Cancer Ther.* 2009;8(2):123-129.

70. Dean-Clower E, Doherty-Gilman AM, Keshaviah A, et al. Acupuncture as palliative therapy for physical symptoms and quality of life for advanced cancer patients. *Integr Cancer Ther.* 2010;9(2):158-167.

71. Deng G, Rusch V, Vickers A, et al. Randomized controlled trial of a special acupuncture technique for pain after thoracotomy. *J Thorac Cardiovasc Surg.* 2008;136(6):1464-1469.

72. Wong RK, Sagar SM, Chen BJ, Yi GY, Cook R. Phase II randomized trial of acupuncture-like transcutaneous electrical nerve stimulation to prevent radiation-induced xerostomia in head and neck cancer patients. *J Soc Integr Oncol.* 2010;8(2):35-42.

73. Simcock R, Fallowfield L, Jenkins V. Group acupuncture to relieve radiation induced xerostomia: a feasibility study. *Acupunct Med.* 2009;27(3):109-113.

74. Mao JJ, Styles T, Cheville A, Wolf J, Fernandes S, Farrar JT. Acupuncture for nonpalliative radiation therapy-related fatigue: feasibility study. *J Soc Integr Oncol.* 2009;7(2):52-58.

75. Molassiotis A, Svlt P, Diggins H. The management of cancer-related fatigue after chemotherapy with acupuncture and acupressure: a randomised controlled trial. *Complement Ther Med.* December 2007;15(4):228-237.

76. Wong R, Sagar S. Acupuncture treatment for chemotherapy-induced peripheral neuropathy – a case series. *Acupunct Med.* 2006;24(2):87-91.

77. Walker EM, Rodriguez AI, Kohn B, et al. Acupuncture versus venlafaxine for the management of vasomotor symptoms in patients with hormone receptor-positive breast cancer: a randomized controlled trial. *J Clin Oncol.* February 2010;28(4):634-640.

78. Ashamalla H, Jiang ML, Guiguis A, Peluso F, Ashamalla M. Acupuncture for the alleviation of hot flashes in men treated with androgen ablation therapy. *Int J Radiat Oncol Biol Phys.* April 2011;79(5):1358-1363.

79. Beer TM, Benavides M, Emmons SL, et al. Acupuncture for hot flashes in patients with prostate cancer. *Urology.* November 2010;76(5):1182-1188.

80. Stone JA, Johnstone PA. Mechanisms of action for acupuncture in the oncology. *Curr Treat Options Oncol.* December 2010;11(3-4):118-127.

81. Pfister DG, Cassileth BR, Deng GE, et al. Acupuncture for pain and dysfunction after head and neck dissection: results of a randomized controlled trial. *J Clin Oncol.* 2010;28(15):2565-2570.

82. Molassiotis A, Sylt P, Diggins H. The management of cancer-related fatigue after chemotherapy with acupuncture and acupressure: a randomized controlled trial. *Complement Ther Med.* 2007;15(4):228-237.

83. Balk J, Day R, Rosenzweig M, Beriwal S. Pilot, randomized, modified, double-blind, placebo-controlled trial of acupuncture for cancer-related fatigue. *J Soc Integr Oncol.* 2009;7(1):4-11.

84. Shen J, Wenger N, Glaspy J, et al. Electroacupuncture for control of myeloablative chemotherapy-induced emesis: a randomized controlled trial. *JAMA.* 2000;284(21):2755-2761.

85. Deng G, Hou BL, Holodny AI, Cassileth BR. Functional magnetic resonance imaging (fMRI) changes and saliva production associated with acupuncture at L1–2 acupuncture point: a randomized controlled study. *BMC Complement Altern Med.* 2008;8:37.

86. Crew KD, Capodice JL, Greenlee H, et al. Randomized, blinded, sham-controlled trial of acupuncture for the management of aromatase inhibitor-associated joint symptoms in women with early-stage breast cancer. *J Clin Oncol.* 2010;28(7):1154-1160.

87. Lu MB, Rosenthal DS. Recent advances in oncology acupuncture and safety considerations in practice. *Curr Treat Options Oncol.* 2010;11:141-146.

88. Baldwin AL, Vitale A, Brownell E, Scicinski J, Kearns M, Rand W. The touchstone process: an ongoing critical evaluation of Reiki in the scientific literature. *Holist Nurs Pract.* September–October 2010;24(5):260-276.

89. Barnes PM, Bloom B, Nahin R. CDC National Health Statistics Report #12. *Complementary and Alternative Medicine Use among Adults and Children.* United States, 2007. Hyattville, MD: National Center for Health Statistics; December 2008.

90. Agdal R, von B Hjelmborg J, Johannessen H. Energy healing for cancer: a critical review. *Forsch Komplementmed.* 2011;18(3)146-154.

91. Pohl G, Seemann H, Zojer N, et al. "Laying on of hands" improves well-being in patients with advanced cancer. *Support Care Cancer.* 2007;15:143-151.

92. Schouten S. Psychic healing and complementary medicine. *Eur J Parapsychol.* 1992-1993;9:35-91.

93. Bishop FL, Barlow F, Walker J, McDermott C, Lewith GT. The development and validation of an outcome measure for spiritual healing: a mixed methods study. *Psychother Psychosom.* 2010;79(6):350-362.

94. Byers T, Nestle M, McTiernan A, et al. American Cancer Society guidelines on nutrition and physical activity for cancer prevention: reducing the risk of cancer with healthy food choices and physical activity. *CA Cancer J Clin.* March–April 2002;52:92-119.

95. Brown JK, Byers T, Doyle C, et al. Nutrition and physical activity during and after cancer treatment: an American Cancer Society guide for informed choices. *CA Cancer J Clin.* 2003;53:268-291.

96. Winningham ML, MacVicar MG. The effect of aerobic exercise on patient reports of nausea. *Oncol Nurs Forum.* 1988;15:447-450.

97. Gianni L, Dombernowsky P, Sledge G, et al. Cardiac function following combination therapy with paclitaxel and doxorubicin: an analysis of 657 women with advanced breast cancer. *Ann Oncol.* 2001;12:1067-1073.

98. Jones LW, Peppercorn J, Scott JM, Battaglini C. Erratum to: exercise therapy in the management of solid tumors. *Curr Treat Options Oncol.* 2010;11:73-86.

99. Holmes MD, Chen WY, Feskanich D, Kroenke CH, Colditz GA. Physical activity and survival after breast cancer diagnosis. *JAMA.* May 2005;293(20):2479-2486.

100. Jones LW, Watson D, Herndon JE. Peak oxygen consumption and long-term all-cause mortality in non-small cell lung cancer. *Cancer.* October 2010;116(20):4825-4832.

101. Jones LW, Peddle CJ, Eves ND, et al. Effects of presurgical exercise training on cardiorespiratory fitness among patients undergoing thoracic surgery for malignant lung lesions. *Cancer.* 2007;110:590-598.

102. Peddle CJ, Jones LW, Eves ND, et al. Effects of presurgical exercise training on quality of life in patients undergoing lung resection for suspected malignancy: a pilot study. *Cancer Nurs.* March–April 2009;32(2):158-165.

103. Speck RM, Courneya KS, Masse LC, Duval S, Schmitz KH. An update of controlled physical activity trials in cancer survivors: a systematic review and meta-analysis. *J Cancer Surviv.* 2010;4:87-100.

104. Segal R, Evans W, Johnson D, et al. Structured exercise improves physical functioning in women with stages I and II breast cancer: results of a randomized controlled trial. *J Clin Oncol.* 2001;19:657-665.

105. Courneya KS, Segal RJ, Mackey JR, et al. Effects of aerobic and resistance exercise in breast cancer patients receiving adjuvant chemotherapy: a multicenter randomized controlled trial. *J Clin Oncol.* 2007;25:4396-4404.

106. Markes M, Brockow T, Resch KL. Exercise for women receiving adjuvant therapy for breast cancer. *Cochrane Database Syst Rev.* 2006;CD005001.

107. Cramp F, Daniel J. Exercise for the management of cancer-related fatigue in adults. *Cochrane Database Syst Rev.* April 2008;2:CD006145.

108. Lowe SS, Watanabe SM, Courneya KS. Physical activity as a supportivecare intervention in palliative cancer patients: a systematic review. *J Support Oncol.* 2009; 7(1):27-34

109. Lee MS, Choi TY, Ernst E. Tai chi for breast cancer patients: a systematic review. *Breast Cancer Res Treat.* 2010;120:309-316.

110. Ernst E. Massage therapy for cancer palliation and supportive care: a systematic review of randomised clinical trials. *Support Care Cancer.* April 2009;17(4):333-337.

111. Gansler T, Kaw C, Crammer C, Smith T. A population based study of prevalence of complementary methods use by cancer survivors: a report from the American Cancer Society's studies of cancer survivors. *Cancer.* 2008;113(5):1048-1057.

112. Kim JI, Lee MS, Kang JW, Choi do Y, Ernst E. Reflexology for the symptomatic treatment of breast cancer: a systematic review. *Integr Cancer Ther.* 2010;Dec;9(4):326-330.

113. Ernst E, Posadzki P, Lee MS. Reflexology: an update of a systematic review of randomized clinical trials. *Maturitas.* 2011;68:116-120.

114. Chiropractic. American Cancer Society. [Online]. http://www.cancer.org/Treatment/TreatmentsandSideEffects/ComplementaryandAlternativeMedicine/ManualHealingandPhysicalTouch/chiropractic. Accessed September 17, 2011.

115. Lawrence DJ, Meeker W, Branson R, Bronfort G. Chiropractic management of low back pain and low back-related leg complaints: a literature synthesis. *J Manipulative Physiol Ther.* November–December 2008;31(9):659-674.

116. Alcantara J, Alcantara JD, Alcantara J. The chiropractic care of patients with cancer: a systematic review of the literature. *Integr Cancer Ther.* 2011; e-pub ahead of print June 10,2011.

117. Evans RC, Rosner AL. Alternatives in cancer pain treatment: the application of chiropractic care. *Semin Oncol Nurs.* August 2005;21(3):184-189.

118. Chang KH, Brodie R. Complementary and alternative medicine use in oncology: a questionnaire survey of patients and health care professionals. *BMC Cancer.* 2011;11:196.

119. Frenkel M, Ben Arye E, Baldwin CD, Sierpina V. Approach to communicating with patients about the use of nutritional supplements in cancer care. *South Med J.* 2005;98:289-294.

120. Ulbricht C, Chao W, Costa D, Rusie-Seamon E, Weissner W, Woods J. Clinical evidence of herb-drug interactions: a systematic review by the Natural Standard Research Collaboration. *Curr Drug Metab.* 2008;9:1063-1120.

121. Ulbricht CE, Chao W. Phytochemicals in the oncology setting. *Curr Treat Options Oncol.* 2010;11:95-106.

122. Amin A, Gali-Muhtasib H, Ocker M, Schneider-Stock R. Overview of major classes of plant-derived anticancer drugs. *Int J Biomed Sci.* 2009;5:1-11.

123. Ernst E, Pittler MH. Efficacy of ginger for nausea and vomiting: a systematic review of randomized clinical trials. *Br J Anaesth.* 2000;84:367-371.

124. Kang SC, Lee CM, Choi H, et al. Evaluation of oriental medicinal herbs for estrogenic and antiproliferative activities. *Phytother Res.* 2006;20:1017-1019.

125. Barton DL, Soori GS, Bauer BA, et al. Pilot study of Panax quinquefolius (American ginseng) to improve cancer-related fatigue: a randomized, double-blind, dose-finding evaluation: NCCTG trial N03CA. *Support Care Cancer.* 2010;18:179-187

126. McLarty J, Bigelow RL, Smith M, Elmajian D, Ankem M, Cardelli JA. Tea polyphenols decrease serum levels of prostate-specific antigen, hepatocyte growth factor, and vascular endothelial growth factor in prostate cancer patients and inhibit production of hepatocyte growth factor and vascular endothelial growth factor in vitro. *Cancer Prev Res (Phila).* 2009;2:673-682.

127. Nakachi K, Suemasu K, Suga K, Takeo T, Imai K, Higashi Y. Influence of drinking green tea on breast cancer malignancy among Japanese patients. *Jpn J Cancer Res.* 1998;89:254-261.

128. Tyagi A, Agarwal C, Dwyer-Nield LD, Singh RP, Malkinson AM, Agarwal R. Silibinin modulates TNF-α and INF-γ mediated signaling in tumorigenic mouse lung epithelial LM2 cells. *Mol Carcinog.* 2011; e-pub ahead of print August 31, 2011.

129. Noh EM, Yi MS, Youn HJ, et al. Silibinin enhances ultraviolet B-induced apoptosis in mcf-7 human breast cancer cells. *J Breast Cancer.* March 2011;14(1):8-13.

130. Kauntz H, Bousserouel S, Gossé F, Raul F. Silibinin triggers apoptotic signaling pathways and autophagic survival response in human colon adenocarcinoma cells and their derived metastatic cells. *Apoptosis.* 2011; e-pub ahead of print July 16, 2011; 16:1042-1053.

131. Cheung CW, Gibbons N, Johnson DW, Nicol DL. Silibinin—a promising new treatment for cancer. *Anticancer Agents Med Chem.* 2010;10:186-195.

132. American Cancer Society. Complementary and alternative medicine. [Online]. http://www.cancer.org/Treatment/TreatmentsandSideEffects/ComplementaryandAlternativeMedicine/HerbsVitaminsandMinerals/mistletoe. Accessed September 17, 2011.

133. Büssing A, Raak C, Ostermann T. Quality of life and related dimensions in cancer patients treated with mistletoe extract (iscador): a meta-analysis. *Evid Based Complement Alternat Med.* 2010;2012:219402; e-pub ahead of print June 14, 2011.

134. Kleijnen J, Knipschild P. Mistletoe treatment for cancer: review of controlled trials in humans. *Phytomedicine.* 1994;1:255.

135. Eisenbraun J, Scheer R, KrÖz M, Schad F, Huber R. Quality of life in breast cancer patients during chemotherapy and concurrent therapy with a mistletoe extract. *Phytomedicine.* January 2011;18(2-3):151-157.

136. Brandeberger M, Simões-Wüst AP, Rostock M, Rist L, Saller R. An exploratory study on the quality of life and individual coping of cancer patients during mistoletoe therapy. *Integr Cancer Ther.* 2012;11(2):90-100.

137. Bar-Sela G, Epelbaum R, Schaffer M. Curcumin as an anticancer agent: review of the gap between basic and clinical applications. *Curr Med Chem.* 2010;17(3):190-197.

138. Wikipedia. Vitamin. [Online]. http://en.wikipedia.org/wiki/Vitamin. Accessed July 18, 2012.

139. Lawson KA, Wright ME, Subar A, et al. Multivitamin use and risk of prostate cancer in the National Institutes of Health-AARP Diet and Health Study. *J Natl Cancer Inst.* 2007;99:754-764.

140. Giovannucci E, Stampfer MJ, Colditz GA, et al. Multivitamin use, folate, and colon cancer in women in the nurses' health study. *Ann Intern Med.* 1998;129:517-524.

141. Eussen SJ, Vollset SE, Igland J, et al. Plasma folate, related genetic variants, and colorectal cancer risk in EPIC. *Cancer Epidemiol Biomarkers Prev.* May 2010;19(5):1328-1340.

142. Feigelson HS, Jonas CR, Robertson AS, McCullough ML, Thun MJ, Calle EE. Alcohol, folate, methionine, and risk of incident breast cancer in the American Cancer Society Cancer Prevention Study II Nutrition Cohort. *Cancer Epidemiol Biomarkers Prev.* February 2003;12(2):161-164.

143. Moertel CG, Fleming TR, Creagan ET, Rubin J, O'Connell MJ, Ames MM. High-dose vitamin C versus placebo in the treatment of patients with advanced cancer who have had no prior chemotherapy. A randomized double-blind comparison. *N Engl J Med.* January 1985;312(3):137-141.

144. Bjelakovic G, Nikolova D, Gluud LL, Simonetti RG, Gluud C. Mortality in randomized trials of antioxidant supplements for primary and secondary prevention: systematic review and meta-analysis. *JAMA.* 2007;297:842-857.

145. Labriola D, Livingston R. Possible interactions between dietary antioxidants and chemotherapy. *Oncology.* 1990;13:1003-1008.

146. Jackson RD, LaCroix AZ, Gass M, et al. Women's health initiative investigators. Calcium plus vitamin D supplementation and the risk of fractures . *N Engl J Med.* 2006; 354:669-683.

147. LaCroix AZ, Kotchen J, Anderson G, et al. Calcium plus vitamin D supplementation and mortality in postmenopausal women: the women's health initiative calcium-vitamin D randomized controlled trial. *J Gerontol A Biol Sci Med Sci.* May 2009;64(5):559-567.

148. Lappe JM, Travers-Gustafson D, Davies KM, Recker RR, Heaney RP. Vitamin D and calcium supplementation reduces cancer risk: results of a randomized trial. *Am J Clin Nutr.* 2007;85:1586-1591.

149. Attia S, Eickhoff J, Wilding G, et al. Randomized, double-blinded phase II evaluation of docetaxel with or without doxercalciferol in patients with metastatic, androgen-independent prostate cancer. *Clin Cancer Res.* 2008; 14:2437-2443.

150. Beer TM, Lemmon D, Lowe BA, Henner WD. High-dose weekly oral calcitriol in patients with a rising PSA after prostatectomy or radiation for prostate carcinoma. *Cancer.* 2003; 97:1217-1224.

151. American Cancer Society. Complementary and alternative medicine. [Online]. http://www.cancer.org/Treatment/TreatmentsandSideEffects/ComplementaryandAlternative Medicine/HerbsVitaminsandMinerals/vitamin-e. Accessed September 17, 2011.

152. National Cancer Institute. The SELECT prostate cancer prevention trial. [Online]http://www.cancer.gov/clinicaltrials/noteworthy-trials/select/Page1. Accessed July 18, 2012.

153. Lawenda BD, Kelly KM, Ladas EJ, Sagar SM, Vickers A, Blumberg JB. Should supplemental antioxidant administration be avoided during chemotherapy and radiation therapy? *J Natl Cancer Inst.* 2008;100:773-783.

154. Mizuta T, Ozaki I, Eguchi Y, et al. The effect of menatetrenone, a vitamin K2 analog, on disease recurrence and survival in patients with hepatocellular carcinoma after curative treatment: a pilot study. *Cancer.* 2006;106:867-872.

155. Habu D, Shiomi S, Tamori A, et al. Role of vitamin K2 in the development of hepatocellular carcinoma in women with viral cirrhosis of the liver. *JAMA.* 2004;292:358-361.

Special Populations

CHAPTER 62 Geriatric Palliative Care

Jessica Israel ■ R. Sean Morrison

In our society, the overwhelming majority of people living with serious illness are elderly. They spend years living with chronic diseases accompanied by multiple coexisting conditions, progressive dependency on others, and heavy care needs met mostly by family members. Abundant evidence suggests that the quality of life in the setting of serious illness is often poor, characterized by inadequately treated physical distress, fragmented care systems, poor to absent communication between doctors and patients and families, and enormous strains on family caregiver and support systems. In this chapter, we focus on the palliative care needs of older adults.

BIOLOGY OF AGING

Body Composition

Aging is a process that converts healthy adults into frail ones with diminished reserves in most physiologic systems and with an exponentially increasing vulnerability to most diseases and death (1). Aging is the most significant and common risk factor for disease in general. The process itself is a mystery, still poorly understood even in this age of advanced biotechnologic capability. Normal aging appears to be a fairly benign process. The body's organ system reserves and homeostatic control mechanisms steadily decline. Commonly, this slow erosion only becomes obvious in times of maximum body stress or serious illness. However, as the process continues, it takes less and less insult for the underlying physiologic weakness to become apparent. It is difficult to differentiate the effects of aging alone from those of concurrent disease or environmental factors. Eventually, a critical point is reached, when the body's systems are overwhelmed, and death ultimately results. Morbidity is often compressed into the last period of life (2).

Substantial changes occur in body composition with aging. These changes become important when related to nutritional needs, pharmacokinetics, and metabolic activity. As adults age, the proportion of bodily lipid doubles and lean body mass decreases. Bones and viscera shrink and the basal metabolic rate declines. Although specific age–associated changes occur in each organ system, changes in body composition and metabolism are highly variable from individual to individual.

Renal Function

The aging kidney loses functioning nephrons. Cross-sectional and longitudinal studies have also demonstrated a decline in creatinine clearance. There is also evidence to show decreased renal plasma flow, decreased tubular secretion and reabsorption, decreased hydrogen secretion, and decreased water absorption and excretion (3). When kidney disease complicates this aging process, the outcome can be highly deleterious.

Underlying renal function is an important issue in geriatric pharmacology. Many medications rely on the kidneys' mechanisms for excretion and their metabolites may accumulate and lead to side effects or toxic injury in an impaired system. Commonly used medications are more likely to damage older kidneys, including nonsteroidal anti-inflammatory drugs (NSAIDs) and intravenous contrast dye (4).

Gastrointestinal and Hepatic Function

The gastrointestinal tract changes less with aging than other body systems, but there are still some deficiencies that may affect medication delivery and breakdown, as well as nutritional status and metabolism. The esophagus may show delayed transit time. The stomach may atrophy and produce less acid. Colonic transit is greatly slowed, whereas small intestinal transit appears unaffected. Pancreatic function is usually well maintained, although trypsin secretion may be decreased.

The liver usually retains adequate function, although there are variable changes seen in its metabolic pathways. The cytochrome P450 system may decline in efficiency and liver enzymes may be less inducible. The most significant change is the sharp decline in demethylization, the process that metabolizes medications such as benzodiazepines in the liver. This change may necessitate dosage adjustments. In addition, drugs that undergo hepatic first–pass metabolism by extraction from the blood may have altered clearance with increasing age because of decreased hepatic blood flow.

Brain and Central Nervous System Changes

The brain and central nervous system slowly atrophy with age. Neurons stop proliferating and are not replaced when they die, resulting in neuronal loss as well as loss of dendritic arborization. There are also some degree of neurotransmitter and receptor loss. The extent of this loss is not well understood.

Age-related changes in pain perception may exist, but their clinical importance is uncertain. Although degenerative changes occur in areas of the central and autonomic nervous system that mediate pain, the relevance of these changes has yet to be determined (5). Clinical observations from elderly patients who report minimal pain and discomfort despite the presence of cardiac ischemia or intraabdominal catastrophe suggest that pain perception may be altered in the elderly. However, experimental data suggest that significant, age-related changes in pain perception probably do not occur (6). Until further studies conclusively demonstrate that the perception of pain decreases with age, stereotyping of most elderly patients as experiencing less pain may lead to inaccurate clinical assessments and needless suffering (5).

DEMOGRAPHY OF SERIOUS ILLNESS IN THE UNITED STATES

The median age at death in the United States is now 78 years and has been associated with a steady and linear decline in age-adjusted death rates since 1940. In 1900, life expectancy at birth was <50 years; a girl born today may expect to live to age 81 and a boy to age 76. Those reaching 65 years can expect to live another 18 years on average and those reaching age 80 can expect to live an additional 8 years. These unprecedented increases in life expectancy (equivalent to that occurring between the Stone Age and 1900) are due primarily to decreases in maternal and infant mortality, resulting from improved sanitation, nutrition, and effective control of infectious diseases. As a result, there has been an enormous growth in the number and health of the elderly. By the year 2030, 20% of the United States' population will be over age 65, as compared with <5% at the turn of the 20th century (7).

Although death at the turn of the 20th century was largely attributable to acute infectious diseases or accidents, the leading causes of death today are chronic illness such as heart disease, cancer, stroke, and dementia. With advances in the treatment of atherosclerotic vascular disease and cancer, many patients with these diseases now survive for years. Many diseases that were rapidly fatal in the past have now become chronic illnesses.

In parallel, deaths that occurred at home in the early part of the 20th century now occur primarily in institutions—68% of all deaths occur in hospitals or nursing homes (8). The reasons for this shift in location of death are complex, but appear to be related to health system and reimbursement structures that promote hospital-based care and provide relatively little support for home care and custodial care services despite the significant care burdens and functional dependency that accompany life-threatening chronic disease in the elderly. The older the patient, the higher the likelihood of death in a nursing home or hospital, with an estimated 76% of persons over 85 years experiencing an institutional death and a similar number spending at least some time in an institution in the year prior to death (8). These statistics, however, hide the fact that most of an older person's last months and years are still spent at home in the care of family members, with hospitalization and/or nursing home placement occurring only near the very end of life. National statistics also obscure the variability in the experience of living with serious illness. For example, the need for institutionalization or paid formal caregivers in the last months of life is much higher among the poor and women. Similarly, persons suffering from cognitive impairment and dementia are much more likely to spend their last days in a nursing home compared with cognitively intact, elderly persons dying from nondementing illnesses.

CARE SYSTEMS FOR OLDER ADULTS WITH SERIOUS ILLNESS

The needs of older adults living with serious illness are not well matched by current models of care. Specifically, multiple studies demonstrate that the personal and practical care needs of patients who are seriously ill and their families are not adequately addressed by routine office visits or hospital and nursing home stays and that this failure results in substantial burdens—medical, psychological, and financial—on patients and their caregivers (9). Neither paid personal care services at home nor nursing home costs for the functionally dependent elderly are covered by Medicare, but instead are paid for approximately equally from out-of-pocket and Medicaid budgetary sources that were originally developed to provide care for the indigent. In the context of chronic progressive disease, the burden of coordinating an array of social and medical services falls on primary physicians and more often, individual families.

In response to the needs of seriously ill older adults and their families, palliative care teams have become increasingly prevalent in United States hospitals and provide comprehensive interdisciplinary care for seriously ill patients and families in collaboration and consultation with primary physicians. Over 80% of hospitals with over 300 beds now report a palliative care team and over two-third of all hospitals report a palliative care team—a steady 140% increase in prevalence since 2000 (10). Hospital palliative care teams have been shown to significantly reduce symptom burden, enhance patient and family satisfaction, and lower costs (Morrison nejm, health affairs, NEJM). Other programs, although less well developed, focused on reducing functional decline and delirium and improving transitions from hospitals also show promising early results (11).

In the ambulatory care setting, programs are less well developed than in hospitals. Hospice services, under the Medicare benefit, are available in most US communities and provide palliative care, primarily at home, for patients with a life expectancy of 6 months or less who are willing to forgo insurance coverage for life-prolonging treatments. Overall, about 40% older adults access their hospice benefit prior to death and median length of stay on hospice is on the order of 3 weeks (12). Reasons for the low rate of utilization of the Medicare Hospice Benefit vary by community but include the inhibiting requirements that patients acknowledge that they are dying in order to access the services, that physicians certify a prognosis of 6 months or less, and that very few hours (usually 4 or less) of personal care home attendants are covered under the benefit. In addition, the fiscal structure of the Medicare Hospice Benefit lends itself well to the predictable trajectory of late-stage cancers, but not so well to the unpredictable chronic course of other common causes of death in the elderly such as congestive heart failure, chronic lung disease, stroke, and dementing illnesses.

Other programs that coordinate care for patients who have complex illnesses, outside of hospice, are becoming increasingly available in many communities—primarily for younger adults or for individuals enrolled in Medicare Advantage (i.e., Medicare managed care plans). These programs typically focus on intensive telephonic case management and have been shown in early studies to improve care for those with serious illness (13). The quality, cost, and extent of the services provided are highly variable.

Finally, comprehensive multidisciplinary home care programs that serve frail older adults have been developed in several specialized settings. The Program of All-Inclusive Care for the Elderly (PACE) is a capitated Medicare and Medicaid benefit for frail older adults that offers comprehensive medical and social services at day health centers, in homes, and at inpatient facilities. Patients enrolled in PACE have higher rates of advance directive completion and lower rates of nursing home admission, hospitalization, and hospital deaths than do patients who do not use the services (ref Morrison NEJM). Similar programs of team-coordinated home-based care exist within the Veterans Administration (VA) (VA home-based primary care and VA palliative care programs). All VA hospitals are required to have both a home-based primary care program for homebound veterans and a palliative care team. Furthermore, under recent VA regulations, all veterans are allowed access to hospice at the same time as they are receiving disease-directed or curative treatments.

In nursing homes, the site of care for many of the most seriously ill and cognitively impaired older adults, incentives promoting palliative care standard are lacking. Indeed, nursing home quality metrics focus on improvement of function and maintenance of weight and nutritional status. Evidence of the decline that accompanies the dying process is typically regarded as a measure of substandard care (14). Therefore, a death in a nursing home is often viewed as evidence particularly by state regulators of poor care rather than an expected outcome for a frail, chronically ill, older person. The financial and regulatory incentives and quality measures that currently exist in long-term care promote tube feeding over spoon feeding and transfer to hospital or emergency department in the setting of acute illness or impending death (Table 62.1). They fail to either assess or reward appropriate attention to palliative measures, including relief of symptoms, spiritual care, and promotion of continuity with concomitant avoidance of brink-of-death emergency room and hospital transfers (15). Although provision of hospice services has been shown to improve quality in nursing homes (16), penetration of hospice services into most nursing homes remains low and increasing federal scrutiny on long-lengths of stay of nursing home residents on the hospice benefit has led to concerns about enrolling this patient population.

TABLE 62.1 Benefits and risks of tube feeding in older adults/nursing home residents	
Benefits of Tube Feeding in Older Adults/ Nursing Home Patients	**Risks of Tube Feeding in Older Adults/Nursing Home Patients**
Improved survival for patients in persistent vegetative state	Dementia patients more likely to be physically restrained
Improved survival for patients with extreme short bowel syndrome or proximal bowel obstruction	Increased risk of aspiration pneumonia, diarrhea, gastrointestinal discomfort, and problems associated with accidental feeding tube removal by the patient
Improved survival *AND* quality of life for patients with bulbar amyotrophic lateral sclerosis	With impaired renal function or in last days of life patient may have choking, increased pulmonary secretions, dyspnea, pulmonary edema, and ascites
Improved survival for patients in acute phase of stroke or head injury	
Improved survival in patients receiving short-term critical care	
Improved nutritional status of patients with advanced cancer undergoing intensive radiation therapy	
No Survival Benefit in patients with dementia	

Table adapted from data summarized in Casarett D, Kapo J, Caplan A. Appropriate use of artificial nutrition and hydration—fundamental principles and recommendations. *N Engl J Med.* 2005;353:2607–2612.

PALLIATIVE CARE NEEDS OF OLDER ADULTS

Although death occurs far more commonly in older adults than in any other age group, remarkably little is known about the course of serious illness in the oldest old, that is, those over age 75. Most research on the experience of living with serious illness has been done in younger populations, and most studies examining pain and symptom management have focused on younger populations. Studies in older adults have focused primarily on patients' preferences for care rather than on the actual care received. Indeed, the largest study to date of the experience of living with a serious illnesses in the United States (Study to Understand Prognoses and Preferences for Outcomes and Risks of Treatments [SUPPORT]) studied the hospital experience of patients with a median age of 66 (17). The median age of death in the United States is 78 years, and many of the oldest old die in nursing homes or at home rather than in hospital. Data from Medicare and state Medicaid registries suggest that expensive and high technology interventions are less frequently applied to the oldest patients, independent of functional status and projected life expectancy. Whereas these discrepancies may reflect patient preferences and indicate appropriate utilization of resources and patient preferences, it is more likely that they represent a form of implicit rationing of resources based on age. The implication is disturbing, considering that half of the highest cost, Medicare enrollees survive at least 1 year (18).

Aside from pain and other sources of physical distress (see Section "Symptom Management: The Challenge of Pain"), the key characteristic that distinguishes the experience of serious illness in the elderly from that experienced by younger groups is the nearly universal occurrence of long periods of functional dependency and need for family caregivers in the last months to years of life. In SUPPORT, the median age of participants was 66 years and 55% of patients had persistent and serious family caregiving needs during the course of their terminal illness (19), and in another study of 988 terminally ill patients, 35% of families had substantial care needs (20). This percentage rises exponentially with increasing age. Although paid care supplements provide the sole source of care in 15% to 20% of patients (transportation, homemaker services, personal care, and more skilled nursing care), the remaining 80% to 85% of patients receive most of their care from unpaid family members (20). Furthermore, most family caregiving is provided by women (spouses and adult daughters and daughters-in-law), placing significant strains on the physical, emotional, and socioeconomic status of the caregivers. Those ill and dependent patients without family caregivers, or those whose caregivers can no longer provide nor afford needed services, are placed in nursing homes. In the United States, this typically occurs after patients exhaust all of their financial savings in order to become eligible for Medicaid. At present, 20% of over the age 85 population reside in a skilled nursing facility, and this number is expected to increase dramatically in the next 50 years (21). Present estimates suggest that the current number of skilled nursing facility beds in the United States will be woefully inadequate for the needs of our aging population.

SYMPTOM MANAGEMENT: THE CHALLENGE OF PAIN

The constellation of symptoms seen in seriously ill, older, adult patients is different from that of young adults. Delirium, sensory impairment, incontinence, dizziness, cough, and constipation are more prevalent in older adults (22). The elderly, on average, have 1.5 more symptoms than younger persons in the year prior to death, and 69% of the symptoms reported for people aged 85 or more lasted more than a year as compared with 39% of those for younger adults (<55 yr) (22).

Studies focusing specifically on the prevalence of pain have shown consistently high levels of untreated or undertreated pain in older adults. In one study of elderly cancer patients in nursing homes, 26% of patients with daily pain received no analgesic at all and 16% received only acetaminophen, a percentage that rose with increasing age and minority status (23). A subsequent study revealed that 41% of patients who were assessed having pain on their first assessment continued to have moderate or excruciating daily pain on their second assessment 60 to 180 days later (24). Studies comparing pain management in cognitively intact versus demented elderly with acute hip fracture also found a high rate of undertreatment of pain in both groups, a phenomenon that worsened with increasing age and cognitive impairment (25,26). Similarly, a study of outpatients with cancer found that age and female sex were predictors of undertreatment, a disturbing observation given the dramatic rise in cancer prevalence with increasing age (27,28). Chronic pain due to arthritis, other bone and joint disorders, and low back pain syndrome is probably the most common cause of distress and disability in the elderly, affecting 25% to 50% of community-dwelling, older adults. It is likely that these symptoms also are consistently undertreated (29). These data suggest that the time before death among elderly persons is often characterized by significant physical distress that is neither identified nor properly treated.

Despite the high prevalence of pain and other symptoms in the elderly, most studies focusing on the assessment and treatment of pain and other symptoms have enrolled younger adults with cancer. It is unclear whether these results can be generalized to a geriatric population. Pain assessment in the elderly is often complicated by the coexistence of cognitive impairment. The assessment and management of pain in the cognitively impaired patient present special challenges to the healthcare professional. The cognitively impaired patient is often unable to express pain adequately, request analgesics, or operate patient-controlled, analgesia devices. This increases the risk of undertreatment. The fear of precipitating or exacerbating a delirious episode by employing opioids in the management of pain may also lead to inadequate pain management.

As with the cognitively intact patient, the initial step in the assessment of pain in the demented individual is to ask the patient. Although patients with severe dementia may be incapable of communicating, many patients with moderate degrees of impairment can accurately localize and grade the severity of their pain (30,31). In the noncommunicative patient, alternative means of assessment must be identified. The need for careful pain assessment in this population of patients is underscored by evidence that suggests that medical professionals undertreat pain in the presence of cognitive impairment (25,26,32) and that pain may be aggravated in the presence of cognitive deficits (30). Untreated pain can result in agitation, disruptive behavior, and may worsen or precipitate a delirious episode (33–35).

Pain assessment in the noncommunicative patient should begin with observation of both nonverbal cues, such as facial expressions (grimacing and frowning) and motor behavior (bracing, restlessness, and agitation) and verbal cues, such as groaning, screaming, or moaning. Data from cognitively intact individuals suggest that nonverbal behaviors correlate with self-reported pain in nondemented patients recovering from surgery (36,37). Pharmacologic therapy should be titrated upward in small, incremental doses until the nonverbal/verbal behavior disappears or side effects become apparent. This approach is particularly useful in the agitated patient whose behavior may well stem from untreated or undertreated pain. The risk of undertreating severe pain is generally more concerning, both medically and ethically, than the risk of worsening delirium with medications. Table 62.2 summarizes available pain assessment tools useful in care of older adults.

Pharmacologic therapy for pain must be modified in older adults. The World Health Organization's analgesic ladder approach may not be appropriate for the elderly. For example, the increased risk of side effects, including renal failure and gastrointestinal bleeding, mandates great caution in the use of NSAIDs. This caution extends to currently available parenteral NSAIDs because of the significantly increased risk of gastrointestinal bleeding, particularly with higher doses and with duration of use >5 days (38–40). The American Geriatrics Society has recommended that opioids be considered as a first-step treatment rather than NSAIDs (29). If NSAIDs are used, careful monitoring of renal function and close observation of the development of gastrointestinal bleeding must be undertaken.

Opioid therapy remains the cornerstone of pain management in palliative care and this is also true for older adults. Some aspects of opioid therapy require special consideration in the elderly. Older adults will have a more pronounced pharmacologic effect after any weight-adjusted opioid dose than younger patients. The analgesia is more intense, and cognitive and respiratory effects, and perhaps constipation, are more severe. This enhanced effect is likely due to a lesser volume of distribution (approximately half that of younger patients), a decreased clearance, and diminished target organ reserve (central nervous system, pulmonary function, and bowel function). Age is the single most important predictor of initial opioid dose requirements for postoperative pain (41). The following formula, based on a review of records of >1,000 adults between ages 20 and 70 undergoing major surgery, provides a rough estimate of the appropriate starting dose in parenteral morphine sulfate equivalents for adult opioid-naive patients (with the exception of the oldest old): average first 24-hour morphine (mg) requirement for patients over 20 years of age = 100 minus the patient's age (41). Other factors that will influence opioid effects, but to a lesser degree than that of age, are body weight, severity of pain, abnormal renal function, nausea/vomiting, and cardiopulmonary insufficiency. After the initial dose determination, drugs should be titrated on the basis of analgesic effect.

There are no data as to appropriate starting doses for analgesia in older adults. A reasonable starting dose may be 30% to 50% of that recommended for a younger adult.

Practically speaking, however, the best advice is almost obvious. In opioid-naive older adults, one should start with the smallest dose available for the product. The key to prescribing a correct regimen is not in the first order you write, but rather, in what happens when this dose becomes effective. In an acute pain syndrome, the reassessment of the patient's level of pain at the right follow-up interval will lead to the appropriate dose titration. An intravenous medication should be effective within 6 to 15 minutes and oral medications within an hour. Reassessing effective analgesia needs to occur frequently in an acute pain crisis.

Several opioids are best avoided in older adults. Meperidine is particularly hazardous as a result of the accumulation of its toxic metabolite, normeperidine, in patients with impaired renal function. Indeed, toxic levels can accumulate in older adults with "normal kidneys" due to age-related changes in creatinine clearance. There are almost no circumstances in which meperidine should be used on older adults. Similarly, pentazocine should also be avoided in older adults because of the increased incidence of delirium and agitation associated with its use. Finally, opioids with long half-lives (e.g., methadone and levorphanol) or opioids with sustained-release preparations (e.g., sustained-release morphine, oxycodone, and hydromorphone and transdermal fentanyl) should be used with caution, rarely be used in opioid-naive geriatric patients, and should probably only be used following steady-state accumulation of shorter acting opioids.

With respect to adjuvant agents, amitriptyline and the other tricyclic antidepressants, although efficacious in some neuropathic pain syndromes, are poorly tolerated in older adults due to their anticholinergic properties. Bowel and bladder dysfunction, orthostatic hypotension resulting in falls, delirium, movement disorders, and dry mouth are very common with these medications. If tricyclics are to be used, then nortriptyline or desipramine is the agent of choice and initial dosages should be very low and dose titration should be undertaken very slowly.

ALZHEIMER DISEASE AND RELATED DEMENTIAS

Irreversible dementia is a frightening and difficult diagnosis for geriatric patients and their families. A diagnosis of dementia means a certain and progressive decline in

TABLE 62.2	Pain assessment tools for older adults
Brief Pain Inventory (BPI) (Charles S. Cleeland PhD)	Originally developed for cancer pain, but validated for nonmalignant pain as well, used widely in research, widely translated into other languages, looks at pain and its impact on function
Checklist of Nonverbal Pain Indicators (CNPI) (Karen S. Feldt PhD RN CS GNP)	Designed specifically for cognitively impaired patients, looks at behavior both at rest and with movement
Faces Pain Scale (FPS) (Daivia Bieri et al.)	Designed originally as a pediatric pain assessment tool but now shown to be effective in older adults. Scale is seven faces, each depicting increasing levels of pain. This scale does not require verbal interaction so is useful in patients with expressive language problems
Functional Pain Scale (FPS) (FM Gloth III MD CMD et al.)	Specifically developed for older adults, has both a subjective and objective component. Looks at a rating of "tolerable" vs. "intolerable" and the impact on function
Numeric Rating Scale (NRS) (Keela A. Herr RN PhD and Linda Garand RN, PhD, CS)	This is a horizontal scale with two versions 1–20 or 0–10. Zero equals no pain, with the higher number being equal to the worst pain one can experience
Pain Assessment in Advanced Dementia Scale (PAINAD) (Victoria Warden RN et al.)	Specifically designed for cognitively impaired patients with advanced disease. Relies on observations of specific behaviors (breathing, facial expressions, vocalizations, consolability, and body language) to determine a level of pain
Pain Thermometer (Keela A. Herr RN PhD and Paula R. Mobily RN PhD)	Uses the visual of a vertical thermometer to rate pain. Pain increases as you move up the thermometer. Can be useful in patients with limited verbal communication and has been used in cognitively impaired patients
Verbal Descriptor Scale (VDS) (Keela A. Herr RN PhD and Linda Garand RN, PhD, CS)	Uses descriptive phases to reflect differing severity of pain. Patient needs to be able to articulate symptoms but the tool is well studied for use in older adults and even those with mild to moderate cognitive compromise
Verbal Numeric Scale (VNS) (Diane M. Young MSN, RN et al.)	Patients verbally rate their pain on a scale of 0–10. Again, 0 equals no pain and 10 is the worst pain imaginable. There is no visual component to this scale

Based on Compilation from the Iowa Geriatric Education Center (www.healthcare.uiowa.edu).

cognitive abilities over time and an eventual loss of independence. Dementia is a progressive, incurable illness, and all treatments are palliative. The average survival after a diagnosis of Alzheimer disease ranges from 7 to 10 years. Patients with dementia require medical care that focuses on preserving dignity and quality of life. Physicians should seek to aggressively manage the symptoms that endanger these goals. This must be done in early stages of the disease, the more moderate stages, and finally the advanced stages. The needs of patients in each stage are different, but the focus is always to preserve dignity and quality of life.

In early dementia, perhaps the most important job for the physician is to recognize and diagnose the disease and then to educate patients and their families about what they can expect. At this stage, patients can still make decisions for themselves. Physicians should ask patients about their preferences for medical treatments in the later stages of their disease and facilitate these important conversations between their patients and caregivers. Specific discussions about life-prolonging treatments, such as artificial nutrition and hydration, should take place. Physicians should ask patients to designate one or more primary decision makers to speak for them in preparation for later stages of disease when they are no longer able to make decisions for themselves. Patients should be encouraged to talk with their designated caregivers and loved ones about their views about advanced medical therapies such as feeding tubes, mechanical ventilation, and cardiopulmonary resuscitation (CPR). Although it is important to explore patients' specific preferences with regard to medical technology, it is equally important to explore the patients' values and goals of medical care: What is most important in their lives? What makes their lives worth living? What religious or spiritual values may be important? There is evidence that early conversations about advance directives help to prepare families for future decision making and may reduce the difficulty that comes with later surrogate decision making (42).

The early stages of Alzheimer disease may be amenable to pharmacologic therapy with cholinesterase inhibitors. Treatment with these medications may improve performance in activities of daily living, modestly improve cognitive function, or slow down the progression of the disease process. Aggressive control of vascular risk factors and the use of aspirin and cholesterol-lowering agents may slow down the progress of vascular dementia. The goals of both types of therapies are to preserve independence for as long as possible.

Many patients with early-stage disease have concurrent psychiatric issues. Depression is especially common, affecting approximately 50% of the early Alzheimer disease population. The symptoms of depression in early disease may be atypical and include indifference, difficulties with emotional engagement, and decreased motivation. Antidepressant therapies are often indicated, and cholinesterase inhibitors may be beneficial. Support groups may also be helpful at this stage of disease, both for patients and their caregivers.

Moderate-stage dementia is the longest stage of the disease. The physician's focus should be keeping the patient's environment safe, treating psychiatric symptoms, and supporting the patient's caregivers. As patients move to this more middle stage of the disease, their need for supervision at home and help with performing activities of daily living become greater. Behavioral disturbances, agitation, and paranoia often occur in concert with increased dependence. These changes may become significant sources of caregiver stress. Palliative measures in moderate-level dementia include recognition and attention to caregiver stress, treatment of behavioral and psychiatric disturbances, and instituting environmental safety modifications. Additionally, patients with a moderate degree of cognitive impairment often exhibit impaired eating behaviors, and physicians must work with patients and their caregivers to meet nutritional demands, as well as modifying food products for easier mealtimes.

Caregiver stress is common, as relatives take on a more active and demanding role in the everyday routines of patients with progressive dementia. Many have never been in the role of primary caregiver for anyone other than their own children. Some primary caregivers may be geriatric patients themselves. Most families will face a high level of financial stress. Unless a patient has access to social services (Medicaid in the United States), out-of-pocket costs for additional help at home, pharmaceutical products, and durable medical equipment are high. Adult day programs may be hard to find, and respite programs are typically expensive. Patients with this degree of cognitive compromise may be difficult to place in nursing homes because often they do not carry other comorbid diagnoses, and the reimbursement rate for pure custodial care is low. Many caregivers leave their jobs or families behind to care for their loved ones. Some need to take on a second job to keep up with the financial burdens.

Caregivers may feel underappreciated because their loved ones fail to acknowledge how hard they are working or the sacrifices they are making. Eventually, patients fail to be able to even recognize who their caregivers are. These very real stresses need to be recognized, acknowledged, and supported. Physicians should question caregivers about fatigue, social isolation, depression, and physical symptoms. They should remind caregivers to take breaks and encourage other family members to help out. Caregiver support groups may also be helpful.

Behavioral disturbances become more frequent as dementia progresses. Although they may occur at any stage of the disease, they are associated with increasing cognitive and functional decline. Symptoms include anxiety, depression, paranoia, delusions, hallucinations, sleep disorders, agitation, and combativeness. The presence of behavioral disturbance, especially paranoia and aggression, can increase the likelihood of nursing home placement. Treatment should be aimed at improving the quality of life of the patient and caregiver and should include both pharmacologic and nonpharmacologic considerations. Careful attention should be given to alternative causes of behavioral disturbance, such as uncontrolled pain, untreated infection, or suboptimal management of concurrent disease. Treatment of underlying medical illness may lead to sustained improvement in both cognitive status and behavior. In addition, the etiology of agitation may be based on basic human needs—hunger, thirst, or the need to change wet or soiled clothing. Identifying the root of the problem may be difficult, as patients with moderate degrees of dementia cannot tell their caregivers what exactly is bothering them. Nevertheless, the presence of a new behavioral disturbance should precipitate a medical evaluation and should not simply be considered a consequence of the underlying dementing illness.

Treating obvious etiologies as well as addressing possible modifications in the patient's care environment can be useful ways to address behavioral disturbances. For example, a careful history may demonstrate that agitated and paranoid behavior occurs at bath time. In this case, perhaps changing the water temperature or moving from a tub to a sponge bath may be less threatening for patients and lead to decreased agitation (43). Evidence suggests that involving patients actively in grooming routines may also decrease agitation. Calm environments, the use of usual routines, favorite pieces of music, and visits from children or pets may all be soothing. Attention to a patient's sleeping patterns is also important. Increasing daytime activities and decreasing daytime napping may help patients sleep better at night.

In addition to these behavioral interventions, low-dose standing or as-needed major tranquilizers, such as haloperidol, risperidone, or olanzapine, may be required to successfully manage behavioral disturbances and prevent hospital admissions. It is important to consider potential cardiovascular risk when prescribing these medications where there is an FDA black box warning of sudden cardiovascular death.

However, when considering this potential toxicity, the prescriber should weigh the risk–benefit ratios. Treating a dignity and quality-of-life-compromising condition at the end of life may have more gravity than the potential risk. Discussion with the patient's family about the issue is important. Bedtime dosing with major tranquilizers or with trazodone may help with sleep disturbances. Benzodiazepines may be associated with paradoxical agitation, excessive somnolence, and falls and should be avoided in most patients.

Advanced dementia is the final stage of this terminal disease. Patients with end-stage dementia are dying. Research has demonstrated a median 6-month survival rate for patients with end-stage dementia, with or without tube feeding, although the range of survival times is wide (44–47). Most patients in this stage of disease are bedbound and nonverbal. Many patients in this stage of disease are placed in a nursing home because of their increasing care demands. Although comfort care and palliation of suffering should be the paramount focus of care, patients with advanced dementia often receive nonpalliative interventions at the end of life, such as tube feedings, CPR, mechanical ventilation, and systemic antibiotics in their final days of life (25,45,46,48,49).

Surrogate decision making in end-stage disease is inevitable. The process is made easier for all involved if, in the early stages of disease, the aforementioned critical discussions of treatment goals and end-of-life preferences have occurred. Caregivers may face multiple, difficult decisions, including emergency surgery, intubation, feeding tubes, and CPR. Even if the advance wishes were well communicated, it may still be difficult for family members to carry them out. Nonetheless, decisions should always be based on previously expressed wishes (if known) and the best interest of the patient with respect to the potential benefits or burdens of the proposed treatment. Physicians should offer caregivers continued support and offer them regular and repeated reviews of the goals of treatment and the expectations that follow interventions.

Comfort measures and the relief of suffering should be the primary palliative goals. Careful attention to potential sources of discomfort, such as pain and concurrent illness, is important. Pain is very commonly overlooked and undertreated in this population. Analgesic therapy should be empiric and preventive if an underlying source exists or the patient faces potentially uncomfortable procedures such as dressing changes or position changes. Physicians should also recognize that patients with advanced dementia may experience more discomfort from routine procedures, such as vital signs monitoring, phlebotomy, finger sticks, and bladder catheterizations, because they cannot understand what is being done to them and why. Unnecessary procedures should be discontinued. Topical anesthetic preparations may make the necessary procedures more bearable.

CONCLUSION

As a result of the unprecedented improvements in maternal and infant mortality and successes in the control, if not cure, of common chronic diseases, most people who die in the United States are old and frail. Conservative projections suggest that in the next 30 years, we will see a dramatic shift in demographics, with over 20% of the United States population being over age 65 in the year 2030. The elderly die of chronic, progressive illnesses (such as end-stage heart and lung disease, cancer, stroke, and dementia). These diseases have unpredictable clinical courses and prognoses, and current care systems are not well adapted to the trajectory of illness or the clinical needs of these group of patients. In contrast to younger adults, older adults often have unrecognized and untreated symptoms, cognitive impairment, and an extremely high prevalence of functional dependency and associated family caregiver burden. It is clear that our current systems of reimbursement are ill equipped to provide primary care with continuity, support for family caregivers, and home care and nursing home services. Because care for a frail, older adult typically includes preventive, life-prolonging rehabilitation and palliative measures in varying proportions and intensity based on the individual patient's needs and preferences, any new models of care will have to be responsive to this range of service requirements. Several "mixed management" models of care are available to address the needs of the frail elderly, including hospital palliative care teams, PACE, and new models of ambulatory care management—primarily for commercially insured or Medicare Advantage enrollees. Future research needs to be targeted at understanding the palliative care needs of older adults, developing medical interventions that address these needs, and developing models and systems of care that will meet the global needs of these patients and their families.

REFERENCES

1. Miller RA. The biology of aging and longevity. In: Hazzard WR, Blass JP, Ettinger WH, et al., eds. *Principles of Geriatric Medicine and Gerontology*. New York, NY: McGraw-Hill; 1999:1-19.
2. Fries J. Aging, natural death and the compression of morbidity. *N Engl J Med*. 1990;303:130.
3. Avorn J, Gurwitz J. Principles of pharmacology. In: Cassell C, Cohen H, Larson E, et al., eds. *Geriatric Medicine*. 3rd ed. New York, NY: Springer; 1997.
4. Perneger TV, Whelton PK, Klag MJ. Risk of kidney failure associated with the use of acetaminophen, aspirin, and nonsteroidal antiinflammatory drugs. *N Engl J Med*. 1994;331:1675-1679.
5. Ferrell B. Pain management in elderly people. *J Am Geriatr Soc*. 1991;39:64-73.
6. Harkins S. Pain perceptions in the old. *Clin Geriatr Med*. 1996;12:435-459.
7. Olshansky SJ. Demography of aging. In: Cassel CK, Cohen HJ, Larson EB, et al., eds. *Geriatric Medicine*. 3rd ed. New York, NY: Springer; 1997.
8. National Vital Statistics System. *Deaths by Place of Death, Age, Race, and Sex: United States, 1999-2005*. Atlanta, GA: Center for Disease Control and Prevention. http://www.cdc.gov/nchs/nvss/mortality/gmwk309.htm. Accessed February 20, 2012.
9. Morrison, RS, Meier DE. Palliative care. *N Engl J Med*. 2004;350:2582-2590.
10. Center to Advance Palliative Care/National Palliative Care Research Center. *America's Care of Serious Illness: A*

State-by-State Report Card on Access to Palliative Care in Our Nation's Hospitals. New York, NY: Center to Advance Palliative Care and the National Palliative Care Research Center; 2012. http://www.capc.org/reportcard/. Accessed Februaruy 20, 2012.

11. Siu AL, Spragens LH, Inouye SK, Morrison RS, Leff B. The ironic business case for chronic care in the acute care setting. *Health Aff (Millwood).* January–February 2009;28(1):113-125.

12. National Hospice and Palliative Care Organization. *NHPCO Facts and Figures. Hospice Care in America.* Alexandria, VA: National Hospice and Palliative Care Organization; 2012. http://www.nhpco.org/files/public/Statistics_Research/2011_Facts_Figures.pdf. Accessed February 20, 2012.

13. Spettell CM, Rawlins WS, Krakauer R, et al. A comprehensive case management program to improve palliative care. *J Palliat Med.* 2009;12:827-832.

14. Keay TJ, Fredman L, Taler GA, et al. Indicators of quality medical care for the terminally ill in nursing homes. *J Am Geriatr Soc.* 1994;42:853-860.

15. Engle VF. Care of the living, care of the dying: reconceptualizing nursing home care. *J Am Geriatr Soc.* 1998;46:1172-1174.

16. Teno JM, Gozalo PL, Lee IC, et al. Does hospice improve quality of care for persons dying from dementia? *J Am Geriatr Soc.* 2011;59:1531-1536.

17. The SUPPORT Principal Investigators. A controlled trial to improve care for seriously ill hospitalized patients. The study to understand prognoses and preferences for outcomes and risks of treatments (SUPPORT). *JAMA.* 1995;274:1591-1598.

18. Lubitz JD, Riley FF. Trends in Medicare payments in the last year of life. *N Engl J Med.* 1993;328:1092-1096.

19. Covinsky KE, Landefeld CS, Teno J, et al. Is economic hardship on the families of the seriously ill associated with patient and surrogate care preferences? SUPPORT Investigators. *Arch Intern Med.* 1996;156:1737-1741.

20. Emanuel EJ, Fairclough DL, Slutsman J, et al. Assistance from family members, friends, paid caregivers, and volunteers in the care of terminally ill patients. *N Engl J Med.* 1999;341:956-963.

21. Ferrell B. Overview of aging and pain. In: Ferrell BR, Ferrell BA, eds. *Pain in the Elderly: A Report of the Task Force on Pain in the Elderly of the International Association for the Study of Pain.* Seattle, WA: IASP Press; 1996.

22. Seale C, Cartwright A. *The Year Before Death.* Brookfield, WI: Ashgate; 1994.

23. Bernabei R, Gambassi G, Lapane K, et al. Management of pain in elderly patients with cancer. *JAMA.* 1998;279:1877-1882.

24. Teno JM, Weitzen S, Wetle T, et al. Persistent pain in nursing home residents. *JAMA.* 2001;285:2081.

25. Feldt KS, Ryden MB, Miles S. Treatment of pain in cognitively impaired compared with cognitively intact older patients with hip-fracture. *J Am Geriatr Soc.* 1998;46:1079-1085.

26. Morrison RS, Siu AL. A comparison of pain and its treatment in advanced dementia and cognitively intact patients with hip fracture. *J Pain Symptom Manage.* 2000;19:240-248.

27. Cleeland CS, Gonin R, Hatfield AK, et al. Pain and its treatment in outpatients with metastatic cancer. *N Engl J Med.* 1994;330:592-596.

28. Stein W. Cancer pain in the elderly. In: Ferrell BR, Ferrell BA, eds. *Pain in the Elderly: A Report of the Task Force on Pain in the Elderly of the International Association for the Study of Pain.* Seattle, WA: IASP Press; 1996.

29. American Geriatrics Society. The management of chronic pain in older persons: AGS panel on chronic pain in older persons. *J Am Geriatr Soc.* 1998;46:635-651.

30. Parmelee P. Pain in cognitively impaired older persons. *Clin Geriatr Med.* 1996;12:473-487.

31. Ferrell BA, Ferrell BR, Rivera LSO. Pain in cognitively impaired nursing home patients. *J Pain Symptom Manage.* 1995;10:591-598.

32. Sengstaken E, King S. The problem of pain and its detection among geriatric nursing home residents. *J Am Geriatr Soc.* 1993;41:541-544.

33. Duggleby W, Lander J. Cognitive status and postoperative pain: older adults. *J Pain Symptom Manage.* 1994;9:19-27.

34. Lynch EP, Lazor MA, Gellis JE, et al. The impact of postoperative pain on the development of postoperative delirium. *Anesth Analg.* 1998;86:781-785.

35. Morrison RS, Magaziner J, Gilbert M, et al. Relationship between pain and opioid analgesics on the development of delirium following hip fracture. *J Gerontol A Biol Sci Med Sci.* 2003;58:76-81.

36. Mateo OM, Krenzischek DA. A pilot study to assess the relationship between behavioral manifestations and self-report of pain in postanesthesia care unit patients. *J Post Anesth Nurs.* 1992;7:15-21.

37. Le Resche L, Dworkin S. Facial expressions of pain and emotions in chronic TMD patients. *Pain.* 1988;35:71-78.

38. Strom BL, Berlin JA, Kinman JL, et al. Parenteral ketorolac and risk of gastrointestinal and operative site bleeding. A postmarketing surveillance study. *JAMA.* 1996;275:376-382.

39. Camu F, Lauwers MH, Vanlersberghe C. Side effects of NSAIDs and dosing recommendations for ketorolac. *Acta Anaesthesiol Belg.* 1996;47:143-149.

40. Maliekal J, Elboim CM. Gastrointestinal complications associated with intramuscular ketorolac tromethamine therapy in the elderly. *Ann Pharmacother.* 1995;29:698-701.

41. Macintyre PE, Jarvis DA. Age is the best predictor of postoperative morphine requirements. *Pain.* 1996;64:357-364.

42. Tilden VP, Tolle SW, Nelson CA, et al. Family decision-making to withdraw life-sustaining treatments from hospitalized patients. *Nurs Res.* 2001;50:105-115.

43. Wells DL, Dawson P, Sidani S, et al. Effects of an abilities-focused program of morning care on residents who have dementia and on caregivers. *J Am Geriatr Soc.* 2000;48:442-449.

44. Meier DE, Ahronheim JC, Morris J, et al. High short-term mortality in hospitalized patients with advanced dementia: lack of benefit of tube feeding. *Arch Intern Med.* 2001;161:594-599.

45. Morrison RS, Siu AL. Survival in end-stage dementia following acute illness. *JAMA.* 2000;284:47-52.

46. Mitchell SL, Kiely DK, Hamel MB, Park PS, Morris JN, Fries BE. Estimating prognosis for nursing home residents with advanced dementia. *JAMA.* 2004;291(22):2734-2740.

47. Luchins DJ, Hanrahan P, Murphy K. Criteria for enrolling dementia patients in hospice [See comments]. *J Am Geriatr Soc.* 1997;45:1054-1059.

48. Ahronheim J, Morrison R, Morris J, et al. Palliative care in advanced dementia: a randomized controlled trial and descriptive analysis. *J Palliat Med.* 2000;3:265-273.

49. Ahronheim JC, Morrison RS, Baskin SA, et al. Treatment of the dying in the acute care hospital. Advanced dementia and metastatic cancer. *Arch Intern Med.* 1996;156:2094-2100.

CHAPTER 63

Palliative Care in Pediatrics

Liza-Marie Johnson ■ Melissa DeLario ■ Justin N. Baker ■ Javier R. Kane

P alliative medicine for children is the art and science of family-centered care aimed at enhancing quality of life, promoting healing, and attending to suffering. Inherent in this definition is the possibility of delivering palliative care in partnership with curative care for children with life-limiting illness or for children who may not die. Many principles already reviewed in other sections of this book are universally applicable across the age spectrum of the dying, so this chapter provides an overview of issues specific to the care of the life-threatened child.

Each year in the United States, approximately 53,000 children die, compared with approximately 2.4 million adults. National Vital Statistics for 2007, published in 2010, demonstrate that accidents remain the number one cause of death in children aged 1 to 19 (1). The second leading cause of death for children for ages 1 to 4 is congenital malformations, deformations, and chromosomal abnormalities; ages 5 to 14 is malignancy; and for ages 15 to 19 is homicide. For infants, the leading causes of death are congenital malformations, deformations, and chromosomal abnormalities, disorders related to short gestation and low birth weight, sudden infant death syndrome, and newborns affected by maternal complications of pregnancy such as uterine rupture. Hundreds of thousands more children are living with life-threatening conditions. Goldman (2) estimated that 50/100,000 children were living with life-threatening illness. Feudtner et al. (3) have done extensive research characterizing the epidemiology of childhood death. They have defined a group of complex chronic conditions (CCCs) "that can be reasonably expected to last at least 12 months (unless death intervenes) and to involve either several different organ systems or one organ system severely enough to require specialty pediatric care and probably some period of hospitalization in a tertiary care center." National data demonstrated that of 1.75 million deaths occurring in the 0 to 24-year-old population from 1979 to 1997, 5% were attributable to cancer CCCs, 16% to non–cancer CCCs, 43% to injuries, and 37% to all other death causes. Non–cancer CCCs accounted for approximately 25% of infant deaths, 20% of childhood deaths, and 7% of adolescent deaths. Death rates from CCCs are declining slowly due to advances in medical care for ill children. Feudtner estimates that each year approximately 15,000 infants, children, adolescents, and young adults might benefit from supportive care services delivered both at home and in the hospital, and that on any given day, approximately 5,000 are living in the last 6 months of their lives, many of whom die in hospitals after prolonged periods of inpatient care and artificial life-sustaining therapies (4,5). A recent retrospective observational study examined hospitalizations in the United States for children with CCCs and found that over time, the use of inpatient resources has increased (6). Additionally, Burns et al. (7) showed consistent increases in hospitalizations for children with CCCs from 1991 to 2005. Children at risk for chronic physical, developmental, behavioral, or emotional conditions account for about 18% of all children but represent 10% of pediatric hospital admissions and 70% of healthcare expenditures (8–10). The results of these studies suggest that more efforts should be focused on ongoing care of these children on both outpatient and inpatient bases. The diseases of childhood which might be appropriate for palliative care are many and include the following:

1. Conditions for which curative or life-prolonging treatment is possible but may fail, such as advanced or progressive malignancy or malignancy with a poor prognosis, or complex and severe congenital or acquired heart disease.
2. Conditions requiring long periods of intensive treatment aimed at prolonging quality of life such as human immunodeficiency virus, cystic fibrosis, severe gastrointestinal disorders, or malformations such as gastroschisis, severe epidermolysis bullosa, severe immunodeficiencies, renal failure when dialysis and/or transplantation are not available or indicated, chronic or severe respiratory failure, or muscular dystrophy.
3. Progressive conditions in which treatment is exclusively palliative from diagnosis such as mucopolysaccharidoses or other storage disorders, progressive metabolic disorders, certain chromosomal abnormalities such as Trisomy 13 or Trisomy 18, or severe forms of osteogenesis imperfecta.
4. Conditions with severe, non-progressive disability, causing extreme vulnerability to health complications such as severe cerebral palsy, extreme prematurity, severe neurologic impairments due to illness or injury, or severe brain malformations. Given the uncertainty of prognosis, many children with these conditions will not fit eligibility criteria for hospice care in the United States, which generally requires a life expectancy of 6 months or less (11).

SUFFERING

Suffering results from a threat to one's physical and psychological self, from a threat to one's relationships with others, and from a threat to one's relationship with a transcendent source of meaning (12). Suffering is a profoundly personal experience and is endurable, and at times even fulfilling, when it becomes meaningful (13). Despite best efforts, children living with chronic, life-threatening, and terminal illnesses experience substantial suffering. The extent, as well type, of suffering has broad-ranging implications in the child's life as a whole and in the family as a functional unit. Understanding the illness experience of patient and families is essential. Parents who recognize that their children have a poor prognosis and believe that their children are suffering from the illness and its treatment are more likely to put greater value on comfort and quality of life as they make care decisions.

Serious illness threatens children's sense of personal integrity and shatters all aspects of their lives. Physical pain and other symptoms cause fear, depression, and isolation. Illness affects their daily activities, sense of well-being, physical strength and agility, and the motives and quality of their relationships. Disease crushes their sense of security and brings fears of the unknown, rejection, and punishment. Children also become confused by the experience of a mixed variety of emotions of anger, anxiety, sadness, loneliness, and isolation in the presence of a threatening situation (14). Children are highly vulnerable to the stress inherent to the experience of severe illness. They have an egocentric view of the world and lack a fully developed repertoire of coping mechanisms, such as problem solving or decision making, which are influenced by age-dependent behavior and cognitive abilities.

Within the physical realm, the published experience speaks best to those with malignant diseases. Recent studies by Wolfe et al. (15) and Collins et al. (16,17) point to the wide variety and high prevalence of symptoms from which children with life-threatening illness suffer. There appears to be significant discrepancies between the reports of parents and physicians regarding the children's symptoms in the last month of life, with parents reporting each symptom more than the physicians. Furthermore, currently available treatments may not be successful in easing suffering associated with these symptoms that can cause significant distress. For children with nonmalignant diseases, some of the more troublesome symptoms might include gastroesophageal reflux, neuroirritability, immobility, incontinence, seizures, muscle spasms, pressure ulcers, contractures, recurrent infections, increased secretions, restlessness, sleep disturbance, and edema. There are few valid and reliable tools available to assess these symptoms and little data to substantiate the use of many of the interventions currently prescribed.

Suffering, for the parents of a child with a life-threatening illness, can also be a multidimensional experience of pain, fear, failure, despair, powerlessness, hopelessness, purposelessness, and vulnerability. Parental anxiety is due in part to the changing parent–child structure, the need to understand the illness experience, become familiar with the hospital environment, adapt to the changing relationships with their child and other family members, and negotiate with professionals about their care (18,19). Parents must also deal not only with the immediate threat of disease on their child's life but also with important additional family stressors during treatment such as lifestyle changes, marital tension, financial strain, loss of self-esteem, and even loss of sleep (20). Furthermore, when confronted with the suffering and possible death of their child, parents frequently recognize their own limitations and mortality. Their perception of life, death, and the world around them is changed dramatically by the reality of the loss of their child. In addition, parents must also satisfy the emotional needs of other children in the family which many times parallel those of the seriously ill child (21). Finally, children and their families may also suffer spiritually. This may be manifested as a sense of isolation and abandonment, a sense of hopelessness and uncertainty about the meaning and ultimate purpose of life.

The American Academy of Pediatrics supports an integrated model of palliative care in which the components of palliative care are offered at diagnosis and continued throughout the course of illness, whether the outcome ends in cure or death (22). Basic principles of pediatric palliative care include the following:

1. All children suffering from chronic, life-threatening, and terminal illnesses are eligible.
2. Care is patient and family centered and is based on continued healing relationships.
3. Care focuses on attending to suffering and enhancing quality of life for the child and family.
4. Care is provided for the child as a unique individual and the family as a functional unit.
5. Care is incorporated into the mainstream of medical care regardless of the curative intent of therapy.
6. Care is not directed at shortening life.
7. Care is coordinated and continuous throughout the illness trajectory and across all settings in which the child receives services.
8. Care is goal directed and consistent with the beliefs and values of the child and his or her caregivers.
9. Care is interdisciplinary and addresses all levels of the patient's and family's illness experience.
10. Advocacy for participation of the child and caregivers in decision making is paramount.
11. Facilitation and documentation of communication are critical tasks of the team.
12. Respite care and support are essential for families and caregivers.
13. Bereavement care should be provided for surviving family members including parents and siblings, for as long as needed.
14. Prognosis for short-term survival and a "Do Not Resuscitate" order are not required for eligibility.

These essentials do not mandate a particular structure for care delivery other than to suggest the function of an interdisciplinary team of health care and allied health care professionals to provide care coordination and to facilitate the delivery of services with the goal to attend suffering, promote healing, and improve quality of life.

INDIVIDUALIZED ADVANCED CARE PLANNING AND COORDINATION

Seriously ill patients and their families must often make difficult care decisions. Healthcare providers must empower them in this process through expert communication, information sharing, and support in the context of a therapeutic alliance. Care providers must communicate openly and honestly about the child's condition and prognosis and help identify realistic goal-directed treatment options. In the presence of advancing illness parents often have an overwhelming desire to continue cure-directed interventions while emphasizing comfort and quality of life (23). Families often need assistance in balancing these dual goals of care and with implementing a care plan that reflects their personal beliefs and values within the framework provided by a complex healthcare system. Much of the fragmentation of services that occurs in modern healthcare systems results from the lack of a coordinating entity. The loss of continuity may be addressed by providing a medical home for these children along with the services of an advanced-illness care coordinator supported by a physician with palliative care experience. Pediatric practices that act as the medical home for children with chronic conditions and provide care coordination are associated with fewer hospitalizations and improved care quality (24). Care coordination may be facilitated by a registered nurse whose primary responsibilities are to enhance communication across settings, facilitate the participation of the patient and family in the decision-making process, ensure that healthcare providers adhere to the goals and principles of palliative care, and honor the patient and family's wishes. The coordinator may advocate for change in the nature of the palliative care interventions according to the stage of disease and the patient and family's expectations, hopes, values, and concerns. The coordinator may also be responsible for ensuring access to proper management of pain and other symptoms, as well as to optimize physical function, and facilitate psychosocial and spiritual support. In our experience, provision of a trained advanced illness care coordinator to facilitate end-of-life communication can help the medical team and family embrace the reality of imminent death, provide effective anticipatory guidance about what to expect as the illness progresses, increase utilization of and length of stay in end-of-life services, facilitate completion of advance directives, and honor the families' preferences for the location of death. The roles provided by a physician advocate and the integration of services facilitated by the advanced care coordinator are essential for maintaining a patient and family centered, relationship-based approach and promotion of palliative care goals (25,26).

ETHICAL ISSUES

Although palliative care is becoming increasingly integrated in the care of children at the end of life, the process of caring for children at this stage is not always without conflict. Conflict may occur between family members, between staff, or between family members and staff when disagreements arise over the goals of care and on what treatments or limitations of treatment are in the best interests of the child. Conflicts may be highly emotional and may result in moral distress. Clinical ethics consultation may be helpful when agreements cannot be achieved on the goals of care. In difficult cases, institutional ethics committees can help resolve conflicts about treatment decisions, provide a forum for discussion of hospital policies, and educate the healthcare community about ethical concepts (27).

Decision-making capacity (DMC) includes the ability to understand and appreciate the risks, benefits, and outcomes of a medical decision as well as understanding the consequences of alternative decisions. Children are considered to have an evolving sense of DMC and thus parents or guardians are considered the best surrogate decision makers to make decisions on behalf of the child (28). As they mature, children form opinions about their health care, particularly children with a significant illness history, and these opinions should be included and valued in the discussion. Whenever possible, caregivers must make an effort to invite children to participate in medical decision making and honor their end-of-life care wishes. This is particularly important for any child, regardless of age, who can understand his or her medical condition, who can communicate his or her preferences, and who is able to reach a reasonable decision and can understand its consequences (28). Children ≥ age 14 should provide assent whenever possible (29,30).

Clinicians assisting families with treatment decisions in palliative care have valuable expertise with these decisions and can provide recommendations among therapies to families, while making it clear that families who select an alternative therapy will not be abandoned. Decision making should be shared and driven by communication between child, parent, and physician (31). Understanding the illness experience from the perspective of the child and family, establishing accurate prognosis and communicating it effectively, setting reasonable goals and establishing a comprehensive advanced-illness care plan are indispensable steps in this process.

Foregoing life-sustaining medical therapies through withholding or withdrawal of artificial life-sustaining interventions is often ethically permissible, but this is a possible source of conflict within a family or with medical staff. Family care conferences and interdisciplinary team meetings to facilitate communication and clarify goals of care are often helpful at resolving conflicts. The ability to provide an intervention (such as artificial nutrition and hydration) is not an obligation to provide that intervention, particularly if the burdens of the therapy are greater than the benefits to the patient and family (32,33). When the risk–benefit ratio of an intervention is unclear, shared decision making may result in a time-limited trial to assess if the intervention is beneficial and compatible with the goals of care. Although some find one morally more distressing than the other, the withholding and withdrawing of an intervention are ethically equivalent and therefore it is permissible to withdraw medical therapies not felt to be compatible with the goals of care, even if withdrawal leads to the patient's natural death (such as removal of a ventilator) (33). In making these difficult decisions the right to self-determination, or autonomy, allows individuals and families to make risk–benefit determinations specific to their personal experiences and value systems. The discontinuation of non-beneficial interventions is within the scope of parental decision-making authority and should not be viewed as inconsistent with a child's best interests. Clinicians should seek to override family wishes only when those wishes clearly conflict with the best interests of a child. Clinical ethics consultation is always advisable in these cases.

Imminently dying children should not be allowed to experience suffering at the end of life. Clinicians have a fiduciary responsibility to their patients and should control symptoms with appropriate medical interventions. The principles that guide the rule of double effect and sedation of highly symptomatic patients with pain or dyspnea in adults also apply in the care of children (34). The goal of therapy is to relieve distressing symptoms and not to hasten death. Consultation with palliative care and pain teams can aid clinicians with symptom management at the end of life and is recommended.

Unfortunately, a small number of children will experience intractable physical suffering that is refractory to traditional medical interventions. Parents of seriously ill children may be willing to try a variety of approaches, some of which may be potentially harmful, hoping for benefit in a desperate situation, particularly when the condition imposes a heavy burden for which mainstream therapies are insufficient (35). Of note, although some alternative medicine practices in the care of seriously ill children may be justified, there are no published guidelines for the use of these practices in children (36). In these rare circumstances, palliative sedation therapy (PST) with medications achieving continuous deep sedation (CDS) can be ethically permissible and numerous case series have demonstrated efficacy in patients for refractory suffering. Propofol is an example of one such medication and has been demonstrated to reduce pain and suffering in pediatric patients (37–39). The indications for PST at the end of life include two core components: the presence of severe suffering refractory to standard palliative management and the primary aim of relief of distress (40). We recommend that traditional therapies be maximized under a time-limited trial and ethics consultation be obtained prior to the initiation of PST in pediatric patients. Used appropriately, PST does not hasten death (41). The use of sedation for existential (emotional) suffering is discouraged (42). Figure 63.1 provides guidelines for clinicians considering PST in an imminently dying patient (Fig. 63.1).

SYMPTOM CONTROL

Pain Assessment and Management

Pain is "an unpleasant sensory and emotional experience associated with actual or potential tissue damage, or described in terms of such damage" (43). Several outstanding and more comprehensive resources are available for pain management in children (44–49). Pain is subjective in nature.

The experience of pain can be modulated by environmental, developmental, behavioral, psychological, familial, and cultural factors. Unrelieved pain for the child can produce fear, mistrust, irritability, impaired coping, and posttraumatic stress symptoms. Parents feel guilt and anger when pain is undertreated and may even lead them to consider euthanasia as a treatment alternative (50). Many children have pain at some time during their course with life-threatening illness; it can be disease related, treatment related, and/or related to psychological distress. Incidental, or traumatic, pain can still occur in a life-threatened child as well.

Pain assessment must be age-appropriate and requires a careful history and physical examination, determination of the primary cause(s) of pain, and evaluation of secondary causes and modulating features. Pain complaints should always be taken seriously; severe pain for a child is a medical emergency. Elements of the pain assessment should include the quality of the pain, region and radiation, severity, temporal factors, and provocative and palliative factors. Additional historical elements include disease stage and context, fear of pain, ability to take medication, prior analgesic use, potential role of disease-specific treatment, reactions of parents and family context, and other nonpain symptoms, including depression and/or anxiety, sleep disturbance, and most important, interference with activities of daily life, including play. Methods of pain assessment must be appropriate to the child's age, situation, emotional resources, developmental level and context, and wishes of the child and family. Ideally, pain assessment, being subjective, should be by self-report in verbal children able to communicate. For children >7 years of age, visual analog or verbal response scales that rate the pain on a horizontal or numeric scale are appropriate. For children aged 3 to 7, several validated, self-report tools are available, including Faces Scale, Oucher, poker chip tool, body maps, and pain thermometers, but more research is needed in this population of young children. The Bieri modification of the Faces Scale has improved morphometrics and score distribution (51–57).

For infants, toddlers, and preverbal children, several observation assessment scales exist, including the r-FLACC, NCCPC-PV, and the Pediatric Pain Profile Tools for the numeric assessment of pain in the cognitively impaired child have also been described (58–61). In general, pain management for children should follow the World Health Organization analgesic ladder (62). Table 63.1 lists some of the more commonly used and available medications for mild, moderate, and severe pain. Particularly for children who cannot swallow pills, the long half-life, low cost, and availability in concentrated liquid formulation make methadone a good choice for long-term analgesia and for preventing opioid withdrawal symptoms (63,64). A short initial and long terminal half-life requires judicious titration to prevent oversedation. Given the toxic metabolite accumulation and the availability of several alternatives, meperidine cannot be recommended and is excluded from the table. Medications for pain should be administered according to a regular schedule. Rescue doses should be provided for intermittent or more severe breakthrough pain. Effective management of procedural pain is as critical as expert anticipation,

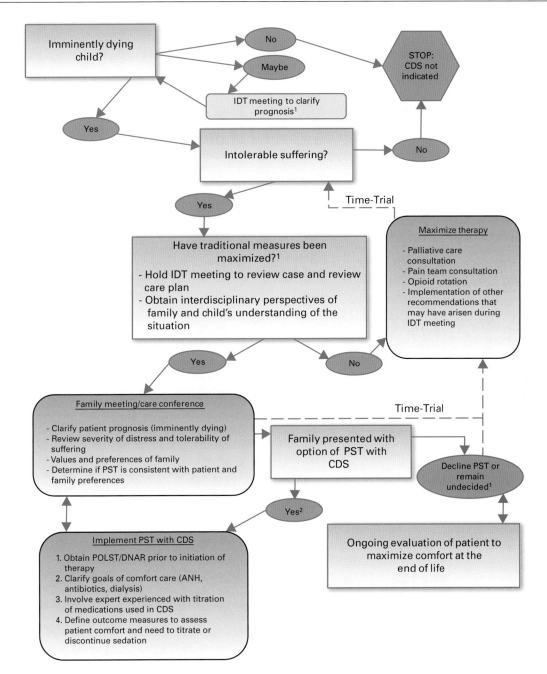

Figure 63.1. Algorithm for possible initiation of palliative sedation therapy (PST) with continuous deep sedation (CDS).

1. Consider ethics consultation if staff cannot agree with prognosis, intolerable suffering, or goals of care and this is causing staff or patient distress.
2. CDS is a rarely utilized intervention. Opportunity for controversy exists if its purpose is misunderstood or if used inappropriately. For this reason we strongly recommend ethics consultation in pediatric patients prior to initiation of PST with CDS.

prevention, and treatment of medication side effects (65,66). Depending on the etiology of the pain being treated, there are many nonopiate adjunct therapies available. Table 63.2 lists some of the more commonly used medications and their indications. For children, in particular, choose the simplest, most effective, least painful route which for most will be oral or sublingual or for those with central venous access, parenteral. Intramuscular injections should be avoided if possible. Rectal administration is possible, and many medications, including nonopiates and opiates as well as medication for nonpain symptoms, can be absorbed rectally. Subcutaneous infusion, popular in adult hospice and palliative medicine,

is possible in children but may be inadvisable for needle-phobic children. Transdermal and inhalational routes may also be used in children, but little pharmacokinetic data are available regarding their use; anecdotally, absorption and/or metabolism of transdermal fentanyl may be faster in children, requiring patch changes every 2 days if breakthrough pain occurs. Promotion of good psychosocial and spiritual care must be partnered with appropriate pharmacology (67). Children should be given choices as often as possible. Behavioral methods, such as deep breathing (blowing bubbles), progressive relaxation, and biofeedback, have a role in pain management for children. Physical methods, such as

TABLE 63.1	Opioid and nonopioid analgesics				
Drug	Initial Dose (mg/kg/dose)	Route	Interval	Maximum Dose	Formulation
Acetaminophen	10–15	p.o./p.r.	q4h	1 g/dose; 4 g/d	T, CT, L, D, S
Ibuprofen	5–10	p.o.	q6h	2.4 g/d; 3.4 g/d (adults)	T, CT, L, D
Choline magnesium trisalicylate	7.5–20	p.o.	b.i.d.–t.i.d.	1.5 g/dose	T, L
Naproxen	5–7	p.o.	q8–12h	1 g/d	T, L
Ketorolac	0.5	p.o., i.v., i.m.	q6h	30 mg/dose i.v., 10 mg/dose p.o.	I, T
Codeine	0.5–1	p.o., s.q., i.m.	q3–4h	60 mg/dose	T, L, I
Tramadol	1–2	p.o.	q6h	100 mg/dose, 400 mg/d	T
Morphine	0.2–0.5	p.o., s.l., p.r.	q3–4h	Titrate	T, L, D, S
	0.1	i.v., s.q., i.m.	q2–4h	Titrate	I
	0.3–0.6 (long-acting)	p.o.	q8–12h	Titrate	SRT
Hydromorphone	0.03–0.08	p.o., p.r.	q3–4h	Titrate	T, L, S
	0.015	i.v., s.q., i.m.	q2–4h	Titrate	I
Methadone	0.2	p.o.	q8–12h	Titrate	T, L
	0.1	i.v., s.q., i.m.	q8–12h	Titrate	I
Fentanyl	0.5–1 µg/kg/h	Transdermal	q48–72h	Titrate	P
	5–15 µg/kg (sedative)	t.m.	q4–6h	Titrate	LO
	1–2 µg/kg	i.v., s.q.	q1–2h	Titrate	I
Oxycodone	0.05–0.15	p.o.	q6h	Titrate	T, L
	0.1–0.3 (long-acting)	p.o.	q12h	Titrate	SRT

CT, chewable tablet; D, drops; I, injection; L, liquid; LO, lozenge; P, patch; S, suppository; SRT, sustained-release tablet; T, tablet or capsule.

touch therapies, including massage, transcutaneous electrical nerve stimulation, physical therapy, heat/cold, and acupuncture and/or acupressure, for example, are helpful adjuncts. Cognitive modalities, including distraction, music, art, play, imagery, and hypnosis, are also effective in children. Studies have demonstrated efficacy of many of these modalities alone or in combination with pharmacologic therapies (68,69).

These therapies should be approached from a family-centered perspective; parents can easily be taught many of these techniques. Providing effective tools for parental involvement in symptom management should increase feelings of control in an often uncontrollable situation.

Respiratory Symptoms

Dyspnea is a term used to describe a feeling of breathlessness. It is a distressing symptom for children and families; it can be a major detriment to comfort and quality of life in advanced disease. In many cases, it is also associated with shorter survival. Possible causes include tumor metastases, pneumonia, effusions, or neuromuscular problems that impair breathing. Measurement of dyspnea is difficult as it is subjective and does not correlate well with respiratory rate, work of breathing, or oxygen level. The Dalhousie Dyspnea Scales have been validated for use in children aged 6 to 18 years (70). In older children, the modified Borg scale or 15-count breathlessness score may be useful (71). Care of patients with dyspnea typically involves treatment of the underlying cause, if possible, oxygen, oral and/or parenteral opiates, and/or benzodiazepines (72). Nebulized morphine does not appear to be superior to other routes of administration in the treatment of dyspnea (73). Some patients may benefit from using a fan with cold air blowing on the face, pulmonary rehabilitation, and chest physiotherapy to mobilize secretions (74–76). Interestingly, the use of supplemental oxygen has not been found to be more beneficial than air inhalation in adults

TABLE 63.2 Adjuvant drugs useful in pediatric pain management

Drug	Initial Dose (mg/kg/dose)	Route	Interval	Maximum Dose	Formulation	Indication
Amitriptyline	0.1	p.o.	q.h.s.	2 mg/kg/d	T, I	Neuropathic pain, depression, sleep disturbance
Nortriptyline	0.2–0.5	p.o.	q.h.s.	3 mg/kg/d	T, L	Neuropathic pain, depression, sleep disturbance
Paroxetine	10 mg/dose	p.o.	q.a.m.	60 mg/d	T, L, SRT	Neuropathic pain, depression
Fluoxetine	0.2	p.o.	q.a.m.	80 mg/d	T, L, SRT, 90 mg/q/wk	Neuropathic pain, depression
Carbamazepine	2.5–5	p.o., p.r.	b.i.d.–q.i.d.	2400 mg/d	T, L, SRT, CT	Neuropathic pain
Valproic acid	5	p.o.	q.d.–t.i.d.	60 mg/kg/d	T, L, SRT	Neuropathic pain
	5	i.v.	q6–8h		I	
	10–15	p.r.	q8h		L	
Clonazepam	0.003–0.01	p.o.	t.i.d.–q.i.d.	0.2 mg/kg/d	T	Neuropathic pain
Gabapentin	5	p.o.	b.i.d.–t.i.d.	2400 mg/d	T, L	Neuropathic pain
Methylphenidate	0.1	p.o.	q4h–q24	60 mg/d	T, SRT	Coanalgesia, decreased sedation with opiates
Dextroamphetamine	0.1	p.o.	q4h–q24	40 mg/d	T, SRT	Coanalgesia, decreased sedation with opiates
Diazepam	0.1–0.2	i.v., i.m.	q2–4h	10 mg/dose	T, L, I	Anxiety, muscle spasm
	0.2–0.3	p.o.	q4–6h	10 mg/dose	T, L	
	0.3–0.5	p.r.	q2–4h	20 mg/dose	I, S	
Midazolam	0.05–0.1	i.v., s.q., i.m.	q2–4h	2.5 mg/dose	I	Anxiety, muscle spasm
	0.2–0.3	Intranasal			I	
	0.25–0.5	p.o.			L	
Lorazepam	0.05	p.o., s.l., p.r., i.v., i.m.	q4–6h	2 mg/dose	T, L, I	Anxiety, muscle spasm
Dexamethasone	Varies by indication	p.o., i.v., i.m., s.q.	q6–12h	10 mg/dose	T, L, I	Bone pain, increased intracranial pressure

CT, chewable tablet; I, injection; L, liquid; S, suppository; SRT, sustained release tablet or capsule; T, tablet or capsule.

with end-stage dyspnea (77). There are no studies to support the use of supplemental oxygen in children at the end of life although practical experience suggests that this treatment may have additional psychological benefits for the parents of the sick child.

Gastrointestinal Symptoms

Gastrointestinal symptoms are commonly seen in children at the end of life. These include nausea and vomiting, constipation, diarrhea, gastroesophageal reflux, and anorexia-cachexia syndrome. These symptoms cause significant distress and diminish function and quality of life (78). In young children, nausea may manifest as inactivity, weakness, irritability, and poor appetite. In older children, self-report is the preferred method of assessment. Nausea and vomiting may be secondary to gastrointestinal illness such as gastroenteritis, constipation, gastric stasis, gastroesophageal reflux, eosinophilic esophagitis, ileus, peritoneal irritation, pancreatitis, obstruction, intussusception, appendicitis, food poisoning, or overfeeding. Pyloric stenosis, necrotizing enterocolitis, Hirschsprung disease, hepatobiliary disease, intestinal malformation, and dietary protein intolerance may be sources of nausea and vomiting in the neonate. Gastritis and gastroparesis may be a source of symptoms in the neurologically impaired child. Other neurologic causes of nausea and vomiting include increased intracranial pressure secondary to brain tumor, subdural hemorrhage, and obstructive hydrocephalus. Middle ear disease or some brain tumors may cause nausea and vomiting from stimulation of the vestibular pathway. Certain medications, including chemotherapy, opioids, antibiotics, nonsteroidal anti-inflammatory agents, and anticholinergics, can cause severe nausea and vomiting. Urinary tract infections, pharyngitis, systemic infections, as well as other illnesses, such as congenital adrenal hyperplasia, inborn errors of metabolism, and Reye's syndrome, can also present with emesis. Anticipatory nausea and vomiting may reflect the presence of anxiety and stress. Postoperative nausea and vomiting is also a common occurrence in children. Unsuspected pregnancy may be a source of nausea and vomiting in adolescent girls. Identification of the source and mechanism of these symptoms is important in order to select the appropriate therapy. Table 63.3 lists some of the antiemetics used in the treatment of children. Prokinetic agents, such as metoclopramide, are useful in the treatment of ileus and intestinal hypomotility. Antihistamines (e.g., diphenhydramine, dimenhydrinate, and meclizine), phenothiazines (e.g., promethazine and chlorpromazine), and butyrophenones (e.g., haloperidol) are useful in the treatment of centrally mediated nausea and vomiting. Ondansetron and granisetron, which are 5-HT3 antagonists, are the treatment of choice in chemotherapy and radiation therapy–induced and postoperative nausea and vomiting. Addition of an oral neurokinin-1 antagonist such as aprepitant can provide superior protection against nausea and vomiting caused by highly emetogenic chemotherapy (79). Corticosteroids have intrinsic antiemetic properties and potentiate the effect of other antiemetics. Cannabinoids have antiemetic properties and may be beneficial to some pediatric patients. Benzodiazepines may reduce anxiety and the likelihood of anticipatory nausea. Nondrug measures for palliation of nausea and vomiting that may enhance the effect of antiemetic drugs include acupuncture, psychological techniques, and transcutaneous electrical nerve stimulation (80).

Constipation may be defined as the passage of small hard feces infrequently and with difficulty. Most cases of constipation in children are considered functional and not associated with a particular physical or biochemical abnormality. In the palliative care setting, however, constipation can often be traced to an organic source. In the child with severe constipation clinicians must learn to recognize encopresis, which may be mistaken by diarrhea, fecal impaction, and intestinal obstruction. On physical examination, clay-like masses may be palpated in a partially distended abdomen and hard stools may be palpated on rectal examination. Opioids, vincristine, and drugs with anticholinergic effects, such as phenothiazines and tricyclic antidepressants, may cause constipation. Other causes include malignant intestinal obstruction and metabolic conditions such as dehydration, cystic fibrosis, hypothyroidism, and hypercalcemia. Spinal cord injuries or other neuromuscular illnesses may be associated with constipation as well. Opioid-induced constipation occurs due to the action of these medications on the peripheral mu receptors in the gastrointestinal tract. This action triggers delayed gastric emptying via constriction of the pyloric sphincter, decreased peristalsis and increased absorption of water and electrolytes from the gastrointestinal tract, and increased anal sphincter tone, all of which contribute to constipation development (81). As in adults, prophylactic measures are the first line of intervention (82). Mobility, adequate fluid intake, and increased fiber in the diet are helpful. Also, children must be encouraged to attempt defecation after meals to take advantage of the gastrocolic reflex. Hospital staff must allow children privacy for defecation and, whenever possible, the use of a commode or lavatory rather than a bedpan should be encouraged. While useful, however, children at the end of life may not be able to take advantage of these options due to decreased oral intake, decreased wakefulness, or altered mobility. Treatment of constipation in children includes a variety of oral laxatives and/or enemas. Patients with hard stools can receive laxatives with predominately softening action such as mineral oil, lactulose, or docusate sodium. If on physical examination the rectum is full of soft feces, a predominantly peristalsis-stimulating agent such as senna or bisacodyl may be indicated. Osmotic laxatives, such as polyethylene glycol or magnesium citrate, and rectal laxatives, such as glycerin suppositories, sodium docusate, or sodium phosphate enemas, can also be used in symptomatic children with severe constipation (83). Maintenance therapy may be necessary for patients with chronic constipation. The use of laxatives in these patients does not lead to dependence. Mineral oil does not cause malabsorption of fat-soluble vitamins and may be used in children as part of a maintenance regimen but should be avoided in neurologically impaired

TABLE 63.3 Antiemetics					
Drug	Initial Dose (mg/kg/dose)	Route	Interval	Maximum Dose	Formulation
Butyrophenones					
Droperidol	0.05–0.06	i.m., i.v.	q4–6h	2.5–5 mg/dose	I
Haloperidol	0.01–0.05	p.o., i.m., i.v., s.q.	q8–12h	0.15 mg/kg/d	T, L, I
Prokinetic agents					
Metoclopramide	0.1–0.2 (postoperative)	p.o., i.m., i.v., s.q.	q6–8h	10 mg/dose	T, L, I
	1–2 (chemo-induced)	p.o., i.v.	q2–4h		
Phenothiazines					
Promethazine	0.25–1.0	p.o., i.m., i.v., p.r.	q4–6h	25 mg/dose	T, L, I, S
Chlorpromazine	0.5–1.0	p.o., p.r.	q4–6h	200 mg/d	T, L, I, S
	0.5–1.0	i.m., i.v.	q6–8h	75 mg/d	
Prochlorperazine	0.1–0.15	p.o., i.m.	q6–8h	2.5 mg/dose	T, L, I, S
Thiethylperazine	10 mg/dose (>12 y)	p.o., i.m., p.r.	q8–24h	10 mg/dose	T, I, S
Antihistamines					
Diphenhydramine	0.5–1.0	p.o., i.m., i.v.	q6–8h	300 mg/d	T, L, I
Dimenhydrinate	0.5–1.0	p.o., i.m., i.v.	q6–8h	150 mg/d	T, CT, L, I
Hydroxyzine	2 mg/kg/d	p.o., i.m.	q6–8h	100 mg/dose	T, L, I
Meclizine	25 mg/dose (>12 y)	p.o.	q12–24h	100 mg/d	T, CT
Trimethobenzamide	5.0	p.o., i.m., p.r.	q6–8h	200 mg/dose	T, I, S
Serotonin antagonists					
Ondansetron	0.1–0.15	p.o., i.v.	t.i.d.	8 mg/dose	T, L, I
Granisetron	0.01–0.02	p.o., i.v.	q.d., b.i.d.	2 mg/d	T, I
Steroids					
Dexamethasone	0.1–0.2	p.o., i.v., s.q.	q4–6h	20 mg/dose	T, L, I
Cannabinoids					
Dronabinol	5 mg/m²	p.o.	q4–6h	20 mg/d	T

CT, chewable tablet; I, injection; L, liquid; S, suppository; T, tablet or capsule.

children at risk for bronchoaspiration. The use of biofeedback in the treatment of constipation has not been clearly defined (84). In patients in whom oral medications are not feasible or tolerated, treatment of constipation proves to be difficult. Recently, the development and FDA approval of subcutaneously administered methylnaltrexone has proven helpful in adults with opioid-induced constipation (85,86). This medication, with the addition of a methyl group to naltrexone, allows the medication to react only with gastrointestinal tract μ-receptors, thus allowing analgesia centrally, but lessening peripheral side effects. This medication improves oral to cecal transit time, thus allowing for easier defection.

As useful as the medication can be in adults, it is not yet FDA approved for use in children. However, there are case reports of its use in both injectable and enteral forms (87).

Diarrhea, one of the most common problems encountered by pediatricians, is defined as the passage of frequent, loose stools. Viral, bacterial, and parasitic infections are among the most common causes of acute diarrhea. Most patients with acute diarrhea have viral gastroenteritis, especially if stools are watery and do not contain either blood or mucus (88). Patients with fever, abdominal cramps, and/or bloody stools most likely have dysentery syndrome and should be treated empirically with trimethoprim/sulfamethoxazole while awaiting results of culture and bacterial susceptibility (89). Diarrhea persisting for longer than 3 weeks is said to be chronic and may be linked to serious organic noninfectious diseases such as anatomic defects, malabsorption syndromes, endocrinopathies, and neoplasms. Dehydration is particularly common in young children with diarrhea and vomiting. Aggressive, prophylactic treatment with hydration solutions (e.g., Pedialyte) and careful follow-up are paramount to prevent serious complications. Products containing salicylates (e.g., bismuth subsalicylate) should be avoided in children. The use of kaolin/pectin and probiotics appear to be a useful adjunct to rehydration solutions (90).

Gastroesophageal reflux is particularly common in children with neurologic impairment, some of whom may require surgical fundoplication to reduce symptoms and decrease the risk of aspiration pneumonia. Useful medications include aluminum hydroxide with or without magnesium hydroxide, calcium carbonate, and H_2-receptor blockers (e.g., ranitidine) and proton pump inhibitors (e.g., omeprazole and lansoprazole) (91).

Anorexia and cachexia can be the result of prolonged illness such as cancer, acquired immunodeficiency syndrome, and pulmonary or cardiac disease. Children receiving cancer treatment may also develop cancer treatment–related cachexia. In patients with advanced disease, particularly solid tumors, anorexia-cachexia syndrome often correlates with poor quality of life and poor outcome. Patients with anorexia-cachexia have diminished caloric intake, increased basal energy expenditure, progressive loss of lean body mass, and weight loss. While decreased oral intake is often a natural development at the end of life, it can cause distress for children and their families due to social associations with food preparation and eating (78). The underlying cause should be delineated in order to choose appropriate treatment, if indicated. For patients experiencing cachexia as a result of prolonged, chronic childhood diseases, megestrol acetate, a synthetic progesterone derivative, appears promising as an agent to reverse the growth failure observed in these patients but may cause symptomatic adrenal suppression requiring treatment with hydrocortisone (92). Cyproheptadine can be used as an appetite stimulant and has been proven helpful to prevent further weight loss in children with cancer-associated cachexia (93). Corticosteroids and cannabinoids may also have a therapeutic role in some patients. While a hypercaloric diet is not sufficient to reverse the syndrome, enteral nutritional supplementation may be appropriate in some cases. Parenteral nutrition support may be appropriate for patients in whom nutritional support is required for a short period of time or in patients for whom the enteral route is not feasible.

Pruritus

Pruritus may be multifactorial in children but is most commonly related to dry skin or to medication side effects, in particular, opiates. There are no standardized assessment tools for pruritus. Physical signs include excoriation, lichenification, and/or erythema. Patients may show behavioral clues such as rubbing of eyes, nose, and/or other skin surfaces. Treatment depends upon the cause; topical therapy with moisturizers and emollients may ameliorate itching associated with dry skin. Systemic corticosteroids may be effective for the severe pruritus associated with progressive lymphomas. For drug-induced pruritus, modification of the drug regimen is the best therapy. If children must be maintained on a medication associated with pruritus, appropriate pharmacotherapy should be instituted, including antihistamines or opiate antagonists such as nalbuphine or low-dose naloxone (94).

Bone Marrow Failure

Bone marrow failure is most often associated with progressive leukemias or solid tumor with marrow involvement. It may lead to fatigue from progressive anemia, infection related to leukopenia, and bleeding as a result of thrombocytopenia. These may diminish the child's ability, and often the parent's willingness, to allow the child to fully participate in the activities of daily living. Decisions regarding interventions must be made based on quality of life goals; parents and providers alike often must be weaned from their adherence to following blood counts. Palliative transfusions may be a part of an overall care plan for a child with end-stage leukemia or other bone marrow disorders. Packed red blood cell may be indicated, for example, for a leukemic child who is still able to go to school, whereas they may not be indicated for an unresponsive, bedbound child. Platelet transfusions may be indicated to control or prevent bleeding. For neutropenic patients, proactive decisions may be made regarding the level of intervention for infection, be it comfort measures only, oral broad-spectrum antibiotics, or parental antibiotics, depending upon parent and child preferences in care. The presence of bone marrow failure impacts the way in which the child receives medical care. Children with leukemia, for example, are less likely than patients with solid tumors to receive hospice care and less likely to have support withdrawn (95).

Urinary Symptoms

Urinary retention is often a side effect of medications with anticholinergic properties, with urinary infection, or in children with metastasizing tumors or spinal cord involvement. Treatments may include medication changes, catheterization, physical measures such as compresses or gentle pressure to the bladder, cholinergic medications such as bethanechol, or opiate antagonists for opiate-induced retention (96).

Fatigue

Fatigue is one of the most prevalent symptoms in children dying with cancer (97). It is a nonspecific symptom that is difficult to measure and describe due to its subjective nature and the lack of confirmed physiologic and laboratory indicators.

Symptoms of fatigue may include physical weakness, mental exhaustion, disruption of sleep, reduced energy, emotional withdrawal, decreased play, or participation in usual activities. Fatigue may be observed in a wide variety of childhood illnesses, including infectious, inflammatory, malignant, and chronic processes, or psychological conditions such as stress, anxiety, and depression. Some medications, including chemotherapeutic regimens used in the treatment of cancer, can cause fatigue and generalized weakness (98).

Fatigue measurement instruments have been developed and tested (99). Common causes of prolonged fatigue, such as anemia, hypothyroidism, sleep disturbances, anxiety, and depression, should be excluded. A good history and physical examination may point to other potential causes that may respond to therapy. If available, treatment should be directed at the medical or psychiatric condition most likely associated with fatigue. In addition, a graded and gradual increase in exercise and rehabilitation may be helpful. Cognitive-behavioral approaches may also be an effective counseling technique to assist the child in switching to a more adaptive coping strategy. Whenever possible, graded reintegration with peer and school activities is recommended. The use of drugs has not been explored well in children. Steroids, transfusion of blood products, thyroxine, recombinant erythropoietin, and methylphenidate have been used in the treatment of fatigue with varying results (100).

Neurologic Symptoms

Some of the more common and distressing neurologic symptoms in children with malignant disease may include seizures, headaches, and sleep disturbances. Children with neurodegenerative disorders or static encephalopathies may suffer from muscle weakness, muscle spasms, contractures, progressive immobility, and loss or nongain of developmental milestones and communication difficulties. An interdisciplinary and proactive approach to these complex symptoms coupled with patient–family education is paramount.

Seizures in children with malignancy are often due to primary or metastatic brain lesions, metabolic disturbances, or as a side effect of chemoradiotherapy or medications. For children with known seizures, maintenance medications are appropriate; for children at risk for seizures, availability of at least one anticonvulsant in the home should be planned. For children unable to take medications orally, as most would be during a generalized seizure, administration of several agents by alternative routes is possible, including valproic acid, phenytoin, pentobarbital, lorazepam, and diazepam rectally, lorazepam sublingually, midazolam and phenobarbital subcutaneously, and fosphenytoin, phenobarbital, and lorazepam intramuscularly. Rectal diazepam gel provides premeasured medication in a convenient dose delivery device: its efficacy and safety in childhood have been demonstrated in randomized clinical trials (101).

Headache, like seizures, is often multifactorial. A careful history and examination of the child will often suggest the cause. Increased intracranial pressure may result in symptoms associated with headache, such as nausea, vomiting, photophobia, lethargy, transient neurologic deficits, and severe irritability, in the preverbal child. Depending on the cause, increased intracranial pressure may be treated with surgery, chemotherapy, radiotherapy, steroids, or expectant management only. Immediate and aggressive use of analgesics, antiemetics, and, often, benzodiazepines is critical for the management of rapidly escalating headache.

For children oversedated from opiates, the addition of adjuvant medications may permit dose reductions. Psychostimulants such as methylphenidate or dexamphetamine have been used empirically to improve the quality of life. The use of long-acting oral preparations or continuous parenteral infusions may reduce periods of increased sedation due to large bolus doses.

Sleep disturbance and insomnia in children are often undetected unless specifically elicited in the history. Problem sleeplessness in children may result from behavioral, circadian, biological, or medical abnormalities. In chronically ill children, the presence of other symptoms, such as pain, dyspnea, and wheezing, and emotional symptoms, such as anxiety, may be contributing factors and should be treated aggressively. Hypnotics are the mainstay of therapy for inadequate sleep; low-dose tricyclic antidepressants, such as amitriptyline, may also be appropriate, particularly for children also presenting with neuropathic pain (102).

In our experience, delirium at the end of life is a common experience frequently unrecognized by pediatric healthcare providers. It is a state of altered consciousness, confusion, and reversal of the sleep–wake cycle that develops acutely and may fluctuate throughout the day. Delirium may be secondary to opioids or anticholinergics, infection, dehydration, renal or liver abnormalities, or psychosocial or spiritual distress. Management involves treating the underlying cause of delirium. Benzodiazepines (i.e., lorazepam) and antipsychotic medications (i.e., haloperidol) are often helpful to manage agitation, mental confusion, and restlessness.

PSYCHOSOCIAL SUPPORT

Family Communication

The death of a child is perhaps the most catastrophic loss a human being can face and is inherently difficult to prepare for. Psychosocial support in palliative care calls for attention to effective communication and informed decision making to assure optimum quality of life and to decrease suffering in all of its dimensions surrounding the death of a child (103). Open, age-appropriate communication helps the sick child deal with uncertainty (104). Good psychosocial care encompasses listening empathically, asking questions, providing honest information, talking about feelings and fears, and identifying hopes and realistic goals of care. Central to the existence of the dying person, adult and child alike, is the need to have meaningful relationships, a sense of completion in one's life, a sense of meaning, and a sense of unconditional love.

The beliefs, attitudes, and functional dynamics of individual family members, the family unit, as well as of the extended community can have a significant influence on the child's experience of his or her illness and possible death. Sick children and their parents need to feel in control of some aspects of their lives. For children, maintaining a sense of normalcy is equally important. Effective interventions are often those that aim to help patients understand their condition, to participate in the decision-making process, and to restore their sense of personal integrity, dignity, autonomy, self-mastery, and self-control. There is evidence of effectiveness for interventions incorporating cognitive-behavioral techniques on variables such as self-efficacy, self-management of disease, family functioning, psychosocial well-being, reduced isolation, social competence, hope, and pain (105). Family support and family therapy are important means of intervention for seriously ill children and their families to improve family function, particularly cohesiveness, conflict resolution, and expression of thoughts and feelings (106). Honest, open age-appropriate communication should also occur with siblings of the ill child. Table 63.4 describes the illness experience according to the child's stage of cognitive development.

The psychological adaptation of the primary caregivers to the challenges of serious illness is important for the mental health of the children (107). Generally speaking, families must be supported in the "letting go" process and supported as they face anticipatory grieving and in their quest to fulfill the universal needs of meaning, purpose, value, self-worth, and a sense of competence in the care of their child (108). Psychosocial interventions in palliative care should encourage honest communication between children, their families, and healthcare professionals and strengthen interpersonal relationships so that they may feel connected and part of each other (109). The palliative care team can gently encourage the patient and the family to act on the opportunities for reconciliation, to express their love for each other, their forgiveness of past transgressions, and their gratitude.

Grief and Bereavement

The death of a child is one of the most intense, painful events that a parent can experience. The untimely loss of a child goes against the expected natural life order of events. Numerous studies have shown that parental grief is more intense and longer lasting than other types of grief (110,111). The loss of a child has been associated with increased risk of negative physical and psychosocial health events such as psychological and physical illness, marital problems, and increased mortality (112–114). Clinically significant depression is present in 20% to 25% of bereaved parents (115). Families with low cohesion, high conflict, and poor conflict resolution report higher intensity of grief and psychosocial morbidity (106).

Bereavement is the objective situation of losing someone significant through death, and the adjustment that follows. Grief refers to the distress resulting from bereavement and includes the complex cognitive, emotional, and social difficulties. Responses to bereavement are influenced by many variables: age and stage of development, gender, history of previous loss or trauma, relationship quality with the deceased, psychiatric history, and the type of loss (anticipated, traumatic, and violent) (116). When loss is unanticipated, it places the bereaved at increased risk for grief complications; with less time to prepare for the end of life, the subset of parents whose children die unexpectedly or suddenly during therapy may be at increased risk for negative grief sequelae. Parents of children who receive stem cell transplant as the last cancer therapy often have little time to recognize their child has no realistic chance of cure and may benefit from ongoing discussions regarding goals and prognosis while undergoing transplant (117). Legacy building is often helpful for families who are adjusting to the anticipated death of a child (118). Members of the care team can facilitate discussions about legacy building between the child and family members in order to help them create legacy items such as memory books, photos, and artwork in order to enable discussions about the impending death and honoring the child's wishes.

Familial relationships, social networks, religion, and culture influence the expression of grief. The ability to make meaning of the loss and articulate positive outcomes of a loved one is fundamental to the grieving process and fosters healing (119). Making meaning after the loss of a child has been shown to take longer than other losses and parents who fail to ultimately make meaning of the loss are at increased risk for poor adjustment (120,121). The inability to make sense of the experience is a risk factor for the development of complicated grief.

Parents who share their problems with others during the illness and have access to psychological support during the last month of their child's life are more likely to work through grief in the long term, particularly if they have the opportunity to discuss their child's condition with the attending staff and other members of the care team (psychologist or social work) (122). Parents appreciate efforts by staff members to support them and commemorate the deceased child and notice when, in contrast, familiar faces or condolence cards are not received (123).

Prolonged grief disorder (PGD), also known as complicated grief, is a distinct constellation of symptoms, different from depression and anxiety, which can predict health outcomes and emotional dysfunction after loss. Complicated grief is an elevated level of grief that persists for more than 6 months after the loss of a loved one and often implies an individual is suffering unresolved symptoms of grief. PGD has been characterized by intense yearning, crying, preoccupation with thoughts of the deceased, disbelief over the death, feeling stunned, and lack of acceptance. The symptoms are more marked and persistent when compared with normal grief. The rate of PGD in bereaved parents varies greatly (10% to 28%) in the literature due to different screening methodologies to identify potential cases (121). Regardless, this is higher than the rate of PGD in other general and naturally bereaved populations (~3% to 7%) and

TABLE 63.4 Illness experience

Infant

Developmental task	Achievement of awareness of being separate from significant others
Impact of illness	Potential distortion of differentiation of self from parent/significant others
Cognitive age/stage	Sensorimotor (birth through 2 y)
Major fears	Separation, strangers
Concept of death	Unable to differentiate death from temporary separation or abandonment
Spiritual interventions	Provide consistent caretakers. Minimize separation from parents and significant others. Decrease parental anxiety, which is projected to infant. Maintain crib/nursery as "safe place" where no invasive procedures are performed. Actively listen to parents, reassure parents of the adequacy of their parenting skills, encourage parental presence. Encourage/facilitate the use of spiritual support system for the family.

Toddler

Developmental task	Initiation of autonomy
Impact of illness	Interference with the development of sense of control and loss of independence
Cognitive age/stage	Preoperational thought (2–7 y): egocentric, magical, little concept of body integrity
Major fears	Separation, loss of control
Concept of illness	Phenomenism (2–7 y): perceives external, unrelated, concrete phenomena as cause of illness, e.g., "being sick because you don't feel well." Contagion: perceives cause of illness as proximity between two events that occurs by "magic," e.g., "getting a cold because you are near someone who has a cold".
Concept of death	Recognizes death in terms of immobility. Often viewed as reversible, temporary, or foreign.
Spiritual interventions	Minimize separation from parents/significant others. Keep security objects at hand. Provide simple, brief explanations. Explain and maintain consistent limits. Encourage participation in daily care, etc. Provide opportunities for play and play therapy. Set limits. Reassure the child that disease is not punishment (by God, Higher Power, or other authority figure).

Preschooler

Developmental task	Creation of sense of initiative
Impact of illness	Interference/loss of accomplishments such as walking, talking, controlling basic bodily functions
Cognitive age/stage	Preoperational thought (3–7 y): egocentric, magical, tendency to use and repeat words the child does not understand, providing own explanations and definitions. Literal translation of words. Inability to abstract.
Major fears	Bodily injury and mutilation; loss of control; the unknown; the dark; being left alone
Concept of illness	Phenomenism; contagion (3–7 y)
Concept of death	Recognizes death in terms of immobility. Often viewed as reversible, temporary, or foreign. Begins to question and develop a mature concept.
Spiritual interventions	Do not underestimate the level of comprehension. Provide simple, concrete explanations. Advance preparation is important; days for major events and hours for minor events. Verbal explanations are usually insufficient, so use pictures, models, actual equipment, and medical play. When appropriate, initiate discussion of love and caring from Higher Power to relieve anxiety and loneliness. Show behavioral qualities of love, trust, respect, caring, and setting of firm limits and disciplining without anger.

(Continued)

TABLE 63.4 Illness experience (*Continued*)

School-age child

Developmental task	Development of a sense of industry
Impact of illness	Potential feelings of inadequacy/inferiority if autonomy and independence are compromised
Cognitive age/stage	Concrete operational thought (7–10+ y): beginning of logical thought but tendency to be literal
Major fears	Loss of control; bodily injury, and mutilation; failure to live up to expectations of important others; death
Concept of illness	Contamination: perceives cause as person, object, or action external to the child that is "bad" or "harmful" to the body, e.g., "getting a cold because you didn't wear a hat." Internalization: perceives illness as having an external cause but being located inside the body, e.g., "getting a cold by breathing in air and bacteria".
Concept of death	Recognizes all the components of irreversibility, universality, nonfunctionality, and causality
Spiritual interventions	Provide choices whenever possible. Stress contact with school or organized religious peer group. Use diagrams, pictures, and models for explanations. Emphasize the "normal" things the child can do. Reassure child he/she has done nothing wrong; hospitalization, etc., is not "punishment." Be alert to anxiety about being punished by deity. Provide appropriate concrete explanations in response to questions regarding spiritual rituals; if appropriate promote prayer and relationship with child's concept of God. Model behaviors that show forgiveness and acceptance.

Adolescent

Developmental task	Achievement of a sense of identity
Impact of illness	Potential alteration/relinquishment of newly acquired roles and responsibilities
Cognitive age/stage	Formal operational thought (11+ y): beginning of ability to think abstractly. Existence of some magical thinking (e.g., feeling guilty for illness) and egocentrism.
Major fears	Loss of control; altered body image; separation from peer group
Concept of illness	Physiologic: perceives cause as malfunctioning or nonfunctioning organ or process; can explain illness in a sequence of events. Psychophysiological: realizes that psychological actions and attitudes affect health and illness.
Concept of death	Speculates on the implications and ramifications of death. Understands effect of death on other people and society as a whole. Future oriented, has difficulty in understanding reality of death as a present possibility.
Spiritual interventions	Allow adolescent to be an integral part of decision making regarding care. Give information sensitively, because this age group reacts to the content of information as well as the manner in which it is delivered. Allow as many choices and as much control as possible. Be honest about treatment and consequences. Stress what the adolescent can do for himself or herself and the importance of cooperation and compliance. Assist in maintaining contact with peer group. Provide answers without bias and enable participation in discussions of illness in terms of philosophical or spiritual beliefs. Encourage contact with friends and use of spiritual rituals if adolescent continues to use them. Observe and document verbalizations of patient's values and beliefs.

Modified from Gibbons MB. Psychosocial aspects of serious illness in childhood and adolescence. In: Armstrong-Dailey A, Zarbock-Goltzer S, eds. *Hospice Care for Children.* New York, NY: Oxford University Press; 1993:62–63. Concept of death from Faulkner KW. Children's understanding of death. In: Armstrong-Dailey A, Zarbock-Goltzer S, eds. *Hospice Care for Children.* New York, NY: Oxford University Press; 1993:9–21. Spiritual interventions from Hart D, Schneider D. Spiritual care for children with cancer. *Semin Oncol Nurs.* 1997;13:263–270.

separation distress (intrusive thoughts about the loss and yearning for the deceased) is not uncommon in parentally bereaved populations (124). Increased parent satisfaction with a child's primary oncologist during the end-of-life period has been associated with lower separation distress and total grief scores (124). Longer time elapsed from the death of a child is associated with lower grief scores suggesting symptoms of grief diminish with time.

Children's Understanding of Death

Most children suffering from a life-limiting illness understand death better than other children their age. From birth to 3 years, children grasp events at the level of feeling and action which corresponds to Piaget's sensorimotor stage of cognitive development. Children at this age may interpret death as a temporary separation or abandonment. Children of ages 3 to 6 years, preoperational stage of cognitive development according to Piaget, view death as a state of immobility, which may be temporary and reversible. The average child becomes aware of death at age 7.5, with the first death usually being an older relative (125). At this age, most children recognize the four major concepts regarding death: irreversibility, finality, inevitability, and causality (126). Between 6 and 12 years of age, Piaget's stage of concrete operations, children begin to realize that people who die are not able to function. As children enter what Piaget calls the stage of formal operations, which usually spans from 12 years of age onward, they develop the ability for abstract reasoning, and their thoughts about death are similar to those of a mature adult. It is again important to note that chronically ill and dying children, given the appropriate explanations, may come to understand concepts of death and dying well beyond that expected for their chronologic age. Stories, games, play, art, and music are among many tools that caregivers have to stimulate communication and help children freely express their thoughts and emotions.

Adolescent patients and siblings can be deeply affected by loss, particularly when the loss is a sibling or close friend. Shock, depression, loneliness, anger, difficulty sleeping, feelings of emptiness, disbelief, hopelessness, vulnerability, fear of intimacy, and guilt are typical adolescent responses to loss (119,127–129). The loss may be associated with depressive symptoms or produce high levels of death anxiety and intense grief (130). Death anxiety occurs because the loss is a tangible reminder of individual mortality and triggers concerns about their own potential for death. There is a time after loss of a loved one when adolescents are, "consumed by their irrevocably changed reality" (131). The more a teen identifies with the deceased, the more likely they are to consider their own mortality (132).

Adolescents can identify factors helpful in coping with loss. Interactions (phone calls and visiting) prior to the loss are helpful to teens, as is learning the cause of death (133). Attending a ritual service fosters public social support and has been shown to be helpful. Emotional support can be found in such things as listening, understanding feelings, or receiving a hug (127,134). Common sources of support used by teens are close friends, family, school teachers, and guidance counselors. Children and adolescents can also experience complicated grief and in these cases professional therapy may be beneficial.

Adjustment Disorder

Chronically ill children who have difficulty coping with the challenges imposed on their lives are often diagnosed as having an adjustment disorder. Children with serious and chronic illness are at increased risk for adjustment disorders (135). The severity of illness, including possible life-limiting illness, does not independently predict a person's adjustment to illness; there are many variables involved in coping with chronic or life-threatening disease (136). Low self-esteem, poor school attendance, and familial variables are mediators of the adjustment response (136). When adjustment disorder is present, it may occur with depressed mood, anxiety, disturbance of conduct, or a combination of these. Identification of children who may have difficulty adjusting is important as most of these children may benefit from appropriate behavioral and cognitive-behavioral therapies.

Anxiety

Anxiety disorders are one of the most prevalent categories of childhood and adolescent psychopathology (137). One of the dilemmas in clinical practice is to define what constitutes an anxiety disorder in comparison with normal anxiety in the presence of stressful life circumstances. Seriously ill children are under considerable personal and family strain and may experience symptoms of anxiety as a manifestation of psychological distress without meeting the criteria for diagnosis of an anxiety disorder. Children who experience difficulty functioning as a result of their anxiety symptoms may have an adaptive disorder. Some of the most common subclinical anxiety symptoms in children include over-concern about competence, excessive need for reassurance, fear of the dark, fear of harm to self or an attachment figure, and somatic complaints. Teenagers may also manifest unrealistic fears, excessive worry about past behavior, and self-consciousness as signs of increased anxiety. Working with the family system is the key way to decrease the anxiety symptoms experienced by the child (138). The aim of the therapy is to disrupt the dysfunctional patterns of interaction that promote family insecurity and to support areas of family competence. Attention to the child–parent relationship is vital to preventing and treating anxiety symptoms. Behavioral therapy, cognitive-behavioral therapy, and psychodynamic psychotherapy are useful therapeutic techniques to help the child and family in the process of coping with the challenges of a life-limiting illness. Commonly selected medications for treating anxiety symptoms include tricyclic antidepressants and selective serotonin reuptake inhibitors. Selection of the medication depends on the presence of comorbidities (139).

Depression

Major depression and dysthymia are common disorders occurring in children and adolescents. Fortunately, although children with medical problems appear to be at slightly elevated risk for depression and have higher rates of maladjustment, most children with chronic disease are not depressed. The clinical picture of depression in children and adolescents varies considerably across different developmental stages. Younger children may show more somatic complaints, auditory hallucinations, temper tantrums, and other behavioral problems. Older children may report low self-esteem, guilt, and hopelessness. The family relationships of youth with depressive symptomatology are frequently characterized by conflict, maltreatment, rejection, and problems with communication, with little expression of positive affect and support (140,141). For children at the end of life, depressive symptoms may occur as a normal reaction to grief and could suggest the need to explore their fears and concerns and find support in their search for meaning and understanding of their disease, suffering, and imminent death.

The most important tool in diagnosis of depression in children is the comprehensive psychiatric evaluation that should be conducted by a trained clinician. Standardized interviews, however, are long and may not be appropriate for children with chronic illness in whom "depressive" symptoms may be related to the illness. Psychiatric symptom checklists derived from these standardized interviews have been developed and can be useful screening tools. The treatment of depressive youth should be provided in the least restrictive treatment setting that is safe and effective for a given patient. Given the developmental and psychosocial context in which depression unfolds, pharmacotherapy alone is usually not sufficient. Treatment may include a combination of cognitive-behavioral therapy, interpersonal therapy, psychodynamic psychotherapy, and other psychotherapies. For patients requiring pharmacotherapy, selective serotonin reuptake inhibitors are the initial treatment of choice (141).

SPIRITUAL SUPPORT

Patients and their families are especially concerned with spirituality in the contexts of suffering, debilitation, and dying. Spirituality is that part of our human nature that enables us to find a sense of meaning in our experiences. Many agree that the key to emotional coping with serious illness and disability is frequently found within the matrix of spirituality. Spirituality gives us meaning and direction and brings a sense of order into our lives. This is equally true for children. Children, as well as adults, ask questions, search for a deeper understanding of their experiences, and express their emotions in response to their own interpretation of reality (142). Children are likely to base their spirituality on the relationship with their parents or other primary caregivers. Children's spirituality matures and evolves out of these

important relationships, which suggests that spiritual care should be offered to the patient as well as his or her family (143). In addition, children often take religious teachings literally and require explanations beyond these literal meanings to assist them in the process of understanding and interpreting their life experiences.

The developmental stages may assist in the determination of appropriate interventions for spiritual care for the seriously ill child (144). Spiritual interventions introduced into the mainstream of medical therapy are directed to help children articulate their questions, express their emotions, and search for creative answers (145). These activities may allow patients and their families to discover meaning and purpose in their experiences, a sense of oneness with life, of belonging to something beyond themselves, of being part of something greater. This spiritual experience of transcendence beyond the self may facilitate coping by providing a sense of order despite the experience of serious illness and death. Many times at this stage, patients and families manifest a deep yearning for life but also a willingness to accept death, and to live their lives in harmony, giving and receiving love. Inadequate staffing, inadequate training of healthcare providers to detect patients' spiritual needs, and being called to visit with patients and families too late to provide all the care that could have been provided have been identified as barriers for effective spiritual care (146). Suggested spiritual interventions are included in Table 63.4.

REFERENCES

1. Heron M, Sutton PD, Xu J, et al. Annual summary of vital statistics. *Pediatrics.* 2010;125:4-15.
2. Goldman A. *Care of the Dying Child.* Oxford: Oxford University Press; 1999.
3. Feudtner C, Hays RM, Haynes G, et al. Deaths attributed to pediatric complex chronic conditions: national trends and implications for supportive care services. *Pediatrics.* 2001;107(6):E99.
4. Feudtner C, DiGiuseppe DL, Neff JM. Hospital care for children and young adults in the last year of life: a population-based study. *BMC Med.* 2003;1(1):3.
5. Feudtner C, Christakis DA, Zimmerman FJ, et al. Characteristics of deaths occurring in children's hospitals: implications for supportive care services. *Pediatrics.* 2002;109(5):887-893.
6. Simon TD, Berry J, Feudtner C, et al. Children with complex chronic conditions in inpatient hospital settings in the United States. *Pediatrics.* 2010;126(4):647-655.
7. Burns KH, Casey PH, Lyle RE, et al. Increasing prevalence of medically complex children in US hospitals. *Pediatrics.* 2010;126(4):638-646.
8. Newacheck PW, Strickland B, Shonkoff JP, et al. An epidemiologic profile of children with special health care needs. *Pediatrics.* July 1998;102(1 pt 1):117-123.
9. Policy statement: organizational principles to guide and define the child health care system and/or improve the health of all children. *Pediatrics.* May 2004;113(5 suppl):1545-1547.
10. Liptak GS, Shone LP, Auinger P, Dick AW, Ryan SA, Szilagyi PG. Short-term persistence of high health care costs in a nationally representative sample of children. *Pediatrics.* October 2006;118(4):e1001-e1009.

11. Himelstein BP, Hilden JM, Boldt AM, et al. Pediatric palliative care. *N Engl J Med*. 2004;350(17):1752-1762.

12. Brenneis JM. Spirituality and suffering. In: Parris WC, ed. *Cancer Pain Management*. Boston, MA: Butterworth–Heinemann; 1997:507-515.

13. Byock IR. The nature of suffering and the nature of the opportunity at the end of life. *Clin Geriatr Med*. 1996;12:237-252.

14. Attig T. Beyond pain: the existential suffering of children. *J Palliat Care*. 1996;12:20-23.

15. Wolfe JW, Grier HE, Klar N, et al. Symptoms and suffering at the end of life in children with cancer. *N Engl J Med*. 2000;342:326-333.

16. Collins JJ, Devine TD, Dick GS, et al. The measurement of symptoms in young children with cancer: the validation of the memorial symptom assessment scale in children aged 7-12. *J Pain Symptom Manage*. 2002;23(1):10-16.

17. Drake R, Frost J, Collins JJ. The symptoms of dying children. *J Pain Symptom Manage*. 2003;26(1):594-603.

18. Contro N, Larson J, Scofield S, et al. Family perspectives on the quality of pediatric palliative care. *Arch Pediatr Adolesc Med*. 2002;156(1):14-19.

19. Meyer EC, Burns JP, Griffith JL, et al. Parental perspectives on end-of-life care in the pediatric intensive care unit. *Crit Care Med*. 2002;30(1):226-231.

20. Durbin M. From both sides now: a parent-physician's view of parent-doctor relationships during pediatric cancer treatment. *Pediatrics*. 1997;100:263-267.

21. Sharpe D, Rossiter L. Siblings of children with a chronic illness: a meta-analysis. *J Pediatr Psychol*. 2002;27(8):699-710.

22. American Academy of Pediatrics. Committee on bioethics and committee on hospital care. Palliative care for children. *Pediatrics*. 2000;106:351-357.

23. Wolfe J, Klar N, Grier HE, et al. Understanding of prognosis among parents of children who died of cancer: impact on treatment goals and integration of palliative care. *JAMA*. November 2000;284(19):2469-2475.

24. Cooley WC, McAllister JW, Sherrieb K, Kuhlthau K. Improved outcomes associated with medical home implementation in pediatric primary care. *Pediatrics*. July 2009;124:358-364.

25. Baker JN, Barfield R, Hinds PS, Kane JR. A process to facilitate decision making in pediatric stem cell transplantation: the individualized care planning and coordination model. *Biol Blood Marrow Transplant*. March 2007;13:245-254.

26. Baker JN, Hinds PS, Spunt SL, et al. Integration of palliative care practices into the ongoing care of children with cancer: individualized care planning and coordination. *Pediatr Clin North Am*. February 2008;55:223-250.

27. American Academy of Pediatrics. Committee on bioethics. Institutional ethics committees. *Pediatrics*. 2001;107:205-209.

28. American Academy of Pediatrics. Committee on bioethics. Guidelines on forgoing life-sustaining medical treatment. *Pediatrics*. 1994;93:532-536.

29. Freyer DR. Care of the dying adolescent: special considerations. *Pediatrics*. 2004;113:381-388.

30. American Academy of Pediatrics. Committee on bioethics. Informed consent, parental permission, and assent in pediatric practice. *Pediatrics*. 1995;95(2):314-317.

31. Feudtner C. Collaborative communication in pediatric palliative care: a foundation for problem-solving and decision-making. *Pediatr Clin North Am*. October 2007;54(5):583-607.

32. American Medical Association. Medical futility in end-of-life care. Report of the council on ethical and judicial affairs. *JAMA*. 1999;281:937-941.

33. Nelson LJ, Rushton CH, Cranford RE, et al. Forgoing medically provided nutrition and hydration in pediatric patients. *J Law Med Ethics*. 1995;23:33-46.

34. Fleischman A. Commentary: ethical issues in pediatric pain management and terminal sedation. *J Pain Symptom Manage*. 1998;15(4):260-261.

35. Angell M, Kassirer JP. Alternative medicine—the risks of untested and unregulated remedies. *N Engl J Med*. 1998;339:839-841.

36. Kemper K, Cassileth B, Ferris T. Holistic pediatrics: a research agenda. *Pediatrics*. 1999;103:902-909.

37. Glover ML, Kodish E, Reed MD. Continuous propofol infusion for the relief of treatment-resistant discomfort in a terminally ill pediatric patient with cancer. *J Pediatr Hematol Oncol*. 1996;18(4):377-380.

38. Tobias JD. Propofol sedation for terminal care in a pediatric patient. *Clin Pediatr*. 1997;36(5):291-293.

39. Anghelescu DA, Hamilton H, Faughnan LG, Johnson LM, Baker JN. Pediatric palliative sedation therapy with Propofol: recommendations based on experience in children with terminal cancer. *J Palliative Med*. June 2012 [Epub ahead of print] PMID: 22731512.

40. Morita T, Tsuneto S, Shima Y. Definition of sedation for symptom relief: a systematic literature review and a proposal of operational criteria. *J Pain Symptom Manage*. 2002;24(4):447-453.

41. Maltoni M, Pittureri C, Scarpi E, et al. Palliative sedation therapy does not hasten death: results from a prospective multicenter study. *Ann Oncol*. 2009;20(7):1163-116.

42. Kirk TW, Mahon MM. National Hospice and Palliative Care Organization (NHPCO) position statement and commentary on the use of palliative sedation in imminently dying terminally ill patients. *J Pain Symptom Manage*. 2010;39(5):914-923.

43. Pain terms: a list with definitions and notes on usage. Recommended by the IASP Subcommittee on Taxonomy. PMID: 460932. *Pain*. 1979;6(3):249-252.

44. Yaster M, Krane EJ, Kaplan RF, et al., eds. *Pediatric Pain Management and Sedation Handbook*. St. Louis, MO: Mosby; 1997.

45. Kraemer FW, Rose JB. Pharmacologic management of acute pediatric pain. *Anesthesiol Clin*. 2009 27(2): 241-268.

46. Ballas SK. Current issues in sickle cell pain and its management. *Hematology Am Soc Hematol Educ Program*. 2007:97-105.

47. Bruera ED, Portenoy RK, eds, *Cancer Pain: Assessment and Management*. 2nd ed. New York, NY: Cambridge University Press; 2010.

48. *Cancer Pain Relief and Palliative Care in Children*. Geneva: World Health Organization; 1998:76.

49. Berde CB, Sethna NF. Analgesics for the treatment of pain in children. *N Engl J Med*. 2002;347(14):1094-1103.

50. Dussel V, Joffe S, Hilden JM, Watterson-Schaeffer J, Weeks JC, Wolfe J. Considerations about hastening death among parents of children who die of cancer. *Arch Pediatr Adolesc Med*. March 2010;164(3):231-237.

51. Wong DL. *Whaley and Wong's Essentials of Pediatric Nursing*. 5th ed. St. Louis, MO: Mosby; 1997.

52. Tomlinson D, von Baeyer CL, Stionson JN, Sung L. A systematic review of faces scales for the self-report of pain intensity in children. *Pediatrics*. 2010;126:e1168.

53. Beyer JE. *The Oucher: A User's Manual and Technical Report*. Evanston, IL: Hospital Play Equipment; 1984.

54. Hester NO, Foster R, Kristensen K. Measurement of pain in children. Generalizability and validity of the pain ladder and the poker chip tool. In: Tyler DC, Krane EJ, eds. *Pediatric*

Pain: Advances in Pain Research and Therapy. Vol 15. New York, NY: Raven Press; 1990:79-84.

55. Finley GA, McGrath PJ. *Measurement of Pain in Infants and Children.* Seattle, WA: IASP Press; 1998.

56. Goodenough B, Addicoat L, Champion GD, et al. Pain in 4- to 6-year-old children receiving intramuscular injections: a comparison of the faces pain scale with other self-report and behavioral measures. *Clin J Pain.* 1997;13(1):60-73.

57. Hicks CL, von Baeyer CL, Spafford PA, et al. The faces pain scale-revised: toward a common metric in pediatric pain measurement. *Pain.* 2001;93(2):173-183.

58. Malviya S, Voepel-Lewis T, Burke C, Merkel S, Tait AR. The revised FLACC observational pain tool: improved reliability and validity for pain assessment in children with cognitive impairment. *Paediatr Anaesth.* 2006;16(3):258.

59. Breau LM, McGrath PJ, Camfield CS, Finley GA. Psychometric properties of the non-communicating children's pain checklist-revised. *Pain.* 2002;99(1-2):349.

60. Hunt AM. A survey of signs, symptoms and symptom control in 30 terminally ill children. *Dev Med Child Neurol.* 1990;32(4):341.

61. Solodiuk J, Curley MA. Pain assessment in nonverbal children with severe cognitive impairments: the Individualized Numeric Rating Scale (INRS). *J Pediatr Nurs.* 2003;18(4):295-299.

62. McGrath PA. Development of the World Health Organization Guidelines on cancer pain relief and palliative care in children. *J Pain Symptom Manage.* 1996;12(2):87.

63. Shir Y, Rosen G, Zeldin A, et al. Methadone is safe for treating hospitalized patients with severe pain. *Can J Anaesth.* 2001;48(11):1109-1113.

64. Siddappa R, Fletcher JE, Heard AM, et al. Methadone dosage for prevention of opioid withdrawal in children. *Paediatr Anaesth.* 2003;13(9):805-810.

65. Young KD. Pediatric procedural pain. *Ann Emerg Med.* 2005;45(2):160-171.

66. Murat I, Gall O, Tourniaire B. Procedural pain in children: evidence-based best practice and guidelines. *Reg Anesth Pain Med.* 2003;28(6):561-572.

67. Howard RF. Current status of pain management in children. *JAMA.* 2003;290(18):2464-2469.

68. Mercadante S. Cancer pain management in children. *Palliat Med.* 2004;18(7):654-662.

69. Uman LS, Chambers CT, McGrath PJ, Kisely S. Psychological interventions for needle-related procedural pain and distress in children and adolescents. *Cochrane Database Syst Rev.* 2006;4:CD005179.

70. McGrath PJ, Pianosi PT, Unruh AM, Buckley CP. Dalhousie dyspnea scales: construct and content validity of pictorial scales for measuring dyspnea. *BMC Pediatr.* 2005;5:33.

71. Prasad SA, Randall SD, Balfour-Lynn IM. Fifteen-count breathlessness score: an objective measure for children. *Pediatr Pulmonol.* 2000;30(1):56-62.

72. Ben-Aharon I, Gafter-Gvili A, Paul M, Leibovici L, Stemmer SM. Interventions for alleviating cancer-related dyspnea: a systematic review. *J Clin Oncol.* 2008;26(14):2396.

73. Bruera E, Sala R, Spruyt O, Palmer JL, Zhang T, Willey J. Nebulized versus subcutaneous morphine for patients with cancer dyspnea: a preliminary study. *J Pain Symptom Manage.* 2005;29(6):613.

74. Galbraith S, Fagan P, Perkins P, Lynch A, Booth S. Does the use of a handheld fan improve chronic dyspnea? A randomized, controlled, crossover trial. *J Pain Symptom Manage.* 2010;39(5):831.

75. Lanken PN, Terry PB, Delisser HM, et al. An official American Thoracic Society clinical policy statement: palliative care for patients with respiratory diseases and critical illnesses. *Am J Respir Crit Care Med.* 2008;177(8):912.

76. Bausewein C, Booth S, Gysels M, Higginson I. Non-pharmacological interventions for breathlessness in advanced stages of malignant and non-malignant diseases. *Cochrane Database Syst Rev.* 2008;2:CD005623.

77. Cranston JM, Crockett A, Currow D. Oxygen therapy for dyspnoea in adults. *Cochrane Database Syst Rev.* 2008;3:CD004769.

78. Santucci G, Mack J. Common gastrointestinal symptoms in pediatric palliative care: nausea, vomiting, constipation, anorexia, cachexia. *Pediatr Clin North Am.* 2007;54:673-689.

79. Hesketh PJ, Grunberg SM, Gralla RJ, et al. The oral neurokinin-1 antagonist aprepitant for the prevention of chemotherapy-induced nausea and vomiting: a multinational, randomized, double-blind, placebo-controlled trial in patients receiving high-dose cisplatin – the Aprepitant Protocol 052 Study Group. *J Clin Oncol.* 2003;21(22):4112.

80. Burish TG, Tope DM. Psychological techniques for controlling the adverse side effects of cancer chemotherapy. Finding from a decade of research. *J Pain Symptom Manage.* 1992;7:287-301.

81. Kyle G. Constipation and palliative care – where are we now? *Int J Palliat Nurs.* January 2007;13(1):6-16.

82. Roma E, Adamidis D, Nikolara R, et al. Diet and chronic constipation in children: the role of fiber. *J Pediatr Gastroenterol Nutr.* 1999;28:169-174.

83. Bell EA, Wall GC. Pediatric constipation therapy using guidelines and polyethylene glycol 3350. *Ann Pharmacother.* 2004;38(4):686-693.

84. Heymen S, Jones KR, Scarlett Y, et al. Biofeedback treatment of constipation: a critical review. *Dis Colon Rectum.* 2003;46(9):1208-1217.

85. Lang L. The food and drug administration approvesmethylnaltrexone bromide for opioid-induced constipation. *Gastroenterology.* 2008;135(1):6.

86. Moss J and Rosow CE. Development of peripheral opioid antagonists: new insights into opioid effects. *Mayo Clin Proc.* 2008;83(10):1116-1130.

87. Lee JM and Mooney J. Methylnaltrexone in treatment of opioid-induced constipation in a pediatric patient. *Clin J Pain.* 2011; E-pub ahead of print August 26, 2011.

88. Clark B, McKendrick M. A review of viral gastroenteritis. [Review] [104 refs] [Journal Article. Review. Review, Tutorial]. *Curr Opin Infect Dis.* 2004;17(5):461-469.

89. Nataro J. Treatment of bacterial enteritis. *Pediatr Infect Dis J.* 1998;17:420-421.

90. Allen SJ, Okoko B, Martinez E, Gregorio G, Dans LF. Probiotics for treating infectious diarrhea. *Cochrane Database Syst Rev.* 2006;2:CD003048.

91. Israel DM, Hassel E. Omeprazole and other proton pump inhibitors: pharmacology, efficacy, and safety, with special reference to use in children. *J Pediatr Gastroenterol Nutr.* 1998;27:568-577.

92. Orme LM, Bond JD, Humphrey MS, et al. Megestrol acetate in pediatric oncology patients may lead to severe, symptomatic adrenal suppression. *Cancer.* 2003;98(2):397-405.

93. Couluris M, Mayer JL, Freyer DR, Sandler E, Xu P, Krischer JP. The effect of cyproheptadine hydrochloride (periactin) and megestrol acetate (megace) on weight in children with cancer/treatment-related cachexia. *J Pediatr Hematol Oncol.* 2008; 30:791-797.

94. Maxwell LG, Kaufmann SC, Bitzer S, et al. The effects of a small-dose naloxone infusion on opioid-induced side effects and analgesia in children and adolescents treated with intravenous patient-controlled analgesia: a double-blind, prospective, randomized, controlled study. *Anesth Analg.* 2005;100(4):953-958.

95. Klopfenstein KJ, Hutchison C, Clark C, et al. Variables influencing end-of-life care in children and adolescents with cancer. *J Pediatr Hematol Oncol.* 2001;23(8):481-486.

96. Yamanishi T, Yasuda K, Kamai T, et al. Combination of a cholinergic drug and an alpha-blocker is more effective than monotherapy for the treatment of voiding difficulty in patients with underactive detrusor. [Clinical Trial. Journal Article. Randomized Controlled Trial]. *Int J Urol.* 2004;11(2):88-96.

97. Hockenberry M. Symptom management research in children with cancer. [Review] [38 refs] [Journal Article. Review. Review, Tutorial]. *J Pediatr Oncol Nurs.* 2004;21(3):132-136.

98. Viner R, Christie D. Fatigue and somatic symptoms. *BMJ.* 2005;330(7498):1012-1015.

99. Hockenberry MJ, Hinds PS, Barrera P, et al. Three instruments to assess fatigue in children with cancer: the child, parent and staff perspectives. *J Pain Symptom Manage.* 2005;25(4):319-328.

100. Mock V, Atkinson A, Barsevick A, et al. National Comprehensive Cancer Network. NCCN Practice Guidelines for cancer-related fatigue. *Oncology.* 2000;14(11A):151-161.

101. Dreifuss FE, Rosman NP, Cloyd JC, et al. A comparison of rectal diazepam gel and placebo for acute repetitive seizures. *N Engl J Med.* 1998;338(26):1869-1875.

102. Sheldon SH. Insomnia in children. *Curr Treat Options Neurol.* 2001;3:37-50.

103. Chesson RA, Chisholm D, Zaw W. Counseling children with chronic physical illness. *Patient Educ Couns.* 2004;55(3):331-338.

104. Beale EA, Baile WF, Aaron J. Silence is not golden: communicating with children dying from cancer. *J Clin Oncol.* 2005;23(15):3629-3631.

105. Barlow JH, Ellard DR. Psycho-educational interventions for children with chronic disease, parents and siblings: an overview of the research evidence base. *Child Care Health Dev.* 2004;30(6):637-645.

106. Kissane DW, Bloch SB, Onghena P, et al. The Melbourne family grief study I: perceptions of family functioning in bereavement. *Am J Psychiatry.* 1996;153:650-658.

107. Johnson G, Kent G, Leather J. Strengthening the parent-child relationship: a review of family interventions and their use in medical settings. *Child Care Health Dev.* 2005;31(1):25-32.

108. Byock I. *Dying Well.* New York, NY: Riverhead; 1997.

109. Kane JR, Hellsten MB, Coldsmith A. Human suffering: the need for relationship-based research in pediatric end-of-life care. *J Pediatr Oncol Nurs.* 2004;21(3):180-185.

110. Rando TA. An investigation of grief and adaptation in parents whose children have died of cancer. *J Pediatr Psychol.* 1983,8:3-20.

111. Middleton W, Raphael B, Burnett P, Martinek N. A longitudinal study comparing bereavement phenomena in recently bereaved spouses, adult children, and parents. *Aust N Z J Psychiatr.* 1998;32:235-241.

112. Li J, Precht DH, Mortensen PB, Olsen J. Mortality in parents after death of a child in Denmark: a nationwide follow-up study. *Lancet.* 2003;361:363-367.

113. Zhang B, El-Jawahri A, Prigerson HG. Update on bereavement research: evidence-based guidelines for the diagnosis and treatment of complicated grief. *J Palliative Med.* 2006:9:1188-1203.

114. Lannen PK, Wolfe J, Prigerson HG, Onelov E, Kreicbergs UC. Unresolved grief in a national sample of bereaved parents: impaired mental and physical health 4 to 9 years later. *J Clin Oncol.* 2008:26(36):5870-5876.

115. McCarthy MC, Clarke NE, Ting CL, Conroy R, Anderson VA, Heath JA. Prevalence and predictors of parental grief and depression after the death of a child from cancer. *J Palliative Med.* 2010:13(11):1321-1326.

116. Genevro JL. Report on bereavement and grief research by the Center for the Advancement of Health. *Death Stud.* 2004;28(6):491-575.

117. Ullrich CK, Dussel V, Hilden JM, Sheaffer JW, Lehmann L, Wolfe J. End-of-life experience of children undergoing stem cell transplantation for malignancy: parent and provider perspectives and patterns of care. *Blood.* 2010;115(19):3879-3885.

118. Foster TL, Gilmer MJ, Davies B, et al. Bereaved parents' and siblings reports of legacies created by children with cancer. *J Pediatr Oncol Nurs.* 2009;26:369.

119. Oltjenbruns KA. Positive outcomes of adolescents' experience with grief. *J Adolesc Res.* 1991;6(1):43-53.

120. Neimeyer RA. Reconstructing meaning in bereavement. In: Watson M, Kissane DW, eds. *Handbook of Psychotherapy in Cancer Care.* Chichester: John Wiley & Sons, Ltd; 2011:241-257.

121. Lichtenthal WG, Currier JM, Neimeyer RA, Keesee NJ. Sense and significance: a mixed methods examination of meaning making after the loss of one's child. *J Clin Psychol.* July 2010;66(7):791-812.

122. Kreicbergs UC, Lannen P, Onelov E, Wolfe J Parental grief after losing a child to cancer: impact of professional and social support on long-term outcomes. *J Clin Oncol.* August 2007;25(22):3307-3312.

123. Macdonald ME, Liben S, Carnevale FA, et al. Parental perspectives on hospital staff members' acts of kindness and commemoration after a child's death. *Pediatrics.* October 2005;116(4):884-890.

124. Kersting A, Brähler E, Glaesmer H, Wagner B. Prevalence of complicated grief in a representative population-based sample. *J Affect Disord.* June 2011;131(1-3):339-343.

125. Morin SM, Welsh LA. Adolescents' perceptions and experiences of death and grieving. *Adolescence.* 1996;31(123):585-595.

126. Wass H. Concepts of death: a developmental perspective. In: Wass H, ed. *Childhood and Death.* Washington, DC: Hospice Foundation of America; 1995.

127. Ringler LL, Hayden DC. Adolescent bereavement and social support: peer losses compared to other losses. *J Adolesc Res.* 2000;15:209-230.

128. Rheingold AA, Smith DW, Ruggiero KJ, Saunders BE, Kilpatrick DG, Resnick HS. Loss, trauma, exposure and mental health in a representative sample of 12-17 year old youth: data from the National Survey of Adolescents. *J Loss Trauma.* 2004;9(1): 10-19.

129. Fanos JH, Nickerson BG. Long-term effects of sibling death during adolescence. *J Adolesc Res.* 1991;6(1): 70-82.

130. Harrison L, Harrington R. Adolescents' bereavement experiences. Prevalence, association with depressive symptoms, and use of services. *Journal Adolesc.* 2001;24:159-169.

131. Hogan N, Desantis L. Basic constructs of a theory of adolescent sibling bereavement. In: Kass D, Silverman PR, Nickman SL, eds. *Continuing Bonds: New Understandings of Grief.* Taylor & Francis Co. Washington, DC: 1996:235-264.

132. Servaty-Seib HL, Pistole MC. Adolescent grief: relationship category and emotional closeness. *Omega.* 2006;54(2):147-167.

133. Schachter S. Adolescent experiences with the death of a peer. *Omega.* 1991;24(1):1-11.

134. Rask K, Kaunonen M, Paunonen-Ilmonen. Adolescent coping with death after the death of a loved one. *Int J Nurs Pract.* 2002;8:137-142.

135. Wallander JL, Thompson RJ. Psychosocial adjustment of children with chronic physical conditions. In: Roberts MC, ed. *Handbook of Pediatric Psychology.* New York, NY: Guilford Press; 1995:124-141.

136. Turkel S, Pao M. Late consequences of chronic pediatric illness. *Psychiatr Clin North Am.* 2007;30:819-835.

137. Bernstein GA, Borchardt CM, Perwien AR. Anxiety disorders in children and adolescents: a review of the past 10 years. *J Am Acad Child Adolesc Psychiatry.* 1996;35:1110-1119.

138. Norberg AL, Lindblad F, Boman KK. Coping strategies in parents of children with cancer. *Soc Sci Med.* 2005;60(5):965-975.

139. American Academy of Child and Adolescent Psychiatry. Work group on quality issues. Practice parameters for the assessment and treatment of children and adolescents with anxiety disorders. *J Am Acad Child Adolesc Psychiatry.* 1997;36:69S-84S.

140. Birmaher B, Ryan ND, Williamson DE, et al. Childhood and adolescent depression: a review of the past 10 years. Part I. *J Am Acad Child Adolesc Psychiatry.* 1996;35:1427-1439.

141. American Academy of Child and Adolescent Psychiatry. Practice parameters for the assessment and treatment of children and adolescents with depressive disorders. *J Am Acad Child Adolesc Psychiatry.* 1998;37:63S-83S.

142. Sommer DR. Exploring the spirituality of children in the midst of illness and suffering. *ACCH Advocate.* 1994;1:7-12.

143. Houskamp BM, Fisher LA, Stuber ML. Spirituality in children and adolescents: research findings and implications for clinicians and researchers. *Child Adolesc Psychiatr Clin N Am.* 2004;13(1):221-230.

144. Heilferty CM. Spiritual development and the dying child: the pediatric nurse practitioner's role. *J Pediatr Health Care.* 2004;18(6):271-275.

145. Stuber ML, Houskamp BM. Spirituality in children confronting death. *Child Adolesc Psychiatr Clin N Am.* 2004;13(1):127-136, viii.

146. Feudtner C, Haney J, Dimmers MA. Spiritual care needs of hospitalized children and their families: a national survey of pastoral care providers' perceptions. *Pediatrics.* 2003;111(1):e67-e72.

CHAPTER 64

Hematopoietic Stem Cell Transplantation and Supportive Care

Nina L. Bray ■ Ann M. Berger

INTRODUCTION

Hematopoietic stem cell transplantation (HSCT) is a process that worldwide more than 50,000 patients undergo each year (1). HSCT refers to the administration of hematopoietic progenitor cells from any source (e.g., bone marrow, peripheral blood, and umbilical cord blood) or donor (e.g., allogeneic and autologous) to reconstitute the bone marrow in efforts to treat disorders such as malignancies, genetic disorders, and bone marrow failure due to other causes.

HSCT is a lengthy process endured by patients and their families with many substantial side effects and complications (Table 64.1). It dramatically changes the lives of these patients and families in many dimensions, and improved transplantation strategies have contributed to survival increments of 10% per decade (2). Patients who survive for 2 years after allogeneic HSCT now have survival rates that exceed 80% at 15 years (3,4), and survival rates approach 70% at 10 years following autologous HSCT (5). However, these patients still have to contend with numerous short- and long-term complications; thus, it is important to increase the emphasis of their care on additional supportive techniques that will bolster them through the process of survival. Our goal is to address the challenges of this process and how the medical community can tackle them. Some of the obstacles these patients face have been dealt with in the topics that are covered in other chapters in this book; thus, this chapter will focus on the specific concerns pertaining to overall quality of life (QOL) enhancement in the holistic supportive care of the HSCT patient.

QUALITY OF LIFE

As we discuss some of the complications and the proposed interventions, it is important to note that patients do not experience these complications in discrete units, but in symptom clusters of varying magnitude and scope (6,7). There are models of these symptom clusters; however, it is of critical importance to recognize these not just as symptoms or clusters of symptoms but to realize that these clusters occur in the wider context of their lives. This realization is critical because it helps the clinician recognize that while each symptom is of great concern at the time of presentation, these symptoms are just a portion of the overall effect on the patient. Specifically, as patients consider the process of HSCT, they question not only what these individual complications will be but also what their QOL will be following transplant. Generally, QOL is difficult to measure as inherently it is a multidimensional, dynamic, and subjective concept that encompasses every dimension of a person's life including good health, adequate housing, employment, personal and family safety, good relationships, education, and enjoyment of leisurely pursuits. As the numbers of survivors increase, it is more and more important to further evaluate and improve QOL, especially as issues related to QOL are routinely cited by cancer survivors as among their greatest concerns (8). However, there is evidence that suggests that transplant physicians consider QOL as a secondary to the curative potential of HSCT, underestimate patient's symptoms, and overestimate QOL (3,9). Patients often describe significantly more distress from their symptoms than are even recognized by their medical providers (10).

Bury (11) describes illness as a "biographical disruption" in which a person's life story is disrupted in the light of their illness, the treatment demands, and the many changes that occur. In this chapter, we hope to emphasize that supportive care of the HSCT patient centers on the patient's life story, relating both to their QOL and their need for holistic supportive care. In covering some of the complications of the process of HSCT, we hope to highlight some of the main factors that affect QOL and propose interventions that can help improve QOL in these patients. In addition, we also hope to help the clinician to better listen and more fully appreciate the stories of our patients so that we can truly help all.

HEALTHCARE TEAM/MULTIDIMENSIONAL MODEL OF CARE

Evaluation of HSCT transplantation is a complex process, it has wide variability across transplant centers, and there are no formal guidelines to conduct pre-HSCT evaluation (12). There is also wide variation in supportive care practices in HSCT (13). From the time patients contemplate the process through the time years later when they are looking back on it, likely forever changed, they experience the effects in all dimensions of their lives—physical, psychological, social, and spiritual (Fig. 64.1). The effects extend beyond these groupings but the model is a useful starting place from which healthcare team can better address and support the patients through the many HSCT complications. This not only requires physicians from nearly every specialty but also nurses from a wide variety of backgrounds, social workers, mental health specialists, pastoral care, nutritionists, and many others. As a team, we can better encompass treatment aimed at helping patients in all aspects of their care.

TABLE 64.1 Complications of hematopoietic stem cell transplant

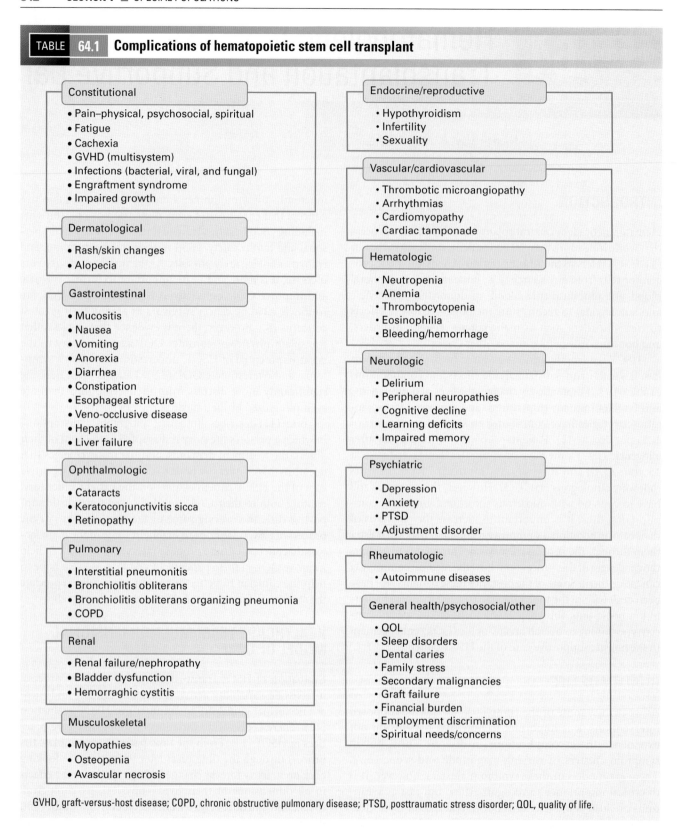

Constitutional
- Pain–physical, psychosocial, spiritual
- Fatigue
- Cachexia
- GVHD (multisystem)
- Infections (bacterial, viral, and fungal)
- Engraftment syndrome
- Impaired growth

Dermatological
- Rash/skin changes
- Alopecia

Gastrointestinal
- Mucositis
- Nausea
- Vomiting
- Anorexia
- Diarrhea
- Constipation
- Esophageal stricture
- Veno-occlusive disease
- Hepatitis
- Liver failure

Ophthalmologic
- Cataracts
- Keratoconjunctivitis sicca
- Retinopathy

Pulmonary
- Interstitial pneumonitis
- Bronchiolitis obliterans
- Bronchiolitis obliterans organizing pneumonia
- COPD

Renal
- Renal failure/nephropathy
- Bladder dysfunction
- Hemorraghic cystitis

Musculoskeletal
- Myopathies
- Osteopenia
- Avascular necrosis

Endocrine/reproductive
- Hypothyroidism
- Infertility
- Sexuality

Vascular/cardiovascular
- Thrombotic microangiopathy
- Arrhythmias
- Cardiomyopathy
- Cardiac tamponade

Hematologic
- Neutropenia
- Anemia
- Thrombocytopenia
- Eosinophilia
- Bleeding/hemorrhage

Neurologic
- Delirium
- Peripheral neuropathies
- Cognitive decline
- Learning deficits
- Impaired memory

Psychiatric
- Depression
- Anxiety
- PTSD
- Adjustment disorder

Rheumatologic
- Autoimmune diseases

General health/psychosocial/other
- QOL
- Sleep disorders
- Dental caries
- Family stress
- Secondary malignancies
- Graft failure
- Financial burden
- Employment discrimination
- Spiritual needs/concerns

GVHD, graft-versus-host disease; COPD, chronic obstructive pulmonary disease; PTSD, posttraumatic stress disorder; QOL, quality of life.

PHYSICAL

Graft-versus-Host Disease

Graft-versus-host disease (GVHD) is one of the most common complications after allogeneic hematopoietic cell transplantation. Acute GVHD is typically defined as a disease that occurs in the first 100 days after transplant and chronic is defined as a disease that occurs after 100 days (14).

It is generally recognized that a temporal distinction is rather arbitrary and that disease manifestations would be a more appropriate means to make the distinction between

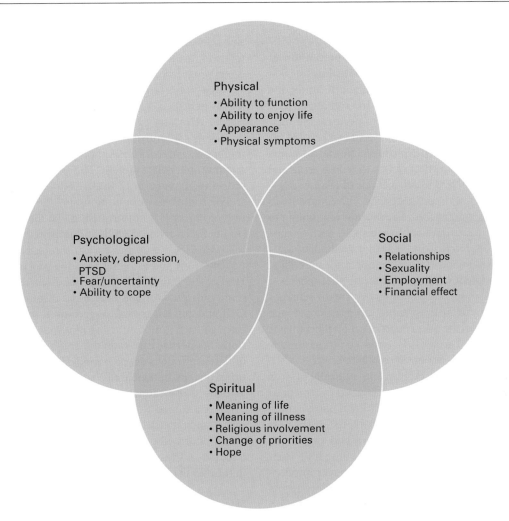

Figure 64.1. Multidimensional model of care. PTSD, posttraumatic stress disorder.

acute and chronic GVHD as they appear to involve different immune cell subsets, involve different cytokine profiles, involve somewhat different host targets, and respond differently to treatment. Accordingly, the NIH Consensus Conference has suggested a more complex categorization of acute and chronic GVHD (15,16). In either case, acute and chronic GVHD have a significant impact on short- and long-term morbidity as well as mortality in patients undergoing HSCT. As a result of the physical and emotional aspects of the transplant process and development of GVHD, QOL in transplant survivors can be adversely affected. The strongest association between reduced QOL and impaired functional status following HSCT is the presence of chronic GVHD (17). For patients with acute GVHD, they had measureable declines in their QOL over the first 6 months after HSCT compared with those with no acute GVHD; however, this effect did not persist at 12 months after HSCT unless the patient developed chronic GVHD (18).

Acute GVHD

Occurring at rates 10% to 80% depending on the study, underlying disease, prophylaxis regimens, and other factors, acute GVHD is the most frequent cause of mortality following allogeneic HSCT due to its clinical toxicity, requirement for intensive immunosuppressive management and associated infections (19–21). It generally develops within 2 to 8 weeks after marrow transplantation. The most common manifestation of acute GVHD is dermatological (21,22) which in most cases accompanies other manifestations in the liver or gastrointestinal tract but each can occur independently.

The rash of acute GVHD is most commonly maculopapular, but can also be morbilliform, or sometimes a confluent erythematous exanthema. It may be pruritic or painful and it may often involve the palms and soles which can help distinguish it from drug eruptions that are usually not in this location (23,24). It can be mild and affect <25% of the body but also can be severe, leading to whole body erythema, desquamation, bullae formation, and sloughing of the skin (25). Patients with severe skin GVHD have similar features and the need for similar treatments as those of severely burned patients. Hepatic GVHD is difficult to diagnose due to a lack of definitive testing and these patients have many other reasons to present with hepatic dysfunction (drug toxicity, TPN, infection, cholelithiasis, veno-occlusive disease, etc.). Gastrointestinal involvement can lead to nausea, anorexia, pain, and watery secretory diarrhea. In more severe cases, it may lead to mucosal denudation causing bloody diarrhea, hemorrhage, protein losing enteropathy, or ileus (26).

There have been many advances in the prevention of acute GVHD but currently immunosuppressive drugs such as methotrexate, cyclosporine, and anti-lymphocyte antibodies are the mainstay in the prevention of GVHD and can be used in conjunction with engineered grafts to decrease the incidence of GVHD (27). Ursodeoxycholic acid can be used for hepatic prophylaxis (28). T-cell depletion of the marrow using anti-T-cell antibodies is an effective way to reduce acute and chronic GVHD but can lead to a higher rate of relapse (29).

Initial treatment is with corticosteroids, with about 40% to 50% of patients responding (30). Patients not responding to corticosteroids are treated with salvage therapies such as anti-thymocyte globulin, interleukin 2 receptor antibodies, anti-CD147 monoclonal antibody, tumor necrosis factor antibodies, mycophenolate mofetil, and extracorporeal photopheresis; however, there are no specific guidelines that are the standard of care (21,31). Many of these agents produce a response to the acute GVHD; however, the risk of infectious mortality remains high as the treatment of acute GVHD leads to further immunosuppression and thus infectious susceptibility.

As these patients can quickly become critically ill, it is important to provide immediate disease-based treatment as outlined above. In addition, organ-specific supportive measures are critically important. Specific therapies for the skin include the use of topical emollient therapy and meticulous wound care, with considerations for care in a burn unit when appropriate and possible. For gastrointestinal tract complications, bowel rest, hyperalimentation, and antimotility agents may be required. In cases of bloody diarrhea, transfusion support may be necessary. Octreotide may help control the secretory component of gastrointestinal GVHD (32). As the majority of patients with steroid-refractory GVHD have a high mortality due to infection (33), systematic monitoring and judicious use of antibiotics for prophylaxis against infectious pathogens are essential.

Chronic GVHD

Chronic GVHD affects 27% to 60% of patients receiving allogeneic transplants from sibling donors and 42% to 72% from those receiving transplants from unrelated donors (34,35). The median onset of chronic GVHD is 4 to 6 months after HSCT (36). The major risk factors for chronic GVHD are human leukocyte antigen disparity, increasing age, and preceding acute GVHD (37,38). Treatment of chronic GVHD is usually less aggressive than that of acute GVHD; however, most of the chronic GVHD patients require prolonged treatment lasting many months to years (20). In addition, combined with the stress of the existing diagnosis, the added stressor of developing chronic GVHD represents the most important cause of non-relapse mortality beyond 2 to 3 months after transplantation. This is usually due to its significant immune dysfunction and the resultant increased infectious susceptibility (21). Detailed grading systems have been developed by the NIH Consensus Conference to classify the severity of chronic GVHD which help predict outcomes

(15,39). Generally, risk factors for worse prognosis are extensive skin involvement, progressive onset of chronic GVHD following acute GVHD, thrombocytopenia at diagnosis, and direct progression from acute GVHD (40).

First-line treatment for chronic GVHD is steroids, and just as in acute GVHD, approximately 50% of patients are steroid-refractory patients which is associated with a worse prognosis. Second-line initial treatments are calcineurin inhibitors, extracorporeal photopheresis, mTOR inhibitors, and mycophenolate mofetil. The assessment of effectiveness of treatment is at 8 to 12 weeks (39).

With all these complications and the resultant prolongation of illness, it is not surprising that the strongest association between reduced QOL and impaired functional status following HSCT is the presence of chronic GVHD (17). These patients continue to battle with the process and effects of HSCT. The individual symptoms discussed below lead to numerous physical and emotional disturbances that effect QOL and thus it is critical to aggressively support each patient through each symptom using innovative and creative solutions. Supportive care should include education, prevention of flares, infectious disease prophylaxis, physical and occupational therapy, nutrition, alleviation of chronic manifestations and effects of treatments, and promotion of coping mechanisms or resources to help patients deal with the psychosocial, sexual, and financial consequences of the disease (41). Below, we will address the skin, oral, ocular, and gynecological manifestations as these are key places where supportive care can aid in the overall care for the chronic GVHD patient.

Skin. The cutaneous manifestations of chronic GVHD are broad, but can be classified into three groups: lichen planus-like lesions, sclerotic skin manifestations, and poikilodermatous changes. Lichenoid chronic GVHD presents as an erythematous papular rash that resembles lichen planus; sclerodermatous GVHD may involve the dermis or muscle fascia leading to dermal fibrosis and fasciitis, while poikilodermatous skin changes appear as patches of mottled pigmentation and telangiectasias (23,25,34). All of these changes can lead to fragile skin with increased risk of erosions and ulceration or the skin can become thickened and tight with resultant detriment to the range of motion and poor wound-healing capacity. Any of these changes can lead to intense pruritus or pain. Hair loss and destruction of sweat glands are common; blistering may occur in severe cases. These symptoms are compounded by the patient's perception of their further worsening appearance, especially if widespread.

Oral and topical steroids serve as the primary treatment for cutaneous chronic GVHD (34,36,42). Petrolatum-based emollients are helpful for those patients with xerotic skin. In addition, topical calcineurin inhibitors (tacrolimus and pimecrolimus), phototherapy, and extracorporeal photopheresis can be helpful. Oral anti-pruritic agents such as antihistamines and tricyclic antidepressants such as doxepin should be used with caution as they can worsen oral and ocular sicca symptoms. Topical hydrocortisone, pramoxine, menthol-based creams/lotions, doxepin cream, or colloidal oatmeal powder bathtub soaks can also be used for short-term relief of intractable pruritus. For patients with thickened/tight skin and decreased range of motion, deep muscle/fascial massage is recommended, as well as daily stretching and referral to physical and/or occupational therapy. Surgical release can be considered in extreme cases. For patients with erosions and ulcerations, topical or oral antimicrobials, wound dressings, and debridement should all be considered. It is also important to instruct patients to take preventive measures such as avoidance of sun exposure, use of sunscreens (SPF > 20 with broad-spectrum UVA and UVB protections), and the use of protective clothing as there is an increased risk of skin cancer in patients with chronic GVHD (2,42–45).

Oral. Almost 80% of patients diagnosed with chronic GVHD demonstrate some degree of oral involvement, making this one of the most common clinical manifestations of chronic GVHD. The clinical findings can include erythema, leukoplakia, lichenoid lesions, ulcers, mucosal atrophy, cicatricial changes, and xerostomia (44,45). These can range from very mild changes to severe ones that can be functionally debilitating and lead to a decreased QOL due to significant pain, weight loss, malnutrition, and the loss of the ability to enjoy food and the process of eating.

Similar to the treatment of skin chronic GVHD, topical high potency corticosteroids are often used for the treatment of oral chronic GVHD (46). Additionally, supportive interventions for patients with oral chronic GVHD include encouraging good oral hygiene and utilizing of topical anesthetic agents, such as viscous lidocaine, to reduce pain and facilitate oral intake. Patients with xerostomia may benefit from salivary stimulants (sugarless gum or candy), oral lubricants or saliva substitutes, and frequent water sipping. Cholinergic agonists to stimulate saliva production (e.g., pilocarpine and cevimeline) may be useful in patients in whom the use of these agents is not contraindicated. Xerostomia can increase the risk of tooth decay, so it is also important to encourage the use of topical fluorides (47). Advise patients to avoid mint-flavored toothpastes and whitening products, as these can further aggravate the oral mucosa.

Ocular. Keratoconjunctivitis sicca is the most frequent presentation of chronic GVHD of the eye (42,48). Other eye chronic GVHD consequences are acute conjunctival inflammation and pseudomembranous and cicatricial conjunctivitis. These can lead to ocular irritation, dry eye syndrome, pain, or visual changes. Topical treatments include artificial tear liquids, ointments, slow dissolving hydroxypropyl methylcellulose, cyclosporine eye drops, cyclosporine eye patches/contacts, serum eye drops, and judicious use of topical steroid drops. Oral medications include cevimeline, pilocarpine, flaxseed oil, and doxycycline. Occlusive eye wear, warm compresses, humidified environments, or specialized contact lenses can also be used. Surgical interventions can also be considered (42,48,49).

Vulvar/Vaginal. Gynecological presentations of chronic GVHD are not as frequently studied as the other complications of

chronic GVHD (50). However, the effects of chronic GVHD on the female reproductive tract can be difficult for women and thus it is important to ask about these issues, assess them, and treat them aggressively or refer to a physician that can do so. Symptoms can include dysuria, dryness, tenderness to touch, and dyspareunia. On examination, there may be erosions and fissures, introital stenosis, resorption of the labia minora, vaginal synechiae, or vaginal narrowing. Treatment includes the avoidance of mechanical and chemical irritants, the use of emollients such as lanolin cream applied to external genitalia, and water-based lubricants internally for the vagina. Short-term use of ultrahigh potency corticosteroid or topical calcineurin ointments can also be tried. In addition, topical and systemic estrogen or hormone treatment can be tried for patients that do not have contraindications. Dilators can be helpful in vaginal GVHD that leads to fibrotic vaginal scarring, and only in extreme cases, surgical interventions should be performed (42,43,50–52). Though they are limited in number, gynecologists with familiarity of GVHD are the best physicians to treat these patients.

PSYCHOLOGICAL

Psychological Effects

An important survey of 600 HSCT survivors was conducted in 2006 by the Bone Marrow Transplant Information Network, which found that 73% of respondents endorsed emotional/psychological health as the most significant issue facing them following transplantation (53). Studies also have shown that biopsychosocial models will better predict cancer treatment–related pain and distress than a strictly biomedical model (54). The transplant process can be psychologically devastating which consequently can be destructive in a patient's personal and family life. Patients that undergo this process have many sources of stress as they are faced with many questions about the process and how they will fare in comparison to the statistics they are given. There undoubtedly will be fear: fear that the transplant will not cure, fear that it might kill, fear of pain, fear of the complications, fear that they will never be the same, fear for their family, etc. Even if they are cured of the disease they had, studies show that HSCT patients have a sense of feeling different from "normal people" despite having physical recovery (55).

These patients have been forever changed by their experience of illness and all the psychosocial changes a prolonged illness can bring. Unfortunately, in 2008, The Institute of Medicine report identified that meeting psychosocial needs of patients and family is the exception rather than the common occurrence in the current healthcare climate (56). This is not an unsurprising finding as the psychological and social issues can be more challenging for the healthcare team than the medical issues (57). We hope that this improves in the future but this will require an increased awareness of these issues as well as a dedicated approach to identifying, recognizing, and treating the reality of the psychosocial distress that endangers these patients. Attention to psychosocial factors in cancer patients before transplantation is important because social support, optimism, and self-efficacy measured prior to HSCT predicted health-related QOL 1 year post-transplantation (58). Not surprisingly, patients with previous psychiatric morbidity such as those patients with anxiety or depression are at risk for poorer health outcomes, longer length of hospital stay, and higher mortality (59–63).

During HSCT, between 37% and 53% of patients experience mental disorders that meet the diagnostic criteria for psychiatric illness (64,65). Mood disturbances occur more frequently in patients undergoing HSCT than in other types of cancer patients (66,67). The most common diagnosis is mixed anxiety and depressive reaction (64). In long-term survivors, defined as those who have survived greater than 1-year post-transplant, 20% to 43% reported clinically significant global psychological distress (68,69). Of HSCT survivors, only a minority consider themselves to have "returned to normal" following HSCT. Discordance between pre-HSCT expectations for returning to normal and current functional status was associated with greater current psychological distress; however, it is important to note that the rates of anxiety, depression, and posttraumatic stress disorder do decline with time after transplant (70,71). Some studies show that treatment-related distress decreases to baseline 5 years posttransplant but there is a wide variability on the trajectory of recovery following HSCT that depends on numerous factors such as physical limitations, social support, and coping styles (69,71–73).

Unfortunately, only about 50% of distressed HSCT survivors receive mental health services due to time limitations, lack of awareness of services available, embarrassment or discomfort associated with the need for mental health services, and physical limitations (74). It is important for clinicians to be aware of these barriers and address them. In addition to medications for psychiatric disturbances, clinicians should encourage patients to use mental health services and complementary services such as guided imagery, life review, relaxation breathing, and healing touch and increase physical activity or even simply go outside and experience sunshine. Clinicians can also further support the patient during regular visits by thorough empathic listening, providing information about both feelings and procedures, reframing negative statements, improving coping strategies, distraction, humor, giving opportunities to discuss fears and losses, arranging meetings with others who have had an HSCT or suggesting an appropriate support group, and including family in all interventions, as appropriate. Reducing fears with these interventions has helped patients maintain hope (75).

Psychological effects of HSCT are not only negative. HSCT patients also report positive sequelae in conjunction with negative sequelae. The concept of posttraumatic growth has been evolving in the past decade, and increasing numbers of studies are being done to evaluate the benefits that come from stressful ordeals such as HSCT (76). Some of these benefits are having a new philosophy of life, having a greater appreciation of life, making changes in personal characteristics or attributes, finding support within the family, improving relationships within the family, and finding help and support from friends. The poorer the patient's prognosis and the more risk associated with the process predicted more positive sequelae. However, just as negative sequelae, positive sequelae diminished with time (74). Predictors of posttraumatic growth are good social support, the ability to approach rather than avoid, young age, less education, greater use of positive re-interpretation or cognitive appraisal sense of mastery, self-efficacy, problem solving, seeking alternative rewards, more stressful appraisal of the experience, and more negatively biased recall of pretransplant levels of psychological distress (66,76,77).

As the concept of posttraumatic growth becomes real, so does the concept of survival and survivorship. Mullan, a physician, faced with his own battle with cancer grappled with his own concept of survivorship and broke it into three phases:

- Acute survival—Surviving the initial diagnosis and treatment.
- Extended survival—The time after treatment ceases and when the patient is most concerned about their disease returning or the treatment not working.
- Permanent survival—When it appears the disease has been permanently eradicated or "cured" and the patient recommences their life but knowing that things have changed (78).

Survivorship is in part a psychological understanding that shows that the process of cancer and its treatment has psychological effects. They can be devastating or they can lead to growth, but regardless, it is important to understand and appreciate that the psyche is forever changed in the process.

SOCIAL

Caregiver Effects

Caregivers are the unsung heroes of the HSCT process. They give invaluable emotional and physical support during the patients' long hospital stays. Their presence alone protects the patients from loneliness and complete isolation. They are also an invaluable, though very ill-defined, part of the healthcare team. Without the caregiver, the healthcare team would be less able to understand the patient's specific and occasionally unspoken needs and, in addition, would not have the help in coaching, guiding, and motivating the patient throughout the long and volatile recovery period.

The presence of a caregiver has been associated with improved survival at 1 year after transplantation versus patients without a dedicated caregiver (79). HSCT caregivers are females in 51% to 72% of cases, the patient's spouse 71% to 90% of the time, with a mean age of 43 to 50 years (39). Predictors of strain in family caregivers are younger age of persons with cancer, younger age of the caregiver, being a female caregiver, and being a spouse rather than a non-spouse. The strain is also most apparent in those of lower socioeconomic status (38). These caregivers are tasked with the responsibility of taking on unfamiliar roles without adequate support, which can lead to the potential for the development of interpersonal conflict within the family because of high levels of stress and the duty of managing multiple roles.

One of the earliest papers about HSCT effects on the family was that of Lesko (80) published in 1994. Factors that were reported to affect better outcomes for caregivers and patients were awareness of the transplant process, preparation, and understanding of probable side effects and toxicities including those that would affect body image and patients' coping abilities. Around this time, the concept of primary caregiver as psychologically a "second-order patient" began to be more widely acknowledged (81). Further studies described five factors that affect caregiver vulnerability during the acute phase of HSCT:

- preexisting stress related to the initial cancer diagnosis;
- the high level of uncertainty associated with the transplant process, especially if treatment is not curative;
- the struggle to maintain one's sense of personal control over the situation;
- the major disruption in the caregiver's personal life; and
- the financial burden and or strain on family resources (82,83).

Multiple complications requiring repeated hospitalizations caused worse outcomes on all fronts. With all these vulnerabilities, it is not incredibly surprising that despite not having to go through the physical process of HSCT, the effects of the patient's illness on the caregiver can cause emotional and functional distress at levels equal to or even greater than that of the patients themselves. They frequently feel that they must "be strong" and be the support and strength to their loved one. They end up suppressing their own emotional responses and are less likely to obtain mental health intervention than the patient (84).

In a 5-year longitudinal study comparing marital satisfaction after HSCT, female spouses that were the caregivers of HSCT recipients reported decreased martial satisfaction from 6 months through 5 years after transplant (85). In another study of QOL in spouse/partner caregivers and HSCT recipients, caregivers and healthy controls reported better physical health than HSCT recipients; however, both partners and recipients reported more depressive symptoms and sleep and sexual problems than controls. Moreover, caregivers reported less social support, decreased dyadic satisfaction and spiritual well-being, as well as more loneliness than both recipients and health controls. Furthermore, caregivers also reported less posttraumatic growth than HSCT recipients (84).

HSCT caregivers in multiple studies have consistently identified early, in-depth education and physical and emotional aspects of care as most important to their well-being (86). Importance of open and early communication in regard to the peritransplant process, expectations for discharge, long-term goals, and overall prognosis has been shown to decrease tension and foster a trusting relationship with the healthcare team (81). Psychoeducational interventions combine the use of written, group, and individual instruction to provide a thorough understanding of the type of care that is expected in terms of medications, adverse effects, symptoms, psychological

support, and procedures to be performed—these interventions aid in satisfying the caregiver's educational needs and feelings of mastery with the transplant process (86,87,88). This is a beginning but more studies need to be done as the process of HSCT transitions from inpatient to outpatient. Will these changes increase or decrease strain on the caregiver? These are important questions, as caregiver presence is vitally important to patient outcomes and the changing trends in medical practice will continue to affect the caregiver.

Sexual Dysfunction/Infertility

Since the 1970s, sexual function has been identified as an important aspect of patient care (89). It may be difficult to discuss due to the sensitive and private nature of the subject, but, when asked, patients acknowledge that this is a significant concern (56). All aspects of the human sexual response can be affected by the transplantation process and this is an important part of many patients' return to normalcy.

There are numerous factors that can lead to sexual dysfunction, such as a changed physique, reduced self-esteem, increased fear/uncertainty, fatigue, impotence, decreased libido, incontinence, infertility, premature ovarian failure/menopause, vaginal dryness, dyspareunia, depression, anxiety, and loss of meaning (90). Sexual dysfunction is a common complaint after transplantation but tends to be more common in women. One study by Syrjala et al. showed that 3 years after transplant, 80% of women reported at least one sexual problem as against 29% of men. Variables that predicted lower sexual satisfaction in men were older age, poorer psychological function, not being married, and lower sexual satisfaction prior to transplant. In contrast, there were no pretransplant predictors for women's posttransplant satisfaction (91). Another study by Syrjala et al. showed that both sexes declined in sexual activity at 6 months after HSCT, but 77% of men recovered by 1 year while only 55% of women did in the same time period (92). This conclusion highlights the importance of posttransplant screening of sexual dysfunction, which is even more important in females. Adult women posttransplant should be evaluated by a gynecologist, and it is likely that many will need hormone replacement therapy, if not contraindicated, to maintain libido, sexual function, and bone density.

The PLISSIT model has been widely available for addressing sexual concerns since 1976 (93). It addresses the best way for clinicians to approach the subject and help both male and female patients with this very private matter. It consists of four major considerations:

P—Permission: Create a comfortable climate that gives permission for patient to discuss sexual concerns, validating sexuality as a legitimate health issue.

LI—Limited Information: Address specific sexual concerns and attempt to correct misinformation.

SS—Specific Suggestions: Offer practical advice on how to deal with specific sexual problems.

IT—Intensive Therapy: Refer to a specialist such as sex therapist, gynecologist, urologist, and psychiatrist if problem is not resolving.

In addition to addressing and supporting patients through their sexual concerns posttransplant, it is extremely important to also address their fertility concerns as loss of fertility can have a significant influence on QOL and is frequently reported as a "loss" by female HSCT recipients (94–96). Some survivors, male and female, have reported that dealing with their loss of fertility was as painful as confronting cancer itself (97). For males, sperm banking is the cornerstone of fertility preservation; however, in one study only 91% of oncologists agreed that sperm banking should be offered to all eligible men. Yet in practice, only 48% offered it at all and those who did so did it less than 25% of the time, citing the difficulty in finding sperm banks, financial implications, and insufficient time (98). Another study showed that when offered, patients do elect for gamete/embryo preservation. After transplant, the collected material is used frequently and pregnancies in partners of male patients were often successful despite prolonged storage times (99). The frequency of pregnancy complications (caesarean section, preterm delivery, and low birth weight) was much higher in female allograft recipients compared with the normal population. This was more pronounced for females that received total body irradiation as part of their conditioning regimens. However, partners of male HSCT recipients had uncomplicated pregnancies (100). Another study reported that HSCT survivors of both genders had a lower prevalence of conception compared with their siblings but if pregnancy did occur, the outcome was likely to be favorable. Increased risk of infertility was reported when the HSCT recipient was female, age at HSCT was >30 years, and with use of total body irradiation in conditioning (101). Numerous studies show no increase in congenital abnormalities in patients that have undergone HSCT (102).

Oncofertility is a new and rapidly growing field and one that should not be ignored as patients approach the perilous process of HSCT (103). There are various options to preserve fertility and they should be fully reviewed with patients before proceeding with the treatment.

Financial Burden

HSCT is a highly technical process that involves many disciplines of care and thus it is very expensive and important to determine financial coverage early in the transplant process. Hematological cancers are significantly more expensive to treat than other common types of cancers (breast, colon, lung, and prostate) (104). There is a wide variation in estimates of cost of the transplant, from ~$30,000 to ~$200,000 depending on the type of transplant, source of stem cells, and whether it can be performed as an outpatient or inpatient basis (105–107). Costs include physician charges, medication cost, blood product and transfusion costs, graft procurement, hospitalization, and laboratory and radiologic investigations. In addition, there are many complications that can occur and thus these complications can further increase the overall cost of the procedure. These complications (graft failure, dialysis, mechanical ventilation, and

prolonged inpatient stay) are the main source of an increase in the total direct costs of HSCT (108). There are numerous indirect costs associated with HSCT such as lost wages and travel costs, as some patients need to travel and stay a significant distance from home. In addition, caregivers separately incur costs of care through money spent directly as well as time lost from work (109). There has been a trend to transition from inpatient to outpatient monitoring posttransplant which is helpful to reduce the cost of HSCT. A study in 2002 showed that the total cost difference between inpatient and outpatient transplant was significant ($40985 vs. $29210); however, a lack of caregivers limits its implementation, no doubt that this is at least partially due to the direct out-of-pocket burden it puts on caregivers (110).

In an ideal healthcare system, this is where insurance coverage would help. Unfortunately, limits on benefits and various types of cost-sharing in insurance plans may quickly lead to high out-of-pocket costs once cancer treatment begins. Some patients report more than $100,000 in medical bills, despite having an insurance policy throughout their treatment (111). In addition, people who depend on their employer for health insurance may not be protected from catastrophically high healthcare costs if they become too sick to work. While cancer patients who are unable to work can usually continue their employer-sponsored insurance coverage for up to 18 months by paying the full premium, that additional cost can be a substantial burden since these patients are typically living on a reduced income. In addition, the HSCT process can last much longer than this especially if there are numerous posttransplant complications. Patients that survive for years after HSCT may have trouble finding affordable insurance and others that try to apply for government programs such as Medicare or Medicaid face long waiting periods and strict eligibility guidelines. Medical costs are increasingly becoming the sole reason for bankruptcy, with a conservative estimate of two-thirds of all bankruptcies having a medical cause despite the fact that >75% of these people do have medical insurance (112). The National Donor Marrow Program (NDMP) provides a booklet titled "Mapping the Maze: A Personal Financial Guide to Blood Stem Cell Transplant" which helps patients through the financial, insurance, and legal obstacles of HSCT which at this time is also available for free download through the NDMP web site (113). Resources such as this are invaluable and of critical importance to helping the patient and caretaker navigate the financial burdens of care.

Undoubtedly, these financial stressors can be significant in the patient's and caregiver's psychosocial distress. Unfortunately, there is a paucity of studies that have assessed the role of the healthcare team in addressing these financial burdens. As patients face the overwhelming process of HSCT, it is important to provide resources for addressing their insurance coverage and limitations of their coverage, and possibly guiding them to other resources that can aid in paying their medical bills. Having a healthcare team member that is familiar with the patient's history, the transplant process, the insurance terminology, and other resources to help raise funds is a very important asset to the patient with yet another overwhelming task associated with their disease. This is especially important as sometimes insurance and cost issues can delay the transplant procedure which then has the possibility of negatively affecting the process itself.

SPIRITUAL

From the beginning of the planning stages through the entire journey of HSCT, this process will bring changes at many levels to the patient and the family. Any life-threatening illness can become a crisis time for the patient and family, which can bring up questions of mortality, the meaning of life, and the meaning of illness and test the bonds of relationships (114). These changes and questions can be even more pronounced in patients undergoing the long arduous process of HSCT. Medicine has a long history of attempting to cure and relieve suffering; however, from diagnosis through treatment and ideally into survivorship, the existential questions can be disconcerting and uncomfortable, thereby adding another dimension of suffering which medicine is not always equipped to address. The search for meaning is ongoing, multifaceted, and may be lived out in a variety of ways. Living with illness and the harsh but powerful treatment it demands brings many changes, some of which lead to a sense of loss of control. The healthcare team while often supportive sometimes fails to see these needs of those they cared for, specifically these deeper spiritual ones (115).

In a small hermeneutic study in 1996 by Steeves, patients were interviewed within the first 100 days of HSCT about the meaning of their lives during and following the transplant. In finding meaning, patients renegotiated their social position in their new situation and tried to reach an understanding of their experiences as a whole (116). The conclusion of the study was a focus on the concept of holism and the importance of listening to the patient perspective. Another study looked at global meaning (the belief that life has a purpose and coherence) and showed that having global meaning was associated with less psychological distress (117). Chronic GVHD patients typically have lower QOL scores; however, a higher level of spiritual well-being was a significant independent predictor of contentment with QOL in these patients (118). *Disappointingly, about 50% of cancer patients report that their spiritual needs are not being supported by a religious community and about 70% report that their spiritual needs are not being supported by the medical system.* Spiritual support by religious communities or the medical system is associated with improvements in patient's QOL (119). If this was any other medical outcome, it would be considered a treatment failure and rapidly addressed. While there is increasing research in this area, it is imperative that this support be addressed more aggressively and more seriously in this fragile population.

As we know that addressing spiritual matters improves patient's QOL, we as clinicians should encourage these behaviors or, at the very least, have someone on the team that can do so. Often patients and families turn to the healthcare team to help directly or indirectly answer these spiritual concerns. Clinicians can easily miss the importance of how that which is not present gives depth, perspective, and clues to the real meaning of social action in clinical encounters (120). People with a religious faith may find it helpful talking to a priest, pastor, imam, rabbi, or other religious leader, while others may find it important to have quiet time to reflect, read, walk in nature, be artistic, spend time with loved ones, or do other things that bring meaning to their lives. We cannot continue to miss the opportunities to further explore these profound concerns (Table 64.2).

The clinician who dares to ask about spirituality imparts a vital message to the patient that they are being cared for by someone who has not forgotten that a broken patient remains a whole person and that healing transcends survival (121). As one approaches this topic, it is central to realize that supportive care is not always about fixing the situation. It is about awareness of the patient's inner life and remembering it does not want to be fixed, but often it wants simply to be seen and heard. In the text, *Sharing the Darkness* by Cassidy, she describes moments that occur when a doctor or nurse is confronted with a painful situation and there seems to be nothing that can be done. However, she implores that if the doctor or nurse can simply stay with that person during the uncomfortable and difficult time, then they will have shared a moment of that person's darkness, which thereby gives support (122). Quinn goes so far as to state that the clinical team member will find it difficult to recognize or support the patient/family in this search if that team member is unaware of their own search to find meaning and their own need for support (115). There are many proponents for further medical education on spirituality needs of self and patient (123,124). In addition, specific courses have been developed for clinicians to explore and support spiritual and

TABLE 64.2	Supporting spiritual distress
• Be present for the patient without the need of "doing" something
• Allowing time, space, and privacy to explore issues
• Asking questions directly and indirectly about meaning
• Watch and listen for cues of spiritual distress
• Being aware of own spirituality
• Caring for self
• Showing humility
• Being aware of the patients culture and religious spiritual needs
• Involving pastoral support/prayer
• Offering use of labyrinths
• Art therapy/mandalas
• Healing touch/Reiki

religious issues confronting critically ill patients and their families (125).

Moving from the numinous to the tangible, there are many discrete treatment plans and modalities that have been shown to be effective in positively affecting the patient's spiritual needs. Art therapy is shown to help patients who have difficult family relationships prior to admission and those who wish to explore existential/spiritual issues (126). The meaning-making intervention is novel psychological intervention that consists of discrete tasks that address the normative distress associated with the search for meaning within the context of cancers of many types (127). Negative spiritual coping is associated with worse outcomes in HSCT patients (128). More studies need to be done but it would make sense that candidly helping patients explore their existential issues can possibly help them improve their coping skills and hopefully lead to improved outcomes and QOL.

CONCLUSION

Support for the HSCT patient and family is greatly needed as the effects of transplantation are far-reaching and profound. In this chapter, we have highlighted only a few of the many physical, psychological, social, and spiritual effects and interventions of HSCT (Table 64.3). It is our hope that in compiling this information in one location, the body of the present research as well as its shortcomings can be viewed and a more unified holistic approach could be developed. This is just the beginning of understanding and supporting patients as they try to maintain their QOL throughout the process of HSCT. The diverse effects and highly individual patient responses often require a team approach that is large and flexible. There are an increasing number of proposals

to incorporate palliative care teams in the management of all patients preparing to endure the process of HSCT (129). Palliative care team expertise in symptom management and holistic care with an interdisciplinary team approach would benefit patients and the HSCT team as they help address the comprehensive care of the HSCT patient. Just as the biomedical cornerstones of care must be addressed to treat the diseases leading to HSCT, early and continuous interventions in supportive physical, psychological, social and spiritual care must become the standard of care in order to effectively treat the patient.

REFERENCES

1. Pasquini MC, Wang Z. Current use and outcome of hematopoietic stem cell transplantation: CIBMTR Summary Slides, 2010. http://www.cibmtr.org. Accessed October 6, 2012.
2. Wingard JR, Vogelsang GB, Deeg HJ. Stem cell transplantation: supportive care and long-term complications. *Hematol Am Soc Hematol Educ Program.* 2002;2002:422-444.
3. Hendrinks MG, Schouten HC. Quality of life after stem cell transplantation: a patient, partner and physician perspective. *Eur J Intern Med.* 2002;13:52-56.
4. Pidala J, Anasetti C, Jim H. Quality of life after allogenic hematopoietic cell transplantation. *Blood.* 2009;114:7-19.
5. Kopp M, Schweigkofler H, Holzner B, et al. EORTC QLQ-C30 and FACT-BMT for the measurement of quality of life in bone marrow transplant recipients: a comparison. *Eur J Haematol.* 2000;65:97-103.
6. Bevans MF, Mitchell SA, Marden S. The symptom experience in the first 100 days following allogeneic hematopoietic stem cell transplantation. *Support Care Cancer.* 2008;16:1243-1254.
7. Kirkova J, Walsh D, Aktas A, Davis MP. Cancer symptom clusters: old concept but new data. *Am J Hosp Palliat Care.* 2010;27:282-288.
8. Baker, F, Denniston M, Smith T, West MM. Adult cancer survivors: how are they faring? *Cancer.* 2005;104:2565-2576.
9. Lee SJ, Joffe S, Kim HT, et al. Physicians' attitudes about quality-of–life issues in hematopoietic stem cell transplantation. *Blood.* 2004;104:2194-2200.
10. Strömgren AS, Groenvold M, Pedersen L, Olsen AK, Spile M, Sjøgren P. Does the medical record cover the symptoms experienced by cancer patients receiving palliative care? A comparison of the record and patient self-rating. *J Pain Symptom Manage.* 2001;21(3):189-196.
11. Bury M. Chronic illness as a biographical disruption. *Soc Health Illn.* 1982;4:167-182.
12. Hamadani M, Craig M, Awan FT, Devine SM. How we approach patient evaluation for hematopoietic stem cell transplantation. *Bone Marrow Transplant.* 2010;45:1259-1268.
13. Lee SJ, Astigarraga CC, Eapen M, et al. Variation in supportive care practices in hematopoietic cell transplantation, *Biol Blood Marrow Transplant.* 2008;14:1231-1238.
14. Schaffer JV. The changing face of graft-versus-host disease. *Semin Cutan Med Surg.* 2006;25:190-200.
15. Filipovich AH, Weisdorf D, Pavletic S, et al. National Institutes of Health consensus development project on criteria for clinical trials in chronic graft-versus-host disease: I. Diagnosis and staging working group report. *Biol Blood Marrow Transplant.* 2005;11:945-956.
16. Griffith LM. Chronic graft vs. host disease: implementation of the NIH consensus criteria for clinical trials. *Biol Blood Marrow Transplant.* 2008;14:379-384.

TABLE 64.3	**Supportive care interventions**
Physical	• Acknowledge patient's distress • Aggressive medication treatment • Aggressive GVHD prevention and treatment • Exercise
Psychological	• Improve communication between healthcare team and patient /family • Individual counseling • Group therapy
Social	• Caregiver support • Financial resources/counseling • Job counseling/retraining
Spiritual	• Spiritual awareness • Asking about spiritual suffering • Providing resources for spiritual issues

17. Baker KS, Fraser CJ. Quality of life and recovery after graft-versus-host disease. *Best Pract Res Clin Haematol.* 2008;21:333-341.

18. Lee SJ, Kim HT, Ho VT, et al. Quality of life associated with acute and chronic graft-vs-host disease. *Bone Marrow Transplantation.* 2006;38:305-310.

19. Joachim Deeg H, Flowers ME. Acute graft-versus-host disease. In: Treleaven J, Barrett AJ, eds. *Hematopoietic Stem Cell Transplantation in Clinical Practice.* Amsterdam: Elsevier Limited; 2009:387-400.

20. Weisdorf D. GVHD the nuts and bolts. *Hematol Am Soc Hematol Educ Program.* 2007:62-67.

21. Jacobsohn DA, Vogelsang GB. Acute graft versus host disease. *Orphanet J Rare Dis.* 2007;2:35.

22. Ferrara JL, Levine JE, Reddy P, Holler E. Graft-versus-host disease. *Lancet.* 2009;373:1550-1561.

23. Saurat JH. Cutaneous manifestations of graft versus host disease. *Int J Dermatol.* 1981;20:249-256.

24. Cutler C, Antin JH. Manifestations and treatment of acute graft-versus-host disease. In: Appelbaum FR, Forman SJ, Negrin RS, Blume KG, eds. *Thomas' Hematopoietic Cell Transplantation: Stem Cell Transplantation.* Ames, IA: Wiley-Blackwell: 2009;1287-1303.

25. Chavan R, el-Azhary R. Cutaneous graft-versus-host disease: rationales and treatment options. *Dermatol Ther.* 2011; 24:219-228.

26. Ross WA. Treatment of gastrointestinal acute graft-versus-host disease. *Curr Treat Options Gastroenterol.* 2005;8:249-258.

27. Barrett AJ, Le Blanc K. Prophylaxis of acute GVHD: manipulate the graft or the environment? *Best Pract Res Clin Haematol.* 2008;21:165-176.

28. Ruutu T, Eriksson B, Remes K, et al. Ursodeoxycholic acid for the prevention of hepatic complications in allogeneic stem cell transplantation. *Blood.* 2002;15:1977-1983.

29. Bron D. Bone marrow transplantation. In: Klastersky J, Schimpff SC, Senn HJ, eds. *Supportive Care in Cancer.* 2nd ed. New York, NY: Marcel Dekker, Inc; 1999:166-185.

30. Saliba RM, de Lima M, Giralt S, et al. Hyperacute GVHD: risk factors, outcomes, and clinical implications. *Blood.* 2007;109:2751-2758.

31. Hsu B, May R, Carrum G, Krance R, Przepiorka D. Use of anti-thymocyte globulin for treatment of steroid-refractory acute graft-versus-host disease: an international practice survey. *Bone Marrow Transplant.* 2001;28:945-950.

32. Ippoliti C, Champlin R, Bugazia N, et al. Use of octreotide in the symptomatic management of diarrhea induced by graft-versus-host disease in patients with hematologic malignancies. *J Clin Oncol.* 1997;15:3350-3354.

33. Bolaños-Meade J, Vogelsang GB. Novel strategies for steroid-refractory acute graft-versus-host disease. *Curr Opin Hematol.* 2005;12:40-44.

34. Lee SJ, Vogelsang G, Flowers ME. Chronic graft-versus-host disease. *Biol Blood Marrow Transplant.* 2003;9:215-233.

35. Socié G, Salooja N, Cohen A, et al. Nonmalignant late effects after allogeneic stem cell transplantation. *Blood.* 2003;101:3373-3385.

36. Lee SJ. Have we made progress in the management of chronic graft-v-host disease? *Best Pract Res Clin Haematol.* 2010;23:529-535.

37. Wagner JL, Seidel K, Boeckh M, et al. De novo chronic graft-versus-host disease in marrow graft recipients given methotrexate and cyclosporine: risk factors and survival. *Biol Blood Marrow Transpl.* 2000;6:633-639.

38. Remberger M, Kumlien G, Aschan J, et al. Risk factors for moderate-to-severe chronic graft-versus-host disease after

39. Wolff D, Schleuning M, von Harsdorf S, et al. Consensus conference on clinical practice in chronic GVHD: second-line treatment of chronic graft-versus-host disease. *Biol Blood Marrow Transplant.* 2011;17:1-17.

40. Akpek G, Zahurak ML, Piantadosi S, et al. Development of a prognostic model for grading chronic graft-versus-host disease. *Blood.* 2001;97:1219-1226.

41. Shlomchik, WD, Lee SJ, Couriel D, Pavletic SZ. Transplantation's greatest challenges: advances in chronic graft-versus-host disease. *Biol Blood Marrow Transplant.* 2007;13:2-10.

42. Couriel DR. Ancillary and supportive care in chronic GVHD. *Best Pract Res Clin Haematol.* 2008;21:291-307.

43. Couriel D, Carpenter PA, Cutler C, et al. Ancillary therapy and supportive care of chronic graft-versus-host disease: national institutes of health consensus development project on criteria for clinical trials in chronic Graft-versus-host disease: V. Ancillary Therapy and Supportive Care Working Group Report. *Biol Blood Marrow Transplant.* 2006;12:375-396.

44. Ratanatharathorn V, Ayash L, Lazarus HM, Fu J, Uberti JP. Chronic graft-versus-host disease: clinical manifestation and therapy. *Bone Marrow Transplant.* 2001;28:121-129.

45. Cowen EW, Hymes SR. Cutaneous manifestations of chronic graft versus host disease. In: Vogelsang GB, Pavletic SZ, eds. *Chronic Graft Versus Host Disease: Interdisciplinary Management.* Cambridge University Press; 2009:169-181.

46. Imanguli MM, Alevizos I, Brown R, Pavletic SZ, Atkinson JC. Oral graft-versus-host disease. *Oral Dis.* 2008;14:396-412.

47. Schubert MM, Sullivan KM. Recognition, incidence, and management of oral graft-versus-host disease. *NCI Monogr.* 1990;9:135-143.

48. Livesey SJ, Holmes JA, Whittaker JA. Ocular complications of bone marrow transplantation. *Eye.* 1989;3:271-276.

49. Kim SK, Smith JA, Dunn JP. Chronic ocular graft versus host disease. In: Vogelsang GB, Pavletic SZ, eds. *Chronic Graft Versus Host Disease: Interdisciplinary Management.* Cambridge: Cambridge University Press; 2009:199-206.

50. Turner ML, Stratton P. Gynecological manifestations of chronic graft versus host disease. In: Vogelsang GB, Pavletic SZ, eds. *Chronic Graft Versus Host Disease: Interdisciplinary Management.* Cambridge: Cambridge University Press; 2009:207-215.

51. Spiryda LB, Laufer MR, Soiffer RJ, et al. Graft-versus-host disease of the vulva and/or vagina: diagnosis and treatment. *Biol Blood Marrow Transplant* 2003;9:760-765.

52. Anderson M, Kutzner S, Kaufman RH. Treatment of vulvovaginal lichen planus with vaginal hydrocortisone suppositories. *Obstet Gynecol.* 2002;100:359-362.

53. McQuellon RP, Andrykowski M. Psychosocial issues in hematopoietic cell transplantation. In: Appelbaum FR, Forman SJ, Negrin RS, eds. *Thomas' Hematopoietic Cell Transplantation: Stem Cell Transplantation,* 4th ed. Oxford: Wiley-Blackwell; 2009:488-501.

54. Schulz-Kindermann F, Hennings U, Ramm G, Zander AR, Hasenbring M. The role of biomedical and psychosocial factors for the prediction of pain and distress in patients undergoing high-dose therapy and BMT/PBSCT. *Bone Marrow Transplant.* 2002;29:341-351.

55. Sherman RS, Cooke E, Grant M. Dialogue among survivors of hematopoietic cell transplantation support-group themes. *J Psychosoc Oncol.* 2005;23:1-24.

56. Adler NE, Page AEK, eds. *Cancer Care for the Whole Patient: Meeting Psychosocial Health Needs.* Institute of Medicine. Washington, DC: The National Academies Press; 2008.

57. Eldredge DH, Nail LM, Maziarz RT, Hansen LK, Ewing D, Archbold PG. Explaining family caregiver role strain following autologous blood and marrow transplantation. *J Psychosoc Oncol.* 2006;24:53-74.

58. Hochhausen N, Altmaier EM, McQuellon R, et al. Social support, optimism, and self-efficacy predict physical and emotional well-being after bone marrow transplantation. *J Psychosoc Oncol.* 2007;25:87-101.

59. Prieto JM, Blanch J, Atala J, et al. Stem cell transplantation: risk factors for psychiatric morbidity. *Eur J Cancer.* 2006;42:514-520.

60. Garcia C Jr, Botega NJ, De Souza CA. A psychosocial assessment interview of candidates for hematopoietic stem cell transplantation. *Haematologica.* 2005;90:570-572.

61. Prieto JM, Blanch J, Atala J, et al. Psychiatric morbidity and impact on hospital length of stay among hematologic cancer patients receiving stem-cell transplantation. *J Clin Oncol.* 2002;20:1907-1917.

62. Goetzmann L, Klaghofer R, Wagner-Huber R, et al. Psychosocial need for counseling before and after a lung, liver or allogenic bone marrow transplant–results of a prospective study. *Z Psychosom Med Psychother.* 2006;52:230-242.

63. Goetzmann L, Klaghofer R, Wagner-Huber R, et al. Quality of life and psychosocial situation before and after a lung, liver or an allogeneic bone marrow transplant. *Swiss Med Wkly.* 2006;136:281-290.

64. Khan AG, Irfan M, Shamsi TS, Hussain M. Psychiatric disorders in bone marrow transplant patients. *J Coll Physicians Surg Pak.* 2007;17:98-100.

65. Fritzsche K, Struss Y, Stein B, Spahn C. Psychosomatic liaison service in hematological oncology: need for psychotherapeutic interventions and their realization. *Hematol Oncol.* 2003;21:83-89.

66. Cooke L, Gemmill R, Kravits K, Grant M., Psychological issues of stem cell transplantation. *Semin Oncol Nurs.* 2009;25:139-150.

67. Andrykowski MA, Henslee PJ, Barnett RL. Longitudinal assessment of psychosocial functioning of adult survivors of allogeneic bone marrow transplantation. *Bone Marrow Transplant.* 1989;4:505-509.

68. Rusiewicz A, DuHamel KN, Burkhalter J, et al. Psychological distress in long-term survivors of hematopoietic stem cell transplantation. *Psycho-Oncology.* 2008;17:329-337.

69. McQuellon RP, Russell GB, Rambo TD, et al. Quality of life and psychological distress of bone marrow transplant recipients: the "time trajectory" to recovery over the first year. *Bone Marrow Transplant.* 1998;21:477-486.

70. Andrykowski MA, Brady MJ, Greiner CB, et al. "Returning to normal" following bone marrow transplantation: outcomes, expectations and informed consent. *Bone Marrow Transplant.* 1995;15:573-581.

71. Sun CL, Francisco L, Baker KS, Weisdorf DJ, Forman SJ, Bhatia S. Adverse psychological outcomes in long-term survivors of hematopoietic cell transplantation: a report from the Bone Marrow Transplant Survivor Study. *Blood.* August 2011 [Epub ahead of print].

72. Syrjala KL, Langer SL, Abrams JR, et al. Recovery and long-term function after hematopoietic cell transplantation for leukemia or lymphoma. *J Am Med Assoc.* 2004;291:2335-2343.

73. Fromm K, Andrykowski MA, Hunt J. Positive and negative psychosocial sequelae of bone marrow transplantation: implications for quality of life assessment. *J Behav Med.* 1996;19:221-240.

74. Mosher CE, DuHamel KN, Rini CM, et al. Barriers to mental health service use among hematopoietic SCT survivors. *Bone Marrow Transplant.* 2010;45:570-579.

75. Cohen MZ, Ley CD. Bone marrow transplantation: the battle for hope in the face of fear. *Oncol Nurs Forum.* 2000;27:473-480.

76. Widows MR, Jacobsen PB, Booth-Jones M, Fields KK. Predictors of posttraumatic growth following bone marrow transplantation for cancer. *Health Psychol.* 2005;24:266-273.

77. Jacobsen PB, Sadler IJ, Booth-Jones M, et al. Predictors of posttraumatic stress disorder symptomatology following bone marrow transplantation for cancer. *J Consult Clin Psychol.* 2002;70:235-240.

78. Mullan F, Seasons of survival: reflections of a physician with cancer. *N Engl J Med.* 1985;313:270-273.

79. Bolwell BJ, Foster L, McLellan L, et al. The presence of a caregiver is a powerful prognostic variable of survival following allogeneic bone marrow transplantation. *Proc Am Soc Hematol.* 2001;98:202A (abstract 845).

86. Chow K, Coyle N. Providing Palliative care to family caregivers throughout the bone marrow transplantation trajectory: research and practice: partners in care. *J Hosp Palliat Nurs.* 2011;13:7-13.

80. Lesko LM. Bone marrow transplantation: support of the patient and his/her family. *Support Care Cancer.* 1994;2:35-49.

81. Lederberg MS. The family of the cancer patient. In: Holland JC, ed. *Psycho-Oncology.* 1st ed. New York, NY: Oxford University Press; 1998:981.

82. Fife BL, Monahan PO, Abonour R, Wood LL, Stump TE. Adaptation of family caregivers during the acute phase of adult BMT. *Bone Marrow Transplant.* 2009;43:959-966.

83. Simon RW. The meanings individuals attach to role identities and their implications for mental health. *J Health Soc Behav.* 1997;38:256-274.

84. Bishop MM, Beaumont JL, Hahn EA, et al. Late effects of cancer and hematopoietic stem-cell transplantation on spouses or partners compared with survivors and survivor-matched controls. *J Clin Oncol.* 2007;25:1403-1411.

85. Langer SL, Yi JC, Storer BE, Syrjala KL. Marital adjustment, satisfaction and dissolution among hematopoietic stem cell transplant patients and spouses: a prospective, five-year longitudinal investigation. *Psycho-Oncology.* 2010;19:190-200.

87. Honea NJ, Brintnall R, Given B, et al. Putting evidence into practice: nursing assessment and interventions to reduce family caregiver strain and burden. *Clin J Oncol Nurs.* 2008;12: 507-516.

88. Grimm PM, Zawacki KL, Mock V, Krumm S, Frink BB. Caregiver responses and needs: an ambulatory bone marrow transplant model. *Cancer Pract.* 2000;8:120-128.

89. Hughes MK. Alterations of sexual function in women with cancer. *Semin Oncol Nurs.* 2008;24:91-101.

90. Quinn, B. Psychologic and supportive care issues in the transplant setting. In: Treleaven J, Barrett AJ, eds. *Hematopoietic Stem Cell Transplantation in Clinical Practice.* Amsterdam: Elsevier Limited; 2009:369-377.

91. Syrjala KL, Roth-Roemer SL, Abrams JR, et al. Prevalence and predictors of sexual dysfunction in long-term survivors of marrow transplantation. *J Clin Oncol.* 1998;16:3148-157.

92. Syrjala KL, Kurland BF, Abrams JR, et al. Sexual function changes during the 5 years after high-dose treatment and hematopoietic cell transplantation for malignancy with case-matched controls at 5 years. *Blood.* 2008;111:989-996.

93. Annon, JS. *Behavioral Treatment of Sexual Problems: Brief Therapy.* New York, NY: Harper & Row; 1976.

94. Hammond C, Abrams JR, Syrjala KL. Fertility and risk factors for elevated infertility concern in 10-year hematopoietic cell transplant survivors and case-matched controls. *J Clin Oncol.* 2007;25:3511-3517.

95. Watson M, Wheatley K, Harrison GA, et al. Severe adverse impact on sexual functioning and fertility of bone marrow transplantation, either allogeneic or autologous, compared with consolidation chemotherapy alone: analysis of the MRC AML 10 trial. *Cancer.* 1999;86:1231-1239.

96. Curbow B, Legro MW, Baker F, Wingard JR, Somerfield MR. Loss and recovery themes of long-term survivors of bone marrow transplants. *J Psychosocial Oncol.* 1993;10:1-20.

97. Schover LR. Motivation for parenthood after cancer: a review. *J Natl Cancer Inst Monogr.* 2005;34:2-5.

98. Schover LR, Brey K, Lichtin A, Lipshultz LI, Jeha S. Oncologists' attitudes and practices regarding banking sperm before cancer treatment. *J Clin Oncol.* 2002;20:1890-1897.

99. Babb A, Farah N, Lyons C, et al. Uptake and outcome of assisted reproductive techniques in long-term survivors of SCT. *Bone Marrow Transplant.* 2012;47:568-73.

100. Salooja N, Szydlo RM, Socie G, et al. Pregnancy outcomes after peripheral blood or bone marrow transplantation: a retrospective survey. *Lancet.* 2001;358:271-276.

101. Carter A, Robison LL, Francisco L, et al. Prevalence of conception and pregnancy outcomes after hematopoietic cell transplantation: report from the Bone Marrow Transplant Survivor Study. *Bone Marrow Transplant.* 2006;37:1023-1029.

102. Loren AW, Chow E, Jacobsohn DA, et al. Pregnancy after hematopoietic cell transplantation: a report from the late effects working committee of the Center for International Blood and Marrow Transplant Research. *Biol Blood Marrow Transplant.* 2011;17:157-166.

103. Woodruff TK. The emergence of a new interdiscipline: oncofertility. *Cancer Treat Res.* 2007;138:3-11.

104. Greenberg D, Earle C, Fang CH, Eldar-Lissai A, Neumann PJ. When is cancer care cost-effective? A systematic overview of cost-utility analyses in oncology. *J Natl Cancer Inst.* 2010;20;102:82-88.

105. Bennett CL, Armitage JL, Armitage GO, et al. Costs of care and outcomes for high-dose therapy and autologous transplantation for lymphoid malignancies: results from the University of Nebraska 1987 through 1991. *J Clin Oncol.* 1995;13:969-973.

106. Hartmann O, Le Corroller AG, Blaise D, et al. Peripheral blood stem cell and bone marrow transplantation for solid tumors and lymphomas: hematologic recovery and costs. A randomized, controlled trial. *Ann Intern Med.* 1997;126:600-607.

107. Lee SJ, Anasetti C, Kuntz KM, Patten J, Antin JH, Weeks JC. The costs and cost-effectiveness of unrelated donor bone marrow transplantation for chronic phase chronic myelogenous leukemia. *Blood.* 1998;92:4047-4052.

108. Majhail NS, Mothukuri JM, Brunstein CG, Weisdorf DJ. Costs of hematopoietic cell transplantation: comparison of umbilical cord blood and matched related donor transplantation and the impact of posttransplant complications. *Biol Blood Marrow Transplant.* 2009;15:564-573.

109. Meehan KR, Fitzmaurice T, Root L, Kimtis E, Patchett L, Hill J. The financial requirements and time commitments of caregivers for autologous stem cell transplant recipients. *J Support Oncol.* 2006:187-190.

110. Frey P, Stinson T, Siston A, et al. Lack of caregivers limits use of outpatient hematopoietic stem cell transplant program. *Bone Marrow Transplant.* 2002;30:741-748.

111. Schwartz K, Claxton G, Martin K, Schmidt C. Spending to survive: cancer patients confront holes in the health insurance system, Kaiser Family Foundation & American Cancer Society, February 2009. http://www.kff.org/insurance/upload/7851.pdf. Accessed October 6, 2012.

112. Himmelstein DU, Thorne D, Warren E, Woolhandler S. Medical bankruptcy in the United States, 2007: results of a national study. *Am J Med.* 2009;122:741-746.

113. Jolley P, Storey J, Richetts J. Mapping the Maze, National Marrow Donor Program, Sept 2011. https://secure.marrow.org/Patient/Support_and_Resources/Resource_Library/Plan_resources/Mapping_the_Maze_-_Complete_Manual_(PDF).aspx. Accessed July 22, 2012.

114. Bolen JS. *Close to the Bone: Life-Threatening Illness and the Search for Meaning.* New York, NY: Touchstone; 1996.

115. Quinn B. Cancer and the treatment: does it make sense to patients? *Hematology.* 2005;10(suppl 1):325-328.

116. Steeves RH. Patients who have undergone bone marrow transplantation: their quest for meaning. *Oncol Nurs Forum.* 1992;19:899-905.

117. Vehling S, Lehmann C, Oechsle K, et al. Global meaning and meaning-related life attitudes: exploring their role in predicting depression, anxiety, and demoralization in cancer patients. *Support Care Cancer.* 2011;19:513-520.

118. Harris BA, Berger AM, Mitchell SA, et al. Spiritual well-being in long-term survivors with chronic graft-versus-host disease after hematopoietic stem cell transplantation. *J Support Oncol.* 2010;8:119-125.

119. Balboni TA, Vanderwerker LC, et al. Religiousness and spiritual support among advanced cancer patients and associations with end-of-life treatment preferences and quality of life. *J Clin Oncol.* 2007;25:555-560.

120. Buetow SA. Something in nothing: negative space in the clinician-patient relationship. *Ann Fam Med.* 2009;7:80-83.

121. Ferrell B. Meeting spiritual needs: what is an oncologist to do? *J Clin Oncol.* 2007;25:467-468.

122. Cassidy S. *Sharing in the Darkness.* London: Darton, Longman and Todd; 1988.

123. Graves DL, Shue CK, Arnold L. The role of spirituality in patient care: incorporating spirituality training into medical school curriculum. *Acad Med.* 2002;77:1167.

124. Barnett KG, Fortin AH 6th. Spirituality and medicine. A workshop for medical students and residents. *J Gen Intern Med.* 2006;21:481-485.

125. Todres ID, Catlin EA, Thiel MM. The intensivist in a spiritual care training program adapted for clinicians. *Crit Care Med.* 2005;33:2733-2736.

126. Gabriel B, Bromberg E, Vandenbovenkamp J, Walka P, Kornblith AB, Luzzato P. Art therapy with adult bone marrow transplant patients in isolation: a pilot study. *Pyscho-Oncology.* 2001;10:114-123.

127. Lee V. The existential plight of cancer: meaning making as a concrete approach to the intangible search for meaning. *Support Care Cancer.* 2008;16:779-785.

128. Sherman AC, Plante TG, Simonton S, Latif U, Anaissie EJ. Prospective study of religious coping among patients undergoing autologous stem cell transplantation. *J Behav Med.* 2009;32:118-128.

129. Chung HM, Lyckholm LJ, Smith TJ. Palliative care in BMT. *Bone Marrow Transplant.* 2009;43:265-273.

CHAPTER 65

Long-Term Survivorship: Late Effects

Debra L. Friedman

INTRODUCTION

During the last several decades, multi-modal therapy for childhood cancer has resulted in markedly improved survival and currently 80% of children are cured. In the United States, there are currently >300,000 survivors of childhood cancer, and it is estimated that 1 in every 620 young adults between the ages of 20 and 39 is a survivor of childhood cancer (1–3). With this improvement in survival, the earlier expectation that a large proportion of childhood cancer survivors will now reach adulthood has become a reality. However, this cure comes at a cost. We have known for some years that the very therapy responsible for this survival can also produce adverse long-term outcomes that may limit survival and reduce survivors' quality of life. Cancer, its treatments, and other factors, such as genetic predisposition and environmental exposures, place survivors of childhood cancer at risk for long-term adverse physiological and psychological sequelae, many of which are not yet evident during the childhood years (4–15).

Although research regarding long-term health-related outcomes has been carried on for over 25 years, changes in therapeutic approaches and increased survivorship mandate the need for ongoing studies that focus on health-related outcomes that are not only limited to a simple analysis of cure but also consider the quality of survivorship. These data can help direct appropriate clinical care for patients and also assist in the development of effective screening to reduce long-term morbidity. In this chapter, we briefly review some of the more common medical and psychosocial conditions for which childhood cancer survivors are at risk, discuss models of care and the need for risk-based monitoring for said health conditions, and provide information on resources available to healthcare providers following childhood cancer survivors. We also address some of the unique issues faced by patients who are diagnosed with cancer during their adolescent and young adult years.

COMMON PHYSIOLOGIC AND PSYCHOSOCIAL SEQUELAE OF CHILDHOOD CANCER

Tables 65.1 and 65.2 display some of the more common late effects associated with radiation and chemotherapy and further details are provided in the section below. Table 65.3 lists the common first-line therapies for the common pediatric cancers.

Cardiovascular

Childhood cancer survivors with a history of exposure to anthracyclines (doxorubicin, daunorubicin, and idarubicin) or thoracic radiotherapy are at risk for long-term cardiac toxicity. Current therapy, which attempts to decrease anthracycline exposure, and modern radiotherapy techniques, which result in a smaller volume of the heart receiving high doses of radiation, are likely to reduce these risks.

Anthracyclines are an important group of therapeutic agents used in the treatment of childhood cancer and approximately 50% of children currently receive anthracycline as treatment for cancer. Anthracycline-related cardiac abnormalities include cardiomyopathy, heart failure, and cardiac death and may be symptomatic or asymptomatic depending on severity. Cardiac abnormalities are reported with increased frequency in females, as well as those treated with doses >200 to 300 mg/m², at a younger age and risk increases from time of exposure (16–30).

The effects of thoracic radiation therapy are difficult to separate from those of anthracyclines because few children undergo thoracic radiation therapy without the use of anthracyclines. However, the pathogenesis of the injury differs, with radiation primarily affecting the fine vasculature of the heart that can present as pericarditis, pancarditis, myopathy, coronary artery disease, myocardial infarction, valve disease, and conduction defects (16,31–33). These cardiac toxic effects are related to age at exposure, time since exposure, total radiation dose, individual radiation fraction size, and the volume of the heart that is exposed.

In addition to direct cardiac toxicity, survivors of childhood acute lymphoblastic leukemia (ALL), the most common malignancy of childhood, are at risk for components of the metabolic syndrome, which include obesity with visceral adiposity, insulin resistance, hypertension, and dyslipidemia (34–38).

Pulmonary

Pulmonary toxicity, which manifests as restrictive defects with fibrosis, may follow exposure to total body radiation as part of hematopoietic cell transplant, thoracic radiotherapy, or exposure to several chemotherapeutic agents, bleomycin, busulfan, and the nitrosoureas (carmustine and lomustine). Risk is largely related to dose (39–42).

TABLE 65.1	Radiation late effects	
System	**Radiation Dose Range**	**Potential Effects**
Neurological	>18 Gy	Precocious puberty and growth hormone deficiency
	>40–60 Gy	Cognitive dysfunction, leukencephalopathy, and second CNS tumors (worsens with increased dose)
		Stroke, ototoxicity, myelitis, blindness, peripheral neuropathy, and pituitary and hypothalamic dysfunction
Eye	10–15 Gy	Cataracts
	>40–50 Gy	Cornea, lacrimal duct, retina, conjunctiva, sclera, and optic neuropathy
Cardiac	>30–40 Gy (may be synergistic with anthracyclines)	Cardiomyopathy
		Pericarditis
		Coronary artery disease
		Valvular disease
Pulmonary	>10 Gy (may be synergistic with bleomycin)	Pulmonary fibrosis
Thyroid	>20 Gy	Overt or compensated hypothyroidism
		Thyroid nodules or cancer
		Hyperthyroidism
Gonadal	>4–12 Gy (20 in younger females)	Ovarian failure
	>1–6 Gy	Oligospermia/azoospermia
	>24 Gy	Leydig cell dysfunction
Second malignancies	>20–30 Gy	Sarcomas
		CNS tumors
		Breast cancer
		Melanoma
		Non–melanoma skin cancer
		Thyroid
Any	Dose dependent	Any organ within the field of radiation may sustain dysfunction or may be at risk for development of a second cancer

CNS, central nervous system.

Gastrointestinal and Hepatic

Gastrointestinal and hepatic effects are rare. Following high doses of radiotherapy for abdominal sarcoma, intestinal fibrosis, obstruction, strictures, colitis, malabsorption, and diarrhea can occur. Similarly, rare are hepatic fibrosis, veno-occlusive disease, and portal hypertension following hepatic radiation or exposure to methotrexate, mercaptopurine, thiopurine, and dactinomycin (43).

Renal

Chronic nephrotoxicity can occur following exposure to cisplatin, carboplatin, ifosfamide, and rarely methotrexate,

TABLE 65.2	Chemotherapy late effects	
System	**Agents and Dose Range**	**Potential Effects**
Neurological	Intrathecal chemotherapy methotrexate (>3 g/m^2)	Cognitive dysfunction Cognitive dysfunction and leukencephalopathy (risk increases with increased dose)
Cardiac	Anthracyclines >200–300 mg/m^2 (less with XRT to chest)	Cardiomyopathy Arrhythmias
Hearing	*Platinums*	Hearing loss
Pulmonary	Bleomycin >200 u/m^2 (less with XRT to chest) Carmustine (BCNU)	Restrictive lung disease
Urological	Cyclophosphamide Ifosfamide	Chronic hemorrhagic cystitis Second bladder cancers Chronic hemorrhagic cystitis
Hepatic	Methotrexate Thioguanine Mercaptopurine Dactinomycin Busulfan	Hepatic dysfunction Veno-occlusive disease (dactinomycin, busulfan, and thioguanine)
Renal	Platinums Ifosfamide	Renal insufficiency or failure Renal electrolyte wasting/insufficiency
Gonadal	Alkylating agents Nitrosoureas	Ovarian failure; early menopause Testicular failure; Leydig cell dysfunction
Second malignancies	Alkylating agents: Mechlorethamine>>others Topoisomerase II inhibitors Platinums Cyclophosphamide	Leukemia Transitional bladder carcinoma

XRT, radiation therapy; BCNU, carmustine.

radiation therapy, or removal of a kidney in the setting of other risk factors. Both glomerular and tubular injuries can be seen and many patients are asymptomatic (44–49).

Endocrine Function and Fertility

Thyroid dysfunction, as manifested by hypothyroidism, hyperthyroidism, goiter, or nodules, is a common delayed effect of radiation therapy for Hodgkin disease, brain tumors, and ALL (50,51). Other endocrine abnormalities can occur following cranial irradiation, including growth hormone deficiency, delayed or precocious puberty, and hypopituitarism (14,52–54). These effects are related to dose, age at time of exposure, and gender.

Alkylating agents are the chemotherapeutic agents that are most responsible for gonadal toxicity. Males retain

endocrine function following higher cumulative doses than do females, but spermatogenesis is highly sensitive to even relatively low doses of alkylating agents, such as cyclophosphamide, ifosfamide, and procarbazine. Passage through puberty and retention of normal male hormonal production and function is possible after relatively high doses of alkylating agent's radiation (55–60). Unlike the situation in males, hormonal function and potential for fertility are synchronous in females. Prepubertal females possess their lifetime supply of oocytes with no new oogonia formed after birth. This may protect them against the effects of chemotherapy and radiation therapy. As the number of oocytes is fixed, and they are extruded during ovulation, risk of menstrual irregularity, ovarian failure, and infertility increases with age at treatment (61–66). Given the high risk of infertility and sterility following childhood cancer treatment, efforts are

TABLE 65.3	Common pediatric cancers and common first-line treatments
Disease	**Treatment**
Acute lymphoblastic leukemia	Cranial and craniospinal radiotherapy (some high risk or central nervous system disease)
	Testicular radiotherapy (only with testicular involvement)
	Vincristine, corticosteroids, asparaginase, daunorubicin, doxorubicin, cyclophosphamide, cytarabine, mercaptopurine, methotrexate, and thiopurine
Acute myeloid leukemia	Daunorubicin, idarubicin, mitoxantrone, cytarabine, etoposide, and thioguanine
Lymphomas	Radiation to involved sites
	Doxorubicin, bleomycin, vincristine, vinblastine, etoposide, prednisone, cyclophosphamide, cytarabine, dexamethasone, rituximab, methotrexate, procarbazine, mechlorethamine, dacarbazine, and mercaptopurine
Central nervous system malignancy	Cranial or craniospinal radiation
	Vincristine, cyclophosphamide, carmustine, lomustine, carboplatin, cisplatin, methotrexate, and etoposide
Soft tissue sarcomas (rhabdomyosarcoma and others)	Radiation to involved sites
	Vincristine, doxorubicin, cyclophosphamide, irinotecan, topotecan, etoposide, ifosfamide, and dactinomycin
Bone sarcomas (osteosarcoma and Ewing sarcoma)	Radiation to involved sites (Ewing only)
	Vincristine, doxorubicin, cyclophosphamide, irinotecan, topotecan, etoposide, ifosfamide, dactinomycin, methotrexate, and cisplatin
Germ cell tumors	Radiation to involved site (rare)
	Cisplatin, carboplatin, etoposide, and bleomycin
Wilms tumor	Radiation to involved sites
	Vincristine, dactinomycin, doxorubicin, cyclophosphamide, carboplatin, and etoposide

underway to help preserve function. This includes reduction in cumulative doses of radiation and chemotherapy as well as ovarian and sperm cryopreservation, which includes some yet experimental and evolving methodologies for women and prepubertal males (67,68).

When fertility is preserved, pregnancy outcomes and health of offspring become of paramount importance. Treatment in females with high doses of radiation can lead to uterine vascular insufficiency, spontaneous abortion, neonatal death, low-birth-weight infants, fetal malposition, and premature labor (69,70). However, outside of these risks, offspring of childhood cancer survivors have not been found to have an excess of birth defects or adverse health outcomes (70–74).

Musculoskeletal Late Effects

Normal cells are affected by radiation therapy in growing children, and this can result in soft tissue hypoplasia, diminution of bone growth, and decreased bone mineral density, the latter of which can also be adversely affected by

corticosteroid use, vitamin D deficiency, and estrogen deficiency. Avascular necrosis is also reported following corticosteroid exposure (75–84).

Neurocognitive and Psychological Late Effects

Neurocognitive dysfunction is most commonly seen following cranial radiotherapy in survivors of ALL or central nervous system tumors and need for special education services is not uncommon. Younger age at the time of treatment and higher dose are associated with increased risk. Treatment intensity and length of treatment can also adversely affect cognitive performance, due to absences from school and psychologic problems. Intrathecal and intravenous methotrexate and oral corticosteroids (dexamethasone > prednisone) may also contribute to cognitive dysfunction, but findings are not consistent across studies (85–97).

Psychological effects of cancer and its treatment are now being recognized because of the efforts of investigators who are examining the adjustment of long-term survivors and their parents and siblings. Findings are very diverse, with some studies among survivors reporting normal function, less risk taking, and post-traumatic growth while many others reporting increases in mental health disorders and symptoms such as stress, distress, anxiety, depression, post-traumatic stress disorder, impaired health-related quality of life (HRQOL), fatigue, and chronic pain (90,98–115).

Subsequent Malignant Neoplasms

Many studies have examined the incidence and spectrum of second malignant neoplasms (SMNs) in childhood cancer survivors. A number of treatment-related risk factors including chemotherapeutic agents and radiotherapy have been identified. Notably, radiation therapy is associated with the development of solid cancers, while alkylating agents and topoisomerase II inhibitors are associated with the development of leukemia (116–133). Unless more is learned about the pathophysiology of SMN and the inter-individual variation in susceptibility, targeted preventive strategies are limited. However, the reduction in dose or elimination of radiation for certain embryonal tumors and the reduction in use and alteration in schedule of certain specific drugs can be expected to have a positive effect. In future, those children who received radiation or chemotherapeutic agents with known carcinogenic effects or cancers associated with genetic risk should be so informed and should be seen regularly by a healthcare provider familiar with their treatment and risks and who can evaluate early signs and symptoms and recommend appropriate screening.

FUNCTIONAL OUTCOMES

As a result of cancer and its treatment, and perhaps in part to the physiologic and psychosocial adverse outcomes for which survivors are at risk, childhood and adolescent cancer survivors are in most, but not all studies are likely not only to require special education services and less likely to marry, but also to divorce and to be gainfully and appropriately employed (92,93,134–143).

RISK-BASED HEALTH CARE AND MODELS OF CARE FOR CHILDHOOD CANCER SURVIVORS

The risk and severity of some, albeit not all, adverse outcomes for which childhood cancer survivors are at risk changes throughout their lifespan (144). Table 65.4 shows the components of survivorship care. To facilitate and standardize risk-based care to prevent, ameliorate, or detect early adverse sequelae of treatment, several evidence-based screening and monitoring guidelines have been established (145–149). In the United States, the Children's Oncology Group (COG)'s "Long-term Follow-up Guidelines for Survivors of Childhood, Adolescent and Young Adult Cancer" is widely used (148). Recommendations for screening and monitoring are based on the therapeutic exposure or modality and modifying risk factors. Level of evidence for the association between the exposure and adverse outcome is provided with

supporting references. Together with these guidelines are >40 detailed "Health Links" focusing on physiologic, psychosocial, and functional areas of health, designed for patients and healthcare providers. These guidelines and health links are available to the public at www.survivorshipguidelines.org.

To facilitate the education of survivors and all of their healthcare providers, a survivorship care plan is recommended for all cancer survivors. While formats differ, the key components include diagnosis, stage, chemotherapy with selected cumulative doses, radiotherapy with dose and site, known co-morbidities, known adverse effects of treatment with long-term implications, and using the COG guidelines, a plan for monitoring for long-term adverse outcomes. Contact information for treating providers and the survivorship team (if different) is also included.

In a survey of 179 of 220 COG institutions, 87% reported providing survivorship care and 68% provided survivors with survivorship care plan. For pediatric survivors, 59% provided care in a specialized late effects program. For adult survivors, 47% of institutions transitioned care to adult providers, while 44% preferred continued follow-up for their adult survivors in the treating institution, although a dedicated adult-based program was not necessarily provided (150).

Childhood cancer is unlike most chronic diseases of childhood (e.g., cystic fibrosis and congenital heart disease) where ongoing, organ-directed treatment is usually required and it is obvious which specialty should take overall charge throughout the lifespan, including the transition to adult care. In contrast most childhood cancer survivors do not require antineoplastic therapy or other "acute care" services traditionally provided by pediatric or medical oncologists. Instead, survivors must be provided with expertise from various specialties to manage long-term complications of prior cancer treatment. To accomplish this, several models have evolved for the care of childhood cancer survivors and vary according to the resources they require and the exact services they can provide; each has advantages and disadvantages (151–153). Figure 65.1 describes some models of care for cancer survivors.

Methods necessary for detection and management of late effects range from simple to sophisticated, depending on the specific abnormality and on the risks conferred by specific therapeutic exposures. For survivors at minimal risk, management may be provided outside of a specialty-oriented medical center by a community-based primary care provider. For patients who are at high risk for, or have already developed, one or more late effects of moderate or greater severity, the involvement of specialized diagnostic equipment and health professionals within a specialty-oriented medical center may be required for all follow-up care or in a consultative fashion as requested by the primary care provider. For those with cognitive impairment or mental health challenges, care should include provision of emotional assessment and support, medical information, and opportunities for linking with allied professional and community resources. Thus, risk-adapted monitoring and management of late effects clearly has an impact on where follow-up should occur and who should participate in that follow-up.

TABLE 65.4	Components of survivorship care

Key Program Components

Multidisciplinary "Core Team" responsible for coordinating care

Access to appropriate diagnostic monitoring

Access to appropriate medical and behavioral consultants

Service Capabilities

Survivor/family education about cancer diagnosis, past treatment, and current health status including complications and recommendations

Preparation of survivorship care plan

Clinical services to include

    Review of diagnosis, treatment, complications, and co-morbidities

    Risk-adapted history and physical examination and laboratory and diagnostic studies

    Psychosocial and functional needs assessment and support

Follow-up and coordination with other healthcare providers

Coordination of referrals and follow-up

Educational and vocational counseling

Financial assistance

Availability between scheduled appointments

Formal transition-of-care preparation and assistance

Means for tracking survivor status beyond transition of care

Additional Desirable Components

Database to assist with clinical care and research activities

Appropriate clinical space for evaluations (ideally outside of acute oncology setting and suitable for teens and adults)

Training opportunities

Collaboration with adult-based services

Maintain follow-up with survivor and healthcare providers to collect data on health outcomes

Availability of assistance post transfer of care

It is well acknowledged that survivors need to be educated about their cancer diagnosis, treatments received, current health status, need for monitoring, and recommended disease prevention practices. As evidenced from several reports from the Childhood Cancer Survivor Study (CCSS), this has been less than universally successful. This cohort of over 14,000 patients, treated between 1970 and 1986, completed self-report questionnaires in the last decade, which included information on a variety of health-related outcomes and behaviors (154). Barriers and obstacles to health care of adult survivors in this cohort were identified in several key areas: the survivor's knowledge and psychological state, the health provider, and the health system itself (155). This is supported by the report of Kadan-Lottick et al., which found that only 35% of the survivors understood that serious health problems could result from past therapies and only 15% reported ever receiving a written record of their cancer diagnosis and treatment (156). Other reports from the CCSS and others found a lower rate of utilizing cancer-screening practices in survivors and suboptimal healthcare utilization among adult survivors (157–161). Patient information has been shown to enhance attitude to follow-up and influence adverse lifestyle behaviors (162,163). The above results suggest that survivors both need and can benefit from information provided to them about their past history and future health concerns.

In the United States, where most health insurance is private and employer-based rather than provided through a national health service, the challenges to employment and the access to insurance and medical care are intertwined. Strategies have been published for decades to assist survivors in gaining access to health insurance coverage and in obtaining work and dealing with discrimination in the workplace (164–166). Access to an experienced medical social worker is helpful in addressing these challenges and

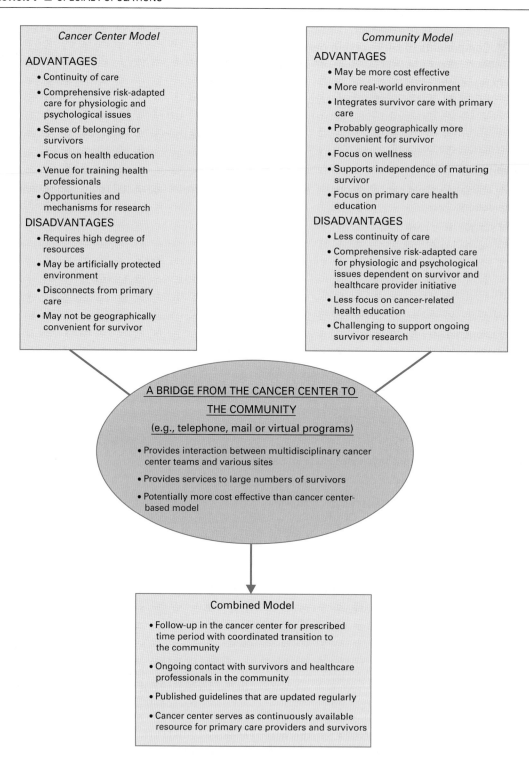

Figure 65.1. Models of care for survivors of childhood cancer.

this has been utilized in some of the models of long-term follow-up (167,168).

Follow-up can be coordinated by the primary oncology team in the oncology clinic, by a dedicated late effects team in the oncology clinic, or by a dedicated late effects team outside of the oncology clinic. A true survivorship clinic in the cancer center is therefore one with a dedicated team of experts providing continuity of care from active treatment

to follow-up and then provide a transition from pediatrics to adult medicine and from the cancer center to the community. Cancer center–based survivor clinics, regardless of the staff or space details, generally provide comprehensive and systematic follow-up, which can benefit survivors in a multitude of ways. There is continuity of care from the acute phase to the follow-up phase of the illness; it can support medical training of professionals who will be providing care to the survivors in the community at a later date; patients develop a sense of the survivor community; health education is a focus of the comprehensive care delivered; physiologic and psychosocial needs can be more easily addressed in an integrated fashion; and survivors have ready access to clinical research studies. Another set of potential models puts the follow-up directly in the community.

In concept and with limited experience, follow-up of at least some childhood cancer survivors can be done successfully by health professionals in typical practices, such as a pediatricians, family medicine specialists, internists, medicine-pediatric specialists, or mid-level providers including advanced practice nurses and physician assistants. There is coordination between the risk-adapted follow-up that the survivor requires and the general primary care that promotes independence on the part of the survivor and their families.

A combination of the cancer center and community models appears to be the most ideal. An example would be follow-up in the cancer center model for a specified time period with transfer of follow-up to a community-based primary care practice with variable levels of continued involvement from the late effects team. The time of transfer could be designed based on combination factors, including risk for developing adverse late effects, complexity of those late effects, psychosocial and developmental issues, and the knowledge demonstrated on the part of the survivor or their family. Involvement of the cancer center clinic could be only advisory at the request of the primary care provider. More optimally, the cancer center late effects team would provide ongoing guidance with respect to monitoring and management of late effects using specified guidelines.

Transition of care for adult survivors of childhood cancer is a process as opposed to an action. Education is required for the survivor, family members, and community or adult-based healthcare providers. Readiness on the part of all parties must be assessed and a transition and transfer plan developed (129). Table 65.5 shows the components of the transition and transfer process.

SURVIVORS OF ADOLESCENT AND YOUNG ADULT CANCER

Survival rates for adolescents and young adults (AYAs) diagnosed with cancer between ages 15 and 39, overall, have not increased since 1975 to 1980, a point at which their survival rates were superior to most other age groups (3,169,170). As outlined in detail by the AYA Oncology Progress Review Group (PRG) sponsored by the National Cancer Institute and the Lance Armstrong Foundation (LAF), specific issues for the AYA age group include lack of primary health care, lack of medical insurance, delays in diagnosis, rare tumors with unknown biologic prognostic factors, access to care, psychosocial and developmental considerations, decreased participation in clinical trials, and a significant burden of adverse long-term effects (171). To improve outcomes for AYA patients, recommendations in the PRG include the creation or modification of assessment tools specific for AYA

TABLE 65.5	Components of transition and transfer to adult-based follow-up

Prior to Transition and Transfer

Review prior disease and treatment

Prepare detailed survivorship care plan

Assess patient and family readiness

Assess financial or insurance barriers

Transition and Transfer

Introduction of process

Clinical evaluation

Updated survivorship care plan

Coordination of transfer with patient, family, adult healthcare team, and subspecialists

Psychosocial support

Written referral to all healthcare providers with survivorship care plan

After Transition and Transfer

Maintain follow-up with survivor and healthcare providers to collect data on health outcomes

Availability of assistance or re-consideration of transfer of care

oncology issues and the report cited the paucity of such tools for assessing HRQOL. Furthermore, the PRG stated that such measures should "span the survivorship continuum, be developmentally appropriate, include co-morbidity assessment and family well-being, and be usable with patients with vary literacy levels and cultural identities (171)."

While studies of AYA patients treated in the medical oncology setting are limited, there is some evidence of impairment of HRQOL in young adult patients treated for prostate, testicular, bone, and breast cancers (172–176).

Adolescence and young adulthood are periods marked with significant changes and challenges, which include physical and sexual maturity, establishment of independence, and development of personal identity (177). Adolescent development is characterized by continued involvement with family and increased involvement in peer and romantic relationships outside of the family. Further, investment in achievement and development of a sense of competence expand beyond school and academic achievement to include involvement in work (178). A cancer diagnosis during adolescence or young adulthood may interrupt the normal developmental process, as the necessary practicalities of treatment may result in less opportunity for independence, decision-making, and social growth (178–183). Disturbance of body image due to the effects of chemoradiotherapy is not unexpected (182). Some studies have shown adolescents to have impaired HRQOL as compared with younger patients, although other studies indicate that older adolescents may have greater perceived control, may be able to demonstrate greater coping strategies, and may utilize cognitive abilities to interpret health status information (184–186).

CONCLUSIONS

Survivorship from childhood, adolescent, and young adult cancer remains high, but the very therapies responsible for this survivorship share the etiologic limelight for adverse long-term medical, psychosocial, and functional sequelae. Cancer, therefore, should now be viewed not as an acute illness, but as a chronic process with acute and long-term components. Survivorship should be considered from the time of diagnosis, and supportive oncology should be provided together with cytotoxic therapy, surgery, and radiation to help patients live with, through, and after a diagnosis of cancer. More research is required to determine the most cost-effective practices for following a growing cohort of cancer survivors with risk adaptation. However, the success in curing children, adolescents, and young adults should not be overshadowed by these challenges.

REFERENCES

1. Hewitt M, Breen N, Devesa S. Cancer prevalence and survivorship issues: analyses of the 1992 National Health Interview Survey. *J Natl Cancer Inst.* 1999;91(17):1480-1486.
2. Jemal A, Siegel R, Xu J, Ward E. Cancer statistics, 2010. *CA Cancer J Clin.* 2010;60(5):277-300.
3. Ries L, Eisner M, Kosary C, et al. Cancer Statistics Review, 1975–2002. SEER; 2005 [updated 2005; cited]; http://seer.cancer.gov/csr/1975_2002/.
4. Friedman DL, Meadows AT. Late effects of childhood cancer therapy. *Pediatr Clin North Am.* 2002;49(5):1083-1106, x.
5. Hudson MM. Survivors of childhood cancer: coming of age. *Hematol Oncol Clin North Am.* 2008;22(2):211-231, v-vi.
6. Hudson MM, Mertens AC, Yasui Y, et al. Health status of adult long-term survivors of childhood cancer: a report from the Childhood Cancer Survivor Study. *JAMA.* 2003;290(12):1583-1592.
7. Hudson MM, Mulrooney DA, Bowers DC, et al. High-risk populations identified in Childhood Cancer Survivor Study investigations: implications for risk-based surveillance. *J Clin Oncol.* 2009;27(14):2405-2414. PMCID: 2677926.
8. Kurt BA, Armstrong GT, Cash DK, et al. Primary care management of the childhood cancer survivor. *J Pediatr.* 2008;152(4):458-466.
9. Oeffinger KC. Childhood cancer survivors and primary care physicians. *J Fam Pract.* 2000;49(8):689-690.
10. Oeffinger KC. Shared care of adult survivors of childhood cancers. *Lancet Oncol.* 2008;9(3):191-193.
11. Oeffinger KC, Hudson MM. Long-term complications following childhood and adolescent cancer: foundations for providing risk-based health care for survivors. *CA Cancer J Clin.* 2004;54(4):208-236.
12. Oeffinger KC, Hudson MM, Landier W. Survivorship: childhood cancer survivors. *Prim Care.* 2009;36(4):743-780.
13. Oeffinger KC, Mertens AC, Hudson MM, et al. Health care of young adult survivors of childhood cancer: a report from the Childhood Cancer Survivor Study. *Ann Fam Med.* 2004;2(1):61-70.
14. Oeffinger KC, Mertens AC, Sklar CA, et al. Chronic health conditions in adult survivors of childhood cancer. *N Engl J Med.* 2006;355(15):1572-1582.
15. Oeffinger KC, Nathan PC, Kremer LC. Challenges after curative treatment for childhood cancer and long-term follow up of survivors. *Hematol Oncol Clin North Am.* 2010;24(1):129-149.
16. Adams MJ, Hardenbergh PH, Constine LS, Lipshultz SE. Radiation-associated cardiovascular disease. *Crit Rev Oncol Hematol.* 2003;45(1):55-75.
17. Adams MJ, Lipshultz SE, Schwartz C, Fajardo LF, Coen V, Constine LS. Radiation-associated cardiovascular disease: manifestations and management. *Semin Radiat Oncol.* 2003;13(3):346-356.
18. Ewer MS, Jaffe N, Ried H, Zietz HA, Benjamin RS. Doxorubicin cardiotoxicity in children: comparison of a consecutive divided daily dose administration schedule with single dose (rapid) infusion administration. *Med Pediatr Oncol.* 1998;31(6):512-515.
19. Green DM, Grigoriev YA, Nan B, et al. Congestive heart failure after treatment for Wilms' tumor: a report from the National Wilms' Tumor Study Group. *J Clin Oncol.* 2001;19(7):1926-1934.
20. Green DM, Hyland A, Chung CS, Zevon MA, Hall BC. Cancer and cardiac mortality among 15-year survivors of cancer diagnosed during childhood or adolescence. *J Clin Oncol.* 1999;17(10):3207-3215.
21. Kremer LC, van Dalen EC, Offringa M, Ottenkamp J, Voute PA. Anthracycline-induced clinical heart failure in a cohort of 607 children: long-term follow-up study. *J Clin Oncol.* 2001;19(1):191-196.
22. Lipshultz SE. Ventricular dysfunction clinical research in infants, children and adolescents. *Prog Pediatr Cardiol.* 2000;12(1):1-28.
23. Lipshultz SE, Landy DC, Lopez-Mitnik G, et al. Cardiovascular status of childhood cancer survivors exposed and unexposed to cardiotoxic therapy. *J Clin Oncol.* 2012;30(10):1050-1057.
24. Lipshultz SE, Lipsitz SR, Mone SM, et al. Female sex and drug dose as risk factors for late cardiotoxic effects of doxorubicin therapy for childhood cancer. *N Engl J Med.* 1995;332(26):1738-1743.
25. Pein F, Sakiroglu O, Dahan M, et al. Cardiac abnormalities 15 years and more after adriamycin therapy in 229 childhood survivors of a solid tumour at the Institut Gustave Roussy. *Br J Cancer.* 2004;91(1):37-44. PMCID: 2364747.
26. van Dalen EC, Michiels EM, Caron HN, Kremer LC. Different anthracycline derivates for reducing cardiotoxicity in cancer patients. *Cochrane Database Syst Rev.* 2006;(4):CD005006.
27. van Dalen EC, Raphael MF, Caron HN, Kremer LC. Treatment including anthracyclines versus treatment not including anthracyclines for childhood cancer. *Cochrane Database Syst Rev.* 2011;(1):CD006647.
28. van Dalen EC, van der Pal HJ, Caron HN, Kremer LC. Different dosage schedules for reducing cardiotoxicity in cancer patients receiving anthracycline chemotherapy. *Cochrane Database Syst Rev.* 2009;(4):CD005008.
29. van der Pal HJ, van Dalen EC, Hauptmann M, et al. Cardiac function in 5-year survivors of childhood cancer: a long-term follow-up study. *Arch Intern Med.* 2010;170(14):1247-1255.
30. van der Pal HJ, van Dalen EC, Kremer LC, Bakker PJ, van Leeuwen FE. Risk of morbidity and mortality from cardiovascular disease following radiotherapy for childhood cancer: a systematic review. *Cancer Treat Rev.* 2005;31(3):173-185.

31. Galper SL, Yu JB, Mauch PM, et al. Clinically significant cardiac disease in patients with Hodgkin lymphoma treated with mediastinal irradiation. *Blood.* 2011;117(2):412-418.

32. Hull MC, Morris CG, Pepine CJ, Mendenhall NP. Valvular dysfunction and carotid, subclavian, and coronary artery disease in survivors of Hodgkin lymphoma treated with radiation therapy. *JAMA.* 2003;290(21):2831-2837.

33. Constine LS. Late effects. In: Halperin EC, Constine LS, Tarbell N, eds. *Pediatric Radiation Oncology.* Philadelphia, PA: Lippincott Williams & Wilkins; 1999.

34. Chow EJ, Pihoker C, Hunt K, Wilkinson K, Friedman DL. Obesity and hypertension among children after treatment for acute lymphoblastic leukemia. *Cancer.* 2007;110(10):2313-2320.

35. Chow EJ, Simmons JH, Roth CL, et al. Increased cardiometabolic traits in pediatric survivors of acute lymphoblastic leukemia treated with total body irradiation. *Biol Blood Marrow Transplant.* 2010;16(12):1674-1681. PMCID: 2975816.

36. Esbenshade AJ, Simmons JH, Koyama T, Koehler E, Whitlock JA, Friedman DL. Body mass index and blood pressure changes over the course of treatment of pediatric acute lymphoblastic leukemia. *Pediatr Blood Cancer.* 2011;56(3):372-378.

37. Jarfelt M, Bjarnason R, Lannering B. Young adult survivors of childhood acute lymphoblastic leukemia: spontaneous GH secretion in relation to CNS radiation. *Pediatr Blood Cancer.* 2004;42(7):582-588.

38. Oeffinger KC, Mertens AC, Sklar CA, et al. Obesity in adult survivors of childhood acute lymphoblastic leukemia: a report from the Childhood Cancer Survivor Study. *J Clin Oncol.* 2003;21(7):1359-1365.

39. Fryer CJ, Hutchinson RJ, Krailo M, et al. Efficacy and toxicity of 12 courses of ABVD chemotherapy followed by low-dose regional radiation in advanced Hodgkin's disease in children: a report from the Children's Cancer Study Group. *J Clin Oncol.* 1990;8(12):1971-1980.

40. Kreisman H, Wolkove N. Pulmonary toxicity of antineoplastic therapy. *Semin Oncol.* 1992;19(5):508-520.

41. Marina NM, Greenwald CA, Fairclough DL, et al. Serial pulmonary function studies in children treated for newly diagnosed Hodgkin's disease with mantle radiotherapy plus cycles of cyclophosphamide, vincristine, and procarbazine alternating with cycles of doxorubicin, bleomycin, vinblastine, and dacarbazine. *Cancer.* 1995;75(7):1706-1711.

42. Nysom K, Holm K, Hertz H, Hesse B. Risk factors for reduced pulmonary function after malignant lymphoma in childhood [comment]. *Med Pediatr Oncol.* 1998;30(4):240-248.

43. Hudson MM. Late gastrointestinal and hepatic effects. In: Schwartz CL, Hobbie W, Constine L, Ruccione K, eds. *Survivors of Childhood and Adolescent Cancer.* Heidelberg: Springer; 2005.

44. Marks LB, Larrier N. Genitourinary. In: Schwartz CL, Hobbie W, Constine L, Ruccione K, eds. *Survivors of Childhood and Adolescent Cancer.* Heidelberg: Springer; 2005.

45. Cassady JR. Clinical radiation nephropathy. *Int J Radiat Oncol Biol Phys.* 1995;31(5):1249-1256.

46. Hutchison FN, Perez EA, Gandara DR, Lawrence HJ, Kaysen GA. Renal salt wasting in patients treated with cisplatin. *Ann Intern Med.* 1988;108(1):21-25.

47. Irwin C, Fyles A, Wong CS, Cheung CM, Zhu Y. Late renal function following whole abdominal irradiation. *Radiother Oncol.* 1996;38(3):257-261.

48. Prasad VK, Lewis IJ, Aparicio SR, et al. Progressive glomerular toxicity of ifosfamide in children. *Med Pediatr Oncol.* 1996;27(3):149-155.

49. Shnorhavorian M, Friedman DL, Koyle MA. Genitourinary long-term outcomes for childhood cancer survivors. *Curr Urol Rep.* 2009;10(2):134-137.

50. Sklar C, Whitton J, Mertens A, et al. Abnormalities of the thyroid in survivors of Hodgkin's disease: data from the Childhood Cancer Survivor Study. *J Clin Endocrinol Metab.* 2000;85(9):3227-3232.

51. Rutter MM, Rose SR. Long-term endocrine sequelae of childhood cancer. *Curr Opin Pediatr.* 2007;19(4):480-487.

52. Schmiegelow M, Lassen S, Poulsen HS, et al. Cranial radiotherapy of childhood brain tumours: growth hormone deficiency and its relation to the biological effective dose of irradiation in a large population based study. *Clin Endocrinol* (Oxf). 2000;53(2):191-197.

53. Chemaitilly W, Sklar CA. Endocrine complications in long-term survivors of childhood cancers. *Endocr Relat Cancer.* 2010;17(3):R141-R159.

54. Armstrong GT, Chow EJ, Sklar CA. Alterations in pubertal timing following therapy for childhood malignancies. *Endocr Dev.* 2009;15:25-39.

55. Thomson AB, Critchley HO, Kelnar CJ, Wallace WH. Late reproductive sequelae following treatment of childhood cancer and options for fertility preservation. *Best Pract Res Clin Endocrinol Metab.* 2002;16(2):311-334.

56. Kenney LB, Laufer MR, Grant FD, Grier H, Diller L. High risk of infertility and long term gonadal damage in males treated with high dose cyclophosphamide for sarcoma during childhood. *Cancer.* 2001;91(3):613-621.

57. Relander T, Cavallin-Stahl E, Garwicz S, Olsson AM, Willen M. Gonadal and sexual function in men treated for childhood cancer. *Med Pediatr Oncol.* 2000;35(1):52-63.

58. Lopez Andreu JA, Fernandez PJ, Ferris i Tortajada J, et al. Persistent altered spermatogenesis in long-term childhood cancer survivors. *Pediatr Hematol Oncol.* 2000;17(1):21-30.

59. Ben Arush MW, Solt I, Lightman A, Linn S, Kuten A. Male gonadal function in survivors of childhood Hodgkin and non-Hodgkin lymphoma. *Pediatr Hematol Oncol.* 2000;17(3):239-245.

60. Howell S, Shalet S. Gonadal damage from chemotherapy and radiotherapy. *Endocrinol Metab Clin North Am.* 1998;27(4):927-943.

61. Chemaitilly W, Mertens AC, Mitby P, et al. Acute ovarian failure in the Childhood Cancer Survivor Study. *J Clin Endocrinol Metab.* 2006;91(5):1723-1728.

62. Friedman DL. The ovary. In: Schwartz CL, Hobbie W, Constine L, Ruccione K, eds. *Survivors of Childhood and Adolescent Cancer.* Heidelberg: Springer; 2005.

63. Meirow D. Reproduction post-chemotherapy in young cancer patients. *Mol Cell Endocrinol.* 2000;169(1–2):123-131.

64. Mertens AC, Ramsay NK, Kouris S, Neglia JP. Patterns of gonadal dysfunction following bone marrow transplantation. *Bone Marrow Transplant.* 1998;22(4):345-350.

65. Sklar CA, Mertens AC, Mitby P, et al. Premature menopause in survivors of childhood cancer: a report from the Childhood Cancer Survivor Study. *J Natl Cancer Inst.* 2006;98(13):890-896.

66. Wallace WH, Shalet SM, Hendry JH, Morris-Jones PH, Gattamaneni HR. Ovarian failure following abdominal irradiation in childhood: the radiosensitivity of the human oocyte. *Br J Radiol.* 1989;62(743):995-998.

67. Lee SJ. Preservation of fertility in patients with cancer. *N Engl J Med.* 2009;360(25):2680; author reply 2-3.

68. Ginsberg JP, Carlson CA, Lin K, et al. An experimental protocol for fertility preservation in prepubertal boys recently diagnosed

with cancer: a report of acceptability and safety. *Hum Reprod.* 2010;25(1):37-41. PMCID: 2794668.

69. Signorello LB, Mulvihill JJ, Green DM, et al. Congenital anomalies in the children of cancer survivors: a report from the Childhood Cancer Survivor Study. *J Clin Oncol.* 2012;30(3):239-245. PMCID: 3269950.

70. Hudson MM. Reproductive outcomes for survivors of childhood cancer. *Obstet Gynecol.* 2010;116(5):1171-83.

71. Boice JD Jr, Robison LL, Mertens A, Stovall M, Green DM, Mulvihill JJ. Stillbirths and male irradiation. *J Radiol Prot.* 2000;20(3):321-322.

72. Boice JD Jr, Tawn EJ, Winther JF, et al. Genetic effects of radiotherapy for childhood cancer. *Health Phys.* 2003;85(1):65-80.

73. Kenney LB, Nicholson HS, Brasseux C, et al. Birth defects in offspring of adult survivors of childhood acute lymphoblastic leukemia. A Childrens Cancer Group/National Institutes of Health Report. *Cancer.* 1996;78(1):169-176.

74. Winther JF, Boice JD Jr., Frederiksen K, et al. Radiotherapy for childhood cancer and risk for congenital malformations in offspring: a population-based cohort study. i. 2009;75(1):50-56. PMCID: 2697125.

75. van Dorp W, van Beek RD, Laven JS, et al. Long-term endocrine side effects of childhood Hodgkin's lymphoma treatment: a review. *Hum Reprod Update.* 2012;18(1):12-28.

76. Wasilewski-Masker K, Kaste SC, Hudson MM, Esiashvili N, Mattano LA, Meacham LR. Bone mineral density deficits in survivors of childhood cancer: long-term follow-up guidelines and review of the literature. *Pediatrics.* 2008;121(3):e705-e713.

77. Ness KK, Mertens AC, Hudson MM, et al. Limitations on physical performance and daily activities among long-term survivors of childhood cancer. *Ann Intern Med.* 2005;143(9):639-647.

78. van der Sluis IM, van den Heuvel-Eibrink MM, Hahlen K, Krenning EP, de Muinck Keizer-Schrama SM. Altered bone mineral density and body composition, and increased fracture risk in childhood acute lymphoblastic leukemia. *J Pediatrs.* 2002;141(2):204-210.

79. Gleeson HK, Darzy K, Shalet SM. Late endocrine, metabolic and skeletal sequelae following treatment of childhood cancer. *Best Pract Res Clin Endocrinol Metab.* 2002;16(2):335-348.

80. Kadan-Lottick N, Marshall JA, Baron AE, Krebs NF, Hambidge KM, Albano E. Normal bone mineral density after treatment for childhood acute lymphoblastic leukemia diagnosed between 1991 and 1998. *J Pediatr.* 2001;138(6):898-904.

81. Vassilopoulou-Sellin R, Brosnan P, Delpassand A, Zietz H, Klein MJ, Jaffe N. Osteopenia in young adult survivors of childhood cancer. *Med Pediatr Oncol.* 1999;32(4):272-278.

82. Cohen LE. Endocrine late effects of cancer treatment. *Endocrinol Metab Clin North Am.* 2005;34(3):769-789, xi.

83. Shusterman S, Meadows AT. Long term survivors of childhood leukemia. *Curr Opin Hematol.* 2000;7(4):217-222.

84. Simmons JH, Chow EJ, Koehler E, et al. Significant 25-hydroxyvitamin D deficiency in child and adolescent survivors of acute lymphoblastic leukemia: treatment with chemotherapy compared with allogeneic stem cell transplant. *Pediatr Blood Cancer.* 2011;56(7):1114-1119. PMCID: 3135735.

85. Armstrong GT. Long-term survivors of childhood central nervous system malignancies: the experience of the Childhood Cancer Survivor Study. *Eur J Paediatr Neurol.* 2010;14(4): 298-303. PMCID: 2885448.

86. Butler RW, Sahler OJ, Askins MA, et al. Interventions to improve neuropsychological functioning in childhood cancer survivors. *Dev Disabil Res Rev.* 2008;14(3):251-258.

87. Mulhern RK, Merchant TE, Gajjar A, Reddick WE, Kun LE. Late neurocognitive sequelae in survivors of brain tumours in childhood. *Lancet Oncol.* 2004;5(7):399-408.

88. Anderson DM, Rennie KM, Ziegler RS, Neglia JP, Robison LR, Gurney JG. Medical and neurocognitive late effects among survivors of childhood central nervous system tumors. *Cancer.* 2001;92(10):2709-2719.

89. Waber DP, Carpentieri SC, Klar N, et al. Cognitive sequelae in children treated for acute lymphoblastic leukemia with dexamethasone or prednisone [see comments]. *J Pediatr Hematol Oncol.* 2000;22(3):206-13.

90. Kahalley LS, Wilson SJ, Tyc VL, et al. Are the psychological needs of adolescent survivors of pediatric cancer adequately identified and treated? *Psychooncology.* 2012.

91. Nathan PC, Schiffman JD, Huang S, et al. Childhood cancer survivorship educational resources in North American pediatric hematology/oncology fellowship training programs: a survey study. *Pediatr Blood Cancer.* 2011;57(7):1186-1190.

92. Mitby PA, Robison LL, Whitton JA, et al. Utilization of special education services and educational attainment among long-term survivors of childhood cancer: a report from the Childhood Cancer Survivor Study. *Cancer.* 2003;97(4):1115-1126.

93. Langeveld NE, Ubbink MC, Last BF, Grootenhuis MA, Voute PA, De Haan RJ. Educational achievement, employment and living situation in long-term young adult survivors of childhood cancer in the Netherlands. *Psychooncology.* 2003;12(3):213-225.

94. Kingma A, Van Dommelen RI, Mooyaart EL, Wilmink JT, Deelman BG, Kamps WA. No major cognitive impairment in young children with acute lymphoblastic leukemia using chemotherapy only: a prospective longitudinal study [comment]. *J Pediatr Hematol Oncol.* 2002;24(2):106-114.

95. Palmer SL, Goloubeva O, Reddick WE, et al. Patterns of intellectual development among survivors of pediatric medulloblastoma: a longitudinal analysis. *J Clin Oncol.* 2001;19(8):2302-2308.

96. Kingma A, van Dommelen RI, Mooyaart EL, Wilmink JT, Deelman BG, Kamps WA. Slight cognitive impairment and magnetic resonance imaging abnormalities but normal school levels in children treated for acute lymphoblastic leukemia with chemotherapy only. *J Pediatr.* 2001;139(3):413-420.

97. Kingma A, Rammeloo LA, van Der Does-van den Berg A, Rekers-Mombarg L, Postma A. Academic career after treatment for acute lymphoblastic leukaemia. *Arch Dis Child.* 2000;82(5):353-357.

98. Phipps S, Peasant C, Barrera M, Alderfer MA, Huang Q, Vannatta K. Resilience in children undergoing stem cell transplantation: results of a complementary intervention trial. *Pediatrics.* 2012;129(3):e762-e770. PMCID: 3289525.

99. Kazak AE, Bosch J, Klonoff EA. Health psychology special series on health disparities. *Health Psychol.* 2012;31(1):1-4.

100. Katz LF, Leary A, Breiger D, Friedman D. Pediatric cancer and the quality of children's dyadic peer interactions. *J Pediatr Psychol.* 2011;36(2):237-247. PMCID: 3107586.

101. Bruce M, Gumley D, Isham L, Fearon P, Phipps K. Post-traumatic stress symptoms in childhood brain tumour survivors and their parents. *Child Care Health Dev.* 2011;37(2):244-251.

102. Zebrack BJ, Donohue JE, Gurney JG, Chesler MA, Bhatia S, Landier W. Psychometric evaluation of the Impact of Cancer (IOC-CS) scale for young adult survivors of childhood cancer. *Qual Life Res.* 2010;19(2):207-218. PMCID: 2906664.

103. Sanders JE, Hoffmeister PA, Storer BE, Appelbaum FR, Storb RF, Syrjala KL. The quality of life of adult survivors of childhood hematopoietic cell transplant. *Bone Marrow Transplant.* 2010;45(4):746-754. PMCID: 2850957.

104. Kazak AE, Derosa BW, Schwartz LA, et al. Psychological outcomes and health beliefs in adolescent and young adult survivors of childhood cancer and controls. *J Clin Oncol.* 2010;28(12):2002-2007. PMCID: 2860405.

105. Recklitis CJ, Licht I, Ford J, Oeffinger K, Diller L. Screening adult survivors of childhood cancer with the distress thermometer: a comparison with the SCL-90-R. *Psychooncology.* 2007;16(11):1046-1049.

106. Patenaude AF, Kupst MJ. Psychosocial functioning in pediatric cancer. *J Pediatr Psychol.* 2005;30(1):9-27.

107. Zebrack BJ, Gurney JG, Oeffinger K, et al. Psychological outcomes in long-term survivors of childhood brain cancer: a report from the Childhood Cancer Survivor Study. *J Clin Oncol.* 2004;22(6):999-1006.

108. Patterson JM, Holm KE, Gurney JG. The impact of childhood cancer on the family: a qualitative analysis of strains, resources, and coping behaviors. *Psychooncology.* 2004;13(6):390-407.

109. Glover DA, Byrne J, Mills JL, et al. Impact of CNS treatment on mood in adult survivors of childhood leukemia: a report from the Children's Cancer Group. *J Clin Oncol.* 2003;21(23):4395-4401.

110. Zebrack BJ, Zeltzer LK, Whitton J, et al. Psychological outcomes in long-term survivors of childhood leukemia, Hodgkin's disease, and non-Hodgkin's lymphoma: a report from the Childhood Cancer Survivor Study. *Pediatrics.* 2002;110(1 Pt 1):42-52.

111. Langeveld NE, Stam H, Grootenhuis MA, Last BF. Quality of life in young adult survivors of childhood cancer. *Support Care Cancer.* 2002;10(8):579-600.

112. Jenney ME, Levitt GA. The quality of survival after childhood cancer. *Eur J Cancer.* 2002;38(9):1241–1250; discussion 51-53.

113. Meeske KA, Ruccione K, Globe DR, Stuber ML. Posttraumatic stress, quality of life, and psychological distress in young adult survivors of childhood cancer. *Oncol Nurs Forum.* 2001;28(3):481-489.

114. Hobbie WL, Stuber M, Meeske K, et al. Symptoms of posttraumatic stress in young adult survivors of childhood cancer. *J Clin Oncol.* 2000;18(24):4060-4066.

115. Kazak AE, Stuber ML, Barakat LP, Meeske K, Guthrie D, Meadows AT. Predicting posttraumatic stress symptoms in mothers and fathers of survivors of childhood cancers. *J Am Acad Child Adolesc Psychiatry.* 1998;37(8):823-831.

116. O'Brien MM, Donaldson SS, Balise RR, Whittemore AS, Link MP. Second malignant neoplasms in survivors of pediatric Hodgkin's lymphoma treated with low-dose radiation and chemotherapy. *J Clin Oncol.* 2010;28(7):1232-1239.

117. Nathan PC, Ness KK, Mahoney MC, et al. Screening and surveillance for second malignant neoplasms in adult survivors of childhood cancer: a report from the Childhood Cancer Survivor Study. *Ann Intern Med.* 2010;153(7):442-451. PMCID: 3084018.

118. Friedman DL, Whitton J, Leisenring W, et al. Subsequent neoplasms in 5-year survivors of childhood cancer: the Childhood Cancer Survivor Study. *J Natl Cancer Inst.* 2010;102(14):1083-1095. PMCID: 2907408.

119. Meadows AT, Friedman DL, Neglia JP, et al. Second neoplasms in survivors of childhood cancer: findings from the Childhood Cancer Survivor Study cohort. *J Clin Oncol.* 2009;27(14):2356-2362. PMCID: 2738645.

120. Goldsby R, Burke C, Nagarajan R, et al. Second solid malignancies among children, adolescents, and young adults diagnosed with malignant bone tumors after 1976: follow-up of a Children's Oncology Group cohort. *Cancer.* 2008;113(9):2597-2604. PMCID: 2765980.

121. Bluhm EC, Ronckers C, Hayashi RJ, et al. Cause-specific mortality and second cancer incidence after non-Hodgkin lymphoma: a report from the Childhood Cancer Survivor Study. *Blood.* 2008;111(8):4014-4021. PMCID: 2288716.

122. Rubino C, Adjadj E, Guerin S, et al. Long-term risk of second malignant neoplasms after neuroblastoma in childhood: role of treatment. *Int J Cancer.* 2003;107(5):791-796.

123. Neglia JP, Friedman DL, Yasui Y, et al. Second malignant neoplasms in five-year survivors of childhood cancer: Childhood Cancer Survivor Study. *J Natl Cancer Inst.* 2001;93(8):618-629.

124. Socie G, Curtis RE, Deeg HJ, et al. New malignant diseases after allogeneic marrow transplantation for childhood acute leukemia. *J Clin Oncol.* 2000;18(2):348-357.

125. Metayer C, Lynch CF, Clarke EA, et al. Second cancers among long-term survivors of Hodgkin's disease diagnosed in childhood and adolescence. *J Clin Oncol.* 2000;18(12):2435-2443.

126. Bhatia S, Yasui Y, Robison LL, et al. High risk of subsequent neoplasms continues with extended follow-up of childhood Hodgkin's disease: report from the Late Effects Study Group. i. 2003;21(23):4386-4394.

127. Veiga LH, Bhatti P, Ronckers CM, et al. Chemotherapy and thyroid cancer risk: a report from the Childhood Cancer Survivor Study. *Cancer Epidemiol Biomarkers Prev.* 2012;21(1):92–101. PMCID: 3253948.

128. Henderson TO, Whitton J, Stovall M, et al. Secondary sarcomas in childhood cancer survivors: a report from the Childhood Cancer Survivor Study. *J Natl Cancer Inst.* 2007;99(4):300-308.

129. Bassal M, Mertens AC, Taylor L, et al. Risk of selected subsequent carcinomas in survivors of childhood cancer: a report from the Childhood Cancer Survivor Study. *J Clin Oncol.* 2006;24(3):476-483.

130. Inskip PD, Curtis RE. New malignancies following childhood cancer in the United States, 1973–2002. *Int J Cancer.* 2007;121(10):2233-2240.

131. Fletcher O, Easton D, Anderson K, Gilham C, Jay M, Peto J. Lifetime risks of common cancers among retinoblastoma survivors. *J Natl Cancer Inst.* 2004;96(5):357-363.

132. Wong FL, Boice JD Jr, Abramson DH, et al. Cancer incidence after retinoblastoma. Radiation dose and sarcoma risk. *JAMA.* 1997;278(15):1262-1267.

133. Eng C, Li FP, Abramson DH, et al. Mortality from second tumors among long-term survivors of retinoblastoma. *J Natl Cancer Inst.* 1993;85(14):1121-1128.

134. Frobisher C, Lancashire ER, Winter DL, Taylor AJ, Reulen RC, Hawkins MM. Long-term population-based divorce rates among adult survivors of childhood cancer in Britain. *Pediatr Blood Cancer.* 2010;54(1):116-122.

135. Nagarajan R, Neglia JP, Clohisy DR, et al. Education, employment, insurance, and marital status among 694 survivors of pediatric lower extremity bone tumors: a report from the Childhood Cancer Survivor Study. *Cancer.* 2003;97(10):2554-2564.

136. Pastore G, Mosso ML, Magnani C, Luzzatto L, Bianchi M, Terracini B. Physical impairment and social life goals among

adult long-term survivors of childhood cancer: a population-based study from the childhood cancer registry of Piedmont, Italy. *Tumori.* 2001;87(6):372-378.

137. Rauck AM, Green DM, Yasui Y, Mertens A, Robison LL. Marriage in the survivors of childhood cancer: a preliminary description from the Childhood Cancer Survivor Study. *Med Pediatr Oncol.* 1999;33(1):60-63.

138. Hays DM, Landsverk J, Sallan SE, et al. Educational, occupational, and insurance status of childhood cancer survivors in their fourth and fifth decades of life. *J Clin Oncol.* 1992;10(9):1397-1406.

139. Lund LW, Schmiegelow K, Rechnitzer C, Johansen C. A systematic review of studies on psychosocial late effects of childhood cancer: structures of society and methodological pitfalls may challenge the conclusions. *Pediatr Blood Cancer.* 2011;56(4):532-543.

140. Kirchhoff AC, Krull KR, Ness KK, et al. Occupational outcomes of adult childhood cancer survivors: a report from the Childhood Cancer Survivor Study. *Cancer.* 2011;117(13):3033-3044.

141. van Dijk J, Oostrom KJ, Huisman J, et al. Restrictions in daily life after retinoblastoma from the perspective of the survivors. *Pediatr Blood Cancer.* 2010;54(1):110-115.

142. van Dalen EC, Kremer LC. Employment status among cancer survivors. *JAMA.* 2009;302(1):33-34; author reply 4-5.

143. Pang JW, Friedman DL, Whitton JA, et al. Employment status among adult survivors in the Childhood Cancer Survivor Study. *Pediatr Blood Cancer.* 2008;50(1):104-110.

144. Hewitt M, Weiner SL, Simone JV. *Childhood Cancer Survivorship: Improving Care and Quality of Life.* Washington, DC: The National Academies Press; 2003.

145. Landier W, Wallace WH, Hudson MM. Long-term follow-up of pediatric cancer survivors: education, surveillance, and screening. *Pediatr Blood Cancer.* 2006;46(2):149-158.

146. Landier W, Bhatia S, Eshelman DA, et al. Development of risk-based guidelines for pediatric cancer survivors: the Children's Oncology Group Long-Term Follow-Up Guidelines from the Children's Oncology Group Late Effects Committee and Nursing Discipline. *J Clin Oncol.* 2004;22(24):4979-4990.

147. Long term follow up of survivors of childhood cancer. A national guideline.[cited]; Available from.

148. Knijnenburg SL, Kremer LC, Versluys AB, Van Der Beek JR, Jaspers MW. Development and evaluation of a patient information website for childhood cancer survivors. *Stud Health Technol Inform.* 2009;150:342-346.

149. Skinner R, Wallace WH, Levitt GA. Long-term follow-up of people who have survived cancer during childhood. *Lancet Oncol.* 2006;7(6):489-498.

150. Eshelman-Kent D, Kinahan KE, Hobbie W, et al. Cancer survivorship practices, services, and delivery: a report from the Children's Oncology Group (COG) nursing discipline, adolescent/young adult, and late effects committees. *J Cancer Surviv.* 2011;5(4):345-357.

151. Friedman DL, Freyer DR, Levitt GA. Models of care for survivors of childhood cancer. *Pediatr Blood Cancer.* 2006;46(2):159-168.

152. Goldsby RE, Ablin AR. Surviving childhood cancer; now what? Controversies regarding long-term follow-up. *Pediatr Blood Cancer.* 2004;43(3):211-214.

153. Prasad PK, Bowles T, Friedman DL. Is there a role for a specialized follow-up clinic for survivors of pediatric cancer? *Cancer Treat Rev.* 2010;36(4):372-376.

154. Robison LL. The Childhood Cancer Survivor Study: a resource for research of long-term outcomes among adult survivors of childhood cancer. *Minn Med.* 2005;88(4):45-49.

155. Mertens AC, Cotter KL, Foster BM, et al. Improving health care for adult survivors of childhood cancer: recommendations from a delphi panel of health policy experts. *Health Policy.* 2004;69(2):169-178.

156. Kadan-Lottick NS, Robison LL, Gurney JG, et al. Childhood cancer survivors' knowledge about their past diagnosis and treatment: Childhood Cancer Survivor Study. *JAMA.* 2002;287(14):1832-1839.

157. Nathan PC, Ford JS, Henderson TO, et al. Health behaviors, medical care, and interventions to promote healthy living in the Childhood Cancer Survivor Study cohort. *J Clin Oncol.* 2009;27(14):2363-2373. PMCID: 2738646.

158. Nathan PC, Greenberg ML, Ness KK, et al. Medical care in long-term survivors of childhood cancer: a report from the Childhood Cancer Survivor Study. *J Clin Oncol.* 2008;26(27):4401-4409. PMCID: 2653112.

159. Oeffinger KC, Nathan PC, Kremer LC. Challenges after curative treatment for childhood cancer and long-term follow up of survivors. *Pediatr Clin North Am.* 2008; 55(1):251-273, xiii.

160. Oeffinger KC, Ford JS, Moskowitz CS, et al. Breast cancer surveillance practices among women previously treated with chest radiation for a childhood cancer. *JAMA.* 2009;301(4):404-414. PMCID: 2676434.

161. Oeffinger KC, Mertens AC, Hudson MM, et al. Health care of young adult survivors of childhood cancer: a report from the Childhood Cancer Survivor Study. *Ann Fam Med.* 2004;2(1):61-70. PMCID: 1466633.

162. Crom DB, Chathaway DK, Tolley EA, Mulhern RK, Hudson MM. Health status and health-related quality of life in long-term adult survivors of pediatric solid tumors. *Int J Cancer Suppl.* 1999;12:25-31.

163. Eiser C, Hill JJ, Blacklay A. Surviving cancer: what does it mean for you? An evaluation of a clinic based intervention for survivors of childhood cancer. *Psychooncology.* 2000;9(3):214-220.

164. Hoffman B. Cancer survivors' employment and insurance rights: a primer for oncologists. *Oncology (Huntingt).* 1999;13(6):841-846; discussion 6, 9, 52.

165. Monaco GP. Socioeconomic considerations in childhood cancer survival. Society's obligations. *Am J Pediatr Hematol Oncol.* 1987;9(1):92-98.

166. Parsons SK. Financial issues in pediatric cancer. In: Pizzo PA, Poplack DG, eds. *Principles and Practice of Pediatric Oncology.* 4th ed. Philadelphia, PA: Lippincott, Williams & Wilkins; 2002.

167. Ross JW. The role of the social worker with long term survivors of childhood cancer and their families. *Soc Work Health Care.* 1982;7(4):1-13.

168. Zebrack BJ, Chesler MA. Managed care: the new context for social work in health care—implications for survivors of childhood cancer and their families. *Soc Work Health Care.* 2000;31(2):89-103.

169. Bleyer A. Adolescent and young adult (AYA) oncology: the first A. *Pediatr Hematol Oncol.* 2007;24(5):325-336.

170. Bleyer A. Young adult oncology: the patients and their survival challenges. *CA Cancer J Clin.* 2007;57(4):242-255.

171. Health NIo, Foundation LA. *Closing the Gap: Research and Care Imperatives for Adolescents and Young Adults with*

Cancer: Report of the Adolescent and Young Adult Oncology Progress Review Group. National Cancer Institute; 2006.

172. Aksnes LH, Hall KS, Jebsen N, Fossa SD, Dahl AA. Young survivors of malignant bone tumours in the extremities: a comparative study of quality of life, fatigue and mental distress. *Support Care Cancer.* 2007;15(9):1087-1096.

173. Compas BE, Beckjord E, Agocha B, et al. Measurement of coping and stress responses in women with breast cancer. *Psychooncology.* 2006;15(12):1038-1054.

174. Jayadevappa R, Bloom BS, Fomberstein SC, Wein AJ, Malkowicz SB. Health related quality of life and direct medical care cost in newly diagnosed younger men with prostate cancer. *J Urol.* 2005;174(3):1059-1064; discussion 64.

175. Kroenke CH, Rosner B, Chen WY, Kawachi I, Colditz GA, Holmes MD. Functional impact of breast cancer by age at diagnosis. *J Clin Oncol.* 2004;22(10):1849-1856.

176. Miyake H, Muramaki M, Eto H, Kamidono S, Hara I. Health-related quality of life in patients with testicular cancer: a comparative analysis according to therapeutic modalities. *Oncol Rep.* 2004;12(4):867-870.

177. Evan EE, Zeltzer LK. Psychosocial dimensions of cancer in adolescents and young adults. *Cancer.* 2006;107(7 suppl):1663-1671.

178. Lerner R, Steinberg L. *Handbook of Adolescence.* 3rd ed. New York, NY: Wiley; 2004.

179. Blum RW. Introduction. Improving transition for adolescents with special health care needs from pediatric to adult-centered health care. *Pediatrics.* 2002;110(6 Pt 2):1301-1303.

180. Madan-Swain A, Brown RT, Foster MA, et al. Identity in adolescent survivors of childhood cancer. *J Pediatr Psychol.* 2000;25(2):105-115.

181. Patterson J, Blum RW. Risk and resilience among children and youth with disabilities. *Arch Pediatr Adolesc Med.* 1996;150(7):692-698.

182. Zebrack BJ, Chesler M. Health-related worries, self-image, and life outlooks of long-term survivors of childhood cancer. *Health Soc Work.* 2001;26(4):245-256.

183. Zebrack BJ, Zeltzer LK. Living beyond the sword of Damocles: surviving childhood cancer. *Expert Rev Anticancer Ther.* 2001;1(2):163-164.

184. Claflin CJ, Barbarin OA. Does "telling" less protect more? Relationships among age, information disclosure, and what children with cancer see and feel. *J Pediatr Psychol.* 1991;16(2):169-191.

185. Jamison RN, Lewis S, Burish TG. Cooperation with treatment in adolescent cancer patients. *J Adolesc Health Care.* 1986;7(3):162-167.

186. Varni JW, Katz ER, Colegrove R Jr, Dolgin M. Perceived social support and adjustment of children with newly diagnosed cancer. *J Dev Behav Pediatr.* 1994;15(1):20-26.

Noreen M. Aziz

BACKGROUND AND SIGNIFICANCE

With continued advances in strategies to detect cancer early and treat it effectively along with the aging of the population, the number of individuals living years beyond a cancer diagnosis can be expected to continue to increase. Statistical trends show that, in the absence of other competing causes of death, 64% of adults diagnosed with cancer today can expect to be alive in 5 years (1–4). Relative 5-year survival rates for those diagnosed as children (age <19 years) are even higher, with almost 79% of childhood cancer survivors estimated to be alive at 5 years and 75% at 10 years (5).

Survival from cancer has seen dramatic improvements over the past three decades, mainly as a result of advances in early detection, therapeutic strategies, and the widespread use of combined modality therapy (surgery, chemotherapy, and radiotherapy) (6–10). Medical and sociocultural factors such as psychosocial and behavioral interventions, active screening behaviors, and healthier lifestyles may also play an integral role in the length and quality of that survival (11).

Although beneficial and often lifesaving against the diagnosed malignancy, most therapeutic modalities for cancer are associated with a spectrum of late complications ranging from minor and treatable to serious or, occasionally, potentially lethal (2,6,12–15). Although living for extended periods of time beyond their initial diagnosis, many cancer survivors often face various chronic and late physical and psychosocial sequelae of their disease or its treatment. Additionally, as the number of survivors and their length of survival expand, long-term health issues specific to cancer survival are also fast emerging as a public health concern. Questions of particular importance to cancer survivors include surveillance for the adverse sequelae, or late and long-term effects, of treatment; the development of new (second) cancers; and recurrence of their original cancer. One-fourth of *late deaths* occurring among survivors of childhood cancer during the extended survivorship period, when the chances of primary disease recurrence are negligible, can be attributed to a treatment-related effect such as a second cancer or cardiac dysfunction (16). The most *frequently observed* medical sequelae among pediatric cancer survivors include endocrine complications, growth hormone deficiency, primary hypothyroidism, and primary ovarian failure. Also included within the rubric of late effects are second cancers arising as a result of genetic predisposition (e.g., familial cancer syndromes) or the mutagenic effects of therapy. These factors may act independently or synergistically. Synergistic effects of mutagenic agents

such as cigarette smoke or toxins such as alcohol are largely unknown (2,6,12).

Therefore, there is today a greater recognition of symptoms that persist after the completion of treatment and that arise years after primary therapy. Both acute organ toxicities such as radiation pneumonitis and chronic toxicities such as congestive cardiac failure, neurocognitive deficits, infertility, and second malignancies are being described as the price of cure or prolonged survival (2,6,12). The study of late effects, originally within the realm of pediatric cancer, is now germane to cancer survivors at all ages because concerns may continue to surface throughout the life cycle (2,6). These concerns underscore the need to follow up and screen survivors of cancer for toxicities such as those mentioned and also to develop and provide effective interventions that carry the potential to prevent or ameliorate adverse outcomes.

The goal of survivorship research is to focus on the *health and life* of a person with a history of cancer *beyond* the acute diagnosis and treatment phase. Survivorship research seeks to examine the causes of, and to prevent and control the adverse effects associated with, cancer and its treatment and to optimize the physiologic, psychosocial, and functional outcomes for cancer survivors and their families. A hallmark of survivorship research is its emphasis on understanding the integration/interaction of multidisciplinary domains.

This chapter presents definitional issues relevant to cancer survivorship; examines late effects of cancer treatment among survivors of pediatric and adult cancer; and articulates gaps in knowledge and emerging research priorities in cancer survivorship research relevant to late effects of cancer treatment. It draws heavily from pediatric cancer survivorship research because a paucity of data continues to exist for medical late effects of treatment for survivors of cancer diagnosed as adults. Research on late effects of cancer treatment began in the realm of pediatric cancer and continues to yield important insights into the impact of cancer therapies among adults.

DEFINITIONAL ISSUES

Fitzhugh Mullan, a physician diagnosed with and treated for cancer himself, first described cancer survivorship as a concept (17). Definitional issues for cancer survivorship encompass three related aspects (2,6):

1. *Who is a cancer survivor?* Philosophically, anyone who has been diagnosed with cancer is a survivor, from the time of

diagnosis to the end of life.[1] Caregivers and family members are also included within this definition as secondary survivors.

2. *What is cancer survivorship?* Mullan described the survivorship experience as similar to the seasons of the year. Mullan recognized three seasons or phases of survival: acute (extending from diagnosis to the completion of initial treatment, encompassing issues dominated by treatment and its side effects); extended (beginning with the completion of initial treatment of the primary disease, remission of disease, or both, dominated by watchful waiting, regular follow-up examinations, and, perhaps, intermittent therapy); and permanent survival (not a single moment; evolves from extended disease-free survival when the likelihood of recurrence is sufficiently low). An understanding of these phases of survival is important for facilitating an optimal transition into and management of survivorship.

3. *What is cancer survivorship research?* Cancer survivorship research seeks to identify, examine, prevent, and control adverse cancer diagnosis and treatment-related outcomes (such as late effects of treatment, second cancers, and quality of life); to provide a knowledge base regarding optimal follow-up care and surveillance of cancer survivors; and to optimize health after cancer treatment (2,6).

Other important definitions include those for long-term cancer survivorship and late versus long-term effects of cancer treatment. Generally, *long-term cancer survivors* are defined as those individuals who are 5 or more years beyond the diagnosis of their primary disease and embody the concept of permanent survival described by Mullan. *Late effects* refer specifically to unrecognized toxicities that are absent or subclinical at the end of therapy and become manifest later with the unmasking of hitherto unseen injury caused by any of the following factors: developmental processes, the failure of compensatory mechanisms with the passage of time, or organ senescence. *Long-term effects* refer to any side effects or complications of treatment for which a patient with cancer must compensate; also known as persistent effects, they begin during treatment and continue beyond the end of treatment. Late effects, in contrast, appear months to years after the completion of treatment. Some researchers classify cognitive problems, fatigue, lymphedema, and peripheral neuropathy as long-term effects, whereas others classify them as late effects (18–21). Chemotherapeutic drugs for which late effects have been reported most frequently include adriamycin, bleomycin, vincristine, methotrexate, and cytoxan (Table 66.1) (22–46).

This chapter focuses largely on the *physiologic* or *medical* long-term and late effects of cancer treatment. Physiologic sequelae of cancer treatment can also be further classified as follows:

1. System specific (e.g., organ damage, organ failure, premature aging, immunosuppression, issues related to compromised immune systems, and endocrine damage)

2. Second malignant neoplasms (such as an increased risk of recurrent malignancy, increased risk of a certain cancer associated with the primary malignancy, and/or increased risk of secondary malignancies associated with cytotoxic or radiologic cancer therapies; this topic is not covered in detail in this chapter as it is reviewed comprehensively elsewhere in this book)

3. Functional changes such as lymphedema, incontinence, pain syndromes, neuropathies, fatigue; cosmetic changes such as amputations, ostomies, and skin/hair alterations; and comorbidities such as osteoporosis, arthritis, and hypertension

REVIEW OF LATE AND LONG-TERM EFFECTS BY ORGAN SYSTEM OR TISSUES AFFECTED[2]

System-Specific Physiologic Sequelae[3]

Cardiac Sequelae

The heart may be damaged by both therapeutic irradiation and chemotherapeutic agents commonly used in the treatment of cancer. Several types of damage have been reported including pericardial, myocardial, and vascular. Cardiac damage is most pronounced after treatment with the anthracycline drugs doxorubicin and daunorubicin, used widely in the treatment of most childhood cancers and adjuvant chemotherapy for breast and many other adult cancers. An additive effect has also been reported when anthracyclines are used in conjunction with cyclophosphamide and radiation therapy. Anthracyclines cause myocardial cell death, leading to a diminished number of myocytes and compensatory hypertrophy of residual myocytes (47). Major clinical manifestations include reduced cardiac function, arrhythmia, and heart failure. Chronic cardiotoxicity usually manifests itself as cardiomyopathy, pericarditis, and congestive heart failure.

Cardiac injury that becomes clinically manifest during or shortly after completion of chemotherapy may progress, stabilize, or improve after the first year of treatment. This improvement may either be of a transient nature or last for a considerable length of time. There is also evidence of a continuum of injury that will manifest itself throughout the lives of these patients (48). From a risk factor perspective, patients who exhibit reduced cardiac function within 6 months of completing chemotherapy are at increased risk for the development of late cardiac failure (49). However, a significant incidence of late cardiac decompensation manifested by cardiac failure or lethal arrhythmia occurring 10 to 20 years after the administration of these drugs has also been reported (50).

In a recent study of Hodgkin's disease (HD) survivors, investigators reported finding cardiac abnormalities in most

---

[1]From the National Coalition for Cancer Survivorship.

[2]Common to both children and adults depending on cancer site and treatment(s) received.
[3]These include organ damage, failure, or premature aging resulting from chemotherapy, hormone therapy, radiation, surgery, or any combination thereof.

TABLE 66.1 **Possible late effects of radiotherapy and chemotherapy**

Organ System	Late Effects/Sequelae of Radiotherapy	Late Effects/Sequelae of Chemotherapy	Chemotherapeutic Drugs Responsible
Bone and soft tissues	Short stature, atrophy, fibrosis, osteonecrosis	Avascular necrosis	Steroids
Cardiovascular	Pericardial effusion, pericarditis; coronary arterial disease	Cardiomyopathy, congestive cardiac failure	Anthracyclines Cyclophosphamide
Pulmonary	Pulmonary fibrosis, decreased lung volumes	Pulmonary fibrosis Interstitial pneumonitis	Bleomycin, BCNU Methotrexate, adriamycin
Central nervous system	Neuropsychological deficits, structural changes, hemorrhage	Neuropsychological deficits, structural changes Hemiplegia, seizure	Methotrexate
Peripheral nervous system		Peripheral neuropathy, hearing loss	Cisplatin, vinca alkaloids
Hematologic	Cytopenia, myelodysplasia	Myelodysplastic syndromes	Alkylating agents
Renal	Decreased creatinine clearance Hypertension	Decreased creatinine clearance Increased creatinine, renal filtration Delayed renal filtration	Cisplatin Methotrexate Nitrosoureas
Genitourinary	Bladder fibrosis, contractures	Bladder fibrosis, hemorrhagic cystitis	Cyclophosphamide
Gastrointestinal	Malabsorption, stricture, abnormal LFT	Abnormal LFT, hepatic fibrosis, cirrhosis	Methotrexate, BCNU
Pituitary	Growth hormone deficiency, pituitary deficiency		
Thyroid	Hypothyroidism, nodules		
Gonadal	Men: risk of sterility, Leydig cell dysfunction	Men: sterility	Alkylating agents
	Women: ovarian failure, early menopause	Women: sterility, premature menopause	Procarbazine
Dental/oral health	Poor enamel and root formation, dry mouth		
Ophthalmologic	Cataracts, retinopathy	Cataracts	Steroids

BCNU, carmustine; LFT, liver function test.
Data from Ganz (12,13) and Aziz (2,6).

of the participants (51). This is an important finding, especially because the sample consisted of individuals who did not manifest symptomatic heart disease at screening and described their health as "good." Manifestations of cardiac abnormalities include the following:

1. Restrictive cardiomyopathy (suggested by reduced average left ventricular dimension and mass without increased left ventricular wall thickness)
2. Significant valvular defects
3. Conduction defects
4. Complete heart block
5. Autonomic dysfunction (suggested by a monotonous heart rate in 57%)
6. Persistent tachycardia and
7. Blunted hemodynamic responses to exercise

The peak oxygen uptake (VO_{2max}) during exercise, a predictor of mortality in heart failure, was significantly reduced (<20 mL/kg/m^2) in 30% of survivors and was correlated with increasing fatigue, increasing shortness of breath, and a decreasing physical component score on the SF-36. Given the presence of these clinically significant cardiovascular abnormalities, investigators recommend serial, comprehensive cardiac screening of HD survivors who fit the profile of having received mediastinal irradiation at a young age.

Congestive cardiomyopathy is directly related to the total dose of the agent administered; the higher the dose, the greater the chance of cardiotoxicity. Subclinical abnormalities have also been noted at lower doses. The anthracyclines doxorubicin and daunorubicin are well-known causes of cardiomyopathy that can occur many years after completion of therapy. The incidence of anthracycline-induced cardiomyopathy, which is dose dependent, may exceed 30% among patients receiving cumulative doses in excess of 600 mg/m^2. A cumulative dose of anthracyclines >300 mg/m^2 has been associated with an 11-fold increased risk of clinical heart failure, compared with a cumulative dose of <300 mg/m^2, the estimated risk of clinical heart failure increasing with time from exposure and approaching 5% after 15 years.

A reduced incidence and severity of cardiac abnormalities was reported in a study of 120 long-term survivors of acute lymphoblastic leukemia (ALL) who had been treated with lower anthracycline doses (90 to 270 mg/m^2), compared with previous reports in which subjects had received moderate anthracycline doses (300 to 550 mg/m^2) (52,53). Twenty-three percent of the patients were found to have cardiac abnormalities, 21% had increased end-systolic stress, and only 2% had reduced contractility. The cumulative anthracycline dose within the 90 to 270 mg/m^2 range did not relate to cardiac abnormalities. The authors concluded that there may be no safe anthracycline dose to completely avoid late cardiotoxicity. A recent review of 30 published studies in childhood cancer survivors found that the frequency of clinically detected anthracycline cardiac heart failure ranged from 0% to 16% (54). In an analysis of reported studies, the type of anthracycline (e.g., doxorubicin) and the maximum dose given in a 1-week period (e.g., >45 mg/m^2) were found

to explain a large portion of the variation in the reported frequency of anthracycline-induced heart failure.

Cyclophosphamide has been associated with the development of congestive cardiomyopathy, especially when administered at the high doses used in transplant regimens. Cardiac toxicity may occur at lower doses when mediastinal radiation is combined with the chemotherapeutic drugs mentioned above. Late onset of congestive heart failure has been reported during pregnancy and rapid growth or after the initiation of vigorous exercise programs in adults previously treated for cancer during childhood or young adulthood as a result of increased afterload and the impact of the additional stress of such events on marginal cardiac reserves. The initial improvement in cardiac function after completion of therapy appears to result, at least in part, from compensatory changes. Compensation may diminish in the presence of stressors such as those mentioned earlier and myocardial depressants such as alcohol.

The incidence of subclinical anthracycline myocardial damage has been the subject of considerable interest. Steinherz et al. (55) found that 23% of 201 patients who had received a median cumulative dose of doxorubicin of 450 mg/m^2 had echocardiographic abnormalities at a median of 7 years after therapy. In a group of survivors of childhood cancer who received a median doxorubicin dose of 334 mg/m^2, it was found that progressive elevation of afterload or depression of left ventricular contractility was present in approximately 75% of patients (47). A recent review of the literature on subclinical cardiotoxicity among children treated with an anthracycline found that the reported frequency of subclinical cardiotoxicity varied considerably across the 25 studies reviewed (frequency ranging from 0% to 57%) (56). Because of marked differences in the definition of outcomes for subclinical cardiotoxicity and the heterogeneity of the patient populations investigated, it is difficult to accurately evaluate the potential long-term outcomes within anthracycline-exposed patient populations or the potential impact of the subclinical findings.

Effects of radiation on the heart may be profound and include valvular damage, pericardial thickening, and ischemic heart disease. Patients with radiation-related cardiac damage have a markedly increased relative risk (RR) of both angina and myocardial infarction (RR 2.56) years after mediastinal radiation for HD in adult patients, whereas the risk of cardiac death is 3.1 (57). This risk was greatest among patients receiving >30 Gy of mantle irradiation and those treated before 20 to 21 years of age. Blocking the heart reduced the risk of cardiac death due to causes other than myocardial infarction (58).

In general, among anthracycline-exposed patients, the risk of cardiotoxicity can be increased by mediastinal radiation (59), uncontrolled hypertension (60,61), underlying cardiac abnormalities (62), exposure to non-anthracycline chemotherapeutic agents (especially cyclophosphamide, dactinomycin, mitomycin C, dacarbazine, vincristine, bleomycin, and methotrexate) (63,64), female gender (65), younger age (66), and electrolyte imbalances such as hypokalemia and hypomagnesemia (67). Previous reports have suggested that doxorubicin-induced cardiotoxicity can be prevented by continuous infusion of the drug (68). However, Lipshultz et al. (69) compared cardiac outcomes in children receiving either bolus or continuous infusion of doxorubicin and reported that continuous doxorubicin infusion over 48 hours for childhood leukemia did not offer a cardioprotective advantage over bolus infusion. Both regimens were associated with progressive subclinical cardiotoxicity, therefore suggesting that there is no benefit from continuous infusion of anthracyclines.

Chronic cardiotoxicity associated with radiation alone most commonly involves pericardial effusions or constrictive pericarditis, sometimes in association with pancarditis. Although a dose of 40 Gy of total heart irradiation appears to be the usual threshold, pericarditis has been reported after as little as 15 Gy, even in the absence of radiomimetic chemotherapy (70,71). Symptomatic pericarditis, which usually develops 10 to 30 years after irradiation, is found in 2% to 10% of patients (72). Subclinical pericardial and myocardial damage, as well as valvular thickening, may be common in this population (73,74). Coronary artery disease has been reported after radiation to the mediastinum, although mortality rates have not been significantly higher in patients who receive mediastinal radiation than in the general population (58).

Given the known acute and long-term cardiac complications of therapy, prevention of cardiotoxicity is a focus of active investigation. Several attempts have been made to minimize the cardiotoxicity of anthracyclines, such as the use of liposomal-formulated anthracyclines, less cardiotoxic analogs, and the additional administration of cardioprotective agents. The advantages of these approaches are still controversial, but there are ongoing clinical trials to evaluate the long-term effects. Certain analogs of doxorubicin and daunorubicin, with decreased cardiotoxicity but equivalent antitumor activity, are being explored. Agents such as dexrazoxane, which are able to remove iron from anthracyclines, have been investigated as cardioprotectants. Clinical trials of dexrazoxane have been conducted in children, with encouraging evidence of short-term cardioprotection (75); however, the long-term avoidance of cardiotoxicity with the use of this agent has yet to be sufficiently determined. The most recent study by Lipshultz et al. reported that dexrazoxane prevents or reduces cardiac injury, as reflected by elevations in troponin T, which is associated with the use of doxorubicin for childhood ALL without compromising the antileukemic efficacy of doxorubicin. Longer follow-up will be necessary to determine the influence of dexrazoxane on echocardiographic findings at 4 years and on event-free survival (76).

Another key emerging issue is the interaction of taxanes with doxorubicin. Epirubicin–taxane combinations are active in treating metastatic breast cancer, and ongoing research is focusing on combining anthracyclines with taxanes in an effort to continue to improve outcomes following adjuvant therapy (77). Clinically significant drug interactions have been reported to occur when paclitaxel is administered with doxorubicin, cisplatin, or anticonvulsants (phenytoin, carbamazepine, and phenobarbital), and pharmacodynamic interactions have been reported to occur with these agents that are sequence- or schedule dependent (78). Because the taxanes undergo hepatic oxidation through the cytochrome P-450 system, pharmacokinetic interactions from enzyme induction or inhibition can also occur. A higher than expected myelotoxicity has been reported. However, there is no enhanced doxorubicinol formation in human myocardium, a finding consistent with the cardiac safety of the regimen (79). Investigators have suggested that doxorubicin and epirubicin should be administered 24 hours before paclitaxel and the cumulative anthracycline dose be limited to 360 mg/m^2, thereby preventing the enhanced toxicities caused by sequence- and schedule-dependent interactions between anthracyclines and paclitaxel (78). Conversely, they also suggest that paclitaxel should be administered at least 24 hours before cisplatin to avoid a decrease in clearance and increase in myelosuppression. With concurrent anticonvulsant therapy, cytochrome P-450 enzyme induction results in decreased paclitaxel plasma steady-state concentrations, possibly requiring an increased dose of paclitaxel. A number of other drug interactions have been reported in preliminary studies for which clinical significance has yet to be established (78).

The human epidermal growth factor receptor (HER)2 is overexpressed in approximately 20% to 25% of human breast cancers and is an independent adverse prognostic factor. Targeted therapy directed against this receptor has been developed in the form of a humanized monoclonal antibody, trastuzumab. Unexpectedly, cardiac toxicity has developed in some patients treated with trastuzumab, and this has a higher incidence in those treated in combination with an anthracycline (80,81). Both clinical and in vitro data suggest that cardiomyocyte HER2/erbB2 is uniquely susceptible to trastuzumab (82). Trastuzumab has shown activity as a single agent in metastatic breast cancer both before chemotherapy and in heavily pretreated patients, and its use in combination with an anthracycline or paclitaxel results in a significant improvement in survival, time to progression, and response (80). The HER2 status of a tumor is a critical determinant of response to trastuzumab-based treatment; those expressing HER2 at the highest level on immunohistochemistry, 3+, derive more benefit from treatment with trastuzumab than those with overexpression at the 2+ level. Interactions between the estrogen receptor and HER2 pathway have stimulated interest in using trastuzumab in combination with endocrine therapy.

Neurocognitive Sequelae

Long-term survivors of cancer may be at risk for neurocognitive and neuropsychological sequelae. Among survivors of childhood leukemia, neurocognitive late effects represent one of the more intensively studied topics. Adverse outcomes are generally associated with whole-brain radiation and/or therapy with high-dose systemic or intrathecal methotrexate or cytarabine (83–85). High-risk characteristics, including higher dose of central nervous system (CNS) radiation, younger age at treatment, and female sex, have been well documented. Results from studies of neurocognitive outcomes are directly responsible for the marked reduction (particularly in younger children) in the use of cranial radiation, which is currently reserved for treatment of very high-risk subgroups or patients with CNS involvement (86).

A spectrum of clinical syndromes may occur, including radionecrosis, necrotizing leukoencephalopathy, mineralizing microangiopathy, and dystrophic calcification, cerebellar sclerosis, and spinal cord dysfunction (87). Leukoencephalopathy has been primarily associated with methotrexate-induced injury of white matter. However, cranial radiation may play an additive role through the disruption of the blood–brain barrier, therefore allowing greater exposure of the brain to systemic therapy.

Although abnormalities have been detected by diagnostic imaging studies, the abnormalities observed have not been well demonstrated to correlate with clinical findings and neurocognitive status (88,89). Chemotherapy- or radiation-induced destruction in normal white matter partially explains intellectual and academic achievement deficits (90). Evidence suggests that direct effects of chemotherapy and radiation on intracranial endothelial cells and brain white matter as well as immunologic mechanisms could be involved in the pathogenesis of CNS damage.

Neurocognitive deficits, as a general rule, usually become evident within several years of CNS radiation and tend to be progressive in nature. Survivors of leukemia treated at a younger age (e.g., <6 years of age) may experience significant declines in intelligence quotient (IQ) scores (91). However, reductions in IQ scores are typically not global, but rather reflect specific areas of impairment, such as attention and other nonverbal cognitive processing skills (92). Affected children may experience information-processing deficits, resulting in academic difficulties. These children are particularly prone to problems with receptive and expressive language, attention span, and visual and perceptual motor skills, most often manifested in academic difficulties in the areas of reading, language, and mathematics. Accordingly, children treated with CNS radiation or systemic or intrathecal therapy with the potential to cause neurocognitive deficits should receive close monitoring of academic performance. Referral for neuropsychological evaluation with appropriate intervention strategies, such as modifications in curriculum, speech and language therapy, or social skills training, implemented in a program tailored for the individual needs and deficits of the survivor should be taken into consideration (93). Assessment of educational needs and subsequent educational attainment have found that survivors of childhood leukemia are significantly more likely to require special educational assistance, but have a high likelihood of successfully completing high school (37,94). However, when compared with siblings, survivors of leukemia and non-Hodgkin's lymphoma (NHL) are at greater risk for not completing high school. As would be anticipated from the results of neurocognitive studies, it has been shown that survivors, particularly

those under 6 years of age at treatment, who received cranial radiation and/or intrathecal chemotherapy were significantly more likely to require special education services and least likely to complete a formal education (86,95,96).

Progressive dementia and dysfunction have been reported in some long-term cancer survivors as a result of whole-brain radiation with or without chemotherapy and occur most often in patients with brain tumor and patients with small cell lung cancer who have received prophylactic therapy. Neuropsychological abnormalities have also been reported after CNS prophylaxis utilizing whole-brain radiation for leukemia in childhood survivors. In fact, cognitive changes in children began to be recognized as treatments for childhood cancer, especially ALL, became increasingly effective. These observations have resulted in changes in treatment protocols for childhood ALL (97,98).

Several recent studies have reported cognitive dysfunction in women treated with adjuvant therapy for breast cancer (99,100). In one study (101), investigators compared the neuropsychological performance of long-term survivors of breast cancer and lymphoma treated with standard-dose chemotherapy who carried the epsilon 4 allele of the apolipoprotein E (APOE) gene with those who carry other APOE alleles. Survivors with at least one epsilon 4 allele scored significantly lower in the visual memory ($P < 0.03$) and the spatial ability ($P < 0.05$) domains and tended to score lower in the psychomotor functioning ($P < 0.08$) domain as compared with survivors who did not carry an epsilon 4 allele. No group differences were found on depression, anxiety, or fatigue. The results of this study provide preliminary support for the hypothesis that the epsilon 4 allele of APOE may be a potential genetic marker for increased vulnerability to chemotherapy-induced cognitive decline.

Although cranial irradiation is the most frequently identified causal factor in both adults and children, current work in adults indicates that cognitive problems may also occur with surgery, chemotherapy, and biologic response modifiers (102–104). These findings need to be validated in prospective studies along with the interaction among treatment with chemotherapeutic agents, menopausal status, and hormonal treatments. Emotional distress has also been related to cognitive issues in studies of patients beginning cancer treatment.

Patients have attributed problems in cognition to fatigue, and others have reported problems with concentration, short-term memory, and problem solving and concerns about "chemobrain" or "mental pause" (105). Comparisons across studies are difficult because of different batteries of neuropsychological tests used; differences among patient samples by diagnosis, age, gender, or type of treatment received; and, finally, inconsistency in the timing of measures in relation to treatment landmarks. Despite these methodological issues, studies have shown impairments in verbal information processing, complex information processing, concentration, and visual memory (106–109).

Current studies indicate that cognitive deficits are often subtle but observed consistently in a proportion of patients, may be durable, and can be disabling (110). Deficits have been observed in a range of cognitive functions. Although underlying mechanisms are unknown, preliminary studies suggest a genetic predisposition. Cognitive impairment may be accompanied by changes in the brain, detectable by neuroimaging. Priorities for future research include the following:

1. Large-scale clinical studies that use both a longitudinal design and concurrent evaluation of patients with cancer who do not receive chemotherapy. Such studies should address the probability and magnitude of cognitive deficits, factors that predict them, and underlying mechanisms
2. Exploration of discrepancies between subjective reports of cognitive dysfunction and the objective results of cognitive testing
3. Studies of cognitive function in patients receiving treatment for diseases other than breast cancer, in both men and women, to address the hypothesis that underlying mechanisms relate to changes in serum levels of sex hormones and/or to chemotherapy-induced menopause
4. Development of interventions to alleviate these problems
5. Development of animal models and the use of imaging techniques to address mechanisms that might cause cognitive impairment

Endocrinologic Sequelae

Thyroid. Radiation exposure to the head and neck is a known risk factor for subsequent abnormalities of the thyroid. Among survivors of HD and, to a lesser extent, survivors of leukemia, abnormalities of the thyroid gland, including hypothyroidism, hyperthyroidism, and thyroid neoplasms, have been reported to occur at rates significantly higher than those found in the general population (111–114). Hypothyroidism is the most common nonmalignant late effect involving the thyroid gland. Following radiation doses above 15 Gy, laboratory evidence of primary hypothyroidism is evident in 40% to 90% of patients with HD, NHL, or head and neck malignancies (113–116). In a recent analysis of 1,791 five-year survivors of pediatric HD (median age at follow-up, 30 years), Sklar et al. (114) reported the occurrence of at least one thyroid abnormality in 34% of subjects. The risk of hypothyroidism was increased 17-fold compared with sibling control subjects, with increasing dose of radiation, older age at diagnosis of HD, and female sex as significant independent predictors of an increased risk. The actuarial risk of hypothyroidism for subjects treated with 45 Gy or more was 50% at 20 years following diagnosis of their HD. Hyperthyroidism was reported to occur in only 5%. Finally, it is important to note that the risk of hypothyroidism in adult patients treated with mantle irradiation for HD is significant. Most of the adult cases occur in the first 5 years, but the risk is lifelong. These issues are of key importance for survivors of adult cancer with a history of radiation therapy for head and neck cancer.

Hormones affecting growth. Poor linear growth and short adult stature are common complications after successful treatment of childhood cancers (117). The adverse effect of CNS radiation on final height as an adult among patients with childhood leukemia has been well documented, with final heights below the fifth percentile occurring in 10% to 15% of survivors (43,118,119). The effects of cranial radiation appear to be related to age and gender, with children younger than 5 years at the time of therapy and female patients being more susceptible. The precise mechanisms by which cranial radiation induces short stature are not clear. Disturbances in growth hormone production have not been found to correlate well with observed growth patterns in these patients (31,120). The phenomenon of early onset of puberty in girls receiving cranial radiation may also play some role in the reduction of final height (33,121). In survivors of childhood leukemia not treated with cranial radiation, there are conflicting results regarding the impact of chemotherapy on final height (122).

Hormonal rationale for obesity. An increased prevalence of obesity has been reported among survivors of childhood ALL (123–125). Craig et al. (126) investigated the relationship between cranial irradiation received during treatment of childhood leukemia and obesity. Two hundred thirteen (86 boys and 127 girls) irradiated patients and 85 (37 boys and 48 girls) nonirradiated patients were enrolled. For cranially irradiated patients, an increase in the body mass index (BMI) Z score at the final height was associated with female sex and lower radiation dose but not with age at diagnosis. Severe obesity, defined as a BMI Z score >3 at final height, was present only in girls who received 18 to 20 Gy irradiation, at a prevalence rate of 8%. Both male and female nonirradiated patients had raised BMI Z scores at latest follow-up, and there was no association with age at diagnosis. The authors concluded that these data demonstrated a sexually dimorphic and dose-dependent effect of cranial irradiation on BMI. In a recent analysis from the Childhood Cancer Survivor Study, Oeffinger et al. (127) compared the distribution of BMI of 1,765 adult survivors of childhood ALL with that of 2,565 adult siblings of survivors of childhood cancer. Survivors were significantly more likely to be overweight (BMI, 25–30) or obese (BMI, 30 or more). Risk factors for obesity were cranial radiation, female gender, and age from 0 to 4 years at diagnosis of leukemia. Girls diagnosed under the age of 4 who received a cranial radiation dose >20 Gy were found to have a 3.8-fold increased risk of obesity.

Gonadal dysfunction. Treatment-related gonadal dysfunction has been well documented in both men and women following childhood malignancies (128). However, survivors of leukemia and T-cell NHL treated with modern conventional therapy are at a relatively low risk of infertility and delayed or impaired puberty. Treatment-related gonadal failure or dysfunction, expressed as amenorrhea or azoospermia, can lead to infertility in both male and female survivors of cancer and may have its onset during therapy (129). Infertility can be transient, especially in men, and may recover over time after therapy. Reversibility is dependent on the dose of gonadal radiation or alkylating agents. Ovarian function is unlikely to recover long after the immediate treatment period because long-term amenorrhea commonly results from loss of ova. Cryopreservation of sperm before treatment is an option for men (130), but limited means are available to preserve ova or protect against treatment-related ovarian failure for women (131–133). A successful live birth after orthotopic auto-transplantation of cryopreserved ovarian tissue has recently been reported (134–137). A reasonable body of research on topics relating to the long-term gonadal effects of radiation and chemotherapy exists (138–161) and provides a basis for counseling patients and parents of the anticipated outcomes on pubertal development and fertility. A detailed review of this topic is beyond the scope of this chapter.

Among survivors of adult cancer, the risk of premature onset of menopause in women treated with chemotherapeutic agents such as alkylating agents and procarbazine or with abdominal radiation therapy is age related, with women older than age 30 at the time of treatment having the greatest risk of treatment-induced amenorrhea and menopause and sharply increased rates with chemotherapy around the age of 40. Tamoxifen has not been associated with the development of amenorrhea so far (162). Cyclophosphamide at doses of 5 g/m^2 is likely to cause amenorrhea in women over 40, whereas many adolescents will continue to menstruate even after >20 g/m^2 (163). Although young women may not become amenorrheic after cytotoxic therapy, the risk of early menopause is significant. Female disease-free survivors of cancer diagnosed at ages 13 to 19 who were menstruating at age 21 were at a fourfold higher risk of menopause compared with controls (140).

Fertility and Pregnancy Outcomes

Fertility. The fertility of survivors of childhood cancer, evaluated in the aggregate, is impaired. In one study, the adjusted relative fertility of survivors compared with that of their siblings was 0.85 (95% confidence interval [CI], 0.78, 0.92). The adjusted relative fertility of male survivors (0.76; 95% CI, 0.68, 0.86) was slightly lower than that of female survivors (0.93; 95% CI, 0.83, 1.04). The most significant differences in the relative fertility rates were demonstrated in male survivors who had been treated with alkylating agents with or without infradiaphragmatic irradiation (164).

Fertility can be impaired by factors other than the absence of sperm and ova. Conception requires delivery of sperm to the uterine cervix and patency of the fallopian tubes for fertilization to occur and appropriate conditions in the uterus for implantation. Retrograde ejaculation occurs with a significant frequency in men who undergo bilateral retroperitoneal lymph node dissection. Uterine structure may be affected by abdominal irradiation. Uterine length was significantly reduced in 10 women with ovarian failure who had been treated with whole abdomen irradiation. Endometrial thickness did not increase in response to hormone replacement therapy in three women who underwent weekly ultrasound examination. In the majority of the women in the study, uterine artery blood flow was undetectable by Doppler ultrasound (165,166). Similarly, four of eight women who

received 1,440 cGy total-body irradiation had reduced uterine volume and undetectable uterine artery blood flow (167). These data are pertinent when considering the feasibility of assisted reproduction for these survivors.

Pregnancy. Most chemotherapeutic agents are mutagenic, with the potential to cause germ cell chromosomal injury. Possible results of such injury include an increase in the frequency of genetic diseases and congenital anomalies in the offspring of successfully treated childhood and adolescent cancer patients. Several early studies of the offspring of patients treated for diverse types of childhood cancer identified no effect of previous treatment on pregnancy outcome and no increase in the frequency of congenital anomalies in the offspring (168–170). However, a study of offspring of patients treated for Wilms' tumor demonstrated that the birth weight of children born to women who had received abdominal irradiation was significantly lower than that of children born to women who had not received such irradiation (171), a finding that was confirmed in several subsequent studies (142,172,173). The abnormalities of uterine structure and blood flow reported after abdominal irradiation might explain this clinical finding.

Prior studies of offspring of childhood cancer survivors were limited by the size of the population of offspring and the number of former patients who had been exposed to mutagenic therapy. Several recent studies that attempted to address some of these limitations did not identify an increased frequency of major congenital malformations (174–179), genetic disease, or childhood cancer (180,181) in the offspring of former pediatric cancer patients, including those conceived after bone marrow transplant (182). However, there are data suggesting a deficit of males in the offspring of the partners of male survivors in the Childhood Cancer Survivor Study cohort (183), as well as an effect of prior treatment with doxorubicin or daunorubicin on the percentage of offspring with a birth weight <2,500 g born to female survivors in the Childhood Cancer Survivor Study who were treated with pelvic irradiation (184).

Pulmonary Sequelae

The *acute* effects of chemotherapy on the lungs may be lethal, may subside over time, may progress insidiously to a level of clinical pulmonary dysfunction, or may be manifested by abnormal pulmonary function tests. Classically, high doses of bleomycin have been associated with pulmonary toxicity. However, drugs such as alkylating agents, methotrexate, and nitrosoureas may also lead to pulmonary fibrosis, especially when combined with radiation therapy. Radiation is thus an important contributor to pulmonary sequelae of chemotherapy (185). Alkylating agents can injure the lung parenchyma, cause restrictive lung disease by inhibiting chest wall growth, and lead to thin anteroposterior chest diameters even 7 years after completion of therapy. Bleomycin may cause pulmonary insufficiency and interstitial pneumonitis (186).

Pulmonary fibrosis can cause late death in the survivorship period. Among children treated for brain tumors with high doses of nitrosourea and radiotherapy, 35% died of pulmonary fibrosis, 12% within 3 years and 24% after a symptom-free period of 7 to 12 years (187). The risk of overt decompensation continues for at least 1 year after cessation of therapy and can be precipitated by infection or exposure to intraoperative oxygen. In terms of long-term outcomes, a recent study noted that 22% of HD patients with normal pulmonary function tests at the end of therapy (three cycles each of Mustargen, Vincristine [Oncovin], Procarbazine, Prednisone [MOPP] and Adriamycin, Bleomycin, Vinblastine, Dacarbazine [ABVD] or two cycles of each plus 2,550 cGy of involved field radiotherapy) developed abnormalities with follow-up of 1 to 7 years.

The long-term outcome of pulmonary toxicity is determined by factors such as the severity of the acute injury, the degree of tissue repair, and the level of compensation possible. Pulmonary dysfunction is usually subclinical and may be manifested by subconscious avoidance of exercise owing to symptoms. Premature respiratory insufficiency, especially with exertion, may also become evident with aging. Recent aggressive lung cancer treatment regimens consisting of surgery, radiation, and chemotherapy may well put patients at high risk for decreased pulmonary function and respiratory symptoms.

Genitourinary Tract

Several drugs such as cisplatin, methotrexate, and nitrosoureas have been associated with both acute and chronic toxicities such as glomerular and tubular injury (188). Glomerular injury may recover over time, whereas tubular injury generally persists. Hemodialysis to counteract the effects of chronic renal toxicity may be warranted for some patients. Ifosfamide may cause Fanconi syndrome with glycosuria, phosphaturia, and aminoaciduria and may affect glomerular filtration. Hypophosphatemia may result in slow growth, with possible bone deformity if untreated.

Radiation therapy may cause tubular damage and hypertension as a result of renal artery stenosis, especially in doses >20 Gy, particularly among children (189). Radiation and chemotherapy may act synergistically, the dysfunction occurring with only 10 to 15 Gy.

The bladder is particularly susceptible to certain cytotoxic agents. Acrolein, a metabolic by-product of cyclophosphamide and ifosfamide, may cause hemorrhagic cystitis, fibrosis, and occasionally diminished bladder volume. An increased risk of developing bladder cancer also exists. Radiation may lead to bladder fibrosis, diminished capacity, and decreased contractility, the severity of which is proportional to dose and area irradiated. The resultant scarring may diminish urethral and ureteric function.

Gastrointestinal/Hepatic

There are few studies describing long-term effects to this system, either due to underdetection or due to a longer latency period than for other organs. Hepatic effects may result from the deleterious effects of many chemotherapeutic agents and radiotherapy. Transfusions may increase the risk of viral hepatitis. Hepatitis C has also been identified in

increasing numbers of survivors, 119 of the 2,620 tested. Of these patients, 24 of 56 who agreed to participate in a longitudinal study underwent liver biopsy. Chronic hepatitis was noted in 83%, fibrosis in 67%, and cirrhosis in 13%. Fibrosis and adhesions are known to occur after radiotherapy to the bowel.

Compromised Immune System

Hematologic and immunologic impairments can occur after either chemotherapy or radiation and are usually acute in nature. They are temporally related to the cancer treatment. Occasionally, persistent cytopenias may persist after pelvic radiation or in patients who have received extensive therapy with alkylating agents. Alkylating agents may cause myelodysplastic syndrome or leukemia as a late sequela. Immunologic impairment is seen as a long-term problem in HD, relating to both the underlying disease and the treatments used. HD patients are also at risk for serious bacterial infections if they have undergone splenectomy.

Peripheral Neuropathies

These effects are particularly common after taxol, vincristine, and cisplatin. However, despite the frequent use of such chemotherapeutic agents, few studies have characterized the nature and course of neuropathies associated with these drug regimens or dose levels (190,191). Peripheral neuropathy may or may not resolve over time, and potential residual deficits are possible. Clinical manifestations include numbness and tingling in the hands and feet years after completion of cancer treatment.

Second Malignant Neoplasms and Recurrence

Second malignant neoplasms occur as a result of an increased risk of second primary cancers associated with the following:

1. Primary malignancy
2. Iatrogenic effect of certain cancer therapies (192–195)

Examples include the development of breast cancer after HD, ovarian cancer after primary breast cancer, and cancers associated with the *HNPCC* gene. Survivors of cancer in childhood have an 8% to 10% risk of developing a second malignant neoplasm within 20 years of the primary diagnosis (196,197); this is attributable to the mutagenic risk of both radiotherapy and chemotherapy (198–211). This increased risk may be further potentiated in patients with genetic predispositions to malignancy (212–218). The risk of secondary malignancy induced by cytotoxic agents is related to the cumulative dose of drug or radiotherapy (dose dependence).

The risk of malignancy with normal aging results from the risk of cumulative cellular mutations. Compounding the normal aging process by exposure to mutagenic cytotoxic therapies results in an increased risk of secondary malignancy, particularly after radiotherapy, alkylating agents, and podophyllotoxins. Commonly cited secondary malignancies include the following:

1. Leukemia after alkylating agents and podophyllotoxins (219)
2. Solid tumors such as breast, bone, and thyroid cancer in the radiation fields in patients treated with radiotherapy (220)
3. Bladder cancer after cyclophosphamide
4. A higher risk of contralateral breast cancer after primary breast cancer
5. Ovarian cancer after breast cancer

A detailed discussion of this significant topic is beyond the scope of this chapter. However, the importance of the risk of breast cancer in women treated with chest irradiation and the importance of second primaries in patients with a prior head and neck cancer cannot be overemphasized.

Ancillary Sequelae

Lymphedema. Lymphedema can occur as a persistent or late effect of surgery and/or radiation treatment and has been reported most commonly after breast cancer treatment, incidence rates ranging between 6% and 30% (221). Lymphedema can occur in anyone with lymph node damage or obstruction to lymphatic drainage. Women undergoing axillary lymph node dissection and high-dose radiotherapy to the axilla for breast cancer are regarded as the highest risk group. Clinically, lymphedema symptoms may range from a feeling of fullness or heaviness in the affected limb to massive swelling and major functional impairment. Recommendations from the American Cancer Society conference on lymphedema in 1998 emphasize the need for additional research on prevention, monitoring, early intervention, and long-term treatment. Treatments suggested encompass multiple treatment modalities including skin care, massage, bandaging for compression, and exercise. Intermittent compression pumps were recommended only when used as an adjunct to manual approaches within a multidisciplinary treatment program, and routine use of medications such as diuretics, prophylactic antibiotics, bioflavonoids, and benzopyrones was discouraged in the absence of additional research. The impact of sentinel node biopsy in lieu of extensive axillary node dissection procedures for breast cancer on the incidence of lymphedema is not known at this time. A recent review by Erickson et al. (222) found that arm edema was a common complication of breast cancer therapy, particularly when axillary dissection and axillary radiation therapy were used, and could result in substantial functional impairment and psychological morbidity. The authors note that although recommendations for "preventive" measures (e.g., avoidance of trauma) are anecdotally available, these measures have not been well studied. They found that nonpharmacologic treatments, such as massage and exercise, have been shown to be effective therapies for lymphedema, but the effect of pharmacologic interventions remains uncertain.

Fatigue. Fatigue has been reported as a persistent side effect of treatment in many studies (95,223–225). This is especially true among patients who have undergone bone marrow transplantation (226). Treatment-related fatigue may be associated with various factors such as anemia, infection, changes in hormonal levels, lack of physical activity, cytokine release, and sleep disorders (227). The impact of exercise interventions on fatigue is a promising area of research. Fatigue is an important influence on quality of life for both the patient and the family and needs to be managed effectively.

Sexuality and intimacy. Sexuality encompasses a spectrum of issues ranging from how one feels about one's body to the actual ability to function as a sexual being and has been reported as a persistent effect of treatment. In a recent study on breast, colon, lung, and prostate cancer survivors, issues related to sexual functioning were among the most persistent and severe problems reported. Preexisting sexual dysfunction may also be exacerbated by cancer and its treatment (228). A detailed discussion of this topic is beyond the scope of this chapter.

Surgical and radiation-induced toxicities. *Surgical* effects include increased risk of infections and physiologic compromise associated with nephrectomy (lifestyle changes to prevent trauma to remaining kidney), splenectomy (increased risk of sepsis resulting from encapsulated bacteria), and limb amputation.

Radiation therapy may especially exert effects on the musculoskeletal system and soft tissues among children and young adults, causing injury to the growth plates of long bones and muscle atrophy, osteonecrosis, and fractures (2,5). Short stature can occur as a result of direct bone injury or pituitary radiation and resultant growth hormone deficiency. Chronic pain, the result of scarring and fibrosis in soft tissues surrounding the joints and large peripheral nerves, is a particularly distressing problem among patients who have received moderately high doses of radiation. Soft tissue sarcomas, skin cancers at previously irradiated sites, and pregnancy loss due to decreased uterine capacity in young girls after abdominal radiation are also possible.

CANCER SURVIVORS, HEALTH-CARE UTILIZATION, AND COMORBID CONDITIONS

Cancer survivors are high health-care utilizers affecting distinct health-care domains (229,230). Data clearly show that cancer survivors are at greater risk for developing secondary cancers, late effects of cancer treatment, and chronic comorbid conditions. Exposures leading to these risks include cancer treatment, genetic predisposition, and/or common lifestyle factors (231–233). Although the threat of progressive or recurrent disease is at the forefront of health concerns for a cancer survivor, increased morbidity and decreased functional status and disability that result from cancer, its treatment, or health-related sequelae are also significant concerns. The impact of chronic comorbid conditions on cancer and its treatment is heightened more so among those diagnosed as adults and those who are elderly at the time of diagnosis.

Presented next is a brief overview of some factors potentiating the risk of chronic comorbid conditions among cancer survivors. A brief discussion of the major comorbid illnesses observed among survivors is also presented.

Metabolic Syndrome-Associated Diseases: Obesity, Diabetes, and Cardiovascular Disease

Obesity is a well-established risk factor for cancers of the breast (postmenopausal), colon, kidney (renal cell), esophagus (adenocarcinoma), and endometrium; therefore, a large proportion of patients with cancer are overweight or obese at the time of diagnosis (234,235). Additional weight gain can also occur during or after active cancer treatment, an occurrence that has been frequently documented among individuals with breast cancer, but recently has been reported among patients with testicular and gastrointestinal cancers as well (227,236). Given data that obesity is associated with cancer recurrence in both breast and prostate cancer and reduced quality of life among survivors, there is compelling evidence to support weight control efforts in this population (14,15,237,238). Also, gradual weight loss has proven benefits in controlling hypertension, hyperinsulinemia, pain, and dyslipidemia and in improving levels of physical functioning, conditions that are reportedly significant problems in the survivor population (14,15,21,239). Accordingly, the ACS Recommendations for Cancer Survivors lists the "achievement of a healthy weight" as a primary goal (14).

Obesity represents one of several metabolic disorders that are frequently manifest among cancer survivors; disorders that are grouped under the umbrella of "the metabolic syndrome" include diabetes and cardiovascular disease (CVD). Insulin resistance is the underlying event associated with the metabolic syndrome, and insulin resistance, co-occurring hyperinsulinemia, or diabetes has been reported as health concerns among cancer survivors (240–242). As Brown et al. (231) observe, diabetes may play a significant role in the increased number of noncancer-related deaths among survivors; however, its role in progressive cancer is still speculative.

Although there is one study that suggests that older breast cancer patients derive a cardioprotective benefit from their diagnosis and/or associated treatments (most likely tamoxifen) (243), most reports indicate that CVD is a major health issue among survivors, evidenced by mortality data that show that half of the noncancer-related deaths are attributed to CVD (10). Risk is especially high among men with prostate cancer who receive hormone ablation therapy, as well as with patients who receive adriamycin and radiation treatment to fields surrounding the heart (244). Although more research is needed to explore the potential benefits of lifestyle interventions specifically within survivor populations, the promotion of a healthy weight through a low saturated fat diet with ample amounts of fruits and vegetables and moderate levels of physical activity is recommended (14,15).

Osteoporosis

Osteoporosis and osteopenia are prevalent conditions in the general population, especially among women. Despite epidemiologic findings that increased bone density and low fracture risk are associated with increased risk of breast cancer (245–253), clinical studies suggest that osteoporosis is still a prevalent health problem among survivors (254–257). Data of Twiss et al. indicate that 80% of older breast cancer patients have T-scores <–1 and therefore had been clinically confirmed with osteopenia at the time of their initial appointment. Other cancer populations, such as premenopausal breast and prostate cancer patients, may possess good skeletal integrity at the onset of their disease, but are at risk for developing osteopenia that may ensue with treatment-induced ovarian failure or androgen ablation.

Decreased Functional Status

Previous studies indicate that functional status is lowest immediately after treatment and tends to improve over time; however, the presence of pain and co-occurring diseases may affect this relationship (258). In the older cancer survivor, regardless of duration following diagnosis, the presence of comorbidity, rather than the history of cancer per se, correlates with impaired functional status (259). Cancer survivors have almost a twofold increase in having at least one functional limitation; however, in the presence of another comorbid condition, the odds ratio increases to 5.06 (95% CI, 4.47–5.72) (260). These findings have been confirmed by other studies in diverse populations of cancer survivors (261–263). A cost analysis by Chirikos et al. (263) indicates that "the economic consequence of functional impairment exacts an enormous toll each year on cancer survivors, their families, and the American economy at large."

GRADING OF LATE EFFECTS

The assessment and reporting of toxicity, based on the toxicity criteria system, plays a central role in oncology. Grading of late effects can provide valuable information for systematically monitoring the development and/or progression of late effects (264). Although multiple systems have been developed for grading the adverse effects[4] of cancer treatment, there is, to date, no universally accepted grading system (3). In contrast to the progress made in standardizing acute effects, the use of multiple late effects grading systems by different groups hinders the comparability of clinical trials, impedes the development of toxicity interventions, and encumbers the proper recognition and reporting of late effects. The wide adoption of a standardized criteria system can facilitate comparisons between institutions and across clinical trials.

Multiple systems have been developed and have evolved substantially since being first introduced more than 20 years ago (265). Garre et al. (266) developed a set of criteria to grade late effects by degree of toxicity as follows: grade 0 (no late effect), grade 1 (asymptomatic changes not requiring any corrective measures and not influencing general physical

---

[4]Any new finding or undesirable event that may or may not be attributed to treatment. Some adverse events are clinical changes or health problems unrelated to the cancer diagnosis or its treatment. A definitive assignment of attribution cannot always be rendered at the time of grading.

activity), grade 2 (moderate symptomatic changes interfering with activity), grade 3 (severe symptomatic changes that require major corrective measures and strict and prolonged surveillance), and grade 4 (life-threatening sequelae). The Swiss Pediatric Oncology Group (SPOG) grading system has not been validated so far. It also ranges from 0 to 4: grade 0, no late effect; grade 1, asymptomatic patient requiring no therapy; grade 2, asymptomatic patient, requires continuous therapy, continuous medical follow-up, or symptomatic late effects resulting in reduced school, job, or psychosocial adjustment while remaining fully independent; grade 3, physical or mental sequelae not likely to be improved by therapy but able to work partially; and grade 4, severely handicapped, unable to work independently (267).

The National Cancer Institute Common Toxicity Criteria system was first developed in 1983. The most recent version, CTCAE v3.0 (Common Terminology Criteria for Adverse Events version 3.0), represents the first comprehensive, multimodality grading system for reporting *both* acute and late effects of cancer treatment. This new version requires changes in the following two areas:

1. Application of adverse event criteria (e.g., new guidelines regarding late effects, surgical and pediatric effects, and issues relevant to the impact of multimodal therapies)
2. Reporting of the *duration* of an effect

This instrument carries the potential to facilitate the standardized reporting of adverse events and a comparison of outcomes between trials and institutions.

It is important to be aware that tools for grading late effects of cancer treatment are available, to validate them in larger populations, and to examine their utility in survivors of adult cancers. Oncologists, primary care physicians, and ancillary providers should be educated and trained to effectively monitor, evaluate, and optimize the health and well-being of a patient who has been treated for cancer. Additional research is needed to provide adequate knowledge about symptoms that persist following cancer treatment or those that arise as late effects, especially among survivors diagnosed as adults. Prospective studies that collect data on late effects will provide much needed information regarding the temporal sequence and timing of symptoms related to cancer treatment. It may be clinically relevant to differentiate between onset of symptoms during treatment, immediately posttreatment, or months later. Continued, systematic follow-up of survivors will result in information about the full spectrum of damage caused by cytotoxic and/or radiation therapy and possible interventions that may mitigate these adverse effects. We also need to examine the role of comorbidities on the risk of, and development of, late effects of cancer treatment among, especially, adult cancer survivors. Guidelines for the practice of follow-up care of survivors of cancer and evaluation and management of late effects need to be developed so that effects can be mitigated when possible. Clearly, survivors can benefit from guidelines established for the primary prevention of secondary cancers as well as for continued surveillance (268,269).

FOLLOW-UP CARE FOR LATE AND LONG-TERM EFFECTS

Optimal follow-up of survivors includes both ongoing monitoring and assessment of persistent and late effects of cancer treatment and the successful introduction of appropriate interventions to ameliorate these sequelae. The achievement of this goal is challenging and inherent in that challenge is the recognition of the importance of preventing premature mortality from the disease and/or its treatment and the prevention or early detection of both the physiologic and psychological sources of morbidity. The prevention of late effects, second cancers, and recurrences of the primary disease requires watchful follow-up and optimal utilization of early detection screening techniques. Physical symptom management is as important in survivorship as it is during treatment, and effective symptom management during treatment may prevent or lessen lasting effects.

Regular monitoring of health status after cancer treatment is recommended, because this should

1. Permit the timely diagnosis and treatment of long-term complications of cancer treatment
2. Provide the opportunity to institute preventive strategies such as diet modification, tobacco cessation, and other lifestyle changes
3. Facilitate screening for, and early detection of, a second cancer
4. Ensure timely diagnosis and treatment of recurrent cancer
5. Permit the detection of functional or physical or psychological disability

There has been no consensus on overall recommendations for routine follow-up after cancer therapy for *all* cancer survivors. A recent review by Kattlove and Winn (270) can help guide oncologists in providing continuing quality care for their patients—care that spans a broad spectrum of medical areas ranging from surveillance to genetic susceptibility. Health promotion is a key concern of patients once acute management of their disease is complete. Increasingly, cancer survivors are looking to their oncology care providers for counsel and guidance with respect to change in lifestyle that will improve their prospects of a healthier life and possibly a longer one as well. Although complete data regarding change in lifestyle among cancer survivors have yet to be determined, and there remains an unmet need for behavioral interventions with proven efficacy in various cancer populations (271), the oncologist can nonetheless make use of extant data and should also be attentive to new developments in the field.

Follow-up care and monitoring for late effects is usually done more systematically and rigorously for survivors of childhood cancer while they continue to be part of the program or clinic where they were treated. The monitoring of adult cancer sites for the development of late effects, particularly outside the oncology practice, is neither thorough nor systematic. It is important that survivors of both adult and childhood cancers be monitored for the late and long-term effects of treatment, as discussed in preceding sections, at regular intervals.

It is now recognized that cancer survivors may experience various late physical and psychological sequelae of treatment and that many health-care providers may be unaware of actual or potential survivor problems (272). Until recently, there were no clearly defined, easily accessible risk-based guidelines for cancer survivor follow-up care. Such clinical practice guidelines can serve as a guide for doctors, outline appropriate methods of treatment and care, and address specific clinical situations (disease-oriented) or use of approved medical products, procedures, or tests (modality oriented). In response to this growing mandate, the Children's Oncology Group has now developed and published its guidelines for long-term follow-up for Survivors of Childhood, Adolescent, and Young Adult Cancers (273). These risk-based, exposure-related clinical practice guidelines are intended to promote earlier detection of and intervention for complications that may potentially arise as a result of treatment of pediatric malignancies and are both evidence based (utilizing established associations between therapeutic exposures and late effects to identify high-risk categories) and grounded in the collective clinical experience of experts (matching the magnitude of risk with the intensity of screening recommendations). Importantly, they are intended for use beginning 2 or more years following the completion of cancer therapy and are not intended to provide guidance for follow-up of the survivor's primary disease.

Of great significance to survivors of adult cancer, using the best available evidence, the American Society of Clinical Oncology (ASCO) expert panels have also identified and developed recommendations for practice for posttreatment follow-up of specific cancer sites (breast and colorectal; source: www.asco.org). In addition, ASCO has also created an expert panel tasked with the development of follow-up care guidelines geared toward the prevention or early detection of late effects among survivors diagnosed and treated as adults.

To facilitate optimal follow-up during the posttreatment phase, the patient's age at diagnosis, side effects of treatment reported or observed during treatment, calculated cumulative doses of drugs or radiation, and an overview of late effects most likely for a given patient given the treatment history should be summarized and kept on file. A copy of this summary should be provided to the patient or to the parent of a child who has undergone treatment for cancer. The importance of conveying this detailed treatment history to primary care providers should be clearly communicated, especially if follow-up will occur in the primary/family care setting. Finally, screening tests that may help detect subclinical effects that could become clinically relevant in the future should be listed.

Recommendations for regular, ongoing follow-up of cancer survivors are summarized in Table 66.2. For the prevention or early detection of second malignant neoplasms occurring as a late effect of treatment, providers should remain ever vigilant for the possibility. A detailed history and physical examination is always appropriate, in conjunction with screening at age-appropriate intervals or as outlined by panel recommendations arrived through consensus.

Physicians, caregivers, and the family must be able to hear and observe what the patient is trying to communicate, reduce fear and anxiety, counter feelings of isolation, correct misconceptions, and obtain appropriate symptom relief. Practitioners inheriting care for child or adult survivors need to understand the effects of cytotoxic therapies on the growing child or the adult at varying stages/ages of life and be knowledgeable about interventions that may mitigate the effects of these treatments.

Patient education should guide lifestyle and choices for follow-up care, promote adaptation to the disease or relevant sequelae, and help the patient reach an optimal level of wellness and functioning, both physical and psychological, within the context of the disease and treatment effects.

REVIEW AND CONCLUSIONS

Our knowledge about the late effects of cancer treatment, in large part, comes from studies conducted among survivors of pediatric cancer. We need to explore further the impact of cancer treatment on late effects in survivors who were adults when diagnosed. We also need to examine the role of comorbidities on the risk of, and development of, late effects of cancer treatment among these adult cancer survivors. Future research must be directed toward identification of risks associated with more recent treatment regimens, as well as the very late occurring outcomes resulting from treatment protocols utilized three or more decades ago. As treatment- and patient-related factors impact the subsequent risk of late occurring adverse outcomes, clear delineation of those survivors who are at high risk for specific adverse outcomes is essential for the rational design of follow-up guidelines, prevention, and intervention strategies.

Each person with cancer has unique needs based on the extent of the disease, effects of treatment, prior health, functional level, coping skills, support systems, and many other influences. This complexity requires an interdisciplinary approach, by all health professionals, that is organized, systematic, and geared toward the provision of high-quality care. This ambience may facilitate the adaptation of cancer survivors to temporary or permanent sequelae of the disease and its treatment.

The sizeable population of cancer survivors presents many important questions related to treatment decisions, the impact of medical effects of cancer treatment on health, and long-term follow-up care needs related to cancer as well as other chronic comorbid conditions. It is critical, if we are to develop effective research priorities and recommendations for clinical care, education, and policy related to care for survivors of cancer, that we note the two following key points:

1. The population of cancer survivors consists of individuals with varying needs and issues—those cured of their disease and no longer undergoing active treatment, as well

TABLE 66.2	Follow-Up Care and Surveillance for Late Effects	
Follow-Up Visit	**Content of Clinic Visit**	**Suggested Evaluative Procedures and Ancillary Actions**
Chemotherapy/treatment cessation visit	1. Review complete treatment history	Develop late effect risk profile
	2. Calculate cumulative dosages of drugs	Summarize all information in previous column
	3. Document regimen(s) administered	Provide copy to patient (or parent if minor child)
	4. Radiation ports, dosage, machine	Instruct that this summary should be provided to primary care or other health-care providers
	5. Document patient age at diagnosis/ treatment	Keep copy of summary in patient chart
	6. Side effects during treatment	
	7. Identify likely late effects	
	8. Baseline "grading" of late effects (Garre or Swiss Pediatric Oncology Group [SPOG])	
General measures at every visit	1. Detailed history	Evaluate symptomatology, patient reports of issues
	2. Complete physical examination	Review any intercurrent illnesses
	3. Review systems	Evaluate for disease recurrence, second neoplasms
	4. Medication, maintenance, prophylactic antibiotics	Systematic evaluation of long-term (persistent) and late effects (see specific measures)
	5. Education: grade point average, school performance	Grade long-term and late effects: Garre or SPOG criteria
	6. Employment history	Complete blood cell, urinalysis; other tests depending on exposure history and late effect risk profile
	7. Menstrual status/cycle	
	8. Libido, sexual activity	
	9. Pregnancy and outcome	
Specific measures to evaluate late effects Relevance differs by:	Growth: includes issues such as short stature, scoliosis, hypoplasia	Monitor growth (growth curve), sitting height, parental heights, nutritional status/diet; evaluate scoliosis, bone age, growth hormone assays, thyroid function; endocrinologist consult; orthopedic consult
1. Age at diagnosis/treatment		
2. Specific drugs, regimens	Cardiac	Electrocardiogram, echo, afterload reduction, cardiologist consult
3. Combinations of treatment modalities		Counsel against isometric exercises if high risk, advice ob/gyn risk of cardiac failure in pregnancy
4. Dosages administered		
5. Expected toxicities (based on mechanics of action of cytotoxic drugs; cell-cycle–dependent; proliferation kinetics)	Neurocognitive	History and examination
		Communicate: school, family, special education
		Compensatory remediation techniques

(Continued)

TABLE 66.2	Follow-Up Care and Surveillance for Late Effects (Continued)	
Follow-Up Visit	Content of Clinic Visit	Suggested Evaluative Procedures and Ancillary Actions
6. Exceptions occur to the theoretical assumption that least susceptible organs/tissues are those that replicate slowly or not at all (vinca, methotrexate, adriamycin)		Neuropsychology consult; computed tomography or magnetic resonance imaging; cerebral spinal fluid; basic myelin protein Written instructions, appointment cards
7. Combinations of radiation/chemotherapy more often associated with late effects	Neuropathy	History/examination: neurologic examination, sensory changes hands/feet, paresthesias, bladder, gait, vision, muscle strength Neurologist consult
	Gonadal toxicity	History for primary vs. secondary dysfunction, gonadal function (menstrual cycle, pubertal development/delay, libido); hormone therapy; interventions (bromocriptine)
		Premature menopause: hormone replacement unless contraindicated; dual-energy x-ray absorptiometry scans for osteoporosis; calcium
		Endocrinologist consult
		Reproductive technologies
	Pulmonary	Chest x-ray; pulmonary function tests; pulmonologist consultation
	Urinary	Urinalysis; blood urea nitrogen/creatinine; urologist if hematuria
	Thyroid	Annual thyroid-stimulating hormone; thyroid hormone-replacement; endocrinologist
	Weight history	Evaluate dietary intake (food diary)/physical activity
		Nutritionist and/or endocrinologist consult
	Lymphedema	History/examination: swelling, sensations of heaviness/fullness
	Fatigue	Rule out hypothyroidism, anemia, cardiac/pulmonary sequelae; evaluate sleep habits
		Evaluate physical fitness and activity levels
		Regular physical activity unless contraindicated
	Surgical toxicity	Antibiotic prophylaxis (splenectomy)
	Gastrointestinal/hepatic	Liver function, hepatitis screen, gastroenterologist consult
	Screening guidelines differ by age	Follow guidelines for age-appropriate cancer screening (mammogram, Pap smear, fecal occult blood test/flexible sigmoidoscopy)
Screening for second malignant neoplasms	Oncologist consult	Mammogram at age 30 if history of mantle radiation for Hodgkin's disease
		Screen for associated cancers in hereditary nonpolyposis colorectal cancer family syndrome
		Screen for ovarian cancer if history of breast cancer and BRCA I and II.
Assess/manage comorbidities	Osteoporosis; heart disease; arthritis, etc.	History/examination; be cognizant of risk; appropriate consult

Evaluations are suggestions only. Relevance will differ by treatment history and late effect risk profile.
Data from Aziz (2,6).

as patients with recurrences or resistant disease requiring ongoing treatment.

2. Regardless of disease status, any survivor may experience lasting adverse effects of treatment (274).

Research conducted with cancer survivors indicates that long-term adverse outcomes are more prevalent, serious, and persistent than expected. However, the late effects of cancer and its treatment in survivors, especially among those who were adults when diagnosed, and/or those belonging to ethnoculturally diverse or medically underserved groups, remain poorly documented (274). In addition, survivors of cancer have significantly poorer health outcomes on multiple burden of illness measures than do people without a history of cancer. These health decrements may occur or continue many years after diagnosis. Comorbid conditions are another major issue for many diagnosed with cancer, yet little is known about the quality of the noncancer-related care received by these survivors (275). It has been reported that it is more likely that survivors would not receive recommended care across a broad range of chronic medical conditions (e.g., angina, congestive heart failure, and diabetes). Quality of life issues in long-term survivors of cancer differ from the problems they face at the time of diagnosis and treatment (273). Interventions with the potential to treat or ameliorate these many and varied late and chronic effects of cancer and its treatment must be developed, evaluated for efficacy, and disseminated.

The larger scientific community has begun to champion the need for cancer survivorship research and to call for solutions that will lead to both increased length and quality of life for all survivors of cancer (276). This demand is reflected in the language of several Institute of Medicine (IOM) reports, PRG documents, and National Cancer Institute bypass budgets. The IOM report on cancer survivors who were adults when diagnosed articulates key areas for research and care delivery, especially with respect to the development of a formal care plan for survivors that integrates, within one document, key treatment-relevant variables, exposures, late effect risks, and management/follow-up care needs (277). The recent IOM report on childhood survivorship cites the need to create and evaluate standards and alternative models of care delivery, including collaborative practices between pediatric oncologists and primary care physicians as well as hospital-based long-term follow-up clinics (278). Another IOM report, Ensuring Quality Cancer Care, recognized that attributes of high-quality care could be linked to optimal outcomes such as enhanced length and quality of survival, and that continued medical follow-up of survivors should include basic standards of care that address the specific needs of long-term survivors.

Survivors of cancer who have completed initial therapy generally require significant amounts of follow-up care during the first 2 years of diagnosis. The frequency and intensity of monitoring diminishes each year thereafter, a dramatic decrease occurring 2 to 5 years posttreatment. Conversely, the risk of late effects and the impact of long-term effects increase with time. This progressive fall-off in cancer- and

noncancer-related medical visits may reflect either a failure of the medical system to convey the risk of adverse, treatment-related sequelae or a manifestation of system-driven barriers (unequal access, disparities in receipt of quality care). Patient-driven factors (fear of recurrence or of findings) are also critical. Not all survivors may be aware of the late effects they may be at risk for. Therefore, physicians and institutions treating them must provide survivors with a discharge summary detailing key treatment/exposure and baseline health information that may be relevant if or when late effects become manifest.

Most of the cancer survivors return to their primary care providers for medical follow-up once treatment ends, many of whom may be unaware of the additional health risks of cancer treatment. Providing education and training is therefore necessary. Extant published international long-term follow-up care guidelines provide a logical basis for informed practice, but are not truly evidence based and must be updated regularly and communicated optimally to providers and survivors to be truly effective and useful (279,280).

Cancer survivors are a vulnerable population due to the impact of cancer and its treatment on various health outcomes and also because of the potential impact of their cancer history on comorbid conditions. Attention may shift away from important health problems not related to cancer or surveillance may become overvigilant. The lack of evidence base that can help tailor optimal care strategies needs to be addressed. The relative roles of primary care providers and specialists in the care of cancer survivors are not clear. Developing and testing interventions that examine outcomes among groups of survivors managed under different follow-up care settings is a critical need.

It is imperative that we achieve an evidence-based understanding of the frequency, content, setting, and experiences of follow-up care received by the broader population of cancer survivors in order to develop standards for such care with a view toward preventing, detecting early, or ameliorating long-term or late effects of cancer and its treatment. Findings from methodologically rigorous studies will improve our understanding of the nature and extent of the burden of illness carried by cancer survivors, yield key information regarding follow-up care, and facilitate future efforts focusing on the development of standards or best practices for such care, especially when notable health disparities might exist.

REFERENCES

1. American Cancer Society. *Cancer Facts and Figures, 2003.* Atlanta, GA: American Cancer Society; 2004.
2. Aziz NM, Rowland J. Trends and advances in cancer survivorship research: challenge and opportunity. *Semin Radiat Oncol.* 2003;13:248-266.
3. Jemal A, Clegg LX, Ward E, et al. Annual report to the nation on the status of cancer, 1875-2001, with a special feature regarding survival. *Cancer.* 2004;101:3-27.
4. Rowland J, Mariotto A, Aziz NM, et al. Cancer survivorship—United States, 1971–2001. *MMWR Morb Mortal Wkly Rep.* 2004;53:526-529.

5. Ries LAG, Smith MA, Gurney JG, et al., eds. *Cancer Incidence and Survival Among Children and Adolescents: United States SEER Program 1975–1995*. NIH Publication 99-4649. Bethesda, MD: National Cancer Institute; 1999.

6. Aziz NM. Long-term survivorship: late effects. In: Berger AM, Portenoy RK, Weissman DE, eds. *Principles and Practice of Palliative Care and Supportive Oncology*. 2nd ed. Philadelphia, PA: Lippincott Williams & Wilkins; 2002:1019-1033.

7. Chu KC, Tarone RE, Kessler LG. Recent trends in U.S. breast cancer incidence, survival, and mortality rates. *J Natl Cancer Inst*. 1996;88:1571-1579.

8. McKean RC, Feigelson HS, Ross RK. Declining cancer rates in the 1990s. *J Clin Oncol*. 2000;18:2258-2268.

9. Ries LAG, Wing PA, Miller DS. The annual report to the nation on the status of cancer, 1973-1997, with a special section on colorectal cancer. *Cancer*. 2000;88:2398-2424.

10. Shusterman S, Meadows AT. Long term survivors of childhood leukemia. *Curr Opin Hematol*. 2000;7:217-220.

11. Demark-Wahnefried W, Peterson B, McBride C. Current health behaviors and readiness to pursue life-style changes among men and women diagnosed with early stage prostate and breast carcinomas. *Cancer*. 2000;88:674-684.

12. Ganz PA. Late effects of cancer and its treatment. *Semin Oncol Nurs*. 2001;17(4):241-248.

13. Ganz PA. *Cancer Survivors: Physiologic and Psychosocial Outcomes*. Alexandria, VA: American Society of Clinical Oncology; 1998:118-123.

14. Schwartz CL. Long-term survivors of childhood cancer: the late effects of therapy. *Oncologist*. 1999;4:45-54.

15. Brown ML, Fintor L. The economic burden of cancer. In: Greenwald P, Kramer BS, Weed DL, eds. *Cancer Prevention and Control*. New York, NY: Marcel Dekker; 1995:69-81.

16. Sklar CA. Overview of the effects of cancer therapies: the nature, scale and breadth of the problem. *Acta Paediatr Suppl*. 1999;88:1-4.

17. Mullan F. Seasons of survival: reflections of a physician with cancer. *N Engl J Med*. 1995;313:270-273.

18. Loescher LJ, Welch-McCaffrey D, Leigh SA. Surviving adult cancers. Part 1: physiologic effects. *Ann Intern Med*. 1989;111:411-432.

19. Welch-McCaffrey D, Hoffman B, Leigh SA. Surviving adult cancers. Part 2: psychosocial implications. *Ann Intern Med*. 1989;111:517-524.

20. Herold AH, Roetzheim RG. Cancer survivors. *Prim Care*. 1992;19:779-791.

21. Marina N. Long-term survivors of childhood cancer. The medical consequences of cure. *Pediatr Clin North Am*. 1997;44:1021-1041.

22. Green DM. Late effects of treatment for cancer during childhood and adolescence. *Curr Probl Cancer*. 2003;27(3):127-142.

23. Mertens AC, Yasui Y, Neglia JP, et al. Late mortality experience in five-year survivors of childhood and adolescent cancer: The Childhood Cancer Survivor Study. *J Clin Oncol*. 2001;19:3163-3172.

24. Robison LL, Bhatia S. Review: late-effects among survivors of leukaemia and lymphoma during childhood and adolescence. *Br J Haematol*. 2003;122:345-356.

25. Boulad F, Sands S, Sklar C. Late complications after bone marrow transplantation in children and adolescents. *Curr Probl Pediatr*. 1998;28:273-304.

26. Bhatia S, Landier W, Robison LL. Late effects of childhood cancer therapy. In: DeVita VT, Hellman S, Rosenberg SA,

eds. *Progress in Oncology*. Sudbury: Jones and Bartlett; 2002:171-213.

27. Dreyer ZE, Blatt J, Bleyer A. Late effects of childhood cancer and its treatment. In: Pizzo PA, Poplack DG, eds. *Principles and Practice of Pediatric Oncology*. 4th ed. Philadelphia, PA: Lippincott Williams & Wilkins; 2002:1431-1461.

28. Hudson M. Late complications after leukemia therapy. In: Pui CG, ed. *Childhood Leukemias*. Cambridge, MA: Cambridge University Press; 1991:463-481.

29. Blatt J, Copeland DR, Bleyer WA. Late effects of childhood cancer and its treatment. In: Pizzo PA, Poplack DG, eds. *Principles and Practice of Pediatric Oncology*. Revised ed. Philadelphia, PA: Lippincott-Raven; 1997:1091-1114.

30. Kirk JA, Raghupathy P, Stevens MM, et al. Growth failure and growth-hormone deficiency after treatment for acute lymphoblastic leukemia. *Lancet*. 1987;1:190-193.

31. Blatt J, Bercu BB, Gillin JC, et al. Reduced pulsatile growth hormone secretion in children after therapy for acute lymphoblastic leukemia. *J Pediatr*. 1984;104:182-186.

32. Silber JH, Littman PS, Meadows AT. Stature loss following skeletal irradiation for childhood cancer. *J Clin Oncol*. 1990;8:304-312.

33. Leiper AD, Stanhope R, Preese MA, et al. Precocious or early puberty and growth failure in girls treated for acute lymphoblastic leukemia. *Horm Res*. 1988;30:72-76.

34. Ogilvy-Stuart AL, Clayton PE, Shalet SM. Cranial irradiation and early puberty. *J Clin Endocrinol Metab*. 1994;78:1282-1286.

35. Furst CJ, Lundell M, Ahlback SO. Breast hypoplasia following irradiation of the female breast in infancy and early childhood. *Acta Oncol*. 1989;28(4):519-523.

36. Meyers CA, Weitzner MA. Neurobehavioral functioning and quality of life in patients treated for cancer of the central nervous system. *Curr Opin Oncol*. 1995;7:197-200.

37. Haupt R, Fears TR, Robeson LL, et al. Educational attainment in long-term survivors of childhood acute lymphoblastic leukemia. *JAMA*. 1994;272:1427-1432.

38. Stehbens JA, Kaleih TA, Noll RB, et al. CNS prophylaxis of childhood leukemia: what are the long-term neurological, neuropsychological and behavioral effects? *Neuropsychol Rev*. 1991;2:147-176.

39. Ochs J, Mulhern RK, Faircough D, et al. Comparison of neuropsychologic function and clinical indicators of neurotoxicity in long-term survivors of childhood leukemia given cranial irradiation or parenteral methotrexate: a prospective study. *J Clin Oncol*. 1991;9:145-151.

40. Ash P. The influence of radiation on fertility in man. *Br J Radiol*. 1990;53:155-158.

41. Didi M, Didcock E, Davies HA, et al. High incidence of obesity in young adults after treatment of acute lymphoblastic leukemia in childhood. *J Pediatr*. 1995;127:63-67.

42. Oberfield SE, Soranno D, Nirenberg A, et al. Age at onset of puberty following high-dose central nervous system radiation therapy. *Arch Pediatr Adolesc Med*. 1996;150:589-592.

43. Sklar C, Mertens A, Walter A, et al. Final height after treatment for childhood acute lymphoblastic leukemia: comparison of no cranial irradiation with 1,800 and 2,400 centigrays of cranial irradiation. *J Pediatr*. 1993;123:59-64.

44. Greendale GA, Petersen L, Zibecchi L, et al. Factors related to sexual function in postmenopausal women with a history of breast cancer. *Menopause*. 2001;8:111-119.

45. Ganz PA, Greendale GA, Petersen L, et al. Managing menopausal symptoms in breast cancer survivors: results of a randomized controlled trial. *J Natl Cancer Inst*. 2000;5:1054-1064.

46. Yancik R, Ganz PA, Varricchio CG, et al. Perspectives on comorbidity and cancer in older patients: approaches to expand the knowledge base. *J Clin Oncol.* 2001;19:1147-1151.

47. Lipshultz SE, Colan SD, Gelber RD, et al. Late cardiac effects of doxorubicin therapy for acute lymphoblastic leukemia in childhood. *N Engl J Med.* 1991;324:808-814.

48. Bu'Lock FA, Mott MG, Oakhill A, et al. Left ventricular diastolic function after anthracycline chemotherapy in childhood: relation with systolic function, symptoms and pathophysiology. *Br Heart J.* 1995;73:340-350.

49. Goorin AM, Borow KM, Goldman A, et al. Congestive heart failure due to adriamycin cardiotoxicity: its natural history in children. *Cancer.* 1981;47:2810-2816.

50. Steinherz LJ, Steinherz PG. Cardiac failure and dysrhythmias 6-19 years after anthracycline therapy: a series of 15 patients. *Med Pediatr Oncol.* 1995;24:352-361.

51. Adams MJ, Lipsitz SR, Colan SD, et al. Cardiovascular status in long-term survivors of Hodgkin's disease treated with chest radiotherapy. *J Clin Oncol.* 2004;22(15):3139-3148.

52. Kremer LCM, van Dalen EC, Offringa M, et al. Anthracycline-induced clinical heart failure in a cohort of 607 children: long-term follow-up study. *J Clin Oncol.* 2001;19:191-196.

53. Sorensen K, Levitt G, Chessells J, et al. Anthracycline dose in childhood acute lymphoblastic leukemia: issues of early survival versus late cardiotoxicity. *J Clin Oncol.* 1997;15:61-68.

54. Kremer LCM, van Dalen EC, Offringa M, et al. Frequency and risk factors of anthracycline-induced clinical heart failure in children: a systematic review. *Ann Oncol.* 2002;13:503-512.

55. Steinherz LJ, Steinherz PG, Tan CT, et al. Cardiac toxicity 4-20 years after completing anthracycline therapy. *JAMA.* 1991;266:1672-1677.

56. Kremer LCM, van der Pal HJH, Offringa M, et al. Frequency and risk factors of subclinical cardiotoxicity after anthracycline therapy in children: a systematic review. *Ann Oncol.* 2002;13:819-829.

57. Hancock SL, Tucker MA, Hoppe RT. Factors affecting late mortality from heart disease after treatment of Hodgkin's disease. *JAMA.* 1993;270:1949-1955.

58. Hancock SL, Donaldson SS, Hoppe RT. Cardiac disease following treatment of Hodgkin's disease in children and adolescents. *J Clin Oncol.* 1993;11:1199-1203.

59. Fajardo L, Stewart J, Cohn K. Morphology of radiation-induced heart disease. *Arch Pathol.* 1968;86:512-519.

60. Minow RA, Benjamin RS, Gottlieb JA. Adriamycin (NSC-123127) cardiomyopathy: an overview with determination of risk factors. *Cancer Chemother Rep.* 1975;6:195-201.

61. Prout MN, Richards MJ, Chung KJ, et al. Adriamycin cardiotoxicity in children: case reports, literature review, and risk factors. *Cancer.* 1977;39:62-65.

62. Von Hoff DD, Layard MW, Basa P, et al. Risk factors for doxorubicin-induced congestive heart failure. *Ann Intern Med.* 1979;91:710-717.

63. Kushner JP, Hansen VL, Hammar SP. Cardiomyopathy after widely separated courses of adriamycin exacerbated by actinomycin-D and mithramycin. *Cancer.* 1975;36:1577-1584.

64. Von Hoff DD, Rozencweig M, Piccart M. The cardiotoxicity of anticancer agents. *Semin Oncol.* 1982;9:23-33.

65. Lipshultz SE, Lipsitz SR, Mone SM, et al. Female sex and drug dose as risk factors for late cardiotoxic effects of doxorubicin therapy for childhood cancer. *N Engl J Med.* 1995;332:1738-1743.

66. Pratt CB, Ransom JL, Evans WE. Age-related adriamycin cardiotoxicity in children. *Cancer Treat Rep.* 1978;62:1381-1385.

67. Pai VB, Nahata MC. Cardiotoxicity of chemotherapeutic agents: incidence, treatment and prevention. *Drug Saf.* 2000;22:263-302.

68. Legha SS, Benjamin RS, Mackay B, et al. Reduction of doxorubicin cardiotoxicity by prolonged continuous intravenous infusion. *Ann Intern Med.* 1982;96:133-139.

69. Lipshultz SE, Giantris AL, Lipsitz SR, et al. Doxorubicin administration by continuous infusion is not cardioprotective: the Dana-Farber 91-01 acute lymphoblastic leukemia protocol. *J Clin Oncol.* 2002;20:1677-1682.

70. Marks RD Jr, Agarwal SK, Constable WC. Radiation induced pericarditis in Hodgkin's disease. *Acta Radiol Ther Phys Biol.* 1973;12:305-312.

71. Martin RG, Ruckdeschel JC, Chang P, et al. Radiation-related pericarditis. *Am J Cardiol.* 1975;35:216-220.

72. Ruckdeschel JC, Chang P, Martin RG, et al. Radiation-related pericardial effusions in patients with Hodgkin's disease. *Medicine.* 1975;54:245-259.

73. Perrault DJ, Levy M, Herman JD, et al. Echocardiographic abnormalities following cardiac radiation. *J Clin Oncol.* 1985;3:546-551.

74. Kadota RP, Burgert EO Jr, Driscoll DJ, et al. Cardiopulmonary function in long-term survivors of childhood Hodgkin's lymphoma: a pilot study. *Mayo Clin Proc.* 1988;63:362-367.

75. Wexler LH. Ameliorating anthracycline cardiotoxicity in children with cancer: clinical trials with dexrazoxane. *Semin Oncol.* 1998;25:86-92.

76. Lipshultz SE, Rifai N, Dalton VM, et al. The effect of dexrazoxane on myocardial injury in doxorubicin-treated children with acute lymphoblastic leukemia. *N Engl J Med.* 2004;351(2):145-153.

77. Gluck S. The expanding role of epirubicin in the treatment of breast cancer. *Cancer Control.* 2002;9(suppl 2):16-27.

78. Baker AF, Dorr RT. Drug interactions with the taxanes: clinical implications. *Cancer Treat Rev.* 2001;27(4):221-233.

79. Sessa C, Perotti A, Salvatorelli E, et al. Phase IB and pharmacological study of the novel taxane BMS-184476 in combination with doxorubicin. *Eur J Cancer.* 2004;40(4):563-570.

80. Jones RL, Smith IE. Efficacy and safety of trastuzumab. *Expert Opin Drug Saf.* 2004;3(4):317-327.

81. Schneider JW, Chang AY, Garratt A. Trastuzumab cardiotoxicity: speculations regarding pathophysiology and targets for further study. *Semin Oncol.* 2002;293(suppl 11):22-28.

82. Schneider JW, Chang AY, Rocco TP. Cardiotoxicity in signal transduction therapeutics: erbB2 antibodies and the heart. *Semin Oncol.* 2001;28:18-26.

83. Meadows AT, Gordon J, Massari DJ, et al. Declines in IQ scores and cognitive dysfunctions in children with acute lymphocytic leukaemia treated with cranial irradiation. *Lancet.* 1981;2:1015-1018.

84. Jankovic M, Brouwers P, Valsecchi MG, et al. Association of 1800 cGy cranial irradiation with intellectual function in children with acute lymphoblastic leukaemia. ISPACC. International Study Group on Psychosocial Aspects of Childhood Cancer. *Lancet.* 1994;344:224-227.

85. Hertzberg H, Huk WJ, Ueberall MA, et al. The German Late Effects Working Group. CNS late effects after ALL therapy in childhood. Part I. Neuroradiological findings in long-term survivors of childhood ALL: an evaluation of the interferences between morphology and neuropsychological performance. *Med Pediatr Oncol.* 1997;28:387-400.

86. Green DM, Zevon MA, Rock KM, et al. Fatigue after treatment for Hodgkin's disease during childhood or adolescence. *Proc Am Soc Clin Oncol.* 2002;21:396a.

87. Price R. Therapy-related central nervous system diseases in children with acute lymphocytic leukemia. In: Mastrangelo R, Poplack DG, Riccardi R, eds. *Central Nervous System Leukemia: Prevention and Treatment.* Boston, MA: Martinus Nijhoff; 1983:71-83.

88. Peylan-Ramu N, Poplack DG, Pizzo PA, et al. Abnormal CT scans of the brain in asymptomatic children with acute lymphocytic leukemia after prophylactic treatment of the central nervous system with radiation and intrathecal chemotherapy. *N Engl J Med.* 1978;298:815-818.

89. Riccardi R, Brouwers P, Di Chiro G, et al. Abnormal computed tomography brain scans in children with acute lymphoblastic leukemia: serial long-term follow-up. *J Clin Oncol.* 1985;3:12-18.

90. Mulhern RK, Reddick WE, Palmer SL, et al. Neurocognitive deficits in medulloblastoma survivors and white matter loss. *Ann Neurol.* 1999;46:834-841.

91. Packer RJ, Sutton LN, Atkins TE, et al. A prospective study of cognitive function in children receiving whole-brain radiotherapy and chemotherapy: 2-year results. *J Neurosurg.* 1989;70:707-713.

92. Peckham VC, Meadows AT, Bartel N, et al. Educational late effects in long-term survivors of childhood acute lymphocytic leukemia. *Pediatrics.* 1988;81:127-133.

93. Moore IM, Packer RJ, Karl D, et al. Adverse effects of cancer treatment on the central nervous system. In: Schwarta CL, Hobbie WL, Constine WL, et al., eds. *Survivors of Childhood Cancer: Assessment and Management.* St. Louis, MO: Mosby; 1994:81-95.

94. Mitby PA, Robison LL, Whitton JA, et al. Utilization of special education services among long-term survivors of childhood cancer: a report from the Childhood Cancer Survivor Study. *Cancer.* 2003;97:1115-1126.

95. Loge JH, Abrahamsen AF, Ekeberg O, et al. Hodgkin's disease survivors more fatigued than the general population. *J Clin Oncol.* 1999;17:253-261.

96. Knobel H, Loge JH, Lund MB, et al. Late medical complications and fatigue in Hodgkin's disease survivors. *J Clin Oncol.* 2001;19:3226-3233.

97. Chessells JM. Recent advances in the management of acute leukaemia. *Arch Dis Child.* 2000;82:438-442.

98. Pui CH. Acute lymphoblastic leukemia in children. *Curr Opin Oncol.* 2000;12:2-12.

99. van Dam FS, Schagen SB, Muller MJ, et al. Impairment of cognitive function in women receiving adjuvant treatment for high-risk breast cancer: high-dose versus standard-dose chemotherapy. *J Natl Cancer Inst.* 1998;90:210-218.

100. Brezden CB, Phillips KA, Abdolell M, et al. Cognitive function in breast cancer patients receiving adjuvant chemotherapy. *J Clin Oncol.* 2000;18:2695-2701.

101. Ahles TA, Saykin AJ, Noll WW, et al. The relationship of APOE genotype to neuropsychological performance in long-term cancer survivors treated with standard dose chemotherapy. *Psychooncology.* 2003;12(6):612-619.

102. Ganz PA. Cognitive dysfunction following adjuvant treatment of breast cancer: a new dose-limiting toxic effect? *J Natl Cancer Inst.* 1998;90:182-183.

103. Hjermstad M, Holte H, Evensen S, et al. Do patients who are treated with stem cell transplantation have a health-related quality of life comparable to the general population after 1 year? *Bone Marrow Transplant.* 1999;24:911-918.

104. Walker LG, Wesnes KP, Heys SD, et al. The cognitive effects of recombinant interleukin-2 therapy: a controlled clinical trial using computerised assessments. *Eur J Cancer.* 1996;32A:2275-2283.

105. Curt GA, Breitbart W, Cella D, et al. Impact of cancer related fatigue on the lives of patients: new findings from the fatigue coalition. *Oncologist.* 2000;5:353-360.

106. Ahles TA, Tope DM, Furstenberg C, et al. Psychologic and neuropsychologic impact of autologous bone marrow transplantation. *J Clin Oncol.* 1996;14:1457-1462.

107. Ahles TA, Silberfarb PM, Maurer LH, et al. Psychologic and neuropsychologic functioning of patients with limited small-cell lung cancer treated with chemotherapy and radiation therapy with or without warfarin: a study by the Cancer and Leukemia Group B. *J Clin Oncol.* 1998;16:1954-1960.

108. Mulhern RK, Kepner JL, Thomas PR, et al. Neuropsychologic functioning of survivors of childhood medulloblastoma randomized to receive conventional or reduced-dose craniospinal irradiation: a Pediatric Oncology Group study. *Clin Oncol.* 1998;16:1723-1728.

109. Raymond-Speden E, Tripp G, Lawrence B, et al. Intellectual, neuropsychological, and academic functioning in long-term survivors of leukemia. *J Pediatr Psychol.* 2000;25:59-68.

110. Tannock IF, Ahles TA, Ganz PA, et al. Cognitive impairment associated with chemotherapy for cancer: report of a workshop. *J Clin Oncol.* 2004;22(11):2233-2239.

111. Shalet SM, Beardwell CG, Twomey JA, et al. Endocrine function following the treatment of acute leukemia in childhood. *J Pediatr.* 1977;90:920-923.

112. Robison LL, Nesbit ME Jr, Sather HN, et al. Height of children successfully treated for acute lymphoblastic leukemia: a report from the Late Effects Study Committee of Childrens Cancer Study Group. *Med Pediatr Oncol.* 1985;13:14-21.

113. Hancock SL, Cox RS, McDougall IR. Thyroid diseases after treatment of Hodgkin's disease. *N Engl J Med.* 1991;325:599-605.

114. Sklar C, Whitton J, Mertens A, et al. Abnormalities of the thyroid in survivors of Hodgkin's disease: data from the Childhood Cancer Survivor Study. *J Clin Endocrinol Metab.* 2000;85:3227-3232.

115. Glatstein E, McHardy-Young S, Brast N, et al. Alterations in serum thyrotropin (TSH) and thyroid function following radiotherapy in patients with malignant lymphoma. *J Clin Endocrinol Metab.* 1971;32:833-841.

116. Rosenthal MB, Goldfine ID. Primary and secondary hypothyroidism in nasopharyngeal carcinoma. *JAMA.* 1976;236:1591-1593.

117. Sklar CA. Growth and neuroendocrine dysfunction following therapy for childhood cancer. *Pediatr Clin North Am.* 1997;44:489-503.

118. Berry DH, Elders MJ, Crist W, et al. Growth in children with acute lymphocytic leukemia: a Pediatric Oncology Group study. *Med Pediatr Oncol.* 1983;11:39-45.

119. Papadakis V, Tan C, Heller G, et al. Growth and final height after treatment for childhood Hodgkin disease. *J Pediatr Hematol Oncol.* 1996;18:272-276.

120. Shalet SM, Price DA, Beardwell CG, et al. Normal growth despite abnormalities of growth hormone secretion in children treated for acute leukemia. *J Pediatr.* 1979;94:719-722.

121. Didcock E, Davies HA, Didi M, et al. Pubertal growth in young adult survivors of childhood leukemia. *J Clin Oncol.* 1995;13:2503-2507.

122. Katz JA, Pollock BH, Jacaruso D, et al. Final attained height in patients successfully treated for childhood acute lymphoblastic leukemia. *J Pediatr.* 1993;123:546-552.

123. Odame I, Reilly JJ, Gibson BE, et al. Patterns of obesity in boys and girls after treatment for acute lymphoblastic leukaemia. *Arch Dis Child.* 1994;71:147-149.

124. Van Dongen-Melman JE, Hokken-Koelega AC, Hahlen K, et al. Obesity after successful treatment of acute lymphoblastic leukemia in childhood. *Pediatr Res.* 1995;38:86-90.

125. Sklar CA, Mertens AC, Walter A, et al. Changes in body mass index and prevalence of overweight in survivors of childhood acute lymphoblastic leukemia: role of cranial irradiation. *Med Pediatr Oncol.* 2000;35:91-95.

126. Craig F, Leiper AD, Stanhope R, et al. Sexually dimorphic and radiation dose dependent effect of cranial irradiation on body mass index. *Arch Dis Child.* 1999;81:500-510.

127. Oeffinger KC, Mertens AC, Sklar CA, et al. Obesity in adult survivors of childhood acute lymphoblastic leukemia: a report from the Childhood Cancer Survivor Study. *J Clin Oncol.* 2003;21:1359-1365.

128. Thomson AB, Critchley HOD, Wallace WHB. Fertility and progeny. *Eur J Cancer.* 2002;38:1634-1644.

129. Lamb MA. Effects of cancer on the sexuality and fertility of women. *Semin Oncol Nurs.* 1995;11:120-127.

130. Brougham MF, Kelnar CJ, Sharpe RM, et al. Male fertility following childhood cancer: current concepts and future therapies. *Asian J Androl.* 2003;5(4):325-337.

131. Wallace WH, Anderson R, Baird D. Preservation of fertility in young women treated for cancer. *Lancet Oncol.* 2004;5(5):269-270.

132. Opsahl MS, Fugger EF, Sherins RJ. Preservation of reproductive function before therapy for cancer: new options involving sperm and ovary cryopreservation. *Cancer J.* 1997;3:189-191.

133. Oktay K, Newton H, Aubard Y, et al. Cryopreservation of immature human oocytes and ovarian tissue: an emerging technology? *Fertil Steril.* 1998;69:1-7.

134. Donnez J, Dolmans MM, Demylle D, et al. Livebirth after orthotic transplantation of cryopreserved ovarian tissue. *Lancet.* 2004;364(9443):1405-1410.

135. Wallace WH, Pritchard J. Livebirth after cryopreserved ovarian tissue autotransplantation. *Lancet.* 2004;364(9451):2093-2094.

136. Bath LE, Tydeman G, Critchley HO, et al. Spontaneous conception in a young woman who had ovarian cortical tissue cryopreserved before chemotherapy and radiotherapy for a Ewing's sarcoma of the pelvis: case report. *Hum Reprod.* 2004;19(11):2569-2572.

137. Wallace WH, Kelsey TW. Ovarian reserve and reproductive age may be determined from measurement of ovarian volume by transvaginal sonography. *Hum Reprod.* 2004;19(7):1612-1617.

138. Chapman RM, Sutcliffe SB, Malpas JS. Cytotoxic-induced ovarian failure in Hodgkin's disease. II. Effects on sexual function. *JAMA.* 1979;242:1882-1884.

139. Waxman JHX, Terry YA, Wrigley PFM, et al. Gonadal function in Hodgkin's disease: long-term follow-up of chemotherapy. *Br Med J.* 1982;285:1612-1613.

140. Byrne J, Fears TR, Gail MH, et al. Early menopause in long-term survivors of cancer during adolescence. *Am J Obstet Gynecol.* 1992;166:788-793.

141. Madsen BL, Giudice L, Donaldson SS. Radiation-induced premature menopause: a misconception. *Int J Radiat Oncol Biol Phys.* 1995;32:1461-1464.

142. Li FP, Gimbreke K, Gelber RD, et al. Outcome of pregnancy in survivors of Wilms' tumor. *JAMA.* 1987;257:216-219.

143. Constine LS, Rubin P, Woolf PD, et al. Hyperprolactinemia and hypothyroidism following cytotoxic therapy for central nervous system malignancies. *J Clin Oncol.* 1987;5:1841-1851.

144. Lushbaugh CC, Casarett GW. The effects of gonadal irradiation in clinical radiation therapy: a review. *Cancer.* 1976;37:1111-1125.

145. Stillman RJ, Schinfeld JS, Schiff I, et al. Ovarian failure in long-term survivors of childhood malignancy. *Am J Obstet Gynecol.* 1981;139:62-66.

146. Wallace WHB, Thomson AB, Kelsey TW. The radiosensitivity of the human oocyte. *Hum Reprod.* 2003;18:117-121.

147. DaCunha MF, Meistrich ML, Fuller LM, et al. Recovery of spermatogenesis after treatment for Hodgkin's disease: limiting dose of MOPP chemotherapy. *J Clin Oncol.* 1984;2:571-577.

148. Narayan P, Lange PH, Fraley EE. Ejaculation and fertility after extended retroperitoneal lymph node dissection for testicular cancer. *J Urol.* 1982;127:685-688.

149. Schlegel PN, Walsh PC. Neuroanatomical approach to radical cystoprostatectomy with preservation of sexual function. *J Urol.* 1987;138:1402-1406.

150. Rowley MJ, Leach DR, Warner GA, et al. Effect of graded doses of ionizing radiation on the human testis. *Radiat Res.* 1974;59:665-678.

151. Speiser B, Rubin P, Casarett G. Aspermia following lower truncal irradiation in Hodgkin's disease. *Cancer.* 1973;32:692-698.

152. Shamberger RC, Sherins RJ, Rosenberg SA. The effects of postoperative adjuvant chemotherapy and radiotherapy on testicular function in men undergoing treatment for soft tissue sarcoma. *Cancer.* 1981;47:2368-2374.

153. Green DM, Brecher ML, Lindsay AN, et al. Gonadal function in pediatric patients following treatment for Hodgkin disease. *Med Pediatr Oncol.* 1981;9:235-244.

154. Sklar C. Reproductive physiology and treatment-related loss of sex hormone production. *Med Pediatr Oncol.* 1999;33:2-8.

155. Shalet SM, Horner A, Ahmed SR, et al. Leydig cell damage after testicular irradiation for lymphoblastic leukaemia. *Med Pediatr Oncol.* 1985;13:65-68.

156. Leiper AD, Grant DB, Chessells JM. Gonadal function after testicular radiation for acute lymphoblastic leukaemia. *Arch Dis Child.* 1986;61:53-56.

157. Sklar CA, Robison LL, Nesbit ME, et al. Effects of radiation on testicular function in long-term survivors of childhood acute lymphoblastic leukemia: a report from the Children Cancer Study Group. *J Clin Oncol.* 1990;8:1981-1987.

158. Chapman RM, Sutcliffe SB, Malpas JS. Cytotoxic-induced ovarian failure in women with Hodgkin's disease. I. Hormone function. *JAMA.* 1979;242:1877-1881.

159. Whitehead E, Shalet SM, Jones PH, et al. Gonadal function after combination chemotherapy for Hodgkin's disease in childhood. *Arch Dis Child.* 1982;57:287-291.

160. Ortin TT, Shostak CA, Donaldson SS. Gonadal status and reproductive function following treatment for Hodgkin's disease in childhood: the Stanford experience. *Int J Radiat Oncol Biol Phys.* 1990;19:873-880.

161. Mackie EJ, Radford M, Shalet SM. Gonadal function following chemotherapy for childhood Hodgkin's disease. *Med Pediatr Oncol.* 1996;27:74-78.

162. Goodwin PJ, Ennis M, Pritchard KI, et al. Risk of menopause during the first year after breast cancer diagnosis. *J Clin Oncol.* 1999;17:2365-2370.

163. Koyama H, Wada T, Nishzawa Y, et al. Cyclophosphamide induced ovarian failure and its therapeutic significance in patients with breast cancer. *Cancer.* 1977;39:1403-1409.

164. Byrne J, Mulvihill JJ, Myers MH, et al. Effects of treatment on fertility in long-term survivors of childhood or adolescent cancer. *N Engl J Med.* 1987;317:1315-1321.

165. Critchley HOD, Wallace WHB, Shalet SM, et al. Abdominal irradiation in childhood: the potential for pregnancy. *Br J Obstet Gynaecol.* 1992;99:392-394.

166. Critchley HOD. Factors of importance for implantation and problems after treatment for childhood cancer. *Med Pediatr Oncol.* 1999;33:9-14.

167. Bath LE, Critchley HO, Chambers SE, et al. Ovarian and uterine characteristics after total body irradiation in childhood and adolescence: response to sex steroid replacement. *Br J Obstet Gynaecol.* 1999;106:1265-1272.

168. Li FP, Fine W, Jaffe N, et al. Offspring of patients treated for cancer in childhood. *J Natl Cancer Inst.* 1979;62:1193-1197.

169. Hawkins MM, Smith RA, Curtice LJ. Childhood cancer survivors and their offspring studied through a postal survey of general practitioners: preliminary results. *J R Coll Gen Pract.* 1988;38:102-105.

170. Byrne J, Rasmussen SA, Steinhorn SC, et al. Genetic disease in offspring of long-term survivors of childhood and adolescent cancer. *Am J Hum Genet.* 1998;62:45-52.

171. Green DM, Fine WE, Li FP. Offspring of patients treated for unilateral Wilms' tumor in childhood. *Cancer.* 1982;49:2285-2288.

172. Byrne L, Mulvihill JJ, Connelly RR, et al. Reproductive problems and birth defects in survivors of Wilms' tumor and their relatives. *Med Pediatr Oncol.* 1988;16:233-240.

173. Hawkins MM, Smith RA. Pregnancy outcomes in childhood cancer survivors: probable effects of abdominal irradiation. *Int J Cancer.* 1989;43:399-402.

174. Hawkins MM. Is there evidence of a therapy-related increase in germ cell mutation among childhood cancer survivors? *J Natl Cancer Inst.* 1991;83:1643-1650.

175. Green DM, Zevon MA, Lowrie G, et al. Pregnancy outcome following treatment with chemotherapy for cancer in childhood and adolescence. *N Engl J Med.* 1991;325:141-146.

176. Nygaard R, Clausen N, Siimes MA, et al. Reproduction following treatment for childhood leukemia: a population-based prospective cohort study of fertility and offspring. *Med Pediatr Oncol.* 1991;19:459-466.

177. Dodds I, Marrett LD, Tomkins DJ, et al. Case-control study of congenital anomalies in children of cancer patients. *Br Med J.* 1993;307:164-168.

178. Kenny LB, Nicholson HS, Brasseux C, et al. Birth defects in offspring of adult survivors of childhood acute lymphoblastic leukemia. *Cancer.* 1996;78:169-176.

179. Green DM, Fiorello A, Zevon MA, et al. Birth defects and childhood cancer in offspring of survivors of childhood cancer. *Arch Pediatr Adolesc Med.* 1997;151:379-383.

180. Mulvihill JJ, Myers MH, Connelly RR, et al. Cancer in offspring of long-term survivors of childhood and adolescent cancer. *Lancet.* 1987;2:813-817.

181. Hawkins JJ, Draper GJ, Smith RA. Cancer among 1,348 offspring of survivors of childhood cancer. *Int J Cancer.* 1989;43:975-978.

182. Sanders JE, Hawley J, Levy W, et al. Pregnancies following high-dose cyclophosphamide with or without high-dose busulfan or total-body irradiation and bone marrow transplantation. *Blood.* 1996;87:3045-3052.

183. Green DM, Whitton JA, Stovall M, et al. Pregnancy outcome of partners of male survivors of childhood cancer. A report from the Childhood Cancer Survivor Study. *J Clin Oncol.* 2003;21:716-721.

184. Green DM, Whitton JA, Stovall M, et al. Pregnancy outcome of female survivors of childhood cancer. A report from the Childhood Cancer Survivor Study. *Am J Obstet Gynecol.* 2002;187:1070-1080.

185. Horning SJ, Adhikari A, Rizk N. Effect of treatment for Hodgkin's disease on pulmonary function: results of a prospective study. *J Clin Oncol.* 1994;12:297-305.

186. Samuels ML, Douglas EJ, Holoye PV, et al. Large dose bleomycin therapy and pulmonary toxicity. *JAMA.* 1976;235:1117-1120.

187. O'Driscoll BR, Hasleton PS, Taylor PM, et al. Active lung fibrosis up to 17 years after chemotherapy with carmustine (BCNU) in childhood. *N Engl J Med.* 1990;323:378-382.

188. Vogelzang NJ. Nephrotoxicity from chemotherapy: prevention and management. *Oncology.* 1991;5:97-112.

189. Dewit L, Anninga JK, Hoefnagel CA, et al. Radiation injury in the human kidney: a prospective analysis using specific scintigraphic and biochemical endpoints. *Int J Radiat Oncol Biol Phys.* 1990;19:977-983.

190. Hilkens PHE, Verweij J, Vecht CJ, et al. Clinical characteristics of severe peripheral neuropathy induced by docetaxel, taxotere. *Ann Oncol.* 1997;8:187-190.

191. Tuxen MK, Hansen SW. Complications of treatment: neurotoxicity secondary to antineoplastic drugs. *Cancer Treat Rev.* 1994;20:191-214.

192. Bhatia S, Robison LL, Meadows AT, LESG Investigators. High risk of second malignant neoplasms (SMN) continues with extended follow-up of childhood Hodgkin's disease (HD) cohort: report from the Late Effects Study Group. *Blood.* 2001;98:768a.

193. van Leeuwen FE, Klokman WJ, Stovall M, et al. Roles of radiotherapy and smoking in lung cancer following Hodgkin's disease. *J Natl Cancer Inst.* 1995;87:1530-1537.

194. Kreiker J, Kattan J. Second colon cancer following Hodgkin's disease. A case report. *J Med Liban.* 1996;44:107-108.

195. Deutsch M, Wollman MR, Ramanathan R, et al. Rectal cancer twenty-one years after treatment of childhood Hodgkin disease. *Med Pediatr Oncol.* 2002;38:280-281.

196. Hawkins MM, Draper GJ, Kingston JE. Incidence of second primary tumors among childhood cancer survivors. *Br J Cancer.* 1984;56:339-347.

197. Meadows AT, Baum E, Fossati-Bellani F, et al. Second malignant neoplasms in children: an update from the Late Effects Study Group. *J Clin Oncol.* 1985;3:532-538.

198. Bhatia S, Robison LL, Oberlin O, et al. Breast cancer and other second neoplasms after childhood Hodgkin's disease. *N Engl J Med.* 1996;334:745-751.

199. Malkin D, Li FP, Strong LC, et al. Germline p53 mutations in a familial syndrome of breast cancer, sarcomas, and other neoplasms. *Science.* 1990;250:1333-1338.

200. Neglia JP, Friedman DL, Yasui Y, et al. Second malignant neoplasms in five-year survivors of childhood cancer: childhood cancer survivor study. *J Natl Cancer Inst.* 2001;93:618-629.

201. Bhatia S, Sather HN, Pabustan OB, et al. Low incidence of second neoplasms among children diagnosed with acute lymphoblastic leukemia after 1983. *Blood.* 2002;99:4257-4264.

202. Neglia JP, Meadows AT, Robison LL, et al. Second neoplasms after acute lymphoblastic leukemia in childhood. *N Engl J Med.* 1991;325:1330-1336.

203. Relling MV, Rubnitz JE, Rivera GK, et al. High incidence of secondary brain tumours after radiotherapy and antimetabolites. *Lancet*. 1999;354:34-39.

204. Hawkins MM, Wilson LM, Stovall MA, et al. Epipodophyllotoxins, alkylating agents, and radiation and risk of secondary leukaemia after childhood cancer. *Br Med J*. 1992;304:951-958.

205. Tucker MA. Solid second cancers following Hodgkin's disease. *Hematol-Oncol Clin North Am*. 1993;7:389-400.

206. Beatty O III, Hudson MM, Greenwald C, et al. Subsequent malignancies in children and adolescents after treatment for Hodgkin's disease. *J Clin Oncol*. 1995;13:603-609.

207. Jenkin D, Greenberg M, Fitzgerald A. Second malignant tumours in childhood Hodgkin's disease. *Med Pediatr Oncol*. 1996;26:373-379.

208. Sankila R, Garwicz S, Olsen JH, et al. Risk of subsequent malignant neoplasms among 1,641 Hodgkin's disease patients diagnosed in childhood and adolescence: a population-based cohort study in the five Nordic countries. Association of the Nordic Cancer Registries and the Nordic Society of Pediatric Hematology and Oncology. *J Clin Oncol*. 1996;14:1442-1446.

209. Wolden SL, Lamborn KR, Cleary SF, et al. Second cancers following pediatric Hodgkin's disease. *J Clin Oncol*. 1998;16:536-544.

210. Green DM, Hyland A, Barcos MP, et al. Second malignant neoplasms after treatment for Hodgkin's disease in childhood or adolescence. *J Clin Oncol*. 2000;18:1492-1499.

211. Metayer C, Lynch CF, Clarke EA, et al. Second cancers among long-term survivors of Hodgkin's disease diagnosed in childhood and adolescence. *J Clin Oncol*. 2000;18:2435-2443.

212. Wrighton SA, Stevens JC. The human hepatic cytochromes P450 involved in drug metabolism. *Crit Rev Toxicol*. 1992;22:1-21.

213. Hayes JD, Pulford DJ. The glutathione S-transferase supergene family: regulation of GST and the contribution of the isoenzymes to cancer chemoprotection and drug resistance. *Crit Rev Biochem Mol Biol*. 1995;30:445-600.

214. Raunio H, Husgafvel-Pursiainen K, Anttila S, et al. Diagnosis of polymorphisms in carcinogen-activating and inactivating enzymes and cancer susceptibility: a review. *Gene*. 1995;159:113-121.

215. Smith G, Stanley LA, Sim E, et al. Metabolic polymorphisms and cancer susceptibility. *Cancer Surv*. 1995;25:27-65.

216. Felix CA, Walker AH, Lange BJ, et al. Association of CYP3A4 genotype with treatment-related leukemia. *Proc Natl Acad Sci USA*. 1998;95:13176-13181.

217. Naoe T, Takeyama K, Yokozawa T, et al. Analysis of genetic polymorphism in NQO1, GST-M1, GST-T1, and CYP3A4 in 469 Japanese patients with therapy-related leukemia/myelodysplastic syndrome and de novo acute myeloid leukemia. *Clin Cancer Res*. 2000;6:4091-4095.

218. Blanco JG, Edick MJ, Hancock ML, et al. Genetic polymorphisms in CYP3A5, CYP3A4 and NQO1 in children who developed therapy-related myeloid malignancies. *Pharmacogenetics*. 2002;12:605-611.

219. Zim S, Collins JM, O'Neill D, et al. Inhibition of first-pass metabolism in cancer chemotherapy: interaction of 6-mercaptopurine and allopurinol. *Clin Pharmacol Ther*. 1983;34:810-817.

220. Hildreth NG, Shore RE, Dvortesky PM. The risk of breast cancer after irradiation of the thymus in infancy. *N Engl J Med*. 1989;321:1281-1284.

221. Petrek JA, Heelan MC. Incidence of breast carcinoma-related lymphedema. *Cancer*. 1998;83(suppl 12):2776-2781.

222. Erickson VS, Pearson ML, Ganz PA, et al. Arm edema in breast cancer patients. *J Natl Cancer Inst*. 2004;93:96-111.

223. Andrykowski MA, Curran SL, Lightner R. Off-treatment fatigue in breast cancer survivors: a controlled comparison. *J Behav Med*. 1998;21:1-18.

224. Broeckel JA, Jacobsen PB, Horton J, et al. Characteristics and correlates of fatigue after adjuvant chemotherapy for breast cancer. *J Clin Oncol*. 1998;16:1689-1696.

225. Greenberg DB, Kornblith AB, Herndon JE, et al. Quality of life for adult leukemia survivors treated on clinical trials of cancer and Leukemia Group B during the period 1971–1988. *Cancer*. 1997;80:1936-1944.

226. Bush NE, Haberman M, Donaldson G, et al. Quality of life of 125 adults surviving 6-18 years after bone marrow transplant. *Soc Sci Med*. 1995;40:479-490.

227. Mock V, Piper B, Escalante C, et al. National comprehensive cancer network. NCCN practice guidelines for cancer-related fatigue. *Oncology (Williston Park)*. 2000;14(11A):151-161.

228. Ganz PA, Schag CAC, Lee JJ, et al. The CARES: a generic measure of health-related quality of life for cancer patients. *Qual Life Res*. 1992;1:19-29.

229. Demark-Wahnefried W, Aziz NM, Rowland JH, et al. Riding the crest of the teachable moment. *J Clin Oncol*. 2005;23(24):5814-5830.

230. Day RW. Future need for more cancer research. *J Am Diet Assoc*. 1998;98:523.

231. Brown BW, Brauner C, Minnotte MC. Noncancer deaths in white adult cancer patients. *J Natl Cancer Inst*. 1993;85:979-997.

232. Meadows AT, Varricchio C, Crosson K, et al. Research issues in cancer survivorship. *Cancer Epidemiol Biomarkers Prev*. 1998;7:1145-1151.

233. Travis LB. Therapy-associated solid tumors. *Acta Oncol*. 2002;41:323-333.

234. Bergstrom A, Pisani P, Tenet V, et al. Overweight as an avoidable cause of cancer in Europe. *Int J Cancer*. 2001;91:421-430.

235. World Health Organization. *IARC Handbook of Cancer Prevention*, Vol 6. Geneva: World Health Organization; 2002.

236. Nuver J, Smit AJ, Postma A, et al. The metabolic syndrome in long-term cancer survivors, an important target for secondary measures. *Cancer Treat Rev*. 2002;28:195-214.

237. Freedland SJ, Aronson WJ, Kane CJ, et al. Impact of obesity on biochemical control after radical prostatectomy for clinically localized prostate cancer: a report by the shared equal access regional cancer hospital database study group. *J Clin Oncol*. 2004;22:446-453.

238. Chlebowski RT, Aiello E, McTiernan A. Weight loss in breast cancer patient management. *J Clin Oncol*. 2002;20:1128-1143.

239. Argiles JM, Lopez-Soriano FJ. Insulin and cancer. *Int J Oncol*. 2001;18:683-687.

240. Bines J, Gradishar WJ. Primary care issues for the breast cancer survivor. *Compr Ther*. 1997;23:605-611.

241. Yoshikawa T, Noguchi Y, Doi C, et al. Insulin resistance in patients with cancer: relationships with tumor site, tumor stage, body-weight loss, acute-phase response, and energy expenditure. *Nutrition*. 2001;17:590-593.

242. Balkau B, Kahn HS, Courbon D, et al. Paris Prospective Study. Hyperinsulinemia predicts fatal liver cancer but is inversely associated with fatal cancer at some other sites: the Paris Prospective Study. *Diabetes Care*. 2001;24:843-849.

243. Lamont EB, Christakis NA, Lauderdale DS. Favorable cardiac risk among elderly breast carcinoma survivors. *Cancer.* 2003;98:2-10.

244. Hull MC, Morris CG, Pepine CJ, et al. Valvular dysfunction and carotid, subclavian, and coronary artery disease in survivors of Hodgkin lymphoma treated with radiation therapy. *JAMA.* 2003;290:2831-2837.

245. Buist DS, LaCroix AZ, Barlow WE, et al. Bone mineral density and endogenous hormones and risk of breast cancer in postmenopausal women (United States). *Cancer Causes Control.* 2001;12:213-222.

246. Buist DS, LaCroix AZ, Barlow WE, et al. Bone mineral density and breast cancer risk in postmenopausal women. *J Clin Epidemiol.* 2001;54:417-422.

247. Cauley JA, Lucas FL, Kuller LH, et al. Bone mineral density and risk of breast cancer in older women: the study of osteoporotic fractures. Study of Osteoporotic Fractures Research Group. *JAMA.* 1996;276:1404-1408.

248. Lamont EB, Lauderdale DS. Low risk of hip fracture among elderly breast cancer survivors. *Ann Epidemiol.* 2003;13:698-703.

249. Lucas FL, Cauley JA, Stone RA, et al. Bone mineral density and risk of breast cancer: differences by family history of breast cancer. Study of Osteoporotic Fractures Research Group. *Am J Epidemiol.* 1998;148:22-29.

250. Newcomb PA, Trentham-Dietz A, Egan KM, et al. Fracture history and risk of breast and endometrial cancer. *Am J Epidemiol.* 2001;153:1071-1078.

251. van der Klift M, de Laet CE, Coebergh JW, et al. Bone mineral density and the risk of breast cancer: the Rotterdam Study. *Bone.* 2003;32:211-216.

252. Zhang Y, Kiel DP, Kreger BE, et al. Bone mass and the risk of breast cancer among postmenopausal women. *N Engl J Med.* 1997;336:611-617.

253. Zmuda JM, Cauley JA, Ljung BM, et al. Study of Osteoporotic Fractures Research Group. Bone mass and breast cancer risk in older women: differences by stage at diagnosis. *J Natl Cancer Inst.* 2001;93:930-936.

254. Schultz PN, Beck ML, Stava C, et al. Health profiles in 5836 long-term cancer survivors. *Int J Cancer.* 2003;104:488-495.

255. Twiss JJ, Waltman N, Ott CD, et al. Bone mineral density in postmenopausal breast cancer survivors. *J Am Acad Nurse Pract.* 2001;13:276-284.

256. Ramaswamy B, Shapiro CL. Osteopenia and osteoporosis in women with breast cancer. *Semin Oncol.* 2003;30:763-775.

257. Diamond TH, Higano CS, Smith MR, et al. Osteoporosis in men with prostate carcinoma receiving androgen-deprivation therapy: recommendations for diagnosis and therapies. *Cancer.* 2004;100:892-899.

258. Ko CY, Maggard M, Livingston EH. Evaluating health utility in patients with melanoma, breast cancer, colon cancer, and lung cancer: a nationwide, population-based assessment. *J Surg Res.* 2003;114:1-5.

259. Garman KS, Pieper CF, Seo P, et al. Function in elderly cancer survivors depends on comorbidities. *J Gerontol A Biol Sci Med Sci.* 2003;58:M1119-M1124.

260. Hewitt M, Rowland JH, Yancik R. Cancer survivors in the U.S.: age, health and disability. *J Gerontol A Biol Sci Med Sci.* 2003;58:82-91.

261. Ashing-Giwa K, Ganz PA, Petersen L. Quality of life of African-American and white long term breast carcinoma survivors. *Cancer.* 1999;85:418-426.

262. Baker F, Haffer S, Denniston M. Health-related quality of life of cancer and noncancer patients in medicare managed care. *Cancer.* 2003;97:674-681.

263. Chirikos TN, Russell-Jacobs A, Jacobsen PB. Functional impairment and the economic consequences of female breast cancer. *Womens Health.* 2002;36:1-20.

264. Trotti A. The evolution and application of toxicity criteria. *Semin Radiat Oncol.* 2002;121(suppl 1):1-3.

265. Hoeller U, Tribius S, Kuhlmey A, et al. Increasing the rate of late toxicity by changing the score? A comparison of RTOG/EORTC and LENT/SOMA scores. *Int J Radiat Oncol Biol Phys.* 2003;55(4):1013-1018.

266. Garre ML, Gandus S, Cesana B, et al. Health status of long term survivors after cancer in childhood. *Am J Pediatr Hematol Oncol.* 1994;16:143-152.

267. Von der Weid N, Beck D, Caflisch U, et al. Standardized assessment of late effects in long term survivors of childhood cancer in Switzerland: results of a Swiss Pediatrics Oncology Group (SPOG) study. *Int J Pediatr Hematol Oncol.* 1996;3:483-490.

268. Brown JK, Byers T, Doyle C, et al. Nutrition and physical activity during and after cancer treatment: an American Cancer Society guide for informed choices. *CA Cancer J Clin.* 2003;53:268-291.

269. Rock CL, Demark-Wahnefried W. Nutrition and survival after the diagnosis of breast cancer: a review of the evidence. *J Clin Oncol.* 2002;20:3302-3316.

270. Kattlove H, Winn RJ. Ongoing care of patients after primary treatment for their cancer. *CA Cancer J Clin.* 2003;53:172-196.

271. Robison LL. Cancer survivorship: unique opportunities for research. *Cancer Epidemiol Biomarkers Prev.* 2004;13:1093.

272. Eshelman D, Landier W, Sweeney T, et al. Facilitating care for childhood cancer survivors: integrating children's oncology group long-term follow-up guidelines and health links in clinical practice. *J Pediatr Oncol Nurs.* 2004;21:271-280.

273. Deimling GT, Kahana B, Bowman KF, et al. Cancer survivorship and psychological distress in later life. *Psychooncology.* 2002;11(6):479-494.

274. Yabroff KR, Lawrence WF, Clauser S, et al. Burden of illness in cancer survivors: findings from a population-based national sample. *J Natl Cancer Inst.* 2004;96(17):1322-1330.

275. Earle CC, Neville BA. Under use of necessary care among cancer survivors. *Cancer.* 2004;101(8):1712-1719.

276. Ferrell BR, Hassey Dow K. Quality of life among long-term cancer survivors. *Oncology (Williston Park).* 1997;11(4):565-568,571; discussion 72, 75-76.

277. Hewitt M, Greenfield S, Stovall E, eds. *From Cancer Patient to Cancer Survivor: Lost in Transition.* Washington, DC: National Academies Press; 2005.

278. Hewitt M, Weiner S, Simone J, eds. *Childhood Cancer Survivorship: Improving Care and Quality of Life.* Washington, DC: National Academies Press; 2003.

279. Taylor A, Blacklay A, Davies H, et al. Long-term follow-up of survivors of childhood cancer in the UK. *Pediatr Blood Cancer.* 2004;42(2):161-168.

280. Wallace WH, Blacklay A, Eiser C, et al. Developing strategies for long-term follow-up of survivors of childhood cancer. *BMJ.* 2001;323:271-274.

Research Issues in Supportive Care and Palliative Care

CHAPTER 67

Outcomes Assessment in Palliative Care

Joan M. Teno

A ccountability has been called the *third revolution* in medical care (1). Healthcare providers are now often faced with new questions. For example, what are the outcomes of palliative care that justify its continued institutional support? Or, what is the evidence for the use of a certain medical intervention for a specific patient? Fundamental to answering these questions are defining quality of care for seriously ill patients and determining how care is measured.

Quality care at the end of life is different than during any other period of time. Dying persons, their families, and healthcare providers are often faced with decisions that involve tradeoffs between length of life and quality of life. Reasonable persons may differ in such decisions. Therefore, preferences and values are important to shaping treatment decisions in ways unlike other time periods. Outcomes assessment for the dying must take this into consideration. In this chapter, a practical approach to examining outcomes, whether it is part of an audit prior to quality improvement efforts or for the ongoing assessment of institutional quality of care, will be discussed.

WHY EXAMINE OUTCOME?

The first response of staff to auditing the quality of care is, "Why?" A typical response is that their work cannot be measured. Yet, audits and ongoing quality monitoring through examining administrative data, reviewing medical records, and/or speaking with dying persons and families lead to important opportunities to improve the quality of care. Simply stated, "If you don't measure it, you won't improve it" (2).

The results of assessing the outcomes of palliative medicine can help create the needed attention to the issue of improving the quality of care. Such tension can create the awareness among healthcare providers of opportunities to improve and enhance their current practices. Examining the outcomes can be critical to detecting early problems with new medications or other unintended consequences from medical interventions. Examining outcomes can guide organizational efforts to improve the quality of care. For example, knowing that one in four persons now die in a nursing home provides important information for the planning of new programs to meet the needs of the dying (3).

WHAT OUTCOMES TO MEASURE?

Reflecting on the thirtieth anniversary of St. Christopher's Hospice, Dame Cicely Saunders said, "We have never lost sight of the values that were so important to David: commitment to openness, openness to challenge, and the absolute priority of patients' own views on what they need" (4). Fundamental to palliative care is meeting the needs and expectations of patients and families. Quality in a 42-year-old with an acute myocardial infarction can be measured by whether interventions have been done that minimize infarct size such as the use of aspirin or percutaneous transluminal angioplasty. The vast majority of persons would want efforts to focus on restoring function under these circumstances. On the other hand, the circumstances of a 42-year-old dying of stage IV lung cancer are quite different. Technological interventions require weighting of their impact on both quality and quantity of life—decisions that require the input of an informed patient.

The importance of preferences is reflected in the Institute of Medicine's (IOM) definition of quality of care: the "degree to which health services for individuals and populations increased the likelihood of desired health outcomes and are consistent with professional knowledge" (5). This definition implies that conceptual models for quality care (as well as instruments measuring quality) must be based on both professional knowledge *and* informed patient preferences. To date, most conceptual models have been built either around expert opinion *or* qualitative data from patients, families, or healthcare providers.

Fortunately, both experts and consumers agree in many ways about what is important for the end-of-life care—physical comfort, emotional support, and autonomy. However, they have significant areas of disagreement as well, for example, unmet needs (Table 67.1). Family members want more information on what to expect and how they can help their dying loved ones. Patients and families emphasize the importance of closure at the end of life, including issues of personal relationships. Families often speak of frustration with a lack of coordination of medical care. It is often not clear who is in charge; different healthcare providers provide conflicting information, and transitions can be fraught with confusion (10).

One conceptual model, patient-focused, family-centered medical care (Table 67.1), is based on a review of existing

| TABLE 67.1 | Comparison of domains of expert, patients, family members, healthcare providers, and proposed combined model in measuring quality of care at the end of life | | | | |

	Expert Opinion		Consumer Opinion		Combined Model
Emanuel and Emanuel (6)	Institute of Medicine approaching death: improving care at the end of life (7)	NHO pathway (8)	Patients with human immunodeficiency virus, renal failure on dialysis, and nursing home residents (9)	Patients, families, and healthcare providers	Bereaved family members	Patient-focused, family-centered medical care (10)
Physical symptoms	Overall quality of life	Safe and comfortable dying	Receiving adequate pain and symptom management	Pain and symptom management	Providing desired physical comfort	Providing desired level of physical comfort and emotional support
Psychological and cognitive symptoms	Physical well-being and functioning	Self-determined life closure	Avoiding inappropriate prolongation of the dying	Clear decision making	Achieving control over healthcare decisions and everyday decisions	Promote shared decision making
Social relationships and support	Psychosocial well-being and functioning	Effective grieving	Achieving sense of control	Preparation for death	Burden of advocating for quality medical care	Focus on the individual which includes closure, respect, and dignity of the patient
Economic demands and caregiving demands	Family well-being and perceptions		Relieving burden	Completion	Educating on what to expect and increasing confidence in providing care	Attend to the needs of the family for information, increasing their confidence in helping with patient care and providing emotional support prior to and after the patient's death
Hopes and expectations			Strengthening relationship	Contributing to others	Emotional support prior to and after the patient's death	Coordination and continuity of care
Spiritual and existential beliefs				Affirmation of the whole person		Informing and educating

Nelson EC, Splaine ME, Batalden PB, et al. Building measurement and data collection into medical practice. *Ann Intern Med.* 1998;128:460–466.

professional guidelines *and* results from focus groups conducted with bereaved family members (10,11). According to this model, institutions and care providers striving to achieve patient-focused, family-centered medical care for the seriously ill patient should:

- provide the desired level of physical comfort and emotional support;
- promote shared decision making, including care planning in advance;
- focus on the individual patient by facilitating situations in which patients achieve their desired levels of control, staff members treat patients with respect and dignity, and patients are aided in achieving their desired levels of closure;
- attend to the needs of caregivers for information and skills in providing care for the patient and provide emotional support to the family before and after the patient's death; and
- coordinate patients across disease trajectory, healthcare providers, and settings of care.

On the basis of this model, a survey intended to be used as part of an initial quality audit of the quality of end-of-life care has been developed and validated. Two surveys have been created including the Consumer Assessment and Reports of End of life Care (CARE) that was used in national mortality followback survey (12). This survey was shortened to create the Brown University Family Evaluation of Hospice Care and has been adopted by National Hospice and Palliative Care Organization with a recent study of "early adopter hospices" showing variation suggesting discriminant validity (13).

WHEN ARE OUTCOMES MEASURED?

The question of when outcomes are measured is an extremely important consideration. Dying is unlike any other period of time. Often, the dying person and her healthcare providers are balancing the hope for longevity versus the need to make appropriate preparation. Although many outcome measures are not clearly linked to disease trajectory and patient readiness, several outcomes are linked to either. For example, issues around closure are clearly linked to the dying person

and family readiness to discuss that the patient is dying. Therefore, the wording of questions and timing of administration of survey must be done in a sensitive manner to reflect where the dying person is in their readiness to discuss existential issues. Other process measures, such as counseling on advance directives or discussion of hospice, should reflect the recommendation of professional guidelines with measures of quality of care to include counterbalancing measures about whether such discussions were done in a sensitive and compassionate manner.

HOW ARE OUTCOMES MEASURED?

Assessment of outcomes refers to measuring the "end results"—the impact or effect of medical care on the dying person and/or the family. Measuring outcomes allows you to judge the effectiveness of medical interventions, innovative programs, and new medications. In addition to examining outcomes, process measures provide important information for quality improvement and examination of the effect of new programs. A *process measure* examines what a service or intervention does for patients and their families. For example, a process measure focuses on whether there is a regular assessment of pain noted in the medical record, while an *outcome measure* examines whether patients report that they received their desired amount of pain relief. Both are important and critical to measure. Ultimately, the quality of medical care is judged by changes in outcome indicators. Yet, an organization will not achieve those outcomes if it does not implement key processes of care that are known to benefit medical care.

Key to choosing an outcome or process measure is the intended use of the quality measures. Table 67.2 notes the four potential uses of measurement tools.

The areas of emphasis and desired characteristics vary for measurement tools intended for different purposes (Table 67.3). For example, the intended audience for quality improvement measures is the institutional and quality improvement team, whereas the intended audience for public accountability is the healthcare purchaser and consumer.

Measurement tools used for public accountability need further evidence that justifies their use. For example, given

TABLE 67.2	**Purposes of quality measures**

1. Quality improvement—measures to provide information for healthcare institutions to reform or shape how care is provided

2. Clinical assessment—measures to guide individual patient management

3. Research—measures that assess the phenomenon of interest

4. Accountability—measures that allow comparison of quality of care for the purposes of quality assurance or for consumer choice between healthcare institutions or practitioners

From Teno JM, Byock I, Field MJ. Research agenda for developing measures to examine quality of care and quality of life of patients diagnosed with life-limiting illness. White paper from the conference on Excellent Care at the End of Life through Fast-Tracking Audit, Standards, and Teamwork (EXCELFAST), September 28–30, 1997. *J Pain Symptom Manage.* 1999;17:75–82.

TABLE 67.3	**Areas of emphasis based on the purpose of quality measure**			
	Purpose of Measure			
	Clinical Assessment	**Research**	**Improvement**	**Accountability**
Audience	Clinical staff	Science community	Quality improvement team and clinical staff	Payers, public
Focus of measurement	Status of patient	Knowledge	Understand care process	Comparison
Confidentiality	Very high	Very high	Very high	Purpose is to compare groups
Evidence base to justify use of the measure	Important and the measure should have face validity from a clinical standpoint	Builds off existing evidence to generate new knowledge	Important	Extremely important in that proposed domain ought to be under control of that institution
Importance of psychometric properties	Important to the individual provider	Extremely important to that research effort	Important within that setting	Valid and responsive across multiple settings

This table was adapted from an article by Solberg LI, Mosser G, McDonald S. The three faces of performance measurement: improvement, accountability, and research. *Jt Comm J Qual Improv.* 1997;23:135–147. On the Three Faces of Performance Measurement: Improvement, Accountability, and Research and reproduced from an article by Teno JM, Byock I, Field MJ. Research agenda for developing measures to examine quality of care and quality of life of patients diagnosed with life-limiting illness. White paper from the conference on Excellent Care at the End of Life through Fast-Tracking Audit, Standards, and Teamwork (EXCELFAST), September 28–30, 1997. *J Pain Symptom Manage.* 1999;17:75–82.

the intended audiences and implications of the use of measurement tools for public accountability, more stringent psychometric properties must be used for these measures. In addition, there must be either normative or empirical research that substantiates a claim that the construct being measured for public accountability is under the control of that healthcare institution.

Typically, measurement tools can review the medical record, examine administrative data (such as death certificate or billing data), or conduct interviews with a patient or a proxy such as a family member. Each potential source of data has strengths and limitations that should be considered when selecting a measurement tool or strategy.

Medical records are legal documents that should reflect the medical care that patients receive. Yet, medical records reflect staff perceptions, and their contents are subject to reporting bias. For example, a nurse may document that a patient understands how to take his/her medications on hospital discharge; this documentation reflects the nurse's perception. Yet, patients and families often report that they did *not* understand that explanation when interviewed after hospital discharge (14). Furthermore, not all discussions are documented in the medical record. Discussions about resuscitation preferences are usually only documented when the patient or family consents to a "do not resuscitate" order. Therefore, a physician and patient may have talked about resuscitation preferences and decided *not* to forgo

cardiopulmonary resuscitation, but there is nothing documented in the medical record because cardiopulmonary resuscitation is the default in most of the US hospitals.

Administrative data, such as death certificate data, billing data, and the Minimum Data Set, are readily assessable information that can provide invaluable information. Examining death certificate data that are published on the Internet (see www.cdc.gov) and available in public use files can provide hospice and palliative programs with information about their "market share," that is, what proportion of persons for whom they provide medical care in a certain geographic area. This information can highlight areas that are underserved and opportunities for program expansion. Users of administrative data need to be aware that it can be inaccurate because of coding problems, key punch errors, or economic incentives to upgrade a patient's condition to get more reimbursement. For example, one prospective cohort study of nursing home residents with advance dementia found that 37% did not have dementia mentioned on their death certificate.

The Minimum Data Set is used in US nursing homes to systematically collect information on more than 300 items on a quarterly basis. This instrument can provide institution-specific and national estimates of outcomes, such as pain management (15). Yet, these data reflect staff perceptions of patients' levels of pain. Therefore, ascertainment bias is an important concern in the use of these data.

Surveys, either self- or telephone administered, provide information directly from the patient and family perspective about the quality of care. Typically, satisfaction measures which ask a person to rate the quality of care with response categories that vary from "poor" to "excellent" have not yielded discriminating information about the quality of care. The respondents' task with these rating questions includes several steps: First, determine whether that event occurred; second, formulate their expectations regarding that aspect of care; and third, choose a category from the response categories. Often, persons have lowered expectations regarding

their medical care, which, at least in part, explains the finding of high satisfaction in the face of indicators of poor quality of care, for example, severe pain (16,17).

Newer methods have begun using either "patient-centered reports" or "preference-based questions" (i.e., unmet needs) to capture the consumer perspective (Fig. 67.1) (18). These methodologies, unlike typical satisfaction questions that rely on rating questions, provide information that guide improvement of the quality of care. For example, knowing that 85% of patients believe a healthcare provider is "very good" does not tell that provider in what ways and

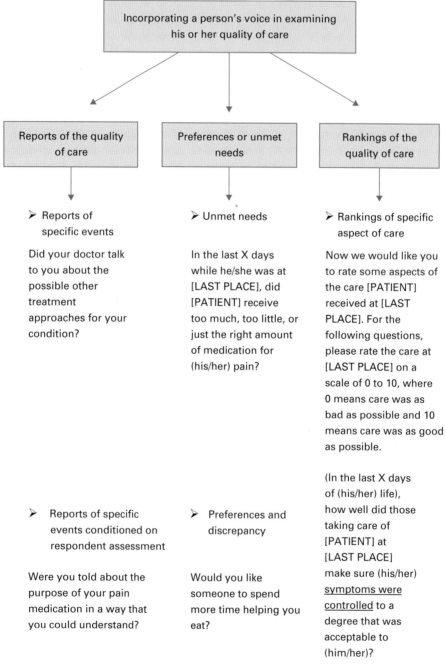

Figure 67.1. Proposed classification scheme for measuring a patient and family voice about the quality of medical care. Adapted from Teno JM. Putting the patient and family voice back into measuring the quality of care for the dying. *Hosp J.* 1999;14(3–4):167–176.

specific processes of care that he/she can improve. On the other hand, knowing that 20% of patients did not understand a provider's directions for taking pain medications does provide a tangible target for improving and enhancing the quality of care. Moreover, patient-centered reports and preference-based questions have strong face validity with healthcare providers. In the future, surveys need to rely on all three methodologies—ratings, patient-centered reports, and preference-based questions—to capture the consumer perspective on the quality of care at the end of life.

WHICH TOOL SHOULD BE USED?

Selecting a measurement tool should be guided by its intended use and the characteristics of the particular tool. The goals of measurement should be clear. As noted in Table 67.3, different psychometric properties (i.e., reliability, validity, and responsiveness of the tool) are needed for different intended uses. In addition, the intended audience is different for each of the four key purposes of measurement listed in Table 67.3. Measurement tools used for accountability, for example, have an intended audience of health insurers, the government, and other such institutions that pay for healthcare services. The focus of measurement is to compare healthcare institutions or plans. Given this purpose, it is very important that there is evidence that what is being measured is under the control of that healthcare institution and that the chosen instrument is reliable, valid, and responsive across the settings.

Reliability is necessary but not sufficient evidence of validity of an instrument or measurement tool. Reliability examines the degree to which the measurement tool is capable of reproducing the same results over time. Therefore, a person should give the same response to a question if asked within a short period of time.

A measurement tool is valid if there is evidence that it measures what it purports to measure. In essence, one is asking whether the measurement tool is reporting the truth. Often, the intent of the measurement tool is to identify a perception or attitude of the respondent. In this case, there is no "gold standard" by which to judge whether the measurement tool is accurately representing the construct that is being measured.

Content validity asks whether the measurement tool examines the correct concepts at face value. Were experts involved as advisors in the creation of the tool? Was the selection of concepts based on a theoretical model? *Construct validity* examines the degree to which the results from that measurement tool are associated with preestablished and known relationships. For example, a measure of overall satisfaction should be associated with consumer choice of healthcare plans.

Responsiveness examines the degree to which a measurement tool changes as a result of interventions or historical events. Often, responsiveness is not reported in the initial validation of a measurement tool. Rather, responsiveness is reported at a later date after the measurement tool has been utilized in intervention studies or research that tracks quality over time.

Over the past several decades, an increasing number of measurement tools have been developed for examining the quality of end-of-life care. A web site maintained by the Center for Gerontology and Health Care Research at Brown University offers a structured literature review of existing instruments that focus on examining palliative care outcomes (see www.chcr.brown.edu/pcoc/toolkit.htm). This web site is a good starting point for selecting measurement tools for quality improvement and research purposes. The site provides published instruments in 10 domains and selects promising instruments for in-depth review, including psychometric properties and response burden.

For a seriously ill and dying population, the time burden on respondents and staff is an important consideration for selecting an instrument. Limiting the scope of domains covered and the number of individual cases for which data are collected can reduce time burden. For an interview respondent—especially a seriously ill patient—it is particularly important to limit the scope of domains that are covered in the interview. For the purpose of quality improvement, you do not need to collect a large number of cases. A small number of cases collected by a random sample can provide invaluable information to guide a quality improvement effort.

HOW IS THE SAMPLE SELECTED?

A fundamental, yet often perplexing, step is deciding who is to be included in the sample. This relates to the "denominator" for the outcome being measured. Simply stated, a rate is composed of a numerator and a denominator. Determining who is in the denominator can be difficult in palliative medicine. For example, three decades ago, most persons would have considered patients with leukemia in childhood to be among those patients with a terminal illness. However, this no longer is the case due to the tremendous strides made in treating cancers in childhood. Researchers and quality improvement teams, then, must make decisions about which patients to include in the overall group of interest (i.e., the denominator).

The difficulty of accurate prognostication is an additional issue. Physicians are often overly optimistic in their prognoses, resulting in uncertainty about patients' actual time before death. Even the best statistical models are inaccurate because they are applying historical information from a previous cohort of similar patients to predict the future. There is a certain error in those estimates. Moreover, new treatments can invalidate even the best estimates by prediction models.

Although the timing of the interview is not as critical for certain domains, such as pain assessment, other domains are very sensitive to the time from death at which the interview takes place. For example, the timing of a discussion about stopping active treatment depends on the patient's prognosis and condition. The difficulty with prognostication also impacts the ability to compare different healthcare units or institutions. It is possible that institutions will interview persons at different time periods prior to death. This situation may result in differences in observed quality measures that reflect timing of the interview more than differences in the quality of care provided.

Given these prognostication issues, an institution may do frequent interviews to capture the same time period from death across patients or relies on retrospective interviews with bereaved family members to collect information on a certain time period. Doing a prospective patient data collection has important advantages. First and foremost, the results could improve the quality of care of that individual patient. Second, the information originates from the patient and not a surrogate. Yet, retrospective interviews with bereaved family members remain an important tool to examine the quality of end-of-life care.

If information is desired about the last week of life, often a family member is the only person that is able to provide a consumer perspective on the quality of end-of-life care delivered to the deceased and his/her family. The advantage of this "mortality followback" approach is that the denominator can be precisely defined, given that demographic information (including next of kin) is reported on death certificates to state-level departments of vital registries. Therefore, data collection can occur quickly without the costs of case finding for the prospective sample of patients. Because of this, mortality followback surveys have been used by both the United Kingdom (19,20) and the United States to collect (21–23) information on the last year of life of decedents, quality of decision making, and the benefits of hospice services.

WHAT ARE THE NEXT STEPS?

The first step in improving the quality of end-of-life care is taking stock—identifying and understanding the opportunities to improve. Simply stated, if you do not measure it, you will not improve it (2). Measuring or conducting an audit is the first step (Fig. 67.2). A metaphor for the audit is the physician review of system. A review of system only provides with a symptom. The next step is to ask further questions and consider ordering diagnostic tests to understand the diagnosis or in the case of audit—the root cause or high leverage process of care where an intervention would improve the quality of care. The second step is to engage stakeholders and define the goal. Engaging stakeholders means to present the results of the audit in a way that does not assign blame, but rather looks for shared opportunities to improve and enhance the quality of care. Key to the success of this second step is raising awareness and developing a shared goal.

The third step is actually improving the quality of end-of-life care through interventions and measuring whether these interventions succeed in creating change. Often, persons believe that education which provides knowledge and impacts attitudes will achieve change. Many times, even knowledge is not sufficient to change behavior. Instead, changes must be made in the processes of care that provide the cues and default pathways that ensure persons will choose the right behavior. Often, this change can be achieved

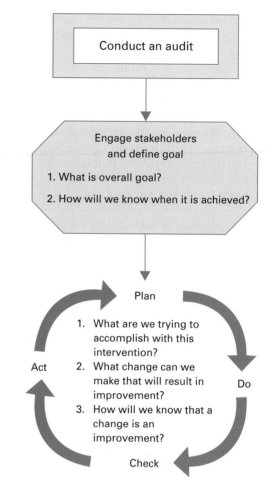

Figure 67.2. Quality improvement model.

through a model of rapid improvement that utilizes multiple plan, do, check, and act (PDCA) cycles (24). PDCA cycles allow testing of interventions first on a small scale (sometimes as small as only one nurse with one patient). From the information learned, the intervention can be refined or a different one can be tested.

Three key questions help to frame the work of the PDCA cycle. First, what is one trying to accomplish with this intervention? Just as an overall goal was identified in step 2 of the quality improvement model, a goal must be stated for each PDCA cycle. Second, what changes can one make that will result in improvement? This may involve brainstorming with a team of colleagues about what interventions can achieve the goal of the cycle. An effort should be made to be creative, yet one should not be afraid to copy the success of others. Third, how will one know that change is an improvement? It is important to choose either a process or outcome variable that examines whether the goal of that cycle is being met and that data are tracked for the goal of that cycle, as well as the overall goal for the improvement effort. Often, a quality improvement team must test multiple interventions and conduct multiple PDCA cycles to achieve the overall goal. Two recent studies suggest that application of rapid cycle quality improvement can result in substantial gains of the quality of pain management in the nursing homes or feeding tube decision making (25, 26).

CONCLUSIONS

Outcomes assessment is key to improving the quality of end-of-life care. At this early stage of development of supportive and palliative care, we urgently need both research and quality improvement efforts that will contribute to the scientific evidence base. Care at the end of life is quite different than care at other time periods. Patients' informed preferences play an even more central role in decision making and outcomes. Not all persons with stage IV lung cancer, for example, will want experimental chemotherapy, and quality indicators must take into account that reasonable persons have different treatment preferences. Hence, measuring the quality of end-of-life care often requires interviews to examine the consumer perspective.

Even at this early stage, there are several promising measurement tools for quality improvement audits, for research, and for accountability. Selection of these measurement tools must be guided by the intended use of the data. The use of measurement tools for accountability carries two key requirements: an evidence base that suggests that the domain of interest is under the control of healthcare providers and demonstration of satisfactory psychometric properties of the tool across settings of care.

With an increased focus on accountability, healthcare providers will need to become familiar with methods to improve the quality of medical care. Measurement plays an important role in quality improvement efforts—from the initial audit that raises awareness of an opportunity to improve to ongoing assessments of whether interventions are achieving their goals. The ideal quality monitoring system for palliative care should strongly link guidelines and proposed quality indicators. Guidelines should be based on both normative and empirical research. Quality indicators can measure information about the structure of a healthcare institution (e.g., availability of certain services and existence of policies) about processes of care (i.e., the interactions of healthcare providers, patients, and family members), and about outcomes of care (i.e., the effectiveness of treatment).

Currently, most quality indicators measure either structure or processes of care. Outcome measures are intuitively more attractive, but they are more difficult to apply because of our limited ability to adjust for differences in patient characteristics and the relatively small numbers of people with a particular condition treated at institutions each year. One argument in favor of collecting process data is that they are a more sensitive measure of quality because adverse outcomes do not occur every time there is an error in the provision of medical care. Furthermore, important outcomes—both positive and negative—often appear months or even years after care has been given. Quality indicators based on measures of structure or process, however, are only as good as their ability to predict outcomes of importance.

ACKNOWLEDGMENTS

This chapter in part is based on a background paper prepared for the National Cancer Policy Board of the IOM. The author acknowledges the helpful comments by Ms. Helen Gelband and Cindy Williams for editorial assistance.

REFERENCES

1. Relman AS. Assessment and accountability: the third revolution in medical care [editorial]. *N Engl J Med.* 1988;319(18):1220-1222.
2. Nelson EC, Splaine ME, Batalden PB, Plume SK. Building measurement and data collection into medical practice. *Ann Intern Med.* 1998;128(6):460-466.
3. Teno JM. Facts on dying: Brown Atlas site of death 1989–1997. http://www.chcr.brown.edu/dying/factsondying.htm. Accessed February 26, 2004.
4. Saunders C, ed. *Monograph in Commemoration of the 30th Anniversary of St. Christopher's Hospice.* London: St. Christopher's Hospice; 2001.
5. Institute of Medicine, ed. *Medicare: A Strategy for Quality Assurance.* Washington, DC: National Academy Press; 1990.
6. Emanuel EJ, Emanuel LL. The promise of a good death. *Lancet.* 1998;351(suppl 2):SII21-SII29.
7. Institute of Medicine, Committee on Care at the End of Life, ed. *Approaching Death: Improving Care at the End of Life.* Washington, DC: National Academy Press; 1997.
8. National Hospice Organization, ed. *A Pathway for Patients and Families Facing Terminal Illness: Self-Determined Life Closure, Safe Comfortable Dying and Effective Grieving.* Alexandria, VA: National Hospice Organization; 1997.
9. Singer PA, Martin DK, Kelner M. Quality end-of-life care: patients' perspectives. *JAMA.* 1999;281(2):163-168.
10. Teno JM, Casey VA, Welch L, Edgman-Levitan S. Patient-focused, family-centered end-of-life medical care: views of the guidelines and bereaved family members. *J Pain Symptom Manage.* Special Section on Measuring Quality of Care at Life's End II. 2001;22(3):738-751.
11. Teno JM, Connor SR. Referring a patient and family to high-quality palliative care at the close of life: "We met a new personality. with this level of compassion and empathy". *JAMA.* 2009;301(6):651-659.
12. Teno JM, Clarridge BR, Casey V, et al. Family perspectives on end-of-life care at the last place of care. *JAMA.* 2004;291(1):88-93.
13. Connor SR, Teno J, Spence C, Smith N. family evaluation of hospice care: results from voluntary submission of data via website. *J Pain Symptom Manage.* 2005;30(1):9-17.
14. Cleary PD, Edgman-Levitan S, Roberts M, et al. Patients evaluate their hospital care: a national survey. *Health Aff (Millwood).* 1991;10(4):254-267.
15. Teno JM, Weitzen S, Wetle T, Mor V. Persistent pain in nursing home residents. *JAMA.* 2001;285(16):2081.
16. Desbiens NA, Wu AW, Broste SK, et al. Pain and satisfaction with pain control in seriously ill hospitalized adults: findings from the SUPPORT research investigations. For the SUPPORT Investigators. Study to understand prognoses and preferences for outcomes and risks of treatment. *Crit Care Med.* 1996;24(12):1953-1961.
17. Quality improvement guidelines for the treatment of acute pain and cancer pain. American Pain Society Quality of Care Committee. *JAMA.* 1995;274(23):1874-1880.

18. Teno JM. Putting the patient and family voice back into measuring the quality of care for the dying. *Hosp J.* 1999;14(3–4):167-176.

19. Cartwright A. Changes in life and care in the year before death 1969–1987. *J Public Health Med.* 1991;13(2):81-87.

20. Addington Hall J, McCarthy M. Regional study of care for the dying: methods and sample characteristics. *Palliat Med.* 1995;9(1):27-35.

21. NCHS. *The National Mortality Followback Survey – Provisional Data, 1993. Public User Data File Documentation.* Hyattsville, MD: Centers for Disease Control and Prevention; 1998.

22. Teno JM, Gozalo PL, Lee IC, et al. Does hospice improve quality of care for persons dying from dementia? *J Am Geriatr Soc.* 2011;59(8):1531-1536.

23. Teno JM, Mitchell SL, Kuo SK, et al. Decision-making and outcomes of feeding tube insertion: a five-state study. *J Am Geriatr Soc.* 2011;59(5):881-886.

24. Langley G, Nolan K, Nolan T, Norman C, Provost L, eds. *The Improvement Guide: A Practical Approach to Enhancing Organizational Performance.* San Francisco, CA: Jossey-Bass Publishers; 1996.

25. Baier RR, Gifford DR, Patry G, et al. Ameliorating pain in nursing homes: a collaborative quality-improvement project. *J Am Geriatr Soc.* 2004;52(12):1988-1995.

26. Rabeneck L, McCullough LB, Wray NP. Ethically justified, clinically comprehensive guidelines for percutaneous endoscopic gastrostomy tube placement. *Lancet.* 1997;349(9050):496-498.

CHAPTER 68

Measurement of Quality of Life Outcomes

Benjamin J. Miriovsky ■ Amy P. Abernethy

BACKGROUND

According to the American Academy of Hospice and Palliative Medicine, the goal of palliative care is "…to prevent and relieve suffering, and to support the best possible quality of life for patients and their families, regardless of their stage of disease or the need for other therapies, in accordance with their values and preferences" (1). Given the centrality of the concept of quality of life (QoL) to palliative and supportive oncology, assessment of QoL is essential, both as part of routine clinical practice and for research purposes (2). Practical uses of routine measurement of QoL include identifying and prioritizing problems, facilitating communication, screening for unidentified problems, encouraging shared decision making, and monitoring change and effectiveness of treatment (3). The last point in this list is particularly important because without tools to systematically assess QoL and evaluate the effectiveness of standard practices or novel interventions, the extent to which the ultimate goals of palliative medicine are realized (i.e., the prevention and relief of suffering) cannot be honestly assessed.

While there is broad consensus about the importance of routine measurement of QoL in palliative medicine (4), there is little consensus about how this is best achieved (5,6), though the recommendations are consistent that patients themselves, without interpretation by third parties, are the best source of information regarding QoL. Such reports taken directly from patients, without other censoring, are referred to as *patient-reported outcomes* (PROs) and form the basis for QoL measurement. There are numerous other types of PROs, especially symptoms, such as pain, nausea, breathlessness, and anxiety, which are often related to QoL, pertinent to palliative and supportive oncology, and best collected via PRO assessment instruments as well. This chapter will broadly discuss terminology in QoL research, the statistical basis, relevant available instruments for palliative medicine, and a framework for selecting among the available instruments.

TERMINOLOGY

In order to understand the basis for disagreement about best practices for measuring QoL, it is prudent to examine currently used definitions for the numerous terms. A thorough, but by no means comprehensive, list of relevant terms and definitions is included for quick reference (Table 68.1). QoL, as defined by the World Health Organization (WHO)

Quality of Life Group, is an individual's "…perception of their position in life in the context of the culture and value systems in which they live and in relation to their goals, expectations, standards and concerns. It is a broad ranging concept affected in a complex way by the person's physical health, psychological state, level of independence, social relationships, personal beliefs and their relationship to salient features of their environment" (13). Despite this definition, research in QoL measurement is complicated (11), with multiple authors having acknowledged that there is still a lack of agreement on the exact definition (5,14,15), and that imprecision and inconsistency persist (11). In fact, the term *QoL* sometimes is used to refer to the general construct related to overall satisfaction with all aspects of an individual's life, while at other times it is used more specifically to reflect those experiences impacted by disease or its treatment (14). There are a number of terms—*functional status, health status, QoL,* and *health-related quality of life (HRQoL)*—that have been used interchangeably in the literature because they overlap to some degree with respect to definition, but in fact, differ in important ways (11). Further discussion on QoL measurement depends upon clarification, to the extent possible, of these terms.

Functional status generally refers to the ability to physically perform tasks related to daily living, such as household activities, personal care, and eating (11), although, in some contexts, the term reflects the ability to perform in expected social roles. Functional status is traditionally assessed by clinicians (e.g., the Karnofsky Performance Status Scale (16), Eastern Cooperative Oncology Group Performance Status Scale (17), and Palliative Performance Scale (18)). *Health status* is a multidimensional concept that is broader than functional status, typically representing an individual's perception about overall state of health, both physical and mental (11). Again, the term can be used for even more general concepts, such as how the perception of the overall state of health influences social roles and spirituality (14).

By definition, QoL is a very subjective concept, yet one that almost everyone can intuitively understand. It also has intuitive meaning to most people, but the meaning undoubtedly varies between individuals. It is this variability that complicates QoL research, as consistent implementation of a single, agreed-upon definition (even though one has been put forward by the WHO) across the spectrum of QoL research is impractical.

Because the term *QoL* extends beyond the scope of health (mental and physical) to include the influence of

TABLE 68.1	Definitions for commonly encountered terms in quality of life measurement

Term	Definition
Ability to detect change	Evidence that a PRO instrument can identify differences in scores over time in individuals or groups who have changed with respect to the measurement concept (7)
Clinician-reported outcome (ClinRO)	Outcomes that are either observed by the physician (e.g., cure of infection and absence of lesions) or require physician interpretation (e.g., radiologic results and tumor response). In addition, ClinROs may include formal or informal scales completed by the physician using information about the patient (8)
Concept	The specific measurement goal or the thing that is measured by a PRO (7)
Conceptual framework	Explicitly defines the concepts measured by the instrument in a diagram that presents a description of the relationships between items, domain (subconcepts), and concepts measured and the scores produced by a PRO instrument (7)
Construct validity	The degree to which what was measured reflects the *a priori* conceptualization of what should be measured (9)
Content validity	The extent to which the instrument actually measures the concepts of interest (10)
Criterion validity	The extent to which the scores of PRO measure reflect the gold standard measure of the same concept (7)
Domain	A subconcept represented by a score of an instrument that measures a larger concept comprised of multiple domains (7)
Health-related quality of life	The subjective assessment of the impact of disease and treatment across the physical, psychological, social, and somatic domains of functioning and well-being (11)
Instrument	A means to capture data (i.e., a questionnaire) plus all the information and documentation that supports its use. Generally, that includes clearly defined methods and instruction for administration or responding; a standard format for data collection; and well-documented methods for scoring, analysis, and interpretation of results in the target population (7)
Item	An individual question, statement, or task (and its standardized response options) that is evaluated by the patient to address a particular concept (7)
Metadata	Structured information that describes, explains, locates, or otherwise makes it easier to retrieve, use, or manage an information source (12)
Patient-reported outcome (PRO)	A measurement based on a report that comes directly from the patient (i.e., study subject) about the status of a patient's health condition without amendment or interpretation of the patient's response by a clinician or anyone else (7)
Proxy-reported outcome	A measurement based on a report by someone other than the patient reporting as if he or she is the patient (7)
Quality of life	An individual's perception of their position in life in the context of the culture and value systems in which they live and in relation to their goals, expectations, standards, and concerns. It is a broad-ranging concept affected in a complex way by the person's physical health, psychological state, level of independence, social relationships, personal beliefs, and their relationship to salient features of their environment (13)
Recall period	The period of time patients are asked to consider in responding to a PRO item or question (7)
Reliability	The ability of an instrument to yield the same result on serial administrations when no change in the concept being measured is expected (10)
Scale	The system of numbers of verbal anchors by which a value or score is derived for an item. Examples include visual analog scales (VAS), Likert scales, and rating scales (7)
Score	A number derived from a patient's response to items in a questionnaire. A score is computed based on a prespecified, validated scoring algorithm and is subsequently used in statistical analyses of clinical results (7)

social, political, economic, and environmental factors on an individual's experience, recent literature within the context of QoL research in medicine has focused on the concept of HRQoL. HRQoL is defined as "…the subjective assessment of the impact of disease and treatment across the physical, psychological, social and somatic domains of functioning and well-being" (11). HRQoL is intended to differentiate between the effects of factors intrinsic to the individual from those related to societal factors, such as political and societal norms (14). With respect to measuring HRQoL, there is some disagreement about which domains, among physical, psychological, and social, are necessary for inclusion. There is agreement, however, that a comprehensive approach to measurement of HRQoL is necessary because of the multidimensional nature of the concept (11).

Acknowledging the preference for the term *HRQoL* in recent literature, and cogent arguments surrounding its use, we prefer QoL in the setting of palliative and supportive oncology, as attempting to compartmentalize HRQoL from QoL is exceedingly difficult and practically trivial in this setting. In the setting of life-threatening illness, health-related aspects touch nearly every aspect of life and are often all encompassing. Thus, further discussions will consistently utilize the term *QoL*, rather than HRQoL. Additionally, because PROs serve as the foundation for QoL measurement, the terms *PRO* and *QoL* instruments are used interchangeably, with PRO instruments reflecting a more general term that may or may not be specifically designed to measure QoL but rather may be specific to other PRO constructs such as symptom assessment.

METHODOLOGICAL BASIS FOR MEASURING QoL

The Importance of Direct Patient Reports

As opposed to traditional evaluations, such as laboratory and imaging data, or even functional status assessments by clinicians, patients themselves are the most appropriate source for QoL measurements, without interpretation by third parties, thus the emphasis on PROs within QoL literature. While direct patient reports are considered the gold standard for QoL measurement, the need for proxy reports of QoL is often necessary in palliative and supportive oncology, where patient's ability to directly complete questionnaires, even in assisted forms, often becomes limited (19–21). In another variation on the theme of direct reporting, caregiver reports—either as proxy reports of patient experience or as reports of caregiver experience with respect to domains such as distress and satisfaction—are an important source of information in palliative medicine. However, such reports are not strictly PROs and are surrogates and cannot serve as the "gold standard" for measuring QoL. Thus, proxy reports and caregiver reports will receive only brief discussion in a later section "Caregiver/Proxy Considerations."

Developing Measurement Tools

There is an extensive body of literature regarding the development and psychometric assessment of PRO and QoL measurement instruments. The methodological basis for psychometric assessment is crucial for research that involves PRO assessments, as it provides important background to understanding and comparing the validity and reliability of various measurement tools. However, such detail is beyond the scope of this text and readers are referred to other excellent texts on these issues (22,23). Even from a clinician's viewpoint, however, it is important to understand some overarching concepts of psychometric analysis; hence, the following sections approach these concepts from the clinician's viewpoint. Practically, an *item* refers to a single question or statement, a *factor* or *subscale* is a collection of items addressing one domain (or subconcept) related to the overarching concept of interest, and an *instrument* refers to the entire collection of items related to the concept of interest (i.e., survey or questionnaire), in addition to the supporting documentation and associated standard procedures (Table 68.1); the terms questionnaire and survey are used interchangeably with instrument.

Instrument Development

In developing an instrument based on direct patient reports to measure QoL, a sound conceptual framework is necessary. In the context of PRO instrument development, a conceptual framework "explicitly defines the concepts measured by the instrument in a diagram that presents a description of the relationships between items, domain (subconcepts), and concepts measured and the scores produced by a PRO instrument" (7). That is, the conceptual framework identifies the factors that influence the concept of interest and how these factors and the concept are related. Typically, the initial conceptual framework is based upon expert opinion and literature review using *a priori* hypotheses. After developing an initial conceptual framework, direct patient input is obtained, typically through focus groups or structured interviews of patients within the population of interest to ensure that the *a priori* hypotheses are consistent with patient's experience and perception. For complex concepts, such as breathlessness, multiple domains impact the overall concept, so identifying appropriate domains and then assessing these is paramount to assessing the overarching concept. The conceptual framework typically evolves over time, with each iterative change moving the framework closer to actual patient experience.

Validity

Validity is one of the key psychometric properties of measurement scales and reflects the extent to which an instrument measures the concept or domain of interest in the target population (14); that is, validity addresses the question "Is the instrument measuring what you think it is measuring?" From a psychometric standpoint, validity has three main forms: content, construct, and criterion validity. *Content validity* describes a qualitative assessment as to whether the items accurately reflect those experiences and perceptions that are important (14). Because it is a qualitative assessment, there is not a formal, standardized metric to score content validity. Rather, the adequacy of content validity is based on expert opinion, literature review, or patient input (14). Content validity has received significant emphasis within the PRO literature, especially recently with the United States Food and Drug Administration (FDA) guidance document for use of PROs in product-labeling claims (7). The FDA guidance document clearly identifies content validity as the psychometric cornerstone for product-labeling claims based on PRO data. *Construct validity* describes the degree to which what was measured reflects the *a priori* conceptualization of what should be measured (9). Subcomponents of construct validity are convergent and discriminant validity, which assess the degree of similarity between measures that are theoretically similar (convergent validity) or the extent to which measures that are theoretically different actually differ (discriminant validity). For example, a new measure of anxiety would be expected to have high convergent validity with the anxiety subscale of the Hospital Anxiety and Depression Scale (24). *Criterion validity* describes the extent to which the scores of PRO instrument reflect the gold standard measure of the same concept (7). Criterion validity is often difficult to assess in the PRO arena because identifying gold standard measures for many PRO concepts is difficult (7), implicitly deemphasizing criterion validity.

Reliability

Reliability describes an instrument's consistency (14) or the ability of an instrument to yield the same result on serial administrations when no change in the concept being measured is expected (10). It is important to note that validity depends upon reliability (i.e., an instrument that measures the concept of interest accurately must do so consistently), but that reliability does not depend upon validity (i.e., the instrument may consistently measure the wrong thing). Within the realm of PROs, reliability is most commonly assessed via test–retest and internal consistency. With test–retest methods, the same subjects complete the same instruments on two occasions. Any differences in responses between the two occasions not attributable to a true change in the experience is attributed to lack of reliability (14), placing great importance on the time interval between testing (10). Reliability can be quantitatively assessed with Cronbach's α, which measures the internal consistency of an instrument. Internal consistency reflects the degree to which items within a scale measure the same concept, in a given population (14). Well-established thresholds for interpreting Cronbach's α are available; in general, coefficient $\alpha > 0.7$ is the minimum acceptable threshold for comparisons between groups (10). The dependence of reliability on the target population supports the importance of reassessing psychometric properties when instruments are introduced to new populations (14).

Ability to Detect Change

The ability of a PRO measure to detect change is intuitively important since many PROs are collected longitudinally. Demonstration of this ability, according to the FDA, requires that changes in the PRO measure parallel changes in other factors that indicate a change in the status of the concept of interest (7). For example, in patients receiving a new treatment for opioid-induced constipation, changes in a PRO measure designed to assess overall bowel health may be linked with the use of certain other bowel products, such as enemas, to establish the ability to detect change. The measure must demonstrate the ability to detect both improvements in health status and losses. Further, it is important to detect changes throughout the range of possible values.

A clinical trial that includes QoL as a primary or secondary outcome should include an explicit statement of the anticipated minimal change that will be considered evidence of meaningful effect; this should align with the minimally important clinical difference. In registry studies or routine care, where longitudinal collection and analysis are critical, understanding the concept of minimally important change detected (25), rather than establishing that number explicitly, may be sufficient. When interpreting results from intervention and observational studies, it is critical to consider the result within the context of the instrument's ability to reliably and validly measure meaningful change, the magnitude of change observed, and the related clinical impact.

Areas of Controversy

The increasing emphasis placed upon content validity has generated some controversy as PRO developers attempt to improve content validity, in part by meticulously wording items and instructions to minimize variations in interpretation between patients (26). However, the ability to improve content validity likely is asymptotic, in that individual variability undoubtedly influences interpretation of questions in ways that are not controllable since responses to an instrument capture the patient's true (and unique) perceptions. There are concerns that in the pursuit of greater content validity, other important characteristics of PRO measures may be underdeveloped or underappreciated (9). For example, in pursuing greater content validity, the constraints placed upon questions may actually limit patient perspective by forcing some degree of conformity or may result in misinterpretation of results. In palliative and supportive oncology, where the patient's experience is the most important outcome, artificially constraining or limiting the range of experiences communicated risks undermining the foundation of the discipline.

Consider a trial of interventions in patients with advanced cancer designed to delay the development of disability. Upon entering the study, a patient rates his disability as severe because his reference point is a previously health state. Four months later, he rates his disability as mild, though on more open-ended questioning, notes he can simply sit on the front porch and watch his grandchildren as he knows that any other activities are unrealistic. Thus, his goal is now to simply make it to the front porch, whereas 4 months prior his goal was to play with his grandchildren. Even though the instrument measures disability from the view of the patient and would thus have adequate content validity, the interpretation regarding the merits of the intervention would be erroneous, as the patient has clearly become more disabled, but has shifted his frame of reference, a fact which is not captured by content validity and becomes invisible as the scope of the instrument's questions narrow in order to refine content validity. Further, the quest for improved content validity may result in measures with marginal content validity being cast aside without consideration of other properties, such as reliability or ability to detect change, highlighting the need for contextual consideration of all the psychometric properties of PRO instruments. Much of this quibbling over fine nuances of instruments and semantics has come at the expense of practical research and clinical implementation; in palliative and supportive oncology, the goal of assessment of QoL through the lens of the patient should be paramount.

COLLECTING QOL DATA

Beyond the psychometric properties of PRO instruments discussed above, one of the most important considerations regarding PRO data is how it will be collected. Central to that decision is the mode of administration. Often, choice of PRO instrument and mode of administration are considered jointly, however, they need not be, as administration methods are generally agnostic to the instrument and simply provide a platform for presenting and collecting information. There are two main ways of collecting PRO data—on paper and electronically.

Paper-Based Methods

Historically, QoL questionnaires were collected via paper forms and paper-based methods still stand as the gold standard for PRO collection. From a practical standpoint, collection of PRO data via paper-based methods is comfortable for both patients and providers. Implementing paper-based PRO collection systems is not limited by unfamiliarity with new technologies or significant upfront capital investment. There is a vast array of existing paper-based PRO instruments across a range of disease states that have been extensively evaluated and are ready for immediate use.

When administering PRO instruments via paper methods, consistency is the guiding principle; items should be presented in the same order for every collection. Patients should complete forms in a confidential space, without fear that "wandering eyes" will see responses. Once forms are completed, they should be reviewed for completeness. Finally, data should be entered into electronic forms using double data entry techniques, to enhance transcription accuracy, ideally augmented with near-real-time exploratory analyses to examine the believability of the data within the clinical

context (27), seeking clarification from patients when data are missing or inconsistent.

However, paper forms have many limitations. They require personnel for sorting, distribution, and collection. This represents an ever-present risk for inconsistencies and a source of ongoing cost. Paper forms collected as part of routine/scheduled clinical visits are generally straightforward, but this approach routinely and systematically misses participants unwilling or unable to attend a clinical appointment. Collection between visits is logistically difficult with paper forms; delivery of the paper forms either requires participants take paper booklets home with them or coordinating timely delivery of booklets through postal services. Certainly, if home visits occur as part of routine care within a palliative and supportive oncology practice, this shortcoming is at least partially mitigated, as more of the responsibility shifts to the healthcare team. Between-visit forms can be distributed and collected directly, without involving postal or delivery services. Regardless, obtaining a reliable date–time stamp for at-home paper-based administration remains a challenge. Relying on at-home paper booklets risks participants completing multiple days of reporting all at once—either in a retrospective manner (i.e., the so-called parking lot effect in which all responses for the past month are completed immediately before a visit while sitting in the parking lot) or a prospective manner (i.e., filling out all the forms immediately upon arriving home from the clinical visit). Paper forms often include illegible or uninterpretable responses and require manual data entry, which is administratively burdensome and subject to transcription errors. Manual entry also generates a lag-time in monitoring response rates, complicating the process of reducing missing data (28). Overall, there is a threshold beyond which the continuing data collection and quality assurance costs of paper-based PROs surpass the upfront technology costs for electronic data capture, making electronic PROs (ePROs) the cheaper and more reliable approach.

Electronic Capture Methods

As personal technology has become portable and inexpensive, interest in electronic capture methods for PRO data has grown. Similar to traditional paper-based collection, electronic collection begins with instrument(s) selection. Integral to the choice of instruments is the choice of platform, as not all instruments are tested across multiple platforms, nor would every instrument be amenable to every platform. Feasibility of ePRO capture has been demonstrated on a variety of platforms (e.g., web-based, laptop/desktop computers, tablet personal computers, interactive voice response system [IVRS], handheld device, and digital pen) and across a spectrum of disease states (29–31). Recently, feasibility of ePRO technology has been demonstrated in hospice and palliative care settings (32–34).

Considering the merits of each demonstrated electronic capture technology within palliative and supportive oncology helps define and target each technology for the most appropriate setting. For ePRO collection using tablet computers or larger handheld devices, clinical appointments or inpatient wards are the most appropriate settings. Patients are provided the device at the time of check-in to clinic or at predetermined times of day (if inpatient), with pre-loaded PRO measures such that patients simply select their response to each item as it is presented. With digital pens, patients select responses on specially designed paper surveys, with responses electronically recorded by the pen. With IVRS, patients call a telephone number and are prompted, via an automated transcript, to select a preferred language and to provide an identifier, and are then guided through the PRO measure, providing verbal responses to each item. Digital pens and IVRS can be implemented in any clinical setting—inpatient ward, outpatient clinic, or from home. Web-based platforms delivered via nearly any Internet-enabled device are also potentially useful in all clinical settings. Access to web-based platforms can be provided at "confidential" computer stations in clinic waiting rooms, or in the exam room itself, as well as from any web-enabled device including home computers, small or large handheld devices, and portable telephones. Regardless of platform, data are transmitted to a central, secure repository immediately upon submission and can be accessed for "real-time" incorporation into routine care, if desired. Factors influencing platform selection include budget and technical support, technology literacy of the target population, collection logistics (in-clinic, between-visit, or combination), and the instrument(s) chosen (28).

As ePRO methods advance, more instruments are being developed exclusively for electronic methods of administration, such as the National Cancer Institute-supported Patient-Reported Outcomes Measurement Information System (PROMIS) (35–37), the Patient-Reported Outcomes version of the Common Toxicity Criteria for Adverse Events (PRO-CTCAE) (38), and the Patient Care Monitor (PCM), version 2 (39). The PROMIS and PRO-CTCAE tools take advantage of electronic functionalities such as skip patterns or computerized adaptive testing, which can reduce the number of items patients have to complete, an important consideration in hospice and palliative medicine, while the PCM also fulfills clinical documentation needs for clinical review of systems and triggers for accompanying patient education.

Compared with paper methods, delivery of ePROs can be automated, minimizing the risk of inconsistent presentation of materials or mishandling paper forms. Electronic methods also eliminate the potential for illegible responses and data transcription errors. Manual entry of paper forms generates a lag-time in monitoring response rates, complicating the process of identifying and reducing missing data, whereas electronic capture facilitates real-time monitoring of response rates and review for missing data (28). Electronic methods also provide immediate and accurate date–time stamps. Additionally, electronic platforms may provide a safer environment for patients to disclose sensitive concerns, such as sexual function (40).

While enthusiasm for electronic capture methods is understandably high, it must be tempered based on several limitations. First, completion of electronically delivered PRO measures requires some level of comfort with and access to newer technologies, which may prove challenging in certain situations. For example, in rural areas, using web-based methods to collect PROs between visits may be impractical due to unpredictable web access, while some geriatric populations may be uncomfortable with tablet or handheld technologies. Second, if an instrument has never been tested on electronic platforms, it may be time-consuming to migrate (the term reflecting transitioning instruments from paper to electronic administration) the instrument, though guidelines for demonstrating equivalence between paper-based and electronic methods were recently established (41). In general, paper to web migration yields between-platform equivalence comparable to the test–retest reliability of the original mode, but this is not always the case and should be tested (42). Finally, electronic methods require greater upfront investment in terms of the hardware and software, electronic storage (meeting appropriate security standards), training, and technical support. Further discussion regarding choosing among various hardware and software options is beyond the scope of this discussion, but discussion of guiding principles can be found in a recent white paper (43).

Practical Considerations

Patient Factors

Any decision to incorporate PROs into the process of care (research or clinical) requires consideration of the burden to the patient the PRO measure(s) represent. The choice between paper and electronic approaches is critical and is influenced by the location, cognitive capacity, and performance status of palliative and supportive oncology patients. Within a setting of routine clinical care, lengthy questionnaires may result in increasing missing data over time, as patients grow weary of serially completing such questionnaires. The capacity to answer lengthy instruments cannot be predicted *a priori* and differs between groups. At Duke Cancer Institute, patients in a variety of solid tumor clinics routinely complete 80 to 86 item instruments without significant fatigue or burnout; median time to complete the survey is 11 minutes, reducing to <8 minutes after several visits in the clinic using the same instrument (39). An upcoming guidance document from the Center for Medical Technology Policy will recommend that, for patients with cancer, completion of PRO instruments takes no more than 20 minutes at the initial visit and less than 10 minutes at subsequent visits (44). Patients should be offered private spaces for completing instruments, to minimize concerns regarding confidentiality, especially for sensitive questions. Instructions should be provided for every item, even if it only frames the recall period. The instrument should be delivered with adequate font size and at appropriate literacy levels. Additionally, physical assistance should be provided if needed.

Clinician Factors

Even within the research setting, assessing the impact of PRO collection on routine care is important. Will the PRO results be made available immediately as part of routine care or only available to research personnel? If data are to be made available to clinicians, are appropriate support services available to assist in managing newly identified concerns or issues? Are there mechanisms to support incorporation of PRO data into clinical care, if it will be made available, or will it be "one more thing" for which clinicians are responsible? What will be the impact of the PRO collection on workflow? What are the risk management concerns? Though often mundane, these factors are important to consider in the implementation phase.

Most recent literature recommends providing clinician feedback of concerning patient-reported information, such as reports of new chest pain (43). The thresholds for triggering a clinical alert, components of the alert message, method of delivering the notice to the clinician, and of verifying clinician acknowledgment must be carefully considered, and preferably standardized (45,46). Ideally, within a rapid-learning healthcare system, these factors could feed forward to help monitor for the response to standardized interventions, supporting continuous improvement in the quality of care delivered. Consider the nausea item of a QoL instrument used during palliative care home visits with standardized thresholds and clinical pathways guiding interventions. As the system accumulates experience with defining refractory nausea and the results of standardized interventions, those clinicians responsible for the nausea clinical pathway receive routine feedback regarding efficacy and can iteratively adapt the system and update the care pathway.

To improve the likelihood that PROs are warmly received, the healthcare team (physicians, mid-level providers, nurses, etc.) should be involved in the development process, especially with respect to integrating the PRO instruments into the clinical workflow. This inclusive implementation process will help shape the perception of the PRO data, in that buy-in from the healthcare team will make the PRO collection process a necessary and desired component of care, rather than simply an extra task to complete (45).

Caregiver/Proxy Considerations

Patients in palliative and supportive oncology represent a unique subset of patients within medicine in that up to 70% of patients with life-limiting illness become unable to complete self-reported surveys (21). In such situations, when the goal of palliative and supportive treatments remains optimizing QoL for both the patient and the family, other measures of QoL are important; how best to obtain surrogate assessments of QoL remains unclear. In most cases, the patient's caregiver, often a family member or close friend, completes a questionnaire (ideally the same as, or very similar to, the one the patient had completed when able). Obviously, such approaches are subject to bias, as caregivers cannot possibly answer the items identically to the patient. In fact, there are numerous studies that indicate moderate, at best, agreement between patient and proxy reports of QoL (19,21,47). Across numerous studies, there seems to be better agreement between patients and proxy reports for more observable domains, such as service utilization, emesis, and

functionality, but proxies tend to underestimate QoL and overestimate pain and distress, when compared with patients (47). For example, in a recent study by Jones et al. (21), both caregiver reports and proxy reports by palliative care physician underestimated QoL, as measured by the McGill Quality of Life scale (MQoL). Disagreements were greater for physical and psychological domains and smaller for spiritual and support domains. The general consensus from a review by McPherson and Addington-Hall and supplemented by the study by Jones et al. is that additional research is needed to better understand how patient and proxy reports differ and how to incorporate proxy reports into routine care (21,47). Acknowledging that proxy reports were only "fair substitutes" for direct patient reports, Kutner et al. (19) advocate for collecting QoL assessment from all possible respondents (patients, caregivers, and healthcare providers) from initial palliative care evaluation, in part to gather as much information about QoL and in part anticipating the decline in patient ability to provide such information. This approach provides individualized correlations between patient and proxy assessment, so that when only proxy assessments are available they can be interpreted as appropriately as possible.

While there is no clear answer as to how to incorporate proxy reports into routine clinical care, direct patient reports of QoL are unquestionably preferred. Further studies regarding factors influencing agreement between patient and proxy reports of QoL are needed and further evaluation of how proxy reports should be used to support clinical decisions within palliative and supportive oncology. Almost all intervention studies within palliative medicine have been driven by direct patient reports (48,49). As such, among adult patients, proxy reports of patient QoL should be used only if the patient's mental or physical condition precludes completing self-assessments.

Pediatric patients represent a special consideration to this general rule, in part because pediatric patients enrolled in palliative care programs have trajectories that are significantly different than adults (50). There has long been concern that children cannot reliably evaluate and self-report QoL; however, emerging methods for questionnaire design have yielded promising results as children begin to self-report QoL (51,52). There is no consensus about the exact manner in which direct patient reports and proxy reports should be integrated into routine care, in part because studies evaluating patient reports of QoL within pediatric populations have not focused on palliative care and in part because the field is still quite new. The current standard for pediatric patients is to collect both direct patient and proxy reports, primarily from parents. Again, it is unclear which of these types of data should be used for clinical decision making, but historically, parent reports have had the most influence (51,52).

Ensuring Quality

Data quality is a keystone to both clinical and research endeavors across all aspects of medicine, including palliative and supportive oncology. Regardless of how data quality is assessed, there are two critical concepts related to PRO data quality. The first relates to missing data. Missing data are anathema to quality data. It degrades the quality of the information and decreases its analytic potential. Within palliative and supportive oncology, missing data will most likely manifest as symptom burden increases, functionality decreases, and death approaches. In order to reduce the chance of missing data, the PROs chosen within this setting should be meaningful, both to patients and clinicians. Furthering this attribute is the incorporation of PRO collection into routine practice, whereby both patients and clinicians expect PRO data and value its collection. Selecting a PRO instrument that minimizes respondent burden, especially since the expectation is for symptom burden to increase and functionality to decrease in this population can also reduce missingness. In most cases, even within palliative and supportive oncology, electronic administration supports real-time, or near-real-time, quality monitoring of information being collected in order to identify patterns of missing data and develop interventions in response to the identified patterns in order to reduce missingness. Additionally, consideration must be given to collecting proxy reports, which must be clearly delineated from true patient reports by the metadata embedded within the database when patients are unable to complete reports themselves (see previous section). *Metadata* are data about data. More precisely, metadata are "…structured information that describes, explains, locates, or otherwise makes it easier to retrieve, use, or manage an information source" (12).

The second issue related to data quality is consistency. While the time frame within palliative and supportive oncology is relatively short, compared with other applications of QoL assessment, the importance of collecting the same data in the same manner longitudinally and systematically is equally important. As available instruments change and evolve, or new ones are developed, there is often pressure (whether internal or external) to implement the updated instruments. However, caution is advised, because changing instruments disrupts the value of longitudinal data collection and may hinder comparisons between groups collected with different instruments. If instruments are changed, such changes should be noted within the metadata embedded within the database. Appropriate metadata are essential to data quality and to help maintain understanding of consistency and changes. For example, consider a palliative care registry where patients may not always able to complete a PRO instrument, even with assistance. The ability of the person to complete the instrument may change over time as cognition wanes. In these settings, proxy reports involving close family or caregivers may become the only available measures and the only available data to be incorporated into registries; therefore, it is essential to identify, via metadata, who is completing the instrument. Further, imagine that the instrument being completed by proxy reporters changes in 2015 compared with what was used in 2011. Metadata need to be able to designate which instrument is being used, including

psychometric features, so that information collected in 2015 can be appropriately compared back with information collected in 2011.

Implementation Issues

Even as the process of selecting the actual PRO instrument evolves, the tasks related to successful implementation must be identified. Here, we briefly outline a practical framework for successful implementation centered on achieving data quality and consistency.

Consistency

Just as with mode of administration, implementing of PRO data collection is best achieved if consistency, specifically procedural consistency, is the central tenet. Standard operating procedures should be established for each site of data collection that clearly defines, as much as possible, how patients, researchers, and clinicians interact with the collection system (paper or electronic). These standard operating procedures should specify training methods and any training materials should be readily accessible and easy-to-use (preferably in both text and video format) (43). Standardization should be viewed as an exercise in simplification, despite its upfront tediousness. Every aspect of the process that can be standardized should be standardized, including the data set itself. All PRO-containing data sets should include metadata that describe key components important for subsequent analyses and end-users, including who completed the instrument (patient or proxy), where it was completed (outpatient clinic, home, inpatient ward, etc.), which version was administered, and a flag for irregularities identified as part of internal quality control.

Another aspect of consistency in this setting reflects administering the same instrument over the life span of the registry. The strength of this recommendation depends partly upon context; for PROs collected as part of research, this consistency is strongly recommended, while if the PROs are collected and embedded within an electronic health record, this recommendation is less stringent. Nevertheless, if the data are collected prospectively, the strong preference is for consistency in PRO instrument administered. Regardless of purpose, collected data should include metadata labels.

Feasibility and Usability

Even the most conceptually sound PRO instrument and administration method may not perform as expected in practice, so the system should be piloted prior to full-scale implementation. Both usability and feasibility should be considered, and testing should be conducted within the target population. As elaborated on www.usability.gov, usability is not a single, one-dimensional property of the interface, but rather a synthesis of 1) Ease of learning—How fast can a user who has never seen the user interface before learn it sufficiently well to accomplish basic tasks?; 2) Efficiency of use— Once an experienced user has learned to use the system, how fast can tasks be accomplished?; 3) Memorability—If a user has used the system before, can the system be used effectively from memory at next use or does the user have to start over again learning everything?; 4) Error frequency and severity—How often do users make errors while using the system, how serious are these errors, and how do users recover from these errors?; and 5) Subjective satisfaction—How much does the user like using the system? The degree of usability testing should match the complexity of the task and is obviously much greater for electronic versus paper-based methods. At a minimum, usability testing for an ePRO system includes documentation of respondents' ability to navigate the electronic platform, follow instructions, and answer questions. Ultimately, the goal is to demonstrate that respondents can complete the computerized instrument as intended. Generally, less than 10 representative patients are required to verify usability. If the system is not usable, then it should be iteratively updated until usable.

Feasibility extends usability and establishes the practical implementation of the software system in the local setting (e.g., clinic, home, and hospital). Assessment approaches are similar and the software goes through iterative updates until feasible. During this process, patients can contribute critical advice for the "help" manual and instruction sets.

The contribution of patient input in usability and feasibility testing is important and cognitive debriefing is an appropriate method for obtaining such input. The debriefing can occur via probing questions from an interviewer (e.g., "What does the instruction 'skip item' mean to you here?") or with think-aloud techniques as respondents complete the questionnaire. The contributions of cognitive debriefing to usability and feasibility testing illuminate how patients interpret questions, and ultimately respond to them, as well as in clarifying instructions.

How to Choose a Platform

As with most other aspects of PROs, the choice of PRO capture method is highly dependent upon the intended use. Both paper-based and electronic platforms offer advantages and disadvantages, as outlined above. Providing an interface familiar to or preferred by particular patients or populations may reduce missing data not at random. In typical clinical practice, one modality will be available, largely for cost and simplicity considerations, but more flexibility may be preferred within a research setting. Modes may be mixed across patients in a study (e.g., each patient selects a specific mode at baseline and continues to report via that mode throughout a study) or within patients (e.g., a patient reports by web until he becomes symptomatically ill, at which point IVRS becomes preferable).

In general, electronic capture is preferred to paper because of its flexibility and its ability to reduce the chance that the PRO data will be missing. In contemporary research, paper methods are usually most cost effective until registries start to grow in size or number of sites. If the study is intentionally small (e.g., less than 100 patients), paper methods

will likely suffice, but as the scope of a study grows, upfront investments in electronic approaches will realize substantial downstream gains in efficiency, cost, and data quality. Regardless of the ultimate choice of administration method, clear documentation of the rationale for the choice and clear evidence of appropriate psychometric assessment are strongly recommended. Assistance with this process may arise from internal expertise (as in many academic institutions) or may rely upon input from a commercial vendor, whose involvement can range from consulting only to nearly full control of the development and implementation process.

EXISTING INSTRUMENTS

The task of evaluating available instruments to measure QoL in palliative and supportive oncology can be daunting, in large part because of the plethora of available instruments. In 2007, a PubMed search for PRO instrument development articles since 1995 resulted in more than 2,000 citations (53). While the following discussion will focus primarily on multidomain instruments, it is important to note that PRO instruments assume a variety of forms: 1) general assessment scales (e.g., QoL); 2) disease-specific scales (e.g., chronic obstructive pulmonary disease, cancer [including scales for individual tumor types], and congestive heart failure); 3) symptom-specific scales (e.g., pain, breathlessness, and distress); 4) evaluations of functioning across a variety of domains (e.g., physical functioning, social functioning, and emotional functioning); 5) scales assessing satisfaction with care received; and 6) other (e.g., adherence with therapy). Some PRO instruments are extensive, with dozens of items related to a single concept (e.g., breathlessness), while others have 80 or more items reflecting many different patient-reported concerns constituting an entire clinical review of systems, and yet others are single-item instruments measuring a single construct in a single question.

It is also important to note that not all PRO instruments assess QoL. There are numerous excellent instruments for symptom assessment in palliative and supportive oncology, such as the Edmonton Symptom Assessment Scale (54), MD Anderson Symptom Index (55), and Memorial Symptom Assessment Scale (56). Such instruments are not included in the following discussion because they were developed for symptom assessment, not QoL evaluation.

An international, multidisciplinary group convened a meeting in 2004 to consider clinical trials in palliative medicine. As part of this meeting, an Outcomes Working Group authored a series of recommendations regarding the role of PROs in palliative medicine clinical trials (57). Among the 12 recommendations, 3 stand out as particularly relevant to this discussion on instrument choice. First, "...measurement should assess multidimensional aspects shown to be important to patients with advanced disease" (57). The authors identified nine domains relevant to palliative medicine clinical trials: symptom management, whole person and maintaining QoL, functional aspects, satisfaction, relationships, decision making and care planning, continuity and communication, family burden and well-being, and quality of death and end-of-life experience (57). In addition to identifying relevant domains, the authors identify instruments appropriate for each domain. Second, "Patient-reported outcomes should be assessed by measures that balance simplicity, parsimony, and psychometric rigor" (57). This recommendation captures much of the above discussion regarding the tension between psychometric characteristics, patient, and clinician factors. It highlights that psychometric properties cannot alone drive the choice of instrument.

Additional guidance for identifying appropriate QoL instruments comes from the WHO Quality of Life Working Group which identified six key domains within QoL: physical, psychological, material, social well-being, environment, and independence (13). Of particular value within palliative and supportive oncology are the emphasis on physical, psychological, social well-being, and independence. There is also growing recognition of the importance of assessing the spiritual/existential domain within palliative and supportive oncology (6).

Several recent reviews have identified numerous QoL instruments either developed for or tested within palliative and supportive oncology (6,58). The systematic review by Albers et al. (6) is noteworthy because of its attention to the psychometric and clinimetric characteristics of the instruments. Within the realm of palliative and supportive oncology, the recall period (e.g., "over the past week" and "during the past month") is an important consideration since QoL may be rapidly changing. There is no uniformly agreed-upon recall period, but Albers et al. argue that 1 week is an appropriate recall period within most palliative care settings.

No single instrument will perfectly meet the needs of a particular implementation, in part explaining the continued proliferation of QoL instruments. For most purposes, selecting an existing instrument is the most practical decision. The following discussion is not intended to be comprehensive in reviewing existing QoL instruments, nor as an endorsement of or recommendation for the included instruments, but is intended to review select instruments that are commonly encountered in the literature and that were developed for or evaluated in patients with life-limiting illness. All instruments presented assess general QoL and are multidimensional, multi-item instruments with established, documented scoring systems. Additionally, the reviewed instruments involve direct patient reports, as opposed to proxy reports or structured interviews (e.g., the Quality at the end-of-life scale [QUAL-E] (59) or the Schedule for the Evaluation of Individual Quality of Life [SEIQoL] (60)). In some cases, specific modifications have been made to broader instruments for palliative medicine populations and in such cases, both the original and modified instruments are discussed.

MQoL Questionnaire

Developed in 1995 specifically for patients with advanced disease, the MQoL contains 17 items (32). There is a single item assessing overall QoL and 16 items graded on a numerical

rating scale from 1 to 10. Domains addressed include physical, psychological, existential, and support. The total score is the mean of the four domain subscores. The MQoL takes 10 to 15 minutes to complete and asks patients to respond to items based on the previous 2 days (32). Psychometric properties have been demonstrated in a variety of disease stages and in populations with variable prognoses, including palliative care and hospice settings. Concern has been raised that the MQoL is insufficiently sensitive for tracking changes in an individual patient longitudinally, but that it can be used to track changes in groups (61). Regardless, the relative simplicity of the MQoL and its common use within the literature make the MQoL a realistic option for routine collection of QoL in palliative and supportive oncology.

More recently, a shortened version of the MQoL, the Cardiff Short Form (MQoL-CSF) was developed, again for specific application within palliative care settings (62). While the original MQoL survey is 17 items in length, the MQoL-CSF consists of only 8 items and uses a numerical rating scale from 1 to 10. The items include one global QoL question, three physical domain items, two psychological domain items, and two items regarding the existential domain (62). When compared with the original MQoL, the MQoL-CSF may be less sensitive to treatment, support, and pain, but demonstrated utility in following patients routinely and longitudinally (62).

Medical Outcomes Study Short-Form Health Survey (SF-36)

The SF-36 has been widely used across a variety of disease states and prognoses, including palliative medicine. Developed by Ware and Sherbourne (63), it has been described as not only a functional status and QoL instrument but also a measure of global health status (58). It is composed of eight subscales, evaluating impacts of physical and emotional problems on physical activities, social activities, and role activities, as well as physical pain, vitality, general mental health, and general health perceptions (47). The SF-36 contains 36 items and can be completed directly by the patient or by an interviewer. Respondents are instructed to answer the question with respect to the prior month. It typically requires less than 10 minutes to complete and has been studied in palliative and supportive oncology (64–68). Within palliative care settings, questions regarding the length of the instrument have been raised, as well as concerns about floor effects. Shorter versions (12- and 8-item surveys) exist but have not been sufficiently studied in palliative care settings.

European Organization for Research and Treatment of Cancer (EORTC) Quality of Life Questionnaire

The EORTC Quality of Life Core Questionnaire (QLQ-C30) was developed in the early 1990s to support efforts at measuring QoL in oncology clinical trials (69). It consists of 30 items and addresses issues related to functionality in physical, role, social, emotional, and cognitive dimensions.

Additionally, it assesses symptom burden through a combination of symptom subscales and single-item symptom measures. Scores for these items are graded on a numerical rating scale from 1 to 4. Finally, there are single-item assessments of overall health and overall QoL over the prior week, graded from 1 to 7 on a numerical rating scale. The recall period for the EORTC QLQ-C30 is 1 week and the instrument generally takes less than 15 minutes to complete. The EORTC QLQ-C30 has been translated to and evaluated in numerous languages. It has demonstrated validity, reliability, and ability to detect change in numerous studies. However, concern has been raised about respondent burden in palliative care settings (i.e., can patients with life-limiting illness complete a 30-item scale?) and that some questions use "normal" activities as benchmarks that may lead to undervaluation of QoL within palliative care populations (70).

In response to some of these concerns, the EORTC developed an instrument specifically for palliative and supportive oncology, the EORTC Quality of Life Questionnaire for Palliative Care (QLQ-PAL15) (71). Compared with the original EORTC QLQ-C30, the QLQ-PAL15 reduces respondent burden with 15 items, compared with 30, taking less than 10 minutes to complete. Also, some items have been reworded to avoid benchmarking activities to normal, making the item more suitable to patients with life-limited illness. Unfortunately, the EORTC QLQ-PAL15 development did not include direct patient input and may overemphasize physical aspects of QoL, while missing existential issues (58). Because the instrument is relatively new, it has not yet generated a significant track record in terms of utilization.

Functional Assessment of Cancer Therapy-General (FACT-G)

The FACT-G instrument consists of 27 items. Developed by Cella et al. (72) to measure QoL in cancer patients, numerous other versions of the instrument have been subsequently developed to evaluate QoL by cancer subtypes (full list available at www.facit.org). The FACT-G assesses physical, social, emotional, and functional domains using a numerical rating scale from 0 to 4. It has demonstrated validity and reliability in cancer patients and its development incorporated direct patient input (72). Its responsiveness to change supports the use for monitoring individual patients, in addition to groups.

In an effort to further build upon the FACT-G, a specific palliative care subscale was created to target palliative care populations and supplement the FACT-G. The combination of the FACT-G and palliative care subscale has undergone formal psychometric evaluation in the form of the Functional Assessment of Chronic Illness Therapy-Palliative Care (FACIT-Pal) (73). The FACIT-Pal supplements the 27-item FACT-G with an additional 19 items. The additional items address physical symptoms prevalent in advanced illness, relationships with family and friends, life closure issues (e.g., "making every day count"), and decision-making abilities (73). The total number of items in the FACIT-Pal makes it longer than most other instruments developed specifically

for patients with advanced illness (e.g., MQoL and EORTC QLQ-PAL15), but, within a research implementation, offers a validated instrument for advanced illness and a formal score for QoL (the FACT-G) that can be compared more broadly and to historical results.

HOW TO CHOOSE THE "RIGHT" PRO INSTRUMENT

There is no "perfect" PRO for any given research or clinical application, making it disingenuous to identify a single PRO instrument as most favorable within the setting of palliative and supportive oncology. Regardless, the critical first step in selecting a PRO instrument is clear and careful definition of the target population, concept to be measured, and intended use (routine clinical care or research). For any given population or context, it is important to have some *a priori* hypotheses and justification for outcomes being measured. For palliative and supportive oncology, justification for inclusion of PROs in routine care or research is intuitive—improving the patient experience is the central tenet of the discipline, emphasizing the importance of systematically collecting patient perspective. Even in palliative and supportive oncology, however, there needs to be a systematic approach to selecting salient outcomes. In some instances, domain-specific instruments (e.g., breathlessness and nausea) may be appropriate, while in other a more general, multidomain instrument measuring QoL may be preferred. Far too frequently the tail wags the dog in the PRO arena; that is, PRO instruments are selected first, prior to identifying outcomes of interest. Consider a clinical trial examining the impact of a new pharmaceutical agent on breathlessness. Clearly, the most important outcome is breathlessness, meaning a PRO instrument for breathlessness, rather than a more general QoL instrument, would be the most appropriate choice. Thus, the importance of rational identification of outcomes of interest early in the process cannot be overemphasized. Such an approach will produce a sound base for evaluating PRO instruments and administration methods.

After clearly defining the population and outcomes of interest, existing PRO instruments that will assess the outcomes of interest can be identified. If a suitable measure is not identified, options include modifying an existing instrument or developing something new. In general, it is preferable to utilize an existing instrument, as developing a new PRO instrument is resource-intensive. After identifying (or developing) a measure, administration mode should be selected. Electronic administration is preferred, but not all instruments have been evaluated using electronic administration, though guidelines for establishing equivalence between paper-based methods and electronic administration exist to help guide the process (41). Important to the scientific basis of the PRO instrument are its psychometric properties. While high content validity is generally viewed as essential, it is possible to effectively use an instrument with modest content validity, depending on the purpose of collecting PRO data, highlighting the importance of understanding and defining its intended use.

For almost every application within palliative and supportive oncology, collection of PRO data is appropriate. Careful planning, in identifying appropriate PRO instruments for inclusion, selecting modes of instrument administration, and implementing the PRO collection system, is essential, but when effective it generally produces more complete data sets that are better positioned to improve the patient experience, which is ultimately the goal of palliative and supportive oncology.

ACKNOWLEDGMENTS

Dr. Abernethy has research funding from the US National Institutes of Health, US Agency for Healthcare Research and Quality, Robert Wood Johnson Foundation, Pfizer, Eli Lilly, Bristol Meyers Squibb, Helsinn Therapeutics, Amgen, Kanglaite, Alexion, Biovex, DARA Therapeutics, Novartis, and Mi-Co. In the last 2 years she has had nominal consulting agreements (<$10,000) with Helsinn, Proventys, Amgen, and Novartis. Dr. Miriovsky has nothing to disclose.

REFERENCES

1. American Academy of Hospice and Palliative Medicine, Center to Advance Palliative Care, Hospice and Palliative Nurses Association, Last Acts Partnership, National Hospice and Palliative Care Organization. National Consensus Project for quality palliative care: clinical practice guidelines for quality palliative care, executive summary. *J Palliat Med.* 2004;7:611-627.

2. Bausewein C, Simon ST, Benalia H, et al. Implementing patient reported outcome measures (PROMs) in palliative care—users' cry for help. *Health Qual Life Outcomes.* April 2011;9(1):27.

3. Higginson IJ, Carr AJ. Measuring quality of life: using quality of life measures in the clinical setting. *BMJ.* May 2001;322(7297):1297-1300.

4. Ferrell B, Connor SR, Cordes A, et al. The National Agenda for Quality Palliative Care: The National Consensus Project and the National Quality Forum. *J Pain Symptom Manage.* June 2007;33(6):737-744.

5. McCabe C, Cronin P. Issues for researchers to consider when using health-related quality of life outcomes in cancer research. *Eur J Cancer Care (Engl).* September 2011;20(5):563-569.

6. Albers G, Echteld MA, de Vet HCW, Onwuteaka-Philipsen BD, van der Linden MHM, Deliens L. Evaluation of quality-of-life measures for use in palliative care: a systematic review. *Palliat Med.* January 2010;24(1):17-37.

7. US Department of Health and Human Services, Food and Drug Administration. Guidance for industry: patient-reported outcome measures: use in medical product development to support labeling claims. 2009. http://www.fda.gov/downloads/Drugs/GuidanceComplianceRegulatoryInformation/Guidances/UCM193282.pdf. Accessed July 26, 2011.

8. Willke RJ, Burke LB, Erickson P. Measuring treatment impact: a review of patient-reported outcomes and other efficacy endpoints in approved product labels. *Control Clin Trial.* December 2004;25(6):535-552.

9. McClimans LM, Browne J. Choosing a patient-reported outcome measure. *Theor Med Bioeth.* February 2011;32(1):47-60.

10. Frost MH, Reeve BB, Liepa AM, Stauffer JW, Hays RD, Mayo/FDA Patient-Reported Outcomes Consensus Meeting Group. What is sufficient evidence for the reliability and validity of patient-reported outcome measures? *Value Health.* October 2007;10(suppl 2):S94-S105.

11. Revicki DA, Osoba D, Fairclough D, et al. Recommendations on health-related quality of life research to support labeling and promotional claims in the United States. *Qual Life Res.* 2000;9(8):887-900.

12. NISO. *Understanding Metadata.* Baltimore, MD: NISO Press; 2004.

13. Kuyken W, Group TW. The World Health Organization Quality of Life assessment (WHOQOL): position paper from the World Health Organization. *Soc Sci Med.* November 1995;41(10):1403-1409.

14. Meyer KB, Clayton KA. Measurement and analysis of patient-reported outcomes. *Methods Mol Biol.* 2009;473:155-169.

15. Jocham HR, Dassen T, Widdershoven G, Halfens R. Quality of life in palliative care cancer patients: a literature review. *J Clin Nurs.* September 2006;15(9):1188-1195.

16. Karnofsky D, Abelmann W, Craver L. The use of the nitrogen mustards in the palliative treatment of carcinoma. With particular reference to bronchogenic carcinoma. *Cancer.* 1948;1:634-656.

17. Zubrod CG, Schneiderman M, Frei E III, et al. Appraisal of methods for the study of chemotherapy of cancer in man: comparative therapeutic trial of nitrogen mustard and triethylene thiophosphoramide. *J Chronic Dis.* January 1960;11(1):7-33.

18. Anderson F, Downing GM, Hill J, Casorso L, Lerch N. Palliative performance scale (PPS): a new tool. *J Palliat Care.* 1996;12(1):5-11.

19. Kutner JS, Bryant LL, Beaty BL, Fairclough DL. Symptom distress and quality-of-life assessment at the end of life: the role of proxy response. *J Pain Symptom Manage.* October 2006;32(4):300-310.

20. Donaldson MS. Taking stock of health-related quality-of-life measurement in oncology practice in the United States. *J Natl Cancer Inst Monographs.* October 2004;2004(33):155-167.

21. Jones JM, McPherson CJ, Zimmermann C, Rodin G, Le LW, Cohen SR. Assessing agreement between terminally ill cancer patients' reports of their quality of life and family caregiver and palliative care physician proxy ratings. *J Pain Symptom Manage.* September 2011;42(3):354-365.

22. Lipscomb J, Gotay CC, Snyder C. *Outcomes Assessment in Cancer.* Cambridge: Cambridge University Press; 2005.

23. Streiner DL, Norman GR. *Health Measurement Scales: A Practical Guide to Their Development and Use.* 4th ed. New York, NY: Oxford University Press; 2008.

24. Snaith RP. The hospital anxiety and depression scale. *Health Qual Life Outcomes.* 2003;1:29.

25. Norman GR, Sloan JA, Wyrwich KW. Interpretation of changes in health-related quality of life: the remarkable universality of half a standard deviation. *Med Care.* May 2003;41(5):582-592.

26. Magasi S, Ryan G, Revicki D, et al. Content validity of patient-reported outcome measures: perspectives from a PROMIS meeting. *Qual Life Res.* 2012;21(5):739-746.

27. Day S, Fayers P, Harvey D. Double data entry: what value, what price? *Control Clin Trial.* February 1998;19(1):15-24.

28. Rose M, Bezjak A. Logistics of collecting patient-reported outcomes (PROs) in clinical practice: an overview and practical examples. *Qual Life Res.* February 2009;18(1):125-136.

29. Abernethy AP, Herndon JE, Wheeler JL, et al. Feasibility and acceptability to patients of a longitudinal system for evaluating cancer-related symptoms and quality of life: pilot study of an

e/Tablet data-collection system in academic oncology. *J Pain Symptom Manage*. June 2009;37(6):1027-1038.

30. Basch E, Artz D, Dulko D, et al. Patient online self-reporting of toxicity symptoms during chemotherapy. *J Clin Oncol*. May 2005;23(15):3552-3561.

31. Salaffi F, Gasparini S, Grassi W. The use of computer touch-screen technology for the collection of patient-reported outcome data in rheumatoid arthritis: comparison with standardized paper questionnaires. *Clin Exp Rheumatol*. April 2009;27(3):459-468.

32. Kamal AH, Bull J, Stinson C, et al. Collecting data on quality is feasible in community-based palliative care. *J Pain Symptom Manage*. November 2011;42(5):663-667.

33. Kallen MA, Yang D, Haas N. A technical solution to improving palliative and hospice care. *Support Care Cancer*. 2012;20(1):167-174.

34. Dy SM, Roy J, Ott GE, et al. Tell us™: a web-based tool for improving communication among patients, families, and providers in hospice and palliative care through systematic data specification, collection, and use. *J Pain Symptom Manage*. October 2011;42(4):526-534.

35. Cella D, Yount S, Rothrock N, et al. The Patient-Reported Outcomes Measurement Information System (PROMIS): progress of an NIH Roadmap cooperative group during its first two years. *Med Care*. May 2007;45(5 suppl 1):S3-S11.

36. Reeve BB, Burke LB, Chiang Y-P, et al. Enhancing measurement in health outcomes research supported by agencies within the US Department of Health and Human Services. *Qual Life Res*. 2007;16(suppl 1):175-186.

37. Garcia SF, Cella D, Clauser SB, et al. Standardizing patient-reported outcomes assessment in cancer clinical trials: a patient-reported outcomes measurement information system initiative. *J Clin Oncol*. November 2007;25(32):5106-5112.

38. Basch EM, Reeve BB, Mitchell SA, et al. Electronic toxicity monitoring and patient-reported outcomes. *Cancer J*. June 2011;17(4):231-234.

39. Abernethy AP, Zafar SY, Uronis H, et al. Validation of the Patient Care Monitor (Version 2.0): a review of system assessment instrument for cancer patients. *J Pain Symptom Manage*. October 2010;40(4):545-558.

40. Dupont A, Wheeler J, Herndon JE, et al. Use of tablet personal computers for sensitive patient-reported information. *J Support Oncol*. April 2009;7(3):91-97.

41. Coons SJ, Gwaltney CJ, Hays RD, et al. Recommendations on evidence needed to support measurement equivalence between electronic and paper-based patient-reported outcome (PRO) measures: ISPOR ePRO Good Research Practices Task Force report. *Value Health*. June 2009;12(4):419-429.

42. Gwaltney CJ, Shields AL, Shiffman S. Equivalence of electronic and paper-and-pencil administration of patient-reported outcome measures: a meta-analytic review. *Value Health*. February 2008;11(2):322-333.

43. Miriovsky BJ, Basch EM, Kulig K, Abernethy AP. Using patient-reported outcomes in registries. In: Gliklich RE, Dreyer NA, eds. *Registries for Evaluating Patient Outcomes: A User's Guide*. 3rd ed. Rockville, MD: Agency for Healthcare Research and Quality; 2012, in press.

44. Center for Medical Technology Policy (CMTP). Effectiveness guidance document: recommendations for incorporating patient-reported outcomes into the design of post-marketing clinical trials in adult oncology. www.cmtpnet.org. May 2012. http://www.cmtpnet.org/wp-content/uploads/downloads/2012/05/PRO-EGD.pdf. Accessed August 2, 2012.

45. Basch E, Abernethy AP. Commentary: encouraging clinicians to incorporate longitudinal patient-reported symptoms in routine clinical practice. *J Oncol Pract*. January 2011;7(1):23-25.

46. Cleeland CS, Wang XS, Shi Q, et al. Automated symptom alerts reduce postoperative symptom severity after cancer surgery: a randomized controlled clinical trial. *J Clin Oncol*. March 2011;29(8):994-1000.

47. McPherson CJ, Addington-Hall JM. Judging the quality of care at the end of life: can proxies provide reliable information? *Soc Sci Med*. January 2003;56(1):95-109.

48. Currow DC, McDonald C, Oaten S, et al. Once-daily opioids for chronic dyspnea: a dose increment and pharmacovigilance study. *J Pain Symptom Manage*. September 2011;42(3):388-399.

49. Abernethy AP, McDonald CF, Frith PA, et al. Effect of palliative oxygen versus room air in relief of breathlessness in patients with refractory dyspnoea: a double-blind, randomised controlled trial. *Lancet*. September 2010;376(9743):784-793.

50. Feudtner C, Kang TI, Hexem KR, et al. Pediatric palliative care patients: a prospective multicenter cohort study. *Pediatrics*. June 2011;127(6):1094-1101.

51. Varni JW, Thissen D, Stucky BD, et al. PROMIS® Parent Proxy Report Scales: an item response theory analysis of the parent proxy report item banks. *Qual Life Res*. October 2011. Epub ahead of print. PubMed ID: 21971875

52. Parsons SK, Fairclough DL, Wang J, Hinds PS. Comparing longitudinal assessments of quality of life by patient and parent in newly diagnosed children with cancer: the value of both raters' perspectives. *Qual Life Res*. 2012;21(5):915-923.

53. Turner RR, Quittner AL, Parasuraman BM, Kallich JD, Cleeland CS, Mayo/FDA Patient-Reported Outcomes Consensus Meeting Group. Patient-reported outcomes: instrument development and selection issues. *Value Health*. October 2007;10(suppl 2):S86-S93.

54. Chang VT, Hwang SS, Feuerman M. Validation of the Edmonton Symptom Assessment Scale. *Cancer*. May 2000;88(9):2164-2171.

55. Cleeland CS, Mendoza TR, Wang XS, et al. Assessing symptom distress in cancer patients: the M.D. Anderson Symptom Inventory. *Cancer*. October 2000;89(7):1634-1646.

56. Portenoy RK, Thaler HT, Kornblith AB, et al. The Memorial Symptom Assessment Scale: an instrument for the evaluation of symptom prevalence, characteristics and distress. *Eur J Cancer*. 1994;30A(9):1326-1336.

57. Mularski RA, Rosenfeld K, Coons SJ, et al. Measuring outcomes in randomized prospective trials in palliative care. *J Pain Symptom Manage*. July 2007;34(1):S7-S19.

58. Granda-Cameron C, Viola SR, Lynch MP, Polomano RC. Measuring patient-oriented outcomes in palliative care: functionality and quality of life. *Clin J Oncol Nurs*. February 2008;12(1):65-77.

59. Steinhauser KE, Clipp EC, Bosworth HB, et al. Measuring quality of life at the end of life: validation of the QUAL-E. *Palliat Support Care*. March 2004;2(1):3-14.

60. O'Boyle C. The Schedule for the Evaluation of Individual Quality of Life (SEIQoL). *Int J Mental Health*. 1994;23:3-23.

61. Cohen SR, Mount BM. Living with cancer: "good" days and "bad" days—what produces them? Can the McGill quality of life questionnaire distinguish between them? *Cancer*. October 2000;89(8):1854-1865.

62. Lua PL, Salek S, Finlay I, Lloyd-Richards C. The feasibility, reliability and validity of the McGill Quality of Life Questionnaire-Cardiff Short Form (MQOL-CSF) in palliative care population. *Qual Life Res*. September 2005;14(7):1669-1681.

63. Ware JE, Sherbourne CD. The MOS 36-item short-form health survey (SF-36). I. Conceptual framework and item selection. *Med Care*. June 1992;30(6):473-483.

64. Gwede CK, Small BJ, Munster PN, Andrykowski MA, Jacobsen PB. Exploring the differential experience of breast cancer treatment-related symptoms: a cluster analytic approach. *Support Care Cancer*. August 2008;16(8):925-933.

65. Berger AM, Lockhart K, Agrawal S. Variability of patterns of fatigue and quality of life over time based on different breast cancer adjuvant chemotherapy regimens. *Oncol Nurs Forum*. September 2009;36(5):563-570.

66. Pidala J, Kurland B, Chai X, et al. Patient-reported quality of life is associated with severity of chronic graft-versus-host disease as measured by NIH criteria: report on baseline data from the chronic GVHD consortium. *Blood*. April 2011;117(17):4651-4657.

67. Möller A, Sartipy U. Predictors of postoperative quality of life after surgery for lung cancer. *J Thorac Oncol*. February 2012;7(2):406-411.

68. Grande GE, Farquhar MC, Barclay SIG, Todd CJ. Quality of life measures (EORTC QLQ-C30 and SF-36) as predictors of survival in palliative colorectal and lung cancer patients. *Palliat Support Care*. September 2009;7(3):289-297.

69. Aaronson NK, Ahmedzai S, Bergman B, et al. The European Organization for Research and Treatment of Cancer QLQ-C30: a quality-of-life instrument for use in international clinical trials in oncology. *J Natl Cancer Inst*. March 1993;85(5):365-376.

70. Bruley DK. Beyond reliability and validity: analysis of selected quality-of-life instruments for use in palliative care. *J Palliat Med*. 1999;2(3):299-309.

71. Groenvold M, Petersen MA, Aaronson NK, et al. The development of the EORTC QLQ-C15-PAL: a shortened questionnaire for cancer patients in palliative care. *Eur J Cancer*. January 2006;42(1):55-64.

72. Cella DF, Tulsky DS, Gray G, et al. The Functional Assessment of Cancer Therapy scale: development and validation of the general measure. *J Clin Oncol*. March 1993;11(3):570-579.

73. Lyons KD, Bakitas M, Hegel MT, Hanscom B, Hull J, Ahles TA. Reliability and validity of the Functional Assessment of Chronic Illness Therapy-Palliative care (FACIT-Pal) scale. *J Pain Symptom Manage*. January 2009;37(1):23-32.

CHAPTER 69

Research Issues: Ethics and Study Design

David Casarett

The goal of good palliative care is to relieve suffering and to improve quality of life. However, it is apparent that access to palliative care is inconsistent, and standards to guide palliative care have not been established clearly. These deficiencies exist, at least in part, because of a lack of solid evidence on which to base clinical decisions (1–3). Therefore, there is an urgent need for research that can provide evidence to define the standard of care and to increase access to quality care.

Recent years have seen a dramatic increase in palliative care research, defined broadly as activities that are designed to contribute to generalizable knowledge (4) about the end-of-life care. This growth has created a heterogeneous field that encompasses both qualitative and quantitative techniques, and descriptive as well as interventional study designs (5). Although the past 10 years have seen impressive growth in all of these areas, this rate of growth appears to be particularly rapid for interventional research, including controlled trials of pain medications (6,7), interventional procedures for pain (8), and other nonpharmacologic interventions to improve a variety of aspects of end-of-life care (9–13).

Despite the valuable knowledge that has been produced by this research, and the promise of important advances in future, its progress has been slowed by a persistent uncertainty about the ethics of these studies (14). Indeed, there have been concerns raised from several quarters about whether patients near the end of life should ever be asked to participate in any form of research (15,16). Others have objected to this extreme position (2,17). Nevertheless, many providers, Institutional Review Boards (IRBs), ethics committees, study sections, and even investigators remain uncertain about the ethical limits of research involving dying patients.

These concerns have considerable intuitive appeal and must be taken seriously. Indeed, it would be unfortunate if the progress of palliative care research were slowed by the sorts of ethical scandals that have threatened other fields of research that involve vulnerable populations, such as those with mental illness (18). However, strict overseeing and tight limits on palliative care research have the potential to do equal damage to the growing field. Therefore, in order to avoid potential scandals, without excessive regulation and overseeing, it will be important that palliative care investigators and clinicians consider these concerns in a fair and balanced way.

This chapter discusses six ethical aspects of palliative care research that investigators and clinicians should consider in designing and conducting palliative care research. These include the following:

1. Whether the study is research or quality improvement (QI)
2. The study's potential benefits to future patients
3. The study's potential benefits to subjects
4. The study's risks to subjects
5. Subjects' decision-making capacity
6. The voluntariness of subjects' choices to participate in the research

Each of these is discussed, as well as the opportunities for each to enhance the ethics of palliative care research.

DEFINING RESEARCH

The first and, arguably, the most important question that palliative care investigators face in designing an ethical study is whether it is research or QI. This decision is extremely important and has profound implications for the study's design, and the ethical standards to which it will be held. For instance, federal law requires most research projects to be reviewed by local IRBs to assure that informed consent is obtained from each subject, that research risks are reasonable in relation to expected benefits, and that the subjects are recruited in an equitable fashion (4). In comparison, there are few widely accepted standards that govern QI.

In many situations, it is clear that a planned study is research. For instance, there is likely to be general agreement that randomized clinical trials comparing one or more pain medications, or population-based studies of symptom prevalence are research, and should be held to the ethical standards for research. However, QI activities often share many of the attributes of research. For instance, both QI and research involve systematic data collection methods, such as surveys and chart reviews. Both apply statistical methods to test hypotheses, to establish relationships between variables, and to evaluate outcomes. Both QI and research are designed to produce knowledge that could benefit patients other than those directly involved in the activity. In practical terms, therefore, QI and research activities are often difficult to distinguish. This can produce confusion and conflicting opinions from IRBs that review study protocols (19).

Unfortunately, the federal regulations that make the distinction between research and QI so important offer little practical assistance in distinguishing between the two types of activities. In those regulations, research is defined as "a systematic investigation, including research development, testing and evaluation, designed to develop or contribute to generalizable knowledge" (4). Although elegant in its simplicity, this definition may prove prohibitively difficult for palliative care investigators to apply. It is often not clear how systematic an activity needs to be in order to be considered research. Nor is it clear how generalizability should be defined or how an investigator's intent should be measured.

In an effort to make the distinction between QI and research clearer, additional criteria have been proposed. These include the degree to which a study deviates from standard care, whether an activity requires identifiable recruitment practices, how individuals are selected to receive a particular intervention, the degree of uncertainty associated with the intervention, and whether the patients involved benefit from the knowledge to be gained (20–22). One of the most recent of these efforts (21) describes a two-step algorithm that investigators may find useful when the existing criterion of an intent to produce generalizable knowledge (4) fails to provide adequate guidance. This algorithm is based on the additional risks or burdens that are imposed by a study and on whether the patients involved in the study will benefit from the knowledge to be gained. Briefly, this algorithm suggests that studies should be considered as research, rather than as QI, if they expose patients to risks in order to generate knowledge that will not benefit them.

This algorithm may prove to be too restrictive, as some have argued (22). Moreover, a recent addition to this debate has presented a convincing argument that too much regulation and oversight of QI carries risks as well (23). In any event, it should not take precedence over existing federal regulations (4). It is at most a guide that palliative care investigators may wish to turn to. When the status of a project is unclear, investigators should also seek guidance from their own IRB.

BENEFITS TO FUTURE PATIENTS: A STUDY'S VALIDITY AND VALUE

Palliative care research is designed to produce knowledge that will advance understanding of end-of-life care. Implicit in this goal is the expectation that this knowledge will eventually improve care for future patients. Therefore, the first ethical aspect of palliative care research that deserves consideration is its potential benefits for future patients. These benefits to others can be described in terms of validity and value.

Validity

First, all studies must be valid. That is, they must use techniques of design and data analysis that peer reviewers can agree as appropriate. In addition, all studies must be designed to produce knowledge that is generalizable. Indeed, generalizability is the cornerstone of the Common Rule's definition of research: "a systematic investigation, including research development, testing, and evaluation, designed to develop or contribute to generalizable knowledge" (4). These

requirements collectively describe a study's validity (24). Validity is a threshold requirement for all research, because it is unethical to expose human subjects to risks in studies that peer reviewers agree cannot adequately answer a research question (25). Therefore, at a minimum, investigators must routinely consider a study's validity.

Value

Above this threshold of validity, palliative care studies may offer more or less importance or "value." Broadly, value can be defined as the likelihood that a study's results will improve the health and well-being of future patients (26). Like validity, value is an important measure of a study design's scientific quality, but it is also a measure of its ethical quality. Value is an essential aspect of a study's ethical design because a central goal of research is to produce knowledge that will ultimately be "important" (4,27), "fruitful" (28), or "valuable" (29). In fact, one reason that subjects participate in clinical research is to produce knowledge that will benefit others (30,31). Because subjects are willing to accept risks and burdens of research at least in part in order to benefit others, investigators have accepted an ethical responsibility to maximize the probability that a study will be able to do so. Therefore, in addition to widely accepted scientific arguments for valuable research, there are compelling ethical arguments as well.

Maximizing Validity and Value in Palliative Care Research

Space does not permit a comprehensive overview of ways in which a palliative care study's validity and value can be assessed and improved. Indeed, such a discussion moves quickly beyond ethics and into the technical language of study design and health measurement. Nevertheless, several broad recommendations are possible.

First, a study's sample size should be adequate to answer the research question that is posed. Problems of underpowered studies, and particularly clinical trials, are both widespread and well described (32). But issues of power and sample size are particularly relevant to pain and symptom research, in which random variation can be quite large (33). To minimize these problems, it may be useful to establish consortia or collaborative groups that can participate in multicenter studies. Such arrangements have been highly effective in promoting research on rare disorders and may be applicable to palliative care research as well, in which investigators are limited and available patients are often sparse.

Second, palliative care investigators can enhance the ethical quality of a study by taking reasonable steps to increase the generalizability of its results. These steps might include sample size calculations that permit subgroup analysis of groups of patients that have typically not been the focus of investigation, such as patients with noncancer diagnoses, or elderly patients. The generalizability of a study's results might also be enhanced by recruiting subjects outside academic medical settings, because preliminary evidence suggests that these patients, and their needs for care, may be different than those who receive care in academic settings (34).

In addition, palliative care investigators can enhance the generalizability, and therefore the value, of their research by making reasonable efforts to include patients who are receiving care at home, and particularly those who are enrolled in a home hospice program. Substantial barriers may make it difficult to include these patients in research. Nevertheless, few data exist to guide the management of home care patients near the end of life, and palliative care investigators can enhance the value of their research by including this population whenever possible (35).

Of course, all of these improvements in generalizability come at a substantial cost. For instance, studies that recruit subjects from several different settings require more elaborate designs for recruitment and follow-up. In addition, investigators who include plans for subgroup analysis in their sample size calculations face rapidly escalating sample size requirements and costs. Nevertheless, steps such as these offer an important way to enhance the value of a palliative care study, and therefore its ethical quality. Therefore, it will also be important that funding agencies understand the ethical importance of generalizability and that generalizability comes with a financial cost.

BENEFITS TO SUBJECTS

Palliative care investigators can also enhance the ethical rigor of a study by maximizing the benefits that it will offer to subjects. Broadly, these benefits can be considered under two categories: benefits to subjects during the study and benefits to future patients from the data that are collected. Each of these is discussed in the subsequent text.

Benefits to Subjects During the Study

Investigators may have several opportunities to maximize potential benefits of research to the subjects who participate. Perhaps the first, at least in an interventional study, is in their choice of an intervention. Ideally, a new intervention to be studied should have a reasonable chance of success. More important, though, if it is to offer subjects a significant potential benefit, an intervention should offer the possibility of a meaningful improvement over other interventions that are available to subjects outside the study. For instance, a pain management algorithm that is expected to reduce cancer pain (36) would only offer potential benefits if it is qualitatively or quantitatively different than those that constitute the usual standard of care. On the other hand, a comparison of two medications that are commercially available, such as topical fentanyl and sustained release morphine, would not offer subjects any potential benefit. This is true even if the study's results offer considerable clinical value (36).

The potential benefits of a study can also be enhanced by choosing an active control design, rather than a placebo (37). If a placebo is used, a study's potential benefits can also be improved by altering the standard 1:1 randomization scheme in a placebo-controlled trial in a way that increases the subjects' chances of receiving an active agent (7). The potential benefits of a placebo-controlled trial can also be enhanced by using a crossover design, so that all subjects are offered potential benefits, if the medication's pharmacokinetic profile makes it possible to avoid carryover effects.

These suggestions should be tempered by two caveats. First, the potential benefits of research are never certain. If they were, a randomized trial would not be ethically acceptable. That is, a legitimate argument for the uncertainty that justifies a clinical trial, or equipoise, could not be made (38). However, investigators generally design studies of interventions for which there is at least some evidence of effectiveness. Therefore, although these potential benefits are not certain, they are more or less likely, and this assessment of likelihood should be considered in the design of pain research.

Second, palliative care studies need not always offer potential benefits. Indeed, many, and perhaps most, will not. Nevertheless, when a study does offer potential benefits, investigators may consider enhancing a study's potential benefits in these ways. The importance of doing so is particularly great if other aspects of a study raise ethical concerns, which might be the case if subjects' decision-making capacity is limited or if the study's risks are substantial.

Benefits from Data Collected During a Study

Although the opportunities to enhance potential benefits described in the preceding text apply largely to studies involving interventions, another opportunity applies equally well, if not better, to research that is descriptive. A common ethical issue in the design of palliative care research, and particularly descriptive research, is the possibility that data gathered may contribute to a subject's care. For instance, data gathered during a descriptive study may identify pain that is inadequately treated (39–41), dissatisfaction with pain management (42,43), or related clinical problems such as depression (44,45).

In anticipation of instances such as these, investigators can design standard operating procedures that help ensure that valuable clinical information is made available to the subject and his/her clinicians. At the least, these procedures should include data about the presence of unrecognized and untreated symptoms, and concurrent disorders like depression. This is arguably an ethical obligation of symptom-oriented research (17). Moreover, these procedures offer a significant opportunity for investigators to enhance the potential benefits of pain research.

Benefits to Subjects after a Study Has Ended

Investigators can also enhance the potential benefits for subjects after a study has ended. These sorts of poststudy benefits are not usually included in assessments of a study's balance of risks and benefits. They are also components of a study's value, because these benefits generally come from the knowledge that the study has produced. Nevertheless, subjects may benefit from the knowledge to be gained from a study if the study's results are applied to their care. Investigators have numerous opportunities to ensure that these results are translated into subjects' care and, by doing so, can enhance the study's potential benefits to subjects.

For instance, subjects in palliative care research can benefit after a study if they learn from the study's aggregate results. This might be the case if a study comparing two pain medications found that one resulted in fewer overall side effects (37). Subjects in the study would benefit from these data because this knowledge should allow them to make a more informed choice among available medications. Subjects might also benefit from results that are specific to them. For instance, if a subject receives two medications in a blinded crossover trial, and prefers one to the other, he or she would be better able to choose between these medications in future clinical situations, armed with the results of a blinded comparison of the two.

Finally, investigators can increase the likelihood that subjects have continued access to medications that are studied. If medications are not available, either due to high cost or because the medication has not yet received regulatory approval, subjects will not benefit (immediately) from the study's results. Therefore, by arranging reduced rate programs or open-label extension phases, investigators can increase a study's potential benefits for subjects by helping to ensure that subjects will benefit from the study's results.

This benefit may be particularly important in palliative care research, because mortality rates in some studies are very high. This means that subjects may not live long enough to see a study medication's approval for clinical use or to see a study's results published and translated into improved care. For this reason, it is especially important that investigators consider mechanisms by which results can be applied to the care of research subjects in a timely fashion.

MINIMIZING RISKS AND BURDENS

Investigators can also enhance a study's ethical soundness by taking steps to minimize a study's risks and burdens. Although the distinction between risks and burdens is not always clear, a rough heuristic is useful. In general, a risk can be considered as the probability of an adverse medical event or undesirable outcome. Risks might include side effects of a medication or increased pain during a study. The term *burden* can be used to describe those unpleasant features of participation in a study that are more certain and which are better thought of as inconveniences. Additional visits to the clinic, time spent filling out questionnaires, or time spent waiting in the clinic might be described as burdens.

Identifying Risks and Burdens

Attention to the ethical design of pain research, and to the minimization of research risks and burdens, requires a clear agreement about how they should be defined. The criteria

by which study risks and burdens are identified and evaluated use the concept of incremental or "demarcated" risks imposed by participation in a study (46). The application of this standard to interventional pain research would mean that investigators designing a trial to compare the effectiveness of two opioids (37) need not go to great lengths to justify the risks of the opioids being evaluated, if subjects in the trial would have received similar medications, with similar risks, off protocol. Of course, the risks of any medication in a clinical trial should be disclosed in the informed consent process (4). Nevertheless, investigators are not under the obligation to minimize or justify these risks as they would be if, for instance, the same medications were being given to patients with mild pain, who would not receive them as part of standard care.

Minimizing Risks: The Choice of Control

Perhaps one of the most contentious and emotional questions in palliative care research (47,48), and indeed in research generally (49–51), is whether a placebo or sham control arm is ethically appropriate. The ongoing debates about the scientific merit of these controls and the competing advantages of active control superiority trials and equivalency trials are beyond the scope of this discussion. However, several general points can be made about the ethics of placebo- and sham-controlled trials. Each of these designs is discussed in the subsequent text.

Broadly, placebos can be defined as interventions that are "ineffective or not specifically effective" for the symptom or disorder in question (52). Increased attention to the ethical issue of placebo controls in recent years has produced a growing consensus that all subjects in a clinical trial should have access to the best available standard of care (53). Therefore in infectious disease research, for instance, all subjects with meningitis would have access to an antimicrobial agent that has proved effective. However, this requirement may be difficult to apply to studies of treatment for pain, other symptoms, or depression, in which the placebo response can be quite substantial. These difficulties are compounded when the symptom being studied is transient, such as incident pain (7).

For these reasons, it may not be practical to prohibit placebos in palliative care research, and a placebo control may be ethically acceptable in several situations. First, placebos are acceptable if subjects receive a placebo in addition to the standard care. For example, subjects might be randomly assigned to receive either an opioid or an opioid plus an adjuvant agent. Second, a placebo arm is justified if the symptom under study has no effective treatment. For example, the transient nature of incident pain often defies adequate treatment on an as-needed basis, and a placebo control might be justified in a randomized controlled trial of a novel agent for the treatment of incident pain. Third, a placebo control is justified if subjects have adequate access to breakthrough or "rescue" treatment. This may in turn alter a trial's end points. For instance, the free use of breakthrough dosing in a trial suggests the possible inclusion of these doses as a study end point either directly (54,55) or as part of a composite end point (6,56).

Concrete recommendations about sham procedures are somewhat more elusive, in part because sham procedures themselves are difficult to define. In general, although sham procedures in palliative care research involve the use of a control procedure such as a nerve block, which is administered in a way that makes it ineffective (8), these procedures create ethical concerns because some subjects, or all subjects, depending on the study's design, are exposed to the risks of the procedure without hope of its benefits (49). Like placebo controls, shams also have a role in research, because the nonspecific therapeutic effects of surgery may be substantial. For instance, Leonard Cobb's research in the 1950s effectively debunked a widely used cardiac procedure that, if it had been widely disseminated, would eventually have put thousands of patients at risk.

Investigators have an opportunity to reduce these concerns substantially in the design of a sham-controlled study. For instance, investigators might conduct these studies in a setting in which the procedure itself (whether sham or real) poses few if any additional or "incremental" risks above and beyond the usual care. Investigators might insert a sham epidural catheter that would then be used for postoperative analgesia (57). When this is not possible, investigators can choose a crossover design, in which subjects are assigned to receive either the sham or the real procedure, followed by the other. This design does not decrease the incremental risks of the sham procedure. However, it does ensure that all subjects who bear the risks of the sham procedure also have access to the real procedures' potential benefits. This crossover sham design has been used in other settings (58) and might be appropriate for pain research when the risks or discomforts of the sham procedure are substantial.

Minimizing Burdens

For the most part, opportunities to minimize burdens are readily apparent. For instance, it seems reasonable wherever possible to minimize surveys, interviews, and additional study visits (59). These are all burdens that investigators routinely consider carefully in designing studies. However, there may be other needs and concerns that may be unique to, or more common in, patients near the end of life.

Although it is intuitively obvious that all research subjects would like to avoid the added time commitment and inconvenience of travel to and from additional appointment, this concern may be especially important to patients near the end of life, for whom long periods of time spent sitting in a car can exacerbate discomfort. Similarly, patients may view surveys and questionnaires not only as time consuming but also as a drain on their energy. Therefore, investigators who conduct palliative care research may have an added reason to minimize the burdens of extra visits and data collection procedures and to rely on telephone data collection strategies whenever possible.

Palliative care investigators may also need to consider the burdens that a study creates for friends and family members who often take on substantial burdens as caregivers (60–63). Although most of the burdens of research participation are borne by the subject, the requirements of time, travel, and perhaps time off from work create burdens for others. Patients may be very sensitive to these burdens and, for some patients with chronic pain, burdens to others can be influential in the decision whether or not to enroll in a study (31). By building flexibility into a study design (e.g., use of brief telephone interviews and multiple options for timing of clinic visits), investigators may be able to reduce the burdens of research participation on others.

ENSURING DECISION-MAKING CAPACITY

Patients who consent to participate in research should have adequate decision-making capacity, which refers to the subjects' ability to understand relevant information, to appreciate the significance of that information, and to reason through to a conclusion that makes sense for them (64). These concerns are parallel concerns in research involving patients with dementia (65), psychiatric illness (66), and patients in the intensive care setting (67). However, deficits in decision-making capacity may create several additional challenges for palliative care investigators.

First, concern about capacity is reasonable given the prevalence of cognitive impairment at the end of life (68,69). Cognitive impairment occurs in 10% to 40% of patients in the final months and in up to 85% of patients in the last days of life (68,69). Cognitive impairment may be difficult to identify in palliative care research because decision-making capacity varies over time (69), and because impairment may result from the experimental or therapeutic medications themselves, such as opioids, benzodiazepines, and corticosteroids (70,71,72). Investigators who conduct trials of medications will encounter these challenges even more frequently if trials are designed to evaluate treatments for delirium, for which impairment is an inclusion criterion (73).

Second, the effects of cognitive impairment on comprehension may be complicated by clinical depression, which occurs in 5% to 25% of patients near the end of life (44,45,74,75). Clinically significant adjustment disorders may be even more common (44). It is possible that these disorders may impair either comprehension or decision making, or both (66), but studies have not yet supported this conclusion.

Third, even in the absence of overt cognitive impairment or depression, it is possible that severe symptoms or affective disorders may impair subjects' ability to understand the risks and benefits of research participation. For some studies, particularly clinical trials, the presence of one or more of these intractable symptoms is an inclusion criterion (76–78). It is possible that severe symptoms may impair comprehension if patients are unable to concentrate on the information offered in the informed consent process (79).

Finally, these challenges may be compounded in prospective studies that require participation over days or weeks. In these studies, even if patients have the capacity to consent at the time of enrollment, they may not retain that capacity throughout the study. Therefore, days or weeks after patients give consent to participate, they may be unable to understand changes in their condition clearly enough to withdraw. The result can be a "Ulysses contract" of sorts, in which research subjects find it easier to enroll than they do to withdraw (80).

None of these challenges is easily remedied. Indeed, it is obstacles such as these that lead some authors to argue that patients near the end of life should not be allowed to enroll in research (15,16). Nevertheless, palliative care investigators have several concrete opportunities to enhance the ethical quality of palliative care research when decision-making capacity is uncertain.

First, at a minimum, investigators whose research involves patients near the end of life who are likely to lack decision-making capacity might institute brief assessments of understanding. Although this strategy cannot assess decision-making capacity, a few simple questions in either open-ended or multiple choice format provide a brief assessment of understanding (80,81,82). In some situations, investigators may wish to assess decision-making capacity more formally using validated instruments (83).

These sorts of safeguards need not be employed in all studies. Instead, their use should be guided by the prevalence of cognitive impairment in a study population and by the balance of risks and benefits that a study offers (35). For instance, when palliative care research involves only interviews or behavioral interventions that pose minimal risks, informal capacity assessments are generally sufficient. "Minimal risks" are defined as those risks that are encountered during a patient's usual care or in everyday life (4). When research poses greater than minimal risks but offers potential benefits, some assessment of understanding may be appropriate. This research includes studies that involve a placebo (7) or invasive interventions such as nerve blocks (84) or epidural catheters (85). When a study that poses greater than minimal risks does not offer potential benefits or is conducted in a population in which the prevalence of cognitive impairment is high (e.g., an inpatient hospice unit), a formal evaluation of capacity should be considered. This research includes studies that involve a placebo when an effective agent is available (6), and some pharmacokinetic/pharmacodynamic studies that required blood samples and prolonged observation, without potential benefits (86).

If a patient does not have the capacity to give consent, a legally authorized representative may be able to give consent for research. This follows from federal guidelines governing research involving children (4) and is justified by the argument that surrogate decision makers should be allowed to consent to research, just as they are allowed to consent to medical therapy. However, as with other research that involves patients without capacity to consent, investigators should be aware of applicable state laws that may restrict or even prohibit surrogate consent for research. In addition, investigators in this field should be alert to possible future changes in federal regulations that have been discussed (87).

If a patient does not have the capacity to consent but is still able to participate in decisions, investigators should obtain assent from the patient and informed consent from the patient's surrogate (88,89). This "dual consent" ensures that patients are as involved in the decision as possible, yet provides the additional protection of a surrogate's consent.

If a patient has decision-making capacity intermittently or is expected to lose capacity, investigators may obtain advance consent. This approach has been used in a study of treatment for delirium, in which informed consent was obtained from patients while they had decision-making capacity (73). Advance consent should be obtained only for specific studies and should be obtained close to the planned start of research, for instance, at the time of hospitalization or enrollment in a hospice or palliative care program.

PROTECTING VOLUNTARINESS

Another way that investigators can enhance the ethical soundness of a study's design is to examine ways in which the subjects' voluntary participation can be protected (90). In general terms, a choice is voluntary if it is made without significant controlling influences (91,92). At first glance, assurances of voluntariness appear to be an issue of informed consent, and in fact for the most part they are. However, a study's design and plan for subject selection and recruitment may have as great an influence on subjects' freedom to refuse research participation as does the informed consent process. In particular, two features of a study's design are relevant. First, a prospective subject's choice must be made with full knowledge of available alternatives (4). Second, his or her choice must be made with the understanding that he or she can withdraw at any time (4). Each of these creates opportunities in a study's design to ensure voluntariness that are discussed in the subsequent text.

Reasonable Alternatives to Participation

First, investigators can make sure that a study recruits subjects from an environment with excellent standards of palliative care. If patients generally receive excellent care, they will be best able to make a free and uncoerced choice about research participation. If, however, patients do not have access to a bare minimum of treatment options and expertise, they may view research participation more favorably, out of desperation.

One solution, albeit a somewhat draconian one, would be to require that palliative care research be conducted only in settings in which patients have access to a full range of services, treatment, and expertise. Although this requirement would reduce the potential for research participation out of desperation, it would effectively limit research to a small number of academic centers, with a possible loss of generalizability (34). Another more practical option might be to include a lead-in phase when clinical pain research is conducted in settings where the standard of care is poor (17). A lead-in phase allows an opportunity to optimize palliative care prior to recruitment. This strategy not only has ethical value but scientific value as well because it provides a uniform baseline prior to randomization.

Opportunities to Withdraw

Investigators can also enhance the ethics of a study's design by ensuring that subjects are able to withdraw at any time. Although a subject's ability to withdraw should be a fundamental aspect of any ethical research (4), there may be unique barriers to withdrawal from palliative care research. For instance, subjects who withdraw from clinical pain research that involves one or more medications will usually need access to a different medication upon withdrawal. This problem may be straightforward in many cases, but can be very challenging if in an interventional study the investigational medication is an opioid, which requires the subject to get a new prescription and get it filled. Most states have created considerable barriers to opioid prescribing, including triplicate prescriptions, which may make it very difficult for a subject to obtain a new prescription and get it filled in a timely manner. If a subject has his or her medication available, the process may be easier. Nevertheless, considerable challenges of calculating an equianalgesic dose remain. For both of these reasons, investigators can enhance the ethical design of pain research by developing mechanisms to ensure that subjects who drop out continue to receive adequate pain treatment with as little interruption as possible.

CONCLUSION

The field of palliative care, and the standard of care that it represents, depends upon rigorous research to provide data that will guide clinical care. Although this research raises substantial ethical questions, these questions need not curtail what promises to be a valuable and highly productive area of research. Of course, the concerns discussed in the preceding text should be taken seriously. To do otherwise is to risk the sorts of ethical missteps that have produced scandals in other fields. Nevertheless, these ethical questions can be addressed through careful planning, and with attention to the adequacy of a study's design, and to the informed consent process.

REFERENCES

1. Symptoms in Terminal Illness: A Research Workshop. Solar Building, Rockville, Maryland, 2006. http://ninr.nih.gov/ninr/wnew/symptoms_in_terminal_illness.html
2. Mount B, Cohen R, MacDonald N, et al. Ethical issues in palliative care research revisited. *Palliat Med.* 1995;9:165-170.
3. Krouse RS, Easson AM, Angelos P. Ethical considerations and barriers to research in surgical palliative care. *J Am Coll Surg.* 2003;196(3):469-474.
4. Department of Health and Human Services. *Protection of Human Subjects.* Title 45 Part 46: Revised. Code of Federal Regulations. 1991 June 18.
5. Corner J. Is there a research paradigm for palliative care? *Palliat Med.* 1996;10:201-208.
6. Dhaliwal HS, Sloan P, Arkinstall WW, et al. Randomized evaluation of controlled-release codeine and placebo in chronic cancer pain. *J Pain Symptom Manage.* 1995;10(8):612-623.
7. Farrar JT, Cleary J, Rauck R, et al. Oral transmucosal fentanyl citrate: randomized, double-blinded, placebo-controlled trial for treatment of breakthrough pain in cancer patients. *J Natl Cancer Inst.* 1998;90(8):611-616.
8. Polati E, Finco G, Gottin L, et al. Prospective randomized double-blind trial of neurolytic coeliac plexus block in patients with pancreatic cancer. *Br J Surg.* 1998;85:199-201.
9. Elliott TE, Murray DM, Oken MM, et al. Improving cancer pain management in communities: main results from a randomized controlled trial. *J Pain Symptom Manage.* 1997;13(4):191-203.
10. de Wit R, van Dam F, Zandbelt L, et al. A pain education program for chronic cancer pain patients: follow-up results from a randomized controlled trial. *Pain.* 1997;73(1):55-69.
11. Kravitz RL, Delafield JP, Hays RD, et al. Bedside charting of pain levels in hospitalized patients with cancer: a randomized controlled trial. *J Pain Symptom Manage.* 1996;11(2):81-87.
12. Teno J, Lynn J, Connors AF Jr, et al. The illusion of end-of-life resource savings with advance directives. *J Am Geriatr Soc.* 1997;45(4):513-518.
13. Bredin M, Corner J, Krishnasamy M, et al. Multicentre randomised controlled trial of nursing intervention for breathlessness in patients with lung cancer. *Br Med J.* 1999;318(7188):901-904.
14. Casarett D, Knebel A, Helmers K. Ethical challenges of palliative care research. *J Pain Symptom Manage.* 2003;25(4):S3-S5.
15. de Raeve L. Ethical issues in palliative care research. *Palliat Med.* 1994;8(4):298-305.
16. Annas GJ. *Some Choice: Law, Medicine, and the Market.* New York, NY: Oxford University Press; 1998.
17. Casarett D, Karlawish J. Are special ethical guidelines needed for palliative care research? *J Pain Symptom Manage.* 2000;20:130-139.
18. Hilts PJ. VA Hospital is told to halt all research. *New York Times.* March 25, 1999.
19. Lynn J, Johnson J, Levine RJ. The ethical conduct of health services research: a case study of 55 institutions' applications to the SUPPORT project. *Clin Res.* 1994;42:3-10.
20. Brett A, Grodin M. Ethical aspects of human experimentation in health services research. *JAMA.* 1991;265:1854-1857.
21. Casarett D, Karlawish J, Sugarman J. Determining when quality improvement activities should be reviewed as research: proposed criteria and potential implications. *JAMA.* 2000;283:2275-2280.
22. Cretin S, Keeler EB, Lynn J, et al. Should patients in quality-improvement activities have the same protections as participants in research studies? *JAMA.* 2000;284:1786.
23. Lynn J, Maily MA, Bottrell M, et al. The ethics of using quality improvement methods in health care. *Ann Intern Med.* 2007;46;666-673.
24. Freedman B. Scientific value and validity as ethical requirements for research: a proposed explication. *IRB Rev Hum Subjects Res.* 1987;9:7-10.
25. Rutstein DR. The ethical design of human experiments. In: Freund PA, ed. *Experimentation with Human Subjects.* New York, NY: George Braziller; 1970:383-401.
26. Casarett DJ, Karlawish JH, Moreno JD. A taxonomy of value in clinical research. *IRB Rev Hum Subjects Res.* 2002;24(6):1-6.
27. Brody BA. *World Medical Association, Declaration of Helsinki. The Ethics of Biomedical Research. An International Perspective.* New York, NY: Oxford University Press; 1998.
28. The Nuremberg Code. Reprinted. In: Brody B. *The Ethics of Biomedical Research. An International Perspective.* New York, NY: Oxford University Press; 1947:213.
29. Freedman B. Placebo-controlled trials and the logic of clinical purpose. *IRB Rev Hum Subjects Res.* 1990;12:1-6.

30. Advisory Committee on Human Radiation Experiments. *Final Report. Vol 061 00000848–9.* Washington, DC: Government Printing Office; 1995.

31. Casarett DJ, Karlawish J, Sankar P, et al. Obtaining informed consent for clinical pain research: patients' concerns and information needs. *Pain.* 2001;92:71-79.

32. Meinert CL. *Clinical Trials. Design, Conduct, and Analysis.* Oxford: Oxford University Press; 1986.

33. Moore RA, Gavaghan D, Tramer MR, et al. Size is everything—large amounts of information are needed to overcome random effects in estimating direction and magnitude of treatment effects. *Pain.* 1998;78:209-216.

34. Casarett D. How are hospice patients referred from academic medical centers different? *J Pain Symptom Manage.* 2001;27:197-203.

35. Casarett D, Kirschling J, Levetown M, et al. NHPCO task force statement on hospice participation in research. *J Palliat Med.* 2001;4:441-449.

36. Du Pen SL, Du Pen AR, Polissar N, et al. Implementing guidelines for cancer pain management: results of a randomized controlled clinical trial. *J Clin Oncol.* 1999;17(1):361-370.

37. Ahmedzai S, Brooks D. Transdermal fentanyl versus sustained-release oral morphine in cancer pain: preference, efficacy, and quality of life. The TTS-Fentanyl Comparative Trial Group. *J Pain Symptom Manage.* 1997;13(5):254-261.

38. Freedman B. Equipoise and the ethics of clinical research. *N Engl J Med.* 1987;317:141-145.

39. Ingham J, Seidman A, Yao TJ, et al. An exploratory study of frequent pain measurement in a cancer clinical trial. *Qual Life Res.* 1996;5(5):503-507.

40. Twycross R, Harcourt J, Bergl S. A survey of pain in patients with advanced cancer. *J Pain Symptom Manage.* 1996;12(5):273-282.

41. Parmelee PA, Smith B, Katz IR. Pain complaints and cognitive status among elderly institution residents. *J Am Geriatr Soc.* 1993;41:517-522.

42. Ward SE, Gordon DB. Patient satisfaction and pain severity as outcomes in pain management: a longitudinal view of one setting's experience. *J Pain Symptom Manage.* 1996;11(4):242-251.

43. Desbiens NA, Wu AW, Broste SK, et al. Pain and satisfaction with pain control in seriously ill hospitalized adults: findings from the SUPPORT research investigations. *Crit Care Med.* 1996;24(12):1953-1961.

44. Derogatis LR, Morrow GR, Fetting J, et al. The prevalence of psychiatric disorders among cancer patients. *JAMA.* 1983;249:751-757.

45. Kathol RG, Mutgi A, Williams J, et al. Diagnosis of depression in cancer patients according to four sets of criteria. *Am J Psychiatry.* 1990;147:1021-1024.

46. Freedman B, Fuks A, Weijer C. Demarcating research and treatment: a systematic approach for the analysis of the ethics of clinical research. *Clin Res.* 1992;40:653-660.

47. Kirkham SR, Abel J. Placebo-controlled trials in palliative care: the argument against. *Palliat Med.* 1997;11(6):489-492.

48. Hardy JR. Placebo-controlled trials in palliative care: the argument for. *Palliat Med.* 1997;11(5):415-418.

49. Macklin R. The ethical problems with sham surgery in clinical research. *N Engl J Med.* 1999;341:992-996.

50. Rothman KJ, Michels KB. The continuing unethical use of placebo controls. *N Engl J Med.* 1994;331:394-398.

51. Temple RT, Ellenberg SS. Placebo-controlled trials and active control trials in the evaluation of new treatments. Part 1: ethical and scientific issues. *Ann Intern Med.* 2000;133:455-463.

52. Shapiro AK, Shapiro E. The placebo: is it much ado about nothing? In: Harrington A, ed. *The Placebo Effect.* Cambridge, MA: Harvard University Press; 1998.

53. World Medical Association International Code of Medical Ethics; amended by the 35th World Medical Assembly; October 1983, 2000; Venice, Italy.

54. Broomhead A, Kerr R, Tester W, et al. Comparison of a once-a-day sustained-release morphine formulation with standard oral morphine treatment for cancer pain. *J Pain Symptom Manage.* 1997;14(2):63-73.

55. Maxon HRD, Schroder LE, Hertzberg VS, et al. Rhenium-186(Sn)HEDP for treatment of painful osseous metastases: results of a double-blind crossover comparison with placebo. *J Nucl Med.* 1991;32(10):1877-1881.

56. Silverman DG, O'Connor TZ, Brull SJ. Integrated assessment of pain scores and rescue morphine use during studies of analgesic efficacy. *Anesth Analg.* 1993;77:168-170.

57. Haak van der Lely F, Burm AG, van Kleef JW, et al. The effect of epidural administration of alfentanil on intra-operative intravenous alfentanil requirements during nitrous oxide-oxygen-alfentanil anaesthesia for lower abdominal surgery. *Anaesthesia.* 1994;49(12):1034-1038.

58. Hahn AF, Bolton CF, Pillay N, et al. Plasma-exchange therapy in chronic inflammatory demyelinating polyneuropathy. A double-blind, sham-controlled, cross-over study. *Brain.* 1996;119(pt 4):1055-1066.

59. Bruera E. Ethical issues in palliative care research. *J Palliat Care.* 1994;10:7-9.

60. Family Caregiving: Agenda for Action, Improving Services and Support for America's Family Caregivers. Washington, DC: National Health Council; 1999.

61. Steele RG, Fitch MI. Needs of family caregivers of patients receiving home hospice care for cancer. *Oncol Nurs Forum.* 1996;23:823-828.

62. Emanuel EJ, Fairclough DL, Slutsman J, et al. Assistance from family members, friends, paid care givers, and volunteers in the care of terminally ill patients. *N Engl J Med.* 1999;341:956-963.

63. Takesaka J, Crowley R, Casarett D. What is the risk of distress in palliative care survey research? *J Pain Symptom Manage.* 2004;28(6):593-598.

64. Grisso T, Appelbaum PS. *Assessing Competence to Consent to Treatment.* New York, NY: Oxford University Press; 1998.

65. Marson DC, Schmitt FA, Ingram KK, et al. Determining the competency of Alzheimer patients to consent to treatment and research. *Alzheimer Dis Assoc Disord.* 1994;8(suppl 4):5-18.

66. Elliott C. Caring about risks: are severely depressed patients competent to consent to research? *Arch Gen Psychiatry.* 1997;54:113-116.

67. Lemaire F, Blanch L, Cohen SL, et al. Working Group on Ethics. Informed consent for research purposes in intensive care patients in Europe—part II. An official statement of the European Society of Intensive Care Medicine. *Intensive Care Med.* 1997;23(4):435-439.

68. Breitbart W, Bruera E, Chochinov H, et al. Neuropsychiatric syndromes and psychological symptoms in patients with advanced cancer. *J Pain Symptom Manage.* 1995;10(2):131-141.

69. Pereira J, Hanson J, Bruera E. The frequency and clinical course of cognitive impairment in patients with terminal cancer. *Cancer.* 1997;79(4):835-842.

70. Bruera E, Franco JJ, Maltoni M, et al. Changing pattern of agitated impaired mental status in patients with advanced cancer: association with cognitive monitoring, hydration, and opioid rotation. *J Pain Symptom Manage.* 1995;10(4):287-291.

71. Bruera E, MacMillan K, Kuchn N, et al. The cognitive effects of the administration of narcotics. *Pain.* 1989;39:13-16.

72. Stiefel FC, Breitbart W, Holland JC. Corticosteroids in cancer: neuropsychiatric complications. *Cancer Invest.* 1989;7:479-491.

73. Breitbart W, Marotta R, Platt MM, et al. A double-blind trial of haloperidol, chlorpromazine, and lorazepam in the treatment of delirium in hospitalized AIDS patients. *Am J Psychiatry.* 1996;153(2):231-237.

74. Brown JH, Henteleff P, Barakat S, et al. Is it normal for terminally ill patients to desire death? *Am J Psychiatry.* 1986;143: 208-211.

75. Massie MJ, Holland JC. Depression and the cancer patient. *J Clin Psychiatry.* 1990;51:12-17.

76. Eisenach JC, DuPen S, Dubois M, et al. The Epidural Clonidine Study Group. Epidural clonidine analgesia for intractable cancer pain. *Pain.* 1995;61(3):391-399.

77. Pappas GD, Lazorthes Y, Bes JC, et al. Relief of intractable cancer pain by human chromaffin cell transplants: experience at two medical centers. *Neurol Res.* 1997;19(1):71-77.

78. Plancarte R, de Leon-Casasola OA, El-Helaly M, et al. Neurolytic superior hypogastric plexus block for chronic pelvic pain associated with cancer. *Reg Anesth.* 1997;22(6):562-568.

79. Kristjanson LJ, Hanson EJ, Balneaves L. Research in palliative care populations: ethical issues. *J Palliat Care.* 1994;10(3):1010-1015.

80. Dresser R. Bound to treatment: the Ulysses contract. *Hastings Cent Rep.* 1984;14:13-16.

81. Miller CK, O'Donnell DC, Searight HR, et al. The deaconess informed consent comprehension test: an assessment tool for clinical research subjects. *Pharmacotherapy.* 1996;16(5):872-878.

82. Penman DT, Holland JC, Bahna GF, et al. Informed consent for investigational chemotherapy: patients' and physicians' perceptions. *J Clin Oncol.* 1984;2:849-855.

83. Grisso T, Appelbaum PS. The MacArthur treatment competence study III. *Law Hum Behav.* 1995;19:149-174.

84. Mercadante S. Celiac plexus block vs. analgesics in pancreatic cancer pain. *Pain.* 1993;52:187-192.

85. Boswell G, Bekersky I, Mekki Q, et al. Plasma concentrations and disposition of clonidine following a constant 14-day epidural infusion in cancer patients. *Clin Ther.* 1997;19(5):1024-1030.

86. Hoffman M, Xu JC, Smith C, et al. A pharmacodynamic study of morphine and its glucuronide metabolites after single morphine dosing in cancer patients with pain. *Cancer Invest.* 1997;15(6):542-547.

87. National Bioethics Advisory Commission. *Research Involving Persons with Mental Disorders That May Affect Decisionmaking Capacity.* Rockville, MD: Author; 1998.

88. High DM, Whitehouse PJ, Post SG, et al. Guidelines for addressing ethical and legal issues in Alzheimer disease research: a position paper. *Alzheimer Dis Assoc Disord.* 1994;8:66-74.

89. High DM. Advancing research with Alzheimer disease subjects: investigators' perceptions and ethical issues. *Alzheimer Dis Assoc Disord.* 1993;7:165-178.

90. Agrawal M. Voluntariness in clinical research at the end of life. *J Pain Symptom Manage.* 2003;25(4):25-32.

91. Beauchamp TL, Childress JF. *Principles of Biomedical Ethics.* 5th ed. Oxford: Oxford University Press, 2001.

92. Faden RR, Beauchamp TL. *A History and Theory of Informed Consent.* New York, NY: Oxford University Press; 1986.

Note: The letters 'f' and 't' following the locators refer to figures and tables respectively.